OCCUPATIONAL THERAPY
Practice Skills for Physical Dysfunction

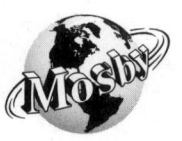

Visit our website at www.mosby.com

OCCUPATIONAL THERAPY
Practice Skills for Physical Dysfunction

Edited by

LORRAINE WILLIAMS PEDRETTI, MS, OTR
Professor Emeritus, Department of Occupational Therapy
San José State University
San José, California

MARY BETH EARLY, MS, OTR/L
Professor, Occupational Therapy Assistant Program
LaGuardia Community College
The City University of New York
Long Island City, New York

FIFTH EDITION

With 53 contributors and 764 illustrations

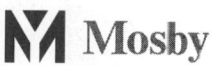 Mosby

A Harcourt Health Sciences Company

St. Louis   London   Philadelphia   Sydney   Toronto

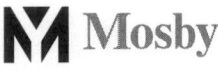

A Harcourt Health Sciences Company

Editorial Director: John Schrefer
Editor: Kellie White
Developmental Editor: Christie Hart
Editor's Assistant: Rebecca Swisher
Project Manager: Patricia Tannian
Production Editor: Larry State
Book Design Manager: Gail Morey Hudson
Cover Designer: Teresa Breckwoldt

FIFTH EDITION

Mosby, Inc.
A Harcourt Health Sciences Company
11830 Westline Industrial Drive
St. Louis, Missouri 63146

Printed in the United States of America

International Standard Book Number
0-323-00765-1

01   02   03   04   05   CL/KPT   9   8   7   6   5   4   3   2   1

Contributors

Carole Adler, BS, OTR
Occupational Therapy Supervisor
Spinal Cord Injury Unit
Therapy Services Division
Santa Clara Valley Medical Center
San José, California

Denis Anson, MS
Assistant Professor
Occupational Therapy Department
College Misericordia
Dallas, Pennsylvania

Diane J. Atkins, OTR, FISPO
Assistant Professor/Coordinator
Amputee Program
The Institute for Rehabilitation and Research (TIRR)
Department of Physical Medicine and Rehabilitation
Baylor College of Medicine
Houston, Texas

Julie Belkin, OTR, CO, MBA
President
3-Point Products, Inc.
Annapolis, Maryland

Estelle B. Breines, PhD, OTR, FAOTA
Program Director, Occupational Therapy
School of Graduate Medical Education
Seton Hall University
South Orange, New Jersey

Wendy Storm Buckner, MHE, OTR/L
Assistant Professor
Department of Occupational Therapy
Medical College of Georgia
Augusta, Georgia

Ann Burkhardt, MA, OTR/L, FAOTA, BCN
Director of Occupational Therapy
New York Presbyterian Hospital
Columbia Presbyterian Center
Associate Professor of Clinical Occupational Therapy
Programs in Occupational Therapy
Columbia University
Professional Associate
Mercy College
Dobbs Ferry, New York

Cindy Maultsby Burt, MS, OTR
Assistant Director of Rehabilitation Services
Sport/Hand/Work Programs
Department of Rehabilitation Services
University of California–Los Angeles
Los Angeles, California

Gordon Umphred Burton, PhD, OTR
Chair and Professor
Department of Occupational Therapy
San José State University
San José, California

Sonia Coleman, MEd, OTR/L
Assistant Professor
Department of Occupational Therapy and Occupational
Science
Towson University
Towson, Maryland

Teru A. Creel, MS, OTR/L
Assistant Professor and Academic Fieldwork Coordinator
Department of Occupational Therapy
Medical College of Georgia
Augusta, Georgia

Jan Zaret Davis, BS, OTR
NDT Occupational Therapy Instructor in Adult Hemiplegia
President, International Clinical Educators, Inc.
Port Townsend, Washington

Elizabeth DePoy, PhD, MSW, OTR
Professor
Department of Social Work
University of Maine
Orono, Maine

Maureen Duncan, BA, BSOT, OTD
Assistant Professor
Department of Occupational Therapy
Creighton University
Omaha, Nebraska

Laura E. Dunlop, OTR/L
Adjunct Instructor
New York University
Department of Occupational Therapy
Clinical Specialist in Pain Management
Private Practice Including Consultation and Supervision
New York, New York

Mary Beth Early, MS, OTR/L
Professor
Occupational Therapy Assistant Program
F. H. LaGuardia Community College
The City University of New York
Long Island City, New York

Joyce M. Engel, PhD, OTR/L, FAOTA
Associate Professor
Department of Rehabilitation Medicine
Division of Occupational Therapy
University of Washington
Seattle, Washington

Diane Foti, MS, OTR
Senior Occupational Therapist
Kaiser Permanente Medical Center
Hayward, California
Lecturer
San José State University
San José, California

Patricia Ann Gentile, MS, OTR/L
Chief Occupational Therapist
The Jamaica Hospital Medical Center and The Brady Institute
of Traumatic Brain Injury
Jamaica, New York

Glen Gillen, MPA, OTR, BCN
Instructor in Clinical Occupational Therapy
College of Physicians and Surgeons
Columbia University
New York, New York

Lynn Gitlow, PhD, OTR/L
Department of Occupational Therapy
Husson College
Bangor, Maine

Coralie H. Glantz, BS, OTR/L, FAOTA
Glantz/Richman Rehabilitation Associates
Riverwoods, Illinois

Carolyn Glogoski, PhD, OTR
Associate Professor
Department of Occupational Therapy
Program in Gerontology
San José State University
San José, California

Sharon A. Gutman, PhD, OTR
Assistant Professor
Department of Occupational Therapy
Long Island University
Brooklyn, New York

Linda Gutterman, BS, OT
Director
Rehabilitation and Holistic Health Service
Village Center for Care AIDS Day Treatment Program
New York, New York

Diane Harlowe, MS, OTR, FAOTA
Associate Lecturer and Administrative Program Specialist
Occupational Therapy Program
University of Wisconsin–Madison
Madison, Wisconsin

Meenakshi B. Iyer, PhD, OTR
Assistant Professor
Department of Physical Therapy
Georgia State University
Atlanta, Georgia
Adjunct Assistant Professor
Department of Physical Therapy
University of Texas Health Science Center at San Antonio
San Antonio, Texas

Janet L. Jabri, MBA, OTR, FAOTA
National Director of Rehabilitation
GCI Rehabilitation Division
Pan Care, Inc.
San José, California

Karen Nelson Jenks, MS, OTR
Occupational Therapist
Community Home Health
Los Gatos, California

Mary C. Kasch, OTR, CHT, FAOTA
Executive Director
Hand Therapy Certification Commission
Kansas City, Missouri

Denise D. Keenan, OTR, CHT
Program Coordinator
IHC Hand Care
Sandy, Utah

Amy Phillips Killingsworth, MA, OTR
Professor
Department of Occupational Therapy
San José State University
San José, California

Regina M. Lehman, MS, OTR/L
Director
Department of Occupational Therapy
Coler-Goldwater Memorial Hospital
Roosevelt Island, New York

Susan M. Lillie, BS, OTR, CDRS
Senior Occupational Therapist
Adaptive Driving Evaluation Program
Department of Therapy Services
Santa Clara Valley Medical Center
San José, California

Maureen Michele Matthews, BS, OTR
Therapy Services Outpatient Program Manager
Santa Clara Valley Medical Center
San José, California

Guy L. McCormack, PhD, OTR, FAOTA
Chairperson and Associate Professor
Department of Occupational Therapy
Samuel Merritt College
Oakland, California

Patricia Ann Morris, OTR, BS
Senior Occupational Therapist
Department of Occupational Therapy/Supportive Services
Wayne State University
Detroit, Michigan

Ed Nickerson, PT, OCS
Senior Physical Therapist
Campus Commons Physical Therapy
Sacramento, California

Lorraine Williams Pedretti, MS, OTR
Professor Emeritus
Department of Occupational Therapy
San José State University
San José, California

Sara A. Pope-Davis, MOT, OTR/L
Occupational Therapist
Memorial Home Care
South Bend, Indiana

Linda Anderson Preston, BS, OTR, BCN
Clinical Specialist
Patricia Neal Outpatient Therapy Center
Roane Medical Center
Harriman, Tennessee

Sandra Utley Reeves, BS, OTR/L
Staff Occupational Therapist
Department of Rehabilitation Services
Shands Hospital at the University of Florida
Gainesville, Florida

Nancy Richman, BS, OTR/L, FAOTA
Glantz/Richman Rehabilitation Associates
Riverwoods, Illinois

Lynda M. Rock, MOT, OTR
Formerly Unit Coordinator
OT/PT Outpatient Services
The Institute for Rehabilitation and Research
Houston, Texas

Charlotte Brasic Royeen, PhD, OTR, FAOTA
Associate Dean for Research
Professor in Occupational Therapy
School of Pharmacy and Allied Health Professions
Creighton University
Omaha, Nebraska

Joyce Shapero Sabari, PhD, OTR, BCN
Associate Professor and Chair
Occupational Therapy Program
State University of New York
Downstate Medical Center
Brooklyn, New York

Winifred Schultz-Krohn, MA, OTR, BCP, FAOTA
Assistant Professor
Department of Occupational Therapy
San José State University
San José, California

Kathleen Barker Schwartz, EdD, OTR, FAOTA
Professor
Department of Occupational Therapy
San José State University
San José, California

Patricia Smith, MS, OTR, FAOTA
Director
Occupational Therapy Assessment and Modification
San José, California

Joan Smithline, BS, PT
Clinical Specialist
Stanford Health Services, Department of Rehabilitation
Services
Stanford, California
Founder, Back On-Line
Work Place Design
Menlo Park, California

Michelle Tipton-Burton, BS, OTR
Occupational Therapy Supervisor
Day Treatment Program
Therapy Services Division
Santa Clara Valley Medical Center
Instructor
San José State University
San José, California

Mary Warren, MS, OTR/L
Director
Visual Independence Program
Eye Foundation of Kansas City
Department of Ophthalmology, School of Medicine
University of Missouri–Kansas City
Kansas City, Missouri

Carol J. Wheatley, MS, OTR/L, CPCRT
Occupational Therapist
Rehabilitation Technology Services
Maryland Rehabilitation Center
Division of Rehabilitation Services
Maryland State Department of Education
Baltimore, Maryland

Lynn Yasuda, MSEd, OTR, FAOTA
Interim Director
Education and Staff Development
Rancho Los Amigos Medical Center
Downey, California

Elizabeth June Yerxa, EdD, LHD, ScD, OTR, FAOTA
Distinguished Professor Emerita
Department of Occupational Science and Occupational
Therapy
University of Southern California
Los Angeles, California

Dedication

To my mother (in memoriam), who taught me compassion.
To my father (in memoriam), who taught me to strive and honored my
    achievements.
To my sister Mary, who nurtured my spirit and my intellect.
To my brother Lawrence, who was my hero and my advocate.
To my brother Julius (in memoriam), who was a role model for holiness,
    goodness, and love.
To my sister Jean, who inspired me to take the risks that made this possible.

Lorraine Williams Pedretti
December 2000

To my mother, who showed me joy in doing and pleasure in creating
To my father, who taught me to question and persevere.

Mary Beth Early
December 2000

Preface

Successful rehabilitation of the adult with physical dysfunction requires the skillful collaboration of many participants: the patient, the family or significant others, and a variety of health care professionals from a range of disciplines. Occupational therapists contribute significantly to the achievement of successful rehabilitation outcomes.

Health care and rehabilitation today look very different than in 1981, when the first edition of this text was published, and they continue to change. Increased pressures for accountability and cost containment have drastically altered the manner in which therapy services are provided and have shifted services away from the hospital and into less expensive settings in the home and community. Funding limitations and health care regulations now force therapists on a regular basis to make difficult choices about the extent, frequency, and duration of treatment. Thus today's occupational therapist must be prepared with a high degree of professionalism, ethical judgment, clinical reasoning skills, creativity, adaptability, and resourcefulness. An appreciation of the greater context in which health care occurs is invaluable.

Since first published in 1981, this text has enjoyed a reputation for being practical, practice oriented, and rich in the technical details that clinicians seek. The editors have sought to preserve this emphasis while also including information about the contemporary context of health care. In the fifth edition of this text the reader is introduced to important changes in practice that have occurred in recent years. Chapters new to this edition include the occupational therapy process, treatment contexts, evidence-based practice, occupational therapy in prevention programs, teaching activities, infection control and safety, occupational performance, leisure activities, functional motion assessment, pain manage-

ment, oncology, special needs of the older adult, and HIV infection and AIDS.

This book is intended as a text for occupational therapy students in baccalaureate and entry-level master's degree programs and as a reference for occupational therapy practitioners. The text has these aims:

1. To introduce the reader to occupational therapy practice in physical dysfunction
2. To prepare the student for occupational therapy practice with adults who have acquired physical disabilities
3. To teach skills necessary for beginning practice in occupational therapy for physical dysfunction
4. To provide a foundation for the development of clinical reasoning skills

The editors have assumed that the reader has mastered foundation concepts in general psychology, anatomy and physiology, neuroanatomy and neurophysiology, kinesiology, human growth and development, medical terminology, conditions of orthopedic and neurological dysfunction, and theories of occupational therapy.

The text is divided into six parts. Part One addresses models for practice, and history and practice trends. Part Two describes occupational therapy process and practice (OT process, treatment contexts, evaluation, treatment planning, evidence-based practice, OT for prevention of injury and physical dysfunction, teaching activities, documentation, and infection control and safety in the treatment environment). Part Three explores occupational performance and covers evaluation and intervention for the performance areas: ADL, mobility, sexuality, work evaluation and work hardening, leisure activities, and assistive technology. Part Four gives a detailed exploration of evaluation and intervention for the performance components.

Topics covered include functional motion assessment, range of motion, muscle strength, motor control, visual deficits, sensory dysfunction, perceptual motor deficits, cognitive dysfunction, social and psychological factors, and pain management. Part Five introduces occupational therapy interventions for the performance components and performance areas. These include therapeutic occupations and modalities, orthotics, and the sensorimotor approaches to treatment. Finally, Part Six provides treatment applications for selected physical disabilities. These include cerebrovascular accident, traumatic brain injury, degenerative neurological diseases, dysphagia, spinal cord injury, neurogenic and myopathic dysfunction, arthritis, hand and upper extremity injuries, hip fractures and lower extremity joint replacement, low back pain, burns, amputations, cardiac and pulmonary diseases, oncology, special needs of older adults, and HIV infection and AIDS. It is not possible to cover all of the physical disabilities that may be acquired in adult life. Those chosen are often encountered in practice and employ principles of treatment that are applicable to similar disabilities.

Each chapter begins with key terms and learning objectives and concludes with review questions. We suggest that the reader preview the key terms and learning objectives before turning to the text of the chapter.

The reader might also survey the headings within the chapter before starting to read. Review questions at the end of chapters are intended to assist the student in mastering content, beginning to develop clinical reasoning skills, achieving learning objectives, and preparing for evaluation of learning. Instructors may wish to use the questions to construct examinations.

Sample case studies are included in each chapter in Part Six. These case studies serve as models of OT intervention for the novice and are not meant to present a comprehensive treatment picture. An appendix at the end of the book includes 12 case studies and a reproducible treatment plan outline that can be used for classroom discussion, homework assignments, and individual and group treatment planning practice. Some of the case studies are based on patients seen in actual practice; however, all identifying information has been changed or deleted.

The terms *patient* and *client* are used in this book to designate the consumer or recipient of occupational therapy services. The use of one term or the other in an individual chapter may reflect the practice context, as well as the preference of the particular contributing author.

Lorraine Williams Pedretti
Mary Beth Early

Acknowledgments

With this edition several new chapter contributors are introduced. Many are nationally and internationally known experts in their disciplines. Administrators, educators, researchers, and master clinicians are represented. Our expert contributors, past and present, are gratefully acknowledged for their excellent work.

Sincere appreciation is extended to Martha Sasser, former Executive Editor, and Amy Christopher, former Developmental Editor, for their guidance and support through the conception and development of the proposal and the manuscript. Kellie White, Executive Editor; Christie Hart, Developmental Editor; Leslie Mosby, Associate Developmental Editor; Christine O'Brien and Rebecca Swisher, Assistant Editors; and Larry State and the production staff are gratefully acknowledged for their continued assistance.

Gratitude is extended to Dr. A. Lee Dellon for reviewing the chapter on sensation and sensory dysfunction and to Maureen Matthews, who graciously took on responsibility for several chapters and who was instrumental in identifying and helping with other contributors.

To those publishers and vendors who permitted us to use material from their publications, we extend our sincere gratitude. Photographers and artists, and the patients and models who posed for photographs, are also gratefully acknowledged.

Finally, special appreciation is extended to our professional colleagues, and to our families, Robert Pedretti, Mark Pedretti, Robert Dehler, and Jeffrey Felipe Dehler, for their ongoing support, patience, and assistance.

Lorraine Williams Pedretti
Mary Beth Early

Contents

CHAPTER 1

Occupational Performance and Models of Practice for Physical Dysfunction

LORRAINE WILLIAMS PEDRETTI
MARY BETH EARLY

KEY TERMS

Occupational performance
Domain of concern
Frame of reference
Performance areas
Performance components
Performance contexts
Occupation
Occupational role
Occupations
Purposeful activity
Adjunctive methods
Enabling activities
Intervention level
Theory
Model of practice
Model of human occupation
Biomechanical model
Motor control model
Rehabilitation model

LEARNING OBJECTIVES

After studying this chapter the student or practitioner will be able to do the following:

1. Define *occupational performance.*
2. Name the performance areas and performance components.
3. Compare the American occupational performance model with the Canadian Model of Occupational Performance.
4. List the intervention levels in the treatment continuum and give examples of the kinds of intervention strategies that are used at each level.
5. Define and compare *frame of reference, theory,* and *conceptual model of practice.*
6. Name and describe four models of practice that are used often to guide treatment intervention for physical dysfunction.
7. List four treatment approaches that are considered within the motor control model.
8. List intervention strategies that are considered part of the rehabilitation model.
9. Describe the kinds of physical dysfunction most likely to be treated using the biomechanical model and the motor control model.

Occupational performance is the domain of concern of occupational therapy (OT). The elements of the occupational performance domain of concern are the performance areas, performance components, and performance contexts,[13] which are described in this chapter.

Also in this chapter, the scope of practice in physical dysfunction is outlined on a continuum within the context of occupational performance. Additionally, a summary is presented of models of practice most often used to guide clinical reasoning in physical disabilities practice.

OCCUPATIONAL PERFORMANCE

Occupational performance describes the content of the OT process and the **domain of concern** in OT practice across specialty areas.[5,13] Work, play, and self-care have always been the core of OT, but the performance components and scope of occupational performance were further developed by a series of task forces and committees of the American Occupational Therapy Association (AOTA) in the 1970s.[5,7,8,10] The current conception of occupational performance was generated from conceptualizations of professional practice and was originally described as a **frame of reference** for practice and for curriculum design in education.[4,5,31] Subsequently, occupational performance terminology was defined and standardized in official documents of the AOTA.[3,10,11,13]

The elements of occupational performance are the **performance areas, performance components,** and **performance contexts.** The performance areas are (1) activities of daily living, (2) work and productive activities, and (3) play or leisure activities. Supporting these performance areas are the performance components: (1) the sensorimotor component, (2) the cognitive integration and cognitive components, and (3) the psychosocial skills and psychological components. Performance of **occupation** occurs within the temporal and environmental contexts[13] in which tasks are performed (Fig. 1-1).

The Canadian Model of Occupational Performance (CMOP) is similar to the American model. It includes performance areas of self-care, productivity, and leisure, and classifies occupation under these categories. The environment consists of physical, social, cultural, and

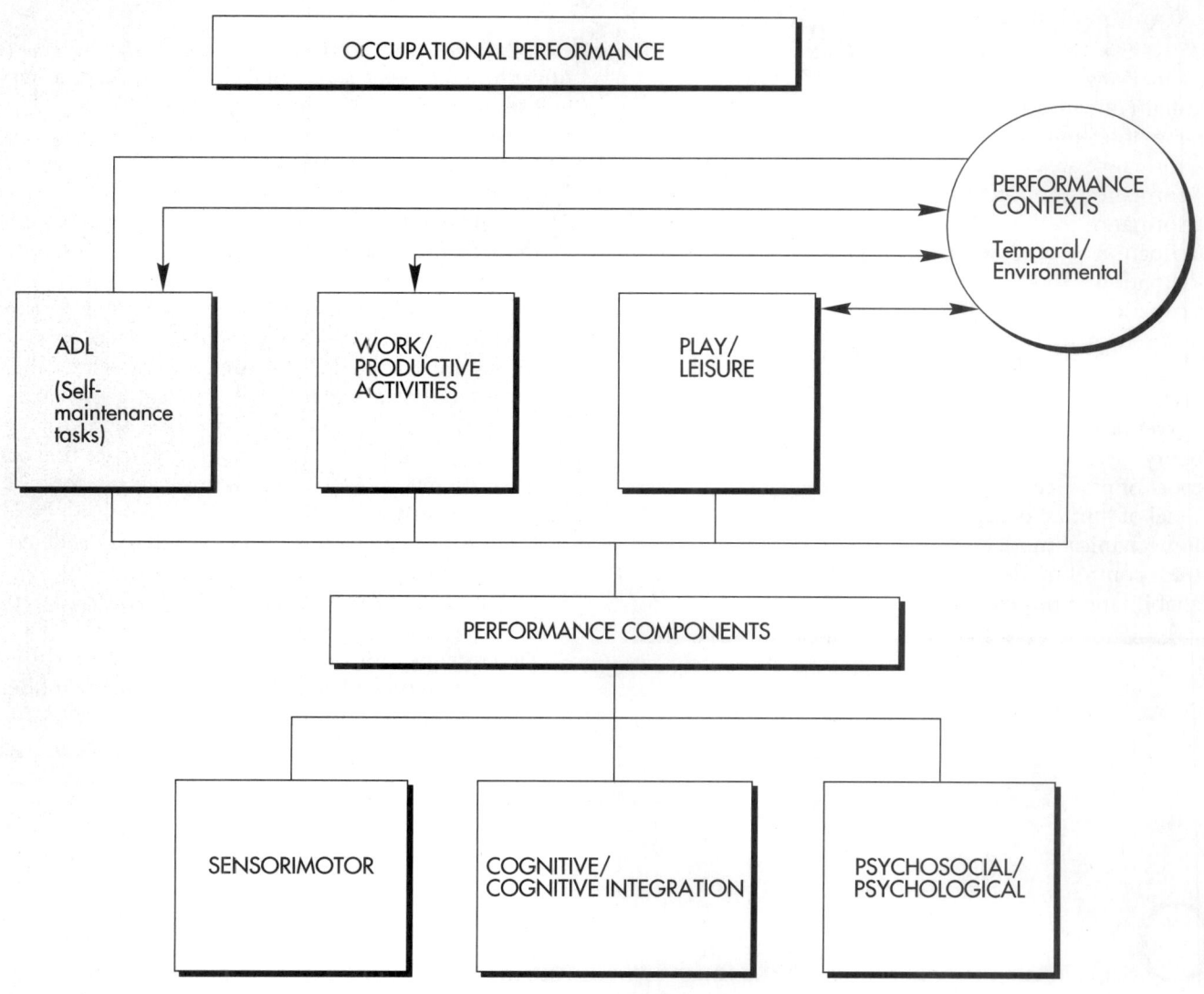

FIG. 1-1

Occupational performance: domain of concern. Based on uniform terminology for occupational therapy, ed 3, *Am J Occup Ther* 48:1047-1054, 1994. (Diagram adapted from the American Occupational Therapy Association: *A curriculum guide for occupational therapy educators,* 1974.)

institutional elements. Occupational performance is described as "the result of interactions between the person, the environment and the occupation. The person is seen as possessing physical, affective, and cognitive performance components, central to which is the essential core of being, the spiritual element."[29] Spirituality as the central core of being is a unique feature of the CMOP (Fig. 1-2).[17,29]

Occupational performance refers to the ability to perform those tasks that make it possible to carry out **occupational roles** in a satisfying manner appropriate for the individual's developmental stage, culture, and environment.[2,4,5,6,32] Occupational roles develop in conjunction with the **occupations** that the individual performs in the society. These include such roles as preschooler, student, parent, homemaker, employee, volunteer, or retired worker.[5,32]

Occupational performance requires learning and practice opportunities specific to life roles and developmental tasks and the use of all performance components. Deficits in task learning experiences, performance components, or impoverished performance contexts may lead to limitations in occupational performance.[5]

Performance Areas

Activities of daily living (ADL), work and productive activities, and play or leisure activities are the performance areas. ADL include the self-maintenance tasks of grooming, hygiene, dressing, feeding and eating, mobility, socialization, communication, and sexual expression. Work and productive activities include home management, care of others, educational activities, and vocational activities. Play and leisure include play exploration and play or leisure performance in age-appropriate activities.[4,13,30]

Performance Components

Performance components are "the learned developmental patterns of behavior which are the substructure and foundation of the individual's occupational performance."[4,5,6] Performance components include (1) the sensorimotor component, (2) the cognitive integration and cognitive components, and (3) the psychosocial skills and psychological components.[4,5,13] Adequate neurophysiological development and integrated functioning of the performance components are basic to an

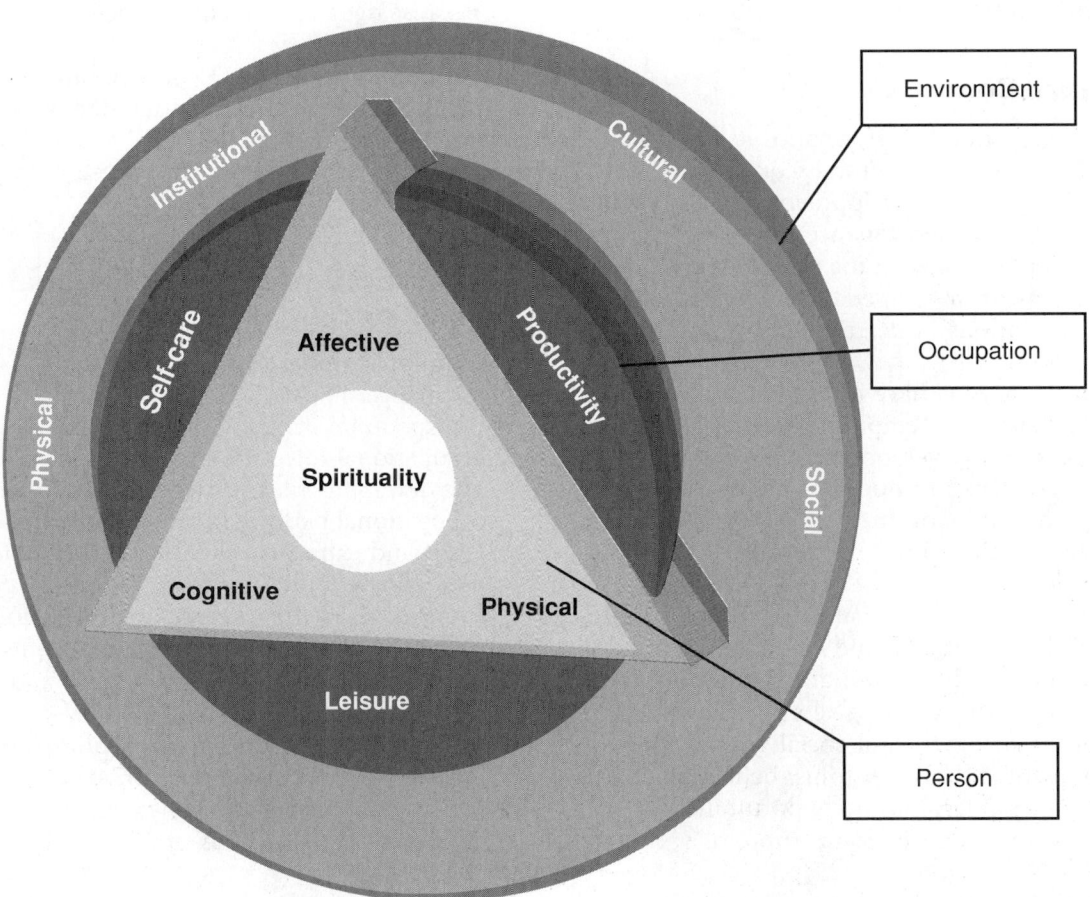

FIG. 1-2
The Canadian Model of Occupational Performance. From *Enabling occupation: an occupational therapy perspective*, 1997. Reproduced with permission, CAOT Publications.

individual's ability to perform occupational tasks or activities in the performance areas.[32]

The sensorimotor component includes three function types: sensory, neuromusculoskeletal, and motor. Sensory functions include sensory awareness and processing and perceptual processing. Neuromusculoskeletal functions include reflex responses, range of motion, muscle tone, strength, endurance, postural control, postural alignment, and soft-tissue integrity. Motor functions include gross coordination, crossing the midline, laterality, bilateral integration, motor control, praxis, fine coordination and dexterity, and oral motor control.[13]

The cognitive integration and cognitive components refer to the ability to use higher brain functions. These components include level of arousal, orientation, recognition, attention span, initiation of activity, termination of activity, memory, sequencing, categorization, concept formation, spatial operations, problem solving, learning, and generalization.[13]

The psychosocial skills and psychological components comprise the abilities for social interaction and emotional processing. In this category are values, interests, self-concept, role performance, social conduct, interpersonal skills, self-expression, coping skills, time management, and self-control.[13]

Performance Contexts

Successful occupational performance occurs in the context of the individual's cultural requirements and is consistent with age and developmental stage.[30] When assessing function in performance areas, the occupational therapist must consider the performance contexts in which the patient must operate. The selection of appropriate interventions is determined, in part, by the performance context.[13]

Performance contexts have both temporal and environmental dimensions. Temporal dimensions include the individual's age, developmental stage or phase of maturation, and stage in important life processes such as parenting, education, or career. Disability status (e.g., acute, chronic, terminal, improving, or declining) must also be considered.[13]

Environmental dimensions are manifested in three frameworks: physical, social, and cultural. The physical environment includes home, buildings, outdoors, furniture, tools, and other objects. The social environment includes significant others and social groups. The cultural environment includes customs, beliefs, standards of behavior, political factors, and opportunities for education, employment, and economic support.[13]

Concerns of Occupational Therapy

The concerns of OT are the performance areas, performance components, performance contexts, and occupational performance itself.[5,13,30,34] To facilitate occupa-

tional performance the OT program may include treatment methods designed for the remediation of deficits or for the compensation for deficits in performance areas, performance components, and performance contexts; in many cases both remediation and compensation are used.[5] In a remediation approach, treatment is focused on improving performance components. It is assumed that improvement in performance components (e.g., strength, visual perception, or cognitive skills) can be expected and, in turn, will lead to improved functioning in performance areas. Examples of remediation strategies are muscle strengthening, sensory reeducation, and cognitive retraining. When improvement is not expected or a remediation approach is not feasible, the compensation approach may be used. The compensation approach focuses on remaining abilities and aims to improve function by adapting or compensating for performance component deficits. Compensatory interventions might include strategies such as adapting methods of task performance to accommodate muscle weakness, providing assistive devices to compensate for limited joint motion, and changing the environment to accommodate limited mobility.[19,22]

Because the achievement of functional independence in performance areas is a core concept of OT theory and the ultimate goal of the OT process, intervention strategies must ultimately be directed to the patient's achievement in performance areas[13,38] when a performance component (e.g., motor skill development) is being addressed.

Assumptions About Occupational Performance

The following are assumptions about occupational performance:

- Occupational performance is essential to satisfactory occupational role fulfillment.
- The development, performance, and maintenance of occupational performance are influenced by intrapersonal and extrapersonal elements. Intrapersonal elements include the temporal aspects of performance contexts, as well as genetic, neurophysiological, and pathological factors. Extrapersonal elements include the physical environment, objects and tools, and social, cultural, and familial elements.
- An appropriate balance in occupational performance is essential for the maintenance of health.
- Appropriate balance changes with chronological and developmental age, life cycle, and life events and circumstances.
- Appropriate balance is personally chosen and may vary widely from individual to individual.
- Failure in development of occupational performance or loss, disruption, or change of occupational roles can arise from intrapersonal or extrapersonal factors.

- Adequate occupational performance is dependent on intact neurophysiological development[32] and the integrated functioning of the sensorimotor, cognitive integration and cognitive, and psychosocial and psychological subsystems of the individual.
- Defect, disease, or injury affecting any performance component may lead to a failure of integration of the performance component subsystems and results in a failure or disruption in the performance areas and thus a failure or disruption in satisfying fulfillment of occupational roles.
- The role of the occupational therapist is to facilitate both an appropriate balance and optimum occupational performance toward the resumption of occupational roles.
- The occupational therapist is concerned with compensation for deficits in the performance areas and remediation of performance components.
- The primary treatment tool of the occupational therapist is **purposeful activity.**
- Other treatment tools of the occupational therapist include **adjunctive methods** and **enabling activities,** described below, that are used to prepare the patient for function in the performance areas.[41]
- Exclusive use of such preparatory methods out of context of the patient's occupational performance is not considered OT.

TREATMENT CONTINUUM IN THE CONTEXT OF OCCUPATIONAL PERFORMANCE

As OT has become less dependent on medical direction, its role has expanded considerably. Occupational therapists have developed and demonstrated competence in many specialized practice areas associated with physical dysfunction. The occupational therapist's concern, from the onset of the illness or injury, is for the patient to become as independent as possible in the performance areas and to resume previous occupational roles or to assume new and satisfying occupational roles. In the treatment of many physical disabilities OT intervention may begin at the time of surgery or in the early stages of acute care and continue through the final stages of rehabilitation. Thus OT can make an important contribution at every level in the treatment continuum.[35]

Fig. 1-3 shows a conceptualization of the treatment continuum in physical disability practice. The continuum consists of four levels of intervention or intervention categories.[15] The levels in the continuum overlap, or can occur simultaneously. The treatment continuum is not a strict step-by-step progression. It addresses the performance components and performance areas of occupational performance and takes the patient through a logical progression from dependence to occupational performance to resumption of valued social and occupational roles. The treatment continuum identifies the concerns of OT practice within the context of occupational performance. Four **intervention levels** in the treatment continuum are described as follows:

Intervention Level One: Adjunctive Methods

Procedures that prepare the patient for occupational performance but are preliminary to the use of purposeful activity are concerns of OT.[14] Level one methods, called **adjunctive methods,** may include exercise, facilitation and inhibition techniques, positioning, sensory stimulation, selected physical agent modalities, and provision of devices such as braces and splints.[41] Level one methods and devices are often used in (but are not limited to) the acute stages of illness or injury. When using these methods the occupational therapist is likely to be most concerned with assessing and remediating performance components. It is important for occupational therapists to plan the progression of treatment so that adjunctive modalities are used as preparation for purposeful activity and are directed toward maximum independence in the performance areas.

Intervention Level Two: Enabling Activities.

Many methods used in OT may not be considered purposeful activity but may be steps toward ability to perform purposeful activities. Such methods are referred to as **enabling activities.** Purposeful activity has an autonomous or inherent goal beyond the motor function required to perform the task[14] and requires the active participation of the patient.[9,12] Many patients are not ready for activity at this performance level.

Occupational therapists have created many enabling devices and methods that simulate purposeful activities, such as sanding boards, skate boards, stacking cones or blocks, practice boards for mastery of clothing fasteners and hardware, driving simulators, work simulators, and tabletop activities such as form boards for training in perceptual-motor skills. Such devices and activities are not likely to be as meaningful to the patient or to stimulate as much interest and motivation as purposeful activities. They may be needed, however, as a preparatory or ancillary part of the treatment program to train patients in specific sensorimotor, perceptual, or cognitive functions necessary for activities in the performance areas.

Such equipment as wheelchairs, ambulatory aids, special clothing, communication devices, environmental control systems, and other assistive devices may also be enabling. These devices can be important for increasing independence in the performance areas and assumption of occupational roles.

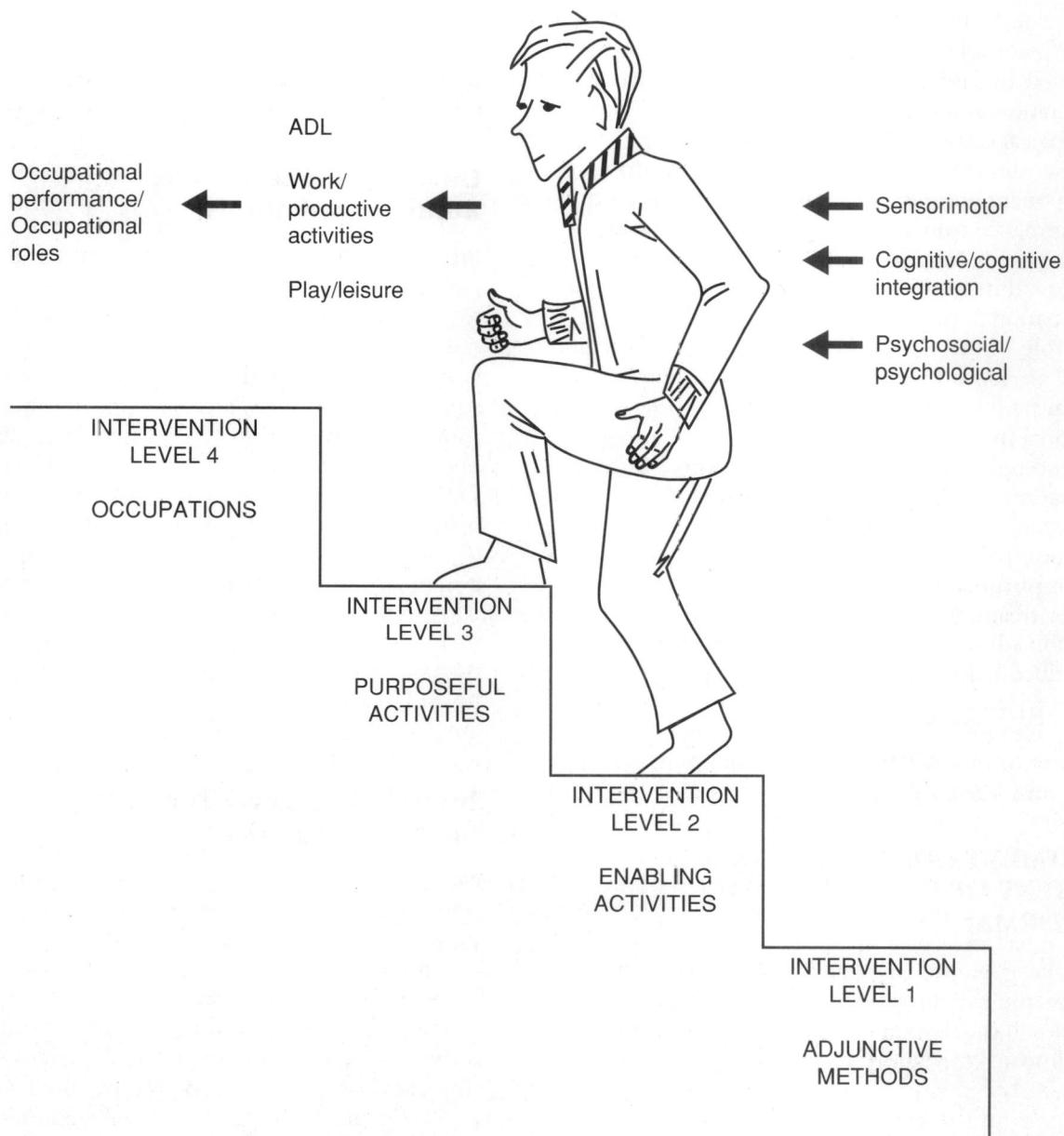

FIG. I-3
Treatment continuum in occupational performance.

At intervention level two the therapist is still concerned with assessment and remediation of performance components and begins to assess and teach activities in the performance areas.

Intervention Level Three: Purposeful Activity

Purposeful activity has been the core of OT since its inception. Purposeful activity includes activities that have an inherent or autonomous goal and are relevant and meaningful to the patient.[14] Purposeful activity is part of the daily life routine and occurs in the context of occupational performance.[12] Examples are feeding, hy-

giene, dressing, mobility, communication, arts, crafts, games, sports, work, and educational activities.

The individual performing the activity determines its purposefulness. Purposefulness is also affected by the context in which the activity is performed. OT practitioners use purposeful activities to evaluate, facilitate, restore, or maintain a person's ability to function in life roles.[12] Purposeful activity is used to enhance functioning in the performance areas. The OT practitioner carries out treatment with purposeful activity in a health care facility, a community agency, or the patient's home. At this level the OT practitioner is concerned primarily with assessing and remediating deficits in the performance areas.

Intervention Level Four: Occupations

The highest stage of the treatment continuum engages the patient in natural **occupations** in his or her living environment and in the community.[15] The patient performs appropriate tasks of ADL, work and productive activities, and play and leisure to his or her maximum level of independence. Involvement in scheduled OT decreases and ultimately ends as the individual resumes and effectively performs valued occupational roles.

CONCEPTUAL SYSTEMS

The practice of OT in physical dysfunction should be guided by a unifying conceptual system. Frames of reference, theories, and models can be used as conceptual systems. These three terms are sometimes used interchangeably, and there is no universal agreement on their definitions.[18] Theories, models, and frames of reference have been described for OT by Fidler,[33] Mosey,[33,34] Reilly,[33] Kielhofner,[24-27,35] Ayres,[33] Llorens,[33] Gilfoyle and Grady,[21] King,[28] Allen,[1] and Schkade and Schultz,[39] among others.

Frame of Reference

According to Mosey,[34] a **frame of reference** is derived from a profession's model and guides interaction with clients. She defined *frame of reference* as "a set of interrelated, internally consistent concepts, definitions, and postulates that provides a systematic description of or prescription for a practitioner's interaction within a particular aspect of a profession's domain of concern."[34] Frames of reference link theory to practice and must meet certain criteria to be considered frames of reference. Mosey saw a frame of reference as a guide rather than a formula for action.[34]

Theory

A **theory** encompasses principles and relationships that predict or explain phenomena under specified conditions.[18] Mosey[34] stated that theory development occurs through direct observation or through speculation about the relationships between events.[34] According to Reed[37] "theory attempts to (1) define and explain relationships between concepts or ideas related to the phenomenon of interest [occupational endeavor in occupational therapy], (2) explain how these relationships can predict behavior or events, and (3) suggest ways that the phenomenon can be changed or controlled."[37] OT theory is concerned with the concepts of person, environment, health, and occupation. OT and other practice professions must have a theoretical base that can be translated into specific guidelines for practice and continuously examined for their effectiveness.[37]

Model

Mosey defined *model* as "the typical way in which a profession perceives itself, its relationship to other professions, and its association with the society to which it is responsible."[34] The model is characterized by "a description of the profession's philosophical assumptions, ethical code, theoretical foundation, domain of concern, legitimate tools, and the nature of and principles for sequencing the various aspects of practice."[34]

Christiansen[18] defined a model as a way of "structuring or organizing knowledge for the purpose of guiding thinking." The purpose of a model is to help the practitioner analyze situations, determine methodologies, and conceive alternatives—in other words, to provide guidelines for practice. The use of a model in practice can be the basis for theory development.[18]

Kielhofner referred to "conceptual models of practice."[24] He stated that the purpose of conceptual models is to provide specific prescriptions for practice. He stated that "a conceptual practice model presents and organizes a number of theoretical concepts used by therapists in their work."[24]

Several **models of practice** are used in OT. Some of these have also been referred to as treatment approaches.[23,36] Each conceptual practice model addresses a specific area of human function and is based on a theory that explains the organization and order of some aspect of human function on which the model focuses. More than one practice model is needed to address the broad range of OT's domain of concern.[24] The practice models summarized below are those considered to be used most often (though not exclusively) and most applicable in physical disabilities practice.

MODELS OF PRACTICE
Model of Human Occupation

The **Model of Human Occupation** (MOHO)[25-27] applies to all aspects of occupational performance, not just the physical. It is a systems model, in which the human being engaged in occupation expresses a complex interaction of aspects that cannot be fully comprehended when viewed separately. Engagement in occupation requires three subsystems intricately linked to produce performance: the *volition subsystem* (personal causation, values, interests), the *habituation subsystem* (habits and roles), and the *performance subsystem* (the skills of the mind, brain, and body working together). Engagement in occupation occurs within the environment, which constantly provides feedback and information that intimately and dynamically influence the three subsystems and their product—occupational performance.

Assessment and intervention within MOHO may address any of the subsystems, or their constituent parts, or the environment, or any combination of these. The concepts defined within the volition subsystem allow the therapist to consider motivational factors. The patient with a weak sense of *personal causation*[26]—feelings of competence and belief in one's own ability to be effective—may respond better to a therapeutic approach that is highly directive and authoritarian than to one that is more collaborative and puts the burden of responsibility on the patient.

The habituation subsystem is relevant to any intervention plan that requires a patient to develop or relearn habits or roles. For example, a consideration of *habit maps*[26]—how habits are constructed and cued by features of the temporal environment—may assist the therapist in creating and refining a compensatory strategy to maximize functional independence in a patient who is relearning grooming routines after a head injury. The concept of *role scripts*[26]—an internalized sense of how a role is understood and how it should be translated into action—may help the therapist analyze how an individual approaches a particular occupational role.

Altering features of the environment to elicit a change in occupational performance is a key principle of MOHO. The following types of change are employed[26]:

1. Purposeful alteration of the physical setting (e.g., adding a ramp)
2. Providing a new object (e.g., equipping the patient with a reacher to grasp objects out of arm's reach)
3. Providing or facilitating a change in social groups (e.g., training the caregiver to break down and cue a sequence such as brushing teeth)
4. Arranging for the patient to experience new occupations (e.g., using a computer to access the internet)

A further principle of intervention in the model of human occupation is that "change is often disorderly."[26] Therapeutic progress is therefore not linear and predictable but may meander and fluctuate as the patient seeks to establish a new balance in occupational performance. The model of human occupation may be useful in combination with any of the models addressed below.

Biomechanical Model

The **biomechanical model** for the treatment of physical dysfunction applies the mechanical principles of kinetics and kinematics to the movement of the human body.[24,36] These mechanical principles deal with the way that forces acting on the body affect movement and equilibrium.[16] Methods of treatment in this model use principles of physics related to forces, levers, and torque.

Examples of biomechanical techniques are joint measurement, muscle strength testing, kinetic activity,

therapeutic exercise, and orthotics. The purposes of the biomechanical methods are to (1) assess specific physical limitations in range, strength, and endurance, (2) restore function of range, strength, and endurance, and (3) reduce deformity.

The biomechanical model is most appropriate for patients who have motor unit or orthopedic disorders but whose central nervous system (CNS) is intact. These patients can control isolated movement and specific movement patterns, but have weakness, low endurance, or joint limitation. Examples of such disabilities are orthopedic dysfunctions, including rheumatoid arthritis, osteoarthritis, fractures, amputations, hand trauma, burns, and motor unit disorders, such as peripheral nerve injuries, Guillain-Barré syndrome, spinal cord injuries, and muscular dystrophy.

Biomechanical methods of evaluation and treatment are directed primarily at restoring sensorimotor components. Many of the adjunctive or enabling techniques and modalities are also biomechanical, and biomechanical principles can also be applied to purposeful activity in the performance areas. For example, the activities of sawing wood, rolling out dough, and vacuuming carpets rely on biomechanical principles for their actions and therapeutic effects when used to improve physical performance.

Before the motor control model of treatment evolved, therapists tried to apply biomechanical principles to patients with damaged central nervous systems and met with many problems as a result. Because biomechanical treatment requires controlled voluntary movement, it is inappropriate for patients who lack such control.

Motor Control Model

The **motor control model** is used with persons who have CNS dysfunction. Four approaches to treatment, variously referred to as the sensorimotor or neurodevelopmental approaches, are included in this model.[24] These four approaches are based on theories of CNS development and motor recovery.[20] The normal CNS produces controlled, well-modulated movement. In the damaged CNS, coordination and well-modulated, controlled movement are not possible. Methods of treatment in sensorimotor approaches use neurophysiological mechanisms to normalize muscle tone and elicit more normal motor responses.[20,42] Some approaches use reflex mechanisms, and the sequence of treatment may be based on the recapitulation of ontogenetic development.[40] Chapters 32 through 36 describe the sensorimotor approaches of Rood, Brunnstrom (movement therapy), Knott and Voss (proprioceptive neuromuscular facilitation), and Bobath (neurodevelopmental treatment).

All of the sensorimotor approaches are directed to motor recovery and improvement of motor performance. They do not consider motivation, arousal, attention, role dysfunction, or temporal adaptation and the influence of these factors on motor behavior.[20]

Sensorimotor treatment principles can also be applied to purposeful activity, as described in Chapters 33 through 36. Sensorimotor treatment methods may be used "to prepare the client or patient for better performance and prevention of disability through self-participation in occupation."[8] When used to precede and enable purposeful activity, and as part of purposeful activity, sensorimotor methods can be a valuable aid in restoring occupational performance.

Rehabilitation Model

The term *rehabilitation* means a return to ability, that is, the return to the fullest physical, mental, social, vocational, and economic usefulness that is possible for the individual. It means the ability to live and work with remaining capabilities.[23] Therefore the focus in the treatment program is on abilities rather than on disabilities. Rehabilitation is concerned with the intrinsic worth and dignity of the individual and with the restoration of a satisfying and purposeful life. The **rehabilitation model** uses measures that enable the patient to live as independently as possible with some residual disability. Its goal is to help the patient learn to work around or compensate for physical, cognitive, or perceptual limitations.[36]

The rehabilitation model is a dynamic process and requires that the patient be a member of the rehabilitation team. It requires ongoing assessment and follow-up to maintain maximum function and therefore must keep pace with advances in methods and equipment (rehabilitation technology), social change, and community resources to provide the best services and opportunities for each patient.[23]

Using this model, OT focuses on performance areas more than on performance components. The aim of the OT program is to minimize disability barriers to role performance. The occupational therapist must assess the patient's capabilities and determine how to overcome the effects of the disability. The treatment methods of the rehabilitation model include modalities such as the following:

- Acquisition of and training in the use of assistive technology
- Adaptive clothing
- Architectural adaptations
- Community transportation
- Home evaluation and adaptation
- Homemaking and child care
- Leisure activities
- Prosthetic training
- Self-care evaluation and training
- Wheelchair management
- Work simplification and energy conservation
- Work-related activities

Frequently the methods of the rehabilitation model are used in combination with methods of the biomechanical or motor control model. Biomechanical or sensorimotor principles can be applied during rehabilitation activities to enhance and reinforce the restoration of the sensorimotor and cognitive components. Further, the treatment program often focuses on performance areas and performance components simultaneously. Thus the combined restoration of sensorimotor, cognitive, and psychosocial functions improves functioning in the performance areas.

SUMMARY

Occupational performance describes the domain of concern for OT practice. The treatment continuum, conceptualized within an occupational performance framework, accommodates a broad spectrum of OT from acute care to long-term rehabilitation. It also encompasses the wide range of modalities used in OT practice for physical disabilities.

The OT practitioner uses a suitable practice model or models to guide clinical reasoning in evaluation and treatment planning. The OT practitioner assesses performance areas, performance components, and performance contexts and then identifies assets, skills, and deficits in the individual's occupational roles and role dysfunction. Guided by the selected practice model or models, OT practitioners select goals, objectives, and intervention strategies designed to restore the patient to his or her maximum level of performance in valued occupational roles.

REVIEW QUESTIONS

1. Briefly outline the elements of the occupational performance domain of concern.
2. Define *model*, *theory*, and *frame of reference*.
3. What is the purpose of a model?
4. What is the difference between a performance area and a performance component? How are they related?
5. Define *occupational role*. Give some examples.
6. Select one of your occupational roles and list all of the tasks in each of the performance areas that are necessary to fulfill that role.
7. List the levels in the treatment continuum and give examples of treatment modalities that might be used in each.
8. Define *enabling activities* as used in this chapter.
9. Relate the MOHO concepts of personal causation, habit map, and role script to one of your occupational roles.

10. Which treatment modalities can be thought of as primarily biomechanical in nature?
11. With which diagnoses is a biomechanical model most likely to be used? Why?
12. For which diagnoses is the motor control model most likely to be effective?
13. How can the sensorimotor approaches be integrated in an occupational performance framework?
14. Describe the rehabilitation model.
15. List six treatment modalities that are within the rehabilitation model
16. How is the rehabilitation model integrated with the other models of practice discussed in this chapter?

REFERENCES

1. Allen C: Activity, occupational therapy's treatment method, *Am J Occup Ther* 41:563-565, 1987.
2. American Occupational Therapy Association: Occupational therapy: its definition and functions, *Am J Occup Ther* 26:204-205, 1972.
3. American Occupational Therapy Association: Position paper: occupational performance: occupational therapy's definition of function, *Am J Occup Ther* 49(10):1019-1020, 1995.
4. American Occupational Therapy Association: *The roles and functions of occupational therapy personnel*, Rockville, Md, 1973, The Association.
5. American Occupational Therapy Association: *A curriculum guide for occupational therapy educators*, Rockville, Md, 1974, The Association.
6. American Occupational Therapy Association: Project to delineate the roles and functions of occupational therapy personnel, Rockville, Md, 1972. Cited in *A curriculum guide for occupational therapy educators*, Rockville, Md, 1974, The Association.
7. American Occupational Therapy Association: Task force on target populations, Association report II, *Am J Occup Ther* 28:231, 1974.
8. American Occupational Therapy Association: Resolution 532-79 (1979), Occupation as the common core of occupational therapy, Representative Assembly minutes, April 1979, Detroit, Mich, *Am J Occup Ther* 33:785, 1979.
9. American Occupational Therapy Association: Purposeful activities, a position paper, *Am J Occup Ther* 37:805, 1983.
10. American Occupational Therapy Association: Occupational therapy product output reporting system and uniform terminology for reporting occupational therapy services. In *Reference manual of the official documents of the American Occupational Therapy Association*, Rockville, Md, 1989, The Association.
11. American Occupational Therapy Association: Uniform terminology for occupational therapy, ed 2, *Am J Occup Ther* 43:808-815, 1989.
12. American Occupational Therapy Association: Position paper: purposeful activity, *Am J Occup Ther* 47:1081-1082, 1993.
13. American Occupational Therapy Association: Uniform terminology for occupational therapy, ed 3, *Am J Occup Ther* 48:1047-1054, 1994.
14. Ayres AJ: Basic concepts of clinical practice in physical disabilities, *Am J Occup Ther* 12:300, 1958.
15. Baird AM, Honis DM, Kozikeowski RA, et al: Intervention for people with physical disabilities: what are occupational therapy practitioners doing? A paper presented in partial fulfillment for the requirements, master of science in occupational therapy, College Misericordia, 1999, Dallas, Pa.(Unpublished).
16. Brunnstrom S: *Clinical kinesiology*, ed 3, Philadelphia, 1972, FA Davis.
17. Canadian Association of Occupational Therapists: *Occupational therapy guidelines for client-centered practice*, Toronto, Canada, 1991, The Association.
18. Christiansen C: Occupational therapy, intervention for life performance. In Christiansen C, Baum C: *Occupational therapy: overcoming human performance deficits*, Thorofare, NJ, 1991, Slack.
19. Culler KH: Home and family management. In Hopkins HL, Smith HD: *Willard & Spackman's occupational therapy*, ed 8, Philadelphia, 1993, JB Lippincott.
20. Di Joseph LM: Independence through activity: mind, body, and environment interaction in therapy, *Am J Occup Ther* 36:740, 1982.
21. Gilfoyle E, Grady A: *Children adapt*, ed 2, Thorofare, NJ, 1989, Slack.
22. Holm MB, Rogers JC, James AB: Treatment of activities of daily living. In Neistadt M, Crepeau EB: *Willard & Spackman's Occupational Therapy*, ed 9, Philadelphia, 1998, JB Lippincott.
23. Hopkins HL, Smith HD, Tiffany EG: Rehabilitation. In Hopkins HL, Smith HD, editors: *Willard & Spackman's occupational therapy*, ed 6, Philadelphia, 1983, JB Lippincott.
24. Kielhofner G: *Conceptual foundations of occupational therapy*, ed 2, Philadelphia, 1997, FA Davis.
25. Kielhofner G, editor: *A model of human occupation*, Baltimore, 1985, Williams & Wilkins.
26. Kielhofner G, editor: *A model of human occupation: theory and application*, ed 2, Baltimore, 1995, Williams & Wilkins.
27. Kielhofner G, Burke JP: A model of human occupation. I. Conceptual framework and content, *Am J Occup Ther* 34:572, 1980.
28. King LJ: Toward a science of adaptive responses, *Am J Occup Ther* 32:429, 1978.
29. Law M et al: *Canadian occupational performance measure*, Ottawa, Canada, 1998, CAOT Publications.
30. Llorens LA: *Application of a developmental theory for health and rehabilitation*, Rockville, Md, 1976, American Occupational Therapy Association.
31. Llorens LA: Personal communication, July 6, 1988.
32. Llorens LA: Performance tasks and roles through the life span. In Christian C, Baum C: *Occupational therapy: overcoming human performance deficits*, Thorofare, NJ, 1991, Slack.
33. Miller BR and associates: *Six perspectives on theory for the practice of occupational therapy*, Rockville, Md, 1988, Aspen Publishers.
34. Mosey AC: *Occupational therapy: configuration of a profession*, New York, 1981, Raven Press.
35. Pedretti LW: The compatibility of treatment methods in physical disabilities with the philosophical base of occupational therapy. Unpublished paper presented to the American Occupational Therapy Association National Conference, Philadelphia, May 13, 1982.
36. Reed KL: *Models of practice in occupational therapy*, Baltimore, 1984, Williams & Wilkins.
37. Reed KL: Theory and frame of reference. In Neistadt ME, Crepeau EB: *Willard & Spackman's occupational therapy*, ed 9, Philadelphia, 1998, JB Lippincott.
38. Rogers JC: The spirit of independence: the evolution of a philosophy, *Am J Occup Ther* 36:709, 1982.
39. Schkade JK, Schultz S: Occupational adaptation: toward a holistic approach for contemporary practice. I. *Am J Occup Ther* 46:829-837. II. *Am J Occup Ther* 46:917-925, 1992.
40. Stockmeyer SA: An interpretation of the approach of Rood to the treatment of neuromuscular dysfunction, *Am J Phys Med* 46:900, 1967.
41. Trombly CA: Include exercise in purposeful activity, *Am J Occup Ther* 36:467, 1982 (letter).
42. Willard HL, Spackman CS, editors: *Occupational therapy*, ed 4, Philadelphia, 1971, JB Lippincott.

CHAPTER 2

History and Practice Trends in the Treatment of Physical Dysfunction

KATHLEEN BARKER SCHWARTZ

KEY TERMS

Moral treatment
Rehabilitation model
Medical model
Reductionism
Arts and crafts movement
Scientific management

LEARNING OBJECTIVES

After studying this chapter the student or practitioner will be able to do the following:
1. Trace the ideas, values, and beliefs that have influenced the development of occupational therapy (OT) as a profession.
2. Understand how the history of the profession has contributed to the opportunities and challenges that physical disabilities practitioners face today.

ROOTS OF OCCUPATIONAL THERAPY

The founders of occupational therapy (OT) shared a belief in the value of occupation. However, they each had somewhat different views of practice, depending on their particular disciplines. William Rush Dunton was a psychiatrist, Herbert J. Hall was a physician, Eleanor Clarke Slagle came from a background in social welfare, Susan Johnson was a former arts and crafts teacher, Thomas Kidner and George Barton were former architects, and Susan Tracey was a nurse. These people were also influenced by ideas and beliefs prevalent during the latter part of the 19th century and the early years of the 20th. The three ideologies that seemed to have most shaped the profession's development were **moral treatment, arts and crafts,** and **scientific management.**

Moral Treatment

Moral treatment originated in 19th-century Europe and was promoted by physicians such as Philippe Pinel and Samuel Tuke. The main features of this philosophy included respect for human individuality, acceptance of the unity of mind and body, and belief that a humane approach using daily routine and occupation could lead to recovery.[5] Moral treatment represented a shift in thinking from a pessimistic viewpoint that labeled the mentally ill as subhuman and incurable to an optimistic one that viewed the mentally ill as capable of reason and able to respond to humane treatment.

Dr. Benjamin Rush, an American advocate of moral treatment, believed that occupations should "engage the mind, and exercise the body: as swinging, riding, walking, sewing, embroidery, bowling, gardening, mechanic arts; to which may be added reading, writing, conversation, etc., the whole to be performed with order and regularity."[28] Dr. Thomas Kirkbride of the Pennsylvania Hospital for the Insane described moral treatment as daily routine to provide "active movements and diversity of occupations" such as agricultural pursuits, carpentry, painting, and manual crafts.[25] Moral treatment as provided in small asylums was initially successful. However, overcrowding and financial difficulties eventually reduced treatment to custodial care.

Building on these ideas half a century later, the famous neuropathologist Adolf Meyer proposed that many illnesses were "problems of adaptation" that could be remediated through involvement in curative occupations.[21] Dunton and Slagle enthusiastically supported this view, and Meyer's philosophy of OT was published in the first issue of the profession's journal. Slagle, who worked with Meyer at Phipps Clinics, developed habit training programs in mental hospitals to reestablish healthy habits of self-care and social behavior.[30]

Arts and Crafts

The rise of the **arts and crafts movement** in the 1890s was in reaction to the perceived social ills created by the Industrial Revolution.[7] The economy was changing from an agrarian to a manufacturing society, so that what had previously been made by hand was now produced in factories. Proponents of the arts and crafts movement asserted that this resulted in a society of dissatisfied workers who were bored by monotonous and repetitive working conditions.

The use of arts and crafts as a therapeutic medium in OT arose from this trend. The arts and crafts approach was based on the belief that craft work improved physical and mental health through exercise and the satisfaction gained from creating a useful or decorative article with one's own hands. According to Johnson, the therapeutic value of handicrafts lay in their ability to provide occupation that stimulated "mental activity and muscular exercise at the same time."[16] Different handicrafts could also be graded for the desired physical and mental effects. Crafts were successfully used by OT reconstruction aides during World War I for the physical and mental restoration of disabled servicemen.[27] For treating tuberculosis, Kidner advocated a graduated approach that began with bedside crafts and habit training and proceeded to occupations related to shop work and ultimately actual work within the institution.[18]

Thus the ideas from the moral treatment and arts and crafts movements became intertwined as a definition of OT evolved to include treatment of individuals with physical and mental disabilities. In its early years OT worked with patients throughout three stages of recovery.[13] During convalescence, patients would engage in bedside occupations that primarily consisted of handicrafts such as embroidery and basket weaving. Once patients were able to get out of bed, they would engage in occupations designed to strengthen both body and mind, such as weaving or gardening, and occupations designed to reestablish basic habits of self-care and communication. When they were almost ready to return to the community, patients would engage in occupations that would prepare them for vocational success, such as carpentry, painting, or manual crafts.

Scientific Management

Frederick Taylor, a prominent engineer, introduced his theory of **scientific management** in 1911.[32] He proposed that rationality, efficiency, and systematic observation could be applied to industrial management and to all other areas of life, including teaching, preaching, and medicine. Progressive reformers of the period advocated that the ideology of scientific management address societal problems such as poverty and illness. These reformers criticized the noisy, dirty asylum of the 19th century and urged that the image of medical care be transformed into the clean, efficient hospital.[15] The idea that knowledge could be developed through research and observation and applied to patient care became an underlying tenet of the science of medicine and ultimately resulted in the development of reliable protocols for surgical and medical interventions.[34]

The founders of OT were attracted to the idea of a scientific approach to treatment. Barton was particularly taken with Taylor's time and motion studies and thought they might provide a model for OT research.[4] Dunton advocated that those who entered the profession be capable of engaging in systematic inquiry in order to further the profession's goals.[10] Similarly, Slagle urged research in OT to validate OT's efficacy.[30] By 1920 the profession was promoting the notion of the "science" of occupation by calling for "the advancement of occupation as a therapeutic measure, the study of the effects of occupation upon the human being, and the dissemination of scientific knowledge on this subject."[8]

There is little in the OT literature of the early 20th century to suggest that OT practice was informed by systematic observation. One exception was the Department of Occupational Therapy at Walter Reed Hospital in Washington, D.C., under the direction of psychologist Bird T. Baldwin.[3] OT reconstruction aides were assigned to the orthopedic ward, where methods of systematically recording range of motion and muscle strength were established. Activities were selected based on an analysis of the motions involved, including joint position, muscle action, and muscle strengthening. Methods of adapting tools were suggested, and splints were fabricated to provide support during the recovery process. Treatment with this systematic approach was more narrowly focused at times but was applied within the context of what Baldwin called "functional restoration," in which OT's purpose was to "help each patient find himself and function again as a complete man [sic] physically, socially, educationally, and economically."[2]

Besides advocating a scientific approach to practice, the scientific management ideology emphasized efficiency and a mechanistic approach to medical care. Using the factory analogy, patients were the product, and nurses and therapists were the factory workers. It was assumed that doctors had the most scientific knowledge and therefore should be positioned at the top of the medical hierarchy. Dunton, a physician himself, seemed to support this arrangement: "The occupational therapist, therefore, has the same relation to the physician as the nurse, that is, she is a technical assistant."[9] As the profession evolved, an emphasis on efficiency and deference to medical authority became problematic for the profession. The focus on science and the resulting growth of the medical model were both beneficial and detrimental to OT practice.

EXPANSION AND SPECIALIZATION
The Rehabilitation Model

The growth of the **rehabilitation model** began after World War II and peaked with the health care industry boom in the early 1970s, following the passage of bills establishing Medicare and Medicaid. Although this growth was initially driven by the need to treat the country's wounded soldiers, care of injured and chronically ill civilians also became a concern.

World War II revived the need for the United States to provide medical care for its wounded soldiers. Many more soldiers survived than in World War I because of recent scientific discoveries such as sulfa and penicillin. The Second World War also served to highlight the value of OT services: "Although occupational therapy started during the last World War, it developed slowly [until] now when doctors are finding this aid to the sick and wounded invaluable."[22]A major effort was launched to reorganize and revitalize the Veterans Administration (VA) hospital system. Departments of physical medicine and rehabilitation were created to bring together all the services needed to care for the large number of war injured. "The theory that handicapped persons can be aided by persons who understand their special needs originated during World War II. The armed services established such hospitals for disabled veterans as the one for paraplegics in Birminham, California. They helped the morale and physical condition of the patients so much that others were built for civilians."[23]

The interdisciplinary approach to care was emulated in the private sector. Demand for medical services increased in the civilian population as the treatment of chronic disability became a priority. Howard Rusk, a prominent voice in the development of rehabilitation medicine, asserted that the critical shortage of trained personnel would impede the country's ability to deliver services to the "5,300,000 persons in the nation who suffer from chronic disability."[17] He cited OT as one of the essential rehabilitation services. In response to the growing demand for rehabilitation services, Congress passed the Hill-Burton Act in 1946 to provide federal aid for the construction of rehabilitation centers. A proviso of the legislation was that rehabilitation centers must "offer integrated services in four areas: medical, including occupational and physical therapy, psychological, social and vocational."[35] The passage of legislation establishing Medicare and Medicaid in 1965 put further demands on rehabilitation services to serve the chronically ill and elderly within health care institutions, as well as the community.

Physical Dysfunction as a Specialty

The creation of a specialty in physical dysfunction came about as a response to the changing demands of the marketplace and its requirement that specialists possess particular kinds of medical knowledge and technological skills.[12] This new specialty began with an increasing focus on occupations that would promote physical strength and endurance: "The Army is death on the old-time invalid occupations of basket weaving, chair caning, pottery and weaving. These are 'not believed to be interesting occupation for the present condition of men in military service,' says an officer from the Surgeon General's office. The stress now is on carpentry, repair work at the hospital, war-related jobs like knitting camouflage nets, and printing."[11]

The scientific approach of joint measurement and muscle strengthening that Baldwin pioneered at the end of World War I was adopted and improved upon. As Claire Spackman wrote, "Communication of new or improved techniques . . . [was] of vital importance. The work of the past had been empirical, now the therapists had the task of . . . becom[ing] highly skilled in the treatment of specific types of cases."[31] According to Spackman, the occupational therapists serving people with physical disability needed to be skilled in teaching activities of daily living (ADL), work simplification and rehabilitation techniques for the handicapped homemaker, and training in the use of upper extremity prostheses. But first and foremost, she asserted, "Occupational therapy treats the patient by the use of constructive activity in a simulated, normal living and/or working situation. . . . Constructive activity is the keynote of occupational therapy."[31]

As the rehabilitation movement helped to establish the importance of OT, it further positioned the profession within the **medical model.** OT was urged to specialize and separate into two distinct fields, physical dysfunction and mental illness. The head orthopedist at Rancho Los Amigos Hospital in Downey, California argued that the separation would result in "strengthened treatment techniques" and thus more credibility among medical doctors. He asserted that "the medical profession in general does not recognize your field as an established necessary specialty."[14] The American Occupational Therapy Association sought closer ties with the American Medical Association to gain more credibility. The following quote indicates the difficulties the profession faced in defining and promoting itself:

> Both occupational and physical therapy have taken some selling—to the medical profession as well as to the public. Many hospitals have still to discover occupational therapy. Some die-hard MDs, reluctant to see its medical implication, still think a lot of it is boondoggling, and there's been a lot of confusion about its function. Occupational therapy is not giving someone something to do just to keep him happy. It is not vocational training. It is not making pretty things to sell. All of these have therapeutic value as morale builders but they're not occupational therapy. As defined by the American Medical Association, occupational therapy is treatment for illness or disability through remedial work activity prescribed by a doctor and directed by trained technicians.[11]

The closer relationship with medicine probably helped the profession gain credibility, at least within the medical model. This alignment had the negative consequences of less autonomy for the profession and a specialized and narrower treatment approach to OT practice.

A CHALLENGE TO OCCUPATIONAL THERAPY PRACTICE
Moral Treatment Versus Medical Model

A cry arose in the late 1960s and in the 1970s from some of the leaders in OT for practice to return to its roots in moral treatment and to forego what Shannon referred to as the "technique philosophy."[29] In his article on what he called "the derailment of occupational therapy," Shannon described two philosophies at odds with each other. One, he asserted, viewed the individual "as a mechanistic creature susceptible to manipulation and control via the application of techniques"; the other, based on the profession's early philosophy of moral treatment, emphasized a holistic and humanistic view of the individual.

Kielhofner and Burke described the situation as a conflict between two paradigms.[20] Early OT practice, they asserted, was based on the paradigm of occupation that had moral treatment as its foundation. This paradigm provided a "holistic orientation to Man [sic] and health in the context of the culture of daily living and its activities." Post-World War II practice, they asserted, was based on the paradigm of **reductionism,** a mode of thinking characteristic of the medical model. This view emphasized the individual's "internal states" and represented a shift in focus to "internal muscular, intrapsychic balance and sensorimotor problems." The authors acknowledged that practice based on the reductionist paradigm "would pave the way for the development of more exact technologies for the treatment of internal deficits"; however, they were concerned it "necessitate[d] a narrowing of the conceptual scope of occupational therapy."[20]

To say that early OT practice was based on the humanistic and holistic philosophy of moral treatment is

to tell only part of the story. As this chapter describes, the founders were influenced by at least two other ideologies, scientific management and arts and crafts, both of which could be placed in the reductionistic paradigm. Scientific management's focus was definitely reductionistic, with its ideas about efficiency and systematic observation. Handicrafts were frequently used in a manner consistent with the medical model when they were prescribed for a particular disability. Indeed, the Committee on Installations and Advice, directed by Dunton, was formed to analyze the most commonly used crafts and to match the therapeutic value of each craft to a particular symptom or disability.[26]

The question arises as to how the founders could have supported competing visions of practice. The answer may be that the models were not considered at that time to be incompatible because the scientific and medical model had not fully taken hold. It appears that in the founding years OT primarily *practiced* moral treatment and *talked about* how practice should also be medical and scientific. When early practitioners were asked to treat patients in order to "restore the functions of nerves and muscles" or to make use of "the affected arm or leg,"[31] they based their treatment on their belief in the importance of occupation, habit training, and their knowledge of crafts. Once knowledge and technologic advances were sufficient and occupational therapists could actually practice using a scientific, medical perspective, it became apparent that the ideas underlying these two paradigms were in conflict.

The physical dysfunction therapist was faced with the problem of how to give treatment that was, on the one hand, holistic and humanistic and, on the other, reductionistic and scientific. Baldwin's answer in 1919 was to see activities such as muscle strengthening and splint fabrication as techniques that contributed to the larger goal of "functional restoration" of the individual's social, physical, and economic well-being.[3] Spackman's answer in 1968 was that the occupational therapist should use "constructive activity in a simulated, normal living and/or working situation. This is and always has been our function."[31] She emphasized the teaching of ADL and work simplification and was critical of treatment that consisted of having patients sand or use a bicycle saw when "constructive activity" was involved.

Another answer to the question of differing paradigms was to move outside the medical model. Bockoven urged OT practitioners in mental health to stop "running dinky little sideshows in large medical institutions" and instead to set up services in the community based on moral treatment. He said, "It is the occupational therapist's inborn respect for the realities of life, for the real tasks of living, and for the time it takes the individual to develop his modes of coping with his tasks, that leads me to urge haste on the profession . . .

to assert its leadership in fashioning the design of human service programs. . . . Don't drop dead, take over instead!"[6] Yerxa urged therapists not to rely solely on doctor's orders: "The written prescription is no longer seen by many of us as necessary, holy or healthy. . . . The pseudo-security of the prescription required that we pay a high price. That price was the reduction of our potential to help clients because we often stagnated at the level of applying technical skills."[36]

Physical Dysfunction Therapists' Response

As practice moved into the 1980s, there was much concern that if therapists did as their critics suggested, they would jeopardize reimbursement as well as referrals. Therapists argued that they were being asked to exclude skills and knowledge they believed were valuable in patient treatment, such as exercise, splinting, and facilitation techniques. They further argued that many patients receiving OT services were initially not at the level of motor capability that would enable them to engage in satisfying occupations. It was proposed that adjunctive techniques such as exercise and biofeedback should be considered legitimate when used to prepare the patient for further engagement in occupation.[33] A study conducted in 1984 by Pasquinelli[24] showed that although therapists valued occupation, they used a wide variety of treatment techniques and approaches, including facilitation and non-activity-oriented techniques. Both Trombly and Ayres argued that instead of attempting to redirect the focus of OT, the profession should include current clinical practices that had proved effective on an empirical and practical basis.[1,33]

PRESENT PRACTICE: INFORMED BY HISTORY

Health care practice at the end of the 20th century is heavily influenced by the efficiency ideology initially introduced by scientific management in the first part of the century. This only emphasizes the importance of integrating the humanistic and scientific in the practice of OT for physical dysfunction.

Early treatment was based on therapists' belief in the importance of occupation, habit training, and their knowledge of crafts. As scientific knowledge and technology advanced, OT defined a role for itself within the rehabilitation model. This resulted in the emergence of physical dysfunction as a specialty within OT. The closer relationship with medicine helped the profession gain credibility; however, it became apparent by the late 1960s that the scientific reductionism of the medical model was at odds with the holistic humanism of moral treatment.

Since the late 1960s, physical dysfunction occupational therapists have been trying to integrate the two views of practice. They have worked to incorporate the humanistic values and yet encourage development of the scientific techniques and procedures that best ensure patient success. Efforts today are directed at evidence-based practice and identifying treatment models that explain and accommodate physical dysfunction OT.[19]

OT's history has shown that although treatment techniques have changed throughout the 20th century, the values and beliefs established in the formative years continue to influence practice. The most enduring belief is this: that occupation as prescribed by OT practitioners promotes health, prevents and remedies dysfunction, and elicits adaptation to the environment. As new treatment techniques and technologies are developed in the future, OT intervention that promotes occupational function will remain consistent with the philosophical base of the profession.

REVIEW QUESTIONS

1. Name the seven founders of occupational therapy, and list the professional background of each.
2. What ideologies shaped the development of occupational therapy in the late 19th and early 20th centuries?
3. What were the main features of the philosophy of moral treatment?
4. Describe the ideas that were the foundations of occupation as a remedy for mental and physical illness.
5. What provoked the rise of the arts and crafts movement?
6. How did the arts and crafts movement influence occupational therapy?
7. Describe scientific management. How did it influence the development of occupational therapy?
8. When did the rehabilitation model evolve? How did the world wars influence the development of the rehabilitation model?
9. How did physical dysfunction become a specialty?
10. What factors influenced occupational therapy to adopt the medical model?
11. What was the apparent conflict between moral treatment and the medical model?
12. What is reductionism?
13. How is the apparent conflict between reductionism and holistic or humanistic treatment being resolved in physical dysfunction practice?

REFERENCES

1. Ayres AJ: Basic concepts of clinical practice in physical disabilities, *Am J Occup Ther* 12:300, 1958.
2. Baldwin BT: Occupational therapy, *Am J Care Cripples* 8:447, 1919.
3. Baldwin BT: *Occupational therapy applied to restoration of function of disabled joints,* Washington, DC, 1919, Walter Reed General Hospital.
4. Barton GE: The movies and the microscope. Manuscript in American Occupational Therapy Archives: Bethesda, Md, c1920.

5. Bing R: Occupational therapy revisited: a paraphrastic journey: 1981 Eleanor Clark Slagle lecture, *Am J Occup Ther* 35:499, 1981.

6. Bockoven JS: Legacy of moral treatment: 1800s to 1910, *Am J Occup Ther* 25:224, 1971.

7. Boris E: *Art and labor: Ruskin, Morris and the craftsman ideal in America*, Philadelphia, 1986, Temple University.

8. Constitution of the National Society for the Promotion of Occupational Therapy, Baltimore, 1917, Sheppard Pratt Hospital Press.

9. Dunton WR: *Prescribing occupational therapy*, Springfield Ill, 1928, Charles C Thomas.

10. Dunton WR: The three "r's" of occupational therapy, *Occup Ther Rehab* 7:345-348.

11. The gift of healing, *Mademoiselle*, pp 114-15, 177-178, 1943.

12. Gritzer G, Arluke A: *The making of rehabilitation*, Berkeley, 1985, University of California Press.

13. Hanson C, Walker K: The history of work in physical dysfunction, *Am J Occup Ther* 46:56, 1992.

14. Higher status near, doctor tells therapists: department scrapbooks, 1955-63, Archives of the Department of Occupational Therapy, San José State University, San José, Calif.

15. Hofstadter R: *The age of reform*, New York, 1969, Knopf.

16. Johnson SC: Instruction in handcrafts and design for hospital patients, *Modern Hosp* 15:1, 69-72, 1920.

17. Lack of trained personnel felt in rehabilitation field, *The New York Times*, Jan 25, 1954.

18. Kidner TB: Planning for occupational therapy, *Modern Hosp* 21:414-428, 1923.

19. Kielhofner G: *Conceptual foundations of occupational therapy*, ed 2, Philadelphia, 1997, FA Davis.

20. Kielhofner G, Burke JP: Occupational therapy after 60 years, *Am J Occup Ther* 31(1):675-689, 1977.

21. Meyer A: The philosophy of occupational therapy, *Arch Occup Ther* 1:1-10, 1922.

22. Occupational therapy classes have outstanding guest speakers from various army and civilian hospitals: department scrapbook, 1943-54, Archives of the Department of Occupational Therapy, San José State University, San José, Calif.

23. OT instructor says San José needs rehabilitation center, *Spartan Daily*, San José, Calif, Feb 9, 1953, San José State College, San José, Calif.

24. Pasquinelli S: *The relationship of physical disabilities treatment methodologies to the philosophical base of occupational therapy*, unpublished thesis, San José State University, 1984.

25. Peloquin SM: Looking back-moral treatment: contexts considered, *Am J Occup Ther* 43:537, 1989.

26. Putnam ML: Report of the committee on installations and advice, *Occup Ther Rehab* 4:57-60

27. Quiroga V: *Occupational therapy: the first 30 years, 1900-1930*, Bethesda, Md, 1995, American Occupational Therapy Association.

28. Reed KL: The beginnings of occupational therapy. In Hopkins HL, Smith HD, editors: *Willard & Spackman's occupational therapy*, ed 8, Philadelphia, 1993, JB Lippincott.

29. Shannon PD: The derailment of occupational therapy, *Am J Occup Ther* 31:229, 1977.

30. Slagle EC: A year's development of occupational therapy in New York State hospitals, *Modern Hosp* 22:98-104, 1924.

31. Spackman CS: A history of the practice of occupational therapy for restoration of physical function: 1917-1967, *Am J Occup Ther* 22:67-71, 1968.

32. Taylor F: *The principles of scientific management*, New York, 1911, Harper.

33. Trombly CA: Include exercise in purposeful activity, *Am J Occup Ther* 36:467, 1982 (letter).

34. Weibe R: *The search for order, 1877-1920*, New York, 1967, Farrar, Straus & Giroux.

35. Workshop on rehabilitation facilities, 1955: department scrapbooks 1955-63, Archives of the Department of Occupational Therapy, San José State University, San José, Calif.

36. Yerxa EJ: 1966 Eleanor Clarke Slagle Lecture: Authentic occupational therapy, *Am J Occup Ther* 21:1-9, 1967.

PART TWO

OCCUPATIONAL THERAPY PROCESS AND PRACTICE

CHAPTER 3

The Occupational Therapy Process— An Overview

MARY BETH EARLY

KEY TERMS

Occupational therapy practitioner
Referral
Screening
Registered occupational therapist
Evaluation
Certified occupational therapy assistant
Intervention planning
Intervention
Reevaluation
Transition services
Discontinuation
Clinical reasoning
Occupational therapy aide
Ethics
Ethical dilemmas
Clinical context

LEARNING OBJECTIVES

After studying this chapter the student or practitioner will be able to do the following:

1. Identify and describe the major stages in the occupational therapy (OT) process.
2. Explain why clinical practice may appear less sequential and orderly than these stages suggest.
3. Describe how clinical reasoning adjusts to consider various factors that may be present in the intervention context.
4. Identify appropriate delegation of responsibility among the various levels of OT practitioners.
5. Discuss ways in which OT practitioners may effectively collaborate with members of other professions involved in patient care.
6. Recognize ethical dilemmas that may occur frequently in OT practice, and identify ways in which these may be addressed and managed.

This chapter introduces the occupational therapy (OT) process, briefly summarizing the stages from referral through discontinuation of service. The chapter aims to acquaint the reader with the complexity and creativity of clinical reasoning as it evolves in the transactions between patient and therapist within the context of the contemporary clinical environment. In so doing, it sets the stage for the chapters that follow. Treatment contexts are covered in more detail in Chapter 4. Chapters 5 and 6 expand on the stages of evaluation and intervention. Chapter 7 presents evidence-based practice. Chapter 8 addresses prevention of disability and health promotion, an aspect of intervention. Chapter 9 provides an overview and detail of teaching activities. Chapter 10 addresses documentation. The present chapter considers the complementary roles of different

OT practitioners, as well as relationships between OT and the other professional disciplines involved in the care of the patient or client with physical dysfunction. Common ethical dilemmas are introduced, and ways to analyze these are presented.

Steps or Stages of the Occupational Therapy Process

The OT process is often presented as a series of discrete stages or steps. These are[9,18]:

1. **Referral:** The physician or other legally qualified professional requests OT services for the patient. Referral may be oral, but a written record is also necessary. Guidelines for referral may vary by state, with some states restricting OT to physician referral.

2. **Screening:** The **registered occupational therapist** (OTR) performs a quick assessment to determine whether OT services would be helpful to this patient. The OTR may perform screening independently or as a member of the health care team.

3. **Evaluation:** The OTR identifies the information to be collected and the areas to be evaluated and selects assessment instruments. The OTR may delegate some parts of the evaluation, such as the administration of selected assessments, to the **certified occupational therapy assistant** (COTA). The data are then analyzed to determine the patient's specific strengths and deficits.

4. **Intervention planning:** Working with the patient, the OT practitioners (OTR and COTA) develop a plan for restoring, improving, or maintaining the patient's ability to function in daily life roles and activities. The OTR is responsible for the plan and for any parts delegated to the COTA. The plan includes client-centered goals and methods for reaching them. The values and goals of the patient are primary; those of the therapist secondary.[8] Cultural, social, and environmental factors are incorporated into the plan. The plan must detail the scope and frequency of the treatment and the anticipated date of completion.

5. **Intervention:** The OT team carries out the treatment plan. The OTR may assign to the COTA significant responsibilities in providing purposeful activities and therapeutic modalities. Nonetheless, the OTR retains the responsibility to direct, monitor, and supervise the intervention and must ascertain that relevant and necessary interventions are provided in an appropriate and safe manner and that documentation is accurate and complete.

6. **Reevaluation:** With the same instruments used in the initial evaluation, OT practitioners again evaluate the patient to determine what changes have occurred since the previous evaluation. This measurement of the outcomes of treatment is critical in showing the effectiveness of the intervention. The intervention plan may be changed, continued, or discontinued, based on the results of the reevaluation.

7. **Transition services:** Working in tandem with the patient, the patient's family, and the treatment team, the OTR and COTA develop a plan for the patient to carry over after leaving the current treatment setting. The discharge may be to the patient's home or to an intermediate care or long-term care facility.

8. **Discontinuation:** The OTR determines whether the patient has reached the established goals or achieved the maximum benefit from OT; alternately, the patient may choose to discontinue service before reaching these limits. The OTR formally discontinues service and creates a discontinuation plan that documents follow-up recommendations and arrangements. Final documentation includes a record of any change in the patient's status from first evaluation through the end of OT services.

Fig. 3-1 shows the relationship between the various stages of the intervention process. When the stages of the intervention process are presented and studied in a linear and sequential manner, the reader may be led to believe that the stages always occur in this sequence. In fact, this is rarely the case. Rather, while the general trend of the stages follows that presented above and in Fig. 3-1 (i.e., referral leading to evaluation leading to intervention planning and then intervention itself), in many clinical settings the stages may be compressed. A single visit may encompass receipt of referral and a brief

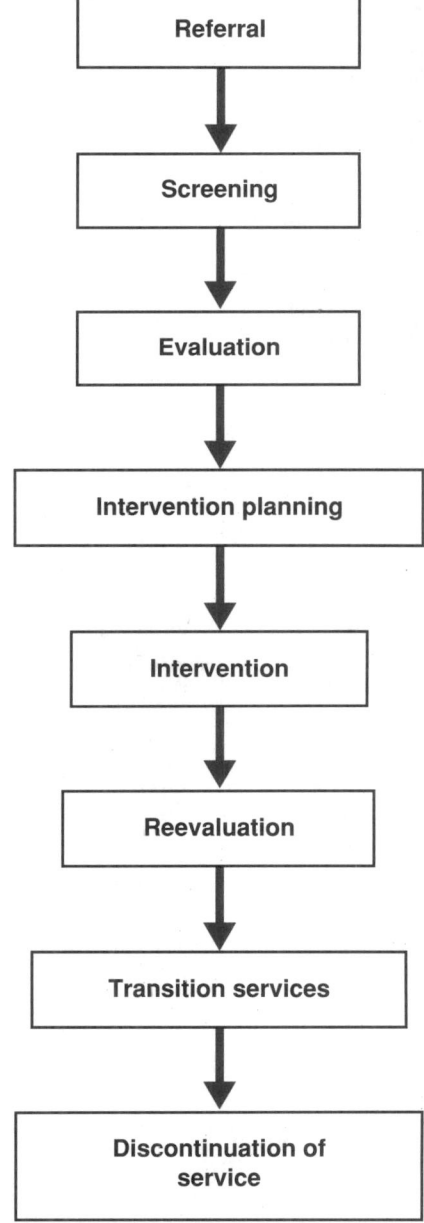

FIG 3-1
Stages or steps in the occupational therapy intervention process.

evaluation and administration of some intervention procedures. Intervention planning may occur within the therapist's mind and may not be documented until after the first intervention has occurred during this initial visit. Further, the therapist may consider transition services on first meeting the patient. This rapid and apparently seamless integration of information and action by the therapist requires knowledge of various theoretical models (see Chapter 1) and practical techniques, along with clinical experience.

Clinical Reasoning in the Intervention Process

Since 1986 the American Occupational Therapy Association (AOTA) has funded a series of studies to examine how occupational therapists think and reason in their work with patients.[14] **Clinical reasoning** can be defined informally as how we think about what we do. Gillette and Mattingly[14] identified two aspects of occupational therapists' clinical reasoning: the *mechanistic* and the *phenomenological*. Mechanistic aspects are closely allied with the practice of medicine and address factors such as how the body works biomechanically. Phenomenological factors address the experience of "being in the world," or the life of the individual as perceived by that person.

Fleming[11] further identified three "tracks" used by the expert clinician to organize and process data: the *procedural*, the *interactive*, and the *conditional*.

- *Procedural reasoning* is concerned with getting things done, with what "has to happen next." This track is closely allied with the mechanistic aspect of reasoning.
- *Interactive reasoning* is concerned with person-to-person interchanges with patients. The therapist uses this track to engage with, to understand, and to motivate the patient. Understanding the patient's point of view is fundamental to this kind of reasoning.
- *Conditional reasoning* is concerned with the contexts in which interventions occur, the contexts in which the patient performs occupations, and the ways in which various factors might affect the outcomes and direction of therapy. Using a "what if?" or conditional approach, the therapist imagines possible scenarios for the patient.

Experienced master clinicians engage simultaneously in all three tracks to develop and modify their plans and actions during all phases of the intervention process. Some of the questions a therapist might consider on each of the three tracks are listed in Box 3-1.

Yet another dimension of expert clinical reasoning was identified by Mattingly.[17] *Narrative reasoning* uses story making or story telling as a way to understand the patient's experience. The patient's explanation or description of life and the disability experience reveals themes that permeate the patient's understanding and that will affect the enactment and outcomes of thera-

peutic intervention. In this sense, narrative reasoning is phenomenological. Narrative reasoning is also used by therapists to plan or "emplot" therapy, to create a story line of what will happen for the patient as a result of therapy. Here the therapist draws on both interactive and conditional tracks, using the patient's words and metaphors to project possible futures for the patient.

Clinical Reasoning in Context

Pressures for cost containment and reduction of unnecessary services have forced therapists to divide their attention between the needs of the client-patient and the practical realities of health care reimbursement and documentation. Thus, on first meeting the patient, the therapist will want to know the anticipated or planned or required date of discharge, as well as the scope of services that will be reimbursed and those that are likely to be denied. Simultaneously, the therapist is assessing and considering the patient, attempting to engage the patient in identifying and planning goals, and weighing the patient's motivation against the interventions that might be possible or useful in the particular situation. Further, the therapist is alert to requirements for documentation and the particular current procedural terminology (CPT) codes that may apply and is thinking

---

BOX 3-1
Questions for the Three-Track Mind

Procedural questions
What is the diagnosis?
What prognosis, complications, and other factors are associated with this diagnosis?
What is the general protocol for assessment and intervention with this diagnosis?
What interventions (adjunctive methods, enabling activities, purposeful activities) might be employed?

Interactive questions
Who is the patient?
What are the patient's goals, concerns, interests, and values?
How does the patient see his or her life story?
How does the illness or disability fit into this life story?
How might I engage this patient?
How can we communicate?

Conditional questions
What are the many contexts of the patient's life? (temporal and environmental contexts, social aspects, cultural aspects, context of therapy and reimbursement issues)
What future(s) can be imagined for the patient? What events could or would shape the future?
How can I engage the patient to imagine, believe in, and work toward a future?

about how to document service accurately and effectively so that reimbursement will not be challenged and so the patient's needs may be adequately addressed.

From first meeting the patient or client, the therapist is guided by the patient's or client's goals and preferences. Client-centered service delivery requires client (or family) involvement and collaboration at all stages of the intervention process.[8] Effectively engaging the client and the family demands cultural sensitivity and an ability to communicate with people of diverse backgrounds. In some cultures, the idea of participating equally in decision making with a health professional may be unknown. Being asked by a therapist to make decisions may feel quite unfamiliar and uncomfortable to the patient. Thus the therapist must assess the person's readiness to collaborate, adjust to the

patient's point of view, and find other ways to ensure that the intervention plan is acceptable to the patient and family.

Some of the many questions addressed by the multilevel thinking process of the occupational therapist are depicted in Fig. 3-2.

Client-Centered Practice: Not Yet a Reality

Involving patients and clients in identifying their own goals and in making decisions about their own care and treatment is highly valued by leaders in the OT profession[13,21,22] and is endorsed by the AOTA in its policy and practice guidelines.[1,9] Despite this expectation, most clinicians involve clients only part of the time, and some therapists do not involve patients or clients at all

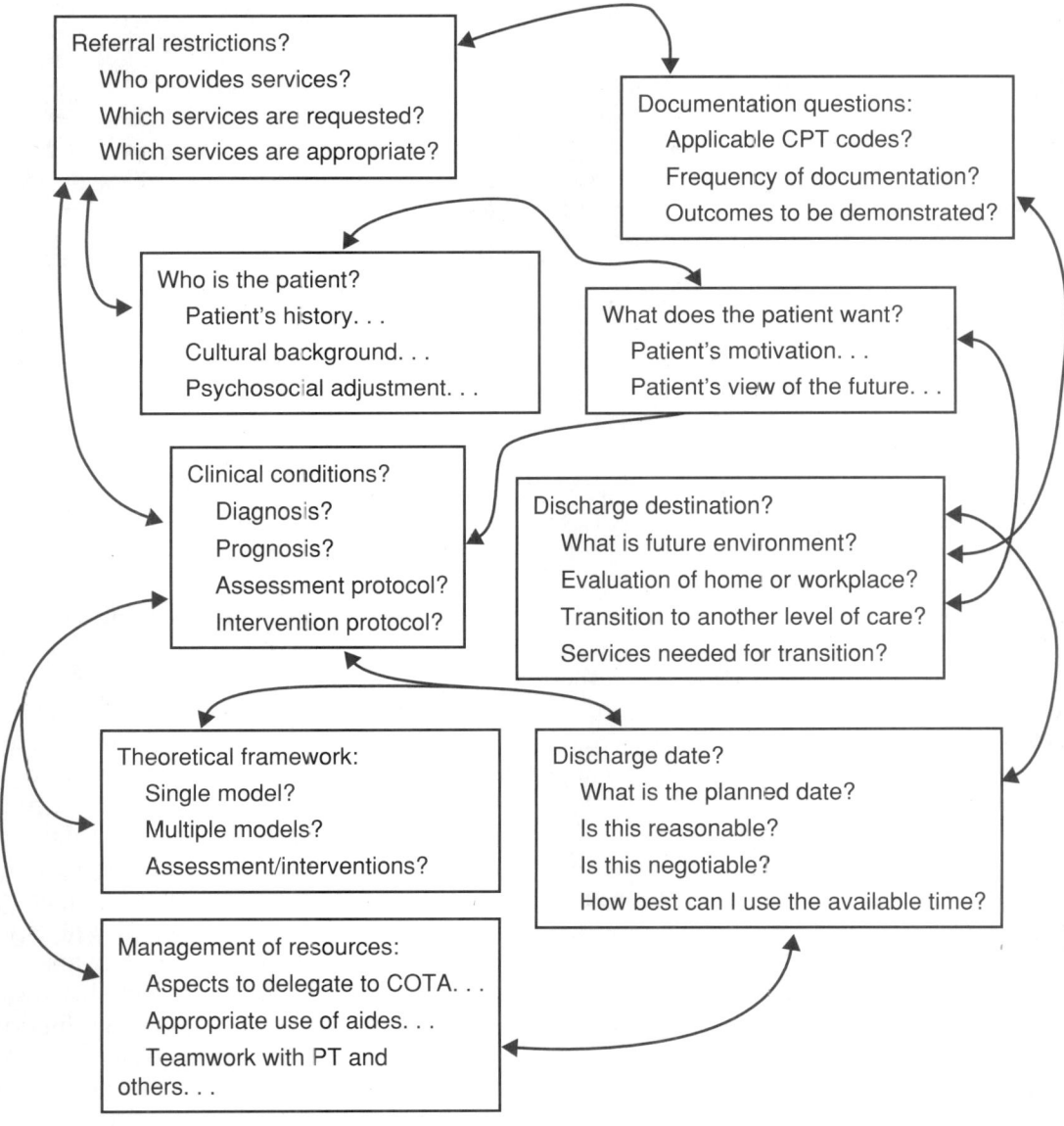

FIG. 3-2
Multilevel thinking of the occupational therapist (arrows show that flow of reasoning process circulates in a multidimensional and open manner, engaging many factors simultaneously).

in making decisions.[19] Some factors proposed as reasons for this are time constraints, beliefs about the client's cognitive level (and ability to comprehend or make decisions), and the person's age (older persons being less likely to be involved by therapists).[19]

As is described further in Chapter 5, effective and comprehensive client involvement begins when the therapist first meets the patient or client. Therapists using a "top-down" assessment model, such as the Canadian Occupational Performance Measure (COPM),[16] initiate assessment by asking clients to identify and choose goals early in the intervention process. Regardless of disability status or perceived limitations in cognitive functioning, every client should be invited to participate in assessment and treatment decisions.

Teamwork Within the Occupational Therapy Profession

The OT profession recognizes and certifies two levels of practitioners, the OTR and the COTA. The AOTA has provided many documents to guide practice and to clarify the relationship between the two levels of practitioner.[3,4,7,9] The OTR who is managing a case or providing services to patients should use the following as a guide:

- Services are to be provided by personnel who have demonstrated service competency.
- In the interests of rendering the best care at the least cost, the OTR may delegate tasks to COTAs and, in some specific instances, to aides or other personnel, provided these providers have the competencies to render such services.
- The OTR retains final responsibility for all aspects of care, including documentation.

OTR-COTA Relationships

To work effectively with COTAs, the OTR must understand the role of the technical-level practitioner. It is common for OTRs to alternately overestimate and underestimate the capabilities of COTAs. In overestimating the training and abilities of COTAs, OTRs might assume that a COTA is a "mini-OTR," believing that the COTA is trained to provide services identical to those of the OTR but perhaps at a lesser pace and level and with a smaller caseload. In underestimating the COTA, the OTR might assume that the COTA is a "glorified aide," capable of performing only concrete and repetitive tasks under the strictest supervision.

The appropriate role of the COTA is complementary to that of the OTR. Employed effectively, the COTA can extend the reach of the OTR by providing therapy services under supervision that ranges from close to general (depending on the practice setting and the experience and service competencies of the COTA).[4] Working together with several COTAs, the OTR will be able to manage a larger caseload and will have the option of introducing more advanced and specialized services (since COTAs provide routine services). Many variations exist. Some services that may be delegated to service-competent COTAs include the following:

1. Administration of selected screening instruments or of assessments such as range of motion (ROM) tests, interviews and questionnaires, activities of daily living (ADL) evaluations, and other assessments that follow a defined protocol.[9]
2. Development of some elements of the intervention plan (e.g., planning for dressing training and planning for kitchen safety training).[9]
3. Provision of intervention services.[9] The COTA, by education and training, is prepared to provide interventions in the areas of ADL, work and productive activities, and play or leisure. With appropriate training and supervision, the COTA can undertake interventions related to performance components.
4. Facilitation of the transition to the next service setting by, for example, making arrangements with or educating family members or contacting community providers.
5. Assistance with the development of a plan for discontinuation of service.
6. Contributions to documentation, record keeping, resource management, quality assurance, selection and procurement of supplies and equipment, and other aspects of service management.
7. Education of the patient, family, or community about OT services.

Occupational Therapy Aides

The OTR may also extend the reach of services by employing aides. AOTA guidelines stipulate that the **OT aide** works only under direction and close supervision of an OT practitioner (OTR or COTA).[8] Aides may perform only specific, selected, delegated tasks. While the COTA may direct and supervise the aide, the OTR is ultimately responsible for the actions of the aide.[8] Tasks that might be delegated to an aide include transporting patients, setting up equipment, preparing supplies, and performing simple and routine patient services for which the aide has been trained. Individual jurisdictions and health care regulatory bodies may restrict aides from providing patient care services; reimbursement may also be denied for some services provided by aides. Where permitted, the OTR may delegate routine tasks to aides to increase productivity.

Teamwork with Other Professionals

Many health care workers collaborate in the care of persons with physical disabilities. Depending on the setting, the OTR may work together with physical therapists, speech and language pathologists, activity therapists, nurses, vocational counselors, psychologists, social workers, pastoral care specialists, orthotists, prosthetists, rehabilitation engineers, vendors of durable medical equipment, and physicians from many different specialties.

Treatment contexts are discussed in Chapter 4; relationships among and expectations of various health care providers are often determined by the context of care. For example, in home care in certain jurisdictions the nurse may be the leader of the team. In settings under the medical model, the physician is most often the leader. Some rehabilitation facilities employ a team approach to assessment and intervention, which reduces duplication of services and increases communication and collaboration. Several individuals from different professions may together perform a single assessment. For example, the OTR may be the lead member of the team in some settings, or may be the director of rehabilitation services. In a team, members adjust scheduling and expectations to accommodate one another's goals and plans.

Many factors affect relationships among professionals across disciplines: the treatment context, reimbursement restrictions, licensure laws and other jurisdictional elements, and the training and experience of the individuals involved. Relationships develop over time, based on experience and interaction and sometimes on personality. Even where formal jurisdictional boundaries may appear to limit roles for OT, informal patterns often develop at variance with the prescribed rules. For example, while in some states physician referral may be required to initiate OT service, physicians may expect the OTR to initiate the referral and actually perform a cursory screening before the physician becomes involved. Some physicians rely on OT staff to identify those patients who are most likely to benefit, and issue referrals at their suggestion.

Another example in which interdisciplinary boundaries may be at variance with actual practice is in the relationships among the rehabilitation specialists of OT, PT, and speech therapy. By formal definition, each discipline has a designated scope of practice, with some areas of overlap and occasional dispute. Nonetheless, it is common for practitioners to share skills and caseloads across disciplines and to train each other to provide less complex aspects of each discipline's care. Two terms used to describe this are *cross-training* and *multiskilling*.

Cross-training is the training of a single rehabilitation worker to provide services that would ordinarily be rendered by several different professions. *Multiskilling* is sometimes used synonymously with cross-training, but may also mean the acquisition by a single health care worker of many different skills. Arguments have been made for and against cross-training and multiskilling.[10,12,20,23] The consumer may benefit by having fewer health care providers and better integration of services. Involving fewer providers may reduce costs. Therapists may benefit by having other practitioners available to cover services on evenings and weekends, and in rural areas where specialized services are not widely available.

The disadvantages cited include the prospect of erosion of professional identity, possible risk to consumers of harm at the hands of less skilled providers, and ceding the control of individual professions to outside parties such as insurers and advocates of competing professions.

Ethics

When studied as part of an OT professional education, **ethics** may seem an idealized and compartmentalized course or topic. Yet clinicians encounter **ethical dilemmas** with surprising frequency. In an ethics survey conducted by Penny Kyler for AOTA in 1997 and 1998,[15] clinician respondents ranked the following as the five most frequently occurring ethics issues confronting them in practice:

1. Cost-containment policies that jeopardize patient care
2. Inaccurate or inappropriate documentation
3. Improper or inadequate supervision
4. Provision of treatment to those not needing it
5. Colleagues violating patient confidentiality[15]

Additional concerns were related to conflict with colleagues, lack of access to OT for some consumers, and discriminatory practice. Further, 21% of clinicians reported they faced ethical dilemmas daily, 31% weekly, and 32% at least monthly.[15]

The AOTA has provided several documents to assist OT practitioners in analyzing and resolving ethical questions: the *Occupational Therapy Code of Ethics*,[6] the *Guidelines to the Occupational Therapy Code of Ethics*,[5] and *Core Values and Attitudes of Occupational Therapy Practice*.[2] While these documents provide a basis for resolving ethical issues, practitioners may find additional resources and support if they also approach institutional ethics committees and review boards for guidance. Kyler[15] also suggests that OT practitioners act to formalize resolutions for recurring questions by engaging with peers and others to analyze and consider courses of action.

To reiterate, OT practitioners should anticipate that they will encounter ethical distress (defined as the subjective experience of discomfort originating in a conflict between ethical principles) frequently in clinical practice. Many approaches may be useful. A plan of action for addressing ethical distress and resolving ethical dilemmas may involve the following:

1. Reviewing AOTA guidelines[2,5,6]

2. Seeking guidance from institutional ethics and review boards
3. Approaching and engaging with colleagues, peers, and the community to identify and debate ethical questions and formalize resolutions

SUMMARY

The occupational therapy process begins with referral and ends with discontinuation of service. While discrete stages can be named and described, the process is more fluid than stepwise, with the stages at times intermingled. This may look confusing to the novice, but it is actually a hallmark of clinical reasoning.

Clinical reasoning simultaneously employs three "tracks": procedural, interactive, and conditional. While logically analyzing how to proceed through the steps of therapy, the therapist also considers how best to interact with the patient. Further, the therapist creates scenarios of possible future situations. The expert clinician seeks to uncover how the patient understands the disability and uses a narrative or story making approach to capture the patient's imagination of how therapy will benefit him or her.

The OT profession endorses client-centered practice, engaging the patient in all stages of decision making, beginning with assessment. To make this ideal a clinical reality requires that the OTR approach every patient as a co-participant and assist the patient in identifying and prioritizing goals and considering and selecting intervention approaches.

The registered occupational therapist and certified OT assistant have specific responsibilities and areas of emphasis within the OT process. The OTR is the manager and director of the process and delegates specific tasks and steps to the qualified COTA. Aides may also be employed to extend the reach of OT services.

Effective practice typically involves interactions with members of other professions. This requires that the OT practitioner consider the treatment context, the scope of practice of other professions, the applicable jurisdictions and health care regulations, and other factors (e.g., culture, personality, and history) that affect the individual situation.

Ethical questions arise with increasing frequency in modern health care. The AOTA provides guidelines and other resources; practitioners are urged to consider institutional and local resources as well, and to take an active role in identifying and resolving ethical concerns.

REVIEW QUESTIONS

1. Name the eight stages in the OT process.
2. Explain why these stages are not always distinct or sequential.
3. Define the terms *mechanistic* and *phenomenological* and give examples to illustrate these contrasting terms.
4. Name the three tracks of clinical reasoning identified by Fleming and give examples of each.
5. What is narrative reasoning and how is it used in occupational therapy?
6. Discuss some of the obstacles to making client-centered practice the norm.
7. Contrast the roles of the OTR and the COTA. List at least six tasks that may be delegated to the COTA.
8. What services may the OT aide be assigned? What are the limits, and why?
9. Visit and observe two different settings in which OT services are offered. Analyze the differences in the two settings in the way members of the different professions work together. Suggest possible reasons for the differences you find.
10. Are you comfortable with the practices of cross-training and multiskilling? Why or why not?
11. Describe an ethical dilemma you have experienced or encountered in the workplace or fieldwork. How did or would you go about resolving the dilemma?

REFERENCES

1. American Occupational Therapy Association: Concept paper: service delivery in occupational therapy, *Am J Occup Ther* 49:1029-1031, 1995.
2. American Occupational Therapy Association: Core values and attitudes of occupational therapy practice, *Am J Occup Ther* 47:1083-1084, 1993.
3. American Occupational Therapy Association: Career exploration and development: a companion guide to the occupational therapy roles document, *Am J Occup Ther* 48:844-851, 1994.
4. American Occupational Therapy Association: Guide for supervision of occupational therapy personnel, *Am J Occup Ther* 49:1027-1028, 1995.
5. American Occupational Therapy Association: Guidelines to the occupational therapy code of ethics, *Am J Occup Ther* 52:881-884, 1998.
6. American Occupational Therapy Association: Occupational therapy code of ethics, *Am J Occup Ther* 48:1037-1038, 1994.
7. American Occupational Therapy Association: Occupational therapy roles, *Am J Occup Ther* 47:1087-1099, 1993.
8. American Occupational Therapy Association: Position paper: use of occupational therapy aides in occupational therapy practice, *Am J Occup Ther* 49:1023-1025, 1995.
9. American Occupational Therapy Association: Standards of practice for occupational therapy, *Am J Occup Ther* 52:866-869, 1998.
10. Collins AL: Multiskilling: a survey of occupational therapy practitioners' attitudes, *Am J Occup Ther* 51:749-753, 1997.
11. Fleming MH: The therapist with the three-track mind, *Am J Occup Ther* 45:1007-1014, 1991.
12. Foto M: Multiskilling: who, how, when, and why? *Am J Occup Ther* 50:7-9, 1996.
13. Fisher AG: Uniting practice and theory in an occupational framework: 1998 Eleanor Clarke Slagle Lecture, *Am J Occup Ther* 52:509-522, 1998.
14. Gillette NP, Mattingly C: Clinical reasoning in occupational therapy, *Am J Occup Ther* 41:399-400, 1987.

15. Kyler P: Issues in ethics for occupational therapy, *OT Practice* 3(8):37-40, 1998.
16. Law M, Baptiste S, Carswell A, et al: *Canadian occupational performance measure,* ed 2, Toronto, 1994, Canadian Association of Occupational Therapists.
17. Mattingly C: The narrative nature of clinical reasoning, *Am J Occup Ther* 45:998-1005, 1991.
18. Moyers PA: The guide to occupational therapy practice, *Am J Occup Ther* 53:247-322, 1999.
19. Northen JG, Rust DM, Nelson CE, et al: Involvement of adult rehabilitation patients in setting occupational therapy goals, *Am J Occup Ther* 49:214-220, 1995.
20. Pew Health Professions Commission: *Health professions education for the future: schools in service to the nation,* San Francisco, 1993, The Commission.
21. Pollock N: Client-centered assessment, *Am J Occup Ther* 47:298-301, 1993.
22. Schlaff C: From dependency to self-advocacy: redefining disability, *Am J Occup Ther* 47:943-952, 1993.
23. Yerxa EJ: Who is the keeper of occupational therapy's practice and knowledge? *Am J Occup Ther* 49:295-299, 1995.

CHAPTER 4

Treatment Contexts

MAUREEN MICHELE MATTHEWS
MICHELLE TIPTON-BURTON

KEY TERMS

Treatment context
Performance context
Temporal
Environmental
Continuum of care
Acute care
Caregiver
Hospice
Inpatient rehabilitation
Acute rehabilitation
Subacute rehabilitation
Residential care
Home health care
Respite
Home- and community-based therapy
Day treatment
Industrial rehabilitation
Work site

LEARNING OBJECTIVES

After studying this chapter the student or practitioner
will be able to do the following:
1. Define, compare, and contrast treatment context
   and performance context.
2. Identify ways in which different treatment contexts
   affect the occupational performance of persons
   receiving occupational therapy (OT) services.
3. Identify the treatment contexts that afford the most
   realistic projections of how the patient will perform
   in the absence of the therapist.
4. Identify environmental and temporal aspects of at
   least three treatment contexts.
5. Describe ways in which the therapist can alter
   environmental and temporal features of contexts to
   obtain more accurate measures of performance.

Individuals with physical disability receive occupational therapy (OT) services in a variety of settings. These may include acute hospitals, acute rehabilitation centers, subacute rehabilitation facilities, skilled nursing facilities, home health, day treatment, community care programs, and work sites. Even within these categories, each facility is different, and each setting represents a different treatment context.

Treatment context refers to the environment in which treatment occurs, an environment that includes the physical setting and the social, economic, cultural, and political situation that surrounds it. Treatment context has many aspects. Some are abstract: government regulations, the economic realities of reimburse-

ment rules, the workplace pressures of critical pathways and other clinical protocols, the range of services that are considered customary and reasonable, and the traditions and culture that the staff have developed over time. In addition, there are physical aspects such as the building itself, the temperature and humidity of the air, the colors and materials that are used, the layout of the space, and the furnishings and lighting. Practitioners must always be aware that context influences patient performance in evaluation and in treatment; treatment context also determines the kinds of therapeutic treatments available.[12] Length of stay (LOS) and limitations on numbers of visits constrain therapists in selecting frames of reference, limiting choices to those that can produce outcomes within the allotted time. Patient performance in one treatment setting may not be a fair indicator of performance in a different treatment context.

This chapter introduces the range in context typically associated with treatment settings and explores the influence of treatment context on patient performance. Suggestions for modifications of the therapeutic environment and clinical approach are given.

RELATIONSHIP OF TREATMENT CONTEXT TO PERFORMANCE CONTEXT

To the patient, especially the patient with an acute condition, the treatment context represents a novel **performance context**. The third edition of the Uniform Terminology of the American Occupational Therapy Association (AOTA) defines performance context as those factors or situations that influence a person's ability to engage in specific performance areas. Performance context has temporal and environmental aspects. The **temporal** aspects of performance context are identified as chronological age, stage of development, life cycle, and disability status. The identified **environmental** aspects of performance are physical, social, and cultural.[1]

The temporal aspects of performance context derive from the patient. In other words, the patient is a certain age and is at a certain life stage. The disability status of the patient (acute, chronic, or terminal) will affect performance and will perhaps change over time. Even though most temporal aspects derive from the patient, the treatment context introduces other temporal factors. For example, perceived control over scheduling of appointments and over the individual's daily life may vary with treatment setting.

The environmental aspects of performance context change as a person moves from location to location (e.g., work to home to gym). A treatment setting is unlike any of these "normal" performance contexts. Each treatment setting has unique physical, social, and cultural circumstances that influence the individual's ability to engage in required performance areas. These environmental features make it difficult to project how the patient will perform in another setting. For example, individuals who are in control in their home environment may abdicate control for even simple decisions in an acute care hospital.[3] The therapist observing a patient passively allowing health care providers to make even routine decisions may come to the (erroneous) conclusion that the patient is generally indecisive and passive.

Each treatment setting provides a different context for treatment decisions by the therapist, as well as a different context for performance by the patient. The following section discusses the main categories of settings

in which OT services are provided to persons with physical disabilities.

CONTINUUM OF HEALTH CARE

The variety of settings from acute hospital to rehabilitation center to day treatment, home health, outpatient, skilled nursing facility, and work sites forms a **continuum of care**, albeit not always in a sequential fashion, for the physically disabled patient. Persons with physical disabilities are referred to OT services for a variety of reasons and may enter the health care system at any point on the continuum. A patient in an acute hospital might be referred for bed mobility, transfers, and self-care retraining. Depending on the severity of the condition and the treatment potential, the patient may later be treated in a rehabilitation or a day treatment program. A home health or outpatient therapist may see the same individual to address unresolved problems. Should the patient return to the workforce, he or she might later benefit from OT at the workplace, specifically an assessment of the workplace and recommendations about modifications to the work environment or job tasks.

Although many OT patients follow the continuum of health care through several treatment settings, a large number receive services in only one of these settings. Depending on the setting, the person who receives OT may be referred to by a unique consumer name or label that implies role and behavioral expectations of the consumer (Box 4-1). These role and behavioral expectations will affect therapist conduct, patient performance, and treatment options.

Inpatient Settings

Settings in which the patient receives nursing and other health care while staying overnight are classified as inpatient settings.

Acute Care Inpatient

Patients in an **acute care** inpatient setting typically have an acute disability. The condition that led to hospitalization is generally new and either is of recent onset or is a new exacerbation of a chronic condition. Acute hospitalization, especially when unplanned, results in a sudden change in the performance contexts of the patient. All previous social roles are left hanging as a person who may have been a parent or **caregiver** becomes a patient. Career and education are interrupted. An individual who had felt in control of his or her destiny becomes controlled by the circumstances of disability and hospitalization.

Financial and family concerns that may have been manageable before the hospitalization must be managed differently. An acute decline in a chronic condition abruptly confronts the patient with a long-term prognosis, an impending future that may have been ignored for years.

Terminally ill patients may also be found in the acute care hospital. For some, adjustment to dying may be just beginning. Other patients may have been ill, may have known the prognosis longer, and may be close to acceptance. Individuals who have been managed in their own home by a **hospice** program may be hospitalized for pain management, placement, or imminent death; in such cases a patient's hospice goals may be compromised by admission to the hospital.

Pain is another factor for many acute care patients. Movement frequently increases pain but is necessary for healing. Pain decreases the patients' ability to attend to tasks, and may increase fear and shorten temper. A therapist unfamiliar with pain levels of patients with acute orthopedic conditions may have difficulty determining when it is appropriate to push the patients to do more and when it is more appropriate to report the pain to the nursing department. The therapist who develops skill in working with patients in pain will be able to facilitate

treatment goals more effectively than one who ignores or coddles patients in pain (see also Chapter 29).

Because of the urgent nature of an acute admission, many patients arrive without a change of clothes. Clothing available to the hospitalized patient is usually limited to hospital pajamas and gowns. Hospital pants, which are ill fitting with no stretch, can be difficult to don and to keep fastened. Dissimilarities between a hospital gown and a shirt can increase performance errors in dressing.

Patient rooms in an acute care hospital are different from those in homes. Flooring, furniture, lighting, and bathroom facilities are designed for providing medical care and comfort to the bed bound or ill. The absence of carpeting in most hospital rooms presents a smooth and slippery surface for transfer training. Obviously, patients will perform this task differently on a carpeted surface. The incidence of falls in the geriatric population is higher in acute hospitals than in the community or skilled nursing facilities.[6]

Although many hospitals have single rooms, being assigned a roommate is a common situation.[3] Screening performed upon assignment typically follows medical concerns (e.g., limiting the spread of infection and locating surgical patients in the same area) and gender. While having a roommate may provide patients with someone to talk to if they feel up to it, the situation may also expose patients to unfamiliar social and cultural circumstances.

Acute hospitalizations are frequently stressful and frustrating for patients. Away from home while ill, subjected to multiple tests and examinations with sleep interrupted by the sounds of the nursing unit or the need for medical intervention, patients are in a socially compromised environment. Concerns as to whether they might be able to return home after the hospitalization, who will help with care, or who is helping care for dependent loved ones may add to the patient's feelings of stress.

Patients are subjected to frequent intrusions and a lack of privacy during acute hospitalization. Physicians, nurses, therapists, technicians, and housekeeping staff arrive unscheduled. Patients may be exposed for the first time to cultures other than their own. Language and cultural barriers may arouse fear and adversely affect patient performance.

Acute care is a troublesome treatment context for therapists, since patient performance is difficult to assess. Performance may be enhanced or reduced by factors in the hospital environment. Because of time constraints, it is often necessary to perform assessments in patient rooms, rather than in areas elsewhere in the medical center that have been designed for the practice of activities of daily living (ADL). Patient performance in self-care may be artificially enhanced by a lack of the extraneous stimuli found in the home and by the physical attributes of hospital equipment. To compensate, the therapist might position the patient's bed flat, eliminate the bed rails, and lower the bed fully to better simulate the patient's home environment.

Bathing ability is difficult to assess if the patient is accustomed to taking baths and a tub is not available to assess transfers or bathing status. Using clinical experience and judgment, the therapist must be able to project from the patient's performance in the hospital what the patient's performance might be at home. Asking the patient how the environment and the performance might vary between home and the acute care hospital can be helpful. However, it is difficult to obtain accurate information about the relative size and placement of features in the home environment while the person is away from home; therefore referral to a home health therapist is often advisable.

The treatment context of the acute care hospital presents unique financial, social, and physical constraints to the acute care therapist. Treatment goals are generally directed toward promoting medical stability or providing for safe, expedient discharge. It is not unusual for the acute care patient to receive OT for the first time on the day of discharge. In this one visit the therapist must communicate the role of OT and assist the patient in identifying problems and assets in the discharge environment. The patient and the family frequently look to the therapist to identify what the patient will need at home. The therapist cannot possibly make this determination without identifying issues and concerns in the discharge environment. The acute care treatment plan for a patient facing imminent discharge may identify durable medical equipment, inpatient rehabilitation, skilled nursing, outpatient, or home health therapy needs. Identification of needs by the therapist does not automatically ensure that the patient will receive the recommended services. By contacting other members of the health care team and communicating concerns, the therapist can help make sure that evaluation recommendations will be implemented.

The occupational therapist must work with the health care team to rapidly identify issues affecting patient progress or discharge. An experienced therapist equipped with knowledge of the resources available among the health care team and in the community promotes swifter recovery and discharges by working with the patient and team to quickly and accurately identify areas of concern and promote solutions for resolution of problems. For example, a therapist who determines that a patient living alone at discharge would be unable to prepare meals might contact the social worker, who would help set up delivery of hot meals to the home. Another example is a therapist who evaluates a patient scheduled for imminent discharge, finding that the patient moves impulsively and lacks insight into the consequences of his or her actions and is confused when performing self-care tasks. In this instance, the therapist may express these concerns to the discharge coordinator or the physician. The social worker might be consulted about family support available, or discharge may be delayed to determine the cause of the patient's cognitive deficits.

Inpatient Rehabilitation Context

Patients may reside in **inpatient rehabilitation** units when they are able to tolerate several (usually 3) hours of therapy per day and are deemed capable of benefiting from rehabilitation. Rehabilitation settings may be classified as acute or subacute (see below) and are less clinically sterile than acute care hospital environments. The disability status of patients in such settings is slightly less acute than in the acute care hospital. Pain, while still present and affecting patient performance, is less intense and more familiar to the patient. Fear of movement while in pain is generally less than in the acute setting. Performance in ADL will reflect the patient's adaptation to pain.

Patients are expected to dress in their typical clothing rather than hospital issue or pajamas. Expectations that the patient eat meals at a table in a dining area (rather than in bed or at bedside) lend a social element that is not present in the acute care hospital and may not have been present in the patient's home.

ACUTE REHABILITATION. When patients are medically stable and able to tolerate 3 hours of combined therapy services, they may be moved along the continuum from acute inpatient to the **acute rehabilitation** setting. Patients still may need acute medical care in the acute rehabilitation environment. Stays in acute rehabilitation generally range from 2 to 3 weeks, with some patients discharged in a few days and others in a matter of months. The usual goal of an acute rehabilitation stay is discharge to a lesser level of care (e.g., a board and care residence or home).

The process of adjustment to disability has begun by the time the patient has entered acute rehabilitation. As the patient begins to participate in physical activities, deficits and strengths have become more defined. An improvement in function from the level at onset of disability may have occurred. This indicates to the patient that the disability is not static.

Rehabilitation centers attempt to room patients of similar diagnosis and age together. In particular, adolescents benefit from this approach, because their psychological development is in an important phase. Issues of being able to make choices for oneself, control one's environment, and separate from childhood into independent adulthood are forming.[7] A rehabilitation team sensitive to these issues can promote independent decision making within an environment and situation that otherwise gives a strong message of loss of control.

In rehabilitation, there is movement away from the role of patient to former and new life roles. Interventions focused on resumption of those roles will facilitate the transition. For parents, introduction of children into the treatment environment can promote a shift away from the patient role and toward the role of parent.

Although bedrooms in acute rehabilitation facilities are similar to those found in acute hospitals, personalizing one's room by bringing in pictures, comforters, and other items from home is encouraged. Rehabilitation patients are expected to dress in street clothes rather than pajamas, which characterize infirmity. Most clothing is easy-to-don leisure wear. A hidden danger is that dressing training in the rehabilitation center may miss critical elements associated with donning less comfortable but necessary clothes such as neckties and panty hose.

Simulated living environments, family rooms, kitchens, bathrooms, and laundry facilities can be found at most rehabilitation centers. These environments may be inaccurate replicas of the performance contexts in which the person will ultimately have to function. For example, laundry machines may be side by side and top loading rather than coin operated and front loading. Kitchens may be wheelchair accessible in the facility but inaccessible in the home. Clutter, noise, and types of appliances will vary from the patient's natural environment.

Access to the community is not generally evaluated in the acute rehabilitation setting because of the inpatient nature of the setting, coordination of multidisciplinary schedules, and locations of applicable community environments relative to the facility. Some urban facilities are able to integrate community training more smoothly because stores, restaurants, and theaters are closer. These amenities are not identical to those that patients use within their own community, and performance will reflect this variance.

Within a rehabilitation center, many patients form new social relationships with individuals who have similar disabilities. The advantages of these relationships are emotional support and encouragement from the progress of others. The chief disadvantage is that patients may form false expectations (both negative and positive) of their own potential.

The culture of rehabilitation facilities is focused on patient performance and goal attainment. The patient's own culture may be compromised in the process of rehabilitation unless the team is sensitive to and adaptable to the patient's perspective. For example, some cultures view hospital settings as a place for respite and passive patient involvement. Engaging patients in ADL performance can be in direct conflict with patient and family expectations. When cultural perspectives clash, unrealistic goals are frequently the result. As is the case in any phase of rehabilitation, goal attainment and patient performance are dependent upon clear communication and identification of goals that are relevant and meaningful to the patient.

There are more similarities than differences in acute and subacute rehabilitation settings. The primary differences found in subacute centers are as follows:

SUBACUTE REHABILITATION. Subacute rehabilitation facilities are found in skilled nursing facilities and other venues that do not provide acute medical care. The equipment available to the therapist for treatment and evaluation in the subacute setting may be comparable to that found in the acute rehabilitation facility, but in most cases is more limited. Lengths of stay are frequently longer in the subacute setting and may last from a few days to several months. The goal in a subacute setting is usually discharge to a lesser level of care.

Treatment can be paced more slowly in a subacute setting because the urgency for quick discharge is not always present. Engaging in 3 hours of therapy per day is not mandatory. Patient endurance will influence the frequency and duration of therapies.

Because many subacute rehabilitation centers are housed in skilled nursing facilities, the patient may have roommates who are convalescing rather than actively participating in a rehabilitation program. Under those circumstances, the social and emotional bonds formed with roommates can be less motivating than in an acute rehabilitation facility.

SKILLED NURSING FACILITIES. A skilled nursing facility (SNF) is an institution that meets Medicare or Medicaid criteria for skilled nursing care, including rehabilitation services. Subacute rehabilitation centers may be housed in SNFs, but occupational therapy services may also be provided to individuals who are not in a subacute program. Many residents (the preferred consumer label for persons who live in long-term care settings) will remain in SNFs for the remainder of their lives; others will be discharged home.[4] Goals may be directed toward independence or toward safe medical management of the resident.

Extreme variations in disability status are present in SNFs. Observing residents who are severely and permanently disabled may lead newly disabled individuals to form negative expectations of their own prognosis and performance. Younger adults placed in SNFs (where most residents are older adults) may feel isolated, which can adversely affect performance.

The physical environment in skilled nursing facilities impedes the natural performance of ADL. Most equipment is medical or utilitarian, except that found in the common areas. ADL practice in a common area is impractical because the area is frequently crowded and compromises privacy and confidentiality. The therapist is challenged to adapt medical equipment to simulate real-life surroundings and must be able to project how actual performance will vary from therapeutic trials.

Friends are less likely to visit in this environment. Feelings of abandonment are not uncommon. Maintaining connections with friends from the outside demands active pursuit of these relations. A strong family commitment can support outside relationships by providing transportation to church and social gatherings.

A common belief in American society is that people go to skilled nursing facilities to live out their final days. Family and friends may expect less of the individual than they would in other settings. A therapist who facilitates identification of realistic and meaningful expectations and goals for the resident can promote a more positive outlook and outcome.

Many skilled nursing facilities are staffed with individuals from other cultures. Language barriers between the residents and staff may further isolate the resident. Incompatibilities in cultural expectations are not uncommon. The occupational therapist can improve communication between residents and staff by educating staff members about each resident's goals and culture.

RESIDENTIAL CARE. Generally, **residential care** facilities are long-term settings that resemble home situations; persons may reside there on a permanent or transitional basis, depending on prognosis.[13] Facilities are staffed 24 hours a day, but therapists and assistants are present for only part of the day. Rehabilitation technicians implement treatment plans. This "real world laboratory" creates an environment that is more conducive to autonomy and independence.

Similarities in the age of residents, their disability status, and even diagnoses are commonly present. The bonds formed typically promote better performance. Cooperative living is the expectation; performance can be enhanced by this standard.

Although the environment is not the resident's own home, it more closely resembles the resident's natural living situation than do other inpatient settings. The therapist can identify key performance issues in this context. Difficulties with evening self-care, follow-through with safety guidelines, problem solving, schedules, and rules are reported to the therapist by the technician. Modifications in treatment can be more easily tailored to promote independence under such close supervision.

HOME HEALTH. Home health care, treatment based in the patient's home, affords the most natural context for treatment. Blue Cross of California defines a meaningful therapeutic outcome as "one in which the activity level achieved by the patient . . . is . . . necessary for the patient to function most effectively at home or work."[15] The patient, returning home from the hospital, begins to resume life roles at home. Fear of the health care provider is frequently decreased at home. The belief that the health care provider will prevent the patient from returning home is eliminated. The patient can begin to view the therapist as an ally for home living.

The therapist and patient meeting in the patient's home take on new roles. A visiting therapist is a guest in the home and is subject to certain social rules associated with guests. For example, following the family customs of removing street shoes may seem odd to a hospital therapist but is standard practice in many home settings. Schedules for meals, waking, and sleeping fall within patient and family control. The home health therapist's schedule is more likely to be dictated by the patient than vice versa.

The physical environment at home is familiar and affords orientation in its familiarity. The confusion that might be experienced in a hospital or clinic setting is reduced. However, the moving of furniture to make things more accessible for the patient may decrease orientation and increase confusion.

Self-care, homemaking, and cooking tasks evaluated in the context of the home define the challenges that the patient meets daily. The clothing, furniture, appliances, and utensils used in everyday life are present. No longer must the therapist project how the patient can get into or out of the bathtub. Rather, the task of bathing can be worked on in its natural context, and patient performance is realistic. Caring for and feeding animals, answering the door safely, and determining a grocery list for the week suddenly become treatment goals and venues.

Social and family support or lack thereof is readily evident to the home health therapist. Individuals who appeared alone and unsupported while hospital inpatients may have a network of friends and family members who lend support at home. Conversely, other individuals who had frequent visitors in the hospital may be abandoned when the realities of disability reach the home setting.

The home health patient typically requires the assistance of a caregiver for some aspects of his or her ADL. Nearly 20% of all family caregivers are employed full-time outside the home.[2] These caregivers are available for only part of the patient's day and will be concerned primarily with the safety of the patient during their absence.

Stress is common among caregivers. **Respite** care, which temporarily places the patient under the care and supervision of an alternative caregiver for a few hours or several days, can provide necessary relief for a caregiver.[2] Caring for a person with a disability in one's home is not an easy task. Box 4-2 identifies practical concerns surrounding the presence of a patient in the home.

The unique culture of the patient and family unit are evident at home. Religious symbols and practices may be brought into therapy by the patient. A desire to kneel, to genuflect, or to light a candle may never have been communicated in other settings, where the context did not evoke these behaviors.

BOX 4-2

Concerns in Caring for a Person with Disability in One's Home

Amount and type of care needed
Long-term versus temporary, intensive supervision or assistance versus minimal, help available to the caregiver, presence of alternative solutions, and personal feelings about the patient and the type of care required (intimate assistance versus household tasks)

Impact on the household
Effect on spouses, children, and others living in the home; possible involvement of family in making decisions

Environmental concerns
Need and possibility of adapting the home, expenses of adaptations

Work and finance
Options for family medical leave; ability and need to quit work; benefits available

Adapted from Visiting Nurses Association of America: *Caregiver's handbook: a complete guide to home medical care*, New York, 1997, DK Publishing.

Viewing the patient's environment firsthand, the therapist can make recommendations for environmental adaptations, see them implemented, and modify those changes as needed to best meet the patient's needs.[10] Physical changes to the home, including moving furniture, dishes, or bathing supplies, should not be undertaken without the permission of the patient. If the patient is in the home of a family member or friend, the permission of the homeowner must also be sought.

Control of the environment in the home falls to the patient and family. Clinicians who fail to ask permission before adapting the environment will rapidly alienate their patients. A throw rug, viewed by the therapist as a tripping hazard, may be a precious memoir from the patient's childhood home. In seeking permission of the patient and family and providing options, the therapist opens communication. An adhesive mat placed beneath the throw rug will provide a safer surface on which to walk. Another possible solution is to hang the rug as a wall tapestry, where it will be more visually prominent and less prone to damage.

Health care workers in the home occasionally encounter ethical dilemmas, often involving safety.[11] The therapist must be able to determine the best mechanism for resolving issues of safety hazards. Fire and health hazards must be discussed and corrected when the safety of the patient or adjacent households is in jeopardy. By broaching the subject diplomatically and di-

rectly, the therapist can address most hazards and accomplish their removal. In a rental situation, the patient may wish to avoid having safety concerns presented to a landlord for fear of eviction. Inclusion of the patient in problem identification and solution generation may not yield the desired results. Consultation with other professionals can prove fruitful in issues of ethics.

Outpatient

Outpatient OT is provided in hospitals and freestanding clinics to patients who reside elsewhere. Outpatients are medically stable and able to tolerate a few hours of therapy and a trip to an outpatient clinic. Although many outpatients are adjusting to a new disability, some persons with long-standing disability may be referred for therapeutic tune-ups and equipment-related issues. Individuals may view themselves either as dependent (the patient role) or as more in control (the client role), depending on the type of problem for which they are referred.

Outpatient therapy schedules are under the control of the patient more frequently than therapy schedules for inpatients are. Transportation issues and pressing family matters necessitate that clinics offer a variety of treatment times from which a patient may choose. Otherwise, the patient may turn to a different clinic or choose to forego therapy.

To evaluate home-based tasks in an outpatient setting the therapist must extrapolate how task performance will vary at home.[14] Similarity or difference relative to home will affect the patient's ability to perform ADL tasks. The physical layout and equipment of outpatient clinics vary and tend to be designed to meet the treatment needs of specific disabilities. Hand therapy programs, for example, will have treatment tables for exercise and activities and areas for splint fabrication. An industrial work area with special exercise equipment such as Baltimore Therapeutic Equipment (BTE), which mimics work tasks, is not uncommon. Less commonly found in the outpatient setting are complete kitchens with cooking equipment and therapeutic apartments with bathing facilities, living rooms, and bedrooms. Hospital-based outpatient programs might have access to homemaking and bathing areas used in the inpatient rehabilitation center.

The context of self-care tasks is rather awkward for outpatients. Patients who have been assisted with bathing and dressing before coming to the clinic may resist working on these same tasks during therapy. The more unnatural and inappropriate a task seems to patients, the less likely that they will perform well and benefit.

The social context found in outpatient programs is quite distinctive. The patient has begun to resume life in the home and community and may be newly aware of problems not previously foreseen or acknowledged. If the therapist is viewed as an ally in resolving problems and promoting a smooth transition to home, the patient or family members may easily disclose concerns. However, if the patient and family fear that the patient will be removed from the home because of an inability to manage there, they may actively hide concerns from the therapist. In the former instance the patient and family view themselves as being in control of the situation. In the latter, control and power are assumed to belong to the health care professional. An outpatient therapist must be skilled in giving control to the patient. Soliciting patient opinion and listening for unspoken needs are two methods for increasing the patient's sense of control.[10] Providing choices for treatment does much to motivate clients and improve performance in tasks.

Each outpatient clinic has its own culture. Some are perceived as clinically more professional, while others have more of an office atmosphere, and still others the flavor of a community center or gym. The culture of the clinic lends a context for performance to the patient. More clinical and professional settings may help some patients feel most comfortable and professionally managed. The same setting might lead other patients to fear failure; a community center atmosphere may be comfortable to these patients.

Home- and community-based therapy

Most clinicians are familiar with home health care. An alternative course for patients with traumatic injuries such as head or spinal cord injuries is a **home- and community-based therapy** program. Treatment is delivered in the home, but that is where the similarity to home health ends. This type of program provides intensive rehabilitation in the patient's own home and community. The client receives comprehensive rehabilitation services and acquires functional skills in daily activities in the normal environments of home, school, work site, and community. This enhances the likelihood of a successful and functional outcome.

For example, a young mother may benefit more from working on realistic meaningful tasks in her home and community than she would in a clinic setting. The patient is performing in her natural physical, social, and cultural environment. Scheduling is within control of the patient, and treatment sessions vary in length and frequency depending on the goals. An all-morning session to work with the client as she moves through her daily routine (e.g., bathing and dressing her child, going grocery shopping, and performing various household chores) would be possible.

Clinically, the therapist must be able to adapt the treatment to the natural social and cultural aspects present in the home. Attempts to alter the natural social and cultural order are ill advised, since things are likely to return to their natural state when the treatment session ends and the therapist leaves.

When practice is necessary for goal attainment, a rehabilitation technician or therapy aide may be charged with carrying out treatment programs set by the therapist. The technician who spends many hours with the patient can provide greater insight in cases when treatment is not succeeding because it interferes with the natural context of the client's lifestyle. Adjusting treatment strategies to adapt to these lifestyle differences will ensure better clinical outcomes.

Day treatment

Day treatment programs are becoming more popular as a way of decreasing the length of inpatient hospitalizations and containing rehabilitation costs. Programs vary, but the underlying philosophy is to provide an intensive interdisciplinary treatment for patients who do not need to be hospitalized.[8] Patients receiving day treatment typically live at home. Most programs offer a team approach. Professionals from all disciplines are engaged cooperatively, sharing their expertise to meet the patient's individual goals.

Many day treatment programs are designed without the traditional time constraints inherent in a more traditional outpatient program. Lengthy community outings and home and work site treatment sessions may be used as a method of attaining goals. A day treatment therapist may have the best opportunity to evaluate and treat patients in all of their natural environments.

Work site therapy programs

Industrial rehabilitation can be conducted in the context of the employee's place of work. **Work site** therapy programs in the workplace are designed to address an employee's therapy needs related to work injury. The injured worker can remain at or return to work for treatment. Work hardening is taken out of the clinic setting and put back in the workplace. This cost-effective approach places the patient back into the work role. Prevention of further injury occurs naturally when employees are treated at the work site.

Treating individuals at their place of work helps them make the transition from the patient role to the role of client or worker. The therapist engaged in the treatment context of the worksite must never compromise the worker's status.[9] The employer and peers must view the employee as a worker rather than as a patient. Maintaining confidentiality can be challenging because the coworkers' curiosity is often aroused by the unfamiliar face of the therapist in the workplace. The therapist must remember never to answer queries that would compromise client-therapist confidentiality. Unsolicited requests from coworkers for medical advice and work site modifications are best referred to that employee's doctor or manager, respectively.

In the work setting the therapist is answerable to the employer as well as the employee, and often also to an insurance company. By encouraging the injured employee to communicate his or her needs for work modification and suggestions for how productivity might be maintained, the therapist will pave the way for a successful transition to work. The therapist must be able to step back from the client, see the needs of the employer, and promote resolution of work-related issues that would interfere with a smooth transition to productive work. Scheduling of therapy visits to the workplace must meet the needs of both the employee and employer. Work site visits should be scheduled in a manner that minimizes stopping or interfering with the natural flow of work.

The financial impact of work modifications will concern the employer. Employers do not have unlimited resources for modifying work environments. Only reasonable and necessary work modifications should be considered. Suggestions for work modifications that have an associated cost should be discussed with the employer and not with the employee. This is unique to the environment of work and one of the rare times in which the patient will not be privy to all of the therapist's recommendations and suggestions. The therapist can suggest work modifications that do not have any cost, but must consider the impact of these modifications on coworkers using the same equipment. As a rule of thumb, modifications that affect workers other than the employee must be discussed with management before they are presented to the employee.

In a traditional clinic setting, a secretary who sustained a repetitive motion injury of her wrist may receive various modalities to control her symptoms of pain and edema and may be educated on joint and tendon protection techniques while performing various movements in a clinic setting. When the secretary is treated in her work environment additional benefits may occur. Joint and tendon protection techniques are applied at work while performing day-to-day work tasks. Since the client's injury occurred at work, it could be exacerbated or prevented at work. See also Chapters 16 and 17 with regard to the role of the occupational therapist with workers and in work settings.

SUMMARY

Treatment context, the environment in which treatment occurs, has temporal and environmental dimensions that affect both the therapist and the person receiving therapy services. Knowing the features of each treatment context and anticipating how the context will affect performance prepares the therapist to best meet patient and client needs. A skilled therapist can

guide the patient via careful questioning toward meaningful and attainable goals. Sensitivity to the unique needs of each individual in each treatment setting is critical.

REVIEW QUESTIONS

1. Identify the temporal and environmental aspects of performance context.
2. Name at least five treatment settings in the continuum of care.
3. Discuss how names applied to various consumer groups affect performance.
4. Identify environmental and temporal aspects of acute hospitalization and identify modifications a therapist can make to adjust performance to more closely mimic that at home.
5. Discuss how control over the schedule promotes a sense of control in patients and clients.
6. Identify persons with whom home modifications must be discussed before they are implemented, and explain why.
7. Identify modifications that should not be discussed with the employee without employer approval, and explain why.
8. Discuss situations that have the potential to compromise patient confidentiality at the work site, and identify appropriate responses.

REFERENCES

1. American Occupational Therapy Association: Uniform terminology for occupational therapy, ed 3, *Am J Occup Ther* 48:1047-1055, 1994.
2. Atchison B: Occupational therapy in home health: rapid changes need proactive planning, *Am J Occup Ther* 51(6):406-409, 1997.
3. Blau SP, Shimberg EF: *How to get out of the hospital alive: a guide to patient power*, New York, 1997, Macmillan.
4. Bausell RX, Rooney MA, Inlander CB: *How to evaluate and select a nursing home*, Beverly, Mass, 1988, Addison-Wesley.
5. Boaz RF: Full-time employment and formal caregiving in the 1980's, *Medical Care* 34(6):524-536, 1996.
6. Chu LW et al: Risk factors for falls in hospitalized older medical patients, *J Gerontol A Biol Sci Med Sci* 54(1):M38-M43, 1999.
7. Dunn W: *Pediatric occupational therapy—facilitating effective service provision*, Thorofare, NJ, 1991, Slack.
8. Gilliand E: The day treatment program: meeting rehabilitation needs for SCI in the changing climate of health care reform, *SCI Nurs* 13(1):6-9, 1996.
9. Haffey WJ, Abrams DL: Employment outcomes for participants in a brain injury reentry program: preliminary findings, *J Head Trauma Rehabil* 6(3):24-34, 1991.
10. Head J, Patterson V: Performance context and its role in treatment planning, *Am J Occup Ther* 51(6):453-457, 1997.
11. Opachich KJ: Moral tensions and obligations of occupational therapy practitioners providing home care, *Am J Occup Ther* 51(6):430-435, 1997.
12. Park S, Fisher AG, Velozo CA: Using the assessment of motor and process skills to compare occupational performance between clinics and home setting, *Am J Occup Ther* 48:697-709, 1994.

13. Proctor D, Kaplan SH: The occupational therapist's role in a transitional living program for head injured clients, *Occup Ther Health Care* 9(1):17-35, 1995.
14. Rogers JC, Holm MB, Stone RG: Evaluation of daily living tasks: the home care advantage, *Am J Occup Ther* 51(6):410-422, 1997.
15. Stewart DL, Albin SH: *Documenting function in physical therapy*, St Louis, 1993, Mosby.

SUGGESTED READING

Heron E: *Tending lives—nurses on the medical front pulse*, New York, 1998, Ballantine.
Visiting Nurses Association of America: *Caregiver's handbook: a complete guide to home medical care*, New York, 1997, DK Publishing.

CHAPTER 5

Occupational Therapy Evaluation and Assessment of Physical Dysfunction

LORRAINE WILLIAMS PEDRETTI
MARY BETH EARLY

KEY TERMS

Evaluation
Assessment
Client-centered practice
Evaluation process
Initial evaluation
Screening
Occupational therapy diagnosis
Clinical reasoning
Informal observation
Formal (structured) observation
Standardized test
Nonstandardized test

LEARNING OBJECTIVES

After studying this chapter the student or practitioner will be able to do the following:
1. Differentiate and define *evaluation* and *assessment*.
2. List and describe the steps in the evaluation process.
3. Know the purposes of occupational therapy (OT) evaluation.
4. Describe the desired outcome of the initial evaluation.
5. Describe four methods of assessment that occupational therapists use.
6. Compare standardized and nonstandardized tests.

Evaluation refers to "the process of obtaining and interpreting data necessary for intervention. This includes planning for and documenting the evaluation process and results." **Assessment** refers "to specific tools or instruments that are used during the evaluation process."[2]

Evaluation is the process of gathering data, identifying problems, formulating hypotheses, and making decisions for treatment interventions.[9,17] The evaluation is carried out using formal and informal screening and other methods, including a review of the medical record, an interview, observation, standardized tests, and nonstandardized tests.[9] In **client-centered practice**, the patient and patient's family participate in decision making, to the extent possible, throughout the **evaluation process**. Evaluations are usually performed at the beginning of treatment, periodically during the term of treatment, and at the end of treatment.[16]

In occupational therapy (OT), evaluation of occupational performance, performance areas, performance components, and performance contexts is the basis for developing treatment objectives and intervention strategies. The OT evaluation should identify occupational problems that are of concern to the patient.[4,16]

An **initial evaluation** takes place before treatment begins, and reevaluation occurs periodically during the course of OT intervention.[15] The results of the initial evaluation are used to identify deficits in performance areas and performance components. Deficits in performance areas are defined as limitations in the ability to perform desired self-care, work and productive activities, or leisure skills. Deficits in performance components are physical, cognitive, or psychosocial impairments that limit adequate and satisfying function in the performance areas. Performance contexts may also be assessed at this time. The occupational therapist must assess the environments in which tasks are to be performed and features of the environment that affect the patient's ability to function optimally.[4]

The initial evaluation is the foundation for selecting treatment objectives and treatment methods.[17] Reevaluation is essential to determining the effectiveness of treatment, modifying treatment to suit the patient's needs, and revising the treatment plan. Reevaluation may lead to the elimination of unattainable goals, the modification of goals that were partially or completely achieved, and the adoption of new goals as additional problems are identified or progress is made.

Evaluation and **assessment** provide therapists with specific methods for determining their effectiveness as a planner and administrator of treatment.[17] Evaluation yields specific information that can be communicated to other members of the rehabilitation team. Furthermore, careful evaluation and assessment can enhance the development of OT instruments, programs, and protocols. Assessment data that are collected systematically may be used for the development of standardized assessments and thus contribute to a better understanding of the assessment and treatment methods that are effective in OT practice.

To evaluate effectively, the therapist must be knowledgeable about the dysfunction, its causes, course, and prognosis; familiar with a variety of assessment tools, their uses, and proper administration; and able to select assessments that are suitable to the patient and the dysfunction. Thus, an understanding of possible dysfunction in performance areas, performance components, and performance contexts is essential, as is a mastery of applicable treatment principles. When performing assessments, the therapist must approach the patient with openness and without preconceived ideas about the individual's limitations or personality. The therapist must have good observation skills and must be able to gain the trust of the patient in a short time.[20]

EVALUATION PROCESS
Screening and Initial Evaluation

The evaluation process (Fig. 5-1) is initiated with **screening**, which includes reviewing the patient's medical record and possibly discussing the patient with other staff.[3]

Following the screening, initial assessments are conducted. The occupational therapist interviews the patient, administers selected screening tests, and makes observations about the patient's physical condition and affective state. The estimated duration of treatment and the need to coordinate treatment with other services can also be determined at this time.[3,15]

The initial evaluation establishes the patient's treatment priorities, describes potential posttreatment circumstances, describes the **occupational therapy diagnosis,** and proposes treatment goals and objectives that can be achieved in a time frame prescribed by the patient's insurance carrier.[16]

Identifying Treatment Model or Models

The next step in the evaluation process is to select an appropriate treatment model or models and the specific assessments that will yield the information needed as the basis for clinical decision making consistent with the selected practice model. For example, for a patient who has rheumatoid arthritis, the therapist is likely to select the biomechanical and rehabilitation models. Using these models, the therapist assesses factors such as joint range of motion (ROM), muscle strength, and physical endurance as well as activities of daily living (ADL), work, and leisure activity performance. In another example, for a patient who had suffered a cerebrovascular accident (CVA) or stroke, the therapist could select the neurodevelopmental model and plan to assess motor control, muscle tone, coordination, and the postural reflex mechanism.

Assessment

After selecting an appropriate treatment model, the therapist assesses occupational performance, performance areas, and performance components. The primary focus of OT is to maximize occupational performance by identifying deficits in occupational performance and providing intervention strategies to eliminate or alleviate such deficits. A top-down approach to evaluation proceeds first with occupation-based assessments and then with the assessment of performance components.

The therapist assesses the patient by using structured interviews, clinical observation, formal and informal observations, standardized tests, and nonstandardized tests. The therapist studies assessment results to identify deficits in the performance areas, performance components, and performance contexts. Identification of deficits is always somewhat provisional, and open to revision because new information may alter the therapist's formulation of the patient's occupational performance problems.

Problem Identification

Data necessary to plan treatment are interpreted and synthesized.[3] Assets are noted and deficits in performance areas, performance components, and performance contexts that necessitate OT intervention are identified. The occupational therapist assesses the individual's occupational roles and role dysfunction and makes an OT

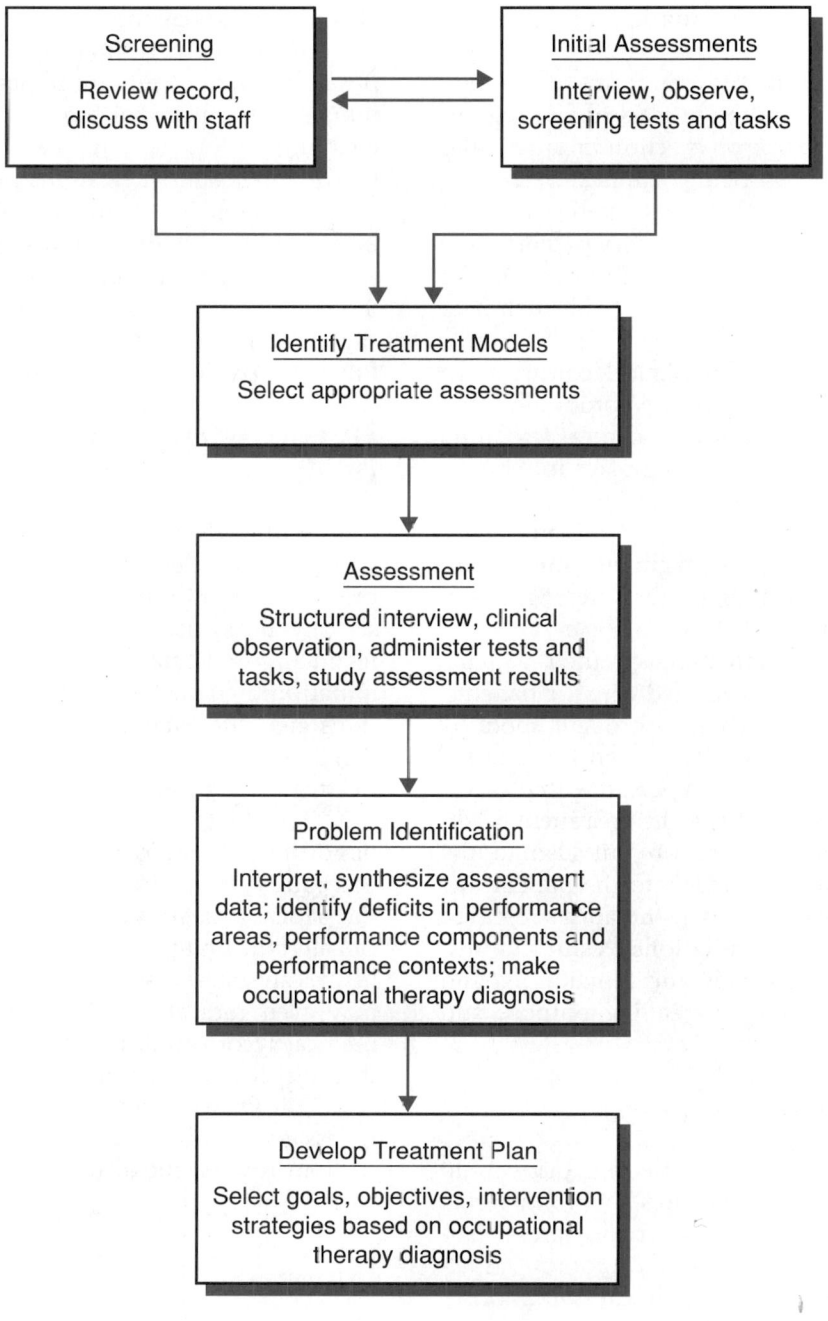

FIG. 5-1
The evaluation process.

diagnosis.[15] The **occupational therapy diagnosis** is a list of occupational performance deficits and performance skills deficits that describes the effects of the patient's medical or psychiatric condition on function in essential and desired life roles.[16]

Developing a Treatment Plan

The final stage of the evaluation process is to develop a treatment plan. Goals, objectives, and evidence-based intervention strategies (see Chapter 7) that will address

the occupational therapy diagnosis (i.e., problems and deficits) are selected in conjunction with the patient and patient's family or significant others.

CLINICAL REASONING

During the evaluation process the therapist uses clinical reasoning and clinical decision making to identify problems and select intervention strategies.[17] **Clinical reasoning**, described in Chapter 3, guides decisions about the collection, classification, and analysis of data and ultimately helps to determine appropriate goals and intervention strategies.[18]

Clinical reasoning includes several forms of thinking and ways of perceiving. It is the process of figuring out how to select the most appropriate action in a particular case for the patient's well-being. Clinical reasoning combines theoretical principles with the knowledge and habitual ways of seeing and doing things that come from experience. Clinical reasoning improves as the therapist gains and applies findings from research data and experience.[12,13]

The simple application of theoretical constructs to arrive at answers to questions about appropriate intervention strategies is only a part of the clinical reasoning process. OT theory provides a starting place for clinical reasoning but cannot provide all the answers for the course of action in a particular case. Because each patient is unique and complex, treatment must be individualized. This requires judgment, creativity, and improvisation.[12,13]

When occupational therapists teach their patients everyday activities they are confronted with the patients' experiences of profound life changes brought about by the disability, the loss of capacities taken for granted, and reorientation to the world as a person with physical and functional limitations. Thus the treatment is directed not only to the dysfunction but also to the human meaning of the dysfunction to the patient. OT treats the "illness experience."[13] The therapist's role is to help patients confront the limitations, "claim the disability," reclaim a changed body and functioning, and develop a new sense of self with meaning, purpose, and value.[12,13]

CONTENT OF THE EVALUATION

During the initial OT evaluation, the therapist should include an assessment of the patient's goals, functional abilities in the occupational performance areas, performance components, and performance contexts as relevant to the individual and the clinical condition.[3,5] The therapist should also assess performance components, paying particular attention to the sensorimotor component and cognitive integration and cognitive components in physical disabilities. The therapist also assesses or observes psychosocial skills and psychological components[5] during the initial visits with the patient. The occupational therapist may need to plan remediation or compensation for these latter components, as well as for the more obvious sensorimotor deficits. Alternatively, the therapist might refer the patient to the appropriate service for remediation, depending on the severity of the problems. The occupational therapist should obtain information about the patient's medical, educational, and work histories, family, and cultural background.[3] The therapist should also assess the patient's environment as a determinant of occupational performance. The social, cultural, and physical environments are all performance contexts that influence occupational functioning. The disabling and enabling factors of the patient's environments and person-environment relationships need to be assessed and considered in treatment planning.[5,11] This information should guide the therapist in selecting appropriate and meaningful treatment objectives and methods. Structuring treatment on the basis of the patient's needs, values, and sociocultural milieu facilitates the patient's full participation in the treatment process.

METHODS OF ASSESSMENT
Medical Records

Data gathered from the medical record are important parts of the evaluation process. The medical record can provide information on the diagnosis, prognosis, medical history, precautions, current treatment regimen, social data, psychological data, and other rehabilitation therapies. Daily notes from nurses and physicians give information about current medications and the patient's reactions and responses to the hospital, treatment regimen, and persons in the treatment facility.[19] Ideally, the occupational therapist will have the opportunity to study the medical record before seeing the patient to begin the evaluation process. Knowing the patient's diagnosis before beginning the evaluation can alert the occupational therapist to problems that are likely, can suggest assessments that might be useful, and may even indicate a likely treatment approach. The medical record indicates problem areas and helps the therapist focus attention on the relevant factors of the case.[16,20] Occasionally, special circumstances make it necessary for the therapist to begin the evaluation without the benefit of the information in the medical record.

Interview

The initial interview is a valuable step in the evaluation process. The interview is a shared experience in which both the therapist and client ask and answer questions. An essential purpose of the interview is for the therapist to hear the client's story and know all of the particulars of the client's situation. These data are the basis for meaningful treatment planning.[10] The occupational therapist gathers information during the interview on how the patient perceives his or her roles, dysfunction, needs, and goals, and the patient can learn about the role of the occupational therapist and OT in the rehabilitation program.[10,20] An important outcome of the initial interview is the development of collaboration, rapport, and trust between therapist and patient.[10]

The initial interview should take place in an environment that is quiet and ensures privacy. The therapist should plan the interview in advance, determining what information must be acquired and preparing some specific questions. The interviewer and patient should set aside a specified period of time for the interview. The first few minutes of the interview may be devoted to getting acquainted and orienting the patient to the OT clinic or service and to the role and goals of OT.

The two essential elements for a successful interview are a solid knowledge base and active-listening skills. The therapist must acquire these abilities through study, practice, and preparation. The therapist's knowledge will influence the selection of questions or topics to be covered in the interview. The interview should cover the areas that are relevant both to OT and to the construction of a meaningful treatment plan. Active listening creates opportunities for genuine communication. The interviewer who listens actively demonstrates respect for and a vital interest in the patient.[1] The therapist tries to understand what the patient is feeling and the meaning of the patient's message. The interview is an opportunity to establish a collaborative therapeutic relationship with the patient.[10]

Throughout the interview the therapist should listen to ascertain the patient's attitude toward the dysfunction. The therapist invites the patient to express what he or she sees as the primary problems and goals for rehabilitation. These may differ substantially from the therapist's judgment and must be given careful consideration when therapist and patient reach the point of setting treatment goals together. As the interview progresses, there should be an opportunity for the patient to ask questions as well. The therapist must have good listening and observation skills to gather the maximum amount of information from the interview. Further, the therapist must have the patience to wait through periods of silence for the patient to consider the questions and formulate responses.

It will probably be necessary to take notes or record the initial interview. The patient should be advised of this method in advance, understand the reasons this is done, know the uses to which the material will be put, and be allowed to read the notes or listen to the tape if he or she desires.[19,20]

During the initial phase of the interview, the therapist should explain the purpose of the interview and how the information will be used. As the interview progresses, the therapist may seek the desired information by asking appropriate questions and guiding the responses and ensuing discussion so that relevant topics are addressed. The occupational therapist may wish to seek information about the patient's family and friends, community and work roles, educational and work histories, leisure and social interests and activities, and the living environment to which the patient will return. The interview can be concluded with a summary of the major points covered, information gained, estimate of problems and assets, and plans for further OT evaluation.

Observation

Some aspects of the evaluation will be based on the occupational therapist's **informal observation** of the patient during the interview and formal observation during the assessment procedures that follow. The occupational therapist will base some of the reevaluation of the patient on observations during treatment.

Informal Observation

The occupational therapist can gain much information by observing the patient as he or she approaches or is approached. What is the posture, mode of ambulation, and gait pattern? How is the patient dressed and groomed? Is there an obvious motor dysfunction? Are there apparent musculoskeletal deformities? What are the facial expression, tone of voice, and manner of speech? How are the hands held and used? Are there pain mannerisms, such as protection of an injured part or grimaces and groans? Are there apparent body odors?

Formal Observation

Occupational therapists use **formal structured observation** to assess performance of self-care, home management, mobility, and transferring (see Chapters 13 and 14). The therapist observes the patient perform these skills in real or simulated environments. The therapist can determine the patient's level of independence, speed, skill, need for special equipment, and the feasibility of further training. The therapist can also observe for the performance component deficits that may be causing difficulties with performance of essential life tasks.

The rapport and trust that develop between the patient and the therapist flow out of the communication between them. The quality of communication in the interview and observation phases of the evaluation process is critical to all subsequent interactions and thus to the effectiveness of treatment. The patient must sense that he or she has been heard and understood by someone who is empathic and who has the necessary knowledge and skills to facilitate rehabilitation. The therapist who is an effective communicator projects self-confidence and confidence in the profession, setting the tone for all future interaction with the patient and enhancing the development of the patient's trust in the therapist and in the potential effectiveness of OT.[20]

Assessments

The evaluation is carried out through **assessments** such as tests and measurements in OT. Relevant and accurate evaluation is critical to decision-making for planning treatment, determining school and community living placement, considering admission to and discharge from clinical programs, and other dispositions that may be based on test results. Thus, in reporting assessment data it is essential that the information be supported by relevant and accurate testing procedures.[7]

Occupational therapists use both standardized and nonstandardized assessments. The development of standardized OT assessments that are grounded in theory has been increasing in recent years.

STANDARDIZED TESTS. Standardized tests include specific instructions for administration and scoring and have statistical evidence of validity and reliability. They are norm referenced—that is, norms are used as standards for interpreting individual test scores. Individual test scores are compared with scores of persons in the norm group.[3,6,7,21]

Occupational therapists have been encouraged to use standardized tests to record information obtained from patients. Using standardized tests can improve the ability to formalize OT evaluation based on quantitative assessment. Results of the initial assessments and follow-up assessments can be reported in a consistent, objective, and reliable manner. This approach requires that occupational therapists increase their knowledge and skill in testing. Use of standardized assessments enhances professional credibility.[22] To use standardized tests effectively, the occupational therapist must have the necessary skills for competent test administration and should follow test protocols carefully.[3]

Many standardized tests designed by professionals in disciplines other than OT are used by occupational therapists to measure achievement, development, intelligence, manual dexterity, motor skills, personality, sensorimotor function, and vocational skills.[6,8] *The Mental Measurements Yearbook,*[14] *Occupational Therapy Assessment Tools: An Annotated Index*[6] *Occupational Performance Assessment,*[9] and *Assessment and Evaluation: An Overview*[19] are excellent sources of information about standardized tests. Current health care journals and psychologic abstracts also provide information about standardized assessments that may be relevant to OT.[7] While it is desirable to have standardized and objective tests in OT, professional judgment and interpretation are always an important part of the evaluation process.[15]

Nonstandardized Assessments

Many assessments that occupational therapists use are **nonstandardized tests.** That is, they have unknown reliability and validity. Many are informal instruments developed by therapists to suit the needs of particular practice settings. Still others are adaptations of standardized assessment instruments that are used with patients other than those for whom they were designed.

Standardized instruments designed by other professionals for their own disciplines are sometimes used by occupational therapists.[8,23]

In contrast to standardized tests, administration and scoring of nonstandardized assessments is more subjective. There may be no specific instructions for administration, criteria for scoring, or information on interpreting results of the assessment.[15] The results and interpretation of nonstandardized tests depend on the clinical skill, experience, judgment, and bias of the evaluator.[7] Some nonstandardized assessments provide instructions for test administration and broad criteria for scoring and interpretation but still require the use of considerable subjective professional judgment.[15] The manual muscle test, described in Chapter 22, is an example of such a test.

SUMMARY

The occupational therapy evaluation is a complex process of data gathering and analysis that yields one or more OT diagnoses that become the starting point for intervention. Evaluation of the patient with physical dysfunction includes an examination of medical records, interview, observation, and the administration of specific formal and informal assessments. The evaluation of the patient is based on an analysis of the data gathered from the assessments. Those data are used to identify problems and assets relevant to the patient's occupational performance and to plan appropriate intervention goals and strategies.

Occupational therapists have developed many useful informal assessments. These include tests, checklists, and rating scales. Some of these have been developed into standardized tests. Occupational therapists have recognized the need to identify and employ discipline-specific assessments to help establish the scientific base of the profession. Many such tests have been designed and introduced in recent years.

Selection of appropriate assessments will depend on the patient's diagnosis, medical history, lifestyle, interests, living situation, needs, values, and environment. Clinical reasoning in the OT evaluation is responsive to information gathered during the evaluation. Thus, the therapist is thoughtful and reflective in selecting treatment objectives, methods, and progression. Decisions reached during evaluation lead to the construction of the treatment plan, discussed in Chapter 6.[20]

REVIEW QUESTIONS

1. Define evaluation and assessment.
2. List four purposes of occupational therapy evaluation.
3. Which skills must the occupational therapist possess to be an effective evaluator?

4. List and describe the steps in the evaluation process.
5. Which specific occupational performance areas and performance components are most likely to be assessed by the occupational therapist when treating patients with physical dysfunction?
6. Describe four methods of assessment that occupational therapists use in the evaluation process.
7. Along with diagnosis and medical data, which other important factors about the patient should be considered by the occupational therapist during the evaluation and in treatment planning?
8. Compare standardized and nonstandardized tests. What are the characteristics of each?
9. What are the criteria for the effective use of standardized tests?

REFERENCES

1. Allen C: The performance status examination: paper presented at the American Occupational Therapy Association annual conference, San Francisco, October 1976. Cited in Hopkins HL, Smith HD, editors: *Willard and Spackman's occupational therapy*, ed 6, Philadelphia, 1983, JB Lippincott.
2. American Occupational Therapy Association: Clarification of the use of the terms assessment and evaluation, *Am J Occup Ther* 49:10, 1072, 1995.
3. American Occupational Therapy Association: Standards of practice for occupational therapy, *Reference manual of the official documents of The American Occupational Therapy Association*. Bethesda, Md, 1996, The Association.
4. American Occupational Therapy Association: Uniform terminology for occupational therapy, third edition. In *Reference manual of the official documents of the American Occupational Therapy Association*, ed 6, Bethesda, Md, 1996, The Association.
5. American Occupational Therapy Association: Uniform terminology for occupational therapy, third edition, *Am J Occup Ther* 48(11):1047-1054, 1994.
6. Asher IE: *Occupational therapy evaluation tools: an annotated index*, ed 2, Bethesda, Md, 1996, American Occupational Therapy Association.
7. Atchison B: Selecting appropriate assessments, *Physical Disabilities Special Interest Section Newsletter* 10:2, 1987. Published by the American Occupational Therapy Association.
8. Bowker A: Standardized tests utilized by therapists in the field of physical disabilities, *Physical Disabilities Special Interest Section Newsletter* 6:4, 1983. Published by the American Occupational Therapy Association.
9. Christiansen C: Occupational performance assessment. In Christiansen C, Baum C, editors: *Occupational therapy: overcoming human performance deficits*, Thorofare, NJ, 1991, Slack.
10. Henry AD: The interview process in occupational therapy. In Neidstadt ME, Crepeau EB: *Willard and Spackman's occupational therapy*, ed 9, Philadelphia, 1998, JB Lippincott.
11. Letts L et al: Person-environment assessment in occupational therapy, *Am J Occup Ther* 48(7):608, 1994.
12. Mattingly C: What is clinical reasoning? *Am J Occup Ther* 45(11):979, 1991.
13. Mattingly C, Fleming MH: *Clinical reasoning*, Philadelphia, 1994, FA Davis.
14. Mitchell JV, editor: *Mental measurements yearbook*, ed 11, Highland Park, NJ, 1992, Rutgers University.
15. Mosey AC: *Occupational therapy, configuration of a profession*, New York, 1981, Raven Press.
16. Neistadt ME: Overview of evaluation. In Neidstadt ME, Crepeau EB: *Willard & Spackman's occupational therapy*, ed 9, Philadelphia, 1998, JB Lippincott.
17. Opacich KF: Assessment and informed decision-making. In Christiansen C, Baum C, editors: *Occupational therapy: overcoming human performance deficits*, Thorofare, NJ, 1991, Slack.
18. Rogers JC, Masagatani G: Clinical reasoning of occupational therapists during the initial assessment of physically disabled patients, *Occup Ther J Res* 4:195, 1982.
19. Smith HD: Assessment and evaluation: an overview. In Hopkins HL, Smith HD, editors: *Willard and Spackman's occupational therapy*, ed 8, Philadelphia, 1993, JB Lippincott.
20. Smith HD, Tiffany EG: Assessment and evaluation: an overview. In Hopkins HL, Smith HD, editors: *Willard and Spackman's occupational therapy*, ed 6, Philadelphia, 1983, JB Lippincott.
21. Tuckman BW: *Conducting educational research*, ed 2, New York, 1978, Harcourt Brace Jovanovich.
22. Watson M Analysis: standardized testing objectives, *Physical Disabilities Special Interest Section Newsletter* 6:4, 1983. Published by the American Occupational Therapy Association.
23. Watts JH et al: The assessment of occupational functioning: a screening tool for use in long-term care, *Am J Occup Ther* 40:231, 1986.

CHAPTER 6

Treatment Planning

LORRAINE WILLIAMS PEDRETTI
MARY BETH EARLY

The purpose of occupational therapy (OT) is to help clients learn or relearn essential occupational performance tasks in the areas of activities of daily living (ADL), work, and play or leisure that will enable them to live as independently as possible. Clients or their insurers fund OT services. They want to see results in as short a time as is reasonable and will pay only for treatment that results in improvements in occupational performance.[8] A well-designed treatment plan is essential to the achievement of these objectives.

A **treatment plan** is the design or proposal for a therapeutic program. Pelland described it as "the core of occupational therapy practice,"[9] and Day described it as the "core of teaching" in the OT internship.[3] The treatment plan is based on patient priorities, a critical analysis of performance deficits identified in the initial evaluation, and the unique circumstances of the individual patient. Occupational therapists also consider their clients' physical and social performance contexts in treatment planning.[8] These factors make OT intervention complex and treatment planning a challenge for therapists.

Effective treatment planning is possible if the therapist has made a thorough and careful evaluation, has reviewed, analyzed, and summarized assessment data, has selected an appropriate practice model or models, has identified treatment goals and objectives, and has chosen appropriate treatment methods. Further, the treatment plan should include ongoing reevaluation and data collection and the restatements of treatment priorities.[2] In short, the treatment plan includes goals and objectives and treatment methods or intervention strategies based on identified problems and indicates how the program should progress.[3] In this chapter the terms *treatment methods* and *intervention strategies* are used synonymously.

Writing a treatment plan is necessary. Writing a plan yields specific objectives outlined in an orderly and sequential manner that will be clear to the therapist, patient, and other concerned persons. The treatment plan guides the therapist to proceed efficiently and provides a standard for measuring the progress of the patient and the effectiveness of the plan.

Practicing therapists sometimes work intuitively, do not write out their treatment plans, and consequently find it difficult to articulate the rationale for the work they have done.[2] Such clinicians may be working in a trial-and-error manner, wasting precious time and money. They may be poorly prepared to defend their course of action to themselves, the patient, the rehabilitation team, an insurance company, or even those involved in potential legal proceedings. They may convey uncertainty in their reports about the patients assigned to them. Absence of a stated treatment plan can also present problems to other staff members who may have to substitute in the absence of the treating clinician.

Perhaps one of the most important purposes for writing a treatment plan is to plan, analyze, and continually reevaluate the proposed course of action. In so doing, the therapist should ask many questions. Some of these are as follows:

1. What are the problems that this patient is experiencing?
2. How does the patient view these problems?
3. In what other ways can the problems be defined?
4. What are the patient's capabilities and assets?
5. What are the patient's limitations and deficits?
6. What does OT have to offer this patient?
7. Which needs does the OT treatment program aim to address?
8. What is or are the most appropriate practice model(s) or treatment approach(es) on which to base the treatment plan?
9. What are the goals of treatment?
10. What are specific treatment objectives?
11. Are the treatment objectives consistent with the patient's needs and personal aspirations?
12. If objectives are not compatible, how should they be modified?
13. Which treatment methods are available to meet the objectives?
14. In what time frame should the patient have met the objectives?
15. What standards shall be used to determine whether the patient has reached an objective?
16. How will the effectiveness of the treatment plan be evaluated?

The sequence of questions may vary, depending on the reasoning process of the therapist, and may change as additional information about the patient is revealed.

Analyzing the course of action through a process of planned and critical reasoning is essential in developing an effective treatment plan. The treatment plan affirms the therapist's competence and the professionalism of OT. It can provide a systematic method for gathering research data. It also helps the therapist document the purposes and effectiveness of OT services.

TREATMENT PLANNING PROCESS

The purpose of OT treatment planning is to identify problems and find solutions so as to promote health, well-being, and optimal functioning in persons who are ill or disabled. Treatment planning is a problem-solving process that follows a logical progression (Fig. 6-1).[4] Hopkins and Tiffany[4] described a problem-solving process and applied it to treatment planning. The steps are as follows:

1. Assess, analyze, and identify problems.
2. Explore prospective solutions and develop treatment goals and objectives.
3. Design and implement a plan of action—the treatment plan.
4. Assess the outcomes of the plan and modify it if necessary.
5. Terminate treatment when the objectives have been achieved or treatment is no longer feasible.[4]

Data Gathering

After the patient is referred for OT services, the therapist must gather data to develop an appropriate treatment plan. Sources for these data are the referral form; the medical record; social, educational, vocational, and play histories; interview of the patient or family and friends; and results of the OT evaluation and those of other services. The details of the evaluation process were outlined in Chapter 5.

Data Analysis and Problem Identification

After gathering the data, the therapist proceeds to data analysis and problem identification. Data are analyzed to identify problems in occupational performance and determine if OT can be employed to alleviate the problems.[10] From a careful analysis of all the data gathered,

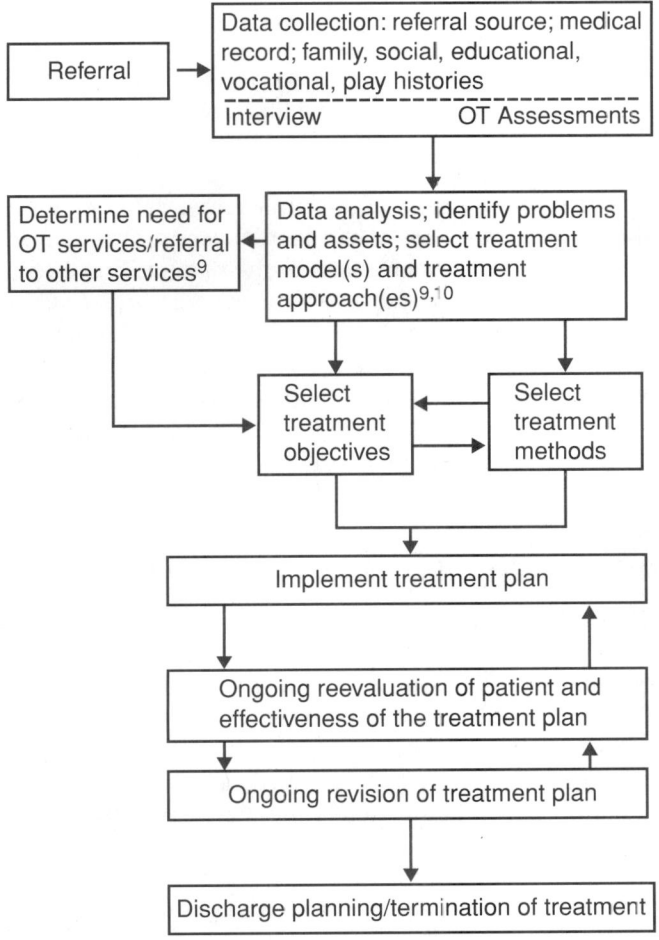

FIG. 6-1
Schematic of the treatment planning process.

support system and living environment that can be considered assets.

Selecting a Practice Model or Treatment Approach

A treatment plan should be based on one or more OT practice models or a specific treatment approach. The model or approach suggests which evaluation procedures, objectives, and methods will be most appropriate.[9,10] The practice model or approach also influences the problem-solving process, since each has its particular philosophy, body of knowledge, evaluation methods, and intervention strategies. However, there is some overlap among models. Each practice model guides the clinical reasoning process of treatment planning in particular ways.[4]

As an example of how the therapist selects a treatment approach and how the approach in turn affects the therapist's reasoning, consider the patient with a fractured arm resulting in limited joint motion and muscle weakness from disuse. For such a patient the therapist might select the biomechanical approach. Evaluation procedures in this approach focus on joint range of motion (ROM) measurement and muscle strength testing. Treatment might involve therapeutic exercise and activities. On the other hand, if the patient has hemiplegia, the therapist might choose the neurodevelopmental (Bobath) approach and evaluate muscle tone and postural mechanisms. Treatment is directed to normalizing tone through positioning, handling techniques, special movement patterns, and facilitating a more normal postural mechanism through activities that demand weight shifts and weight bearing. See Chapter 1 for a discussion of practice models and treatment approaches.

Selecting and Writing Treatment Goals and Objectives

Treatment goals and objectives are statements of what needs to happen or what is desirable to happen for the patient. They are written to address the problems identified in the OT evaluation. After the therapist gathers data and selects a practice model and one or more treatment approaches, some general kinds of intervention strategies that would facilitate the patient's rehabilitation may come to mind. For example, after the evaluation it may be apparent that the patient could benefit from training in activities of daily living (ADL). Having ideas for methods can facilitate the selection and writing of treatment objectives. Writing objectives and selecting treatment methods actually are concurrent and mutually dependent elements of the treatment planning process.

Goals
Goals are general statements that describe global or general changes in function at some time in the future.

the therapist develops a list of problems that forms the basis of the treatment plan. Deficits in the performance areas and performance components that may be amenable to OT intervention are noted. Limitations that require intervention by other professional services should be communicated through the appropriate referral process.

The therapist must also consider how **assets** in the patient and the patient's social and living environments can be used to enhance progress toward independence. Assets are the strengths in the patient's situation that can contribute to the achievement of treatment objectives. Good physical conditioning before disability, absence of concomitant medical problems, good psychological coping skills, a positive outlook, and determination are examples of personal assets. A supportive partner, family and friends, an accessible living environment, adequate financial resources for equipment or home modification, and good support services available in the patient's community are all factors in the patient's

For example, a goal might be: *The patient will be independent in self-care.* Since self-care encompasses many activities, it is not possible to achieve this goal without many specific subordinate objectives.

Objectives

Objectives are steps toward achieving goals. An example of an objective toward reaching the goal of self-care independence is: *The patient will transfer to and from the toilet without assistance.* The following narrative will focus on writing objectives.

A treatment objective is a statement of intent describing a proposed change in a patient. The statement clearly conveys the change in function, performance, or behavior that the patient will demonstrate when the treatment has been successfully completed. Whenever possible, the therapist should select objectives and plan the treatment program in conjunction with the patient. The therapist and patient select objectives that are attainable within the time frame of the treatment program. Treatment methods relevant to those objectives are also selected. Objectives should reflect the patient's needs and priorities and be consistent with both the general goals stated on the referral and those determined by the evaluation. The objectives should aim toward occupational performance within the context that is customary or expected for the individual patient. OT objectives should complement those of other rehabilitation services. Evaluation of progress examines the extent to which the selected objectives have been achieved.

Novice therapists may wonder whether it is really necessary to state such detailed objectives, especially when the course of treatment seems obvious. When clearly defined objectives have not been stated, there is no sound basis for selecting appropriate intervention strategies or for evaluating the effectiveness of the treatment program. It is important to state objectives to measure the degree to which the patient is able to perform in the desired manner.

Writing Treatment Objectives

The method for writing treatment objectives, described below, is based on models for writing competency-based educational objectives described by Mager and Kemp.[6,7]

A comprehensive objective conveys an idea of what the patient's performance will be like when the objective has been achieved. The idea conveyed is identical to the one the therapist and the patient have in mind. It succeeds in communicating their intent and describes the terminal behavior of the patient well enough to preclude misinterpretation. A comprehensive treatment objective has three elements.

TERMINAL BEHAVIOR. Terminal behavior represents the physical changes, kind of behavior, or performance skill that the patient is expected to display.[7]

The terminal behavior is composed of an action verb and the subject or object being acted upon. For example: "To remove the blouse." *Remove* is the action verb, and the *blouse* is the object of the action.

CONDITIONS. Conditions are the circumstances required for the performance of the terminal behavior. The conditions answer such questions as "Is special equipment necessary?" "Are assistive devices required?" "Are supervision, assistance, or verbal cues essential?" "Are special environmental arrangements needed?"[6,7] For example, the following condition might answer such a question: "If given verbal cues, the patient will remove the blouse." This indicates that the patient will be able to remove the blouse only when someone is present to provide verbal cues. This represents a special circumstance that enables adequate performance of the terminal behavior: *to remove the blouse.*

Patients can achieve many treatment objectives without any special devices, equipment, environmental modification, cues, or human assistance. Therefore, a statement of conditions is not necessary in many instances. It is an optional element of the objective and should be used only when some special circumstance is required to enable the performance of the terminal behavior. (Note that the intervention strategy and the time frame in which the treatment program is to take place are *not* conditions.)

CRITERION. The criterion is the performance standard or degree of competence the patient is expected to achieve, stated in measurable or observable terms.[6,7] The criterion answers such questions as "how much," "how often," "how well," "how accurately," "how completely," and "how quickly."[6] If it is possible to estimate the patient's potential level of competence, it is important to include a criterion or performance standard in the objective. This is the only way the therapist can determine the achievement of the stated terminal behavior with certainty. Like conditions, the criterion is an optional element in the treatment objective. Although stating a performance standard is desirable, it is not always necessary or possible.

Muscle grades, increases in range of motion (ROM), degree of competence in task performance, and speed of performance are some examples of criteria. Although stating the length of the treatment program in an objective is sometimes necessary to satisfy reimbursement agencies, length of treatment is *not* a criterion.

Sample Objectives

The following are some sample treatment objectives and an analysis of their elements:

1. *Given assistive devices, the patient will eat independently in 30 minutes.* In this objective, the terminal behavior is the statement, "the patient will eat."

Here, the object of the action verb *eat* does not need to be explicitly stated, since the consumption of food is implicit. The condition is *given assistive devices*. This statement indicates the special circumstances (the devices) that will make eating possible. The performance standards are *independently in 30 minutes*. This statement reflects that the patient will be able to eat without human assistance and will achieve eating of a meal within 30 minutes. Depending on the situation, this statement may require further refinement and specificity. For example, the kinds of devices and the kinds of foods could be specified.

2. *The ROM of the left elbow flexion will increase.* As written, this objective is a good statement of terminal behavior. It indicates the kind of change in physical function that is expected as a result of the treatment program. Conditions are not necessary, since no special circumstances are needed for the patient to demonstrate or perform the increased ROM. However, the objective does need a criterion because the amount of increase in ROM is not stated, making progress difficult to measure. The objective can be reworded like this: "The ROM of left elbow flexion will increase from 115° to 135° so that eating finger foods is possible." This adds the criteria of degrees of ROM to be increased and of an observable activity that uses full elbow flexion.

3. *The patient will operate the control systems of the left above-elbow prosthesis without hesitation while performing bilateral ADL.* In this objective, "operate the control systems" is the terminal behavior. "Operate" is the action verb, and "control systems" are the objects of the action. This is the skill (behavior) that is expected as a result of the prosthetic training program. Conditions are not necessary, because the desired goal is for the patient to be able to perform this skill under any circumstances. "Without hesitation" and "while performing bilateral ADL" are the criteria. The level of skill in performance is observable. Further refinement of this objective might indicate exactly which bilateral activities are to be performed, such as buttoning a shirt, cutting meat, or tying shoes.

4. *Given assistive devices, the patient will dress herself in 30 minutes or less.* "The patient will dress" is the terminal behavior. It is the action verb, and the implicit objects involved with the action are the patient's clothes. The availability of assistive devices is a necessary condition for this patient to perform this task, and so the statement of conditions, "given assistive devices," is needed. The criterion or performance standard is stated in terms of speed and indicates that dressing in 30 minutes is a reasonable expectation for this patient. Further refinement of this objective might include the kinds of clothing and the kinds of assistive devices, or standards of neatness, if these are important for the patient's situation and values.

5. *Given setup of mobile arm supports and assistive devices, the patient will feed himself independently.* The statement: "patient will feed himself" is the terminal behavior. The mobile arm supports and assistive devices and their setup constitute the conditions for this behavior. The criterion for performance under these conditions is "independently," which indicates that once the equipment and devices are provided and properly set up, the task of eating can be performed without further human assistance.

There are many variables and unknown factors in the performance and functions of persons with physical dysfunction. Therefore, the degree to which they can benefit from, participate in, or succeed at rehabilitation programs cannot be predicted with certainty. This sometimes makes it difficult for therapists to write comprehensive treatment objectives. However, the therapist should attempt to write such objectives, using past experience with similar patients and knowledge gained during the evaluation process to describe desired terminal behavior, conditions, and criteria for each treatment objective. If this is not possible, it is recommended that a specific statement of terminal behavior be used until applicable conditions and criteria become apparent. The stated terminal behaviors can then be modified to become comprehensive objectives as treatment progresses.

Selecting Intervention Strategies

When goals and objectives have been identified, the **intervention strategies** that can help patients achieve them are selected. This is probably one of the most difficult steps in the treatment planning process. It is based on the selected practice model(s) and the clinical reasoning of the therapist, in collaboration with the patient.

For example, with a patient who has muscle weakness, the biomechanical approach might be selected. The objective is increasing muscle strength. A graded therapeutic activity or exercise program would be the method of choice to reach this objective.

In OT practice, many factors influence the selection of intervention strategies. Some of those that should be considered are the following:

1. The patient's interests, psychosocial needs, and vocational goals[5]
2. The patient's physical and sociocultural environment
3. The roles the patient will assume on return to the community
4. The general goals (in terms of functional outcomes) for the patient

5. Activities or exercises that are useful and meaningful to the patient that can be used in the treatment program[5]
6. Precautions or contraindications that affect the OT program
7. The prognosis for physical and functional recovery
8. The results of the OT evaluation and those of other services
9. Other treatment the patient is receiving
10. The goals of treatment in other services, and how OT goals relate to these other goals
11. How much energy the patient expends in other therapies
12. The state of the patient's general health
13. Ways in which treatment can be graded to meet the patient's changing needs as progression or regression occurs
14. Special equipment or adaptations of therapeutic equipment needed for the patient to perform maximally

When intervention strategies are selected, it should be clear to others reading the treatment plan exactly how they will be used to reach specific objectives. Sometimes several methods may be needed to achieve one objective, or the same methods may be used to reach several objectives.

Implementing the Treatment Plan

When at least some objectives and treatment methods have been selected, the treatment plan is implemented. The patient engages in the procedures that have been designed to ameliorate problems and capitalize on assets (i.e., the patient's personal strengths and the positive aspects of the patient's physical, social, and living environment). A comprehensive treatment plan may evolve over a period of time. For example, while a protracted assessment (e.g., of ADL) is in progress, the patient may have begun a program of therapeutic activity to strengthen specific muscle groups. Therefore, as the assessment is being completed, new problems may be identified and additional objectives and methods may be added to the treatment plan.

Reevaluating the Patient and the Treatment Plan

Once the treatment plan is implemented, the therapist conducts an ongoing evaluation of its effectiveness through continuous observation and reevaluation. The therapist must be an alert observer and ask the following questions: (1) Are the objectives realistic and suitable to the patient's needs and capabilities? (2) Are the methods most appropriate for achieving the treatment objectives? (3) Does the patient relate to the treatment methods and see them as worthwhile and meaningful?

In addition to these observations, the therapist may use the same assessments that were used during the initial evaluation to reevaluate performance skills and performance components. Gains or losses may then be compared to evaluation data recorded at the outset. This validates the treatment plan and provides the objective evidence of change that is required for reimbursement.

Scrutinizing the treatment plan in this way will enable the therapist to modify the plan as the need arises. The criterion for determining the effectiveness of the plan is the progress of the patient toward the stated objectives.

Revising the Treatment Plan

The information gained from observations and reevaluation of the patient, as previously outlined, may necessitate some revision or modification of the initial treatment plan. For example, the patient's progress may be significant enough that it is beneficial to increase the duration, complexity, or resistance of the activity. Conversely, a gradual decline of physical function in degenerative diseases may necessitate a reduction in resistance, duration, and complexity of activity. This is a common adjustment in conditions for which maintenance of optimal function is the primary objective.

If the patient is unable to see the therapeutic program as helpful or meaningful, a change in treatment approaches and methods may be necessary. On the other hand, if the patient is highly motivated, the plan can sometimes be accelerated. The initial plan is continually revised according to the patient's needs and progress. This process of reevaluation, revision, and reimplementation of the treatment plan goes on throughout the course of the therapeutic program.[9,10]

Discharge Planning and Terminating Treatment

Ultimately, the whole treatment program is directed to preparing the patient to return home or to another suitable living arrangement. Discharge planning actually occurs throughout the treatment program. All treatment is directed to preparing the patient to return to the community. Often therapy will continue on a less intensive basis at home or in another living environment.

Discharge Planning

As the treatment program in the primary health care facility is progressing, **discharge planning** should be initiated. This is a team effort that involves the patient, the family, and all rehabilitation specialists concerned with the patient's care. Preparation for discharge includes considering medical conditions, providing assistive devices and mobility equipment, planning a home activity or exercise program, and making a home visit to assess architectural barriers in the environment. Discharge planning should include patient education and education and training of caregivers for a smooth transition. Arrangement for home care therapies and referral to appropriate community agencies is another important aspect of discharge planning.[11]

The psychological preparation of the patient and family members is essential. They may not be emotionally prepared for or functionally capable of managing the transition to the new environment. Generalizing learning from the health care facility to the home may be difficult for the patient. The family may not know the patient's capabilities or how best to give assistance. Providing emotional support, education, training, counseling, and information about resources to the patient and the family is helpful in easing the transition. The family needs information about the following:

- The patient's ADL status and performance expectations
- Solutions to accessibility problems in the home, workplace, and community
- Information on home modification
- How to obtain, use, and care for assistive devices or mobility equipment

- Community resources such as emergency care, self-help groups, respite care, and independent living centers[12]

Maintaining contact with the primary care facility as a resource for information or further treatment can be reassuring and helpful.[1]

Terminating Treatment

Termination of treatment involves a final evaluation of the patient. The clinician should clearly indicate objectives achieved, partially achieved, or not achieved in the treatment program. The discharge summary is written on the basis of these data and indicates the expected future performance of the patient. Termination can affirm the success of the treatment program. In reality, however, termination is not always achieved. Patients may be discharged before objectives of treatment are met and treatment is concluded.[4] The patient may be referred to another facility or to home care where another therapist assumes the continuity of the treatment program. Careful communication between therapists and agencies is necessary to ensure a smooth transition and continuity of care (see Chapter 4 for more information on this point).

TREATMENT PLAN MODEL

Case _____

PERSONAL DATA

Name _____ Age _____

Diagnosis _____ Disability _____

Treatment goals stated in the referral _____

PRACTICE MODEL(S)/TREATMENT APPROACH(ES)

O.T. Evaluation
Occupational performance
Performance areas
  1. Activities of daily living
  2. Work and productive activities
  3. Play or leisure activities
Performance contexts
  1. Physical aspects
  2. Temporal aspects
  3. Sociocultural aspects
Performance components
  1. Sensorimotor
  2. Cognitive integration and cognitive
  3. Psychosocial skills and psychological

Evaluation Summary
Problem List
Assets
Treatment Plan Outline
  1. Problem
  2. Objective
  3. Methods
  4. Grading

FIG. 6-2
Treatment plan model.

SUMMARY

A treatment plan is a proposal for the therapeutic program. It is based on the client's priorities and problems identified in the OT initial evaluation. Written treatment plans are important for describing the treatment program to others, measuring progress objectively, and analyzing and reevaluating the course of action. The treatment plan documents the effectiveness of OT services.

Treatment planning follows a systematic process. After the initial OT evaluation the occupational therapist identifies problems, explores and identifies potential solutions, selects goals and objectives, chooses treatment strategies, and assesses the outcomes of the plan. Preparation for termination of treatment is an ongoing process in the treatment plan.

TREATMENT PLAN MODEL

The treatment plan model is useful for teaching and learning treatment planning during academic preparation. It may be modified for clinical use (Fig. 6-2). The student is presented with a hypothetical case study or an actual patient and is directed to complete the treatment plan, using the *Treatment Planning Guide* shown in Box 6-1. If given a hypothetical (rather than actual) patient, the student is directed to complete the "Evaluation Summary" section of the treatment plan according to knowledge of the particular diagnosis and its resultant disability. See the Appendix on p.1021 for additional case studies that can be used for treatment planning practice. A sample treatment plan developed according to this model follows below.

BOX 6-1   TREATMENT PLANNING GUIDE

The treatment planning guide is a reference for filling out a treatment plan for either an actual or a hypothetical patient.

PERSONAL DATA

Fill in the requested information from the medical record or case study.

Name_____

Age_____

Diagnosis _____

Disability_____

Treatment aims stated in the referral _____

PRACTICE MODEL AND APPROACH

State the practice model or treatment approach on which the treatment plan is based. More than one may be necessary.

OT EVALUATION

From the list below, select the performance areas and performance components that should be evaluated.

Performance Areas

Self-care
- ❏ Feeding
- ❏ Dressing
- ❏ Hygiene
- ❏ Transferring
- ❏ Community mobility

Work and productive activities
- ❏ Work habits and attitudes
- ❏ Potential work skills
- ❏ Work tolerance
- ❏ Home management
- ❏ Child care

Play and leisure
- ❏ Past and present leisure interests and play activities
- ❏ Modes of relaxation

Performance Components

Sensorimotor
- ❏ Muscle strength
- ❏ Range of motion

- ❏ Physical endurance
- ❏ Standing tolerance
- ❏ Walking tolerance
- ❏ Sitting balance
- ❏ Involuntary movement
- ❏ Movement speed
- ❏ Level of motor development
- ❏ Equilibrium and protective responses
- ❏ Coordination and muscle control
- ❏ Spasms
- ❏ Spasticity
- ❏ State of motor recovery (stroke patient only)
- ❏ Postural reflex mechanism
- ❏ Functional movement patterns
- ❏ Hand function
- ❏ Swallowing and cranial nerve functions
- ❏ Sensation—touch, pain, temperature, proprioception, taste, smell
- ❏ Body schema
- ❏ Motor planning

Continued

BOX 6-1   TREATMENT PLANNING GUIDE—cont'd

- ❑ Stereognosis
- ❑ Visual perception
  - ❑ Visual fields
  - ❑ Spatial relations
  - ❑ Position in space
  - ❑ Figure/background
  - ❑ Perceptual constancy
  - ❑ Visual-motor coordination
  - ❑ Depth perception
  - ❑ Perception of vertical/horizontal elements
  - ❑ Eye movements
- ❑ Functional auditory perception

Cognitive/cognitive integration
- ❑ Memory
- ❑ Judgment
- ❑ Safety awareness
- ❑ Problem-solving ability
- ❑ Motivation
- ❑ Sequencing
- ❑ Rigidity
- ❑ Abstract thinking
- ❑ Functional language skills
  - ❑ Comprehension of speech/writing
  - ❑ Ability to express ideas
  - ❑ Reading
  - ❑ Writing
- ❑ Functional mathematical skills
  - ❑ Mental calculations
  - ❑ Written calculations

Psychosocial/psychological skills
- ❑ Self-identity
- ❑ Self-concept
- ❑ Coping skills
- ❑ Maturity (development level)
- ❑ Adjustment to disability
- ❑ Reality functioning
- ❑ Interpersonal skills—dyadic and group interactions

EVALUATION SUMMARY
Summarize findings from assessments.

PROBLEM LIST
Identify and list the problems that require occupational therapy intervention.

ASSETS
List the assets of the patient and his or her situation that can be used to enhance progress toward maximum independence.

OBJECTIVES
Write specific treatment objectives in comprehensive form. Each should relate to a specific problem in the problem list and be identified by the corresponding number.

METHODS OF TREATMENT
Describe in detail appropriate treatment methods for the patient.

GRADATION OF TREATMENT
Briefly state how treatment methods will be graded to enhance the patient's progress.

BOX 6-2   SAMPLE TREATMENT PLAN

CASE STUDY
Mrs. R. is 49 years old. She has two sons. One is 26 years old and married, and the other is 17. Mrs. R. is divorced. She and her younger son live with her married son, his wife, and their 4-year-old boy. Before the onset of her illness, Mrs. R. lived in an apartment with her younger son.

Mrs. R. had Guillain-Barré syndrome six months ago. She has been left with residual weakness of all four extremities. Some additional gains in strength are anticipated, but full recovery is not expected. Mrs. R. uses a standard wheelchair for mobility.

Mrs. R. appears thin and frail. She speaks in a weak voice and appears to be passive and discouraged. She feels she cannot accomplish anything. Mrs. R. does not communicate with her daughter-in-law, and there are conflicts between the couple and Mrs. R. concerning the management of the teenage son. Mrs. R. feels unable to assert her authority as his mother or to express her needs and feelings. The disability has brought about the loss of her independence and has changed her role in relation to her younger son.

Her daughter-in-law reported that Mrs. R. is dependent for self-care, never attempts to help with homemaking, and isolates herself in her room much of the time. She believes that her mother-in-law

is capable of more activity "if only she would try." She says she is willing to allow Mrs. R. to do some of the household work.

Mrs. R. was referred for OT services as an outpatient for restoration or maintenance of motor functioning and increased independence in ADL and home management.

TREATMENT PLAN
Personal Data
Name: Mrs. R.
Age: 49
Diagnosis: Guillain-Barré syndrome
Disability: Residual weakness, upper and lower extremities
Treatment aims stated in referral: Restoration or maintenance of motor functioning and increased independence in ADL, home management, and leisure activities.
Practice Models
Biomechanical, rehabilitative
OT Assessments
Performance Areas
Self-care
Home management
Leisure skills

BOX 6-2   SAMPLE TREATMENT PLAN—cont'd

Performance Contexts
Physical aspects
Temporal aspects
Sociocultural aspects
Performance Components
Sensorimotor
Muscle strength
Active and passive ROM
Physical endurance
Movement speed
Coordination
Functional movement
Sensation (touch, pain, thermal, proprioception)
Cognitive/Cognitive Integrative
Judgment
Safety awareness
Motivation
Psychosocial/psychological skills
Coping skills
Adjustment to disability
Social skills
Interpersonal relationships

EVALUATION SUMMARY
Performance Areas
ADL: Mrs. R. manages some personal care such as washing her face, hair care, and tooth care. She needs some assistance with dressing and has difficulty with buttons and zippers. She requires an adaptive toothbrush and needs assistance in toilet transferring and showering.

Work and Productive Activities: Mrs. R. does not perform any home management tasks but is potentially capable of light activities such as table setting, dusting, and folding clothes. Mrs. R.'s daughter-in-law is willing to allow her mother-in-law some household activities if understanding about their respective roles can be established.

Leisure Skills: Mrs. R. spends a lot of time alone in her room. Her activities are limited to reading and watching television. Before the onset of her disability she liked visiting friends, shopping, and tending planter boxes on her outdoor patio.

Performance Contexts
Physical aspects: The home is a one-level spacious ranch-style house. There are two steps up to the entry. Mrs. R.'s son has built a ramp next to the steps for wheelchair access. Mrs. R.'s bedroom is at the rear of the home and looks out on the backyard garden. Her bedroom is large enough to accommodate the wheelchair, and there is a rear exit at the end of the hallway, a short distance from her bedroom. The bedroom was previously used as a guest room and sewing room by Mrs. R.'s daughter-in-law. The bathroom is next to Mrs. R.'s bedroom and is wheelchair accessible. It has a tub and shower combination that is enclosed by a shower curtain.

Temporal aspects: Mrs. R. has been divorced for 9 years. She has had a few relationships since her divorce, but none was serious. Mrs. R. had planned to support her son until the time he went to work or college. She looked forward to increased independence and more involvement with her leisure activities and community charitable organizations. Mrs. R. tended to have

periods of mild depression before her illness but otherwise seemed well adjusted.

Sociocultural aspects: Mrs. R. is from a large Italian Catholic family. Her parents were first-generation Americans and retained many of the cultural practices of the "old country." Mrs. R. enjoyed cooking special ethnic foods such as pasta dishes and Italian desserts. Her participation in church was mainly at holidays. She was not a member of a particular parish and did not belong to any church organizations. Since the onset of her disability, Mrs. R. has not done any cooking, nor has she attended church on holidays. She has avoided family gatherings.

Performance Components
Sensorimotor
Physical Endurance: Mrs. R.'s physical endurance is limited to 1 hour of light upper-extremity activity before she needs a rest. She uses a wheelchair for energy conservation and propels it using both arms and legs.

Coordination: Slight incoordination is evident during fine hand activities such as buttoning, applying makeup, or using eating utensils.

Strength/ROM: Muscle testing revealed that all muscles are the same grades bilaterally: scapula and shoulder muscles are F+ to G (3+ to 4); elbow and forearm muscles are F+ to G (3+ to 4); wrist and hand musculature is graded F+ (3+). Trunk muscles are G (4); all muscles of the hip are G (4), except adductors and external rotators, which are F+ (3+). Knee flexors and extensors are G (4). Ankle plantar flexors and dorsiflexors are F (3), and all foot muscles are F− (3−) to P (2). PROM of all joint motions is within normal limits.

Sensation: Sensory modalities of touch, pain, temperature, and proprioception are intact

Cognitive/Cognitive Integrative
No cognitive deficits were observed.

Psychosocial Skills/Psychological
Mrs. R. seems discouraged about her disability. She feels she cannot accomplish anything and tends to stay in her room alone. The living arrangement is less than ideal. There are communication problems and conflicts about the supervision of the teenage son. The disability has brought about the loss of Mrs. R.'s independence and has changed her roles as homemaker and mother. She feels unable to assert her authority as mother of her 17-year-old or to express her needs and feelings

PROBLEMS
1. Self-care dependence
2. Homemaking dependence
3. Dependent transferring
4. Isolation, apparent depression
5. Reduced social interaction
6. Muscle weakness
7. Low physical endurance
8. Mild incoordination

ASSETS
Potential for good living situation
Presence of able-bodied adults who can assist
Potential for some further sensorimotor recovery

Continued

BOX 6-2   *SAMPLE TREATMENT PLAN—cont'd*

Good sensation
Some functional muscle strength
Good joint mobility

Intervention Strategies

PROBLEM 1

Self-care dependence

Objective

Given assistive devices, Mrs. R. will be able to dress herself independently within 20 minutes.

Method

Putting on bra: using a back-opening stretch bra, pass bra around waist so that opening is in front and straps are facing up; fasten bra in front at waist level; slide fastened bra around at waist level so that cups are in front; slip arms through straps and work straps up over shoulders; adjust cups and straps. *Putting on shirt*: place loose-fitting blouse on lap with back facing up and neck toward knees; place arms under back of blouse and into arm holes; push sleeves up onto arms past elbows; gather back material up from neck to hem with hands and duck head forward and pass garment over head; work blouse down by shrugging shoulders and pulling into place with hands; use button hook to fasten front opening. *Putting on underpants and slacks*: sitting on bed or in wheelchair, cross legs, reach down, and place one opening over foot; cross opposite leg, place other opening over foot; uncross legs, work pants up over feet and up under thighs (a dressing stick may be used to pull pants up if leaning forward is difficult); shift hips from side to side and work pants up as far as possible over buttocks; stand, if possible, and pull pants to waist level, then sit and pull zipper up with pre-fastened zipper pull; use Velcro at waist closure on slacks. *Putting on socks*: seated and using stretch socks, cross one leg, place sock over toes, and work sock up onto foot and over heel; cross other leg and repeat. *Putting on shoes*: using slip-on shoe with Velcro fasteners, use procedure for socks.

Gradation

Progress to more difficult tasks such as pantyhose, tie shoes, dresses, pullover garments.

PROBLEM 2

Homemaking dependence

Objective

Given assistive devices, Mrs. R. will perform light homemaking activities.

Methods

Using a dust mitt, patient dusts furniture surfaces easily reached from wheelchair, such as lamp tables and coffee table; sits at sink to wash dishes; practices folding small items of clothing such as panties, nylons, and children's underwear while sitting at kitchen table; have Mrs. R.'s daughter-in-law observe activities at treatment facility; work out an acceptable list of activities and a schedule with both women. Discuss how Mrs. R. could make some contributions to home management routines; ask Mrs. R. to keep activity diary, noting any performance difficulties and successes for review at next visit.

Gradation

Increase number of household responsibilities. Increase time spent on household activities.

PROBLEMS 4, 5

Isolation, depression, reduced social interaction

Objective

Mrs. R. will reduce time spent alone from 6 waking hours to 3 waking hours.

Method

Establish an acceptable graded activity schedule between Mrs. R. and son and daughter-in-law; include homemaking tasks and socialization with family through playing games, watching TV, preparing and eating meals, and conversing; family members encourage Mrs. R. to be with them but to be accepting if she refuses; have Mrs. R. keep activities diary for review; determine how time is spent and discuss how it could be more productive and enjoyable. Initiate leisure activity, such as tending potted house plants; arrange with the family to have one of Mrs. R.'s friends come to visit.

Gradation

Increase time spent out of own room; include friends, neighbors, and family in household social activities; plan a community outing for shopping or lunch; include outdoor gardening such as tending herbs in raised containers.

PROBLEM 6

Muscle weakness

Objective

Muscle strength of shoulder flexors will increase from F+ (3+) to G (4).

Method

1. *Activities*: reaching for glasses in overhead cupboard and placing them on the table, replacing glasses in cupboard when dry; rolling out pastry dough on a slightly inclined pastry board; wiping table, counter, and cupboard doors, using a forward push-pull motion; Turkish knotting project with weaving frame set vertically in front of her and tufts of yarn on right and left sides, at hip level.

2. Light progressive resistive exercise to shoulder flexion: patient is seated in a regular chair, wearing a weighted cuff above each elbow that is one half the weight of her maximum resistance. Lifts arms alternately through 10 repetitions and then rests. Repeated using three quarters maximum resistance, then full resistance.

Gradation

Increase activities, resistance, number of repetitions, and length of time as strength improves.

PROBLEM 6

Muscle weakness

Objective

Strength of wrist flexors and extensors and finger flexors will increase from F+ (3+) to G (4).

Method

1. *Activities to improve finger flexors*: tearing lettuce to make a salad; hand washing panties and hosiery. Progress to kneading soft clay or bread dough.

2. *Light, progressive resistive exercises for wrist flexors and extensors*: patient is seated, side to table, with pronated forearm resting on the table and hand extended over edge of table; a hand cuff, with small weights equal to one half of her maximum resistance

BOX 6-2   SAMPLE TREATMENT PLAN—cont'd

attached to the palmar surface, is worn on the hand; patient extends the wrist through full range of motion against gravity for 10 repetitions, then rests. Exercise is repeated, using three quarters maximum resistance and then full resistance. The same procedure is used to exercise wrist flexors, except that the forearm is supinated on the table, and the weights are suspended from the dorsal side of the hand cuff

Gradation

Increase hand activities, resistance, repetitions, and time.

REVIEW QUESTIONS

1. Define *treatment plan*.
2. Why write a treatment plan?
3. Why base the treatment plan on a specific practice model or approach?
4. List the steps in developing a treatment plan.
5. List, define, and give examples of the three elements of a comprehensive treatment objective.
6. If a comprehensive objective cannot be written, which one element would be *most* important to identify first?
7. List six factors to consider when selecting treatment methods.
8. Is it necessary to develop a complete comprehensive treatment plan before treatment can begin?
9. Why might it be necessary to change the initial treatment plan?
10. What is the criterion that is used to evaluate the effectiveness of a treatment plan?
11. How does the therapist know when to modify or change the plan?
12. What are some of the concerns and preparations for termination of treatment?

REFERENCES

1. Baum C: Identification and use of environmental resources. In Christiansen C, Baum C: *Occupational therapy, overcoming human performance deficits*, Thorofare, NJ, 1991, Slack.
2. Christiansen C: Occupational therapy: intervention for life performance. In Christiansen C, Baum C: *Occupational therapy, overcoming human performance deficits*, Thorofare, NJ, 1991, Slack.
3. Day D: A systems diagram for teaching treatment planning, *Am J Occup Ther* 27:239, 1973.
4. Hopkins HL, Tiffany EG: Occupational therapy—a problem solving process. In Hopkins HL, Smith HD: *Willard & Spackman's occupational therapy*, ed 8, Philadelphia, 1993, JB Lippincott.
5. Hopkins HL et al: Therapeutic application of activity. In *Willard & Spackman's occupational therapy*, ed 6, Philadelphia, 1983, JB Lippincott.
6. Kemp JE: *The instructional design process*, New York, 1985, Harper & Row.
7. Mager RF: *Preparing instructional objectives*, ed 2 (rev), Belmont, Calif, 1984, David S. Lake.
8. Neistadt ME: Overview of treatment. In Neistadt ME, Crepeau EB: *Willard & Spackman's occupational therapy*, ed 9, Philadelphia, 1998, JB Lippincott.
9. Pelland MJ: A conceptual model for the instruction and supervision of treatment planning, *Am J Occup Ther* 41:351, 1987.
10. Smith HD: Assessment and evaluation: an overview. In Hopkins HL, Smith HD, editors: *Willard & Spackman's occupational therapy*, ed 8, Philadelphia, 1993, JB Lippincott.
11. Spencer EA: Functional restoration: preliminary concepts and planning. In Hopkins HL, Smith HD, editors: *Willard & Spackman's occupational therapy*, ed 8, Philadelphia, 1993, JB Lippincott.
12. Versluys HP: Family influences. In Hopkins HL, Smith HD: *Willard & Spackman's occupational therapy*, ed 8, Philadelphia, 1993, JB Lippincott.

CHAPTER 7

A Model of Evidence-Based Practice for Occupational Therapy

ELIZABETH DEPOY
LYNN GITLOW

KEY TERMS

Scientific inquiry
Evidence-based practice
Thinking processes
Action processes
Inductive reasoning
Deductive reasoning
Statement of problem
Problem mapping
Need statement
Goal
Objective
Process objective
Outcome objective
Specificity

LEARNING OBJECTIVES

After studying this chapter the student or practitioner will be able to do the following:

1. Articulate the need for evidence-based practice.
2. List in sequence the steps of evidence-based practice and detail the content and process of each step.
3. Distinguish between problem statements and need statements.
4. Analyze and map problems.
5. Identify needs based on empirical evidence.
6. Translate need statements into goals and objectives.
7. Distinguish between process objectives and outcome objectives.
8. Develop interventions based on goals and objectives.
9. Articulate process and outcome success criteria based on goals and objectives.
10. Specify evidence that will be used to investigate success criteria.
11. Develop and execute sound plans to assess objective achievement.
12. Based on assessment, determine the extent to which the needs were met and the problem was resolved.

The importance of empirical analysis and identification of the problems and needs that occupational therapy (OT) practitioners address has been emphasized at local and national levels over the past two decades. Educators, scholars, and practitioners increasingly discuss and encourage the use of theoretically grounded and supported OT interventions and the development of solid evidence of successful outcome of practice. Current evidence-based OT practice is needed at multiple levels (individual, group, community, agency, and government) if OT is to be a viable and valued profession that will flourish in the competitive environment of managed care and fiscal scarcity. Evidence-based practice involves the integration of **scientific inquiry** into all domains of OT practice. This chapter provides a framework through which readers may understand and learn the systematic, research-based thinking and action processes necessary to conduct all or part of the sequence of evidence-based practice.[6] The chapter begins with identification and clarification of the problems that OT addresses and proceeds with intervention development, culminating in outcomes assessment.

WHAT IS EVIDENCE-BASED PRACTICE AND WHY IS IT NEEDED?

Evidence-based practice is defined as "the integration of critical, analytic, scientific thinking and action processes throughout all phases and domains of OT practice." Let us look at this definition more closely. First, we distinguish thought and action from each other. In systematic inquiry, it is essential for the thinking sequence and rationale to be presented clearly. **Thinking processes** are composed of the reasoning sequence and logic that OT practitioners use to conceptualize treatment and specify desired outcomes. Thinking processes involve the selection of a theoretical framework in which the OT practitioner plans the steps necessary to assess problems, evaluate treatment, specify desired outcomes, and plan a research strategy to determine and systematically demonstrate the degree to which outcomes were met for an individual receiving OT services. Sometimes we are not fully aware of our thought processes, but they are there nonetheless and are the foundation of evidence-based practice, as we will see later in this chapter.

Action processes are the specific behaviors involved in implementing thinking processes.[6] Action processes are behavioral steps. In evidence-based practice, these steps are founded on scientific inquiry such that any claim is supported with empirically derived information.

Evidence-based practice is not a new phenomenon in OT practice. Rather, it is an approach to practice that is informed by systematic thinking, action, and assessment. Although evidence-based practice is not research in itself, it is the application of research thinking and action to the conceptualization, enactment, and investigation of the process and outcome of intervention. "An evidence-based OT practice uses research evidence together with clinical knowledge and reasoning to make decisions about interventions that are effective for a specific client(s)."[12]

What is meant by *evidence?* This question is not easily answered. Synonyms for evidence include terms such as *documentation, indication, sign, proof, authentication,* and *confirmation.* In this chapter, we will define *evidence* as *information that is used to support a claim.* In this case, the claim is that OT interventions are beneficial. What information would be acceptable to us as evidence to support the claim about OT interventions? In the professional world, belief is insufficient. We must look at information that is obtained or developed through systematic inquiry.

The model we propose in this chapter builds upon basic professional knowledge and skills to guide the reader through each of the steps of evidence-based practice. At this point, the reader may be asking why evidence-based practice is even needed. Let us briefly turn to this point before going on with the model.

The emphasis on documenting the value of OT intervention is not new. Our professional organizations have been concerned for a long time with promoting the development of educational programs and methods to ensure that practitioners have the skills and knowledge to document the value of their interventions. For example, in 1965 the American Occupational Therapy Foundation (AOTF) was established. The Foundation's purpose in supporting research was to document the potency of occupation in restoring, maintaining, and enhancing health.[2] In 1998, the American Occupational Therapy Association (AOTA) Representative Assembly approved a document titled *Research Competencies for Occupational Therapy.* These competency guidelines provide the support educators need to emphasize the inclusion of basic research skills at all levels of education. Incorporation of basic research competence in all OT curricula provides a foundation for every practitioner to appreciate and participate in evidence-based practice.[1] In 1999, the AOTA and AOTF committed $300,000 to develop the Center for Outcomes Research and Education (CORE), which will focus its research on new developments in outcomes measurement.[2]

Increasingly, cost containment drives service delivery. Thus empirical evidence of the cost effectiveness, quality, processes, and outcome of OT services has become essential for the survival of the profession in current and future health care markets.[3] Practitioners must be conversant with and capable of evidence-based practice if they are to demonstrate the efficacy of OT to multiple audiences, both internal and external to the profession.

Within the profession, OT practitioners use the information obtained from evidence-based practice not only to improve the processes and outcomes of their practices, but also to engage in informed thinking when choosing among possible interventions. A recent study of practitioners' perceptions of evidence-based practice suggests that OT practitioners view scientific literature as a valuable resource when supporting the effectiveness of OT interventions in conversations with persons other than clients. However, for informing intervention choice, practitioners tended to consult and depend on trusted personal sources.[7] Evidence-based practice systematically guides practitioners in determining which interventions are effective to produce desired outcomes, which interventions need to be improved, and what kinds of new knowledge need development. Additionally, having credible evidence to demonstrate that the interventions OT practitioners use produce desirable outcomes provides concrete feedback to the consumer.[11,15] Finally, by systematically evaluating new interventions, OT practitioners can provide evidence for advancing new clinical practices in the profession.

Pressures and demands on health practitioners from external sources render evidence-based practice even more critical for three reasons. First, the location of service delivery and the time allowed for service delivery are in flux. Long-term hospital stays and treatments in acute care settings are being replaced by community-based treatment,[4] and the length of time for delivery of treatment is shortening as third-party payers demand more efficient and cost-effective health care. Evidence-based practice guides the practitioner in choosing the most cost-effective intervention without sacrificing quality in a fiscally driven health care environment. Second, by systematically examining the processes and outcomes of current practice, OT practitioners can provide an evidentiary basis for clinical thinking and action, which then can be presented to consumers, other professionals, insurers, and policy makers. Third, systematic inquiry transcends professional boundaries. Therefore evidence-based practice provides a basis for discussion with other members of the health care team. It is no secret that OT practitioners have always had difficulty in clearly describing what they do to those outside the profession. Moreover, OT practitioners have typically placed more emphasis on providing direct services than on publishing studies that document the results or that attribute successful outcomes to OT intervention. In today's increasingly complex and competitive health care environment, OT practitioners must clearly demonstrate their contribution to achieving clinical outcomes. It is particularly critical to do this if referral sources are to understand the benefits of OT to diverse client groups.[9]

As we proceed through the model of evidence-based practice, we will draw your attention to the skills and knowledge you already possess that are relevant to this conceptual approach. Let us now turn to the philosophical foundation and steps of the model.

Theoretical and Logical Foundations of Evidence-Based Practice

Evidence-based practice is grounded in logic and the systematic thinking that undergirds all research thinking processes. Inductive and deductive reasoning form the basis for these thinking processes. Moreover, the two major research design traditions, naturalistic and experimental-type inquiry, are based on these logic structures.[6] Therefore OT practitioners must understand them and use them to guide thinking and action and to support claims regarding the outcomes of OT intervention.

Inductive reasoning is a thinking process whereby one begins with seemingly unrelated data and links these data together by discovering relationships and principles within the data set. Inductive reasoning leads us to select naturalistic strategies, those in which theory is derived from gathered evidence rather than tested by scientific experimentation. Among the methods used in naturalistic design are interview, observation, and textual analysis.[6] Data are collected and themes that emerge from repeated examination of the data are named, defined, and placed in a theoretical context.

Deductive reasoning begins with a theory and reduces the theory to its parts, which are then verified or discounted through examination. Deductive reasoning provides the foundation for experimental-type research, in which theories or parts are stated in measurable terms and objective measurement forms the basis of all inquiry. Strategies used in deductive traditions include sampling, measurement, and statistical analysis. Because the rules of logic guide thinking, one can easily follow thinking processes and identify the basis on which guesses, claims, decisions, and pronouncements are made and verified.

Complementarity With Contemporary Practice Models

Although it may seem difficult at first to engage in the formal, logical thinking processes that undergird research, we do it every day. Let us look at how the decision-making skills we use in OT practice mirror the logical thinking processes that form the foundation of evidence-based practice. Box 7-1 presents the steps of evidence-based practice, and Table 7-1 illustrates the relationship between clinical decision-making and evidence-based thinking processes.

BOX 7-1
Framework of Steps in Evidence-Based Practice

- Identification and clarification of the problem to be addressed by the intervention
- Understanding of need—what is needed to resolve all or part of the problem?
- Goals and objectives to address the need
- Intervention to achieve the goals and objectives
- Process and outcome assessment to examine success of an intervention.

TABLE 7-1
Relationship Between Clinical Reasoning and Evidence-Based Practice

Clinical Decision Making	Evidence-Based Practice
Referral to OT	Problem definition
Evaluation and assessment of patient or client (OT diagnosis)	Need statement
Process and outcome objectives	Goals and objectives
OT intervention	Intervention
Reassessment of process and outcomes	Empirical assessment

Sequence of Evidence-Based Practice
Our model of evidence-based practice has five steps, as listed in Box 7-1. The process begins with a conceptualization of the problem to be addressed. This leads to the question, "What exactly is a problem?"

Statement of the Problem
Although we often see problems as entities existing outside ourselves, problems are contextually embedded in personal and cultural values. A **statement of the problem** is a statement of value, a statement of what is not desired or of what should be improved. Although it seems simple to specify a problem, we often see problems stated in terms of a preferred solution; this limits our options in analyzing problem components and solutions. Moreover, in evidence-based practice, problem statements must be derived from credible, systematically generated knowledge, including scholarly literature and inquiry. The following case serves as an example:

Jennifer is an OT who has just evaluated a client with carpal tunnel syndrome. Jennifer specifies the client's problem as "limited hand strength." This problem statement suggests only one solution—to increase hand strength. By systematic inquiry, Jennifer can expand her analysis of the problem to "limited hand strength does not allow the client to participate in work or self-care activity," which allows her to generate additional potential solutions. For example, the client may take the following measures: look for alternative work, increase hand strength, work with adaptive equipment, adapt the environment, and so forth. By expanding a problem statement, the OT practitioner moves beyond the obvious primary difficulty and its solution and can capture the breadth of focus of the problem as revealed by systematically derived evidence from literature, the client, or others.[12] If the client did not want to work on hand strength, but saw the solution as seeking alternative employment, the therapist would have missed the essence of the client's problem and thus would have selected inappropriate interventions and outcomes. Thus it is critical to include the client and other sources of knowledge beyond practitioner guessing in formulating the problem statement.

There are many ways to identify problems. **Problem mapping** is a method in which one expands a problem statement beyond its initial conceptualization by asking two questions repeatedly: (1) What caused the problem? and (2) What are the consequences of the problem? Let us apply the problem mapping method to the statement, "Jane has limited short-term memory." To conduct problem mapping, we first need to conceptualize the problem as a river. Making the original statement of the problem is analogous to stepping into the river and picking up one rock. As we look upstream, we see causes of the problem, and as we look downstream, we see the problem's consequences. How does this work? See Fig. 7-1 to look at the problem map. Each box above the initial problem contains a possible answer to the question of what caused the problem. Once we determine first-level causes of the problem, we ask, "What caused the cause of the problem?" and so on, until we reach cultural and social value statements. Keep in mind that the knowledge that is used to identify causes and consequences must be generated from credible, research-based sources such as empirical studies and well-tested theory.[8]

Below the initial problem statement, we repeatedly ask the question, "What is the consequence of the problem?" As with the upstream map, this question about the consequences of consequences is repeated until we reach the effect of the problem on ourselves. Thus the problem map expands the problem statement from documented cultural, social, and environmental causes to personal effect and suggests many different sites or targets for intervention. The problem map is a valuable tool that can help broaden the scope of OT intervention systematically beyond the level of the individual.

As you might imagine from this example of Jane, many causes and consequences of problems cannot be resolved by OT intervention. While many OT practitioners will likely expand their efforts into political action or other areas at some point in their careers, others will

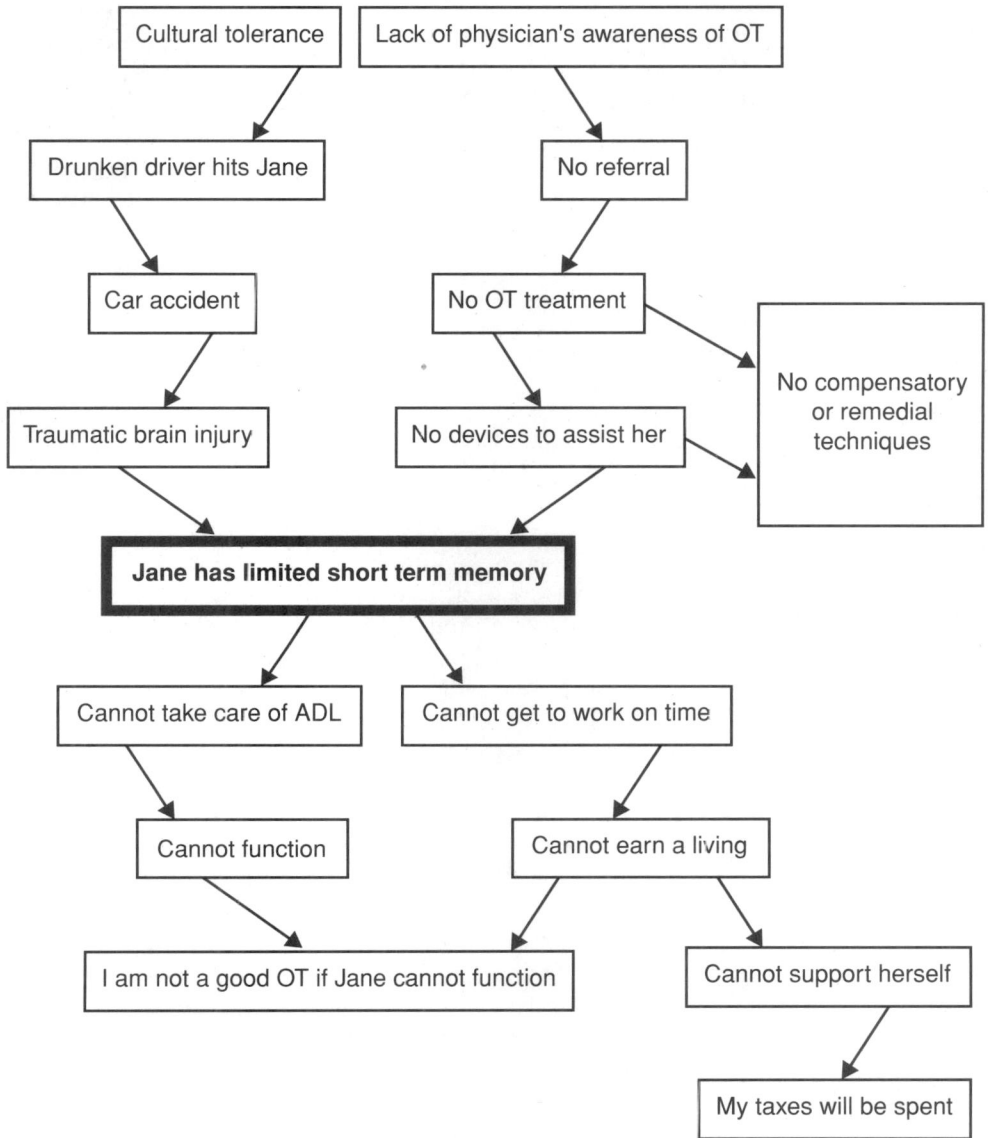

FIG. 7-1
Problem map.

look for clinical interventions that can improve the functional independence of individuals. Jane's problem map suggests numerous points of intervention for clinical OT in cognitive remediation, compensatory training, and provision of assistive devices and services such as assistive technology (AT). Two theory- and knowledge-based performance areas on which the OT practitioner might focus intervention are (1) for Jane to work on self-care and (2) to address strategies that will enable Jane to arrive at work on time. The OT practitioner could also make a referral to a social service agency for Jane, who might be eligible for Social Security disability income; thus the OT practitioner would intervene at the level of Jane's inability to support herself financially. In addition, as we look at the expanded problem, the OT practitioner may also want to intervene on the macro

level by promoting stricter legislation and cultural "zero tolerance" of drunk driving, perhaps by educating adolescents and young adults.

Consider the initial problem statement focusing on Jane's limited short-term memory. This is not a problem that can be resolved by an OT practitioner as it is stated. Therefore the OT practitioner must reconceptualize and restate the problem so that he or she can intervene in meaningful and systematically documentable ways within OT's professional role. Problem mapping or other logical, evidence-based problem identification techniques help in examining and analyzing problems beyond their initial presentation and identifying the strength of the evidence on which problems are analyzed. In evidence-based practice, problem analysis and a careful statement of the part of the problem to be addressed are critical if the rest of the steps are to be implemented. Including data from the client's perspective in the process will help to formulate the problem in a way that is meaningful and relevant for the client. Furthermore, clarifying the problem will help the therapist ascertain what is needed to resolve the part of the problem that will be addressed.

Now let us move to the next step of evidence-based practice, determining need.

Ascertaining Need

After problem mapping, the next step is ascertaining need. In this step, one must clarify exactly what is needed to resolve the problem. Let us examine the distinction between *problem* and *need*. As discussed earlier, a *problem* is a value statement about what is desired. For a problem to be relevant to OT practitioners, it must concern improvement or maintenance of occupational performance. Thus the problem area on the map that the OT practitioner would target for resolution would be delimited and guided by the professional and theoretical domains of OT concern. A **need statement** is a systematic, evidence-based claim, linked to all or part of a problem, that specifies what conditions and actions are necessary to resolve the part of the problem to be addressed. Thus the identification of need involves collecting and analyzing information such as assessment data and the client interview to ascertain what is necessary to resolve a problem.

At this needs assessment stage of the evidence-based practice sequence, the one may already have information on which to formulate need or may collect data in a systematic fashion to clearly delimit and identify need. A need statement should specify **who** is the target of the problem, **what** changes are desired, **what degree of change** is desired, and **how** one will recognize that the change has occurred. The need statement must be based on empirically derived data already contained in the literature or documentation or revealed in a needs assessment inquiry. Can you see that the need statement uses the research process to define the next steps of specifying goals and objectives, determining the intervention, and specifying the evaluative criteria to determine the success of an intervention?

Let us advance our example from our problem statement again. As already mentioned, the problem as stated (limited short-term memory) is not a problem that can be resolved by an OT practitioner. Yet it is common for referrals for OT intervention to identify problems such as this one. Thus the use of a problem map or similar problem analysis strategy is not only a reasonable thinking tool, but also is essential if we are to define the nature of our interventions more clearly and thereby document the unique contributions and outcomes of OT. We thus choose to reason about the causes and consequences of the problem to identify

whether an area exists in which Jane would require specialized OT intervention. As we mapped the problem, we found that OT did indeed have a critical role to play in Jane's treatment. Her ability to engage in meaningful occupational performance is impaired in that she is unable to manage her time and be punctual as a result of her limited short-term memory.

Given the problem statement, the therapist conducts a research-based needs assessment to determine what is necessary to resolve the part of the problem that therapist will address, to set goals and objectives to guide the selection of intervention, and to determine what processes and outcome should be expected.

Using a systematic approach to data collection, the OT practitioner uses naturalistic techniques, including an interview and systematic observation of Jane, to ascertain Jane's desires and skills. The OT practitioner also administers a standardized cognitive assessment and an occupational performance assessment. In this instance the OT practitioner is integrating qualitative and quantitative inquiry strategies to document a complete understanding of need and to provide the empirical basis for clinical decisions, as well as expected outcomes. One of the tools that the OT practitioner may use to collect data is the Canadian Occupational Performance Measure (COPM). This criterion-referenced measure is used to identify client-perceived problem areas in daily functioning in the areas of self-care, productivity, and leisure. By means of a semistructured interview format, the COPM may be used to assess the performance components the client identifies as interfering with the client's ability to function in a particular area.[3] The data from the COPM are credible, comparative, and accepted as scientific evidence in the research world. See Chapters 5 and 13 for further information regarding the COPM.

Systematic assessment reveals that Jane identifies returning to her job as a saleswoman in a boutique as her most important goal. Additionally, the results of the COPM interview reveal that Jane is not satisfied with her ability to manage her time or her ability to be punctual and that she perceives these two issues as the greatest barriers to achieving her desired goal of return to work. She recognizes that her impaired short-term memory will affect her ability to do other work-related tasks, but she reports being most concerned about time management and promptness.

Standardized testing indicates that Jane's short-term memory is impaired but that her capacity to respond appropriately to external cues remains intact. Additionally, Jane's performance on the Wisconsin Card Sorting Test reveals that she is able to solve problems and that she demonstrates abstract reasoning. The Wisconsin Card Sorting Test is a standardized cognitive assessment of executive function that was developed to assess problem solving, abstract reasoning, and the ability to shift cognitive strategies.[10] Standardized testing also demonstrates that Jane is able to learn new behaviors with specific, well-structured practice in the environment in which she will function. Based on this empirically generated information, the therapist and Jane have a sound and credible basis for deciding that the intervention will be directed to the need to find and teach Jane compensatory strategies for time management and promptness. Further, Jane indicated in her social history interview that she is married and that her husband would be supportive in helping her get to work. Based on this information generated from naturalistic inquiry, the therapist and Jane decide to include Jane's husband in the intervention and to work first in Jane's home environment and then transfer her treatment to the work environment. Can you see from this example how evidence-based practice both provides the guidance and the documentation for clinical decisions and suggests future steps in the intervention and outcome assessment processes? Anyone who observes the intervention process can easily see the rationale for decisions and actions. Credible, research-based knowledge is structured in a manner that provides a clear reasoning trail.

The desired outcomes are implicit in the need statement, which provides a basis for formulating measurable outcomes of intervention. What is needed is home-based and then work site–based OT intervention to assist Jane with time management and promptness, as a skill to facilitate her return to work. The evidence for targeting this intervention, and for the goals and objectives to follow, is clear and specified, as is the desired outcome.

Let us consider a different type of need statement that illustrates why evidence-based practice requires systematic inquiry.

George, an OT practitioner, is asked by an employer to address a problem involving several computer operators whose ability to perform their jobs has been impaired or lost as a result of neck pain. After constructing a problem map, based on literature about causes and consequences of neck pain, George formulates a need statement based on two areas that he believes will address the problem: instruction in proper body mechanics and instruction in a regularly scheduled upper body stretching routine. He begins his intervention by teaching proper body mechanics and upper body stretching techniques to the computer operators, but the problem is not resolved. The computer operators continue to be unable to do their jobs and their complaints of neck pain continue. George' intervention is not successful in resolving the problem for which he was hired.

What was missing from George's reasoning? He based his problem map on educated but preconceived guesses without fully assessing the situation. Had he conducted an empirically based needs assessment that included systematic interview, testing, and observation of the workers in the process, he might have found that the monitors were too high for the operators and the chair heights were not adjustable. Thus the intervention he chose of body mechanics instruction and upper body stretching may have been viable in some situations but did not address the specific needs, which had not been accurately assessed. Had he used inquiry skills to ascertain the needs rather than guessing the needs and then jumping from the problem to the intervention, he would quickly have identified the appropriate target areas.

In any needs assessment, formal research strategies or well-conducted *a priori* studies are useful for identifying and documenting needs. For individual clinical problems, strategies of single case design are indicated to reveal a comprehensive clinical assessment to guide and test the efficacy of intervention decisions for a client. For program development, the therapist may want to use "group" (also called nomothetic) designs, such as survey, interview, or standardized testing strategies, to yield needed information on which to support a needs claim. Naturalistic inquiry or integrated method may be valuable to ascertain the perspectives of client groups whose problems and needs the therapist knows little about. Many excellent research texts exist from which to build research knowledge. (See the recommended reading at the end of this chapter.)

The next step in the process of evidence-based practice is translating the needs into goals and objectives.

Goals and Objectives

Goals and *objectives* are two words with which OT practitioners are familiar, since the words are used to structure treatment. In evidence-based practice, goals and objectives emerge from the need statement and are essential not only for structuring intervention, but also for specifying how the process and outcome of intervention will be examined and supported.

A definition of the two terms is helpful. According to Bloom and associates,[5] **goals** "are statements about what clients and relevant others would like to happen or do or to be." In other words, a goal is a vision statement about future desires that is delimited by the need that it addresses. **Objectives** are statements about both how to reach a goal and how to determine if all or part of the goal has been reached. The objective sets up the systematic approach to attaining the goal as well as the empirical measurement or assessment thereof.[13]

There are two basic types of objectives: process and outcome. **Process objectives** define concrete steps necessary to attain a goal. Process objectives are those interventions or services that will be provided or structured by the OT practitioner.[12] **Outcome objectives** define the criteria that must occur or exist to determine that all or part of the goal has been reached; outcome objectives further specify how the criteria will be demonstrated. Outcome objectives indicate that a change has taken place as a result of participation in the OT process.[12]

To develop goal and objective statements in this model of evidence-based practice, the therapist examines the need carefully, including the evidence to support the need. The therapist formulates conceptual goal and objective statements that imply how the process and outcomes of intervention will be assessed. Goals are overall conceptual statements about what is desired; objectives are statements that are operationalized (i.e., stated in terms of how they will be measured). Both are based on empirically generated knowledge from the needs assessment.

Let us now return to Jane to illustrate evidence-based goals and objectives. From the problem and need statements, we have determined that an overall goal for Jane's intervention is to develop, teach, and have Jane learn compensatory strategies for promptness and time management so she can improve her performance in these areas and return to work. Based on the evidence given in the needs assessment, the OT intervention will be carried out at first in Jane's home with her husband participating, and then a transition will be made to the workplace.

One critical element of goal setting in evidence-based practice is **specificity**. The following example takes the previous treatment goal and uses it to write specific goal and objective statements:

GOAL NO. 1: JANE WILL IMPROVE HER PROMPTNESS TO BE ABLE GET TO WORK ON TIME (PERFORMANCE) AND TO HER SATISFACTION. The objectives we will use to attain this goal include the following:

1. Jane will be presented with assistive technology supports and services and catalogues of assistive devices from which she can select those she thinks will be most useful for her to achieve the goal.
2. Given a choice of a variety of assistive devices (e.g., alarm watches, paging devices, and clocks), Jane will choose one or more devices to use as an external cue provider for promptness.
3. Jane will select one daily activity at home for which she needs an external promptness cue.
4. With assistance from the OT practitioner, Jane and her husband will configure the device to cue Jane to attend to this daily event.
5. Jane's husband will monitor her promptness and provide feedback to Jane and the therapist regarding the effectiveness of the assistive device in meeting the goal.
6. Once Jane has demonstrated that she can promptly attend to her schedule at home, she will begin to use the promptness cue to arrive at work on time and to her satisfaction.
7. Once Jane has demonstrated that she can arrive at work on time, the therapist will work with Jane at the work site so that she can use the device to attend promptly to her work schedule to her and her employer's satisfaction.
8. Using the most effective strategy and devices, Jane will improve her promptness sufficient to work and sufficient for her satisfaction.

GOAL NO. 2: COLLABORATIVELY ESTABLISH, TEACH, AND HAVE CLIENT DEMONSTRATE LEARNING OF A COMPENSATORY STRATEGY THAT SHE WILL USE TO MANAGE HER TIME AT WORK (PERFORMANCE) TO HER SATISFACTION. The objectives we will use to attain this goal include the following:

1. Jane will be supplied with catalogues and assistive devices from which to select a time management strategy.
2. Jane will select the device or devices that she will use as compensatory strategies for time management.
3. Jane and her husband will be trained to use the device.
4. Jane will practice using the device until she is able to manage her time to her and her husband's satisfaction.

Once these two goals are reached in the home environment, goals and objectives specific to the workplace will be established and therapy will be transferred to the work environment.

As you can see by reading these goals and objectives, they are not new ideas but rather very directive, conceptual statements based on an empirical understanding of need. As we will see in the section on process and outcome assessment, stating the goals and objectives as demonstrated above determines what will be examined to ascertain treatment success.

Intervention

Specific goals and objectives help to define intervention strategies and identify success markers. The **process objectives** specify the treatment steps and sequence. Ongoing systematic assessment of process objectives monitors completion of actions within a time frame. Periodic assessment of client progress on outcome objectives provides empirical evidence of client progress to both the client and the therapist. Based on intermediate and ongoing data collection activities, intervention can continue as planned, be revised in response to evidence, or be terminated before desired outcomes are reached.

Once intervention is terminated, final process and outcome assessment are conducted. Let us examine the final step of evidence-based practice.

Process and Outcome Assessment

To review, the process objectives are those that specify the steps of intervention and the outcome objectives are those that delineate the desired outcome. In Box 7-2, process objectives are identified with a **"P"** and outcome objectives are identified with an **"O."** These objectives

BOX 7-2
Goals, Objectives, Evidence, and Success Criteria

Goal No. 1: Jane will improve her promptness to be able to get to work on time (performance) and to her satisfaction.

1. **(P)** Jane will be supplied with catalogues and assistive devices from which to select those that she thinks will be most useful for her to achieve the goal.

   Criterion for success: completion of activity

   Evidence: notes of each session documenting progress toward goal

2. **(P)** Given a variety of assistive devices (e.g., alarm watches, paging devices, and clocks), Jane will choose a device to use as an external cue provider for promptness.

   Criterion for success: selection of device

   Evidence: notes of each session documenting progress toward goal

3. **(P)** Jane will select one activity at home for which she needs an external promptness cue.

   Criterion for success: selection of activity

   Evidence: notes of each session documenting progress toward goal

4. **(O)** With assistance from the OT, Jane and her husband will configure the device to cue Jane to attend to this daily event.

   Criterion for success: demonstration of completion of objective by Jane and her husband

   Evidence: progress notes indicating mastery of task

5. **(P)** Jane's husband will monitor her promptness and provide feedback to Jane and the therapist regarding the effectiveness of the assistive device in meeting the goal.

   Criterion for success: daily record of Jane's promptness supplied to her each evening after dinner

   Evidence: husband's written time charts

6. **(O)** Using the most effective strategy and devices, Jane will improve her promptness sufficient to work and sufficient for her satisfaction.

   Criterion for success: significant improvement in Jane's promptness.

   Evidence: COPM score on this item, compared with COPM score on pretest on this item.

Goal #2 Collaboratively establish, teach, and have client demonstrate learning of a compensatory strategy that she will use to manage her time at work (performance) to her satisfaction.

1. **(P)** Jane will be supplied with catalogues and assistive devices from which to select a time management strategy.

   Criterion for success: completion of activity

   Evidence: notes of each session documenting progress toward goal

2. **(P)** Jane will select the device or devices that she will use as compensatory strategies for time management.

   Criterion for success: completion of activity

   Evidence: notes of each session documenting progress toward goal

3. **(P)** Jane and her husband will be trained to use the device

   Criterion for success: completion of training

   Evidence: notes of each session documenting progress toward goal

4. **(O)** Jane will practice using the device until she is able to manage her time to her and her husband's satisfaction.

   Criterion for success #1: significant improvement in Jane's satisfaction from pretest on related COPM score

   Criterion for success #2: report from Jane's husband of significant satisfaction with Jane's time management now as compared with before

   Evidence: COPM score and husband's self-report

P, Process; *O,* outcome.

can be assessed by using both quantitative and naturalistic techniques and by applying systematic inquiry to examine whether objectives have been attained. To brush up on inquiry, we suggest that you consult one of the many excellent research method texts, some of which we list at the end of this chapter. You also may want to work collaboratively with other OT practitioners, professionals, and clients to select measures and assessment strategies to provide evidence of successful completion of objectives.

To carry out outcome assessment of Jane's intervention, a pre-post test design is selected. Although Jane's intervention will be measured multiple times, only the change

from beginning to end will be used for outcome assessment. To assess outcome, the therapist will use ongoing documentation of objective completion. Box 7-2 illustrates how each objective will be assessed.

Reexamine the table now in light of the need statement. The links among needs, goals and objectives, and process and outcome have been clearly illustrated. Each step of evidence-based practice emerges and is anchored in the previous step. Moreover, systematic inquiry provides the specificity and empirical evidence supporting the extent to which the intervention resolved the part of the problem that was identified as falling within the OT domain.

SUMMARY

This chapter presents research-based thinking and action as valued tools in OT practice. A model of evidence-based practice in which research rigor informs a sequence of systematically linked steps in reasoning and action is proposed. This model begins with a clear problem statement that guides all of the remaining steps. Naturalistic and experimental research traditions are applied to clinical decision making to guide the subsequent steps of identifying and documenting need, positing goals and objectives, selecting intervention, and assessing the efficacy of the process and outcomes of intervention.

In closing, we encourage you to perform deliberately each of the steps of evidence-based practice and to find a personal style for using empirical evidence in professional practice. Evidence-based practice is not only a valuable approach in direct intervention, but also provides the empirical foundation for knowledge building and intervention development in the OT profession.

REVIEW QUESTIONS

1. List three reasons why OT practitioners need to use evidence-based practice to demonstrate the efficacy of OT practice to external audiences.
2. Name and describe each of the steps in the model of evidence-based practice.
3. Compare the steps in the model of evidence-based practice with the steps in the clinical reasoning process.
4. Using a potential OT client as a case study, select a problem and develop a problem map.
5. Pose strategies to ascertain the need based on your problem statement.
6. Identify the need for your client based on your problem statement.
7. What is the difference between goals and objectives, and what is their relationship?
8. How do goals and objectives relate to need?
9. How do goals and objectives relate to a problem?
10. Identify goals for your client.
11. What are the two types of objectives described in this chapter, and what are the differences between them?
12. Based on your goals for your client, identify at least two process objectives and two outcome objectives. Include criteria for success and evidence in your objectives.
13. Chose at least two interventions to achieve the goals and objectives you have established in question 12.
14. Identify process and outcome assessment to examine the success of your interventions.

REFERENCES

1. American Occupational Therapy Foundation Academic Development Committee, Research Advisory Council: *Research Competencies for Occupational Therapy*, 1999, the Foundation. On line at "http://www.aotf.org/html/research_competencies_for_occu.html"
2. American Occupational Therapy Foundation: *About AOTF*, 1999, the Foundation. On-line at "http://www.aotf.org/html/about_aotf.html."
3. Baum C: Occupation-based practice, prevention, and policy: issues for the new millennium. Paper presented at the Strategic Thinking Meeting, AOTA conference, Indianapolis, Ind, 1999.
4. Bergman A: Devolution continues: disability policy for the new millenium. Paper presented at the Leadership Seminar, Orono, Me, 1998.
5. Bloom M, Fischer J, Orme JG: *Evaluating practice: guidelines for the accountable professional*, ed 2, Boston, Mass, 1998, Allyn & Bacon.
6. DePoy E, Gitlin L: *Introduction to research: understanding and using multiple strategies*, St Louis, 1998, Mosby.
7. Dubouloz C, Egan M, Vallerand J: Occupational therapists' perceptions of evidence-based practice, *Am J Occup Ther* 53(5):445-453, 1999.
8. Egan M, Dubouloz C, Von Zweck C, et al: The client-centered evidence-based practice of occupational therapy, *Can J Occup Ther* 65(3):136-143, 1998.
9. Fine S: Surviving the health care revolution: rediscovering the meaning of "good work." In Scott AH, editor: *New frontiers in psychosocial occupational therapy*, New York, 1998, Harworth Press.
10. Haase B: Cognition. In Van Dusen J, Brunt D, editors: *Assessment in occupational therapy and physical therapy*, Philadelphia, 1997, WB Saunders.
11. Jacobs K: Alignment: leading health care by sharing common dreams, *Am J Occup Ther* 53(5):429-433, 1999.
12. Law M, Baum C: Evidence-based occupational therapy, *Can J Occup Ther* 65(3):131-135, 1998.
13. Letts L, Law M, Pollack N, et al: *A programme evaluation workbook for occupational therapists: an evidence-based practice tool*, Ottowa, 1999, Canadian Association of Occupational Therapists.
14. Ottenbacher K, Christiansen CH. Occupational performance assessment. In Christiansen CH, Baum CM, editors: *Occupational therapy: enabling function and well-being*, ed 2, Thorofare, NJ, 1997, Slack.
15. Tickle-Degnan L: Communication with clients about treatment outcomes: the use of meta-analytic evidence in collaborative treatment planning, *Am J Occup Ther* 52(7):526-530, 1998.

RECOMMENDED READING

Alter C, Even W: *Evaluating your practice: a guide to self-assessment*, New York, 1990, Springer-Verlag.
Campbell DT, Stanley JC: *Experimental and quasi-experimental design*, Chicago, 1963, Rand-McNally.
DeVellis RF: *Scale development: theory and applications*, Newbury Park, Calif, 1991, Sage.
Glaser B, Strauss A: *Grounded theory: strategies for qualitative research*, New York, 1967, Aldine.
Kane RL: *Understanding health care outcomes research*, Gaithersburg, Md, 1997, Aspen.
Knoke D, Bohrnstedt GW: *Basic social statistics*, Itasca, Ill, 1991, Peacock.
McDowell I, Newell C: *Measuring health: a guide to rating scales and questionnaires*, ed 2, New York, 1996, Oxford University Press.
Miles MB, Huberman AM: *Qualitative data analysis: a source book of new methods*, Newbury Park, Calif, 1984, Sage.
Miller D: *Handbook of research design and social measurement*, Newbury Park, Calif, 1991, Sage.
Munro BH: *Statistical methods for health care research*, ed 3, Philadelphia, 1998, JB Lippincott.

Ottenbacher K: *Evaluating clinical change: strategies for occupational and physical therapists*, Baltimore, 1986, Williams & Wilkins.

Patton M: *Qualitative evaluation and research methods*, ed 2, Newbury Park, Calif, 1990, Sage.

Pyrczak F: *Success at statistics*, Los Angeles, 1996, Pyrczak Publishing.

Reason P, Rowan J, editors: *Human inquiry: a sourcebook for new paradigm research*, New York, 1981, John Wiley & Sons.

Royeen C, editor: *Clinical research handbook*, Thorofare, NJ, 1989, Slack.

Royse DD, Thyer BA: *Program evaluation: an introduction*, ed 2, Chicago, 1996, Nelson Hall.

Shaffir WB, Stebbins RA, editors: *Experiencing fieldwork: an inside view of qualitative research*, Newbury Park, Calif, 1991, Sage.

Strauss A: *Qualitative analysis for social scientists*, New York, 1987, Cambridge University Press.

Yin RK: *Case study research*, Newbury Park, Calif, 1989, Sage.

CHAPTER 8

Occupational Therapy for Prevention of Injury and Physical Dysfunction

DIANE HARLOWE

KEY TERMS

Primary prevention
Secondary prevention
Tertiary prevention
Secondary conditions
Risk factors
Risk assessment
Falls prevention
Ergonomics
Well elderly study
ROM Dance Program
FAST: Families and Schools Together

LEARNING OBJECTIVES

After studying this chapter the student or practitioner will be able to do the following:

1. Discuss the involvement of occupational therapy (OT) in the prevention of injury and physical dysfunction, as related to political, social, economic, and health care financing trends during the last four decades of the 20th century.
2. Describe important considerations for the future expansion of OT roles in prevention.
3. Define primary, secondary, and tertiary preventions and discuss the roles played by OT practitioners at each level.
4. Describe three key factors in the practice of prevention in OT.
5. Identify roles that OT practitioners play in primary, secondary, and tertiary prevention of falls.
6. Define ergonomics and describe the roles that occupational therapists play in the prevention of injuries in the workplace.
7. Provide a general description of the interventions provided in "The Well Elderly Study Occupational Therapy Program," and discuss implications of the results of research.
8. Describe the ROM Dance program and discuss methods for integrating ROM Dance exercise and relaxation techniques in clinical practice.
9. Discuss the American Occupational Therapy Association's (AOTA's) initiatives in preventing youth violence, and describe the FAST program.

This chapter provides a brief history of the role of occupational therapy (OT) in the prevention of injuries and physical dysfunction, as related to general trends in health care financing. Primary, secondary, and tertiary interventions are defined, and key factors in the provision of effective prevention services are identified. Tertiary prevention techniques for specific physically disabling conditions are not covered here, since other portions of this text provide extensive information in this area. Prevention of falls, workplace injuries, and ergonomics are highlighted. In addition, three innovative primary and secondary intervention programs are summarized. Practitioners are urged to maximize day-to-day opportunities to more fully integrate prevention activities into practice.

BRIEF HISTORY OF PREVENTION MODEL IN OCCUPATIONAL THERAPY

One of the basic assumptions of the OT profession is that individuals develop and maintain health and prevent dysfunction through occupational performance. The philosophical base statement of the American Occupational Therapy Association (AOTA) asserts that "Occupational therapy is based on the belief that purposeful activity (occupation) . . . may be used to prevent and mediate dysfunction."[1] Reitz[39] stated that, "Since its inception, occupational therapy has recognized the importance of both preventive action and the promotion of wellness." Prevention of disability has been defined by the AOTA as "any activity intended to keep specific diseases or disabling conditions from occurring or worsening." Promoting health and wellness is the basis of prevention efforts and should be the cornerstone of all therapeutic intervention."[2] The ability to integrate these factors into one's clinical reasoning so as to select appropriate assessments and develop an effective treatment plan is the art and the science of occupational therapy preventive intervention.

During the past four decades the prevention model has been explored in the OT literature.[16] Varied roles and services appropriate for OT practitioners have been described. Direct involvement in preventive intervention, as opposed to remediation and compensation (see Table 8-1), has been dramatically affected by the changing trends in health care financing and reimbursement trends.

During the 1960s most occupational therapists were employed in long-term care institutions. Such settings often maintained statistics on service provision, but a productivity monitor was unheard of, and the cost of OT was seldom computed or charged directly to the patient. Although the majority of services provided were remedial, compensatory, or diversional, some aspects emphasized prevention.[51] The following OT prevention roles in physical disabilities were identified in 1969 by Wilma West[52]:

TABLE 8-1
Occupational Therapy Intervention Approaches

Intervention Approaches	Focus of Intervention
Remediation and Restoration	
Changing the biologic, physiologic, psychologic, or neurologic process	Restoring or remediating impairments in performance components
Teaching and training	Establishing new skills, habits, or behaviors in performance components
Compensation and Adaptation	
Changing the task	Adapting the task requirements, procedures, task objects
Changing the context	Modifying or adapting the task environment
Disability Prevention	
Primary prevention	Occupations that prevent health problems
Secondary prevention	Safe task methods and task objects
Tertiary prevention	Safe occupational performance
Health Promotion	
Lifestyle redesign	Purposeful and meaningful occupations Balance of rest, work, play and leisure Healthy interaction with the environment

From Moyers PA: *Am J Occup Ther* 53: 274, 1999. Used with permission of the American Occupational Therapy Association.

- Preventing deformity, weakness, and loss of motion, as in physical dysfunction
- Preventing accidents by teaching safety practices, and preventing strains through instruction in proper body mechanics
- Preventing dependency, for a broad range of handicapping conditions, through the teaching of abilities for daily living
- Preventing the need for institutional care, for the elderly or incapacitated, through adaptations of the home
- Preventing invalidism of cardiac patients with energy-saving devices and procedures
- Preventing vocational misfits, in terms of interest, attitude, or skill, through prevocational exploration and evaluation

■ Preventing misunderstanding and mistreatment of children with aberrant motor performance or social behavior, by counseling their parents, siblings, and teachers.[52]

In the early 1970s, Lela Llorens[28] edited a book of collected papers highlighting the shift in the practice of OT from a remedial, institutionally based, medical model to a health-oriented preventive model practiced in the community. At that time, providing OT in a private clinic or the public school system was considered nontraditional. It was also not uncommon for patients with a physically disabling condition such as stroke to be detained in an acute care hospital for months before being transferred to a rehabilitation unit or hospital, where they might receive their first visit from an occupational therapist. At the start of the decade OT was seldom available in acute care to prevent a disabling condition's potential secondary effects such as contractures, decubiti, and depression. At that time, Medicare reimbursed hospitals and physicians on a fee-for-service basis, creating a monetary incentive to maintain patients in the acute care setting for lengthy periods. As hospital administrators began to realize that Medicare would reimburse charges for OT, the availability of acute care OT for physical disabilities increased, as did OT's involvement in preventive intervention. The goal to "shift our point of entry"[28] was realized in diverse ways, and by expanding the availability of services in the community, therapists were able to focus on more primary and secondary levels of prevention (Box 8-1). In 1979, AOTA published an official position paper that identified and illustrated OT's expanding roles in the area of primary and secondary levels of prevention.[1]

In 1984 Medicare reimbursement for acute care hospitalization shifted to a Diagnostic Related Grouping (DRG) system that fiscally reinforced shortened lengths of stay. This provided unexpected opportunities for occupational therapists who were able to market their skills in facilitating patients' independent functioning in self-care, an important factor in decreasing lengths of stay. OT functional evaluations and discharge recommendations became more valued, in part because of the financial losses that hospitals incurred if patients were readmitted shortly after discharge. It became increasingly important to identify patients at risk for falls both during and after hospitalization. If a patient required readmission for a fall-related injury, procedures might not be reimbursed if the fall was determined to be precipitated by a premature discharge. Since most falls occurred during functional activity, occupational therapists became actively involved in this aspect of prevention, both in the hospital and through home safety evaluations after discharge. Competitive marketing of emerging health care systems through community-based health education and wellness programs also increased OT involvement in prevention since occupational therapists were recruited to design and often implement outreach preventive health education. The ROM dance program[19,20] discussed in this chapter was created as a result of such an initiative.

During the 1990s the emerging dominance of health maintenance organizations (HMOs) and preferred provider organizations (PPOs) had some positive effects on OT involvement in prevention. These HMOs and PPOs have a vested interest in prevention activities at all levels because keeping people well is more profitable under these systems than is remediating health problems that could have been prevented. During the past decade, OT literature has reflected the increasing importance of prevention, and Rothman and Levine[40] have published an extensive text titled *Prevention Practice: Strategies for Physical Therapy and Occupational Therapy* that focuses on incorporating the prevention of physical dysfunction into daily practice. It emphasizes "an expanded view of the roles of physical and occupational therapists . . . practicing in so-called 'rehabilitation' [where OT practitioners] interact with clients who are experiencing multichronicity. For example, we may develop a plan of care related specifically to a pathologic condition such as a hip fracture. . . . However, that same client may also have a history of coronary heart failure, chronic obstructive pulmonary disease, and diabetes. In effect, the presence of multichronicity obligates us to be alert to make preventive interventions at any point along the health service spectrum."[40]

OT literature also articulated the need for occupational therapists to expand awareness of and involvement in prevention activities on the local, state, and national levels. Kniepmann[27] provided a review of some key national initiatives and resources and discussed their implications for OT. She noted that, "Occupational therapists must identify ways to move into the

BOX 8-1
Levels of Prevention

Primary prevention
■ Employed before a critical event occurs
■ Goal: Reduce incidence of disorder

Secondary prevention
■ Keep mild disorders from becoming severe ones
■ Avert disorder with an "at risk" individual, group, or population

Tertiary prevention
■ Keep serious disorders from producing permanent disability
■ Maximize function and minimize detrimental effects of a disabling condition

day-to-day settings where health habits, illness, and injury occur. . . . A major challenge for occupational therapists is to find innovative, effective, and economical ways to 'move upstream' by transferring the knowledge and skill base of occupational therapy to address all levels of prevention. . . . Occupational therapists can act as consultants, program planners, staff trainers/educators, researchers, community health advisors, primary care providers, policy makers, case managers, and advocates—for individuals, groups, and communities."[27]

FORECASTING THE FUTURE OF PREVENTION IN OCCUPATIONAL THERAPY

Looking forward to the first decade of the new millennium, Baum and Law[4] state that, "As the health system changes its focus to persons' long-term health needs, issues surrounding occupation become central to promoting health and reducing the cost of chronic disability." Realizing the goal of reducing the cost of chronic disability is one of the potential benefits of cost containment and managed care because it creates a context for the reimbursement of preventive OT services. This theoretical opportunity creates the challenge to "package" OT services in a manner that fits into the shifting health care delivery systems. It is also a challenge for those reflecting on current practice in the OT literature to identify and work within new models of delivery of preventive care. One example of an emerging model of care is "disease management."[4] This ". . . is a comprehensive, integrated approach to care and reimbursement . . . [which] attempts to encompass the entire course of a disease, whether it is in an acute phase or remission and whether the care is delivered in the hospital, the home, or the community. This approach also considers the consequences of the condition across time. The purpose of disease management is to help people develop healthy behaviors not only to improve their health, but also to cut health care costs associated with secondary conditions. In the United States, nurses and health educators are carrying out much of this work."[4] Many opportunities exist for occupational therapists to provide services within such a model, especially with the management of rheumatic diseases and those that frequently result in physical disability and dysfunction, such as diabetes.

Looking ahead, "Occupational therapists must continue to identify high-risk populations and to design prevention services that promote healthy outcomes."[16] One high-risk population is the large aging portion of the workforce. Combined with the expected increase in disabled workers, the advancing age of the workforce will increase risk factors for work-related injuries and resulting physical dysfunction. The desire to reduce disability

and its associated costs will challenge employers to seek effective prevention programs, and OT workplace services such as those reviewed in this chapter should expand dramatically. In the future, we may see increasing numbers of referrals to OT by physicians who are concerned that aging patients' physical or mental status may impair driving ability, which could pose a threat to public safety. Another societal concern is preventing youth violence, which is a serious risk factor for injury and physical dysfunction. We hope that occupational therapists will be able to garner grant funding from the armories of the "wars" on drugs and crime to develop, implement, and research activity-based programs for preventing youth violence within high-risk populations. Such a program, FAST, is described later in this chapter.

It is highly desirable that occupational therapists expand their scope of services to new settings and become increasingly involved in prevention planning and legislation on the local, state, and national levels. Nevertheless, therapists' natural and immediate concern will be the clients already in their care. The clinical reasoning questions regarding prevention will always be, What risks does this client face? What interventions could be used to prevent these risks? What funding is available? Will consumers adopt these recommendations and take responsibility for implementation?

PREVENTIVE INTERVENTION IN OCCUPATIONAL THERAPY

The 1999 *Guide to Occupational Therapy Practice*[36] includes "disability prevention" as one of the four categories of interventions employed by OT (Table 8-1). The Guide describes disability prevention by OT practitioners as preventing the occurrence of "impairments, activity limitations, and participant restrictions. . . ."[36] It also refers to three levels of intervention, described as follows.

Primary Prevention

Primary prevention is employed before a critical event occurs. It involves protecting individuals or groups who are not at any greater risk from the negative effects of identified health hazards than is the general population. The goal of primary prevention is to reduce the incidence of disorder by altering the environment or by making the individual or group less susceptible to stress. Public health programs and interventions that support and protect "the health and well-being of the society at large"[27] are considered primary prevention. An example of community-wide primary prevention of physical disability is the passage of laws that require the use of seat belts to prevent injuries caused by motor vehicle accidents. Other examples include statewide laws and programs to promote the use of helmets to prevent head injuries while using motorcycles and bicycles.

The occupational therapist providing services for primary prevention of physical dysfunction may focus on consumer education regarding risk factors for injuries caused by accidents or habitual stresses such as repetitive motions. An important goal is to facilitate understanding of the linkages between one's occupational behavior and the risks for injury. OT may also assist consumers in clarifying their values about health and in acquiring the knowledge, habits, and attitudes needed for preventive intervention. OT primary prevention also includes altering the environment or providing other interventions to reduce susceptibility to injury or physical dysfunction.

Secondary Prevention

The goal of **secondary prevention** is keeping mild disorders from becoming severe. Secondary prevention is most often practiced with individuals or groups that have been identified as at risk for a severe dysfunction. Intervention is provided to assist in preventing a disorder or retarding its progression to a more serious or chronic condition. Such activities may include screening, early diagnosis, appropriate referral, prompt treatment, consultation, and community-based and home health care.

An example of secondary prevention of physical dysfunction in OT clinical services is providing instruction in joint protection, body mechanics, and work simplification techniques to clients with a newly diagnosed condition that has the potential to be physically disabling, such as rheumatoid arthritis. Occupational therapists are also directly engaged in activities to reduce or eliminate architectural barriers that restrict employment and mobility for people with physical disabilities. The current trend is for occupational therapists to provide home safety evaluations for frail, elderly clients recently discharged from acute care hospitals or rehabilitation or extended care facilities; this also would be considered secondary prevention. The client is identified as being at risk for falls, and the OT safety evaluation and therapeutic intervention are intended to reduce the risk of future falls that might result in a physically disabling injury.

Tertiary Prevention

The goal of **tertiary prevention** is to prevent a serious disorder from producing permanent disability. OT tertiary prevention aims to reduce the barriers to desired occupational performance among physically disabled individuals within present or future performance contexts. Tertiary prevention includes the provision of a wide range of rehabilitative services to improve functional performance, prevent declines in performance,

and assist in attaining desired productivity and participation in community life. Occupational therapists are considered experts in tertiary prevention, since the main goal of this level is to maximize function and minimize the detrimental effects of a disabling condition.

KEY FACTORS IN PRACTICE OF PREVENTION IN OCCUPATIONAL THERAPY

"Prevention is anticipatory action based upon knowledge."[53] The knowledge essential to clinical reasoning and judgments about appropriate preventive intervention in OT patient care is grounded in three key areas. To develop an appropriate plan for intervention, knowledge of the following areas should be integrated with data gained from a client-centered assessment of occupational performance:

1. *Awareness of preventive intervention opportunities and resources.* Therapists who are committed to implementing preventive intervention must be vigilant in maintaining a current awareness of new clinical resources and service and reimbursement pathways as they emerge. Knowledge of current research on the efficacy of intervention techniques is also important for effective practice of prevention. The OT practitioner must empower clients and their families to acquire appropriate knowledge, skills, and equipment needed to incorporate preventive practices into their lifestyles. This is as important as maintaining an awareness of the opportunities that arise to provide preventive intervention services in one's current practice.

2. *Early identification and awareness of risk factors.* Identifying risks is the first step in planning for the prevention of **secondary conditions,** which are defined as pathology, impairments, or functional limitations that derive from the primary disabling condition. Individuals with disabling conditions have a "narrow margin of health"[42] and are at risk for accidents, injuries, and secondary conditions that unnecessarily increase the severity of the disability and that require attention to prevent.[42] Maintaining a current awareness of the risk factors encountered by the population served is critical to planning preventive intervention strategies within the scope of an occupational therapist's practice. Many clinics have developed structured formats for evaluation of an individual's functional performance components related to specific diagnoses. Equally helpful would be a **risk assessment** checklist of risks and **risk factors** that an individual with a specific diagnosis would be expected to encounter in the future. Checklists may include the risk of falls, contractures, decreased endurance, decubiti, and driving risks, among other conditions. Such an assessment could be used to

guide consumer education and discharge planning. In fact, a therapist's ability to effectively communicate knowledge of risk factors and methods of prevention to the client and family may be the key to facilitating healthy behavioral change. Consumers who fully understand the risks they face are much more likely to implement recommendations. Therefore the consumers' level of knowledge and beliefs should be assessed; limited knowledge could be considered a risk factor (Box 8-2).

3. *Assessment of consumers' health belief risk factors.* The health belief model was developed and expanded to help therapists understand and predict adoption of preventive health behaviors in response to specific health risks.[23] This model asserts that a number of factors predict whether consumers are likely to implement recommendations to adopt preventive health behaviors. The predictive factors relate to the consumers' assessment of the relative importance of the risk factors, the value of the recommendations for prevention, and the consumers' ability to carry out the recommendations.[23,27] Consumers' judgments are often unconscious or not expressed to the therapist. Therefore the consumers' implementation of a recommendation may be sabotaged by an unconscious belief, and a therapist's effectiveness may depend on the ability to perceive and address such unexpressed concerns. Box 8-2 provides a proposed format for structuring an assessment of consumers'

BOX 8-2
Assessing Clients' Attitudes Regarding Health Risks and Preventive Intervention

Personal threat assessment
What is the chance that this (identified risk) can happen to me?
If it does, how bad will it be?

Personal cost-benefit analysis
Will the short and long-term benefits of following the therapist's recommencation be worth what it will cost me and my family in terms of such things as money, effort, social status, and self-concept?

Belief in self-efficacy
Do I have what it takes (e.g., self-discipline, determination, knowledge, and skill) to pull it off?

Belief in resources
Can the people and structures within my environments adapt and support these lifestyle changes?
What new resources will be available to assist in following this recommendation?

ability to understand the risks they face and their beliefs about the need to implement preventive recommendations. Assisting consumers in addressing these questions will help in developing a collaborative, client-centered plan of care.

APPLYING PRINCIPLES OF PREVENTIVE INTERVENTION

Since the principles of prevention are applicable to such a broad scope of physically disabling conditions, only a few specific areas are used as examples.

Prevention of Falls

Falls are a major source of physical dysfunction and mortality among the well elderly and physically disabled populations.[13] Preventing accidental falls by senior citizens has been a national health priority, and considerable research with implications for OT practice has been conducted in this area.[49,50] One study indicated that reported falls were reduced by 60% after a community-based program to reduce hazards in the home environments of senior citizens.[37] The interventions used in this study were similar to those typically provided by occupational therapists performing home safety assessments and modifications, such as securing rugs and electrical cords, removing clutter, and installing hand rails, grab bars, and nonskid strips. An extensive review of the literature on the intrinsic and extrinsic factors related to falls[44] in the elderly population was provided by Holliday, Cott, and Torresin[20] and Cook and Miller.[12] Intrinsic risk factors include poor balance, gait impairment, muscle weakness, decreased range of motion (ROM), visual and other sensory impairments, chronic disease, physical disability, blood pressure changes, cognitive impairment, and side effects of medications.

Falls often occur during occupational performance. Occupational therapists are providing a wide range of services in prevention of primary, secondary, and tertiary falls in diverse settings.

Primary prevention of falls can involve such activities as controlling environmental hazards or providing educational services to the well elderly[12] who are no more at risk for falls than their age mates. I participated in an example of the latter at a number of Wisconsin state-funded "Senior Expos." This annual event draws thousands of seniors who participate in educational programming designed to appeal to their interests and needs, especially in the areas of prevention and health promotion. Prevention of falls in the home has been a popular topic. In addition to providing information on risk factors, adaptive equipment, and environmental modifications, occupational therapists have emphasized the relationship between falls and occupational behavior. Presentations have involved examples of fall hazards encountered by therapists providing OT services through the home health organization that sponsors the presentations. Since many healthy participants are in attendance because of their concern for the safety of infirm or disabled friends and relatives, these lectures have been an excellent opportunity to market OT home safety assessment services.

An OT home safety assessment is a secondary prevention program most frequently provided to clients who are at a greater risk for falls because of recent discharge from a hospital or nursing home. An occupational behavior model is used to assess the person (intrinsic risk factors), environment (extrinsic risk factors), and occupation fit. One important risk factor is the area of consumer attitudes (Box 8-2). Therefore the therapist assists clients and their families in conducting a personal threat assessment by highlighting the interaction of primary risk factors during specific high-risk activities such as going to the bathroom in the middle of the night. This provides an opportunity to examine values and conduct a cost-benefit analysis about such simple environmental or behavioral strategies as leaving a light on. A new behavior such as leaving a light on may conflict with strong values and ingrained habituation systems. Considerable therapeutic skill is needed to reinforce the client's belief in self-efficacy to implement recommendations. Framing the change as a challenge is often helpful because this acknowledges the effort required and facilitates mobilization of resources. For example, if a family expresses the value of conserving money, it may be helpful to engage in a brainstorming session on how to acquire recommended adapted devices at the lowest cost. This approach is valued by those who are in other disciplines in the home health organization and prefer to delegate this aspect of care to OT practitioners, who usually complete the service in one to three sessions. This approach also provides an excellent opportunity to identify other aspects of care that can be provided by an OT practitioner.

Service on multidisciplinary fall prevention teams in hospitals and nursing homes is another important contribution made by OT practitioners. A quality improvement team at St. Mary's Hospital Medical Center in Madison, Wisconsin, created a hospital-wide program to identify acute care patients who met preestablished fall risk criteria. The admitting nurse administered a falls assessment. Certain high-risk trigger factors generated automatic referrals to OT and physical therapy. One of the most important risk factors identified was a positive orthostatic test, which consists of a 20- to 30-mm change in a patient's blood pressure while the patient is making the transition from lying to standing. Patients with this or other risk factors wore green-tinted hospital identification bracelets so that all employees were alerted to the risk for falls. Patients in this program received increased physical and cognitive activity to maintain strength and alertness, were monitored during transfers, and were provided standby assistance during toileting whenever possible. The team implementing this program found that the slippers given to patients were impeding ambulation because of the tacky tread, so new slippers were ordered for use throughout the hospital. Since a review of hospital data indicated that falls occurred when patients attempted to scale guard rails on the bed for toileting, the use of guard rails was decreased. The team's occupational therapist proposed the use of female urinals, which were adopted throughout the hospital. In addition, OT supplied each unit with a box of video tapes of old comedies and Lawrence Welk shows, music audio tapes, long-handled reachers, games, and hand exercise equipment to lend to patients and their families during admission; this was very well received. Additional prevention activities included monitoring the environment for hazards and initiating improvements. The hospital is gathering data to assess the effectiveness of this approach.

Tertiary prevention is provided to clients who experience falls on a recurrent basis. All too often, the problem of repeated falls for elderly or disabled individuals is not addressed effectively. One high-incidence factor is the presence of a high-level spinal cord injury. It is not uncommon for individuals with long-term spinal cord injuries to incur physical injuries, including fractures, as a result of caretaker error in assisting with transfers. The strength of postural bones is compromised by not bearing weight, causing individuals with spinal cord injury to be more susceptible to fracture. This situation is further complicated by the frequent turnover of caregivers employed as personal assistants. OT literature emphasizes the importance of providing employer education to individuals and families responsible for hiring and training personal assistants.[5] OT interventions include client and caregiver education and training concerning risk factors and interventions to prevent falls, but this education is not provided consistently. Transfer training of newly employed personal assistants might be enhanced if the development of training videos were routinely incorporated into the rehabilitation program. Videos should be developed within the environment where the patient is likely to be functioning on a long-term basis. Simple, clear, and concise instructions with a viewing time of no more than 15 minutes would facilitate frequent use. A brief explanation of the hazards and precautions may be helpful in preventing future injury. Maintaining or providing an extra copy of the tape may also facilitate long-term use of such a valuable prevention resource. Another resource that is helpful to OT practitioners is Morse's "Preventing Patient Falls,"[35] which includes the Morse Fall Scale and strategies for prevention.

"A Matter of Balance" is an award-winning prevention program designed to reduce the fear of falling and increase the activity level of elders.[7,43] This community-based intervention provides nine 2-hour group sessions that include activities to address physical, social, and cognitive factors involved in the fear of falling. The program is based on the premise that the fear of falling can lead to reductions in activity, mobility, and physical conditioning, which may increase risk. Results of a randomized controlled trial of 434 older adults showed that after 1 year, participants reported less fear of falling and greater fall management than control subjects. Other findings included a better mean score on the total sickness Impact Profile and scales for physical conditioning, mobility range, and social behavior.

Ergonomics and Prevention of Injuries in the Workplace

Ergonomics is the science of workplace design. Increasingly, occupational therapists are involved in ergonomics and prevention of injuries in the workplace. AOTA's official statement on "Occupational Therapy Services in Work Practice"[3] states that OT practitioners "play an important role in promoting optimal levels of work performance for all individuals. . . . Occupational therapy practitioners provide work-related services in many settings, including . . . acute care and rehabilitation facilities, industrial and office environments, work evaluation and work hardening programs, sheltered work programs, school-to-work transition programs, psychiatric treatment centers, programs for the elderly, educational systems, and home environments."[3] The AOTA statement provides guidelines for the provision of individual OT services to achieve goals in work disability prevention and management programs.

AOTA has also published a resource titled *Preventing and Treating Carpal Tunnel Syndrome*,[54] with clear descriptions and illustrations that can be helpful for consumer education. Topics include description of the syndrome, testing methods, and exercises and tools to remediate and help prevent carpal tunnel syndrome. A list of risk factors includes maintaining a constant grip on tools, working in a cold environment, performing highly repetitive jobs, using poor body mechanics, and working at a keyboard for extended periods. A variety of treatment techniques are explored, such as use of heat, stretch, joint mobilization, edema management, and splinting. Although geared for the individual, information in this resource may be used effectively in corporate education and prevention programs.

Corporate interest in establishing fitness and injury prevention programs has increased, and the cost of self-insurance and reduction of purchased insurance have been influential.[21] The Occupational Safety and Health Administration (OSHA) proposal to set workplace ergonomic standards has stimulated many corporations to increase services. New standards would require employers to have a plan to prevent ergonomic injuries and pay for treatment.[8,38] Occupational therapists have responded to the proactive corporate climate in unique, creative, and effective ways. Occupational therapists affiliated with Bellin Memorial Hospital in Green Bay, Wisconsin, market their occupational health services[6] to local industry on a fee-for-service basis. Among the program elements they offer are the following:

1. Preemployment functional testing to screen for propensities for carpal tunnel syndrome, back injuries, and lifting problems, as related to specifications of the job description
2. Acute treatment of work-related injuries
3. Return-to-work programs
4. Functional capacity evaluations
5. On-site services, including work hardening and a video analysis of the ergonomic job site assessment
6. Task analysis for job descriptions to assist in complying with guidelines of the Americans with Disabilities Act
7. Education programs in cumulative trauma disorders, back injury prevention, office ergonomics, stretching, exercise, and high-risk factors for job duties

Another innovative service was developed by occupational therapist Michael Melnick, who provides consultation to industry. One of Melnick's clients reported that "costs for injuries dropped by 80% three years after Melnick redesigned factory workstations in St. Paul and Philadelphia [and] Minnesota Power went from having 10 or 12 back injuries a year to being cited by the Minnesota Safety Council for 1 million work hours without a 'medical attention back injury.'"[24] Another successful model was described by Hanson,[17] who reported on an ergonomic intervention program in a Florida acute care hospital, with occupational therapists playing a central role. The occupational therapist conducted work site analyses for injured workers and recommended improvements for the work environment. Patient handling was found to be the highest risk factor for sustaining work-related injury. New ergonomic patient lifting and transfer equipment was purchased, and the occupational therapist was involved in training nurses in use of the equipment and evaluating their responses. OT plays a key role in assessing work tasks in this setting and offering environmentally sound improvement options. King and colleagues[26] describe OT preventive intervention for workers in a child care program. Carayon and Smith[9] provide a thorough literature review and practical guidelines to prevent strain in computerized workplaces, and Claiborne and Williams[10] illustrate the importance of addressing the person, environment, and task performance fit when providing ergonomic computer workstations for individual clients.

Ergonomics in the workplace will take on a new dimension in the near future. In addition to expanding involvement of the elderly population in the workforce, a much greater percentage of the disabled population will be employed than ever before, as a result of recent initiatives. The Wisconsin-based "Pathways to Independence" is the largest of the 12 federally funded state programs designed to support employment of individuals in four disability groups: physical disabilities, mental illness, developmental disabilities, and acquired immune deficiency syndrome/human immunodeficiency virus (AIDS/HIV). This complex pilot program is designed to eliminate the most significant barriers to employment that result from public support policies. More than 6.6 million Americans have a permanent disability and receive income support from Social Security Disability Income (SSDI) or Supplemental Security Income (SSI). Less than 1% of SSI or SSDI beneficiaries leave those programs each year as a result of paid employment. Beneficiaries claim that one of the most important barriers to paid employment is the potential loss of Medicaid and Medicare. These individuals cannot afford to work because under current policies their coverage is jeopardized if they earn more than $500 per month for 9 months. Pathways to Independence will provide these individuals with a clear-cut guarantee of continued health coverage and will also provide comprehensive assistance in achieving their employment goals.[15] The program is designed to increase tax revenues through the employment of large numbers of disabled individuals. The implications for the therapist are enormous, since these individuals could benefit greatly from the OT services in the workplace. The OT profession must monitor these national trends as they emerge to ensure optimum deployment of OT services, including prevention.

RESEARCH ON OCCUPATIONAL THERAPY PREVENTION PROGRAMS

One of the goals of the AOTA is to facilitate research on the efficacy of OT services, including preventive intervention programs. Although the OT literature reveals a range of OT prevention programs, two are highlighted in this chapter because they focus on primary and secondary prevention with targeted adult populations who may be at risk for injury and physical dysfunction.

Well Elderly Study Occupational Therapy Program

One of the most notable occupational therapy efficacy studies of the 1990s was a rigorous experimental test of a preventive occupational therapy intervention.[12] The University of Southern California's **Well Elderly Study** Occupational Therapy Program was "found to be highly successful in enhancing the physical and mental health, occupational functioning, and life satisfaction of multi-

cultural, community-dwelling elders. . . . The treatment . . . emphasized the therapeutic process of lifestyle redesign in enabling the participants to actively and strategically select an individualized pattern of personally satisfying and health promoting occupations."[22]

The 361 participants were randomly assigned to three study groups for 9 months. The first group received preventive OT, the second group was involved in a social activities program led by nonprofessionals, and the third group served as the control group and did not receive any services. The OT intervention included a 2-hour weekly group session involving 8 to 10 participants. This was supplemented by a 1-hour monthly individual session with the therapist. The aim of treatment was to reduce the health risks of older adulthood, and the participants were encouraged to use occupation in a personalized way to adapt to their specific challenges associated with aging. The program consisted of a series of eight "occupational self-analysis" content areas, which included the following:

1. *Introduction to the power of occupations* reviewed the physical, social, emotional, cognitive, and temporal meaning and ritual dimensions of occupations. This was related to the way in which participants' occupational choices affected their past, present, and future experience of well-being.
2. *Aging, health, and occupation* explored expanded concepts of health and wellness and involved a self-analysis. Elders generated their own list of "25 Ways to Stay Healthy," in which participants included such divergent elements as amusement, creation of love and support, maintenance of a positive mind-set, exercise, and diet. Various tools were introduced to improve health, such as skill development in reading nutritional labels, games and puzzles for mental alertness, and the ROM Dance that is described later. The coordinator of the USC Well Elderly Study said, "We chose to use the ROM Dance for our program because the technique is framed within the context of occupation. The music and visual imagery encouraged relaxation, and we found the gentle movement to be especially helpful for seniors with arthritis."[34] Many participants discovered new occupations (e.g., using public transportation) or reinitiated old ones (e.g., table tennis). The focus of this content area was to position the participant "to begin to thoughtfully weave his or her occupations into a coherent, personalized health promoting pattern."[22]
3. The *transportation* content area helped participants explore their individualized obstacles and inhibitory fears and assisted them in gaining a broader knowledge, experience, and skill base to help them develop an image of themselves as urban travelers.
4. *Safety* education included videos and lectures on crime prevention and the actual practice of community protection techniques during the OT outings.

Home safety stressed prevention of falls and burglary, and each participant conducted a personal home evaluation and experimented with techniques and equipment to improve safety and body mechanics.

5. The *social relationships* content area covered changes caused by loss, relocation, or disability and the effect of the changes on occupational routines. Program involvement facilitated the expansion of participants' social relationships.

6. *Cultural awareness* allowed participants to open new doors of cross-cultural understanding within the context of occupation. The intent of this was to address the unexpected outcome of a preliminary study detailing the extent to which interpersonal clashes between elderly members of different ethnic groups impeded healthy living. This content area included outings to multicultural museums, celebration of holidays, meals, music, and even elevator etiquette.

7. *Finances* included exploration of how to optimize occupational experiences and enjoyment of life on a marginal income.

8. The *Integrative Summary: Lifestyle Redesign Journal* allowed each participant to crystallize his or her occupational analysis by creating a book of ideas, pictures, and memories gathered during the 9-month program. It was hoped that the book would contribute to long-term retention of the occupational knowledge and adaptive patterns participants had attained.

The results of the study showed that the elders who received OT exhibited fewer declines in physical health, physical and social functioning, vitality, mental health, and life satisfaction than those assigned to the nonprofessionally led activity or control groups. These favorable outcomes led to the conclusion that preventive OT is capable of reducing the health risks of older adulthood, including the primary risk of physical dysfunction.[22]

Maintaining Physical Mobility: The ROM Dance Program

The **ROM Dance Program** (Fig. 8-1) is a preventive exercise and relaxation intervention that was created in 1981 by Diane Harlowe and Tricia Yu. The 7-minute ROM Dance incorporates whole-body range of motion with the movement principles of T'ai Chi Ch'uan. It is performed while listening to soothing music and lyrics that employ the archetypal images of healing: warm water, sunlight, and friendship. The ROM Dance was created as one of the three main elements of a preventive arthritis education program. The program consisted of eight weekly 90-minute sessions that also included relaxation and pain management techniques and education on joint protection, energy conservation, work

simplification, splints, and coping techniques. Long-term efficacy studies demonstrated the therapeutic effects of the ROM Dance Program for ambulatory adults with rheumatoid arthritis.[48-50]

The ROM Dance is an example of a preventive intervention technique that can be incorporated easily into clinical practice. Since its creation the ROM Dance has been used with and adapted for adults and children with a wide variety of painful or limiting conditions. A series of video and audio tapes have been developed to facilitate ease of use. In addition to the original Sunlight version, tapes are available for the Seated ROM Dance, adapted for those who use wheelchairs, and the Moonlight Version, adapted for those with lupus and sun sensitivity. A reclining version is under development for individuals confined to bed. Harlowe and Yu[18,19] provide lesson plans for teaching the ROM Dance in a series of health education classes, and Johnson, Searles, and McNamara[24] provide a detailed description for use in home health. The text, video tape, and audio tape resources are designed for self-instruction, and continuing education programs are also available for OT practitioners. These resources assist in using the ROM Dance throughout a continuum of care, as well as throughout the management of a disease.

FUTURE INITIATIVES IN PREVENTION

AOTA is acting to increase future roles for OT in prevention. One example is in the area of prevention of youth violence, an increasingly important risk factor for injuries that result in physical dysfunction. A paper titled *Occupational Therapy's Role in Preventing Youth Violence*[14] reviews the scope of the problem and the qualifications of OT practitioners to play an important role in prevention. Since youth violence is currently considered a grave public health problem in the United States, considerable funding has been earmarked for the development, implementation, and research of programs that target prevention of youth violence. One of the many ways that AOTA is addressing this issue is by seeking funding to evaluate OT's role in the implementation of the program described below.[41]

Prevention of Youth Violence: FAST Program

One highly successful, activity-based program that is well suited for involvement in and referral to by OT practitioners is titled **Family and Schools Together (FAST).** This well-researched program was created by Lynn McDonald, MSW, PhD, in 1988 and was showcased at the 1998 White House Conference on School Safety. FAST addresses youth violence by enhancing relationships with families, peers, teachers, school staff, and other members of the community. The program is a secondary prevention

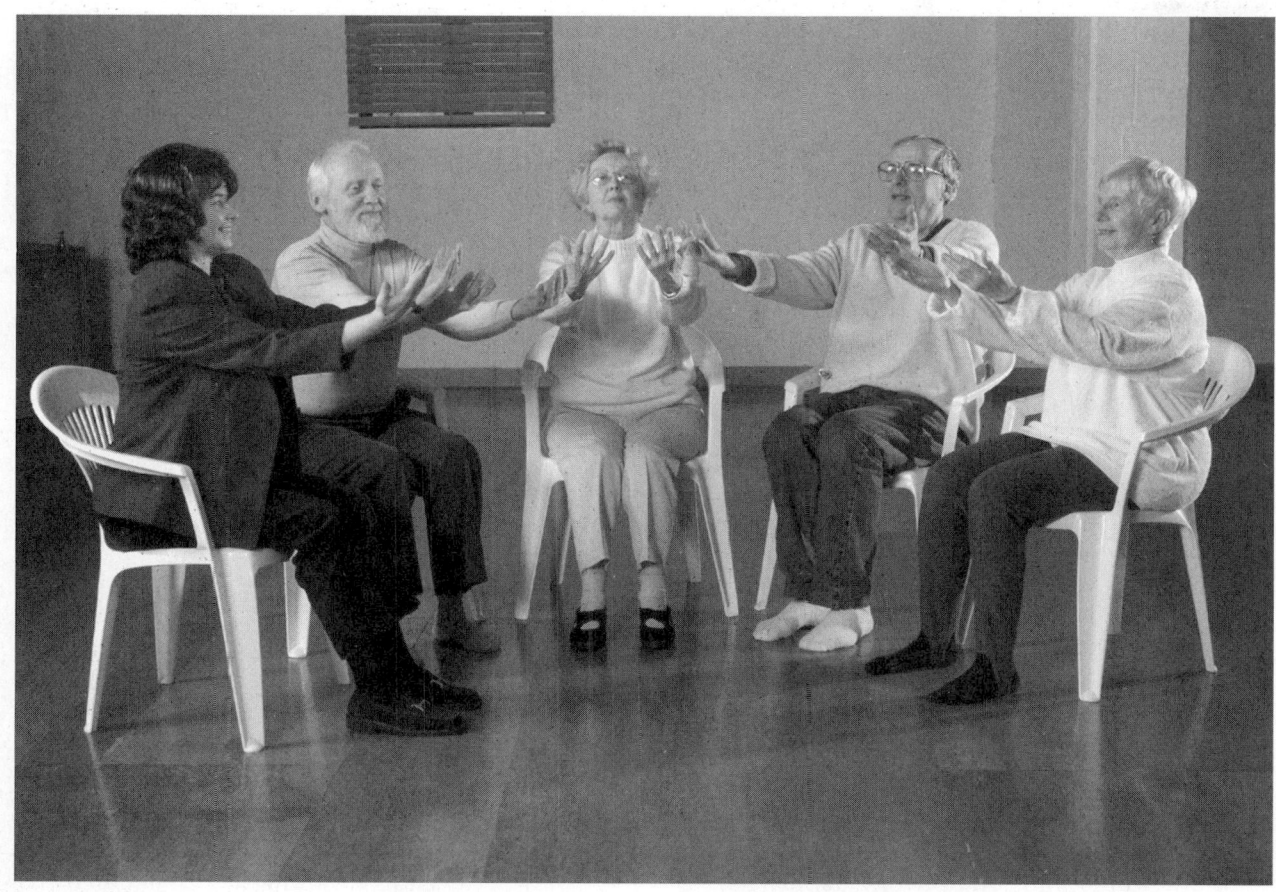

A

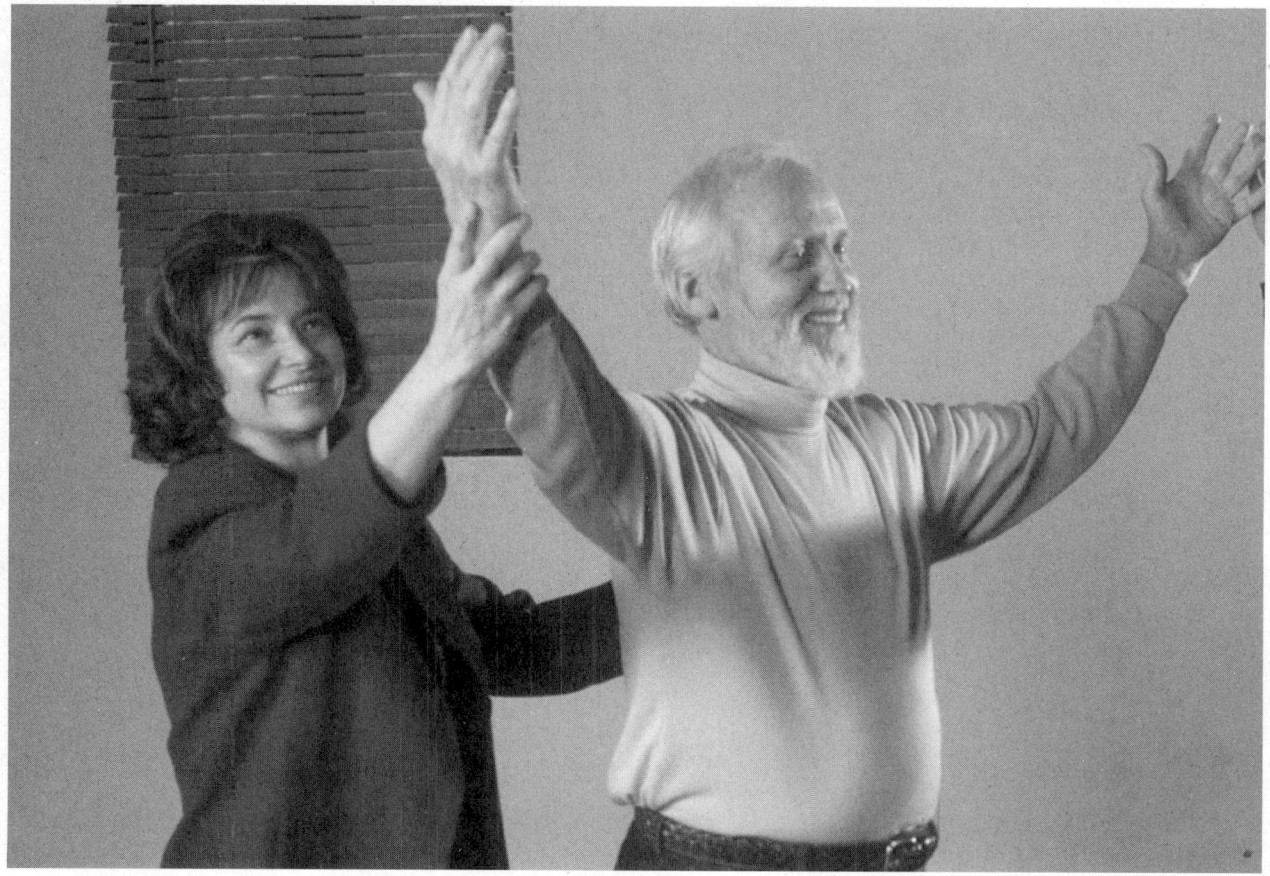

B

FIG. 8-1
Therapist instructing ROM dance. **A,** Dance instructed to a group. **B,** Assisting a client with alignment. (Photos by William J. Fritsch.)

strategy for children ages 4 to 14 who have been identified as at-risk through a school-based screening. The intent is to intervene early to prevent children from dropping out of school and becoming delinquent or violent. After 10 years of development and research, FAST was available in more that 450 schools in 31 states and 5 countries. Currently, it is also being provided to all interested families in three inner-city schools in Chicago and to a Native American tribe on a reservation in Wisconsin. A wide variety of funding sources have supported the program's cost per family of $1,200 for 86 hours of service delivered in over 30 sessions over a time span of 2 years.[30]

FAST is composed of three main elements: identification and outreach, multifamily activity sessions, and ongoing, monthly parent-run meetings for 2 years. During the outreach phase, an experienced FAST parent is paired with a professional to visit homes of identified children and their primary caretakers, who are often isolated and stressed and have a low income. The entire self-defined family is invited to join 10 to 15 other families for 8 to 10 weekly group meetings that comprise the second element of the program. Group sessions are composed of carefully crafted, structured, interactive activities that are repeated each week to establish ritual. Activities include:

1. A FAST welcome and creation of a family flag directed by the parent
2. A meal where the parent delegates a child to serve their family
3. A family drawing and talking game where the parent ensures each family member has a turn and inquires positively about others
4. A "feeling charades" game with the parent directing family members to "act out" or guess from selected feeling cards
5. Peer activities such as buddy time followed by a parent self-help group that builds an informal social support network in age-appropriate groupings
6. Parent-child special play time during which the parent is nondirective and nonjudgmental, following the child's lead for 15 uninterrupted minutes, with active coaching from the FAST team
7. A fixed lottery and meal preparation with each family highlighted as a "big winner," then responsible for cooking the meal the next week, thus encouraging reciprocal and respectful support
8. A closing circle and final ritual to build traditions across families and community members . . .[29]

Structured into these activities are opportunities for families to "behaviorally rehearse requests for compliance from the child in gradually more complex behaviors without using coercion; organizing family communication through systematic turn-taking with positive inquiry; repeated observation, identification, expression and labeling practices of eight basic emotions among family members; appropriate use and delegation of

parental power; playing responsively to create 'goodness of fit,' and supporting the child's delayed gratification."[33] During involvement in the entire program, parents spend 15 minutes a day in special play and peer support. Thus the program successfully affects the families' habituation systems (see Model of Human Occupation in Chapter 1), which may be one of the main factors contributing to its success.

The third element of the program begins after families graduate from the weekly sessions and join an ongoing, school-based collective of families who meet once a month for 2 years. This provides ongoing opportunities for community building and networking, which are valuable protective factors.

The efficacy with which this program uses activities to build protective factors for at-risk youth warrants attention and involvement from OT practitioners who may, in turn, enhance the intervention. Studies on evaluation of the effect of FAST on youth functioning include measures for conduct disorder and anxiety and withdrawal (factors identified as underlying mental health correlates predictive of violent behavior). One study involving 104 FAST children showed a statistically significant reduction in measures for both conduct disorder and anxiety withdrawal from the pretest to the posttest.[32] In another study of 197 children, parents and teachers reported statistically significant reductions of behaviors reflecting conduct disorder and anxiety withdrawal.[31] In the aforementioned studies, improvements were also shown in measures for attention span, socialized aggression, and motor excess. Six-month and 2-year follow-up data suggest that gains were maintained over time.[30] These results demonstrate FAST's effectiveness at reducing behaviors that can contribute to poor functioning in the school, social, and home environments where youth violence is apt to occur.

SUMMARY

OT prevention activities have expanded steadily during the past four decades. Possibilities for continued growth in this area are greater than ever before. Contemporary health care values are more firmly rooted in prevention, and occupational therapists are demonstrating the value of the profession's unique approach to intervention. With predictable and ongoing shifts in funding mechanisms, identifying opportunities to meet the needs of potential client populations will continue to be a challenge. Nevertheless, history predicts the future, and the adaptability and creativity inherent to the OT thought process will help in expanding the scope of OT prevention services in the decades to come. Accidents and activities that cause injury and physical dysfunction occur within the context of occupation, and prevention will continue to be a major focus of concern for occupational therapy.

REVIEW QUESTIONS

1. How does clinical reasoning facilitate the identification and provision of OT preventive intervention for clients receiving OT services?
2. Describe disability prevention in OT.
3. Why would the provision of instruction in joint protection and energy conservation to a client with inflammatory rheumatoid arthritis be classified as secondary prevention?
4. What is the first step in planning for the prevention of secondary conditions for OT clients who have a physical disability?
5. Summarize the main points of the "Health Belief Model," and describe how these issues affect the likelihood that an OT client will follow through on recommendations for preventive intervention.
6. How would an occupational therapist go about assessing clients' attitudes regarding health risks and preventive intervention?
7. Identify services provided by OT practitioners in primary, secondary, and tertiary prevention of falls.
8. How might an OT practitioner make use of research data on the risks for falls?
9. What is ergonomics?
10. Describe roles played by occupational therapists in preventing injuries in the workplace.
11. Why will ergonomics take on a new dimension in the future, and what are the implications for the practice of OT in this area?
12. Describe the eight occupational self-analysis content areas in the Well Elderly Study Occupational Therapy Program, and summarize the results of each.
13. For what population was the ROM Dance exercise and relaxation program originally developed, and in what ways has it been adapted for broader use?

REFERENCES

1. American Occupational Therapy Association, AOTA Representative Assembly minutes: The philosophical base of occupational therapy, *Am J Occup Ther* 33:780-813, 1979.
2. American Occupational Therapy Association, Commission on Practice: Occupational therapy in the promotion of health and the prevention of disease and disability: position paper, *Am J Occup Ther* 43(12):806, 1989.
3. American Occupational Therapy Association, Commission on Practice: Statement: occupational therapy services in work practice, position paper, *Am J Occup Ther* 46(12):1086-1088, 1992.
4. Baum CM, Law M: Occupational therapy practice: focusing on occupational performance, *Am J Occup Ther* 51(4):277-288, 1997.
5. Baum C, LaVesser P: Caregiver assistance: using family members and attendants. In Christiansen C, editor: *Ways of living: self care strategies for special needs*, Bethesda, Md, 1994, American Occupational Therapy Association.
6. Bellin Occupational Health: *Rehabilitation*, unpublished program description, Green Bay, Wisc, 1995.
7. Boston University Roybal Center for Enhancement of Late Life Function: *A matter of balance*, program described online at www.bu.edu/roybal.
8. Cancio LI, Cashman TM: Self-reported cumulative trauma symptoms among hospital employees: analysis of an upper-extremity symptom survey, *Am J Occup Ther* 53(2):227-230, 1999.
9. Carayon P, Smith RO: Physical and mental strain in computerized workplaces: causes and remedies. In Rothman J, Levine R, editors: *Prevention practice: strategies for physical therapy and occupational therapy*, Philadelphia, 1992, WB Saunders.
10. Claiborne D, Williams K: Cost-effective ergonomics, *OT Practice* September 1998, pp 47-48.
11. Clark F, Azen SP, Zemke R, et al: Occupational therapy for independent-living older adults: a randomized controlled trial, *JAMA* 278:1321-1326, 1997.
12. Cook A, Miller PA: Prevention of falls in the elderly. In Larson KO, Stevens-Ratchford RG, Pedretti L, et al: *ROTE: the role of OT with the elderly*, ed 2, Bethesda, Md, 1996, American Occupational Therapy Association.
13. Czaja SJ: Safety and security of the elderly: implications for smart house design, *Int J Technol Aging* 1(1):49-48, 1988.
14. Daunhauer L, Jacobs K: Occupational therapy's role in preventing youth violence. Available online at www.aota.org/nonmembers/area8/links/link02.asp.
15. Department of Health and Family Services of Wisconsin: *Pathways to independence*. Available online at www.dhfs.state.wi.us.
16. Grossman J: A prevention model for occupational therapy, *Am J Occup Ther* 45(1):33-41, 1991.
17. Hanson CS: Ergonomics in health care, *Am J Occup Ther* 51(8):701-703, 1996.
18. Harlowe D, Yu PB: *The ROM Dance: a range of motion exercise and relaxation program*, Madison, Wisc, 1992, St. Mary's Hospital Medical Center and University of Wisconsin, Madison.
19. Harlowe D, Yu P: *ROM Dance instructional materials*, material online at www.romdance.com, Uncharted Country Mind/Body Resources
20. Holliday PJ, Cott CA, Torresin WD: Preventing accidental falls by the elderly. In Rothman J, Levine R, editors: *Prevention practice: strategies for physical therapy and occupational therapy*, Philadelphia, 1992, WB Saunders.
21. Isernhagen SJ: Corporate fitness and prevention of industrial injuries. In Rothman J, Levine R, editors: *Prevention practice: strategies for physical therapy and occupational therapy*, Philadelphia, 1992, WB Saunders.
22. Jackson J, Carlson M, Mandel D, et al: Occupation in lifestyle redesign: the well elderly study occupational therapy program, *Am J Occup Ther* 52(5):326-336, 1998.
23. Janz NK, Becker MN: The health belief model: a decade later, *Health Educ* 11:1-48, 1984.
24. Johansson C: The "back guy" conquers corporate culture, *OT Week*, July 1998, pp 10-11.
25. Johnson J, Searles L, McNamara S: In-home geriatric rehabilitation: improving strength and function, *Top Geriatric Rehabil* 8(3):51-64, 1993.
26. King PM, Gratz R, Scheuer G, et al: The ergonomics of child care: conducting worksite analyses, *Work*, 25-32, 1996.
27. Kniepmann K: Prevention of disability and maintenance of health. In Christiansen CH, Baum CM, editors: *Occupational therapy: enabling function and well-being*, ed 2, Thorofare, NJ, 1997, Slack.
28. Llorens L: *Consultation in the community: occupational therapy in child health*, Dubuque, Iowa, 1973, Kendall/Hunt Publishing.
29. McDonald L, Billingham S, Conrad T, et al: Families and schools together (FAST): integrating community development with clinical strategies, *Families in Society* March, 1997.
30. McDonald L, Howard D: Families and schools together, *Office of Juvenile Justice and Delinquency fact sheet* 88: December 1998.
31. McDonald L, Payton E, Sayger T, et al: Increasing protective factors for mental health in Head Start children through outreach and multifamily FAST groups, *National Head Start Research Conference*, Washington, DC, 1998.

32. McDonald L, Sayger TV: Impact of a family and school-based prevention program on protective factors for high-risk youth, *Drugs and Society* 12:61-85, 1998.

33. McDonald L, Sayger T, Payton E, Whitfield H: Systematically building multiple protective factors to increase Head Start children's mental health: the evaluated and replicated multifamily FAST program, *Summary of conference proceedings, Head Start's Fourth National Research Conference*, 1998.

34. McKean L: ROM Dance is a therapeutic intervention in OT well elderly lifestyle redesign study, *ROM Dance Newsletter* 1:1, 1999.

35. Morse JM: *Preventing patient falls*, Thousand Oaks, Calif, 1997, Sage Publications.

36. Moyers PA: Guide to occupational therapy practice, *Am J Occup Ther* 53: 247-322, 1999.

37. Plautz B, Beck DE, Selmar C, et al: Modifying the environment: a community-based injury-reduction program for elderly residents, *Am J Prev Med* 12(4) (suppl):33-38, 1996.

38. Occupational Safety and Health Administration guidelines. Online at www.osha.gov.

39. Reitz SM: A historical review of occupational therapy's role in preventive health and wellness, *Am J Occup Ther* 46(1):50-55, 1992.

40. Rothman J, Levine R, editors: *Prevention practice: strategies for physical therapy and occupational therapy*, Philadelphia, 1992, WB Saunders.

41. Scheinholtz M: *Evaluating occupational therapy's role in implementing the FAST program*, Bethesda, Md, 2000, American Occupational Therapy Association (unpublished).

42. Tarlov A, Pope A: *Disability in America: toward a national agenda for prevention*, Washington, DC, 1991, Institute of Medicine, National Academy Press

43. Tennstedt S, Howland J, Lachman M: A randomized controlled trial of a group: intervention to reduce fear of falling and associated activity restriction in older adults, *J Gerontol B Psychol Sci Soc Sci* 53B:384-392, 1998.

44. Tideiksaar R: Falls in nursing home residents, *Long-Term Care Forum*, Fall 1991, pp 12-14.

45. U.S. Department of Health and Human Services, Public Health Services: *Healthy people 2000—national health promotion and disease prevention objectives*, DHHS Publication No. (PHS) 91-50212, Washington, DC, 1991, US Government Printing Office.

46. US Department of Health and Human Services, National Conference on the Prevention of Primary and Secondary Disabilities: *Building partnerships towards health–reducing the risks for disability*, Atlanta, 1991, Centers for Disease Control and Prevention.

47. Vanderschmidt HF, Koch-Weser D, Woodbury PA: *Handbook of clinical prevention*, Baltimore, 1987, Williams & Wilkins.

48. Van Deusen J, Harlowe D: One-year follow-up results of ROM Dance research, *Occup Ther J Res* 8(1):53-54, 1988.

49. Van Deusen J, Harlowe D: A comparison of the ROM Dance home exercise rest program with traditional routines, *Occup Ther J Res* 7:349-361, 1987.

50. Van Deusen J, Harlowe D: The efficacy of the ROM Dance Program for adults with rheumatoid arthritis, *Am J Occup Ther* 41:90-95, 1987.

51. West W: The occupational therapist's changing responsibility to the community, *Am J Occup Ther* 21(5):312-316, 1967.

52. West W: The growing importance of prevention, *Am J Occup Ther* 23(3), 1969.

53. Wiemer R: Some concepts of prevention as an aspect of community health, *Am J Occup Ther* 26(1):312-316, 1972.

54. Williams R: *Preventing and treating carpal tunnel syndrome*, Baltimore, 1994, American Occupational Therapy Association.

CHAPTER 9

Teaching Activities in Occupational Therapy

JOYCE SHAPERO SABARI

KEY TERMS

Activity analysis
Activity adaptation
Activity synthesis
Training versus learning
Skill acquisition
Skill retention
Skill generalization
Closed tasks
Open tasks
Procedural versus declarative learning
Implicit and explicit learning processes
Strategy
Metacognition
Intrinsic and extrinsic feedback
Knowledge of performance feedback
Knowledge of results feedback
Contextual interference
Blocked and random practice schedules
Whole versus part practice
Practice context

LEARNING OBJECTIVES

After studying this chapter the student or practitioner will be able to do the following:
1. Identify a variety of situations in which occupational therapists analyze, adapt, and synthesize activities.
2. Discuss specific outcome goals for which occupational therapists teach activities.
3. Distinguish between training and learning in terms of therapeutic goals and intervention strategies.
4. Analyze how therapeutic interventions will differ, depending on the various types of learning processes a client needs to develop.
5. Apply current knowledge about factors that influence the teaching-learning process to occupational therapy interventions.
6. Implement occupational therapy treatment designed to promote active strategy development.
7. Provide appropriate instruction, feedback, and practice tailored to individual tasks and client goals.
8. Promote generalization of learning to real-life situations through effective approaches to teaching activity.

ACTIVITY: A CRITICAL COMPONENT OF OCCUPATIONAL THERAPY INTERVENTION

Occupational therapists are activity experts. Regardless of diagnosis or treatment setting, enhanced activity performance is an ultimate goal of occupational therapy (OT) intervention. In addition, activity performance often serves as a tool in the intervention process to help clients meet their OT goals.[10]

In the context of intervention for clients with physical disabilities, occupational therapists do the following:
1. Analyze activities
2. Adapt activities
3. Synthesize activities
4. Teach activities

Activity Analysis, Adaptation, and Synthesis

Occupational therapists perform an **activity analysis** for the activities that clients are required or wish to perform. One reason for such analysis is to determine an activity's long-range effect on the client's health. A detailed assessment of an activity's ergonomic effects on musculoskeletal function enables the therapist to recommend or institute appropriate adaptations to the environment and the procedure in order to prevent repetitive stress injuries. Analysis of an activity's energy requirements provides a foundation for adaptations designed to maximize the client's cardiovascular and muscular endurance capabilities.

A second reason occupational therapists analyze activities is to determine the extent to which specific performance components are needed. After this analysis the therapist determines which performance component deficits are contributing to the client's difficulties performing selected activities in specific contexts. Next, the therapist determines the client's potential to improve these performance components. If there is realistic potential for improvement, the occupational therapist develops a program to improve the performance components. The ultimate goal is that the client will use the enhanced skills and be able to perform the identified activities, as well as a myriad of unanticipated tasks.

At times a review of medical data and evaluation findings indicates a low potential for improvement in an identified performance component. In these situations occupational therapists teach performance of selected activities with adaptations that enable individuals to engage in desired occupations despite continuing limitations in performance components.

Activity adaptation is the modification of well-recognized tasks. Occupational therapists are skilled at adapting the context, materials, or rules of familiar activities to achieve two general goals. First, therapists adapt activities to make performance easier or safer, based on knowledge of individual clients' available performance components and health risks. Second, therapists adapt activity features when activity engagement is designed as a therapeutic challenge to help the client develop improved function in selected performance components.

Activity synthesis is the development of new and often unfamiliar activities. As with activity adaptation, occupational therapists synthesize new activities for two general purposes. First, a newly synthesized activity may be designed to create a unique option for accomplishing a given occupation or satisfying specific rule requirements. Second, synthesized activities such as short-term games or novel challenges provide therapeutic opportunities for clients to practice meeting performance component goals.

Students and therapists who are reading this text have already learned the foundations of activity analysis, adaptation, and synthesis in previous OT course work. The goal of this chapter is to introduce principles and guidelines to enhance the effectiveness of teaching activities in the context of occupational therapy intervention.

When and Why Occupational Therapists Teach Activities

A significant portion of OT intervention entails teaching activities. When cognitive impairments limit an individual's ability to remember procedures and precautions associated with tasks of daily living, occupational therapists reteach familiar activities.

New ways of performing familiar activities are taught to clients with a wide spectrum of illnesses, injuries, and disabilities. Often, these new procedures are taught to help clients compensate for short- or long-term performance component impairments or restrictions. In other situations the new procedures are designed to enhance the activity's safety for clients with specified risks or vulnerabilities. An office worker is taught new strategies for using her computer to prevent repetitive stress injury and reduce musculoskeletal pain. A client recovering from coronary bypass surgery learns new ways of performing familiar activities to minimize cardiovascular demands. After hip replacement surgery a client learns alternative methods that allow him or her to continue performing daily tasks within the constraints of temporary orthopedic contraindications. A client with balance impairments caused by neuromuscular disease learns to perform upright activities in ways that will minimize the risk of falls.

Occupational therapists teach new activities for meeting medical or therapeutic goals. Persons with newly acquired disabilities and illnesses need to learn activities that were not in their previous repertoire of required tasks. Often they must learn to perform these tasks within the constraints of performance component limitations. Such activities range from managing a bowel and bladder routine after spinal cord injury to self-administering insulin injections with hemiparesis. Performing home exercise routines, managing personal care attendants, maneuvering a wheelchair, using assistive technology, and donning orthotic devices are other examples of these activities.

Finally, occupational therapists teach activities that will serve as therapeutic challenges to help individuals improve performance components. Before engaging in a board game that will elicit repetitive, resisted muscle contractions, the client who is recovering from a peripheral nerve injury needs to learn how the activity should be performed. The therapist teaches the client how to position his or her body, the game board, and the game pieces so that the activity will have the maximum therapeutic impact. Before beginning a kitchen activity that has been designed to provide balance and cognitive challenges to a client coping with residual impairments from a brain injury, the therapist teaches the client the salient features of the therapeutic task. This may include adaptations that enhance the activity's relevant challenges to the client's performance components, as well as strategic recommendations for maximizing performance.

When occupational therapists teach activities, the ultimate goal is functional task performance. At the very least this requires that the client learn to perform the activity outside of the treatment setting and apart from the therapist's supervision. The goals of teaching will vary, depending on the severity of each individual's physical and cognitive limitations. If caregiver supervision will always be needed, it is the therapist's responsibility to include caregivers in the process of activity learning. For clients who expect to resume independent function, the therapist's teaching methods must ensure generalization of learning to a variety of contexts and related tasks. Furthermore, a successful occupational therapist uses learning principles that are appropriate to meeting the selected goals.

PRINCIPLES OF TEACHING ACTIVITY

Occupational therapists structure the environment, the task goals, and interactions with each client to maximize the teaching-learning process (Fig. 9-1).

Types of Learning Processes

Training Versus Learning Outcomes

The goal of **training** is for the client to memorize a prescribed solution to a selected task challenge, whereas the goal of **learning** is for the client to develop his or her own solution, which can be applied in a variety of situations.[5] Based on each client's abilities and role demands, the occupational therapist determines whether the teaching goal will be to promote training or learning. Both training and learning entail **skill acquisition** and **skill retention** (Table 9-1).

Skill acquisition occurs during initial instruction and practice. **Skill retention,** which is demonstrated after the initial practice session, is often referred to as *carryover.* A major distinction between training and learning is that **skill generalization** is an outcome of learning, but not of training. When the occupational therapist chooses a training approach, task practice must occur in the actual setting in which the individual plans to perform the task. Unless the person actively develops a personal performance strategy, there is no evidence that skill acquisition and retention can be transferred to contexts other than the training situation.[9,21,23]

Frequently, the OT goal is that a client will generalize, or transfer, skills learned in the therapy setting and use them in multiple real-life contexts. Several principles presented later in this chapter guide the therapist's teaching strategies when generalization of learning is the outcome goal.

Gentile's Taxonomy of Task Categories

One scheme for classifying activities is based on two dimensions of task-related environmental features. First, the supporting surfaces and task objects may be either stationary or in motion. Second, the environmental features may vary between one performance of the task to the next or remain unchanged between trials.[3] Occupational therapists can use this task classification system to guide the choice of teaching strategies.[16]

The use of repetitive practice (training) as a strategy for learning is effective only with **closed tasks,** or activities in which the supporting surfaces and task objects are stationary and do not vary between performance trials. Most daily activities, however, necessitate adaptation to changing environmental conditions in different situations and at different times. In Gentile's taxonomy, these are categorized as variable motionless tasks. For example, motor requirements for drinking beverages will vary, depending on the type of mug, cup, or glass that is used, as well as on how much the container is filled. Independent dressing requires that a person achieve mastery over putting on clothing of varying styles, dimensions, and fabrics.

Open tasks are characterized by an unpredictable motion of supporting surfaces or task objects during task performance. These activities necessitate the appropriate timing of responses, as well as spatial anticipation of where relevant objects will be moving. For example, when sitting in a moving train, a passenger must maintain balance when the supporting surface is moving unpredictably. When crossing a street, an individual must anticipate the speed and rhythm of both pedestrians and oncoming traffic. When playing most ball games, competitors must predict the speed and direction of the ball to position themselves in the right place at the right time. Research has shown that the skills required for

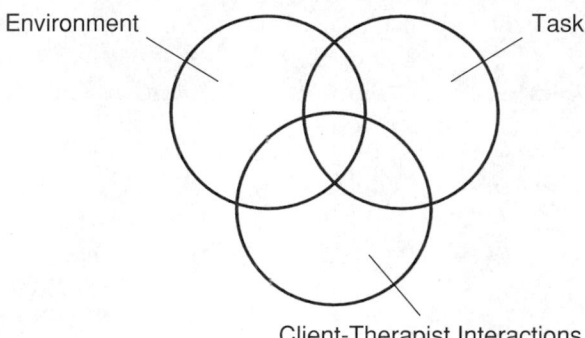

Fig. 9-1
Teaching-learning process in occupational therapy.

| TABLE 9-1 |
| Stages of Skill Development |

Training	Learning
Stage one: skill acquisition	Stage one: skill acquisition
Stage two: skill retention	Stage two: skill retention
	Stage three: skill generalization

successful open-task performance cannot be learned through repetitive practice in a stationary environment.[6]

Procedural Versus Declarative Learning

A popular categorization of memory[24] has been adapted[19] to represent the degree to which awareness, attention, or other cortical processes are used during skill acquisition, retention, and performance. **Declarative learning** is needed for tasks in which language skills are used to organize and practice complex sequences of action. Learning a new recipe or a multistep dance routine may require that a person be able to consciously express the processes to be performed. Mental rehearsal is an effective technique for enhancing declarative learning. During mental rehearsal the individual practices the sequence by reviewing it silently or articulating the process orally or in writing.

Procedural learning is accomplished without a significant language component and is effective when learning tasks that are typically performed automatically. Procedural learning is developed through task practice in a series of varying contexts. An individual learns to maneuver a wheelchair through a process of procedural learning. Verbal instruction alone is of little value. Rather, a person learns the procedures for performing this novel motor activity through opportunities, while sitting in the wheelchair, to experiment with different combinations of arm or arm and leg movements to achieve propulsion in a variety of directions and speeds. It is the occupational therapist's responsibility to determine whether procedural or declarative learning is most appropriate for each specific goal and individual.

Implicit Versus Explicit Learning Processes

Gentile[4] proposes that individuals use two distinct but interdependent processes during the acquisition of functional motor skills. An **explicit learning process,** which is consciously driven, guides the kinematics of the movement. Gentile hypothesizes that people use an explicit process to develop a "ballpark" match between the shape or direction of their movements and the environmental requirements for achieving the goal. External feedback is likely to have a beneficial effect on the explicit learning process.

An **implicit learning process** guides the kinetics of the movement, or the dynamics of force generation. This aspect of movement requires appropriate selection of muscle contraction patterns, determined by accurate predictions of how external forces will affect the movement. Gentile hypothesizes that "the refinement of force dynamics is due to a self-organizing process of implicit learning."[4] This self-organizing process may take longer to develop than explicit learning. Furthermore, implicit learning lies beyond conscious awareness and is unlikely to be augmented by external feedback.

Factors That Influence the Teaching-Learning Process

The literature about skill development presents several concepts that are helpful in guiding occupational therapists when teaching activities to clients (Box 9-1).

Learner's Active Participation

Learning is an active process. Although passive interventions such as massage or physical manipulation may be useful procedures for achieving some OT goals, they do not contribute to the learning process. Clients are most likely to learn new skills when they are active participants in setting and clearly understanding the outcome goals. When declarative learning is the appropriate mechanism for both the task and the client, it may be helpful for the therapist to periodically ask the client to rephrase the objectives and procedures for task performance.

Strategy Development

Strategies are organized plans or sets of rules that guide action in a variety of situations.[15] *Motor strategies* include the vast repertoire of kinematic and kinetic linkages that underlie performance of skilled, efficient movement. *Cognitive strategies* include the multiple and varied tactics people use to facilitate processing, storage, retrieval, and manipulation of. *Interpersonal strategies* help in social interactions with other individuals. *Coping strategies* allow people to adapt constructively to stress.

Strategies provide individuals with foundational skills that can be adapted to the ever-changing demands of occupations within the infinite variations of multiple environments. Thus learning is more likely to be generalized to new situations when people are given opportunities to develop foundational strategies.[21] People develop strategies through a process of encountering problems, implementing solutions, and monitoring the effects of these solutions. Occupational therapists use

---

BOX 9-1

Factors That Support Generalization of Learning

Active participation
Strategy development
Externally focused instruction
Intrinsic feedback
Practice conditions
    Contextual interference
    Random practice schedules
    Naturalistic contexts
    Whole-task practice

activities to help clients develop useful strategies by structuring tasks, within a safe environment, that provide individuals with opportunities to try out different solutions to the challenges that arise.[14]

Self-awareness and self-monitoring skills are critical prerequisites to a person's ability to generate and apply appropriate strategies. **Metacognition** is the knowledge and regulation of personal cognitive processes and capacities.[8] It includes an awareness of personal strengths and limitations and the ability to evaluate task difficulty, plan ahead, choose appropriate strategies, and shift strategies in response to environmental cues.

Toglia's dynamic interactional model[22,23] for individuals with cognitive impairments after brain injury emphasizes the importance of metacognition. Self-review of performance and guided planning for tackling the challenges of future tasks are key factors in the therapeutic process.

Although metacognition is typically discussed in relation to improving cognitive skills, self-awareness and monitoring of relevant performance components may be equally important prerequisites to developing effective motor, interpersonal, and coping strategies. Specifically, intervention directed toward helping clients develop enhanced awareness of body kinematics and alignment may be an important component to motor learning.[1]

Instruction

Therapeutic instruction provides cues that orient the client to selected performance guidelines. Instruction can be presented verbally, visually, or tactokinesthetically.

Verbal instruction related to activity performance may be most useful when words are kept to a minimum. Particularly when clients exhibit language or other cognitive impairments, excessive banter from a therapist may distract clients from attending to relevant visual and somatosensory cues from the environment and from their own bodies.

Visual instruction may be provided through the therapist's own performance of the task. In addition, photographs and line drawings provide powerful visual cues about optimal postural alignment or the appropriate sequence required for task performance.

Somatosensory instructions provide cues through tactile and kinesthetic channels. Manual guidance[2] is often an effective technique for providing specific instructions about the recommended direction and speed (kinematics) of a functional movement. Manual guidance may be more effective than verbal or visual instructions when procedural, rather than declarative learning, is the outcome goal.

Regardless of the sensory channel, instructions for learning may elicit either an internal or an external focus of attention.[28] A considerable amount of research evidence[18,28] suggests that body-related instructions (an internal focus) are less effective than instructions related to the effect of a performer's action on the environment (an external focus). Occupational therapists are particularly skillful at structuring therapeutic tasks so that a critically selected effect of a movement, rather than a feature of the movement itself, becomes the instructional focus. For example, when the performance component goal is to promote scapular abduction to improve the efficiency of forward reach, better outcomes are achieved when clients with traumatic brain injury are instructed to externally focus on reaching to control a game panel, as compared with when they are instructed to internally focus on how far they can reach an arm forward.[20] Similarly, Nelson and colleagues[11] have shown that treatment designed to improve coordinated forearm pronation-supination is more effective in stroke rehabilitation when clients are instructed to externally focus on turning an adapted dice-thrower in the context of a game, as compared with when they are instructed to internally focus on the movement itself. Wu and colleagues[27] found that intervention to improve symmetrical posture in adults with hemiplegia had significantly better outcomes when an external focus of attention, integrated into wood sanding and bean bag toss games, was elicited by the activity synthesis and therapeutic instruction.

Feedback

Feedback, or information about a response,[12] can be intrinsic or extrinsic, concurrent or terminal, and can provide knowledge of performance or results. **Intrinsic feedback** is a result of an individual's proprioceptive, tactile, vestibular, visual, and auditory sensory systems. A person learning to use a computer keyboard first uses visual feedback to see if his or her fingers are positioned properly and if he or she is depressing the correct keys. Quickly, the individual progresses to relying on tactile and proprioceptive feedback about finger alignment and keystrokes. This frees the individual to look at the manuscript while typing.

Extrinsic feedback is information from an outside source. The typed manuscript, as projected on the monitor or printed on hard copy, provides extrinsic feedback about the results of the typist's actions. Another person can provide extrinsic feedback about task performance by giving information to the typist about body alignment, hand positioning, and key selection. Although extrinsic feedback may be helpful early in the learning process, the typist will achieve greater independence and efficiency in computer activities by developing the ability to continue learning through intrinsic, rather than extrinsic, feedback.

Occupational therapists often work with clients whose sensory recognition or processing abilities have been impaired. In these situations, extrinsic feedback from a therapist or technological device can provide useful supplementary information to facilitate early awareness and learning.

Therapists need to remember that inaccurate feedback provides confusing information to clients about the outcome of their attempts at task performance. Clear differences between praise for effort and positive verbal feedback about performance must be established.

Technological feedback mechanisms include electromyographic and electrogoniometric biofeedback systems, as well as digital displays of pertinent kinetic or cardiovascular data on computerized exercise equipment. These feedback systems provide information that is more timely, more consistent, and more accurate than feedback from a human therapist. However, true generalization of learning can never occur unless a person learns to generate and respond to intrinsic feedback. Therefore, extrinsic feedback must be gradually decreased if the client's goal is independent performance in a wide variety of unanticipated task situations.

Concurrent feedback, provided in an ongoing fashion during task performance, may be intrinsic or extrinsic. Terminal, or summary, feedback is given after task completion. There are no published studies that compare the effectiveness of concurrent and terminal feedback.

KNOWLEDGE OF PERFORMANCE AND KNOWLEDGE OF RESULTS. Knowledge of performance feedback (KP) is information about the processes used during task performance.[19] Performance factors of interest to occupational therapists include kinetic and kinematic components of movement, as well as specific cognitive and interpersonal strategies. KP may play a role in dynamically guiding performance as it occurs. **Knowledge of results feedback (KR)** is feedback about the outcome of an action in terms of accomplishing an intended goal.[19] KR can serve as a basis for more effective performance in future trials. In the computer keyboard example presented earlier, KP was illustrated by the typist's intrinsically generated information about finger alignment and keystrokes, as well as by the extrinsically generated feedback about these performance factors that was provided by another person. KR was illustrated by the information about typing accuracy, as provided by the soft copy or print version of the text the typist produced. Typing speed, measured in words per minute, also provides KR.

Extrinsic KR has been more widely studied than KP; however, most published research has been related to normal subjects performing contrived tasks in laboratory settings. Results of laboratory research with normal subjects supports the view that intrinsic feedback is more critical than extrinsic feedback to skill generalization. Studies have shown that frequent, accurate, immediate KR tends to promote improved performance during the acquisition phase of learning, but poorer

performance during the retention and transfer stages.[17,26] Similarly, bandwidth KR, in which feedback is provided only when the performance response is outside a given range of acceptable performance, leads to better generalization of learning.[26] Schmidt[18] hypothesizes that, when limited KR is provided during acquisition, individuals are forced to rely on relevant cues provided by intrinsic mechanisms to improve their performance on future trials. Thus they tend to depend less on extrinsic feedback.

How can occupational therapists help clients develop effective intrinsic feedback mechanisms? First, therapists can provide clients with effective models of action[2] and awareness of what proprioceptive and tactile feedback should accompany appropriate performance strategies.[13] Therapists can achieve this with clear visual and proprioceptive instruction through manual guidance, visual modeling, and understandable figures or photographs. Next, therapists can provide clients with active opportunities to perform tasks under varying contextual conditions. In addition, therapists strive to achieve a balance between providing extrinsic feedback and requiring that clients continually assess their own performance. Finally, therapists help clients actively set their own goals and determine strategies for improving future task performance.

Practice Conditions

Practice is a powerful component of the occupational therapy process. The ways in which a therapist structures the practice conditions can influence a client's success in meeting performance goals.

CONTEXTUAL INTERFERENCE. Contextual interference refers to factors in the learning environment that increase the difficulty of initial learning. Limited KR is one example of contextual interference that has already been discussed. As shown by studies of KR, these factors tend to promote more effective retention and generalization. One explanation for this finding is that a high level of contextual interference forces a person to "use multiple and variable processes to overcome the difficulty of practice."[29] Furthermore, people develop more elaborate memory representations of the underlying strategies that were used for task achievement during the acquisition phase of learning.

BLOCKED AND RANDOM PRACTICE SCHEDULES. Blocked and random practice schedules are examples of low and high contextual interference, respectively. During **blocked practice,** clients practice one task until they master it. This is followed by practice of a second task until it is also mastered. In **random practice,** clients attempt multiple tasks or variations of a task before they have mastered any one of the tasks. A random practice schedule may be used in an OT program designed to teach wheelchair transfer skills. The client is introduced to several transfer situations and asked to practice each of them during the course of a single session. For example, the client will practice moving between the wheelchair and a therapy mat, between wheelchair and chair, and between a toilet and the wheelchair. Blocked practice schedules are generally chosen when training is the long-term goal. However, when a client shows potential to generalize learning, a random practice schedule is preferred.

WHOLE VERSUS PART PRACTICE. Therapists may intuitively believe that it will be easier for a client to learn small segments of a task before learning how to perform the task in its entirety. However, breaking a task into its component parts for teaching purposes is useful only if the task can naturally be divided into recognizable units.[25] This is because continuous skills (or whole task performance) are easier to remember than discrete responses.[18] For example, once a person has learned to ride a bicycle, he or she will retain this motor skill even without practicing for many years. On the other hand, segmented laboratory-type motor skills may be acquired easily but are less likely to be retained over time. Therapists are advised to teach such tasks in their entirety rather than in artificial segments. For example, for best retention and generalization, it is better to teach putting on a shirt as a complete task than to practice a different portion of the task during each therapy session. If it is difficult for a client to master all the steps at once, the therapist may provide cuing or manual guidance for selected aspects of the task. This way, the client experiences completion of the task on each trial, and the therapist gradually gives less assistance as practice sessions continue.

PRACTICE CONTEXTS. Only closed tasks[4] are always performed under identical environmental conditions. All other activities necessitate that the individual demonstrate versatility of performance. Practice under variable contexts enhances generalization of learning and helps the individual achieve this versatility. For example, wheelchair mobility is practiced on a variety of indoor and outdoor surfaces. Self-feeding is practiced with a variety of utensils and types of food. Furthermore, if self-feeding is a particularly difficult challenge for a client because of severe physical or cognitive limitations, OT feeding practice will occur in a variety of environments— alone in one's hospital room or home kitchen, as well as in group settings, such as a cafeteria or a restaurant.

SUMMARY

Occupational therapists analyze, adapt, synthesize, and teach activities to clients with physical disabilities. The

purposes of activity-based intervention are to enhance specific activity performance and help clients improve performance components that will enable them to perform a vast number of anticipated and unanticipated tasks. Occupational therapists reteach familiar activities, teach new ways of performing familiar activities, teach new activities for meeting therapeutic goals, and teach activities that will serve as therapeutic challenges to help clients improve performance components.

Occupational therapists implement a variety of teaching strategies designed to promote skill acquisition, retention, and generalization. Teaching methods are based on principles developed from research on learning and are selectively chosen on an individual basis. Different principles will be integrated into OT treatment, based on a variety of factors:

1. Whether training or learning is the outcome goal
2. The type of task an individual needs to learn
3. The learning processes associated with the task goals

Active participation and strategy development are key features of effective learning. Occupational therapists maximize the learning process by (1) helping clients develop self-awareness and self-monitoring skills, (2) providing effective instruction tailored to individual needs, (3) implementing feedback strategies that augment each individual's learning goals, and (4) conducting therapeutic interventions in practice contexts that maximize skill generalization and task performance in each client's expected real-life environment.

REVIEW QUESTIONS

1. Provide examples, other than those described in the chapter, of how occupational therapists analyze, adapt, synthesize, and teach activities in interventions for clients with physical disabilities.
2. What is the difference between skill acquisition, retention, and generalization? Apply these terms to describe the learning stages in a client you have observed.
3. What is the difference between closed tasks, variable motionless tasks, and open tasks? How will teaching methods differ between these types of tasks?
4. When are declarative learning and procedural learning processes used? How will teaching methods differ when declarative or procedural processes are required?
5. How can occupational therapists help clients develop metacognitive skills? Why are these skills important in the learning process?
6. In which situations is extrinsic feedback valuable to the therapeutic process? What are some advantages and disadvantages to providing extrinsic feedback to clients?

7. How will a therapist structure a therapeutic activity to present instructions that elicit an external, rather than an internal, focus of attention?

8. What is the difference between KP and KR feedback? Give an example of how KP feedback can be provided by using an external, rather than an internal, focus of attention.

9. Why does contextual interference contribute to generalization of learning? Think of an example, other than those described in the chapter, of how contextual interference can be incorporated into an OT session.

10. Differentiate between random and blocked practice schedules. In which situations would each of these practice schedules be chosen?

11. Provide examples of how a therapist might structure whole practice versus part practice. In which situations might each of these types of practice be appropriate?

12. In which ways can occupational therapists enhance the variability of practice contexts? Give practical examples of how occupational therapists working in inpatient settings can provide treatment in natural contexts.

REFERENCES

1. Carr JH, Shepherd RB: *Neurological rehabilitation: optimizing motor performance*, Oxford, Eng,1998, Butterworth Heinemann.

2. Carr JH, Shepherd RB: *A motor relearning program for stroke*, ed 2, Rockville, Md, 1987, Aspen.

3. Gentile AM: Implicit and explicit processes during acquisition of functional skills, *Scand J Occup Ther* 5:7-16, 1998.

4. Gentile AM: A working model of skill acquisition with application to teaching, *Quest* 17:3-23, 1972.

5. Higgins S: Motor skill acquisition, *Phys Ther* 71(2):123-139, 1991.

6. Higgins JR, Spaeth RK: Relationship between consistency of movement and environmental condition, *Quest* 17:61-69, 1972.

7. Jarus T: Motor learning and occupational therapy: the organization of practice, *Am J Occup Ther* 48(9):810-816, 1994.

8. Katz N, Hartman-Maier A: Metacognition: the relationships of awareness and executive functions to occupational performance. In Katz N, editor: *Cognition and occupation in rehabilitation: cognitive models for intervention in occupational therapy*, Bethesda, Md, 1998, American Occupational Therapy Association.

9. Magill RA: *Motor learning: concepts and applications*, ed 4, Madison, Wis, 1993, Brown & Benchmark.

10. Moyers P: The guide to occupational therapy practice, *Am J Occup Ther* 53(3):247-322, 1999.

11. Nelson DL et al: The effects of an occupationally embedded exercise on bilaterally assisted supination in persons with hemiplegia, *Am J Occup Ther* 50(8):639-646, 1996.

12. Poole J: Application of motor learning principles in occupational therapy, *Am J Occup Ther* 45(6):530, 1991.

13. Ryerson S, Levit K: *Functional movement reeducation*, New York, 1997, Churchill Livingstone.

14. Sabari J: Using activities as challenges to facilitate development of functional skills. In Hinojosa J, Blount ML, editors: *Activities, the texture of life: describing purposeful activities*, Bethesda, Md, 2000, American Occupational Therapy Association.

15. Sabari J: Application of learning and environmental strategies to activity based treatment. In Gillen G, Burkhardt A, editors: *Stroke rehabilitation: a function-based approach*, St Louis, 1998, Mosby.

16. Sabari J: Motor learning concepts applied to activity-based intervention with adults with hemiplegia, *Am J Occup Ther* 45(6):523-530,1991.

17. Salmani AW, Schmidt RA, Walter CB: Knowledge of results and motor learning: a review and critical reappraisal, *Psych Bull* 95: 355-386, 1984.

18. Schmidt RA: *Motor performance and learning: principles for practitioners*, Champaign, Ill, 1992, Human Kinetics.

19. Shumway-Cook A, Woollacott M: *Motor control: theory and practical applications*, Baltimore, 1995, Williams & Wilkins.

20. Sietsema JM et al: The use of a game to promote arm reach in persons with traumatic brain injury, *Am J Occup Ther* 47( ):19-24, 1993.

21. Singer RN, Cauraugh JHL: The generalizability effect of learning strategies for categories of psychomotor skills, *Quest* 37:103-119, 1985.

22. Toglia J: A dynamic interactional model to cognitive rehabilitation. In Katz N, editor: *Cognition and occupation in rehabilitation: cognitive models for intervention in occupational therapy*, Bethesda, Md, 1998, American Occupation Therapy Association.

23. Toglia JT: Generalization of treatment: a multicontext approach to cognitive perceptual impairment in adults with brain injury, *Am J Occup Ther* 45(6):505-515, 1991.

24. Tulving E: *Elements of episodic memory*, Oxford, Eng, 1983, Clarendon Press.

25. Winstein CJ: Designing practice for motor learning clinical implications. In Lister MJ, editor: *Contemporary management of motor control problems: proceedings of the II STEP conference*, Alexandria, Va, 1991, Foundation for Physical Therapy.

26. Winstein CJ: Knowledge of results and motor learning—implications for physical therapy, *Phys Ther* 71(2):140-149, 1991.

27. Wu SH, Huang HT, Lin CF, et al: Effects of a program on symmetrical posture in patients with hemiplegia: a single-subject design, *Am J Occup Ther* 50(1):17-23, 1996.

28. Wulf G, Hob M, Prinz W: Instructions for motor learning: differential effects of internal versus external focus of attention, *J Motor Behav* 30(2):169-179, 1998.

Documentation of Occupational Therapy Services

MAUREEN MICHELE MATHEWS
JANET L. JABRI

KEY TERMS

Referral
Database
Baseline
Premorbid functional status
Performance baseline
Initial evaluation report
Occupational therapy file
Permanent legal medical record
Reassessment
Interim assessment report
Discharge summary
Progress note
Subjective Objective Assessment Plan (SOAP)
Occupational Therapy Sequential Client Care Record (OTSCCR)
Problem-Oriented Medical Record (POMR)
Automated documentation systems

LEARNING OBJECTIVES

Study of this chapter will allow the student or clinician to do the following:

1. Briefly describe what is meant by documentation of occupational therapy services.
2. Identify when the documentation process is initialized.
3. Identify at least five purposes of documentation.
4. Briefly summarize the content of the initial evaluation report.
5. Explain how goals are established.
6. Identify the importance of patient inclusion in goal setting.
7. Explain how the treatment plan is established, including its relationship to problems and goals.
8. Describe the contents of an interim assessment report.
9. Identify the key elements of a discharge summary.
10. Identify the four components of a SOAP note.
11. Describe the OTSCCR documentation system and its relationship to the problem-oriented medical record.
12. Describe how the Problem-Oriented Medical Record is structured.
13. List the advantages and disadvantages of an automated documentation system.
14. Identify six documentation guidelines that help ensure that the therapist meets legal and ethical obligations

Documentation of occupational therapy (OT) refers to all information recorded about the patient from the time of referral to the time of discharge from OT. Documentation is initiated upon receipt of the referral and includes acknowledgment of the referral, initial evaluation, progress notes, periodic interim reassessments, and a discharge summary. Justifications for assistive technology may also be included in OT documentation. Backup documentation, not usually entered into the medical record, may include evaluation test results, checklists, or patient worksheets. Backup documentation is typically kept in the OT therapy file. The medical record contains pertinent information about the patient's status, progress, and performance.

There is no standard or single method within the profession for documenting OT services. Funding agencies and treatment facilities may prescribe the types of records kept and reports to be written.[4,9] Regardless of the method of documentation, it is critical that all entries be clear, concise, objective, accurate, and complete. Inaccuracies in the medical record may lead to miscommunication and result in inappropriate treatment. Documentation is part of a legal record; omissions or errors in documentation may cause doubts about the accuracy of the entire record.[3] The occupational therapist is responsible for ensuring that all documentation requirements are met in a timely fashion.

Documentation directed toward patient-centered goals that are meaningful to the patient and agreeable to the clinician can effectively meet most purposes for documentation. To engage the patient in the establishment of mutually agreeable goals, the therapist must explain the purposes of OT, ask questions and solicit information that identifies patient concerns and desires for therapeutic outcomes, and help the patient and family identify realistic expectations of therapy. The process of engaging patients in goal setting, although time consuming, can provide a framework for OT treatment and documentation while engaging the patient in the therapeutic process.[12]

PURPOSES OF DOCUMENTATION

Documentation is the major avenue through which health care providers communicate about a client or patient to others. A broad target audience, each with its own purpose, reviews the medical record. Effective documentation serves many purposes, including the following:

1. Communicating patient status and response to treatment to the physician and other health care team members
2. Promoting continuity of treatment when staff changes occur

3. Providing clear, objective data about the patient on which future treatment can be based
4. Providing justification to utilization reviewers for continued treatment
5. Ensuring payment by third-party payers for services
6. Complying with the law and aiding in litigation
7. Providing a method to ensure patient rights and advocacy
8. Interpreting the treatment program to the patient, family, and other concerned individuals or agencies
9. Evaluating the effectiveness of OT intervention
10. Ensuring facility accreditation from such organizations as the Joint Commission for the Accreditation of Healthcare Organizations (JCAHO) or the Commission for Accreditation of Rehabilitation Facilities (CARF)
11. Providing data for research and advancement of the profession of occupational therapy
12. Facilitating training and student education programs[3,4,8,9]

RECORDS AND REPORTS
Permanent Legal Record

The permanent legal record contains defined information from the entire treatment team. The documents in a particular record are considered the only official information related to that particular patient or client. Each facility determines the contents of this record, which may be based on requirements set by internal systems, licensing agencies, accrediting bodies, and third-party payers. This record will be used within the facility by the treatment team to understand the full patient treatment picture, by utilization reviewers to determine justification for continued treatment, and by quality assurance teams to assess overall patient outcomes and services. This record may also be used by third-party payers to determine payment for services, by the court system for litigation, and by outside agencies for continued treatment or services after discharge from the facility.

The OT documents contained in the permanent legal record consist of the physician's referral, initial evaluation, ongoing progress notes, interim reassessments, and the discharge summary. These items provide a concise summary of all tests and observations, treatment goals, and treatment plans and measurements of progress toward the established goals. In addition, the occupational therapist may be required to provide entries in other sections of the permanent record, such as the interdisciplinary care plan or the patient care conference note.

Records and Reports Process and Formats
Referral

OT evaluation and treatment are usually initiated by receipt of a patient (client) **referral** (Fig. 10-1). This

2/1/2000 - Occupational Therapy referral received.
Evaluation initiated.
Report to follow.

FIG. 10-1
Sample of referral receipt.

referral is generally, but not always, received from the physician and may specify the reason the referral was requested. When a physician's referral is required, it should include the following: the OT treatment diagnosis and onset date, precautions, the date of any recent change in level of function, a request for evaluation and any other specific treatment orders, the physician's signature, and the date.[1] The first entry into the permanent record may be an acknowledgment of receipt of the referral and the initial plan of action. The response time is established by each facility but is usually within 24 to 48 hours of receipt of the referral.

Initial Evaluation

The initial evaluation is a three-step process. The first step is to gather information about the patient and identify the patient's **premorbid functional status**. The second step is to complete the assessment and establish a baseline of current patient performance. The final step is to use the information obtained in steps one and two and apply clinical reasoning skills to draw sound conclusions and establish the treatment goals and plan.

Step 1: Building the General Information Database

The therapist begins the initial evaluation process by reviewing data obtained from the permanent record. He or she also interviews referring sources, the patient, and family members and observes patient performance and behavior to build a general information **database**. This database includes the patient's name and address, important phone numbers, information on family members, third-party payers (both primary and secondary), and family, educational, and work histories. In addition, the database contains pertinent medical, physical, and mental status information related to specific primary and secondary diagnoses, as well as other related information about prior levels of function. Expected treatment outcomes and discharge plans are also pertinent to the database. Information obtained will be integrated into the initial evaluation. Nonessential information may be kept in the OT file for reference during treatment. During the interview process the cli-

nician educates the client about the role of OT and facilitates the identification of mutually agreeable functional goals. These goals will form the framework for all documentation.[12]

Step 2: Establishing the Performance Baseline

The second step in the initial evaluation involves assessments and tests to establish the **performance baseline**. Accuracy in the administration of tests and recording of test results is critical. Future evaluation results will be compared with initial findings to determine progress. The degree of improvement may determine the course, duration, and extent of treatment approved by the physician and third-party payers.

The **occupational therapy file** should contain detailed results of all evaluations completed. This file augments the permanent medical record and contains detailed information and test results. The items in the file may include: (1) range of motion (ROM) measurements, (2) manual muscle testing, sensory testing, and perceptual and cognitive evaluation results, and (3) activities of daily living (ADL), functional mobility, home management, vocational, and avocational assessment findings. A summary of normative data and an organized presentation of abnormal findings are typically delineated in the permanent legal record.

Step 3: Establishing the Treatment Plan

The final step involves using the data gathered in the previous two steps to establish a clear plan of action. Drawing on goals important to the client, the clinician identifies problems amenable to OT intervention, defines goals more clearly, and establishes a plan of treatment to accomplish those goals. The refined problems, plans, and goals are reintroduced to the client to verify that the course of action is agreeable.

Initial Evaluation Report

Initial evaluation report formats vary greatly from setting to setting. Most facilities have printed forms that the therapist fills in; others require a complete narrative report. There are pros and cons for either format. Forms ensure that information is complete. The subheadings trigger a written response for all evaluation areas. A form's limited space encourages brevity and conciseness. In general, the form saves time, and most team members find it faster for gleaning needed information. The form also presents a ready format for computer keyboard input. Using forms makes it easier to gather aggregate data for use in outcome studies. The form may not meet the specialized documentation needs of all diagnoses, however, or provide sufficient space for important information not covered in the subheadings. A form may also elicit more information than is needed to capture the clinical picture.

SANTA CLARA **VALLEY** MEDICAL CENTER

Santa Clara Valley Medical Center
751 South Bascom Avenue
San José, California 95128

OCCUPATIONAL THERAPY EVALUATION

☐ Initial ☐ Interim ☐ Discharge

Name: Room #
Chart #: Acct. #:
DOB: Age: M F
Date of onset:
Date of referral:
Date O.T. initiated:
Reason for consult:

OCCUPATIONAL THERAPY

Medical Hx/Dx:

Precautions:

Social Hx:

Clinical Status (ROM, Strength, Sensation, Other):

Functional Status (Mobility, Transfers, Self care):

Equipment/Splinting/Positioning Needs:

Problems: Goals/Recommendations:

Frequency/Duration:

__________ OTR __________ Date __________ M.D. __________ Date

4124 REV | 7/87 Disposition: Medical Chart - Perm Canary - To Division File SCVMC 6041-53-12

FIG. 10-2
Occupational therapy evaluation form. From Therapy Services Division, Santa Clara Valley Medical Center, San José, Calif.

The greatest advantage of the narrative format is its adaptability to the special needs of the individual patient. However, the narrative format generally takes longer to complete and to read and is prone to errors of omission because the form does not provide clinicians with prompts to cover all subjects.

The initial evaluation, whether it is in form (Fig. 10-2) or narrative format, can be divided into several distinct sections as follows: (1) general information, which includes the patient's identifying information, medical history, and prior level of function; (2) clinical evaluation and interpretation; (3) functional status assessment; and (4) evaluation summary, which includes problem identification, objectives and goals, and treatment plan.

General Information

The first section of a report in the narrative format consists of basic identifying information about the patient. This includes the patient's name, the medical record or account number, the referring physician, and the referral and evaluation dates. This section of the report details pertinent medical history, including the primary treatment diagnosis and any related secondary diagnoses with their onset dates. The general information section should list any precautions or contraindications to be observed during treatment. The patient's prior level of function, prior living situation, and previous vocational and leisure activities level of function are also noted (Fig. 10-2).

Clinical Evaluation

The clinical evaluation section is a synopsis of evaluation results (Fig. 10-2). It is helpful to relay standardized results or use standardized rating scales for easy interpretation by others. Standardized scales also ensure reliable replication of the evaluation process at reassessment and discharge times. The evaluations performed will depend upon the specific diagnosis. For example, a patient with a brain injury may require a physical assessment (ROM, motor function, and sensory), as well as perceptual and cognitive testing. For a mental disorder such as depression, the assessment may focus primarily on behavior and cognitive parameters.

Functional Status Assessment

The functional status assessment section covers the evaluation of the functional performance of the patient. The clinical evaluation results have substantial bearing on these assessments; a standardized scale is imperative to ensure reliability of results through the treatment process. The scope of this OT assessment will depend on the defined roles of the department within the facility. In the sample form (Fig. 10-2), bed mobility, transfers, and daily living skills are assessed. A "levels of assistance" scale is provided in Table 10-1.

Evaluation Summary

The evaluation summary is the most important section of the report. In this section, the previously recorded information is analyzed and a problem list is developed. The problems listed are those that might impede the patient's efforts to attain maximal independence. It should be noted that the list might include problems that OT intervention would not directly affect (e.g., a spouse's disability or financial constraints). These problems will influence the treatment approach taken by the

TABLE 10-1
Definitions of Levels of Assistance

Level of Assistance	Abbreviation	Definition
Independent	Ind.	Patient requires no assistance or cueing in any situation. Patient is trusted in all situations 100% of the time to do the task safely.
Supervision	Sup.	Caregiver is not needed to provide hands-on guarding but may need to give verbal cues for safety.
Contact guard/standby	Con. Gd./Stby	Caregiver must provide hands-on contact guard or be within arm's length for the patient's safety.
Minimum assistance	Min.	Caregiver provides physical and cueing assistance in 25% of the task.
Moderate assistance	Mod.	Caregiver assists the patient with 50% of the task; assistance can be physical and cueing.
Maximum assistance	Max.	Caregiver assists the patient with 75% of the task; assistance can be physical and cueing.
Dependent	Dep.	Patient is unable to assist in any part of the task; caregiver performs 100% of the task for the patient physically and cognitively.

Adapted from Occupational therapy evaluation form, Therapy Services Division, Santa Clara Valley Medical Center, San José, Calif.

occupational therapist. Using this problem list, the therapist must set realistic and functional therapy goals. The goals are predictions of the patient outcome. The therapist must apply theoretical knowledge and clinical reasoning skills to predict one or more treatment outcomes for the patient. Establishing goals that are meaningful, realistic, and mutually agreeable to the patient and therapist is the most critical part of the initial evaluation process. These initial goals are the indicators that will be used to measure the effectiveness of the therapy intervention and the success for the patient.

Therapy goals can be subdivided into *goals* and *objectives*. *Goals* are the maximal predicted outcomes expected for a patient after the full treatment program has been completed. *Objectives* describe the level of function expected after a predesignated period of treatment intervention, usually 1 week or 1 month. Each goal must reflect a measurable, realistic, and functional outcome for the patient. For example, a long-term goal for a patient currently requiring maximum assistance for eating might read, "Using modified utensils, the patient will eat independently." An objective (1-week or short-term goal) might read, "The patient will require modified assistance for eating, using adapted utensils."

Finally, a treatment plan must be established. The treatment plan indicates the treatment interventions that the therapist will employ to help the patient achieve predetermined goals. This plan establishes the treatment frequency and duration. Daily eating retraining and upper extremity functional strengthening for 2 weeks may be a treatment plan established to achieve increased independence in eating.

The summary section may also include a discharge plan once therapy has been completed, as well as a checkbox to note that the goals have been discussed and reflect those of the patient and family. Finally, a physician's review of the plan and verifying signature may be necessary.

Interim Assessment Report

If treatment occurs over an extended time, it may be necessary to complete a full reassessment. The format of the reassessment is often the same as that of the initial evaluation. The main difference is that this report reflects the changes from the initial evaluation results to the present clinical findings. The interim report reflects progress made toward the predicted goals and is a measure of success of the treatment intervention. The new evaluation results may present an opportunity for revising initial goals and treatment timelines. Interim assessments are an important tool for the ongoing utilization review process. They allow the therapist to justify continued treatment intervention by clearly outlining the effectiveness and efficiency of the treatment that has occurred.

Discharge Summary Report

At the completion of the treatment regimen, a **discharge summary** is necessary. The format of the summary can be the same as that used for the initial evaluation and interim assessments. This summary describes the final status of the patient at the time of discharge from the particular setting. Documentation of progress from the initial assessment to the time of discharge must be objective, accurate, and understandable. Key elements required in a discharge summary include identification of goals attained, a statement of goals not attained and why they were not attained, and discharge recommendations. Additional interventions and follow-up care needed to ensure ongoing improvement or maintenance of function should be clearly defined in the discharge recommendations.

The discharge summary is a key document because it reflects all progress and accomplishments achieved in the case. The data can be used for many purposes. Quality assurance committees may use the data to evaluate the effectiveness of the treatment. The data may also be used for outcome studies to prove the efficacy of treatment within certain diagnostic categories. In addition, insurance payers may use the report to determine payment for the service, and other service agencies such as outpatient clinics may use the data to help establish goals and treatment plans in the new treatment setting.

Progress Note

Progress notes may be required on a per-treatment, daily, or weekly basis. Generally, daily notes are very brief and reflect treatment provided, patient response to the treatment, and progress noted. Revision of the treatment plan and goals is not always necessary (Fig. 10-3).

Weekly progress notes are more thorough and should summarize the treatment provided, the treatment frequency, the patient's response to treatment, and progress toward goals or lack of progress, with justification. The objectives should be updated and the treatment plan revised. The new objectives and treatment plans are established to reflect the expected outcome for the following week's treatment regimen (Fig. 10-4).

Patient was seen for dressing retraining. Patient required moderate assistance for upper body dressing and maximal assistance for lower body dressing. Plan to continue w/ established treatment plan.

FIG. 10-3
Brief daily note sample.

Patient has been seen daily for dressing retraining. Patient has progressed from moderate to minimal assistance needed in dressing upper body and from maximal to moderate assistance required in lower body dressing. ROM limitations, left neglect, and decreased endurance are primary contributors to functional deficits. The patient will progress to standby assistance for upper body dressing and to minimal assistance in lower body dressing in one week.

FIG. 10-4
Weekly progress note sample.

Problem:	Assisted dressing.
Progress:	Patient now dresses upper body with minimal assistance and lower body with moderate assistance. Last week patient required moderate assistance for upper body dressing and maximal assistance for lower body dressing.
Program:	ADL retraining.
Plan:	Achieve standby assistance in upper body and minimal assistance in lower body dressing in one week.

FIG. 10-6
Problem-focused problem notes sample.

S:	Patient states he can put on shirt by himself.
O:	Patient required assistance of therapist to orient shirt correctly and guide shirt over shoulders. Moderate assistance was needed to start items over feet and to clear clothing over hips. Previously needed moderate assistance for donning shirt and maximal assistance for lower body dressing.
A:	Visual spatial deficits and poor endurance inhibit independence.
P:	Continue guided dressing training with emphasis on paced activity. Patient to require standby assistance in upper body dressing and minimal assistance for lower body dressing in one week.

FIG. 10-5
SOAP notes sample.

Various styles or formats for progress notes are used to ensure consistency of the content of the notes. SOAP notes are one of the most frequently used formats. The acronym stands for Subjective (the patient's view of the problem), Objective (the clinical findings about the problem), Assessment (relevant data from reevaluations), and Plan (therapeutic interventions and goals) (Fig. 10-5).[9] This method of recording information is based on the system designed by Weed[10] in the Problem-Oriented Medical Record. Another format for short daily notes states the problem, progress, description of the treatment program, and future plans (Fig. 10-6). Still another possibility is to enter similar information in a format dictated by a computerized documentation system.

JUSTIFICATION FOR ASSISTIVE TECHNOLOGY

Occupational therapists are frequently called on to help justify the use of assistive technology, such as bath equipment, wheelchairs, and environmental controls. When justifying such equipment, clinicians must familiarize themselves with the unique requirements of the third-party payer. A medical insurance company might consider use of equipment justified if it will eliminate dependency. The vocational rehabilitation agency may require that use of the equipment allow the client to realize vocational potential or be able to return to work. For the educational system, the key issues would be access to education or improved ability to learn. Justification of the need for equipment in terms acceptable to the third-party payer is critical to securing payment for assistive technologies.[5]

OCCUPATIONAL THERAPY FILE

It is common practice for the OT services to maintain separate departmental files. Supporting records, notes, and worksheets, as well as copies of documentation prepared for the permanent medical record, can be found in such files. Supporting data may include test results such as range of motion forms, treatment checklists, samples of the patient's writings, ADL checklists, informal team conference notes, treatment plan approaches, and other supporting materials that guide treatment. The supporting data form the framework that will become part of the permanent medical record.

The OT file improves treatment efficiency and provides other advantages. The permanent medical record is used by many team members and is not always readily available for review; the therapy record is more available for updating of data and clarification of earlier treatment procedures and findings. The OT file provides detailed information to a substitute clinician in the absence of the primary therapist, ensuring continuity of treatment. The record is also available for review during formal and informal conferences or during any treatment session.

QUALITY OF DOCUMENTATION CONTENT

The quality of the documentation content is of the utmost importance. Documentation must be well organized, objective, and accurate and must contain only pertinent information. Conciseness and brevity are dictated by time constraints for both the writer and the reader. The therapist must consider who will read the report, which may influence what needs to be reported and how the report will be written.[2] The target audience, be it other clinicians, insurance payers, or a lay person, will influence the use of medical terminology or medical abbreviations, as well as the amount of detail provided for the reader's understanding.

The content of documentation is governed by law. Laws have been enacted to ensure quality care and cost containment. The written record is the primary means of justifying appropriate treatment by the appropriate clinician in the most cost-effective environment. To preserve the rights of the patient, the record must be factual and include no value judgments that might be prejudicial to the patient.[6,11]

Health records may be used in litigation for settling insurance claims and may be examined by third-party payers, fiscal intermediaries, and other utilization review boards.[6,11] The review of the records is governed by principles of ethical practice in relation to confidentiality, and the records are under strict control of the physician or health care agency. No privileged information, oral or written, can be released without the signed consent of the patient.[3] In addition, the patient has the right to know what is in the record and can ask to see it. The physician is responsible for providing the information in the manner he or she sees fit. Each facility has procedures outlining how a patient might look at the medical record. The therapist should follow the facility's procedures if a patient asks to view the medical record.

It is important to remember that the legal written record is the only acceptable proof of the treatment intervention. If something is not written, in the eyes of outside reviewers (e.g., third-party payers or jurors) it did not happen. Box 10-1[6] provides documentation guidelines to help ensure that the therapist meets legal and ethical obligations.

REPORTING SYSTEMS
Problem-Oriented Medical Record

The Problem-Oriented Medical Record (POMR) was devised by Dr. Lawrence L. Weed at Case Western Reserve University.[10] It provides a computer-compatible model that follows a systematic progression from evaluation to progress reporting. It is a problem-solving model that is readily accepted by occupational therapists and can be implemented in any setting. It offers a method by which evaluation and treatment standards can be documented and enforced.[7]

The POMR encourages an interdisciplinary model in which all health care services integrate information into one document. The database is composed of physical, social, and demographic information contained in one report. From this database, a problem list is formulated and kept at the front of the record. The list serves as an index to all problems and may also include anticipated problems. Each problem is numbered and named, and these designations remain the same for each hospitalization of the patient. All of the treatment plans must be titled and numbered according to the problem list, then dated and signed. To illustrate how the POMR works, by reading all of the notes that refer to problem three, the health care worker can learn what each service is contributing to the patient's total rehabilitation at any given time.

All progress notes are dated, numbered, and titled according to the problem to which they refer. All progress notes are recorded in the same section of the chart, following the previously mentioned SOAP outline. Progress notes are written whenever a staff member has relevant information to record. The frequency of entries to the record may reflect policies of the treatment facility, the acuteness of the patient's condition, or the need for continued evaluation.[7] The record concludes with a problem-oriented discharge summary.

The POMR facilitates communication among health disciplines because all progress notes are intermixed and all personnel are bound by the same criteria for recording. All service providers are up to date on progress in other areas, and treatment can be ad-

---

BOX 10-1

Documentation Guidelines

1. Date all entries for accurate sequencing of the treatment.
2. Document missed treatments.
3. Document at the time of the treatment so the entry will completely and accurately reflect the treatment session.
4. Document in specific facts rather than in general terms.
5. Do not point blame to other care providers in the record.
6. Do not change a legal record after the fact without clarifying the time and nature of the change.

From Acquaviva J, editor: *Effective documentation for occupational therapy*, ed 2, Rockville, Md, 1998, American Occupational Therapy Association.

justed accordingly. The patient can be educated about his or her condition and progress in an organized manner that focuses on the problems from an interdisciplinary approach. The POMR allows documentation adequate for quality assurance and third-party payer requirements, specifically with regard to coordination of care across disciplines. The POMR offers a recording system that can improve the standards of documentation.[7]

OCCUPATIONAL THERAPY SEQUENTIAL CLIENT CARE RECORD

The Occupational Therapy Sequential Client Care Record (OTSCCR) created by Llorens[4] is unique to OT. Rather than using medical or psychologic reporting systems, it is organized according to a theoretical framework consistent with the characteristics, goals, and objectives of OT. As the field of OT has developed, increased attention has been given to measuring the quality of care, achieving autonomy in decision making, providing accountability to patients and funding agencies, and assuming professional responsibility for services. Llorens described the client care record as the "key document for determining quality and effectiveness of care."[4] The OTSCCR system combines the theoretical framework of Llorens' Occupational Therapy Developmental Analysis, Evaluation, and Intervention Schedule with the scientific method of the POMR for documenting care in OT. The OTSCCR includes a database, information about the evaluation process, problem identification, an OT plan, progress notes, and a discharge summary. It is based on the developmental frame of reference and occupational performance model, and data are recorded and analyzed according to the performance areas and performance components of the occupational performance model. The OTSCCR documents factual information about the client based on actual behavior. It is designed to span the time the client is served by OT from admission to discharge. It is retained by the OT department for use in preparing reports and communicating with the client and other interested persons or agencies.[4]

Automated Documentation Systems

The availability of therapy documentation software has increased. These systems range from primary documentation formats to integrated systems that provide not only basic documentation but also billing mechanisms, administrative tracking information, and protocols for generating outcome data.

The ultimate advantage of using an automated system is that it saves time, not only in documentation but also in collating data for outcome studies and other required administrative reports. In addition, data-

handling abilities are far more advanced and accurate than with manual systems. Disadvantages of automated systems include the following:

1. Difficulty of securing a system that meets all the needs of the program or requests from outside agencies
2. Cost of hardware sufficient for the needs of the facility
3. Cost of training
4. Unwillingness of staff to accept the system
5. Difficulty of maintaining patient confidentiality
6. Insufficient access for all users[8]

SUMMARY

Documentation of OT services consists of written records and reports that contain pertinent information about the patient's status, progress, and performance. The occupational therapist is responsible for keeping accurate records to document the patient's evaluation results, the identified problems, the treatment goals and plan, and the patient's progress toward the established plan.

Documentation is necessary for administrative, reimbursement, communication, quality assurance, educational, and legal purposes. Documentation is essential in justifying the necessity and expense of treatment. Accurate and objective documentation creates a record of the efficacy of OT.

OT documentation includes the referral, evaluation data, initial evaluation, progress notes, interim reassessments, and the discharge summary. Records and reports should reflect clear, concise, accurate, and objective information about the patient. To prevent misinterpretation and misunderstanding, the report writer must consider the reader of the documents. Documentation should be well organized and developed according to an agreed-on system for internal consistency of the record. Most important, documentation should reflect a treatment plan that has engaged the patient in the therapeutic process by the establishment of therapeutically meaningful and mutually agreeable goals.

REVIEW QUESTIONS

1. What is meant by documentation of OT services?
2. When is the documentation process initialized?
3. List at least five purposes of documentation.
4. What is the difference in content between the OT file and the permanent legal record? What kinds of documents are contained in each?
5. Briefly summarize the content of the initial evaluation report and explain how goals are established.
6. How is the treatment plan developed?
7. What is contained in an interim assessment report?
8. What is contained in the discharge summary report?

9. List two formats for progress notes.
10. What should be considered in justifying assistive technology?
11. Why is accurate, complete, and concise documentation important?
12. Describe the POMR and OTSCCR recording systems.
13. What are the advantages of an automated documentation system?

REFERENCES

1. Allen C, Foto M, Moon T, et al: Understanding the medical review process. In Acquaviva J, editor: *Effective documentation for occupational therapy*, ed 2, Rockville, Md, 1998, American Occupational Therapy Association.
2. Baum CM, Luebben AJ: *Prospective payment systems*, Thorofare, NJ, 1981, Slack.
3. Gleave GJ: Medical records and reports. In Willard HS, Spackman SC, editors: *Occupational therapy*, ed 4, Philadelphia, 1971, JB Lippincott.
4. Llorens LA: *Occupational therapy sequential client care record manual*, Laurel, Md, 1982, Ramsco Publishing.
5. Luebben AJ: Documentation for assistive technology. In Acquaviva J, editor: *Effective documentation for occupational therapy*, ed 2, Rockville, Md, 1998, American Occupational Therapy Association.
6. McCann KD, Steich T: Legal issues in documentation: fraud, abuse, and confidentiality. In Acquaviva J, editor: *Effective documentation for occupational therapy*, ed 2, Rockville, Md, 1998, American Occupational Therapy Association.
7. Potts LR: The problem oriented record: implications for occupational therapy, *Am J Occup Ther* 26:6(288), 1972.
8. Robertson S: Why we document. In Acquaviva J, editor: *Effective documentation for occupational therapy*, ed 2, Rockville, Md, 1998, American Occupational Therapy Association.
9. Tiffany EG: Psychiatry and mental health. In Hopkins HL, Smith HD, editors: *Willard and Spackman's occupational therapy*, ed 6, Philadelphia, 1983, JB Lippincott.
10. Weed LL: *Medical records, medical education and patient care*, Chicago, 1971, Year Book Medical Publishers.
11. Wells C: The implications of liability: guidelines for professional practice, *Am J Occup Ther* 23:1(18), 1969.
12. Wilson D: If I had known then what I know now. In Acquaviva J, editor: *Effective documentation for occupational therapy*, ed 2, Rockville, Md, 1998, American Occupational Therapy Association.

CHAPTER 11

Infection Control and Safety Issues in the Clinic

WENDY STORM BUCKNER

KEY TERMS

Acquired immune deficiency syndrome
Antiseptic
Apnea
Arterial monitoring line
Autoclave
Endotracheal tube
Catheter
Fistula
Fowler's position
Human immunodeficiency virus
Hyperalimentation
Immunization
Infusion pump
Intravenous
Isolation
Nasogastric tube
Total parenteral nutrition
Universal precautions
Dyspnea

LEARNING OBJECTIVES

After studying this chapter the student or practitioner will be able to do the following:

1. Recognize the role of occupational therapy personnel in preventing accidents.
2. Identify recommendations for safety in the clinic.
3. Describe preventive positioning for patients with lower extremity amputations, total hip replacements, rheumatoid arthritis, burns, and hemiplegia.
4. Describe the purposes of special equipment.
5. Identify precautions when treating patients who require special equipment.
6. Identify universal precautions and explain the importance of following them with all patients.
7. Describe proper techniques of hand washing.
8. Recognize the importance for all health care workers to understand and follow isolation procedures used in patient care.
9. Identify procedures for handling patient injuries.
10. Describe guidelines for handling various emergency situations.

The occupational therapist must make sure patients remain safe within the health care setting. Medical technology and cost control pressures have made it necessary for rehabilitation professionals to treat seriously ill patients early in their illness and for shorter periods. These situations increase the potential for injuries to the patients. Occupational therapy (OT) personnel are legally liable for negligence if a patient is injured because staff failed to follow proper procedures.[4] This chapter reviews specific safety precautions for use with a variety of patients. It identifies precautions to consider when encountering equipment commonly used with patients. Guidelines for handling various emergency situations are reviewed. The chapter is only an overview and cannot substitute for training in specific procedures used in many facilities. In addition to following these procedures, the occupational therapist should teach patients and their families applicable techniques that the families can follow at home.

SAFETY RECOMMENDATIONS FOR THE CLINIC

Prevention of accidents and subsequent injuries begins with consistent application of basic safety precautions for the clinic:

1. Wash your hands for at least 30 seconds[3] before and after treating each patient to reduce cross-contamination.
2. Make sure space is adequate to maneuver equipment. Avoid placing patients where they may be bumped by equipment or passing personnel. Keep the area free from clutter.
3. Do not attempt to transfer patients in congested areas or in areas where your view is blocked.
4. Routinely check equipment to be sure it is working properly.
5. Make sure the furniture and equipment in the clinic are stable. When not using items, store them out of the way of the treatment area.
6. Keep the floor free of cords, scatter rugs, litter, and spills. Ensure that the floors are not highly polished, because polished floor may be very slippery.
7. Do not leave patients unattended. Use restraint belts properly to protect patients when they are not closely observed.
8. Have the treatment area and supplies ready before the patient arrives.
9. Allow only properly trained personnel to provide patient care.
10. Follow the manufacturer's and facility's procedures for handling and storing potentially hazardous material. Be sure such materials are marked and stored in a place that is in clear view. Do not store such items above shoulder height.
11. Clearly label emergency exits and evacuation routes.
12. Have emergency equipment, such as fire extinguishers and first aid kits, readily available.

PREVENTIVE POSITIONING FOR SPECIFIC DIAGNOSES

Many patients require proper positioning to prevent complications and maintain function. Staying in one position for a long time can lead to the development of contractures and bedsores (decubitus ulcers).

Specific patient conditions such as impaired sensation, paralysis, poor skin integrity, poor nutrition, impaired circulation, and spasticity require special attention. Inspect the patient's skin, especially bony prominences over the sacrum, ischium, trochanters, elbows, and heels. Reddened areas may develop from pressure within 30 minutes. Other indicators of excessive pressure are complaints of numbness or tingling and localized swelling.

Pillows, towel rolls, or similar devices may be used to provide comfort and stability but should be used cautiously to prevent secondary complications. The following examples of patient conditions demonstrate the need for specific positioning techniques. It is important to review these principles with both the patient and the caregiver.

Patients with *lower extremity amputations (above-knee)* should avoid hip flexion and hip abduction. Limit the length of time the patient may sit to 30 minutes per hour. When the patient is supine, do not elevate the stump on a pillow for more than a few minutes. Prone lying is recommended to help avoid contracture of the hip flexor muscles.

Patients with *lower extremity amputations (below-knee)* should avoid prolonged hip and knee flexion to prevent contractures. Limit the length of time the patient may sit to 30 minutes per hour. When the patient is supine, do not elevate the stump on a pillow for more than a few minutes. When the stump is elevated, keep the knee in extension. Instruct the patient to keep the knee extended throughout the day. Again, prone lying is recommended.

Patients with *total hip replacements* should avoid positions of instability. For the posterolateral approach, this includes hip adduction, internal rotation, and flexion over 90°. For the anterolateral approach, positions to avoid include adduction, external rotation, and excessive hyperextension.

To prevent contractures because of muscle spasticity, patients with *hemiplegia* should avoid the following positions for prolonged periods: shoulder adduction and internal rotation, elbow flexion, forearm supination or pronation, wrist flexion, finger and thumb flexion and adduction, hip and knee flexion, hip external rotation, and ankle plantar flexion and inversion. Both the arm and leg should be moved through the available range of motion several times per day.

Patients with *rheumatoid arthritis* should avoid prolonged immobilization of the joints of the affected extremity. *Gentle* active or passive range of motion of the joints should be performed several times per day, providing the joints are not acutely inflamed.

As *burns* heal, scars and contractures are likely to form. Therefore it is important to avoid prolonged static positions of the joints affected by the burn or skin graft, especially positions of comfort. The positions comfortable to the patient do not produce the needed stress or tension to the wound, which must be kept mobile. When the burn is located on the flexor or adductor surface of a joint, positions of flexion and adduction should be avoided. Passive or active exercise should be performed frequently on both the involved and uninvolved joints. The patient will probably have to endure a great amount of pain to restore normal joint function.

PRECAUTIONS WITH SPECIAL EQUIPMENT

Before seeing a patient at bedside, the OTR should contact the nursing department to determine whether they have any specific instructions regarding positioning. For example, a patient may need to follow a turning schedule and may be limited in the length of time allowed to remain in one position. If the patient's current position in bed is not suitable for treatment, the treatment might be rescheduled. Other options would be to temporarily change the position of the patient or to treat the patient as much as possible in the current position. If the patient's position is changed, the patient should be returned to the preferred position at the end of treatment.

Hospital Beds

Two of the beds most commonly used in hospitals are the standard manually operated and electrically operated beds. Both beds are designed to make it easier to support the patient and to change a patient's position. Other, more specialized beds are needed for more traumatic cases. Whatever type is used, the bed should be positioned so that the patient is easily accessed and the therapist can use good body mechanics (see Chapter 14).

Most *standard adjustable beds* are adjusted by means of electrical controls attached to the head or the foot of the bed or to a special cord that allows the patient to operate the controls. The controls are marked according to their function and can be operated with the hand or foot. The entire bed can be raised and lowered, or the upper portion of it can be raised while the lower portion remains unchanged. When the upper portion is raised slightly, the patient's position is referred to as **Fowler's position**. Most beds allow the lower portion to be adjusted to provide knee flexion, with associated hip flexion.

Side rails are attached to most beds as a protective measure. Some rails are lifted upward to engage the locking mechanism, whereas others are moved toward the upper portion of the bed until the locking mechanism is engaged. If a side rail is used for patient security, the OTR should be sure the rail is locked securely before leaving the patient. The rail should be checked to ensure it does not compress, stretch, or otherwise interfere with any IV or other tubing.

A *turning frame* (e.g., Stryker wedge frame) has front and back frames that are covered with canvas. The support base allows elevation of the head or foot ends of the frames or of the entire bed. One person can easily turn the patient horizontally from prone to supine or from supine to prone. This bed is used most frequently with patients who have spinal cord injuries and require immobilization. The turning frame allows access to the patient and permits the patient to be moved from one place to another without being removed from the frame. Because of the limited number of possible positions, the skin of patients using this type of bed should be monitored frequently.

The *circular turning frame (Circ-o-lectric bed)* has a front and a back frame attached to two circular supports. The frames on which the patient is positioned move the patient vertically from supine to prone or from prone to supine. The circular support frames are moved by an electric motor and can be stopped at any point within their half-circle range. The patient or other persons can use a control switch to adjust the position. The circular turning bed has uses similar to the Stryker frame and also provides the benefit of frequent position changes to relieve skin pressure. However, a patient is still at risk for skin problems because of the pressure forces that may occur when the bed is turned or rotated vertically. Patients may experience symptoms of motion sickness such as vertigo, nausea, or hypotension when being turned.

The *air-fluidized support bed (Clinitron)* is an expensive bed that contains 1600 pounds of silicone-coated glass beads called microspheres. Heated, pressurized air flows through the beads to suspend a polyester cover that supports the patient. When set in motion, the microspheres develop the properties associated with fluids. Patients feel as if they are floating on a warm waterbed. The risk for skin problems is reduced because of the minimal contact pressure between the patient's body and the polyester sheet. This bed is used with patients who have several infected lesions or who require skin protection and whose position cannot be altered easily. Care should be taken to prevent puncturing the polyester cover (which would allow the microspheres to be expelled).

Ventilators

Ventilators (respirators) move gas or air into the patient's lungs and are used to maintain adequate air exchange when normal respiration is decreased. Two frequently used types of ventilators are the *volume-cycled ventilators* and the *pressure-cycled ventilators*. Both ventilators deliver a predetermined volume of gas (air) during inspiration and allow for passive expiration. The gas delivered by the ventilator usually will be induced into the patient through an **endotracheal tube** (ET). When the tube is in place, the patient is *intubated*. Insertion of the ET will prevent the patient from talking. When the ET is removed, the patient may complain of a sore throat and may have a distorted voice for a short period. It is important to avoid disturbing, bending, kinking, or occluding the tubing or accidentally disconnecting the ventilator tube from the ET. The patient who uses a ventilator may participate in various bedside activities, including sitting and ambulation. Make sure the tubing is sufficiently long to allow the activity to be performed. Because the patient will have difficulty talking, ask questions that can be answered with head nods or other nonverbal means. A patient using a ventilator may have a lower tolerance for activities and should be monitored for signs of respiratory distress such as a change in the respiration pattern, fainting, or blue lips.

Monitors

Various monitors are used to observe the physiologic state of patients who need special care. Therapeutic activities can be performed by patients who are being monitored, provided care is taken to prevent disruption of the equipment. Many of the units have an auditory and a visual signal that are activated by a change in the patient's condition or position or by a change in the function of the equipment. It may be necessary for a nurse to evaluate and correct the cause of the alarm unless the OTR has received special instruction.

The *electrocardiogram* (EKG or ECG) monitors the patient's heart rate, blood pressure, and respiration rate. Acceptable or safe ranges for the three physiologic indicators can be set in the unit. An alarm is activated when the upper or lower limits of the ranges are exceeded or if the unit malfunctions. A monitoring screen provides a graphic and digital display of the values so that health care staff can observe the patient's responses to treatment.

The *pulmonary artery catheter* (PAC) (e.g., Swan-Ganz catheter) is a long, plastic intravenous tube that is inserted into the internal jugular or the femoral vein and passed through to the pulmonary artery. It provides accurate and continuous measurements of pulmonary artery pressures and will detect subtle changes in the patient's cardiovascular system, including responses to medications, stress, and activity. Activities can be performed with the PAC in place, providing they do not interfere with the location of the catheter's insertion. For example, if the catheter is inserted into the subclavian vein, elbow flexion should be avoided and shoulder motions restricted.

The *intracranial pressure (ICP) monitor* measures the pressure exerted against the skull by brain tissue, blood, or cerebrospinal fluid (CSF). It is used to monitor ICP in patients with a closed head injury, cerebral hemorrhage, brain tumor, or overproduction of cerebrospinal fluid. Some of the complications associated with this device are infection, hemorrhage, and seizures. Two of the more commonly used ICP monitoring devices are the ventricular catheter and the subarachnoid screw. Both are inserted in a hole drilled in the skull. Physical activities should be limited when these devices are in place. Activities that would cause a rapid increase in ICP, such as isometric exercises, should be avoided. Positions to avoid include neck flexion, hip flexion greater than 90 degrees, and the prone position. The patient's head should not be lowered more than 15 degrees below horizontal. Care must be taken to avoid disturbing the plastic tube.

The **arterial monitoring line** (A line) is a catheter that is inserted into an artery to continuously measure blood pressure or to obtain blood samples without repeated needle punctures. Treatment can be provided with an A line in place, but care should be taken to avoid disturbing the catheter and inserted needle.

Feeding Devices

Special feeding devices may be necessary to provide nutrition for patients who are unable to ingest, chew, or swallow food. Some of the more commonly seen devices are the nasogastric tube, gastric tube, and intravenous feedings.

The **nasogastric (NG) tube** is a plastic tube inserted through a nostril, terminating in the patient's stomach. The tube may cause the patient to have a sore throat or an increased gag reflex. The patient will not be able to eat food or drink fluids through the mouth while the NG tube is in place. Movement of the patient's head and neck, especially forward flexion, should be prevented.

The *gastric tube (G tube)* is a plastic tube inserted through an incision in the patient's abdomen directly into the stomach. The tube should not be disturbed or removed during treatment.

Intravenous feeding, total parenteral nutrition (TPN), or **hyperalimentation** devices permit infusion of large amounts of nutrients needed to promote tissue growth. A catheter either is inserted directly into the subclavian vein or is passed into the subclavian vein after being inserted into another vein. The catheter may be connected to a semipermanently fixed cannula or sutured at the point of insertion. The OTR should carefully observe the various connections to be certain they are secure before and after treatment. A disrupted or loose connection may result in the development of an air embolus, which could be life threatening.

The system usually includes an **infusion pump**, which will administer fluids and nutrients at a preselected, constant flow rate. An audible alarm will be activated if the system becomes imbalanced or when the fluid source is empty. Treatment activities can be performed as long as the tubing is not disrupted, disconnected, or occluded and as long as undue stress to the infusion site is prevented. Motions of the shoulder on the side of the infusion site may be restricted, especially abduction and flexion.

Most **intravenous (IV) lines** are inserted into superficial veins. Various sizes and types of needles or catheters are used, depending on the purpose of the IV therapy, the infusion site, the need for prolonged therapy, and site availability. Care should be taken during treatment to prevent any disruption, disconnection, or occlusion of the tubing. The infusion site should remain dry, the needle should remain secure and immobile in the vein, and no restraint should be placed above the infusion site. For example, a blood pressure cuff should not be applied above the infusion site. The total system should be observed to be certain it is functioning properly when treatment begins and ends. If the infusion site is in the antecubital area, the elbow should not be flexed. The patient who ambulates with an IV line in place should be instructed to grasp the IV support pole so that the infusion site will be at heart level. If the infusion site is allowed to hang lower, blood flow may be affected. Similar procedures to maintain the infusion site in proper position should be followed when the patient is treated while in bed or at a treatment table. Activities involving elevation of the infusion site above the level of the heart for a prolonged period should be avoided. Problems related to the IV system should be reported to nursing personnel. Simple procedures such as straightening the tubing or removing an object that is occluding the tubing may be performed by the properly trained therapist.

Catheters

A urinary **catheter** is used to remove urine from the bladder when the patient is unable to satisfactorily control retention or release. The urine is drained through plastic tubing into a collection bag, bottle, or urinal. Any form of trauma, disease, condition, or disorder affecting the neuromuscular control of the bladder sphincter may necessitate the use of a urinary catheter. The catheter may be used temporarily or for the remainder of the patient's life.

A urinary catheter can be applied internally *(indwelling catheter)* or externally. Female patients require an indwelling catheter inserted through the urethra and into the bladder. Males may use an *external catheter.* A condom is applied over the shaft of the penis and is held in place by an adhesive applied to the skin or by a padded strap or tape encircling the proximal shaft of the penis. The condom is connected to a drainage tube and bag.

When patients with urinary catheters are treated, several precautions are important. Disruption or stretching of the drainage tube should be prevented, and no tension should be placed on the tubing or the catheter. The bag must not be placed above the level of the bladder for more than a few minutes. The bag should not be placed in the patient's lap when the patient is being transported. The production, color, and odor of the urine should be observed. The following observations should be reported to a physician or nurse: foul-smelling, cloudy, dark, or bloody urine, or a reduction in the flow or production of urine. The collection bag must be emptied when it is full.

Infection is a major complication for persons using catheters, especially for those using indwelling catheters. Everyone involved with the patient should maintain cleanliness during treatment. The tubing should be replaced or reconnected only by those properly trained. Treatment settings in which patients with catheters are

routinely treated have specific protocols for catheter care.

Two types of internal catheters that are frequently used are the *Foley catheter* and *suprapubic catheter.* The Foley catheter is a type of indwelling catheter that is held in place in the bladder by a small balloon inflated with air, water, or sterile saline solution. For removal of the catheter, the balloon is deflated and the catheter is withdrawn. The suprapubic catheter is inserted directly into the bladder through incisions in the lower abdomen and the bladder. The catheter may be held in place by adhesive tape, but care should be used to avoid its removal, especially during self-care activities.

INFECTION CONTROL

Infection control procedures are used to prevent the spread of disease and infection among patients, health care workers, and others. They are designed to interrupt or establish barriers to the infection cycle. **Universal precautions** (Box 11-1 and Fig. 11-1) were first established by the Centers for Disease Control and Prevention (CDC) to protect the health care worker from infectious agents such as the **human immunodeficiency virus** (HIV) and diseases such as **acquired immune deficiency syndrome** (AIDS) and hepatitis B. However, to

---

BOX 11-1
Summary of Universal Precautions

1. Use extreme care to prevent injuries caused by sharp instruments.
2. Cover minor, nondraining, noninfected skin lesions with an adhesive bandage.
3. Report infected or draining lesions and weeping dermatitis to your supervisor.
4. Avoid personal habits (e.g., nailbiting) that increase the potential for oral mucous membrane contact with body surfaces.
5. Perform procedures involving body substances carefully to minimize splatters and aerosols.
6. Cover environmental surfaces with moisture-proof barriers whenever splattering with body substances is possible.
7. Wash hands regularly, especially after gloves are worn.
8. Avoid unnecessary use of protective clothing. Use alternate barriers whenever possible.
9. Wear gloves to touch the mucous membrane or nonintact skin of any patient and whenever direct contact with body substances is anticipated.
10. Wear protective clothing (e.g., gown, mask, and goggles) when splashing of body substances is anticipated.

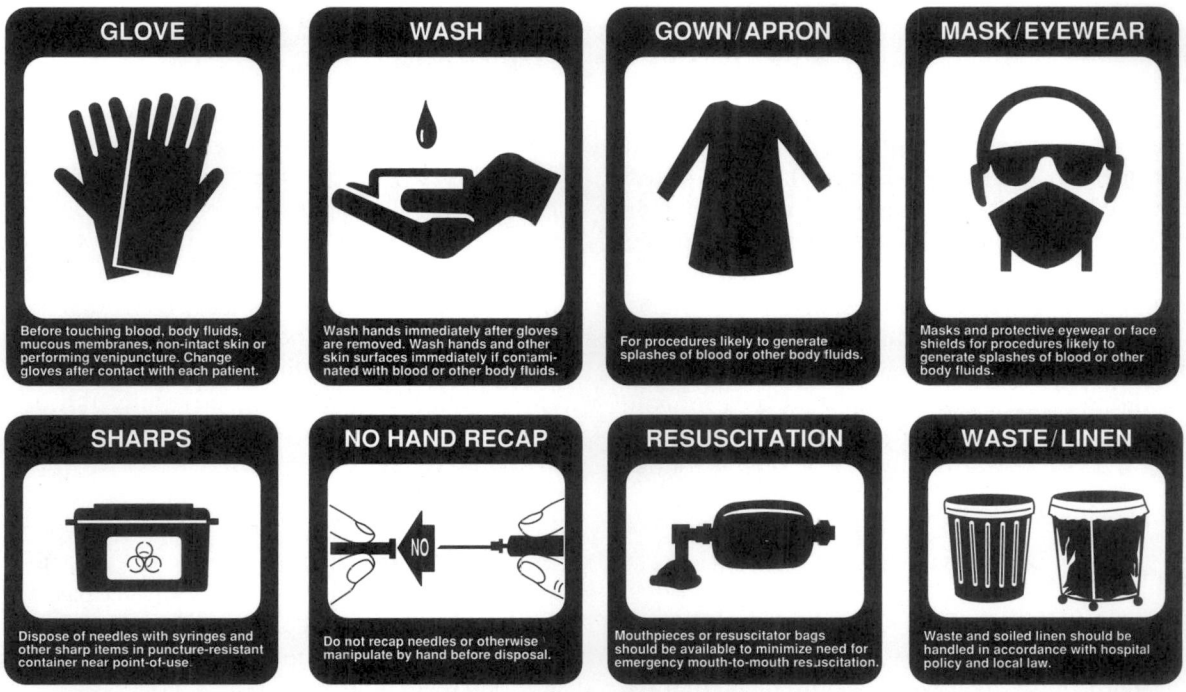

Universal Precautions apply to blood, visibly bloody fluid, semen, vaginal secretions, tissues and to cerebrospinal, synovial, pleural, peritoneal, pericardial and amniotic fluids.

FIG. 11-1
Universal blood and body fluid precautions. (Courtesy Brevis Corp., Salt Lake City, Utah.)

be effective, they must be used with all patients, not just those identified as infected.

The Occupational Safety and Health Administration (OSHA) has issued regulations to protect the employees of health care facilities. All health care settings must do the following to comply with federal regulations:

1. Educate employees on the methods of transmission and the prevention of hepatitis B and HIV.
2. Provide safe and adequate protective equipment and teach employees where the equipment is located and how to use it.
3. Teach employees about work practices used to prevent occupational transmission of disease, including, but not limited to, universal precautions, proper handling of patient specimens and linens, proper cleaning of body fluid spills (Fig. 11-2), and proper waste disposal.
4. Provide proper containers for the disposal of waste and sharp items, and teach employees the color coding system used to distinguish infectious waste.
5. Post warning labels and biohazard signs (Fig. 11-3).
6. Offer the hepatitis B vaccine to employees who are at substantial risk of occupational exposure to the hepatitis B virus.
7. Provide education and follow-up care to employees who are exposed to communicable disease.

OSHA has also outlined the responsibilities of health care employees. These responsibilities include the following:

1. Using protective equipment and clothing provided by the facility whenever the employee contacts, or anticipates contact, with body fluids
2. Disposing of waste in proper containers, applying knowledge and understanding of the handling of

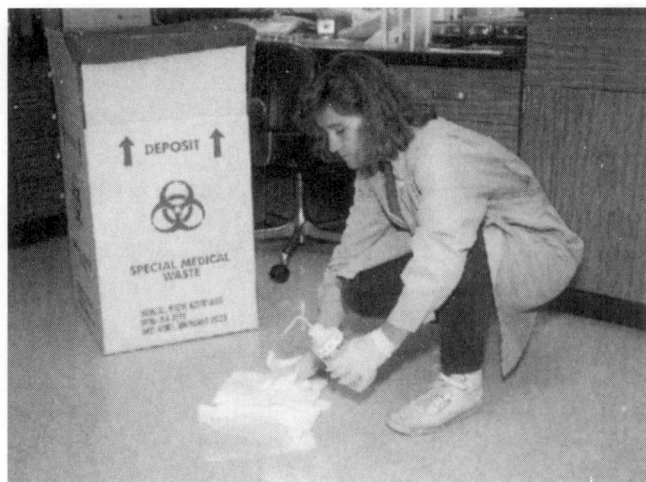

FIG. 11-2
Spills of body fluids must be cleaned up by a gloved employee, using paper towels, which should then be placed in an infectious waste container. Afterward, 5.25% sodium hypochlorite (household bleach) diluted 1:10 should be used to disinfect the area. (From Zakus SM: *Clinical procedures for medical assistants*, ed 3, St Louis, 1995, Mosby.)

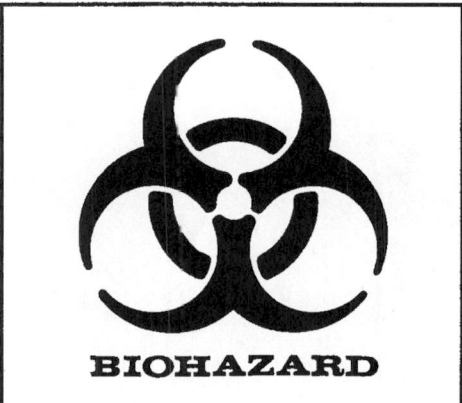

FIG. 11-3
Biohazard label. (From Zakus SM: *Clinical procedures for medical assistants*, ed 3, St Louis, 1995, Mosby.)

infectious waste, and using color-coded bags or containers

3. Disposing of sharp instruments and needles into proper containers without attempting to recap, bend, break, or otherwise manipulate them before disposal
4. Keeping the work environment and patient care area clean
5. Washing hands immediately after removing gloves and at any other times mandated by hospital or agency policy
6. Immediately reporting any exposures such as needle sticks or blood splashes or any personal illnesses to immediate supervisor and receiving instruction about any further follow-up action

Although it is impossible to eliminate all pathogens from an area or object, the likelihood of infection can be greatly reduced. The largest source of preventable patient infection is contamination from the hands of health care workers. Hand washing (Box 11-2 and Figs. 11-4 to 11-7) and the use of gloves are the most effective barriers to the infection cycle. Additional measures include wearing caps, face masks, and gowns and properly disposing of sharp instruments, contaminated dressings, and bed linens.

In the clinic, general cleanliness and proper control of heat, light, and air are also important for infection control. Spills should be cleaned up promptly. Work areas and equipment should be kept free from contamination.

To decontaminate is to "remove, inactivate, or destroy blood-borne pathogens on a surface or item to the point where they are no longer capable of transmitting infectious particles and the surface or item is rendered safe for handling, use, or disposal."[2] Items to be sterilized or decontaminated should first be cleaned thoroughly to remove any residual matter. Sterilization

BOX 11-2
Technique for Effective Hand Washing

1. Remove all jewelry, except plain band-type ring. Remove watch or move it up. Provide complete access to area to be washed.
2. Approach the sink and avoid touching the sink or nearby objects.
3. Turn on the water and adjust it to a lukewarm temperature and a moderate flow to prevent splashing.
4. Wet your wrists and hands with your fingers directed downward and apply approximately 1 teaspoon of liquid soap or granules.
5. Begin to wash all areas of your hands (palms, sides, and backs), fingers, knuckles, and between each finger, using vigorous rubbing and circular motions (Fig. 11-4). If wearing a band, slide it down the finger a bit and scrub skin underneath it. Interlace fingers and scrub between each finger.
6. Wash for at least 30 seconds, keeping the hands and forearms at elbow level or below, with hands pointed down. Wash longer if you have treated a patient known to have an infection.
7. Rinse hands well under running water.
8. Wash wrists and forearms as high as contamination is likely.
9. Rinse hands, wrists, and forearms under running water (Fig. 11-5).
10. Use an orangewood stick or nail brush to clean under each fingernail at least once a day when starting work and each time hands are highly contaminated. Rinse nails well under running water (Fig. 11-6).
11. Dry your hands, wrists, and forearms thoroughly with paper towels. Use a dry towel for each hand. The water should continue to flow from the tap as you dry your hands.
12. Use another dry paper towel to turn water faucet off (Fig. 11-7). Discard all towels in an appropriate container.
13. Use hand lotion as necessary.

Modified from Zakus SM: *Clinical procedures for medical assistants*, ed 3, St Louis, 1995 Mosby.

is used to destroy all forms of microbial life, including highly resistant bacterial spores. An **autoclave** is used to sterilize items by steam under pressure. Ethylene oxide, dry heat, and immersion in chemical sterilants are other methods of sterilization.

A variety of disinfectants may be used to clean environmental surfaces and reusable instruments. When liquid disinfectants and cleaning agents are used, gloves should be worn to protect the skin from repeated or prolonged contact. The CDC, local health department, or hospital infection control department can provide information about the best product and method to use.

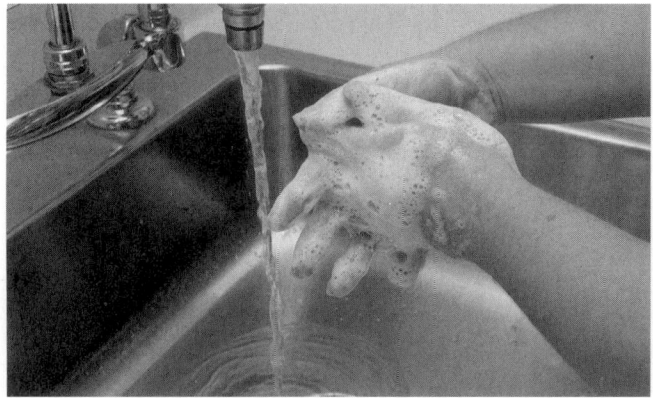

FIG. 11-4
Handwashing technique. Interlace fingers to wash between them. Create a lather with soap. Keep hands pointed down. (From Zakus SM: *Clinical procedures for medical assistants*, ed 3, St Louis, 1995, Mosby.)

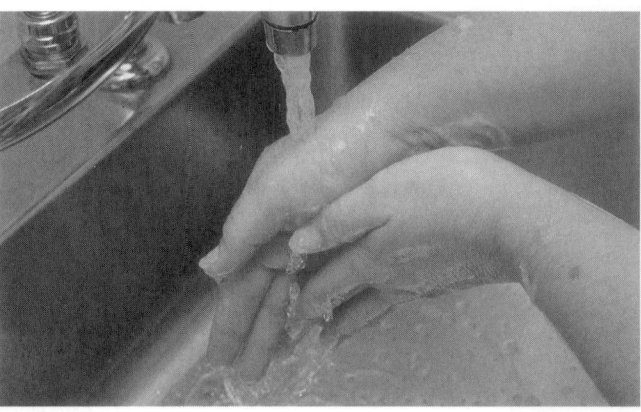

FIG. 11-5
Rinse hands well, keeping fingers pointed down. (From Zakus SM: *Clinical procedures for medical assistants*, ed 3, St Louis, 1995, Mosby.)

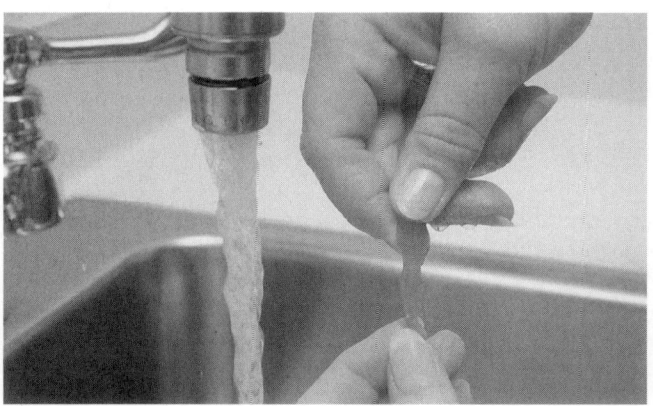

FIG. 11-6
Use blunt edge of an orangewood stick to clean under the fingernails. (From Zakus SM: *Clinical procedures for medical assistants*, ed 3, St Louis, 1995, Mosby.)

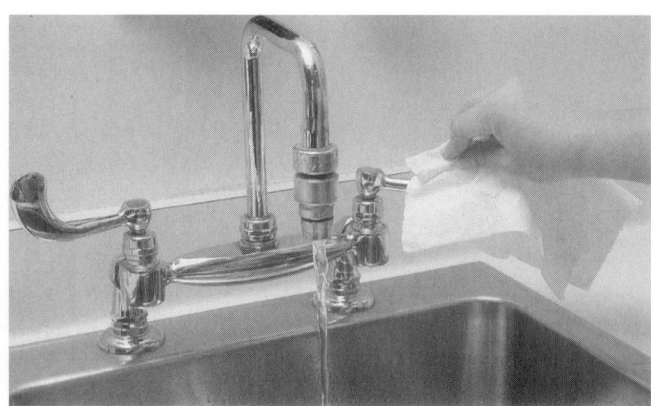

FIG. 11-7
After drying your hands, turn water faucet off, using a dry paper towel. (From Zakus SM: *Clinical procedures for medical assistants*, ed 3, St Louis, 1995, Mosby.)

Instruments and equipment used to treat a patient should be cleaned or disposed of according to institutional or agency policies and procedures. Contaminated reusable equipment should be placed carefully in a container, labeled, and returned to the appropriate department for sterilization. Contaminated disposable items should be placed carefully in a container, labeled, and disposed of.

Contaminated or soiled linen should be disposed of with minimal handling, sorting, and movement. It can be bagged in an appropriate bag and labeled before transport to the laundry, or the bag can be color coded to indicate the type or condition of linen it contains. Other contaminated items such as toys, magazines, personal hygiene articles, dishes, and eating utensils should be disposed of or disinfected. They should not be used by others until they have been disinfected.

Therapists should routinely clean and disinfect personal items such as pens, keys, and clipboards because these objects are touched frequently and may become contaminated.

Isolation Systems

Isolation systems are designed to protect a person or object from becoming contaminated or infected by transmissible pathogens. Various isolation procedures are used in different institutions. It is important for all health care workers to understand and follow the isolation approach used in their facilities so protection can be ensured.

Generally, a patient is isolated from other patients and the hospital environment when he or she has a transmissible disease. Isolation involves placing the

---

STRICT ISOLATION

VISITORS: REPORT TO NURSES' STATION BEFORE ENTERING ROOM

1. Masks are indicated for all persons entering the room.
2. Gowns are indicated for all persons entering the room.
3. Gloves are indicated for all persons entering the room.
4. HANDS MUST BE WASHED AFTER TOUCHING THE PATIENT OR POTENTIALLY CONTAMINATED ARTICLES AND BEFORE TAKING CARE OF ANOTHER PATIENT.
5. Articles contaminated with infective material should be discarded or bagged and labeled before being sent for decontamination and reprocessing.

FIG. 11-8
Strict isolation procedures sign. Card will be color-coded yellow and placed on or next to the door of the patient's room.

RESPIRATORY ISOLATION

VISITORS: REPORT TO NURSES' STATION BEFORE ENTERING ROOM

1. Masks are indicated for those who come close to the patient.
2. Gowns are not indicated.
3. Gloves are not indicated.
4. HANDS MUST BE WASHED AFTER TOUCHING THE PATIENT OR POTENTIALLY CONTAMINATED ARTICLES AND BEFORE TAKING CARE OF ANOTHER PATIENT.
5. Articles contaminated with infective material should be discarded or bagged and labeled before being sent for decontamination and reprocessing.

FIG. 11-9
Respiratory isolation procedures sign. Card will be color-coded blue and placed on or next to the door of the patient's room.

---

patient in a room either alone or with one or more patients with the same disease to reduce the possibility of transmitting the disease to others. Specific infection control techniques must be followed by all who enter the patient's room. These requirements are listed on a color-coded card and placed on or next to the door of the patient's room. Strict isolation and respiratory isolation procedures are shown in Figs. 11-8 and 11-9. Protective clothing, including gown, mask, cap, and gloves, may be needed. When leaving the patient, the caregiver must remove the garments in the proper sequence.

Occasionally, a patient's condition (e.g., burns or a systemic infections) make him or her more susceptible to infection. This patient may be placed in *protective isolation*. In this approach, persons entering the patient's room may have to wear protective clothing to prevent the transmission of pathogens to the patient. The sequence and method of donning the protective garments are more important than the sequence used to remove them.

INCIDENTS AND EMERGENCIES

Occupational therapists should be able to respond to a variety of medical emergencies and to recognize when it is better to get assistance from the most qualified individual available, such as a doctor, emergency medical technician, or nurse. This should be relatively easy in a hospital but may require an extended period if the treatment is conducted in a patient's home or outpatient clinic. It is a good idea to keep emergency telephone numbers readily available. The therapist will need to determine at the time of the incident whether it is wiser to ask for assistance before or after beginning emergency care. In most cases, it will be best to call for assistance before initiating emergency care, unless the delay is life threatening to the patient.

Consistently following safety measures will prevent many accidents. However, the therapist should always be alert to the possibility of an injury and expect the unexpected to happen. Most institutions have specific policies and procedures to follow. In general, the therapist should do the following when there is an injury to a patient:

1. Ask for help. Do not leave the patient alone. Prevent further injury to the patient and provide emergency care.
2. When the emergency is over, document the incident according to the institution's policy. Do not discuss the incident with the patient or significant others or express information to anyone that might indicate negligence.[3]
3. Notify the supervisor of the incident and file the incident report with the appropriate person within the organization.

Falls

The therapist can prevent injuries from falls by remaining alert and reacting quickly when patients lose their balance. Proper guarding techniques must be practiced. In many instances it is wise to resist the natural impulse to keep the patient upright. Instead, the therapist can carefully assist the patient to the floor or onto a firm object.

If a patient begins to fall forward, the following procedure should be used: Restrain the patient by firmly holding the gait belt. Push forward against the pelvis and pull back on the shoulder or anterior chest. Help the patient stand erect once it is determined there is no injury. The patient may briefly lean against you for support. If the patient is falling too far forward to be kept upright, guide the patient to reach for the floor slowly. Slow the momentum by gently pulling back on the gait belt and the patient's shoulder. Step forward as the patient moves toward the floor. Tell the patient to bend the elbows when the hands contact the floor to help cushion the fall. The patient's head should be turned to one side to avoid injury to the face.

If the patient begins to fall backwards, the following procedure should be used: Rotate your body so one side is turned toward the patient's back and widen your stance. Push forward on the patient's pelvis and allow the patient to lean against your body. Then assist the patient to stand erect. If the patient falls too far backward, to stay upright continue to rotate your body until it is turned toward the patient's back and widen your stance. Instruct the patient to briefly lean against your

body or to sit on your thigh. You may need to lower the patient into a sitting position on the floor using the gait belt and good body mechanics.

Burns

Generally, only minor, first-degree burns are likely to occur in occupational therapy. These can be treated with basic first aid procedures. Skilled personnel should be contacted for immediate care if the burn has any charred or missing skin or shows blistering. The following steps should be taken for first-degree burns in which the skin is only reddened:

1. Rinse or soak the burned area in cold (not iced) water.
2. Cover with a clean or sterile dressing or adhesive bandage. In some instances a moist dressing will be more comfortable for the patient.
3. Do not apply any cream, ointment, or butter to the burn because this will mask the appearance and may lead to infection or a delay in healing.

Bleeding

A laceration may result in minor or serious bleeding. The objectives of treatment are to prevent contamination of the wound and to control the bleeding. The following steps should be taken to stop the bleeding:

1. Wash your hands and apply protective gloves. Continue to wear protective gloves while treating the wound.
2. Place a clean towel or sterile dressing over the wound and apply direct pressure to the wound. If no dressing is available, use your gloved hand.
3. Elevate the wound above the level of the heart to reduce blood flow to the area.
4. In some instances the wound can be cleansed with an **antiseptic** or by rinsing it with water.
5. Encourage the patient to remain quiet and avoid using the extremity.
6. If there is arterial bleeding (demonstrated by spurting blood), it may be necessary to apply intermittent, direct pressure to the artery, above the level of the wound. The pressure point for the brachial artery is on the inside of the upper arm, midway between the elbow and armpit. The pressure point for the femoral artery is in the crease of the hip joint, just to the side of the pubic bone.
7. Do not apply a tourniquet unless you have been trained to do so.

Shock

Patients may experience shock as a result of excessive bleeding, as a reaction to the change from a supine to an upright position, or as a response to excessive heat.

Signs and symptoms of shock include pale, moist, and cool skin, shallow and irregular breathing, dilated pupils, a weak or rapid pulse, and dizziness or nausea. Shock should not be confused with fainting, which would result in a slower pulse, paleness, and perspiration. Patients who faint will generally recover promptly if allowed to lie flat. If a patient exhibits symptoms of shock, the following actions should be taken:

1. Determine the cause of shock and correct it if possible. Monitor the patient's blood pressure and pulse rate.
2. Place the person in a supine position, head slightly lower than the legs. If there are head and chest injuries or if respiration is impaired, it may be necessary to keep the head and chest slightly elevated.
3. Do not add heat, but prevent loss of body heat if necessary by applying a cool compress to the patient's forehead and covering the patient with a light blanket.
4. Keep the patient quiet and do not allow exertion.
5. After the symptoms are relieved, gradually return the patient to an upright position and monitor the patient's condition.

Seizures

Seizures may be caused by a specific disorder, brain injury, or medication. The OTR should be able to recognize a seizure and take appropriate action to keep the patient from getting hurt. A patient having a seizure will usually become rigid for a few seconds and then begin to convulse with an all-over jerking motion. The patient may turn blue and may stop breathing for up to 50 to 70 seconds. A patient's sphincter control may be lost during or at the conclusion of the seizure, so the patient may void urine or feces involuntarily. When a patient shows signs of entering a seizure, the following steps should be taken:

1. Place the person in a safe location and position away from anything that might cause injury. *Do not* attempt to restrain or restrict the convulsions.
2. Assist in keeping the patient's airway open, but do not attempt to open the mouth by placing any object between the teeth. Never place your finger or a wooden or metal object in the patient's mouth, and do not attempt to grasp or position the tongue.
3. If the patient's mouth is open, place a soft object between the teeth to prevent the patient from accidentally biting his or her tongue. A tongue depressor wrapped with several layers of gauze and fastened with adhesive tape or a sturdy cloth object may be used.
4. When the convulsions subside, turn the person's head to one side as a precaution against vomiting.

5. After the convulsions cease, have the patient rest. It may be helpful to cover the patient with a blanket or screen to provide privacy.
6. Get medical help.

Insulin-Related Illnesses

Many patients seen in occupational therapy have insulin-related episodes. It is important for the OTR to be able to differentiate between the conditions of hypoglycemia (insulin reaction) and hyperglycemia (acidosis) as shown in Table 11-1.

An *insulin reaction* can be caused by too much systemic insulin, the intake of too much food or sugar, or too little physical activity. If the patient is conscious, some form of sugar (e.g., candy or orange juice) should be provided. If the patient is unconscious, glucose may have to be provided intravenously. The patient should rest, and all physical activity should be stopped. This condition is not as serious as acidosis, but the patient should be given the opportunity to return to a normal state as soon as possible.

Acidosis can lead to a diabetic coma and eventual death if not treated. It should be considered a medical emergency requiring prompt action, including assistance from qualified personnel. The patient should not be given any form of sugar. Usually, an injection of insulin is needed, and a nurse or physician should provide care as quickly as possible.

Respiratory Distress

Dyspnea control postures may be used to reduce breathlessness in patients in respiratory distress. The

TABLE 11-1
Warning Signs and Symptoms of Insulin-Related Illnesses

	Insulin Reaction	Acidosis
Onset	Sudden	Gradual
Skin	Moist, pale	Dry, flushed
Behavior	Excited, agitated	Drowsy
Breath odor	Normal	Fruity
Breathing	Normal to shallow	Deep, labored
Tongue	Moist	Dry
Vomiting	Absent	Present
Hunger	Present	Absent
Thirst	Absent	Present

patient must be responsive and have an unobstructed airway. The *high-Fowler's position* (Fig. 11-10) may be used for patients in bed. The head of the bed should be in an upright position at a 90° angle. If available, a footboard should be used to support the patient's feet. The *orthopneic position* (Fig. 11-11) may be used for patients who are sitting or standing. In either case the patient bends forward slightly at the waist and supports the upper body by leaning the forearms on a table or counter.

Choking and Cardiac Arrest

All health care practitioners should be trained to treat patients who are choking or suffering from a cardiac arrest. Specific training courses are offered by both the American Heart Association and the American Red Cross. *The following information is presented as a reminder of the basic techniques and is not meant to be substituted for training.*

The urgency of choking cannot be overemphasized. Immediate recognition and proper action are essential. When assisting a conscious adult or a child who is more than 1 year old, the following steps should be taken:

1. Ask the patient, "Are you choking?" If the patient can speak, or cough effectively, *do not* interfere with the patient's own attempts to expel the object.
2. If the patient is unable to speak, cough, or breathe, check the mouth and remove any visible foreign object.
3. If the patient is unable to speak or cough, position yourself behind the patient. Clasp your hands over the patient's abdomen, slightly above the umbilicus but below the diaphragm.
4. Use the closed fist of one hand, covered by your other hand, to give three or four abrupt thrusts against the person's abdomen by compressing the abdomen in and up forcefully (Heimlich maneuver). Continue to apply the thrusts until the obstruction becomes dislodged or is relieved or the person becomes unconscious.

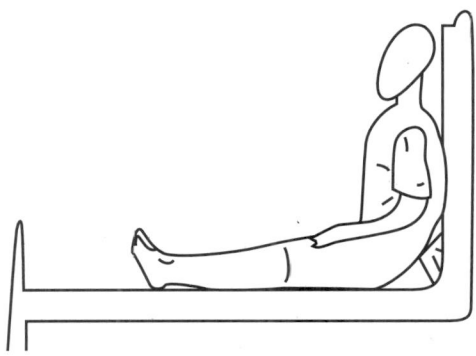

FIG. 11-10
High-Fowler's position.

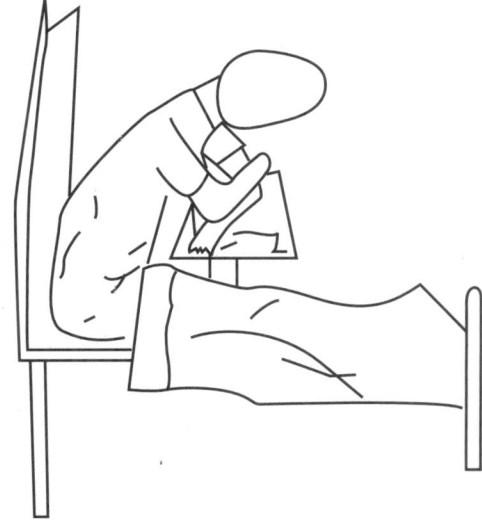

FIG. 11-11
Orthopneic position.

5. Seek medical assistance.

When assisting an unconscious adult or child who is more than 1 year old, the following steps should be taken:

1. Place the person in a supine position and call for medical help.
2. Open the person's mouth and use your finger to attempt to locate and remove the foreign object (finger sweep).
3. Open the airway by tilting the head back and lifting the chin forward. Attempt to ventilate using the mouth-to-mouth technique. If unsuccessful, deliver up to five abdominal thrusts (Heimlich maneuver), repeat the finger sweep, and attempt to ventilate. It may be necessary to repeat these steps. Be persistent and continue these procedures until the object is removed or medical assistance arrives.

It may be necessary to initiate cardiopulmonary resuscitation (CPR) techniques to stabilize the person's cardiopulmonary functions after the object has been removed. The following procedures are recommended for CPR[1]:

1. Determine the patient's condition by gently shaking the patient and asking, "Are you all right?" or, "How do you feel?"
2. If there is no response, place the patient in a supine position on a firm surface. Open the patient's airway by lifting up on the chin and pushing down on the forehead to tilt the head back.
3. Check for respiration by observing the chest or abdomen for movement, listen for sounds of breathing, and feel for breath by placing your cheek close to the person's mouth. If no sign of breath is present, the patient is not breathing, and you should initiate breathing techniques.

4. Pinch the patient's nose closed and maintain the head tilt to open the airway. Place your mouth over the patient's mouth and form a seal with your lips. Perform two full breaths, then evaluate the circulation. Some persons prefer to place a clean cloth over the patient's lips before initiating mouth-to-mouth respirations. If available, a plastic intubation device can be used to decrease the contact between the caregiver's mouth and the patient's mouth and any saliva or vomitus.

5. Palpate the carotid artery for a pulse. If there is no pulse, you must begin external chest compressions.

6. To initiate chest compressions, kneel next to the patient, place the heel of one hand on the inferior portion of the sternum just proximal to the xiphoid process, and place your other hand on top of the first hand. Position your shoulders directly over the patient's sternum, keep your elbows extended, and press down firmly, depressing the sternum approximately $1\frac{1}{2}$ to 2 inches with each compression. Relax after each compression, but do not remove your hands from the sternum. The relaxation and compression phases should be equal in duration. This can be accomplished by mentally counting "one thousand one," "one thousand two," "one thousand three," and so on for each phase.

7. If you perform all CPR procedures without assistance, you should perform 15 chest compressions and then perform two breaths. You must compress at the rate of 80 to 100 times per minute. Continue these procedures until qualified assistance arrives or the patient is able to sustain independent respiration and circulation. If you are alone, attempt to gain assistance from other persons by calling loudly for help. If a second person is present, the person should contact an advanced medical assistance unit before beginning to assist with CPR. In most instances the patient will require hospitalization and evaluation by a physician. (*Note:* Extreme care must be used to open the airway of a person who may have experienced a cervical spine injury. In such cases, use the chin lift, but avoid the head tilt. If the technique does not open the airway, the head should be tilted slowly and gently until the airway is open.)

These procedures are appropriate to use for adults and for children 8 years of age and older. Performing CPR is contraindicated if patients have clearly expressed their desire for "do not resuscitate" (DNR). This information should be clearly documented in the medical chart. A pamphlet or booklet containing diagrams and instructions for CPR techniques (Fig. 11-12) can be obtained from most local offices of the American Heart Association or from a variety of web sites.

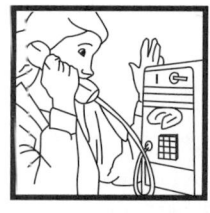

STEP 1

CALL 911

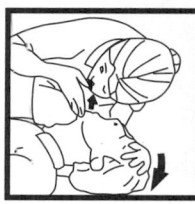

STEP 2

TILT HEAD, LIFT CHIN, CHECK BREATHING

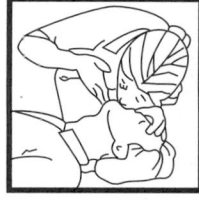

STEP 3

GIVE TWO BREATHS

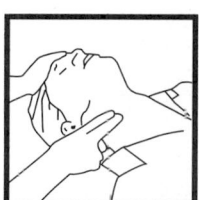

STEP 4

CHECK PULSE

STEP 5

POSITION HANDS IN THE CENTER OF THE CHEST

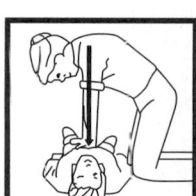

STEP 6

FIRMLY PUSH DOWN TWO INCHES ON THE CHEST 15 TIMES

CONTINUE WITH TWO BREATHS AND 15 PUMPS UNTIL HELP ARRIVES

FIG. 11-12
Standard CPR. (From www.learncpr.org/pocket.html.)

SUMMARY

All occupational therapy personnel have a legal and professional obligation to promote safety for self, the patient, visitors, and others. The OTR should be prepared to react to emergency situations quickly, decisively, and calmly. The consistent use of safe practices helps reduce accidents for both patients and workers and reduces the length and cost of treatment.

RECOMMENDED READINGS

Information on infection control can be obtained from the CDC, OSHA, and the Environmental Protection Agency (EPA).

Information on first aid, choking, and CPR can be obtained from most local offices of the American Heart Association and from the American National Red Cross. In addition, information on emergency procedures may be found at a variety of web sites.

REVIEW QUESTIONS

1. Why is it important to teach the patient and significant others guidelines for handling various emergency situations?
2. Describe at least four behaviors you can adopt to improve patient safety.
3. Describe the consequences of improper positioning of patients.
4. Describe positions to avoid for patients with above- and below-knee lower extremity amputations, total hip replacements, hemiplegia, rheumatoid arthritis, and burns.
5. Define the following: IV line, A line, NG tube, TPN or hyperalimentation, and ventilator.
6. Describe universal precautions.
7. Why is it important to follow universal precautions with all patients?
8. Demonstrate the proper technique for handwashing.
9. How should you respond to a patient emergency?
10. Describe how you would help a patient who is falling forward and one who is falling backward?
11. Which emergency situations might require getting advanced medical assistance and which situations could a therapist handle alone?

REFERENCES

1. Adult basic life support, *JAMA* 268(16):2184-2198, 1992.
2. Occupational Safety and Health Administration: Occupational exposure to blood-borne pathogens: final rule, *Federal Register* 56:64175, 1991.
3. Pierson FM: *Principles and techniques of patient care*, ed 2, Philadelphia, 1999, WB Saunders.
4. Steich TJ: Malpractice and occupational therapy personnel, *Occup Ther News* 39(6):8, 1985.
5. Zakus SM: *Clinical procedures for medical assistants*, ed 3, St Louis, 1995, Mosby.

CHAPTER 12

Occupational Performance

MARY BETH EARLY

KEY TERMS

Occupation
Occupational performance areas
Performance components
Performance context
Identity
Client-centered evaluation and intervention
Narrative interviews
Canadian Occupational Performance Measure
Occupational Performance History Interview, Version II
Activity Configuration
Remediation
Compensation
Environmental modification
Environmental management

LEARNING OBJECTIVES

Study of this chapter will enable the student or practitioner to do the following:

1. Define *occupation*.
2. Provide a detailed analysis of the complex nature of occupation.
3. Describe methods used to elicit occupational information from patients and clients.
4. Discuss the importance of occupation in the formation and maintenance of a sense of identity.
5. Discuss approaches for evaluating occupational performance.
6. Explain how to set client-centered goals related to occupational performance.
7. Compare and contrast various approaches to improve occupational performance.
8. Identify ways to measure progress in reaching occupational performance goals.

This chapter introduces the chapters on the occupational performance areas (activities of daily living, work, and leisure) and on specific aspects of occupational performance (mobility, sexuality, the Americans With Disabilities Act, and assistive technology) that are of particular concern to persons who have physical disabilities. The present chapter frames the content of Part Three and advises the student and reader to keep the focus on occupation when evaluating and treating persons with physical dysfunction.

OCCUPATION AND PHYSICAL DYSFUNCTION

The American Occupational Therapy Association (AOTA) has defined **occupation** as "the ordinary and familiar things that people do every day."[1] The ability to pursue and perform a person's customary occupations is taken for granted so long as a person is well. Injury and disease may disrupt occupation temporarily, but most people seek or are referred for the services of an occupational therapist only when they encounter significant difficulty resuming or enacting (carrying out) occupations that are important to them.

On meeting the patient, how should the occupational therapist approach occupation? How does the therapist evaluate difficulties in occupational performance? Are there preferred methods for the therapist to assist a person to engage in occupations? These are some of the questions that will be considered in this chapter.

ANALYZING OCCUPATIONAL PERFORMANCE

According to the *Uniform Terminology*, third edition,[3] occupations may be classified within three **occupational performance areas:** activities of daily living (ADL), work and productive activities, and play and leisure. Further, performance in occupations may be considered in terms of the **performance components,** the underlying skills or functions (such as muscle strength, balance, or memory) that support the ability to perform. Occupation also occurs within a **performance context,** which has temporal and environmental dimensions. (The reader is encouraged to review Chapter 1 for further detail on the organization of occupational performance.)

The patient with a physical problem who is referred for occupational therapy almost always has obvious deficits in performance components. These deficits (limited range of motion [ROM], reduced muscle strength, impaired balance, and perceptual difficulties) may be so prominent as to distract both patient and therapist from considering occupation itself. However, interventions that seek to improve performance component function without evaluating and improving occupational performance cannot be considered occupational therapy. Thus, even when it seems obvious that the patient needs (for example) to improve sitting balance and increase active ROM and muscle strength in the right upper extremity, the therapist is required to look at the "bigger picture" of occupational functioning—not just occupational functioning in general, but the specific and highly individual functioning desired and required for that individual in his or her chosen and valued occupations.

HIDDEN DIMENSIONS OF OCCUPATION

Occupations have personal meaning, as well as cultural, temporal, psychologic, social, spiritual, and symbolic dimensions.[2,5] Clark and associates[6] state that occupation is "chunks of meaningful activity in which humans engage." The examples given are "dressing, attending a party, gardening, watching television, making love, and preparing a meal."[6] Occupation must be viewed as complex, highly specific, having symbolic attributes, and often charged with emotion.

Nelson[13] makes a distinction between occupational form and occupational performance. *Occupational form* has an objective nature, independent of the person engaged in the occupation. Occupational form is influenced by sociocultural and physical characteristics. Thus, it is not a *medium* such as weaving or cooking, but a *form* such as weaving on a Navajo blanket loom in a hogan or cooking chapatis on a cookfire fueled by cow patties. *Occupational performance* is the action that is structured or elicited by the occupational form.[13] Each occupational performance is a unique enactment of the occupational form.

Occupational performance depends on the individual's (1) perception of occupational form and (2) sense of purpose in this performance.[13] Does the form have meaning to the individual? This affects quality of performance and, indeed, whether performance is initiated and sustained.

Does the occupational form elicit purpose from the individual? What is the nature of this purpose? Purpose must come from the actor, not from outside (i.e., from the therapist). For example, the purpose may be to create something, to fulfill a duty, to please someone else, or to get money. Each performance influences subsequent performances[13] and also affects the individual in a variety of ways.

Breines[4] observed that the purpose of occupation is to make a difference and to have an effect on the world. The therapist's role is, then, to facilitate performance for those who are unable to perform.[4]

Occupations contribute to a person's sense of **identity.** People frequently define who they are by their occupation and their abilities. This is true not only of occupations that are "jobs," but also of leisure and daily living occupations. A person may say, "I am a homemaker," and also "I am a left-midfielder" or "I drive everywhere, and I don't even know where the bus routes are."

Identity is significantly challenged by the inability to perform occupational roles. Dickerson and Oakley[9] found that persons with physical disabilities living in the community reported that they did not expect to resume roles of student, worker, or hobbyist. They noted that treatment of physical dysfunction traditionally focuses on functional restoration (of performance components used in daily living tasks) and not on the less tangible goals of performing in occupational roles.

Competence in occupations is highly valued and central to feelings of self-worth. Taking pride in performance of even mundane tasks is the norm. Consider the following statements that indicate valuing of occupational competence. A 3-year-old declares, "I get dressed all by myself!" A taxi driver says, "I keep my car very clean and neat. My customers always comment." An 80-year-old proudly states, "I still garden 4 hours every day, up and down, on my hands and knees, everything."

Context modifies occupational performance. Expectations and relative valuing of occupational performance are set not just by the individual, but also by the culture, the family, and society in general. This becomes important when the therapist envisions the future occupational performance of a patient. The therapist must find out whether it is important to the patient and family that the patient perform the particular occupation. Further, the therapist must learn the contextual elements (e.g., environment and objects) that will frame the performance of the occupation.

OBTAINING INFORMATION ABOUT OCCUPATIONAL PERFORMANCE

How does the therapist collect data about the occupational performance of a patient with physical dysfunction? Occupational performance is assessed by the patient's self-report, by the report of an informed family member or caregiver, and by naturalistic and structured observation of occupational performance tasks that are important to the patient.

Evaluation of occupational performance necessitates that the patient be asked to identify problems, needs, and priorities. In traditional settings, it may appear that protocol dictates the use of particular forms to assess specific components of performance (e.g., joint ROM). Such forms will not reveal the particular occupational experiences that cause distress. On the other hand, **interviewing** the patient, whether formally using a structured interview format, or less formally in the course of other assessments, will elicit those tasks and areas that the patient finds most troublesome. Beginning with these troublesome and valued tasks is a more direct route to meaningful functional outcomes.

The therapist gathers information about how the patient spends and manages time and perceives his or her own occupational performance. **Narrative interviews** invite patients to speak at length, expanding on their occupational experiences and revealing their feelings and understanding of present and past occupational difficulties. Mallinson, Kielhofner, and Mattingly[11] note that patients may use themes relating to

momentum and entrapment. They may say, for example, that they felt "stuck" or "trapped" or that "it was hard to get going."

Structured interviewing tools such as the Canadian Occupational Performance Measure,[8] Activity Configuration,[7,14] and the Occupational Performance History Interview[10] may be used. (See Table 12-1 for these and others.)

Interview-Based Assessments of Occupational Performance

The **Canadian Occupational Performance Measure** (COPM) is a standardized, semistructured interview that has specific instructions and methods for administering and scoring. It encompasses the areas of self-care, productivity, and leisure and is designed to "detect change in a client's self-perception of occupational performance over time."[8] It measures self-perception of occupational performance, is client centered, and can be used with a variety of disabilities and all developmental stages.[8]

The COPM asks clients to identify issues in occupational performance, rate their problems in terms of importance, and self-rate their level of functioning. The COPM yields self-report scores of performance and of satisfaction. The scores on the COPM are not norm referenced. Instead, they are referenced to the unique problems of each individual patient. The comparison of the individual's scores from assessment to reassessment

TABLE 12-1
Interview-Based Assessments of Occupational Performance

Assessment	Description
Activity Configuration*§	Semi-structured interview yielding data on education, work, leisure, and values, as well as a daily schedule. Interview also elicits occupational roles and balance of activities.
Assessment of Occupational Functioning (AOF)‖	Screening tool, interview format. Measures occupational functioning. Related to Model of Human Occupation (MOHO). Developed for long-term care settings.
Canadian Occupational Performance Measure (COPM)‡	Interview-based rating scale of client's perception of occupational performance and satisfaction with performance. Multiple ratings over time yield outcome data.
Occupational Performance History Interview, Version 2†	Semistructured interview with rating scales for occupational identity, occupational competence, and impact of environment or context. Also includes creation of time line from life history of patient.

*Cykin S: *Occupational therapy: toward health through activities,* Boston, 1979, Little, Brown
†Kielhofner G, Mallinson T, Crawford C, et al: *A user's manual for the occupational performance history interview,* version 2, Chicago, 1998, University of Illinois at Chicago.
‡Law M, Baptiste S, Carswell A, et al: *Canadian occupational performance measure,* ed 3, Ottawa, Ontario, 1998, CAOT Publications
§Watanabe S: *The activities configuration,* 1968 Regional Institute on the Evaluation Process, New York, 1968, American Occupational Therapy Association.
‖Watts JH, Kielhofner G, Bauer DF, et al: The assessment of occupation functioning: a screening tool for use in long term care, *Am J Occup Ther* 40(4):231-240, 1986.

is viewed as the most appropriate measure of change and progress.[8] The COPM targets client-identified problems and is intended to facilitate treatment collaboration between client and therapist.[12]

The **Occupational Performance History Interview, Version II** (OPHI-II),[10] includes a semistructured interview, rating scales, and a life history narrative. The life history narrative invites the patient to tell his or her life story and explain how and why the various events occurred. This contributes to the storytelling, storymaking process of narrative reasoning (see Chapter 3) and helps the therapist view the disability from the patient's perspective.

The COPM and the OPHI-II each require 45 to 60 minutes to administer and score, but this time is justified by the functional data yielded. Either may be used as a starting point for assessment and intervention related to occupational performance.

The **Activity Configuration** (Fig. 12-1) yields information about the patient's values, educational history, work history, leisure interests and activities, vocational interests, and plans.[7,14] From the activity configuration, the therapist can construct a daily schedule of activities, a list of life roles, and an analysis of activity balance in the person's life. As with the COPM and the OPHI-II, administration of the activity configuration is time consuming but worthwhile because it yields rich and detailed data. See Table 12-1 for other interview-based assessments.

Performance-Based Assessment of Occupational Performance

Interview instruments yield important data concerning patient and family perception of the patient's occupational performance. Interviews must be augmented by direct observation of patient performance, so that the therapist can evaluate the safety, accuracy, efficiency, and completeness of the performance. Many structured assessment instruments are available for assessing specific areas of occupational performance, and these are described in their corresponding chapters (see Chapters 13 to 16 and 19).

Notwithstanding the value of these structured assessments, naturalistic observation is sometimes more relevant to the needs of a particular individual in a specific performance context. Consider, for example, the needs of a multiple amputee who must don an unusual orthopedic appliance, or another person who must manage to get up onto a toilet that is in a tight and awkward corner. In these cases the patient's performance on a standard ADL evaluation may miss entirely the specific occupational performances most likely to cause difficulty. It is the therapist's responsibility to carefully review the goals of the patient and make sure that the evaluation sufficiently addresses areas of concern.

Assessment of Occupational Performance When Referral Is More Restricted

Where therapy services require referral or doctor's orders, the therapist must start from the deficit noted in the original order but is also obliged to consider the patient more globally. In other words, the challenge may be to find a way to identify and obtain permission to address other occupational performance areas and tasks that are troublesome to the patient, without exceeding the spirit of the original order.

SETTING GOALS RELATED TO OCCUPATIONAL PERFORMANCE

Goals must be defined jointly by the patient and the therapist. These goals must identify steps toward realizing occupations that are valued by the patient. The therapist will be skilled at refining the client's broad goal statements into treatment objectives that are achievable, understandable, observable, measurable, and stated in behavioral terms. Thus the therapist can help the patient who says, "I want to go home" to identify and work toward a more immediate (but related) objective such as, "The patient will transfer from wheelchair to toilet without assistance." Using a client-centered approach, the therapist can develop a succession of goals leading to the "big goal." The therapist thus creates "the big picture" of "where we are going with therapy" and can remind the patient of the importance and place of the immediate goal.

The therapist must avoid setting goals that indicate functional restoration in the absence of an occupational dimension. A goal statement such as, "Increase elbow flexion by 20°" focuses on functional restoration but does not say why this is important. The therapist provides an occupational dimension and a functional context by writing instead, "Increase elbow flexion by 20° so that patient can eat finger foods independently." See Chapter 6 for further examples of goal statements.

TREATING DEFICITS IN OCCUPATIONAL PERFORMANCE

Deficits in occupational performance are addressed by a variety of methods detailed in Chapters 13 through 19. These methods are based on the following broad concepts and principles:

1. *Occupational performance deficits are rarely amenable to direct remediation.* In other words, while a muscle (e.g., biceps brachii) can be strengthened through exercise and graded resistance, performance of more complex occupational tasks (e.g., feeding self with a spoon) may require more than practice and repetition. **Remediation** *is* useful to alleviate performance component dysfunction that may limit occupational

---

ACTIVITY CONFIGURATION AND DAILY SCHEDULE: OUTLINE FOR INTERVIEW

Background Information

Patient's name _____ Patient's age _____ Patient's sex _____

Patient's life stage _____

Educational History
1. Highest educational level achieved
2. Location and type of schools (e.g., public, private, parochial)
3. Subjects of greatest interest
4. Subjects of least interest
5. Average grades achieved
6. Likes and dislikes about school
7. Leisure interests during school years
8. Social groups to which subject belonged
9. Educational level of parents, siblings
10. Future educational plans
11. Career aspirations

Work History
1. Most recent work or job performed
2. Previous jobs
3. Special job training (past, present)
4. Likes and dislikes about jobs, past and present
5. Most preferred jobs (real or imagined)
6. Preferences for working alone or with others
7. Works alone or with others
8. Socializes with coworkers (on the job, off the job)
9. Job supervisor
10. Type of supervision received (close, distant)
11. Most effective or desirable type of supervision
12. Plans for future work or job changes

Leisure Interests and Activities
1. Interest in sports, games, hobbies (specify)
2. Participation in sports, games, hobbies (when, how long)
3. Other leisure interests that would be pursued given adequate time
4. Are leisure skills considered important to life? Why or why not?

Values and Cultural Influences
1. Cultural group with which the patient identifies
2. Describe cultural customs which are important (e.g., celebrations, holiday festivals, foods, religious practices, garments, family traditions)
3. Health practices unique to this culture; special beliefs about health and illness; respective roles of ill and well members of family; if raised in another country, attitudes toward health care system in United States; experiences with United States health care system
4. Describe things (concrete and abstract) that are most valued (e.g., cars, jewels, toys, pictures, family traditions, honesty, integrity, fairness). Why are they valuable?

Daily Schedule
Construct a daily schedule for a typical weekday and typical weekend day in the patient's life. Give details for hour-by-hour activities.

Life Roles
List all occupational roles of the patient (e.g., worker, father, brother, sportsman, gardener).

Life Balance
Approximate percent of time spent by the patient in each of the performance areas of self-maintenance, home and child management, work, and play and leisure.

FIG. 12-1

Activity configuration/daily schedule. Outline for interview. (Adapted from Cynkin: *Occupational therapy: toward health through activities,* Boston, 1979, Little, Brown.)

performance. In terms of functional outcomes, remediation is valuable *only* if it improves the ability to perform desired occupations.

2. *Adaptation of tools, equipment, and methods may improve performance, but adaptations must be acceptable to the patient and family.* Much adaptive equipment for feeding, hygiene, bathing, grooming, personal care, work, and leisure is available commercially to therapists and also directly to consumers. People are sensitive to appearances and reject adaptive equipment because they believe it stigmatizes them. This applies not just to equipment, but also to methods. Most activities can be done in many ways other than the one that seems customary. For example, a person with a recent hip replacement who finds it difficult to place and retrieve food bowls for pets from their customary location (on the floor) might adapt by placing the bowls on the countertop. However, sanitary concerns may make this solution unacceptable. The therapist must help the patient identify acceptable solutions.

3. **Compensation** *by the individual or by a caregiver may be necessary to enable performance.* When customary procedures (those normally employed by the able bodied) are prevented or rendered awkward by disability, the patient may use a different method, or the deficit in performance may be compensated for by the actions of another person. Consider, for example, a cognitively impaired individual who must be left alone during the day while the caregiver is at work. This patient can still have a hot lunch if the caregiver prepares it in advance, leaves it on a specific accessible shelf in the refrigerator, and provides simple directions for reheating it in an accessible microwave oven.

4. *Modifying the environment or features of the environment may be used to enable performance.* Obvious **environmental modifications** such as wheelchair ramps, keyboard supports, and grab bars are only the beginning. Many less obvious but equally helpful modifications are possible, such as removing area rugs, positioning frequently used items closer, and switching items from left to right or vice-versa, depending on dominance. Any modifications must be agreeable to the patient, family, and others in the situation (e.g., if in a workplace, then to employer and other employees).

5. *Patients and caregivers can contribute ideas to improve performance and will often arrive at creative and workable solutions.* An important therapist role is to facilitate and empower problem identification and problem solving by patients and caregivers.

MEASURING PROGRESS TOWARD OCCUPATIONAL PERFORMANCE GOALS

Progress is easy to measure when goals and objectives are carefully designed to be achievable, understandable, observable, and measurable and are stated in behavioral terms. Direct observation (either naturalistic or structured), using the same assessment procedures employed in the initial evaluation, is the accepted method of measuring progress. Immediately upon the patient's reaching a goal or objective, the therapist must identify or (if the goal has already been identified) refine the next goal or objective. Selection and discussion of objectives and methods should be done in collaboration with the patient. Motivation is enhanced when the therapist maintains an ongoing sense of forward momentum and progress toward "the big goals" the patient has identified.

SUMMARY

Occupational therapists assist individuals who are experiencing impaired ability to carry out desired daily occupations. Occupations are multidimensional and complex; therapy must focus on the occupational goals the patient identifies as important. A top-down, client-centered approach is recommended, employing a narrative interview assessment that yields statements of patient goals and patient perceptions of problems and obstacles. Development of intermediate objectives and selection of methods and approaches must include the patient. Although it is necessary to break down long-term goals into smaller steps or objectives, each step must lead toward success in occupational performance. Continual reassessment and setting of new goals maintain a sense of forward momentum and increase motivation. Therapy does not end when the therapist has helped the patient reach his or her highest functional level. Therapy includes helping patients acquire a sense of occupational competence and identity regardless of how their present functional level compares with their prior level or with "the norm."

REVIEW QUESTIONS

1. What is occupation? How would you define occupation when speaking to a patient?
2. Choose a favorite occupation. Describe the occupational form. Analyze a recent occupational performance, including the following dimensions: physical, cultural, temporal, psychologic, social, spiritual, and symbolic.
3. Using the occupation named in question 2, analyze an occupational performance by someone other than yourself.
4. How are occupation and identity related? List your occupations. Describe how your perception of self might change if you could not perform these occupations.
5. What methods are used for evaluating occupational performance?
6. What is the COPM and what does it yield?
7. What is the OPHI-II and what does it yield?

8. What is the Activity Configuration and what does it yield?
9. Contrast structured and naturalistic observation. In what situations would you prefer one over the other?
10. Describe the procedure and criteria for setting goals related to occupational performance.
11. How can one measure progress toward goals in occupational performance?

REFERENCES

1. American Occupational Therapy Association: Position paper: occupation, *Am J Occup Ther* 49:1015-1018, 1995.
2. American Occupational Therapy Association: Statement-fundamental concepts of occupational therapy: occupation, purposeful activity, and function, *Am J Occup Ther* 51:864-866, 1997.
3. American Occupational Therapy Association: Uniform terminology, ed 3, *Am J Occup Ther* 48:1047-1054, 1994.
4. Breines EB: Making a difference: a premise of occupation and health, *Am J Occup Ther* 43:51-52, 1989.
5. Canadian Association of Occupational Therapists: *Occupational therapy guidelines for client-centred practice*, Toronto, 1991, the Association.
6. Clark FA. Parham D, Carlson ME, et al: Occupational science: academic innovation in the service of occupational therapy's future, *Am J Occup Ther* 45:300-310, 1991.
7. Cynkin S: *Occupational therapy: toward health through activities*, Boston, 1979, Little, Brown.
8. Law M, Baptiste S, Carswell A, et al: *Canadian occupational performance measure*, ed 3, Ottawa, Ontario, 1998, CAOT Publications.
9. Dickerson AE, Oakley F: Comparing the roles of community-living persons and patient populations, *Am J Occup Ther* 49:221-228, 1995.
10. Kielhofner G, Mallinson T, Crawford C, et al: *A user's manual for the occupational performance history interview*, version 2, Chicago, 1998, Model of Human Occupation Clearinghouse, University of Illinois at Chicago.
11. Mallinson T, Kielhofner G, Mattingly C: Metaphor and meaning in a clinical interview, *Am J Occup Ther* 50:338-346, 1996.
12. Neistadt ME: Teaching clinical reasoning as a thinking frame, *Am J Occup Ther* 52:221-229, 1998.
13. Nelson DL: Occupation: form and performance, *Am J Occup Ther* 42:633-641, 1988.
14. Watanabe S: The activities configuration, *1968 Regional Institute on the Evaluation Process, New York Report RAS-123-&-68*, Rockville, Md, 1968, American Occupational Therapy Association.

CHAPTER 13

Activities of Daily Living

DIANE FOTI

KEY TERMS

Activities of daily living
Instrumental activities of daily living
Top-down approach
Bottom-up approach
Maximal level of independence
Levels of independence
Home assessment
Accessibility
Medication management
Backward chaining
Assistive technology

LEARNING OBJECTIVES

After reading this chapter the student or practitioner will be able to do the following:
1. Define ADL and I-ADL.
2. Name two standardized tests of ADL.
3. Describe a bottom-up versus top-down approach to evaluation.
4. Define levels of independence.
5. Explain the usual procedures for ADL and I-ADL assessments.
6. Explain the benefits of a home evaluation.
7. Explain how to record and summarize results of the ADL assessment and training program.
8. Discuss various methods of teaching ADL.
9. Discuss considerations for selecting adaptive equipment.
10. Describe, perform, and teach ADL techniques for individuals with limited ROM and strength, incoordination, paraplegia, quadriplegia, and low vision.

Activities of daily living (ADL) and instrumental activities of daily living (I-ADL) are tasks of self-care, functional mobility, functional communication, home management, and community living that enable an individual to achieve personal independence.[16,20] Evaluation and training in the performance of these important life tasks have long been important aspects of occupational therapy (OT) programs in virtually every type of health care service. Loss of ability to care for personal needs and to manage the environment can result in loss of self-esteem and a deep sense of dependence. Family roles are also disrupted, requiring partners to assume the function of caregiver when one loses the ability to perform ADL or I-ADL independently.[30]

The role of OT is to assess ADL and I-ADL performance skills, determine problems that interfere with independence, determine treatment objectives, and provide training to increase independence. The OT practitioner may also be involved in removing or reducing physical, cognitive, social, and emotional barriers that are interfering with performance. The need to learn new methods or use assistive devices to perform daily tasks may be temporary or permanent, depending on the particular dysfunction and the prognosis for recovery.

DEFINITIONS OF ADL AND I-ADL

Daily activities can be separated into two areas: **activities of daily living** (ADL) and **instrumental activities**

BOX 13-1
Activities in ADL and I-ADL

Activities of Daily Living (ADL)

Self-Care
Grooming
Oral hygiene
Toilet hygiene
Dressing
Feeding and eating
Medication routine
Health maintenance
Emergency response
Community mobility

Functional Mobility
Bed mobility
Wheelchair mobility
Transfers
Functional ambulation

Functional Communication
Writing
Typing/computer use
Telephoning
Augmentative communication devices

Environmental Hardware
Keys
Faucets
Light switches
Windows/doors
Telephone
Computer

Instrumental Activities of Daily Living (I-ADL)

Home Management
Clothing Care
Cleaning
Meal preparation
Money management
Household maintenance
Care of others

Community Living Skills
Shopping
Access to recreation

Environmental Hardware
Vacuum cleaner
Can opener
Stove/oven
Refrigerator
Microwave

Modified from American Occupational Therapy Association: Uniform terminology for occupational therapy, third edition, *Am J Occup Ther* 48(11):1047-1054, 1994.

of daily living (I-ADL). ADL require basic skills, whereas I-ADL require more advanced problem-solving skills, social skills, and more complex environmental interactions. ADL tasks include functional mobility, self-care, functional communication, management of environmental hardware and devices, and sexual expression.[2] I-ADL tasks include home management and community living skills (Box 13-1). Home management is classified with work and productive activities in the Occupational Performance Model.

EVALUATION OF PERFORMANCE AREAS

ADL is one of the major performance areas in the occupational performance model discussed in Chapter 1. A comprehensive evaluation of performance skills should include assessment of the client's abilities and limitations in (1) ADL or self-maintenance, (2) work and pro-

ductive activities, and (3) play and leisure. The role of the OT practitioner is to facilitate skill in performance of these essential tasks of living. It is important to help the individual with a disability to balance activity in each of these three performance areas according to his or her personality, skills, limitations, needs, cultural values, and lifestyle.

The therapist may consider using a **top-down approach** to the evaluation process in order to understand the client's occupational history and interests. A top-down approach may include the charting of a daily or weekly schedule (see Chapter 12), an activities configuration, an interest checklist, or an occupational role history.[10,14,30,33,40] The activities configuration protocol can be used to gather data about the client's values, education, work history, and vocational interests and plans. The interest checklist can be used to determine the degree of interest in five categories of activities—manual skills, physical sports, social recreation, ADL, and cultural and educational activities.[30] The occupational role history is used to indicate the balance between work and leisure roles.[14] Although the interest checklist and the occupational role history were developed for a psychiatric population, they can be adapted for application to clients with a physical dysfunction.

A **bottom-up approach** to the evaluation process focuses on identifying problems in specific performance components. This approach may fail to identify how a performance component deficit affects the client's occupational performance.[15] For example, a therapist determines that a client has impaired fine motor control. A general evaluation may indicate that the client has difficulty with simple tasks such as tying shoes and buttoning clothes. After completing an interest checklist and occupational role history, the occupational therapist also determines that the fine motor control deficit will affect the client's job as a computer operator and limit her ability to continue with a hobby of jewelry making. Although these two approaches to evaluation are discussed separately, a skilled clinician blends the two in practice. Once a functional deficit is identified, the performance component deficit that causes the functional deficit is identified. The therapist can then determine if it is possible to improve or provide remediation for the performance component or if a compensatory method will be needed to improve occupational performance.

An interview and performance evaluation can yield a well-rounded picture of the client's occupational performance. Deficits and imbalances in occupational performance will be apparent. The performance evaluation is fundamental to the development of a comprehensive treatment plan. The performance evaluations to be addressed in this chapter are for ADL and I-ADL. Work evaluation is assessment of specific work skills using real or simulated work situations[21] and is discussed in Chapter 16. Leisure activities are discussed in Chapter 18.

CONSIDERATIONS IN ADL AND I-ADL EVALUATION AND TRAINING

The ADL/I-ADL evaluations include a performance evaluation, assessment of performance components, and evaluation of the client's psychosocial and physical environment. Physical performance components such as strength, range of motion (ROM), coordination, sensation, and balance should be assessed to determine the potential for remediation and possible need for adaptive equipment. Perceptual and cognitive functions should be assessed to determine the potential for learning ADL skills. General mobility in bed or wheelchair or ambulation should also be assessed and are discussed in more detail in Chapter 14.

In addition to these relatively concrete and objective assessments, the occupational therapist should be familiar with the client's culture and the culture's values in relation to self-care, the sick role, family assistance, and independence. The values of the client and the client's peer group and culture should be important considerations in selecting objectives and initial activities in the ADL program. The demands of time and energy for the balance of activities in the client's day may influence how many ADL can be performed independently.

The environment to which the client will return is an important consideration. Will the client live alone or with his or her family or a roommate? Will the client go to a skilled nursing facility or to a board and care home, and will the client go permanently or temporarily? Will the client return to work and community activities? The type and amount of assistance available in the home environment must be considered if the caregiver is to receive training to provide assistance and supervision.

The finances available for assistant care, special equipment, and home modifications are important considerations. For example, a wheelchair-bound client who is wealthy may be willing and able to make major modifications in the home, such as installing an elevator, lowering kitchen counters, widening doorways, and replacing carpeting to accommodate a wheelchair lifestyle. A client with fewer financial resources may need the assistance of an occupational therapist in making less costly modifications, such as removing scatter rugs and door sills, installing a ramp at the entrance, and attaching a handheld shower head to the bathtub faucet.

The ultimate goal of any ADL and I-ADL training program is for the client and family to learn to adapt to the life changes that necessitated a referral to the occupational therapist. For the individual who values independence, the goal may be to achieve the **maximal level of independence**. It is important to note that this level is different for each client. For the client with mild muscle weakness in one arm, complete independence in ADL may be the maximal. In contrast, for the individual with a high-level quadriplegia, self-feeding, oral hygiene, and communication activities with devices and assistance may be the maximal level of independence that can be expected.

For the individual whose culture does not value independence as highly as does Western culture, the occupational therapist may focus primarily on teaching the client and family to adapt. The focus would be on family training and identifying the activities of highest value to the client. The potential for independence depends on each client's unique personal needs, values, capabilities, limitations, and social and environmental resources.

ADL AND I-ADL ASSESSMENT

Assessment of ADL and I-ADL is initiated with an interview, using a checklist as a guide for questioning and selection of performance activities. Several types of ADL and I-ADL checklists and standardized tests are available. They all cover similar categories and performance tasks.[8] The use of a standardized test will ensure a more objective assessment and provide a standard means of measurement. A standardized assessment tool can be used at a later time for reevaluation, and some assessments allow for comparison to a norm group. Asher[4] has developed an annotated index of assessment tools, which can be used as a resource for selecting appropriate tools for evaluation. Some examples of standardized ADL and I-ADL assessments are listed in Table 13-1. The occupational therapist should review the literature periodically to learn about new assessments developed by occupational therapists and about those that have been developed as interdisciplinary assessments, such as the Functional Independence Measure (FIM).[39]

General Procedure

When data have been gathered about the client's physical, psychosocial, and environmental resources, the feasibility of ADL assessment or ADL training should be determined by the occupational therapist in concert with the client, supervising physician, and other members of the rehabilitation team. In some instances, ADL training should be delayed because of limitations of the client or in favor of more immediate treatment objectives that require the client's energy and participation.

The interview may serve as a screening device to help determine the need for further assessment by observation of performance. This need is determined by the therapist based on knowledge of the client, the dysfunction, and previous assessments. A partial or complete performance evaluation is invaluable in assessing ADL performance. The interview alone can lead to inaccurate assumptions. The client may recall performance before the onset of the dysfunction, may have some confusion or memory loss, and may overestimate or underestimate individual abilities because there has been little opportunity to perform routine ADL since the onset of the physical dysfunction.

Ideally, the occupational therapist assesses performance when and where the activities usually take place.

For example, a dressing assessment could be arranged early in the morning in the treatment facility when the client is dressed by nursing personnel, or in the client's home. Self-feeding assessment should occur at regular meal hours. If this timing is not possible, the assessment may be conducted during regular treatment sessions in the OT clinic under simulated conditions. Requiring the client to perform routine self-maintenance tasks at irregular times in an artificial environment may contribute to a lack of carryover, especially for clients who have difficulty generalizing learning.

The therapist should select relatively simple and safe tasks from the ADL and I-ADL checklist and should progress to more difficult and complex items, including some that involve safety measures. The ADL assessment should not be completed at one time because this approach would cause fatigue and create an artificial situation. Tasks that would be unsafe or obviously cannot be performed should be omitted and the appropriate notation made on the assessment form (see Chapter 20).

During the performance assessment the therapist should observe the methods the client is using or attempting to use to accomplish the task and try to determine causes of performance problems. Common causes include weakness, spasticity, involuntary motion, perceptual deficits, cognitive deficits, and low endurance. If problems and their causes can be identified, the therapist has a good foundation for establishing training objectives, priorities, methods, and the need for assistive devices.

Other important aspects of this assessment that should not be overlooked are the client's need for respect and privacy and the ongoing interaction between the client and the therapist. The client's feelings about having his or her body viewed and touched should be respected. Privacy should be maintained for toileting, grooming, bathing, and dressing tasks. The therapist with whom the client is most familiar and comfortable may be the appropriate person to conduct ADL assessment and training. As the therapist interacts with the client during performance of daily living tasks, it may be possible to elicit the client's attitudes and feelings about the particular tasks, priorities in training, dependence and independence, and cultural, family,

TABLE 13-1
Examples of Standardized Assessments for ADL and I-ADL

ADL Assessments	I-ADL Assessments	Measures ADL and I-ADL
Klein-Bell ADL Scale[22]	Assessment of Motor and Process Skills (AMPS)[13]	Canadian Occupational Performance Measure (COPM)[25]
Functional Independence Measure (FIM)[39]	Kitchen Task Assessment (KTA)[5]	Kohlman Evaluation of Living Skills (KELS)[24]

and personal values and customs regarding performance of ADL.

Recording Results of ADL Assessment

During the interview and performance assessment the therapist makes appropriate notations on the checklists. If a standardized assessment is used, the standard terminology identified for that assessment is used to describe or measure performance. Nonstandardized tests may include separate checklists for self-care, home management, mobility, and home environment assessments. When describing **levels of independence,** occupational therapists often use terms like *maximum, moderate,* and *minimal assistance.* These quantitative terms have little meaning to health care professionals unless they are defined or supporting statements are included in progress summaries to give specific meanings for each. It also should be specified whether the level of independence refers to a single activity, a category of activities such as dressing, or all ADL. In designating levels of independence, an agreed-on performance scale should be used to mark the ADL checklist. The following general categories and their definitions are suggested:

1. *Independent:* can perform the activity or activities without cueing, supervision, or assistance, with or without assistive devices, at normal or near normal speeds

---

CASE STUDY 13-1

CASE STUDY—"J.V."

J.V. is a 72-year-old married woman who suffered a cerebral thrombosis resulting in a cerebrovascular accident (CVA) 3 months ago. She lives in a modest home with her husband. J.V. was active before her CVA, volunteering 10 hours a week at a local charity thrift store, walking a mile a day with friends, and caring for her husband, who is diabetic and has poor vision. She was independent with all of the indoor home management activities. She and her husband have a gardener, but J.V. enjoyed gardening with potted plants.

The CVA resulted in an ataxic gait, mild dysarthria (slurred speech), dysphagia (swallowing deficit), and slight hand incoordination. J.V. is easily frustrated and concerned about how she and her husband will manage, since her adult children live 5 hours away. She was referred to occupational therapy for evaluation and training in ADL and I-ADL and for treatment of dysphagia.

The initial evaluation involved an interview with the client and her husband, use of the Kitchen Task Assessment, and an ADL performance evaluation. The evaluation was completed in a 1-hour session. J.V. became restless after 15 minutes, but with redirection continued to attend to the tasks. J.V. is independent with eating, upper body dressing, and grooming while seated. J.V. is independent with toileting. She has been receiving maximum assistance for lower body dressing and bathing. She has difficulty with handwriting, use of the telephone, and handling keys. She requires moderate assistance to walk, using a front-wheeled walker (FWW), but is independent with wheelchair mobility on flat surfaces. Her visual fields are intact. She has no visual-spatial deficit. Her upper extremity strength and range of motion are WNL (within normal limits). Hand coordination is mildly impaired, as demonstrated with moderate difficulty pushing buttons on the phone and shoe tying. She is able to stand while holding on to a stable surface but cannot use her hands for a task while standing.

Results of the Kitchen Task Assessment[5] demonstrated deficits in organization of the task, at which point she required physical assistance. J.V. is highly motivated and has the potential to do simple, hot meal preparation and basic self-care independently, except for showering, for which she requires supervision.

A swallow assessment demonstrated moderately impaired tongue coordination and minimal delay with a swallow. J.V. has already modified her diet by selecting very soft foods and slightly thickened liquids.

Progress Report

J.V. has attended occupational therapy two times a week for 4 weeks. She is generally cooperative and motivated, although periodically she becomes discouraged as she continues to have an ataxic gait and requires the use of the wheelchair for independent mobility. Treatment has focused on lower extremity dressing, oral-motor exercises to improve swallowing, and simple meal preparation. J.V. has made significant progress in the treatment program. She has progressed from maximum assistance with lower extremity dressing to independent while seated. She has improved from chair-level grooming to standing with one-hand stabilization while using the other to brush her hair and teeth. Progress has been made from maximum assistance with bathing to supervised with transfer to a shower seat. From moderate difficulty with use of phone, she has progressed to independent and from dependent with oral-motor exercises she has progressed to supervised. J.V. is now independent in cold meal preparation after initially requiring maximum assistance.

J.V. continues to require a soft diet and slightly thickened liquids because of swallowing difficulties. She is consistent with use of safety techniques for swallowing. She continues to have impaired hand coordination but is learning compensatory techniques to adapt her method of performing various ADL tasks as demonstrated with her progress in ADL.

Occupational therapy has coordinated treatment and goals with the physical therapist and social worker. The therapist has recommended that the social worker refer the client's husband to a low vision center for evaluation, since he was dependent on his wife and never received instruction in low vision training. His independence will relieve some of J.V.'s burden of care giving.

Occupational therapy will focus on hot meal preparation, bed making, and exploring leisure interests with gardening, along with continuing to work toward improvement of oral-motor and hand coordination.

2. *Supervised:* can perform the activity alone but needs someone available for safety
3. *Minimal assistance:* supervision, cueing, or less than 20% physical assistance
4. *Moderate assistance:* supervision, cueing, and 20% to 50% physical assistance
5. *Maximal assistance:* supervision, cueing, and 50% to 80% physical assistance
6. *Dependent:* can perform only one or two steps of the activity or very few activities independently, may fatigue easily and perform very slowly, may require elaborate equipment and devices to perform basic skills such as feeding, needs more than 80% physical assistance

These definitions are broad and general. They can be modified to suit the approach of the particular treatment facility.

Information from the ADL assessment is summarized succinctly for inclusion in the client's permanent records so that interested professional coworkers can refer to it. A sample case study, with ADL and home management checklists, and summaries of an initial assessment and progress report are included in Figs. 13-1 and 13-2. When reviewing these, the reader should keep in mind that the assessment and progress summaries relate only to the ADL portion of the treatment program.

INSTRUMENTAL ACTIVITIES OF DAILY LIVING
Home Management Assessment

Home management tasks are assessed similarly to self-care tasks. First the client should be interviewed to elicit a description of the home and of former and present home management responsibilities. Tasks the client needs to perform when returning home, as well as those that he or she would like to perform, should be ascertained during the interview. If the client has a communication disorder or a cognitive deficit, aid from friends or family members may be enlisted to get the information needed. The client may also be questioned about his or her ability to perform each task on the activities list. The assessment is much more meaningful and accurate if the interview is followed by a performance assessment in the ADL kitchen or apartment of the treatment facility or in the client's home if possible.

The therapist should select tasks and exercise safety precautions consistent with the client's capabilities and limitations. The initial tasks should be simple one- or two-step procedures that are not hazardous, such as wiping a dish, sponging a table top, and turning the water on and off. As the assessment progresses, tasks graded in complexity and involving safety precautions should be performed, such as making a sandwich and a cup of coffee and vacuuming the carpet.

Home management skills apply to women, men, and sometimes adolescents and children. Individuals may live independently or share home management responsibilities with their partners. In some homes it is necessary for a role reversal to occur after the onset of a physical disability, and the partner who usually stays at home may seek employment outside the home, while the disabled individual remains at home.

If a client will be home alone, there are several basic ADL and I-ADL skills needed for safety and independence. Minimal ADL skills include independence with toileting and transfers, allowance for rest periods, and use of the telephone or special call system in case of emergency. Minimal I-ADL skills required to stay at home alone include the ability to (1) prepare or retrieve a simple meal, (2) employ safety precautions and exhibit good judgment, (3) take medication, and (4) get emergency aid if needed. The occupational therapist can assess potential for remaining at home alone through the activities of home management assessment. Safety management as listed in Box 13-1 is part of the home management assessment.

A child with a permanent disability also needs to be considered for assessment and training for I-ADL skills as he or she develops and matures with a growing need for independence.

Home Assessment

When discharge from the treatment facility is anticipated, a **home assessment** should be carried out to facilitate the client's maximal independence in the living environment. Ideally, the physical and occupational therapists should perform the home assessment together. During the home visit, the client and family members or housemates must be present. Budget and time factors may not allow two professional workers to go to the client's home, however. Therefore either the physical or occupational therapist should be able to perform the assessment, or the assessment may be referred to the home health agency that will provide home care services to the client.

The client and a family member should be interviewed to determine the client's and family's expectations and the roles the client will assume in the home and community. The cultural or family values regarding a disabled member may influence role expectations and whether independence will be encouraged. Willingness and financial ability to make modifications in the home can also be determined.[38]

Sufficient time should be scheduled for the home visit so that the client can demonstrate the required transfer and mobility skills. The therapist may also wish to ask the client to demonstrate selected self-care and home management tasks in the home environment. During the assessment the client should use the ambulation aids and any assistive devices that he or she is accustomed to using. The therapist should bring

Text continued on pg. 136

OCCUPATIONAL THERAPY DEPARTMENT
ACTIVITIES OF DAILY LIVING

Name *JV*   Age *72*   Diagnosis *CVA*

Disability *ataxia; dysarthria; dysphagia; hand incoordination*

Activity Precautions *none*

Mode of Ambulation *w/c; FWW with mod A*   Hand Dominance *R*

Previous Functional Level *Independent*

Social / home environment *Pt. is caregiver to husband; lives in own home*

Grading Key:
- I   =   Independent
- S   =   Supervised
- Min A = Minimal Assistance
- Mod A = Moderate Assistance
- Max A = Maximum Assistance
- D   =   Dependent
- N/A   =   Not applicable
- N/T   =   Not tested

TRANSFERS AND AMBULATION

Date	1/29	2/24		Remarks
Tub or Shower	Mod A	S		2° to slippery surfaces
Toilet	I	I		
Wheelchair	I	I		
Bed and Chair	I	I		
Ambulation	Mod A	Min A		FWW
Wheelchair Mgt.	I	I		on flat surfaces
Car	N/T	S		

FUNCTIONAL BALANCE

Date	1/29	2/24		Remarks
Sitting	I	I		
Standing	Mod A	S		Must use hands for balance
Walking	Mod A	Min A		FWW

EATING

Date	1/29	2/24		Remarks
Butter bread	I	I		
Cut meat	I	I		With effort and built-up handle
Eat with spoon	I	I		
Eat with fork	I	I		
Drink w/ straw	I	I		
Drink w/ glass	I	I		
Drink w/ mug	I	I		
Pour from pitcher	N/T	I		

UNDRESS

Date	1/29	2/24		Remarks
Underwear	Max A	I		
Slip/undershirt	I	I		
Dress	N/A	N/A		
Skirt	N/A	N/A		
Blouse/Shirt	Min A	I		Difficulty with buttons
Slacks/Jeans	Max A	I		
Necktie	N/A	N/A		

FIG. 13-1

ADL evaluation form. (Adapted from *Activities of daily living evaluation form 461-1*, Hartford, Conn, 1963, The Hartford Easter Seal Rehabilitation Center.)

UNDRESS (continued)

Date	1/29	2/24		Remarks
Nylons	N/T	N/A		
Housecoat/Robe	Min A	I		To pull robe up
Jacket	I	I		
Belt/Suspenders	N/A	N/A		
Hat	N/T	I		
Coat	N/T	I		
Sweater	I	I		
Mittens/Gloves	N/T	I		
Glasses	I	I		
Brace	N/A	N/A		
Shoes	Max A	I		
Socks	Max A	I		
Boots	Max A	N/T		

DRESS

Date	1/29	2/24		Remarks
Underwear	Max A	I		
Slip/undershirt	I	I		
Dress	N/A	N/A		
Skirt	N/A	N/A		
Blouse/Shirt	Min A	I		Difficulty with buttons
Slacks/Jeans	Max A	I		
Necktie	N/A	N/A		
Nylons	N/T	N/A		
Housecoat/Robe	Max A	I		To pull robe DOWN
Jacket	I	I		
Belt/Suspenders	N/A	N/A		
Hat	N/T	I		
Coat	N/T	I		
Sweater	I	I		
Mittens/Gloves	N/T	I		
Glasses	I	I		
Brace	N/A	N/A		
Shoes	Max A	I		
Socks	Max A	I		
Boots	Max A	N/T		

FASTENERS

Date	1/29	2/24		Remarks
Button	Min A	I		
Snap	Min A	I		
Zipper	I	I		
Hook and eye	N/A	N/A		
Untie Shoes	Max A	I		
Velcro	N/A	N/A		

HYGIENE

Date	1/29	2/24		Remarks
Blow nose	I	I		
Wash face/hands	I	I		While seated
Wash upper body	I	I		While seated
Wash lower body	Max A	I		
Brush teeth	I	I standing		While seated
Brush dentures	N/A	N/A		

FIG. 13-1, cont'd
ADL evaluation form. (Adapted from *Activities of daily living evaluation form 461-1*, Hartford, Conn, 1963, The Hartford Easter Seal Rehabilitation Center.)

Continued

HYGIENE (continued)

Date	1/29	2/24		Remarks
Brush/comb hair	/	/ standing		While seated
Curl hair	N/A	N/A		
Shave	N/A	N/A		
Apply makeup	N/T	/		
Clean fingernails	N/T	/		
Trim nails	N/T	S		
Apply deodorant	/	/		While seated
Shampoo hair	Min A	/		needs items in reach
Use toilet paper	/	/		
Use tampons/napkins	N/A	N/A		

MEDICATION MANAGEMENT

Date	1/29	2/24		Remarks
Identify proper medication	N/T	/		
Open bottle	N/T	/		
Handle pills	N/T	/		needs pill organizer
Manage syringe	N/T	Min A		did this for husband before CVA
Draw medication	N/T	Min A		

COMMUNICATION

Date	1/29	2/24		Remarks
Verbal	/	/		dysarthric
Read	/	/		
Hold book	/	/		
Turn page	/	/		
Write	Mod A	/		Poor legibility
Use telephone	Mod A	/		
Type/keyboard	N/T	N/T		
Handle mail	N/T	N/T		

COMBINED PERFORMANCE ACTIVITIES

Date	1/29	2/24		Remarks
Open/close door	Max A	/		
Remove/replace objects	/	/		
Carry objects while walking/wheeling	Max A	/		from wheelchair
Retrieve object from floor	Max A	/		with reacher

OPERATE

Date	1/29	2/24		Remarks
Light switches	/	/		
Doorbell	/	/		
Door locks/handles	/	/		from wheelchair
Faucets	/	/		from wheelchair
Shades/curtains	N/T	N/T		
Open/close window	N/T	N/T		
Hang up garment	N/T	/		from wheelchair

SUMMARY OF EVALUATION RESULTS

SENSORY STATUS

Date	1/29		2/24				Remarks
Intact (IN) or Impaired (IM)	IN	IM	IN	IM	IN	IM	
Touch	✓	.	✓				

FIG. 13-1, cont'd
ADL evaluation form. (Adapted from *Activities of daily living evaluation form 461-1*, Hartford, Conn, 1963, The Hartford Easter Seal Rehabilitation Center.)

SENSORY STATUS (continued)

Date	1/29		2/24				Remarks
Intact (IN) or Impaired (IM)	IN	IM	IN	IM	IN	IM	
Pain	✓		✓				
Temperature	✓		✓				
Proprioception		✓		✓			
Stereognosis	✓		✓				
Visual Fields	✓		✓				

PERCEPTUAL/COGNITIVE

Date	1/29		2/24				Remarks
Intact (IN) or Impaired (IM)	IN	IM	IN	IM	IN	IM	
Follows directions	✓		✓				
Orientation	✓		✓				
Memory	✓		✓				
Attention span		✓	✓				Needed redirection after 15 min
Problem solving		✓	✓				KTA — problems with organization
Visual spatial	✓		✓				
Left/right discrimination	✓		✓				
Motor planning	✓		✓				

FUNCTIONAL RANGE OF MOTION

Date	1/29		2/24				Remarks
Intact (IN) or Impaired (IM)	IN	IM	IN	IM	IN	IM	
Comb hair	✓		✓				
Feed self	✓		✓				
Fasten buttons	✓		✓				Impaired coordination
Pull up back of pants	✓		✓				
Zip zipper	✓		✓				
Tie shoes	✓		✓				ROM WNL; impaired balance
Reach self	✓		✓				From wheelchair
Stoop	✓		✓				Balance impaired

STRENGTH: indicate muscle grade

Date	1/29		2/24				Remarks
Left (L) or right (R)	L	R	L	R	L	R	
Head/neck	WNL	WNL	WNL	WNL			
Shoulder flexion	WNL	WNL	WNL	WNL			
Shoulder extension	WNL	WNL	WNL	WNL			
Elbow flexion	WNL	WNL	WNL	WNL			
Elbow extension	WNL	WNL	WNL	WNL			
Supination	WNL	WNL	WNL	WNL			
Pronation	WNL	WNL	WNL	WNL			
Wrist extension	WNL	WNL	WNL	WNL			
Wrist flexion	WNL	WNL	WNL	WNL			
Gross grasp	WNL	WNL	WNL	WNL			

COORDINATION

Date	1/29		2/24				Remarks
Left (L) or right (R)	L	R	L	R	L	R	
Fine motor	IM	IM	IM				2/24 slightly improved; pt. is compensating for deficits
Gross U.E.	IM	IM	IM				

FIG. 13-1, cont'd

ADL evaluation form. (Adapted from *Activities of daily living evaluation form 461-1,* Hartford, Conn, 1963, The Hartford Easter Seal Rehabilitation Center.)

OCCUPATIONAL THERAPY DEPARTMENT
ACTIVITIES OF HOME MANAGEMENT

Name _JV_   Date _1/29 (Initial eval)_

Address _Anytown, USA_

Age _72_   Role in family _wife, caregiver_

Diagnosis _CVA_

Activity Precautions _none •_

DESCRIPTION OF HOME

Owns home _X_   Apartment _____   Board & Care _____

No. of rooms _7_	Bathroom description _____	
No. of floors _1_	_Small 27" wide door_	
Stairs _3 to enter_	_Tub – Shower combination_	
Elevator _N/A_	_closed sink_	

Will client be required to perform the following activities? If not, who will perform? x = yes

Meal preparation	_X_	
Serving	_X_	
Wash dishes	_X_	
Shopping		_will need assist as she isn't driving_
Child care	_N/A_	
Laundry	_X_	
Housecleaning		_will hire housekeeper_
Pet care	_X_	
Sewing	_no_	
Hobbies	_X_	_volunteer work_

Does the client really like housework? _yes_

Grading Key:
- I = Independent
- S = Supervised
- Min A = Minimal Assistance
- Mod A = Moderate Assistance
- Max A = Maximum Assistance
- D = Dependent
- N/A = Not applicable
- N/T = Not tested

MEAL PREPARATION

Date	1/29	2/24		Remarks
Manage faucets	S	I		to stand
Handle stove controls	S	S		
Open packages	S	I		
Carry items	Max A	I		from wheelchair
Open cans	N/T	I		
Open jars	N/T	I		
Handle milk carton	I	I		
Empty garbage	N/T	N/T		
Retrieve refrigerator items	S	I		
Reach cupboards	S	I		
Peel vegetables	N/T	I		
Cut safely	N/T	I		

FIG. 13-2

Activities of home management. (Adapted from *Activities of home management form,* Occupational Therapy Department, University Hospital, Ohio State University, Columbus.)

MEAL PREPARATION (continued)

Date	1/29	2/24		Remarks
Break eggs	N/T	N/T		
Use electric mixer	N/T	N/T		
Use toaster	N/T	I		
Use coffee maker	N/T	I		
Use microwave	N/T	I		
Manage oven	N/T	S to Min A		
Pour hot water	N/T	S		

SET UP/CLEAN UP FOR MEAL PREPARATION

Date	1/29	2/24		Remarks
Set table	S	I		From wheelchair
Carry items to table	Max A	I		with wheelchair
Load-empty dishwasher	N/T	I		
Wash dishes	Mod A	I		
Wash pots and pans	Mod A	I		Fatigued rapidly
Wipe counters/stove	S	I		to stand
Wring out dishcloth	S	I		

CLEANING ACTIVITIES

Date	1/29	2/24		Remarks
Pick up object from floor	N/T	I		
Wipe spills	N/T	S		
Make bed	N/T	N/T		
Use dust mop	N/T	N/T		
Dust high surfaces	N/T	N/T		
Dust low surfaces	N/T	N/T		
Mop floor	N/T	N/T		
Sweep	N/T	N/T		
Use dust pan	N/T	N/T		
Vacuum	N/T	N/T		
Clean tub and toilet	N/T	N/T		
Change sheets	N/T	N/T		
Carry pail of water	N/T	N/T		
Carry cleaning tools	N/T	N/T		

LAUNDRY/CLEANING ACTIVITIES

Date	1/29	2/24		Remarks
Do hand washing	N/T	I		
Wring out clothes	N/T	I		
Hang clothing	N/T	S		
Carry laundry to and from washer and dryer	N/T	N/T		
Manage controls on appliances	N/T	I		
Use washing machine	N/T	I		
Retrieve clothes from dryer	N/T	S		
Iron	N/T	N/T		

HEAVY HOUSEHOLD ACTIVITIES, WHO WILL DO THESE?

Date	1/29	2/24		Remarks
Clean stove and oven	N/T	D		
Clean refrigerator	N/T	Mod A		
Shopping	N/T	Mod A		

FIG. 13-2, cont'd

Activities of home management. (Adapted from *Activities of home management form,* Occupational Therapy Department, University Hospital, Ohio State University, Columbus.) *Continued*

HEAVY HOUSEHOLD ACTIVITIES, WHO WILL DO THESE?
LAUNDRY/CLEANING ACTIVITIES (continued)

Date	1/29	2/24		Remarks
Put away groceries	N/T	Mod A		
Wash windows	N/T	D		
Change light bulbs	N/T	D		
Wash bathtub	N/T	D		
Maintain smoke alarms	N/T	D		
Recycle/compost	N/T	Mod A		

MISCELLANEOUS LAUNDRY/CLEANING ACTIVITIES

Date	1/29	2/24		Remarks
Retrieve newspaper	N/T	/		Needs reacher
Retrieve mail	N/T	N/T		
Feed pet	N/T	/		with reacher
Manage pet waste	N/T	D		
Let pet in and out	N/T	/		
Reach thermostat	N/T	/		
Thread needle/knot	N/T	N/T		
Sew on button	N/T	N/T		
Use scissors	N/T	N/T		
Water houseplants	N/T	N/T		

WORK HEIGHTS (Indicate best height)   1/29 - evaluation

Ironing	N/A
Cutting	Wheelchair level approx 31"
Dish washing	standard sink adequate
General work	37"
Maximal depth of counter (reach)	16" (for side reach)
Maximal height of work surface	37"
Maximal reach for high cupboards	43"
Maximal reach for low cupboards	9"
Best height for chair	20-23"

SUGGESTIONS FOR HOME MODIFICATION:

- Transfer tub bench / bathtub mat / grab bar in shower
- Shower hose
- 3 in 1 commode for use at night beside bed & over toilet during day
- Widen bathroom door to 32"

FIG. 13-2, cont'd
Activities of home management. (Adapted from *Activities of home management form*, Occupational Therapy Department, University Hospital, Ohio State University, Columbus.)

a tape measure to measure the width of doorways, the height of stairs, the height of the bed, and other dimensions.

The therapist can begin by explaining the purposes and procedure of the home assessment to the client and others present, if this has not been done before the visit. The therapist can proceed to take the required measurements while surveying the general arrangement of rooms, furniture, and appliances. It may be helpful to sketch the size and arrangement of rooms for later reference and attach these sketches to the home assessment checklist (Fig. 13-3). For more information on a variety of checklists, see Letts and associates.[26] Next, the client demonstrates mobility and transfer skills and essential self-care and home management tasks. The client's ability to use the entrance to the home and to transfer to and from an automobile, if it is to be used, should be included in the home assessment.

HOME EVALUATION CHECKLIST

Name_____ Date_____

Address_____

Diagnosis_____

Mobility Status
- ❑ ambulatory, no device ❑ walker
- ❑ cane ❑ wheelchair

_____

Exterior

Home located on
- ❑ level surface
- ❑ hill

Type of House
- ❑ owns house ❑ mobile home
- ❑ apartment ❑ board and care

Number of floors
- ❑ one story ❑ split level
- ❑ two story

Driveway surface
- ❑ inclined ❑ smooth
- ❑ level ❑ rough

Is the DRIVEWAY negotiable? ❑ yes ❑ no
Is the GARAGE accessible? ❑ yes ❑ no

_____

Entrance

Accessible entrances
- ❑ front ❑ side
- ❑ back

Steps
- number _____
- height of each _____
- width _____
- depth _____

Are there HANDRAILS? ❑ yes ❑ no

If yes, where are they located? ❑ left ❑ right

HANDRAIL height from step surface? _____

If no, how much room is available for HANDRAILS? _____

Are landings negotiable? ❑ yes ❑ no

Briefly describe any problems with LANDINGS:_____
_____

Ramps ❑ yes ❑ no
- ❑ front ❑ back
- height _____
- width _____
- length _____

Are there HANDRAILS? ❑ yes ❑ no
If yes, where are they located? ❑ left ❑ right height_____
If no ramp, how much room is available for one? _____

Porch
- width _____
- length _____
- Level at threshold? ❑ yes ❑ no

Door
- width _____
- threshold height _____ Negotiable? ❑ yes ❑ no
- ❑ swing in
- ❑ swing out
- ❑ sliding

_____

Interior

Living Room

Is furniture arranged for easy maneuverability? ❑ yes ❑ no

Is frequently used furniture accessible ❑ yes ❑ no

Type of floor covering: _____

Comments _____

Hallways

Can wheelchair or walking aide be maneuvered in hallway? ❑ yes ❑ no
- hall width _____
- door width _____

Sharp turns ❑ yes ❑ no

Steps? ❑ yes ❑ no
- number

Are there HANDRAILS? ❑ yes ❑ no
If yes, where are they located? ❑ left ❑ right height_____

Bedroom
- ❑ single
- ❑ shared

Is there room for a W/C? ❑ yes ❑ no

Door
- width _____
- threshold height _____ Negotiable? ❑ yes ❑ no
- ❑ swing in
- ❑ swing out

Bed
- ❑ twin
- ❑ double
- ❑ queen
- ❑ king
- ❑ hospital bed

Overall height _____ Accessible? ❑ yes ❑ no

Would hospital bed fit into room if needed? ❑ yes ❑ no

Clothing:

Are drawers accessible? ❑ yes ❑ no
- ❑ on right ❑ on left

Is closet accessible? ❑ yes ❑ no
- ❑ on right ❑ on left

Comments: _____

Bathroom

Door:
- width _____
- threshold height _____ Negotiable? ❑ yes ❑ no

Tub:
- height, floor-rim _____
- height, tub bottom rim _____
- tub width inside _____
- glass doors? ❑ yes ❑ no
- width of tub doors _____
- overhead shower? ❑ yes ❑ no
- Is tub accessible? ❑ yes ❑ no

Stall Shower: ❑ yes ❑ no
- door width
- height of bottom rim _____
- accessible? ❑ yes ❑ no

Sink:
- height _____
- faucet type _____
- ❑ open
- ❑ closed
- accessible? ❑ yes ❑ no

Toilet:
- height from floor _____
- location of toilet paper _____
- distance from toilet to side wall L _____
- R _____

Grab bars: ❑ yes ❑ no
- Location _____

Comments: _____

Kitchen

Door:
- width _____
- threshold height _____ Negotiable? ❑ yes ❑ no

Stove:
- height _____
- Location of controls ❑ front ❑ back
- Is stove accessible for use? ❑ yes ❑ no

Oven:
- Height from floor to door hinge & door handle _____
- Location of oven _____

Sink:
- Will w/c fit underneath? ❑ yes ❑ no
- Type of faucets _____

Cupboards:
- accessible from w/c? ❑ yes ❑ no

Refrigerator:
- hinges on ❑ left ❑ right
- accessible from w/c? ❑ yes ❑ no

Switches / Outlets:
- accessible? ❑ yes ❑ no

Kitchen Table:
- height from floor _____
- accessible? ❑ yes ❑ no

Comments: _____

Laundry

Door:
- width _____
- threshold height _____ Negotiable? ❑ yes ❑ no

Steps: ❑ yes ❑ no
- number _____
- height _____
- width _____

Are there HANDRAILS? ❑ yes ❑ no

If yes, where are they located? ❑ left ❑ right height_____

FIG. 13-3

Home visit checklist. (Adapted from *Occupational/physical therapy home evaluation form*, San Francisco, 1993, Ralph K. Davies Medical Center, and *Occupational therapy home evaluation form*, Albany, Calif, 1993, Alta Bates Hospital.)

Continued

Washer:
- ❏ Topload
- ❏ Front load
- accessible?   ❏ yes   ❏ no

Dryer:
- ❏ Topload
- ❏ Front load
- accessible?   ❏ yes   ❏ no

Safety

Throw rugs
- ❏ yes   ❏ no
- Location _____

Phone
- accessible?   ❏ yes   ❏ no
- Location _____

Emergency phone numbers
- ❏ yes   ❏ no
- Location _____

Mailbox
- accessible?   ❏ yes   ❏ no
- Location _____

Thermostat
- accessible?   ❏ yes   ❏ no
- Location _____

Electric Outlets / switches
- accessible?   ❏ yes   ❏ no

Imperfect floor?
- ❏ yes   ❏ no
- Location _____

Sharp Edged furniture?
- ❏ yes   ❏ no
- Location _____

Insulated hot water pipes: ❏ yes   ❏ no
- Location _____

Cluttered areas?
- ❏ yes   ❏ no
- Location _____

Fire extinguisher?
- ❏ yes   ❏ no
- Location _____

Equipment present: _____
_____
_____

Problem list: _____
_____
_____
_____

Recommendations for modifications: _____
_____
_____
_____
_____

Equipment Recommendations: _____
_____
_____

FIG. 13-3, cont'd
Home visit checklist. (Adapted from *Occupational/physical therapy home evaluation form,* San Francisco, 1993, Ralph K. Davies Medical Center, and *Occupational therapy home evaluation form,* Albany, Calif, 1993, Alta Bates Hospital.)

During the performance assessment the therapist should observe safety factors, ease of mobility and performance, and limitations imposed by the environment. If the client needs assistance for transfers and other activities, the caregiver should be instructed in the methods that are appropriate. The client may also be instructed in methods to improve maneuverability and simplify performance of tasks in a small space.

At the end of the assessment the therapist can make a list of problems, modifications recommended, and additional safety equipment and assistive devices needed. The most common changes are the following[38]:

1. Installation of a ramp or railings at the entrance to the home
2. Removal of scatter rugs, extra furniture, and bric-a-brac
3. Removal of doorsills
4. Addition of safety grab bars around the toilet and bathtub
5. Rearrangement of furniture to accommodate a wheelchair
6. Rearrangement of kitchen storage
7. Lowering of the clothes rod in the closet.

Access into the bathroom and maneuvering with a wheelchair or walker are common problems. Frequently a bedside commode is recommended until a bathroom can be made accessible or modified to allow independence with toileting (Fig. 13-4). Shower seats can be used in the tub, if a client can transfer over the edge of the tub, and also may be used in a shower. A transfer tub bench (Fig. 13-5) is recommended for individuals who cannot safely or independently step over the edge of the tub. Installation of a hand-held shower hose increases access to the water and also eliminates risky turns and standing while bathing.

When the home assessment is completed, the therapist should write a report summarizing the information on the form and describing the client's performance in the home. The report should conclude with a summary of the environmental barriers and the client's functional limitations encountered. Recommendations should include equipment or alterations needed with specific details about size, building specifications, costs, and sources. Recommendations may also include further functional goals to improve independence in the individual's home environment.

The therapist should carefully review all recommendations with the client and family. This review should be done with tact and diplomacy in a way that gives the client and family options and the freedom to refuse them or consider alternative possibilities. Family finances may limit implementation of needed changes. The social worker may be involved in working out funding for needed equipment and alterations, and the client should be made aware of this service when cost is discussed.[38]

The therapist should include recommendations regarding the feasibility of the client's discharge to the

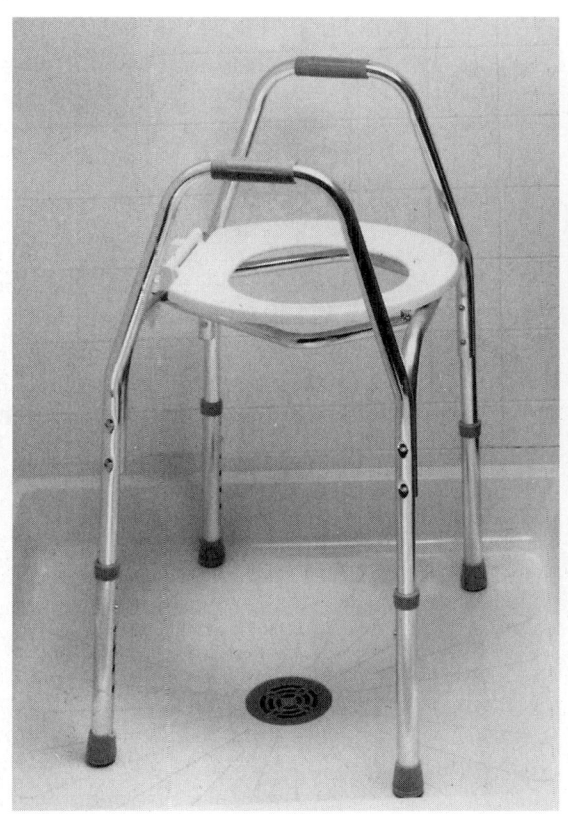

A

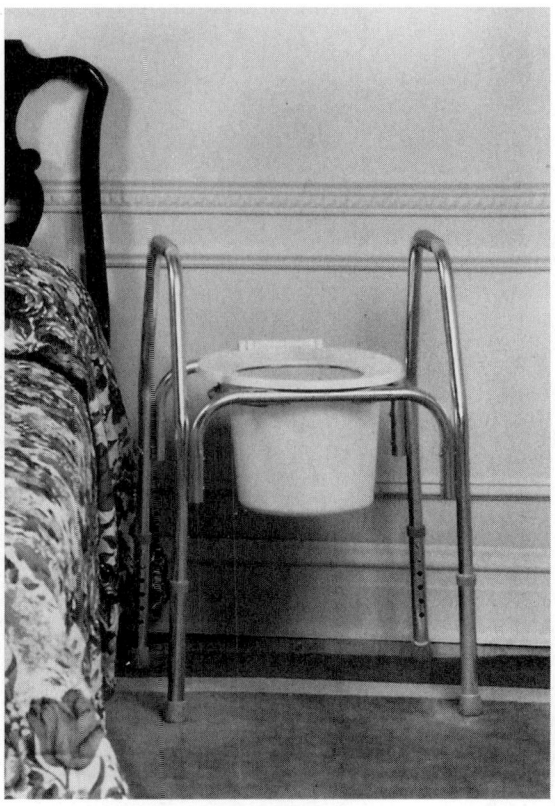

B

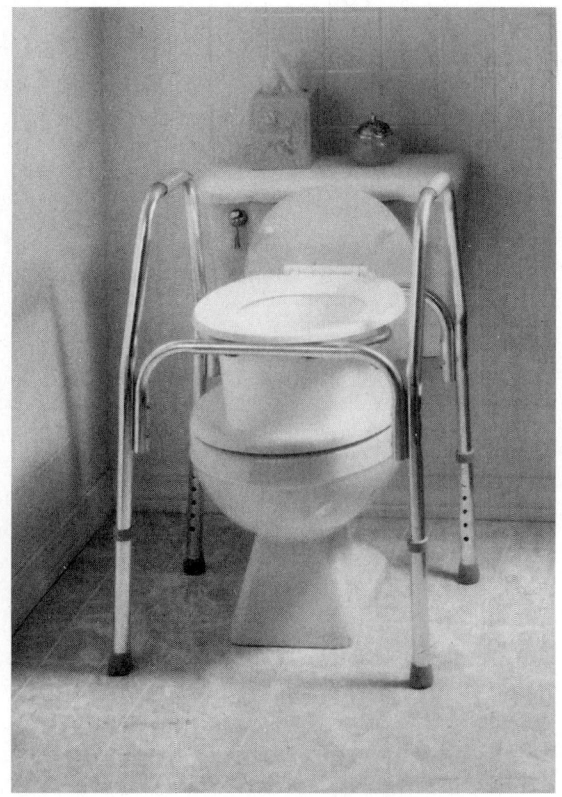

C

FIG. 13-4
All-purpose commode. **A,** In shower. **B,** At bedside. **C,** Over toilet. (Courtesy Sammons Preston.)

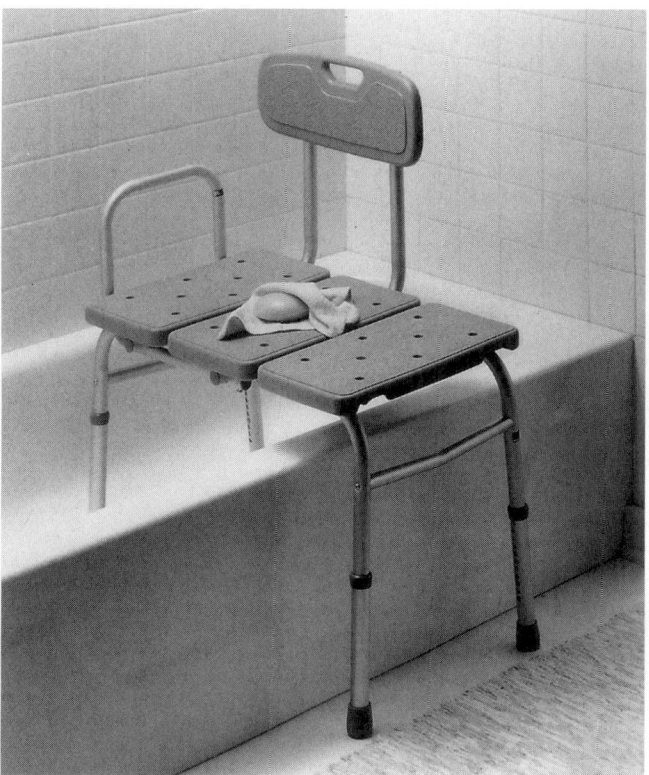

FIG. 13-5
Transfer tub bench. (Courtesy Sammons Preston.)

home environment or remaining in or managing the home alone, if applicable. If there is a question regarding the client's ability to return home safely and independently, the home assessment summary should include the functional skills the client needs to return home.

If a home visit is not possible, much of the information can be gained by interviewing the client and family member(s) following a trial home visit. The family member or caregiver may be instructed to complete the home visit checklist and provide photographs or sketches of the rooms and their arrangements. Problems encountered by the client during the home visit should be discussed and the necessary recommendations for their solution made, as described earlier.[38]

Money and Financial Management

If the client is to resume management of money and financial matters independently, a cognitive and perceptual assessment that accurately tests these skills should be implemented. Because some persons with physical disabilities also have concurrent involvement of cognition and perception, the level of impairment should be determined. Caregivers may require training if the role of financial manager is new and must be assumed. The client may be capable of handling only small amounts of money or may need retraining in activities that require money management, such as shopping, balanc-

ing a checkbook, or making a budget. If a physical limitation is involved, the therapist may introduce adaptive writing devices to allow the client to handle the paperwork aspects of money management.

Community Mobility

Some clients are fortunate enough to be able to drive and to adapt their own vehicle or purchase an adapted van (see Chapter 14). The client who does not meet these criteria must learn to use public transportation or to get around the community on foot or in a wheelchair. In this case, the occupational therapist must assess the client's physical, perceptual, cognitive, and social capabilities to be independent and safe with community mobility.

Physical capabilities to be considered are (1) whether the client has the endurance to be mobile in the community without fatigue and (2) whether the client is sufficiently independent with the walker, cane, crutch, or wheelchair skills and transfers needed to go beyond the home environment. These skills include managing uneven pavement, curbs, and inclines and crossing the street. Other skills to be evaluated before considering community mobility are how to (1) handle money, (2) carry objects in a wheelchair or with a walker, and (3) manage toileting in a public rest room.

Cognitive skills include the ability to be geographically oriented; if taking a bus, to know how to read a schedule and map or know how to get directions; and to have good problem-solving skills if a problem should occur in the community. If the disability is new, the client may be developing new social skills. At first, these skills will be stretched to the limit once the client is out in the community—for example, learning how to be assertive to get an accessible table at a restaurant, obtaining assistance with unreachable items in the grocery store, and becoming comfortable with a new body image within the able-bodied community.

The therapist should also assess the client's community environment. For example, is the neighborhood safe enough for an individual who might be vulnerable because of physical limitations? What is the terrain like? Are there curb cut-outs? Are the sidewalks smooth and even? How far away are the closest store and bus stop?

Accessibility of community transportation should also be considered. Some communities have door-to-door cab and van service, which have certain restrictions. Some of these restrictions include the need to arrange transportation 1 week in advance, the ability to get out the front door and to the curb independently, and the ability to transfer independently into the vehicle. If a public bus is to be used by the client, he must learn how to use the electric lifts and how to lock a wheelchair into place. Because not all bus stops are wheelchair accessible, the neighboring bus stops should be surveyed.

Community mobility requires preplanning by the occupational therapist and the client, accurate assessment of the client's abilities, and knowledge of potential physical, cognitive, and social barriers that may be encountered. A valuable resource by Armstrong and Lauzen, *Community Integration Program*,[3] provides practical treatment protocols to establish a community living skills program. Attaining independence in community mobility is worth the investment because it allows the client to expand life tasks beyond those in the home and interact with the community.

Medication Management and Health Maintenance

Medication management and health maintenance include the client's ability to understand the medical condition and make decisions to maintain good health. The client's ability to handle medications, know when to call a physician, and know how to make a medical appointment is a practical aspect of health management. The evaluation of the client's ability to perform these activities may be completed solely by the occupational therapist but will probably include other team members such as the nurse and the physician.

Performance components must be assessed in light of the skills required for each task. The OT assessment can be helpful in determining which aspects of the task need to be modified for the client to be independent. For example, the occupational therapist can work jointly with a nurse to ensure that a client with hemiplegia and diabetes can manage insulin shots. The OT evaluation considers the client's cognitive and perceptual abilities to make judgments about drawing the insulin out of the bottle, measuring the insulin, and injecting the insulin. Physical concerns include how to stabilize the insulin bottle and handle the syringe with one hand. Other medication management may involve how the client is able to open the medication and measure it, if the medication is a liquid. The occupational therapist may also evaluate and train the client in other skills that affect health management. Examples include using the phone, finding the appropriate phone numbers, and providing the needed information to make a medical appointment.

Health maintenance is an issue for the client and entire health care team. The occupational therapist plays an important role because of the scope of the ADL and I-ADL assessments, which may identify and help resolve problems related to health maintenance.

ADL AND I-ADL TRAINING

If it is determined after an assessment that ADL and I-ADL training are to be initiated, it is important to establish appropriate short- and long-term goals, based on the assessment and on the client's priorities and potential for independence. The following sequence of training for self-care activities is suggested: feeding, grooming, continence, transfer skills, toileting, undressing, dressing, and bathing. This sequence is based on the normal development of self-care independence in children.[38] It provides a good guide but may have to be modified to accommodate the specific dysfunction and the capabilities, limitations, and personal priorities of the client.

The occupational therapist should estimate which ADL and I-ADL tasks are possible and which are impossible for the client to achieve. The therapist should explore with the client the use of alternative methods of performing the activities and the use of any assistive devices that may be helpful. He or she should determine for which tasks the client requires assistance and how much should be given. It may not be possible to estimate these factors until training is under way.

The ADL and I-ADL training program may be graded by beginning with a few simple tasks and gradually increasing the number and complexity of tasks. Training should progress from dependent to assisted to supervised to independent, with or without assistive devices.[38] The rate at which grading can occur depends on the client's potential for recovery, endurance, skills, and motivation.

Methods of Teaching ADL

The therapist must tailor methods of teaching the client to perform daily living tasks to suit each client's learning style and ability. The client who is alert and grasps instructions quickly may be able to perform an entire process after a brief demonstration and oral instruction. Clients who have perceptual problems, poor memory, and difficulty following instructions of any kind need a more concrete, step-by-step approach, reducing the amount of assistance gradually as success is achieved. For these clients it is important to break down the activity into small steps and progress through them slowly, one at a time. A slow demonstration of the task or step by the therapist in the same plane and in the same manner in which the client is expected to perform is helpful. Oral instructions to accompany the demonstration may or may not be helpful, depending on the client's receptive language skills and ability to process and integrate two modes of sensory information simultaneously.

Touching body parts to be moved, dressed, bathed, or positioned, passive movement of the part through the desired pattern to achieve a step or a task, and gentle manual guidance through the task are helpful tactile and kinesthetic modes of instruction (see Chapter 9). These techniques can augment or replace demonstration and oral instruction, depending on the client's best avenues of learning. It is necessary to perform a step or complete a task repeatedly to achieve skill, speed, and retention of learning. Tasks may be repeated several times during the same training session if time and the client's physical and emotional tolerance allow, or they may be repeated daily until the desired retention or level of skill is achieved.

The process of **backward chaining** can be used in teaching ADL skills. In this method the therapist assists the client until the last step of the process is reached. The client then performs this step independently, which affords a sense of success and completion. When the last step is mastered, the therapist assists until the last two steps are reached and the client then completes these two steps. The process continues, with the therapist offering less and less assistance and the client performing successive steps of the task, from last to first, independently. This method is particularly useful in training clients with brain damage.[38]

Before beginning training in any ADL, the therapist must prepare by providing adequate space and arranging equipment, materials, and furniture for maximal convenience and safety. The therapist should be thoroughly familiar with the task to be performed and any special methods or assistive devices that will be used in its performance. The therapist should be able to perform the task, as he or she expects the client to perform it, skillfully. After preparation the activity is presented to the client, usually in one or more of the modes of guidance, demonstration, and oral instruction described earlier. The client then performs the activity either along with the therapist or immediately after being shown, with the amount of supervision and assistance required. Performance is modified and corrected as needed, and the process is repeated to ensure learning.

Because other staff or family members are frequently the individuals reinforcing the newly learned skills, family training is critical to reinforce learning and ensure that the client carries over the skills from previous treatment sessions. In the final phase of instruction, when the client has mastered one or more tasks, he or she is asked to perform them independently. The therapist should check performance in progress and later arrange to check on the adequacy of performance and carryover of learning with nursing personnel, the caregiver, or the supervising family members.[18]

Recording Progress in ADL Performance

The ADL checklists used to record performance on the initial assessment usually have one or more spaces for recording changes in abilities and the results of reassessment during the training process. The sample checklist given earlier in this chapter is so designed and filled in (Fig. 13-1). If a standardized assessment is used during the initial evaluation, it should be used in the reevaluation process to determine the level of progress the client has made.

Progress is usually summarized for inclusion in the medical record. The progress record should summarize changes in the client's abilities and current level of independence and should also estimate the client's potential for further independence, attitude, motivation for ADL training, and future goals for the ADL program. The information about the client's level of assistance needed for ADL and I-ADL will help with the discharge planning. For example, if a client continues to require moderate assistance with self-care, he or she may need to hire an attendant, or the occupational therapist may justify ongoing treatment when the client has potential for further independence.

Assistive Technology and Adaptive Equipment

Assistive technology is defined as any item, piece of equipment, or product system, whether acquired commercially, off the shelf, modified, or customized, that is used to increase or improve functional capabilities of individuals with disabilities. This is a definition provided in PL (Public Law) 100-47, the Technical Assistance to the States Act, in the United States.[9] The terms *assistive technology*, *adaptive equipment*, and *assistive devices* are generally used interchangeably throughout the profession. Adaptive equipment is used to compensate for a physical limitation, to promote safety, and to prevent joint injury. Physical limitations may include a loss of muscle strength, loss of range of motion (ROM), incoordination, or sensory loss. An example of using adaptive equipment to improve safety is the use of a bed or door alarm to alert a caregiver that a patient with impaired cognition is wandering. The use of adaptive equipment to prevent joint injury is indicated for the person with rheumatoid arthritis.

Before recommending a piece of adaptive equipment, the OT practitioner must complete a thorough assessment to determine the client's functional problems and causes of the problems. The OT practitioner may also consider practical solutions first, before settling on adaptive equipment as the solution. Some practical solutions would be to avoid the cause of the problem, use a compensatory technique or alternative method, get assistance from another person, or modify the environment. An example of these considerations is the following case study:

Mrs. S. is 75 years old and living in a nursing home. The occupational therapist receives a referral for a self-feeding assessment because the client has recently lost weight and the nursing aides are reporting that she needs assistance with eating. The nurse mentioned that she thought Mrs. S. needed a built-up handle utensil to eat.

The OT assessment included observation of Mrs. S eating lunch in her usual location (in her room with use of an over-bed table), physical assessment (MMT, ROM, sensation, coordination), gross cognitive and perceptual assessments, and an interview with Mrs. S. The results indicated Mrs. S had problems with sitting properly in her wheelchair. The over-bed table was too high and limited her ability to reach the plate. Her strength, ROM, coordination, and sensation were within normal limits, except that bilateral shoulder flexors and abductors were F- (3-). Mrs. S's cognition and perception were adequate to relearn simple self-care tasks.

Treatment involved working on wheelchair positioning, lowering the over-bed table, and then teaching the client how to use a compensatory technique of elbow propping to bring her hand to her mouth during eating. The OT assessment did not indicate a need for adaptive equipment at this time; instead, the environment was adapted, wheelchair positioning modified, and a compensatory method taught.

If the results of the assessment had indicated that Mrs. S. had a weak grasp and hand incoordination, a built-up handle utensil and plate guard might have been used to promote independence with self-feeding.

Other factors to consider when selecting adaptive equipment are whether the disability is short term or long term, the client's tolerance for gadgets, the client's feelings about the device, and the cost and upkeep of the equipment.

SPECIFIC ADL TECHNIQUES

In many instances, specific techniques to solve specific ADL problems are not possible. Sometimes the occupational therapist has to explore a variety of methods or assistive devices to reach a solution. It is occasionally necessary for the therapist to design a special device, method, splint, or piece of equipment to make a particular activity possible for the client to perform. Many of the assistive devices available today through rehabilitation equipment companies were first conceived and made by occupational therapists and clients. Many of the special methods used to perform specific activities also evolved through the trial-and-error approaches of therapists and their clients. Clients often have good suggestions for therapists, because they live with the limitation and are confronted regularly with the need to adapt the performance of daily tasks.

The purpose of the following summary of techniques is to give the reader some general ideas about how to solve ADL problems for specific classifications of dysfunction. The focus is on compensatory strategies involving changing the method in which an activity is performed, changing the environment, or using an assistive device. If the client has the potential for improvement of specific deficits, treatment that includes remediation should be considered. The references at the end of this chapter provide more specific instruction in ADL

methods. The following categories of physical deficits are addressed in this chapter:

- ADL for the person with limited ROM or strength
- ADL for the person with incoordination
- ADL for the person with hemiplegia or use of only one upper extremity
- ADL for the person with paraplegia
- ADL for the person with quadriplegia
- ADL for the person with low vision

The following ADL and I-ADL are addressed with each of the physical deficits listed above:

- Dressing activities
- Eating activities
- Hygiene and grooming activities
- Communication and environmental adaptations
- Mobility and transfer skills
- Home management activities

ADL for the Person With Limited ROM or Strength

The major problem for persons with limited joint ROM is compensating for the lack of reach and joint excursion through such means as environmental adaptation and assistive devices. Individuals who lack muscle strength may require some of the same devices or techniques to compensate and to conserve energy. Some adaptations and devices are outlined here.[28,32,35,38]

Lower Extremity Dressing Activities

1. Use dressing sticks with a neoprene-covered coat hook on one end and a small hook on the other (Fig. 13-6) for pushing and pulling garments off and on feet and legs.
2. For socks, use a commercially available sock aid (Fig. 13-7).
3. Eliminate the need to bend to tie shoelaces or to use finger joints in this fine motor activity by using elastic shoelaces or other adapted shoe fasteners. Use Velcro-fastened shoes.
4. Use reachers (Fig. 13-8) for picking up socks and shoes, arranging clothes, removing clothes from hangers, picking up objects on the floor, and donning pants.

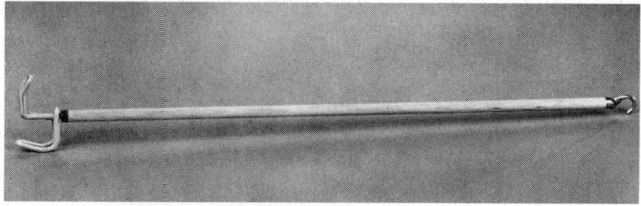

FIG. 13-6
Dressing stick or reacher. (Courtesy Sammons Preston.)

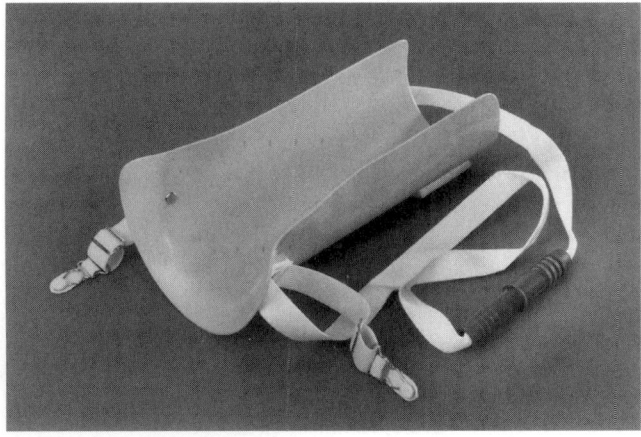

FIG. 13-7
Sock aid. (Courtesy Sammons Preston.)

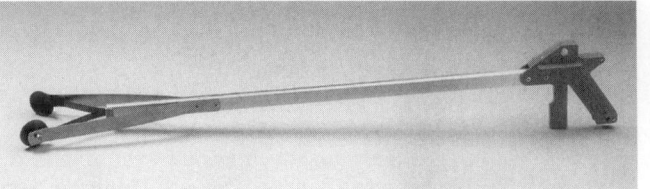

FIG. 13-8
Extended handled reacher.

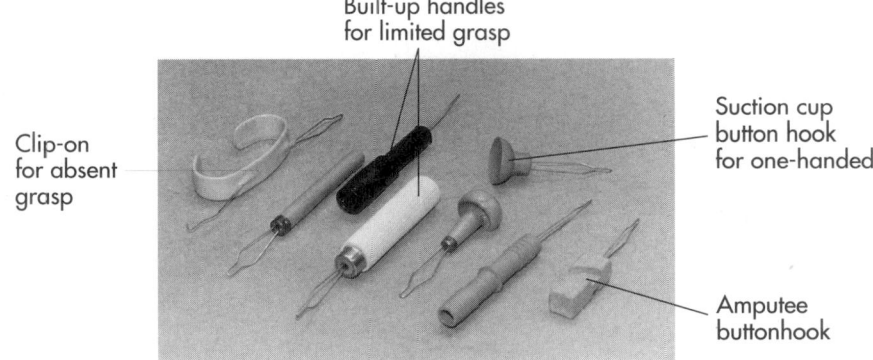

FIG. 13-9
Buttonhooks to accommodate limited or special types of grasp or amputation.

Upper Extremity Dressing Activities

1. Use front-opening garments that are one size larger than needed and made of fabrics that have some stretch.
2. Use dressing sticks (Fig. 13-6) to push a shirt or blouse over the head.
3. Use larger buttons or zippers with a loop on the pull tab.
4. Replace buttons, snaps, hooks, and eyes with Velcro or zippers (for those clients who cannot manage traditional fastenings).
5. Use one of several types of commercially available buttonhooks (Fig. 13-9) if finger ROM is limited.

Eating Activities

1. Use built-up handles on eating utensils that can accommodate limited grasp or prehension (Fig. 13-10).
2. Elongated or specially curved handles on spoons and forks may be needed to reach the mouth. A swivel spoon or spoon-fork combination can compensate for limited supination (Fig. 13-11).
3. Long plastic straws and straw clips on glasses or cups can be used if neck, elbow, or shoulder ROM limits hand-to-mouth motion or if grasp is inadequate to hold the cup or glass.
4. Universal cuffs or utensil holders can be used if grasp is very limited and built-up handles do not work (Fig. 13-12).
5. Plate guards or scoop dishes may be useful to prevent food from slipping off the plate.

Hygiene and Grooming Activities

1. A hand-held flexible shower hose for bathing and shampooing hair can eliminate the need to stand in the shower and offers the user control of the direction of the spray. The handle can be built up or adapted for limited grasp.
2. A long-handled bath brush or sponge with a soap holder (Fig. 13-13) or long cloth scrubber can allow the user to reach legs, feet, and back. A wash mitt (Fig. 13-14) and soap on a rope can aid limited grasp.

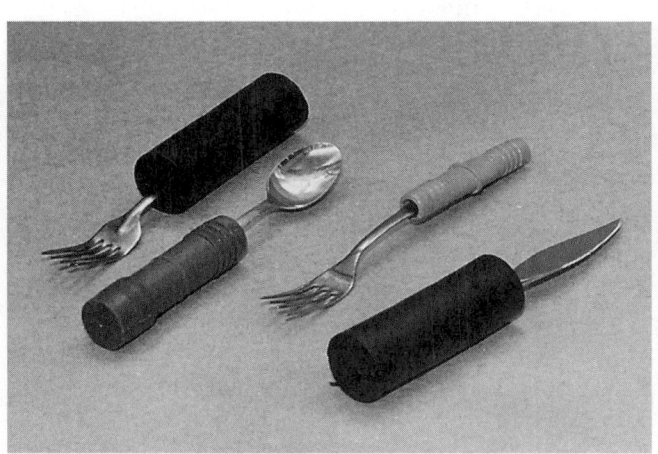

FIG. 13-10
Eating utensils with built-up handles.

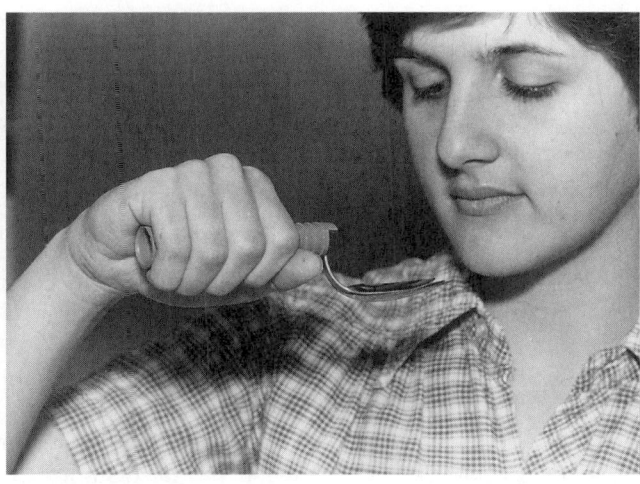

FIG. 13-11
Swivel spoon compensates for limited supination or incoordination.

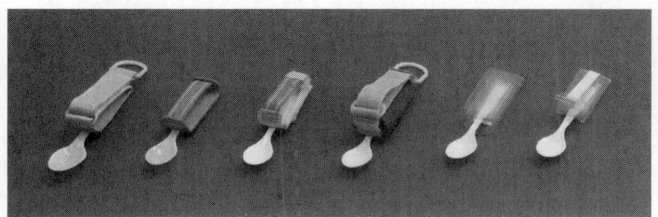

FIG. 13-12
Utensil holders and universal cuffs. (Courtesy Sammons Preston.)

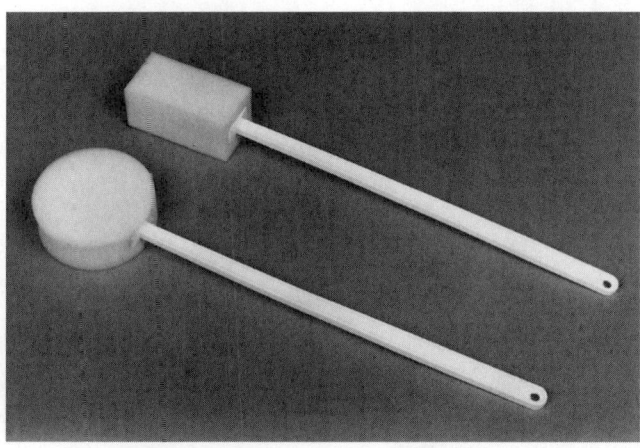

FIG. 13-13
Long-handled bath sponges. (Courtesy Sammons Preston.)

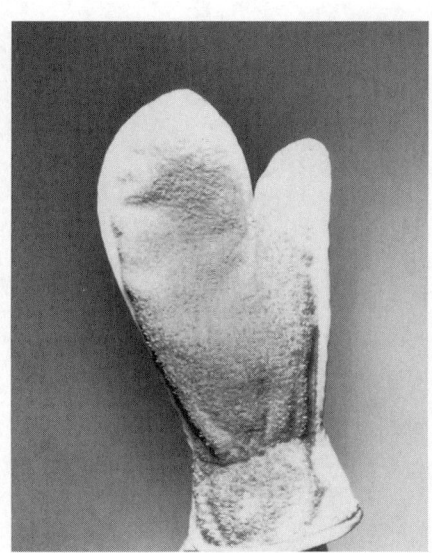

FIG. 13-14
Terry cloth bath mitt. (Courtesy Sammons Preston.)

3. A wall-mounted hair dryer may be helpful. This device is useful for clients with limited ROM, upper extremity weakness, incoordination, or use of just one upper extremity. The dryer is mounted to allow the user to manage his or her hair with one arm or position himself or herself to compensate for limited ROM.[12]

4. Long handles on a comb, brush, toothbrush, lipstick, mascara brush, and safety or electric razor may be useful for clients with limited hand-to-head or hand-to-face movements. Extensions may be constructed from inexpensive wooden dowels or pieces of PVC pipe found in hardware stores.

5. Spray deodorant, hair spray, and spray powder or perfume can extend the reach by the distance the material sprays. Special adaptations may be required by some persons to operate the spray mechanism (Fig. 13-15).

6. Electric toothbrushes and a Water-Pik may be easier to manage than a standard toothbrush.

7. A short reacher can extend reach for using toilet paper. Several types of toilet aids are available in catalogues that sell assistive devices.

8. Dressing sticks can be used to pull garments up after using the toilet. An alternative is the use of a long piece of elastic or webbing with clips on each end that can be hung around the neck and fastened to pants or panties, preventing them from slipping to the floor during use of the toilet.

9. Safety rails (Fig. 13-16) can be used for bathtub transfers, and safety mats or strips can be placed in the bathtub bottom to prevent slipping.

10. A transfer tub bench (Fig. 13-5), shower stool, or regular chair set in the bathtub or shower stall can eliminate the need to sit on the bathtub bottom or stand to shower, thus increasing safety.

11. Grab bars can be installed to prevent falls and ease transfers.

Communication and Environmental Hardware Adaptations

1. Extended or built-up handles on faucets can accommodate limited grasp.

2. Telephones should be placed within easy reach, or portable phones can be used and kept with the client. A clip-type receiver holder (Fig. 13-17), extended receiver holder, or a speaker phone may be necessary. A dialing stick is helpful if individual finger movements are not possible.

3. Built-up pens and pencils can be used to accommodate limited grasp and prehension. A Wanchik writer and several other commercially available or custom-fabricated writing aids are possible (Fig. 13-18).

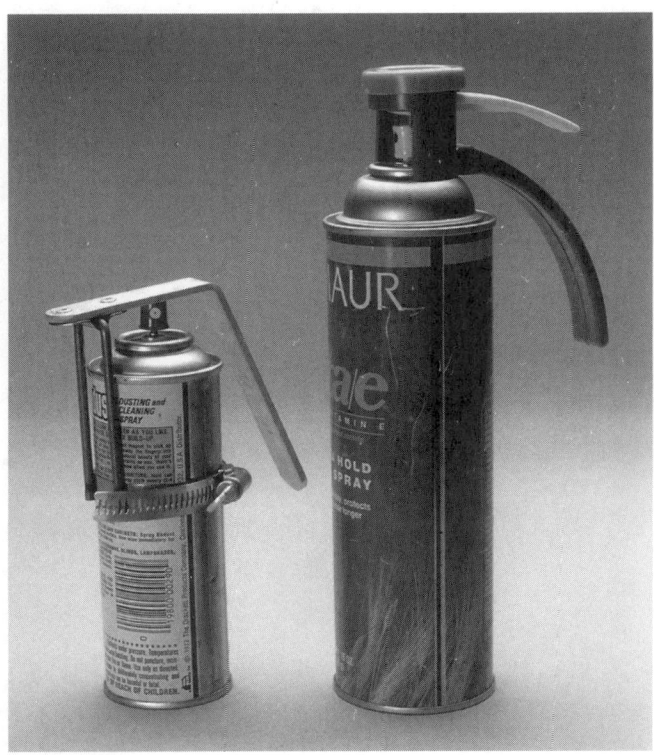

FIG. 13-15
Spray can adapters. (Courtesy Sammons Preston.)

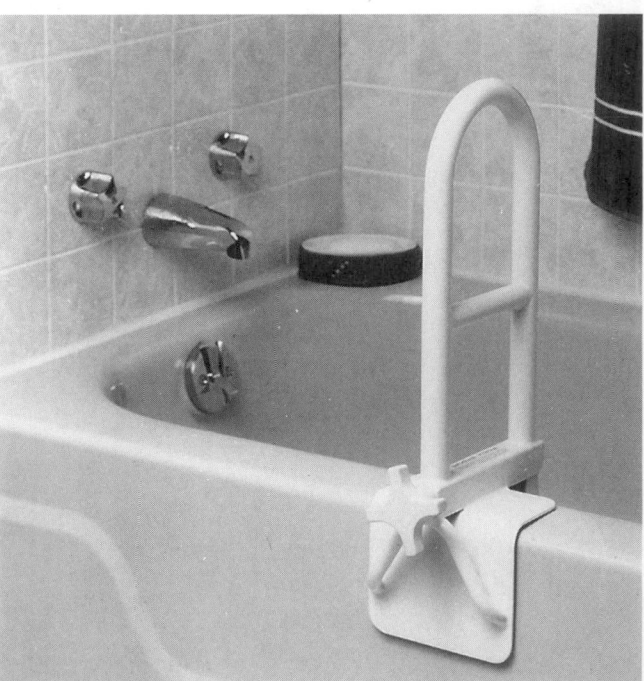

FIG. 13-16
Bathtub safety rail. (Courtesy Sammons Preston.)

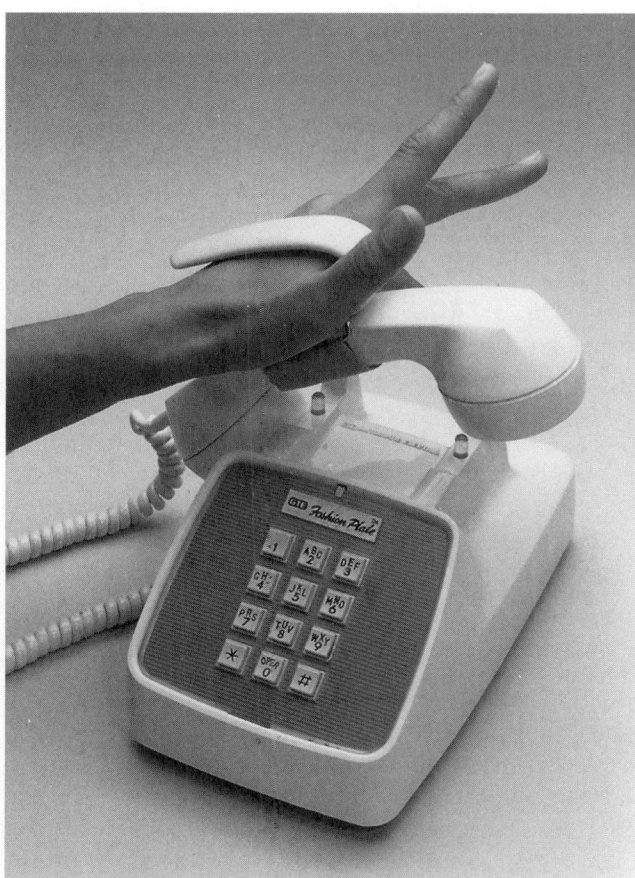

FIG. 13-17
Telephone clip holder. (Courtesy Sammons Preston.)

4. Personal computers, word processors, and book holders can facilitate communication for those with limited or painful joints.
5. Lever-type doorknob extensions (Fig. 13-19), car door openers, and adapted key holders can compensate for hand limitations.

Mobility and Transfer Skills

The individual who has limited ROM without significant muscle weakness may benefit from the following assistive devices:

1. A glider chair that is operated by the feet can facilitate transportation if hip, hand, and arm motion is limited.
2. Platform crutches can prevent stress on hand or finger joints and can accommodate limited grasp.
3. Enlarged grips on crutches, canes, and walkers can accommodate limited grasp.
4. A raised toilet seat can be used if hip and knee motion is limited.
5. A walker with padded grips and forearm troughs can be used if marked hand, forearm, or elbow joint limitations are present.
6. A walker or crutch bag or basket can facilitate the carrying of objects.

Home Management Activities

Home management activities can be facilitated by a wide variety of environmental adaptations, assistive devices, energy conservation methods, and work simplification techniques.[23,35] The principles of joint protection are essential for those with rheumatoid arthritis. These principles are discussed in Chapter 43. The following are suggestions to facilitate home management for persons with limited ROM:

1. Store frequently used items on the first shelves of cabinets, just above and below counters or on counters where possible.

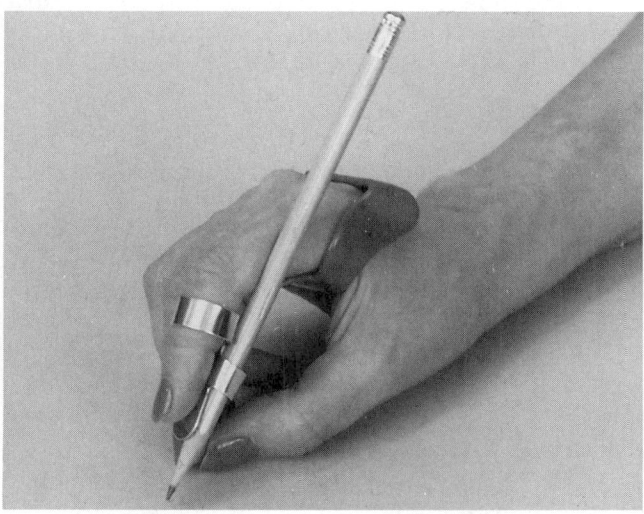

FIG. 13-18
Wanchik writing aid. (Courtesy Sammons Preston.)

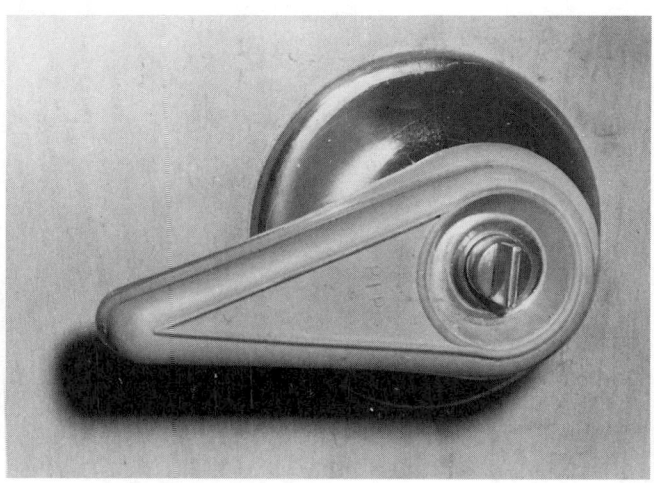

FIG. 13-19
Rubber doorknob extension. (Courtesy Sammons Preston.)

2. Use a high stable stool to work comfortably at counter height, or attach a drop-leaf table to the wall for planning and meal preparation area if a wheelchair is used.
3. Use a utility cart of comfortable height to transport several items at once.
4. Use reachers to get lightweight items (e.g., a cereal box) from high shelves.
5. Stabilize mixing bowls and dishes with nonslip mats.
6. Use lightweight utensils, such as plastic or aluminum bowls and aluminum pots.
7. Use an electric can opener and an electric mixer.
8. Use electric scissors or adapted loop scissors to open packages (Fig. 13-20).
9. Eliminate bending by using extended and flexible plastic handles on dust mops, brooms, and dustpans.
10. Use adapted knives for cutting (Fig. 13-21).
11. Use pull-out shelves to organize cupboards and eliminate bending.
12. Eliminate bending by using a wall oven, countertop broiler, microwave oven, and convection oven.
13. Eliminate leaning and bending by using a top-loading automatic washer and elevated dryer.

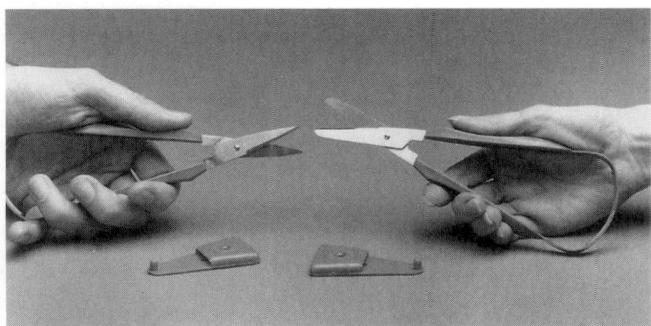

FIG. 13-20
Loop scissors. (Courtesy Sammons Preston.)

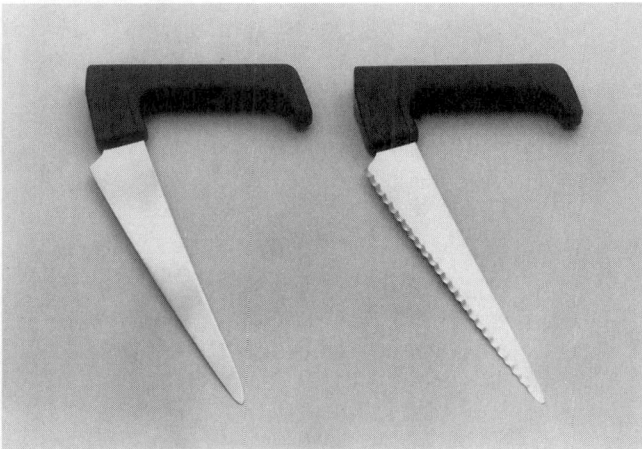

FIG. 13-21
Right-angle knife. (Courtesy Sammons Preston.)

Wheelchair users can benefit from front-loading appliances.
14. Use an adjustable ironing board to make it possible to sit while ironing, or eliminate ironing with the use of permanent press clothing.
15. Elevate the playpen and diaper table and use a bathinette or a plastic tub on the kitchen counter for bathing to reduce the amount of bending and reaching by the ambulatory parent during child care. The crib mattress can be in a raised position until the child is 3 or 4 months of age.
16. Use larger and looser fitting garments with Velcro fastenings on children.
17. Use a reacher to pick up clothing and children's toys.
18. Use a comforter instead of a top sheet and blanket to increase the ease of making the bed.

ADL for the Person With Incoordination

Incoordination in the form of tremors, ataxia, or athetoid or choreiform movements can be caused by a variety of central nervous system (CNS) disorders, such as Parkinson's disease, multiple sclerosis, cerebral palsy, and head injuries. The major problems encountered in ADL performance are safety and adequate stability of gait, body parts, and objects to complete the tasks.[28,38]

Fatigue, emotional factors, and fear may influence the severity of incoordinated movement.[28] The client must be taught appropriate energy conservation and work simplification techniques along with appropriate work pacing and safety methods to prevent the fatigue and apprehension that could increase incoordination and affect performance.

Stabilizing the arm reduces some of the incoordination and may allow the individual to accomplish gross and fine motor movements without assistive devices. A technique that can be used throughout all ADL tasks is the stabilization of the involved upper extremity. This technique is accomplished by propping the elbow on a counter or table top, pivoting from the elbow, and only moving the forearm, wrist, and hand in the activity. When muscle weakness is not a major deficit for the individual with incoordination, the use of weighted devices can help with stabilization of objects. A Velcro-fastened weight can be attached to the client's arm to decrease ataxia, or the device being used (e.g., eating utensils, pens, and cups) can be weighted.[38]

Dressing Activities

To avoid balance problems, the client should attempt to dress while sitting on or in bed or in a wheelchair or chair with arms. The following adaptations can reduce dressing difficulties:

1. Use of front-opening garments that fit loosely can facilitate their donning and removal.
2. Use of large buttons, Velcro, or zippers with loops on the tab can facilitate opening and closing fasteners. A buttonhook with a large, weighted handle may be helpful.
3. Elastic shoelaces, Velcro closures, other adapted shoe closures, and slip-on shoes eliminate the need for bow tying.
4. Trousers with elastic tops for women or Velcro closures for men are easier to manage than trousers with hooks, buttons, and zippers.
5. Using brassieres with front openings or Velcro replacements for the usual hook and eye may make it easier to don and remove this garment. A slipover elastic-type brassiere or bra-slip combination also may eliminate the need to manage brassiere fastenings. Regular brassieres may be fastened in front at waist level, then slipped around to the back and the arms put into the straps, which are then worked up over the shoulders.
6. Men can use clip-on ties.[1,38]

Eating Activities

Eating can be a challenge for clients with problems of incoordination. A lack of control during eating is not only frustrating, but can also cause embarrassment and social rejection. It is important to make eating safe, pleasurable, and as neat as possible. The following are some suggestions for achieving this goal:

1. Use plate stabilizers, such as nonskid mats (Dycem), suction bases, or even damp dishtowels.
2. Use a plate guard or scoop dish to prevent pushing food off the plate. The plate guard can be carried away from home and clipped to any ordinary dinner plate (Fig. 13-22).
3. Prevent spills during the plate-to-mouth excursion by using weighted or swivel utensils to offer stability.

Weighted cuffs may be placed on the forearm to decrease involuntary movement (Fig. 13-23).

4. Use long plastic straws with a straw clip on a glass, or use a cup with a weighted bottom to eliminate the need to carry the glass or cup to the mouth, thus avoiding spills. Plastic cups with covers and spouts may be used for the same purpose.[28,38]
5. Use a resistance or friction feeder similar to a mobile arm support, which was shown by Holser and associates[13] to help control patterns of involuntary movement during feeding activities of adults with cerebral palsy and athetosis. These devices may help many clients with severe incoordination to achieve some degree of independence in feeding. The device is available in adaptive equipment catalogs and is listed as a Friction Feeder MAS (Mobile Arm Support) Kit.

Hygiene and Grooming Activities

Stabilization and handling of toilet articles may be achieved by the following suggestions:

1. Articles such as a razor, lipstick, and a toothbrush may be attached to a cord if frequent dropping is a problem. An electric toothbrush may be more easily managed than a regular one.
2. Weighted wrist cuffs may be helpful during the finer hygiene activities, such as hair care, shaving, and applying make-up.[38]
3. A wall-mounted hair dryer described earlier for clients with limited ROM can also be useful for clients with incoordination.
4. An electric razor, rather than a blade razor, offers stability and safety.[38] A strap around the razor and hand can prevent dropping.

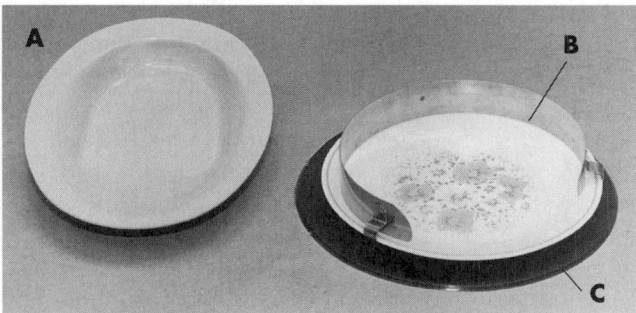

FIG. 13-22
A, Scoop dish. **B,** Plate with plate guard. **C,** Nonskid mat.

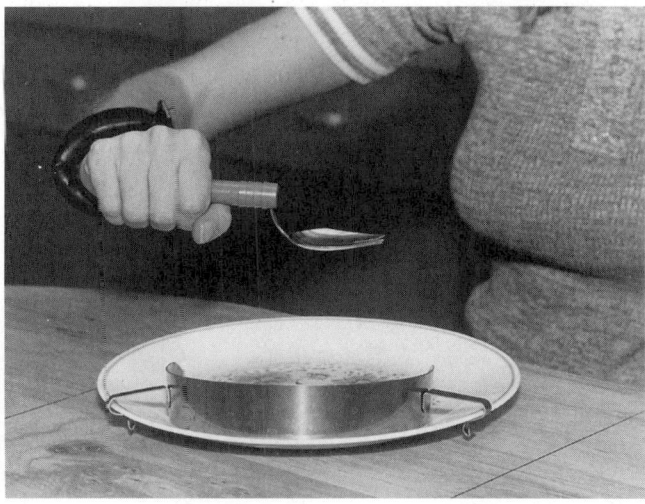

FIG. 13-23
Weighted wrist cuff and swivel utensil can sometimes compensate for incoordination or involuntary motion and limited supination.

5. A suction brush attached to the sink or counter can be used for nail or denture care (Fig. 13-24).

6. Soap should be on a rope. It can be worn around the neck or hung over a bathtub or shower fixture during bathing to keep it within easy reach. A bath mitt with a pocket to hold the soap can be used for washing to eliminate the need for frequent soaping and rinsing and wringing a washcloth. A leg from a pair of pantyhose with a bar of soap in the toe may be tied over a faucet to keep soap within reach and will stretch for use. Liquid soap with a soft nylon scrubber may be used to minimize the handling of soap. Bath gloves can be worn and liquid soap applied to eliminate the dropping of the soap and washcloth.[38]

7. An emery board or small piece of wood with fine sandpaper glued to it can be fastened to the table top for filing nails.[38] A nail clipper can be stabilized in the same manner.

8. Large roll-on deodorants are preferable to sprays or creams.[38]

9. Sanitary pads that stick to undergarments may be easier to manage than tampons.[38]

10. Nonskid mats should be used inside and outside the bathtub during bathing. Their suction bases should be fastened securely to the floor and bathtub before use. Safety grab bars should be installed on the wall next to the bathtub or fastened to the edge of the bathtub. A bathtub seat or shower chair provides more safety than standing while the individual is showering or transferring to a bathtub bottom.[38] Many clients with incoordination require supervisory assistance during this hazardous activity. Sponge bathing while seated at a bathroom sink may be substituted for bathing or showering several times a week.

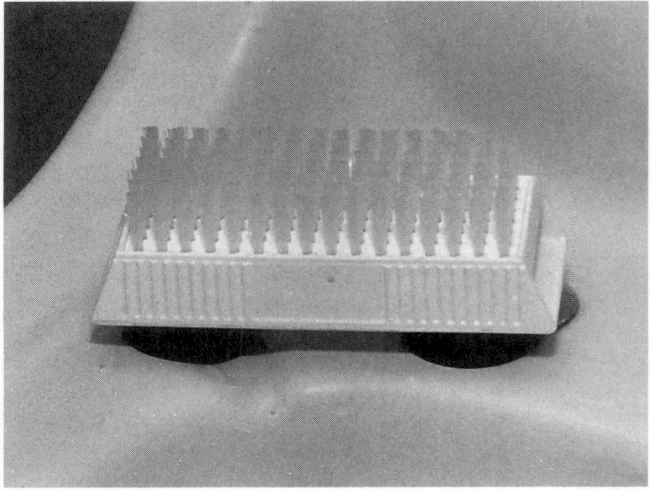

FIG. 13-24
Suction brush attached to bathroom sink for dentures or fingernails. Can also be used in kitchen to wash vegetables and fruit.

Communication and Environmental Hardware Adaptations

1. Doorknobs may be managed more easily if adapted with lever-type handles or covered with rubber or friction tape (Fig. 13-19).

2. Large button phones, speaker phones, or a holder for a telephone receiver may be helpful.

3. Writing may be managed by using a weighted, enlarged pencil or pen. A personal computer with a keyboard guard is a helpful aid to communication. A computer mouse may frequently be substituted for the keyboard.[38] A voice-recognition program may be used with a personal computer to minimize use of the keyboard or mouse.

4. Keys may be managed by placing them on an adapted key holder that is rigid and offers more leverage for turning the key. Inserting the key in the keyhole may be difficult, however, unless the incoordination is relatively mild.

5. Extended lever-type faucets are easier to manage than knobs that turn and push-pull spigots. In order to prevent burns during bathing and kitchen activities, the person with incoordination should turn cold water on first and add hot water gradually.

6. Lamps that can be turned on and off with a wall switch, a light, or a signal-type device can eliminate the need to turn a small switch.

Mobility and Transfers

Clients with problems of incoordination may use a variety of ambulation aids, depending on the type and severity of incoordination. Clients with degenerative diseases sometimes need help to recognize the need for and to accept ambulation aids. This problem may mean moving gradually from a cane to crutches to a walker, and finally to a wheelchair for some persons. The following suggestions can improve stability and mobility for clients with incoordination:

1. Instead of lifting objects, slide them on floors or counters.

2. Use suitable ambulation aids.

3. Use a utility cart, preferably a heavy, custom-made cart that has some friction on the wheels.

4. Remove door sills, throw rugs, and thick carpeting.

5. Install banisters on indoor and outdoor staircases.

6. Substitute ramps for stairs wherever possible.

Home Management Activities

It is important for the occupational therapist to carefully assess performance of homemaking activities to determine (1) which activities can be done safely, (2) which activities can be done safely if modified or adapted, and (3) which activities cannot be done adequately or safely and should be assigned to someone else. The major problems are stabilization of foods and equipment to prevent spilling and accidents and the safe handling of appliances, pots, pans, and household tools to prevent cuts, burns, bruises, electric shock, and falls. The following are suggestions for the facilitation of home management tasks[23,28,38]:

1. Use a wheelchair and wheelchair lapboard, even if ambulation is possible with devices. The wheelchair saves energy and increases stability if balance and gait are unsteady.

2. If possible, use convenience and prepared foods to eliminate as many processes (e.g., peeling, chopping, slicing, and mixing) as possible.

3. Use easy-opening containers or store foods in plastic containers once opened. A jar opener is also useful.

4. Use heavy utensils, mixing bowls, and pots and pans to increase stability.

5. Use nonskid mats on work surfaces.

6. Use electrical appliances such as crock pots, electric fry pans, toaster-ovens, and microwave or convection ovens because they are safer than using a range-top stove.

7. Use a blender and countertop mixer because they are safer than handheld mixers and easier than mixing with a spoon or whisk.

8. If possible, adjust work heights of counters, sink, and range to minimize leaning, bending, reaching, and lifting, whether the client is standing or using a wheelchair.

9. Use long oven mitts, which are safer than pot-holders.

10. Use pots, pans, casserole dishes, and appliances with bilateral handles because they may be easier to manage than those with one handle.

11. Use a cutting board with stainless steel nails (Fig. 13-25) to stabilize meats and vegetables while

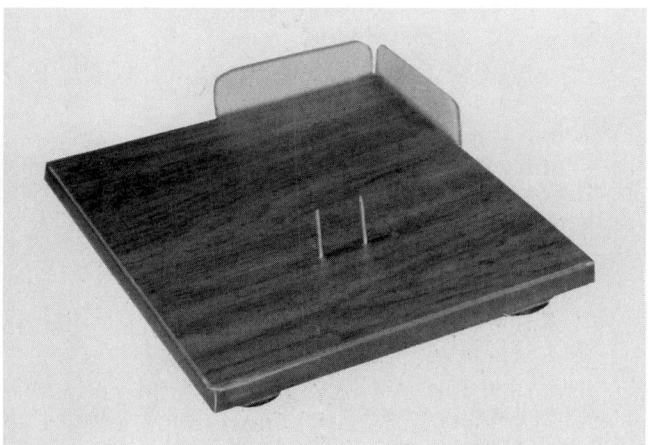

FIG. 13-25
Cutting board with stainless steel nails, suction cup feet, and corner for stabilizing bread is useful for patients with incoordination or use of one hand. (Courtesy Sammons Preston.)

cutting. When the board is not in use, the nails should be covered with a large cork. The bottom of the board should have suction cups or should be covered with stair tread, or the board should be placed on a nonskid mat to prevent slippage when in use.

12. Use heavy dinnerware, which may be easier to handle because it offers stability and control to the distal part of the upper extremity. (On the other hand, unbreakable dinnerware may be more practical if dropping and breakage are problems.)

13. Cover the sink, utility cart, and countertops with protective rubber mats or mesh matting to stabilize items.

14. Use a serrated knife for cutting and chopping because it is easier to control.

15. Use a steamer basket or deep-fry basket for preparing boiled foods to eliminate the need to carry and drain pots containing hot liquids.

16. Use tongs to turn foods during cooking and to serve foods because tongs may offer more control and stability than a fork, spatula, or serving spoon.

17. Use blunt-ended loop scissors to open packages.

18. Vacuum with a heavy upright cleaner, which may be easier for the ambulatory client. The wheelchair user may be able to manage a lightweight tank-type vacuum cleaner or electric broom.

19. Use dust mitts for dusting.

20. Eliminate fragile knickknacks, unstable lamps, and dainty doilies.

21. Eliminate ironing by using no-iron fabrics or a timed dryer or by assigning this task to other members of the household.

22. Use a front-loading washer, a laundry cart on wheels, and premeasured detergents, bleaches, and fabric softeners.

23. Sit when working with an infant and use foam-rubber bath aids, an infant bath seat, and a wide, padded dressing table with Velcro safety straps to offer enough stability for bathing, dressing, and diapering an infant. (Child care tasks may not be possible unless the incoordination is mild.)

24. Use disposable diapers with tape or Velcro fasteners, because they are easier to manage than cloth diapers and pins.

25. Do not feed the infant with a spoon or fork unless the incoordination is very mild or does not affect the upper extremities. This task may need to be performed by another household member.

26. Children's clothing should be large, loose, and made of nonslippery stretch fabrics, and should have Velcro fastenings.

27. Use front infant carriers or strollers for carrying.

ADL for the Person With Hemiplegia or Use of Only One Upper Extremity

Suggestions for performing daily living skills apply to persons with hemiplegia, unilateral upper extremity amputations, and temporary disorders such as fractures, burns, and peripheral neuropathic conditions that can result in the dysfunction of one upper extremity.

The client with hemiplegia needs specialized methods of teaching, and many such clients have greater difficulty learning and performing one-handed skills than do those with orthopedic or lower motor neuron dysfunction. Because the trunk and leg are involved, as well as the arm, ambulation and balance difficulties may exist. Sensory, perceptual, cognitive, and speech disorders may be present in a mild to severe degree. These disorders affect the ability to learn and retain learning and performance. Finally, the presence of apraxia sometimes seen in this group of clients can have a profound effect on the potential for learning new motor skills and remembering old ones. Therefore the client with normal perception and cognition and the use of only one upper extremity may learn the techniques quickly and easily.[38] The client with hemiplegia needs to be assessed for sensory, perceptual, and cognitive deficits to determine the potential for ADL performance and to establish appropriate teaching methods to facilitate learning.

The major problems for the one-handed worker are reduction of work speed and dexterity, and stabilization to substitute for the role normally assumed by the nondominant arm.[28,38] The major problems for the individual with hemiplegia are balance and precautions relative to sensory, perceptual, and cognitive losses.

Dressing Activities

If balance is a problem, the client should dress while seated in a locked wheelchair or sturdy armchair. Clothing should be within easy reach. A reacher may be helpful for securing articles and assisting in some dressing activities. Assistive devices should be used minimally for dressing and other ADL. Compensatory techniques are preferable. For the client with hemiplegia, dressing techniques that employ neurodevelopmental (Bobath) treatment principles are discussed in Chapter 36. The following one-handed dressing techniques* can facilitate dressing for persons with use of only one upper extremity. A general rule is to begin with the affected arm or leg first when donning clothing. Start with the unaffected extremity when removing clothing.

SHIRTS. One of the three following methods can be used to manage front-opening shirts. The first method can also be used for jackets, robes, and front-opening dresses.

METHOD I

Donning Shirt. See Fig. 13-26.

1. Grasp the shirt collar with normal hand and shake out twists (Fig. 13-26, *A*).

2. Position shirt on lap with inside up and collar toward chest (Fig. 13-26, *B*).
3. Position sleeve opening on affected side so opening is as large as possible and close to affected hand, which is resting on lap (Fig. 13-26, *C*).
4. Using normal hand, place affected hand in sleeve opening and work sleeve over elbow by pulling on garment (Fig. 13-26, *D1, D2*).
5. Put normal arm into its sleeve and raise arm to slide or shake sleeve into position past elbow (Fig. 13-26, *E*).
6. With normal hand, gather shirt up middle of back from hem to collar and raise shirt over head (Fig. 13-26, *F*).
7. Lean forward, duck head, and pass shirt over head (Fig. 13-26, *G*).
8. With normal hand, adjust shirt by leaning forward and working shirt down past both shoulders. Reach in back and pull shirt tail down (Fig. 13-26, *H*).
9. Line up shirt fronts for buttoning and begin with bottom button (Fig. 13-26, *I*). Button sleeve cuff of affected arm. Sleeve cuff of unaffected arm may be pre-buttoned if cuff opening is large. Button may be sewn on with elastic thread or sewn onto a small tab of elastic and fastened inside shirt cuff. A small button attached to crocheted loop of elastic thread is another option. Slip button on loop through buttonhole in garment so that elastic loop is inside. Stretch elastic loop to fit around original cuff button. This simple device can be transferred to each garment and positioned before shirt is put on. Loop stretches to accommodate width of hand as it is pushed through end of sleeve.[37]

Removing Shirt

1. Unbutton shirt.
2. Lean forward.
3. With normal hand, grasp collar or gather material up in back from collar to hem.
4. Lean forward, duck head, and pull shirt over head.
5. Remove sleeve from normal arm and then from affected arm.

METHOD II

Donning Shirt. Clients who get their shirts twisted or have trouble sliding the sleeve down onto the normal arm can use method II.

1. Position shirt as described in method I, steps 1 to 3.
2. With normal hand, place involved hand into the sleeve opening and work sleeve onto hand, but do not pull up over elbow.
3. Put normal arm into sleeve and bring arm out to 180° of abduction. Tension of fabric from normal arm to wrist of affected arm will bring sleeve into position.

---

*Summarized from *Activities of daily living for clients with incoordination, limited range of motion, paraplegia, quadriplegia, and hemiplegia,* Cleveland, 1989, Metro Health Center for Rehabilitation, Metro Health Medical Center, Unpublished.

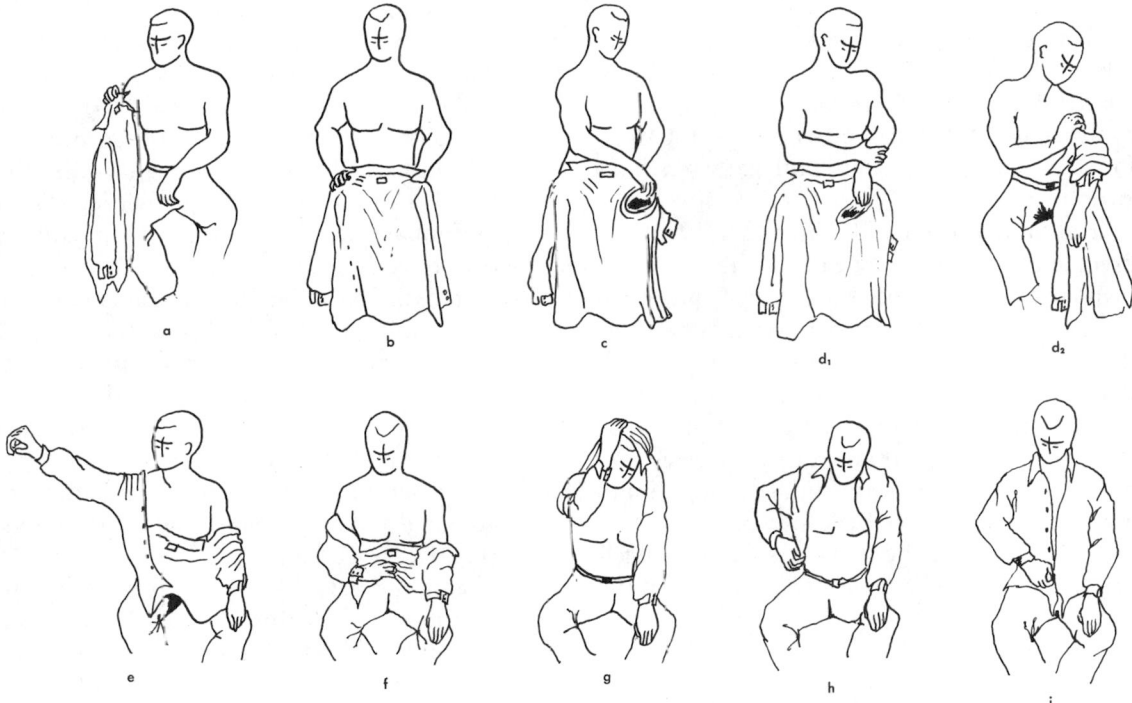

FIG. 13-26
Steps in donning a shirt: method I. (Courtesy Christine Shaw, Metro Health Center for Rehabilitation, Metro Health Medical Center, Cleveland, Ohio.)

4. Lower arm and work sleeve on affected arm up over elbow.
5. Continue as in steps 6 through 9 of method I.
   Removing Shirt
1. Unbutton shirt.
2. With normal hand, push shirt off shoulders, first on affected side, then on normal side.
3. Pull on cuff of normal side with normal hand.
4. Work sleeve off by alternately shrugging shoulder and pulling down on cuff.
5. Lean forward, bring shirt around back, and pull sleeve off affected arm.
   ### METHOD III
   Donning Shirt. See Fig. 13-27.
1. Position shirt and work onto arm as described in method I, steps 1 to 4.
2. Pull sleeve on affected arm up to shoulder (Fig. 13-27, *A*).
3. With normal hand, grasp tip of collar that is on normal side, lean forward, and bring arm over and behind head to carry shirt around to normal side (Fig. 13-27, *B*).
4. Put normal arm into sleeve opening, directing it up and out (Fig. 13-27, *C*).
5. Adjust and button as described in method I, steps 8 and 9.
   Removing Shirt. The shirt may be removed using the procedure described previously for method II.

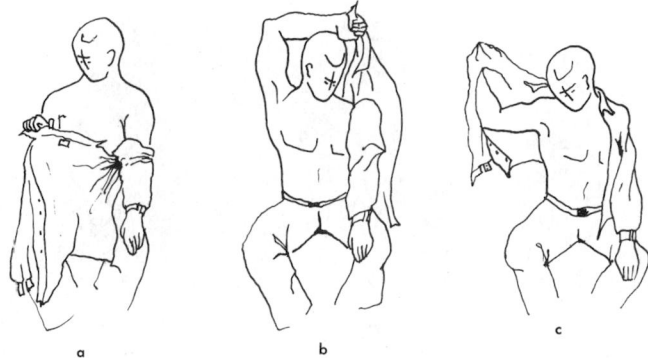

FIG. 13-27
Steps in donning a shirt: method III. (Courtesy Christine Shaw, Metro Health Center for Rehabilitation, Metro Health Medical Center, Cleveland, Ohio.)

Variation for Donning Pullover Shirt
1. Position shirt on lap, bottom toward chest and label facing down.
2. With normal hand, roll up bottom edge of shirt back up to sleeve on affected side.
3. Position sleeve opening so it is as large as possible and use normal hand to place affected hand into sleeve opening. Pull shirt up onto arm past elbow.
4. Insert normal arm into sleeve.
5. Adjust shirt on affected side up and onto shoulder.

6. Gather shirt back with normal hand, lean forward, duck head, and pass shirt over head.
7. Adjust shirt.

Variation for Removing Pullover Shirt

1. Gather shirt up with normal hand, starting at top back.
2. Lean forward, duck head, and pull gathered back fabric over head.
3. Remove from normal arm and then affected arm.

Trousers may be managed by one of the following methods, which may be adapted for shorts and women's panties as well. It is recommended that trousers have a well-constructed button fly front opening, which may be easier to manage than a zipper. Velcro may be used to replace buttons and zippers. Trousers should be worn in a size slightly larger than worn previously and should have a wide opening at the ankles. They should be put on after the socks have been put on but before the shoes are put on. If the client is dressing in a wheelchair, feet should be placed flat on the floor, not on the footrests of the wheelchair.

TROUSERS

METHOD I

Donning Trousers. See Fig. 13-28.

1. Sit in sturdy armchair or in locked wheelchair (Fig. 13-28, *A*).

2. Position normal leg in front of midline of body with knee flexed to 90°. Using normal hand, reach forward and grasp ankle of affected leg or sock around ankle (Fig. 13-28, *B1*). Lift affected leg over normal leg to crossed position (Fig. 13-28, *B2*).
3. Slip trousers onto affected leg up to position where foot is completely inside trouser leg (Fig. 13-28, *C*). Do not pull up above knee, or difficulty will be encountered in inserting normal leg.
4. Uncross affected leg by grasping ankle or portion of sock around ankle (Fig. 13-28, *D*).
5. Insert normal leg and work trousers up onto hips as far as possible (Fig. 13-18, *E1* and *E2*).
6. To prevent trousers from dropping when pulling pants over hips, place affected hand in pocket or place one finger of affected hand into belt loop. If able to do so safely, stand and pull trousers over hips (Fig. 13-28, *F1* and *F2*).
7. If standing balance is good, remain standing to pull up zipper or button (Fig. 13-28, *F3*). Sit down to button front (Fig. 13-28, *G*).

Removing Trousers

1. Unfasten trousers and work down on hips as far as possible while seated.
2. Stand, letting trousers drop past hips, or work trousers down past hips.

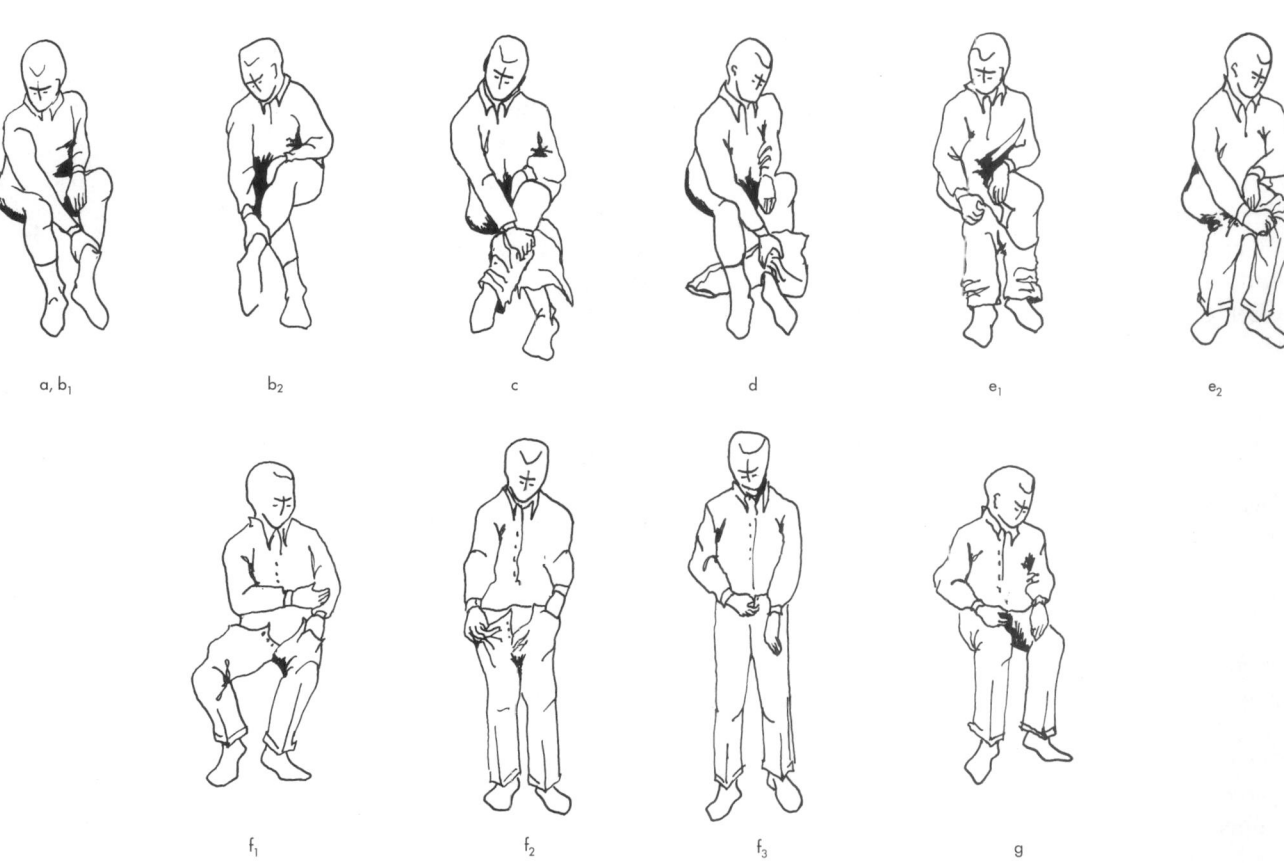

a, b₁   b₂   c   d   e₁   e₂

f₁   f₂   f₃   g

FIG. 13-28

Steps in donning trousers: method I. (Courtesy Christine Shaw, Metro Health Center for Rehabilitation, Metro Health Medical Center, Cleveland, Ohio.)

3. Remove trousers from normal leg.
4. Sit and cross affected leg over normal leg, remove trousers, and uncross leg.

METHOD II

Donning Trousers. Method II is used for clients who are in wheelchairs with brakes locked and footrests swung away, who are in sturdy, straight armchairs positioned with the back against the wall, and for clients who cannot stand independently.

1. Position trousers on legs as in method I, steps 1 through 5.
2. Elevate hips by leaning back against chair and pushing down against the floor with normal leg. As hips are raised, work trousers over hips with normal hand.
3. Lower hips back into chair and fasten trousers.

Removing Trousers

1. Unfasten trousers and work down on hips as far as possible while sitting.
2. Lean back against chair, push down against floor with normal leg to elevate hips, and with normal arm work trousers down past hips.
3. Proceed as in method I, steps 3 and 4.

METHOD III

Donning Trousers. Method III is for clients who are in a recumbent position. It is more difficult to perform than those methods done sitting. If possible, the bed should be raised to a semireclining position for partial sitting.

1. Using normal hand, place affected leg in bent position and cross over normal leg, which may be partially bent to prevent affected leg from slipping.
2. Position trousers and work onto affected leg first, up to the knee. Then uncross leg.
3. Insert normal leg and work trousers up onto hips as far as possible.
4. With normal leg bent, press down with foot and shoulder to elevate hips from bed. With normal arm, pull trousers over hips or work trousers up over hips by rolling from side to side.
5. Fasten trousers.

Removing Trousers

1. Hike hips as in putting trousers on in method III, step 4.
2. Work trousers down past hips, remove unaffected leg, and then remove affected leg.

BRASSIERE

DONNING BRASSIERE

1. Tuck one end of brassiere into pants, girdle, or skirt waistband and wrap other end around waist (wrapping toward affected side may be easiest). Hook brassiere in front at waist level and slip fastener around to back (at waistline level).
2. Place affected arm through shoulder strap, and then place normal arm through other strap.
3. Work straps up over shoulders. Pull strap on affected side up over shoulder with normal arm. Put normal arm through its strap and work up over shoulder by directing arm up and out and pulling with hand.
4. Use normal hand to adjust breasts in brassiere cups.

Note: It is helpful if the brassiere has elastic straps and is made of stretch fabric. If there is some function in the affected hand, a fabric loop may be sewn to the back of the brassiere near the fastener. The affected thumb may be slipped through the loop to stabilize the brassiere while the normal hand fastens it. All elastic brassieres, prefastened or without fasteners, may be put on by adapting method I for pullover shirts described previously. Front-opening bras may also be adapted with a loop for the affected hand with some gross arm function.

REMOVING BRASSIERE

1. Slip straps down off shoulders, normal side first.
2. Work straps down over arms and off hands.
3. Slip brassiere around to front with normal arm.
4. Unfasten and remove.

NECKTIE

DONNING NECKTIE. Clip-on neckties are attractive and convenient. If a conventional tie is used, the following method is recommended:

1. Place collar of shirt in "up" position and bring necktie around neck and adjust so that smaller end is at desired length when tie is completed.
2. Fasten small end to shirt front with tie clasp or spring clip clothespin.
3. Loop long end around short end (one complete loop) and bring up between "V" at neck. Then bring tip down through loop at front and adjust tie, using ring and little fingers to hold tie end and thumb and forefingers to slide knot up tightly.

REMOVING NECKTIE. Pull knot at front of neck until small end slips up enough for tie to be slipped over head. Tie may be hung up in this state and replaced by slipping it over head around upturned collar, and knot tightened as described in step 3 of donning phase.

SOCKS OR STOCKINGS

DONNING SOCKS OR STOCKINGS

1. Sit in straight armchair or in wheelchair with brakes locked, feet on the floor, and footrest swung away.
2. With normal leg directly in front of midline of body, cross affected leg over normal leg.
3. Open top of stocking by inserting thumb and first two fingers near cuff and spreading fingers apart.
4. Work stocking onto foot before pulling over heel. Care should be taken to eliminate wrinkles.
5. Work stocking up over leg. Shift weight from side to side to adjust stocking around thigh.
6. Thigh-high stockings with an elastic band at the top are often an acceptable substitute for panty hose, especially for the nonambulatory individual.
7. Panty hose may be donned and doffed as a pair of slacks, except that the legs would be gathered up one at a time before placing feet into the leg holes.

REMOVING SOCKS OR STOCKINGS

1. Work socks or stockings down as far as possible with normal arm.
2. Cross affected leg over normal one as described in step 2 of process of putting on socks or stockings.
3. Remove sock or stocking from affected leg. Dressing stick may be required by some clients to push sock or stocking off heel and off foot.
4. Lift normal leg to comfortable height or to seat level and remove sock or stocking from foot.

SHOES

If possible, select slip-on shoes to eliminate lacing and tying. If an individual uses an ankle-foot orthosis (AFO) or short leg brace, shoes with fasteners are usually needed.

1. Use elastic laces and leave shoes tied.
2. Use adapted shoe fasteners.
3. Use one-handed shoe-tying techniques (Fig. 13-29).
4. It is possible to learn to tie a standard bow with one hand, but this requires excellent visual, perceptual, and motor planning skills along with much repetition.

ANKLE-FOOT ORTHOSIS. The individual with hemiplegia who lacks adequate ankle dorsiflexion to walk safely and efficiently frequently uses an ankle-foot orthosis (AFO). It can be donned in the following manner.

METHOD I. See Fig. 13-30.

1. Sit in straight armchair or wheelchair with brakes locked and feet on the floor (Fig. 13-30, *A*). The fasteners are loosened and tongue of the shoe pulled back to allow the AFO to fit into the shoe (Fig. 13-30, *B*).

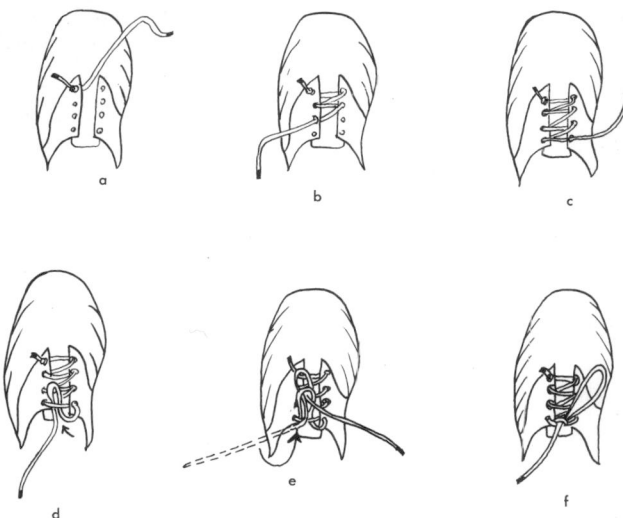

FIG. 13-29
One-hand shoe-tying method. (Courtesy Christine Shaw, Metro Health Center for Rehabilitation, Metro Health Medical Center, Cleveland, Ohio.)

2. AFO and shoe are placed on the floor between the legs but closer to the affected leg, facing up (Fig. 13-30, *C*).
3. With the unaffected hand, lift the affected leg behind the knee and place toes into the shoe (Fig. 13-30, *D*).
4. Reach down with unaffected hand and lift AFO by the upright. Simultaneously use the unaffected foot against the affected heel to keep the shoe and AFO together (Fig. 13-30, *E*).
5. The heel will not be pushed into the shoe at this point. With the unaffected hand, apply pressure directly downward on the affected knee to force the heel into the shoe, if leg strength is not sufficient (Fig. 13-30, *F*).
6. Fasten Velcro calf strap and fasten shoes (Fig. 13-30, *G*). The affected leg may be placed on a footstool to assist with reaching shoe fasteners.
7. To fasten shoes, one-handed bow-tying may be used; elastic shoelaces, Velcro-fastened shoes, or other commercially available shoe fasteners may be required if the client is unable to tie shoes.

METHOD II. Steps 1 and 2 are the same as the positioning required for donning pants.

1. Sit in sturdy armchair or in locked wheelchair.
2. Position normal leg in front of midline of body with knee flexed to 90°. Using normal hand, reach forward and grasp ankle of affected leg or sock around ankle. Lift affected leg over normal leg to crossed position.
3. The fasteners are loosened and tongue of the shoe pulled back to allow the AFO to fit into the shoe; Velcro fastener on upright is unfastened.
4. Using normal hand, hold heel of shoe and work over toes of affected foot and leg. Once toes are in shoe, work top part of AFO around the calf.
5. Pull heel of shoe onto foot with hand or place foot on floor, place pressure on knee, and push heel down into shoe.
6. Fasten Velcro calf strap and fasten shoes.

REMOVING ANKLE-FOOT ORTHOSIS
Variation I

1. While seated as for donning an AFO, cross affected leg over normal leg.
2. Unfasten straps and laces with normal hand.
3. Push down on AFO upright until shoe is off foot.

Variation II

1. Unfasten straps and laces.
2. Straighten affected leg by putting normal foot behind heel of shoe and pushing affected leg forward.
3. Push down on AFO upright with hand and at same time push forward on heel of AFO shoe with normal foot.

Eating Activities

The main problem encountered by the one-handed individual is managing a knife and fork simultaneously for cutting meat. This problem can be solved by the use

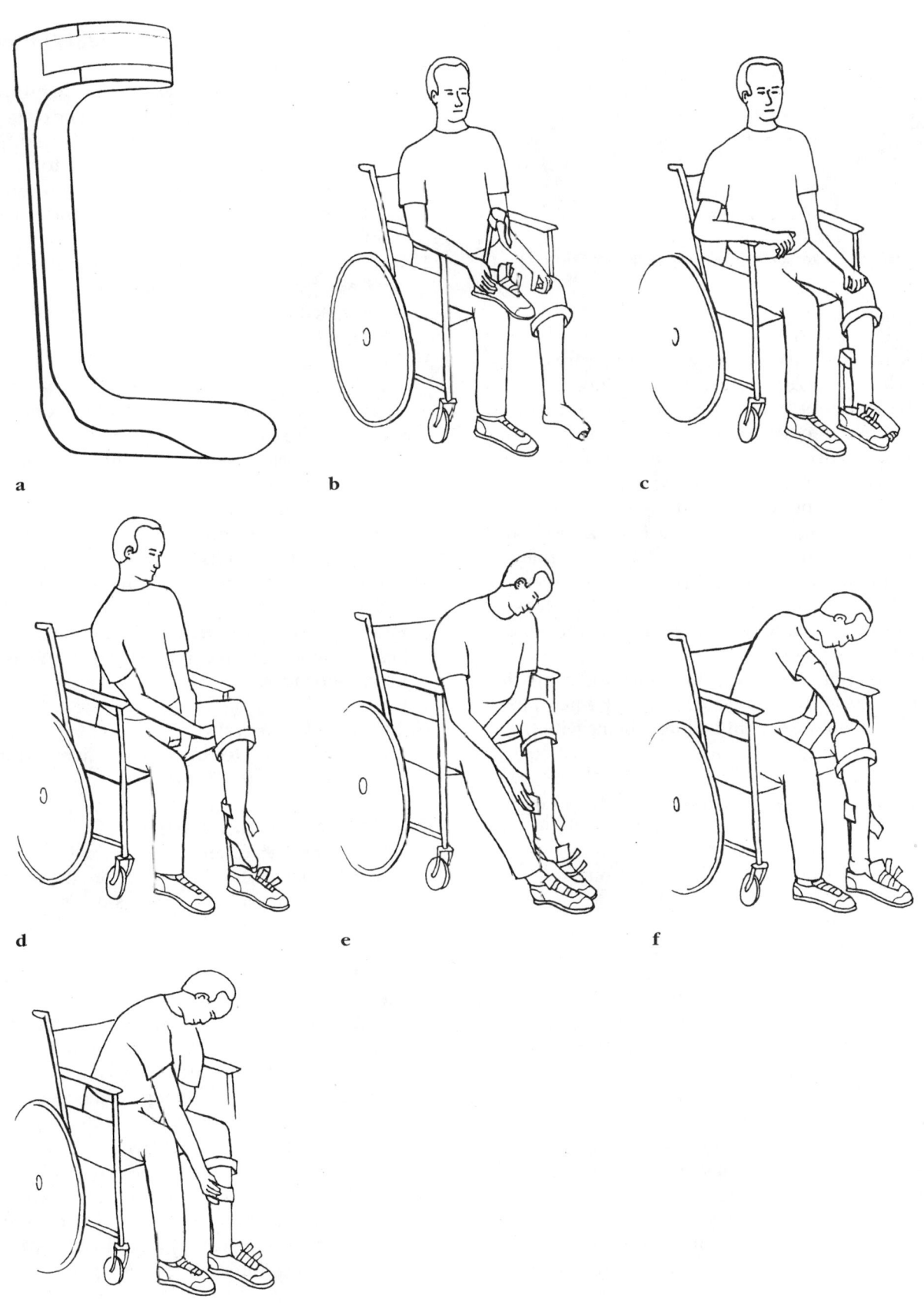

a

b

c

d

e

f

g

FIG. 13-30
Steps in donning ankle-foot orthosis (AFO).

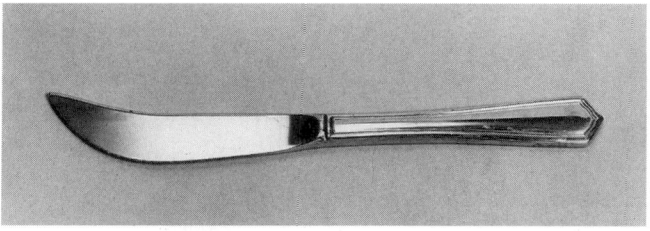

FIG. 13-31
One-handed rocker knife. (Courtesy Sammons Preston.)

of a rocker knife for cutting meat and other foods (Fig. 13-31). This knife cuts with a rocking motion rather than a back-and-forth slicing action. Use of a rocking motion with a standard table knife or a sharp paring knife may be adequate to cut tender meats and soft foods. If such a knife is used, the client is taught to hold the knife handle between the thumb and the third, fourth, and fifth fingers, and the index finger is extended along the top of the knife blade. The knife point is placed in the food in a vertical position, and then the blade is brought down to cut the food. The rocking motion, using wrist flexion and extension, is continued until the food is cut.

The occupational therapist should keep in mind that one-handed meat cutting involves learning a new motor pattern. This skill may be difficult for clients with hemiplegia and apraxia.

Hygiene and Grooming Activities

Clients with the use of one hand or one side of the body can accomplish hygiene and grooming activities by using assistive devices and alternative methods. The following are suggestions for achieving hygiene and grooming with one hand:

1. Use an electric razor rather than a safety razor.
2. Use a shower seat in the shower stall or a transfer tub bench in a bathtub-shower combination. Also use a bath mat, wash mitt, long-handled bath sponge, safety rails on the bathtub or wall, soap on a rope or suction soap holder, and suction brush for fingernail care.
3. Sponge bathe while sitting at the lavatory, using the wash mitt, suction brush, and suction soap holder. The uninvolved forearm and hand may be washed by placing a soaped washcloth on the thigh and rubbing the hand and forearm on the cloth.
4. Use a wall-mounted hair dryer. Such a device frees the unaffected upper extremity to hold a brush or comb to style the hair during blow-drying.[12]
5. Care for fingernails as described previously for clients with incoordination.
6. Use a suction denture brush for care of dentures. The suction fingernail brush may also serve this purpose (Fig. 13-22).

Communication and Environmental Hardware Adaptations

1. The primary problem with writing is stabilization of the paper or tablet. This problem can be overcome by using a clipboard, paperweight, or nonskid surface such as Dycem or by taping the paper to the writing surface. In some instances the affected arm may be positioned on the table top to stabilize the paper passively.
2. If dominance must be shifted to the nondominant extremity, writing practice may be necessary to improve speed and coordination. One-handed writing and typing instruction manuals are available.
3. Book holders may be used to stabilize a book while reading or holding copy for typing and writing practice. A soft pillow will easily stabilize a book while the person is seated in an easy chair.
4. The telephone is managed by lifting the receiver to listen for the dial tone, setting it down, pressing the keys, and lifting the receiver to the ear. To write while using the telephone, a stand or shoulder telephone receiver holder must be used. A speakerphone can also leave hands free to take messages. One-touch dialing using preprogrammed phone numbers eliminates pressing as many keys, simplifies sequencing, and may help compensate for memory deficits.

Mobility and Transfers

Principles of transfer techniques for clients with hemiplegia are described in Chapter 14.

Home Management Activities

Many assistive devices are available to facilitate home management activities. Various factors determine how many home management activities can realistically be performed, which methods can be used, and how many assistive devices can be managed. These factors include (1) whether the client is disabled by the loss of function of one arm and hand, as in amputation or a peripheral neuropathic condition, or (2) whether both arm and leg are affected along with possible visual, perceptual, and cognitive dysfunctions, as in hemiplegia. The references listed at the end of this chapter provide details of home management with one hand. The following are some suggestions for home management for the client with use of one hand[23]:

1. Stabilizing items is a major problem for the one-handed homemaker. Stabilize foods for cutting and peeling by using a cutting board with two stainless steel or aluminum nails in it. A raised corner on the board stabilizes bread for making sandwiches or spreading butter. Suction cups or a rubber mat under the board will keep it from slipping. A nonskid surface or rubber feet may be glued to the bottom of the board (Fig. 13-25).

2. Use sponge cloths, nonskid mats or pads, wet dish-cloths, or suction devices to keep pots, bowls, and dishes from turning or sliding during food preparation.

3. To open a jar, stabilize it between the knees or in a partially opened drawer while leaning against the drawer. Break the air seal by sliding a pop bottle opener under the lid until the air is released, then use a Zim jar opener (Fig. 13-32).

4. Open boxes, sealed paper, and plastic bags by stabilizing between the knees or in a drawer as just described, and cut open with household shears. Special box and bag openers are also available from ADL equipment vendors.

5. Crack an egg by holding it firmly in the palm of the hand. Hit it in the center against the edge of the bowl. Then using the thumb and index finger, push the top half of the shell up and use the ring and little finger to push the lower half down. Separate whites from yolks by using an egg separator, funnel, or large slotted spoon.

6. Eliminate the need to stabilize the standard grater by using a grater with suction feet, or use an electric countertop food processor instead.

7. Stabilize pots on the counter or range for mixing or stirring by using a pan holder with suction feet (Fig. 13-33).

8. Eliminate the need to use hand-cranked or electric can openers, which necessitate the use of two hands, by using a one-handed electric can opener.

9. Use a utility cart to carry items from one place to another. For some clients a cart that is weighted or constructed of wood may be used as a minimal support during ambulation.

10. Transfer clothes to and from the washer or dryer by using a clothes carrier on wheels.

11. Use electrical appliances, such as a lightweight electrical hand mixer, blender, and food processor, that can be managed with one hand and save time and energy. Safety factors and judgment need to be evaluated carefully when electrical appliances are considered.

12. Floor care becomes a greater problem if, in addition to one arm, ambulation and balance are affected. For clients with involvement of only one arm, a standard dust mop, carpet sweeper, or upright vacuum cleaner should present no problem. A self-wringing mop may be used if the mop handle is stabilized under the arm and the wringing lever operated with the normal arm. Clients with balance and ambulation problems may manage some floor care from a sitting position. Dust mopping or using a carpet sweeper may be possible if gait and balance are fairly good without the aid of a cane.

These are just a few of the possibilities for solving home management problems for one-handed individuals. The occupational therapist must evaluate each client to determine how the dysfunction affects performance of homemaking activities. One-handed techniques take more time and may be difficult for some clients to master. Activities should be paced to accommodate the client's physical endurance and tolerance for one-handed performance and use of special devices. Work simplification and energy conservation techniques should be employed. New techniques and devices should be introduced on a graded basis as the client masters first one technique and device and then

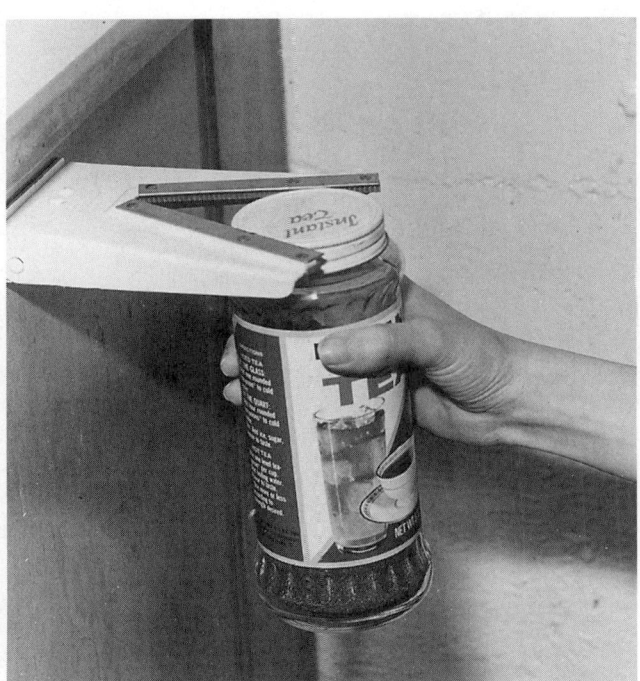

FIG. 13-32
Zim jar opener.

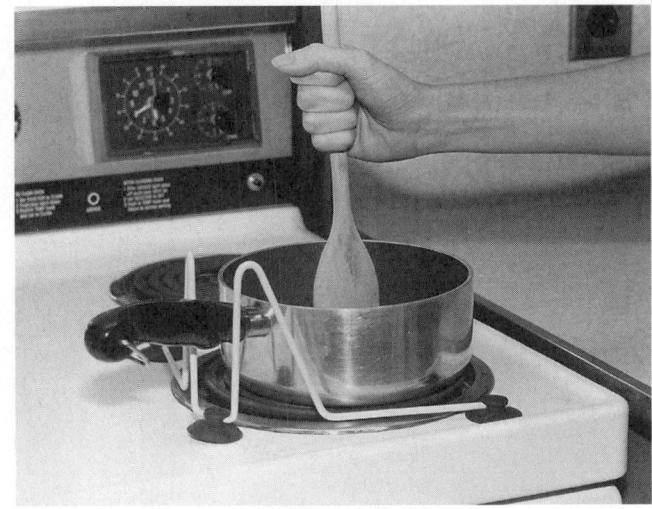

FIG. 13-33
Pan stabilizer.

another. Family members need to be oriented to the client's skills, special methods used, and work schedule. The therapist, with the family and client, may facilitate the planning of homemaking responsibilities to be shared by other family members and the supervision of the client, if that is needed. If special equipment and assistive devices are needed for ADL, it is advisable to acquire these through the health agency, if possible. The therapist can then train the client and demonstrate use of the equipment to a family member before these items are used at home. After training, the occupational therapist should provide the client with sources to replace items independently, such as a consumer catalogue of adaptive equipment.

ADL for the Person With Paraplegia

Clients who are confined to a wheelchair need to find ways to perform ADL from a seated position, to transport objects, and to adapt to an environment designed for standing and walking. Given normal function in the upper extremities, the wheelchair ambulator can probably perform independently. The client should have a stable spine, and mobility precautions should be clearly identified.

Dressing Activities*

It is recommended that wheelchair-bound clients put on clothing in this order: stockings, undergarments, braces (if worn), trousers or slacks, shoes, shirt, or dress.

TROUSERS

DONNING TROUSERS. Trousers and slacks are easier to fasten if they button or zip in front. If braces are worn, zippers in side seams may be helpful. Wide-bottom slacks of stretch fabric are recommended. The procedure for putting on trousers, shorts, slacks, and underwear is as follows:

1. Use side rails or a trapeze to pull up to sitting position, back supported with pillows or headboard of the bed.
2. Sit on bed and reach forward to feet, or sit on bed and pull knees into flexed position.
3. Holding top of trousers, flip pants down to feet.
4. Work pant legs over feet and pull up to hips. Crossing ankles may help get pants on over heels.
5. In semireclining position, roll from hip to hip and pull up garment.
6. A long-handled reacher may be helpful for pulling garment up or positioning garment on feet if there is impaired balance or range of motion in the lower extremities or trunk.

---

*Summarized from *Activities of daily living for clients with incoordination, limited range of motion, paraplegia, quadriplegia, and hemiplegia,* Cleveland, 1989, Metro Health Center for Rehabilitation, Metro Health Medical Center, Unpublished.

REMOVING TROUSERS. Remove pants or underwear by reversing procedure for putting on. Dressing sticks may be helpful for pushing pants off feet.

SOCKS OR STOCKINGS. Soft stretch socks or stockings are recommended. Panty hose that are slightly large may be useful. Elastic garters or stockings with elastic tops should be avoided because of potential skin breakdown. Dressing sticks or a stocking device may be helpful to some clients.

DONNING SOCKS OR STOCKINGS

1. Put on socks or stockings while seated on bed.
2. Pull one leg into flexion with one hand and cross over the other leg.
3. Use other hand to slip sock or stocking over foot and pull sock or stocking on.

REMOVING SOCKS OR STOCKINGS. Remove socks or stockings by flexing leg as described for donning, pushing sock or stocking down over heel. Dressing sticks may be needed to push sock or stocking off heel and toe and to retrieve sock.

SLIPS AND SKIRTS. Slips and skirts slightly larger than usually worn are recommended. A-line, wraparound, and full skirts are easier to manage and look better on a person seated in a wheelchair than narrow skirts.

DONNING SLIPS AND SKIRTS

1. Sit on bed, slip garment over head, and let it drop to waist.
2. In semireclining position, roll from hip to hip and pull garment down over hips and thighs.

REMOVING SLIPS AND SKIRTS

1. In sitting or semireclining position, unfasten garment.
2. Roll from hip to hip, pulling garment up to waist level.
3. Pull garment off over head.

SHIRTS. Fabrics should be wrinkle-resistant, smooth, and durable. Roomy sleeves and backs and full shirts are more suitable styles than closely fitted garments.

DONNING SHIRTS. Shirts, pajama jackets, robes, and dresses that open completely down the front may be put on while the client is seated in wheelchair. If it is necessary to dress while in bed, the following procedure can be used:

1. Balance body by putting palms of hands on mattress on either side of body. If balance is poor, assistance may be needed or bed backrest may be elevated. (If backrest cannot be elevated, one or two pillows may be used to support back.) With backrest elevated, both hands are available.
2. If difficulty is encountered in customary methods of applying garment, open garment on lap with collar toward chest. Put arms into sleeves and pull up over

elbows. Then hold on to shirttail or back of dress, pull garment over head, adjust, and button.

REMOVING SHIRTS
1. Sitting in wheelchair or bed, open fastener.
2. Remove garment in usual manner.
3. If usual manner is not feasible, grasp collar with one hand while balancing with other hand. Gather material up from collar to hem.
4. Lean forward, duck head, and pull shirt over head.
5. Remove sleeves, first from supporting arm and then from working arm.

SHOES

DONNING SHOES. If an individual has sensory loss and is at risk for bruising during transfers, shoes should be donned in bed.

Variation I
1. In sitting position on bed, pull one knee at a time into flexed position with hands.
2. While supporting leg in flexed position with one hand, use free hand to put on shoe.

Variation II
1. Sit on edge of bed or in wheelchair for back support.
2. Bend one knee up to flexed position, while supporting leg with arm, and slip shoe onto foot with free hand.

Variation III
1. Sit on edge of bed or in wheelchair for back support.
2. Cross one leg over other and slip shoe onto foot.
3. Put foot on footrest and push down on knee to push foot into shoe.

REMOVING SHOES
1. Flex or cross leg as described for appropriate variation.
2. For variations I and II, remove shoe with one hand while supporting flexed leg with other hand.
3. For variation III, remove shoe from crossed leg with one hand while maintaining balance with other hand, if necessary.

Eating Activities

Eating activities should present no special problem for the wheelchair-bound person with good to normal arm function. Wheelchairs with desk arms and swing-away footrests are recommended so that it is possible to sit close to the table.

Hygiene and Grooming

Facial and oral hygiene and arm and upper body care should present no problem. Reachers may be helpful for securing towels, washcloths, make-up, deodorant, and shaving supplies from storage areas, if necessary. Special equipment is needed for using tub baths or showers. Transfer techniques for toilet and bathtub are discussed in Chapter 14. The following are suggestions for facilitating bathing activities:

1. Use a hand-held shower hose and keep a finger over the spray to determine sudden temperature changes in water.
2. Use long-handled bath brushes with soap insert for ease in reaching all parts of the body.
3. Use soap bars attached to a cord around the neck, or use liquid soap.
4. Use shower chairs or bathtub seats.
5. Increase safety during transfers by installing grab bars on wall near bathtub or shower and on bathtub.
6. Fit bathtub or shower bottom with nonskid mat or adhesive material.
7. Remove doors on the bathtub and replace with a shower curtain to increase safety and ease of transfers.

Communication and Environmental Hardware Adaptations

With the exception of reaching difficulties in some situations, use of the telephone should present no problem. Short-handled reachers may be used to grasp the receiver from the cradle. A cordless telephone can eliminate reaching, except when the phone needs recharging. The use of writing implements, typewriter, tape recorder, and personal computer should be possible. Managing doors may present some difficulties. If the door opens toward the person, it can be opened by the following procedure:

1. If doorknob is on right, approach door from right and turn doorknob with left hand.
2. Open door as far as possible and move wheelchair close enough so that it helps keep door open.
3. Holding door open with left hand, turn wheelchair with right hand and wheel through door.
4. Start closing door when halfway through.

If the door is very heavy and opens out or away from the person, the following procedure is recommended[7]:
1. Back up to door so knob can be turned with right hand.
2. Open door and back through so that big wheels keep it open.
3. Also use left elbow to keep door open.
4. Wheel backward with right hand.

Mobility and Transfers

Principles of transfer techniques are discussed in Chapter 14.

Home Management Activities

When homemaking activities are performed from a wheelchair, the major problems are work heights, adequate space for maneuverability, access to storage areas, and transfer of supplies, equipment, and materials from place to place. If funds are available for kitchen remodeling, lowering counters and range to a comfortable height for wheelchair use is recommended. Such extensive adaptation is often not feasible, however. The following are some suggestions for home management[23]:

1. Remove cabinet doors to eliminate the need to maneuver around them for opening and closing. Frequently used items should be stored toward the front of easy-to-reach cabinets above and below the counter surfaces.

2. If entrance and inside doors are not wide enough, use a device to reduce wheelchair width or make doors slightly wider by removing strips along the door jambs. Offset hinges can replace standard door hinges and increase the door jamb width by 2 inches (Fig. 13-34).

3. Use a wheelchair cushion to increase the user's height so that standard height counters may be used.

4. Use detachable desk arms and swing-away detachable footrests to allow the wheelchair user to get as close as possible to counters and tables and also to stand at counters, if that is possible.

5. Transport items safely and easily with a wheelchair lap board. The lap board may also serve as a work surface for preparing food and drying dishes. It also protects the lap from injury from hot pans and prevents utensils from falling into the lap (Fig. 13-35).

6. Fasten a drop-leaf board to a bare wall, or install a slide-out board under a counter to provide a work surface that is a comfortable height in a kitchen that is otherwise standard.

7. Fit cabinets with custom- or ready-made lazy susans or pull-out shelves to eliminate the need to reach to rear space (Fig. 13-36).

8. Ideally, ranges should be at a lower level than standard height. If this arrangement is not possible, place the controls at the front of the range, and hang a mirror angled at the proper degree over the range so that the homemaker can see contents of pots.

9. Substitute small electric cooking units and microwave ovens for the range if the range is not safely manageable.

10. Use front-loading washers and dryers.

11. Vacuum carpets with a carpet sweeper or tank-type cleaner that rolls easily and is lightweight or self-propelled. A retractable cord may be helpful for preventing tangling of cord in wheels.

ADL for the Person With Quadriplegia

In general, persons with muscle function from spinal cord levels C7 and C8 can follow many of the methods

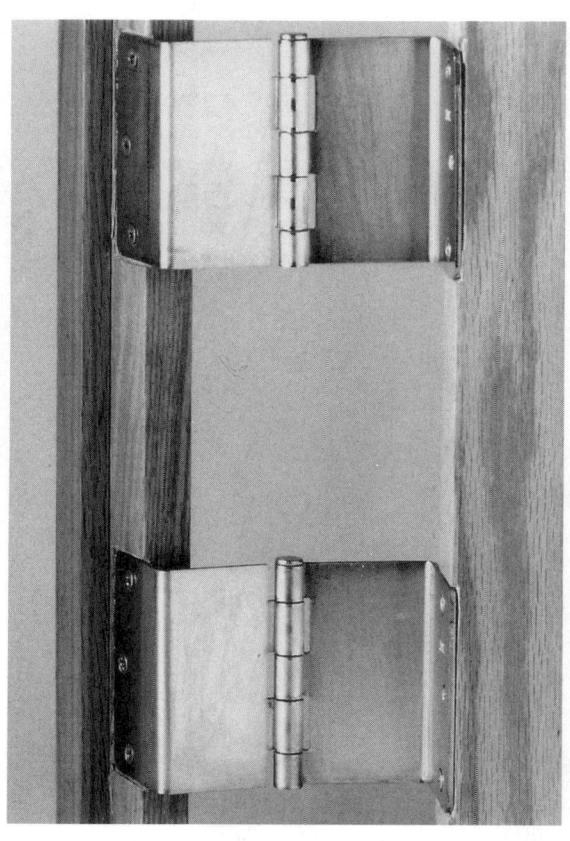

A

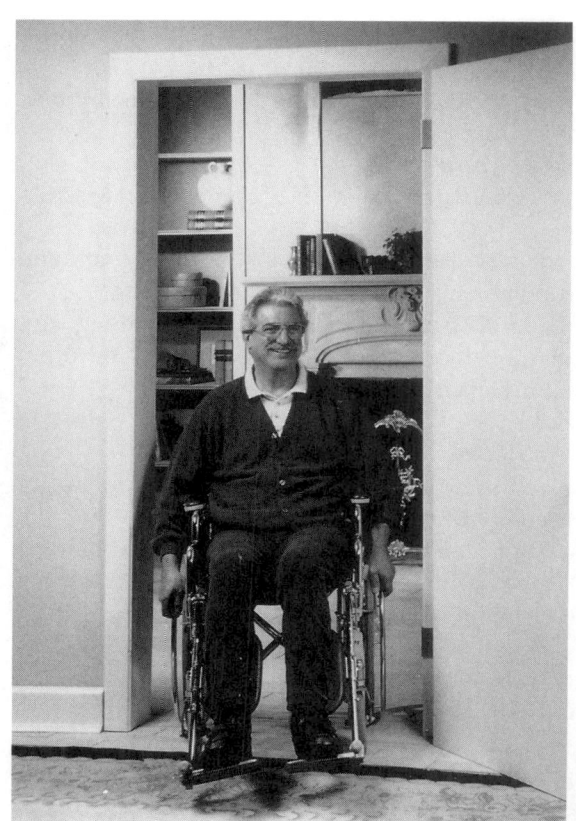

B

FIG. 13-34
A, Offset door hinges. **B,** Offset hinges widen doorway for wheelchair user. (Courtesy Sammons Preston.)

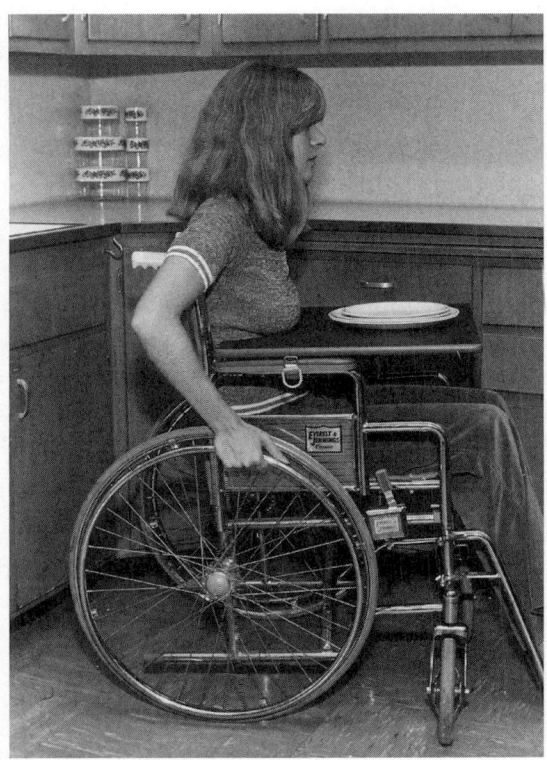

FIG. 13-35
Wheelchair lapboard is used to transport items.

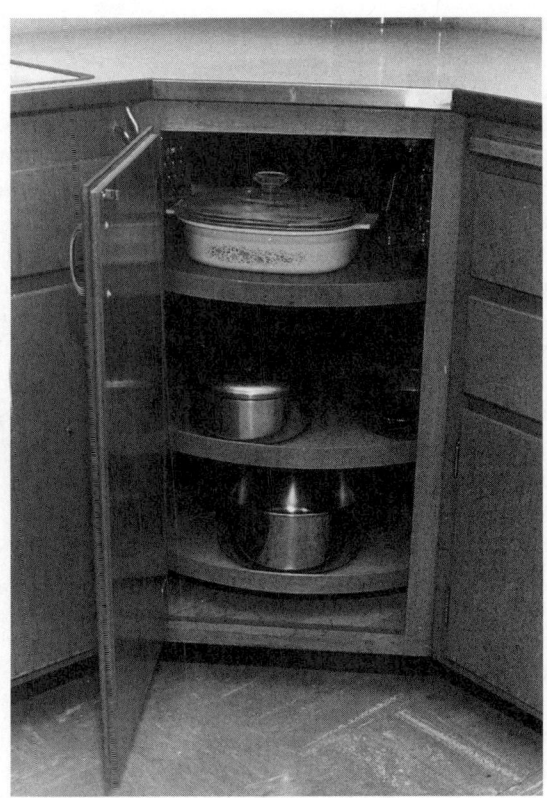

FIG. 13-36
Lazy Susan in kitchen storage cabinet.

just described for paraplegia, except for fine motor tasks such as buttoning or typing. Individuals with muscle function from C6 can be relatively independent with adaptations and assistive devices, whereas those with muscle function from C4 and C5 will require considerable special equipment and assistance. Clients with muscle function from C6 may benefit from the use of a wrist-driven flexor hinge splint. Externally powered splints and arm braces or mobile arm supports are recommended for C3, C4, and C5 levels of muscle function.[1]

Dressing Activities

Training in dressing can be commenced when the spine is stable.[6,36] *Minimum criteria* for upper extremity dressing are as follows:

1. Fair to good muscle strength in deltoids, upper and middle trapezii, shoulder rotators, rhomboids, biceps, supinators, and radial wrist extensors
2. ROM of 0° to 90° in shoulder flexion and abduction, 0° to 80° in shoulder internal rotation, 0° to 30° in external rotation, and 15° to 140° in elbow flexion
3. Sitting balance in bed or wheelchair, which may be achieved with the assistance of bed rails, electric hospital bed, or wheelchair safety belt
4. Finger prehension achieved with adequate tenodesis grasp or wrist-driven flexor-hinge splint

Additional criteria for dressing the lower extremities are as follows[36]:

1. Fair to good muscle strength in pectoralis major and minor, serratus anterior, and rhomboid major and minor
2. ROM of 0° to 120° in knee flexion, 0° to 110° in hip flexion, and 0° to 80° in hip external rotation
3. Body control for transfer from bed to wheelchair with minimal assistance
4. Ability to roll from side to side, balance in side-lying, or turn from supine position to prone position and back
5. Vital capacity of 50% or better

Dressing is *contraindicated* if any of the following factors are present[6,36]:

1. Unstable spine at site of injury
2. Pressure sores or tendency for skin breakdown during rolling, scooting, and transferring
3. Uncontrollable muscle spasms in legs
4. Less than 50% vital capacity

SEQUENCE OF DRESSING. The recommended sequence for training to dress is to put on underwear and trousers while still in bed, then transfer to a wheelchair and put on shirts, socks, and shoes.[36] Some clients may wish to put the socks on before the trousers because socks may help the feet slip through the trouser legs more easily.

EXPECTED PROFICIENCY. Clients with spinal cord lesions at C7 and below can achieve *total dressing*, which includes dressing skills for both the upper and lower extremities. Clients with lesions at C6 can also achieve total dressing, but lower extremity dressing may be difficult or impractical in terms of time and energy for these clients. Clients with lesions at C5 to C6 can achieve upper extremity dressing, with some exceptions. It is difficult or impossible for these clients to put on a brassiere, tuck a shirt or blouse into a waistband, or fasten buttons on shirt fronts and cuffs. Factors such as age, physical proportions, coordination, concomitant medical problems, and motivation will affect the degree of proficiency in dressing skills that can be achieved by any client.[6]

TYPES OF CLOTHING. Clothing should be loose and have front openings. Trousers need to be a size larger than usually worn to accommodate the urine collection device or leg braces if worn. Wrap-around skirts and incontinence pads are helpful for women. The fasteners that are easiest to manage are zippers and Velcro closures. Because the client with quadriplegia often uses the thumb as a hook to manage clothing, loops attached to zipper pulls, undershorts, and even the back of the shoes can be helpful. Belt loops on trousers are used for pulling and should be reinforced. Brassieres should have stretch straps and no wires in them. Front-opening brassiere styles can be adapted by fastening loops and adding Velcro closures; back-opening styles can have loops added at each side of the fastening.

Shoes can be one-half size to one size larger than normally worn to accommodate edema and spasticity and to avoid pressure sores. Shoe fasteners can be adapted with Velcro, elastic shoelaces, large buckles, or flip-back tongue closures. Loose woolen or cotton socks without elastic cuffs should be used initially. Nylon socks, which tend to stick to the skin, may be used as skill is gained. If neckties are used, the clip-on type or a regular tie that has been preknotted and can be slipped over the head may be manageable for some clients.[6,36]

TROUSERS AND UNDERSHORTS
DONNING TROUSERS AND UNDERSHORTS
1. Sit on bed with bed rails up. Trousers are positioned at foot of bed with trouser legs over end of bed and front side up.[36]
2. Sit up and lift one knee at a time by hooking right hand under right knee to pull leg into flexion, then put trousers over right foot. Return right leg to extension or semiextended position while repeating procedure with left hand and left knee.[6] If unable to maintain leg in flexion by holding with one arm or through advantageous use of spasticity, use a dressing band. This device is a piece of elasticized webbing that has been sewn into a figure-eight pattern, with one

small loop and one large loop. The small loop is hooked around the foot and the large hoop is anchored over the knee. The band is measured for individual client so that its length is appropriate to maintain desired amount of knee flexion. Once the trousers are in place, knee loop is pushed off knee and dressing band is removed from foot with dressing stick.[11]
3. Work trousers up legs, using patting and sliding motions with palms of hands.
4. While still sitting, with pants to midcalf height, insert dressing stick in front belt loop. Dressing stick is gripped by slipping its loop over wrist. Pull on dressing stick while extending trunk, returning to supine position. Return to sitting position and repeat this procedure, pulling on dressing sticks and maneuvering trousers up to thigh level.[36] If balance is adequate, an alternative is for client to remain sitting and lean on left elbow and pull trousers over right buttock, then reverse process for other side. Another alternative is for client to remain in supine position and roll to one side; throw opposite arm behind back; hook thumb in waistband, belt loop, or pocket; and pull trousers up over hips. These maneuvers can be repeated as often as necessary to get trousers over buttocks.[6]
5. Using palms of hands in pushing and smoothing motions, straighten the trouser legs.
6. In supine position, fasten trouser placket by hooking thumb in loop on zipper pull, patting Velcro closed, or using hand splints and buttonhooks if there are buttons or a zipper pull for zippers.[6,36]

VARIATION. Substitute the following for step 2: Sit up and lift one knee at a time by hooking right hand under right knee to pull leg into flexion, then cross the foot over the opposite leg above the knee. This position frees the foot to place the trousers more easily and requires less trunk balance. Continue with all other steps.

REMOVING TROUSERS AND UNDERSHORTS
1. Lying supine in bed with bed rails up, unfasten belt and placket fasteners.
2. Placing thumbs in belt loops, waistband, or pockets, work trousers past hips by stabilizing arms in shoulder extension and scooting body toward head of bed.
3. Use arms as described in step 2 and roll from side to side to get trousers past buttocks.
4. Coming to sitting position and alternately pulling legs into flexion, push trousers down legs.[36]
5. Trousers can be pushed off over feet with dressing stick or by hooking thumbs in waistband.

CARDIGANS OR PULLOVER GARMENTS. Cardigan and pullover garments include blouses, vests, sweaters, skirts, and front-opening dresses.[6,36] Upper extremity dressing is frequently performed in the wheelchair for greater trunk stability. The procedure for putting on these garments is as follows:

DONNING CARDIGANS OR PULLOVER GARMENTS

1. Position the garment across thighs with back facing up and neck toward knees.
2. Place both arms under back of garment and in armholes.
3. Push sleeves up onto arms, past elbows.
4. Using a wrist extension grip, hook thumbs under garment back and gather material up from neck to hem.
5. To pass garment over head, adduct and externally rotate shoulders and flex elbows while flexing head forward.
6. When garment is over head, relax shoulders and wrists and remove hands from back of garment. Most of material will be gathered up at neck, across shoulders, and under arms.
7. To work garment down over body, shrug shoulders, lean forward, and use elbow flexion and wrist extension. Use wheelchair arms for balance, if necessary. Additional maneuvers to accomplish task are to hook wrists into sleeves and pull material free from underarms, or lean forward, reach back, and slide hand against material to aid in pulling garment down.
8. Garment can be buttoned from bottom to top with aid of button hook and wrist-driven flexor hinge splint if hand function is inadequate.

REMOVING CARDIGANS OR PULLOVER GARMENTS

1. Sit in wheelchair and wear wrist-driven flexor hinge splints. Unfasten buttons (if any) while wearing splints and using buttonhook. Remove splints for remaining steps.
2. For pullover garments, hook thumb in back of neckline, extend wrist, and pull garment over head while turning head toward side of raised arm. Maintain balance by resting against opposite wheelchair armrest or pushing on thigh with extended arm.
3. For cardigan garments, hook thumb in opposite armhole and push sleeve down arm. Elevation and depression of shoulders with trunk rotation can be used to get garment to slip down arms as far as possible.
4. Hold one cuff with opposite thumb while elbow is flexed to pull arm out of sleeve.

BRASSIERE (BACK-OPENING)

DONNING BRASSIERE

1. Place brassiere across lap with straps toward knees and inside facing up.
2. Using a right-to-left procedure, hold end of brassiere closest to right side with hand or reacher and pass brassiere around back from right to left side. Lean against brassiere at back to hold it in place, while hooking thumb of left hand in a loop that has been attached near brassiere fastener. Hook right thumb in a similar loop on right side and fasten brassiere in front at waist level.
3. Hook right thumb in edge of brassiere. Using wrist extension, elbow flexion, shoulder adduction, and

internal rotation, rotate brassiere around body so that front of brassiere is in front of body.
4. While leaning on one forearm, hook opposite thumb in front end of strap and pull strap over shoulder, then repeat procedure on other side.[6,36]

REMOVING BRASSIERE

1. Hook thumb under opposite brassiere strap and push down over shoulder while elevating shoulder.
2. Pull arm out of strap and repeat procedure for other arm.
3. Push brassiere down to waist level and turn around as described previously, to bring fasteners to front.
4. Unfasten brassiere by hooking thumbs into the adapted loops near the fasteners.

Alternatives for a back-opening bra are (1) a front-opening bra with loops for using a wrist extension grip or (2) a fully elastic bra that has no fasteners and can be donned like a pullover sweater.

SOCKS

DONNING SOCKS

1. Sit in wheelchair, or on bed if balance is adequate, in cross-legged position with one ankle crossed over opposite knee.
2. Pull sock over foot with wrist extension grip and patting movements with palm of hand.[6,36]
3. If trunk balance is inadequate and cross-legged position cannot be maintained, balance by propping foot on stool, chair, or open drawer, while opposite arm is around upright of wheelchair. Using a wheelchair safety belt or leaning against wheelchair armrest on one side are options to maintain balance.
4. Use stocking aid or sock cone (Fig. 13-7) to assist in putting on socks while in this position. Powder sock cone (to reduce friction) and apply sock to cone by using thumbs and palms of hands to smooth sock out on cone.
5. With the cord loops of sock cone around the wrist or thumb, throw cone beyond foot.
6. Maneuver cone over toes by pulling cords using elbow flexion. Insert foot as far as possible into cone.
7. To remove cone from sock after foot has been inserted, move heel forward off wheelchair footrest. Use wrist extension (of hand not operating sock cone) behind knee and continue pulling cords of cone until it is removed and sock is in place on foot. Use palms to smooth sock with patting and stroking motion.[36]
8. Two loops can also be sewn on either side of the top of the sock so that thumbs can be hooked into the loops and the socks pulled on.

REMOVING SOCKS

1. While sitting in wheelchair or lying in bed, use a dressing stick or long-handled shoehorn to push sock down over heel. Cross the legs if possible.
2. Use dressing stick with cup hook on end to pull sock off toes.[7]

SHOES

DONNING SHOES

1. Use same position for donning socks as for putting on shoes.
2. Use long-handled dressing aid and insert aid into tongue of shoe. Place shoe opening over toes. Remove dressing aid from shoe and dangle shoe on toes.
3. Using palm of hand on sole of shoe, pull shoe toward heel of foot. One hand is used to stabilize leg while other hand pushes against sole of shoe to work shoe onto foot. Use thenar eminence and sides of hand for this pushing motion.
4. With feet flat on floor or on wheelchair footrest and knees flexed 90°, place a long-handled shoehorn in heel of shoe and press down on flexed knee.
5. Fasten shoes.[36]

REMOVING SHOES

1. Sitting in wheelchair with legs crossed as described previously, unfasten shoes.
2. Use shoehorn or dressing stick to push on heel counter of shoe, dislodging it from heel. Shoe will drop or can be pushed to floor with dressing stick.[36]

Eating Activities

Eating may be assisted by a variety of devices, depending on the level of muscle function.[1] An injury at C5 or above necessitates mobile arm supports or externally powered splints and braces. A wrist splint and universal cuff may be used together if a wrist-driven flexor hinge splint is not used. The universal cuff holds the eating utensil, and the splint stabilizes the wrist. A nonskid mat and a plate with plate guard may provide adequate stability of the plate for pushing and picking up food (Fig. 13-37).

The spoon plate is an option for independent feeding for clients with high spinal cord injuries. The plate is a portable device that can be adjusted in height to the level of the client's mouth. The plate is made of a high-temperature thermoplastic and is formed over a mold that has a rim bowled to the approximate depth and length of a spoon. The client rotates the device with mouth and neck control. Food is removed from the rim of the plate with the mouth. Successful use of the device depends on adequate oral control, head and trunk control, and motivation. The reader is referred to the original source for information on making or obtaining this device.[41] Also available for clients who have no use of their upper extremities is the electric self-feeder, which requires only slight head motion and is activated by a chin switch (Fig. 13-38).

A regular or swivel spoon-fork combination can be used when there is minimal muscle function (C4 to C5). A long plastic straw with a straw clip to stabilize it in the cup or glass eliminates the need for picking up these drinking vessels. A bilateral or unilateral clip-type holder on a glass or cup makes it possible for many persons with hand and arm weakness to manage liquids without a straw.

Built-up utensils may be useful for those with some functional grasp or tenodesis grasp. Food may be cut with a quad-quip knife if arm strength is adequate to manage the device (Fig. 13-39).

Hygiene and Grooming

1. Use a shower or bathtub seat and transfer board for transfers.
2. Extend reach by using long-handled bath sponges with loop handle or built-up handle.
3. Eliminate need to grasp washcloth by using bath mitts or bath gloves.

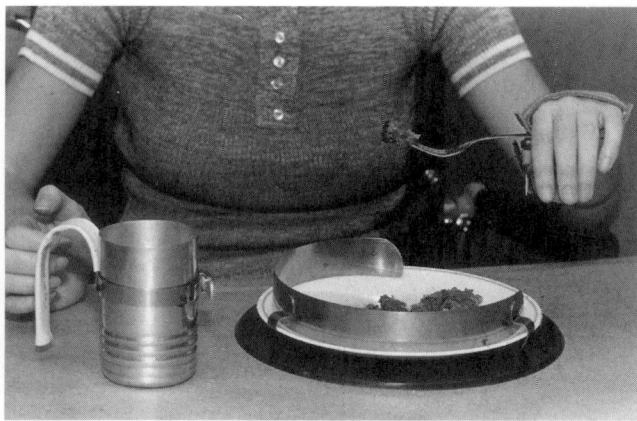

FIG. 13-37
Self-feeding with aid of universal cuff, plate guard, nonskid mat, and clip-type cup holder to compensate for absent grasp.

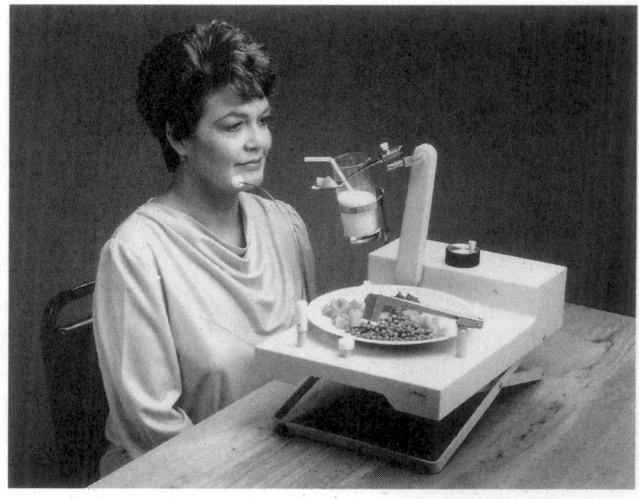

FIG. 13-38
Electric self-feeder. (Courtesy Sammons Preston.)

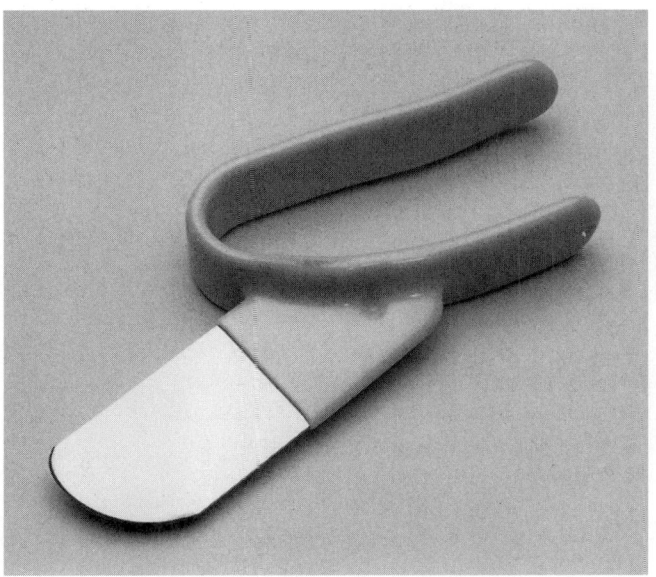

FIG. 13-39
Quad-quip knife.

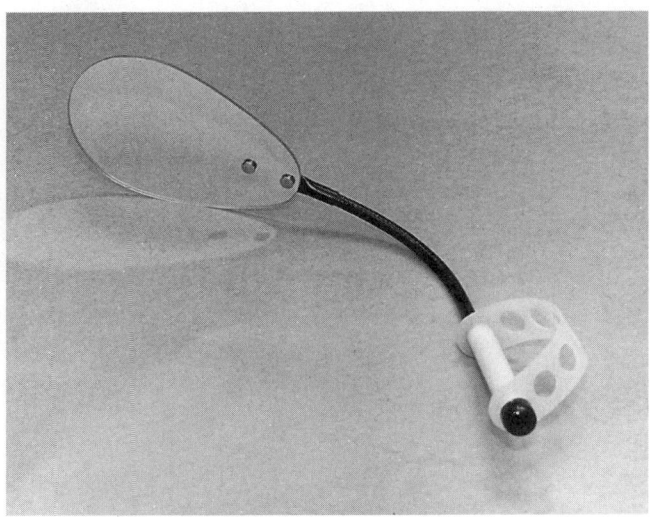

FIG. 13-40
Skin inspection mirror.

4. Hold comb and toothbrush with a universal cuff.[1]
5. Use a wall-mounted hair dryer. Use a universal cuff to hold brush or comb for hair styling while using this mounted hair dryer.[12]
6. Use a clip-type holder for electric razor.
7. Persons with quadriplegia can use suppository inserters to manage bowel care independently.
8. Use skin inspection mirror with long stem and looped handle for independent skin inspection (Fig. 13-40). Devices and methods selected must be adapted according to the degree of weakness of each client.
9. Adapted leg-bag clamps to empty catheter leg-bags are also available for individuals with limited hand function. Elastic leg-bag straps may also be replaced with Velcro straps.

Communication and Environmental Hardware Adaptations

1. Turn pages with an electric page-turner, mouth stick, or head wand if hand and arm function are inadequate (Fig. 13-41).
2. For typing, writing, operating a tape recorder, and painting, insert pen, pencil, typing stick, or paintbrush in a universal cuff that has been positioned with the opening on the ulnar side of the palm for typing (Fig. 13-42).
3. Touch telephone keys with the universal cuff and a pencil positioned with eraser down. The receiver may need to be stationed in a telephone arm and positioned for listening or adapted with a telephone clip holder (Fig. 13-17). Special adaptations are available to substitute for the need to replace the receiver in the cradle. For clients with no arm function, a speaker phone can be used along with a mouth-stick to push the button to initiate a call. The operator assists with dialing.
4. Use personal computers, word processors, or electric typewriters. A computer mouse may be substituted for use of the keyboard. A variety of different mouse designs and sizes are available. Speech recognition programs are available for individuals with little or no arm movement.
5. Built-up pencils and pens or special pencil holders are needed for clients with hand weakness. The Wanchik writer is an effective adaptive writing device (Fig. 13-18).
6. Sophisticated electronic communications devices operated by mouth, pneumatic controls, and head controls are available for clients with no function in the upper extremities.[38]
7. Kelly[19] describes a cassette tape holder and two mouth-sticks that allow C3, C4, or C5 quadriplegic clients to operate a tape recorder or radio independently. The first mouth-stick, with a friction tip, is used to depress the operating buttons and adjust the volume and selector dials of the radio. The second mouth-stick is used to move the cassettes from the cassette holder to the tape recorder and to remove the cassettes from the recorder. The cassette tape stand has eight levels and is designed to hold eight tapes. The reader is referred to the original source for specifications on construction of these devices and to develop methods for a client to be able to manage a CD player.[19]
8. Environmental controls allow for easy operation from a panel designed to run multiple devices such as televisions, radios, lights, telephones, intercoms, and hospital beds (see Chapter 19).

FIG. 13-41
Wand mouth stick is provided by Sammons Preston, An Ability-One Company.

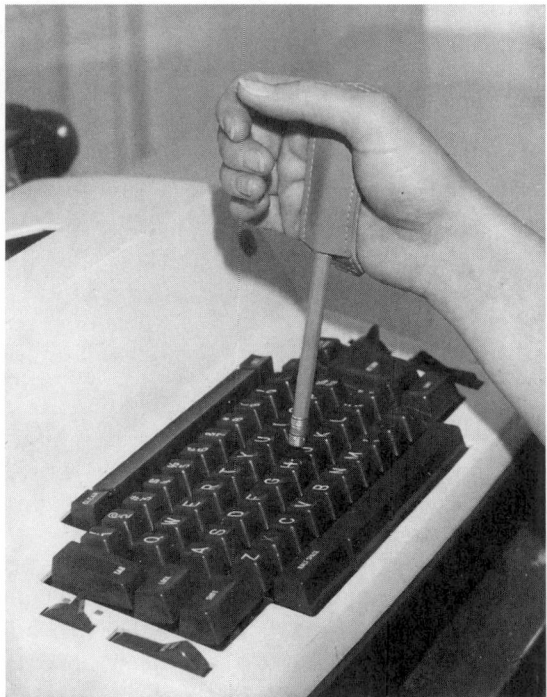

FIG. 13-42
Typing with aid of utensil holder and typing stick.

Mobility and Transfers

Principles of wheelchair transfer techniques for the individual with quadriplegia are discussed in Chapter 14. Mobility depends on degree of weakness. Electric wheelchairs operated by hand, chin, or pneumatic controls have greatly increased the mobility of persons with severe upper and lower extremity weakness. Vans fitted with wheelchair lifts and stabilizing devices permit such clients to be transported to pursue community, vocational, educational, and leisure activities with an assistant. In addition, adaptations for hand controls have made it possible for many clients with function of at least C6 level to drive independently.

Home Management Activities

Clients with muscle function of C6 or better may be independent for light homemaking with appropriate devices, adaptations, and safety awareness. Many of the suggestions for wheelchair maneuverability and envi-

ronmental adaptation outlined for the paraplegic apply here as well. In addition, clients with upper extremity weakness need to use lightweight equipment and special devices. The *Mealtime Manual for People With Disability and the Aging* compiled by Judith Lannefeld Klinger[23] contains many excellent specific suggestions that apply to homemakers with weak upper extremities.

ADL for the Person With Low Vision

The environmental modifications described in the following section are appropriate when performing ADL for all persons with low vision.

Lighting and Magnifiers

1. Improve lighting by aiming light at the work area, not into the eyes.
2. Reduce glare by having adjustable blinds, sheer curtains, or tinted windows. Wearing dark glasses indoors may also reduce glare.
3. Maximize contrast by providing a work surface that is in contrast to the task. For example, serve a meal on a white plate if the table is dark. Paint a white edge on a dark step. Replace white wall switches with black to contrast with the wall.
4. Simplify figure-ground perception by clearing pathways and eliminating clutter.
5. Work in natural light by placing a chair by a window.[34,42]
6. Use magnifiers with lights. These come in a variety of sizes and degrees of magnification. Specialists in low vision can determine the appropriate degree of magnification needed. Some magnifiers are portable, others are attached to stands to do needle work or fine work, and others are sheets of plastic to magnify an entire page of print.[27]

Dressing Activities

1. Light closet to improve acuity. Hang matching clothes together.
2. Pin socks together when placing them in the washer and dryer so they will stay matched.

Eating Activities

1. Provide high contrast. Ensure that plates contrast with table surface or place mats. Avoid patterned tablecloths.
2. Arrange food on the plate in a clockwise fashion and orient the person with low vision to the arrangement.

Hygiene and Grooming Activities

1. Reduce clutter in bathroom drawers and cabinets.
2. Use electric razor.
3. Use magnified mirrors.
4. Use high-contrast bath mat in bathtub.
5. Install high-contrast grab bars in shower.

Communication and Environmental Hardware Adaptations

1. Use talking watches or clocks to tell time.
2. Use talking scale to determine weight.
3. Use large-print magnification screen on computer.
4. Technology for reading print is changing rapidly. Become familiar with the various types of adaptations for reading print.[27]
5. Use high-contrast door knobs. Paint the door frame a color that contrasts highly with the door to improve ease of identifying the door.[34]
6. Use speaker phones, preprogrammed phone numbers, or phone with large print and high contrast numbers. Identify phone buttons with contrasting tape or Velcro dot to teach client how to turn phone on and which buttons to push.
7. Use writing guides to write letters, checks, or signatures.[27]
8. To read, use books on tape or Talking Books.

Mobility and Transfer Skills

Mobility is eased with the clearing of pathways and the minimizing of clutter and furniture. Lighting in hallways and entryways is also needed. The person with low vision needs to optimize visual scanning abilities by learning to turn and position the head frequently when mobile or participating in an activity.[42] The OT practitioner may need to refer a client to a specialist in low vision who is specifically trained in teaching mobility to persons with low vision or legal blindness.

Home Management Activities

A variety of devices are available to compensate for low vision while managing the home. Organization and consistency are critical to the safe and efficient performance of home management tasks. Family members need to remember to replace items where they were found and not reorganize items without assistance from the person with low vision.

1. For safety, place cleaning supplies separate from food supplies.
2. Eliminate extra hazardous cleaning supplies and replace with one multipurpose cleanser. Place this cleaning agent in a uniquely shaped bottle or in a specific location.
3. Mark appliance controls with high-contrast tape or paint to identify start and stop buttons or positions. Place Velcro tabs to mark frequently used positions on dials (e.g., on the 350° position for stove or for the wash and wear cycle on the washer or dryer).
4. Label cans by using rubber bands to attach index cards with bold, dark print to each can. When the can is used, the card may be placed into a stack to create a shopping list.

5. Indicate number of minutes needed for microwave cooking by placing rubber bands on the items. Two rubber bands would indicate that the item should be cooked for 2 minutes. Assistance will be needed for initial setup.
6. Use liquid level indicator to determine when hot liquid reaches 1 inch from top of cup or container.[27]
7. Use cutting guides or specially designed knives to cut meat or bread.[27]
8. Use a tape recorder to make reminder lists or grocery lists.

Medication Management

1. Use medication organizer to organize pills.
2. For diabetic management, there are many different products available for individualized evaluation of the client (e.g., syringe magnifiers, talking or large-print glucometers, and a device to count the insulin dosages).
3. Use talking scales to evaluate weight.[31]

Money Management

1. Use a consistent method of folding money to identify denominations, as in the following example:

$1.00	Keep flat
$5.00	Fold in square half
$10.00	Fold lengthwise
$20.00	Fold in half and then lengthwise.

2. Keep different denominations in different sections of the wallet. Learn to recognize coins by size and type of edge (smooth or rough).[42]

SUMMARY

ADL and I-ADL are tasks of self-maintenance, mobility, communication, home management, and community living skills that enable a person to function independently and assume important occupational roles.

ADL is one of the performance areas in the occupational performance model. Occupational therapists routinely assess performance in ADL to determine clients' levels of functional independence. Interview and observation of performance are used to carry out the assessment. Results of the assessment and ongoing progress are recorded on one of many available ADL checklists or with a standardized assessment, the content of which is summarized for the permanent medical record.

Treatment is directed at training in independent living skills with activities such as eating, dressing, mobility, home management, communication, and community living skills. The occupational therapist can include in the treatment program special equipment and many methods for performing ADL with specific functional problems.

REVIEW QUESTIONS

1. Define ADL and I-ADL. List three classifications of tasks that may be considered in each category.
2. What is the role of OT in restoring ADL and I-ADL independence?
3. List at least three activities that are considered self-care skills, three functional mobility skills, three functional communication skills, three home management skills, and three community living skills.
4. List three factors that the occupational therapist must consider before commencing ADL performance assessment and training. Describe how each could limit or affect ADL performance.
5. What is the ultimate goal of the ADL and I-ADL training program?
6. Discuss the concept of maximal independence, as defined in the text.
7. List the general steps in the procedure for ADL assessment.
8. Describe how the occupational therapist can use the ADL checklist.
9. List the steps in the activities of home management assessment.
10. What is the purpose of the home assessment?
11. List the steps in the home assessment.
12. Who should be involved in a comprehensive home assessment?
13. What kinds of things are observed in a home assessment?
14. How does the therapist record and report results of the home assessment and make the necessary recommendations?
15. How does the occupational therapist, with the client, select ADL and I-ADL training objectives after an assessment?
16. Describe three approaches to teaching ADL skills to a client with perception or memory deficits.
17. List the important factors to include in an ADL progress report.
18. Describe the levels of independence, as defined in the text.
19. Give an example of a health and safety management issue.
20. Give three examples of adaptations that may be helpful for the person with low vision.

EXERCISES

1. Demonstrate the use of at least three assistive devices mentioned in the text.
2. Teach another person to don a shirt, using one hand.
3. Teach another person how to don and remove trousers, as if he or she had hemiplegia.
4. Teach another person how to don and remove trousers, as if the legs were paralyzed.

5. Prepare a meal using only one hand and write about your experience.

REFERENCES

1. *Activities of daily living for patients with incoordination, limited range of motion, paraplegia, quadriplegic, and hemiplegia,* Cleveland, 1968 (rev 1989), Metro Health Center for Rehabilitation, Metro Health Medical Center (unpublished).
2. American Occupational Therapy Association: Uniform terminology for occupational therapy—third edition, *Am J Occup Ther* 48(11):1047-1054, 1994.
3. Armstrong M, Lauzen S: *Community integration program,* ed 2, Washington, 1994, Idyll Arbor.
4. Asher IE: *Occupational therapy assessment tools: an annotated index,* ed 2, Bethesda, Md, 1996, American Occupational Therapy Association.
5. Baum C, Edwards D: Cognitive performance in senile dementia of the Alzheimer's type: the kitchen task assessment, *Am J Occup Ther* 47:431-436, 1993.
6. Bromley I: *Tetraplegia and paraplegia: a guide for physiotherapists,* ed 2, London, 1981, Churchill Livingstone.
7. Buchwald E: *Physical rehabilitation for daily living,* New York, 1952, McGraw-Hill.
8. Christiansen C: Occupational performance assessment. In Christiansen C, Baum C, editors: *Occupational therapy: overcoming human performance deficits,* Thorofare, NJ, 1991, Slack.
9. Cook AM, Hussey SM: Electronic assistive technologies in occupational therapy practice. In Pedretti LW, editor: *Occupational therapy: practice skills for physical dysfunction,* ed 4, St Louis, 1996, Mosby.
10. Cynkin S, Robinson AM: *Occupational therapy and activities health: toward health through activities,* Boston, 1990, Little, Brown.
11. Easton LW, Horan AL: Dressing band, *Am J Occup Ther* 33:656, 1979.
12. Feldmeier DM, Poole JL: The position-adjustable hair dryer, *Am J Occup Ther* 41:246, 1987.
13. Fisher AG: *Assessment of motor and process skills (AMPS),* Fort Collins, Colo, 1995, Three Star Press.
14. Florey LL, Michelman SM: Occupational role history: a screening tool for psychiatric occupational therapy, *Am J Occup Ther* 36:301, 1982.
15. Gray JM: Putting occupation into practice: occupation as ends, occupation as means, *Am J Occup Ther* 52:354, 1998.
16. Guerette P, Moran W: ADL awareness, *Team Rehab Report,* June, 1994.
17. Holser P, Jones M, Ilanit T: A study of the upper extremity control brace, *Am J Occup Ther* 16:170, 1962.
18. Hopkins HL, Smith HD, Tiffany EG: Therapeutic application of activity. In Hopkins HL, Smith HD, editors: *Willard and Spackman's occupational therapy,* ed 6, Philadelphia, 1983, JB Lippincott.
19. Kelly SN: Adaptations for independent use of cassette tape recorder/radio by high-level quadriplegic patients, *Am J Occup Ther* 37:766, 1983.
20. Kemp BJ, Mitchell JM: Functional assessment in geriatric mental health. In JE Birren et al. editors: *Handbook of mental health and aging,* ed 2, San Diego, 1992, Academic Press.
21. Kester DL: Prevocational and vocational assessment. In Hopkins HL, Smith HD, editors: *Willard and Spackman's occupational therapy,* ed 6, Philadelphia, 1983, JB Lippincott.
22. Klein RM, Bell B: Self care skills: behavioral measurement with Klein-Bell ADL Scale, *Arch Phys Med Rehabil* 63(7):335-338, 1982.
23. Klinger JL: *Mealtime manual for people with disabilities and the aging,* Thorofare, NJ, 1997, Slack.
24. Kohlman-Thomson L: *The Kohlman evaluation of living skills (KELS),* ed 3, Bethesda, Md, 1993, American Occupational Therapy Association.

25. Law ML, Baptiste S, Carswell A, et al: *Canadian occupational performance measure (COPM)*, ed 3, Ottawa, 1998, CAOT Publications ACE.

26. Letts L, Law M, Rigby P, et al: Person-environment assessments in occupational therapy, *Am J Occup Ther* 48:608-618, 1994.

27. *The Lighthouse catalog*, New York, The Lighthouse.

28. Malick MH, Almasy BS: Activities of daily living and homemaking. In Hopkins HL, Smith HD, editors: *Willard and Spackman's occupational therapy*, ed 7, Philadelphia, 1988, JB Lippincott.

29. Malick MH, Almasy BS: Assessment and evaluation: life work tasks. In Hopkins HL, Smith HD, editors: *Willard and Spackman's occupational therapy*, ed 6, Philadelphia, 1983, JB Lippincott.

30. Matsusuyu J: The interest checklist, *Am J Occup Ther* 23:323, 1969.

31. *Maxi aids and appliances for independent living*, Farmingdale, NY, Maxi Aids.

32. Melvin JL: *Rheumatic disease: occupational therapy and rehabilitation*, ed 2, Philadelphia, 1982, FA Davis.

33. Moorhead L: The occupational history, *Am J Occup Ther* 23:329, 1969.

34. Orr AL: *Issues in aging and vision: a curriculum for university programs and in-service training*, New York, 1998, American Foundation for the Blind Press.

35. The Professional Manual Subcommittee of the Educational Committee, Allied Health Professional Section of Arthritis Foundation: *Arthritis manual for allied health professionals*, New York, 1973, The Arthritis Foundation.

36. Runge M: Self-dressing techniques for clients with spinal cord injury, *Am J Occup Ther* 21:367, 1967.

37. Sokaler R A buttoning aid, *Am J Occup Ther* 35:737, 1981.

38. Trombly CA: Activities of daily living. In Trombly CA, editor: *Occupational therapy for physical dysfunction*, ed 2, Baltimore, 1983, Williams & Wilkins.

39. Uniform Data System for Medical Rehabilitation: *Functional independence measure (FIM)*, Buffalo, NY, 1993, State University of New York at Buffalo.

40. Watanabe S: *Activities configuration: regional institute on the evaluation process*. Final report. RSA-123-T-68, New York, 1968, American Occupational Therapy Association.

41. Wykoff E, Mitani M: The spoon plate: a self-feeding device, *Am J Occup Ther* 36:333, 1982.

42. Yano E: *Working with the older adult with low vision: home health OT interventions*, Presentation at Kaiser Permanente Medical Center Home Health Department, Hayward, Calif, 1998.

CHAPTER 14

Mobility

TERU A. CREEL
CAROLE ADLER
MICHELLE TIPTON-BURTON
SUSAN M. LILLIE

KEY TERMS

SECTION 1
Functional Ambulation
Functional ambulation
Gait training
Pathological gait
Ambulation aids

SECTION 2
Wheelchair Assessment and Transfers
Rehabilitation technology supplier
Durable medical equipment
Spasticity
Contractures
Skin breakdown
Vital capacity
Medical necessity
Body mechanics
Positioning mass
Pelvic tilt

SECTION 3
Transportation, Community Mobility, and Driving Assessment
Transportation
Paratransit
Americans With Disabilities Act
Specialized training
Clinical evaluations
Cognition
Driver competence
Vision
Perception
Assistive technology
Primary controls
Secondary controls
On-road evaluation
Driver training

LEARNING OBJECTIVES

After studying each section the student or practitioner will be able to do the following:

Section 1
1. Define functional ambulation.
2. Discuss the role of the occupational therapy (OT) practitioner in functional ambulation.
3. Identify appropriate interventions to promote functional ambulation within OT treatment.
4. Identify safety issues in functional ambulation.
5. Recognize basic lower extremity orthotics and ambulation aids.

Section 2
1. Identify the components necessary to perform a wheelchair evaluation.
2. Understand the process of wheelchair measurement and prescription completion.
3. Identify wheelchair safety considerations.
4. Follow guidelines for proper body mechanics.
5. Apply principles of proper body positioning.
6. Identify the steps necessary in performing various transfer techniques.
7. Identify considerations necessary to determine the appropriate transfer method based on the patient's clinical presentation.

Section 3
1. Recognize transportation as a valued skill.
2. Recognize how occupational roles affect the evaluation process and equipment selection.
3. Identify safety issues in driver evaluation.
4. State the purpose of passenger and driver evaluation.
5. Understand the complexity of the driver referral and evaluation process.
6. List the recommended practice components for the driver evaluator.
7. Discuss the effect the loss of a driver's license has on both the individual and society.

Walking, climbing stairs, traveling within one's neighborhood, and driving a car are so universal and customary that most people would not consider these to be complex activities. The basic capacities to move within the environment, to reach objects of interest, to explore one's surroundings, and to come and go at will appear natural and easy. For persons with disabilities, however, mobility is rarely taken for granted or thought of as automatic. A disability may prevent a person from using the legs to walk or using the hands to operate controls of motor vehicles. Cardiopulmonary and medical conditions may limit aerobic capacity or endurance, requiring the person to take frequent rests and to curtail walking to cover only the most basic of needs, such as toileting. Deficits in motor coordination, flexibility, and strength may seriously impair movement and may make difficult any activities that require a combination of mobility (e.g., walking or moving in the environment) and stability (e.g., holding the hands steady as one must when carrying a cup of coffee or a watering can).

Occupational therapy (OT) practitioners help persons with mobility restrictions to achieve maximum access to environments and objects of interest to them. Typically, OT practitioners provide remediation and compensatory training. In so doing, therapists must analyze the activities most valued and environments most used by their clients and must consider any future changes that can be predicted from an individual's medical history, prognosis, and developmental status.

This chapter guides the practitioner in evaluation and treatment of persons with mobility restrictions. Three main topics are explored. The first section addresses **functional ambulation,** which combines the act of walking within one's immediate environment (i.e., home or workplace) with other activities chosen by the individual. Feeding pets, preparing a meal and carrying it to a table, and doing simple housework are tasks that may involve functional ambulation. Functional ambulation may be conducted with aids such as walkers, canes, or crutches.

The second section concerns wheelchairs, their selection, measurement, fitting, and use. For many persons with disabilities, mobility becomes possible only with a wheelchair and specific positioning devices. Consequently, individual evaluation is needed to select and fit this essential piece of personal medical equipment. Proper training in ergonomic use will allow the wheelchair-dependent individual many years of safe and comfortable mobility. Safe and efficient transfer techniques based on the individual's clinical status are introduced in this chapter. Attention is also given to the body mechanics required to safely assist an individual.

The third section covers community mobility, which for many in the United States of America is synonymous with driving. Increased advocacy by and for persons with disabilities has improved access and has yielded an increasing range of options for adapting motor vehicles for individual needs. Public transportation has also become increasingly accessible. Driving is a complex activity, requiring multiple cognitive and perceptual skills. Evaluation of individuals with medical conditions and physical limitations is thus important for the safety of the disabled person and the public at large.

Mobility is an aspect of OT practice that requires close coordination with other health care providers, particularly physical therapists and providers of durable medical equipment. Improving and maintaining the functional mobility of persons with disabilities can be one of the most gratifying practice areas. Consumers experience tremendous energy and empowerment when they are able to access and explore wider and more interesting environments.

SECTION 1
Functional Ambulation

TERU A. CREEL

Functional ambulation is a goal for many OT clients. Functional ambulation, a subcomponent of functional mobility, is the purposeful application of the mobility training taught to the client to enable movement from one position or place to another. Functional ambulation involves achieving a goal such as carrying a plate to the table or carrying groceries from the car to the house. If the individual is using an assistive aid to ambulate and simultaneously has a need to carry an object, solving the problem is more complex. Functional ambulation is applicable for individuals with a variety of diagnoses, such as lower extremity amputation, cerebrovascular accident, acquired brain injury, or total hip replacement.

Functional mobility allows collaboration between the occupational therapist and the physical therapist. Together, the OT practitioner and the physical therapy (PT) practitioner provide the most appropriate technique and ambulation aid for use during functional ambulation. The physical therapist performs **gait training** (the treatments used to improve walking and ameliorate deviations from normal gait) and makes recommendations for ambulation aids. The occupational therapist applies these recommendations during functional activities and provides feedback to the PT practitioner regarding functional outcomes using the recommended techniques and devices.

BASICS OF AMBULATION

Ambulation or bipedal locomotion is a very complex function. Locomotion is the act of getting from one place to another. For two-legged and four-legged animals, gait is the means of achieving locomotion. Leonard[4] stated the following:

> The central nervous system (CNS) somehow must generate the locomotor pattern, generate appropriate propulsive forces, modulate changes in center of gravity, coordinate multi-limb trajectories, adapt to changing conditions and changing joint positions, coordinate visual, auditory, vestibular and peripheral afferent information, and account for the viscoelastic properties of muscles.[4]

The OT practitioner should have a basic understanding of ambulation terminology and techniques and of assistive aids commonly used during functional ambulation.

Locomotion is the act of getting from one place to another. Gait is the means of achieving this action. Gait training is treatment used to improve gait.

The individuals seen by the OT-PT team may exhibit **pathological gait** because of biomechanical or neurophysiological deficits. Problems noted may include decreased walking velocity, decreased weight bearing, increased swing time of the affected lower extremity, or an abnormal base of support. Functional deficits may include unsafe ambulation and insufficient energy. As the physical therapist evaluates the causes of the gait problems, orthotics and ambulatory aids may be recommended. It is important that the OT practitioner reinforce the gait training by following the appropriate recommendations.

The OT practitioner should be familiar with basic lower extremity (LE) orthotics. Should it be determined that the individual has abnormal posture of the ankle, an ankle-foot orthosis (AFO) may be recommended. An AFO, according to *Mosby's Medical, Nursing, and Allied Health Dictionary*,[1] is a protective external device, commonly made of lightweight thermoplastic splinting material and applied to the ankle area to protect or compensate for joint instability. Should it be determined that the individual has knee collapse or hyperextension, an external means of knee control such as a knee-ankle-foot orthosis (KAFO) may be recommended. A KAFO includes offset knee joints and a rigid AFO.[2]

An **ambulation aid** may be recommended for use during ambulation to compensate for impaired balance, decreased strength, pain during weight bearing on one or both lower extremities, or absence of a lower extremity. An ambulation aid may be needed to help with fracture healing, to enhance body functions, or to improve functional mobility.[6]

Ambulation aids are numerous. Basic ambulation aids, from those providing the most support to the least, are a walker, crutches, a single crutch, bilateral canes, and a single cane.[6] The individual may begin ambulation with an aid that provides maximal support or stability and then may be progressed to an aid that provides less support or stability. Once again, it is essential that the OT practitioner communicate with the physical therapist to be kept abreast of any changes in the individual's ambulation aids and the use of such aids.

The basic ambulation techniques recommended by the physical therapist will vary from client to client, depending on the individual's goals, strengths, and weaknesses. General techniques may be applied to various clients based on the clinical judgment of the physical therapist. The OT practitioner reinforces the physical therapist's recommendations, incorporating these general techniques into functional ambulation activities.

During functional ambulation on a level surface, the OT practitioner is positioned slightly behind and to one side of the client. The therapist may position himself or herself to the stronger or weaker side of the client, based on the recommendations and preference of the physical therapist. The therapist maintains contact with the client by using the gait belt. The therapist places his or her feet in an anterior-posterior position, with the outermost foot positioned between the client's lower extremity and the ambulation aid, and the innermost foot posterior to the patient's nearest lower extremity.[6] During ambulation, the therapist moves with (in the same direction as) the client. The therapist's outermost lower extremity moves with the ambulation aid, and the therapist's inside foot moves forward with the client's lower extremity.

FUNCTIONAL AMBULATION

Functional ambulation integrates ambulation into activities of daily living (ADL) and instrumental activities of daily living (I-ADL). Using an occupation-based approach, the OT practitioner assesses the client's abilities within the performance context. What role(s) does the client desire to perform? What tasks does this role require of the client? Based on the answers to these questions, the occupational therapist plans for functional mobility activities with the goal of confident and safe functional ambulation in valued occupational roles and tasks.

When assessing the individual's needs based on roles and desired tasks, the OT practitioner performs a **task analysis,** analyzing the relationship between the client and his or her occupations and environment.[7] A task analysis serves the purpose of determining goals and targeting health outcomes. The task analysis identifies and examines meaningful and purposeful occupations.[5] Table 14-1 provides guidelines for such an analysis as it relates to functional ambulation.

TABLE 14-1

Functional Mobility Analysis

SITUATION: 53-year-old homemaker with ankle amputation ambulating with a cane	
Task Analysis Approach	**Example**
1. Identify the task(s) and specify the long- and short-term goals.	**Task:** Meal preparation; **LTG:** To prepare meal for family; **STG:** To prepare muffins from a mix
2. Gather necessary information concerning:	Necessary information specific to this client:
a. The *action*, including classification of the action and the movement	What motor skills are needed for this activity? What is the client's endurance level?
b. The *environment*, including the influence of both direct and indirect conditions	What are the environmental conditions for conducting this task? What supplies, people, and setting are required?
c. The *client*, including his or her interests, abilities, and whether the minimal prerequisite skills for success are present	What information is known about the client? Interests and activities? What are the strengths and weaknesses from the OT assessment?
d. The *prerequisite skills* or performance components required of the client	What performance components are needed for functional ambulation to successfully bake muffins?
e. The *expectations* of outcome and movement	Client will successfully bake muffins while ambulating with cane
3. Develop a strategy to make up for any deficits identified in #2.	Strategy: What adaptations will be necessary to accommodate availability of unilateral UE to carry supplies because of use of an ambulation aid?
4. Plan the intervention strategy based on the preceding information concerning the individual-activity-environment interaction.	Arrange supplies on countertop near oven to limit need for long distances of ambulation while carrying objects; use countertop or wheeled cart to transport bowls, pans, and other items.
5. Effect the strategy. a. Observe task and performance of the patients. b. Record what happened: What was the outcome and what was the approach and effect of the movement solution?	Implement the task with the client. Observe and record outcomes.
6. Evaluate the observation. a. Compare *expectations* and *what happened*. b. Provide feedback based on the comparison above and assist the patient in making decisions about the next attempt. c. With the client, plan the next activity.	Evaluate: Was client successful in baking muffins? Provide feedback to the client. Plan next activity with client.

Adapted from Higgins JR, Higgins S: The acquisition of locomotor skill. In Craik RL, Oatis CA, editors: *Gait analysis: theory and application,* St Louis, 1995, Mosby.

PRACTICAL INSTRUCTION AND SAFETY

Before beginning functional ambulation, evaluation, or training, the OT practitioner should know basic client information. The therapist reviews the medical record or pertinent notes reporting the client's current status and precautions. As part of this review, the therapist confers with the PT team member regarding the client's current ambulatory status, gait techniques, and ambulation aids or orthosis to be used. Throughout the activity, the therapist reinforces the prescribed ambulation techniques and aids.

Another key to safe and successful functional ambulation is awareness of the client's endurance level. How easily does the client fatigue? What distance is the client able to ambulate? With this information in mind, the therapist can plan ahead for the functional ambulation activity. If the client may fatigue easily, the therapist may have a wheelchair, chair, or stool readily available for use at appropriate intervals or in case of need.

To prepare the client for functional ambulation, the therapist begins with safe and appropriate footwear. The client should don nonskid shoes that fit well to avoid slipping. To increase the client's sense of security and to prevent a loss of balance or falls, the client should be instructed to avoid slippers or ill-fitting shoes or stocking feet.

The client's physiological responses should be monitored during the functional ambulation activity. The therapist should be aware of the client's precautions and respond appropriately. Physiological responses may include a change in breathing patterns, perspiration, reddened skin, a change in mental status, and decreased responsiveness.

During functional ambulation, the OT practitioner should be positioned slightly behind and to one side of the individual. Rather than grasping the individual's clothing, the therapist should maintain contact with the individual by using a gait belt to grasp with one hand, leaving the other hand free to assist with the functional activity.

The therapist should think ahead to be prepared for the unexpected. As with monitoring for fatigue level, the therapist must be prepared in case the unplanned occurs. Preparation includes having a wheelchair, walker, chair, or stool available should the activity need to be adjusted to a lower level of difficulty. Being prepared for the unexpected also involves watching for any obstacles or moving objects that may come into the path of the client, such as other individuals and therapists.

The occupational therapist must not leave the client unattended during functional ambulation, because the client may be unstable and a fall could result. The area being used should be cleared of potential safety hazards. The therapist should be certain that the area to be used for functional ambulation is free of any potential risks such as obstacles and that the floor is dry. Box 14-1 provides a summary of these important points.

FUNCTIONAL AMBULATION APPLICATION

There are numerous opportunities for functional ambulation based on the individual and the specific requirements of the client's roles and desired tasks to be performed. Several typical functional ambulation activities follow. The activities may be modified for the individual clients. Functional ambulation may be incorporated during ADL, work and productive activities, and play or leisure activities.

Kitchen Ambulation

Functional ambulation may occur during meal preparation and cleanup within a kitchen. The OT practitioner must apply the gait training techniques established by the physical therapist in combination with the treatment plan to accomplish meal preparation and cleanup tasks. For example, if the client has left hemiplegia and is ambulating with a quad-cane, the OT practitioner must problem solve to determine how the client will successfully accomplish the meal preparation activity. In this example, the therapist may guide the individual to ambulate to the left of the oven door so as to be able to open the oven door using the unaffected right upper extremity. The same concept should be kept in mind for opening cabinet doors or drawers or refrigerator doors.

Transporting items such as food, plates, and eating utensils during functional ambulation invites creative problem-solving on the part of the occupational therapist, particularly when the client is using an ambulation aid (Figs. 14-1 and 14-2). Walker baskets, rolling carts,

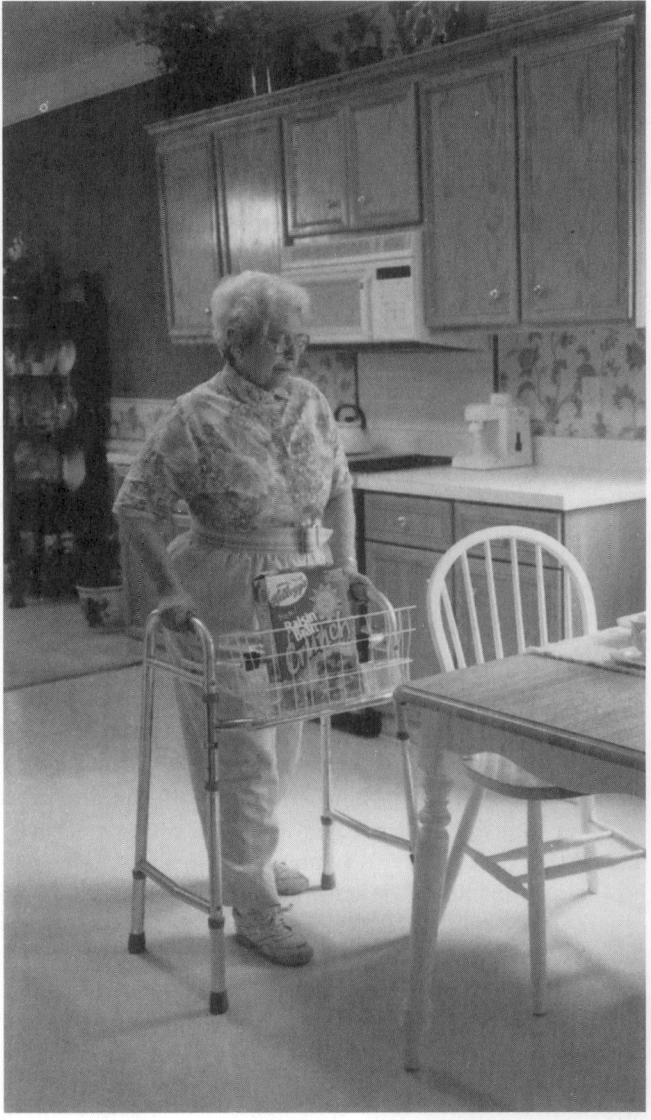

FIG. 14-1
Functional ambulation with a walker and walker basket.

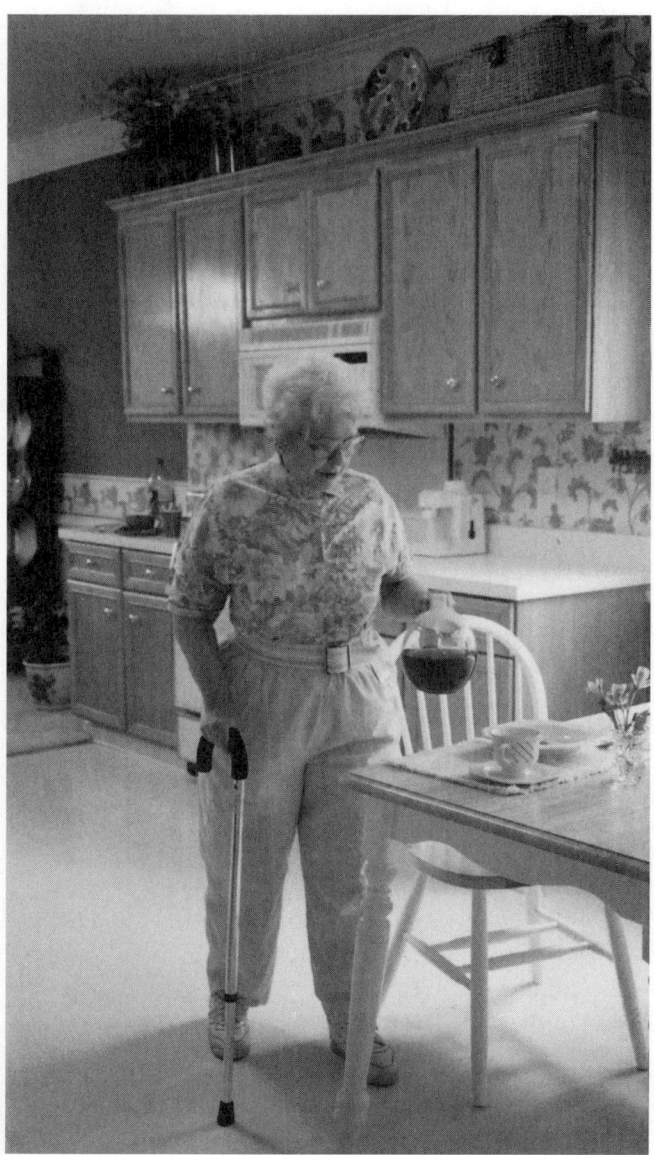

FIG. 14-2
Functional ambulation with a straight cane.

manner. First, approach as close to the sink as possible. This enables the client to perform grooming and hygiene activities. If the walker has a walker basket or if a countertop or cabinets prohibit the client from positioning himself or herself close enough to use the sink safely, the client may need to cautiously maneuver the walker to one side, then carefully move forward toward the sink.

Ambulation to the toilet is another opportunity for OT intervention. The transfer to the toilet should be anticipated upon entering the bathroom, and the client should be guided toward the toilet. Upon parallel alignment in front of the toilet, guide the client to maneuver himself or herself and the ambulation aid by pivoting to position the client to be able to sit on the toilet. Guide the client to pivot the least distance possible, to prevent losing balance. If the toilet is to the left of the client, pivot clockwise approximately 90°. If the toilet is on the right, pivot counterclockwise.

With ambulation to the edge of the bathtub or shower, the use of the bathtub or shower should be anticipated upon entering the bathroom. The client should be guided toward the tub edge. Whether the client is ambulating with a walker, crutches, or cane or with no ambulation aid, the client should be aligned to prepare for a safe transfer as the client nears the edge. If a transfer tub bench, shower chair, or other equipment is necessary for the client, the client should be guided to position himself or herself before the transfer, limiting the risk of losing balance by using a technique requiring the least distance or extraneous movement.

Home Management Ambulation

Functional ambulation within the house during home management activities such as clothing care, cleaning, and household maintenance is another area for OT intervention. With clothing care, functional ambulation may be necessary during sorting, laundering, and storing of clothing. Cleaning, including picking up, vacuuming, sweeping and mopping floors, and dusting and making beds, is an ideal activity for including ambulation where appropriate. Household maintenance, which includes maintaining the home, yard, garden, appliances, and vehicles, may also incorporate functional ambulation. As with any OT intervention, the client should be consulted to determine the home management activity most valued by the client before beginning the functional activity.

Making the bed is an example of a homemaking activity. If the client uses a cane during ambulation, the client may stabilize himself or herself with the cane while using the other arm to straighten and pull up sheets and bedcovers. The client then moves around the bed to the other side to repeat the process. The client should be careful, because he or she may lose balance

or the use of countertops may be appropriate in these situations. Any such adaptation should be discussed to determine if the client finds it acceptable.

Bathroom Ambulation

Functional ambulation to the sink, toilet, or edge of the bathtub or shower is an important concern for OT. Great care should be taken during functional ambulation within the bathroom because of the many risks associated with water and hard surfaces. Spills on the floor and loose bath mats present tripping hazards. It is essential to educate clients about these dangers.

Functional ambulation to the sink, using a walker in this example, may be performed in the following while bending and straightening from bed height to a standing position throughout the activity.

Adaptations may be made to perform functional ambulation activities during household maintenance tasks such as yard work. For example, a client using a walker, crutches, or a cane may carefully ambulate, with assistance as needed, to the location in the yard needing weeding or pruning. Small yard tools may be carried in a walker basket or in a plastic shopping bag hung over the arm. During stationary activities such as weeding or pruning, the client may use a gardening stool. A stool may be used and moved to the next location as the yard work progresses.

SUMMARY

Functional ambulation is the purposeful application of the mobility training taught to the client to enable movement from one position or place to another. Functional ambulation is applicable for clients with a variety of diagnoses, both biomechanical and neurological, across the age span.

Functional ambulation is an area in which the OT and PT practitioners have an opportunity to collaborate. The physical therapist provides the gait training and ambulation aid recommendations, and the OT practitioner reinforces and integrates these recommendations during purposeful activities.

Functional ambulation may be incorporated during ADL, work and productive activities, and play or leisure activities. The OT practitioner may have an opportunity to incorporate functional ambulation frequently during I-ADL.

SECTION 2
Wheelchair Assessment and Transfers

CAROLE ADLER
MICHELLE TIPTON-BURTON

WHEELCHAIRS

A wheelchair can be the primary means of mobility for someone with a permanent or progressive disability such as cerebral palsy, brain injury, spinal cord injury, multiple sclerosis, or muscular dystrophy. It may be needed as a temporary means of mobility by someone with a short-term illness or orthopedic problem. In addition to mobility, the wheelchair can substantially influence the total body positioning, skin integrity, overall function, and general well-being of the patient. Regardless of the diagnosis of the patient's condition, the occupational therapist must understand the complexity of wheelchair technology, available options and modifications, the evaluation and mea-

suring process, the use and care of the wheelchair, and, importantly, the process by which this equipment is funded.

Wheelchairs have evolved considerably in recent years, with significant advances made in powered and manual wheelchair technology by manufacturers and service providers. Products are constantly changing. Many of the improvements result from user and therapist recommendations.

Occupational therapists and physical therapists, depending on their respective roles at their treatment facilities, are usually responsible for evaluating, measuring, and selecting a wheelchair and seating system for the patient. They also teach wheelchair safety and mobility skills. The constant evolution of technology and variety of manufacturers' products make it advisable to include an experienced, knowledgeable, and certified **rehabilitation technology supplier (RTS)** on the ordering team. The RTS is a **durable medical equipment (DME)** supplier who is proficient in ordering custom items and can offer an objective and broad mechanical perspective on the availability and appropriateness of the options being considered. The RTS will be the patient's resource for insurance billing, repairs, and reordering when returning to the community.

Whether the patient requires a noncustom rental wheelchair for temporary use or a custom wheelchair for use over many years, an individualized prescription clearly outlining the specific features of the chair is needed to ensure optimal performance, mobility, and enhancement of function. A wheelchair that has been prescribed by an inexperienced or nonclinical person is potentially hazardous to the patient. An ill-fitting wheelchair can, in fact, contribute to unnecessary fatigue, skin breakdown, and trunk or extremity deformity and can inhibit function.[4] A wheelchair is an extension of the patient's body and should act to facilitate rather than inhibit good alignment, mobility, and function.

WHEELCHAIR EVALUATION

The therapist has considerable responsibility in recommending the wheelchair appropriate to meet not only immediate needs, but also long-term needs. When evaluating for a wheelchair, the therapist must know the patient and have a broad perspective of the patient's clinical, functional, and environmental needs. Careful evaluation of physical status must include the following: the specific diagnosis, prognosis, and current and future problems (e.g., age, spasticity, loss of range of motion [ROM], muscle weakness, and reduced endurance) that may affect wheelchair use. Functional use of the wheelchair in a variety of environments must be considered. Box 14-2 lists questions to ask before making specific recommendations.

All data must be considered before recommendations are made. Before the final prescription is prepared, collected information must be analyzed for an understanding of advantages and disadvantages of recommendations based on the patient's condition and how all specifics will integrate to provide an optimally effective mobility system.

The therapist must develop a good working relationship with the equipment supplier (RTS) and the reimbursement sources to facilitate payment of the most appropriate mobility system for the patient. Oral and written skills must be developed to communicate clearly the medical necessity, appropriateness, and cost-effectiveness of each item throughout the assessment and recommendation process.

To ensure that payment for the wheelchair is authorized, the therapist should have an in-depth awareness of the patient's insurance benefits and must provide documentation with thorough justification of the medical necessity of the wheelchair and any additional modifications. Therapists must explain clearly why particular features of a wheelchair are being recommended. They must be aware of standard versus "up charge" items, the cost of each item, and how these items will affect the end product.

WHEELCHAIR ORDERING CONSIDERATIONS

Before determining a specific brand and specifications of a wheelchair and the wheelchair's specifications, the therapist should carefully analyze the following sequence of evaluation considerations.[1,4,7]

Propelling the Wheelchair

The wheelchair may be propelled in a variety of ways, depending on the physical capacities of the user. If the patient is capable of self-propulsion using his or her arms on the rear wheels of the wheelchair, it should be assumed that there is sufficient bilateral grasp, arm strength, and physical endurance to maneuver the chair independently over varied terrain throughout the day.[7] An assortment of push rims is available to facilitate self-propelling, depending on the user's arm and grip strength. A patient with hemiplegia may propel a wheelchair using the unaffected arm and the ipsilateral leg to maneuver the wheelchair.

If independence in mobility is desired, a power wheelchair should be considered for those who have minimal or no use of the upper extremities or limited endurance. Power chairs are also preferred in situations involving inaccessible outdoor terrain.[7] They have a wide variety of features and can be programmed, driven by foot, arm, head, or neck, or pneumatically controlled. Given today's sophisticated technology, assuming intact cognition and perception, even a person with the most severe physical limitations is capable of independently driving a power wheelchair.

If the chair is to be propelled by the caregiver, consideration must be given to ease of maneuverability and handling, as well as to the positioning and mobility needs of the patient.

Regardless of the method of propulsion, serious consideration must be given to the effect the chair has on the patient's current and future mobility and positioning needs. In addition, lifestyle and environment, available resources such as ability to maintain the chair, transportation options, and available reimbursement sources are major determining factors.

RENTAL VERSUS PURCHASE

The therapist should estimate how long the patient will need the chair and whether the chair should be rented or purchased, which will affect the type of chair being considered. This decision is based on several clinical and functional issues. A rental chair is appropriate for short-term or temporary use, such as when the patient's clinical picture, functional status, or body size is changing. Rental chairs may be necessary when the permanent wheelchair is being repaired. A rental wheelchair also may be useful when the patient has difficulty accepting the idea of using a wheelchair and needs to experience it initially as a temporary piece of equipment. Often the eventual functional outcome is unknown. In that case a chair can be rented for several months until a reevaluation determines whether a permanent chair will be necessary.[1]

A permanent wheelchair is indicated for the full-time user and for the patient with a progressive need for a wheelchair over a long period. It may be indicated when custom features are required and also when body size is changing, such as in the growing child.[1]

Frame Style

Once the method of propulsion and the permanence of the chair have been determined, there are several wheelchair frame styles to consider. The frame style must be selected before specific dimensions and brand names can be determined. The therapist needs to be aware of the various features, the advantages and disadvantages of each, and how these features will affect the patient in every aspect of his of her life, from both a short- and long-term perspective.

WHEELCHAIR SELECTION

The following questions regarding patient needs should be considered carefully before the specific type of chair is determined:[1]

Manual Versus Electric Wheelchair (Fig. 14-3)

Manual Wheelchair (Fig. 14-3, A)
- Does the user have sufficient strength and endurance to propel the chair?
- Does manual mobility enhance functional independence and cardiovascular conditioning of the wheelchair user?
- Does the user demonstrate insufficient cognitive ability to propel an electric wheelchair safely?
- Will the caregiver be propelling the chair at any time?

Electric Wheelchair (Fig. 14-3, B)
- Does the user demonstrate insufficient endurance and functional ability to propel a manual wheelchair independently?
- Does the user demonstrate progressive functional loss, making powered mobility an energy-conserving option?

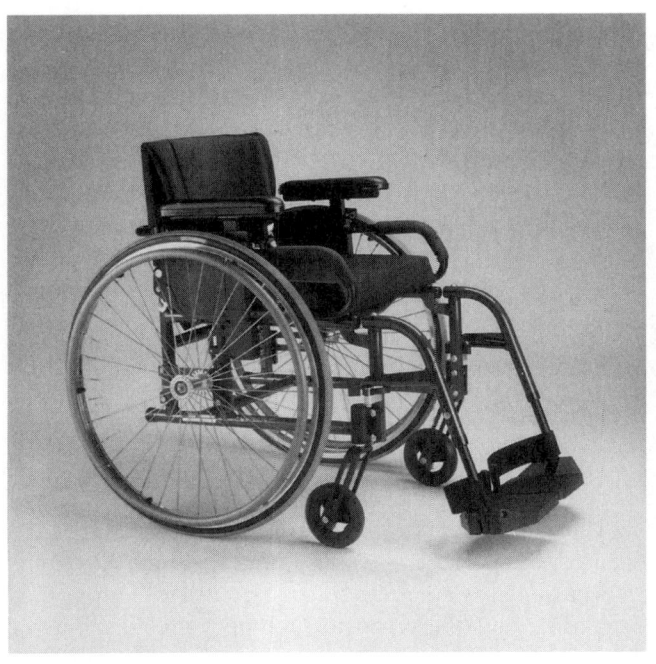

A

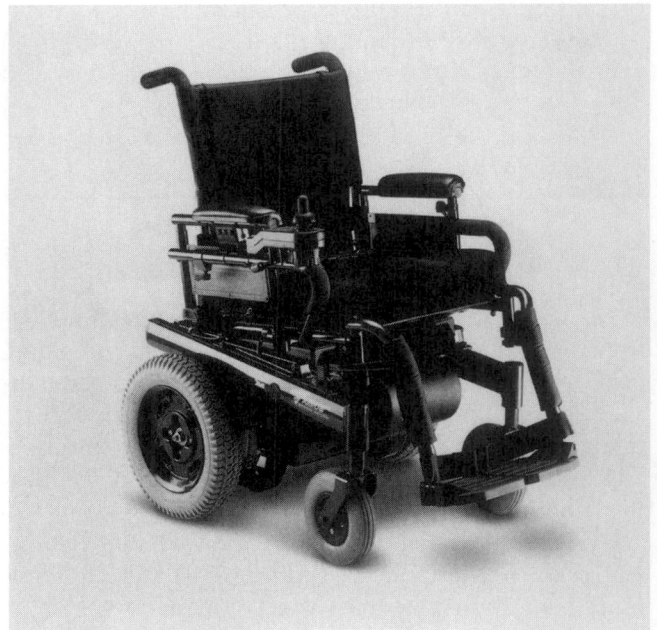

B

FIG. 14-3
Manual versus electric wheelchair. **A,** Rigid frame chair with swing-away footrests. **B,** Power-driven wheelchair with hand control. (**A** courtesy of Quickie Designs; **B** courtesy of Invacare Corporation.)

- Is powered mobility needed to increase independence at school, at work, and in the community?
- Does the user demonstrate cognitive and perceptual ability to operate a power-driven system safely?
- Does the user or caregiver demonstrate responsibility for care and maintenance of equipment?
- Is a van available for transportation?

Manual Recline Versus Power Recline Versus Tilt Wheelchairs (Fig. 14-4)

Manual Recline Wheelchair (Fig. 14-4, A)
- Is the patient unable to sit upright because of hip contractures, poor balance, or fatigue?
- Is a caregiver available to assist with weight shifts and position changes?
- Is relative ease of maintenance a concern?
- Is cost a consideration?

Power Recline Versus Tilt (Fig. 14-4, B and C)
- Does the patient have the potential to operate independently?
- Are independent weight shifts and position changes indicated for skin care and increased sitting tolerance?
- Does the user demonstrate safe and independent use of controls?

- Are there resources for care and maintenance of the equipment?
- Does the user have significant **spasticity** that is facilitated by hip and knee extension during the recline phase?
- Does the user have hip or knee **contractures** that prohibit his or her ability to recline fully?
- Will a power recline or tilt decrease or make more efficient use of caregiver time?
- Will a power recline or tilt reduce the need for transfers to the bed for catheterizations and rest periods throughout the day?
- Will the patient require quick position changes in the event of hypotension and/or dysreflexia?
- Has a reimbursement source been identified for this costly add-on feature?

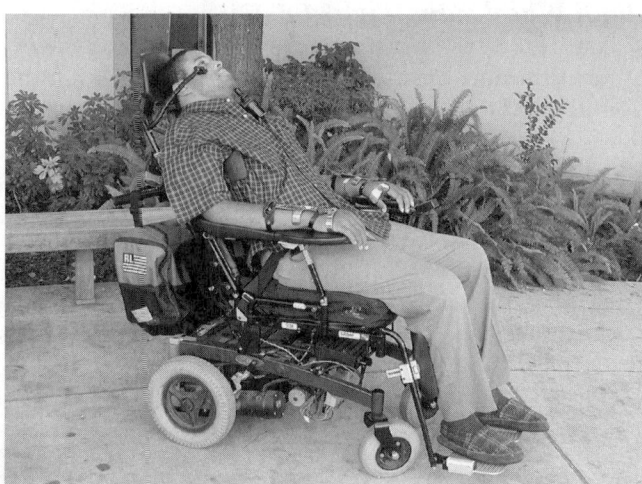

B

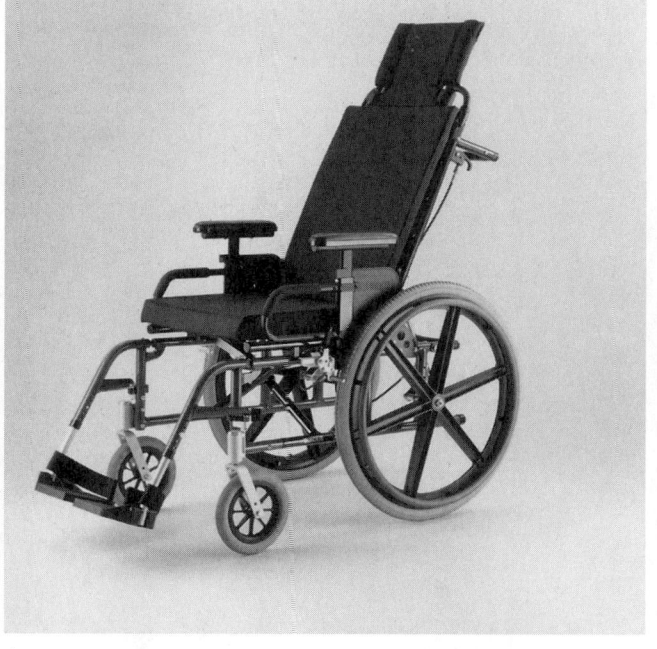

A

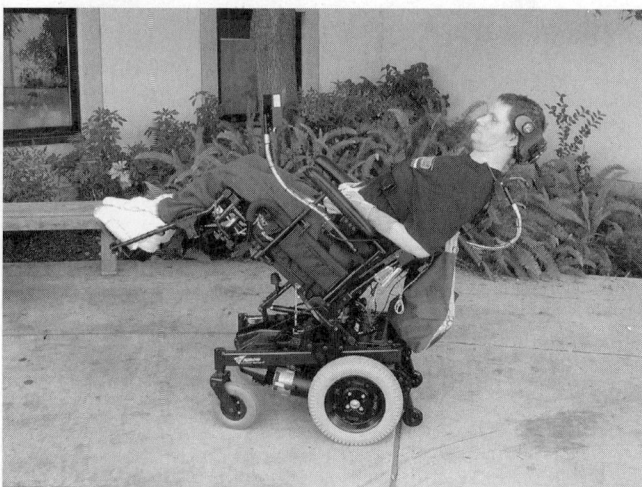

C

FIG. 14-4

Manual recline versus power recline wheelchair. **A,** Reclining back on folding frame. **B,** Low-shear power recline with collar mount chin control on electric wheelchair. **C,** Tilt system with head control on electric wheelchair. (**A** courtesy of Quickie Designs; **B** and **C** courtesy of Luis Gonzalez, SCVMC.)

Folding Versus Rigid Manual Wheelchairs (Fig. 14-5)

Folding Wheelchairs (Fig. 14-5, A)

- Does the patient prefer a traditional-looking chair?
- Is the folding frame needed for transport, storage, or home accessibility?
- Which footrest style is necessary for transfers, desk clearance, and other daily living skills? Elevating footrests may be available only on folding frames.
- Is the patient or caregiver able to load and fit the chair into necessary vehicles?

Equipment suppliers should have knowledge and a variety of brands available. Frame weight can range between 28 and 50 pounds depending on size and accessories. Frame adjustments and custom options depend on the model.

Rigid Wheelchair (Fig. 14-5, B)

- Does the user or caregiver have the upper extremity function and balance to load and unload the non-folding frame from a vehicle if driving independently?
- Will the user benefit from the improved energy efficiency and performance of a rigid frame?

Footrest options are limited and the frame is lighter (20 to 35 pounds). Features include an adjustable seat angle, rear axle, caster mount, and back height. Efficient frame design maximizes performance. There are options in frame material composition, frame colors, and aesthetics. These chairs are usually custom ordered; availability and expertise are usually limited to custom rehabilitation technology suppliers.

Lightweight (Folding or Nonfolding) Versus Standard Weight (Folding) Wheelchairs

Lightweight Wheelchairs: Under 35 Pounds (Fig. 14-5, A)

- Does the user have the trunk balance and equilibrium necessary to handle a lighter frame weight?
- Does the lighter weight enhance mobility by reducing the user's fatigue?
- Will the user's ability to propel the chair or handle parts be enhanced by a lighter weight frame?
- Are custom features (e.g., adjustable height back, seat angle, and axle mount) necessary?

Standard Weight Wheelchairs: Over 35 Pounds (Fig. 14-6)

- Does the user need the stability of a standard weight chair?
- Does the user have the ability to propel a standard weight chair?
- Can the caregiver manage the increased weight when loading the wheelchair and fitting into a vehicle?
- Will the increased weight of parts be unimportant during daily living skills?

Custom options are limited, and these wheelchairs are usually less expensive (except heavy-duty models required for users over 250 pounds).

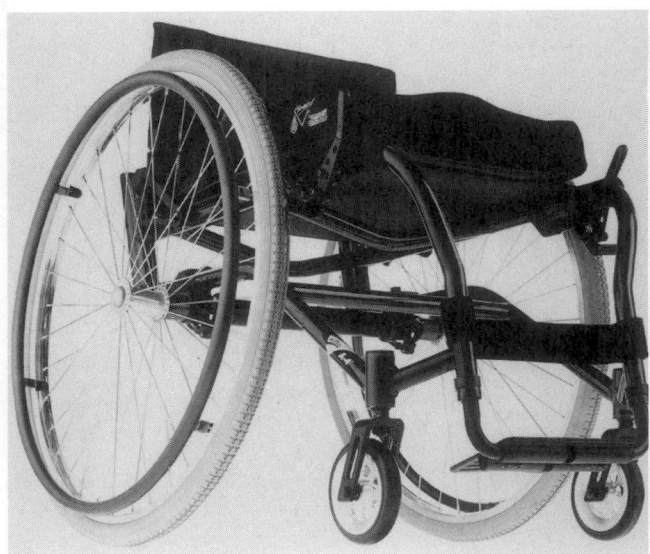

A

B

FIG. 14-5
Folding versus rigid wheelchair. **A,** Lightweight folding frame with swing-away footrests. **B,** Rigid aluminum frame with tapered front end and solid foot cradle. (**A** courtesy of Quickie Designs; **B** courtesy of Invacare Corporation.)

Standard Available Features Versus Custom, Top-of-the-Line Models

The price range, durability, and warranty within a specific manufacturer's model line must be considered.

Standard Available Features
- Is the chair required only for part-time use?
- Does the user have a limited life expectancy?
- Is the chair needed as a second or transportation chair, used only 10% to 20% of the time?
- Will the chair be primarily for indoor or sedentary use?
- Is the user dependent on caregivers for propulsion?
- Will the chair be propelled only by the caregiver?
- Are custom features or specifications not necessary?
- Is substantial durability unimportant?

For standard wheelchairs, a limited warranty is available on the frame. These chairs may be indicated because of reimbursement limitations. Limited sizes and options and adjustability are available. These cost considerably less than custom wheelchairs.

Custom and "Top-of-the-Line" Models
- Will the patient be a full-time user?
- Is there a likely prognosis for long-term use of the wheelchair?

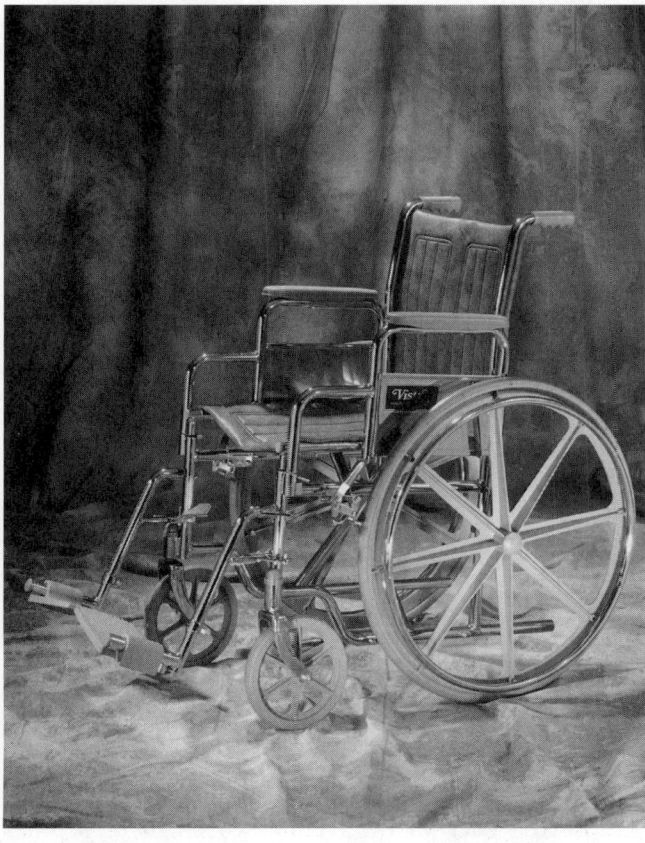

FIG. 14-6
Standard folding frame (over 35 pounds) with swing-away footrests. (Courtesy of Everest & Jennings, Inc.)

- Will this be the primary wheelchair?
- Is the user active both indoors and outdoors?
- Will this frame style improve prognosis for independent mobility?
- Is the user a growing adolescent, or does he or she have a progressive disorder requiring later modification of the chair?
- Are custom features, specifications, or positioning devices required?

Top-of-the-line wheelchair frames usually have a lifelong warranty. A variety of specifications, options, and adjustments are available. Many manufacturers will work with therapists and providers to solve a specific fitting problem. Experience is essential in ordering top-of-the-line and custom equipment.

WHEELCHAIR MEASUREMENT PROCEDURES (FIG. 14-7)

The patient is measured in the style of chair and with the seat cushion that most closely resembles those being ordered. If the patient will wear a brace or body jacket or need any additional devices in the chair, these should be in place during the measurement. Observation skills are important during this process. Measurements alone should not be used. The therapist should "eyeball" the entire body position every step of the way.[1,6]

Seat Width (Fig. 14-7, A)
Objectives
1. Distributing the patient's weight over the widest possible surface.

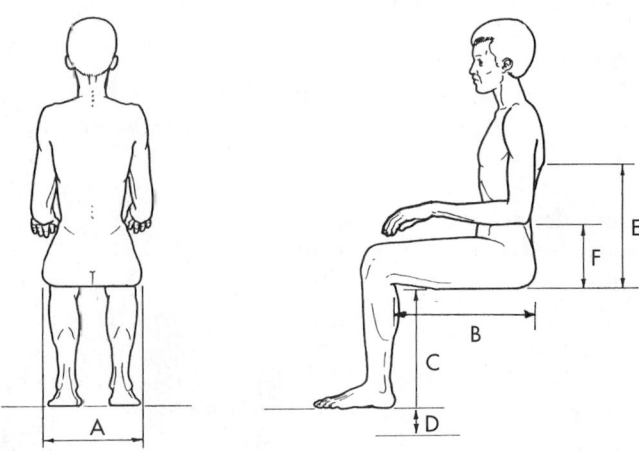

FIG. 14-7
What and where to measure. **A,** Seat width. **B,** Seat depth. **C,** Seat height from floor. **D,** Footrest clearance. **E,** Back height. **F,** Armrest height. (Adapted from Wilson A, McFarland SR: *Wheelchairs: a prescription guide,* Charlottesville, Va, 1986, Rehabilitation Press.)

2. Keeping the overall width of the chair as narrow as possible.

Measurement

Measure across the widest part of either the thighs or hips while the patient is sitting in a chair comparable to that expected.

Wheelchair Clearance

Add $\frac{1}{2}$ to 1 inch on each side of the hip or thigh measurement taken. Consider how increasing the overall width of the chair will affect accessibility.

Checking

Place the flat palm of the hand between the patient's hip or thigh and the wheelchair skirt and armrest.

Considerations

User's potential weight gain or loss
Accessibility of varied environments
Overall width of wheelchair

Seat Depth (Fig. 14-7, B)

Objective

The objective is to distribute the body weight along the sitting surface by bearing weight along the entire length of the thigh to just behind the knee. This approach is necessary to help prevent pressure sores on the buttocks and lower back and for optimal muscle tone normalization throughout the body.

Measurement

Measure from the rear of the buttocks to the inside of the bent knee; the seat edge clearance needs to be 1 to 2 inches less than this measurement.

Checking

Check clearance behind the knees to prevent contact of the front edge of the seat upholstery with the popliteal space.

Considerations

Braces or back inserts that may be pushing the patient forward.
Postural changes throughout the day from fatigue or spasticity.
Thigh length discrepancy; the depth of the seat may be different for each leg.
If considering a power recliner, assume the patient will slide forward slightly throughout the day and make depth adjustments accordingly.
Seat depth may need to be shortened to allow independent propulsion with the lower extremities.

Seat Height from Floor and Foot Adjustment (Fig. 14-7, C, and D)

Objectives

1. Supporting the patient's body while maintaining the thighs parallel to the floor (Fig. 14-5, C)
2. Elevating the foot plates to provide ground clearance over varied surfaces and curb cuts (Fig. 14-7, D)

Measurements

Measure the top of the seat post to the floor and the popliteal fossa to the bottom of the heel.

Wheelchair Clearance

The patient's thighs are kept parallel to the floor so the body weight is distributed evenly along the entire depth of the seat. The lowest point of the footplates must clear the floor by at least 2 inches.

Checking

Slip fingers under the patient's thighs at the front edge of the seat upholstery. *Note:* A custom seat height may be needed to obtain footrest clearance. An inch of increased seat height raises the footplate 1 inch.

Considerations

If the knees are too high, increased pressure at the ischial tuberosities puts the patient at risk for skin breakdown and pelvic deformity.
Sitting too high off the ground can impair the patient's center of gravity, seat height for transfers, and visibility if driving a van from the wheelchair.

Back Height (Fig. 14-7, E)

Objective

Providing back support consistent with physical and functional needs. The chair back should be low enough for maximal function and high enough for maximal support.

Measurements

For full trunk support, measure from the top of the seat post to the top of the shoulders. For minimum trunk support, the top of the back upholstery should permit free arm movement, not irritate the skin or scapulae, and provide good total body alignment.

Checking

Ensure that the patient is not being pushed forward because the back of the chair is too high or leaning backward over the top of the upholstery because the back is too low.

Considerations

Adjustable-height backs (usually offer a 4-inch range)

Adjustable upholstery

Lumbar support or another commercially available or custom back insert to prevent kyphosis, scoliosis, or other long-term trunk deformity

Arm Height (Fig. 14-7, *F*)

Objectives

1. Maintaining posture and balance
2. Providing support and alignment for upper extremities
3. Allowing change in position by pushing down on armrests

Measurements

With the patient in a comfortable position, measure from the seat post to the bottom of a bent elbow.

Wheelchair Clearance

The height of the top of the arm rest should be 1 inch higher than the height from the seat post to the patient's elbow.

Checking

The patient's posture should look correct. The shoulders should not slouch forward or be subluxated or forced into elevation when the patient is in a normal sitting posture, with flexed elbows slightly forward on armrests.

Considerations

Other uses of armrests, such as increasing functional reach or holding a cushion in place

Certain styles of armrests can increase the overall width of the chair.

Whether armrests are necessary at all

The patient's ability to remove and replace the armrest from the chair independently

Review all measurements against standards for a particular model of chair. Manufacturers have lists of the standard dimensions available and the cost for custom modifications.

The goals of pediatric wheelchair ordering, as of all wheelchair ordering, should be obtaining a proper fit and facilitating optimal function. Rarely does a standard wheelchair meet the fitting requirements of a child. The selection of size is variable; therefore custom seating systems specific to the pediatric population are available. A secondary goal is to consider a chair that will accommodate the child's growth.

For children under 5 years of age a decision must be made about whether to use a stroller base or a stan-dard wheelchair base. Considerations are the child's ability to propel the chair relative to the developmental level and the parent's preference for a stroller or a wheelchair.

Many variables must be considered when customizing a wheelchair frame. An experienced RTS or the wheelchair manufacturer should be consulted to ensure that a custom request will be successful.

ADDITIONAL SEATING AND POSITIONING CONSIDERATIONS

A wheelchair evaluation is not complete until the seat cushion, back support, and any other positioning devices and the integration of those parts are carefully thought out, regardless of the diagnosis. It is essential that the therapist appreciate the effect that optimal body alignment has on skin integrity, tone normalization, overall functional ability, and general well-being (Fig. 14-8).[1]

The following are the goals of a comprehensive seating and positioning assessment.

Prevention of Deformity

Providing a symmetrical base of support preserves proper skeletal alignment and discourages spinal curvature and other body deformities.

Tone Normalization

By providing proper body alignment, as well as bilateral weight bearing and adaptive devices as needed, tone normalization can be maximized.

Pressure Management

Pressure sores can be caused by improper alignment and an inappropriate sitting surface. The proper seat cushion can provide comfort, assist in trunk and pelvic alignment, and create a surface that minimizes pressure, heat, moisture, and shearing, the primary causes of **skin breakdown.**

Promotion of Function

Pelvic and trunk stability is necessary to free the upper extremity for participation in all functional activities, including wheelchair mobility and daily living skills.

Maximum Sitting Tolerance

Wheelchair sitting tolerance will increase as support, comfort, and symmetrical weight-bearing are provided.

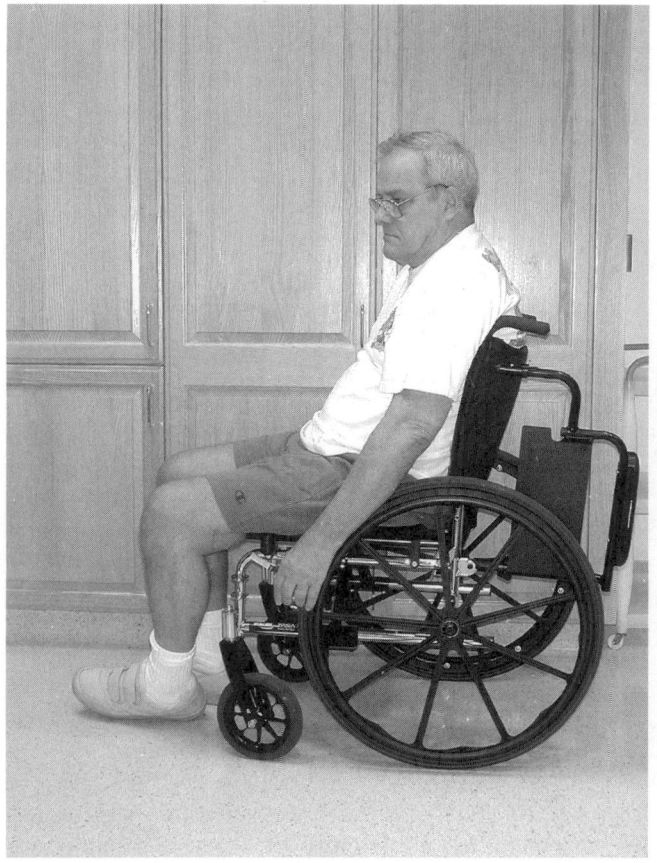

A

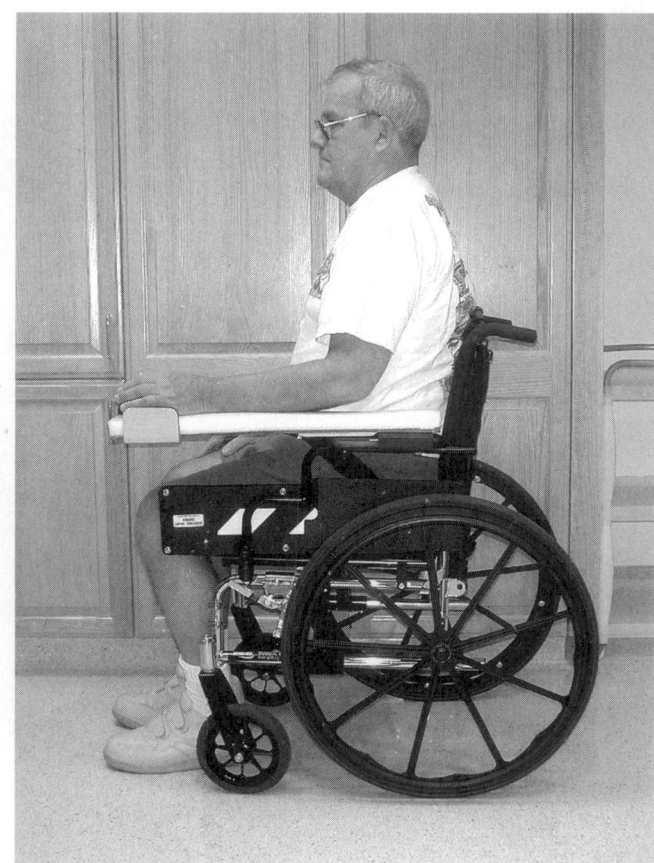

B

FIG. 14-8
A, Stroke patient seated in wheelchair. Poor positioning results in kyphotic thoracic spine, posterior pelvic tilt, and unsupported affected side. **B,** Stroke patient seated in wheelchair with appropriate positioning devices. Seat and back insert facilitate upright midline position with neutral pelvic tilt and equal weight bearing throughout.

Optimal Respiratory Function

Support in an erect, well-aligned position can decrease compression of the diaphragm and thus increase **vital capacity**.

Provision for Proper Body Alignment

Good body alignment is necessary for prevention of deformity, normalization of tone, and promotion of movement. The patient should be able not only to propel the wheelchair, but also to move around within the wheelchair.

A wide variety of seating and positioning equipment is available for all levels of disability. Custom modifications are continually being designed to meet a variety of patient needs. In addition, technology in this area is ever growing, and interest in wheelchair technology as a professional specialty also is growing. However, the skill of clinicians in this field ranges from extensive to negligible. Although it is an integral aspect of any wheelchair

evaluation, the scope of seating and positioning equipment is much greater than can be addressed in this chapter. The suggested reading list at the end of this chapter gives additional resources.

ACCESSORIES

Once the measurements and the need for additional positioning devices have been determined, a wide variety of accessories are available to meet a patient's individual needs. It is extremely important to understand the function of each accessory and how an accessory interacts with the rest of the chair and with seating and positioning equipment.[1,7]

Armrests come in fixed, flip-up, detachable, desk, standard, reclining, and tubular styles. The fixed armrest is a continuous part of the frame and is not detachable. It limits proximity to table, counter, and desk surfaces and prohibits side transfers. Flip-up, detachable desk and standard-length arms are removable and allow side-approach transfers. Reclining arms are attached to the

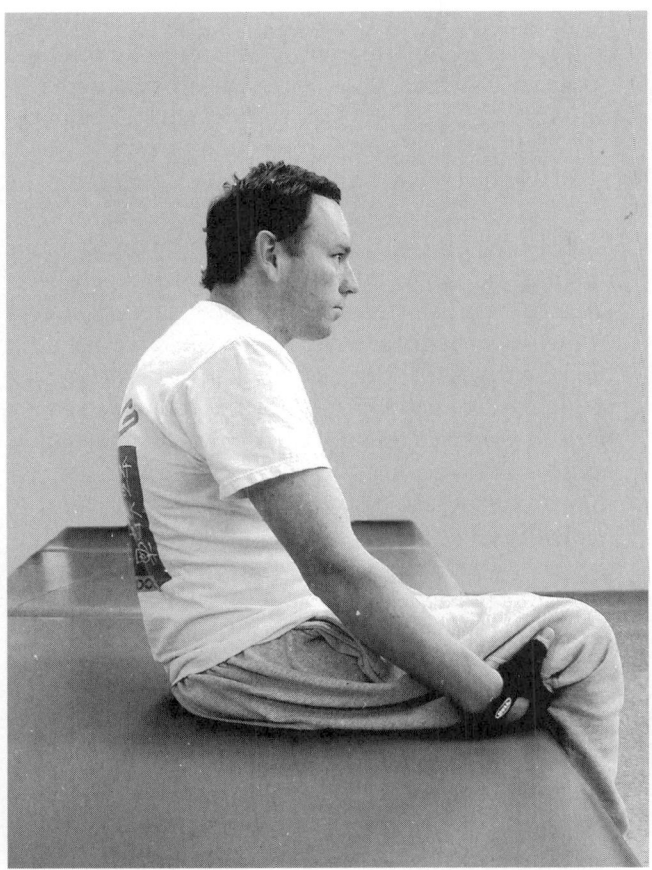

C

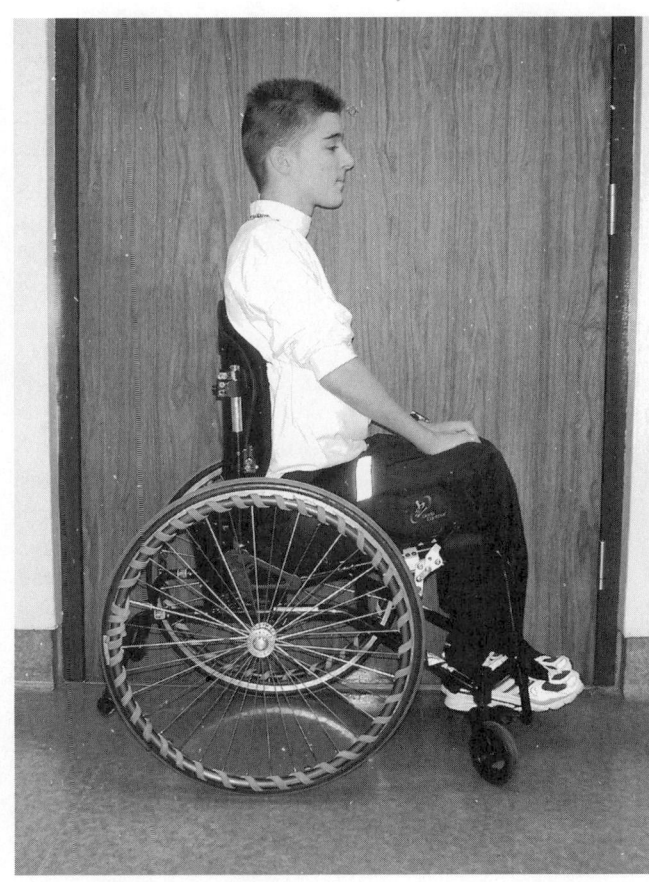

D

FIG. 14-8, cont'd

C, Spinal cord-injured patient sitting with back poorly supported results in posterior pelvic tilt, kyphotic thoracic spine, and absence of lumbar curve. **D,** Spinal cord-injured patient with rigid back support and pressure-relief seat cushion, resulting in erect thoracic spine, lumbar curve, and anterior tilted pelvis.

back post and recline with the back of the chair. Tubular arms are available on lightweight frames.

Footrests may be fixed, swingaway detachable, solid cradle, and elevating. The fixed footrests are attached to the wheelchair frame and are not removable. These footrests prevent the person from getting close to counters and may make some types of transfers more difficult. The swingaway detachable footrests can be moved to the side of the chair or removed entirely. This allows a closer approach to bed, bathtub, and counters, and when the footrests are removed, reduces the overall wheelchair length and weight for easy loading into a car. Detachable footrests lock into place on the chair with a locking device.[7] A solid cradle footrest is found on rigid, lightweight chairs and is not removable. Elevating leg rests are available for patients with such conditions as lower-extremity edema, blood pressure changes, and orthopedic problems.

The footplates may have heel loops and toe straps to aid in securing the foot on the footplate.[7] A calf strap can be used on a solid cradle or when additional support behind the calf is necessary. Other accessories are seat belts, various brake styles, brake extensions, anti-tip devices, caster locks, arm supports, and head supports.

PREPARING THE PRESCRIPTION

Once specific measurements and the need for modifications and accessories have been determined, the wheelchair prescription must be completed. It should be concise and specific so that everything requested can be accurately interpreted by the DME supplier, who will be submitting a sales contract for payment authorization. Before-and-after pictures can be helpful in illustrating **medical necessity**. It is important that the requirements for payment authorization from a particular reimbursement source are known so that medical necessity can be demonstrated. The therapist must be aware of the cost of everything being requested and of the reason each item is necessary. Payment may be denied if clear reasons are not given to substantiate the need for every item and modification requested.

Before the wheelchair is delivered to the patient, the therapist should check the chair to the specific prescription and ensure that all specifications and accessories are correct. When a custom chair has been ordered, it is recommended that the patient be fitted by the ordering therapist to ensure that the chair fits and that it provides all the elements that were expected when the prescription was generated.

WHEELCHAIR SAFETY

Elements of safety for the wheelchair user and the caregiver are as follows:

1. Brakes should be locked during all transfers.
2. The patient should never stand on the foot plates, which are placed in the "up" position during most transfers.
3. In most transfers, it is an advantage to have footrests swung away if possible.
4. If a caregiver is pushing the chair, he or she should be sure that the patient's elbows are not protruding from the armrests and that the patient's hands are not on the hand rims. If approaching from behind to assist in moving the wheelchair, the caregiver should inform the patient of this intent and check the position of the patient's feet and arms before proceeding.
5. To push the patient up a ramp, he or she should move in a normal, forward direction. If the ramp is negotiated independently, the patient should lean slightly forward while propelling the wheelchair up the incline.[8]
6. To push the patient down a ramp, the caretaker should tilt the wheelchair backward by pushing the foot down on the tipping levers to its balance position, which is a tilt of approximately 30°. Then the caregiver should ease the wheelchair down the ramp in a forward direction, while maintaining the chair in its balance position. The caregiver should keep his or her knees slightly bent and the back straight.[8] The caregiver may also move down the ramp backward while the patient maintains some control of the large wheels to prevent rapid backward motion. This approach is useful if the grade is relatively steep. Ramps with only a slight grade can also be managed in a forward direction if the caregiver maintains grasp and pull on the hand grips and the patient again maintains some control of the big wheels to prevent rapid forward motion. If the ramp is negotiated independently, the patient should move down the ramp facing forward while leaning backward slightly and maintaining control of speed by grasping the hand rims. The patient can descend a steep grade by traversing the ramp to slow the chair. Gloves may be helpful to reduce the effect of friction.[8]
7. A caregiver can manage ascending curbs by approaching them forward, tipping the wheelchair back, and pushing the foot down on the tipping levers, thus lifting the front casters onto the curb and pushing forward. The large wheels then are in contact with the curb and roll on with ease as the chair is lifted slightly onto the curb.
8. To descend the curb using a forward approach, the wheelchair is tilted backward and the large wheels are rolled off the curb in a controlled manner while the front casters are tilted up. When the large wheels are off the curb, an assistant can slowly reduce the tilt of the wheelchair until the casters are once again on the street surface. The curb may also be descended using a backward approach. An assistant can move himself or herself and the chair around as the curb is approached and pull the wheelchair to the edge of the curb. Standing below the curb, the assistant can guide the large wheels off the curb by slowly pulling the wheelchair backward until it begins to descend. After the large wheels are safely on the street surface, the assistant can tilt the chair back to clear the casters, move backward, lower the casters to the street surface, and then turn around.[8]

With good strength and coordination, many patients can be trained to manage curbs independently. To mount and descend a curb, the patient must have a good bilateral grip, arm strength, and balance. To mount the curb, the patient tilts the chair onto the rear wheels and pushes forward until the front wheels hang over the curb, then lowers them gently. The patient then leans forward and forcefully pushes forward on the hand rims to bring the rear wheels up on the pavement. To descend a curb, the patient should lean forward and push slowly backward until the rear and then the front wheels roll down the curb.[3]

The ability to lift the front casters off the ground and balance on the rear wheels ("pop a wheelie") is a beneficial skill and expands the patient's independence in the community with curb management and in rural settings with movement over grassy, sandy, or rough terrain. Patients who have good grip, arm strength, and balance usually can master this skill and perform safely. The technique involves being able to tilt the chair on the rear wheels, balance the chair on the rear wheels, and move and turn the chair on the rear wheels. The patient should not attempt to perform these maneuvers without instruction and training in the proper techniques, which are beyond the scope of this chapter. Specific instructions on teaching these skills can be found in the references.[3]

TRANSFER TECHNIQUES

Transferring is the process of a patient's moving from one surface to another. This process includes the sequence of events that must occur both before and after the move, such as the pretransfer sequence of bed mobility and the posttransfer phase of wheelchair positioning. Assuming that a patient has some physical or cognitive limitations, it will be necessary for the therapist to assist in or supervise a transfer. Many therapists are unsure of the transfer type and technique to employ or feel perplexed when a particular technique does not succeed with the patient. It is important to remember that each patient, therapist, and situation are different. This chapter does not include an outline of all techniques but presents the basic techniques with generalized principles. Each transfer must be adapted for the particular patient and his or her needs. The discussion in this chapter includes directions for some transfer techniques that are most commonly employed in practice. These techniques are the stand pivot, bent pivot, and one-person and two-person dependent transfers.

Preliminary Concepts

The therapist must be aware of the following concepts when selecting and carrying out transfer techniques to ensure safety for both the patient and self:

1. The therapist should be aware of the patient's assets and limitations, especially the patient's physical, cognitive, perceptual, and behavioral abilities and deficits.
2. The therapist should know his or her own physical abilities and limitations and whether he or she can communicate clear, sequential instructions to the patient (and if necessary to the long-term caregiver of the patient).
3. The therapist should be aware of and use correct moving and lifting techniques.

Guidelines for Using Proper Mechanics

The therapist should be aware of the following principles of basic **body mechanics**[2]:

1. Get close to the patient or move the patient closer to you.
2. Square off with the patient (face head on).
3. Bend knees; use your legs, not your back.
4. Keep a neutral spine (not bent or arched back).
5. Keep a wide base of support.
6. Keep your heels down.
7. Don't tackle more than you can handle; ask for help.
8. Don't combine movements. Avoid rotating at the same time as bending forward or backward.

The therapist should consider the following questions before performing a transfer:

1. What medical precautions affect the patient's mobility or method of transfer?
2. Can the transfer be performed safely by one person, or is assistance required?
3. Has enough time been allotted for safe execution of a transfer? Are you in a hurry?
4. Does the patient understand what is going to happen? If not, does he or she demonstrate fear or confusion? Are you prepared for this limitation?
5. Is the equipment that the patient is being transferred to and from in good working order and in a locked position?
6. What is the height of the bed (or surface) in relation to the wheelchair? Can the heights be adjusted?
7. Is all equipment placed in the correct position?
8. Is all unnecessary bedding and equipment moved out of the way so that you are working without obstructions?
9. Is the patient dressed properly in case you need to use a waistband to assist? If not, do you need a transfer belt or other assistance?
10. What are the other components of the transfer, such as leg management and bed mobility?

It is important for the therapist to be familiar with as many types of transfers as possible so that each situation can be resolved as it arises.

Many classifications of transfers exist, based on the amount of therapist participation. Classifications range from *dependent*, in which the patient is unable to participate and the therapist moves the patient, to *independent*, in which the patient moves independently while the therapist merely supervises, observes, or provides input for appropriate technique as related to the patient's disability.

Before attempting to move a patient, the therapist must understand the biomechanics of movement and the effect the patient's center of **positioning mass** has on transfers.

Principles of Body Positioning

Pelvic Tilt

Generally, after the acute onset of a disability or prolonged time spent in bed, patients assume a posterior **pelvic tilt** (i.e., a slouched position with lumbar flexion). In turn, this posture moves the center of mass back toward the buttocks. The therapist may need to verbally cue or assist the patient into a neutral or slightly anterior pelvic tilt position to move the center of mass forward over the center of the patient's body.[5]

Trunk Alignment

It may be observed that the patient's trunk alignment is shifted to either the right or the left side. If the therapist assists in moving the patient while the patient's weight is shifted to one side, the movement could throw both the patient and the therapist off balance. The patient may need verbal cues or physical assistance to come to and maintain a midline trunk position before and during the transfer.

Weight Shifting

The transfer is initiated by shifting the patient's weight forward, removing weight from the buttocks. This movement allows the patient to stand, partially stand, or be pivoted by the therapist. This step must be performed regardless of the type of transfer.

Extremity Positioning

The patient's feet must be placed firmly on the floor with ankles stabilized and with knees aligned at 90° of flexion over the feet. This position allows the weight to be shifted easily onto and over the feet. Heels should be pointing toward the surface to which the patient is transferring. The patient should either be barefoot or have shoes on to prevent slipping out of position. The feet can easily pivot in this position, and the risk of twisting or injuring an ankle or knee is minimized.

Upper Extremities

The patient's arms must be in a safe position or in a position in which he or she can assist in the transfer. If one or both of the upper extremities is nonfunctional, the arms should be placed in a safe position that will not be in the way during the transfer (e.g., in the patient's lap). If the patient has partial or full movement, motor control, or strength, he or she can assist in the transfer either by reaching toward the surface to be reached or by pushing off from the surface to be left. The therapist's decision is based on prior knowledge of the patient's motor function.

Preparing Equipment and Patient for Transfer

The transfer process includes setting up the environment, positioning the wheelchair, and helping the patient into a pretransfer position. The following is a general overview of these steps.

Positioning the Wheelchair

1. Place the wheelchair at approximately a 30° angle to the surface to which the patient is transferring.
2. Lock the brakes.
3. Place both of the patient's feet firmly on the floor, hip width apart and with knees over the feet.
4. Remove the armrest closer to the bed.
5. Remove the wheelchair seatbelt.

Bed Mobility in Preparation for Transfer

Rolling the Hemiplegic Patient

1. Before rolling the patient, you may need to put your hand under the patient's scapula on the weak side and gently mobilize it forward to prevent the patient from rolling onto the shoulder, potentially causing pain and injury.
2. Assist the patient in clasping the strong hand around the wrist of the weak arm, and lift upper extremities toward the ceiling.
3. Flex the patient's knees.
4. You may assist the patient to roll onto his or her side by moving the arms, then the legs, and by holding one hand at the scapula area and the other at the hip, guiding the roll.

Side-Lying to Sit Up at the Edge of Bed

1. Bring the patient's feet off the edge of the bed.
2. Stabilize the patient's lower extremities.
3. Shift the patient's body to an upright sitting position.
4. Place the patient's hands on the bed at the sides of his or her body to help maintain balance.

Scooting to the Edge of the Bed

When working with a patient who has stroke or traumatic brain injury, walk the patient's hips toward the edge of the bed. Shift the patient's weight to the unaffected side, position your hand behind the opposite buttock, and guide the patient forward. Shift the patient's weight to the affected side and repeat the procedure if necessary. Move forward until the patient's feet are flat on the floor.

In the case of an individual with spinal cord injury, grasp the patient's legs from behind the knees and pull the patient forward, placing the patient's feet firmly on the floor and being sure that the ankles are in a neutral position.

STANDING PIVOT TRANSFERS

The standing pivot transfer requires the patient to be able to come to a standing position and pivot on one or both feet. It is most commonly used with patients who have hemiplegia, hemiparesis, or a general loss of strength or balance.

Wheelchair to Bed or Mat Transfer (Fig. 14-9)

1. Help the patient scoot to the edge of the surface and put his or her feet flat on the floor. The patient's ankles should be pointed toward the surface to which the patient is transferring.
2. Stand on the patient's affected side with hands either on the patient's scapulae or around the patient's waist or hips. Stabilize the patient's foot and knee with your own foot and knee. Provide assistance by guiding the patient forward as the buttocks are lifted up and toward the transfer surface (Fig. 14-9, A).
3. The patient either reaches toward the surface to which he or she is transferring or pushes off the surface from which he or she is transferring (Fig. 14-9, B).

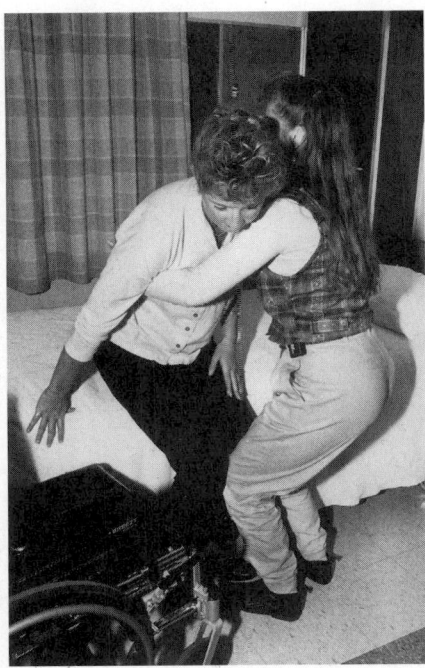
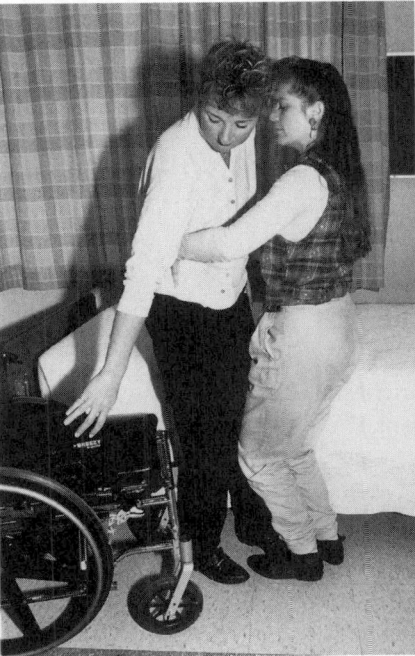
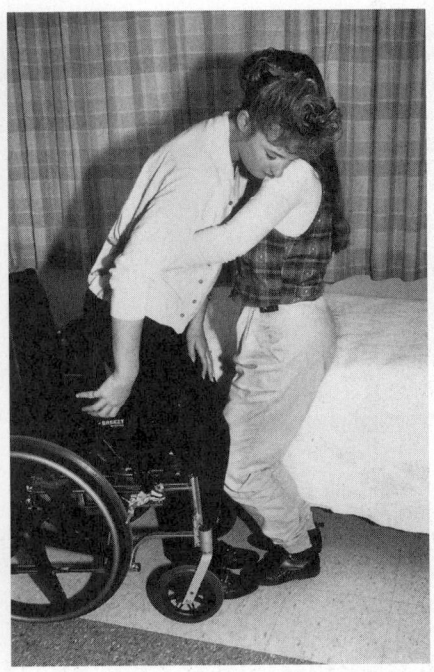

A   B   C

FIG. 14-9
Standing pivot transfer; wheelchair to bed, assisted. **A,** Therapist stands on patient's affected side and stabilizes patient's foot and knee. She assists by guiding patient forward and initiates lifting buttocks up. **B,** Patient reaches toward transfer surface. **C,** Therapist guides the patient toward transfer surface. (Courtesy of Luis Gonzalez, SCVMC.)

4. Guide the patient toward the transfer surface and gently help him or her down to a sitting position (Fig. 14-9, C).

Variations: Standing and/or Stepping Transfer

A standing and/or stepping transfer is generally used when a patient can take small steps toward the surface goal and not just pivot toward the goal. The therapist's intervention may range from physical assistance to accommodate for potential loss of balance to facilitation of near normal movement, equal weight bearing, and maintenance of appropriate posture for patients with hemiplegia or hemiparesis. If a patient demonstrates impaired cognition or a behavior deficit, including impulsiveness and poor safety judgment, the therapist may need to provide verbal cues or physical guidance.

SLIDING BOARD TRANSFERS

Sliding board transfers are best used with those who cannot bear weight on the lower extremities and who have paralysis, weakness, or poor endurance in their upper extremities. The patient should have good upper extremity strength for this transfer. It is most often employed with persons who have lower extrem-

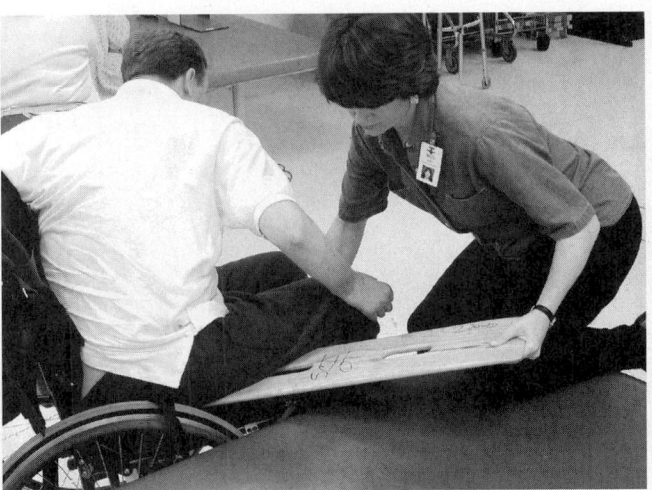

FIG. 14-10
Positioning sliding board. Lift leg closest to transfer surface. Place board midthigh between buttocks and knee, angled toward opposite hip. (Courtesy of Luis Gonzalez, SCVMC.)

ity amputations or individuals with spinal cord injuries.

Method (Fig. 14-10)

1. Position and set up the wheelchair as previously outlined.

2. Lift the leg closer to the transfer surface. Place the board midthigh between the buttocks and knee, angled toward the opposite hip. The board must be firmly under the thigh and firmly on the surface to which the patient is transferring.
3. Block the patient's knees with your own knees.
4. Instruct the patient to place one hand on the edge of the board and the other hand on the wheelchair seat.
5. Instruct the patient to lean forward.
6. The patient should transfer his or her upper body weight in the direction opposite to which he or she is going. The patient should use both arms to maneuver along the board. The patient uses upper extremity strength and trunk balance to scoot along the sliding board.
7. Help the patient by putting your hands on the patient's buttocks or scapulae and helping the patient either shift weight forward or slide across the board, as needed.

BENT PIVOT TRANSFER: BED TO WHEELCHAIR (FIG. 14-11)

The bent pivot transfer is used when the patient cannot initiate or maintain a standing position. A therapist often prefers to keep a patient in the bent knee position to maintain equal weight bearing, provide optimal trunk and lower extremity support, and perform a safer and easier therapist-assisted transfer.

Procedure

1. Help the patient scoot to the edge of the bed until both of the patient's feet are flat on the floor. Grasp the patient around the waist or hips, or even under the buttocks if a moderate or maximal amount of assistance is required.
2. Guide the patient's trunk into a midline position.
3. Shift the weight forward from the buttocks toward and over the patient's feet (Fig. 14-11, *A*).
4. Have the patient either reach toward the surface he or she is transferring to or push from the surface he or she is transferring from (Fig. 14-11, *B*).
5. Assist the patient by guiding and pivoting the patient around toward the transfer surface (Fig. 14-11, *C*).

Depending on the amount of assistance required, the pivoting portion can be done in two or three steps, with the therapist repositioning himself or herself and the patient's lower extremities between steps. The therapist has a variety of choices of where to hold or grasp the patient during the bent pivot transfer, depending on the weight and height of the patient in relation to the therapist and the patient's ability to assist in the transfer. Variations include using both hands and arms at the waist, or trunk, or one or both hands under the buttocks. *The therapist never grasps under the patient's weak arm or grasps the weak arm, an action that could cause significant injury because of weak musculature and poor stability around the shoulder girdle.* The choice is made with consideration to proper body mechanics. Trial and error of technique is

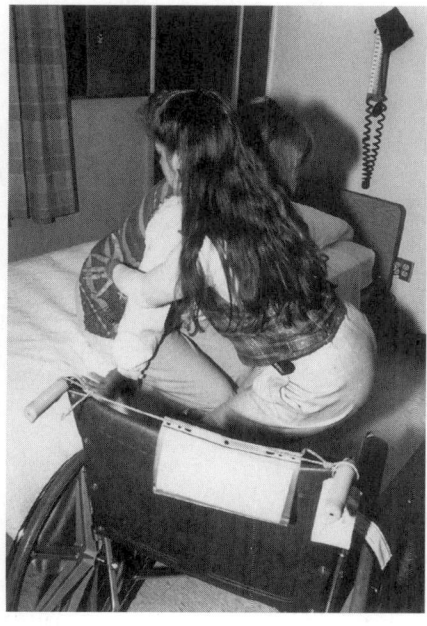 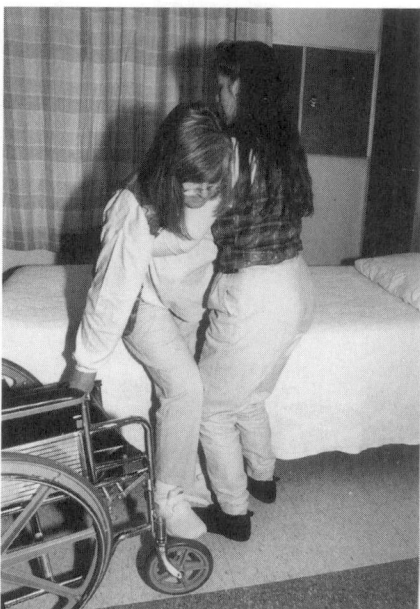 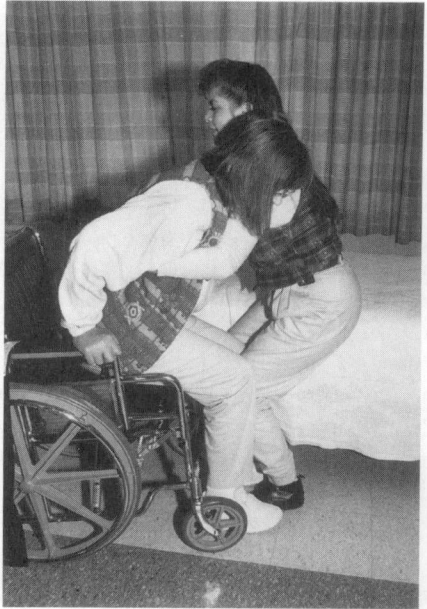

A   B   C

FIG. 14-11
Bent pivot transfer; bed to wheelchair. **A,** Therapist grasps patient around trunk and assists in shifting patient's weight forward over feet. **B,** Patient reaches toward wheelchair. **C,** Therapist assists patient down toward sitting position. (Courtesy Luis Gonzalez, SCVMC.)

advised to allow for optimal facilitation of patient independence, safety, and the therapist's proper body mechanics.

DEPENDENT TRANSFERS

The dependent transfer is designed for use with the patient who has minimal to no functional ability. If this transfer is performed incorrectly, it is potentially hazardous for both therapist and patient. This transfer should be practiced with able-bodied persons and initially used with the patient only when another person is available to assist.[2]

The purpose of the dependent transfer is to move the patient from surface to surface. The requirements are that the patient be cooperative and willing to follow instructions. The therapist should be keenly aware of correct body mechanics, as well as his or her own physical limitations. With heavy patients, it is always best to use the two-person transfer or at least to have a second person available to spot the transfer.

One-Person Dependent Sliding Board Transfer (Fig. 14-12, A-F)

The procedure for transferring the patient from wheelchair to bed is as follows:

1. Set up the wheelchair as described previously.
2. Position the patient's feet together on the floor, directly under the knees, and swing the outside footrest away. Grasp the patient's legs from behind the knees, and pull the patient slightly forward in the wheelchair so that the buttocks will clear the big wheel when the transfer is made (Fig. 14-12, A).
3. Place a sliding board under the patient's inside thigh, midway between the buttocks and the knee, to form a bridge from the bed to the wheelchair. The sliding board is angled toward the patient's opposite hip.
4. Stabilize the patient's feet by placing your own feet laterally around the patient's feet.
5. Stabilize the patient's knees by placing your own knees firmly against the anterolateral aspect of the patient's knees (Fig. 14-12, B).

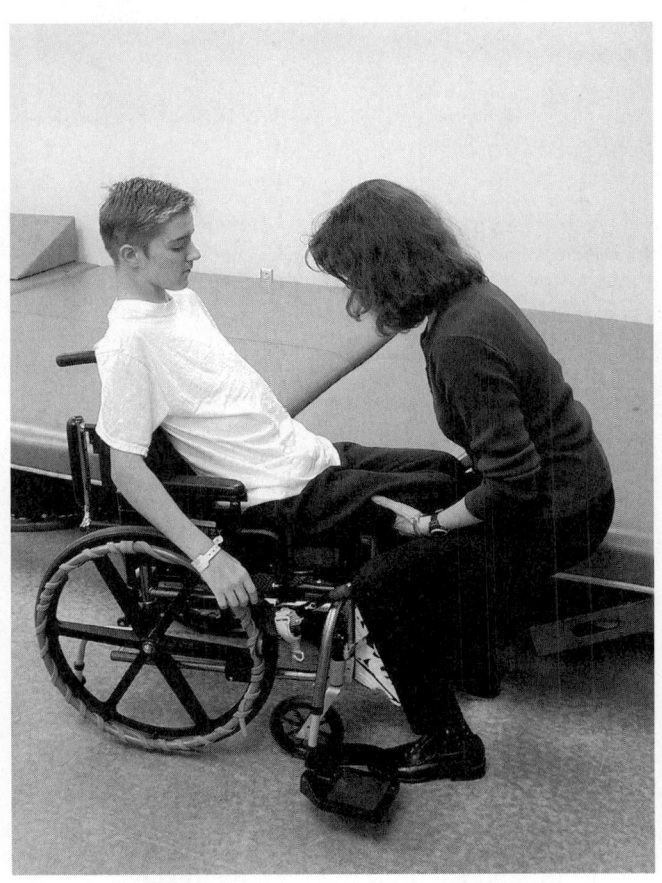

A

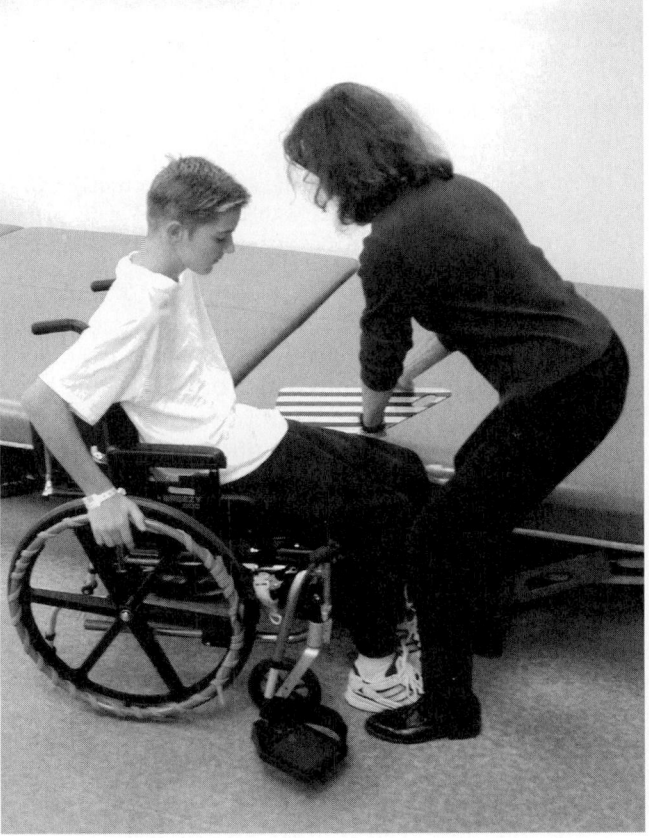

B

FIG. 14-12
One-person dependent sliding board transfer. **A,** Therapist positions wheelchair and patient and pulls patient forward in chair. **B,** Therapist stabilizes patient's knees and feet after placing sliding board.   *Continued*

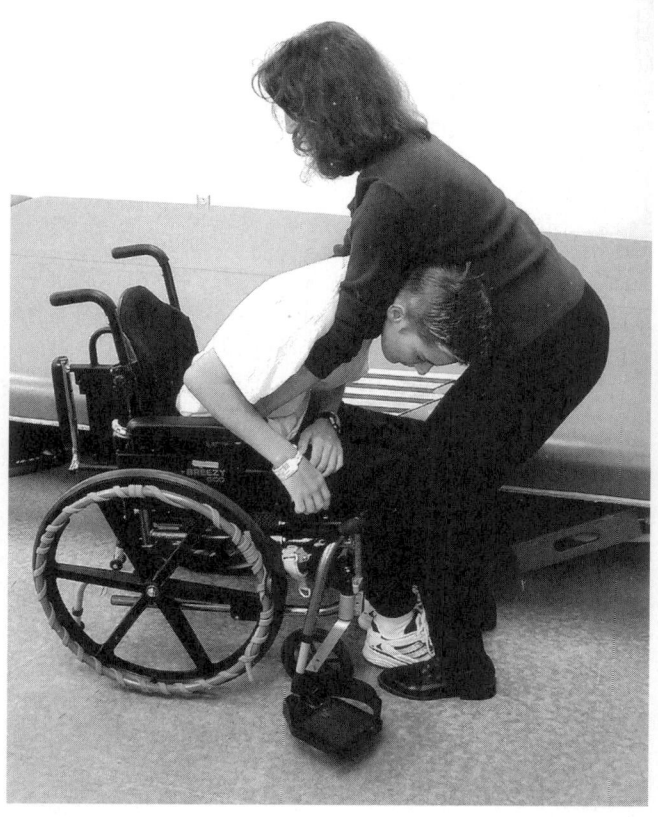

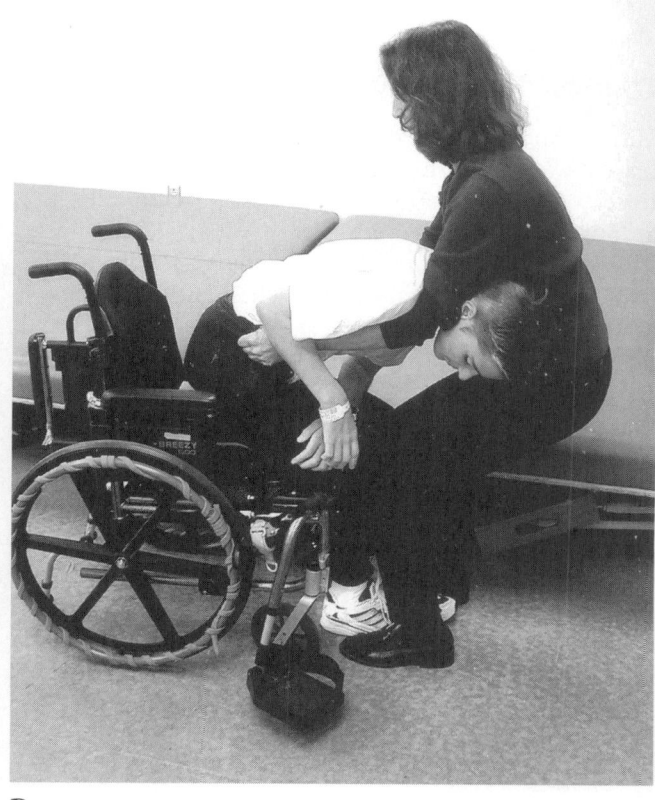

C

D

FIG. 14-12, cont'd

One-person dependent sliding board transfer. **C,** Therapist grasps patient's pants at lowest point of buttocks. **D,** Therapist rocks with patient and shifts patient's weight over patient's feet, making sure patient's back remains straight. (Courtesy of Luis Gonzales, SCVMC.)

6. Help the patient lean over the knees by pulling him or her forward from the shoulders. The patient's head and trunk should lean opposite the direction of the transfer. The patient's hands can rest on the lap.

7. Reach under the patient's outside arm and grasp the waistband of the trousers or under the buttock. On the other side, reach over the patient's back and grasp the waistband or under the buttock (Fig. 14-12, C).

8. After your arms are positioned correctly, lock them to stabilize the patient's trunk. Keep your knees slightly bent and brace them firmly against the patient's knees.

9. Gently rock with the patient to gain some momentum, and prepare to move after the count of three. Count to three aloud, with the patient. On three, holding your knees tightly against the patient's knees, transfer the patient's weight over his or her feet. You must keep your back straight to maintain good body mechanics (Fig. 14-12, D).

10. Pivot with the patient and move him or her onto the sliding board (Fig. 14-12, E). Reposition yourself and the patient's feet and repeat the pivot until the patient is firmly seated on the bed surface, per-

pendicular to the edge of the mattress and as far back as possible. This step usually can be achieved in two or three stages (Fig. 14-12, F).

11. You can secure the patient on the bed by easing him or her against the back of an elevated bed or on the mattress in a side-lying position, then by lifting the legs onto the bed.

The one-person dependent sliding board transfer can be adapted to move the patient to other surfaces. It should be attempted only when therapist and patient feel secure with the wheelchair-to-bed transfer.

Two-Person Dependent Transfers

Bent Pivot: With or Without a Sliding Board Bed to Wheelchair (Fig. 14-13)

A bent pivot transfer is used to allow increased therapist interaction and support. It allows the therapist greater control of the patient's trunk and buttocks during the transfer. This technique can also be employed during a two-person dependent transfer. It is often used with neurologically involved patients because trunk flexion and equal weight bearing are often desirable with this

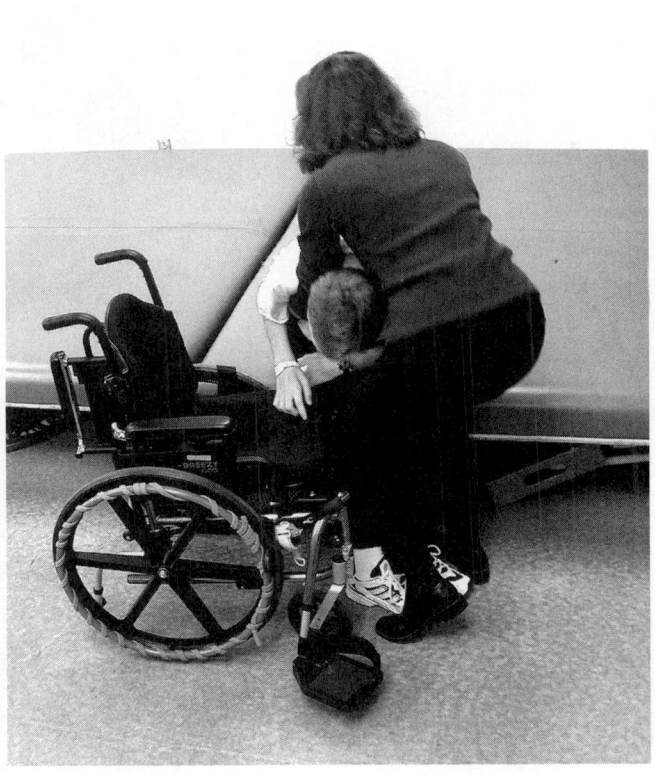

E

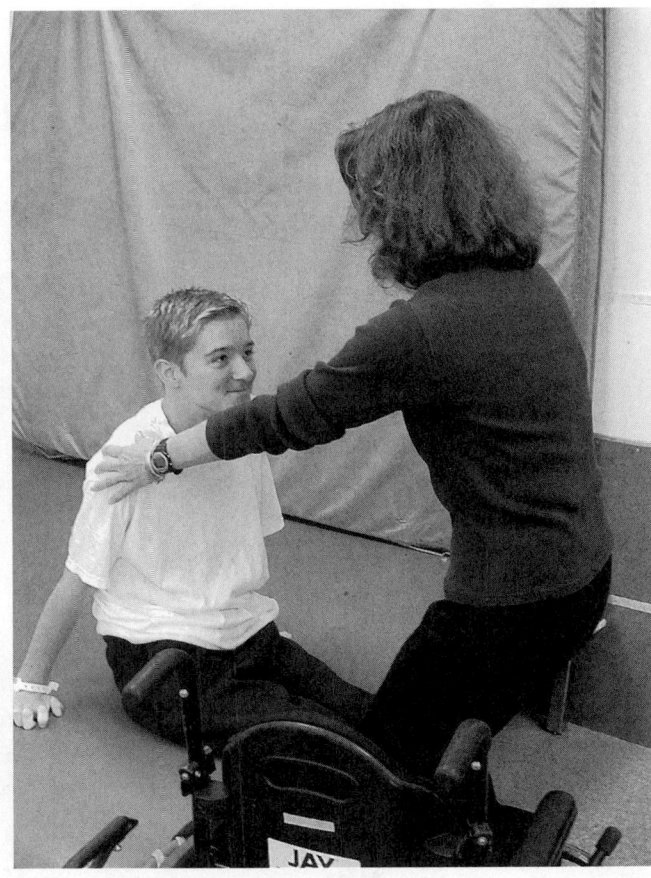

F

FIG. 14-12, cont'd
One-person dependent sliding board transfer. **E,** Therapist pivots with patient and moves patient onto sliding board. **F,** Patient is stabilized on bed. (Courtesy of Luis Gonzales, SCVMC.)

diagnosis. The steps in this two-person procedure are as follows:

1. Set the wheelchair up as described previously.
2. One therapist assumes a position in front of the patient and the other in back.
3. The therapist in front assists in walking the patient's hips forward until the feet are flat on the floor.
4. The same therapist stabilizes the patient's knees and feet by placing his or her knees and feet lateral to each of the patient's.
5. The therapist in back positions himself or herself squarely behind the patient's buttocks, grasping either the patient's waistband or placing his or her hands under the buttocks. Maintain proper body mechanics (Fig. 14-13, A).
6. The therapist in front moves the patient's trunk into a midline position, grasps the patient around the waist or hips, and guides the patient to lean forward and shift his or her weight forward, over the feet and off the buttocks. The patient's head and trunk should lean in the direction opposite the transfer. The patient's hands can rest on the lap (Fig. 14-13, B).

7. As the therapist in front shifts the patient's weight forward, the therapist in back shifts the patient's buttocks in the direction of the transfer. This can be done in two or three steps, making sure the patient's buttocks land on a safe, solid surface. The therapists reposition themselves and the patient to maintain safe and proper body mechanics (Fig. 14-13, C).
8. The therapists should be sure they coordinate the time of the transfer with the patient and one another by counting to three aloud and instructing the team to initiate the transfer on three.

Mechanical Lift Transfer

Some patients, because of body size, degree of disability, or the health and well-being of the caregiver, require the use of a mechanical lift. A variety of mechanical lifting devices can be used to transfer patients of any weight (Fig. 14-14, A and B). A properly trained caregiver, even one who is considerably smaller than the patient, can learn to use the mechanical lift safely and independently.[8] The patient's physical size, the environment in which the lift will be used, and the uses to which the lift

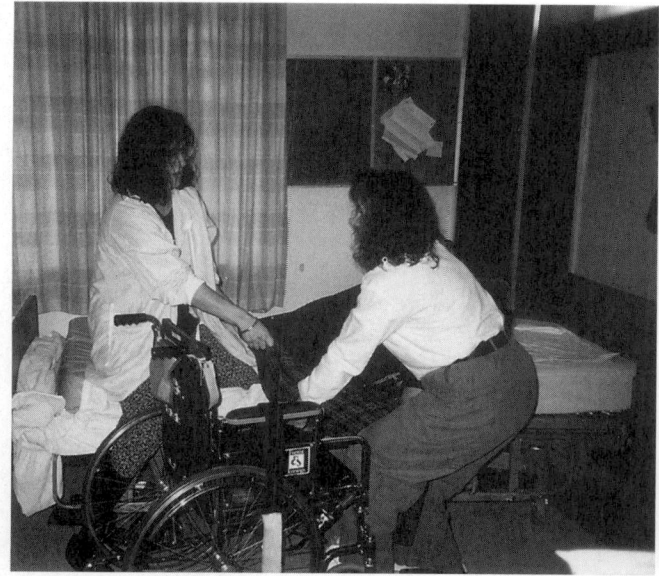

A

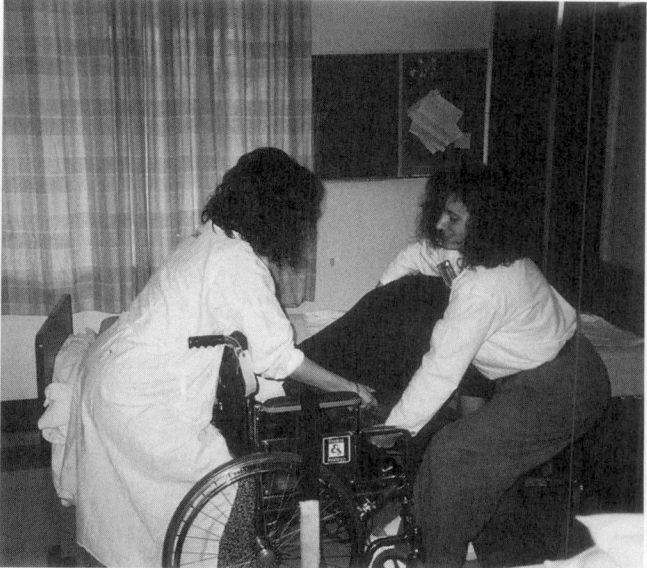

B

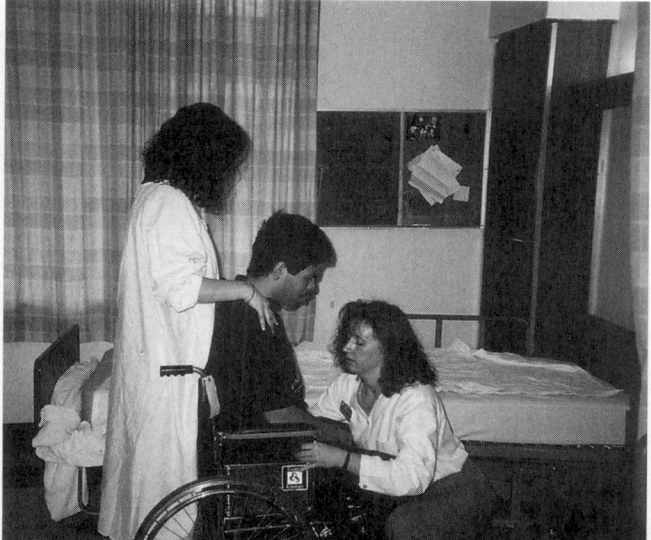

C

FIG. 14-13

Two-person dependent transfer, bed to wheelchair. **A,** One therapist positions self in front of patient, blocking feet and knees. The therapist in back positions self behind patient's buttocks and assists by lifting. **B,** Person in front rocks patient forward and un-weights buttocks as the back therapist shifts buttocks toward wheelchair. **C,** Both therapists position patient in upright, midline position in wheelchair. Seat belt is secured and positioning devices are added. (Courtesy Luis Gonzales, SCVMC.)

will be put must be considered to order the appropriate mechanical lift. The patient and caregiver should demonstrate safe use of the lift to the therapist before the therapist prescribes it.

TRANSFERS TO HOUSEHOLD SURFACES
Sofa or Chair (Fig. 14-15)

Wheelchair-to-sofa and wheelchair-to-chair transfers are similar to wheelchair-to-bed transfers; however, a few unique concerns should be assessed. The therapist and patient need to be aware that the chair may be light and not as stable as a bed or wheelchair. When transferring to the chair, the patient must be instructed to reach for the seat of the chair. The patient should not reach for

the armrest or back of the chair because this action may cause the chair to tip over. When moving from a chair to the wheelchair, the patient should use a hand to push off from the seat of the chair as he or she comes to standing. Standing from a chair is often more difficult if the chair is low or the seat cushions are soft. Dense cushions may be added to increase height and provide a firm surface to which to transfer.

Toilet

In general, wheelchair-to-toilet transfers are difficult because of the confined space in most bathrooms and the inability and lack of support of a toilet seat. The therapist and patient should attempt to position the

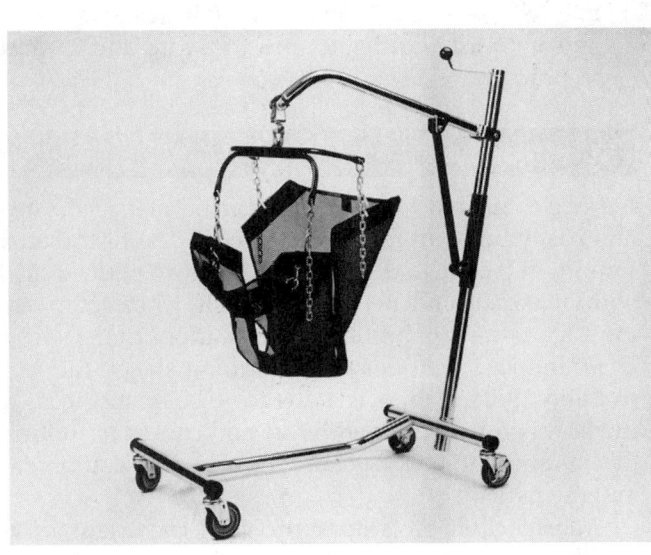

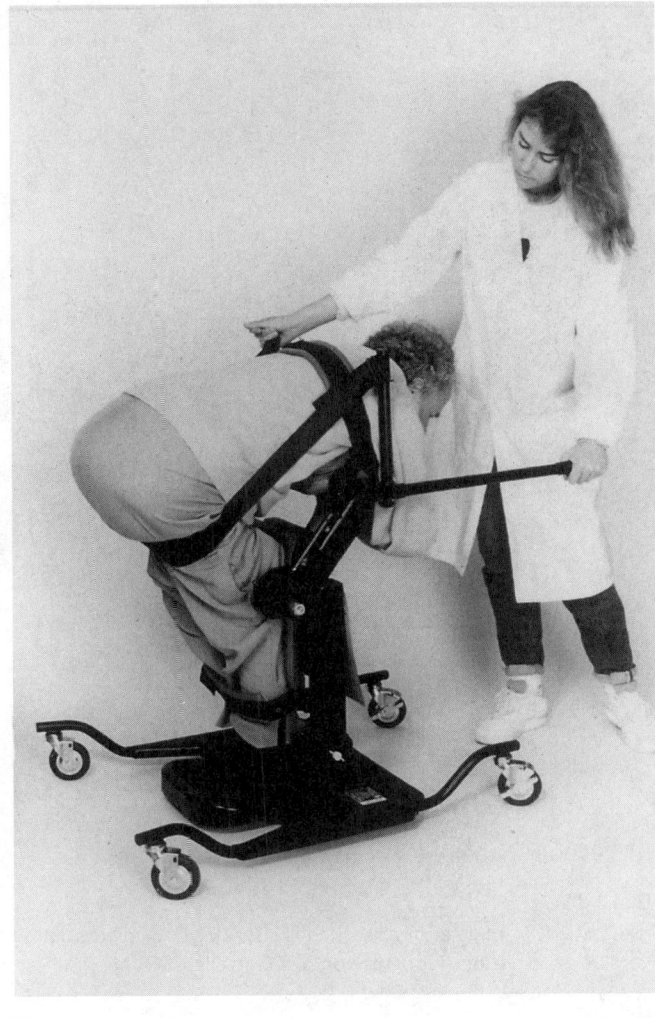

A   B

FIG. 14-14
A, Traditional boom-style mechanical lift. **B,** Patient lift useful in transferring individuals with spinal cord injury. (**A** courtesy of Trans-Aid Lifts, Sunrise Medical; **B** courtesy of EZ-Pivot, Rand-Scott.)

wheelchair next to or at an appropriate angle to the toilet. The therapist should analyze the space around the toilet and wheelchair to ensure no obstacles are present. Adaptive devices such as grab bars and raised toilet seats can be added to increase the patient's independence during this transfer. (Raised toilet seats are poorly secured to toilets and may be unsafe for some patients.) The patient can use these devices to support himself or herself during transfers and maintain a level surface to which to transfer.

Bathtub

The occupational therapist should be cautious when assessing or teaching bathtub transfers because the bathtub is considered one of the most hazardous areas of the home. Transfers from the wheelchair to the bottom of the bathtub are extremely difficult and used with patients who have good bilateral strength and

motor control of the upper extremities (e.g., patients with paraplegia and lower extremity amputation). A commercially produced bath bench or bath chair or a well-secured straight-back chair is commonly used by therapists for seated bathing. Therefore, whether a standing-pivot, bent-pivot, or sliding board transfer is performed, the technique is similar to a wheelchair-to-chair transfer. However, the transfer may be complicated by the confined space, the slick bathtub surfaces, and the bathtub wall between the wheelchair and the bathtub seat.

If a standing-pivot transfer is employed, it is recommended that the locked wheelchair be placed at a 45° angle to the bathtub if possible. The patient should stand, pivot, sit on the bathtub chair, and then place the lower extremities into the bathtub.

If a bent-pivot or sliding board transfer is used, the wheelchair is placed next to the bathtub with the armrest removed. The transfer tub bench may be used,

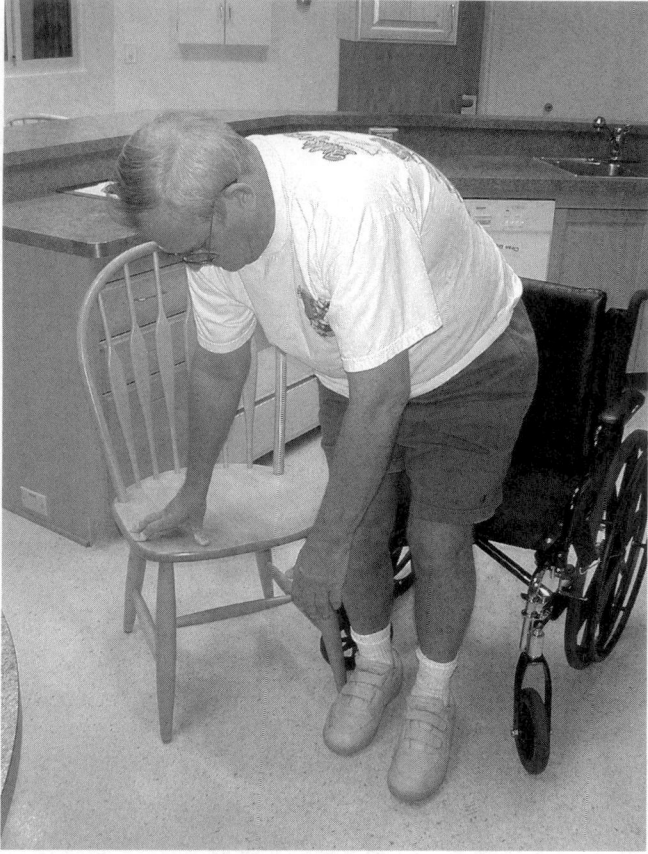

FIG. 14-15
Stroke patient in midtransfer reaches for seat of chair, pivots, and lowers body to sitting. (Courtesy of Luis Gonzales, SCVMC.)

which removes the need for a sliding board. This approach allows the wheelchair to be placed right next to the bench, allowing a safe and easy transfer of the buttocks to the seat. Then the lower extremities can be assisted into the bathtub.

In general, the patient may exit by first placing one foot securely outside the bathtub on a nonskid floor surface and then performing a standing or seated transfer back to the wheelchair.

CAR TRANSFERS

A car transfer is often the most challenging for therapists because it involves trial-and-error methods to develop a technique that is not only safe, but also easy for the patient and caregiver to carry out. The therapist often uses the patient's existing transfer technique. The patient's size, degree of disability, and vehicle style (two-door versus four-door) must be considered. These factors will affect level of independence and may necessitate a change in the usual technique to allow a safe, easy transfer.

In general, it is difficult to get a wheelchair close enough to the car seat, especially with four-door vehicles. The following are some additional considerations when making wheelchair-to-car transfers:

1. Car seats are often much lower than the standard wheelchair seat height, which makes the uneven transfer much more difficult, especially from the car seat to the wheelchair.
2. Occasionally, patients have orthopedic injuries that necessitate the use of a brace such as a halo body jacket or lower extremity cast or splint. The therapist often must alter technique to accommodate these devices.
3. The therapist may suggest use of the sliding board for this transfer, to compensate for the large gap between transfer surfaces.
4. Because uphill transfers are difficult and the level of assistance may increase for this transfer, the therapist may choose a two-person assist instead of a one-person assist transfer to ensure a safe and smooth technique.

SUMMARY

A wheelchair that fits well and can be managed safely and easily by its user and caregiver is one of the most important factors in the patient's ability to perform ADL with maximal independence.[6] Each wheelchair user must learn the capabilities and limitations of the wheelchair and safe methods of performing all self-care and mobility skills. If there is a caregiver, he or she needs to be thoroughly familiar with safe and correct techniques of handling the wheelchair, positioning equipment, and the patient.

Transfer skills are among the most important activities that must be mastered by the wheelchair user. The ability to transfer increases the possibility of mobility and travel. However, transfers can be hazardous. Safe methods must be learned and followed.[8] Several basic transfer techniques are outlined in this chapter. Additional methods and more detailed training and instructions are available, as cited previously.

It should be recognized that many wheelchair users with exceptional abilities have developed unique methods of wheelchair management. Although such innovative approaches may work well for the person who has devised and mastered them, they cannot be considered basic procedures that everyone can learn.[8]

SECTION 3
Transportation, Community Mobility, and Driving Assessment

SUSAN M. LILLIE

IMPORTANCE OF TRANSPORTATION

Mobility is a universal need at any age. Special transportation needs may have been present at birth or may have been caused later by illness or a motor vehicle accident or fall. When basic mobility needs such as visits to the grocery store, pharmacy, and physician cannot easily be met, too often the result is social isolation, depression, and diminishment or loss of life roles.[5,9]

For those with mobility restrictions, accessible **transportation** is essential to quality of life, enabling individuals to engage in meaningful activities and roles, to benefit from social and emotional interactions, and to increase independence. In essence, accessible transport allows people to maintain their self-respect.

Different systems of transportation can be categorized as either public or private. Each system has benefits and limitations. The therapist is uniquely suited to assist persons with disabilities in meeting their needs through both the public transportation system and use of a private vehicle.

PUBLIC TRANSPORTATION

Provided by public and private agencies, public transportation "provides the general public with a general or special service on a regular and continuing basis."[10] Public transportation includes two key systems—fixed route and paratransit.

Fixed route systems use defined routes and designated stops and run on a schedule. The **paratransit** system, sometimes known as the dial-a-ride system, provides demand-response service within a prescribed geographical area; vehicle dispatch occurs only in response to a rider's request.

Inconvenience and fear for personal safety are frequently cited as a barrier to the use of public transportation[5,9] and must be addressed to increase its viability among the disabled populations.

Transportation Improvements: Americans With Disabilities Act

The **Americans With Disabilities Act (ADA)** of 1990 bans discrimination in public transportation. The ADA regulates buses, trains, ships, and other means of transportation that use both fixed and demand-response systems. The ADA does not regulate air travel, public school transportation at the K-12 level, or privately owned over-the-road buses, which have a raised passenger compartment over a baggage storage area.[10]

Newly purchased or leased buses must be modified with a 30-inch-wide by 48-inch-long platform lift, securements for mobility aid devices, priority seating, and a host of other features designed to facilitate navigation of the transportation system by disabled persons.

The ADA also regulates paratransit, which is designated for disabled persons unable to access or navigate a fixed route system.[10] Paratransit is designed to provide the disabled person with the same essential transit coverage that is available to the able-bodied rider. To be

compliant, a transit agency must meet minimum service area and service requirements. The ADA also specifies only curb-to-curb service, although door-to-door service may be provided. One associate or attendant is able to accompany a person with a disability on the paratransit vehicle.

Treatment Implications for Fixed Transit

Because the actual usable space on an ADA-compliant lift varies by manufacturer and lift model, the therapist cannot assume that a mobility aid device will automatically be compatible with an ADA-compliant platform lift.

Knowing platform lift and end flap dimensions is critical when ordering a power wheelchair or scooter. For example, when a power wheelchair's footrests are lower than the lift's end flap or roll stop, the functional length of the wheelchair can exceed 48 inches and will not fit onto an ADA-compliant lift. Scooters, which generally can fit on the lift platform, may be unable to negotiate the tight turn required either to enter the coach or park in the designated area. When a specific power wheelchair or scooter is incompatible with the local transit system, paratransit and private transportation systems are the only transportation options.

Fixed-route training includes common elements such as navigating between the designated stop and destination, flagging the bus, boarding and exiting the bus, dealing with the fare box, and handling spontaneously occurring situations. Bus fleets often have a variety of bus designs, including different lift locations, which necessitates learning different boarding techniques.

Treatment Implications for Paratransit

Awareness of local paratransit service features enables the therapist to provide appropriate transportation interventions. Curb-to-curb service places more physical, visual, perceptual, and cognitive demands on a rider than door-to-door service. The rider must navigate from the drop-off point to the final destination and may need more training for this. Contingency planning and orientation and training in the use of the reservation system may also be needed.

Another characteristic of the paratransit system is that rider trips are combined to fill vehicles. Travel takes much longer than with private transportation and can pose hardships to riders with certain medical symptoms, such as urinary urgency and frequency problems or pain with prolonged immobility. It is also important to know that drop-off points may not have amenities such as restrooms, phone access, food, or water; there are even occasions when miscommunication or errors arise, delaying or inadvertently canceling a ride. As with fixed transit, the unaccompanied paratransit rider needs a certain degree of resourcefulness and problem-solving skill to navigate the system safely and efficiently.

PRIVATE TRANSPORTATION
Passengers and Drivers

Private transportation relies on consumer vehicles that are privately owned by passengers and/or drivers. The advantages of private transportation include 24-hour availability of a personally owned vehicle, immediate origin-to-destination travel, the flexibility to add or delete destinations on a given trip, and a strong sense of control over one's life. The primary disadvantages are that the individual is responsible for his or her own access needs and that a high level of responsibility is required for ongoing maintenance and repair for both the vehicle and its modifications. Individuals preferring the convenience of private transportation must also plan for replacement costs of the vehicle, including any equipment or vehicle upgrades needed to keep pace with future changes in function.

Passenger Evaluations

Passenger evaluations should not be overlooked as a treatment intervention. A trained therapist can significantly improve the safety of the caregiver and the person being transported. Supplemental trunk and head support are needed when an individual has inadequate motor control or strength to overcome gravitational or centrifugal forces in a moving vehicle. Occupant restraint systems provide safety by securing the wheelchair and passenger to the vehicle to prevent unwanted movement or injury.

When a patient is using respiratory equipment such as a ventilator or portable suction device, a backup power supply should be recommended as an essential life-saving modification. An *inverter* is a device that converts DC, 12-volt car battery power to AC, 110-volt household power, providing an alternate, plug-in source of power for respiratory equipment should the batteries fail. Young children may also need specialized products or modifications to accommodate a permanent or temporary disability.

DRIVER EVALUATION PROGRAM
Driving: Relevance to Society

Driving is an essential ADL in most locations in the United States, playing a pivotal role in personal independence, employment,[30] and aging in place. A driver's license symbolizes a rite of passage to adulthood for the teenager, independence to pursue leisure activities and employment opportunities for the adult, and wellness and competence for the mature driver. The ability to drive is regarded as instrumental in obtaining and maintaining an independent lifestyle[5] and in aging in place.[9]

Specialized Training Needs for the Therapist

Driving is a complex task, requiring continuous integration of visual, motor, cognitive, and perceptual skills at a high level of functioning.[20] A driver must continually search, identify, predict, decide, and execute driving decisions in response to the surrounding environment.[14]

Driving presents a greater possibility of personal and public harm than does any other ADL. It is essential that therapists receive **specialized training,** because none is provided within basic OT education. Therapists must be mindful of the industry standard for other professionals who provide driver training—a standard that usually involves state licensing as a driver instructor. Therapists need to seek basic and equivalent driver education and training through recognized entities, such as universities or state-approved courses, in order to provide quality services, teach proper driver education techniques, and minimize on-road risk and liability exposure. One measure of entry-level knowledge is the Association for Driver Rehabilitation Specialists' (ADED) driver certification process (Box 14-3). The Certified Driver Rehabilitation Specialist (CDRS) requires passage of an examination that covers driver education, disabilities, and adaptive driving education.

BOX 14-3
Additional Resources

Websites for pertinent associations

AAA Foundation for Traffic Safety
Publishers of consumer pamphlets and products
http://www.aaafts.org

ADED, the Association for Driver Rehabilitation Specialists
CDRS information, disability fact sheets, bulletin board for driver evaluators
http://www.driver-ed.org

American Association of Retired Persons
Information and publication on older driver issues
http://www.aarp.org

National Mobility Equipment Dealers Association
Product manufacturers and equipment installers
http://www.nmeda.org

National Highway Traffic Safety Administration
Airbag on-off switch and consumer information
http://www.nhtsa.dot.gov

Occupational Therapists and Driving

Occupational therapists make up the overwhelming majority of professionals conducting driver evaluations for the disabled population.[13] The State of California Department of Rehabilitation recommends that occupational therapists conducting driving evaluations have a minimum of 2 years of experience in physical disabilities and knowledge of adaptive equipment, driving systems, and equipment vendors.[26] Knowledge and training in implications of medical conditions and disease processes, ADL, adaptive devices, and occupational theory make OT practitioners uniquely qualified to provide quality driver rehabilitation services. The experienced OT assistant (OTA) may also acquire the specialized training needed to properly conduct driver evaluations. Vehicle entry and exit training, phone screenings, on-road evaluation, and driver training are other roles appropriate for the OTA. Achieving CDRS status or status as a state-licensed driver instructor provides even further opportunities.

Even at the national level of government, therapists are recognized as having unique skills for driver rehabilitation. The National Highway Traffic Safety Administration (NHTSA) is looking to therapists to provide future services for older adult drivers. Working in partnership with both the ADED and the American Occupational Therapy Association (AOTA), NHTSA hopes to increase the availability of driver evaluation training materials, workshops, and programs. With nearly 27 million baby boomers turning 65 in the year 2010, the need to train additional therapists is significant.[9]

Driving Program Structure

Driving programs are provided in private industry as well as in hospital-based settings. In some states the Department of Vocational Rehabilitation sets up its own driving program, hiring therapists to conduct evaluations and training. Some programs do not have trained staff to conduct on-road evaluations but rather provide these services by contracting with licensed driver instructors from outside the program. Other programs provide **clinical evaluations** or screening services, which can identify driving-related impairments that may not have been evident in other ADL or productive work activities.

Pre-program screenings can benefit drivers by providing the information needed for making informed choices. As one client stated after hearing that the projected cost for the evaluation, training, and equipment in a high-tech van would exceed $100,000, "That would buy me a lot of rides." This client chose not to pursue driving.

Program structure depends greatly on referral sources, payment sources, and available equipment and vehicles. Worker's compensation, vocational rehabilitation programs, school systems, private insurance, Medicaid, and Medicare are primary potential sources for funding. Al-though driver evaluations are not routinely covered, approvals for service are becoming more common.

Purpose of a Driving Evaluation

Driving competence can be disrupted by a single disability, multiple medical conditions, or factors of aging. Even experienced drivers are susceptible to these conditions. Driver evaluations provide a safe arena in which to observe driving performance under real conditions and determine what restorative, compensatory, or preventive interventions may be needed for safe driving.

Recommended Practices

Comprehensive services in a driver evaluation program should include clinical, stationary, and on-road performance testing in a special evaluation vehicle (Fig. 14-16).[8,15,25,26]

Recommended practices from ADED include a clinical evaluation followed by (1) an on-the-road evaluation in an actual driving environment, (2) subsequent vehicle modification recommendations and wheelchair measurements, (3) recommended driver training and education, and (4) a final fitting.[2] The State of California's Department of Rehabilitation guidelines also mandate that the recommendations for adaptive equipment be made only when a driver can demonstrate the ability to use the equipment or a similar device in a behind-the-wheel assessment.[27] An on-road evaluation is critical; the context of an actual driving environment is the key to preventing costly and potentially life-threatening mistakes.

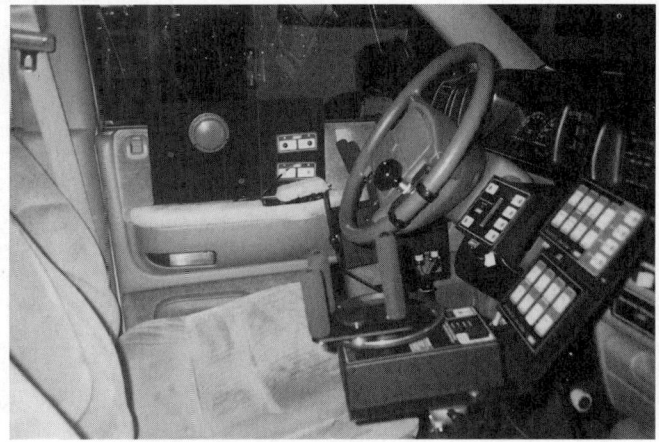

FIG. 14-16
Evaluation van equipped with Electronic Mobility Controls (EMC), including a left-side electronic gas-brake with wrist support, left elbow secondary control button, 7-inch remote steering wheel with a tripin device, and membrane switch consoles for functions such as electric gear shift, ramp, and windows.

Referral Process

Healthcare professionals, including physicians, therapists, and case managers, help determine which individuals could benefit from a driver evaluation. The referral process is complex and cannot always be completed in a seamless fashion (Fig. 14-17).

Each program needs to set criteria for accepting a referral for driver evaluation. The following are items generally included as part of the criteria:

1. Receipt of a physician's referral or prescription for evaluation
2. Receipt of a patient's medical records

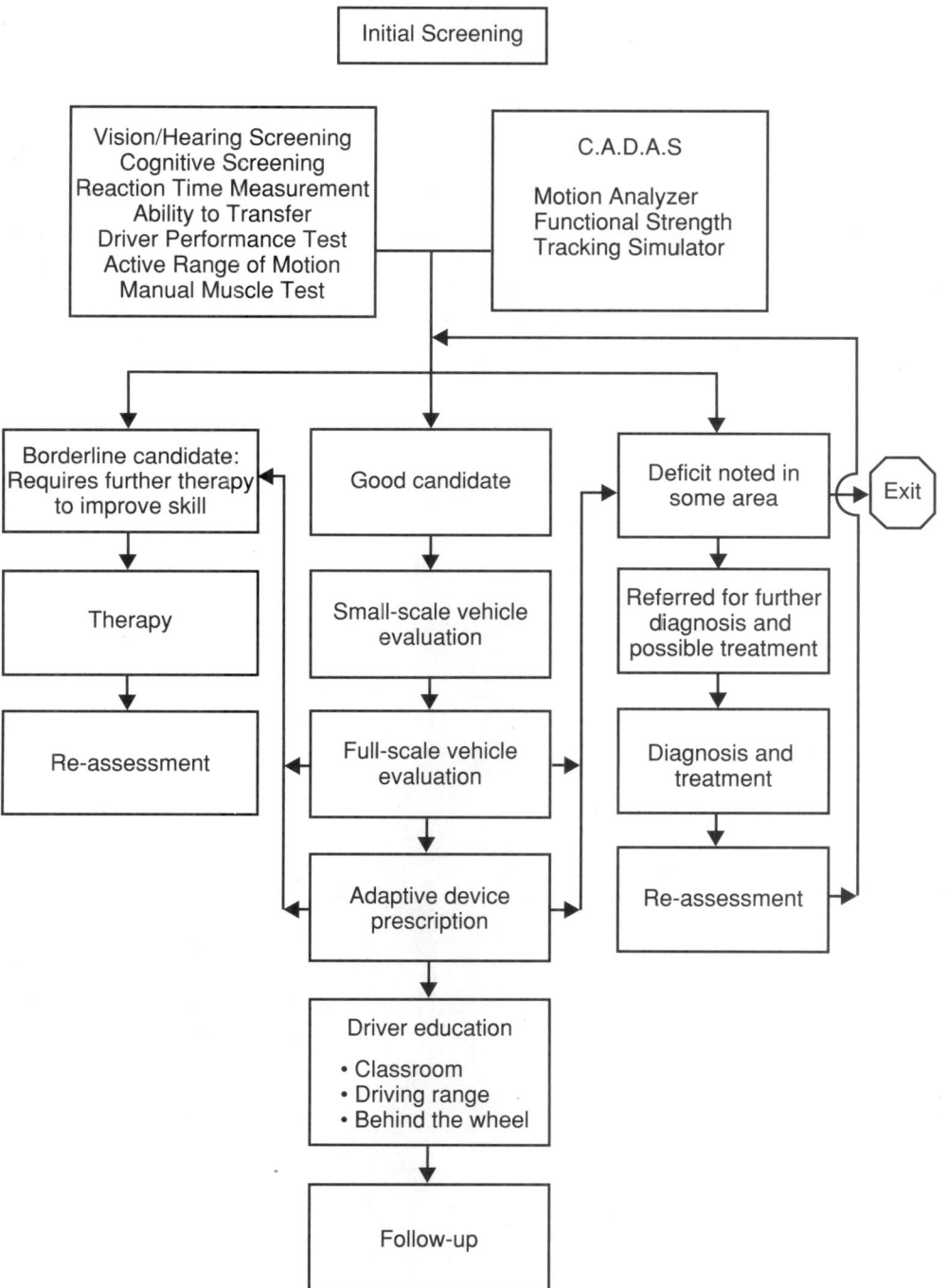

FIG. 14-17

A flow chart detailing the complexity of the driver evaluation referral process. (From Hale PN, Shipp M: Driver assessment, education and training for the disabled. In *Proceedings of the 10th annual RESNA conference*, Washington, DC, 1987, RESNA Press.)

3. Proof that the patient has a valid driver's license or driving permit
4. Confirmation of a source of payment

A referral to a qualified driver evaluation is recommended when (1) there are concerns about the driver's safety, judgment, or competence; (2) physical limitations impair the driver's ability to use a normal driving pattern or equipment; or (3) the driver has a neurological, neuromuscular, or visual impairment.

DRIVING EVALUATIONS AND DISABILITIES
Spinal Cord Injuries

A driving evaluation for the client with a spinal cord injury focuses on the following items:
1. The client's method of mobility
2. The client's transfer ability, wheelchair management, and trunk stability
3. The presence of spasticity in the client
4. The client's available strength and ROM
5. The client's positioning at the driver's station

Most paraplegics and some C7-8 quadriplegics can drive a car that has the following modifications (Fig. 14-18):
1. Hand controls for the accelerator and brake
2. A specially designed steering device

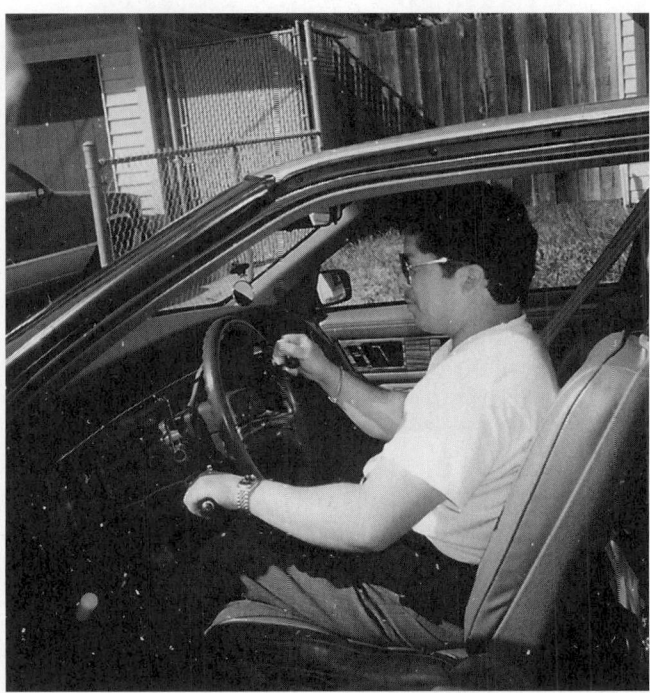

FIG. 14-18
Basic setup for paraplegic includes spinner knob steering device for right-hand steering, push right-angle pull hand control to operate accelerator and brake, extended brake handle to set parking brake, and horn switch relocated to hand control.

3. Accessible horn, dimmer, and wiper controls
4. A parking brake extension

An extensively modified van may be needed when transfers are overly exerting or when assistance is required for a transfer.[25] If a person needs to drive from the wheelchair, additional wheelchair modifications may be needed for trunk stability. Structural modifications to the van (e.g., a raised door, raised roof, or lowered floor) may be necessary to accommodate the wheelchair and driver.[16] Thanks to current technologies, some clients with C4-5 quadriplegia are able to drive with extensive evaluation and training.

Neurological Conditions

Acquired or traumatic brain injuries, cerebral palsy, and other neurological conditions cause disturbances in voluntary movement, muscle tone, **cognition,** perception, and even vision, potentially affecting driving safety.[8] The ability to physically operate the vehicle, make traffic decisions, and respond to the surrounding driving environment may be mildly or severely impaired. Equipment and training are based on the areas affected. Unresolved or poor insight greatly reduces chances of safe driving, since impairments cannot be successfully treated or compensated for unless they are first recognized. Chapter 27 provides additional information on cognition.

Neuromuscular Conditions

The neuromuscular diseases (polio, muscular dystrophy, and multiple sclerosis) impair motor control, endurance, and joint stability. Multiple sclerosis and some forms of muscular dystrophy can affect cognition, perception, and vision. Each diagnosis has a strikingly different pattern of symptoms and progression, and only certain parts of the body may be affected. To the extent possible, the recommended equipment must meet both current and anticipated future needs. Drivers may ambulate with or without devices, push a wheelchair, or use a scooter or even a power wheelchair. Driving equipment is just as varied.

Older Drivers—A Growing Population

The driving ability of older adults changes as they age, but most remain safe drivers. Most **older drivers** adapt by gradually limiting their driving, such as by omitting travel during rush hour and the evening.[18] Others experience an abrupt change in driver status because of a medical event such as a stroke. Lacking specific training, the physician may be reluctant to address **driver competence** in the older adult, fearing that such discussions might permanently destroy even long-standing physician-patient relationships.[22,23]

To date, research has not identified the skills or qualities that make an older driver competent, rendering large-scale epidemiological screening difficult.[9,12,18,19,28] Older adults with multiple medical conditions are probably most at risk and in need of driver evaluation and intervention.

When assessing the older adult with limited driving competence, the therapist should consider graded licensing, which permits driving under certain limitations (e.g., dawn to dusk or no freeway). A recommendation for a graded license extends the older adult's ability to function independently.[1]

Theoretical Constructs

Occupational role and activity analysis frameworks provide a strong foundation for a thorough driver evaluation. The therapist assesses performance components individually. During the on-road test, the therapist then evaluates the client's ability to perform component skills in an integrated fashion, within the performance context of actual driving conditions.

Occupational role theory is also helpful in driver assessment. Occupational roles may carry specific needs related to transportation equipment and parking environments. A construction site inspector may enter or exit a vehicle over 10 times daily and thus may need to consider a transfer seat or using a wheelchair in a van. A certified public accountant audits businesses that may have parking structures or covered parking, thus necessitating that the accountant's minivan not exceed certain height restrictions. In each example the selection of the vehicle and its modifications are based largely on occupational roles.

DRIVING EVALUATION COMPONENTS
Clinical Assessment

The clinical assessment is also referred to as a screening or predriving evaluation. The clinical assessment can be performed solely by the occupational therapist[25,26] or by many members of the rehabilitation team together.[7] Used to identify strengths and impairments related to driving, the clinical assessment begins with a review of medical information, medication and side effects, episodes of seizure or loss of consciousness, mobility status, social history, vocational history, driving history, and purpose of the evaluation. The interview process often results in unexpected, pertinent findings related to the driver evaluation.

It should be clear whether a patient's condition is stable or improving. A history should be taken to determine and document the rate of progression; without this information, it is difficult to establish adequate safety margins to accommodate future changes in condition.

Visual Functioning

A comprehensive **vision** screening is important because vision is the primary sense used to gather information needed for driving-related decision making. Vision testing is completed before other testing to eliminate impaired acuity as a factor. A comprehensive vision screening includes near and far acuities, phoria or alignment, saccades, oculomotor pursuits, range of motion, convergence, and field of vision.[6,11,25,27] Glare recovery is relevant to assess for the older adult evaluation.

Physical Measurements

Muscle strength, active ROM, grip, and reaction time are frequently cited as the basic abilities that must be measured.[26,27,29] Head and trunk control, sitting and standing balance (dynamic and static), and coordination are also important. When neurological disturbances are present, quality of selective movement, muscle tone, and muscle fatigue should be included as well.

Force readings with a torque wrench or Chatillon scale provide data that help determine the level of resistance required for steering or braking, which helps in more complex modifications for driving.

COGNITIVE AND VISUAL-PERCEPTUAL SKILLS

The driver must have adequate, reliable **perception** of a rapidly changing environment, blending both cognitive and visual-perceptual skills. Cognitive areas requiring assessment include selective and sustained attention, initiation, decision making, safety judgment, problem solving and planning, insight, and the ability to shift focus at will.

The ability to multitask or divide attention is also a critical driving skill.[23] Multitasking is the simultaneous performance and monitoring of two or more equally important activities, such as maintaining lane positioning while turning one's head for a visual traffic check.

Visual-perceptual components include visual organization, visual searching and scanning, spatial relations, directionality, and visual processing speed.[15,16,29] Visual memory is also important in driving.

Recommendations for driver's license status should not be made on the basis of test scores alone. There is still no clear evidence that any one test identifies at-risk drivers or predicts driving competence.[12,20] Properly used and selected, however, cognitive and visual-perceptual testing helps the driver evaluator identify impairments, improve behind-the-wheel risk management, and plan treatment for driver rehabilitation.

Vehicle Options

Car Considerations

A basic level of service for the majority of driving programs is the car evaluation. A car is generally appropriate if a person can enter and exit the vehicle and load mobility equipment devices independently. The standard car recommendation is a four-door, midsize vehicle with power steering, power brakes, and an automatic transmission.

If loading a manual wheelchair into a car is not feasible, independence can sometimes be obtained by using a mechanical device such as a car top loader. Limited ambulators may be able to continue using their standard minivan, sport utility vehicle, or truck with the assistance of a power hoist (Fig. 14-19).

Van Considerations

Drivers must choose between full-size vans and minivans. Providing information on the differences between minivans and full-size vans, including accessibility, ground clearance, load capacity, durability, and cost, enables clients to make educated choices that suit their needs, budget, and lifestyle. In any van, wheelchair drivers' needs are more complex and they require more highly skilled evaluation than other drivers because of increased variables that affect driving performance and equipment selection.

Full-size vans require an automatic mechanical lift for the wheelchair or scooter. Mechanical lifts can be mounted on the rear or side of a full-size van or the side of a minivan. Lifts fall into two basic styles, platform-style lifts and rotary or swing in-style lifts (Fig.

14-20). Each lift has unique characteristics that must be considered.[21]

Minivans have fully automatic mechanical side ramps for independent exit and entry (Fig. 14-21). Minivans have limited interior space but much appeal because they drive like a car, are easier to park, and get better gas mileage.

STATIONARY ASSESSMENT

The stationary component of the assessment involves an evaluation of the pre-driving activities and the equipment setup in the static position. Stationary performance alone is inadequate to predict either on-road performance or final equipment needs. The stationary evaluation results in determination of a proposed driving setup adjusted for a driver. If subsequent on-road results are not satisfactory, the stationary process is repeated with the next level of equipment. This trial-and-error approach is an expected and necessary step in **assistive technology** evaluation.[8]

Predriving Tasks

Predriving tasks include achieving mobility to the vehicle, inserting and turning a key (or keyless entry operation), opening and closing the door, entering and exiting the vehicle, loading and unloading mobility devices (e.g., cane, walker, and wheelchair), adjusting the driver seat, adjusting the mirrors, and fastening the seatbelt (and chest strap when needed). Adaptive devices to facilitate independence in predriving tasks include special key holders, loops for lower extremity management, a strap to extend reach for wheelchair loading, and modifications for independent retrieval of the seatbelt.

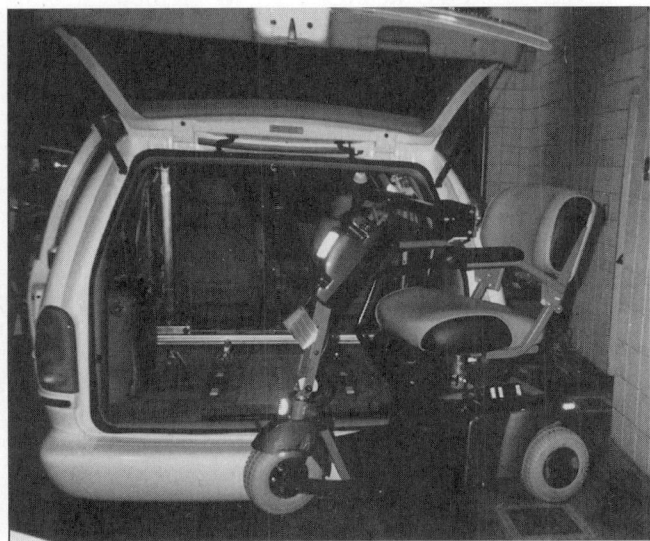

FIG. 14-19
The Curbsider, by Bruno, hoists a scooter or fully assembled power wheelchair, up to 250 pounds, from the sidewalk and lifts it into the back of a standard minivan.

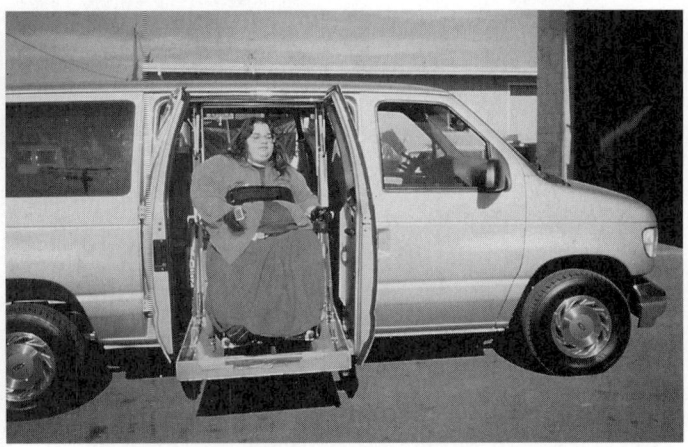

FIG. 14-20
Platform-style lift can be located at side or rear of van. Additional entry headroom, obtained through lowered floor, provides client adequate field of view when driving from power wheelchair.

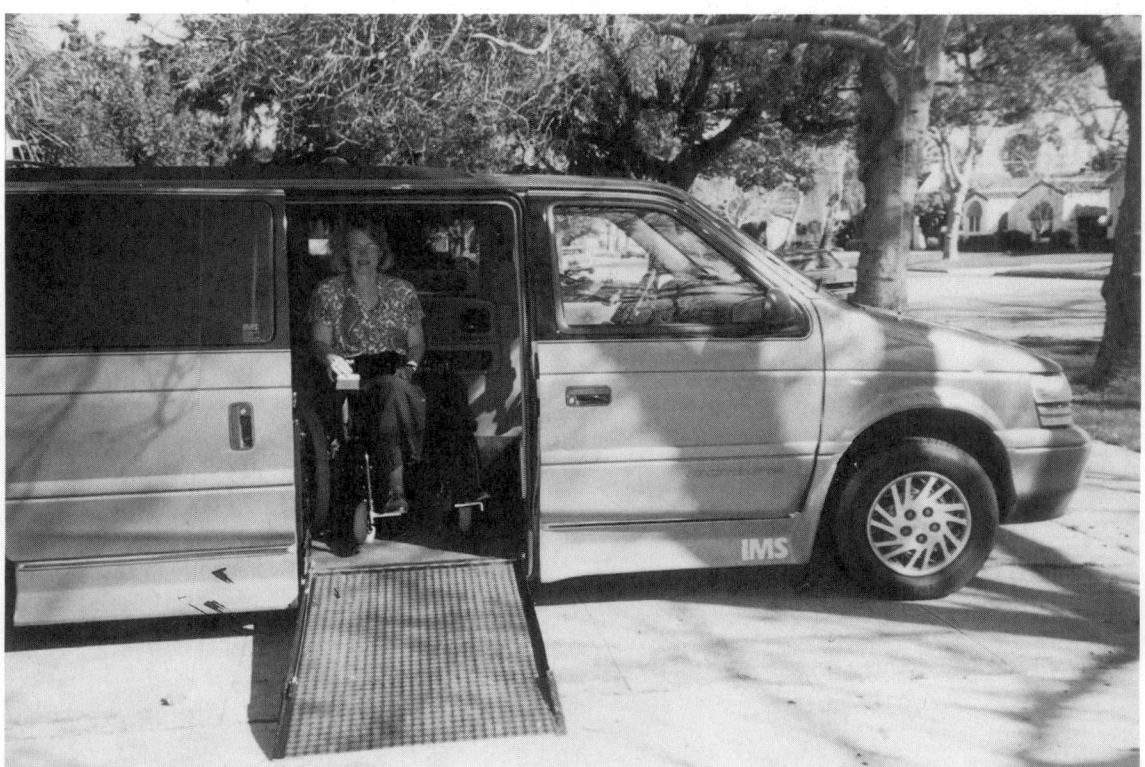

FIG. 14-21
Minivan conversion with side ramp access and lowered 10-inch floor. The vehicle can be lowered to decrease the ramp angle for easier entry and exit.

Primary Control Setup

The first step in the primary control assessment phase is to position the driver to obtain optimal upper extremity function, proper field of view, and trunk stability. Poor trunk stability may necessitate special positioning devices. The upper torso support or chest strap is a commonly used positioning device.[3,4] Equipment setups then begin with the **primary controls**—those devices that control the steering, accelerator, and braking of a vehicle.

Steering Control

When a driver cannot use two hands to steer, a steering device is recommended. One-handed steering by palming the wheel provides inadequate control, especially in sharp, fast turns and evasive maneuvers. The use of adaptive steering devices—the spinner knob, V-grip, tripin, palmar cuff, or amputee ring—improves control of the steering wheel (Fig. 14-22).[8]

A new, critical step in steering assessment developed as a result of airbags. The distance between a driver's sternum to the center of the steering wheel must be a minimum of 10 inches, as recommended by the NHTSA, to prevent serious injury or death from airbag inflation.[17]

More involved steering modifications include extended steering columns, steering wheels with smaller diameters, and reduced levels of steering resistance. High-tech options include a 7-inch remote steering wheel that can be placed anywhere, shown in Fig. 14-16. The final level of current driving technology includes the unilever and joystick systems, which combine steering, acceleration, and brake operations on a single lever. Van modifications, especially at this final level, necessitate extensive additional training for the driver. Only after the stationary steering setup is determined does the process move to the accelerator and brake controls.

Accelerator and Brake Controls

Modified accelerator and brake controls can be installed in most vehicles. Simple modifications such as pedal extensions can be installed on both the accelerator and brake pedals to compensate for limited reach. More drivers need extended pedals with airbags because maintaining proper distance from the airbag prevents fully reaching the accelerator and brake pedals.

With a significant right hemiplegia, the right foot is unable to operate the standard pedals. A left-sided accelerator pedal can be placed to the left of the standard gas pedal to compensate for this condition.

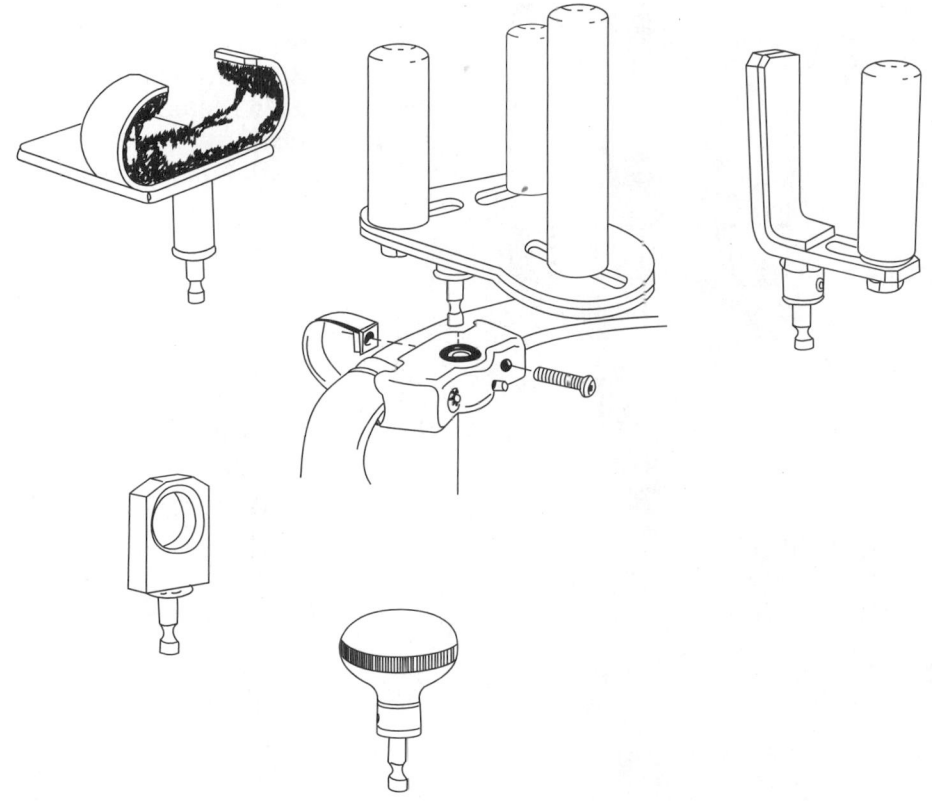

FIG. 14-22
These steering devices accommodate a variety of hand and upper extremity impairments. (Courtesy of Mobility Products and Design.)

When the driver lacks adequate motor control in the lower extremities or when the driver's lower extremities are paralyzed, a device called a "hand control" allows the driver to operate the accelerator and brake pedals with an upper extremity. Hand controls use rotary, push-pull, push-pull down, or push-rocker motions to activate the accelerator and the brake. High-tech accelerator and brake controls have servo motors activated by vacuum, hydraulic, or electronic means and require minimal strength and ROM. Trunk stability is even more critical if such controls are used (Fig. 14-23).

Secondary Controls

All other controls are **secondary controls.** There are four secondary controls that a driver must be able to activate at will when the vehicle is in motion—turn signal indicators, horn, dimmer, and windshield wipers.[24] These can be activated through a variety of switches that either can be placed on the hand control or can be controlled through elbow motion.

On-Road Assessment

Once the driver has been set up with primary controls in the evaluation vehicle, the ability to use these controls must be assessed through actual driving. This assessment is commonly referred to as the behind-the-wheel or on-road portion of the evaluation. The current industry standard is to accept the on-road driving test as the optimal measure of driving competence.[6,12,18,19,26] The **on-road evaluation** should be a minimum of 45 minutes long and no longer than 2 hours of actual driving time. A shorter period is inadequate for obtaining required information.

The driving instructor orients a driver in the use of adaptive driving equipment, maintains vehicle control by intervening for safety when necessary, and directs the route. A score sheet is recommended. Driving performance scores should reflect physical management of the vehicle, ability to use the adaptive equipment,[1] interaction with other traffic, adherence to rules of the road, and safety judgment.[12,25,28]

Driving Route

Driving routes used in assessment should incorporate a sampling of road conditions, traffic patterns, and unusual settings common to the local region. The driving route initially should allow the driver time to become familiar with the evaluation vehicle and adaptive equipment in a low-stimulation environment. This period of learning and accommodation will be longer for the novice or apprehensive driver. The assessment route

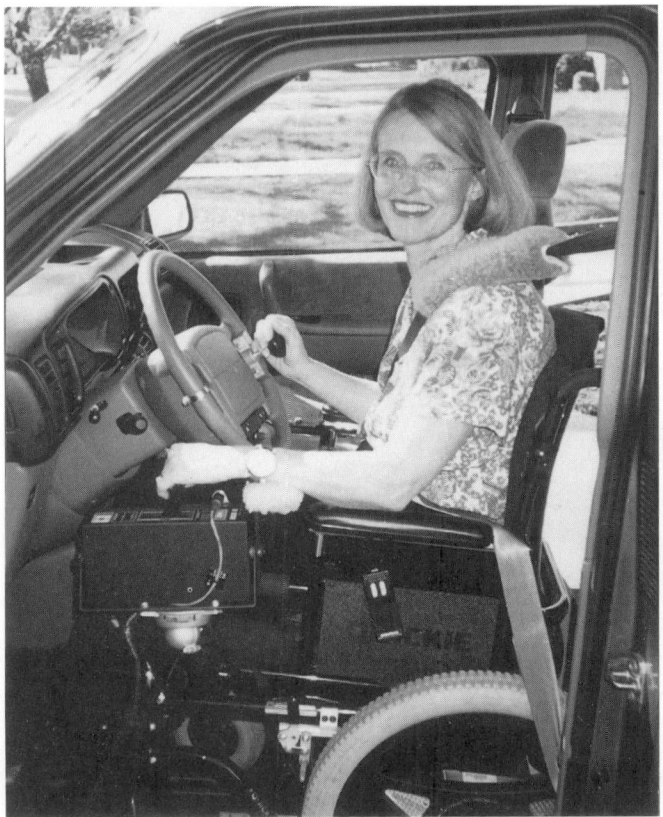

FIG. 14-23
Because of the progression of multiple sclerosis, client changed from driving a car with her feet to driving from her wheelchair using EMC's electronic gas-brake in a minivan. The device, in combination with low-effort steering, successfully reduced fatigue and pain while driving.

should progress through faster and more congested traffic and various traffic conditions to elicit information on the driver's skills in a wide variety of conditions. "Bailout" points are needed along the route for safety.

Driver Recommendations and Interventions

After the driving test is completed, the driving team reviews the results with the driver. Asking the driver for feedback before reviewing results provides a valuable perspective on the driver's insight. Involvement with professional organizations helps the therapist obtain knowledge to develop criteria for various recommendations. (See Box 14-3 for more information.)

The comprehensive driving report should contain a summary of the clinical assessment and a statement of the client's potential to be a safe and independent driver. The report should specify the type of vehicle necessary, the modifications needed, information about mobility equipment, dealer sources for providing the modifications, and other pertinent information. The report should include recommendations on the type of follow-up services required, what to look for, and who is best suited to provide the follow-up services. The report should also estimate the amount (duration, frequency and total length) of driver training needed, what specific areas of training should be emphasized, and where the training is available.[2,25]

Driver Training

Driver training is a key part of the comprehensive driver evaluation process and assistive technology delivery system.[8] Those with cognitive and perceptual impairments will often need to relearn driving behaviors or implement compensatory skills to obtain consistent driving performance, even though adaptive equipment may not be needed.[8] The use of high-tech equipment also necessitates extensive training, with a greater focus on the vehicle control and recovery, especially in unexpected situations and at high speeds.

Follow-Up Services

Follow-up services include midfit and final fitting sessions in the newly modified vehicle. A quality assurance and safety measure, follow-up service ensures that the equipment is located and adjusted to meet the client's functional needs. Follow-up service is important because delivery of the system to a driver marks the first time the system has been operated and adjustment is almost always needed.[8] An on-road session is recommended to make sure adjustments are adequate for function when dynamic forces within the driving environment come into play (Fig. 14-24).

Unsafe Driver

One of the most difficult tasks facing a driver evaluator is notifying a driver candidate that he or she is not able to drive safely. Such decisions need to be carefully reviewed and then communicated to the driver with compassion and understanding. Referring the driver to the motor vehicle department for a photo ID card in exchange for the driver's license and immediately providing materials on alternative transportation can prove helpful at a difficult time.

LEGAL ISSUES AND PUBLIC POLICY
State Laws Pertaining to Therapists

Therapists and physicians need to be aware of their **state's laws** concerning medical conditions and driving. Most states do not require the reporting of medical conditions, seizures, or loss of consciousness to the motor vehicle department.[19,28] Instead, most states rely on voluntary reporting of medical conditions by the driver who has the condition. Although some states advocate

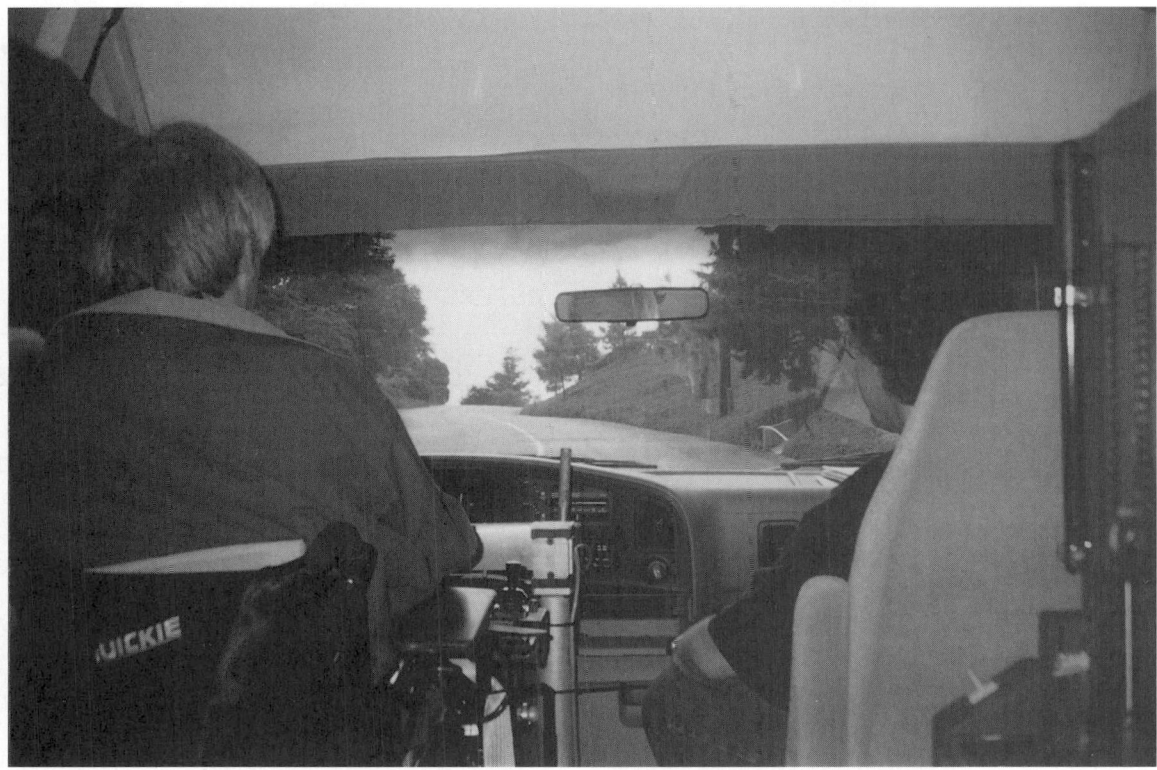

FIG. 14-24
Client, who must negotiate a steep hill near his home, completes a follow-up evaluation in his new Driving Systems, Inc. (dSi), unilever. A drive test in the foothills resulted in additional adjustments to the system before vehicle delivery.

reporting by the family, physician, or law enforcement officials, not all states provide immunity for such reporting. Once identified to the motor vehicle department, the patient undergoes a license review that varies from state to state.

SUMMARY

Community mobility, whether achieved by using public transportation or by driving one's own vehicle, is an important ADL. Individual evaluation, with consideration of valued occupational roles and local transportation options, provides a foundation for intervention. Many possibilities exist, given the range of ADA-mandated services, as well as available assistive technology, for assisting mobility-restricted individuals to move freely within their communities.

REVIEW QUESTIONS

SECTION 1

1. Define functional ambulation. List three activities of daily living or instrumental activities of daily living in which functional ambulation may occur.
2. Who provides gait training?

3. What is the role of the OT practitioner in functional ambulation?
4. How do the OT and PT practitioners collaborate in functional ambulation?
5. List and describe safety issues for functional ambulation.
6. Name five basic ambulation aids in order of most supportive to least supportive.
7. Discuss why great care should be taken during functional ambulation within the bathroom.
8. List at least three diagnoses for which functional ambulation may be appropriate as part of OT services.
9. What purpose does a task analysis serve in preparation for functional ambulation?
10. What suggestions could be made regarding carrying items during functional ambulation when an ambulation aid is used?

SECTION 2

1. What is the objective in measuring seat width?
2. What is the danger of having a wheelchair seat that is too deep?
3. What is the minimal distance for safety from the floor to the bottom of the wheelchair step plate?

4. List three types of wheelchair frames and the general uses of each.
5. Describe three types of wheelchair propulsion systems and tell when each would be used.
6. What are the advantages of detachable desk arms and swing-away footrests?
7. Discuss the factors for consideration before wheelchair selection.
8. Name and discuss the rationale for at least three general wheelchair safety principles.
9. Describe or demonstrate how to descend a curb in a wheelchair with the help of an assistant.
10. Describe or demonstrate how to descend a ramp in a wheelchair with the help of an assistant.
11. List four safety principles for correct moving and lifting technique during wheelchair transfers.
12. Describe or demonstrate the basic standing-pivot transfer from a bed to a wheelchair.
13. Describe or demonstrate the wheelchair-to-bed transfer, using a sliding board.
14. Describe the correct placement of a sliding board before a transfer.
15. In what circumstances would you use a sliding board transfer technique?
16. List the requirements for patient and therapist to perform the dependent transfer safely and correctly.
17. List two potential problems and solutions that can occur with the wheelchair-to-car transfer.
18. When is the mechanical lift transfer most appropriate?

SECTION 3

1. What are the differences between public and private transportation?
2. What are the treatment implications for transportation training on fixed routes? For paratransit?
3. Who should be referred for a driver evaluation?
4. What are the elements of vision screening for driving?
5. Which physical capacities are evaluated in the pre-driving assessment?
6. What cognitive skill is most predictive of poor driver safety and outcome?
7. Why is palming the wheel not advisable for steering? How does a steering device assist the disabled driver?
8. If a car is selected as the vehicle of choice, what type is usually recommended?
9. How long should the behind-the-wheel evaluation session be?
10. How would the experience level of a driver or diagnosis of a driver's condition affect the session length or total number of sessions needed?

11. Why is driver training recommended?
12. What legal issues must be considered by the occupational therapist performing a driving assessment?
13. How can the OTA be utilized in a driver evaluation program?
14. What additional credentials can therapists obtain in the field of driver rehabilitation?

REFERENCES

SECTION 1

1. Anderson KN, editor: *Mosby's medical, nursing and allied health dictionary*, ed 5, St Louis, 1998, Mosby.
2. Esquenazi A, Hirai B: Gait analysis in stroke and head injury. In Craik RL, Oatis CA, editors: *Gait analysis: theory and application*, St Louis, 1995, Mosby.
3. Higgins JR, Higgins S: The acquisition of locomotor skill. In Craik RL, Oatis CA, editors: *Gait analysis: theory and application*, St Louis, 1995, Mosby.
4. Leonard CT: The neurophysiology of human locomotion. In Craik RL, Oatis CA, editors: *Gait analysis theory and application*, St Louis, 1995, Mosby.
5. Moyers PA: Scope of occupational therapy, *Am J Occup Ther* 53(3):258-262, 1999.
6. Pierson FM: *Principles and techniques of patient care*, Philadelphia, 1994, WB Saunders.
7. Watson DE: *Task analysis: an occupational performance approach*, Bethesda, Md, 1997, American Occupational Therapy Association.

SECTION 2

1. Adler C: *Wheelchairs and seat cushions: a comprehensive guide for evaluation and ordering*, San Jose, Calif, 1987, Santa Clara Valley Medical Center, Occupational Therapy Department.
2. Adler C, Musik D, Tipton-Burton M: *Body mechanics and transfers: multidisciplinary cross training manual*, San Jose, Calif, 1994, Santa Clara Valley Medical Center.
3. Bromley I: *Tetraplegia and paraplegia: a guide for physiotherapists*, ed 3, London, 1985, Churchill Livingstone.
4. Pezenik D, Itoh M, Lee M: Wheelchair prescription. In Ruskin AP: *Current therapy in physiatry*, Philadelphia, 1984, WB Saunders.
5. Santa Clara Valley Medical Center, Physical Therapy Department: *Lifting and moving techniques*, San Jose, Calif, 1985, Santa Clara Valley Medical Center.
6. *Wheelchair prescription: measuring the patient* (Booklet no. 1), Camarillo, Calif, 1979, Everest & Jennings.
7. *Wheelchair prescription: wheelchair selection*, (Booklet no. 2), Camarillo, Calif, 1979, Everest & Jennings.
8. *Wheelchair prescription: safety and handling* (Booklet no. 3), Camarillo, Calif, 1983, Everest & Jennings.
9. Wilson AB, McFarland SR: *Wheelchairs: a prescription guide*, Charlottesville, Va, 1992, Rehabilitation Press.

SUGGESTED READINGS

Adler C: Equipment considerations. In Whiteneck et al: *Treatment of high quadriplegia*, New York, 1988, Demos Publications.
Bergen A, Presperin J, Tallman T: *Positioning for function*. Valhalla, NY, 1990, Valhalla Rehabilitation Publications.
Davies PM: *Steps to follow: a guide to the treatment of adult hemiplegia*, New York, 1985, Springer-Verlag.

Ford JR, Duckworth B: *Physical management for the quadriplegic patient*, Philadelphia, 1974, FA Davis.

Gee ZL, Passarella PM: *Nursing care of the stroke patient: a therapeutic approach*, Pittsburgh, Pa, 1985, A.R.E.N. Publications.

Hill JP, editor: *Spinal cord injury: a guide to functional outcomes in occupational therapy*, Rockville, Md, 1986, Aspen.

Outcomes following traumatic spinal cord injury: clinical practice guidelines for health-care professionals, consortium for spinal cord medicine, 1999, Paralyzed Veterans of America.

SECTION 3

1. American Association of Retired Persons: *Graduated driver licensing creating mobility choices*, Pub No D15109, Washington, DC, 1993, The Association.
2. Association of Driver Rehabilitation Specialists: Recommended practices for driver rehabilitation services. In *Members resource guide*, Edgerton, Wisc, 1996, The Association.
3. Babirad J: Considerations in seating and positioning severely disabled drivers, *Assist Technol* 1:31-37, 1989.
4. Blanc C, Hunt JT: Getting in gear, *Team Rehab Report* 33-39, August, 1994.
5. Beverly Foundation: *Community effectiveness in safeguarding at-risk senior drivers*, Interim Report, Pasadena, Calif, February, 1998, The Foundation.
6. Bouska MJ, Gallaway M: Primary visual deficits in adults with brain damage: management in occupational therapy, *Occup Ther Pract* 3(1):1-11, 1991.
7. Breske S: The drive for independence, *Adv/Rehabil* 3(8):10-19, 1994.
8. Cook AM, Hussey SM: *Assistive technologies: principles and practice*, St Louis, 1995, Mosby.
9. Eberhard J: *A national perspective on older adult transportation: safe mobility for life.* Presented at Older Adults and Transportation: The New Millennium Regional Forum, Los Angeles, July 22, 1999.
10. Golden M et al: *Explanation of the contents of the Americans With Disabilities Act of 1990*, Washington, DC, 1990, Disability Rights Education and Defense Fund.
11. Hopewell CA: Head injury rehabilitation: adaptive driving after TBI. In Burke WH et al, editors: *The HDI professional series on traumatic brain injury*, No 5, Houston, 1988, HDI.
12. Janke MK: *Age-related disabilities that may impair drivers and their assessment*, Sacramento, 1994, State of California Department of Motor Vehicles.
13. Kalina T: Starting a driver rehabilitation program, *Work* 8:229-238, 1997.
14. Kaplan W: The occupation of driving: legal and ethical issues, *Physical Disabilities Special Interest Quarterly* 22:1-3, 1999.
15. Latson LF: Overview of disabled drivers' evaluation process, *Physical Disabilities Special Interest Section Newsletter* 10(4), 1987.
16. Linden M, Sprigle S: Development of instrumentation and protocol to measure the dynamic environment of a modified van, *J Rehabil Res Dev* 33(1):23-29, 1999.
17. National Highway Traffic Safety Administration: *Air bags and on-off switches: information for an informed decision*, Pub No DOT HS 808 629, Washington, DC, 1999, US Department of Transportation.
18. Odenheimer GL: *Cognitive dysfunction and driving abilities*, Presentation to the annual meeting of the American Geriatrics Society, Atlanta, May 18, 1990.
19. Odenheimer GL et al: Performance-based driving evaluation of the elderly driver: safety, reliability, and validity, *Gerontol Med Sci* 49(4):M153-M159, 1994.
20. Owen MM, Stressel DL: Motor-free visual perception test as a screening tool for driver evaluation and rehabilitation readiness, *Physical Disabilities Special Interest Section Quarterly* 22:3-4, 1999.
21. Perr A, Barnicle K: Van lifts: the ups and downs and ins and outs, *Team Rehabil Rep* 49-53, 1993.
22. Persson D: The elderly driver: deciding when to stop, *Gerontologist* 33(1): 88-91, 1993.
23. Reuben DB, St George P: Driving dementia: California's approach to a medical and policy dilemma, *West J Med* 164:111-121, 1996.
24. Roush L, Koppa R: *A survey of activation importance of individual secondary controls in modified vehicles*, 1992, Human Factors Program, Safety Division, Texas Transportation Institute, Texas A & M University.
25. Sabo S, Shipp M: *Disabilities and their implications for driving*, Ruston, 1989, Louisiana Tech University Center for Rehabilitation Sciences and Biomedical Engineering.
26. State of California Department of Rehabilitation, Mobility Evaluation Program: *Statement of assurances for providers of driver evaluation services*, Downey, 1990.
27. Strano CM: Driver evaluation and training of the physically disabled driver: additional comments, *Physical Disabilities Special Interest Section Quarterly* 10(4), 1987.
28. Summary of proceedings of the Conference on Driver Competency Assessment, CAL-DMV-RSS-91-132, Sacramento, 1993, State of California Department of Motor Vehicles, Program and Policy Administration, Research and Development Section.
29. Taira ED, editor: *Assessing the driving ability of the elderly*, Binghamton, NY, 1989, Hayworth Press.
30. Taylor H, Harris L: N.O.D. survey of Americans with disabilities: the new competitive advantage: expanding the participation of people with disabilities in the American work force. Reprinted from *Business Week*, May 20, 1994, Washington, DC, National Organization on Disability.

CHAPTER 15

Sexuality and Physical Dysfunction

GORDON UMPHRED BURTON

KEY TERMS

Sensuality
Sexuality
Self-perception
Emasculation
Sexual harassment
Sexual values
Sexual history
New body
Sexual abuse
Erogenous
Vaginal atrophy
Reflexogenic erection
Sexually transmitted diseases
Autonomic dysreflexia
Permission, limited information, specific suggestions, and intensive therapy
Basic sex education

LEARNING OBJECTIVES

After studying this chapter the student or practitioner will be able to do the following:

1. Justify sexuality as a concern of the occupational therapist.
2. List at least five possible reactions of the person with physical disability to his or her sexuality.
3. List some attitudes and assumptions that the able-bodied population may make about the sexuality of people with physical disability.
4. Discuss how sexuality and sensuality are related to self-esteem and a sense of attractiveness.
5. Define sexual harassment and describe how to handle a situation in which clients harass staff in the treatment facility.
6. Describe the effects that such items as mobility aids and splints can have on sexuality.
7. List signs of potential sexual abuse of adults.
8. List at least two treatment goals that are designed to improve sexual functioning.
9. Discuss ways in which the occupational therapist can provide a safe environment for discussing sexual issues.
10. Describe how sexual values can be communicated.
11. List at least five effects that physical dysfunction can have on sexual functioning and possible solutions for each.
12. Discuss the potential hazards of birth control.
13. List the potential complications of pregnancy and childbirth for a woman with disability.
14. Discuss methods of sex education.
15. Define PLISSIT.

Sensuality and **sexuality** are important aspects of everyone's activities of daily living (ADL) and directly relate to the quality of each person's life. As an ADL, sexual functioning is in the domain of occupational therapy (OT). Occupational therapists work with clients in all areas related to sensuality and sexuality (Box 15-1).

Physical limitations may cause the client to question his or her ability to experience sexual pleasure. With the onset of physical disability, the client undergoes a significant change in the commonly held roles and practices of the able-bodied population.[6,36,45] The individual with disability may be regarded by able-bodied persons as asexual, an object of pity, and unattractive.[3,25] Being perceived as unattractive and possibly unlovable can cause the client to believe that he or she can never be intimate with anyone. Holding this belief can lead the client and related others to a sense of despair.

Charlifue and associates[7] and Kettl and associates[24] found that females with acquired spinal cord injuries reported feeling less than half as attractive after they had acquired the disability, even though spinal cord injury is a disability in which there is little observable physical change in body appearance. These studies showed that there was a major decrease in the **self-perception** of attractiveness. Another study found that with the advent of a disability, males felt a loss of their sense of masculinity and sensed a threat to the male role.[35]

These are just a few examples of the feelings and perceptions that affect the sensuality and sexuality of the person who has a physical disability. To accomplish comprehensive rehabilitation with the client, the occupational therapist and other health professionals must address self-perception, beliefs, and needs related to sexuality. This chapter examines issues related to sexuality and sensuality with physical disability.

REACTIONS TO SEXUALITY AND DISABILITY

The many obstacles encountered by people with disability should not interfere with the expression of sensuous and sexual needs. As an informed professional, each therapist can help the adult client eliminate unnecessary obstacles, overcome anxieties, and appreciate personal uniqueness. The expression of sexuality or sensuality is a sign of self-confidence, self-validation, and a sense of being lovable. When a person acquires a disability or is born with a disability, he or she can feel less positive about self and less lovable.[34,35]

Sexuality can symbolize how a person is dealing with the world. If a person feels inadequate as a sexual, sensual, and lovable human being, the motivation to pursue other avenues of life can be affected. When an individual has a negative self-image, coping with life's problems is difficult. Because sexuality is often used as a barometer of how one feels about oneself, it is productive for the therapist to help the client feel as positive as possible about his or her physical and personal qualities. A healthy attitude toward one's sexuality enhances motivation for all aspects of therapy. The therapist must try to help the client adjust self-perceptions enough to function positively in life.

Sexuality has been found to be a predictor of marital satisfaction, adjustment to physical disability, and success of vocational training. In society, people are often judged by physical attractiveness.[36] In Western civilization, physical intimacy is closely associated with love. Therefore, if a person perceives himself or herself as incapable of expressing sensuality or sexuality, it is possible that he or she feels incapable of loving and being loved. Without the capability of loving and being loved, there may be a sense of isolation and of being valueless.[4,32,34]

Adaptive devices such as braces, wheelchairs, and communication aids can be a detriment to one's perceived attractiveness and sexuality. For example, it may be hard to perceive oneself as sexual when there is an indwelling catheter or when braces are worn. By discussing the effects of these devices on social interaction, the client can get some ideas about how to handle difficult situations when they arise.[1,28,32,47]

The treatment goals are to facilitate an increase in self-esteem and enable the client to feel lovable. The therapist's role is to foster feelings of self-worth and productivity and to help minimize feelings of worthlessness and hopelessness.[4,15,34,36] Feeling lovable engenders a sense of self-worth, attractiveness, sensuality, sexuality, and being capable of intimacy. Achieving this goal enhances the development of a healthy and realistic life balance (Fig. 15-1).

BOX 15-1

Factors Related to Sexuality and Sensuality

- Quality of life
- Role delineation
- Cultural aspects
- Impulse control
- Energy conservation
- Muscle weakness
- Hypertonicity and hypotonicity
- Appreciation of body
- Psychosocial issues
- Range of motion
- Joint protection
- Motor control
- Cognition
- Increased or decreased sensation

SEXUALITY AND DISABILITY

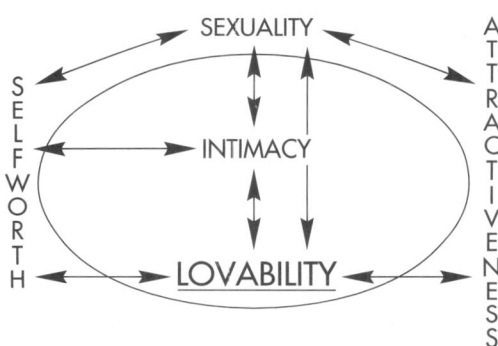

FIG. 15-1
Sexuality and disability.

Whether sex is still possible is a concern that arises after the onset of physical disability. This concern is often set aside in the immediacy of coping with the adjustment to hospital life and activities that make up the daily routine. But the concern is not forgotten. A common complaint made about medical staff by people with disabilities is that the staff never deal with or let people with disability deal with the topic of their sexuality. People with disabilities feel that if their sensuality and sexuality are negated, a significant facet of their personhood is negated. This lack of acceptance causes the person with a disability to lose the feeling that he or she is treated as a whole person.

For both men and women with disabilities, the increased dependence on an able-bodied partner results in a decrease in sex life.[14] One possible explanation is that the able-bodied partner is less inclined to be aroused when he or she has just bathed the partner or assisted the partner with toileting. The therapist must be sensitive to the possibility of these perceptions and help the client deal appropriately with the feelings they evoke.

The client's sense of masculinity or femininity may be threatened by the disability.[29,35,38] Men who have recently acquired a disability report that they feel emasculated.[35,38] Feelings of **emasculation** can be reinforced by physical limitations. For example, lifting weights may no longer be possible, sports participation might not be possible without adaptations, and attendance at sporting events may be limited by lack of access. The necessity to look up at others from a wheelchair and ask for assistance can engender feelings of dependency.

A man with a disability may react to feelings of dependency and emasculation[35] by flirting to prove his masculinity. The client may attempt to flirt or make passes at a therapist. Because it is estimated that up to 10% of the population is homosexual, the therapist can expect that at some time there may be sexual advances from clients of the same sex.

Women experience many of the same feelings but probably interpret and react to them in a different way. Women with disability report feeling unattractive and undesirable. This can lead to despair if a woman feels that she cannot achieve some of her major goals in life. Thus, the female client may flirt to see if she is still attractive to others.

It is important for the therapist to realize that the client is seeking confirmation of his or her sexuality. The therapist should not be surprised by flirtations or sexual advances and should deal with them in a positive and professional manner. All of the therapist's interactions should be directed toward creating an environment that promotes the client's self-esteem, positive and appropriate sexuality, and adjustment to disability.

When responding to the client, the therapist should be alert to the client's current sexuality issues to prevent doing further damage to the client's sense of self. If the therapist rejects or ridicules the client, the client might hesitate to attempt such confirmation of personal attractiveness in future situations that are more socially appropriate. If the therapist rejects the client, the client might deduce that if someone who is familiar with persons who have disabilities is rejecting, then one who is unfamiliar with them would not be likely to be accepting either.

Inappropriate sexual advances, **sexual harassment,** or exploitation of either the therapist or the client cannot be permitted.[30,41] Behavior is considered harassment when it causes the therapist to feel threatened, intimidated, or treated as a sexual object. If sexual harassment is allowed, it can be damaging to the client and to staff morale.[18] The therapist should provide direct feedback explaining that he or she feels offended and that the behavior is inappropriate and must cease. All of the staff should be informed and develop and implement a plan to modify the client's behavior if it persists.

Therapeutic Communication

Conversations regarding sexuality can be good occasions for discussing personal feelings and perceptions. One way to approach discussion of intimate matters is by asking the client how she will perform breast self-examination with her disability. A male client can be asked how he will perform self-examination of the testicles. If the treatment facility does not have information about these examinations, the client can obtain them from the local Planned Parenthood Association. Each of these activities falls into the domain of health maintenance and may not have been discussed by health team members. This interaction will set the stage for discussion of other personal matters, impress upon the client the necessity for concern about personal health, and reaffirm the client's sexual identity.

Clients often feel safe asking the occupational therapist about sexual matters related to their disabilities.

because the therapist deals with other intimate activities such as bathing, dressing, and toileting. It is also important to discuss sexual hygiene as an ADL. The trust built up in the relationship encourages this communication. The therapist should be prepared with information and resources. The therapist does not need to know everything or be a sex counselor but should see that the client gets the necessary information or referral.

The occupational therapist is the most appropriate professional to solve some problems, such as motor performance needed for sexual activity.[8] For example, discussing positioning to reduce pain or spasticity or to enable the client to more comfortably engage in sexual relations will help the client deal with problems before they occur.[11,26,32]

During all aspects of the rehabilitation process, the client needs to work on communication with the therapist, staff, and his or her sexual partner. The therapist can facilitate this process simply by giving the client permission to discuss feelings and potential problems, especially sexual problems. The client needs to learn how to accurately communicate sexual needs, desires, and position options to a partner, either verbally or nonverbally, to have a mutually satisfactory sexual relationship.[24] Each client will have unique problems or issues that are related to the nature of the disability. An example is a client with Parkinson's disease in whom the lack of facial expression impedes the nonverbal communication of intimacy. The client can be taught to communicate feelings verbally that were previously conveyed with facial expressions.

Discussion of sexuality is a way to explore feelings of dependency, identity, attractiveness, and unattractiveness. Communication must be established regarding the feelings of sexual role changes. If a client's perceived roles are threatened, this situation should be dealt with as early as possible in treatment. If it is not, the effects could persist throughout the client's life.

VALUES CLARIFICATION

Sexual values of the client, the partner, and the therapist must be examined for the therapist to interact with the client in the most effective and positive manner.[3,13,29,32,36] Many professional schools do not train health care workers on the subject of sexuality and disability.[3,17,38,42] In-service training can be arranged to help the staff be aware of the sexual needs of people with disability.[16,24] Books, articles, videotapes, and training packets are available for professional education.[5,12,13,38]

Unless the staff is educated about the significance of sexuality and related issues, they could have negative feelings about dealing with these matters.[3,5,42,46] If the therapist is not aware of the thoughts and feelings of all of the individuals involved, the therapist could make in-

correct assumptions that have negative results.[11] One of the most direct ways of gaining information is by taking a **sexual history**.[11,38,39] The purpose of a sexual history is to learn how a person thinks and feels about sex and bodily functions as well as to discover the needs of those concerned.[11,27,38] According to some researchers, many individuals with a disability had a sexual dysfunction before they acquired the physical disability. Taking the sexual history can help to identify such a problem.[28]

SEXUAL HISTORY

When taking a sexual history, the therapist should create an environment that will allow for confidentiality, comfort, and self-expression. In early intervention, the therapist should ask about the client's concerns regarding contraception, safe sex, homosexuality, masturbation, sexual health, aging, menopause, and physical changes.

Following are some questions that could be asked. All questions should not be asked at the same time, nor would all questions be asked of every client.

- How did you first find out about sexuality?
- When and how did you first learn about heterosexuality and homosexuality?
- Who furnished you with information about sexuality when you were young?
- Were you ready for the information when you first heard about sexuality?
- How important is sexuality at this time in your life?
- How would you describe your sexual activities at this time?
- How do you feel sexuality expresses your feelings and meets your needs and those of others?
- If you could change aspects of your current sexual situation, what would you change and how would you change it?
- What concerns do you have about birth control, disease control, and sexual safety?
- What physical, medical, or drug-related concerns do you have relating to your sexuality?
- Have you ever been pressured, threatened, or forced into a sexual situation?
- Which sexual practices have you engaged in, in the past (e.g., oral, anal, and genital)?
- Do you consider certain sexual activities "kinky"? How do you feel about participating in such activities?
- How important do you think sexuality will be in your future?
- What concerns do you have about your sexuality?
- Are there questions or concerns that you have regarding this interview?

After taking the sexual history, the therapist can often ascertain whether there is guilt connected with the sex act, body parts, or sexual alternatives (such as masturbation, oral sex, sexual positions, or sexual devices). For example, some clients report feelings of guilt or fear in relation to having sex after a heart attack or a stroke—fear that sex can cause a stroke or guilt at the notion that it might have caused the first episode. Another fear is that the partner will not accept the presence of catheters, adaptive equipment, or scars. Performance is often an issue. "Can the person with a disability do it?" is the question asked by able-bodied persons and persons with disability alike.

The therapist can furnish the necessary information by (1) directing the client to other professionals, (2) providing magazines and books that discuss the subject, (3) showing movies, or (4) suggesting role models. The therapist must be tactful and remember that the client is probably questioning his or her own values and previous notions about sexuality. Personal care such as toileting, personal hygiene, menstrual hygiene, bathing, and birth control are all issues that can evoke reflection on values regarding sex and body image.

Self-care issues usually are not emphasized enough during acute illness and rehabilitation. Discussing such issues once or twice is not enough. The circumstances and environment in which these issues are discussed should also be considered. The therapist must create an environment that will allow personal discussions to occur. A personal conversation cannot take place in a crowded treatment room, during a rushed and impersonal treatment session, or with a therapist with whom there is not a good personal rapport. Building rapport is a problem in health care facilities in which therapists are frequently rotated or work on a per-diem basis.

A discussion of feelings will also help the client explore his or her **new body** or adapt to ongoing degeneration of the body if there is a progressive disability. These conversations may take place while other therapeutic activities are in progress, so that billing insurers for time is not a barrier.

SEXUAL ABUSE

The **sexual abuse** of adults with disabilities is a considerable problem.[1,40,42,46] Some people who have disabilities have reported being approached by pimps representing prostitution rings that specialize in providing people with disabilities for their customers. Clients should be made aware of the possibility of this type of exploitation. Others have reported that medical staff took inappropriate liberties with them and that attendants on whom they depended demanded sexual favors. Clients can and should report such abuse to Adult Protective Services. The therapist also must report cases of suspected sexual abuse. The client may be reluctant to report abuse because of a concern that it will not be possible to get another aide or that, during the time it takes to hire another aide, essential assistance will not be available. These are major problems for a person who is dependent on others for care.

Therapists usually do not suspect caregivers, medical staff, aides, transportation assistants, or volunteers of sexual abuse, but the therapist should be alert to signs of possible abuse even from these sources.[37] It is a fact of life that some individuals prey on adults and children with disabilities and are drawn to the health fields with this motive.[1] The therapist should watch for signs of potential abuse, such as clients usually being upset after interacting with a specific person, caregivers taking clients off alone for no apparent reason, excessive touching in a sensual manner by caregivers, the client being agitated when around a particular individual, and the client being overly compliant with a specific individual.

Therapists must increase their awareness of what constitutes sexual abuse. Children with disabilities have long been expected to undress and be examined or treated as part of their medical care. This treatment is sometimes necessary, but the preferences and dignity of the client should be respected at all times. A person of any age should not be forced to endure humiliation.

The therapy session should help the client develop a sense of personal ownership of his or her body. This goal may be neglected when working with adults and is often neglected in working with children. For example, a child who believes that he or she does not have the right to say no to being touched, who cannot physically resist unwanted advances, and who may not be able to communicate that abuse has taken place makes a good victim.[1]

The therapist should ask permission before touching the client and should touch with respect and maintain the client's sense of dignity. If the therapist does not ask permission to touch a client, the client can lose the sense of control over being touched by others. The therapist should guard against communicating this notion to the client.

Naming body parts and body processes is a good way of helping clients take charge of their bodies. Once the body parts and processes are named, using correct terminology rather than slang, there is the possibility for the client to communicate and to relate in an appropriate manner.[1,10,31,39] The use of the proper terms has the effect of helping the client view the body in a more positive way, whereas slang tends to communicate negative images.[39]

EFFECTS OF PHYSICAL DYSFUNCTION

Specific physical problems that may create difficulties in sexual performance for people with disabilities and their partners and suggestions for management of the problems are outlined below and summarized in Table 15-1.

TABLE 15-1
Conditions and Possible Effects on Sexual Functioning

								Symptom							Poor		
Diagnosis	Anxiety/Fear	Contrac-tures	Cultural Barriers	Decreased Libido	Depres-sion	Impo-tence	Inconti-nence	Limited ROM	Loss of Mobility	Loss of Sensa-tion	Low En-durance	Medica-tion	Paralysis/Spasticity	Body Image	Tremor	Catheter/Ostomy
Ampu-tations	X	X	X		X				X	X				X		
Arthritis	X	X	X	X	X			X	X		X	X		X	X	
Burns	X	X	X		X			X	X	X	X		X	X		
Cardiac disease	X		X	X	X	X			X		X	X		X		
Cerebral palsy	X	X	X		X		X	X	X	X	X		X	X	X	X
CVA	X	X	X	X	X	X	X	X	X	X	X	X	X	X	X	X
Diabetes	X		X	X	X	X		X	X	X	X			X	X	
Hand injury	X	X	X		X				X					X		
Head injury	X	X	X	X	X†	X	X	X	X	X	X	X	X	X	X	X
Musculo-skeletal	X	X	X		X		X	X	X	X	X	X	X	X	X	
Spinal cord injury	X	X	X	X	X	X	X	X	X	X	X	X	X	X	X	X

X, possible involvement. *CVA*, cerebrovascular accident. *ROM*, range of motion.
*Fear of medication as possible causes.
†Increased or decreased.

Hypertonia

Hypertonia can increase when muscles are stretched. To prevent quick stretching of muscles involved in a movement pattern, motion should be performed slowly. It is advisable to incorporate rotation into the movement to break up the spasticity. Slow rocking can be used to inhibit hypertonic musculature. Gentle shaking or slow stroking (massage) can also be inhibitory. Heat or cold can also be used to inhibit tone. Clients with hypertonia should review options for different positions in which to have sexual intercourse. Alternative ways of dealing with personal hygiene (e.g., toileting, inserting tampons, gynecological examinations, and birth control) may also need to be explored in relation to hypertonicity.

Hypotonia

Clients with low muscle tone (hypotonia) need physical support during sexual activity. Pillows, towels, or bolsters may be used to support body parts, allowing for endurance and protecting the body from overstretching and fatigue. Sexual positions that allow support of the joints involved should be explored. The client and his or her partner should also explore their attitudes about the positions.

Low Endurance

Prolonged sexual activity can be intolerable because of low physical endurance. Some techniques for dealing with low endurance are employing principles of work simplification to sexual activity, using timing to engage in sex when the client has the most energy, and assuming positions in which sexual performance uses less energy.

Loss of Mobility and Contractures

Limited mobility and contractures prohibit many movement patterns and limit the number of positions for sex. Activity analysis must be done to find positions that will allow sexual activity. This system often requires creative problem solving on the part of the client, the partner, and the responsible professional counselor.

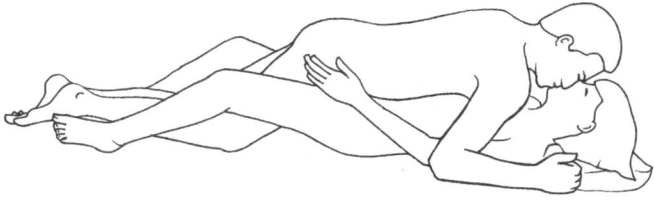

FIG. 15-2
This position places pressure on female's bladder and requires hip abduction but little energy expenditure for her.

Joint Degeneration

Conditions such as arthritis can cause pain, damage to the joints, and contractures. Avoiding stress and repetitive weight bearing on the joints can decrease joint damage. Activity analysis is needed to reduce joint stress and excessive weight bearing on the joints. It is necessary to find a position, such as that shown in Fig. 15-2, that takes weight and stress off the knees or hips. A position with limited hip adduction might not be acceptable for the client, in which case a side-lying position may be more acceptable. If hip abduction is limited, the woman should avoid positions such as those shown in Figs. 15-2, 15-5, and 15-9.

Pain

Pain limits the enjoyment of sexual activities.[21] There is usually a time of day at which pain is diminished and energy is at its highest. Sexual activities can be scheduled for such times. After pain medication has taken effect, many people find that sexual activity is possible. Communication between partners is especially important when pain is involved. An unaffected partner who does not understand the negative effects of pain may believe that the affected partner is not considering his or her personal needs. A referral to a counselor who understands the effects of pain can help work out emotional aspects of this problem. The occupational therapist can help the client think of acceptable ways of meeting the partner's sexual needs without causing pain. Masturbation and mutual masturbation with sexual fantasy are possible ways of meeting sexual

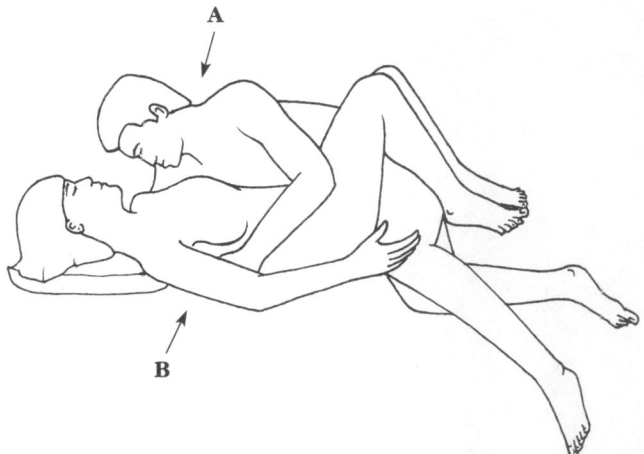

FIG. 15-3
Vaginal entry of B requires no hip abduction, and hip flexion tightness would not impede performance. Energy requirements for both parties is minimal. Bladder pressure, catheter safety, and stoma appliance safety should not be an issue in this position for B. This position may be recommended if B has back pain or is paralyzed, especially if roll is used to support lumbar spine.

needs in these circumstances. In this way the partners are interacting and neither person feels isolated.

Loss of Sensation

The loss of sensation can affect the sexual relationship in several ways. The lack of **erogenous** sensation in the affected area can block proper warning that an area is being abraded (e.g., the vagina not being sufficiently lubricated) or damaged (e.g., bladder or even bones if the partner is on top and being too forceful). A lack of sensation may be a sign of disruption of the reflex loop responsible for sensation and erections in the male and sensation and lubrication in the female.

Aging and Sexuality

With aging, changes take place that can affect sexuality. Menopause and the resulting hormonal changes cause **vaginal atrophy** and slower reactions to sexual stimulation. In the male, greater stimulation may be needed to develop and maintain an erection, and reaction time between erections may be greater. Partners can be informed of ways to increase stimulation and can be helped to understand that it is the quality, not the quantity, of sexual activity that is important in the relationship. The client should be made aware of the maturation process and its normal effect on sexuality so that the disability is not blamed for all of the problems.

Isolation

The environment is composed of objects, persons, and events. In all activities there is an interaction between the person and environment. Some of the objects with which people with disabilities interact are wheelchairs, braces, canes, crutches, and splints. These objects are all hard, cold, and angular. They can communicate a hard exterior and a fragile interior and can convey the notion that there is no softness, that it is not safe to hug, and that a person in a wheelchair or in braces or on crutches can get hurt or toppled if touched. As a result of these ideas, the individual with a disability may feel isolated by the appliances.

Some people tend to withdraw from the objects around the client. This may reinforce the client's notion of a lack of sensuousness and increase the client's sense of isolation. Clients often feel isolated and different from the "normal" population. This phenomenon is more common among clients who have been out of the health care facility for a period of time. In the early phases of the disability, the therapist and the client can role-play about how to deal with a new partner or how to explain equipment used, such as a catheter. This approach may help ease the client's fears and increase the client's comfort with such issues. At the same time the therapist is com-

municating that sex may be a possibility in the future. It should be pointed out to clients that there has never been a time in human history that people with disabilities did not exist in society, that they are a part of society, and that it is not "abnormal" to have disability. All people who live long enough will acquire a disability to a greater or lesser extent at some time.

Medication

Potential side effects of medication are impotence, delayed sexual response, or other problems. Diuretics and antihypertensives can cause impotence, decreased libido, and loss of orgasm. Tranquilizers and antidepressants can contribute to decreased libido and even impotence in some individuals.[38] Side effects of medication should be discussed with the physician and the pharmacist to see whether medications can be altered or changed. If they cannot, acknowledging that the problem is organic can be helpful to the client.

Performance Anxiety

At times of great emotional stress, a male client might find that the erection is inhibited. This problem can

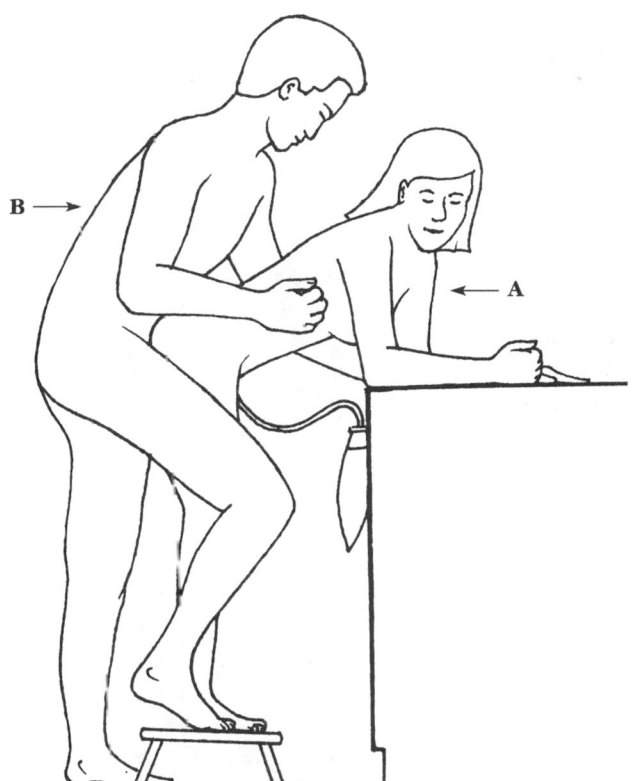

FIG. 15-4
Partner A needs little hip abduction but good strength. Partner B may find decreased strain on his back. Hip, knee, or ankle joint degeneration would preclude this position for either partner.

lead to increased anxiety in relation to sexuality and create a cycle of dysfunctional inhibition. It can be helpful for the client and his partner to take the focus off erection and genital intercourse and focus on sensuality and making each other feel good. A massage is one possibility that will allow for more normal physiological reactions. If this approach does not work, a trained counselor may be needed to help deal with the problem, if it has been determined that the problem is not organic in nature.

Skin Care

The person with a disability should be informed that positioning modifications might be needed to protect the skin, prevent skin breakdown, and increase pleasure. If a sexual position causes repeated rubbing on the skin, this friction can cause abrasions and result in skin damage. The therapist and client can discuss methods to prevent the friction—through an alternative position, for example. Pressure on bony prominences or pressure exerted in a specific area by a partner can also cause problems with skin irritation and must be avoided.

Lubrication

Stimulating natural lubrication in female clients is important. It might be overlooked in a woman with paralysis because she may not be able to feel the stimulation or lack of natural lubrication. There should be stimulation to cause reflexive lubrication even when the woman does not feel it. Without proper lubrication, damage may occur without awareness of the problem. If needed, artificial water-based lubricants (such as K-Y Jelly) should be introduced. The individual should be warned that only water-based lubricants are appropriate because petroleum-based lubricants can cause irritation and can attack latex condoms, causing condom failure. This is a major concern, since the female partner is more likely than the male to become infected with the human immunodeficiency virus (HIV) in any given heterosexual encounter.

Erection

Many men regard the ability to achieve an erection as one of the most significant signs of masculinity.[35] If awareness of sensory stimulation to the penis is blocked by the sensory loss associated with paralysis and the male client does not try to stimulate a reflexogenic erection, he might believe that he is impotent. This is not necessarily true, and the client may go through much needless anguish. The client should be encouraged to explore his body. Rubbing the penis, the thighs, or the anus can be effective ways to evoke a **reflexogenic erection.** Even rubbing the big toe has been reported by some men with quadriplegia to stimulate an erection. If

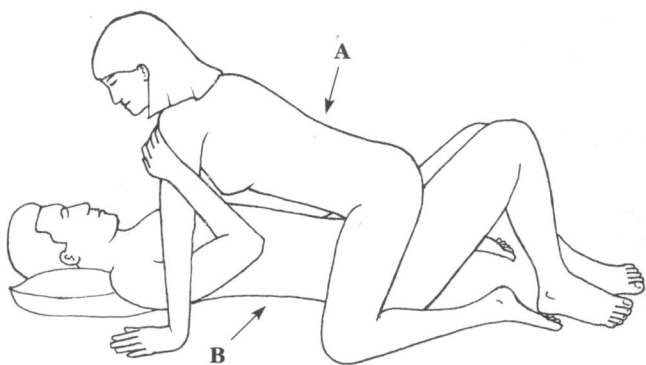

FIG. 15-5

Person *A* must have hip abduction, balance, and endurance but pressure is off of bladder and stoma. If catheter is used it would be unrestricted. Back pain may be avoided by keeping trunk vertical. Person *B*'s hip flexors could be contracted. If low back pain is a problem, legs should be flexed and roll placed under low back. If stoma appliance is used, this position would prevent interference. If low endurance is a problem, this position can be used effectively for *B*.

the normal reflex arc is interrupted, it is usually not possible to achieve an erection, and alternative methods must be explored.

Alternative methods can be forms of sex that do not require an erect penis, such as using a vibrator or trying oral or digital sex. If the client feels that penile intercourse is the only acceptable method, there are other possibilities.* Injections of hormones that stimulate erections can be used, but this practice might have adverse reactions or lead to problems if the client does not have good judgment or lacks hand dexterity. The use of a vacuum tube is sometimes effective and is one of the less invasive techniques.[39] Surgical implants can be used but have disadvantages, such as the possibility of infection and skin breakdown. With a physician's prescription the use of Viagra is a possibility for some clients.

Birth Control

The client should consult with his or her physician in weighing the pros and cons of various methods of birth control. People with disabilities must consider a number of factors when planning birth control.[8,9,19,26,31] Since most disabling conditions do not impair fertility (especially for women), it is important for the client to be aware of birth control and potential complications of the use of birth control.

Condoms require good use of the hands. An applicator can be adapted in some cases, but someone with good hand dexterity must assemble the device beforehand. Diaphragms are not very feasible for people who

---

An excellent discussion of these alternatives can be found in *Sexuality and Disability* 12:1, 1994.

have poor hand function unless the partner does have hand function and both parties feel comfortable about inserting the diaphragm as part of foreplay. The contraceptive sponge also requires good use of hands.

Using birth control pills can increase the risk of thrombosis, especially when the client is paralyzed or has impaired mobility. If the client has decreased sensation, the intrauterine device (IUD) can result in complications from bleeding, cramping, puncturing of the uterus, or infection. The use of spermicides requires good control of the hands or the assistance of the partner who has normal hand function. In using any method of birth control, the client must always be concerned with decreasing the chance of infection and with practicing safe sex.

Adaptive Aids

There might be a need to make use of adaptive aids, especially if the client lacks hand function. One aid is a vibrator for foreplay or masturbation.[17] Special devices have been adapted for men and women.[11,26,31] Pillows may be used for positioning, and other equipment may be used for clients who have special needs. The therapist must prepare the client for the concept of using sexual aids before suggesting the option to the client. For example, the therapist can suggest that the client privately explore the sensation that the vibrator produces in the lower extremities. The client might discover the possible use of the vibrator for sexual stimulation or at least, when told how it can be used, may be more open to the idea of using a vibrator as a sexual aid.

Safe Sex

The issue of safe sex has increased considerably since the advent of acquired immune deficiency syndrome (AIDS). Safe sex is important to protect against all forms of **sexually transmitted diseases** (STDs).[19] Clients need to be advised that this is an important issue. If there is a sensory impairment in and around the genital area, the person might not be aware of an abrasion or infection. Having any genital irritation or infection allows easy entrance for STDs. The person with disability must be informed of the increased risk for HIV and STDs so that extra caution can be taken.

Hygiene

Catheter care is a concern, especially when hand function is impaired. Questions may be raised regarding how or if a person with an indwelling catheter can have sex. Sex is possible for both men and women, but some precautions should be taken. If the catheter becomes kinked or closed off (which will definitely happen in the case of a catheterized man having vaginal intercourse), pressure should not be placed on the bladder. The bladder should be fully voided before sexual activity. Urine flow should be restricted for as short at time as possible and no more than 30 minutes. Damage to the bladder and kidneys could result if these precautions are not followed. The client should not drink fluids for at least 2 hours before sex to prevent the bladder filling during this time. Sexual positions that avoid placing pressure on the bladder should be used (Figs. 15-3 to 15-10). Many of the same positions can be used if the client uses a stoma appliance.

A person with an impairment of bowel or bladder function may have an occasional episode of incontinence during sexual activities. If the client and the therapist discuss this possibility and how to deal with it, some embarrassment can be averted when it occurs. The client and therapist can do role-playing to explore various scenarios such as, "You are planning intimacy

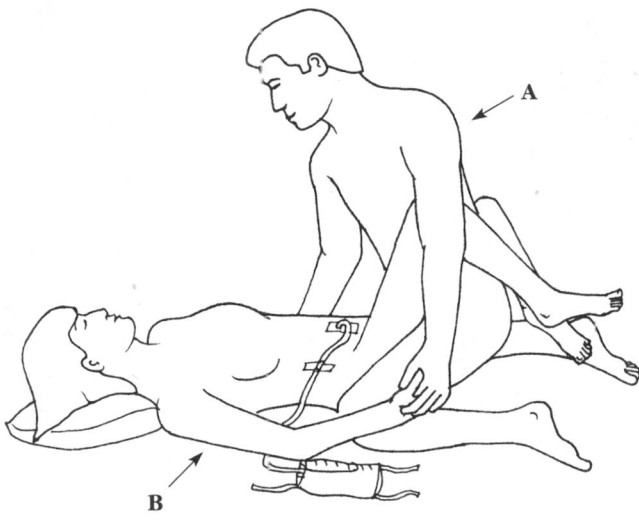

FIG. 15-6
This position keeps pressure off bladder, lessens chance of tubing becoming bent, reduces pressure on back (especially if small roll is used under low back), and does not require B to use much energy. Legs do not need to be as high as is shown, but if hip flexors are contracted, this position may be comfortable.

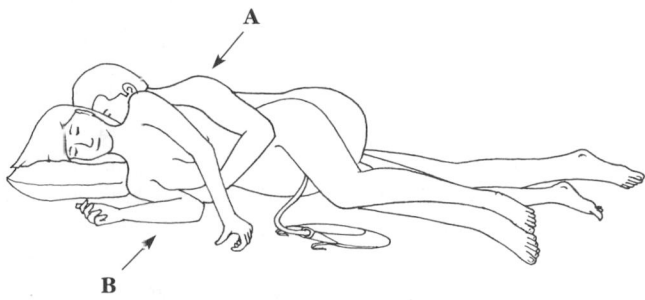

FIG. 15-7
Partner B need not expend much energy in this position. Both partners may avoid swayback in this position. Either person may have hemiparesis. Person B will not need hip abduction, and pressure on stoma bag may be avoided.

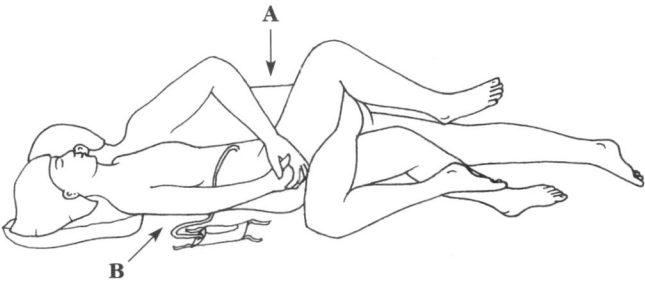

FIG. 15-8
This position can be used if either partner has hemiparesis. If low endurance is a problem, this position can be used. Person A may avoid swayback in this position.

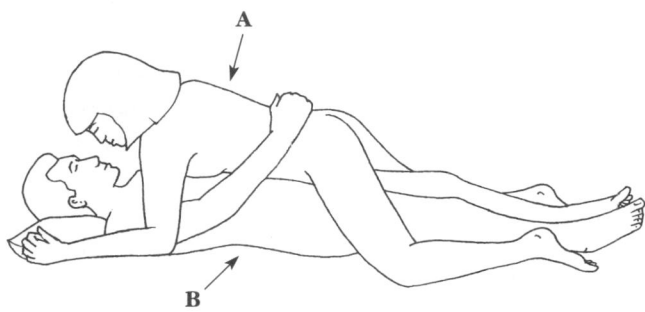

FIG. 15-9
Partner B can be paralyzed or have limited range of motion. His back may need roll for support, and he must be concerned with pressure on his bladder.

with a new partner. How will you explain your catheter and appliances to the person?" These might be awkward conversations for the therapist and the client, but dealing with these issues beforehand is usually easier than waiting for the situation to arise. Such topics must be approached with caution and discretion.

Pregnancy, Delivery, and Child Care

Before becoming pregnant, women must weigh the risks and benefits of pregnancy, childbirth, and child care. Complications of pregnancy might affect the client's function and mobility. These include the potential for respiratory or kidney problems. The effect of the increased body weight on transfers, an increased possibility of **autonomic dysreflexia,** and the need for increased bladder and bowel care should all be considered when pregnancy is contemplated.[44] Labor and delivery can present some special problems, such as a lack of awareness of the beginning of labor contractions. Induction of labor might be contraindicated if a person has a spinal cord injury at T6 or above and the medical staff is not trained to deal with the respiratory problems or dysreflexia that can result. After delivery, the parent with disability will need to have modifications made to

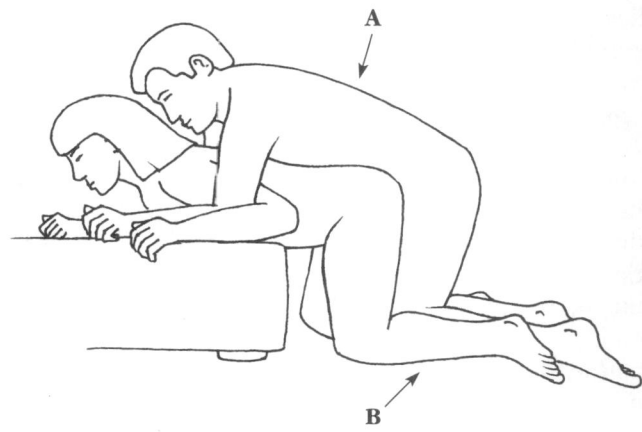

FIG. 15-10
Rear vaginal entry of B, who does not need much energy because of support and little or no abduction of hips. Flexion tightness of hips does not affect performance. Because of weight on B's knees, hips, and back, as well as inevitable repetitive movement at hips, this would not be a good position for individuals with back, hip, or knee joint degeneration.

the wheelchair. The client will need consultations to achieve an optimal level of function in the parenting role.[19]

METHODS OF EDUCATION

The following techniques or approaches have been used effectively to deal with the emotional aspects of sex education of people with disability.

Repeat Information

Mentioning sexual issues just once is not enough. Most people, whether they have disability or not, need to hear information more than once. This fact is especially true for people who are in crisis or who are in the process of adjustment. Too much information, or more than is asked for, should not be offered at one time. Whenever possible, the therapist should try to say something positive in every conversation. Holding out hope for the restoration of function or alternative function is important. The therapist should not assume that the client understands all of the information. To verify that the information is understood, the therapist should invite the client to ask questions and to paraphrase what has been said.

Discovery of the "New" Body

With any disability, the client's body image and perception of the body are altered. In effect, the client has a new body and must find altered ways of moving, interpreting sensations, and performing ADL. A large part of the therapeutic experience is directed toward helping the client discover how to use this new body as effectively as possible. The therapist can facilitate this discovery of the new body by creating situations that encourage awareness of the body through the input of sensation and function.[28] The client alone or with his or her sexual partner can accomplish this awareness through exercises that encourage exploration of the body. Exercises such as the gentle tapping or rubbing of a specific area can be developed to see if there is sensation or if the stimulation causes a change in muscle tone. Many people with a disability such as paralysis report that they have experienced nongenital orgasms[24] by stimulating other new erogenous areas, often in the area just above where sensation starts to appear. The therapist may suggest ways to use this sensation or change in tone in ADL or may ask the client to think of ways this change in tone could be used, such as triggering reflex leg extension to help putting on pants. This discussion will stimulate problem solving by the client.

PLISSIT

The acronym **PLISSIT** stands for *permission, limited information, specific suggestions, and intensive therapy.* PLISSIT is a progressive approach to guide the therapist in helping the client deal with sexual information.[2] *Permission* refers to allowing the client to feel new feelings and experiment with new thoughts or ideas regarding sexual functioning. *Limited information* refers to explaining what effect the disability can have on sexual functioning. An explanation with great detail is not usually necessary early in the counseling process. The next level of information is providing *specific suggestions.* It might be in the therapist's domain to give specific suggestions on dealing with specific problems that relate to the disability, such as positioning. This is the highest level of input the average occupational therapist should attempt without advanced education and training in sexual counseling. Intensive therapy should be reserved for the rare client who has an abnormal coping pattern in dealing with sexuality. An extensive counseling background is needed to provide intensive therapy.

Activity Analysis

To assess the client's positioning needs, the therapist must analyze the components of the particular activity. This analysis entails looking at the physical, psychological, social, cultural, and cognitive components of the client's functioning. The activity analysis should be implemented using an objective and professional perspective. The therapist must realize that the sex act itself, if there is one, is only a small part of the act of making love and should be treated as just one more ADL that must be analyzed and with which the client needs professional assistance. The therapist must also remember

that not all partners had sex on a daily, weekly, or even yearly basis before the onset of the disability. The therapist's values and biases should not be imposed on the client. Same-sex partners, multiple partners, masturbation, or a preference for no sexual activities are some of the client's practices that could evoke bias.

Basic Sex Education

Some clients need **basic sex education** if they didn't have the information before the onset of disability. Some clients may not have been informed because of the disability, or they may be misinformed about sexual practices.[1,8] Research has shown that people with hearing impairments have substantially less information regarding sex than do those without hearing impairments.[43] If the occupational therapist is not the one to educate the client or the client's partner, the therapist should anticipate the need for information and have knowledge of the resources available for the client to acquire the information. It is not advisable to recommend only books about sexuality and people with disabilities. Such books are useful, but their focus on the disability may be discouraging to some. Books written for the able-bodied, such as *The Hite Report on Male Sexuality,*[23] *The Hite Report,*[22] and *How to Satisfy a Woman Every Time,*[20] can be helpful. These books will not only give the client an understanding of sex, but will also show the client that he or she is normal, while minimizing the focus on the disability. Excellent books written for individuals with disabilities also can be recommended. Some of these are *Choices: A Guide to Sexual Counseling with the Physically Disabled,*[31] *Reproductive Issues for Persons with Physical Disabilities,*[19] *The Sensuous Wheeler,*[33] *Sexuality and the Person with Traumatic Brain Injury,*[18] *Sex and Back Pain,*[21] *Sexuality and Disabilities,*[29] *Sexual Function in People with Disability and Chronic Illness,*[38] and *Enabling Romance.*[26]

SUMMARY

Occupational therapists are concerned with the sexuality of their clients because sexuality is related to self-esteem and influences the adjustment to disability and because sexual functioning is an activity of daily living. As with other ADL, a physical dysfunction can necessitate some change in performance of sexual activities. Education, counseling, and activity analysis can be used to solve many common sexual problems confronted by persons with physical dysfunction.

Occupational therapists can provide information and referrals to clients who are concerned with sexual issues. Trained therapists can provide counseling. Issues of sexual function, sexual abuse, and values need to be considered in providing sex education and counseling. Through activity analysis and problem solving, physical limitations that affect sexual functioning can usually be managed. A wide variety of sexual practices, modes of sexual expression, and expressions of sensuality are possible. The client needs the opportunity to explore her or his needs and acceptable options to meet those needs. The occupational therapist is one of the members of the rehabilitation team who has something to offer the client in the area of rehabilitation and sexuality and sensuality.

REVIEW QUESTIONS

1. List at least five areas related to sensuality or sexuality that are usually the concerns of the occupational therapist.
2. What are some common attitudes of the able-bodied population about the sexuality of persons with physical dysfunction?
3. How do these attitudes affect the disabled person's perception of self and attitudes toward his or her own sexuality?
4. How is sexuality related to self-esteem and a sense of attractiveness?
5. Describe some typical questions for taking a sexual history. How can these questions be used to clarify values about sexuality?
6. How do mobility aids and assistive devices affect sexual functioning? How can this concern be managed?
7. What are some signs of potential sexual abuse of adults?
8. What are some suggestions for dealing with the following physical symptoms during sexual activity: hypertonia, low endurance, joint degeneration, and loss of sensation.
9. List some medications that may cause sexual dysfunction.
10. Discuss some issues and precautions relative to birth control for the woman with a physical disability.
11. How is a catheter managed during sexual activity?
12. What are some potential problems in pregnancy, delivery, and child care?
13. Discuss some techniques for educating a person about sexual issues.
14. How should sexual harassment of staff members by clients be handled?

REFERENCES

1. Andrews AB, Veronen LJ: Sexual assault and people with disabilities, *J Soc Work Human Sexuality* 8(2):137-159, 1993.
2. Annon JS: *The behavioral treatment of sexual problems,* vol 1-2, Honolulu, 1974, Enabling Systems.
3. Becker H, Stuifbergen A, Tinkile M: Reproductive health care experiences of women with physical disabilities: a qualitative study, *Arch Phys Med Rehabil* 78(12) (Suppl 5):S26-S33, 1997.
4. Blum RW: Sexual health contraceptive needs of adolescents with chronic conditions, *Arch Pediatr Adolesc Med* 151(3):330-337, 1997.
5. Boyle PS: Training in sexuality and disability: preparing social workers to provide services to individuals with disabilities, *J Soc Work Human Sexuality* 8(2):45-62, 1993.
6. Braithwaite DO: From majority to minority: an analysis of cultural change from able-bodied to disabled, *Int J Intercultural Relations* 14:465-483, 1990.
7. Charlifue SW, Gerhart KA, Menter RR, et al: Sexual issues of women with spinal cord injuries, *Paraplegia* 30(3):192-199, 1992.
8. Choquet M, Du Pasquier Fediaevsky L, Manfredi R, National Institute of Health and Medical Research (INSERM), Unit 169, Villejuif, France: Sexual behavior among adolescents reporting chronic conditions: a French national survey, *J Adolesc Health* 20(1):62-67, 1997.
9. Cole SS, Cole TM: Sexuality, disability, and reproductive issues for persons with disabilities. In Haseltine FP, Cole SS, Gray DB, editors: *Reproductive issues for persons with physical disabilities,* Baltimore, 1993, Paul H Brooks.
10. Cole SS, Cole TM: Sexuality, disability, and reproductive issues through the life span, *Sexuality and Disability* 11(3):189-205, 1993.
11. Cole TM: Gathering a sex history from a physically disabled adult, *Sexuality and Disability* 9(1):29-37, 1991.
12. Cornelius DA, Chipouras S, Makas E, et al: *Who cares? A handbook on sex education and counseling services for disabled people,* Baltimore, 1982, University Park Press.
13. Ducharme S, Gill KM: Sexual values, training, and professional roles, *J Head Trauma Rehabil* 5(2):38-45, 1991.
14. Edwards DF, Baum CM: Caregivers' burden across stages of dementia, *Occup Ther Practice* 2(1):13-31, 1990.
15. Froehlich J: Occupational therapy interventions with survivors of sexual abuse, *Occup Ther in Health Care* 8(2-3):1-25, 1992.
16. Gender AR: An overview of the nurse's role in dealing with sexuality, *Sexuality and Disability* 10(2):71-70, 1992.
17. Goldstein H, Runyon C: An occupational therapy education module to increase sensitivity about geriatric sexuality, *Phys Occup Ther Geriatrics* 11(2):57, 1993.
18. Griffith ER, Lemberg S: *Sexuality and the person with traumatic brain injury: a guide for families,* Philadelphia, 1993, FA Davis.
19. Haseltine FP, Cole SS, Gray DB: *Reproductive issues for persons with physical disabilities,* Baltimore, 1993, Paul H Brooks.
20. Hayden N: *How to satisfy a woman every time,* New York, 1982, Bibli O'Phile.
21. Hebert L: *Sex and back pain,* Bloomington, Minn, 1987, Educational Opportunities.
22. Hite S: *The Hite report,* New York, 1976, Macmillan.
23. Hite S: *The Hite report on male sexuality,* New York, 1981, Knopf.
24. Kettl P, Zarefoss S, Jacoby K, et al: Female sexuality after spinal cord injury, *Sexuality and Disability* 9(4):287-295, 1991.
25. Krause JS, Crewe NM: Chronological age, time since injury, and time of measurement: effect on adjustment after spinal cord injury, *Arch Phys Med Rehabil* 72:91-100, 1991.
26. Kroll K, Klein EL: *Enabling romance,* New York, 1992, Harmony Books.
27. Lefebvre KA: Sexual assessment planning, *J Head Trauma Rehabil* 5(2):25-30,1990.
28. Lemon MA: Sexual counseling and spinal cord injury, *Sexuality and Disability* 11(1):73-97, 1993.
29. Mackelprang R, Valentine D: *Sexuality and disabilities: a guide for human service practitioners,* Binghamton, NY, 1993, Haworth Press.
30. McComas J, Hebert C, Giacomin C, et al: Experiences of students and practicing physical therapists with inappropriate patient sexual behavior, *Phys Ther* 73(11):762-769, 1993.
31. Neistadt ME, Freda M: *Choices: a guide to sex counseling with physically disabled adults,* Malabar, Fla, 1987, Krieger.
32. Nosek M, Rintala D, Young M, et al: Psychological and psychosocial disorders: sexuality issues for women with physical disabilities, *Rehabilitation Research and Development Progress Reports* 34:244-245, 1997.

33. Rabin BJ: *The sensuous wheeler*, Long Beach, Calif, 1980, Barry J Rabin.

34. Rintala D, Howland C, Nosek M, et al: Dating issues for women with physical disabilities, *Sexuality and Disability* 15(4):219-242, 1997.

35. Romeo AJ, Wanlass R, Arenas S: A profile of psychosexual functioning in males following spinal cord injury, *Sexuality and Disability* 11(4):269-276, 1993.

36. Sandowski C: Responding to the sexual concerns of persons with disabilities, *J Soc Work Human Sexuality* 8(2):29-43,1993.

37. Scott R: Sexual misconduct, *PT Magazine Phys Ther* 1(10):78, 1993.

38. Sipski M, Alexander C: *Sexual function in people with disability and chronic illness*, Gaithersburg, Md, 1997, Aspen Publishing.

39. Smith M: Pediatric sexuality: promoting normal sexual development in children, *Nurse Pract* 18(8):37-44, 1993.

40. Sobsey D, Randall W, Parrila RK: Gender differences in abused children with and without disabilities, *Child Abuse Negl* 21(8):707-720, 1997.

41. Stockard S: Caring for the sexually aggressive patient: you don't have to blush and bear it, *Nursing* 21(11):72-73, 1991.

42. Suris JC, Resnick MD, Cassuto N, et al: Sexual behavior of adolescents with chronic disease and disability, *Adolesc Health* 19(2):124-131, 1996.

43. Swartz DB: A comparative study of sex knowledge among hearing and deaf college freshmen, *Sexuality and Disability* 11(2):129-136, 1993.

44. Verduyn WH: Spinal cord injured women, pregnancy, and delivery, *Sexuality and Disability* 11(3):29-43, 1993.

45. Yim SY, Lee IY, Yoon SH, et al: Quality of marital life in Korean spinal cord injured patients, *Spinal Cord* 36(12):826-831, 1998.

46. Young ME, Nosek MA, Howland C, et al: Prevalence of abuse of women with physical disabilities, *Arch Phys Med Rehabil* 78(12)(suppl 5):S34-S38, 1997.

47. Zani B: Male and female patterns in the discovery of sexuality during adolescence, *J Adolesc* 14:163-178, 1991.

SUGGESTED READINGS

Gregory MF: *Sexual adjustment: a guide for the spinal cord injured*, Bloomington, Ill, 1993, Accent On Living.

Kempton W, Caparulo F: *Sex education for persons with disabilities that hinder learning: a teacher's guide*, Santa Barbara, Calif, 1989, James Stanfield.

Leyson JF: *Sexual rehabilitation of the spinal-cord-injured patient*, Totowa, NJ, 1991, Humana Press.

Mackelprang R, Valentine D: *Sexuality and disabilities: a guide for human service practitioners*, Binghamton, NY, 1993, Haworth Press.

Sandowski C: *Sexual concern when illness or disability strikes*, Springfield, Ill, 1989, Charles C Thomas. In *Resources for people with disabilities and chronic conditions*, ed 2, Lexington, Ky, 1993, Resources for Rehabilitation.

Shortridge J, Steele-Clapp L, Lamin J: Sexuality and disability: a SIECUS annotated bibliography of available print materials, *Sexuality and Disability* 11(2):159-179, 1993.

Sipski M, Alexander C: *Sexual function in people with disability and chronic illness*, Gaithersburg, Md, 1997, Aspen.

Sobsey D, Gray S, editors: *Disability, sexuality, and abuse*, Baltimore, 1991, Paul H Brooks.

ADDITIONAL RESOURCES

American Association of Sex Education Counselors and Therapists
435 N. Michigan Avenue, Suite 1717, Chicago, IL 60611
(312) 644-0328

Association for Sexual Adjustment in Disability
PO Box 3579, Downey, CA 90292

Coalition on Sexuality and Disability
122 East Twenty-third Street, New York, NY 10010
(212) 242-3900

Sex Information and Education Council of the United States (SIECUS)
130 West Forty-second Street, Suite 2500, New York, NY 10036
(212) 819-9770

Sexuality and Disability Training Center
University of Michigan Medical Center
Department of Physical Medicine and Rehabilitation
1500 E. Medical Center Drive, Ann Arbor, MI 48109
(313) 936-7057

The Task Force on Sexuality and Disability of the American Congress of Rehabilitation Medicine
5700 Old Orchard Road, Skokie, IL 60077
(708) 966-0095

CHAPTER 16

Work Evaluation and Work Hardening

CINDY MAULTSBY BURT

KEY TERMS

Work therapy
Work injury prevention
Work hardening
Industrial injuries
Job modification
Work samples
Work simulation
Work conditioning
Physical tolerances
Secondary gains
Job analysis
Critical job demands
Work tolerance baseline
Functional capacity evaluations
Work tolerance screenings
Body mechanics

LEARNING OBJECTIVES

After studying this chapter the student or practitioner will be able to do the following:

1. Discuss the role of occupational therapy in the development of work therapy programs.
2. Identify occupational therapists instrumental in the development of work therapy services.
3. Identify settings in which work hardening services are currently provided and discuss the advantages and disadvantages of each setting.
4. Describe the work hardening process.
5. Identify the goals of work hardening.
6. Identify socioeconomic and psychological issues that can have an effect on successful completion of a work hardening program.
7. Identify components of a job analysis.
8. Outline a plan for completing a functional capacity evaluation.
9. Develop a work hardening plan based on a job analysis and functional capacity evaluation of an injured worker.
10. Describe an appropriate work hardening milieu.

In American society, identity and self-worth are closely tied to one's role as a competitive wage earner. Inability to perform in the worker role can lead to role reversals within the family and to lifestyle changes caused by economic hardship, forced inactivity and dependence, depression, and maladaptive psychosocial responses. These problems can become barriers to returning to work, resulting in permanent disability with high economic and social costs. Restoring the worker role can reduce these costs for both the individual and society.

The importance of work as a life role within an industrial society was recognized early in the development of occupational therapy (OT). In its early years, OT was described as "any activity, mental or physical, medically prescribed and professionally guided to aid a patient in the recovery from a disease or injury."[33] After World War I, the focus of OT was the rehabilitation of wounded veterans to help them achieve functional levels necessary to gain employment. Today, **work therapy** has expanded to a full range of industrial therapy services. The **work injury prevention** and management spectrum includes acute treatment, job analysis, job placement, functional capacity evaluation, work hardening, and work conditioning.

Occupational therapists have played a major role in the development of work evaluation and work retraining services. This chapter reviews the historical role of OT in work therapy, describes current models of practice, and presents the work therapy process.

HISTORY OF OCCUPATIONAL THERAPY INVOLVEMENT

Work hardening has been a core component of work therapy throughout the evolution of occupational therapy and practice.[46] In the 1800s, patients with tuberculosis were prescribed graded exercise and work tolerance activities as part of a medical regimen that also included good food and fresh air. Functional activities, including woodworking and graded clerical tasks, were added in the final stages of treatment. Activities were designed to increase physical and emotional tolerances necessary for return to work.[46]

In 1919, George Barton stated that the purpose of work was to divert the mind, exercise the body, and relieve the monotony and boredom of illness.[58] World War I reconstruction workers, the first occupational therapists, taught crafts in military hospitals as "work cure." Their goal was to rehabilitate wounded veterans to help them achieve the functional level necessary to sustain employment.[63] Crafts were regarded as therapeutic modalities used to foster a sense of intrinsic productivity and fulfillment.[31]

Programs of "habit training" with the goal of restoring work habits impaired by disease or accident were implemented in the 1920s. The federal Vocational Rehabilitation Act of 1923 required the inclusion of OT in general hospitals serving persons with **industrial injuries** and illnesses. This legislation marked the beginning of the formal involvement of OT in the vocational rehabilitation movement.[31]

The psychiatric literature of the 1940s described work hardening as a program to prepare the patient for return to competitive life after the sheltered environment of the hospital. Realistic work environments were used, including the hospital laundry, barber shop, and carpentry shop. Personality traits considered important for harmonious working, such as cooperation and friendliness, were evaluated.[56]

Physical disability practice literature in the 1940s also stressed the importance of realistic work experiences for return to productive employment. Treatment programs allowed **job modification** to accommodate variation in worker traits such as speed or productivity while maintaining quality standards.[45]

In the 1950s, a program at Massachusetts General Hospital incorporated the first use of objective evaluation of progress.[74] Objective strength measures were used to track improvements and measure outcomes.

Amendments to the federal Vocational Rehabilitation Act in 1954 provided for the establishment of prevocational services within medical facilities. These amendments increased the prominence of the profession in the vocational rehabilitation field.[31]

In the 1950s, Lillian Wegg was the first health care professional to describe a multidisciplinary program involving an occupational therapist, vocational counselor, physician, and industrial engineer. Work hardening activities included newly evolving **work samples,** work tests, and job simulations. Formal discharge reports provided recommendations for adaptive equipment, modified work schedules, and potential job placement.[75] Wegg revised and expanded components of the program during the next decade, moving away from a medical model and closer to a vocational model. Work hardening was regarded as a vocationally oriented program with the purpose of improving deficient work habits and skills.[76] A physician's prescription was no longer required for referral. Wegg's approach was mirrored by occupational therapist Florence Cromwell. Cromwell emphasized the evaluation of work habits, intellectual and attitudinal factors, and work quality issues such as safety.[19]

Many OT work programs in the 1950s followed the leadership of Wegg and Cromwell and emphasized realistic work and the production of marketable work products. Patients worked in hospital or community settings, producing items for sale while building self-esteem, developing work habits, and increasing physical tolerances.[41]

In the 1970s, work hardening emerged as a primary industrial injury management service.[76] Chronic pain, particularly low back pain, became a major focus of therapeutic intervention. Programs adopted a multidisciplinary approach incorporating medicine, therapy, psychology, vocational counseling, and rehabilitation engineering.[21,24,26] Behavioral factors received increased attention. Abnormal illness behaviors, depression, excessive anger, lack of responsibility, and submaximal effort were found to be important factors for projecting return to competitive employment.[54]

In the 1980s, work hardening programs incorporated the use of standardized **work simulation** equipment. Computerized equipment provided precise objective information to measure such factors as effort, force, and endurance. Therapists combined realistic work activities with high-tech equipment to measure and analyze results.[8]

In 1989, the Commission on Accreditation of Rehabilitation Facilities (CARF) drafted work hardening standards requiring an interdisciplinary approach.[12] These standards were updated in 1992.[13] Work hardening was defined as "a highly structured, goal oriented, individualized treatment program designed to maximize a person's ability to return to work."[12] Interdisciplinary in nature and comprehensive in scope, work hardening used work, defined as real or simulated job tasks, as the treatment modality. Job tasks were combined with injury-specific strengthening and flexibility training in a supportive environment to develop behaviors necessary for successful return to competitive employment.

CURRENT MODELS OF WORK HARDENING PRACTICE

The worker role remains a major focus of OT intervention. Any activity that contributes to the goods and services of society, whether paid or unpaid, is considered a work activity. Work must be purposeful and have meaning for both the individual and society. Engaging in work is considered a productive activity and, as such, a goal of OT intervention.[8,14]

Today's work hardening program models draw on the historical role of work while integrating a variety of current concepts and principles.[17] These include occupational and career development models, medical intervention models, ergonomic and anthropomorphic principles, and technology.[64]

The *Work Hardening Guidelines* were published by the American Occupational Therapy Association (AOTA) in 1986, summarizing the use of basic OT practice principles.[2] These guidelines gave a basic structure for services provided in a variety of settings and encompassed several frames of reference represented in OT practice. In 1992, the *Work Practice Statement* was developed by AOTA to further clarify the role of OT in the rehabilitation process of injured workers.[2]

Work hardening is one of many industrial therapy services. Industrial therapy is diverse and involves a wide range of professionals. These include, but are not limited to, occupational therapists, physical therapists, physicians, occupational health nurses, vocational counselors, safety or risk engineers, and insurance case managers. Industrial therapy services provided by occupational therapists include, but are not limited to, job analysis, functional capacity evaluations, and work retraining, including **work conditioning** and work hardening. Work conditioning is limited to the physical components of flexibility, strength, coordination, and endurance for return to work. The behavioral and vocational components of the return-to-work process are not integrated within the work conditioning process. Work hardening is a multidisciplinary, comprehensive program combining work simulation with strengthening and behavioral components.[2,4,26]

Work conditioning is most often provided as part of the acute medical phase of the rehabilitation process. It is frequently provided as part of the traditional acute care therapy program. Work hardening services are generally provided in the later part of the medical phase of the rehabilitation process, after traditional physical or occupational therapy is completed. The goals of work hardening are closely tied to the requirements of the worker's preinjury job. When return to the original job is not feasible, the worker must be retrained for new employment and enters the vocational rehabilitation phase of the industrial therapy process. Rehabilitation may be more complex and difficult in this phase because of worker fears, forced career changes, and difficulty entering an unfamiliar work environment as a novice worker.

Occupational therapists traditionally have provided industrial therapy services in a hospital or rehabilitation facility. Current practice has expanded this list of service locations to include the provision of services at the injured worker's work site.[53,59] These on-site programs have many benefits. They provide immediate access to rehabilitation services, facilitate early return to work, and allow convenient scheduling and access to therapy while working. Communication between injured employees, supervisors, and care providers is facilitated. On-site programs control employee access to services and are useful in managing both the quality and the cost of care. Positive effects on morale can also result if employees view the program as concerned with their welfare.

The recent expansion of hospital-based industrial programs to community-based, on-site facilities reflects the transition of services to community settings. OT educators and leaders have promoted this transition for the last two decades. On-site industrial programs may include acute treatment, work conditioning, work hardening, functional capacity evaluations, preemployment screenings, and wellness and prevention programs. Occupational therapists have the training and expertise to continue leading the expansion of work services into these new settings. In the continuum of industrial services, work hardening can restore worker function when provided as part of either a hospital-based or an on-site industrial program.

GOALS OF WORK HARDENING

Work hardening goals are focused on the ultimate objective of maximizing the individual worker's ability to return to work. Goals include (1) attaining optimal **physical tolerances** and abilities, (2) maximizing cognitive and psychosocial functioning, (3) developing appropriate worker behaviors, (4) reducing fear and increasing confidence for the resumption of productive work, and (5) identifying problems that may necessitate placement in an alternative job.

POTENTIAL BARRIERS TO SUCCESSFUL WORK HARDENING OUTCOMES

Several physiological and psychological factors may interfere with the attainment of work hardening goals. These potential barriers to success must be recognized and addressed as part of the intervention plan.

Age and Gender

Age and gender have been shown to affect the potential risk of injury and return-to-work status. Older workers and female workers are less skilled than younger workers and male workers in dynamic balance, climbing, and lifting ability.[35] This places older workers and female workers at higher risk of injury than their younger, male counterparts. Once injured, these individuals may be more challenging to rehabilitate and more susceptible to reinjury.[35] In a retrospective study of over 24,000 Michigan workers' compensation cases, the relative risk of back injury was demonstrated to be higher for women than for men in white-collar occupations.[38] Age was determined to be a barrier to work for individuals with rheumatoid arthritis.[65]

Secondary Gains

Injured workers can derive benefits known as **secondary gains** as a result of a work-related injury. The injured worker can perceive disability payments and the potential for financial gain, time off from work, avoidance of responsibility, or sympathy and attention received from others as secondary gains. These secondary gains can delay recovery.[32,36,37,46] Role changes within the family structure may be incentives for family members to reinforce the injured worker's sick role.[54] A newly employed wife might like her new role as breadwinner and reinforce her husband's sick role. A father may suddenly have time to spend with his family and wish to avoid returning to work.

Litigation

Injured workers with pending litigation frequently improve at a slower rate than workers not involved in the legal system.[24] Financial opportunities, including unemployment benefits, welfare benefits, and workers' compensation, can all adversely influence return to work.[32]

Delayed Intervention

Successful completion of a work hardening program is related to the length of time the client has had the disability before program initiation. The longer the period of disability, the less likely that the individual will successfully return to work.[55]

Confidence Level

Positive relationships and meaningful work tasks have been found to increase self-confidence and motivation for return to work. The level of worker confidence in his or her ability to do the same quantity and quality of work as coworkers is an important factor affecting motivation for return to work.[37]

Employer Attitudes

The successful return to work of an injured worker can be affected by an employer's attitudes and relationships with workers. Employers often fear possible reinjury and reduced productivity of returning injured workers.[54] These fears can reduce the motivation for employers to assist injured workers with the return-to-work process. Employees who reported poor relationships with their supervisors had higher injury rates than employees reporting good relationships with their managers.[77]

Culture

Cultural norms and personal attitudes toward work can be critical factors in successful work injury rehabilitation. The value of work within a culture can be crucial in motivating workers to return to work.

Pain

Chronic pain is defined as pain lasting longer than 6 months. Chronic pain can result in psychological disturbances, including insomnia, anxiety, depression, and feelings of helplessness.[36,37,44,54] Psychosocial problems, including alcohol and drug abuse, weight fluctuations, difficulties with relationships, and sexual dysfunction, can result from these disturbances.[36]

Alcohol and Drug Abuse

A high incidence of alcohol and drug abuse is frequently reported among workers with high pain levels. Abuse can precede the injury, be related to attempts to control pain, or result from attempts to reduce or avoid stress. Participation and success can be negatively affected by active drug abuse behavior.

WORK HARDENING PROCESS

Work hardening provides a holistic and realistic link between an injured worker's physical capacities and limitations and essential physical job demands. The development of an individualized work hardening program begins with a specific **job analysis** to determine critical job duties. The ability of an injured worker to perform these duties must then be determined by completing a baseline work tolerance evaluation. Finally, information from the job analysis and the baseline work tolerance evaluation is consolidated to develop an individualized work hardening program. Functional limitations can then be specifically addressed with a work hardening program designed to develop the tolerances required for completing critical job duties.

Step One: Job Analysis

The occupational therapist must clearly understand an injured worker's specific job requirements to plan a meaningful, relevant, and measurable program for the worker. This understanding is gained through a job analysis. Based on **critical job demands,** the job analysis provides the foundation for development of a work hardening plan. A job analysis includes detailed information on all critical job tasks, including physical work demands and the use of equipment, tools, and materials. Physical job demands include walking, balancing, climbing, standing, sitting, crouching, bending, lifting, carrying, pushing and pulling, reaching, handling, and fingering. Sensory components (e.g., vision, hearing, and smell) and environmental conditions (e.g., noise, cold, heat, dust fumes, and vibration) are important considerations. Unique psychosocial demands such as the need to interact effectively with angry customers or tolerance of distracting environments should be considered if they are critical job functions.

The increased reporting of work-related musculoskeletal disorders has made it necessary to identify all high-risk job factors, including frequency, force, duration, posture, and exposure to vibration and cold. Development of worker tolerance for activities involving these factors is imperative for a successful return to work.

The work hardening therapist does not have to complete the job analysis if an employer, insurance carrier, rehabilitation nurse, vocational counselor, or other professional involved in the case has already done so. If the job analysis is available, the therapist can review and validate primary job functions with both employer and employee.

If a job analysis is not available, the therapist should visit the work site to observe primary job tasks. Occupational therapists are qualified by their basic training to perform these on-site job task analyses. However, additional expertise and training is often needed to adequately complete medical and legal documentation requirements. Several government publications can serve as references to assist the therapist in developing a document suitable for legal purposes. These include the *Dictionary of Occupational Titles,*[66] *Revised Handbook for Analyzing Jobs,*[67] and *A Guide to Job Analysis.*[38] A simplified sample of a job analysis form is shown in Fig. 16-1.

JOB ANALYSIS

Job Title ________ Employee ________
Location ________
Work Hours ________ to ________ Days ________ Overtime Per Wk ________
General Job Description:

Equipment, tools, work aids:

Primary job functions:

Time spent:
Standing ________ hrs Sitting ________ hrs Inside ________ hrs Outside ________ hrs

ACTIVITY	YES	NO	REPETITIVE (Frequency)	CONTINUOUS (# Hours)	COMMENTS
Stoop/Bend					
Squat/Crouch					
Kneel					
Climb					
Crawl					
Reach Overhead					
Manipulate/Finger					
Grasp					

LIFT/CARRY	HRS/REPS/POSITION	LIFT/CARRY	HRS/REPS/POSITION
0-10 lbs		11-20 lbs	
21-50 lbs		Over 50 lbs	

Environmental Conditions: (check if present)
Cold ________ Dampness ________ Heat ________ Dust/Fumes ________ Noise ________
Psychological Requirements:

________ Analyst ________ Date

FIG. 16-1
Sample job analysis form.

Step Two: Establishing Work Tolerance Baseline

Determination of the worker's current level of functioning is as important as the job analysis in individual program planning. All pertinent physical, cognitive, and behavioral factors must be included in an assessment of the worker's functional abilities. A factor is pertinent if it is (1) a requirement of the job and (2) subject to impairment as a result of the injury. Medical conditions such as diabetes, hearing loss, and hypertension are important if they are relevant for task performance.

The **work tolerance baseline** can be established using a variety of assessment instruments. Both commercial and facility-specific assessment systems are available and are known by a variety of names, including **functional capacity evaluations,** physical capacity evaluations, **work tolerance screenings,** or work capacity evaluations. The purpose of the evaluation is to provide a systematic process for observing, measuring, analyzing, and recording the ability of an injured worker to perform specific job tasks.

CARF has listed components that should be included in the work tolerance baseline evaluation.[12] These include functional work capacity and musculoskeletal, cardiovascular, cognitive, vocational, behavioral, and attitudinal status. The AOTA Commission on Practice *Official Statement on Work Practice Services* expands these components to include consideration of the injured worker's age, interests, values, culture, and motivation for change.[14]

A **work tolerance baseline evaluation** should include the following components:

- *Medical history.* An efficient evaluation process includes a review of relevant medical records, information concerning both current and past injuries, medical interventions received, and relevant medical conditions such as cardiac status and diabetes. Any orthopedic conditions such as previous fractures and soft tissue problems and any psychiatric conditions and treatment are important to consider. Work restrictions must be obtained from the referring source and noted.

- *Worker interview.* The worker's perception of the injury, work history, functional abilities, education, pain level, and vocational goals can be obtained through an initial interview. This interview provides the evaluator with insight into the worker's attitude, fear of reinjury, motivation for rehabilitation, and vocational goals. Program goals and rules should be established with the worker at this time.

- *Job description with critical job demands.* A job analysis identifies critical job demands. If a job analysis is unavailable, the evaluator can ask the worker to describe job functions and can validate this information with the employer or case manager. In this situation, the therapist can also obtain generic job descriptions with physical work demands from the *Dictionary of Occupational Titles*[66] to help determine critical job demands.

- *Pain assessment.* The location, type, quality, and intensity of pain must be determined during the work tolerance baseline evaluation. The frequency of pain, activities that increase or reduce pain, and techniques used for pain control, including modalities and medications, are important. Many pain questionnaires and charts are available for clinical use. These include topographic pain representations or "pain drawings," analog pain scales, and pain rating scales such as the McGill-Melzack Pain Questionnaire.[27] Chapter 29 provides a further discussion of pain assessment.

- *Physical assessment.* The physical assessment is used to evaluate the worker's abilities to perform critical job duties as described in the job analysis. These can include, but are not limited to, functional range of motion, strength, endurance, sensation, coordination, and dexterity. The physical assessment compares physical functions of the worker to critical job demands, identifying any discrepancies. Because many injured workers are involved in litigation, it is important to use standardized evaluation tools whenever possible. The evaluator should complete a basic work tolerance screening of physical abilities before assessing specific physical abilities to make sure the injured worker is physically capable of completing the baseline work tolerance evaluation. The screening should include generalized testing of range of motion, gross manual muscle testing, sensory screening, and testing of general ability to complete required movements in a safe manner.[79]

The physical assessment includes the following areas of focus:

- *Work postures and mobility.* Flexibility is evaluated to determine functional range of motion of the trunk and lower and upper extremities. Postural strength can be evaluated using the Krause-Weber Test.[41] The VALPAR Work Sample #9 (Whole Body Range of Motion)[73] is used to measure gross body movements as they relate to the functional ability to perform work tasks.

- *Strength.* A variety of standardized and functional tests may be used to measure strength. Dynamometers and pinch gauges are used to measure hand strength. The Baltimore Therapeutic Equipment (BTE) Quest System and Work Simulator,[5] Cybex II,[21] Lido WorkSet,[43] ERGOS,[78] WEST 2A,[48] and WEST 4A[50] are several commercially available devices used to measure strength. Endurance can be evaluated with such devices as the Upper Body Ergometer,[23] Fitron/Lifecycle,[22] and treadmill. Endurance is observed throughout the evaluation. An evaluation of cardiovascular function can be completed as a premeasure and postmeasure test during the endurance testing using a treadmill or the Upper Extremity Ergometer.[23]

- *Sensation.* The evaluation of sensation is vital for workers with hand injuries. The Semmes-Weinstein Monofilament Test (Von-Frey Monofilaments) is used to determine tactile discrimination.[62] Other considerations include edema and coordination. The Schultz Upper Extremity Pain Assessment is a comprehensive test of hand function used by many clinicians.[60,61]

- *Coordination.* Coordination and dexterity tests are used to determine the worker's ability to complete physical work tasks such as handling, manipulating, and fingering. Commonly used tests include the Crawford Small Parts Dexterity Test,[15] Bennett Hand-Tool Dexterity Test,[6] Purdue Pegboard,[69] and the Minnesota Rate of Manipulation Test.[1] Work samples such as the VALPAR #1 Small Tools Mechanical,[70] VALPAR #4 Upper Extremity Range of Motion,[71] and VALPAR #8 Simulated Assembly[72] and the BTE Bolt Box[4] are used to measure upper extremity coordination and dexterity.

- *Lifting, reaching, and carrying.* Lifting, reaching, and carrying tasks are inherent in most jobs. The worker's ability to lift on a frequent or infrequent basis is determined by work simulation or with specific work samples. Floor, knee, waist, shoulder, and overhead level lifting abilities should be assessed, along with one- and two-handed lifting ability. Carrying tasks are assessed in terms of weight loads by distance and time. Reaching is reported in terms of frequency and location or position (e.g., frequently reaches above head). Monitoring **body mechanics** of the worker is imperative during this assessment to prevent reinjury. Work samples such as the WEST 2A,[48] VALPAR Work Sample #9 (Whole Body Range of Motion),[73] and WEST 3 (Comprehensive Weight System)[49] can assess lifting, reaching, and carrying abilities. Frequent lift tests include the Progressive Inertial Lift Evaluation (PILE)[51] and the EPIC 1 Lift Capacity.[47] Lifting and carrying are considered primary physical job factors along with pushing and pulling. Physical job factors are divided into five levels of physical demands, including sedentary, light, medium, heavy, and very heavy work. These levels are specifically outlined in the *Dictionary of Occupational Titles*[66] and the *Revised Handbook for Analyzing Jobs*.[67]

■ *Pushing and pulling.* Pushing and pulling tasks should simulate actual work conditions such as surface friction, handle height, and incline angles. Push-pull sleds can simulate tasks that involve moving and conveying equipment and materials on carpet, linoleum, or concrete floors. A Chatillon force gauge can test actual push-pull force generated.[11] Comparisons of actual force can be made against specific tasks if measures required to complete the tasks are given in terms of pounds of force.

■ *Stooping, bending, kneeling, and crawling.* Stooping, bending, and kneeling can be assessed by observing the patient's completion of simulated work tasks or samples such as the VALPAR #9 (Whole Body Range of Motion)[73] or the WEST 2A.[48] The ability to crawl can be assessed in a simulated work environment if it is considered a primary work demand.

■ *Sitting and standing.* The therapist can observe the functional ability to sit and stand throughout the functional capacity evaluation. The initial interview and dexterity tests provide the evaluator with opportunities to observe the worker in a variety of positions over a long period. Sitting and standing tolerances can be observed while the worker is performing functional tasks.

■ *Work task simulation.* Critical job demands of the worker's job are evaluated using work task simulation and work samples. Job demands may include the use of tools, materials handling, or activities that require repetitive movement or maintenance of prolonged postures (Fig. 16-2). The therapist should also evaluate pertinent environmental factors such as vibration, cold, noise, dust, and heat. A variety of clinic-made devices can be used to simulate work demands. These devices include birdcages, boxes, sleds, and pipe tree assemblies. Standardized work samples are also widely used to evaluate the ability to complete work tasks. Work samples can be used to evaluate single worker traits or clusters of traits. Many of the WEST and VALPAR samples measure clusters of traits, such as strength, endurance, and range of motion, that are inherent in a job. Therapists must use task analysis to

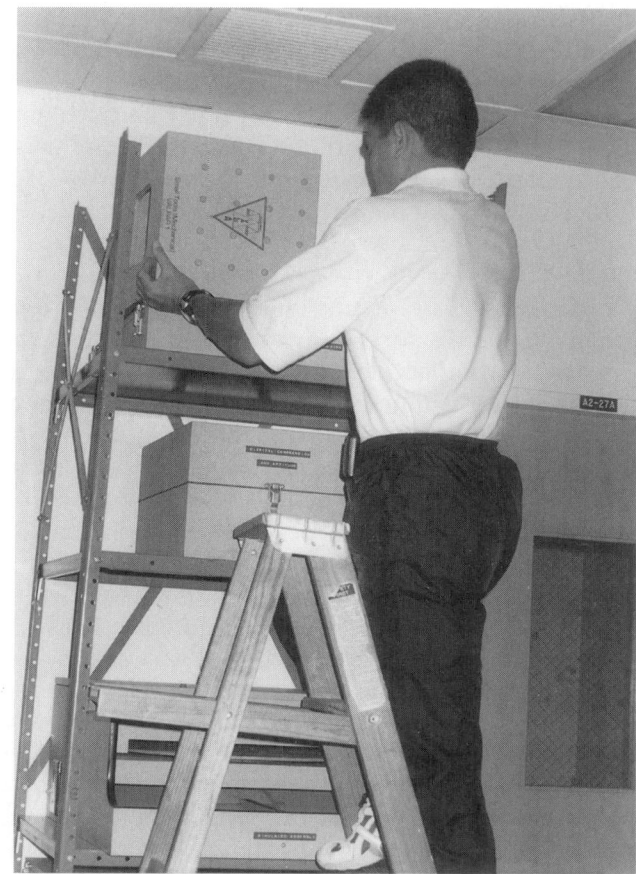

FIG. 16-2
Reaching and climbing.

determine specific problem areas when evaluating a worker during completion of a cluster trait work sample.

When they are used to assess worker performance and potential for return to work, baseline work tolerance evaluations must be based on valid clinical research to ensure that they will stand up in court if challenged. A variety of products are available, with widely differing levels of objective research backing their development, including programs designed by Matheson,[46] Blankenship,[7] and Isernhagen.[35] Proprietary systems including both equipment and training are also available and include the Functional Capacities Assessment by Polinsky Medical Rehabilitation Center,[57] the Matheson Function Capacity Evaluation,[46] and the KEY Functional Assessment.[39] Jacobs published a comprehensive review of work assessments in the second edition of *Occupational Therapy, Work-Related Programs and Assessments*.[37] Selection of a system should be based on individual needs, as well as financial and time constraints.

The final step in the work tolerance baseline evaluation process is summarizing the worker's functional abilities and identifying problems that interfere with work performance. Issues such as pain behaviors, symptom magnification, limited materials handling skills, poor posture and body mechanics, and level of active participation are important to identify. Recommendation for work hardening is made by comparison of the results of the work tolerance baseline evaluation with job-specific duties.

The work tolerance baseline evaluation can be used for a variety of purposes. The evaluation can establish the baseline for work hardening or help to determine safe return-to-work levels, establish modified work duties, or identify a disability rating.[60]

Evaluations range in length from several hours to several days, depending on their purpose. Evaluations establishing baselines for work hardening programs are 3 to 6 hours long and are usually completed on the first or second day of treatment. Assessing other factors such as general aptitudes and worker traits may require a longer time to permit sufficient observation and evaluation.

Step 3: Individual Work Hardening Plan

After the job analysis and functional capacity evaluation are completed, an individualized work hardening plan is developed. To be successful, the plan should determine specific work goals and function as a contract between the worker and the therapist. The goals and interests of the worker and questions of the referring agency are considered essential. The following are examples of typical work hardening goals:

- *Increase duration of daily participation.* The worker's program should begin at a comfortable level that is based on the findings of the functional capacity evaluation. As tolerance for activity improves, hours of participation increase incrementally until they reach the level required for full participation in work duties.
- *Increase physical tolerances to the level of critical job demands.* Work activities requiring identified tolerances should be introduced in graded fashion and replicate, as closely as possible, the actual tasks required for the worker's job.
- *Improve body mechanics and postures.* The therapist may teach and coach the worker to integrate postural awareness and body mechanics skills into functional movement and activities. Newly learned skills are practiced and reinforced in all phases of the program.
- *Develop pain management strategies.* The worker must be encouraged to explore strategies for managing pain so that functional performance is maximized. The therapist should note pain behaviors and give feedback to the worker. A fear of movement because of pain may lead to dysfunctional pain behaviors, such as bracing, guarding, rigidity, rubbing and holding of affected body parts, and other abnormal postures.[8,10] These abnormal postures can lead to increased muscle tension, resulting in increased pain, leading to more tension, and finally becoming a cycle

that is difficult to interrupt. Chronic pain syndromes can develop if this cycle is not broken. The treating physician may be consulted regarding alteration of medication regimens or substitution of other pain control methods.

- *Develop problem-solving skills for self-management at the work site.* Injured workers often have poor judgment and lack the ability to set reasonable limits. Injured workers must learn to recognize and work safely within tolerance levels and to ask for assistance when indicated to prevent reinjury.[7]
- *Facilitate appropriate worker behaviors.* Punctuality and attendance issues should be addressed as needed. Maladaptive patterns such as sleeping late must be eliminated. The worker must develop appropriate interaction skills with supervisors and peers if these skills are deficient. To meet competitive worker levels, it is important to monitor and improve work behaviors, including task completion, quality standards, and productivity.

Real or simulated work tasks are the primary treatment modalities used to develop physical tolerances in a work hardening program. Work tasks and activities selected must be based on the worker's specific job demands and functional deficits as established in the functional capacity evaluation.

It is not always possible to duplicate every job task in the work hardening setting. Activities that require similar physical and cognitive levels of function can be substituted for actual work tasks. Although it is not feasible for a worker to replace automobile mufflers in a standard work hardening setting, it is possible to design a simulated activity requiring tool use in a prolonged overhead reaching position.

Work hardening activities must be compatible with the worker's beginning level of function and must be progressed safely in graded increments until function reaches the level required for work reentry. Symptoms associated with the injury must be managed as the worker reaches competitive work levels.

A good work hardening program includes training in body mechanics and materials handling techniques to protect the worker from further injury (Fig. 16-3). The therapist must teach back-injury prevention, pacing techniques, and safety principles in a manner consistent with the worker's level of education and background. The worker must apply the principles taught to his or her job demands and practice the principle consistently while performing job tasks. Skills must become automatic and be integrated into all daily life tasks.

Work Hardening Milieu

Work hardening programs can be found in a variety of settings, ranging from hospitals to industrial settings. These include outpatient facilities, workshops, private practices, rehabilitation centers, industrial medical

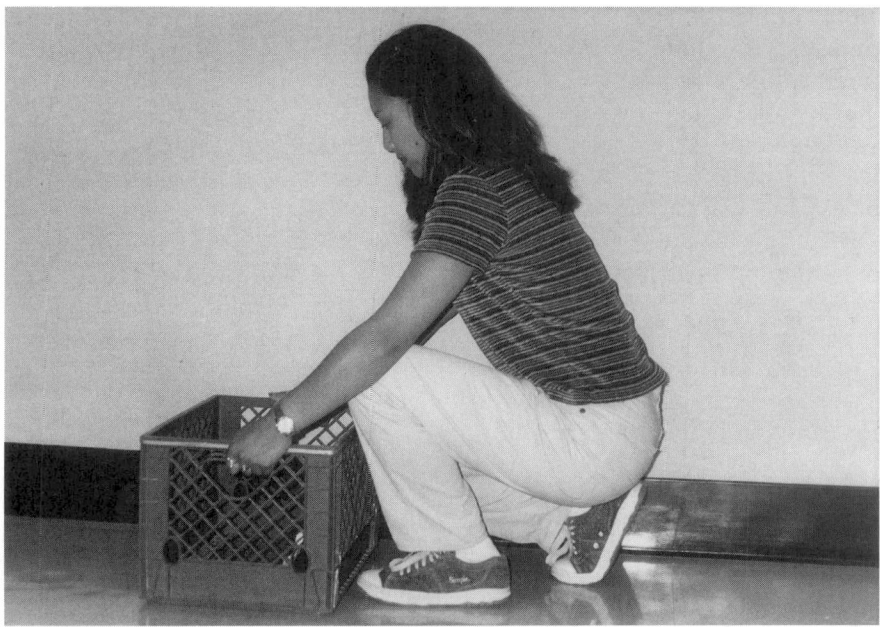

FIG. 16-3
Training in proper body mechanics.

programs, and on-site industrial services within factories and work environments. Regardless of setting, a work hardening facility must replicate a realistic work environment, providing actual and simulated work tasks. Using work that is relevant and meaningful is vital in helping the injured worker understand and accept his or her abilities and limitations.

A realistic work hardening program replicates actual work schedules and environmental conditions. A typical program duplicates the work schedule of the worker, including work breaks, meal breaks, and split shifts if appropriate. It is important to simulate environmental aspects such as working inside versus outside and exposure to dust and noise.

Work hardening services are best presented in a group format with a number of workers present who may be facing similar difficulties and fears. The desire to be competitive with one's peers can be invaluable in facilitating the rehabilitation process. An atmosphere of peer understanding and support can also be beneficial to the worker. The therapist should offer necessary support while making suggestions for compensatory techniques, providing adaptive tools, and reinforcing new learning and skills.

Work hardening programs typically range from 2 to 6 weeks in duration. Continual progress toward return-to-work goals should be observed throughout the program. Services are terminated when goals are met or when measurable progress toward goals is not demonstrated or expected. The therapist should consider referral to other services in the industrial rehabilitation continuum

if measurable improvements are not demonstrated and if these services are likely to be beneficial.

Reporting Results

Work hardening professionals must be skilled at completing objective, quantifiable, and defensible reports. Program results must be reported in accordance with facility protocols and accrediting agency requirements and must include measurable progress toward specific goals. Progress reports must be clear, concise, free of technical jargon, and submitted to referral agencies in a timely manner.[63] Periodic case conferences may be used to promote interdisciplinary communication and coordination.

Referral sources require that a discharge report be submitted at the end of work hardening services. Recommendations may include the use of adaptive equipment, modified work techniques, and any other reasonable accommodations to help the injured worker return to his or her previous level of employment.

SUMMARY

Occupational therapy has been involved in work hardening since the beginnings of the profession in the early 1900s. The profession's use of holistic concepts, task analysis, and activities as therapeutic modalities are reasons for its successful history and pivotal role in work programs. Occupational therapists are trained in physical, cognitive, and behavioral sciences and have the skills necessary to play a vital role in industrial therapy. Industrial therapy continues to be a growing area of occupational therapy practice.

CASE STUDY 16-1

CASE STUDY—J.D.

J.D., a 36-year-old brick mason, sustained a lumbar spine strain while lifting a bag of cement mix. He was referred for work hardening to regain the physical ability required for his job. A job analysis identified the following critical job demands: (1) the ability to lift and carry masonry materials weighing up to 85 pounds on a frequent basis for distances of up to 50 feet; (2) the ability to stoop, crouch, and reach horizontally and vertically on a frequent basis for up to 8 hours; (3) the ability to stand and walk intermittently during an 8-hour work day.

During the functional capacity evaluation, J.D. demonstrated ability to lift and carry 30 pounds on an occasional basis for up to 25 feet, stoop, crouch and reach horizontally and vertically on a frequent basis for 2 hours, and stand and walk intermittently during a 4-hour period without exhibiting overt pain behaviors. Pain behaviors observed after this time included the holding of painful body parts, limping, and awkward posturing.

The work hardening plan addressed J.D.'s goals of gradually increasing tolerances for heavy-duty lifting and carrying, working in a stooped or crouched position while reaching horizontally and vertically, and standing and walking. Additional goals included improving J.D.'s pain tolerances and reducing identified pain behaviors. Specific tasks were assigned to simulate lifting and carrying heavy loads, working in a crouched or stooped position, and standing and walking intermittently. Twice daily stretching and conditioning activities were assigned to promote more natural movements. He was given frequent coaching and support to promote proper body mechanics while reducing his anxiety about anticipated pain.

J.D. made consistent gains towards his goals during the 6 weeks of his program. At six weeks, all goals were met. He was discharged from the work hardening program and successfully returned to work as a brick mason.

REVIEW QUESTIONS

1. Identify three prominent leaders of the occupational therapy profession who advocated the use of work as therapy.
2. When did occupational therapists first use work as a treatment modality?
3. Why is a job analysis a necessary component of the work hardening process?
4. What is the relationship of critical job demands to the functional capacity evaluation and the work hardening plan?
5. Name five intervening socioeconomic and psychological issues that can interfere with successful return to work.
6. What are the three steps in the work hardening process and how are they related to each other?
7. What type of tasks or activities should be used to develop physical tolerances in a work hardening program?
8. Describe the various settings and components of a work hardening program.
9. Discuss at least five goals that a work hardening plan could include.
10. What should the therapist do to protect the worker from further injury during the work hardening process?
11. When should a work hardening program be terminated?

REFERENCES

1. American Guidance Service: *Minnesota rate of manipulation test,* Circle Pines, Minn, 1992, American Guidance Service.
2. American Occupational Therapy Association: *Work hardening guidelines,* Rockville, Md, 1992, The Association.
3. American Physical Therapy Association: *Guidelines for programs for injured workers,* Alexandria, Va, 1995, The Association.
4. *BTE Bolt Box,* Hanover, Md, 1994, Baltimore Therapeutic Equipment.
5. *Quest System,* Hanover, Md, 1994, Baltimore Therapeutic Equipment.
6. Bennett G: *Bennett hand tool dexterity test,* San Antonio, 1981, Psychological Corporation.
7. Bettencourt CM, Carlstrom P: Using work simulations to treat adults with back injuries, *Am J Occup Ther* 40(1):12, 1986.
8. Bing R: Work is a four-letter word: a historical perspective. In Hertfelder S, Gwin C, editors: *Work in progress: occupational therapy in work programs,* Rockville, Md, 1989, American Occupational Therapy Association.
9. Blankenship K: *Blankenship functional capacity evaluation,* Macon, Ga, 1986, Blankenship Corp.
10. Caruso LA, Chan DE: Evaluation and management of the patient with acute back pain, *Am J Occup Ther* 40:347, 1986.
11. Chatillon J: *Chatillon force gauge,* Greensboro, NC, 1991, John Chatillon and Sons.
12. Commission on Accreditation of Rehabilitation Facilities: *Standards manual for organizations serving people with disabilities,* Tucson, Ariz, 1989, The Commission.
13. Commission on Accreditation of Rehabilitation Facilities: *Standards manual for organizations serving people with disabilities,* Tucson, Ariz, 1992, The Commission.
14. Commission on Practice: *Occupational therapy services in work practice: official statement,* Bethesda, Md, 1992, American Occupational Therapy Association.
15. Crawford JE, Crawford DM: *Crawford small parts dexterity test,* San Antonio, 1981, Psychological Corporation.
16. Cromwell F: A procedure for pre-vocational evaluation, *Am J Occup Ther* 13:1, 1959.
17. Cromwell F: Work-related programming in occupational therapy: its roots, course and prognosis. In Cromwell F, editor: *Occupational therapy in health care,* New York, 1985, Haworth Press.
18. Curry R: Understanding patients with chronic pain in work hardening programs, *Work programs special interest section newsletter* (American Occupational Therapy Association) 3:1, 1989.
19. Curry R: Understanding patients with chronic pain in work hardening programs, *Work programs special interest section newsletter* (American Occupational Therapy Association) 3:3, 1989.

20. Curry R: Understanding patients with chronic pain in work hardening programs, *Work programs special interest section newsletter* (American Occupational Therapy Association) 4:1, 1990.
21. *Cybex II*, Ronkonkoma, NY, 1992, Cybex.
22. *Fitron Lifecycle*, Ronkokoma, NY, 1992, Cybex.
23. *Upper Body Ergometer*, Ronkokama, NY, 1992, Cybex.
24. Deyo RA: The role of the primary care physician in reducing work absenteeism and costs due to back pain, *O Med: State of the Art Reviews* 3:17, 1988.
25. Filan SL: The effect of workers' or third-party compensation on return to work after hand surgery, *Med J Aust* 2:80, 1996.
26. Fisher T: Work conditioning is not work hardening, *Special Interest Section Newsletter* (American Occupational Therapy Association) 7:3, 1993.
27. Flower A et al: An occupational therapy program for chronic back pain, *Am J Occup Ther* 35:243, 1981.
28. Gard G, Sandberg AC: Motivating factors for return to work, *Physiother Res Int* 2:100, 1998.
29. Gluck JV, Oleinick A: Claim rates of compensable back injuries by age, gender, occupation, and industry: do they relate to return-to-work experience? *Spine* 14:1572, 1998.
30. Greenberg SN, Bello RP: The work hardening program and subsequent return to work of the client with low back pain, *J Orthop Sports Phys Ther* 24:37, 1996.
31. Harvey-Krefting L: The concept of work in occupational therapy: a historical review, *Am J Occup Ther* 39(5):301-307, 1985.
32. Heck C: Job site analysis for work capacity programming, *Physical Disabilities Special Interest Section Newsletter* (American Occupational Therapy Association) 10:2, 1987.
33. Hopkins H: An introduction to occupational therapy. In Hopkins HL, Smith HD, editors: *Willard and Spackman's occupational therapy*, Philadelphia, 1993, JB Lippincott.
34. Hunter SJ et al: Predicting return to work: a long-term follow-up of railroad workers after low back injuries, *Spine* 21:2319, 1998.
35. Isernhagen SJ: *Work injury: management and prevention*, Rockville, Md, 1988, Aspen.
36. Jacobs K: *Occupational therapy: work related programs and assessment*, Boston, 1985, Little, Brown.
37. Jacobs K: *Occupational therapy: work related programs and assessments*, ed 2, Boston, 1991, Little, Brown.
38. *Guide to job analysis*, Indianapolis, 1991, JIST Works.
39. *Key Functional Assessment*, Minneapolis, 1987, KEY Systems.
40. Key G: Introduction to industrial therapy. In Key G, editor: *Industrial therapy*, St Louis, 1994, Mosby.
41. Kraus H: *Backache, stress and tension: cause, prevention and treatment*, New York, 1965, Simon & Schuster.
42. Lacerte M, Wright GR: Return to work determination, *Phys Med Rehabil State Art Rev* 4:283, 1992.
43. *Lido Workset*, Sacramento, Calif, 1993, Loredan Biomedical.
44. Loeser JD, Egan KJ: *Managing the chronic pain patient*, New York, 1989, Raven Press.
45. Main C: The modified somatic perception questionnaire (MSPQ), *J Psychosom Res* 27:503, 1983.
46. Matheson LN et al: Work hardening: occupational therapy in industrial rehabilitation, *Am J Occup Ther* 39:314, 1985.
47. Matheson R et al: *EPIC 1*, Keene, Ohio, 1994, Roy Matheson and Associates.
48. Matheson R et al: *WEST 2A whole body range of motion and lifting station*, Keene, Ohio, 1994, Roy Matheson and Associates.
49. Matheson R et al: *WEST 3 comprehensive weight system*, Keene, Ohio, 1994, Roy Matheson and Associates.
50. Matheson R et al: *WEST 4A upper body strength and fatigue tolerance*, Keene, Ohio, 1994, Roy Matheson and Associates.
51. Mayer TG et al: Progressive isoinertial lifting evaluation I and II, *Spine* 13:998, 1988.
52. Melzack R: The McGill pain questionnaire: major properties and scoring method, *Pain* 1:277, 1975.
53. Miller D: Industrial therapy: diverse and dynamic, *OT Practice* 11:36, 1998.
54. Ogden-Niemeyer LO, Jacobs K: *Work hardening: state of the art*, Thorofare, NJ, 1989, Slack.
55. Ogden-Niemeyer LO et al: Work hardening: past, present, and future: the work programs special interest section national work-hardening outcome study, *Am J Occup Ther* 48:327, 1994.
56. Phelan LB: Role of manual arts therapy in a neuropsychiatric hospital, *J Rehabil* 14:3, 1949.
57. *Functional Capacities Assessment*, Duluth, Minn, 1992, Polinsky Medical Rehabilitation Center.
58. Reed K: The beginnings of occupational therapy. In Hopkins HL, Smith HD, editors: *Willard and Spackman's occupational therapy*, Philadelphia, 1993, JB Lippincott.
59. Sadusky J: The new industrial revolution, *Rehabil Manage* April/May 1999.
60. Schultz KS: The Schultz structured interview for assessing upper extremity pain, *Occup Ther Health Care* 1:69, 1984.
61. Schultz KS: *Schultz upper extremity pain assessment*, Glenwood Springs, Colo, 1993 , Upper Extremity Technology.
62. Semmes J, Weinstein S: *Semmes-Weinstein Monofilament Test*, Houston, 1994, Research Designs.
63. Smith PC, Bohmfalk JS: *Work related programs in occupational therapy*, New York, 1985, Haworth Press.
64. Smith PC, McFarlane B: *A work hardening model for the 80's: proceedings of the national forum on issues in vocational assessment*, Menomonie, Wis, 1984, Materials Development Center.
65. Straaton KV et al: Barriers to return to work among persons unemployed due to arthritis and musculoskeletal disorders, *Arthritis Rheum* 1:101, 1996.
66. Superintendent of Documents: *Dictionary of occupational titles*, ed 4, Washington, DC, 1991, US Government Printing Office.
67. Superintendent of Documents: *Revised handbook for analyzing jobs*, Washington, DC, 1991, US Government Printing Office.
68. Taylor SE: Industrial rehabilitation. In Hopkins HL, Smith HD, editors: *Willard and Spackman's occupational therapy*, Philadelphia, 1993, JB Lippincott.
69. Tiffin J: *Purdue pegboard*, Chicago, 1968, Science Research Associates.
70. *VALPAR #1 Small tools mechanical*, Tucson, Ariz, 1988, VALPAR Corporation.
71. *VALPAR #4 Upper extremity range of motion*, Tucson, Ariz, 1988, VALPAR Corporation.
72. *VALPAR #8 Simulated assembly*, Tucson, Ariz, 1988, VALPAR Corporation.
73. *VALPAR #9 Whole body range of motion*, Tucson, Ariz, 1988, VALPAR Corporation.
74. Watkins AL: Prevocational evaluation and rehabilitation in a general hospital, *JAMA* 171:4, 1959.
75. Wegg L: Role of the occupational therapist in vocational rehabilitation, *Am J Occup Ther* 11:4, 1957.
76. Wegg L: Essentials of work evaluation, *Am J Occup Ther* 14:65, 1960.
77. Wood DJ: Design and evaluation of a back injury prevention program within a geriatric hospital, *Spine* 12:77, 1987.
78. *Ergos*, Tucson, Ariz, 1990, Work Recovery.
79. Wright R: Putting functional capacity evaluations into your practice, *OT Practice* 6:32, 1998.

CHAPTER 17

Americans With Disabilities Act: Accommodating Persons With Disabilities

PATRICIA SMITH

KEY TERMS

Reasonable accommodation
Essential function
Ergonomics
Participatory ergonomics
Administrative control
Job restructuring
Architectural barrier
Accessibility

LEARNING OBJECTIVES

After studying this chapter the student or practitioner will be able to do the following:

1. List the types of disabilities and conditions that qualify a person for protection under the ADA.
2. Recognize and define specific terms as they are used in the law.
3. Discuss the process for determining essential functions of job.
4. Recognize reasonable accommodations that are possible and appropriate for employment settings.
5. Describe the role of participatory ergonomics in the provision of reasonable accommodations.
6. Describe the step-by-step process of evaluating a building for accessibility.

It is estimated that 43 million Americans have physical or mental disabilities. This number is expected to increase as the population ages. Many of these people were employed before the onset of disability, but few returned to their former place of employment or to a new employment setting. Although the majority of people with disabilities want to work, two thirds of all disabled Americans between the ages of 16 and 64 are not working.[7]

Barriers to the employment of people with disabilities and to their use of transportation, public services, and telecommunications have significant economic and social costs. When barriers are removed, society benefits from the skills, talents, and purchasing power of these workers, who are able to lead more productive and fulfilling lives.

HISTORY OF LEGISLATION

The Civil Rights Act of 1964 prohibited discrimination against handicapped persons who were (1) beneficiaries of programs or activities receiving federal funds or (2) employees of federal contractors or (3) federal employees. The Americans With Disabilities Act (ADA), signed into law on July 26, 1990, gives persons with disabilities civil rights protection similar to that provided to all persons on the basis of race, sex, national origin, age, and religion.[2] The ADA does not preempt any federal, state, or local law that provides greater or equal protection for the rights of persons with disabilities. The ADA guarantees equal opportunity for persons with disabilities in public accommodations such as employment, transportation, state and local government services, and telecommunications.

The ADA provides for monetary and injunctive relief, back pay, future pay, lost benefits, and attorneys' fees for persons proving discrimination. In addition to compensation for actual dollar losses, damages might include awards for emotional pain and suffering and for loss of enjoyment of life. An employer who is shown to have acted with malice and indifference to these federally protected rights may also be subject to fines of up to $300,000 if the employer has more than 500 employees. Smaller employers are also subject to large fines if they do not make good faith efforts to comply with the law.

AMERICANS WITH DISABILITIES ACT

The ADA comprises five sections, called *titles*.[2] Title I concerns employment, Title II concerns public services, Title III covers public accommodations, Title IV relates to telecommunications, and Title V deals with a wide range of other topics concerning implementation of the law. As of July 26, 1992, Title I applies to employers with 25 or more employees, and as of July 26, 1994, it affects employers with 15 or more employees.

The ADA is broad and inclusive in its provisions. It encompasses many areas of intervention appropriate for occupational therapists. The U.S. Equal Employment Opportunity Commission (EEOC) has clearly defined and described the employment provisions in the *Technical Assistance Manual of the Employment Provisions (Title I) of the Americans with Disabilities Act.*[14] Any occupational therapy (OT) practitioner who is interested in providing services in regard to this portion of the ADA should obtain and become familiar with this publication and associated documents and resources.

TERMS USED IN THE LAW

A person with a disability is defined as someone who has a physical or mental impairment that "substantially limits" one or more "major life activities"; has a record of such an impairment; or is regarded as having such an impairment. According to the ADA, an impairment is a physiological or mental disorder. A physical condition, such as pregnancy, that is not the result of a physiological disorder is not an impairment. Similarly, personality traits such as poor judgment or a quick temper are not impairments. Environmental, cultural, or economic disadvantages such as a prison record or a lack of education also are not qualifying impairments.[2] An illustrative example given by the EEOC is that dyslexia, a specific learning disability, is an impairment, whereas an inability to read because of dropping out of school is not considered an impairment.

An impairment is a disability only if it substantially limits one or more major life activities. To be considered disabled, a person must be unable to perform or be significantly limited in the ability to perform an activity, compared with an average person in the general population. Major life activities are activities that an average person can perform with little or no difficulty. Examples of major life activities listed in the law include walking, speaking, breathing, performing manual tasks, seeing, hearing, learning, caring for oneself, working, sitting, standing, lifting, and reading.

Three factors should be considered in determining whether an impairment constitutes substantial limitation: the nature and severity of the limitation, the length or expected length of the limitation, and permanence or expected effect. All of these factors are considered, because simply identifying the name of the condition or the diagnosis does not indicate whether it is substantially limiting to the life of an individual. An individual would be protected under the ADA if he or she has two or more impairments that together cause substantial limitation, even if neither one substantially limits a major life activity by itself.

Other classes of individuals are covered by the provisions of the act. Persons who have successfully completed or are participating in a drug rehabilitation program or have otherwise been successfully rehabilitated and are no longer engaged in the illegal use of drugs are covered on the basis of past addiction. The intent of this provision is to protect people from discrimination based on myths, stereotypes, and fears about disability.

Persons who have a record of a disability or who are regarded as having a disability are protected by the ADA, even if they are not currently limited in a major life activity.[2] This provision brings up a host of possible scenarios. The law protects people with a history of cancer, heart disease, mental illness, or other conditions whose illnesses are cured, controlled, or in remission. The law also protects people who have been erroneously classified as having a disability or who have had a disability misdiagnosed. The perception of disability also entitles a person to protection. Facial scars, for instance, may create the perception of disability and thus carry protection under the law.

TITLE I: EMPLOYMENT PROVISIONS OF THE ADA

A goal of legislators in drafting the bill was to ensure that qualified individuals would have equal access to the rights and privileges of employment. Title I specifically states that it is against the law to discriminate against qualified job applicants or employees on the basis of disability. This protection covers all areas of employment, including the job application process, testing, hiring, job assignment, promotion, discharge, wages, job training, disciplinary actions, leave, benefits, and several other aspects of employment.

As defined by the ADA, a qualified individual with a disability is an individual with a disability who meets the skill, experience, education, and other job-related requirements of a position held or desired and who, with or without reasonable accommodation, can perform the essential functions of the job.[2,14] For an individual to be deemed substantially limited in working, he or she need not be totally unable to work. The individual must be significantly restricted in the ability to perform a broad range of jobs compared with average persons with similar training, skills, and abilities.

Persons Not Covered by Title I of the ADA

Current illegal drug use does not qualify a person for protection under the ADA. The act specifically states that the following are not covered disabilities: transvestitism, transsexualism, pedophilia, exhibitionism, voyeurism, gender identity disorders, compulsive gambling, kleptomania, and pyromania.

Specific Provisions of the Employment Title

The primary intent of the ADA is to allow qualified persons with disabilities to participate in the work force to the same degree as those without disabilities. It is not a preference law, nor is it a quota law. Qualified persons with disabilities must have equal access to employment opportunities, provided they are able to perform the "essential functions of a job with or without reasonable accommodation."[2]

By definition, a person with a disability cannot perform tasks in the same manner as people without a disability; he or she needs some type of accommodation. The ADA requires **"reasonable accommodation,"** meaning that the accommodation is effective for accomplishment of the task.[2] These accommodations can take many forms, such as a restructuring of the job, an alteration of the work schedule, the provision of a signing interpreter, the provision of assistive aids or equipment, the widening of doors, and a host of other modifications. However, the obligation of the employer does not extend to providing items that may be for the personal benefit of the individual, on or off the job, such as a personal attendant.

The ADA also states that making accommodations must not pose an "undue hardship" for the employer.[2] This means that the employer is not required to provide an accommodation that poses substantial difficulty or expense. An accommodation that is unduly expensive, extensive, substantial, or disruptive or that fundamentally alters the nature of operation of the business would be deemed a hardship. For example, a dance club would not be required to accommodate a visually impaired employee by raising the light level because

to do so would fundamentally alter the nature of the business.

Several other concepts must be understood to appreciate the effect of this law. An employer is not required to accommodate an applicant or employee if doing so would pose a "direct threat" to the health and safety of the individual or others in the workplace and if this threat cannot be eliminated or reduced by reasonable accommodation. This threat must create "a significant risk of substantial harm," according to EEOC regulations. The risk of harm must be determined individually, considering severity, duration, and imminence of the potential harm. For example, if there has never been a fire in the building, it is not lawful to cite concern for fire evacuation safety in denying employment to a person who uses a wheelchair. The law states that considerations of "direct threat" must rely on objective, factual evidence and not on subjective perceptions, irrational fears, patronizing attitudes, or stereotypes.[2] This presents another opportunity for OT practitioners to educate employers about the true nature of functional limitations a person with a disability may or may not have.

Once a threat is identified, the employer must evaluate whether the threat poses a significant risk of substantial harm. For individuals with mental or emotional disabilities, the employer must identify the specific behaviors on the part of the individual that pose the direct threat. It is obviously the intent of the federal law that persons with disabilities not be denied employment because of risks that are not truly significant and threatening.

Occupational therapists are always concerned about the safety and health of persons with disabilities. Therapists must take care to ensure that individuals are not barred unfairly in any way from employment because of overly protective concern for their safety and well-being. The requirement to accommodate reasonably applies again to this area of employment. An employer must consider whether a reasonable accommodation might sufficiently reduce or eliminate the potential risk of harm. If no accommodation is possible, the employer is not required to hire the individual. For example, an employer may be seeking to hire someone for a carpentry position. An essential function of this position is the use of power saws and other potentially dangerous equipment. For this position, the employer would not be required to hire an individual who has narcolepsy and unexpectedly loses consciousness.

The concept of *essential functions* is new to many employers who traditionally write job descriptions that describe the means to accomplishing the end product. In a 1981 case filed under the Rehabilitation Act, the U.S. Postal Service required each employee to be able to use both arms when performing the job of distribution clerk. One employee with limited mobility of one arm demonstrated that he was able to perform the essential function of lifting and moving mail, although with one arm rather than two. In this case the court found that the essential function was lifting and moving mail, not using two arms, and the employee was determined to be a qualified individual with a disability.[1]

The term **essential function** means the fundamental job duties of the employment position. In determining the essential functions of a job, the employer must consider all relevant evidence. This evidence includes: (1) the employer's judgment as to which functions are essential; (2) a written job description prepared before interviewing applicants for a job; (3) the amount of time spent performing the function; (4) the consequences of not requiring a person to perform the function; (5) the terms of collective bargaining agreements; and (6) the experience of people who have performed and currently perform similar jobs.

A function cannot be deemed essential if it is in reality marginal or peripheral. For instance, a secretary may be requested to drive to the post office to buy stamps, but this task may be an incidental one that could be performed by another employee and is not essential to the position of secretary. The example of an airline pilot is often used to illustrate the reason for considering all relevant evidence and not just certain aspects such as the amount of time spent performing the function. An airline pilot may spend only 5% of the work shift landing and taking off, but this function is certainly essential for pilots. Likewise, a firefighter may only occasionally carry an unconscious person from a burning building, but the consequences of not requiring performance of this function would be serious.

Employers are permitted to use physical agility tests, medical examinations, aptitude and ability tests, and tests for illegal drug use. There must be no disparate impact—that is, the test must not screen out and discriminate against persons with disabilities.[2] It is not permissible, for instance, to give a written test to a person with the specific learning disability dyslexia unless reading itself is an essential function of the job.

If testing is required for employment, all persons being considered for the job category must be tested in the same manner. It is not permissible to require a medical examination or screening of physical ability only for persons with disabilities. Reasonable accommodation is required in the testing process and testing environment, if notice of the need for accommodation is received before administration of the test.

It is not permissible to require testing or examination or ask questions about disability before an offer of employment is made. The offer of employment may be rescinded upon results of the examination or inquiry. Aside from testing, the employer is permitted to ask the applicant to describe or demonstrate how a job-related function would be performed with or without accommodation. Physical agility tests are not considered medical; therefore they may be given at any point in the application or employment process. However, if a determination of employment is based on the results of such tests, the tests must be related to the job and consistent with business necessity.

Opportunities for Occupational Therapists to Assist Employers

Given the broad provisions of Title I of the ADA, it is apparent that employers, physicians, workers' compensation insurance carriers, and other parties involved in the employment of persons with disabilities may need special expertise to fulfill their obligations lawfully. One important mandate is that the employer show good faith efforts to comply with the law. Many employers lack the in-house knowledge and resources to meet this obligation. The unique training of occupational therapists, especially pertaining to functional performance, adaptation, daily life activities, and knowledge of community resources, equips them well to provide assistance. Several activities that may be unfamiliar to practitioners are not so much new as they are different applications of therapists' skills.

Determination of Essential Functions

The ADA requires employers to examine the precise functional physical activities required to perform work-related tasks. It is the right and responsibility of the employer to determine which functions of their employees' jobs are essential, though they may seek the assistance of an occupational therapist to understand the precise physical nature of the essential functions.

To determine the physical demands of essential functions, a specialized type of task or job analysis is performed. The *Essential Function Analysis Worksheet* is a systematic way to perform this type of task analysis.[8] For each essential function of the job, a worksheet is completed by the occupational therapist in collaboration with the employer and possibly with input from employees currently doing the job (Fig. 17-1). As with many areas of the ADA, terms are used precisely. *Bending* refers to stooping and bending forward at the waist while keeping the knees straight. *Squat* (also called crouch) refers to lowering oneself toward the floor while bending the knees. *Kneel* refers to working at floor or ground level, placing weight on one or both knees. *Climb* includes ladders, stairs, scaffolding, and the like. *Pull/push* refers to pushing objects away from the body or pulling objects toward the body, such as when pushing a cart or pulling a chain hoist. *Using foot controls* may include driving, as well as activating foot switches. *Hand manipulation* refers to gross hand grasp or manipulation, while *fine finger manipulation* denotes precise finger use and may include the use of small tools and parts.

ESSENTIAL FUNCTION ANALYSIS WORKSHEET

Employer Name _____ Date of Analysis _____

Address of Job Site _____

Job Title _____ Hours per Week _____

1. General job description

   _____

2. Essential function _____

   _____

3. Time spent doing essential function

Activity	Total hours doing the activity											Hour continuous performance?	Can it be modified?	
	0	<1	1	2	3	4	5	6	7	8	>8		Yes	No
Sit														
Stand														
Walk														
Bend														
Squat														
Kneel														
Climb														
Push/Pull														
Use Foot Controls														
Reach above Shoulders														

4. Hand manipulation required [ ]yes [ ]no [ ]right [ ]left [ ]both [ ]intermittent [ ]continuous
   Total time continuous _____ Can function be modified? [ ]yes [ ]no

5. Fine manipulation required [ ]yes [ ]no [ ]right [ ]left [ ]both [ ]intermittent [ ]continuous
   Total time continuous _____ Can function be modified? [ ]yes [ ]no

6. Lift [ ]<1 lb [ ]1-10 lbs [ ]11-20 lbs [ ]21-30 lbs [ ]31-40 lbs [ ]41-50 lbs [ ]51-75 lbs
   [ ]76-100 lbs [ ]> 100 lbs [ ]intermittent [ ]continuous Total time continuous _____
   Can function be modified? [ ]yes [ ]no

7. Carry [ ]<1 lb [ ]1-10 lbs [ ]11-20 lbs [ ]21-30 lbs [ ]31-40 lbs [ ]41-50 lbs [ ]51-75 lbs
   [ ]76-100 lbs [ ]> 100 lbs [ ]intermittent [ ]continuous Total time continuous _____
   Can function be modified? [ ]yes [ ]no

8. Psychological requirements

9. Employer confirmation signature _____ Date _____

10. Analysis performed by _____ Date _____

FIG. 17-1

Essential Function Analysis Worksheet. (From Isom R, Boyle K, Smith P: *ADA compliance system*, Athens, Ga, 1993, Elliot & Fitzpatrick.)

The therapist should indicate on the form how much time is spent continuously doing the activity at any one time (i.e., without taking a break or changing or alternating activity). If the work is done intermittently with other activities, the therapist should indicate the maximum period of continuous performance at any one time.

During the process of analyzing the essential functions, the therapist also gathers information about whether a function can be modified and how this might be accomplished. This is discussed further in the later section of the chapter pertaining to reasonable accommodation and participatory ergonomics.

A task analysis for ADA purposes must be focused on the precise nature of activities, such as weights of loads handled, hand functions, duration of effort, and number of repetitions of physical movements. When performing the essential function analysis, the therapist must understand the distinction between the process used for production of a product and the physical activity required for that production process. For instance, although a job function may be to load boxes of machine parts into a truck, this may not require manually lifting the box with two hands, carrying the box using its handles, and climbing into the truck. In other words, it should not be assumed that manual lifting, using the handles, and climbing are essential functions. In contrast, using the hands to type on a computer keyboard may be an essential function for a secretary. Each job needs to be analyzed separately to determine these factors accurately. An example of a completed worksheet pertaining to one of the essential functions of the job of delivery driver illustrates how a single function is analyzed and documented (Fig. 17-2). After each essential function of a job has been analyzed and documented in this way, all of the worksheets pertaining to the job are combined and become a comprehensive document for use by the employer—a document that serves as evidence of good faith compliance with the ADA.

Employers may think that all functions of their jobs are essential, when in reality some functions can be distributed among other workers, some can be eliminated or combined, and some are marginal, not essential, functions. This situation presents another opportunity for an occupational therapist to help employers understand the true nature of their jobs from the standpoint of physical, cognitive, and mental requirements.

Elimination of Discriminatory Questions, Language, and Behaviors

Human resources personnel and hiring managers may not be familiar with preferred terminology with respect to persons with disabilities and may be insensitive to issues of nondiscriminatory language. The therapist may assist the employer in purging employment applications, interview procedures, and other employment practices of discriminatory language, both overt and subtle. All employment documents should be free of negative wording such as the following: *confined to a wheelchair, wheelchair-bound, victim of, suffering from, afflicted with,* and *crippled.*

The ADA encourages self-identification by persons with disabilities. Occupational therapists may train hiring personnel to practice nondiscriminatory behaviors and procedures. Persons unaccustomed to interacting with individuals with disabilities may benefit from role-playing, mock interviewing, and the provision of information about various disabilities and their sequelae. For instance, hiring personnel need to know that HIV and AIDS are not contracted by casual contact and that to deny equal employment opportunities to qualified persons with these disorders constitutes illegal discrimination.

Occupational therapists may wish to develop a handbook of basic tips and suggestions for communicating with people who have hearing impairments and distribute this handbook to managers and coworkers. Among the general principles included in the handbook should be talking directly to the hearing-impaired person and maintaining eye contact, even when an attendant or interpreter is present. Managers and coworkers should be reminded that although the communication skills of people with speech and hearing impairments may be weak, this weakness is not a measure of intelligence or self-confidence. The handbook should also remind managers and coworkers to keep their voices at normal volume and not to raise or exaggerate the tone of their voices, when speaking to speech- and hearing-impaired individuals.

Language used in training materials should be free of jargon. Information should be presented with the intent to inform objectively, rather than to depict persons with disabilities as deserving of pity or as fortunate and "chosen." Community resources and social service agencies can be tapped for information and referral. Disability advocacy groups in the community may be pleased to come to the work site and address groups of employees. Special interest organizations such as the Arthritis Foundation, Cancer Society, Heart Association, and many others can usually provide pamphlets and speakers.

Integration of employees can be fostered by forming work groups to promote contact between workers with disabilities and their coworkers. Assigning tasks to a work group rather than to an individual encourages mainstreaming and reduces the social isolation that frequently occurs for persons with disabilities.[1] Removing the mystique of disability and promoting comfort in the interview situation and everyday working environment can be especially beneficial for all involved.

ESSENTIAL FUNCTION ANALYSIS WORKSHEET

Employer Name __All American Office Place__   Date of Analysis __5/22/1992__

Address of Job Site __10129 Bay Blvd. San Francisco, CA 94134__

Job Title __Delivery Driver__   Hours per Week __40__

1. General job description

    Deliver office supplies and small equipment to customers in local counties.

2. Essential function __Load, unload and deliver office supplies and small equipment.__

3. Time spent doing essential function

Activity	0	<1	1	2	3	4	5	6	7	8	>8	Hour continuous performance?	Can it be modified? Yes	No
Sit		X												X
Stand		X												X
Walk		X											X	
Bend		X												X
Squat		X												X
Kneel	X													
Climb		X											X	
Push/Pull		X												X
Use Foot Controls	X													
Reach above Shoulders	X													

4. Hand manipulation required   [x]yes   [ ]no   [ ]right   [ ]left   [x]both   [x]intermittent   [ ]continuous
   Total time continuous __less than 1 hr.__   Can function be modified?   [ ]yes   [x]no

5. Fine manipulation required   [ ]yes   [x]no   [ ]right   [ ]left   [ ]both   [ ]intermittent   [ ]continuous
   Total time continuous _____   Can function be modified?   [ ]yes   [ ]no

6. Lift   [ ]<1 lb [ ]1-10 bs [ ]11-20 lbs [ ]21-30 lbs [x]31-40 lbs [ ]41-50 lbs [ ]51-75 lbs
   [ ]76-100 lbs [ ]> 100 lbs [x]intermittent [ ]continuous Total time continuous __30 min.__
   Can function be modified?   [x]yes   [ ]no

7. Carry   [ ]<1 lb [ ]1-10 lbs [ ]11-20 lbs [ ]21-30 lbs [x]31-40 lbs [ ]41-50 lbs [ ]51-75 lbs
   [ ]76-100 lbs [ ]> 100 lbs [x]intermittent [ ]continuous Total time continuous __30 min.__
   Can function be modified?   [x]yes   [ ]no

8. Psychological requirements

9. Employer confirmation signature _____   Date _____

10. Analysis performed by _____   Date _____

FIG. 17-2

Partially completed Essential Function Analysis Worksheet. (From Isom R, Boyle K, Smith P: *ADA compliance system*, Athens, Ga, 1993, Elliot & Fitzpatrick.)

Medical Inquiries, Examinations, and Post-Offer Screenings

When an employee is ready to return to work after an injury or illness, the employer may require passage of a job-related examination (sometimes referred to as a fitness-for-duty exam) as a condition of returning to work. The examination must evaluate only the ability to perform the essential functions of the job with or without reasonable accommodation.

The employer may also require passage of an examination by job applicants; however, different regulations apply for a new applicant than for a returning employee. An applicant for a job may be required to participate in an examination only after a conditional offer of employment has been made. Such an applicant examination or screening of physical ability does not have to be related to the job. However, if a person with a disability is screened out, the reason for disqualification must be related to the job and of business necessity. The job-related screening activity must be a valid and legitimate measure of qualification for a specific job. If a test or activity does not relate to the essential functions of the specific job, it is not consistent with business necessity. All persons applying for the job must be examined, irrespective of disability. An employer may give follow-up tests or examinations if the initial examination indicates a problem that may affect job performance.[6]

The post-offer screening should be preceded by a thorough essential function analysis to ensure that the screening is based on the physical and mental requirements of performing the essential functions of the job. The screening protocol should be matched to the specific job and should include the physical requirements of each essential function, the frequency with which each function is performed, and the use of customary tools, protective clothing, or equipment such as a helmet or gloves. The screening protocol also should replicate the work environment as much as possible. Chapter 16 provides further information about developing a similar protocol, referred to as a "Work Tolerance Screening." The screening may be performed in a clinical setting or at the work site. The screening also may be quite brief if only a select number of essential functions are included. This would be the case if only a few functions present substantial challenges in terms of physical functional performance. It is important to remember that a screening is a measure of current performance and does not predict risk of future injury.

Reasonable Accommodation Investigation and Participatory Ergonomics

The ADA requires that persons with disabilities be accommodated to ensure their equal opportunity to be considered for a job, to enable them to perform the essential functions of a job, and to participate in all privileges of employment.[2] ADA regulations require a systematic investigation of reasonable accommodations to achieve this goal.[14] The investigation is to be conducted on an individual basis and should include the participation of the person with the disability. The occupational therapist who is familiar with ergonomic interventions will recognize that this is an ideal opportunity to incorporate an ergonomic perspective to facilitate the fit between the worker and the job.

Ergonomics is the study of the relationship between the worker and the work environment. It is concerned with the problems and processes involved in designing and, in some cases, modifying the environment for effective and suitable human working and living. Participation of the person who is occupied in the environment has been called **participatory ergonomics.** This practice maximizes the chance that the worker's motivations, preferences, and beliefs will be considered and incorporated into any ergonomic solutions. To leave out these elements invites a lack of cooperation and perhaps ultimate failure of the intervention or accommodation. Occupational therapists are especially skilled in communicating with people with disabilities and encouraging their inclusion and participation.

The ADA mandates the provision of an effective accommodation—not necessarily the best solution, but one that will enable a qualified employee to perform the essential functions to meet employer standards of production, quality, and safety.[2] The EEOC has given several examples of possible accommodations.[14] Providing physical access to the work site is a fairly obvious accommodation. The employer should remove structural barriers to any areas where the employee will perform the essential functions of the job, as well as to adjacent areas such as rest rooms, break rooms, lunch rooms, recreational spaces, and any other areas an employee may expect to use. More suggestions about barrier removal for physical access are given later in this chapter as they pertain to Title III of the ADA.

When reasonable accommodation strategies are being developed, the simplest and least costly should be considered first. For instance, the therapist should first investigate whether there is a way to modify how the function is performed, a strategy referred to as an **administrative control.** This strategy satisfies the needs of the worker with disability and the employer's business needs at the same time. Energy conservation techniques may be appropriate for many people and should usually be considered. If these simple interventions are not sufficient, it may be necessary to consider modifying tools or purchasing equipment and aids. Buying commercially available equipment and aids rather than those that are custom made is less expensive. Custom-made devices and assistive technology may be necessary when these previous administrative and ergonomic solutions are not adequate. Employers who are not knowledgeable about other creative and cost-effective solutions often have the perception that the more expensive options are the only ones available.

Job restructuring is another reasonable accommodation that may be considered. This approach includes examining an essential function analysis and rearranging, adding, or deleting requirements in terms of tasks performed. This step may involve combining several tasks the individual with disability is able to perform or removing tasks that cannot be performed and transferring them to another employee. Perhaps the job can be modified so that the hours of work are flexible to allow needed breaks in the day, or perhaps the job may be changed to part time. All of these changes are considered possible and desirable accommodations in the view of the EEOC.

Another accommodation might be reassigning a person with a disability to a vacant position. The ADA does not require the employer to create a position; however, the employer is required to consider placement of the person in a vacant position if one is available. The occupational therapist may assist the employer in determining appropriate vacant positions within the company and evaluating the functional abilities of candidates to perform the essential functions of the available positions. What may appear appropriate to the employer because it is light in nature may be inappropriate for a given individual because of the precise nature of the activities required.

Modifying equipment, providing assistive aids, and training in adaptive methods can also constitute reasonable accommodation. Products designed for other purposes can be combined in creative and new ways. The Job Accommodation Network (JAN) is a service of the President's Committee on Employment of People with Disabilities[9] JAN provides information about resources and reasonable accommodations. By sending follow-up questionnaires to callers who have used JAN services, the organization has been able to compile data about the costs of accommodations. JAN determined that two thirds of accommodations cost less than $500. In a 1982 study for the Department of Labor by Berkeley Planning Associates, it was found that half of all accommodations cost nothing and more than two thirds cost less than $100.[9] Many products that are readily available for consumer use are extremely useful for persons with disabilities. For example, telephones with oversize buttons are thought of as decorative and trendy, but they are also useful for persons with visual or motor impairments.

Occupational therapists are becoming increasingly proficient in locating and applying assistive technology. Detailed information about assistive technology can be found in Chapter 19. Title I of the ADA pertains only to employment issues; in these cases the concern of the clinician is confined to assistive technology for job performance rather than for other areas of functioning such as personal care. The employer's responsibility does not usually extend to durable medical equipment such as wheelchairs. Ethical dilemmas may arise for occupational therapists about employee needs for such personal care equipment; however, it is essential for the OT practitioner working in this area of practice to maintain focus on the rights and responsibilities of the employer, as well as those of the person with a disability.[13]

Persons with psychiatric disabilities may need any of the types of accommodation already discussed, as well as other types of accommodations to enable them to be successfully employed. Interpersonal communication may be especially difficult. It may be helpful to train supervisors to provide written instructions or feedback for the person who becomes anxious and confused when given spoken instructions. Added time, structure, and organization may be helpful. Removing distraction may be useful and readily achievable by positioning room dividers or facing workstations away from open areas. Extra support and reassurance may be necessary for the person reentering the work force after psychiatric hospitalization.

TITLE II OF THE ADA: PUBLIC SERVICES

Title II of the law pertains to all state and local government activities, services, and programs, including courts, police and fire departments, town meetings, and employment offices.[2] Unlike section 504 of the Rehabilitation Act of 1973, which covers only programs receiving federal funds, Title II extends to all the activities of state and local governments, whether or not they receive federal funds. This title prohibits state and local governments from denying participation in any service, program, or activity on the basis of disability. All programs, services, and activities must be integrated and must not have unnecessary eligibility standards or rules that deny participation to persons with disabilities.

Newly constructed buildings and alterations to existing facilities must be structured to ensure access. New buses and rail vehicles must also be accessible. Effective communication must be ensured.[2] Occupational therapists may have opportunities in this area similar to those afforded by Title III. A more complete explanation of potential opportunities is presented later in this chapter.

TITLE III: PUBLIC ACCOMMODATIONS

Title III of the ADA covers all buildings used by the public, such as restaurants, hotels, theaters, retail stores, museums, libraries, parks, private schools, day care centers, and facilities used by social service agencies and health care service providers. This section of the law requires that existing facilities remove **architectural**

barriers where such removal is "readily achievable," a standard that has been defined as "easily accomplishable and able to be carried out without too much difficulty or expense."[2] Barriers must be removed to allow access to the premises and use of the facilities, including: parking areas, walkways, ramps, entrances, display racks, signage, doors, alarms, restrooms, toilet stalls, grab bars, and other features. If a barrier cannot readily be removed, other methods of providing access may be substituted. Examples include providing curb service or a drive-up window, providing home delivery, having employees retrieve items that are beyond reach, and moving certain activities to accessible areas of the facility.

Title III also mandates access to communication. Persons with disabilities must be given the opportunity to see, hear, and understand what is occurring in the environment.[2] Facilities remodeled after January 26, 1992, must be readily accessible and usable by persons with disabilities to the "maximum extent feasible." Specific requirements apply to "key conveniences." These are listed as the path of travel to the altered area (e.g., curb cuts, ramps, doors, and elevators), rest rooms, telephones, and drinking fountains. These key conveniences must be accessible to the maximum extent feasible unless the cost and scope is "disproportionate to the cost of the overall alteration."[2]

New facilities must be "readily accessible to and usable by" persons with disabilities, regardless of cost. Certain implementation dates and exceptions apply to new construction. Detailed information about compliance can be found in the Americans with Disabilities Act Accessible Guidelines for Building and Facilities.[2]

The mandates of Title II and Title III create numerous opportunities for occupational therapists to be of assistance. Whereas Title II mandates access for persons with disabilities to travel to their destinations, Title III requires access for them to participate fully once they arrive. Various references have been and are being developed to provide specific guidelines regarding accessibility.[11,12,14]

General principles of accessibility are part of the basic training of occupational therapists. The process of determining appropriate solutions begins with an analysis of the tasks to be performed or accessibility that is desired, often referred to as an *accessibility audit*. An audit of the facilities may have been performed previously and should be obtained if available. The therapist should perform an audit if none has been done previously. Information from the audit forms the basis of the services and recommendations to be provided.

Step-by-Step Audit of Facilities

The therapist should begin an audit by clearly indicating the physical activities required for access to the facility, determining such things as the means of travel,

strength requirements, and dexterity demands. Next, the therapist performs an analysis of the person with disability and his or her capabilities and limitations with respect to particular tasks. The therapist should keep in mind that persons with disabilities are experts about their own needs and capabilities and possible solutions to their problems.

When the therapist is beginning an audit of **accessibility,** it is helpful to think in terms of the sequential steps taken by an individual seeking access to a facility or service. Upon arriving at the facility, the individual must approach the entrance. If arriving by private vehicle, the person will need a drop-off spot or parking area. The individual must have a means to enter the facility. Once inside, the individual must continue past a receptionist or building directory and may pass through corridors, stairs, and an elevator.

All of the activities and movements in and about the facility should be determined and noted in this systematic manner so that any barriers become evident. The therapist may be accompanied on this excursion by the person with disability and by persons familiar with the facility and the access alternatives that may be feasible. Perhaps another route is more suitable or a different entrance door is more easily used. It must be kept in mind that facilities for persons with disabilities must be enabling and not discriminatory or segregated. For instance, access via a freight elevator on the loading dock is not usually considered a suitable entrance for a person who uses a wheelchair.

General standards of accessibility have been developed by various organizations and regulatory agencies. These standards are reviewed and revised periodically. The most current information can usually be obtained from local sources such as the building department of the city or county. If local regulations are more stringent than the ADA, the local regulations take precedence. Some general sequential guidelines are presented here as a basis for beginning to think about opportunities for occupational therapists to contribute in this area.

Step 1: Entering the Building

Parking spaces or a drop-off zone should be located near an accessible building entrance and connected to that entrance by walkways. Handicapped parking spaces should be designated and reserved. Parking spaces should be 12 feet wide and have an access aisle for loading and unloading. Curb cuts should be textured and should meet the street surface with as little lip as possible. Walkways and ramps should be sloped at no more than 2° to the side (cross slope) and 5° in rise and have a nonslip surface. A handrail should be provided on at least one side; railing on both sides is preferred. The rail should extend beyond the top and bottom of the ramp.

Ramps to doorways should have a 5-foot level surface at the top and bottom. Entrance doors should have at least 32 inches of clear opening and should be power operated or easy to grasp and to push or pull open. Doors in a series should have adequate space between them to permit door swing into the space. Revolving doors and turnstiles are not considered accessible entrances. Appropriate directional signs pointing to the nearest accessible entrance should be posted on any entrance doors that are not accessible.[10]

Step 2: Building Interiors

All essential areas should be accessible without requiring the individual to leave the building or negotiate steps. Corridors should be at least 48 inches wide and free of obstructions such as drinking fountains, supporting columns, telephones, and decorative plants. Floors should have a hard, nonslip surface or low-pile carpet. If public telephones are provided, at least one should be mounted not more than 48 inches high. Drinking fountains, if available, should be no more than 36 inches high to the level of water flow. The path of travel in all areas, such as between desks, should be adequate in width. Identifying signs and labels should be of sufficient size and color contrast for easy viewing. The use of tactile letters and numbers and Braille letters is advisable, as is an auditory signal in elevators to identify the floor level. Elevator controls should not exceed a height of 60 inches. Interior doors to public areas should have at least 30 inches of clear opening. Any stairs should be amply lit and should not have abrupt or open risers that may catch toes or braces.[10]

Step 3: Rest Rooms

Rest rooms present special challenges in terms of providing for safety, especially because they are often small. In general, each building should have a minimum of one rest room for women and one for men that are accessible to persons using wheelchairs. All doors and passageways should be wide enough to permit a wheelchair to make any required turns. Toilet stalls should be of sufficient width to permit a front or side transfer. Handrails should be appropriately located and capable of supporting a 250-pound load. Dispensers, hand dryers, and other fixed items should not impede movement and should be positioned for easy reach, generally not higher than 48 inches. Mirrors should be full length or tilted downward. Sinks should have easy-to-operate handles and knee clearance underneath the fixture. Drains and hot water pipes should be insulated to prevent burns.[10]

Step 4: Other Considerations

All areas of facilities used by the public should be free of barriers to physical movement and impediments to hearing, seeing, and understanding the business being conducted. Unique or unusual environments must be carefully inspected and questioned. For instance, if voice communication must occur through an opening in a glass security window, is there some way to augment communication for the user who is seated or very short in stature? Is there appropriate provision for persons using crutches or walkers to enjoy a sporting event from the grandstand? It is important to consider energy expenditure of persons with disabilities, as well as the needs of elderly persons who may have decreased endurance. The opportunity to sit and rest may be essential for participating in activities.[3]

All of these issues of access and accommodation require expert and sensitive advice from trained professionals such as occupational therapists. The therapist often can recommend low-cost modifications for upgrading existing facilities. The occupational therapist may also give advice during the design phase of new construction. Further information about minimal requirements for access can be found in recently published guidelines and local government publications, as well as on Internet sites dealing with these areas.

Additional information also can be obtained from the online service maintained by the American Occupational Therapy Association. The ADA/Assistive Technology/Home Modification Resource Network is an online list of occupational therapists who specialize in promoting the ADA. Technical advances such as voice-synthesized direction signs and traffic signals, infrared sensors in buildings, and other devices are being developed and are becoming increasingly prevalent.

TITLE IV: TELECOMMUNICATION

Title IV requires that all intrastate and interstate telephone companies establish relay systems for use by hearing- and speech-impaired persons 24 hours per day. These services must be available at no additional cost. This title also requires that television public service announcements produced or funded by the federal government include closed captioning.

SUMMARY

The ADA mandates a broad range of services to ensure equal opportunities for persons with disabilities. The act's various titles, particularly the portions pertaining to employment and to access to public services and facilities, encourage participation in society by the estimated 43 million persons with disabilities in the United States. As employers, public agencies, and services strive to comply with the provisions of the ADA, many exciting opportunities are created for knowledgeable occupational therapists.

The therapist's basic training must be augmented with a thorough study of the law and its regulations and interpretations. To this base of knowledge should be added (1) experience with persons with all types of qualifying disabilities and (2) expertise in ergonomic accommodations to compensate for the impairments that may be associated with these disabilities. Finally, the therapist must understand the business and human resources needs of employers. Armed with this knowledge and experience, occupational therapists are uniquely qualified to provide consulting and direct services to aid in compliance with the ADA.

CASE STUDY 17-1

CASE STUDY—MR. G.

Mr. G. has a congenital orthopedic condition and requires the use of a wheelchair. He is a technical writer and has accepted a position with a new employer. The company is located in a historic building that cannot be extensively modified.

Mr. G. arrives at work by car, enters the building unassisted, and takes the elevator to his floor. He cannot reach the elevator buttons and cannot open the door to his company suite. His cubicle is fully accessible for him; however, he has difficulty using the telephone because he tires of holding the receiver for prolonged periods.

In collaboration with Mr. G. and his employer, the occupational therapist developed and fabricated a small reaching device to use for pressing the elevator buttons. Mr. G. carries the device with him. The door to his company suite is made of glass and is too heavy for him to open. A receptionist is always seated in the lobby. An arrangement was made for the receptionist to open the door for Mr. G. each morning and evening. A doorbell-type buzzer was installed outside the door, and Mr. G. uses the buzzer to ring the reception desk when he desires access. Because Mr. G. works in an open cubicle, it was decided that a speaker telephone would not be feasible; however, a lightweight headset will enable him to use the telephone hands-free. With these simple, low-cost accommodations, Mr. G. is able to perform the essential functions of his job as a technical writer.

REVIEW QUESTIONS

1. Does the ADA pertain to small employers or only to very large employers?
2. What qualifies a person for protection under the ADA?
3. What is meant by "substantially limits a person"?
4. What are the major life activities to which the law refers?
5. Can a person be prevented from participating in a job if the supervisor has any concern about his or her ability to safely perform the job?
6. What six categories of evidence should be considered in determining the essential functions of a job?
7. How can a person with a specific learning disability be tested for ability to perform the essential functions of a job?
8. How can occupational therapists help employers develop employment application forms and interview questions that comply with the ADA?
9. What are some of the ways qualified persons with disabilities can be accommodated if they are unable to perform an essential function of a job?
10. Must all job applicants or only applicants with disabilities be required to pass a screening of physical ability before they begin a new job?
11. Does public access to buildings apply only to government facilities, or does it also apply to buildings owned by private parties?
12. Access is required to what parts of the building?
13. How should an occupational therapist plan an evaluation of a building for accessibility?
14. Are telecommunications companies required to provide any particular services according to the ADA? If so, what are those accommodations?

REFERENCES

1. American Management Association: Special report: ADA in action, *HR focus, special report,* 1992.
2. Americans With Disabilities Act of 1990 (PL 101-336), 42 U.S.C. 12101, *Federal register,* 56:144, 35543-35691, 1990.
3. Bachelder JM, Hilton CL: Implications of the Americans With Disabilities Act of 1990 for elderly persons, *Am J Occup Ther* 48:73, 1994.
4. Carbine M, Schwartz G: *Strategies for managing disability costs,* Washington, DC, 1987, Washington Business Group on Health.
5. Civil Rights Act of 1991 (PL 101-166), 42 U.S.C., *Congressional Record* 137:191, 1991.
6. Ellexson M: ADA compliance: to screen or not to screen? Work Programs Special Interest Section Newsletter, American Occupational Therapy Association 8:1, 1994.
7. International Center for the Disabled: ICD survey of disabled Americans: bringing disabled Americans into the mainstream, New York, 1986, The Center.
8. Isom R, Boyle K, Smith P: *ADA compliance system,* Athens, Ga, 1993, Elliot & Fitzpatrick.
9. Job Accommodation Network: *The truth about accommodations,* Morgantown, W Va, 1994, The Network.
10. National Rehabilitation Association: *Revised manual for accessibility,* Alexandria, Va, 1988, The Association.
11. National Rehabilitation Hospital-ADA Compliance Program: *Answers to questions commonly asked by hospitals and health care providers: ADA,* Washington, DC, 1993, The Hospital.
12. President's Committee on Employment of People With Disabilities: *ADA and the health professions,* Washington DC, 1993, U.S. Government Printing Office.
13. Rein J: Reasonable accommodation in the workplace, *Work programs special interest section newsletter,* 1992, American Occupational Therapy Association.
14. U.S. Equal Employment Opportunity Commission: *Technical assistance manual of the employment provisions of the Americans With Disabilities Act,* Washington DC, 1992, Equal Employment Opportunities Commission.

CHAPTER 18

Leisure Activities

CORALIE H. GLANTZ

NANCY RICHMAN

KEY TERMS

Recreation
Leisure
Coordinated leisure
Complementary leisure
Social roles

LEARNING OBJECTIVES

After studying this chapter the student or practitioner will be able to do the following:

1. Discuss the benefits of leisure for adults.
2. Contrast various forms of leisure.
3. Identify factors that may interfere with leisure exploration and activity.
4. Describe a comprehensive leisure evaluation.
5. Identify specific strategies to promote leisure activity for persons with disabilities.

RECREATION AND LEISURE IN ADULT LIFE

Leisure takes on different aspects of importance throughout the adult years. For young adults, issues of time and financial resources, as well as extensive work and family responsibilities, may limit access to meaningful leisure. Until very recent years, adults with physical disabilities would have had difficulty finding the adaptations necessary to continue with past leisure pursuits or develop new interests. The aging process affects leisure pursuits with the decline in physical abilities, sensory changes, and the perceptions of not being as capable at an endeavor as in previous years. However, as one expert reminds seniors, "If we draw on our own resources to eat right, exercise, and keep active and involved, our older years can be the most rewarding years. Our later years must be infused with expectations and meaningful activity based on our past successes, not on self-pity over past failures. The secret of successful aging is more than being able to tap the resources in our community but we must tap the resiliency of our own spirit."[2]

Adult play is classified as *recreation* and *leisure*. **Recreation** regenerates energy to support the worker role.[13] **Leisure** is freely selected activity pursued simply for the pleasure of the activity, with a minimum of social role obligations and freedom from constraint.[4] Activities that are not clearly work or leisure are called *coordinated leisure* and *complementary leisure*.[13] **Coordinated leisure** is work-related activity that has the element of being freely chosen; reading a professional journal is an example of coordinated leisure. **Complementary leisure** is role related. Involvement in a professional association relates to the work role; being a scout leader relates to community and family roles.[4]

Activity provides for structure and routine in daily life and is individualized. Routine and structure establish a secure base for need fulfillment and support social roles when there is a balance of work and play.[12] This balance enables people to use time effectively and adapt to life changes as they arise. Leisure skills may be developed and incorporated into the changing pattern of daily activity. Both work and play generate **social roles,** which support involvement in a stimulating, caring network of family and friends. Social roles in leisure fill needs for belonging and affection and generate a positive sense of well-being. Active involvement in leisure keeps people feeling young and interested in life.

Leisure activities can be an arena in which to vent feelings and drives in a socially acceptable way. These activities can provide an avenue for people to satisfy their individual needs: the need to express or create, the need to have a sense of achievement, the need for relatedness to others and to the environment, the need to render some socially useful service, and the need to belong and be considered part of a community. Leisure activities give people an opportunity to be productive and contributing members of society, to have identities and to see themselves as unique individuals, to gain recognition, and to have new experiences. People act out their life's roles and succeed or fail in satisfying their needs through their work and their leisure activities.

PRINCIPLES OF WORKING WITH THE OLDER ADULT

When the medical model guides treatment decisions, social and occupational roles are not generally considered. The focus is on diagnosing a specific disease; personal mobility, independent living skills, and other social factors may not be addressed. Dealing with the aging process and subsequent institutionalization reduces opportunities for individuals to exert control over many daily tasks, including choices and opportunities for leisure tasks. This often leads to a decreased sense of competence, decreased motivation, and depression.

Since occupational therapy (OT) is directed at an older adult's ability to function independently in all aspects of daily living, whether work, self-care, play, or leisure, the therapist should be involved in the evaluation of the client's lifelong interests, priorities in pursuit of those interests, and physical, psychosocial, and cognitive ability to pursue those interests. Achieving successful outcomes in the pursuit of leisure activities may require and elicit coordination between the individual's sensory motor, cognitive, and psychosocial systems in the context of interpersonal, cultural, and environmental conditions.[11]

EVALUATION AND INTERVENTION FOR LEISURE ACTIVITIES

To ensure successful performance of leisure activity, the OT practitioner needs a comprehensive approach to evaluation. The important components include the following:

- Demographic material
- Social information
- Educational history
- Occupational history
- Military involvement
- Community and church involvement
- Typical daily routine
- Interests and hobbies
- Mealtime interests
- Abilities
- Sensorimotor components
- Cognitive components
- Psychosocial components

PROBLEM IDENTIFICATION AND GOAL SETTING

The evaluation process must identify any problems that would inhibit successful participation in the chosen leisure activities. Once the overt problem is identified, the OT practitioner must explore the components of the problem and their causative factors and determine whether environmental issues complicate the problem. Thorough problem identification is the most important step in finding solutions and thereby empowering the client to participate successfully in the leisure activity. Within this process the individual and the therapist must collaborate in goal setting and become invested in the accomplishment of the goal.

CULTURAL INFLUENCES

As the OT practitioner determines these activities that had been meaningful to the client, he or she must be aware of the client's culture. This includes knowing what value or lack of value is placed on leisure. The client's values can dictate what tasks are important and how to incorporate these tasks in goal setting. Leisure pursuits may then be adapted to fit the needs of the individual receiving service and be incorporated into the treatment plan to stimulate cognitive awareness and perceptual processing abilities.

COMMUNITY RESOURCES

When a disability challenges an individual's work skills and the individual does not have well-developed leisure interests, the therapist is even more challenged to facilitate involvement in leisure to satisfy needs. A wide variety of community recreation activities are available, encompassing many areas of interest for physically challenged adults. Theater, concert, and dining groups that provide accessible transportation open new opportunities. The availability of active and passive sporting events, including sailing, skiing, and swimming pools with special lifts and well-controlled water temperature, has dramatically changed accessibility of these pursuits. Public transportation is more readily available to meet the needs of people with disabilities as they pursue leisure activities. Therapy must address the ability to take part in community-based leisure activities, starting with the identification of resources and the development of skills to get to the activity and participate in the activity. Clients must achieve security in these abilities if they are to tolerate the extreme risk taking that participation may involve.

DISENGAGEMENT OF THE ELDERLY

A literature review focusing on social gerontology, OT, and quality-of-life issues reveals that disengagement is frequently a function of depression. "Rolelessness," "uselessness," and "old age" as a devalued status cause stress and loss of life satisfaction. Isolation occurs, bringing deterioration of the sensory receptors, and symptoms of dementia may appear. As these changes occur, the person's sense of self begins to change and is influenced by the kind of valuing and social labeling he or she experiences. Productivity is related to life satisfaction,[14] and the loss of productive roles may precipitate a decline in other areas. The person may begin to view self as deficient and incompetent.

WELLNESS CONCEPT

Activity is orienting and physically, socially, and educationally stimulating. Leisure activities can (1) minimize losses, (2) provide development of compensatory techniques that allow increased effectiveness and support competence, and (3) help maintain self-esteem and prevent an individual from being thrown into the vortex of a degenerative spiral of senility. Building on existing strengths, adaptations, and coping mechanisms, the OT practitioner can facilitate the development of leisure skills that will improve health and life satisfaction for the aging person. Leisure activities can contribute to successful adaptation to old age through the establishment of new roles and valued activities. These activities must be those that participants find personally meaningful and that allow individuals to focus on strengths that deemphasize limitations. Deane Davis, when he was the 84-year-old former governor of Vermont, put this idea in modern vernacular: "There's a vast difference between aging and growing old. There's not much you can do about aging . . . but there's a whole lot you can do about growing old." Davis knew a man who was so ready to die that he never bought green bananas. "That's not the way to live. Go out and buy green bananas. Make sure every single day is full of life, full of adventure, and full of function. Life is acting, thinking, doing, being, and growing."[2]

ACTIVITY ANALYSIS

OT education addresses activity analysis and synthesis, which enables the therapist, in collaboration with the client, to design occupational experiences that offer the individual opportunities for effective action. These activities are considered purposeful because they assist and build on the individual's abilities and lead to achievement of personal goals.[11]

An OT practitioner analyzes activity from two major perspectives. First, the practitioner examines an activity to identify its component parts and determine which skills are necessary to complete the task. Second, he or she examines the activity within the context in which it must be performed. The practitioner considers the interpersonal and environmental components, including the individual's age, occupational roles, cultural background, interests, and gender, that affect the performance of the activity. All this information considered together allows the OT practitioner to synthesize (i.e., adapt, grade, and combine) activities for therapeutic purposes[11] so as to allow the client to succeed in his or her chosen leisure time activity.

ABILITY AND INTEREST EVALUATION: LOOKING AT PERFORMANCE AREAS

Practitioners teach skills that relate to performance components and occupational performance areas; if this is not entirely successful, they adapt the task and the environment to facilitate performance. Throughout a purposeful activity, the OT practitioner modifies the setting, the method of personal interaction, and the physical handling[11] to achieve success in pursuit of the leisure time activity. Practitioners of OT also use supportive or assistive devices or techniques to ensure success. Such techniques or devices are considered to facilitate or prepare for the performance of purposeful activity and are used to enhance the effectiveness of an activity.[10,15] The successful performance of leisure activity can promote feelings of personal competence and enable persons to achieve mastery of their environment.[6]

MOTIVATION: MATCHING INTERESTS AND ABILITIES

The process of motivation begins with an identification of the individual's abilities, strengths, and interests through the evaluation. Once identified, these items are matched with the type and task demands of an activity. Matching by evaluation and analysis of the components and context of that activity, OT practitioners can create opportunities for individuals to be successful and find satisfaction in the task. Success is an important motivator, as are individual needs and values. The therapist must identify what is important to an individual at this particular time of life. OT practitioners cannot motivate people directly but can stimulate them to become motivated by their own needs and desires. Practitioners can adjust the environment to set the stage for a person to self-motivate. To cause a person to do something, the therapist must cause them to want to do it. Stirring up interest and desire leads to mental and physical motion. The therapist becomes the force or influence in the process. Pleasure and satisfaction come from the person's accomplishment, and the involvement becomes self-motivating.

THERAPEUTIC USE OF SELF

The therapist's means of helping the person to become motivated will often set the stage for the future action. Each person must be approached differently, and each approach to the same person also may need to be different. The practitioner of OT must be sincere in what he or she does and says; the practitioner cannot "fudge" this. The first contact with a person will often set the stage for future participation in the leisure activity the practitioner is presenting. The practitioner must "make haste slowly" because older persons may be resistant to change and slow to accept new leisure ideas. They need time to think and react. The therapist must remember that progress comes by inches and be sure that each inch is in the direction the therapist wants to go.

The attitudes of the therapist and the older person are vital. The therapist must be encouraging, must conceal any concerns but still be sincere, and must avoid blaming the client for failures while at the same time giving pleasure and individual satisfaction. The elder must maintain a positive attitude, satisfy individual needs, and motivate himself or herself in order to pursue and enjoy leisure activities.

VARIED SETTINGS FOR LEISURE ACTIVITIES

Occupational therapists may be involved with the geriatric client in many medical and social settings. The practitioner's involvement with leisure will vary in scope and intensity in each setting. At any given time, 95% of all elders will reside in the community. Settings in which the client may receive some leisure interventions include home health care services, adult day care, senior centers, and outpatient rehabilitation. The geriatric client may move through different aspects of the system: a rehabilitation hospital or rehabilitation unit of a hospital, subacute care, a long-term transitional hospital, a nursing home, assisted living, or a retirement home.

Leisure routines are an important aspect in any and all settings in which an elderly person may be living or receiving treatment or other services. Practitioners of OT can sometimes be reimbursed by Medicare for one to two visits for leisure evaluation and program planning in the home health setting. However, it is recommended that the development of a leisure-based program be combined with other activities, particularly ones involving ADL skills or physical components that occur during a treatment session focusing on leisure routines. The practitioner should document both the physical and leisure components of the activity.[1]

GROUP PROCESS

The OT practitioner can use group skills and leadership expertise to help members of a group achieve need satisfaction. Many of the individual's needs that were previously mentioned, especially the needs to belong and to have meaningful relationships with others, may be satisfied through group dynamics and task or social roles. Those roles may include the following.[3]

Task Roles

- The initiator-contributor, who suggests new ideas
- The information seeker, who asks for clarification of facts
- The opinion seeker, who asks for clarification of opinions
- The information giver
- The opinion giver
- The elaborator, who spells out suggestions
- The coordinator, who clarifies relationships
- The evaluator-critic, who compares the accomplishments of the group to a standard
- The energizer, who gets things moving
- The procedural recognizer, who performs routine tasks

Social Roles

- The encourager, who praises and accepts contributions
- The harmonizer, who mediates differences
- The compromiser, who changes behavior to maintain harmony
- The standard setter, who expresses standards
- The group observer, who interprets and presents information about what is happening
- The follower, who goes along with the group

CATEGORIES OF LEISURE ACTIVITIES

Participation in leisure activities may take place in large groups, small groups, or individually. The activities may be classified as arts and crafts, active recreation, social recreation, religious, intellectual or educational, community, or service to others, to name just a few. Each can offer many psychosocial and physical benefits, such as the following.

Psychosocial Benefits

- Increased sense of self-worth
- Release of hostility and aggression
- Shared control of self and environment
- Experience of choice
- Increased socialization
- Development of leadership
- Practice in adaptive behavior and coping skills
- Increased attention span
- Adjustment to living arrangements
- Increased tolerance of groups and other people
- Experience of intellectual stimulation

Physical Benefits

- Increased circulation
- Promotion of gross, fine, bilateral, and eye-hand coordination
- Provision of vestibular stimulation
- Provision of sensory stimulation
- Promotion of motor planning
- Improvement or maintenance of perceptual abilities
- Maintenance or improvement of adaptive and coping skills
- Increased strength, range of motion, and physical tolerance
- Improved balance
- Provision of opportunity to grade activities

CONSULTATION TO ACTIVITY PROGRAMS

Acting as consultants, occupational therapists can help develop activity programs throughout the whole continuum of geriatric care. Therapists have many roles. Knowledge and experience enable OT practitioners to give professional advice and guidance and make recommendations. Therapists' expertise is used to recognize and solve problems, and these abilities may be critical to their success as consultants.[5] The ability to communicate and to work with people in order to facilitate change is vital. A thorough understanding of the rules and regulations governing the setting is also a necessity. One of the functions of the consultant therapist is to evaluate the physical environment, the programs, and the staff. In this capacity therapists may have the roles of educator and trainer and may develop programs. They must be flexible and have the knowledge to adjust to the needs of the individual setting. To be a successful consultant, the OT practitioner must have many special at-

tributes, including expertise in the needs of the elderly, a capacity for self-direction, the ability to focus on tasks, the composure needed to remain objective, and the interpersonal skills to negotiate effectively.

As consultants, OT practitioners must make recommendations to improve services to the client; however, they do not have the authority to enforce the implementation of those recommendations. All recommendations and activities should be documented for each consultation visit. The occupational therapist's holistic educational background, coupled with experience, is valuable preparation for the role of consultant. Knowledge of the process of aging and the focus on quality-of-life issues for all people, including those with dementia, is indispensable.[7]

DEMENTIA CARE AND LEISURE SKILLS

Activity involvement in dementia care must be defined as broadly as possible, so as to include the entire interaction between the individual and the environment. The environment defined in its broadest terms includes the physical, social, and cultural environments. All tasks that give people meaning and purpose are included in the concept of activity. These tasks include routine and overlearned procedures that everyone performs without much thought, as well as leisure pursuits. All daily events are defined as activities.

When OT practitioners are involved with activities in a dementia-specific setting, they need to apply the broad definition of activity involvement as they involve staff in meeting the clients' needs. Activities are now defined as any task or encounter. Hellen[9] states, "Anything residents do or are involved with is their activity at that moment. Using activities as a frame around all that the resident does allows a freedom for entertaining numerous possibilities. Shifting focus from doing an activity for the resident to one of *doing with* the resident or allowing them independent involvement stimulates wellness." With this philosophy, OT practitioners can help increase clients' self-esteem.

Dementia-related activity focuses on what an individual can do rather than on what he or she cannot do. A diagnosis of Alzheimer's disease suggests that the person cannot learn. Nonetheless, if the occupational therapist evaluates the person's specific abilities and alters the task and how it is presented so as to use abilities and avoid deficits, the task can often be accomplished successfully.

Depression, which is common especially in the earlier stages of Alzheimer's disease, may contribute to an apparent inability to accomplish tasks. Stress is another factor that may influence the achievement of tasks. A vicious circle may develop in which dysfunction leads to stress and stress leads to depression and further dysfunction. Identification of the specific causative factors leading to stress is the important first step in developing a holistic focus. A reduction in the number or intensity of incidents that increase stress can result in more successful involvement with activities of any kind. The most common stress-related incidents are those that magnify losses. These incidents include losses of the familiar, such as routines, environment, relationships, communication skills, privacy, dignity, and abilities. Providing obvious and easily identifiable purposes for tasks while offering familiar, overlearned activities that target procedural memory may increase opportunities for success and thus reduce stress. Supportive one-to-one interaction and multisensory input may improve communication. Other helpful strategies include limiting decision-making and reducing time demanded for attention to task. Individualizing tasks and breaking them down into manageable steps with proper cueing may allow the person to complete the tasks successfully. Organization, consistency in routines, calmness, and reduction in inappropriate distractions are especially important for the person with dementia.[8]

PROBLEM BEHAVIORS AFFECTING ACTIVITY PARTICIPATION

Behavior affects performance. Problem behaviors must be managed through careful analysis, which includes the following questions:

1. What is the behavior?
2. Why it is a problem?
3. When it is a problem?
4. Where it is a problem?
5. To whom it is a problem?

Perhaps the most critical question is, "What situations precede the problem behavior—what is the possible cause or antecedent?" Alleviation of the possible antecedent or satisfaction of needs associated with the behavior may prevent the situation from arising. For example, if a person finds large groups overstimulating, activities should be done one-on-one or in small groups. If a person identifies too closely with characters in a television show, soap operas on television are not a good leisure activity for that person. If messy activities cause a catastrophic reaction, finger painting would not be the activity of choice. If there is no outlet for excess energy and the person paces or wanders, the therapist must channel the energy into an acceptable activity and plan activities that incorporate rather than accentuate the negative aspects of the behavior. If the individual cannot initiate an activity independently and boredom causes problem behaviors, the individual must be constantly redirected to activities that accommodate those decreased attending skills.[8]

SUMMARY

Leisure activities are important to all people. Work and play situations provide opportunities to act out life's roles and succeed or fail in satisfying needs. When needs cannot be satisfied through work, leisure activities provide alternatives. Leisure experiences must gratify the needs and be directed toward the goals of a specific individual.

The OT practitioner has the ability to administer assessments and analyze data regarding performance areas, performance components, and performance context. He or she can then relate these findings to an individual's priority of needs and interests and thereby help the individual succeed in chosen leisure occupation.

Idleness and lack of purposeful activity are great enemies of aged persons with physical limitations that necessitate adaptation and intervention to enable participation. Idleness does much more than kill time. It kills initiative and self-respect and increases feelings of defeatism. Absence of meaningful occupation encourages mental and physical deterioration and invalidism. The OT practitioner can stimulate occupational performance and help individuals to function at their highest possible levels so they may live life to the fullest.

REVIEW QUESTIONS

1. Name five needs that can be satisfied through leisure occupation.
2. Name eight important components of a comprehensive evaluation.
3. Why is it important for the client to be involved in setting his or her own goals?
4. Why is the client's cultural background important?
5. What does the therapist need to address in determining access to community-based leisure activities?
6. From what two major perspectives does the OT practitioner analyze activity?
7. How can a therapist motivate a person?
8. Name five psychosocial benefits and five physical benefits of leisure activities
9. What are some roles and responsibilities of a consultant?
10. What authority does the consultant possess?
11. What components of the OT educational curriculum prepare a therapist to be a consultant?
12. What two factors influence achievement of tasks for the person with dementia?
13. In dealing with problem behaviors, what aspects of the behavior must the therapist analyze?
14. How can the therapist help a person with dementia achieve success at a task?

15. What type of activity could the therapists suggest for a person with excess energy who paces and wanders?
16. What can absence of meaningful occupation lead to?

REFERENCES

1. American Occupational Therapy Association Commission on Practice Home Health Task Force: *Guidelines for occupational therapy practice in home health*, Bethesda, Md, 1995, The Association.
2. Averyt AC, Furst E, Hummel DD: *Successful aging: a source book for older people and their families*, New York, 1987, Ballantine Books.
3. Benne KD, Sheats P: Functional roles of group members, *Social Issues* 4(2):42-47, 1948.
4. Crepeau EL: Module III treatment approaches: activity programming, *Role of occupational therapy with the elderly*, Rockville, Md, 1986, American Occupational Therapy Association.
5. Epstein CF: Consultation: communicating and facilitation. In Blair J, Gray M, editors: *The occupational therapy manager*, rev ed, Rockville, Md, 1992, American Occupational Therapy Association.
6. Fidler GS, Fidler JW: Doing and becoming: purposeful action and self-actualization, *Am J Occup Ther* 32:305-310, 1979.
7. Glantz CH, Richman N: *Effective OT intervention for the elderly within the continuum of care*, Bethesda, Md, 1997, American Occupational Therapy Association.
8. Glantz CH, Richman N: *Special care household*, Riverwoods, Ill, 1990, Glantz/Richman Rehabilitation Associates.
9. Hellen C: *Alzheimer's disease activity-focused care*, Newton, Mass, 1992, Andover Medical Publishers.
10. Henderson A, Cermak S, Costner W, et al: The issue is: occupational science is multidimensional, *Am J Occup Ther* 45:370-372, 1991.
11. Hinojosa J, Sabari J, Pedretti L: *Purposeful activity: a position paper*, 1992, American Occupational Therapy Association.
12. Keilhofner G: Temporal adaptations, *Am J Occup Ther* 31:235-242, 1977.
13. Kimmel D: *Adulthood and aging*, New York, 1974, John Wiley & Sons.
14. Kleemeir RW: *A part of daily life: Alzheimer's caregivers simplify activities and the home* (Video and Resource Book), Bethesda, Md, 1994, American Occupational Therapy Federation and American Occupational Therapy Association.
15. Pedretti LW, Pasquinelli S: A frame of reference for occupational therapy in physical dysfunction. In Pedretti LW, Zoltan B, editors: *Occupational therapy practice skills for physical dysfunction*, St Louis, 1990, Mosby.

RECOMMENDED READING

Allen CK: Activity, occupational therapy treatment method, *Am J Occup Ther* 41(9):563-575, 1987.
Alzheimer's Association: *Alzheimer care strategies: partners in quality care*, Conference proceedings, Chicago, Ill, 1993, The Association.
Alzheimer's Association: *Guidelines for dignity: goals of specialized Alzheimer/dementia care in residential settings*, Chicago, Ill, 1992, The Association.
Bell G: Role set orientations and life satisfaction. In Gubrium JF, editor: *Times, roles and self in old age*, New York, 1976, Human Sciences Press.
Borg RM, Kennedy S, Smith B: *Bringing out the best-dementia programming and activities*, Partners in Caregiving: The Dementia Services Program, Winston-Salem, NC, 1994, Bowman Gray School of Medicine of Wake Forest University, Department of Psychiatry and Behavioral Medicine.

Born B: *Occupational therapy and long term care position paper*, Rockville, Md, 1993, American Occupational Therapy Association.
Cornelius E, Perschbacker R, Reublinger V, et al: Resident assessment protocol: activities. In *Resident assessment instrument training manual and resource guide*, for use with the Health Care Financing Administration's minimum data set, resident assessment protocols and Utilization Guidelines, Nantick, Mass, 1987, Elliot Press.
Cynkin S: *Occupational therapy: toward health through activities*. Boston, 1979, Little, Brown.
Edinberg MA: *Talking with your aging parents*, Boston, Mass, 1987, Shambhala Publications.
Davis NB, Teaff JD: Facilitative role continuity of the elderly through leisure programming, *Ther Rec J* 14(2):32-36, 1980.
Fuller E: The biology of aging, *Generations, J Am Soc Aging*, 16(4) 1992.
Fuller K: Current ethical issues in aging, *Generations, J Am Soc Aging* 18(4), 1994.
Fuller K: Frontline workers in long-term care, *Generations, J Am Soc Aging* 18(3), 1994.
Fuller K: Technology and aging: developing and marketing new products for older people, *Generations, J Am Soc on Aging* 19(1), 1995.
Glantz CH, Richman N: *Occupational therapy: a vital link to the implementation of OBRA*, Bethesda, Md, 1991, American Occupational Therapy Association.
Glantz CH, Richman N: *Empowerment through wellness*, Riverwoods, Ill, 1992, Glantz/Richman Rehabilitation Associates.
Glantz CH, Richman N: The wellness model in long-term care facilities, *Quest, the Journal of the Illinois Health Care Association*, 1993 Legislative Session, Illinois Health Care Association.
Glantz CH, Richman N: *Enhancing rehabilitation services for older people*, Detroit, 1994, Seventh Annual Continuing Education Program on Issues in Aging, Wayne State Institute of Gerontology, Detroit, Michigan.
Goldberg A, Carrol D, Dobrof R: *How to start and manage a group activities and respite program for people with Alzheimer's disease and their families, a guide for community-based organizations*, New York, 1991, Brookdale Foundation Group, The Brookdale Center on Aging of Hunter College.
Gubrium JF: *The myth of the golden years: a socio-environmental theory of aging*, Springfield, Ill, 1973, Charles C Thomas.
Jaffee EG, Epstein C: *Occupational therapy consultation: theory, principles and practice*, St Louis, 1992, Mosby.
Jenny S, Oropeza M: *Memories in the making—a program of creative art expression for Alzheimer patients*, Orange County, Calif, 1993, Alzheimer's Association.
Keiber DA, Thompson SR: Leisure behavior and adjustment to retirement: implications for post retirement education, *Ther Recreation J* 14(2): 5-17. 1980.
Keilhofner G: A model of human occupation. 3, Benign and vicious cycles, *Am J Occup Ther* 34:572-581, 1980b.
Morris A, Hunt G: *A part of daily life: Alzheimer's caregivers simplify activities and the home* (Video and Resource Book), Bethesda, Md, 1994, American Occupational Therapy Federation and American Occupational Therapy Association.
Parker RA, Downe GR: Recreation therapy: a model for consideration, *Ther Rec J* 15(3):22-26, 1981.
Petty BJ, Moeller TP, Campbell RZ: Support groups for elderly persons in the community, *Gerontologist* 15(6):522, 1976.
Rathbone-McCuan S, Levenson J: The impact of socialization therapy in a geriatric day care setting, *Gerontologist* 15:338-342, 1975.
Risberg G, McCullough VE: *Tough: a personal workbook*, Oak Park, Ill, 1987, Open Arms Press.
Rogers JC: *Occupational therapy services for persons with Alzheimer's disease and other dementias (position paper)*, Rockville, Md, 1986 (reprinted 1993), American Occupational Therapy Association.

Rowles GD: *Prisoners of space? Exploring the geographical experience of older people,* Boulder, Colo, 1978, Westview Press.

Sheridan C: *Failure-free activities for the Alzheimer's patient,* Oakland, Calif, 1987, Cottage Books.

Thews T, Reaves AM, Henry RS: *Dementia care & respite services program, Now what? A handbook of activities for adult day programs,* Winston-Salem, NC, 1993, Bowman Gray School of Medicine of Wake Forest University.

Tickle LS, Yerxa EJ: Need satisfaction of older persons living in the community and in institutions. 1, The environment, *Am J Occup Ther* 1981a.

Zogola J: *Doing things: a guide to programming activities for persons with Alzheimer's disease and related disorders,* Baltimore, 1987, John Hopkins University Press.

CHAPTER 19

Assistive Technology

DENIS ANSON

KEY TERMS

Assistive technology
Rehabilitation technology
Universal design
Human Activity Assistive Technology
Human Environment Technology Interface
Human Interface Assessment
Electronic aids to daily living
Power switching
X-10 system
Infrared
Feature control
Subsumed devices
Augmentative and alternative communications
User control system
Message composition system
Message transmission system
Graphical communication
Physical keyboard
Virtual keyboard
Pointing systems
Dynamic display
Eye-tracking
Morse code
Speech input
Scanning input
Rate enhancement
Prediction
Compression/expansion
Screen enlargement programs
Speech output
Tactile output

LEARNING OBJECTIVES

After studying this chapter the student or practitioner will be able to do the following:
1. Describe the range of assistive technology options currently available for persons with physical disabilities.
2. Discuss and compare three different theoretical models for the interface between humans and technology.
3. Identify common solutions for enabling control of daily living devices through technology.
4. Discuss options for augmentative and alternative communications.
5. Analyze input and output options for assistive technologies and match these to the needs of consumers.

Any discussion of **assistive technology** should begin with a description of the general limits of the topic. This is difficult because the legal definitions of assistive technology are not uniform. Assistive technologies are sometimes included in the category of **rehabilitation technology.** In other cases, rehabilitation technology is considered an aspect of assistive technologies. A third category, technologies that employ **universal design,** doesn't seem to fit into either of the first two categories.

TOWARD DEFINING ASSISTIVE TECHNOLOGY

The category into which an enabling technology falls depends largely on its application, not on a specific device being used. What is merely a convenience for some people may be an assistive technology for others. For purposes of this discussion, the following categories and definitions will apply.

Rehabilitation Technology

The term **rehabilitation technology** should be used to identify those technologies that are intended to restore an individual to a previous level of function after the onset of a pathologic condition. Rehabilitative technologies are generally intended to be used within a therapy setting by trained professionals over a short time. Because they are meant to be used by trained professionals, these technologies may have fairly complex or cryptic controls. It is expected that the professional will have significant training before applying these technologies. The professional guiding the use of such technologies is expected to ensure their correct application and to protect the safety of the individual using the device. Physical agent modalities such as ultrasound, diathermy, paraffin, and functional electric stimulation are examples of rehabilitative technologies. When these technologies have done their job, the client will have better intrinsic function and use of the technology will be discontinued.

Assistive Technology

Assistive technologies help a person with a disability perform tasks. More specifically, assistive technologies allow a person who has a disability to perform tasks that an able-bodied person can perform without technological assistance. Such devices may be designed specifically for a person with a disability or designed for a mass market and subsequently used by a person with a disability. An able-bodied person may prefer to use a technology (such as a television remote control) to perform a task, but this does not rise to the level of as-sistive technology so long as task performance is possible without the technology.

Assistive technologies replace or support an impaired function of the user but do not change the intrinsic functioning of the individual. For example, a wheelchair replaces the function of walking but does not teach the user to walk. Similarly, forearm crutches support independent standing but do not, of themselves, improve strength or bony integrity and so will not change the ability of the user to stand without them.

The design of assistive technologies reflects their intended use over prolonged periods by individuals with limited training and possibly with limited cognitive skills. Assistive technology must not inflict harm on the user through casual misuse. The controls of the device must be readily understood; some training may be necessary to use the device, but the need for retraining should be minimal. An effective assistive technology device should not require deep understanding of its principles and functions to be useful.

Assistive technology devices go home with the client; rehabilitation technology devices generally remain in a clinic. Some technologies may overlap categories, since they may be used differently with different clients. For example, clinicians may use assisted communication as a tool to train unassisted speech for their clients; in this case the technology is rehabilitative. However, assisted communication may also be used to support or replace speech for clients who will not be able to resume speech; in this case the technology is assistive.

Universal Design

Universal design is the newest category of technology. The principles of universal design were published by the Center for Universal Design at North Carolina State University in 1997, and their application is still limited.[4] The concept of **universal design** is simple: if devices are designed with the needs of people with disabilities in mind, they will be more usable for all users, with and without disabilities.

In some cases the universal design philosophy could make assistive technology unnecessary. A can opener that has been designed for one-handed use by a busy housewife also will be usable by the cook who has had a cerebrovascular accident (CVA) and now has the use of only one hand. Another example is that of electronic books now under development that will include features to allow them to be used as "talking books." The goal of this technology is to provide a hands-free, eyes-free interface so that commuters can use the books while driving. However, the same interface will meet the needs of the individual who is blind and *cannot* see the screen or who has mobility limitations and *cannot* operate the manual controls. No further adaptation would be necessary because the product's design already accommodates the special needs of the person with a disability.

THREE MODELS OF ASSISTIVE TECHNOLOGY INTERFACE

Assistive technology interface is the relationship between assistive technology, the user, and the environment. Three models deal with this relationship: the human activity assistance technology model of Cook and Hussey,[5] the human environment technology interface model of Roger Smith, and the human interface assessment model of Anson. On casual examination, the three models appear to be quite different; however, all three models examine the same elements in differing degrees of detail, and nest within one another.

Human Activity Assistive Technology

The **human activity assistive technology (HAAT)** model by Cook and Hussey[5] (Fig. 19-1) emphasizes the importance of the person, the activity, and the context in the selection of assistive technology. Specifically, one using this model considers the context of the person who will be using the technology, the activity that the technology will be used to perform, and the environment in which the technology will be used. Changes in any of these components can require a change of technology, since the overall conditions may no longer fit correctly.

The standard representation of the model, Fig. 19-1, fails to clarify that the technology enables the activity

for the person. Removing the technology portion of the figure will result in an incomplete image but does not appear to remove the person from the activity. A modified representation of this model might look somewhat different (Fig. 19-2). The modified HAAT model shows that assistive technologies may link the person and the activity and may make the activity possible. Removing the assistive technology may separate the person from performing the activity.

Human Enviroment Technology Interface

Roger Smith's **human environment technology interface (HETI)** model[6] (Fig. 19-3) focuses in more detail on the interface between the human and the assistive technology. This model shows that human use of assistive technology requires a complete cycle of performance. The human must receive sensory input from the environment about the task to be performed. Through cognitive processing, the human decides on a course of action and produces an output. The motor output of the human serves as input to the assistive technology; through internal processing the assistive technology produces a performance that should match the desired action of the human. The technology performs the action, which is apparent to the human, and the cycle begins anew. If the cycle is to be complete, the human must be able to observe the action of the technology and produce the motor output that the technology

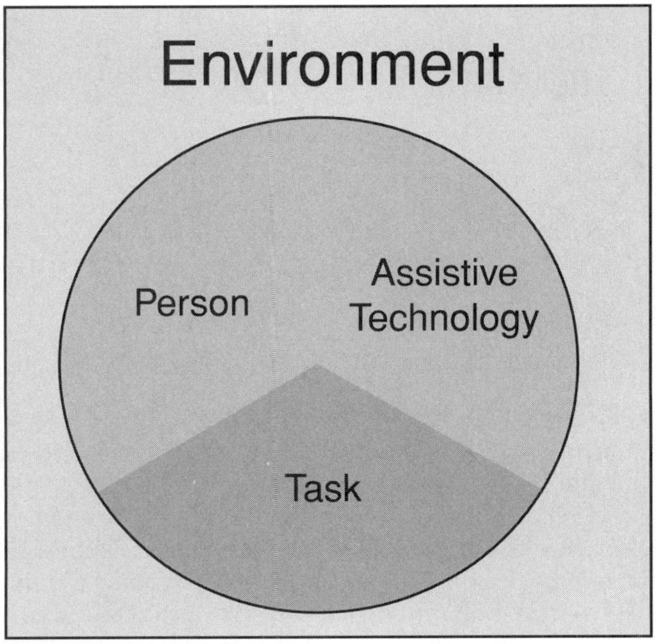

FIG. 19-1
HAAT model.

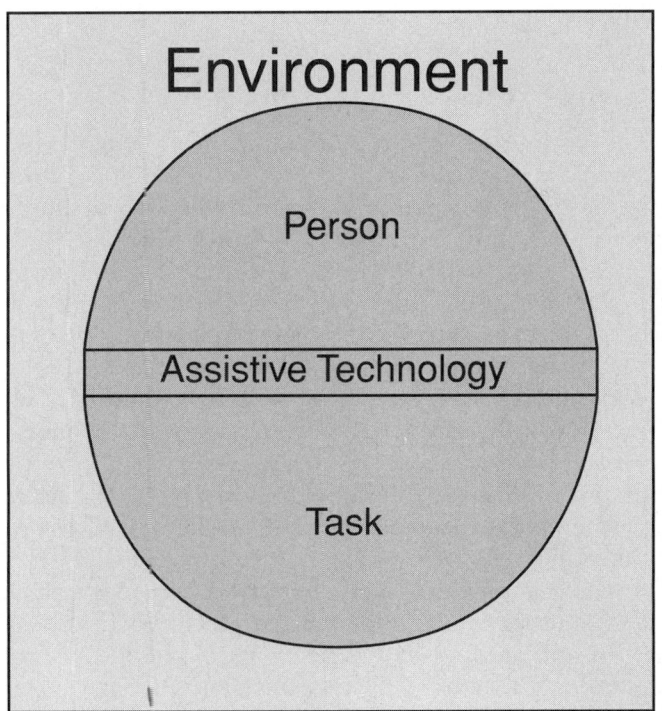

FIG. 19-2
Modified HAAT model.

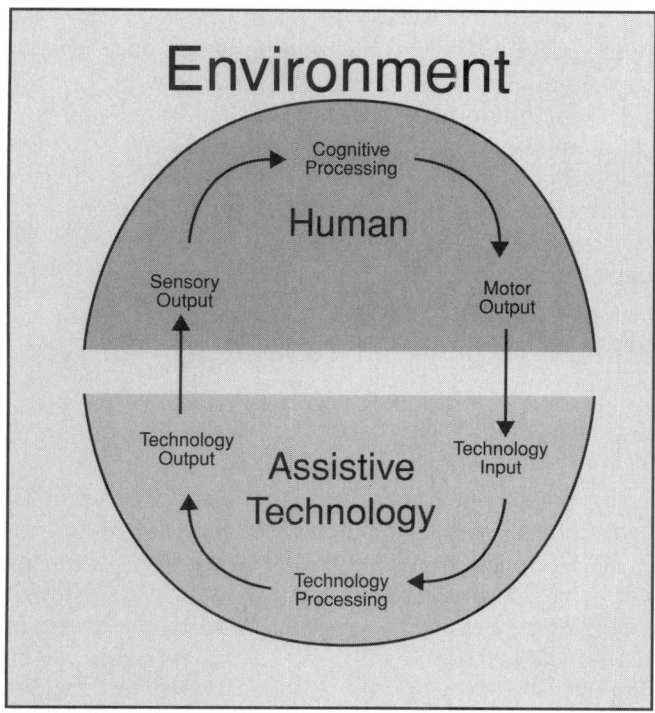

FIG. 19-3
HETI model.

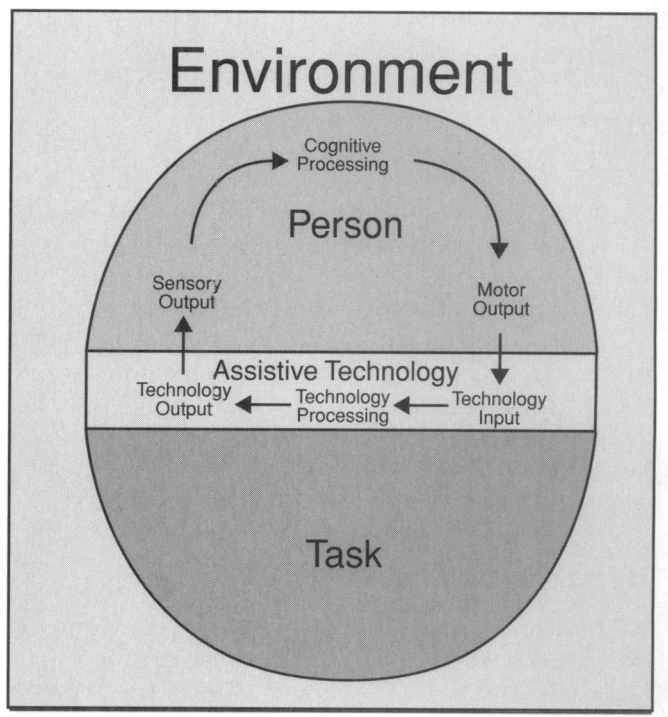

FIG. 19-4
HAAT/HETI model.

input expects; otherwise, the assistive technology will not be functional.

The HETI model is a detailed look at one aspect of the HAAT model, the interface between the human and the assistive technology. The two models are integrated in Fig. 19-4.

Human Interface Assessment

Anson's **human interface assessment (HIA)** model is a still more detailed look at the skills and abilities of the human in motor output and sensory input, with some consideration of cognitive processing. This model (Fig. 19-5) looks in detail at the abilities of the human in Smith's model to match these abilities with the demands of assistive technologies.[1] The HIA model suggests that assistive technology is required *only* when the demands of a task exceed the skills and abilities of an individual; this is so even when a functional limitation exists. However, an assistive technology device may be used to bridge the gap between demands and abilities whenever task demands exceed the native abilities of the individual.

The HIA provides for guided assessment of the skills and abilities of the intended user and matches those skills and abilities to the demands of the technology under consideration. The assessment of abilities in sensory perception, cognitive processing, and motor output yields data that are compared with the input and output capabilities of assistive technologies. Careful

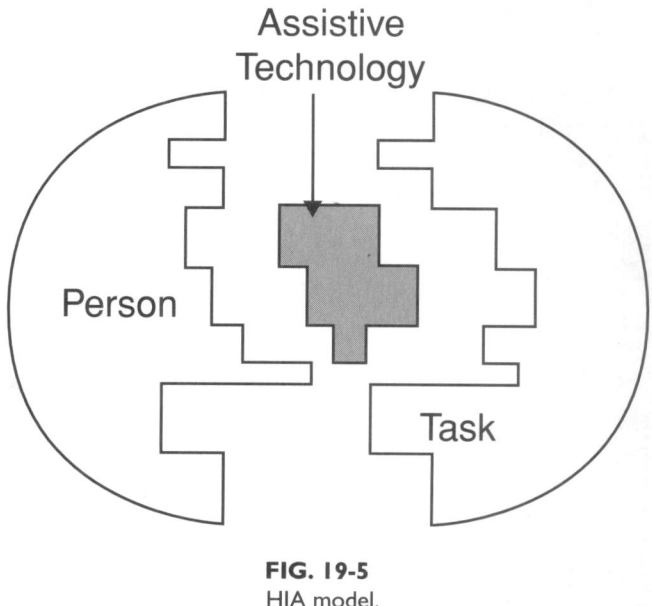

FIG. 19-5
HIA model.

matching is necessary if assistive technologies are to provide effective interventions for individuals.

As Fig. 19-6 shows, the HAAT, HETI, and HIA models are actually nested examinations of the relationship between a person, an activity, the environment, and the assistive technology that makes it possible for the person to perform the activity. These three models examine different portions of the relationship between humans and activities and are complementary to each other.

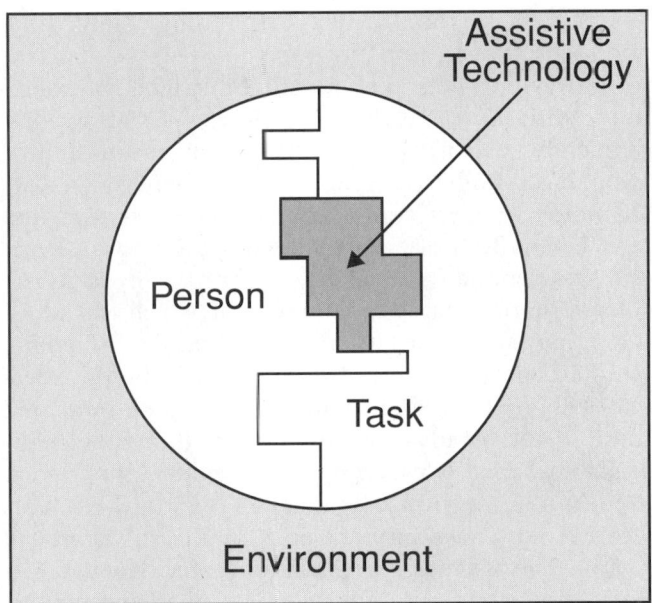

FIG. 19-6
Combining the HAAT and HETI and HIA models.

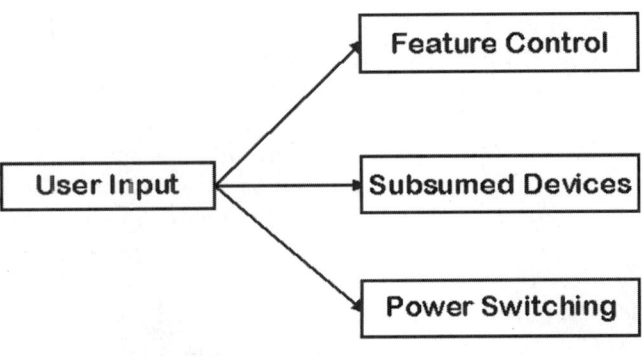

FIG. 19-7
Classification of EADL by control options.

TYPES OF ELECTRONIC ENABLING TECHNOLOGIES

It is useful to categorize assistive technologies by the particular situations or general uses in which they are applied. This chapter deals only with electronic assistive technologies, which in their primary applications may be considered to fall into one of three categories: electronic aids to daily living, alternative and augmentative communications, and general computer applications.

Electronic Aids to Daily Living

Electronic aids to daily living (EADL) are devices that can be used to control electrical equipment in the client's environment. Many therapists and rehabilitation engineers have learned to call items in this class of device "environmental control units," although technically this terminology should be reserved for furnace thermostats and similar controls. The more generic EADL applies not only to control of lighting and temperature, but also to control of radios, televisions, telephones, and other electrical and electronic devices in the client's environment.

EADL systems may be classified further in terms of the degree and types of control they provide to the user. These classifications are *simple power switching, control of device features,* and *subsumed devices* (Fig. 19-7).

Power Switching

The simplest EADL provide only **power switching** of the electrical supply for devices in a room. The switch adaptations for switch-adapted toys provided to children with severe disabilities would formally be considered EADL. Primitive EADL systems may be as simple as a set of electrical switches and outlets in a box, connected to devices within a room via extension cords. Such primitive devices may be unsafe. Extension cords pose safety hazards to people in the environment through the risk of falls (tripping over the extension cords) and fires (overheated or worn cords). Further, the devices may match inadequately the needs of consumers. Because of these limitations, EADL technology moved toward remote switching technologies.

Second-generation EADL systems use various remote control technologies to switch power by remote control to electrical devices in the environment. The technologies employed include ultrasonic pulses, infrared light, and electrical signals propagated through the electrical circuitry of the home. All of these switching technologies remain in use, and some are used for much more elaborate control systems. Only power switching is discussed here.

The most prevalent power-switching EADL control system is that produced by the X-10 Corporation.* The **X-10 system** uses electrical signals sent over the wiring of a home to control power modules that are plugged into wall sockets in series with the device to be controlled. (In a series connection the power module is plugged into the wall and the remotely controlled device is plugged into the power module.) The X-10 system supports up to 16 channels of control, with up to 16 modules on each, for a total of up to 256 devices controlled by a single system.

The signals used to control X-10 modules will not travel through the home's power transformer, so users in single-family dwellings will not interfere with devices in a neighbor's home. This is not necessarily true in an apartment setting, where it is possible for two X-10

---

*Retail Sales Division, 15200 52nd Avenue South, Seattle, WA, 98188-2335; Phone: (205) 241-3285; Fax: (206) 242-4644.

users to inadvertently control each other's devices. The general setup of early X-10 modules was intended to control up to 16 devices on an available channel so that such interference would not occur. In some apartments the power within a single unit may be on different "phases" of the power supplied to the building. (These phases are required to provide 220-volt power for some appliances.) If this is the case, the X-10 signals from a controller plugged into one phase will not cross to the second phase of the installation. A special "phase cross-over" is available from X-10 to correct this problem.

X-10 modules can be used with special lighting modules to dim and brighten room lighting. These modules work only with incandescent lighting but add a degree of control beyond simple switching. For permanent installation the wall switches and receptacles of the home may be replaced with X-10–controlled units. Because X-10 modules do not prevent local control, these receptacles and switches work like standard units, with the added advantage of remote control.

After their introduction in the late 1970s, X-10 modules revolutionized the field of EADL. Before this, remote switching was a difficult and expensive endeavor, restricted largely to applications for people with disabilities and to industrial applications. The X-10 system, however, was intended as a convenience for able-bodied people who did not want to walk across a room to turn on a light. Because the target audience was able to perform the task without remote switching, the technology had to be inexpensive enough that it was easier to pay the cost than get out of a chair. X-10 made it possible for an able-bodied person to remotely control electrical devices for under $100, in contrast to disability-related devices that could cost as much as several thousand dollars. Interestingly, the almost universal adoption of X-10 protocols by disability-related EADL has not led to sudden price drops in the disability field, so many clinicians continue to adapt mass-market devices for individuals with disabilities.

Feature Control

As electronic systems have become more pervasive in the home, simple switching of lights and coffee pots no longer meets the needs of the individual with a disability who wants to control the immediate environment. Wall current control allows a person with a disability to turn radios and televisions on and off but provides no control of features beyond that. A person with a disability may want to surf cable channels as much as an able-bodied person with a television remote control. When advertisements are blaring from the speakers, a person with a disability may want to turn down the sound or tune to another radio station. Although most consumer electronic devices are now delivered with a remote control (generally using infrared signals), most of these remote controls are not usable by a person with a dis-

ability because they require fine motor control and good sensory discrimination.

To provide a person with a disability with control of the features of home electronic devices, EADL systems frequently have hybrid capabilities. A means of directly switching power to remote devices, often using X-10 technology, allows control of devices such as lights, fans, and coffee pots, as well as electrical door openers and other specialty devices. To this capability is added some form of **infrared** remote control, which will allow the EADL system to mimic the signals of standard remote control devices. This control will be provided either (1) by the manufacturer of the device, programming in the standard sequences for all commercially available VCRs, televisions, and satellite decoders or (2) through teaching systems, in which the EADL "learns" the codes beamed at it by the conventional remote. The advantage of the latter approach is that the EADL can learn any codes, even those that have not yet been invented. The disadvantage is that the controls must be taught, requiring more setup and configuration time for the user and caregivers.

Hope for better and simpler control of home audiovisual devices is on the horizon. In November 1999, a consortium of eight home electronics manufacturers released a set of guidelines for home electronics. These guidelines are called HAVi.* The HAVi specification will allow compliant home electronics to communicate so that any HAVi device can control the operation of all of the HAVi devices sharing the standard. A single remote control will be able to control all of the audiovisual devices in the home through a single interface. The Infrared Data Association (IrDA)† is working on specifications focusing purely on infrared controls. The IrDA standard will allow an infrared remote control to control features of computers, home audiovisual equipment, and appliances with a single, standard protocol. Having a single standard for home electronics will allow much easier design of EADL systems for people with disabilities.

The relationship between EADL and computers is one interesting aspect of **feature control** by EADL. Some EADL systems include features that allow the user to control a personal computer. Other EADL are designed to accept control inputs from a personal computer. The goal in both cases is to use the same input method to control a personal computer as to control the EADL. In general, the control demands of an EADL system are much less stringent than are those of a computer. An input method that is adequate for EADL control may be tedious for general computer control. A system that allows fluid control of a computer will not

---

*http://www.havi.org/home.html
†http://www.irda.org/about/index.asp

be strained by the further need to control an EADL. The proper source of control will probably have to be decided on a case-by-case basis. This topic is discussed further in the section on augmentative communications.

Subsumed Devices

The incorporation of an available consumer technology into an EADL is termed a **subsumed device**. Modern EADL frequently incorporate common devices such as the telephone. Because of the pervasiveness of telephones, incorporating telephone electronics into the EADL is less expensive than inventing special systems to control a standard telephone.

Many EADL systems include a speakerphone that allows the user to originate and answer telephone calls using the electronics of the EADL as the telephone. Because of the existing standards, these systems are generally analog, single-line telephones, electronically similar to those found in the typical home. Many business settings now use multiline sets, which are not compatible with home telephones. Some businesses are converting to digital interchanges, which are also incompatible with conventional telephones. Because of this, the telephone built into a standard EADL may not meet the needs of a client with a disability in an office setting. Before recommending an EADL as an access solution for a client in the workplace, the therapist should determine whether the system is compatible with the telecommunications systems in that environment.

Other systems designed for individuals with disabilities are so difficult to control remotely that the EADL must generate an entire control system. For example, hospital bed controls have no provisions for remote control but should be usable by a person with a disability. Some EADL systems can be used as hospital bed controllers. This is important for the client who, for reasons of limited endurance or mobility, must spend a significant portion of the day in bed. These systems allow the user to adjust head and foot height independently, extending the time the user can be independent of assistance for positioning. As with telephone systems, different brands of hospital beds use different styles of controls. The clinician must match the controls provided by the EADL with the inputs required for control of the bed.

Control of EADL

EADL systems are designed to allow the individual with limited physical capability to control devices in the immediate environment. As such, the method used to control the EADL must be within the capability of the client. Since these controls have many features in common with other forms of electronic enablers, the control strategies are discussed later in a separate section.

Augmentative and Alternative Communications

The term **augmentative and alternative communications (AAC)** is used to describe systems that supplement (augment) or replace (alternative) communication by voice or gestures between people. Formally speaking, AAC incorporates all assisted communication, including tools, such as pencils and typewriters, used to communicate over time (as in leaving a message for someone who will arrive at a location after you leave) or over distance (sending a letter to Aunt May). However, as used in assistive technology, AAC denotes the use of technology to allow communication by a person with a disability in ways that an able-bodied individual would be able to accomplish without assistance. Thus using a pencil to write a letter to Aunt May would not be an example of AAC for a person who is unable to speak, since an able-bodied correspondent would use the same technology (pencil and paper) for the same purpose (social communication). However, when a nonvocal person uses a pencil to tell the doctor about sharp pains in the right leg, the pencil is considered an AAC device, since an able-bodied person would talk about the pains.

AAC devices range from extremely low technology to extremely high technology. In hospital intensive care units, low-tech communication boards (Fig. 19-8) can allow a person using a respirator to communicate basic needs. A low-tech communication board can allow a client to deliver basic messages or spell out more involved messages in a fashion that can be learned quickly. For a person with the capacity for only yes or no responses, another person can indicate the rows of the board one at a time, asking if the desired letter is in the row. When the correct row is selected, the assisting person can move across a row until the person with the disability indicates the correct letter. This type of communication is inexpensive and quick to teach, but slow to use. It is adequate when communication needs are

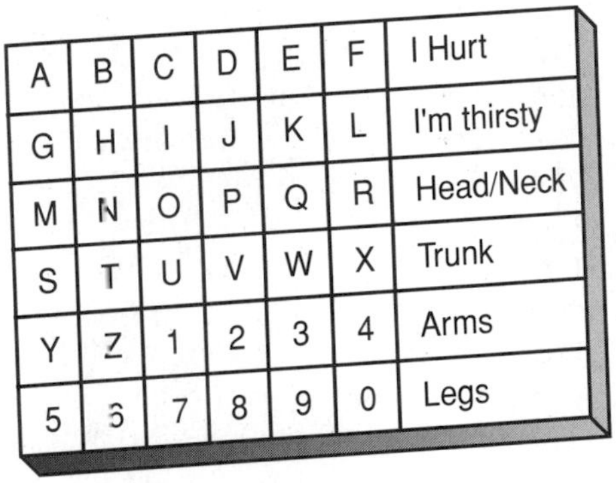

FIG. 19-8
A communication board.

limited but will not serve for long-term or fluent communication needs.

Clinicians frequently recommend electronic AAC devices to meet the communication needs of a person who will be nonvocal for a long time. In selecting a communication device, the clinician must consider the type of communication the individual will use, as well as the settings in which communication will take place.

Light[6] describes four types of human communication: expression of needs and wants, information transfer, social closeness, and social etiquette. In the intensive care setting noted above, most communication will occur at the first two levels. The individual with disability will want to express basic needs of hunger, thirst, and relief of pain. He or she will wish to communicate with the doctor providing care and convey information about where it hurts and whether treatment seems to be working. In work or school settings, more communication is needed to convey information. For example, a student participating in a classroom discussion may want to be able to describe the troop movements in the Battle of Gettysburg. In math class the student may need to present a proof involving oblique and parallel lines. Such an information exchange may be spontaneous, when the person is called on in class, or planned, as in a formal presentation. In a social or interpersonal setting, communication has a markedly different flavor. Teenagers may spend hours on the telephone, exchanging very little "information" but communicating shared feelings and concerns. At a faculty tea much of the communication is formulaic, such as, "How are you today?" Such queries are not intended as questions about medical status but are simply recognition of another's presence and an indication of wishing that person well. The planning and fluency of communication in each domain are substantially different, and the demands on AAC systems in each type of communication are likewise different.

An AAC system used solely for expression of needs and wants can be fairly basic. The vocabulary used in this type of communication is limited; because the expressions tend to be fairly short, the communication rate is not of paramount importance. In some cases the entire communication system is a buzzer used to indicate that the individual is in need and to summon a caregiver. The low-tech communication systems described earlier may meet basic communication needs for individuals whose physical skills are limited to eye blinks or directed eye movement.

Low-tech devices may enable expression of more complex ideas. For example, a therapist became aware that a client with aphasia wanted to communicate something. Since no AAC was available for this client, the therapist began attempting to guess what the client wanted to communicate. After exhausting basic needs ("Do you need a drink? Do you need to use the bathroom?"), the therapist was floundering. Over the next 20 minutes the client was able to communicate that the client's ears were the same shape as Cary Grant's! Even a basic communication aid, such as the ICU aid described above, would have allowed much faster transfer of this information.

Most development in AAC seems to focus on communication of basic needs and transfer of information. Information transfer presents some of the most difficult technological problems because the content of information to be communicated cannot be predicted. The designer of an AAC device probably would not anticipate the need to discuss the shape of Cary Grant's ears during vocabulary selection. To meet such needs, AAC devices must have the ability to generate any concept possible in the language being used. Making these concepts available for fluent communication is the ongoing challenge of AAC development.

Social communication and social etiquette present significant challenges for users of AAC devices. Although the information content of these messages tends to be low and based on convention, the dialog should be varied and spontaneous. Some AAC systems have provision for preprogrammed messages that can be retrieved for social conversation, but providing both fluency and variability of social discourse through AAC remains a challenge. Current devices allow somewhat effective communication of wants. These devices are not nearly so effective in discussing dreams.

Parts of AAC Systems

In general, electronic AAC systems have three components: a user control system, a message composition system, and a message transmission system (Fig. 19-9). The **user control system** allows the user to generate messages and control the device. The **message composition system** allows the user to construct messages to be communicated to others. The **message transmission system** allows the communication partner to receive the message from the user. The issues of user control of AAC devices are essentially the same as those for other electronic assistive technologies and are discussed with access systems in general.

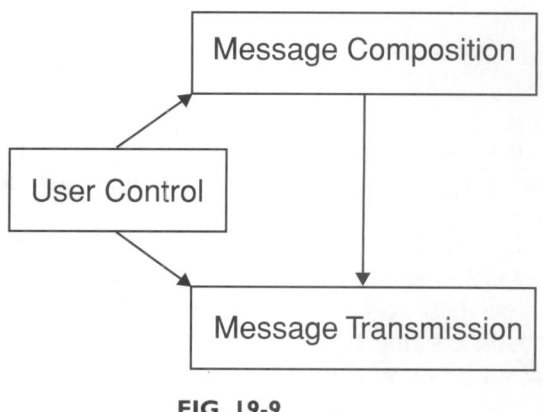

FIG. 19-9
Components of AAC systems.

MESSAGE COMPOSITION. In natural communication, most of the time, a person plans a message before speaking. An AAC device should allow the user to construct, preview, and edit utterances before they become apparent to the communication partner. This gives the user of an AAC device the ability to think before speaking. It also allows compensation for the rate difference between message composition via AAC and communication between able-bodied individuals.

Able-bodied individuals typically speak between 150 and 175 words per minute.[8] Augmentative communication rates are more typically 10 to 15 words per minute, resulting in a severe disparity between the rate of communication construction and expected rate of reception. Although the input techniques discussed offer some improvement in message construction rates, the rate of message assembly using AAC is such that many listeners will lose interest before an utterance can be delivered. If words are spaced too far apart, an able-bodied listener may not be able to assemble them into a coherent message.

The message construction area of an AAC device allows the individual to assemble a complete thought and then transmit it as a unit. A typical AAC device includes a display in which messages can be viewed before transmission. This area allows the communicator to review and edit the message that is being composed before transmitting it to the communication partner. This has two beneficial effects: the communicator can select words with care before communicating them, and the communication partner does not have to be constantly attentive to the conversation.

Communication between able-bodied people generally happens quickly enough to hold attention. When an able-bodied person is communicating with a person using an AAC device, the time between utterances may be too long to hold the attention. The able-bodied person may focus and not be able to maintain attention to the conversation. If messages come as units, the communication partner can respond to a query and then busy himself or herself in another activity while the communicator composes the next message. This is not unlike having a conversation via e-mail.

MESSAGE TRANSMISSION. When the communicator has finished composing a message, it can be transmitted to the communication partner. The means of transmission varies with the device and the setting. Some AAC devices use printed transmission exclusively. The message may be printed on paper tape, standard typewriter paper, or an electronic display that is made visible to the communication partner. Other systems use audible communication, speaking the message aloud by means of speech synthesis. There is a tendency to think of voice output as more appropriate than text, since able-bodied people generally communicate by

voice. In settings such as a classroom discussion, voice communication may be the most appropriate method of communication. In other settings, such as a busy sidewalk or a noisy shop, voice output may be drowned out or unintelligible and printed output may result in more effective communication. In a setting where speaking may disturb others, printed output may again be the transmission method of choice.

In settings in which speaking is the preferred method of communication, voice quality must be considered. Early AAC devices used voices that, to novice listeners, were only slightly more understandable than the communicator's unassisted voice. As speech synthesis technology has improved, AAC voices generally have become more intelligible. The high-quality voices of modern speech synthesizers have vastly improved intelligibility but continue to provide only a narrow range of variation and vocal expression. Although the AAC user has the option of deciding what she or he wants to sound like, the choices are few.

Communication Structure

Communications to be augmented may be categorized in terms of their intent, as well as in the content as Light[7] proposed. At the top level, communications may be categorized, with the conditions discussed above, as primarily oral or primarily written. In these cases, the categorization would be based on the mode of communication that typically would be used by an able-bodied person, not on the form that is being used by the augmented communicator.

SPOKEN OR VOICED COMMUNICATIONS. One category of spoken communication is conversation. Conversation implies a two-way exchange of information. This includes face-to-face communication with a friend, oral presentation when question-and-answer sessions are included, small group discussions, and conversation over a telephone. In all of these cases rapid communication is required and the user is expected to compose and respond immediately. If the composition rate is too slow, communication will break down and the conversation will cease. The augmented communicator may use "telegraphic" speech styles, but this results in primitive language that may be taken to indicate poor cognition.

Another form of spoken communication is the oral presentation in which no question-and-answer component is included or in which such a component is considered separately. In these cases the augmented communicator has ample time to prepare communications before delivery. An entire presentation may be stored in a communication device before the time of delivery. Although the time taken to prepare the message may be long in such cases, this does not inhibit the delivery of the message, as long as the device has adequate storage for the entire presentation. Stephen Hawking orally presents papers at conferences, just as his colleagues do, in spite of his use of an AAC device. However, his ability to respond to questions is severely constrained.

GRAPHICAL COMMUNICATIONS. The category of **graphical communications** includes all forms of communication that are mediated by graphic symbols. This includes writing using paper and pencil, typewriter, computer or word processor, calculator, or drawing program. Within the realm of graphical communications, a wide range of conditions and intents of communication may influence the devices selected for the user.

One type of graphical communication is note taking. Note taking is a method of recording information as it is being transmitted by a speaker, so that the listener can recall it later. The intended recipient of this form of communication is the person who is recording the notes. It is a violation of social convention to ask the speaker to speak more slowly to accommodate the note taker, so a note-taking system must allow rapid recording of information. However, since the listener is also the intended recipient, notes can be cryptic and may be meaningless to anyone other than the note taker.

Messaging is a form of graphical communication that shares many characteristics with note taking. Although the intended recipient is another person, shared abbreviations and nongrammatical language are common in messaging. The language that is common in adolescent e-mail (Fig. 19-10) is barely recognizable as English but is a form of graphical messaging that communicates to its intended audience. Messaging does not demand the speed of input of note taking, since encoding and receiving are not linked in time.

The most language-intensive form of graphical communication is formal writing. This includes writing essays for school, writing for publication, and writing business letters or contracts. Formal writing differs from the previously discussed forms of graphical communication in that it must follow the rules of written grammar. The communicator is expected to spend significant time and effort in preparing a formal written

document, and the abbreviations used in note taking and messaging are not allowed.

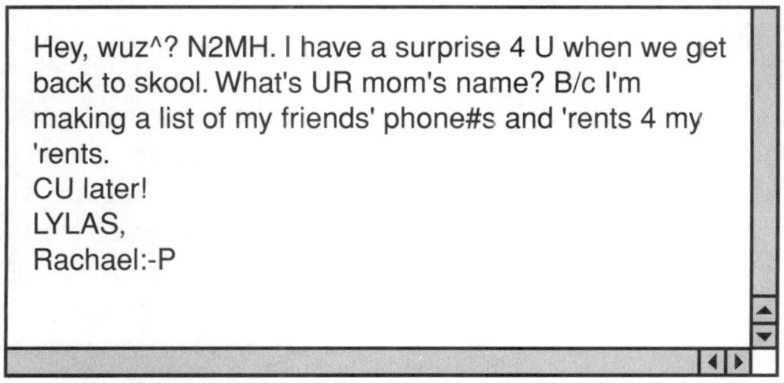

The most difficult formal communication for AAC may be mathematical notation. The early target of AAC devices was narrative text as used in messaging and written prose. Such language is commonly linear and can be composed in the order in which it is to be read. Mathematical expressions, on the other hand, may be two dimensional and nonlinear. Simple arithmetic, such as "$2 + 2 = 4$," is not excessively difficult. But algebraic expressions such as

$$x = \frac{-b \pm \sqrt{b^2 - 4ac}}{2a}$$

can be much more difficult for an AAC device to create. A relatively basic calculus equation, such as

$$\sum_{n=1}^{+\infty} \frac{(-1)^{n+1} \cdot 1 \cdot 3 \cdot 5 \cdots (2n-1)}{2 \cdot 4 \cdot 6 \cdots 2n} x^n$$

can be impossible to write, much less solve, for the user of an AAC device. While current technology allows prose construction with some facility, an AAC user will have marked difficulty with higher mathematics.

General Computer Access

The third category of electronic enabler is general computer access. Computer use is ubiquitous among able-bodied individuals. It is an assistive technology for individuals with a wide range of disabilities because it allows them to perform tasks for which they have no alternative method. Computers can be used to write messages or to research school subjects. For the person with a print impairment the computer can provide access to printed information either through electronic documents or through the use of optical character recognition, which can convert the printed documents into electronic documents. Once a document is stored electronically, it can be presented as large type for the person with a visual acuity limitation or read aloud for the person who is blind or profoundly learning disabled. Computers can allow the manipulation of "virtual objects" to teach mathematical concepts, form constancy, and spatial relations skills that are commonly learned by manipulation of physical objects. Personal digital assistants (PDAs) may be merely useful for the busy executive but may be the only means available for a person with attention deficit disorder to get to meetings on time. For the executive a PDA is a convenience, but for the person with ADHD it is an assistive technology.

Individuals using computers can locate, organize, and present information at levels of complexity not possible without electronic aids. Through the emerging area of cognitive prosthetics, computers can be used to augment attention and thinking skills in people with

---

Hey, wuz^? N2MH. I have a surprise 4 U when we get back to skool. What's UR mom's name? B/c I'm making a list of my friends' phone#s and 'rents 4 my 'rents.
CU later!
LYLAS,
Rachael:-P

FIG. 19-10
Example of messaging encryption in adolescent e-mail.

cognitive limitations. Computer-based biofeedback can monitor and enhance attention to task. Research in temporal processing deficits has led to the development of computer-modified speech programs that can be used to enhance language learning and temporal processing skills.[8,11]

Beyond such rehabilitative applications, the performance-enhancing characteristics of the conventional computer can allow a person with physical or performance limitations to participate in activities that would otherwise be too demanding. An able-bodied person might be annoyed at having to retype a document to accommodate editing changes; thus the cut-and-paste abilities of the computer are a convenience. A person with a disability may lack the physical stamina to complete the task without the cut-and-paste abilities of the computer. For the person with a disability the computer is an assistive technology because the task is impossible without it. Applications of the computer for a person with a disability include all the applications an able-bodied person would use. Additionally, computers may be used as cognitive prosthetics for the person with a disability.

CONTROL TECHNOLOGIES

All of the electronic enabling technologies discussed in this chapter depend on the ability of the individual to control them. Although functions of the various devices differ, the control strategies have common characteristics. Most electronic devices were designed for use by able-bodied persons. Controls of assistive technologies may be categorized by the ways in which they are adapted from standard controls. Electronic controls may be divided into three broad categories: input adaptations, output adaptations, and performance enhancements.

Input to Assistive Technologies

A wide range of input strategies are available to control electronic enablers; these can be more easily understood by considering them in subcategories. Different authors have created different taxonomies to categorize input strategies. The categorization presented here is one variation. For our purposes input strategies will be classified as those using physical keyboards, those using virtual keyboards, and those using scanning techniques.

Physical Keyboards
Physical keyboards typically provide an array of switches, with each switch having a unique function. On more complex keyboards modifier keys may change the base function of a key, usually to a related function. Physical keyboards appear on a wide range of electronic devices, including typewriters, computers, calculators,

telephones, and microwave ovens. In these applications, sequences of keys are used to generate meaningful units such as words, checkbook balances, telephone numbers, and the cooking time for a baked potato. Other keyboards are designed so that pressing a key results in immediate action. For example, the television remote control has keys that switch power or raise volume when pressed.

Physical keyboards can be adapted in a variety of ways. For example, most alphanumeric keyboards are arranged in the pattern of the conventional typewriter. Fig. 19-11 illustrates a conventional computer keyboard from myKey. This pattern was designed, for reasons relating to mechanical limitations, to slow down the user. Most individuals with disabilities do not need artificial restraints to slow them down, so this pattern of keys is seldom optimal for assistive technologies. Alternative keyboard patterns include the Dvorak Two-Handed, Dvorak One-Handed, and Chubon (Fig. 19-12).[1] These patterns offer improvements in efficiency of typing, which may allow a person with a disability to perform for functional periods of time.

The standard keyboard is designed to respond immediately when a key is pressed and, in the case of computer keyboards, to repeat when held depressed. This design benefits the individual with rapid fine motor control but penalizes the individual with delayed motor response. Fortunately, on many devices the response of the keyboard can be modified. "Delayed acceptance" provides a pause between the instant a key is pressed and the instant the key-press takes effect. Releasing the key during this pause will prevent the key from taking effect. If carefully calibrated, this adaptation can allow a person to type with fewer mistakes, resulting in higher accuracy and, sometimes, higher productivity.

The scale of the standard keyboard provides a balance between the fine motor control and range of

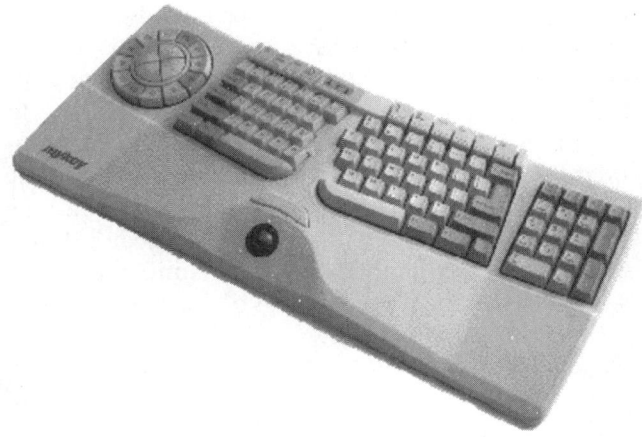

FIG. 19-11

Physical keyboard with adaptive features—the myKey keyboard.

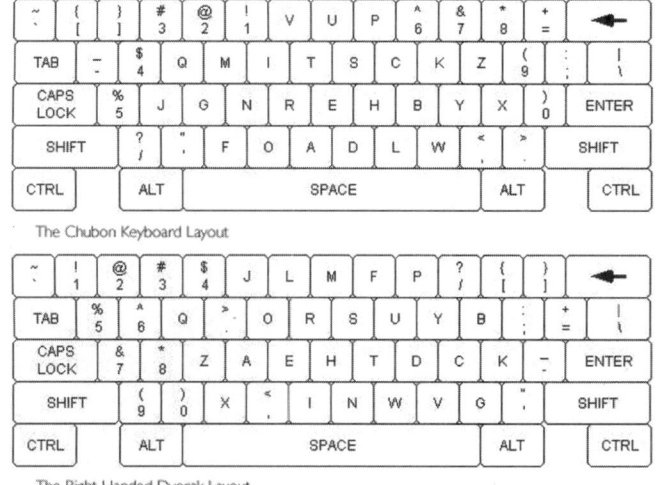

FIG. 19-12
Alternative keyboard patterns.

motion (ROM) of an able-bodied individual. The client with limitations in either ROM or motor control may find the conventional keyboard difficult to use. If the client has limitations in motor control, a keyboard with larger keys or additional space between keys may allow independent control of the device. This adaptation may also assist the person with a visual limitation. However, providing an equivalent number of options on larger keys increases the size of the keyboard, which may make it unusable for a person with limitations in ROM.

To accommodate limitations in ROM, the keyboard controls can be reduced in size. Smaller controls, placed closer together, will allow selection of the full range of options with less demand for joint movement. However, the smaller controls will be more difficult to target for the person with limited motor control. A mini-keyboard is usable only by a person with good fine motor control and may be the only scale of keyboard usable by a person with limited ROM.

A keyboard can be designed with fewer options to accommodate both limited ROM and limited fine motor control. Many augmentative communication devices can be configured with 4, 8, 32, or 64 keys on a keyboard of a single size. Modifier or "paging" keys can allow access to the full range of options for the keyboard, but with an attendant reduction in efficiency. In this approach the person uses one or more keys of the keyboard to shift the meanings of all of the other keys of the keyboard. Unless this approach is combined with a dynamic display, the user must remember the meanings of the keys.

Virtual Input Techniques

When an individual lacks the motor control to use an array of physical switches, a **virtual keyboard** may be used. Virtual keyboards provide the functionality of a physical keyboard system, allowing the user to directly select from the array of options through a unique action, but without physical switches demanding motor action. Instead, the meaning of the "selection" action may be encoded spatially, via pointing, or temporally, via sequenced actions.

POINTING SYSTEMS. The use of **pointing systems** is analogous to the use of a physical keyboard with a physical pointer such as a head-stick or mouth-stick. In these systems a graphical representation of a keyboard is presented to the user, who makes selections by pointing to a region of the graphical keyboard and performing a selection action. The selection action is typically either the operation of a single switch (e.g., clicking the mouse) or the act of holding the pointer steady for a period of time.

The pointer used for pointing systems may consist of a beam of light projected by the user, the reflection of a light source from the user, or sound waves received by a microphone that the user carries. Changing the orientation or position of the sensor moves an indicator over the graphical image of the keyboard, informing the user of the current meaning of the selection action.

Several augmentative communication systems now use a **dynamic display** on which the graphical keyboard can be changed as the user makes selections, so that the meaning of each location of the keyboard changes as a message is composed. Dynamic displays free the user from having to remember the current meaning of a key or decode a key with multiple images on it.

Pointing systems behave very much like physical keyboard systems, and many of the considerations of physical keyboards apply. The key size must balance the demands for fine motor control with the ROM available to the client. The keyboard pattern should be selected to enhance, not hinder, function. The selection technique should facilitate intentional selections while minimizing accidental actions.

The current state-of-the-art pointing system uses eye-tracking input. **Eye-tracking** systems generally are based on reflected infrared light from the surface of the eye. In general, these systems require extreme stability in the physical location of the eye and the camera observing the reflections. Traditionally, this has meant that the user must hold his or her head extremely still for the system to be usable. Because of cost considerations, this input method has not been a reasonable option for a person who could produce head movement, so the requirement of head stabilization has not been a major issue. However, there may be changes in these requirements as eye-gaze moves into mainstream technologies.

The first mainstream products that incorporated eye-tracking were hand-held camcorders, which had eye-tracking built into the view-finder. By tracking the portion of the screen being focused on, this eye-tracking allowed the camera to focus on the part of the display that was of special interest to the person taking the video.

Two divergent approaches to eye-tracking exist in mainstream products. In the first approach, personal computer developers are exploring eye-tracking as a means of detecting the action that the user would like to perform. This tracking would allow the computer to anticipate the needs of the user. To work as a mainstream product, the system must be able to track the user's gaze anywhere in front of the computer monitor. Development of the technology to allow free movement while tracking eye gaze is delaying the introduction of such products.

The second approach to using eye-tracking is more similar to video cameras with built-in eye tracking; these worked because the camera was held to the eye and moved with the eye. An eye-tracking system would be much easier to use if it were small enough to be head mounted because the system would remain in fixed relationship to the eyes. Currently, systems that combine head-mounted displays with eye-tracking are being made available for the development of future products. A number of possibilities are opened by this combination. For example, a head-mounted display might project a control system that the user looked *at* to control devices, and looked *through* for other activities. With binocular eye-tracking combined with head-tracking, an EADL system might be constructed that would allow the user to control devices simply by *looking* at them. Currently, no affordable, easy-to-use, and effective eye-gaze input systems exist. Now that engineers of mainstream devices have discovered this technology, it will probably become less costly and more effective in the future.

SWITCH ENCODING INPUTS. The individual who lacks the ROM or fine motor control necessary to use a physical or graphical keyboard may be able to use a switch encoding input method. In switch encoding, a small set of switches (from one to nine) is used to directly access the functionality of the device. The meaning of the switch may depend on the length of time it is held closed, as in Morse code, or on the immediate history of the switch set, as in the tongue touch keypad.

In **Morse code,** a very small set of switches is used to type. In single-switch Morse, a short switch closure produces an element called a "dit," which is typically written as an "*." A long switch closure produces the "dah" element, which is written as a "-." Formally, a "long switch closure" is three times longer than a short switch closure, a system that can be adjusted to the needs of the individual. Patterns of switch closures produce the letters of the alphabet, number, and punctuation. Pauses longer than five times the short switch closure indicate the end of a character. Two-switch

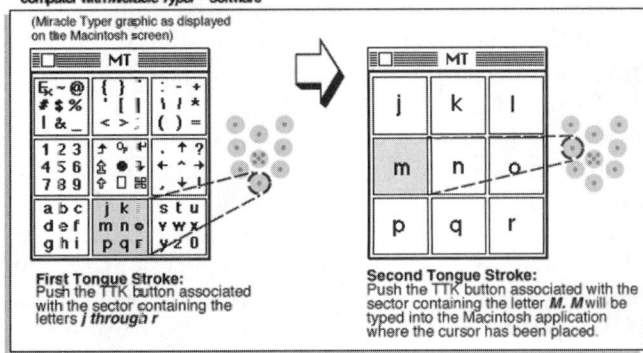

How to type the letter *M* with 2 tongue strokes using the *UCS 1000* and the Apple® Macintosh computer with *Miracle Typer™* software

First Tongue Stroke:
Push the TTK button associated with the sector containing the letters *j through r*

Second Tongue Stroke:
Push the TTK button associated with the sector containing the letter *M. M* will be typed into the Macintosh application where the cursor has been placed.

FIG. 19-13
MiracleTyper enabling character selection by selection history.

Morse is similar, except that two switches are used: one to produce the "dit" element and a second to produce the "dah." Because the meaning of the switches is unambiguous, it is possible for the dit and dah to be the same length, potentially doubling typing speed. Three-switch Morse breaks the time dependence of Morse by using a third switch to indicate that the generated set of dits and dahs constitutes a single letter.

Morse code is a highly efficient method of typing for a person with severe motor control limitations and has the advantage over other virtual keyboard techniques of eventually becoming completely automatic. Many Morse code users indicate that they do not "know" Morse code. They think in words, and the words appear on the screen, just as happens in touch-typing. Many Morse code users type at speeds approaching 25 words per minute, making this a means of functional writing. The historical weakness of Morse has been that each company creating a Morse interface for assistive technology has used slightly different definitions of many of the characters. To address this issue, and to promote application of Morse code, the Morse 2000 organization has created a "standard" for Morse development, which is available on the World Wide Web at http://www.uwec.edu/academic/hss-or/Morse2000/MorseSpecification.doc.[9]

Another variant of switch encoding involves switches that monitor their immediate history for selection. The Tongue Touch Keypad from newAbilities* uses a set of nine switches on a keypad, which is built into a mouthpiece that resembles a dental orthotic, and an on-screen keyboard (Fig. 19-13).

When the keypad is in typing mode, the first switch selection selects a group of nine possible characters, and the second switch action selects a specific character. This approach to typing is somewhat more efficient than

*newAbilities System Inc., 470 San Antonio Rd., Suite G, Palo Alto, CA 94306. http://members.aol.com/UCS1000/home.htm

Morse physically but does require the user to observe the screen to know the current switch meaning.

A different approach to switch encoding is provided by the T9 keyboard.* In this novel interface, each key of the keyboard has several letters on it but the user types as if only the desired character were present. The keyboard software determines from the user's input what word might have been intended. The "disambiguation process" used in the T9 keyboard allows a high degree of accuracy in determining which character the user intended and also allows rapid learning of the keyboard. This input technology is potentially compatible with the pointing systems described earlier in this chapter, providing an excellent balance of target size and available options. Fig. 19-14 shows the T9 keyboard on a Palm Pilot.

SPEECH INPUT. For many, **speech input** has a magical allure. What could be more natural than to speak to an EADL or computer and have one's wishes carried out? When first introduced by Dragon Systems† in 1990, large vocabulary speech input systems were enormously expensive and, for most, of limited utility. Although highly dedicated users were able to type using their voices in 1990, almost no one with the option of the keyboard would choose to use voice for daily work. These early systems required the user to pause between each word so that the input system could recognize the units of speech. Ten years later, the technology has evolved to allow continuous speech, with recognition accuracy greater than 90%. (The companies producing speech products claim accuracy of greater than 95%.) Although this advance in speech technology is remarkable, it does not mean that speech input is the control of choice for people with disabilities, for a number of reasons.

Speech recognition requires consistent speech. Although it is not necessary that the speech be absolutely clear, the user must say words the same way each time for an input system to recognize them. Because of this, the majority of people with speech impairments cannot use a speech input system effectively; slurring and variability of pronunciation will result in a low recognition rate.

A high degree of vigilance is needed during training and use of speech input. Before current speech technology devices can be used, they must be "trained" to understand the voice of the intended user. To do this, the system presents text to the potential user, who must read it into the microphone of the recognition system. If the user lacks the cognitive skills to respond appropri-

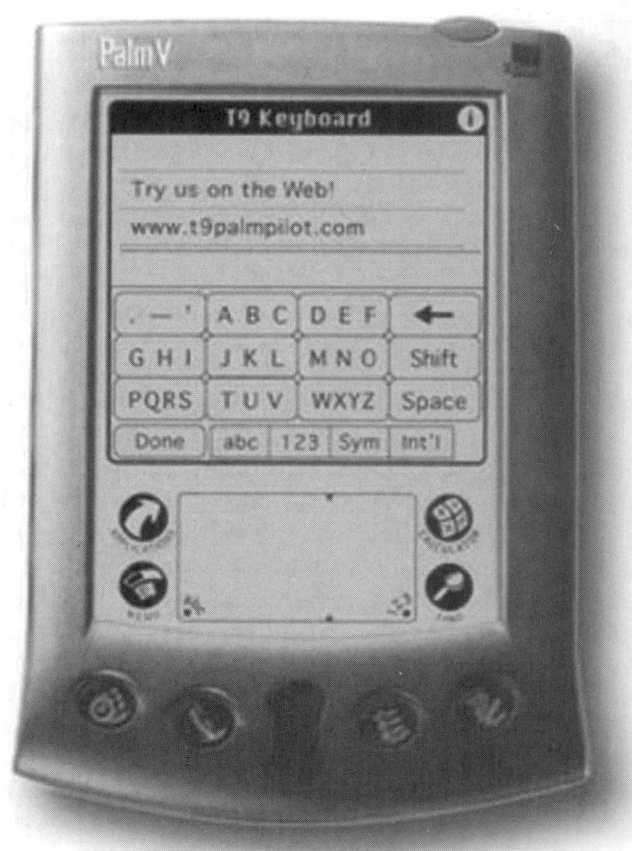

FIG. 19-14

T9 keyboard on a Palm Pilot. (From Tegic Communications.)

ately to the presented cues, the training process will be difficult. A few clinicians have reported success in training students with learning disabilities or other cognitive limitations to use speech input systems, but in general the success rate is poor. Even after training, the user must watch carefully for misrecognized words and correct them at the time the error is made. Modern speech recognition systems depend on context for their recognition. Each uncorrected error slightly changes the context until the system can no longer recognize the words being spoken. Spell-checking a document will not help the user find misrecognized words, since each word on the screen is a correctly spelled word—it just may not be the word the user intended.

Speech input is intrusive. One person in a shared office space talking to a computer will reduce the productivity of every other person in the office. If everyone in the office were talking to their computers, the resulting noise would be intolerable. Many offices have banned speech input for settings where data entry is being performed because of the confusion and errors produced by hearing numbers spoken while trying to focus on other numbers. Speech input is effective for a person who works or lives alone but is not a good input method for most office or classroom settings.

---

*Tegic Communications, 2001 Western Avenue, Suite 250, Seattle, WA 98121. http://www.tegic.com

†Dragon Systems, Inc., 320 Nevada Street, Newton, MA 02460; Phone: +1-617- 965-5200, Fax: +1-617-965-2374.

The type of speech system used depends on the device being controlled. For EADL systems, discrete speech (e.g., "Lights—On") provides an acceptable level of control. The number of options is relatively small, and there is seldom a need for split-second control. Misrecognized words are unlikely to cause difficulty. However, text generation for narrative description places higher demands on the user for input speed and transparency and may call for a continuous input method. Other computer applications, however, may work better with discrete than with continuous input methods. Databases and spreadsheets typically have many small input areas, with limited information in each. These applications are much better suited to discrete speech than continuous speech.

The "holy grail" of speech recognition is a system that will recognize any speaker, with an accuracy better than 99%. Developers of current speech systems say that, based on advances in processor speed and speech technologies, this level of usability should be possible within about 5 years. However, developers have been making the same prediction (within 5 years) for the past 10 years! Modern speech recognition systems are vastly better than those available 10 years ago and are also available at just over 1% of the cost of the early systems. However, even with these improvements, they still are not preferable to the conventional keyboard for most users.

Scanning Input Methods

For the individual with limited cognition or motor control, a variant of row-column scanning is sometimes used. In **scanning input,** the system to be controlled sequentially offers choices to the user and the user indicates assent when the correct choice is offered. Typically such systems first offer groups of choices. When a group is selected, the system offers the items of the group sequentially. Because early systems presented the items as part of a grid and offered the items a row at a time, such systems are commonly referred to as "row-column" scanning even when no rows or columns are present.

Scanning input allows selection of specific choices with limited physical effort. Generally, the majority of the user's time is spent waiting for the desired choice to be offered, so the energy expenditure is relatively small. Unfortunately, the overall time expenditure is usually relatively large. When the system has only a few choices from which to select, as in most EADL systems, scanning is a viable input method. The time spent waiting while the system scans may be a minor annoyance, but the delay in turning on a light a few seconds from now rather than immediately is relatively acceptable. EADL systems are used intermittently throughout the day, rather than continuously, so the delays over the course of the day are acceptable in many cases. For AAC or computer systems, however, the picture is very different.

In either application the process of composing thoughts may require making hundreds or thousands of selections in sequence. The cumulative effect of the pauses in row-column scanning slows productivity to the point that functional communication is difficult and may be impossible. Certainly, when productivity levels are mandated, the communication rate available with scanning input will not be adequate.

Rate Enhancement Options

For EADL systems, rate of control input is relatively unimportant. As noted previously, the number of control options is relatively limited, and rarely are selections severely time constrained. However, the number of selections to be made in sequence is high with AAC and computer control systems, and rate is frequently very important. Because a person with a disability typically cannot make selections at the same rate as an able-bodied person, **rate enhancement** technologies may be used to increase the information transmitted by each selection.

In general, language can be expressed in one of three ways: letter-by-letter spelling, prediction, and compaction and expansion. Of these, the latter two options allow enhancement of language generation rates.

LETTER-BY-LETTER SPELLING. Typical typing uses letter-by-letter representation and is relatively inefficient. For each language and alphabet, there is a balance between the number of characters used to represent a language and the number of elements in a message. English, using the conventional alphabet, averages about six letters (selections) per word (including the spaces between words). When represented in Morse code, the same text will require roughly 18 selections per word. By comparison, the basic Chinese vocabulary can be produced using a single ideogram per word. However, thousands of ideograms exist. In general, having a larger number of characters in an alphabet allows each character to convey more meaning but may make the selection of each specific character more difficult.

Many AAC systems use an expanded set of "characters" in the form of pictograms or icons that represent entire words and may be selected by the user. Such "semantic compaction" allows a large vocabulary to be used within a device but requires a system of selection that may add complexity to the device. For example, a device may require the user to select a word group (e.g., food) before selecting a specific word (e.g., hamburger) from the group. Using subcategories, it is theoretically possible to access a vocabulary of over 2 million words on a 128-key keypad with just three selections.

PREDICTION. Because messages in a language tend to follow similar patterns, significant savings of effort are possible by using **prediction** technology. Two types of prediction are used in language: word completion and word or phrase prediction.

In word completion a communication system (AAC or computer based) will present one or more options to the user after each keystroke, suggesting words that the user might be typing. When the appropriate word is presented by the prediction system, the user may select that word directly rather than continuing to spell out the word. Overall, this strategy may reduce the number of selections. However, it may not improve typing speed. Anson[2] demonstrated that when the user was typing from copy using the keyboard, typing speed was *reduced* in direct proportion to the frequency of using word prediction. The burden of constantly scanning the prediction list overwhelms the potential speed savings of word completion systems under these conditions. However, when the user is typing using an on-screen keyboard or scanning system, with which he or she must scan the input array in any case, word completion does appear to increase typing speed as well as reduce the number of selections made.

Because most language is similar in structure, it is also possible, in some cases, to predict the word that will be used following a specific word. For example, after a person types his or her first name, the surname will often follow. When this prediction is possible, the next word may be generated with a single selection. When combined with word completion, next-word prediction has the potential to decrease the typing effort substantially. However, in many cases this potential is unrealized. Even when provided with next-word prediction, many users become so involved in spelling words that they ignore the predictions even when the predictions are accurate. The cognitive effort of switching between "typing mode" and "list scanning" mode may be greater than the physical benefit of not having to spell a word out.

COMPRESSION AND EXPANSION. **Compression and expansion** strategies allow limited sets of commonly used words to be stored in unambiguous abbreviations. When these abbreviations are selected, either letter by letter or through word completion, the abbreviation is dynamically replaced by the expanded form of the word or phrase.

Because the expansion can be many selections long, this technology offers enormous potential to save energy and time. However, the potential savings are realized only when the person remembers to use the abbreviation rather than the expanded form of a word. Because of this limitation, abbreviations must be carefully selected. Many abbreviations are already in common use and can be stored conveniently. Most people will refer to the television by the abbreviation "TV," which requires just 20% of the selections to represent. With an expansion system, each use of "TV" can automatically be converted to "television" with no addi-

tional effort of the user. Similarly, "TTFN" might be used to store the social message, "Ta-ta for now."

Effective abbreviations will be unique to the user, rather than generally understood. An example of an effective form of abbreviation is the set of language shortcuts commonly used in note taking. These abbreviations form a shorthand unique to the individual, allowing complex thoughts to be represented on the page quickly in the course of a lecture. A clinician should work carefully with the client to develop abbreviations that will be useful and easily remembered.

Another form of "abbreviation" that is less demanding to create involves correction of common spelling errors. For either students or adult writers who have cognitive deficits that influence spelling skills, expansions can be created to automatically correct misspelled words. In these cases the "abbreviation" is the way that the client generally misspells the word and the "expansion" is the correct spelling of the word. Once a library of misspelled words is created, the individual is relieved of the need to worry about the correct spelling. Some maintain that this form of adaptation will discourage the individual from ever learning correct spelling. In cases where the client is still developing spelling skills, this is probably a valid concern and the adaptation should not be used. But for the individual with a cognitive deficit in which remediation is not possible, accommodation through compression and expansion technology is a desirable choice.

None of the control technologies will allow a person with a disability to produce messages at the same rate as an able-bodied person. However, individually and collectively, these technologies can make message generation significantly more efficient and accurate than it would be without them. The techniques are not mutually exclusive. Icons can be predicted using "next word" techniques. Abbreviations can be used in conjunction with word-completion and word-prediction technologies.

Output Options

As noted earlier, the control of assistive technologies involves a cycle of both human output and human input, matched to technology input and technology output. Individuals who have sensory limitations may have difficulty controlling assistive technologies (or common technologies) because they are unable to perceive the messages that are being sent to them by the technology. Adaptations of the output of the technology may be needed for these individuals. These adaptations generally depend on one of three sensory modalities: vision, hearing, or tactile sensation.

Visual Output

The default output of many types of electronic technology is visual. Computer screens are designed to resemble the printed page. AAC systems have input that "looks" like a keyboard, and the systems typically provide a graphical message composition area. EADLs use display panels and lighted icons to show the current status of controlled devices. The user must have visual acuity at nearly normal levels for perception of all of these controls. When the client has some vision but that vision is limited, some adaptations may be required.

COLORS AND CONTRAST. Many types of visual impairment affect the ability to separate foreground and background colors. In addition, bright background colors can produce a visual glare that makes the foreground difficult to perceive. In accommodating visual deficits, the clinician should explore the colors that the client easily perceives and those that the client has difficulty perceiving. For most people, background colors should be muted, soft colors that do not produce strong visual response. On the other hand, icons and letters may be represented in colors that provide visual contrast with the background. Very bright or strident colors should be avoided with both background and icons or letters. The specific colors and contrast levels needed by the user must be selected on an individual basis.

IMAGE SIZE. Visual acuity deficits and display size constraints present difficulty in output displays. Typically, a person with 20/20 vision can easily read text presented in letters about $1/6$ of an inch high. (This is equivalent to a page printed in a 12-point font.) On a typical display, between 100 and 150 words of text, or a similar number of icons, may be presented for selection at one time. If the user has lower visual acuity, the letter and icon size must be increased to accommodate that loss of acuity. However, the display of larger icons necessitates displaying either fewer letters at a time or increasing the display size. For people with severe visual limitations, it would be impractical to display all choices at once.

Screen enlargement programs typically overcome the limitation in display size by enlarging a portion of the full screen and moving this expanded portion to the area most likely of interest to the user. The visual effect of this is similar to viewing the screen through a magnifying glass that the user moves over the display. Most programs can be configured to follow the text insertion point, the mouse pointer, or other changes on the display. Navigation is a serious weakness with all such programs. When the user can see only a small portion of the screen at a time, the landmarks that are normally available to indicate the layout of the text on a page may be invisible because they are not in the field of view. Any screen enlargement program must provide a means the client can use to orient to the location on the screen.

AAC systems can accommodate the needs of a person with low visual acuity by using precisely the same techniques that are used for the person with limited fine motor control. The keyboard of the device can be configured with fewer, larger keys, each of which has a

larger symbol to represent its meaning. However, as with keyboards for those with physical limitations, the result is either fewer communication options or a more complex interface for the user. Also, these accommodations do not adapt the size of the message composition display, which may be inaccessible to the user with visual limitations.

Speech Output

It is important to keep the difference between *voice input* and *voice output* clearly in mind. In *voice input*, the user speaks and the spoken word is converted into commands within the assistive technology. In *voice output*, the device communicates with the user by auditory means, converting printed words or commands into voice. Voice output technology has been in existence for much longer than voice input and is a more mature technology—not perfect, but more mature.

The demands of voice output are varied, depending on the application and the intended listener. In general, systems can be categorized as either those in which a second person is the listener or those in which the user is the listener.

SECOND PERSON AS LISTENER. Most voice output used in AAC applications is intended to be understood by a person who may have little experience with synthetic voices. For example, the AAC user at the corner market buying 2 pounds of hamburger for dinner will communicate with a butcher who will have had very little experience with synthetic voice. When asking for directions on the street corner, the AAC's voice will be competing with the sounds of trucks and busses while attempting to communicate with a listener who probably has little prior experience.

To be understandable by novice listeners in real-world environments, a synthetic voice should be as clear and as "human sounding" as possible. The voice will be easily understood to the extent that it sounds like what the listener expects to hear. Ideally, the voice would provide appropriate inflection in the spoken material and would be able to convey emotional content. Current AAC systems do not convey emotional content well, but high-end voices do sound very much like human speakers. Under adverse conditions, these devices will remain less understandable than a human speaker, because facial and lip movements (that provide additional cues as to the sounds being produced) do not accompany synthetic voices.

USER AS LISTENER. When synthetic voice is used for computer access or EADLs, the voice quality does not need to be as "human sounding." For either use, the user has the opportunity to learn to understand the voice in training. In EADL applications, relatively few utterances need be produced, and these can be designed to sound as different from each other as possible so that there is little chance of confusion. General voice output for an entire language is somewhat more difficult, however, because many words sound similar and can be easily confused.

For general text reading, the primary issue is voicing speed. As noted earlier, humans generally talk at a rate of between 150 and 175 words per minute. However, most humans also read between 300 and 400 words per minute. A person who depends on a human-sounding voice for reading printed material will be limited to reading at less than half the speed of able-bodied readers. To be an effective text access method, synthetic voice must be understandable at speeds in excess of 400 words per minute. This requires significant training, since untrained people without disabilities can't understand speech at such speeds. With training, however, **speech output** is a useful way for a person to access printed material.

Synthetic speech is a useful tool in two cases: when it replaces voice for a person with a disability and when the user is not able to use vision to access the technology. AAC devices using voice provide the most "normal" face-to-face communication available. In most conditions, able-bodied people communicate by voice. People with disabilities generally want to communicate in similar fashion. The other application of voice is "eyes-free" control. In the mass market for able-bodied consumers these applications include the presentation of information over the telephone, while driving, or in other settings where a visual display might be difficult to use. All of these situations are important for people with disabilities as well.

Persons with print impairments also may find value in assistive technologies using voice. Print impairments include conditions that result in very low vision and blindness, as well as conditions that result in the inability to translate visual stimuli to language and those that make manipulation of printed materials difficult.

Voice output technology may be a poor choice for people who are developing language skills. Because English is an irregular language, with many letter combinations making similar sounds, it is almost impossible to learn spelling by listening to the sound of words. As such, children who are blind from birth may not be good candidates for speech output as the primary language access method because the structure of words is lost when the words are converted to speech. For these children and for many others, tactile access is a better tool.

Tactile Output

The oldest method for individuals with visual deficits to access printed material is Braille. In 1829, Louis Braille developed the idea of adapting a military system that allowed aiming artillery in darkness and writing secret messages, to provide a method of reading for students at the National Institute for the Young Blind in Paris.[3] Over time, this original system has been extended to allow communication of music, mathematics, and computer code to readers without vision. Basic Braille uses an array of six dots to represent letters and numbers. However, traditional Braille is only usable for static text, such as printed books. Dynamic information cannot be represented by raised dots on a sheet of paper.

Technology access requires the use of refreshable Braille. Refreshable Braille displays use a set of piezoelectric pins to represent Braille letters. Changing electrical signals to the display move the pins up and down, allowing a single display to represent different portions of a longer document.

Braille is not widely used among individuals who are blind. By some estimates, only 10% of the blind population know and use Braille. It is not usable by those who have limited tactile sensation in addition to blindness. In spite of this, Braille is a skill that probably should be taught to a person who is blind. Most Braille readers are employed; most people who are blind but do not read Braille are not employed. While Braille may not be an essential skill for employment, the ability to learn Braille certainly correlates with the ability to hold a job.[3]

SUMMARY

Assistive technologies provide a means for persons with disabilities to perform tasks that would otherwise be difficult or impossible for them to perform. The development and increased availability of universal design has improved access and ease of use for persons with disabilities, as well as for the "temporarily able-bodied." This chapter has introduced several models for approaching assistive technology. The reader is asked to consider the interface between a person, a technology, an environment, and a task. Various technologies that are current state of the art have been described. These cover the categories of electronic aids to daily living (EADL), augmentative and alternative communications (AAC), and general computer applications and control technologies.

An occupational therapist should always keep in mind that although disability makes few things impossible, it makes many things more difficult. Disability may make some tasks sufficiently hard that they are "not worth it." The goal of rehabilitation is to make those tasks possible. Assistive technology can make many things easier for the person with a disability. When they are easier, many things that were previously not worth the effort can become reasonable to attempt. Assistive technology will never remove the functional limitation. However, it can compensate for that functional limitation and enable ability.

REVIEW QUESTIONS

1. Contrast rehabilitation technology with assistive technology.
2. Discuss the role of universal design in improving technology options for persons with physical impairments.
3. Contrast the three models of HAAT, HETI, and HIA.
4. Identify and describe at least three EADL that are suitable for persons with physical impairments.
5. Indicate some of the technologies that can be used for power switching.
6. Discuss the importance of feature control. Analyze the difficulties and solutions in providing feature control to persons with physical impairments.
7. Discuss several different augmentative and alternative communication devices in terms of their benefits and their limitations.
8. Contrast message composition and message transmission. Identify features that are important in each.
9. Contrast aural and graphical communications in terms of their demands on the user and on the technology.
10. Give some examples of options for input devices. Identify situations in which each would be appropriate and situations in which each would be unworkable.
11. How do prediction and compression and expansion work?
12. The author suggests that prediction technologies may not save time in the way originally envisioned by their designers. What is the reason for this?
13. List considerations that would apply in selecting output options.
14. How would a therapist go about selecting colors and contrast for a visual output display? What factors are important?
15. Braille is the oldest system of tactile input for persons with vision loss, and yet the author advocates its continued use. Why?

REFERENCES

1. Anson DK: *Alternative computer access: a guide to selection,* Philadelphia, 1997, FA Davis.
2. Anson DK: The effect of word prediction on typing speed, *Am J Occup Ther* 47(11):1039-1042, 1993.
3. Canadian National Institute for the Blind: Braille Information Centre. Available online at "http://www.cnib.ca/braille_information/louis_braille.htm." May 1999, the Institute.
4. Center for Universal Design: *Principles of universal design.* Available online at "http://www.design.ncsu.edu:8120/cud/univ_design/princ_overview.htm."
5. Cook AM, Hussey SM: *Assistive technologies: principles and practice,* St Louis, 1995, Mosby.
6. Smith RO: Technological approaches to performance enhancement. In Christiansen C, Baum C, editors: *Occupational therapy: overcoming human performance deficits,* Thorofare, NJ, 1991, Slack Publishers.
7. Light J: Interaction involving individuals using augmentative and alternative communication systems: state of the art and future directions, *Augmentative Altern Communication* 4(2):66-82, 1988.
8. Merzenich M, Jenkins W, Johnston P, et al: Temporal processing deficits of language-learning impaired children ameliorated by training, *Science* 271(5245):77-81, 1996.
9. Miller GA: *Language and speech,* San Francisco, 1981, Freeman.
10. Morse 2000: *Development specification: Morse code input system for the Windows 2000 operating system,* Available online at "http://www.uwec.edu/academic/hss-or/Morse2000/MorseSpecification.doc."
11. Tallal P, Miller S, Bedi G, et al: Language comprehension in language-learning impaired children improved with acoustically modified speech, *Science* 271(5245):81-84, 1996.

CHAPTER 20

Functional Motion Assessment

AMY PHILLIPS KILLINGSWORTH
LORRAINE WILLIAMS PEDRETTI

KEY TERMS

Functional motion assessment
Individual activity analysis
Objective activity analysis
Clinical observation

LEARNING OBJECTIVES

After reading this chapter the student or practitioner will be able to do the following:

1. Define functional motion assessment.
2. Describe why it is desirable to assess motor function through observation of activity performance.
3. State two circumstances under which assessment of performance components is indicated.
4. Define individual activity analysis, or "dynamic performance analysis."
5. Describe why it is not possible to do an accurate objective activity analysis.
6. List at least three questions that can guide the clinical observation and clinical reasoning of the occupational therapy practitioner while conducting a functional motion assessment.
7. List factors other than range of motion (ROM), strength, and motor control that can affect motor performance.
8. Discuss how information gained from the functional motion assessment differs from that gained during assessment of performance components.
9. State the minimum level of strength required throughout the lower extremity for normal stance and positioning.
10. Compare levels of muscle strength and associated endurance in the upper extremities.
11. List activities that can be used to assess functional motion in the upper extremities and in the lower extremities.

Many physical disabilities cause limitations in joint range of motion (ROM), muscle strength, or motor control. These physical impairments result in movement limitations that can cause slight to substantial deficits in occupational performance and prevent pursuit of self-care, work, leisure, and social activities. The **functional motion assessment** is a way of assessing ROM, strength, and motor control available for task performance by observing the patient during performance of functional activities (activities of daily living [ADL], work, or leisure activities).

Since the primary responsibility of the occupational therapist is to assess occupational performance, identify performance problems, and plan treatment strategies that will improve occupational performance, sensorimotor limitations first should be assessed through observation of functional activities. When improvement of performance components is a goal of the intervention program, assessment of performance components may be indicated to make an objective assessment of physical limitations and gains (Chapters 21 to 23).

Sensory, perceptual, cognitive, and psychosocial impairments can also affect motor function. These components must be considered in any performance evaluation (Chapters 24 to 29). However, this chapter is limited to consideration of motor function (i.e., ROM, strength, and motor control) during the functional motion assessment.

Except for a few diagnoses, comprehensive assessments of ROM, muscle strength,[5] and motor control are seldom necessary. For example, performing a full ROM assessment or manual muscle test is time consuming, can be tiring to the client, and may duplicate other services.

CLINICAL OBSERVATON

In occupation-based practice, muscle strength, ROM, and motor control can be observed during the performance of ordinary ADL.[4] For example, while assessing ADL, the therapist can observe for performance difficulties and movement patterns that may signal limited ROM, muscle weakness, muscle imbalance, poor endurance, limited motor control, and compensatory motions used for function.

Essentially, when observing a patient perform selected tasks, the occupational therapist is doing an **individual activity analysis** or "dynamic performance analysis"[7] to diagnose the occupational performance problems of that patient. Because people perform the same task in a variety of ways and because there are so many variables in task performance, it is not possible to do an **objective activity analysis,** one that can be applied universally, and describe the sensorimotor requirements of the myriad of ADL. The purpose of obser-

vation is to understand the patient's occupational performance problems in the context of the interaction between the person, the task, and the environment.[3]

The therapist's scientific knowledge of the particular dysfunction and an analysis of the ways in which activities are generally performed influence the assessment of performance problems and aid in the development of plans to remediate those problems.[3]

The following are questions to guide the **clinical observation** and clinical reasoning processes:

1. Does the patient have adequate ROM to perform the task?
   a. Where are the joint limitations?
   b. What are some possible causes of the limitations?
   c. Are there true ROM limitations or are apparent limitations actually caused by decreased muscle strength?
2. Does the patient have enough strength to perform the task?
   a. In which muscle groups is there apparent weakness?
   b. If strength appears inadequate to perform a task because the patient cannot complete the ROM, is there truly muscle weakness or is there actually limited ROM?
3. Does the patient have enough motor control to perform the task?
   a. Is the movement smooth and rhythmic?
   b. Is movement slow and difficult (e.g., as seen in spasticity and rigidity)?
   c. Are there extraneous movements when the patient performs the task (e.g., tremors, athetoid, or choreiform movements)?

The observing therapist must also consider the patient's understanding of the instructions and perception of task importance, as well as the possibility of sensory, perceptual, and cognitive deficits. An analysis of the results of the functional motion assessment may indicate that formal assessment of performance components is needed. For example, this assessment may be needed to differentiate muscle weakness from limited ROM or to quantify (with a muscle grade) muscle weakness in specific muscle groups.

Assessing ROM, strength, and motor control by observing the patient perform functional activities can aid in selecting meaningful treatment goals relative to improving occupational performance. The therapist can ask the patient about his or her ability to perform the tasks of daily living but should also observe the patient performing such activities as dressing, walking, standing, and sitting to make an accurate assessment.[2]

Joint ROM, manual muscle testing, and motor control assessments (Chapters 21, 22, and 23) will give the therapist specific information about the function of the musculoskeletal, neurophysiological, and sensorimotor systems. Although the tests require minimum to maximum active output by the client, the therapist will not be able to determine the client's ability to integrate these systems to perform specific goal-directed tasks based on the results of these assessments. Rather, the therapist will have information about movements of a specific limb or a combination of limbs. Under carefully controlled conditions the therapist will know about the flexibility of the components of the joint and the strength of muscles to create movements, such as flexion, abduction, and external rotation. However, the patient's motor performance capabilities are not measured by these assessments. For example, the manual muscle test cannot measure muscle endurance (number of times the muscle can contract at its maximum level), motor control (smooth rhythmic interaction of muscle function), and the patient's ability to use the muscles for functional activities.[1] While observing a patient performing functional activities, it would be most helpful if a therapist could also estimate the client's existing ROM, muscle strength, and motor control.

FUNCTIONAL MOTION ASSESSMENT

The activities listed in the following sections for the functional motion assessment are suggested as a general starting place for the student or beginning practitioner. Only upper and lower extremity activities are included. Movements of the face, mouth, neck, and spine are beyond the scope of this chapter. Many more activities could be suggested in each category. The reader is referred to *Musculoskeletal Assessment*, second edition, by Hazel M. Clarkson[2] for a comprehensive and detailed discussion of musculoskeletal assessment and its functional application.

Lower Extremity

Because of the somewhat stereotypical movements of the lower extremity, the arrangement of the large muscle groups, and the nature of the overall functions of weight bearing and ambulation, assumptions can be made about muscle strength during functional activities. For example, to assume a normal stance pattern, ambulate without any compensatory gait patterns, or position the lower extremities (without the assistance of the upper extremities) during dressing, a minimum of F+ muscle strength is required in the musculature of the hips, knees, ankles, and feet. If muscle strength in the lower extremities is only F throughout the lower extremity, ambulation without aids will not be possible.[8] Good to normal muscle strength is required for the endurance to perform the small postural adjustments needed for maintained standing, repetitive movement patterns inherent in walking, and the lifting, maneuvering, and balancing on the lower limbs that usually occur during dressing.

Hip Complex

The hip joints support the body weight. Each joint acts as a fulcrum when a person is standing on one leg. Hip movement makes it possible to move the body closer to or farther from the ground, bring the foot closer to the trunk, and position the lower limb in space.[2]

During functional activities, lumbar-pelvic movements accompany hip movement, which extends the functional capabilities of the hip joint. The hip is capable of flexion, extension, adduction, abduction, and internal and external rotation.[2]

FLEXION AND EXTENSION. Full flexion and extension are required for many ADL. Standing requires full hip extension. Squatting, bending to tie a shoelace with the foot on the ground, and toenail care done with the foot on the edge of the chair all require full or near full hip flexion. Other activities that require moderate to full flexion and extension are donning panty hose or socks, bathing the feet in a bathtub, ascending and descending stairs, and sitting and rising in a standard chair.[2]

ABDUCTION AND ADDUCTION. Most ordinary ADL do not require full ranges of abduction and adduction. The main function of the hip abductors is to keep the pelvis level when one foot is off the ground. For ADL, hip abduction may be used when stepping sideways into a shower or bathtub, donning trousers when sitting, squatting to pick up an object, or sitting with the foot across the opposite thigh.[2]

Hip adduction brings the foot across the front of the body. An individual uses this motion when kicking a ball, moving an object on the floor with the foot, or crossing one thigh over the other for donning or removing shoes and socks.[2]

INTERNAL AND EXTERNAL ROTATION. Internal rotation occurs when a person is pivoting medially on one foot. When a person is sitting, there is internal rotation when the person reaches to the lateral side of the foot for washing or donning socks. Internal rotators are active in walking.[2]

External rotation with hip flexion and abduction brings the foot across the opposite thigh for donning shoes or socks, or for foot hygiene.[2]

Knee

The knee joint supports the body weight. With the foot fixed on the ground, knee flexion lowers the body toward the ground and knee extension raises the body. If the foot is off the ground, as in sitting, the knee and hip are used to orient the foot in space.[2]

Daily living activities that require moderate to full ranges of knee flexion and extension are standing and walking, squatting to lift an object from the floor, crossing the ankle of one foot over the thigh of the opposite leg, sitting down and rising from a chair, and dressing the feet.

Ankle and Foot

The foot is a flexible base of support when a person is on rough terrain. It functions as a rigid lever during terminal stance in the walking pattern. It absorbs shock when transmitting forces between the ground and the leg. The foot and ankle function to elevate the body from the ground when the foot is fixed. Dorsiflexion and plantar flexion occur at the ankle joint. Foot inversion and eversion occur at the subtalar joint.[2]

PLANTAR FLEXION. Full plantar flexion is used when a person is rising on the toes to reach upward to a high shelf. Some plantar flexion is used to depress the accelerator in an automobile or control pedal on a sewing machine and when donning socks or shoes.

DORSIFLEXION. Full range of dorsiflexion is needed to descend stairs. Dorsiflexion is used in such activities as positioning the foot to cut the toenails or tying shoe laces.[2]

INVERSION AND EVERSION. Inversion and eversion function to provide flexibility when an individual is walking on uneven ground. Inversion is used when the foot is crossed over the opposite thigh and the sole is inspected.[2]

Upper Extremity

By simply observing a patient engaging in functional activities, the therapist cannot as easily make general assumptions about muscle strength in the upper extremities as in the lower extremities. There are three reasons why this is the case: the variety of ways in which the upper extremity can be positioned to complete any given task (i.e., there is not one right way to do the task), the complexity of motor patterns possible requiring gross motor and fine motor skill, and the dependency of the distal joints and musculature on the more proximal joints for positioning.

If several people are observed donning shirts, it will be apparent that different techniques are used by each. One person may lift the arm out to the side, increasing shoulder abduction as the shirt is drawn onto the arm. Another person might prefer to dress with the arm more in front of the body, thus positioning the humerus in flexion. A third person might hyperextend the humerus as the shirt is pulled on. The difficulty, of course, is determining exactly how much ROM and muscle strength are minimally required at all of the joints involved when so many options are available to perform one task.

In the first two examples of donning a shirt, the musculature of the shoulder complex would certainly have to create more tension than if the humerus were in the adducted position. It would be inappropriate for the therapist to instruct the client on how to don the shirt if the therapist's goal was to attain some information regarding the client's level of independence in dressing and secondarily to make assumptions about ROM and muscle strength.

The important thing to remember when observing a client perform functional motion tasks with the upper extremities is that even when it is not obvious or readily apparent, the muscles of the shoulder complex are contracting with varying degrees of tension. They may have to contract with enough force to position the hand in space and maintain it there, as when a person is combing hair. At other times the humerus must be held close to the body to provide a stable base from which the forearm, wrist, and hand can maneuver, as when hitting the keys on a keyboard, cutting food with a knife, or writing. It would be an inaccurate assumption that the extremity is just hanging passively at the side when, in fact, the static contractions around the proximal joints make it possible for the musculature of the distal extremity to work effectively. Conversely, the shoulder complex may have to be a moving unit, as opposed to a positioning one, as when moving groceries from a countertop to shelves in a kitchen cabinet.

General guidelines exist for assessing strength for function in the upper extremities. With good to normal endurance the patient with good (G) to normal (N) muscle strength throughout the upper extremity will be able to perform all ordinary ADL without undue fatigue.[6] Ordinary ADL are considered here to be all self-maintenance tasks, mobility, and vocational roles, except for strenuous labor. The patient with fair plus (F+) muscle strength usually will have low endurance and will fatigue more easily than a patient with G to N strength. The patient will be able to perform many ordinary ADL independently but may need frequent rest periods. The patient with muscle grades of fair (F) will be able to move parts against gravity and perform light tasks that require little or no resistance.[4,6] Low endurance is a significant problem and will limit the amount of activity that can be done. The patient with low endurance probably will be able to eat finger foods and perform light hygiene if given the time and rest periods needed to reach the goals.[6] Poor (P) strength is considered below functional range, but the patient with poor strength will be able to perform some ADL with mechanical assistance and can maintain ROM independently.[6] Patients with muscle grades of trace (T) and zero (0) will be completely dependent and unable to perform ADL without externally powered devices. Some activities will be possible with special controls on equipment, such as electric wheelchairs, electronic communication devices, and hand splints.[6]

Individuals use a variety of motor patterns when performing a functional task, and no one way is the right way to perform the task. These facts make it impossible for the therapist to predetermine the level of muscle strength, amount of ROM, and degree of motor control needed in the upper extremity to perform any given task. Individual styles of moving, numerous possibilities for compensatory movements when faced with loss of joint flexibility, poor endurance, lack of motor control, impaired sensation, and pain are all factors that may affect the client's ability to generate tension in a muscle or muscle group and sustain muscle activity.

Shoulder Complex

The shoulder complex is the most mobile joint complex in the body. Its function is to move the arm in space and position the hand for function. The shoulder complex is composed of the acromioclavicular, sternoclavicular, scapulothoracic, and glenohumeral joints and the muscles, ligaments, and other structures that move and support these joints. In the performance of functional activities, scapular, clavicular, and trunk motions normally accompany glenohumeral motion. These associated movements increase the range of glenohumeral motion for function. The shoulder complex functions in a coordinated manner that is accomplished through scapulothoracic and glenohumeral movement. This coordinated function is called *scapulohumeral rhythm.* Thus movements at the shoulder are actually combinations of several joint motions and are dependent on scapulohumeral rhythm in the performance of any given activity.[2]

SHOULDER FLEXION AND ABDUCTION WITH SCAPULA UPWARD ROTATION (OVERHEAD MOVEMENTS). Activities such as placing an object (e.g., book, box, or cup) on an overhead shelf or reaching overhead to pull on a light cord require these movements.[2]

SHOULDER EXTENSION AND ADDUCTION WITH SCAPULA DOWNWARD ROTATION. Activities such as reaching back for toilet hygiene, swinging the arm backward for throwing a ball, and reaching backward to put an arm through the sleeve of a coat require these movements.[2]

HORIZONTAL ADDUCTION AND ABDUCTION. These movements allow the arm to be moved around the body. Reaching the opposite axilla or opposite ear for hygiene activities, opening and closing a sliding door, combing the opposite side of the hair, and reaching the upper back while bathing are some activities that use horizontal adduction and abduction.[2]

INTERNAL AND EXTERNAL ROTATION. Some degree of either internal or external rotation accompanies every glenohumeral motion. The ROM varies in various positions of the arm. Full range of external rotation is required for reaching the back of the head for combing or washing hair. External rotation is often as-sociated with supination when the elbow is extended, as when rotating a doorknob in a clockwise direction.[2]

Internal rotation is used when buttoning a shirt, eating, and drinking from a cup. Full range of internal rotation with scapulothoracic motion is used to reach into a back pocket, fasten a bra, put a belt through the belt keepers on trousers, or do toilet hygiene. Internal rotation is often associated with forearm pronation, as when putting a pillow behind the low back, turning a screwdriver to unfasten a screw, rotating a doorknob in a counterclockwise direction, and pouring water from a vessel.[2]

EXTENSION AND ADDUCTION. Extension and adduction are used to return the arm to the side of the body from shoulder flexion and abduction, as after reaching overhead. These motions are also used when quick movement or force is required, as when an individual is closing a vertically oriented window, crutch walking, or pushing off to rise from an armchair.[2]

FLEXION AND ADDUCTION. Flexion and adduction are used in activities that require reaching the same side of the body, such as washing the cheek or ear and combing hair on the same side. Slight shoulder flexion with adduction is used for hand-to-mouth activities and putting on an earring back.

Elbow and Forearm

Elbow and forearm movements serve to place the hand for function. Elbow flexion moves the hand toward the body and elbow extension moves the hand away from the body. Forearm pronation or supination usually accompanies elbow flexion and extension. Pronation and supination position the hand precisely for the requirements of the given activity. The elbow and forearm support skilled and forceful movements of the hand that are used during performance of ADL and work activities.[2]

Full or nearly full range of elbow flexion, usually with some humeral flexion and forearm supination, is used to bring food to the mouth, hold a telephone receiver, place an earring on the ear, and reach the neck level of a back zipper.

Full range of elbow extension, usually with pronation, is used when an individual is reaching to the feet to tie shoes, throwing a ball overhand, and using the arms to push off from a chair. Many other ADL require less than full range of these movements.[2]

Wrist and Hand

The wrist controls the length-tension relations of the extrinsic muscles of the hand. It positions the hand relative to the forearm for touch, grasp, or manipulation of objects. Wrist extension and ulnar deviation are most important in performance of ADL.[2] It is possible to perform some ADL when there is a loss of wrist ROM by using compensatory movements of the proximal joints.

The primary functions of the hand are to grasp and manipulate objects and to discriminate sensory information about objects in the environment. The arches of the hand make it possible to adapt the hand to the shape of the object being manipulated.

Power grip and precision grip are the bases of all hand activities. Power grip is used when force is required for grasping, such as holding a hammer handle, a full glass, or the handle of a purse or suitcase. Precision grip is used when an object is pinched and when it is being manipulated between the thumb and one or more fingers. Precision grip is used for holding a pencil, moving checkers or chess pieces, turning a key, threading a needle, and opening the cap of a medicine bottle. (See Chapter 31, Section 1, for a full discussion of prehension patterns).[2]

SUMMARY

Many physical disabilities cause deficits in ROM, strength, and motor control that limit occupational performance. The occupational therapist is primarily responsible for assessing occupational performance, identifying performance problems, and planning treatment that will improve the patient's occupational performance.

Because people perform the same activity in a variety of ways, the level of ROM, strength, or motor control needed to do a task is variable. Assessment of physical limitations can be made through observation of a patient's performance of activities. Therefore, the therapist must observe the patient performing selected tasks in the person-task-environment interaction.[3]

While assessing the patient's ability to perform ADL, work, or leisure activities, the therapist should observe for sensorimotor problems. An analysis of the results of observation may indicate that an assessment of performance components is needed. Questions to guide clinical observation and clinical reasoning and suggested activities to assess function of the upper and lower extremities are outlined in this chapter.

REVIEW QUESTIONS

1. Define functional motion assessment.
2. In occupation-based practice, how are sensorimotor functions first assessed?
3. What is meant by individual activity analysis?
4. Why is it not possible to do an objective activity analysis?
5. List three major questions that can guide the clinical observation and clinical reasoning of the occupational therapy practitioner when doing a functional motion assessment.
6. Which factors, other than strength, ROM, and motor control, can affect the functional motion assessment?
7. How is the information gained from assessment of performance components different from that gained in a functional motion assessment?
8. What is the minimum level of strength required throughout the lower extremity for normal stance and positioning?
9. List some activities that can be used to assess functional motion in the lower extremities: hip, knee, ankle, and foot.
10. Compare levels of muscle strength with endurance in the upper extremities.
11. List some activities that can be used to assess functional motion in the upper extremities: shoulder complex, elbow and forearm, and wrist and hand.

REFERENCES

1. Clarkson HM: *Musculoskeletal assessment*, ed 2, Philadelphia, 2000, Lippincott, Williams & Wilkins.
2. Cole JH, Furness AL, Twomey LT: *Muscles in action*, New York, 1988, Churchill Livingstone.
3. Crepeau EB: Activity analysis: a way of thinking about occupational performance. In Neistadt ME, Crepeau EB: *Willard and Spackman's occupational therapy*, ed 9, Philadelphia, 1998, Lippincott.
4. Crepeau EB, editor: *Willard & Spackman's occupational therapy*, ed 9, Philadelphia, 1998, Lippincott.
5. Daniels L, Worthingham C: *Muscle testing*, ed 5, Philadelphia, 1986, WB Saunders.
6. Hislop H, Montgomery J: *Daniels and Worthingham's muscle testing*, ed 6, Philadelphia, 1995, WB Saunders.
7. Killingsworth A: *Basic physical disability procedures*, San Jose, Calif, 1987, Maple Press.
8. Polatajko HJ, Mandich A, Martini R: Dynamic performance analysis: a framework for understanding occupational performance, *Am J Occup Ther* 54(1):65-72.

CHAPTER 21

Joint Range of Motion

LORRAINE WILLIAMS PEDRETTI

KEY TERMS

Range of motion
Active range of motion
Passive range of motion
End-feel
Joint measurement
Axis
Palpation
Goniometer
Two-joint muscle
Stationary bar
Movable bar
Functional range of motion

LEARNING OBJECTIVES

After studying this chapter the student or practitioner will be able to do the following:

1. Define active, passive, and functional ROM.
2. List the purposes of measuring ROM.
3. Name two methods used to screen for ROM limitations.
4. Name disabilities for which joint measurement is often an assessment tool.
5. Describe how ROM measurements are used to select treatment goals and methods.
6. Describe how to establish ROM norms for the patient with unilateral involvement.
7. Describe what the therapist should do before actually measuring the joints with the goniometer.
8. Describe proper positioning of the therapist and how to support limbs.
9. List precautions and contraindications for joint measurement.
10. List and describe the steps in the joint measurement procedure in correct order.
11. Describe how to record results of the joint measurement.
12. Measure all the joints of a normal practice subject, using the 180-degree method and correct procedure.
13. Describe at least three treatment methods that can be used to increase ROM.

Joint **range of motion** (ROM) is the amount of movement that is possible at a joint.[3] It is the arc of motion through which a joint passes. When the joint is moved by the muscles that act on the joint, it called **active range of motion** (AROM). When the joint is moved by an outside force such as the therapist, it is called **passive range of motion (PROM)**.[3] In normal individuals, PROM is slightly greater than AROM because of the slight elasticity of soft tissue.[3,9] If PROM is significantly more than AROM for the same joint motion, it is likely that there is muscle weakness.[12]

Decreased ROM can cause limited function and interfere with the performance of self-care, vocational, leisure, and social activities. The functional motion test

(Chapter 20), screening tests, and measurement of joint ROM with a goniometer can all be used to assess ROM. The primary concern of the occupational therapist is whether ROM is adequate to perform necessary and desired life activities.

Methods used to screen ROM limitations are observation of AROM and PROM. For the former, the therapist asks the patient to perform all the active movements that occur at the joint.[3] For the latter, the therapist moves the joint passively through all of its motions. The purpose of this is to estimate ROM, detect limitations, and observe quality of movement, **end-feel**, and the presence of pain.[3] The therapist can then decide where precise ROM measurement is indicated.

JOINT MEASUREMENT

Joint measurement is an assessment tool often used for physical disabilities that cause limited joint motion. These include skin contracture caused by adhesions or scar tissue; arthritis, fractures, burns, and hand trauma; the displacement of fibrocartilage or the presence of other foreign bodies in the joint; bony obstruction or destruction; and soft tissue contractures, such as tendon, muscle, or ligament shortening. Limited ROM can also be secondary to spasticity, muscle weakness, pain, and edema.[8,12]

ROM measurements help the therapist select treatment goals, appropriate treatment modalities, positioning techniques, and other strategies to reduce limitations. Specific purposes for measuring ROM are to determine limitations that interfere with function or may produce deformity, determine additional range needed to increase functional capacity or reduce deformity, determine the need for splints and assistive devices, measure progress objectively, and record progression or regression.

Normal ROM varies from one person to another. The therapist can establish norms for each individual by measuring the analogous uninvolved part if possible.[3,4] Otherwise, the therapist uses average ranges listed in the literature as a guide.[3] The therapist should check records and interview the patient for the presence of fused joints and other limitations caused by old injuries. Joints should not be forced when resistance is met on passive ROM. Pain may limit ROM, and crepitation may be heard on movement in some conditions.

PRINCIPLES AND PROCEDURES IN JOINT MEASUREMENT

Before measuring ROM, the therapist should be familiar with average normal ROMs, joint structure and function, normal end-feels, recommended positioning for self and patient, and bony landmarks related to each joint and joint **axis**.[3,4,9] The therapist should be skilled in correct positioning and stabilization for measurements, **palpation**, alignment and reading of the **goniometer**, and accurate recording of measurements.[9] For the most reliable measurements, the same therapist should assess and reassess the patient at the same time of day, using the same instrument and the same measurement protocol.[3]

Visual Observation

The joint to be measured should be exposed, and the therapist should observe the joint and adjacent areas.[3] The therapist asks the patient to move the part through the available ROM, if muscle strength is adequate, and observes the movement.[4] The therapist should look for compensatory motions, posture, muscle contours, skin color and condition, and skin creases and compare the joint with the noninjured part, if possible.[3] The therapist should then move the part through its range to see and feel how the joint moves and to estimate ROM.

Palpation

Feeling the bony landmarks and soft tissue around the joint is an essential skill, gained with practice and experience. The pads of the index and middle fingers are used for palpation. The thumb is sometimes used. The therapist's fingernails should not make contact with the patient's skin. Pressure is applied gently but firmly enough to detect underlying muscle, tendons, or bony structures. For joint measurement, the therapist must palpate to locate bony landmarks for placement of the goniometer.[3]

Positioning of Therapist and Support of Limbs

The therapist's position varies, depending on the joints being measured. When fingers or wrist joints are being measured, the therapist may sit next to or opposite the patient. When the larger joints of the upper or lower extremity are being measured, the therapist may stand next to the patient on the side being measured. The patient may be seated or lying down. The therapist needs to employ good body mechanics in posture and in lifting and moving heavy limbs. The therapist should use a broad base of support and stand with the head upright, keeping the back straight. The feet should be shoulder width apart with the knees slightly flexed. The therapist's stance should be in line with the direction of movement. The limb should be supported at the level of its center of gravity, approximately where the upper and middle third of the segment meet. The therapist's hands should be in a relaxed grasp that conforms to the contours of the part. The therapist can provide additional support by resting the part on his or her forearm.[3]

Precautions and Contraindications

In some instances, measuring joint ROM is contraindicated or should be undertaken with extreme caution. It is contraindicated if there is a joint dislocation or unhealed fracture, immediately following surgery of any soft tissue structures surrounding joints, in the presence of myositis ossificans, or if there might be ectopic ossifiction.[3]

Joint measurement must always be done carefully. Extreme caution is needed in the following situations:
1. The patient has joint inflammation.
2. The patient is taking either medication for pain or muscle relaxants.
3. The patient has osteoporosis, hypermobility, or subluxation of a joint.
4. The patient has hemophilia.
5. The patient has a hematoma.
6. The patient has just had an injury to soft tissue.
7. The patient has a newly united fracture.
8. The patient has undergone prolonged immobilization.
9. Bony ankylosis is suspected.[3]

End-Feel

Passive ROM is normally limited by the structure of the joint and surrounding soft tissues. Thus ligaments, the joint capsule, muscle and tendon tension, contact of joint surfaces, and soft tissue approximation may limit the end of a particular ROM. Each of these structures has a different end-feel as the therapist moves the joint passively through the ROM. End-feel is the normal resistance to further joint motion because of stretching of soft tissue, stretching of ligaments and joint capsule, approximation of soft tissue, and bone contacting bone. End-feel is normal when full ROM is achieved and the motion is limited by normal anatomical structures. Abnormal end-feel occurs when the ROM is increased or decreased or when ROM is normal but structures other than normal anatomy stop the ROM.[3] Practice and sensitivity are required for the therapist to detect different end-feels and to distinguish the normal from the abnormal.[3,9]

Normally, end-feel is hard, soft, or firm. An example of hard end-feel is bone contacting bone when the elbow is passively extended and the olecranon process contacts the olecranon fossa. Soft end-feel can be detected on knee flexion when there is soft tissue apposition of the posterior aspects of the thigh and calf. A firm end-feel has a firm or springy sensation that has some give, as when the ankle is dorsiflexed with the knee in extension and the ROM is limited by tension in the gastrocnemius muscle.[3]

In pathological states, end-feel is abnormal when passive ROM is increased or decreased or when PROM is normal but movement is stopped by structures other than normal anatomy.[3] Practice and experience are required to detect end-feel accurately. Normal end-feel for each joint is noted with the directions for joint measurement that are listed in the following sections.

Two-Joint Muscles

When the ROM of a joint that is crossed by a **two-joint muscle** is measured, the ROM of the joint being measured may be affected by the position of the other joint because of passive insufficiency.[3] That is, joint motion is limited by the length of the muscle. A two-joint muscle feels taut when it is at its full length over both joints it crosses and before it reaches the limits of the normal ROM of both joints.[7] For example, when the wrist is in full extension, passive finger extension is normally limited because of the passive insufficiency of the finger flexors that cross the wrist and finger joints. When the joints crossed by two-joint muscles are being measured, it is necessary to place the joint not being measured in a neutral or relaxed position to place the two-joint muscle on slack. For example, when finger extension is being measured, the wrist should be placed in the neutral position to avoid full stretch of the finger flexors over all of the joints they cross. Similarly, when hip flexion is being measured, the knee should also be flexed to place the hamstrings in the slackened position.[3]

METHODS OF JOINT MEASUREMENT
The 180° System

In the 180° system of joint measurement, 0° is the starting position for all joint motions. For most motions the anatomical position is the starting position. The body of the measuring instrument, the goniometer, is a half-circle protractor with an axis and two arms. It is superimposed on the body in the plane in which the motion is to occur. The axis of the instrument is aligned with the axis of the joint. All joint motions begin at 0° and increase toward 180°.[3,5,9] The 180° system is used most often and is the one used later in this chapter to describe procedures for joint measurement.

The 360° System

The 360° system of joint measurement is used less frequently than the 180° system. The goniometer is a full-circle, 360° protractor with two arms. Movements occurring in the coronal and sagittal planes are related to the full circle. When the body is in the anatomical position, the circle is superimposed on it in the same plane in which the motion is to occur, with the joint axis as the pivotal point. "The 0° (360°) position will be overhead and the 180° position will be toward the feet."[5] Thus, for example, shoulder flexion and abduction are movements that proceed toward 0°, and shoulder adduction and extension proceed toward 360°. The average normal ROM for shoulder flexion is 170°. Therefore, in the 360° system, the movement would start at 180° and progress toward 0° to 10°. The ROM recorded would be 10°. On the other hand, shoulder extension that has a normal ROM of 60° would begin at 180° and progress toward 360° to 240°, and 240° would be the ROM recorded.[5] The total ROM of extension to flexion would be 240° to 10°—that is, 230°.[5,6]

Some motions cannot be related to the full circle. In these instances, a 0° starting position is designated, and the movements are measured as increases from 0°. These motions occur in a horizontal plane around a vertical axis. They are forearm pronation and supination, hip internal and external rotation, wrist radial and ulnar deviation, and thumb palmar and radial abduction (carpometacarpal flexion and extension).[5]

GONIOMETERS

Goniometers are usually made of metal or plastic, come in several sizes and types, and are available from medical and rehabilitation equipment companies.[5,9,11] The word **goniometer** is derived from the Greek *gonia*, which means angle, and *metron*, which means measure.[9,13] Thus, *goniometer* literally means "to measure angles."

The universal goniometer (Fig. 21-1) consists of a body, a **stationary (proximal) bar**, and a movable (distal) bar.[3,9] The stationary bar is attached to the body of the goniometer. The body is a half-circle or a full-circle protractor printed with a scale of degrees from 0° to 180° for the half-circle and 0° to 360° for the full-circle goniometer.[3,4] The **movable bar** is attached at the center, or axis, of the protractor and acts as a dial. As the movable bar rotates around the protractor, the dial points to the number of degrees on the scale.

Two scales of figures are printed on the half circle. Each starts at 0° and progresses toward 180°, but in opposite directions. Because the starting position in the 180° system is always 0° and increases toward 180°, the outer row of figures is read if the bony segments being measured are end to end, as in elbow flexion. The inner row of figures is read if the bony segments being measured are alongside one another, as in shoulder flexion.

Fig. 21-1 shows five styles of goniometers. The first (Fig. 21-1, *A*) is a full-circle goniometer that has calibrations for both the 360° and the 180° systems printed on its face. This goniometer has longer arms and is convenient for use on the large joints of the body. Fig. 21-1, *B*, shows a half-circle instrument used for the 180° system. This goniometer is radiopaque and could be used during radiographic examinations if necessary. Its dial is notched at two places for accurate motion reading, regardless of whether the convexity of the half circle is directed toward or away from the direction of motion. Thus the evaluator does not have to reverse the goniometer, obscuring the scale. A special finger goniometer is shown in Fig. 21-1, *D*. Its arms are short and flattened. It is designed to be used over the finger joint surfaces rather than on their lateral aspects, as is done in most of the larger joint motions. Small plastic goniometers are shown in Fig. 21-1, *C* and *E*. These are inexpensive and easy to carry. The longer one can be used with both large and small joints. The smaller is simply a larger one that has been cut for use as a finger goniometer. The dials of transparent goniometers are marked or notched in two places.

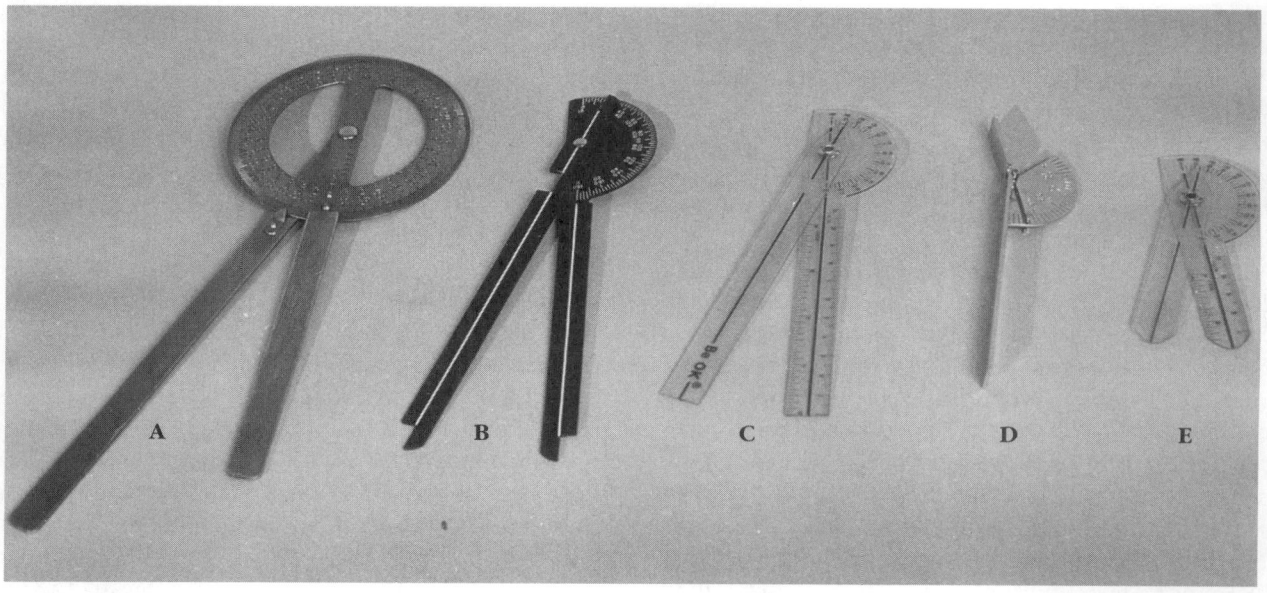

FIG. 21-1
Types of goniometers.

One important feature of the goniometer is the fulcrum. The nut or rivet that acts as the fulcrum must move freely, yet must be tight enough to remain where it was set when the goniometer is removed following joint measurement.[4] For easy, accurate readings, some goniometers have a locking nut that is tightened just before the goniometer is removed.[5]

Other types of goniometers are available. Some have a fluid indicator that provides the reading after the motion is completed.[5] Others can be attached to a body segment and have dials that register ROM. There are special goniometers for cervical and spine ROM measurements and for forearm rotation.[11] A tape measure or metric scale may also be used on some joints by measuring the distance between two segments—for example, the distance between the chin and chest when measuring cervical flexion and extension, the distance between the center of the tips of two fingers for finger abduction, and the distance between the thumb tip and little finger tip for opposition.[3]

RECORDING MEASUREMENTS

When using the 180° system, the evaluator should record the number of degrees at the starting position and the number of degrees at the final position after the joint has passed through the maximum possible arc of motion.[9] Normal ROM always starts at 0° and increases toward 180°. When it is not possible to start the motion at 0° because of a limitation of motion, the ROM is recorded by writing the number of degrees at the starting position followed by the number of degrees at the final position.[3] For example, elbow ROM limitations can be noted as follows:

Normal: 0° to 140°

Extension limitation: 15° to 140°

Flexion limitation: 0° to 110°

Flexion and extension limitation: 15° to 110°

Abnormal hyperextension of the elbow may be recorded by indicating the number of degrees of hyperextension below the 0° starting position with a minus sign, followed by the 0° position and then the number of degrees at the final position.[9] For example:

Normal: 0° to 140°

Abnormal hyperextension: −20° to 0° to 140°

There are alternative methods of recording ROM. The evaluator is advised to learn and adopt the particular method required by the health care facility.

A sample form for recording ROM measurements is shown in Fig. 21-2. Average normal ROM for each joint motion is listed on the form and in Table 21-1. When measurements are being recorded, every space on the form should be filled in. If the joint was not tested, "NT" should be entered in the space.[3]

It should be noted that scapula movement accompanies movements of the shoulder (glenohumeral) joint as outlined. Range of glenohumeral joint motion is highly dependent on scapula mobility, which gives the shoulder its flexibility and wide ranges of motion. Although it is not possible to measure scapula movement with the goniometer, the evaluator should assess scapula mobility by observation of active motion or by passive movement before proceeding with shoulder joint measurements. Scapular ROM is noted as "full" or "restricted."[3] If scapula motion is restricted, as when musculature is in a state of spasticity or contracture, and the shoulder joint is moved into extreme ranges of motion (for example, above 90 degrees of flexion or abduction), glenohumeral joint damage can result.

When joint measurements may be performed in more than one position (e.g., as in shoulder internal and external rotation), the evaluator (E) should note on the record in which position the measurement was taken. The "E" should also note any pain or discomfort experienced by the subject (S), the appearance of protective muscle spasm, whether active or passive ROM was measured, and any deviations from recommended testing procedures or positions.[9]

RESULTS OF ASSESSMENT AS BASIS FOR TREATMENT PLANNING

After joint measurement, the therapist should analyze the results in relation to the patient's life role requirements. The therapist's first concern should be to correct ROM that is below functional limits. Many ordinary ADL do not require full ROM. **Functional ROM** refers to the amount of joint range necessary to perform essential ADL without the use of special equipment. The first concern of treatment is trying to increase any ROM that is limiting performance of self-care and home-maintenance tasks to functional levels.[8] For example, a severe limitation of elbow flexion affects eating and oral hygiene. Therefore it is important to increase elbow flexion to nearly full ROM for function. Likewise, a severe limitation of forearm pronation affects eating, washing the body, telephoning, child care, and dressing. Because sitting comfortably requires hip ROM of at least 0° to 100°, a first goal might be to increase flexion to 100° if it is limited. Of course, if additional ROM can be gained, the therapist should plan the progression of treatment to increase the ROM to the normal range.

Some ROM limitations may be permanent. The role of the therapist in such cases is to work out methods to compensate for the loss of ROM. Possibilities include assistive devices such as a long-handled comb, brush, or shoe horn, a device to apply stockings, or adapted methods of performing a particular skill. See Chapter 13 for further suggestions of ADL techniques for those with limited ROM.

In many diagnoses, such as burns and arthritis, the loss of ROM can be anticipated. The goal of treatment is

JOINT RANGE MEASUREMENTS

Patient's name _____ Chart no. _____

Date of birth _____ Age _____ Sex _____

Diagnosis _____ Date of onset _____

Disability _____

LEFT						RIGHT		
3	2	1	SPINE			1	2	3
			Cervical spine					
			Flexion	0-45				
			Extension	0-45				
			Lateral flexion	0-45				
			Rotation	0-60				
			Thoracic and lumbar spine					
			Flexion	0-80				
			Extension	0-30				
			Lateral flexion	0-40				
			Rotation	0-45				
			SHOULDER					
			Flexion	0 to 170				
			Extension	0 to 60				
			Abduction	0 to 170				
			Horizontal abduction	0-40				
			Horizontal adduction	0-130				
			Internal rotation	0 to 70				
			External rotation	0 to 90				
			ELBOW AND FOREARM					
			Flexion	0 to 135-150				
			Supination	0 to 80-90				
			Pronation	0 to 80-90				
			WRIST					
			Flexion	0 to 80				
			Extension	0 to 70				
			Ulnar deviation	0 to 30				
			Radial deviation	0 to 20				
			THUMB					
			MP flexion	0 to 50				
			IP flexion	0 to 80-90				
			Abduction	0 to 50				
			FINGERS					
			MP flexion	0 to 90				
			MP hyperextension	0 to 15-45				
			PIP flexion	0 to 110				
			DIP flexion	0 to 80				
			Abduction	0 to 25				
			HIP					
			Flexion	0 to 120				
			Extension	0 to 30				
			Abduction	0 to 40				
			Adduction	0 to 35				
			Internal rotation	0 to 45				
			External rotation	0 to 45				
			KNEE					
			Flexion	0 to 135				
			ANKLE AND FOOT					
			Plantar flexion	0 to 50				
			Dorsiflexion	0 to 15				
			Inversion	0 to 35				
			Eversion	0 to 20				

FIG. 21-2
Form for recording joint ROM measurement.

to prevent joint limitation with splints, positioning, exercise, activity, and application of the principles of joint protection.

Limited ROM, its causes, and the prognosis for increasing ROM will suggest treatment approaches. Some of the specific methods used to increase ROM are discussed elsewhere in this text (see Chapters 30 and 31). These include stretching exercise, resistive activity and exercise, strengthening of antagonistic muscle groups, activities that require active motion of the affected joints through the full available ROM, splints, and positioning. To increase ROM, the physician may perform surgery or may manipulate the part while the patient is under anesthesia. The physical therapist may use joint mobilization techniques such as manual stretching with heat and massage.[8]

PROCEDURE FOR MEASURING PASSIVE ROM

Average normal ROM for each joint motion is listed in Table 21-1, in Fig. 21-2, and before each of the following procedures for measurement. The reader should keep in mind that these are averages and ROM may vary considerably from one individual to another. Normal ROM is affected by age, gender, and other factors such as lifestyle and occupation.[9] Therefore the subject (S) in the illustrations may not always demonstrate the average ROM listed for the particular motion.

In the illustrations, the goniometer is shown in such a way that the reader can most easily see its positioning. However, the evaluator (E) may not always be in the best position for the particular measurement. For the purposes of clear illustration, E is necessarily shown off to one side and may have one hand, rather than two, on the instrument. Many of the motions require that E actually be in front of S or that E's hands obscure the goniometer. How E holds the goniometer and supports the part being measured is determined by factors such as the position of S, amount of muscle weakness, presence or absence of joint pain, and whether active or passive ROM is being measured. Both E and S should be positioned for the greatest comfort, correct placement of the instrument, and adequate stabilization of the part being tested to effect the desired motion in the correct plane.

General Procedure—180° Method of Measurement[3,9]

1. S should be comfortable and relaxed in the appropriate position (described below) for the joint measurement.
2. Uncover the joint to be measured.
3. Explain and demonstrate to S what you are going to do, why, and how you expect him or her to cooperate.
4. If there is unilateral involvement, assess the PROM on the analogous limb to establish normal ROM for S.

5. Establish and palpate bony landmarks for the measurement.
6. Stabilize joints proximal to the joint being measured.
7. Move the part passively through ROM to feel joint mobility and end-feel.
8. Return the part to the starting position.
9. To measure the starting position, place the goniometer just over the surface of and lateral to the joint. Place the axis of the goniometer over the axis of the joint, using the designated bony prominence or anatomical landmark. Place the stationary bar on or parallel to the longitudinal axis of the proximal or stationary bone and the movable bar on or parallel to the longitudinal axis of the distal or moving bone. To prevent the indicator on the movable bar from going off the protractor dial, always face the curved side away from the direction of motion, unless the goniometer can be read after movement in either direction.
10. Record the number of degrees at the starting position and remove the goniometer. Do not attempt to hold the goniometer in place while moving the joint through ROM.
11. To measure PROM, hold the part securely above and below the joint being measured and gently move the joint through ROM. Do not force the joints. Watch for signs of pain and discomfort. (Note: PROM may also be measured by asking S to move actively through ROM and hold the position. Then E moves the joint through the final few degrees of PROM).
12. Reposition the goniometer and record the number of degrees at the final position.
13. Remove the goniometer and gently place the part in resting position.
14. Record the reading at final position and any notations on the evaluation form.

DIRECTIONS FOR JOINT MEASUREMENT—180° SYSTEM

SPINE
Cervical Spine

Measurements of neck movements are the least accurate, because there are few bony landmarks and much soft tissue overlying bony segments.[4] A radiographic examination is the best means to make an accurate measurement of the specific joints.[10] Measurements may be taken with a tape measure to record the distance between the chin and chest for flexion and extension, chin and shoulder for neck rotation, and mastoid process and shoulder for lateral flexion.[3]

Approximate estimates of cervical flexion, extension, rotation, and lateral flexion may be made by using the

TABLE 21-1
Average Normal Range of Motion (180° Method)

Joint	ROM	Associated Girdle Motion	Joint	ROM
Cervical Spine			**Wrist**	
Flexion	0° to 45°		Flexion	0° to 80°
Extension	0° to 45°		Extension	0° to 70°
Lateral flexion	0° to 45°		Ulnar deviation (adduction)	0° to 30°
Rotation	0° to 60°		Radial deviation (abduction)	0° to 20°
Thoracic and Lumbar Spine			**Thumb**	
Flexion	0° to 80°		DIP Flexion	0° to 80°-90°
Extension	0° to 30°		MP flexion	0° to 50°
Lateral flexion	0° to 40°		Adduction, radial and palmar	0°
Rotation	0° to 45°		Palmar abduction	0° to 50°
			Radial abduction	0° to 50°
			Opposition	Thumb pad to touch pad of little finger
Shoulder			**Fingers**	
Flexion	0° to 170°	Abduction, lateral tilt, slight elevation, slight upward rotation	MP flexion	0° to 90°
Extension	0° to 60°	Depression, adduction, upward tilt	MP hyperextension	0° to 15°-45°
Abduction	0° to 170°	Upward rotation, elevation	PIP flexion	0° to 110°
Adduction	0°	Depression, adduction, downward rotation	DIP flexion	0° to 80°
Horizontal abduction	0° to 40°	Adduction, reduction of lateral tilt	Abduction	0° to 25°
Horizontal adduction	0° to 130°	Abduction, lateral tilt	**Hip**	
Internal rotation		Abduction, lateral tilt	Flexion	0° to 120° (bent knee)
Arm in abduction	0° to 70°		Extension	0° to 30°
Arm in adduction	0° to 60°		Abduction	0° to 40°
External rotation		Adduction, reduction of lateral tilt	Adduction	0° to 35°
Arm in abduction	0° to 90°		Internal rotation	0° to 45°
Arm in adduction	0° to 80°		External rotation	0° to 45°
Elbow			**Knee**	
Flexion	0° to 135°-140°		Flexion	0° to 135°
Extension	0°			
			Ankle and Foot	
Forearm			Plantar flexion	0° to 50°
Pronation	0° to 80°-90°		Dorsiflexion	0° to 15°
Supination	0° to 80°-90°		Inversion	0° to 35°
			Eversion	0° to 20°

Data adapted from American Academy of Orthopaedic Surgeons: *Joint motion: method of measuring and recording,* Chicago, 1965, The Academy; Esch D, Lepley M: *Evaluation of joint motion: methods of measurement and recording,* Minneapolis, 1974, University of Minnesota Press.
DIP, Distal interphalangeal; *MP,* metacarpophalangeal; *PIP,* proximal interphalangeal.

goniometer or by estimating the number of degrees of motion, using a fixed axis and estimating the arc of motion from that point (see Figs. 21-3 to 21-10).[1,4]

Cervical Flexion
0° to 45° (Fig. 21-3).

POSITION OF THE SUBJECT. Sitting or standing erect.

MEASUREMENT. S is asked to flex the neck so that the chin moves toward the chest. The number of degrees of motion may be estimated, or E may measure the number of inches or centimeters from the chin to the sternal notch.[1,3,9] If a goniometer is used, the axis is placed over the angle of the jaw. E grasps the corner of the protractor, which is positioned with the arc upward, and steadies his or her arm by resting it against S's shoulder. The arms of the goniometer are aligned with a tongue depressor, which S is holding between the teeth. As S performs neck flexion, the movable bar of the goniometer is adjusted downward to align with the new position of the tongue depressor.[4,9]

Cervical Extension
0° to 45° (Fig. 21-4).

POSITION OF THE SUBJECT. Sitting or standing erect.

MEASUREMENT. S is asked to extend the neck as if to look at the ceiling, so that the back of the head approaches the thoracic spine. The number of degrees of

motion may be estimated or the number of inches or centimeters from the chin to the sternal notch may be measured.[3] If a goniometer is used, the axis is placed over the angle of the jaw. E grasps the corner of the protractor, which is now positioned with the arc downward, and steadies his or her arm against S's shoulder. The movable bar of the goniometer is moved upward to align with the tongue depressor as the S extends the neck.[4,9]

Lateral Flexion
0° to 45° (Fig. 21-5).

POSITION OF THE SUBJECT. Sitting or standing erect.

MEASUREMENT. S is asked to flex the neck laterally without rotation, moving the ear toward the shoulder. The number of degrees of motion may be estimated, or E may measure the number of inches or centimeters between the mastoid process and the acromion process of the shoulder.[1,3] If a goniometer is used, the axis is placed over the spinous process of the seventh cervical vertebra. The stationary bar may be over the shoulder and parallel to the floor so that the motion begins at 90°, or it may be aligned with the thoracic vertebra for a starting position of 0°. The movable bar is aligned with the external occipital protuberance.[1,9]

Cervical Rotation
0° to 60° (Fig. 21-6).

POSITION OF THE SUBJECT. Lying supine or seated.

MEASUREMENT. S is asked to rotate the head to right or left without rotating the trunk. The amount of rotation may be estimated in degrees from the neutral position,[1] or a tape measure may be used to measure the distance from the tip of the chin to the acromion process of the shoulder. The measure is taken first in the anatomical position and then again after the neck has been rotated.[3] In the lying position, if a goniometer is used, it is set at 90° and the axis is placed over the vertex of the head. The stationary bar is held steady, parallel to the floor or to the acromion process on the side being tested. The movable bar is aligned with the tip of the nose.[4,9]

Thoracic and Lumbar Spine
Flexion
0° to 80° and + 4 inches (Fig. 21-7).

POSITION OF THE SUBJECT. Standing erect.

MEASUREMENT. Four methods of estimating the range of spinal flexion are as follows: measuring trunk forward flexion in relation to the longitudinal axis of the

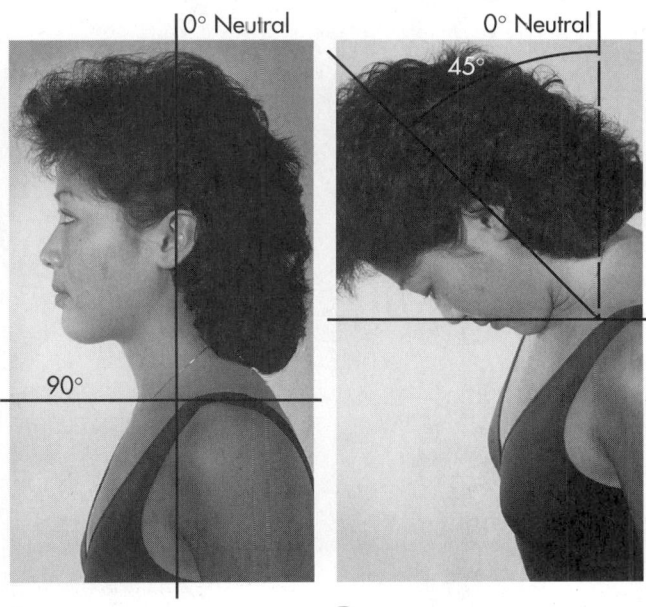

FIG. 21-3
Cervical flexion. **A,** Starting position. **B,** Final position.

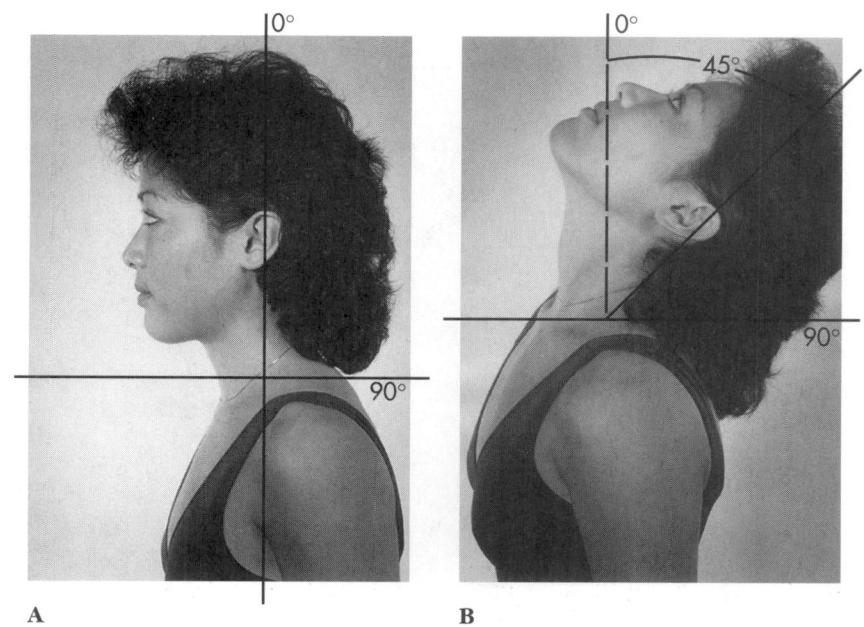

FIG. 21-4
Cervical extension. **A,** Starting position. **B,** Final position.

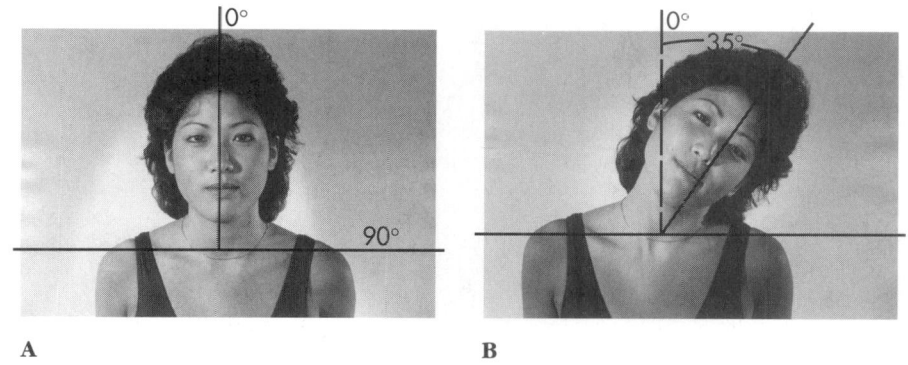

FIG. 21-5
Cervical lateral flexion. **A,** Starting position. **B,** Final position.

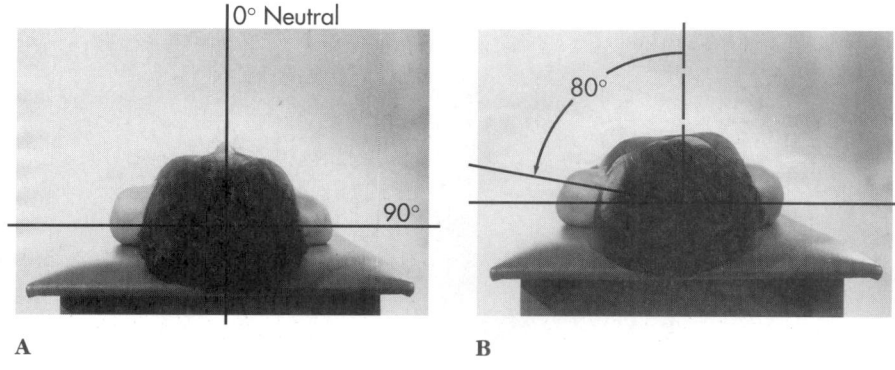

FIG. 21-6
Cervical rotation. **A,** Starting position. **B,** Final position.

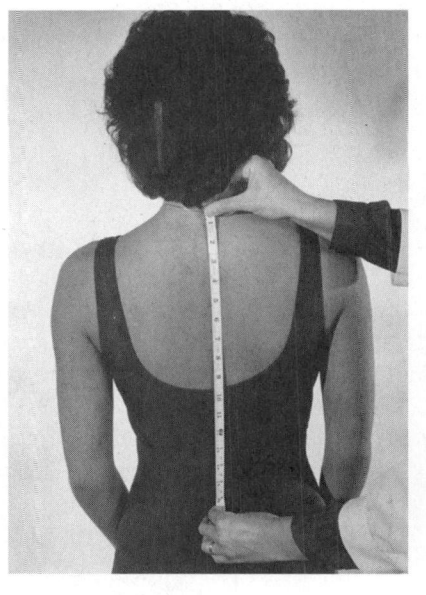

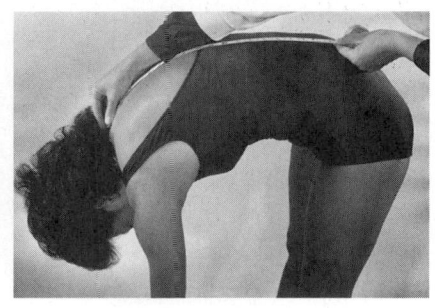

A   **B**

FIG. 21-7
Spine flexion. **A,** Starting position. **B,** Final position.

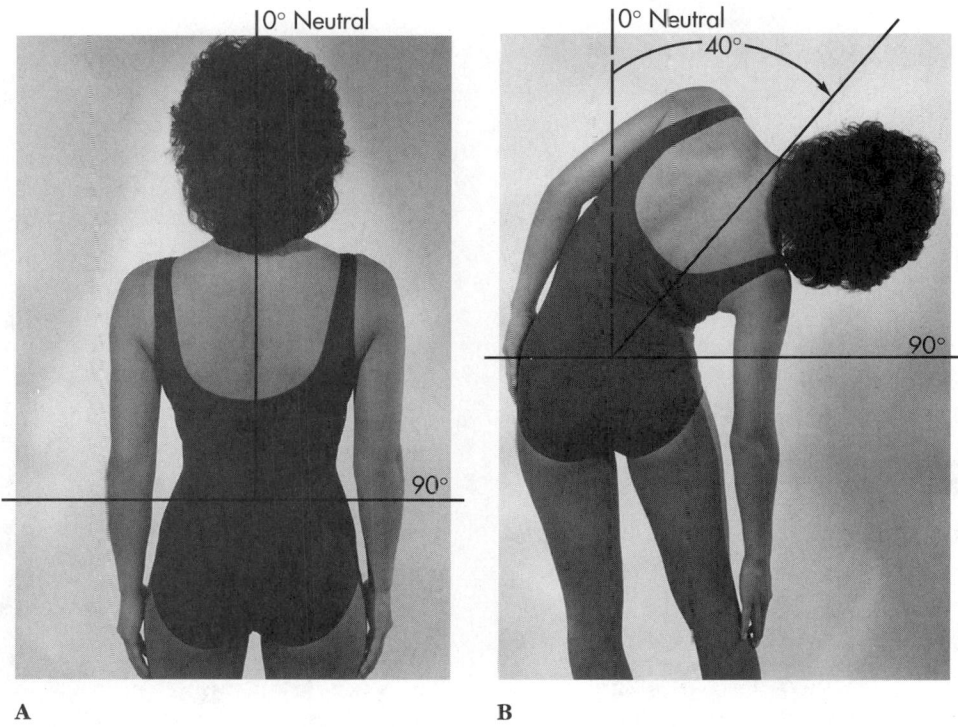

A   **B**

FIG. 21-8
Spine lateral flexion. **A,** Starting position. **B,** Final position.

body (E must hold the pelvis stable with the hands and observe any change in S's normal lordosis); recording the level of the fingertips along the front of S's leg; measuring the number of inches or centimeters between S's fingertips and the floor; and measuring the length of the spine from the seventh cervical vertebra to the first sacral verte-

bra when S is erect and again after S has flexed the spine (Fig. 21-7).[3,9] The fourth is probably the most accurate of these clinical methods.[1] In a normal adult, average increase in length in forward flexion of the spine is 4 inches (10 cm).[3] If S bends forward at the hips with a straight back, no difference in length will occur.

Lateral Flexion

0° to 40° (Fig. 21-8).

POSITION OF THE SUBJECT. Standing erect.

MEASUREMENT. Several methods may be used to estimate the range of lateral flexion of the trunk. The steel tape measure may be held in place during the motion and used to estimate the number of degrees of lateral inclination of the trunk compared with the vertical position. Other methods include estimating the position of the spinous process of C7 in relation to the pelvis (Fig. 21-8); measuring the distance of the fingertips from the knee joint in lateral flexion; measuring the distance between the tip of the third finger and the floor[3]; and using a long-arm goniometer, placing the axis on S1, the stationary bar perpendicular to the floor, and the movable bar aligned with C7.[1,9]

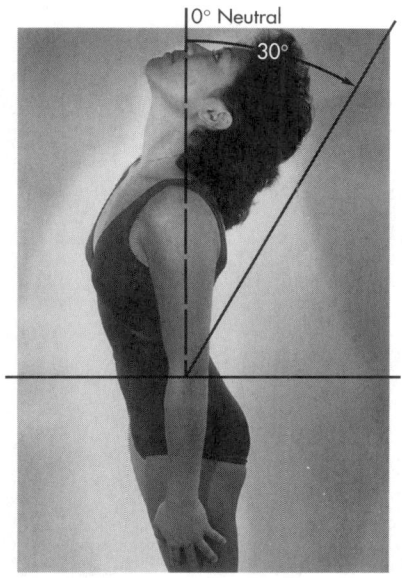

FIG. 21-9
Spine extension.

Extension

0° to 30° (Fig. 21-9).

POSITION OF THE SUBJECT. Standing erect or lying prone.

MEASUREMENT. S is asked to bend backward while maintaining stability of the pelvis. If necessary, E stabilizes the pelvis from the anterior when the measurement is taken in the standing position. The range of extension is estimated in degrees from the vertical, using the superior iliac crest as the pivotal point in relation to the spinous process of C7. With S in the lying position, a pillow is placed under the abdomen and S's hands are placed at shoulder level on the treatment table. The pelvis is stabilized with a strap or by an assistant, and S extends the elbows to raise the trunk from the table. A perpendicular measurement is taken of the distance between the suprasternal notch and the supporting surface at the end of the ROM.[3]

Rotation

0° to 45° (Fig. 21-10).

POSITION OF THE SUBJECT. Lying supine or standing.

MEASUREMENT. S is asked to rotate the upper trunk while maintaining neutral position of the pelvis. E may fix the pelvis firmly to maintain the neutral position. This step is especially important if S is in the standing position. This motion is recorded in degrees, using the center of the crown of the head as a pivotal point and the arc of motion made by the shoulder as it moves upward or forward.

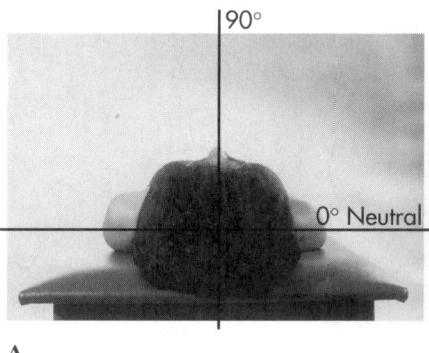
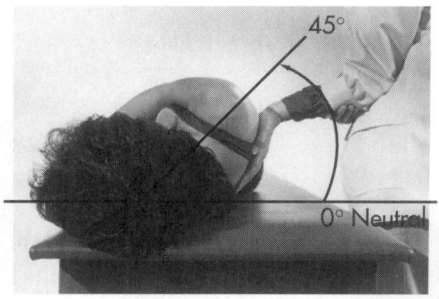

FIG. 21-10
Spine rotation. **A,** Starting position. **B,** Final position.

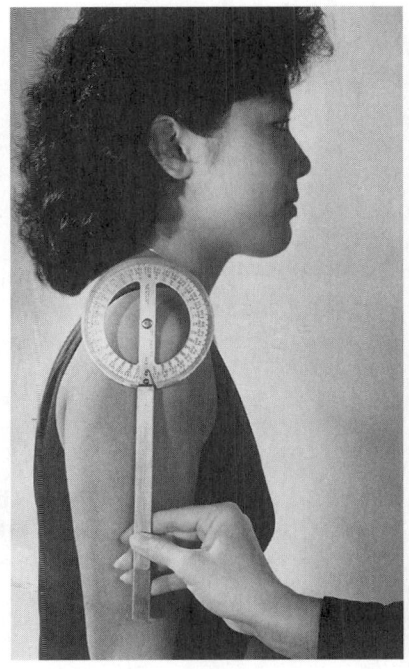 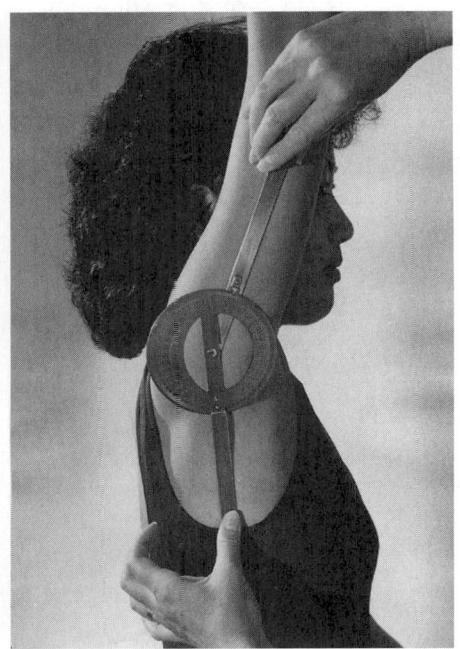

A   **B**

FIG. 21-11
Shoulder flexion. **A,** Starting position. **B,** Final position.

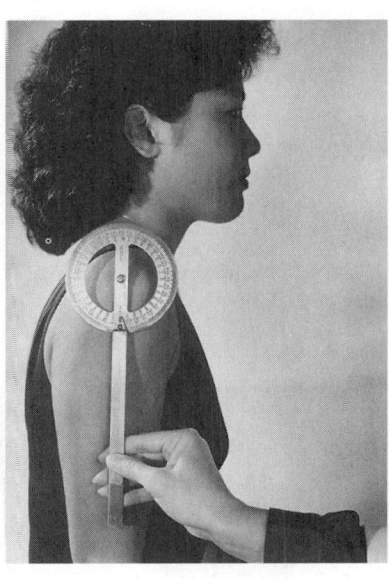 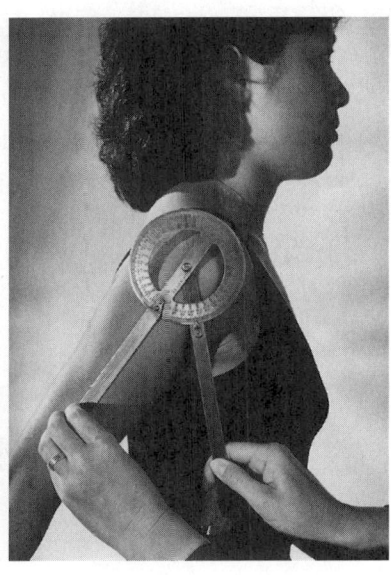

A   **B**

FIG. 21-12
Shoulder extension. **A,** Starting position. **B,** Final position.

UPPER EXTREMITY[1-3,5,9,10]
Shoulder

Flexion
0° to 170° (Fig. 21-11).

POSITION OF THE SUBJECT. Seated or supine with the humerus in neutral rotation.

POSITION OF GONIOMETER. The axis is in the center of the humeral head, just distal to the acromion process on the lateral aspect of the humerus. The stationary bar is parallel to the trunk, and the movable bar is parallel to the humerus. Note that when the shoulder is flexed, the axis point moves upward and backward to the posterior surface of the shoulder. Thus, to take the measurement of the final position, E should place the goniometer on the lateral surface of the shoulder, aligned with the imaginary axis through the center of the humeral head, which is just slightly superior to the crease formed by the deltoid mass.

END-FEEL. Firm.[3]

Extension
0° to 60° (Fig. 21-12).

POSITION OF THE SUBJECT. Seated or prone, with no obstruction behind the humerus and the humerus in neutral rotation.

POSITION OF GONIOMETER. Same as for flexion, but the axis point remains the same for starting and final positions. Movement should be accompanied by a slight upward tilt of the scapula. Excessive scapular motion should be avoided.

END-FEEL. Firm.[3]

Abduction
0° to 170° (Fig 21-13).

POSITION OF THE SUBJECT. Seated or lying prone, with the humerus in adduction and external rotation. Measure on the posterior surface.

POSITION OF GONIOMETER. The axis is on the acromion process on the posterior surface of the shoulder. The stationary bar is parallel to the trunk, and the movable bar is parallel to the humerus.

END-FEEL. Firm.[3]

Internal Rotation
0° to 60° (Fig. 21-14).

POSITION OF THE SUBJECT (USED IF ABDUCTION CANNOT BE ACHIEVED). Seated with humerus adducted against trunk, elbow at 90° and forearm at midposition and perpendicular to body.[3]

POSITION OF GONIOMETER. The axis is on the olecranon process of the elbow, and the stationary bar and movable bar are parallel to the forearm.

Internal Rotation (Alternative Position)
0° to 70° (Fig. 21-15).

POSITION OF THE SUBJECT (USED IF THERE IS NO DANGER OF POSTERIOR DISLOCATION AND ABDUCTION IS POSSIBLE). Prone or supine with the humerus abducted to 90°, the elbow flexed to 90°, and the forearm in pronation, perpendicular to the floor.

POSITION OF GONIOMETER. The axis is on the olecranon process of the elbow, and the stationary bar and movable bar are parallel to the forearm.

END-FEEL. Firm.[3]

External Rotation
0° to 80° (Fig. 21-16).

POSITION OF THE SUBJECT (USED IF ABDUCTION IS NOT POSSIBLE). Seated, the humerus adducted, the elbow at 90°, and the forearm in midposition, perpendicular to the body.

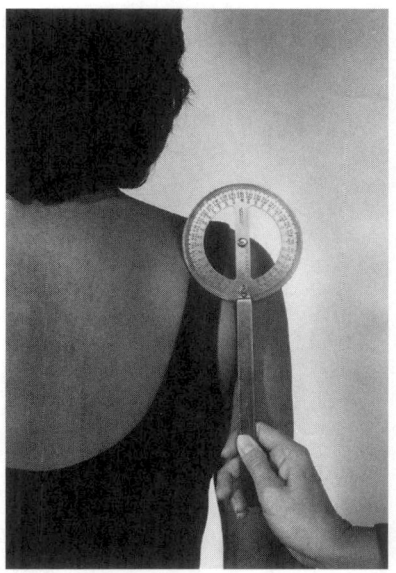
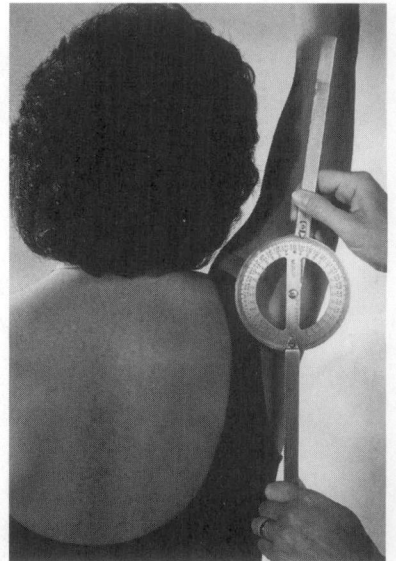

FIG. 21-13
Shoulder abduction. **A,** Starting position. **B,** Final position.

A

B

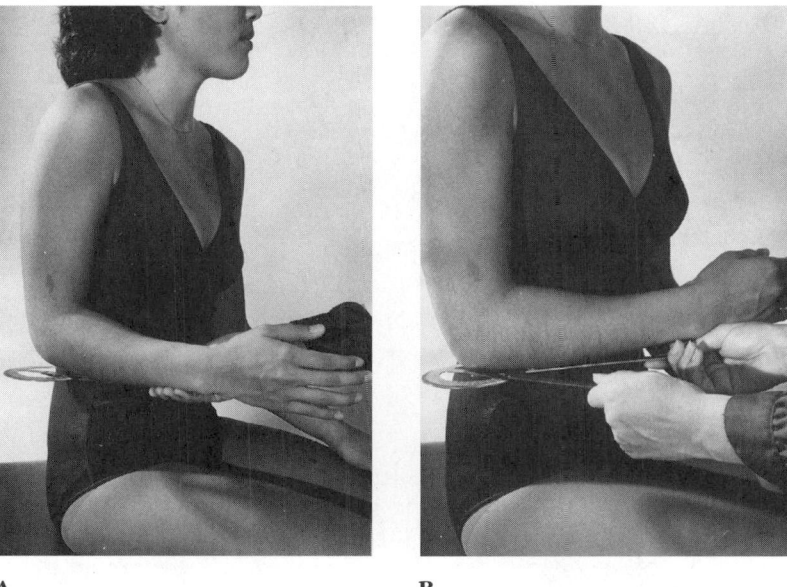

FIG. 21-14
Shoulder internal rotation, shoulder adducted. **A,** Starting position. **B,** Final position.

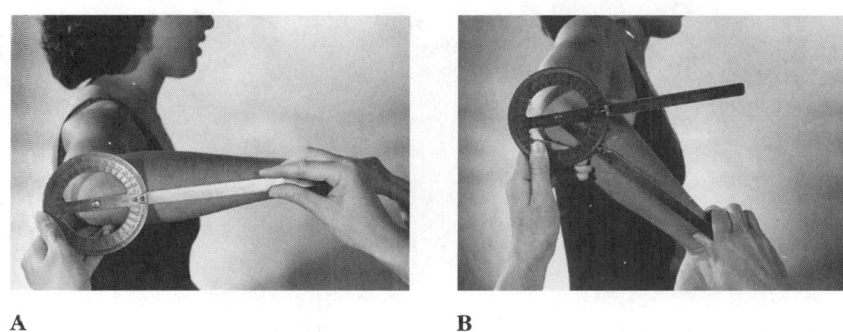

FIG. 21-15
Shoulder internal rotation, shoulder abducted (alternative position). **A,** Starting position. **B,** Final position.

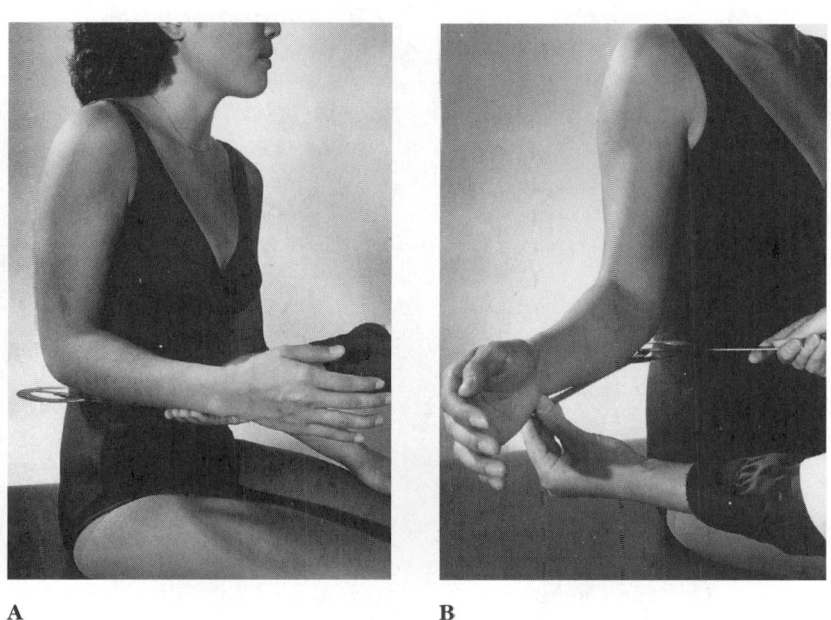

FIG. 21-16
Shoulder external rotation, shoulder adducted. **A,** Starting position. **B,** Final position.

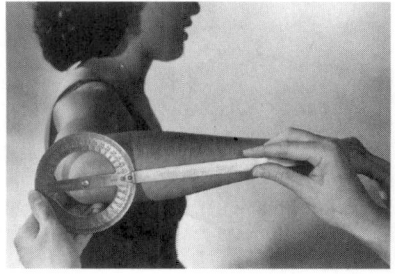 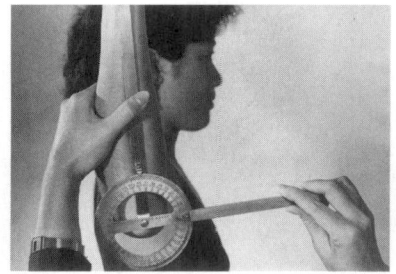

A   B

FIG. 21-17
Shoulder external rotation, shoulder abducted (alternative position). **A,** Starting position. **B,** Final position.

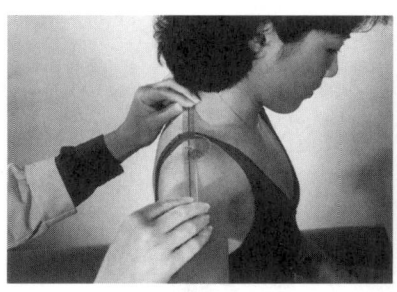 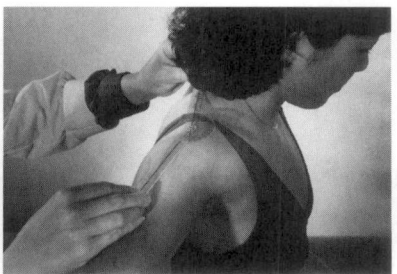

A   B

FIG. 21-18
Shoulder horizontal abduction. **A,** Starting position. **B,** Final position.

POSITION OF GONIOMETER. The axis is on the olecranon of the elbow. The stationary bar and movable bar are parallel to the forearm.[3]

External Rotation (Alternative Position)
0° to 90° (Fig. 21-17).

POSITION OF SUBJECT (USED IF THERE IS NO DANGER OF ANTERIOR DISLOCATION OF THE HUMERUS).[3] Seated or supine with the humerus abducted to 90°, the elbow flexed to 90°, and the forearm pronated.

POSITION OF GONIOMETER. The axis is on the olecranon process of the elbow, and the stationary bar and movable bar are parallel to forearm.

END-FEEL. Firm.[3]

Horizontal Abduction
0° to 40° (Fig. 21-18).

POSITION OF SUBJECT. Seated erect with the shoulder to be tested abducted to 90°, the elbow extended, and the palm facing down. The therapist may support the arm in abduction.[3]

POSITION OF GONIOMETER. The axis is over the acromion process. The stationary bar is parallel over the shoulder toward the neck, and the movable bar is parallel to the humerus on the superior aspect.

END-FEEL. Firm.[3]

Horizontal Adduction
0° to 130° (Fig. 21-19).

POSITION OF SUBJECT AND GONIOMETER. Same as for horizontal abduction.

END-FEEL. Firm or soft.[3]

Elbow

Extension to Flexion
0° to 135°–150° (Fig. 21-20).

POSITION OF SUBJECT. Standing, sitting, or supine with the humerus adducted and externally rotated and the forearm supinated.

POSITION OF GONIOMETER. The axis is placed over the lateral epicondyle of the humerus at the end of the elbow crease. The stationary bar is parallel to the midline of the humerus, and the movable bar is parallel to the radius. After the movement has been completed, the position of the elbow crease changes in relation to

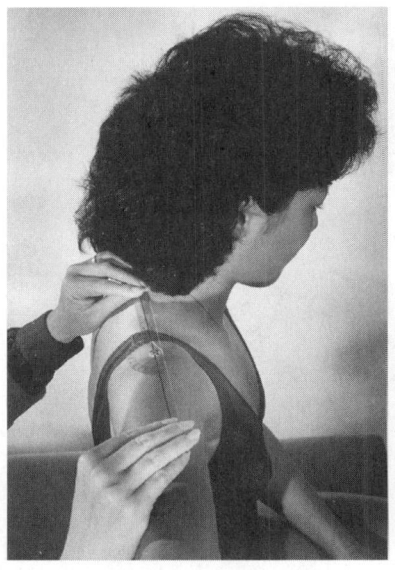 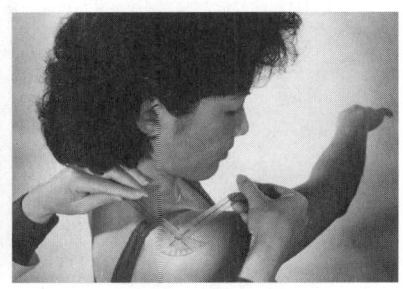

A   B

FIG. 21-19
Shoulder horizontal adduction. **A,** Starting position. **B,** Final position.

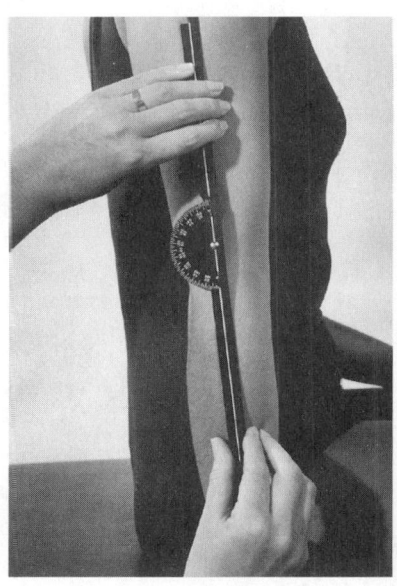 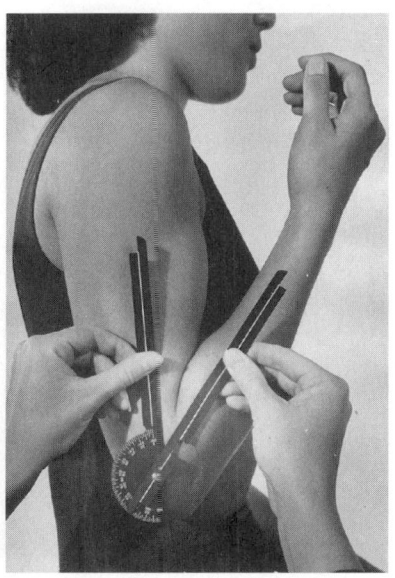

A   B

FIG. 21-20
Elbow flexion. **A,** Starting position. **B,** Final position.

the lateral epicondyle because of the rise of the muscle bulk during the motion. The axis of the goniometer should be repositioned so that it is over, although it will not be directly on, the lateral epicondyle.

END-FEEL. Soft, hard, and firm: flexion. Hard or firm: extension and hyperextension.[3]

Forearm

Supination

0° to 80° or 90° (Fig. 21-21).

POSITION OF THE SUBJECT. Seated or standing with the humerus adducted, the elbow at 90°, and the forearm in midposition.

POSITION OF GONIOMETER. The axis is at the ulnar border of the volar aspect of the wrist, just proximal to the ulna styloid. The movable bar is resting against the volar aspect of the wrist, and the stationary bar is perpendicular to the floor. After the forearm is supinated, the goniometer should be repositioned so that the movable bar rests squarely across the center of the distal forearm.

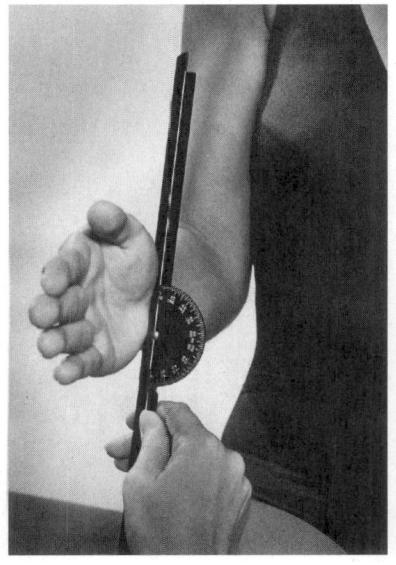
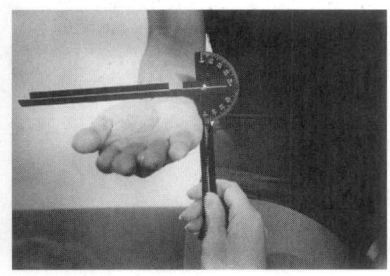

A   B

FIG. 21-21
Forearm supination. **A,** Starting position. **B,** Final position.

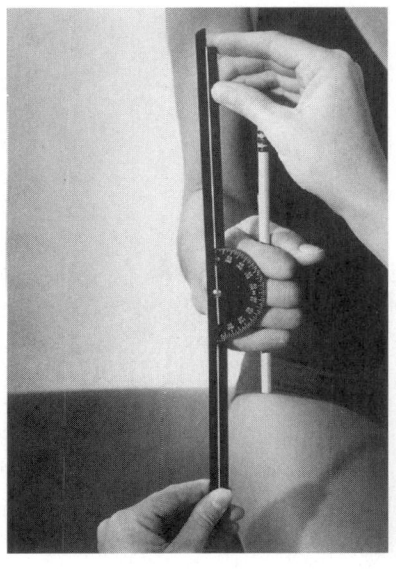
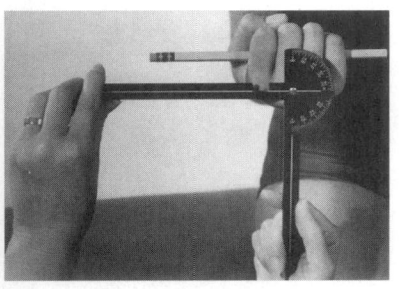

A   B

FIG. 21-22
Forearm supination (alternate method). **A,** Starting position. **B,** Final position.

Supination (Alternative Method)
0° to 80° or 90° (Fig. 21-22).

POSITION OF THE SUBJECT. Seated or standing with the humerus adducted, the elbow at 90°, and the forearm in midposition. Place a pencil in S's hand so it is held perpendicular to the floor.

POSITION OF GONIOMETER. The axis is over the head of the third metacarpal, and the stationary bar is perpendicular to the floor. The movable bar is parallel to the pencil.

END-FEEL. Firm.[3]

Pronation
0° to 80° or 90° (Fig. 21-23).

POSITION OF THE SUBJECT. Seated or standing with the humerus adducted, the elbow at 90°, and the forearm in midposition.

POSITION OF GONIOMETER. The axis is at the ulnar border of the dorsal aspect of the wrist, just proximal to the ulna styloid. The movable bar is resting

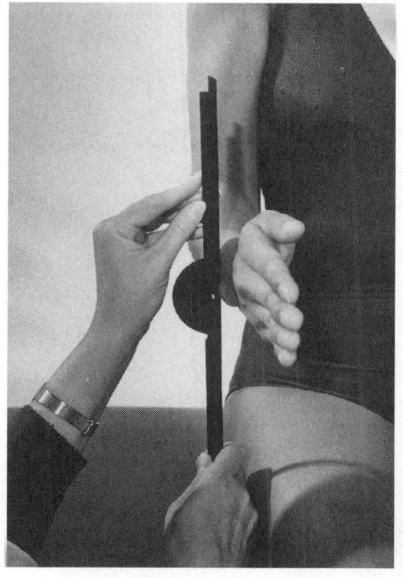

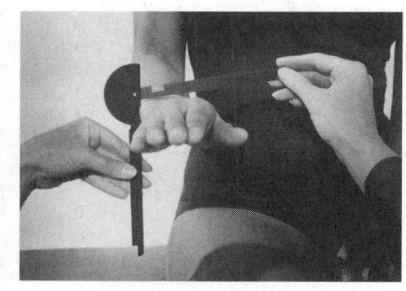

A   B

FIG. 21-23
Forearm pronation. **A,** Starting position. **B,** Final position.

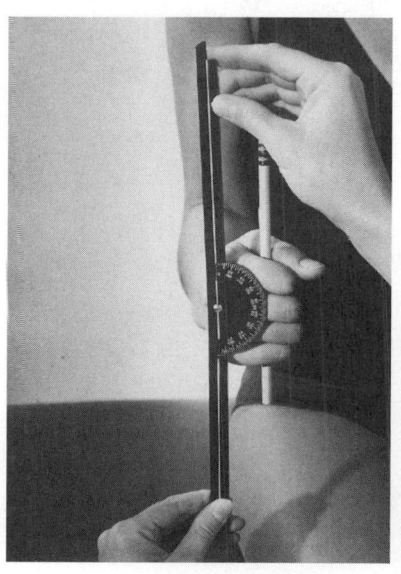

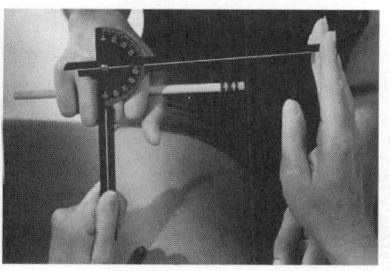

A   B

FIG. 21-24
Forearm pronation (alternate method). **A,** Starting position. **B,** Final position.

against the dorsal aspect of the wrist, and the stationary bar is perpendicular to the floor. After the forearm is pronated, reposition the goniometer so that the movable bar rests squarely across the center of the dorsum of the distal forearm.

Pronation (Alternative Method)
0° to 80° or 90° (Fig. 21-24).

POSITION OF THE SUBJECT. Seated or standing with the humerus adducted, the elbow at 90°, and the forearm in midposition. A pencil is placed in the hand so that it is held perpendicular to the floor.

POSITION OF GONIOMETER. The axis is over the head of the third metacarpal, the stationary bar is perpendicular to the floor, and the movable bar is parallel to the pencil.

END-FEEL. Hard to firm.[3]

Wrist

Flexion
0° to 80° (Fig. 21-25).

POSITION OF THE SUBJECT. Seated with the forearm in midposition and the hand and forearm resting on a table on the ulnar border. The fingers are relaxed or extended. This measurement may also be taken with the forearm pronated and resting on a table.[3]

POSITION OF GONIOMETER. If the wrist is measured with the forearm in midposition, the axis is on the lateral aspect of the wrist just distal to the radial styloid in the anatomical snuffbox. The stationary bar is parallel to the radius, and the movable bar is parallel to the metacarpal of the index finger. If this wrist is measured with the forearm pronated, the axis is placed at the wrist just beneath the ulna styloid, the movable bar is aligned with the fifth metacarpal, and the stationary bar is aligned with the ulna.[3]

END-FEEL. Firm.[3]

Extension
0° to 70° (Fig. 21-26).

POSITION OF THE SUBJECT AND GONIOMETER. The same as for wrist flexion, except that the fingers should be flexed.

END-FEEL. Firm or hard.[3]

Ulnar Deviation
0° to 30° (Fig. 21-27).

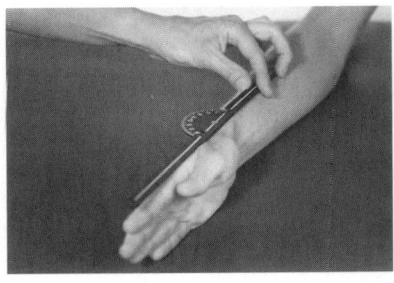
A

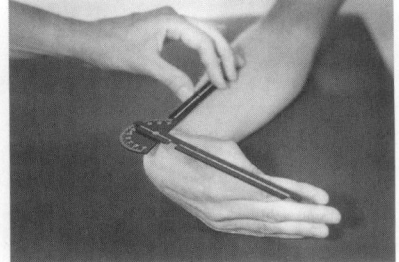
B

FIG. 21-25
Wrist flexion. **A,** Starting position. **B,** Final position.

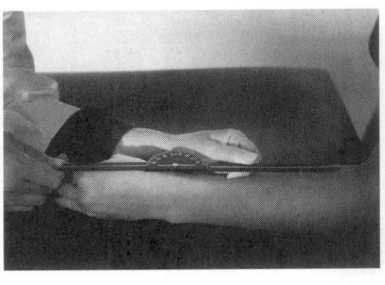
A

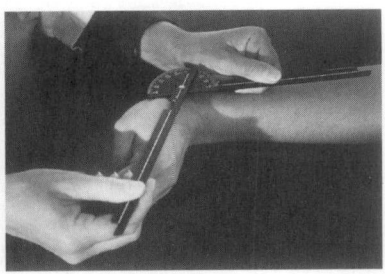
B

FIG. 21-26
Wrist extension. **A,** Starting position. **B,** Final position.

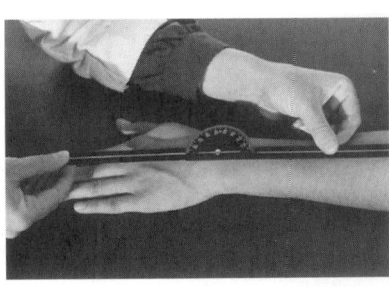
A

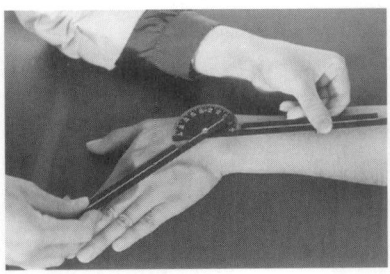
B

FIG. 21-27
Wrist ulnar deviation. **A,** Starting position. **B,** Final position.

POSITION OF THE SUBJECT. Seated with the forearm pronated, the wrist at neutral, the fingers relaxed in extension, and the palm of the hand resting flat on the table surface.

POSITION OF GONIOMETER. The axis is on the dorsum of the wrist at the base of the third metacarpal, over the capitate bone. The movable bar is parallel to the third metacarpal, and the stationary bar is over the midline of the dorsal forearm.

END-FEEL. Firm.[3]

Radial Deviation
0° to 20° (Fig. 21-28).

POSITION OF THE SUBJECT AND GONIOMETER. Same as for ulnar deviation.

END-FEEL. Firm or hard.[3]

Fingers

Metacarpophalangeal Flexion
0° to 90° (Fig. 21-29).

POSITION OF THE SUBJECT. Seated with the elbow flexed, the forearm in midposition, the wrist at 0° neutral, and the forearm and hand supported on a firm surface on the ulnar border.

POSITION OF GONIOMETER. The axis is centered on the dorsal aspect of the metacarpophalangeal (MP) joint. The stationary bar is on top of the metacarpal, and the movable bar is on top of the proximal phalanx.

END-FEEL. Hard or firm.[3]

Metacarpophalangeal Joint Hyperextension
0° to 15°–45° (Fig. 21-30).

POSITION OF THE SUBJECT. Seated with the forearm in midposition, the wrist at 0° neutral, the IP joints relaxed or in flexion, and the forearm and hand supported on a firm surface on the ulnar border.

POSITION OF GONIOMETER. The axis is over the lateral aspect of the MP joint of the index finger. The stationary bar is parallel to the metacarpal, and the movable bar is parallel to the proximal phalanx. The fifth finger MP joint may be measured similarly. ROM of the third and fourth fingers can be estimated by comparison.

An alternative is to place the goniometer on the volar aspect of the hand. With use of the edge of the goniometer, the axis is aligned over the MP joint being measured, the stationary bar is parallel to the metacarpal, and the movable bar is parallel to the proximal phalanx.

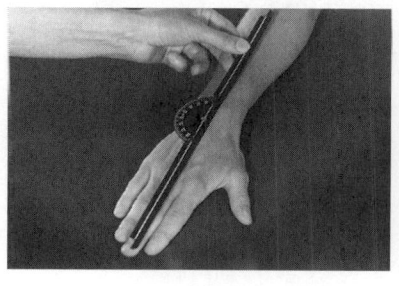

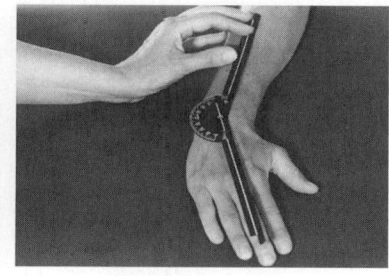

A   B

FIG. 21-28
Wrist radial deviation. **A,** Starting position. **B,** Final position.

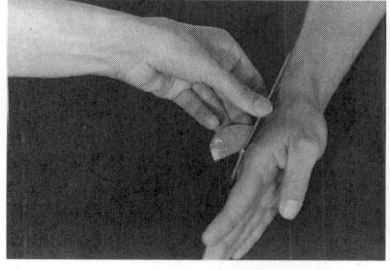
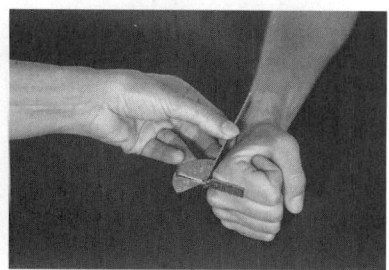

A   B

FIG. 21-29
Metacarpophalangeal flexion. **A,** Starting position. **B,** Final position.

END-FEEL. Firm.[3]

Metacarpophalangeal Abduction
0° to 25° (Fig. 21-31).

POSITION OF THE SUBJECT. Seated with the forearm pronated, the wrist at 0° neutral deviation, the fingers straight, and the hand resting on a firm surface.

POSITION OF GONIOMETER. The axis is centered over the MP joint being measured. The stationary bar is over the corresponding metacarpal, and the movable bar is over the proximal phalanx.

END-FEEL. Firm.[3]

Proximal Interphalangeal Flexion
0° to 110° (Fig. 21-32).

POSITION OF THE SUBJECT. Seated with the forearm in midposition, the wrist at 0° neutral, and the forearm and hand supported on a firm surface on the ulnar border.

POSITION OF GONIOMETER. The axis is centered on the dorsal surface of the proximal interphalangeal (PIP) joint being measured. The stationary bar is placed

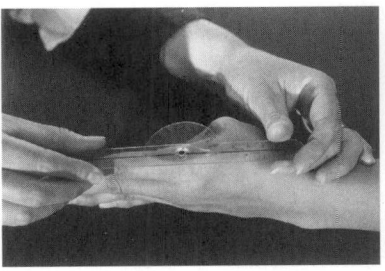
A

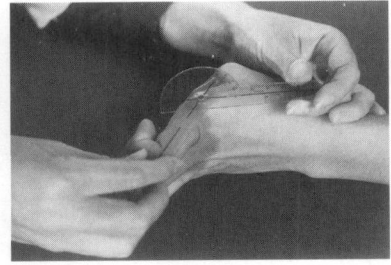
B

FIG. 21-30
Metacarpophalangeal hyperextension. **A,** Starting position. **B,** Final position.

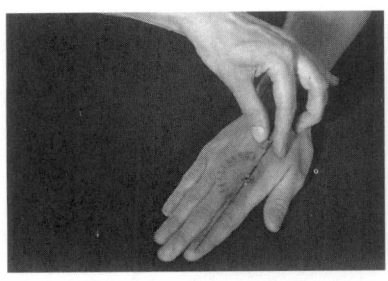
A

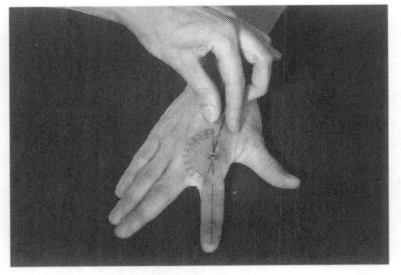
B

FIG. 21-31
Metacarpophalangeal abduction. **A,** Starting position. **B,** Final position.

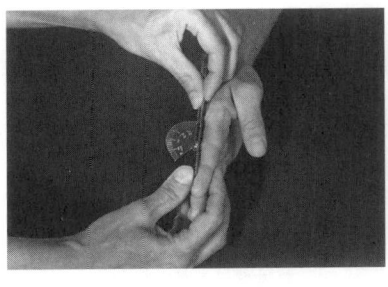
A

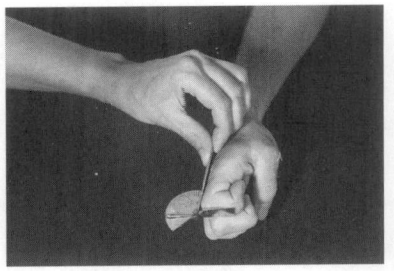
B

FIG. 21-32
Proximal interphalangeal flexion. **A,** Starting position. **B,** Final position.

over the proximal phalanx, and the movable bar is over the distal phalanx.

ALTERNATIVE METHOD. Measurement with a ruler can also be taken. The IP and MP joints of the fingers are flexed toward the palm. A ruler is used to measure from the pulp of the middle finger to the proximal palmar crease.[3]

END-FEEL. Usually hard; may be soft or firm.[3]

Distal Interphalangeal (DIP) Flexion
0° to 80° (Fig. 21-33).

POSITION OF THE SUBJECT. Seated with the forearm in midposition, the wrist at 0° neutral, and the forearm and hand supported on the ulnar border on a firm surface.

POSITION OF GONIOMETER. The axis is on the dorsal surface of the distal interphalangeal (DIP) joint. The stationary bar is over the middle phalanx, and the movable bar is over the distal phalanx.

ALTERNATIVE METHOD. With the MP joints in 0° extension, S flexes the IP and PIP joints toward the palm. With a ruler, a measurement is taken from the pulp of the middle finger to the distal palmar crease.[3]

END-FEEL. Firm.[3]

Thumb

Metacarpophalangeal Flexion
0° to 50° (Fig. 21-34).

POSITION OF THE SUBJECT. Seated with the elbow flexed, the forearm in 45° of supination, the wrist at 0° neutral, the MP and IP joints in extension, and the hand and forearm supported on a firm surface.

POSITION OF GONIOMETER. The axis is on the dorsal surface of the MP joint. The stationary bar is over the thumb metacarpal, and the movable bar is over the proximal phalanx.

END-FEEL. Hard or firm.[3]

Interphalangeal Flexion
0° to 80°–90° (Fig. 21-35).

POSITION OF THE SUBJECT. Same as described for PIP and DIP finger flexion.

POSITION OF GONIOMETER. The axis is on the dorsal surface of the IP joint. The stationary bar is over the proximal phalanx, and the movable bar is over the distal phalanx.

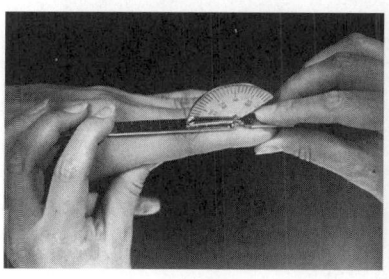 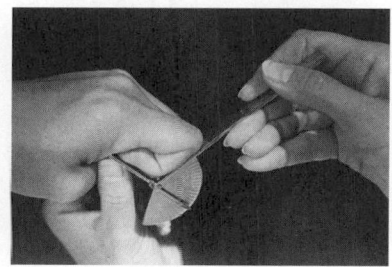

A   B

FIG. 21-33
Distal interphalangeal flexion. **A,** Starting position. **B,** Final position.

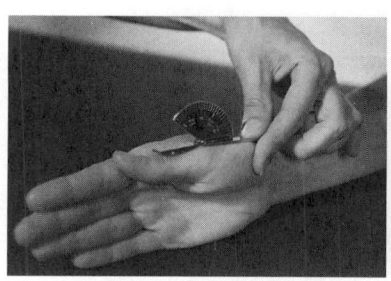 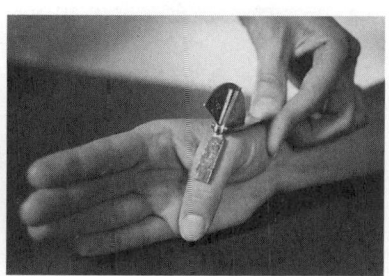

A   B

FIG. 21-34
Thumb Metacarpophalangeal flexion. **A,** Starting position. **B,** Final position.

Radial Abduction (Carpometacarpal Extension)
0° to 50° (Fig. 21-36).

POSITION OF THE SUBJECT. Seated with the forearm pronated and the hand palm down, resting flat on a firm surface.

POSITION OF GONIOMETER. The axis is over the carpometacarpal (CMC) joint at the base of the thumb metacarpal. The stationary bar is parallel to the radius, and the movable bar is parallel to the thumb metacarpal.

Radial Abduction (Alternative Method)
0° to 50° (Fig. 21-37).

POSITION OF THE SUBJECT AND GONIOMETER. S is positioned the same as described in the first method. The axis is over the CMC joint at the base of the thumb metacarpal. The stationary and movable bars are together and parallel to the thumb and the first metacarpals. Neither will be directly over these bones.

END-FEEL. Firm.[3]

Palmar Abduction (Carpometacarpal Flexion)
0° to 50° (Fig. 21-38).

POSITION OF THE SUBJECT. Seated with the forearm at 0° midposition, the wrist at 0°, and the forearm

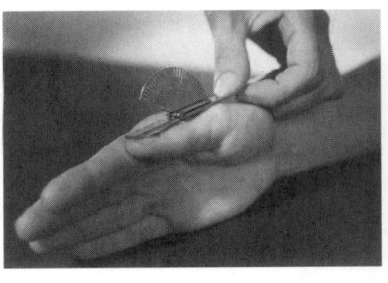
A

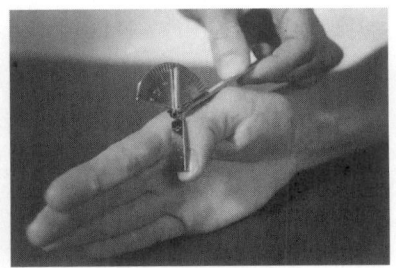
B

FIG. 21-35
Thumb interphalangeal flexion. **A,** Starting position. **B,** Final position.

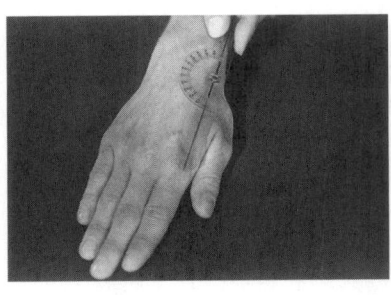
A

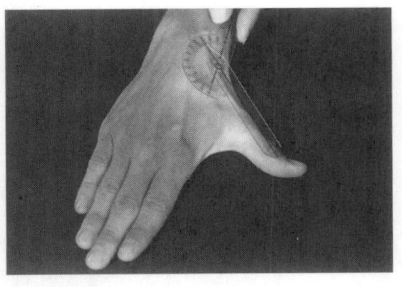
B

FIG. 21-36
Thumb radial abduction. **A,** Starting position. **B,** Final position.

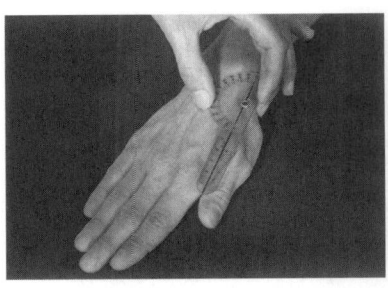
A

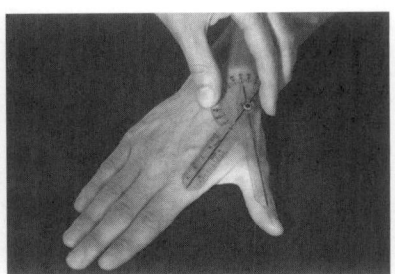
B

FIG. 21-37
Thumb radial abduction (alternative method). **A,** Starting position. **B,** Final position.

and hand resting on the ulnar border. The thumb is rotated so that it is at right angles to the palm of the hand.

POSITION OF GONIOMETER. The axis is at the junction of the thumb and index finger metacarpals. The stationary bar is over the radius, and the movable bar is parallel to the thumb and index finger metacarpals.

Palmar Abduction (Alternative Method)
0° to 50° (Fig. 21-39).

POSITION OF THE SUBJECT AND GONIOMETER. S is positioned the same as described in the first method. The axis is at the junction of the thumb and index finger metacarpals. The stationary and movable

bars are lined up together, parallel to the thumb and the index finger metacarpals.

END-FEEL. Firm.[3]

Opposition
Deficits in opposition may be recorded by measuring the distance between the centers of the pads of the thumb and the fifth finger with a centimeter ruler (Fig. 21-40).

END-FEEL. Soft or firm.[3]

LOWER EXTREMITY[3,5,6,9]
Hip
Flexion
0° to 120° (Fig. 21-41).

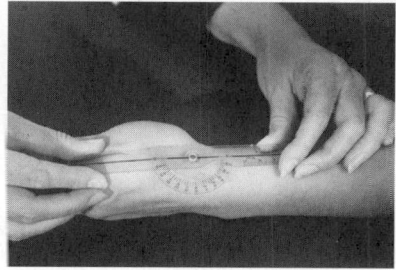
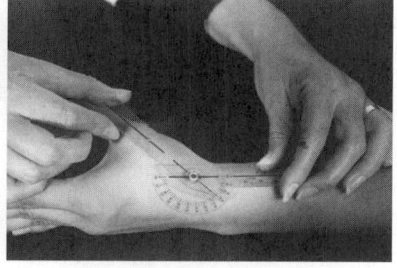

A   B

FIG. 21-38
Palmar abduction. **A,** Starting position. **B,** Final position.

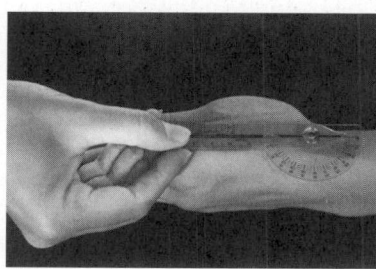
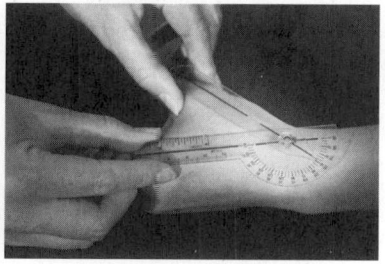

A   B

FIG. 21-39
Palmar abduction (alternative method). **A,** Starting position. **B,** Final position.

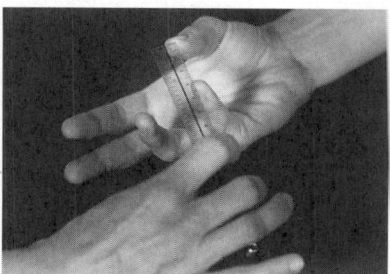

FIG. 21-40
Thumb opposition to fifth finger.

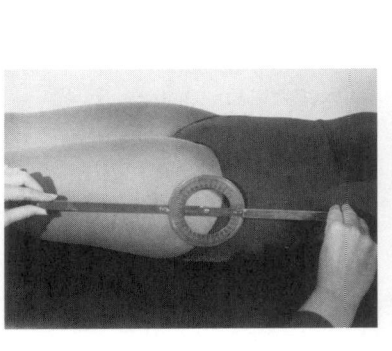
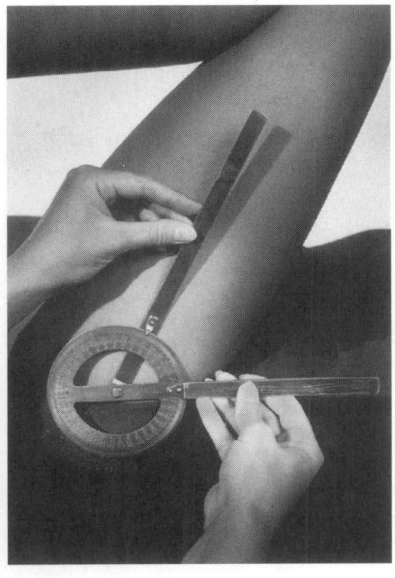

A   B

FIG. 21-41
Hip flexion. **A,** Starting position. **B,** Final position.

POSITION OF THE SUBJECT. Supine, lying with the hip and knee in 0° neutral extension and rotation.

POSITION OF GONIOMETER. The axis is on the lateral aspect of the hip, over the greater trochanter of the femur. The stationary bar is centered over the middle of the lateral aspect of the pelvis, and the movable bar is parallel to the long axis of the femur on the lateral aspect of the thigh. The knee is bent during the motion.

END-FEEL. Soft.[3]

Extension (Hyperextension)
0° to 30° (Fig. 21-42).

POSITION OF THE SUBJECT. The subject is prone, lying with the hip and knee at 0° neutral extension and rotation and the feet over the end of the table.

POSITION OF GONIOMETER. Same as for hip flexion.

END-FEEL. Firm.[3]

Abduction
0° to 40° (Fig. 21-43).

POSITION OF THE SUBJECT. The subject is supine, lying with the legs extended and the hip in 0° neutral rotation. The pelvis is level.

POSITION OF GONIOMETER. The axis is placed on the anterior superior iliac spine. The stationary bar is placed on a line between two anterior superior iliac spines, and the movable bar is parallel to the longitudinal axis of the femur over the anterior aspect of the thigh. Note that the starting position is at 90° for this measurement, and that the recording of the measurement should be adjusted by subtracting 90° from the total number of degrees obtained in the arc of joint motion.

END-FEEL. Firm.[3]

Adduction
0° to 35° (Fig. 21-44).

POSITION OF THE SUBJECT AND GONIOMETER. The subject is supine, lying with the hip and knee of the leg to be tested in extension and neutral rotation. The leg not being tested should be abducted. The goniometer is positioned the same as for hip abduction.

END-FEEL. Firm or soft.[3]

Internal Rotation
0° to 45° (Fig. 21-45).

POSITION OF THE SUBJECT. The subject is seated with the hip in 0° neutral rotation and the hip and knee flexed to 90°. The knee is flexed over the end of the treatment table. A small roll or towel may be placed

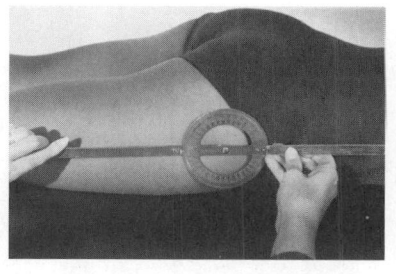 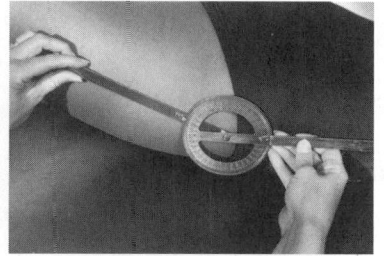

A   B

FIG. 21-42
Hip extension. **A,** Starting position. **B,** Final position.

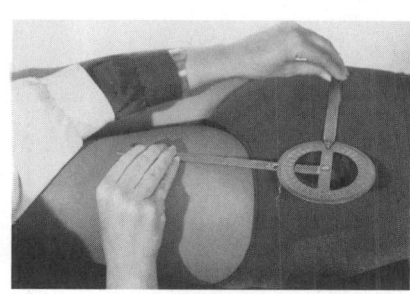 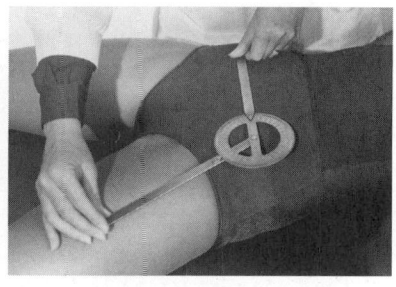

A   B

FIG. 21-43
Hip abduction. **A,** Starting position. **B,** Final position.

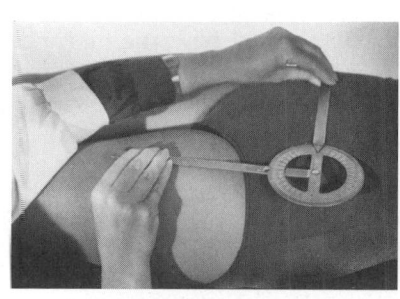 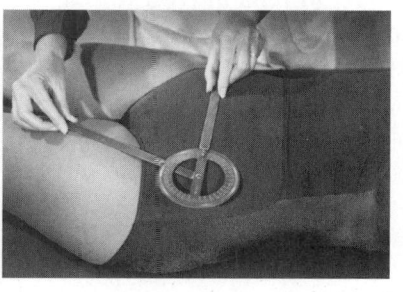

A   B

FIG. 21-44
Hip adduction. **A,** Starting position. **B,** Final position.

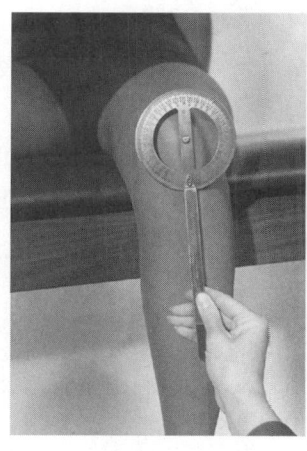 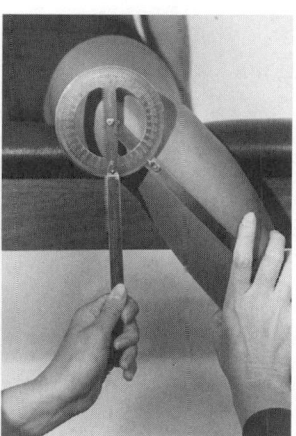

A   B

FIG. 21-45
Hip internal rotation. **A,** Starting position. **B,** Final position.

under the distal end of the femur to maintain it in a horizontal plane. The contralateral hip is abducted, and the foot may be supported on a stool.

POSITION OF GONIOMETER. The axis is on the center of the patella. The stationary and movable bars are parallel to the longitudinal axis of the tibia on the anterior aspect of the lower leg. The stationary bar remains in this position, perpendicular to the floor, while the movable bar follows the tibia as the hip is rotated.

END-FEEL. Firm.[3]

External Rotation
0° to 45° (Fig. 21-46).

POSITION OF THE SUBJECT AND GONIOMETER. The subject is seated with the hip in 0° neutral rotation and the hip and knee of the leg to be tested flexed to 90°. The other leg should be (1) flexed at the knee so that the lower leg is back under the table or (2) flexed at the hip and knee so that the foot is resting on the table. These positions allow the motion to take place without obstruction. The trunk should remain erect during the performance of the motion. The goniometer is positioned as for internal rotation.

END-FEEL. Firm.[3]

Knee

Extension-Flexion
0° to 135° (Fig. 21-47).

POSITION OF THE SUBJECT. The subject should be prone or supine, lying with the knees and hips extended and the hip in 0° neutral rotation.

POSITION OF GONIOMETER. With the subject in the prone position, the axis is centered on the lateral aspect of the knee joint at the lateral epicondyle of the femur. The stationary bar is on the lateral aspect of the thigh, parallel to the longitudinal axis of the femur. The movable bar is parallel to the longitudinal axis of the fibula, aligned with the lateral malleolus, on the lateral aspect of the leg.

END-FEEL. Soft.[3]

Ankle

Dorsiflexion
0° to 15° (Fig. 21-48).

POSITION OF THE SUBJECT. The subject should be lying supine or seated with the knee flexed at least

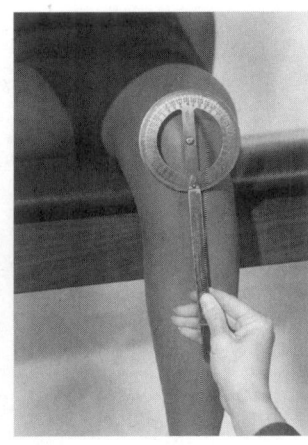 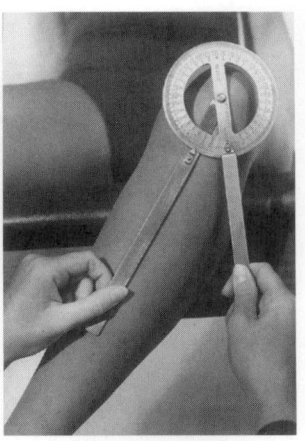

A   B

FIG. 21-46
Hip external rotation. **A,** Starting position. **B,** Final position.

30°. The ankle is at 90° neutral position and the foot is in 0° of inversion and eversion.

POSITION OF GONIOMETER. The axis is placed below the medial malleolus.[3] The stationary bar is parallel to the longitudinal axis of the tibia and the movable bar is parallel with the first metatarsal. (This measurement may also be taken on the lateral side of the foot). Note that measurement begins at 90°, so 90° must be subtracted when recording the joint measurement.

END-FEEL. Firm or hard.[3]

Plantar Flexion
0° to 50° (Fig. 21-49).

POSITION OF THE SUBJECT AND GONIOMETER. Same as for dorsiflexion.

END-FEEL. Firm or hard.[3]

Inversion
0° to 35° (Fig. 21-50).

POSITION OF THE SUBJECT. The subject is supine with the knee and hip extended and in 0° neutral rotation, the ankle in the 90° neutral position, and the foot extended over the edge of the table. A small roll is placed under the knee to maintain slight flexion. The alternative position is sitting with the knee flexed to 90°, the leg over the edge of the supporting surface, and the ankle in 90° neutral position.

POSITION OF GONIOMETER. The axis is placed at the lateral border of the foot near the heel. The stationary bar is parallel to the longitudinal axis of the fibula on the lateral aspect of the leg. The movable bar is parallel to the plantar surface of the heel.

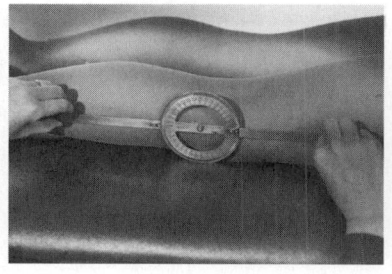 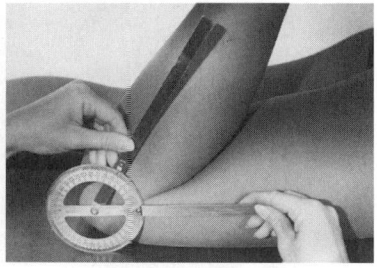

A   B

FIG. 21-47
Knee flexion. **A,** Starting position. **B,** Final position.

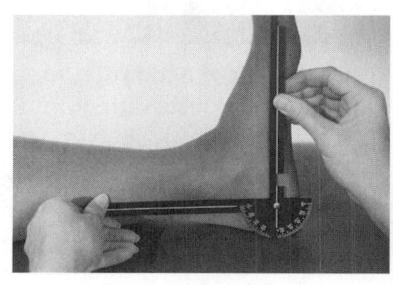 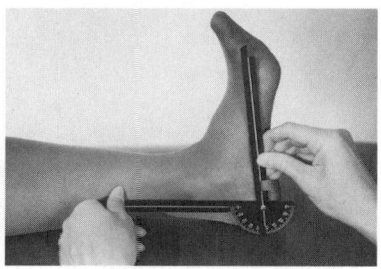

A   B

FIG. 21-48
Ankle dorsiflexion. **A,** Starting position. **B,** Final position.

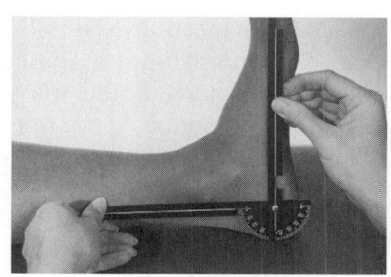 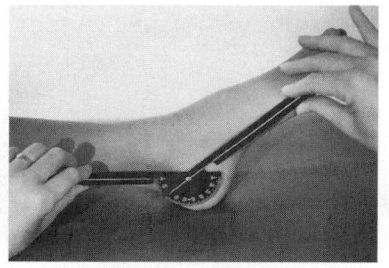

A   B

FIG. 21-49
Ankle plantar flexion. **A,** Starting position. **B,** Final position.

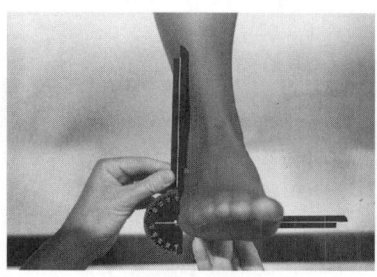 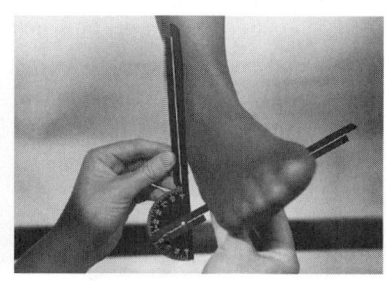

A   B

FIG. 21-50
Ankle inversion. **A,** Starting position. **B,** Final position.

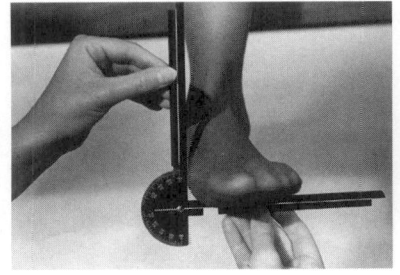
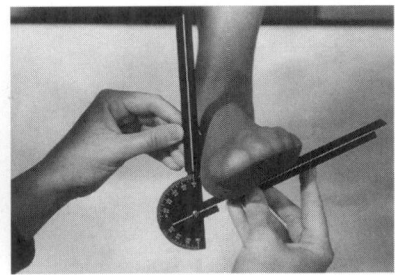

A   B

FIG. 21-51
Ankle eversion. **A,** Starting position. **B,** Final position.

END-FEEL. Firm.[3]

Eversion
0° to 20° (Fig. 21-51).

POSITION OF THE SUBJECT. Same as for inversion.

POSITION OF GONIOMETER. The axis is on the medial border of the foot, just proximal to the metatarsophalangeal joint. The stationary bar is parallel to the longitudinal aspect of the fibula on the medial aspect of the lower leg. The movable bar is parallel to the plantar surface of the sole. Note that measurements for inversion and eversion both begin at 90°. Therefore this amount must be subtracted from the total when measurements are recorded.

END-FEEL. Hard or firm.[3]

SUMMARY

Joint measurement is used to evaluate ROM in persons whose physical dysfunction affects joint mobility. Measurements of ROM are used in setting treatment goals, selecting treatment methods, and making objective assessments of progress.

Before measuring ROM, the OT practitioner should know the principles of joint measurement. The procedure for measuring joint ROM involves correct positioning for patient and therapist, exposure of joints to be measured, palpation, appropriate stabilization and handling of parts, and correct placement of the goniometer at the beginning and end of the ROM.

Directions and illustrations for measuring all of the major joint motions in the neck, trunk, and upper and lower extremities are included in this chapter. The content is designed for the development of the fundamental techniques of joint measurement. The reader is referred to the references for more comprehensive treatment of the topic.[3,9]

REVIEW QUESTIONS

1. Describe general rules for positioning the goniometer when measuring joint ROM.
2. With which diagnoses is joint measurement likely to be used?
3. List and discuss four purposes of joint measurement.
4. Is formal joint measurement necessary for every patient? If not, how may ROM be assessed?
5. What is meant by *palpation*? How is palpation done?
6. In observing joints and joint motions, what should the therapist look for?
7. List at least five precautions or contraindications to joint measurement.
8. What is meant by *end-feel*?
9. When measuring a joint crossed by a two-joint muscle, how should the OT practitioner position the joint not being measured?
10. List the steps in the procedure for joint measurement.
11. How is joint ROM measurement recorded on the evaluation form?
12. List the average normal ROM for elbow flexion, shoulder flexion, finger MP flexion, hip flexion, knee flexion, and ankle dorsiflexion.
13. Describe how to read the goniometer when using the 180-degree system of joint measurement.
14. What is meant by *functional range of motion*?
15. List three treatment methods that could be used to increase ROM.

EXERCISES

1. Measure all of the upper extremity joint motions of a normal subject. Record the findings on the form in Figure 21-2.
2. Repeat the first exercise, but S should play the role of someone with several joint limitations.
3. Observe joint motions used in ordinary ADL (e.g., self-care and home management). Estimate the functional ranges of motion for the following joint

motions: shoulder flexion, external rotation, internal rotation, abduction, elbow flexion, wrist extension, hip flexion and extension, knee flexion, and ankle plantar flexion.

REFERENCES

1. American Academy of Orthopaedic Surgeons: *Joint motion: method of measuring and recording,* Chicago, 1965, The Academy.
2. Baruch Center of Physical Medicine: *The technique of goniometry* (unpublished manuscript), Richmond, Va, Medical College of Virginia.
3. Clarkson HM: *Musculoskeletal assessment, joint range of motion and manual muscle strength,* ed 2, Philadelphia, 2000, Lippincott, Williams & Wilkins.
4. Cole T: Measurement of musculoskeletal function: goniometry. In Kottke FJ, Stillwell GK, Lehmann JF, editors: *Krusen's handbook of physical medicine and rehabilitation,* ed 3, Philadelphia, 1982, WB Saunders.
5. Esch D, Lepley M: *Evaluation of joint motion: methods of measurement and recording,* Minneapolis, 1974, University of Minnesota Press.
6. Hurt SP Considerations of muscle function and their application to disability evaluation and treatment: joint measurement, reprinted from *Am J Occup Ther* 1:69, 1947; 2:13, 1948.
7. Kendall FP, McCreary EK: *Muscles, testing and function,* ed 3, Baltimore, 1983, Williams & Wilkins.
8. Killingsworth A: *Basic physical disability procedures,* San Jose, Calif, 1987, Maple Press.
9. Norkin CC, White DJ: *Measurement of joint motion: a guide to goniometry,* Philadelphia, 1985, FA Davis.
10. Rancho Los Amigos Hospital: *How to measure range of motion of the upper extremities* (unpublished manuscript), Rancho Los Amigos, Calif, the Hospital.
11. Sammons Preston Ability One: Rehabilitation Catalog 2000, Bolingbrook, Ill.
12. Smith HD: Assessment and evaluation: an overview. In Hopkins HL, Smith HD, editors: *Willard and Spackman's occupational therapy,* ed 8, Philadelphia, 1993, JB Lippincott.
13. Thomas CL, editor: *Taber's cyclopedic medical dictionary,* ed 13, Philadelphia, 1977, FA Davis.

CHAPTER 22

Muscle Strength

LORRAINE WILLIAMS PEDRETTI

KEY TERMS

Screening test
Against gravity
Gravity-decreased
Resistance
Manual muscle test
Muscle grades
Endurance
Available ROM
Muscle coordination
Palpate
Substitution

LEARNING OBJECTIVES

After studying this chapter the student or practitioner will be able to do the following:

1. Describe screening tests for muscle strength assessment.
2. Identify what is measured by the manual muscle test (MMT).
3. List diagnoses for which the MMT is appropriate and those for which it is not appropriate, with the rationale for each.
4. List the steps of the manual muscle testing procedure in correct order.
5. Describe the limitations of the MMT.
6. Define muscle grades by name, letter, and number.
7. Administer a manual muscle test, using the directions in this chapter, on a normal practice subject.
8. Describe how the results of the muscle strength assessment are used in treatment planning.

Many physical disabilities cause muscle weakness. Slight to substantial limitations of occupational performance can result from loss of strength, depending on the degree of weakness and whether the weakness is permanent or temporary. If improvement is expected, the occupational therapist must assess the muscle weakness and plan treatment that will enable occupational performance and increase strength.

CAUSES OF MUSCLE WEAKNESS

A loss of muscle strength is a primary symptom of or direct result of the following diseases or injuries:

1. The lower motor neuron disorders, such as peripheral neuropathies and peripheral nerve injuries, spinal cord injury (because those muscles innervated at the level[s] of the lesion generally have a lower motor neuron paralysis), Guillain-Barré syndrome, and cranial nerve dysfunctions
2. Primary muscle diseases, such as muscular dystrophy and myasthenia gravis
3. Neurological diseases in which the lower motor neuron is affected, such as amyotrophic lateral sclerosis or multiple sclerosis

Disabilities in which a loss of muscle strength is caused by disuse or immobilization rather than being a direct effect of the disease process include burns, amputation, hand trauma (unless there is an accompanying nerve injury), arthritis, fractures, and a variety of other orthopedic conditions.

Muscle weakness can restrict or prevent the pursuit of self-care, vocational, leisure, and social activities. These limitations are assessed by observation of performance (see Chapter 20), screening tests, and manual muscle testing, when indicated.

SCREENING TESTS

Screening tests are useful for observing areas of strength and weakness and for determining which areas require specific manual muscle testing.[6,9,10,14] The screening tests can help the therapist avoid unnecessary testing or duplication of services.[10] The tests are used by occupational therapists in some health care facilities where manual muscle testing is the responsibility of the physical therapy service.

Screening may be accomplished by the following means:

1. Examination of the medical record for results of previous muscle test and range of motion (ROM) assessments
2. Observing the patient entering the clinic and moving about
3. Observing the patient perform functional activities such as removing an article of clothing and shaking hands with the therapist[6,10]
4. Performing a gross check of bilateral muscle groups[10]

The last method can be performed while the subject is comfortably seated in a sturdy chair or wheelchair. The subject is asked to perform the motions **against gravity** (movements away from the floor), or in the **gravity-decreased** plane (parallel to the floor) if moving against gravity is not possible. Active range of motion (AROM) is observed and **resistance** (application of force) can be given to the test motions to obtain a gross estimate of strength.

MANUAL MUSCLE TEST

The **manual muscle test** (MMT) is a means of evaluating muscle strength. The MMT measures the maximal contraction of a muscle or muscle group.[6] The criteria used to measure strength are evidence of muscle contraction, amount of ROM through which the joint passes when the muscle contracts, and amount of resistance against which the muscle can contract. Gravity is considered a form of resistance.[6,7,9] The MMT is used to determine amount of muscle power and to record gains and losses in strength.

Purposes of Manual Muscle Testing

The specific strength measurement of individual muscles through manual muscle testing can be essential for diagnosis of some neuromuscular conditions, such as peripheral nerve lesions and spinal cord injury. In peripheral nerve or nerve root lesions the pattern of muscle weakness may help determine which nerve or

nerve roots are involved and whether the involvement is partial or complete. Careful evaluation can help determine the level(s) of spinal cord involvement.[11] Along with sensory evaluation, the MMT can therefore be an important diagnostic aid in neuromuscular conditions.

The purposes for assessing muscle strength are to determine the amount of muscle power available and thus establish a baseline for treatment, to discern how muscle weakness is limiting performance of activities of daily living (ADL), to prevent deformities that can result from imbalances of strength, to determine the need for assistive devices as compensatory measures, to aid in the selection of activities within the patient's capabilities, and to evaluate the effectiveness of treatment.[12]

Methods of Assessment

Muscle strength can be assessed in several ways. The most precise method is a test of individual muscles. In this procedure the muscle is carefully isolated through proper positioning, stabilization, and control of the movement pattern and its strength is graded. This type of muscle testing is described by Kendall and McCreary[11] and Cole, Furness, and Twomey.[8] Another and perhaps more common method of manual muscle testing is to assess the strength of groups of muscles that perform specific motions at each joint. This type of testing was described by Daniels and Worthingham[9] and Hislop and Montgomery[10] and, for the most part, is the form that is presented later in this chapter.

The functional motion assessment described in Chapter 20 and screening tests described above are also used to assess muscle strength. These tests are not as precise as the MMT, and their purpose is to make a general evaluation of muscle strength and to determine areas of weakness, performance limitations, and the need for more precise testing.

Results of Assessment as a Basis for Treatment Planning

When planning treatment for the maintenance or improvement of strength, the occupational therapist considers several factors in the clinical reasoning process before determining treatment priorities, goals, and modalities. The results of the muscle strength assessment will suggest the progression of the treatment program. What is the degree of weakness? Is it generalized or specific to one or more muscle groups? Are the **muscle grades** generally the same throughout, or is there significant disparity in muscle grades? If there is disparity, is there an imbalance of strength between the agonist and antagonist muscles that necessitates protection of the weaker muscles during treatment and ADL? When there is substantial imbalance between an agonist and antagonist muscle, treatment goals may be directed toward strengthening the weaker group while maintaining the strength of the stronger group. Muscle imbalance may also suggest the need for an orthosis to protect the weaker muscles from overstretching while recovery is in progress. Examples of such orthoses are devices such as the bed footboard to prevent overstretching of the weakened ankle dorsiflexors and the wrist cock-up splint to prevent overstretching of weakened wrist extensors.

Muscle grades will suggest the level of therapeutic activity or exercise that can help to maintain or improve strength. Is the weakness mild (G range), moderate (F to F+), or severe (P to 0)?[12] Muscles graded F−, for example, could be strengthened by active assisted exercise or light activity against gravity. Muscles graded P likewise will require activity or exercise in the gravity-decreased plane, with little or no resistance, to increase strength. Further discussion of appropriate exercise and activity for specific muscle grades appears in Chapter 30.

The **endurance** of the muscles (i.e., how many repetitions of the muscle contraction are possible before fatigue sets in) is an important consideration in treatment planning. A frequent goal of the therapeutic activity program is to increase endurance, as well as strength. Because the MMT does not measure endurance, the therapist should assess endurance by engaging the patient in periods of exercise or activity graded in length to determine the amount of time that the muscle group can be used in sustained activity. There is usually a correlation between strength and endurance. Weaker muscles will tend to have less endurance than stronger ones. When selecting treatment modalities for increasing endurance, the therapist may elect not to tax the muscle to its maximal ability but rather to emphasize repetitive action at less than the maximal contraction to increase endurance and prevent fatigue.[12]

Sensory loss, which often accompanies muscle weakness, complicates the ability of the patient to perform in an activity program. If there is little or no tactile or proprioceptive feedback from motion, the impulse to move is decreased or lost, depending on the severity of the sensory loss. Thus the movement may appear weak and ineffective even when strength is adequate for performance of a specific activity. With some diagnoses, a sensory reeducation program (see Chapter 25) may be indicated to increase the patient's sensory awareness and feedback from the part. In other instances the therapist may elect to teach compensation techniques for the sensory loss. These techniques include the use of mirrors, video playback, and biofeedback, which can be used as adjuncts to the strengthening program.

Another important consideration in the therapist's clinical reasoning is the diagnosis and expected course of the disease. Is strength expected to increase, decrease, or remain about the same? If strength is expected to increase, what is the expected recovery period? What is the

effect of exercise or activity on muscle function? Will too much activity delay the progress of recovery? If muscle power is expected to decrease, how rapid will the progression be? Are there factors to be avoided, such as a vigorous activity or exercise program, that can accelerate the decrease in strength? If strength is declining, is special equipment practical and necessary? How much muscle power is needed to operate the equipment? How long will the patient be able to operate a device before a decrease in muscle power makes it impracticable?[12]

The therapist should assess the effect of the muscle weakness on the ability to perform ADL, which can be observed during the ADL assessment. Which tasks are most difficult to perform because of the muscle weakness? How does the patient compensate for the weakness? Which tasks are most important for the patient to be able to perform? Is special equipment necessary or desirable for the performance of some ADL, such as the mobile arm support (Chapter 31) for independence in eating (Chapter 31)?

If the patient is involved in a total rehabilitation program and receiving several other health care services, the activity and exercise programs must be synchronized and well balanced to meet the patient's needs rather than the needs of the professionals, their schedules, and possibly their competition. The occupational therapist needs to be aware of the nature and extent of the programs in which the patient is engaged in physical therapy, recreation therapy, and any other services. Ideally, the health care team should plan the exercise and activity programs together to ensure that they complement one another. The therapist must consider the following questions: What is the patient doing in each of the therapies? How long is each treatment session? Are the goals of all of the therapies similar and complementary, or are they divergent and conflicting? Is the patient being overfatigued in the total program? Are the various treatment sessions in rapid succession, or are they well spaced to meet the patient's need for rest periods?

On the basis of these considerations and others pertinent to the specific patient, the occupational therapist can select enabling and purposeful activities designed to maintain or increase strength, improve performance of ADL, and enable the use of special equipment, while protecting weak muscles from overstretching and overfatigue.

Relationship Between Joint Range of Motion and Muscle Weakness

One of the criteria used to grade muscle strength is the joint range of motion (ROM) of the joint on which the muscle acts—that is, did the muscle move the joint through complete, partial, or no ROM? Another criterion is the amount of resistance that can be applied to the part once the muscle has moved the joint through the partial or complete AROM. In this context, ROM is not necessarily the full average normal ROM for the given joint; rather, it is the ROM available to the individual patient. When the therapist measures joint motion (discussed in Chapter 21), it is the passive ROM (PROM) that is the measure of the range available to the patient. PROM, however, is not an indication of muscle strength.

When performing muscle testing, the occupational therapist must know the patient's **available ROM** (PROM) to assign muscle grades correctly. It is possible that PROM would be limited or less than the average for a joint motion but that the muscle strength would be normal. Therefore it is necessary for the therapist either to have measured joint ROM or to move joints passively to assess available ROM before administering the muscle test. For example, the patient's PROM for elbow flexion may be limited to 0° to 110° because of an old fracture. If the patient can flex the elbow joint to 110° and hold against moderate resistance during the muscle test, the muscle would be graded G(4). In such cases the examiner should record the limitation with the muscle grade—for example, 0° to 110°/G.[9] Conversely, if the patient's available ROM for elbow flexion is 0° to 140°, and he or she can flex the elbow against gravity through only 110°, the muscle would be graded F− because the part moves through only partial ROM against gravity. When the therapist determines the patient's available ROM before performing the muscle test, he or she can grade muscle strength on that basis rather than by using the average normal ROM as the standard.

Limitations of the Manual Muscle Test

The limitations of the MMT are that it cannot measure muscle endurance (the number of times the muscle can contract at its maximum level),[6] **muscle coordination** (the smooth rhythmic interaction of muscle function), or motor performance capabilities of the patient (the use of the muscles for functional activities).[8]

The MMT cannot be used accurately with patients who have spasticity caused by upper motor neuron disorders such as cerebrovascular accident (stroke) or cerebral palsy. In these disorders muscles are often hypertonic. Muscle tone and ability to perform movements are influenced by primitive reflexes and the position of the head and body in space. Also, movements tend to occur in gross synergistic patterns that make it impossible for the patient to isolate joint motions, which is demanded in the manual muscle testing procedures.[2,3,6,7,13]

The MMT is not appropriate for patients with upper motor neuron disorders such as CVA (stroke), cerebral palsy, or head injury. In these disorders muscles are hypertonic. Muscle tone and ability to perform movement

are influenced by primitive reflexes and the position of the head and body in space. Also, movements tend to occur in gross synergistic patterns that make performance of isolated joint motion, required in the MMT, impossible.[2,3,6,7,13] However, when administered during the final recovery stage when spasticity and synergy patterns have disappeared and the patient has achieved isolated control of voluntary muscle function, the MMT may reveal some residual weakness. In these instances, some assessment of strength can be of value in designing a treatment program. (See Chapter 23 for methods of evaluating motor function of patients with upper motor neuron disorders.)

Contraindications and Precautions

Assessment of strength using the MMT is contraindicated when the patient has inflammation or pain in the region to be tested; a dislocation or unhealed fracture; recent surgery, particularly of musculoskeletal structures; or myositis ossificans.[7]

Special precautions must be taken when resisted movement could aggravate the patient's condition, as might occur with osteoporosis; subluxation or hypermobility of a joint; hemophilia or any type of cardiovascular risk or disease; abdominal surgery or an abdominal hernia; and fatigue that exacerbates the patient's condition.[6,7]

Knowledge and Skill of the Examiner

The validity of the MMT depends on the examiner's knowledge and skill in using the correct testing procedure. Careful observation of movement, careful and accurate palpation, correct positioning, consistency of procedure, and experience of the examiner are critical factors in accurate testing.[9-11]

To be proficient in manual muscle testing, the examiner must have detailed knowledge about all aspects of muscle function. Joints and joint motions, muscle innervation, origin and insertion of muscles, action of muscles, direction of muscle fibers, angle of pull on the joints, and the role of muscles in fixation and substitution are important considerations. The examiner must be able to locate and feel contraction of (**palpate**) the muscles, recognize whether the contour of the muscle is normal, atrophied, or hypertrophied, and detect abnormal movements and positions. The examiner must use consistent methods in the application of test procedures. Knowledge and experience are necessary to detect substitutions and to interpret strength grades with accuracy.[10,11]

It is necessary for the examiner to acquire skill and experience in testing and grading muscles of normal persons of both genders and of all ages. Many factors affect muscle strength. The age, gender, and lifestyle of the subject, the muscle size, and type and speed of contraction, the effect of previous training for the testing situation, the joint position during the muscle contraction, previous training effect, time of day, temperature, and fatigue all can affect muscle strength.[6,7] Experience can help the examiner differentiate strength grades if these factors are taken into account.[14]

GENERAL PRINCIPLES OF MANUAL MUSCLE TESTING
Preparation for Testing

If several tests are to be administered, they should be organized to avoid frequent repositioning of the subject.[10] The examiner should observe contour of the part, comparative symmetry of the muscle on both sides, and any apparent hypertrophy or atrophy. During PROM the examiner can estimate muscle tone. Is there lesser or greater than normal resistance to passive movement? During AROM, the examiner can observe quality of movement, such as movement speed, smoothness, rhythm, and any abnormal movements such as tremors.[14]

Correct positioning of the subject and the body part is essential to effective and correct evaluation. The subject should be positioned comfortably on a firm surface. Clothing should be arranged or removed so that the examiner can see the muscle or muscles being tested. If the subject cannot be placed in the correct position for the test, the examiner must adapt the test and use clinical judgment in approximating strength grades.[14] In addition to correct positioning, test validity depends on careful stabilization, palpation of the muscles, and observation of movement.[9]

Gravity Influencing Muscle Function

Gravity is a form of resistance to muscle power. It is used as a grading criterion in tests of the neck, trunk, and extremities. This means that the muscle grade is based on whether a muscle can move the part against gravity.[11] Movements against gravity are in a vertical plane (that is, away from the floor or toward the ceiling) and are used with grades F (3), G (4), and N (5). Movements against gravity and resistance are performed in a vertical plane with added manual or mechanical resistance and are used with F+ (3+) to N (5) grades. Tests for the weaker muscles (O, T [1], P [2], and P+ [2+] grades) are often performed in a horizontal plane (that is, parallel to the floor) to reduce the resistance of gravity on muscle power. This position has been referred to as the gravity-eliminated, **gravity-decreased,** or gravity-lessened test position.[9,11,14] "Gravity eliminated" is the common term to designate this position.[14] Because the effect of gravity on muscle function cannot be eliminated completely, "gravity-decreased" or "gravity-

lessened" may be more accurate terms. The term "gravity-decreased" is used in this chapter.[9,11]

In many muscle tests the effect of gravity on the ability to perform the movement must be considered in grading muscle power. It is of lesser importance, however, in tests of the forearm, fingers, and toes because the weight of the part lifted against gravity is insignificant compared with the muscle strength.[9,11] Therefore the examiner may choose to do the tests for F (3) to N (5) in the gravity-decreased plane. In other tests, positioning for movements in the gravity-decreased position or the against-gravity position may not be feasible. For example, in the test for scapula depression, positioning to perform the movement against gravity would require the subject to assume an inverted position. In individual cases, positioning for movement in the correct plane may not be possible because of confinement to bed, generalized weakness, trunk instability, immobilization devices, and medical precautions. In these instances the examiner must adapt the positioning to the patient's needs and modify the grading using clinical judgment. If tests of the forearm, fingers, and toes are done against gravity rather than in the gravity-decreased plane, the standard definitions of muscle grades can be modified when muscle grades are recorded. The partial ROM against gravity is graded P (2), and the full ROM against gravity is graded F (3).[9] Such modifications in positioning and grading should be noted by the examiner when results of the muscle test are recorded.

For consistency in procedure and grading, the gravity-decreased positions and against-gravity positions are used in the MMTs described later, except where the positioning is not feasible or would be awkward or uncomfortable for the subject. Modifications in positioning and grading have been cited with the individual tests.

Muscle Grades

Although the definitions of the muscle grades are standard, the assignment of muscle grades during the MMT depends on the clinical judgment, knowledge, and experience of the examiner,[9] especially when determining slight, moderate, or maximal resistance. Age, gender, body type, occupation, and leisure activities all influence the amount of resistance that a particular subject can take.[9,11] Normal strength for an 8-year-old girl will be considerably less than for a 25-year-old man, for example. Additionally, strength tends to decline with age, and full resistance to the same muscle group will vary considerably from an 80-year-old man to a 25-year-old man.[7,11] Therefore, the amount of resistance that can be applied to grade a particular muscle group as N (5) or G (4) varies from one individual to another.[9,11]

The amount of resistance that can be given also varies from one muscle group to another. Muscle strength is relative to the cross-sectional size of the muscle. Larger muscles have greater strength.[7,9] For example, the flexors of the wrist are larger and therefore have more power and can take much more resistance than the abductors of the fingers. The examiner must consider the size and relative power of the muscles and the leverage used when giving resistance.[12] The amount of resistance applied should be modified accordingly. When only one side of the body is involved in the dysfunction causing the muscle weakness, the examiner can establish the standards for strength by testing the unaffected side first.

Because weak muscles fatigue easily, the results of muscle testing may not be accurate if the subject is tired. There should be no more than three repetitions of the test movement because fatigue can result in grading errors if the muscle becomes tired as a result of low endurance.[7,8] Pain, swelling, or muscle spasm in the area being tested may also interfere with the testing procedure and accurate grading. Such problems should be recorded on the evaluation form.[14] Psychological factors must be considered in interpreting muscle strength grades. When interpreting strength, the examiner must assess the motivation, cooperation, and effort put forth by the subject.[9]

In the MMT, muscles are graded according to the criteria listed in Table 22-1.[6,9,10,15]

The purpose of using "plus" or "minus" designations with the muscle grades is to "fine grade" muscle strength. These designations are likely to be used by the experienced examiner. Two examiners testing the same individual may vary up to a half grade in their results, but there should not be a whole grade difference.[14]

Substitutions

The brain thinks in terms of movement and not in terms of contraction of individual muscles.[9] Thus a muscle or muscle group may attempt to compensate for the function of a weaker muscle to accomplish a movement. These movements are called trick movements or **substitutions**.[6,7,11] Substitutions can occur during the MMT. To test muscle strength accurately, it is necessary for the therapist to give careful instructions, to eliminate substitutions in the testing procedure by correct positioning, stabilization, and palpation of the muscle being tested, and to ensure careful performance of the test motion without extraneous movements. To prevent substitutions, the correct position of the body should be maintained and movement of the part performed without shifting the body or turning the part.[6,7,11] The examiner must palpate contractile tissue (muscle fibers or tendon) to detect tension in the muscle group under examination. It is only through correct palpation that the examiner can be certain that the motion observed is not being performed by substitution.[6,9] Undetected trick movements can mask the patient's problems and could result in inaccurate treatment planning.[6]

In the tests that follow, possible substitutions are described at the end of the directions. The examiner should be familiar with these substitutions to detect

TABLE 22-1
Muscle Grades and Their Definitions

Number Grade	Word/Letter Grade	Definition
0	Zero (0)	No muscle contraction can be seen or felt.
1	Trace (T)	Contraction can be observed or felt, but there is no motion.
2−	Poor minus (P−)	Part moves through incomplete ROM with gravity decreased.
2	Poor (P)	Part moves through complete ROM with gravity decreased.
2+	Poor plus (P+)	Part moves through less than 50% of available ROM against gravity or through complete ROM with gravity decreased against slight resistance.[9]
3−	Fair minus (F−)	Part moves through more than 50% of available ROM against gravity.[9]
3	Fair (F)	Part moves through complete ROM against gravity.
3+	Fair plus (F+)	Part moves through complete ROM against gravity and slight resistance.
4	Good (G)	Part moves through complete ROM against gravity and moderate resistance.
5	Normal (N)	Part moves through complete ROM against gravity and maximal resistance.

them and correct the procedure. Detecting substitutions is a skill gained with time and experience.

Procedure for Manual Muscle Testing

Testing should be performed according to a standard procedure to ensure accuracy and consistency. The tests that follow are each divided into these steps: (1) position, (2) stabilize, (3) palpate, (4) observe, (5) resist, and (6) grade.

First the subject (S) should be positioned for the specific muscle test. The examiner (E) should position himself or herself in relation to S. Then E stabilizes the part proximal to the part being tested to eliminate extraneous movements, isolate the muscle group, ensure the correct test motion, and eliminate substitutions. E should then demonstrate or describe the test motion to S and ask S to perform the test motion and return to the starting position. E makes a general observation of the form and quality of movement, looking for substitutions or difficulties that may require adjustments in positioning and stabilization. E then places his or her fingers for palpation of one or more of the prime movers, or its tendinous insertion, in the muscle group being tested and asks S to repeat the test motion. E again observes the movement for possible substitution and the amount of range completed. When S has moved the part through the available ROM, E asks S to hold the end position. E removes the palpating fingers and uses the free hand to resist in the direction opposite that of the test movement. For example, when elbow flexion is tested, E applies resistance in the direction of extension. E usually must maintain stabilization when resistance is given. Manual muscle tests use the "break test"; that is, the resistance is applied after S has reached the end of the available ROM.[10]

S should be allowed to establish a maximal contraction (set the muscles) before the resistance is applied.[9,12] In most tests E applies the resistance near the distal segment to which the muscle is attached after preparing S by giving the command to hold. Resistance should be applied gradually in a direction opposite to the line of pull of the muscle or muscle group being tested.[10] The break test should not evoke pain, and resistance should be released immediately if pain or discomfort occurs.[9] Finally, E grades the muscle strength according to the preceding standard definitions of muscle grades. This procedure is used for the tests of strength of grades F+ (3+) and above. Resistance is not applied for tests of muscles from F (3) to 0. Slight resistance is sometimes applied to a muscle that has completed the full ROM in the gravity-decreased plane to determine if the grade is P+. Fig. 22-1 shows a sample form for recording muscle grades.

The following directions do not include tests for the face, neck, and trunk. Refer to the references for these tests, as well as a comprehensive treatment of the topic of manual muscle testing.[6, 8-11]

MANUAL MUSCLE TESTING OF THE UPPER EXTREMITY
Motion

Scapula elevation, neck rotation, and lateral flexion.

Muscles[9]	Innervation: nerve, nerve roots[9,11]
Upper trapezius	Accessory nerve (CN 11), C2-4
Levator scapula	Dorsal scapular nerve, C3-5

Procedure for Testing Grades Normal (N or 5) to Fair (F or 3)[9,10]
1. *Position:* S seated erect with arms resting at sides of body. E stands behind S toward the side to be tested.
2. *Stabilize:* A chair back can offer stabilization to the trunk, if necessary.
3. *Palpate:* The upper trapezius parallel to the cervical vertebrae, near the shoulder-neck curve.[9]
4. *Observe:* Elevation of the scapula as S shrugs the shoulder toward the ear and rotates and laterally flexes the neck toward the side being tested at the same time (Fig. 22-2, A).[11]
5. *Resist:* With one hand on top of the shoulder toward scapula depression and with the other hand on the side of the head toward derotation and lateral flexion to the opposite side (Fig. 22-2, B).[11]

Procedure for Testing Grades Poor (P or 2), Trace (T or 1), and Zero (0)[9]
1. *Position:* S lying prone with head in midposition. E stands opposite the side being tested.
2. *Stabilize:* The weight of the trunk on the supporting surface is adequate stabilization.
3. *Palpate:* The upper trapezius, as described in the previous procedure, while observing S elevate the shoulder being tested. Because of the positioning, the neck rotation and lateral flexion components are omitted for these grades (Fig. 22-2, C).
4. *Grade:* According to standard definitions of muscle grades.

Substitutions: Rhomboids and levator scapula can elevate the scapula if the upper trapezius is weak or absent. In the event of substitution, some downward rotation of the acromion will be observed during the movement.[4,12,15]

Motion

Scapula depression, adduction, and upward rotation.

Muscles[1,4]	Innervation[6,7]
Lower trapezius	Spinal accessory nerve, C3,4
Middle trapezius	
Serratus anterior	Long thoracic nerve, C5-7

MUSCLE EXAMINATION

Patient's name _____ Chart no. _____

Date of birth _____ Name of institution _____

Date of onset _____ Attending physician _____ MD

Diagnosis: _____

LEFT										RIGHT			
				Examiner's initials									
				Date									
			NECK	Flexors			Sternocleidomastoid						
				Extensor group									
			TRUNK	Flexors			Rectus abdominis						
				Rt. ext. obl. / Lt. int. obl.	Rotators		{ Lt. ext. obl. / { Rt. int. obl.						
				Extensors			{ Thoracic group / { Lumbar group						
				Pelvic elev.			Quadratus lumb.						
			HIP	Flexors			Iliopsoas						
				Extensors			Gluteus maximus						
				Abductors			Gluteus medius						
				Adductor group									
				External rotator group									
				Internal rotator group									
				Sartorius									
				Tensor fasciae latae									
			KNEE	Flexors			{ Biceps femoris / { Inner hamstrings						
				Extensors			Quadriceps						
			ANKLE	Plantar flexors			{ Gastrocnemius / { Soleus						
			FOOT	Invertors			{ Tibialis anterior / { Tibialis posterior						
				Evertors			{ Peroneus brevis / { Peroneus longus						
			TOES	MP flexors			Lumbricales						
				IP flexors (first)			Flex. digit. br.						
				IP flexors (second)			Flex. digit. l.						
				MP extensors			{ Ext. digit. l. / { Ext. digit. br.						
			HALLUX	MP flexor			Flex. hall. br.						
				IP flexor			Flex. hall. l.						
				MP extensor			Ext. hall. br.						
				IP extensor			Ext. hall. l.						

Measurements:

Cannot walk	Date	Speech
Stands	Date	Swallowing
Walks unaided	Date	Diaphragm
Walks with apparatus	Date	Intercostals

KEY

5	N	Normal	Complete range of motion against gravity with full resistance.
4	G	Good*	Complete range of motion against gravity with some resistance.
3	F	Fair*	Complete range of motion against gravity.
2	P	Poor*	Complete range of motion with gravity eliminated.
1	T	Trace	Evidence of slight contractility. No joint motion.
0	O	Zero	No evidence of contractility.
S or SS			Spasm or severe spasm.
C or CC			Contracture or severe contracture.

*Muscle spasm or contracture may limit range of motion. A question mark
should be placed after the grading of a movement that is incomplete from
this cause.

Continued

FIG. 22-1

Muscle examination. (Adapted from March of Dimes Birth Defects Foundation.)

LEFT   RIGHT

					Examiner's initials					
					Date					
				SCAPULA	Abductor	Serratus anterior				
					Elevator	Upper trapezius				
					Depressor	Lower trapezius				
					Adductors	Middle trapezius / Rhomboids				
				SHOULDER	Flexor	Anterior deltoid				
					Extensors	Latissimus dorsi / Teres major				
					Abductor	Middle deltoid				
					Horiz. abd.	Posterior deltoid				
					Horiz. add.	Pectoralis major				
					External rotator group					
					Internal rotator group					
				ELBOW	Flexors	Biceps brachii / Brachioradialis				
					Extensor	Triceps				
				FOREARM	Supinator group					
					Pronator group					
				WRIST	Flexors	Flex. carpi rad. / Flex. carpi uln.				
					Extensors	Ext. carpi rad. l. & br. / Ext. carpi uln.				
				FINGERS	MP flexors	Lumbricales				
					IP flexors (first)	Flex. digit. sub.				
					IP flexors (second)	Flex. digit. prof.				
					MP extensor	Ext. digit. com.				
					Adductors	Palmar interossei				
					Abductors	Dorsal interossei				
					Abductor digiti quinti					
					Opponens digiti quinti					
				THUMB	MP flexor	Flex. poll. br.				
					IP flexor	Flex. poll. l.				
					MP extensor	Ext. poll. br.				
					IP extensor	Ext. poll. l.				
					Abductors	Abd. poll. br. / Abd. poll. l.				
					Adductor pollicis					
					Opponens pollicis					
				FACE						

Additional data:

FIG. 22-1, cont'd
Muscle examination. (Adapted from March of Dimes Birth Defects Foundation.)

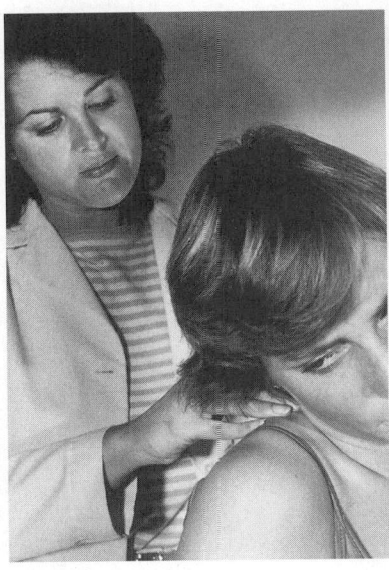 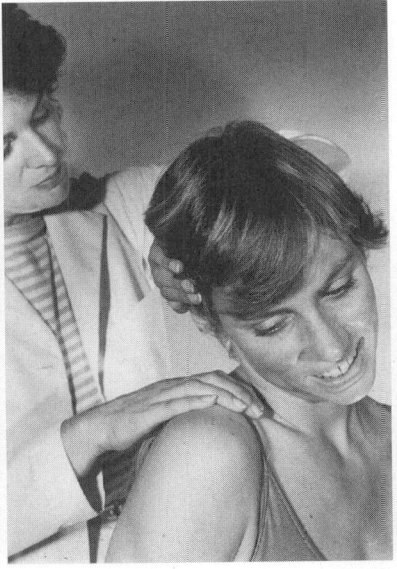 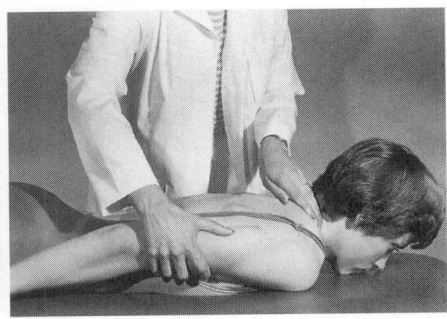

A   B   C

FIG. 22-2
Scapula elevation. **A,** Palpate and observe. **B,** Resist. **C,** Gravity-decreased position.

Procedure for Testing Grades N (5) to F (3)

1. *Position:* S lying prone with arm positioned overhead in 120° to 145° of abduction and resting on the supporting surface. The forearm is in midposition with the thumb toward the ceiling.[10] E stands next to S on the opposite side[7,9] or on the same side.[10]

2. *Stabilize:* The weight of the body is adequate stabilization. This test is given in the gravity-decreased position, because it is not feasible to position S for the against-gravity movement (head down).

   If the deltoid is weak, the arm may be supported and passively raised by E while S attempts the motion.[9]

3. *Palpate:* The lower trapezius distal to the medial end of the spine of the scapula and parallel to the thoracic vertebrae, approximately at the level of the inferior angle of the scapula.[9]

4. *Observe:* S lift the arm off the supporting surface to ear level.[10] During this movement, there is strong downward fixation of the scapula by the lower trapezius (Fig. 22-3, *A*).[9]

5. *Resist:* At the lateral angle of the scapula, toward elevation and abduction (Fig. 22-3, *B*).[9] Resistance may be given on the humerus just above the elbow in a downward direction if shoulder and elbow strength are adequate.[10,11]

Procedure for Testing Grades P (2), T (1), and 0

1. *Position and stabilize:* As described for previous test. No stabilization is required. E may support S's arm if posterior deltoid and triceps are weak.[10]

2. *Palpate and observe:* Same as described for previous test (Fig. 22-3, *C*).

3. *Grade:* Grade P if patient completes full scapular ROM without the weight of the arm.[10]

   Substitutions: Middle trapezius or rhomboids may substitute.[6] Rotation of the inferior angle of the scapula toward the spine is evidence of substitution.[15]

Motion

Scapula abduction and upward rotation.

Muscles[9,11]	Innervation[9,11]
Serratus anterior	Long thoracic nerve, C5-7

Procedure for Testing Grades N (5) to F (3)

1. *Position:* S lying supine with the shoulder flexed to 90° and slightly abducted, elbow extended or fully flexed. E stands next to S on the side being tested.[6,7,9,11]

2. *Stabilize:* The weight of the trunk or over the shoulder.[6]

3. *Palpate:* The digitations of the origin of the serratus anterior on the ribs, along the midaxillary line and just distal and anterior to the axillary border of the scapula.[6,9] Note that muscle contraction may be difficult to detect in women and overweight subjects.

4. *Observe:* S reach upward as if pushing the arm toward the ceiling, abducting the scapula (Fig. 22-4, *A*).[6,9]

5. *Resist:* At the distal end of the humerus and push arm directly downward toward scapula adduction (Fig. 22-4, *B*).[6,7,9] If there is shoulder instability, E should support the arm and not apply resistance. In this instance only a grade of F (3) can be tested.[7]

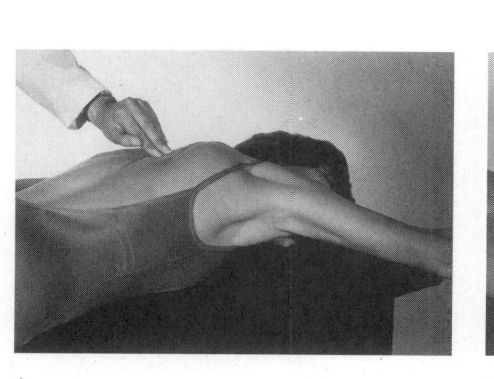
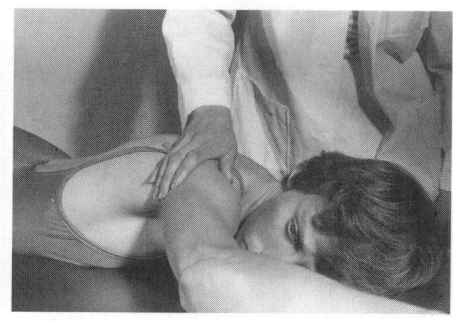
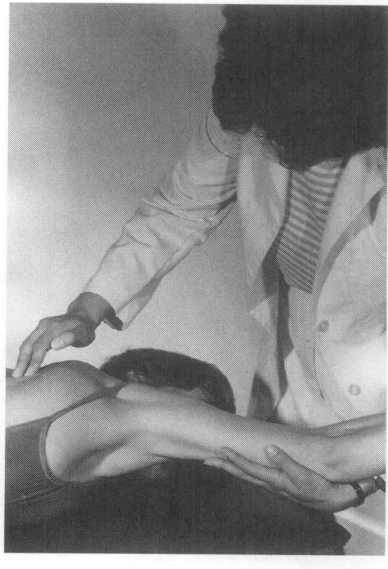

A   B   C

FIG. 22-3
Scapula depression. **A,** Palpate and observe. **B,** Resist. **C,** Test for grades P to O.

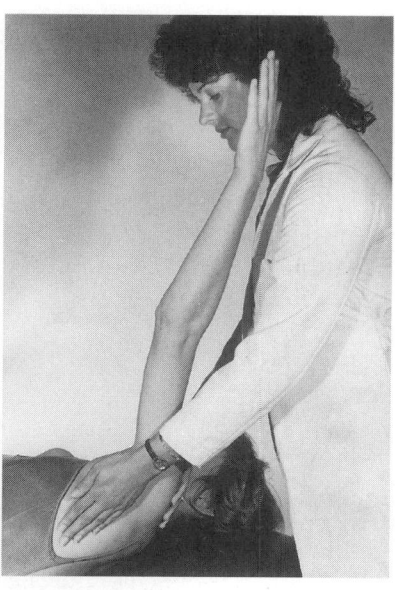
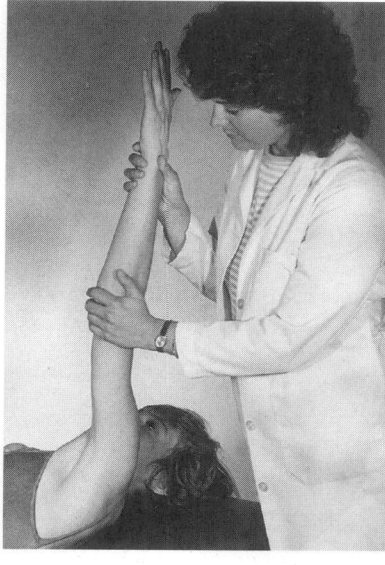
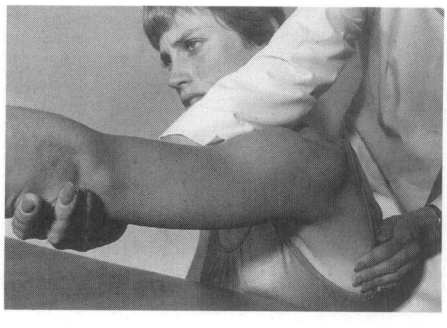

A   B   C

FIG. 22-4
Scapula abduction. **A,** Palpate and observe. **B,** Resist. **C,** Gravity-decreased position.

Procedure for Testing Grades P (2), T (1), and 0

1. *Position:* S seated with the arm supported by E in 90° of shoulder flexion and the elbow extended.[6,9]
2. *Stabilize:* Over the shoulder to be tested.
3. *Palpate:* As described in the previous section.
4. *Observe:* For abduction of the scapula as the arm moves forward (Fig. 22-4, *C*).[9] Weakness of this muscle produces "winging" of the scapula.[8]
5. *Grade:* According to standard definitions of muscle grades.

Substitutions: The pectoralis major and minor may pull the scapula forward into abduction at its insertion on the humerus; the upper and lower trapezius and contralateral trunk rotation may also substitute.[6] E observes for humeral horizontal adduction followed by scapula abduction.[7,12]

Motion

Scapula adduction.

Muscles[9,11]	Innervation[6,9]
Middle trapezius	Spinal accessory nerve, C3,4
Rhomboids	Dorsal scapular nerve, C4,5

Procedure for Testing Grades N (5) to F (3)

1. *Position:* Lying prone with the shoulder abducted to 90° and externally rotated and the elbow flexed to 90°, shoulder resting on the supporting surface. E stands on the side being tested.[9-11]
2. *Stabilize:* The weight of the trunk on the supporting surface is usually adequate stabilization, or over the midthorax to prevent trunk rotation if necessary.
3. *Palpate:* The middle trapezius between the spine of the scapula and the adjacent vertebrae in alignment with the abducted humerus.
4. *Observe:* S lift the arm off the table. Observe movement of the vertebral border of the scapula toward the thoracic vertebrae (Fig. 22-5, A).
5. *Resist:* At the vertebral border of the scapula toward abduction (Fig. 22-5, B).[6,7,9,10]

Procedure for Testing Grades P (2), T (1), and 0

1. *Position and stabilize:* As described for the previous test, but E now supports the weight of the arm by cradling under the humerus and forearm.[12] S may also be positioned sitting erect, with arm resting on a high table and the shoulder midway between 90° flexion and abduction.[9] E stands behind S in this instance.
2. *Palpate and observe:* The middle trapezius. Ask E to bring the shoulders together as if assuming an erect posture. Observe scapula adduction toward the vertebral column (Fig. 22-5, C).
3. *Grade:* According to standard definitions of muscle grades.
   Substitutions: The posterior deltoid can act on the humerus and produce scapula adduction.[6] Observe for humeral extension being used to initiate scapula adduction. Rhomboids may substitute, but scapula will rotate downward.[7,12,15]

Motion

Scapula adduction and downward rotation.

Muscles[7,8]	Innervation[6-8]
Rhomboids major and minor	Dorsal scapular nerve, C4,5
Levator scapula	
Middle trapezius	Spinal accessory nerve, C3,4

Procedure for Testing Grades N (5) to F (3)

1. *Position:* S lying prone with the head rotated to the opposite side; the arm on the side being tested is placed in shoulder adduction and internal rotation, with the elbow slightly flexed and the dorsum of the hand resting over the lumbosacral area of the back.[6,10] E stands opposite the side being tested.[7,8,9]
2. *Stabilize:* The weight of the trunk on the supporting surface offers adequate stabilization.[7,11]
3. *Palpate:* Rhomboid muscles between the vertebral border of the scapula and the 2nd to 5th thoracic vertebrae.[9,11] (They may be more easily discerned toward the lower half of the vertebral border of the scapula, because they lie under the trapezius muscle.)
4. *Observe:* S raise the hand up off the back while maintaining the position of the arm.[7,10] During this

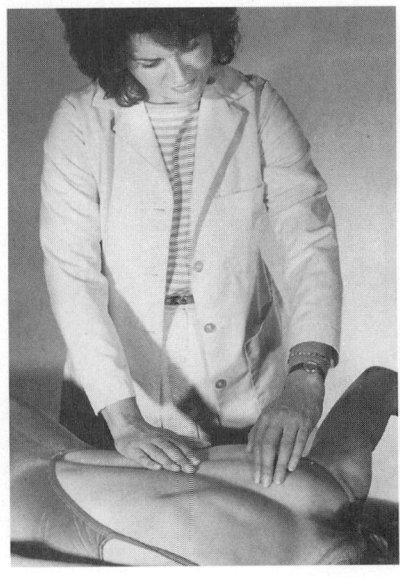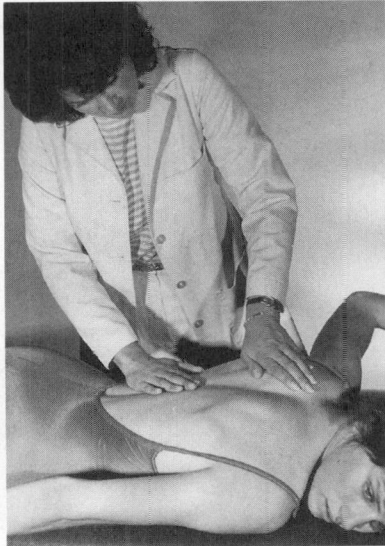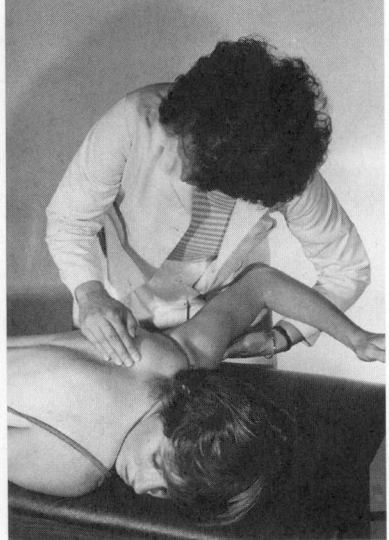

A   B   C

FIG. 22-5
Scapula adduction. **A,** Palpate and observe. **B,** Resist. **C,** Test for grades P to O.

motion, the anterior aspect of the shoulder must lift from the table surface. Observe scapula adduction and downward rotation while the shoulder joint is in some extension (Fig. 22-6, *A*).[9]

5. *Resist:* Over the scapula toward abduction and upward rotation[6] (Fig. 22-6, *B*).

Procedure for Testing Grades P (2), T (1), and 0

1. *Position:* S sitting erect with the arm positioned behind the back in the same manner described for the previous test. E stands behind S, a little opposite the side being tested.[9]
2. *Stabilize:* Trunk by placing one hand over the shoulder, opposite the one being tested, to prevent trunk flexion and rotation.
3. *Palpate:* The rhomboids as described above.
4. *Observe:* Scapula adduction and downward rotation as S lifts the hand away from the back (Fig. 22-6, *C*).
5. *Grade:* According to standard definitions of muscle grades.

Substitutions: Middle trapezius, but the movement will not be accompanied by downward rotation.[10] The posterior deltoid acting to perform horizontal abduction or glenohumeral extension can produce scapula adduction through momentum. Scapula adduction would be preceded by extension or abduction of the humerus.[12,15] The pectoralis minor could tip the scapula forward.[7]

Motion

Shoulder flexion.

Muscles[9]	Innervation[6,9]
Anterior deltoid	Axillary nerve, C5,6
Coracobrachialis	Musculocutaneous nerve, C5-7

Procedure for Testing Grades N (5) to F (3)

1. *Position:* S seated, with the arm relaxed at the side of the body and the hand facing backward.[10] A straight-backed chair may be used to offer trunk support. E stands on the side being tested and slightly behind S.[7,9,15]
2. *Stabilize:* Over the shoulder being tested, but allow the normal abduction and upward rotation of the scapula that occurs with this movement.[9,10]
3. *Palpate:* The anterior deltoid just below the clavicle on the anterior aspect of the humeral head.[7]
4. *Observe:* S flex the shoulder joint to 90° of flexion (parallel to the floor) (Fig. 22-7, *A*).[6,9,10]
5. *Resist:* At the distal end of the humerus downward toward shoulder extension (Fig. 22-7, *B*).[6,7,8,10]

Procedure for Testing Grades P(2), T(1), and 0

1. *Position:* S in side-lying position. The side being tested is superior. If S cannot maintain weight of the arm against gravity, E can support it.[6,10] If the side-lying position is not feasible, S may remain seated, and the test procedure described above can be performed with the grading modified.[9]
2. *Palpate and observe:* The same as described for the previous test. The arm is moved toward the face to 90° of shoulder flexion (Fig. 22-7, *C*).
3. *Grade:* According to standard definitions of muscle grades. If the seated position was used for the tests of

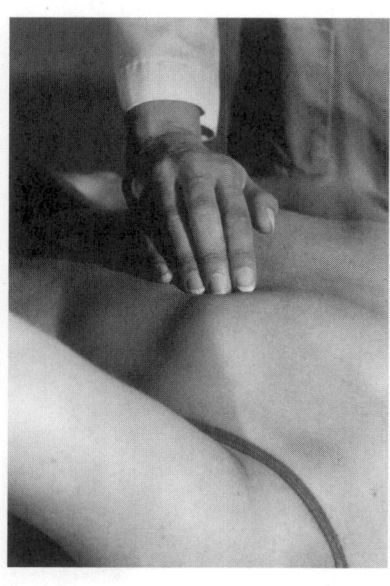 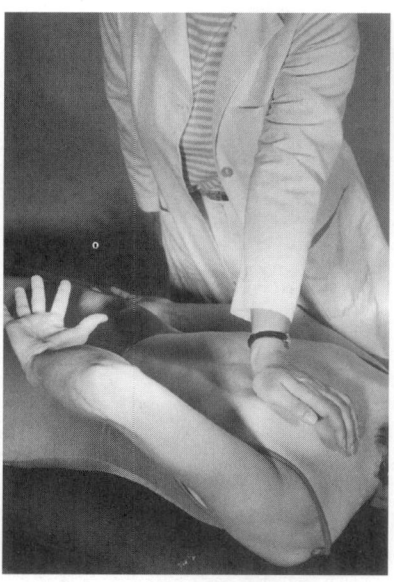 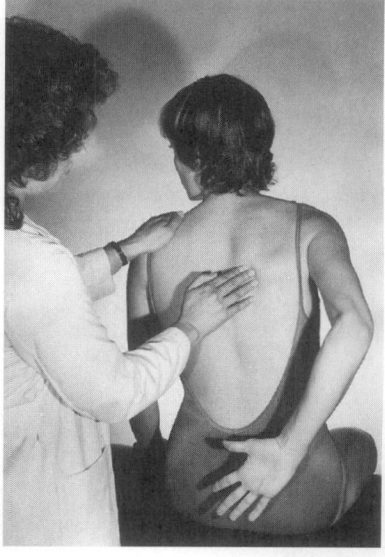

A   B   C

FIG. 22-6
Scapula adduction and downward rotation. **A,** Palpate and observe. **B,** Resist. **C,** Gravity-decreased position.

grades poor to zero, partial ROM against gravity should be graded poor.[9,10]

Substitutions: Clavicular fibers of the pectoralis major can perform flexion through partial ROM while performing horizontal adduction. The biceps brachii may flex the shoulder, but the humerus will first be rotated externally for the best mechanical advantage. The upper trapezius will assist flexion by elevating the scapula. Observe for flexion accompanied by horizontal adduction, external rotation, or scapula elevation.[10,12,15]

Note: Arm elevation in the plane of the scapula, about halfway between shoulder flexion and abduction, is called *scaption.* This movement is more commonly used for function than either shoulder flexion or abduction. Scaption is performed by the deltoid and supraspinatus muscles It is tested similarly to shoulder flexion, described earlier, except that the arm is elevated in a position 30° to 45° anterior to the frontal plane.[6,10]

Motion

Shoulder extension.

Muscles[4,9,11]	Innervation[6,9]
Latissimus dorsi	Thoracodorsal nerve, C6-8
Teres major	Lower subscapular nerve, C5-7
Posterior deltoid	Axillary nerve, C5,6

Procedure for Testing Grades N (5) to F (3)

1. *Position:* S lying prone, with the shoulder joint adducted and internally rotated so that the palm of the hand is facing up.[6,7,10] E stands on the opposite side or on the test side.
2. *Stabilize:* Over the scapula on the side being tested.
3. *Palpate:* The teres major along the axillary border of the scapula. The latissimus dorsi may be palpated slightly below this point or closer to its origins parallel to the thoracic and lumbar vertebrae.[7,9] The posterior deltoid may be found over the posterior aspect of the humeral head (Fig. 22-8, *A*).
4. *Observe:* S extending the shoulder joint.
5. *Resist:* At the distal end of the humerus in a downward and outward direction, toward flexion and slight abduction (Fig. 22-8, *B*).[6,7,9-11]

Procedure for Testing Grades P (2), T (1), and 0

1. *Position:* S in the side-lying position; E stands behind S.[6]
2. *Stabilize:* Over the scapula. If S cannot maintain the weight of the part against gravity, E should support S's arm.[6] If the side-lying position is not feasible, S may remain in the prone lying position and the test may be performed as described for the previous test with modified grading.[9]
3. *Palpate:* The teres major or latissimus dorsi as described for the previous test.

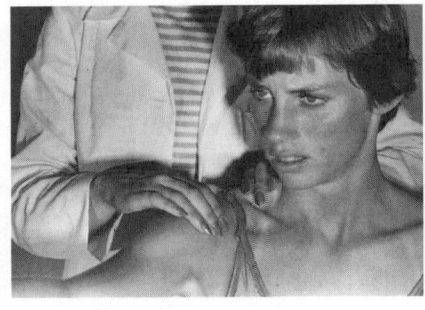
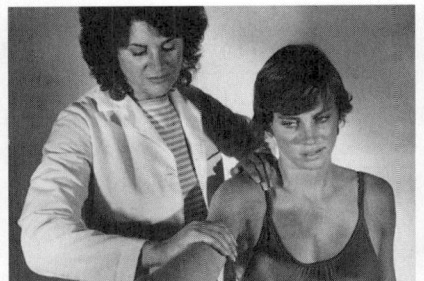
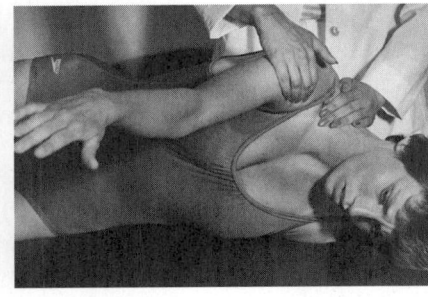

A B C

FIG. 22-7
Shoulder flexion. **A,** Palpate and observe. **B,** Resist. **C,** Gravity-decreased position.

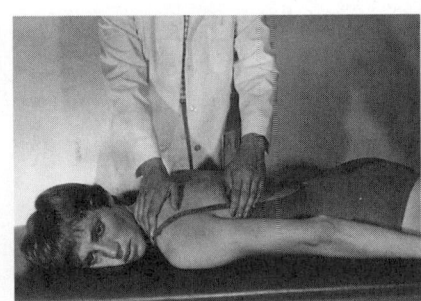
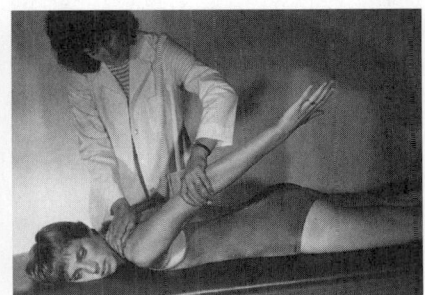
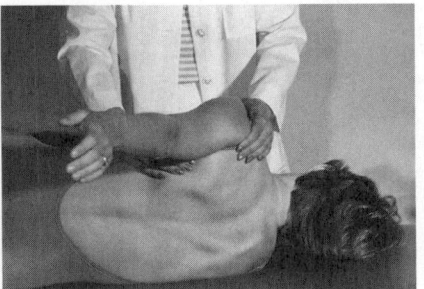

A B C

FIG. 22-8
Shoulder extension. **A,** Palpate and observe. **B,** Resist. **C,** Gravity-decreased position.

4. *Observe:* S extend the arm backward in a plane parallel to the floor (Fig. 22-8, *C*).
5. *Grade:* According to standard definitions of muscle grades. If the test for grades poor to zero was done in the prone-lying position, completion of partial ROM should be graded poor.[9]

Substitutions: Scapula adduction can substitute. Observe for flexion of the shoulder or adduction of the scapula preceding extension of the humerus.[12]

Motion

Shoulder abduction to 90°.

Muscles[9,11]	Innervation[9]
Middle deltoid	Axillary nerve, C5,6
Supraspinatus	Suprascapular nerve, C5

Procedure for Testing Grades N (5) to F (3)

1. *Position:* S seated, with arms relaxed at the sides of the body. The elbow on the side to be tested should be slightly flexed and the palms facing toward the body. E stands behind S.[6,7,10]
2. *Stabilize:* Over the scapula on the side to be tested.[6,9,11]
3. *Palpate:* The middle deltoid over the middle of the shoulder joint from the acromion to the deltoid tuberosity.[6,9,11,12] The supraspinatus is too deep to palpate.[6]
4. *Observe:* S abduct the shoulder to 90°. During the movement, S's palm should remain down and E should observe that there is no external rotation of the shoulder or elevation of the scapula.[6,9-12] (Fig. 22-9, *A*).
5. *Resist:* At the distal end of the humerus toward adduction (Fig. 22-9, *B*).[10]

Procedure for Testing Grades P (2), T (1), and 0

1. *Position:* S in supine position, lying with the arm to be tested resting at the side of the body, palm facing in and the elbow slightly flexed. E stands in front of the supporting surface toward the side to be tested.[9,10]

2. *Stabilize:* Over the shoulder to be tested.
3. *Palpate and observe:* The same as described for the previous test. E asks S to bring the arm out and away from the body, abducting the shoulder to 90° (Fig. 22-9, *C*).
4. *Grade:* According to standard definitions of muscle grades.

Substitutions: The long head of the biceps may attempt to substitute. Observe for elbow flexion and external rotation accompanying the movement.[10] The anterior and posterior deltoids can act together to effect abduction. The upper trapezius may attempt to assist. Observe for scapula elevation preceding the movement.[7,12,15]

Motion

Shoulder external rotation.

Muscles[4,9,11]	Innervation[4,9,11]
Infraspinatus	Suprascapular nerve, C5,6
Teres minor	Axillary nerve, C5,6

Procedure for Testing Grades N (5) to F (3)

1. *Position:* S lying prone, with the shoulder abducted to 90° and the humerus in neutral (0°) rotation, elbow flexed to 90°. Forearm is in neutral rotation, hanging over the edge of the table, perpendicular to the floor.[6-8,10] E stands in front of the supporting surface, toward the side to be tested.[9,11]
2. *Stabilize:* At the distal end of the humerus by placing a hand under the arm on the supporting surface to prevent shoulder abduction.[7,11]
3. *Palpate:* The infraspinatus muscle just below the spine of the scapula on the body of the scapula[6] or the teres minor along the axillary border of the scapula.[9]
4. *Observe:* S rotate the humerus so that the back of the hand is moving toward the ceiling (Fig. 22-10, *A*).[6,7,9-11]
5. *Resist:* On the distal end of the forearm toward the floor in the direction of internal rotation (Fig. 22-10, *B*).[6,9-11] Apply resistance gently and slowly to prevent

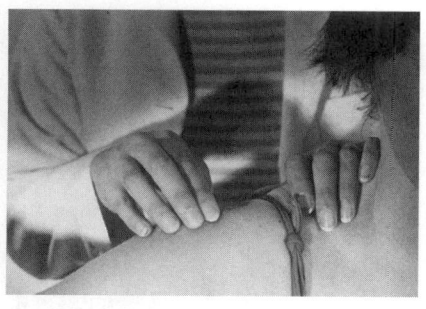   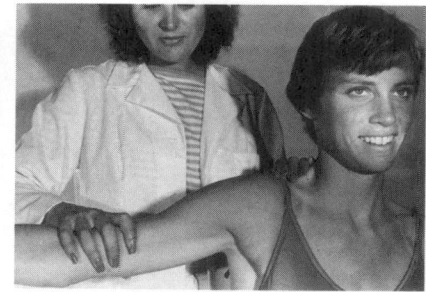   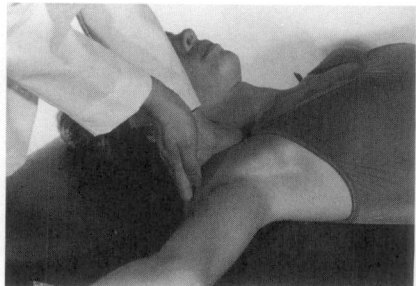

A   **B**   **C**

FIG. 22-9
Shoulder abduction. **A,** Palpate and observe. **B,** Resist. **C,** Gravity-decreased position.

injury to the glenohumeral joint, which is inherently unstable.[10]

Procedure for Testing Grades P (2), T (1), and 0

1. *Position:* S seated, with arm adducted and in neutral rotation at the shoulder. The elbow is flexed to 90° with the forearm in neutral rotation. E stands in front of S toward the side to be tested.[6,7]
2. *Stabilize:* Arm against the trunk at the distal end of the humerus to prevent abduction and extension of the shoulder, and over the shoulder to be tested.[5,7,15] The hand stabilizing over the shoulder can be used to palpate the infraspinatus simultaneously.
3. *Palpate:* The infraspinatus and teres minor as described for previous test.
4. *Observe:* S move the forearm away from the body by rotating the humerus while maintaining neutral rotation of the forearm (Fig. 22-10, C).[6,15]
5. *Grade:* According to standard definitions of muscle grades.

   Substitutions: If the elbow is extended and S supinates the forearm, the momentum could aid external rotation of the humerus. Scapular adduction can pull the humerus backward and into some external rotation. E should observe for scapula adduction and initiation of movement with forearm supination.[12,15]

Motion

Shoulder internal rotation.

Muscles[9,11,12]	Innervation[4,5,9]
Subscapularis	Subscapular nerve, C5,6
Pectoralis major	Medial and lateral pectoral nerves, C5-T1
Latissimus dorsi	Thoracodorsal nerve, C6-8
Teres major	Subscapular nerve, C5-7

Procedure for Testing Grades N (5) to F (3)

1. *Position:* S lying prone with the shoulder abducted to 90° and the humerus in neutral rotation, the elbow flexed to 90°. A rolled towel may be placed under the humerus. The forearm is perpendicular to the floor. E stands on the side to be tested, just in front of S's arm.[6-8,10]
2. *Stabilize:* At the distal end of the humerus by placing a hand under the arm and on the supporting surface, as for external rotation.[6,7,9,11]
3. *Palpate:* The teres major and latissimus dorsi along the axillary border of the scapula toward the inferior angle.
4. *Observe:* S internally rotate the humerus, moving the palm of the hand upward toward the ceiling (Fig. 22-11, A).[6,9]
5. *Resist:* At the distal end of the volar surface of the forearm anteriorly toward external rotation (Fig. 22-11, B).[7,9-11]

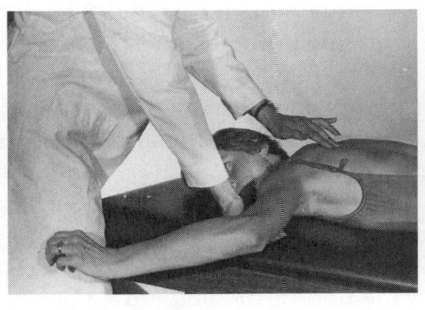 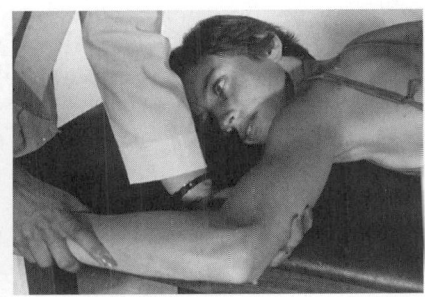 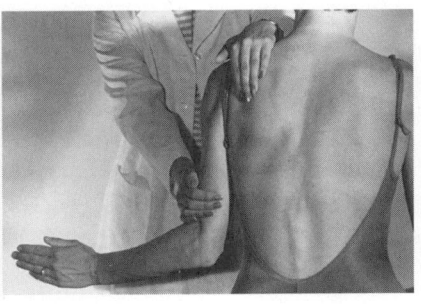

A   B   C

FIG. 22-10
Shoulder external rotation. **A,** Palpate and observe. **B,** Resist. **C,** Gravity-decreased position.

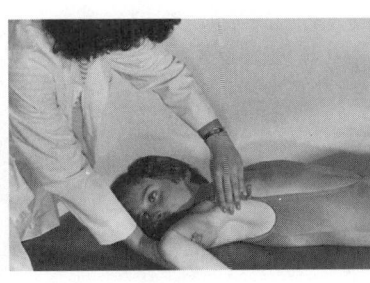 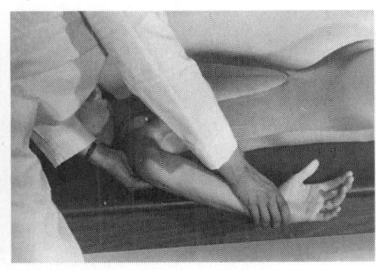 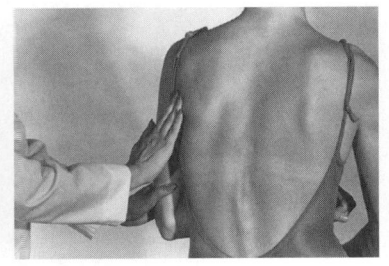

A   B   C

FIG. 22-11
Shoulder internal rotation. **A,** Palpate and observe. **B,** Resist. **C,** Gravity-decreased position.

Procedure for Testing Grades P (2), T (1), and 0

1. *Position:* S seated, with the shoulder adducted and in neutral rotation, elbow flexed to 90° with the forearm in neutral rotation. E stands on the side to be tested.[6,15]
2. *Stabilize:* Arm at the distal end of the humerus against the trunk to prevent abduction and extension of the shoulder.
3. *Palpate:* The teres major and latissimus dorsi, as described for the previous test.
4. *Observe:* S move the palm of the hand toward the chest, internally rotating the humerus (Fig. 22-11, *C*).

    Substitutions: If the trunk is rotated, gravity will act on the humerus, rotating it internally.[6] E should observe for trunk rotation. When the elbow is in extension, pronation of the forearm can substitute.[10,12,15]

Motion

Shoulder horizontal abduction.

Muscles[4,9,12]	Innervation[9,10]
Posterior deltoid	Axillary nerve, C5,6
Infraspinatus	Suprascapular nerve, C5,6

Procedure for Testing Grades N (5) to F (3)

1. *Position:* S prone, with the shoulder abducted to 90° and in slight external rotation, elbow flexed to 90°, and forearm perpendicular to the floor. E stands on the side being tested.[11,12]
2. *Stabilize:* Over the scapula.[6,9]
3. *Palpate:* The posterior deltoid below the spine of the scapula and distally toward the deltoid tuberosity on the posterior aspect of the shoulder.[9]
4. *Observe:* S horizontally abduct the humerus, lifting the arm toward the ceiling (Fig. 22-12, *A*).[10]
5. *Resist:* Just proximal to the elbow obliquely downward horizontal adduction (Fig. 22-12, *B*).[6,10,11]

Procedure for Testing Grades P (2), T (1), and 0

1. *Position:* S seated, with the arm in 90° abduction, the elbow flexed to 90 degrees and the palm down, sup-

ported on a high table or by E.[6,10] If a table is used, powder may be sprinkled on the surface to reduce friction.
2. *Stabilize:* Over the scapula.
3. *Palpate:* The posterior deltoid, as described for the previous test.
4. *Observe:* S pull arm backward into horizontal abduction (Fig. 22-12, *C*).
5. *Grade:* According to standard definitions of muscle grades.

    Substitutions: Latissimus dorsi and teres major may assist the movement if the posterior deltoid is very weak. Movement will occur with more shoulder extension rather than at the horizontal level. Scapula adduction may produce slight horizontal abduction of the humerus, but trunk rotation and shoulder retraction would occur.[6,12,15] The long head of the triceps may substitute. Maintain some flexion at the elbow to prevent this.[10]

Motion

Shoulder horizontal adduction.

Muscles[4,10,12]	Innervation[4,9,10]
Pectoralis major	Medial and lateral pectoral nerves, C5-T1
Anterior deltoid	Axillary nerve, C5,6
Coracobrachialis	Musculocutaneous nerve, C6,7

Procedure for Testing Grades N (5) to F (3)

1. *Position:* S supine, with the shoulder abducted to 90°, elbow flexed or extended. E stands next to S on the side being tested or behind S's head.[4,6,7,9,10]
2. *Stabilize:* The trunk by placing one hand over the shoulder on the side being tested to prevent trunk rotation and scapula elevation.
3. *Palpate:* Over the insertion of the pectoralis major at the anterior aspect of the axilla.[6]
4. *Observe:* S horizontally adduct the humerus, moving the arm toward the opposite shoulder to a position of 90° of shoulder flexion.[11] If S cannot maintain elbow extension, E may guide the forearm to prevent the hand from hitting S's face (Fig. 22-13, *A*).

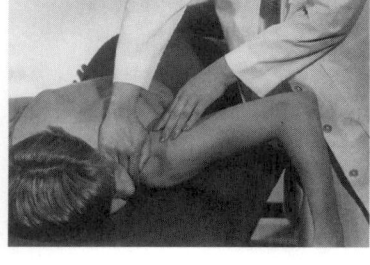 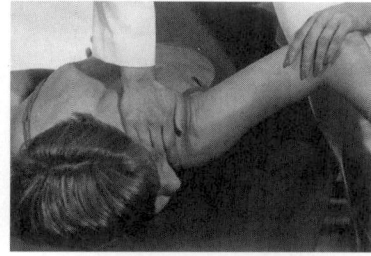 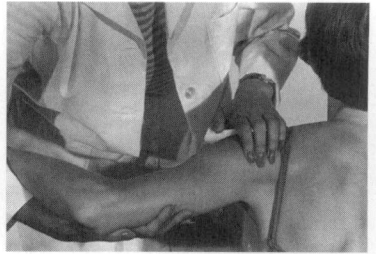

A   B   C

FIG. 22-12
Shoulder horizontal abduction. **A,** Palpate and observe. **B,** Resist. **C,** Gravity-decreased position.

5. *Resist:* At the distal end of the humerus, in an outward direction toward horizontal abduction (Fig. 22-13, B).[6,7,9]

Procedure for Testing Grades P (2), T (1), and 0

1. *Position:* S seated next to a high table with the arm supported in 90° of shoulder abduction and slight flexion at the elbow.[4,10,15] Powder may be sprinkled on the supporting surface to reduce the effect of resistance from friction during the movement, or E may support the arm.[6]
2. *Stabilize:* Over the shoulder on the side being tested, using the stabilizing hand simultaneously to palpate the pectoralis major muscle.[6]
3. *Palpate:* The pectoralis major, as described for the previous test.
4. *Observe:* S horizontally adduct the arm toward the opposite shoulder, in a plane parallel to the floor (Fig. 22-13, C).

Substitutions: Muscles may substitute for one another. If the pectoralis major is not functioning, the other muscles will perform the motion, which will be considerably weakened.[12] Contralateral trunk rotation, the coracobrachialis, or short head of the biceps may substitute.[6]

Motion

Elbow flexion.

Muscles[9,10,11]	Innervation[10,11]
Biceps brachii	Musculocutaneous nerve C5,6
Brachialis	
Brachioradialis	Radial nerve C5,6

Procedure for Testing Grades N (5) to F (3)

1. *Position:* S sitting, with the arm adducted at the shoulder and extended at the elbow, held against the side of the trunk. The forearm is supinated to test for the biceps, primarily (Forearm should be positioned in pronation to test for the brachialis, primarily, and in midposition to test for brachioradialis).[9,10] E

stands next to S on the side being tested or directly in front of S.
2. *Stabilize:* The humerus in adduction.
3. *Palpate:* The biceps brachii over the muscle belly, on the middle of the anterior aspect of the humerus. Its tendon may be palpated in the middle of the antecubital space.[6,7,9] (Brachioradialis is palpated over the upper third of the radius on the lateral aspect of the forearm, just below the elbow. The brachialis may be palpated lateral to the lower portion of the biceps brachii, if the elbow is flexed and in the pronated position.[12])
4. *Observe:* S flex elbow, hand toward the face. E should observe for maintenance of forearm in supination (when testing for biceps) and for relaxed or extended wrist and fingers (Fig. 22-14, A).[6,12]
5. *Resist:* At the distal end of the volar aspect of the forearm, pulling downward toward elbow extension (Fig. 22-14, B).[7,9,11]

Procedure for Testing Grades P (2), T (1), and 0

1. *Position:* S supine, with the shoulder abducted to 90° and externally rotated, elbow extended, and forearm supinated. E stands at the head of the table on the side being tested. (S may also be seated, side being tested resting on the treatment table, which is at axillary height, humerus in 90° abduction, elbow extended, and forearm in neutral position.)[7]
2. *Stabilize:* The humerus. The stabilizing hand can be used simultaneously for palpation here.
3. *Palpate:* The biceps as described for the previous test.
4. *Observe:* S flex the elbow, the hand toward the shoulder.[9] Watch for maintenance of forearm supination and relaxation of the fingers and wrist (Fig. 22-14, C).[12]
5. *Grade:* According to standard definitions of muscle grades.

Substitutions: The brachioradialis will substitute for the biceps, but the forearm will move to midposition during flexion of the elbow. Wrist and finger flexors may assist elbow flexion, which will be preceded by finger

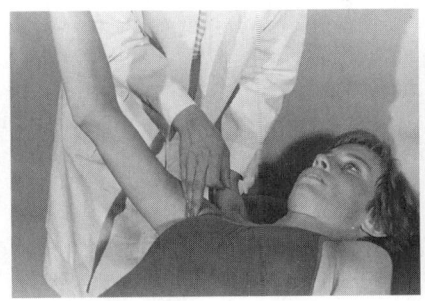 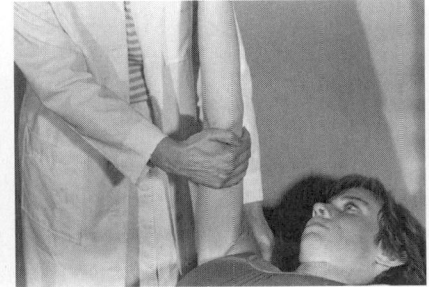 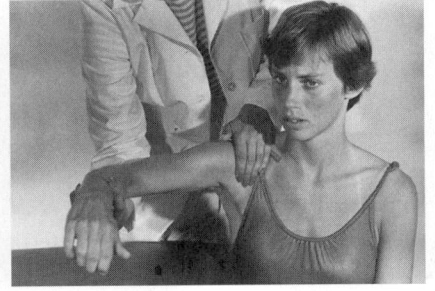

A   B   C

FIG. 22-13
Shoulder horizontal adduction. **A,** Palpate and observe. **B,** Resist. **C,** Gravity-decreased position.

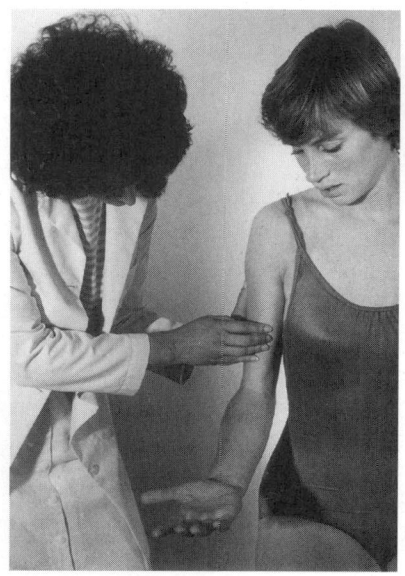 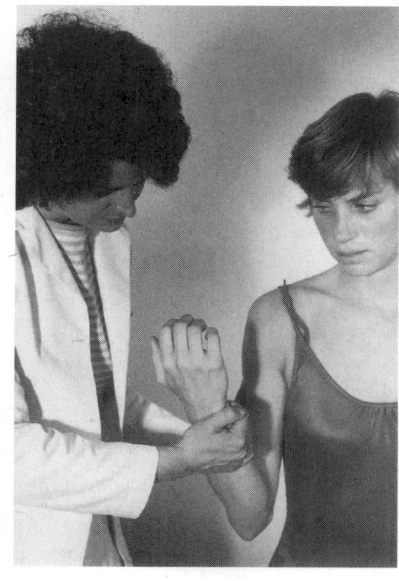 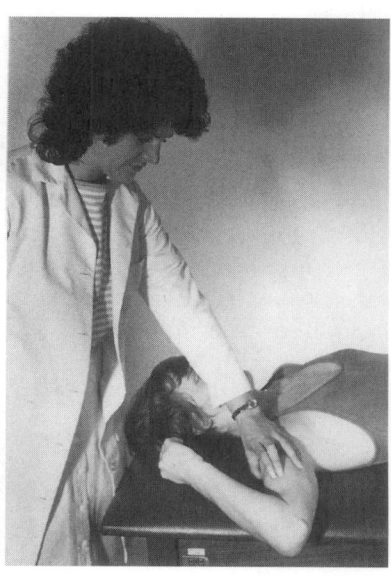

A   B   C

FIG. 22-14
Elbow flexion. **A,** Palpate and observe. **B,** Resist. **C,** Gravity-decreased position.

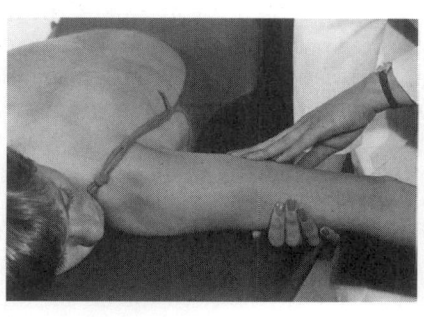 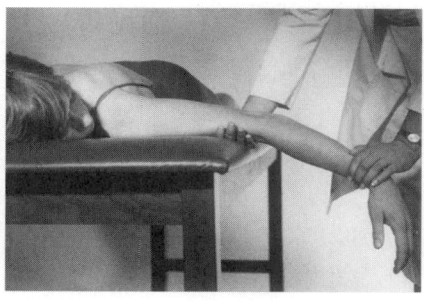 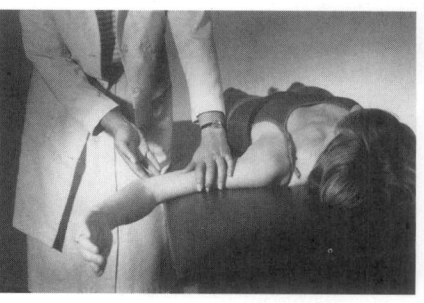

A   B   C

FIG. 22-15
Elbow extension. **A,** Palpate and observe. **B,** Resist. **C,** Gravity-decreased position.

and wrist flexion.[9,10,12] The pronator teres may assist. Forearm pronation during the movement may be evidence of this substitution.[12]

Motion

Elbow extension.

Muscles[6,9,10]	Innervation[9-11]
Triceps	Radial nerve, C6-8
Aconeus	Radial nerve, C7,8

Procedure for Testing Grades N (5) to F (3)

1. *Position:* S prone, with the humerus abducted to 90°, the elbow flexed to 90°, and the forearm in neutral rotation and perpendicular to the floor. E stands next to S, just behind the arm to be tested.[7,11,15]
2. *Stabilize:* The humerus by placing one hand for support under it, between S's arm and the table.[10,11]

3. *Palpate:* The triceps over the middle of the posterior aspect of the humerus or the triceps tendon just proximal to the olecranon process on the dorsal surface of the arm.[6,7,9,12]
4. *Observe:* S extend the elbow to just less than maximum range. The wrist and fingers remain relaxed (Fig. 22-15, *A*).
5. *Resist:* At the distal end of the forearm into elbow flexion. Before resistance is given, be sure that the elbow is not locked. Resistance to a locked elbow can cause joint injury (Fig. 22-15, *B*).[6,9]

Procedure for Testing Grades P (2), T (1), and 0

1. *Position:* S supine, with the humerus abducted to 90° and in external rotation, the elbow fully flexed, and the forearm supinated. E is standing next to S, just behind the arm to be tested.[9] An alternate position is with S seated, shoulder abducted to 90° in neutral

rotation, elbow flexed, and forearm in neutral position, supported by E.[7,10]

2. *Stabilize:* The humerus by holding one hand over the middle or distal end to prevent shoulder motion.
3. *Palpate:* The triceps as described for the previous test.
4. *Observe:* S extend the elbow, moving the hand away from the head (Fig. 22-15, *C*).
5. *Grade:* According to standard definitions of muscle grades.

Substitutions: Finger and wrist extensors may substitute for weak elbow extensors. Observe for finger and wrist extension preceding elbow extension. When upright, gravity and eccentric contraction of the biceps will effect elbow extension from the flexed position,[12] scapula depression, and shoulder external rotation, aided by gravity.[6]

Motion

Forearm supination.

Muscles[4,9,10]	Innervation[6,9,10]
Biceps brachii	Musculocutaneous nerve, C5,6
Supinator	Radial nerve, C5-7

Procedure for Testing Grades N (5) to F (3)

1. *Position:* S seated, with the humerus adducted, the elbow flexed to 90°, and the forearm pronated. E stands in front of S or next to S on the side to be tested.[6,7,9,10]
2. *Stabilize:* The humerus just proximal to the elbow.[6,9]
3. *Palpate:* Over the supinator muscle on the dorsal-lateral aspect of the forearm, below the head of the radius. The muscle can be best felt when the radial muscle group (extensor carpi radialis and brachioradialis) are pushed up out of the way.[4] E may also palpate the biceps on the middle of the anterior surface of the humerus.[6,7]
4. *Observe:* S supinate the forearm, turning the hand palm up. Because gravity assists the movement, after the 0° neutral position is passed, the therapist may apply slight resistance equal to the weight of the forearm(Fig. 22-16, *A*).[6,7]
5. *Resist:* By grasping around the dorsal aspect of the distal forearm with the fingers and heel of the hand, turning the arm toward pronation(Fig. 22-16, *B*).[6]

Procedure for Testing Grades P (2), T (1), and 0

1. *Position:* S seated, shoulder flexed to 90° and the upper arm resting on the supporting surface, elbow flexed to 90°, and the forearm in full pronation in a position perpendicular to the floor.[6,7,15] E stands next to S on the side to be tested.
2. *Stabilize:* The humerus just proximal to the elbow.[6]
3. *Palpate:* The supinator or biceps as described for the previous test.
4. *Observe:* S supinate the forearm, turning the palm of the hand toward the face (Fig. 22-16, *C*).
5. *Grade:* According to standard definitions of muscle grades.

Substitutions: With the elbow flexed, external rotation and horizontal adduction of the humerus will effect forearm supination. With the elbow extended, shoulder external rotation will place the forearm in supination. The brachioradialis can bring the forearm from full pronation to midposition. Wrist and thumb extensors,

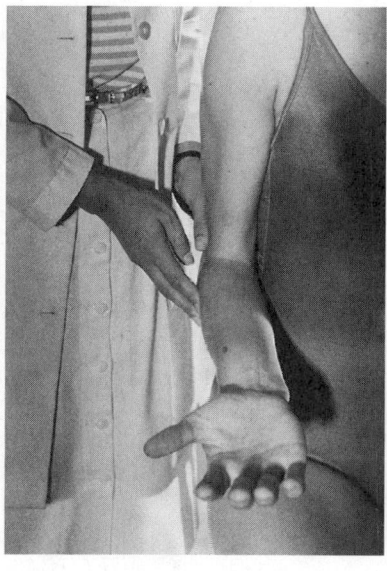   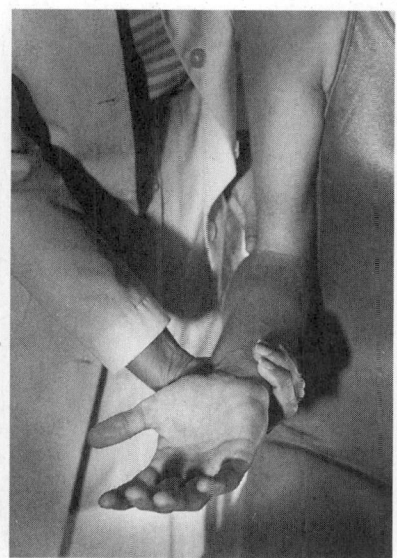   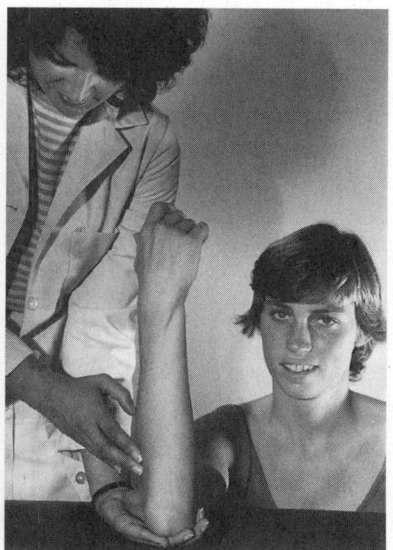

A   B   C

FIG. 22-16
Forearm supination. **A,** Palpate and observe. **B,** Resist. **C,** Gravity-decreased position.

assisted by gravity, can initiate supination. E should observe for external rotation of the humerus, supination to midline only, and initiation of motion by wrist and thumb extension.[10,12,15]

Motion

Forearm pronation.

Muscles[4,10,12]	Innervation[10,11]
Pronator teres	Median nerve, C6,7
Pronator quadratus	Median nerve, C6-8

Procedure for Testing Grades N (5) to F (3)
1. *Position:* S seated, with the humerus adducted, the elbow flexed to 90°, and the forearm in full supination. E stands beside S on the side to be tested.[6,7,9,10]
2. *Stabilize:* The humerus just proximal to the elbow to prevent shoulder abduction.[6,7,9,11]
3. *Palpate:* The pronator teres on the upper part of the volar surface of the forearm, medial to the biceps tendon and diagonally from the medial condyle of the humerus to the lateral border of the radius.[7,9,11,12]
4. *Observe:* S pronate the forearm, turning the hand palm down (Fig. 22-17, *A*).[9] Slight resistance may be applied after the arm has passed midposition to compensate for the assistance of gravity after that point.[6]
5. *Resist:* By grasping over the dorsal aspect of the distal forearm using the fingers and heel of the hand and turn toward supination (Fig. 22-17, *B*).

Procedure for Testing Grades P (2), T (1), and 0
1. *Position:* S seated, shoulder flexed to 90°, elbow flexed to 90°, and the forearm in full supination. The upper arm is resting on the supporting surface and the forearm is perpendicular to the floor.[15] E stands next to S on the side to be tested.
2. *Palpate:* Palpate the pronator teres as described for the previous test.
3. *Observe:* S pronate the forearm, turning the palm of the hand away from the face (Fig. 22-17, *C*).
4. *Grade:* According to standard definitions of muscle grades.
   Substitutions: With the elbow flexed, internal rotation and abduction of the humerus will produce apparent forearm pronation. With the elbow extended, internal rotation can place the forearm in a pronated position. Brachioradialis can bring the fully supinated forearm to midposition. Wrist flexion, aided by gravity, can effect pronation.[6,7,9,10,12,15]

Motion

Wrist extension with radial deviation.

Muscles[9-11]	Innervation[6,10]
Extensor carpi radialis longus (ECRL)	Radial nerve, C5-7
Extensor carpi radialis brevis (ECRB)	Radial nerve, C6-8
Extensor carpi ulnaris (ECU)	

Procedure for Testing Grades N (5) to F (3)
1. *Position:* S seated or supine, with the forearm resting on the supporting surface in pronation, the wrist at neutral, and the fingers and thumb relaxed. E sits opposite S or next to S on the side to be tested.[9,11]
2. *Stabilize:* Over the volar or dorsal aspect of the distal forearm.[6,9,11]

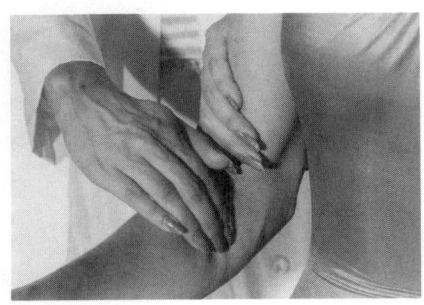

A

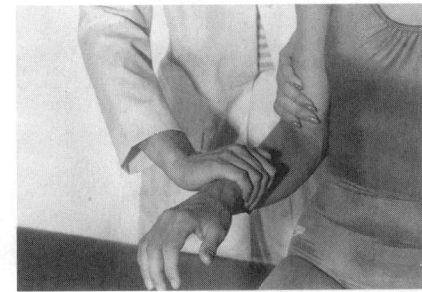

B

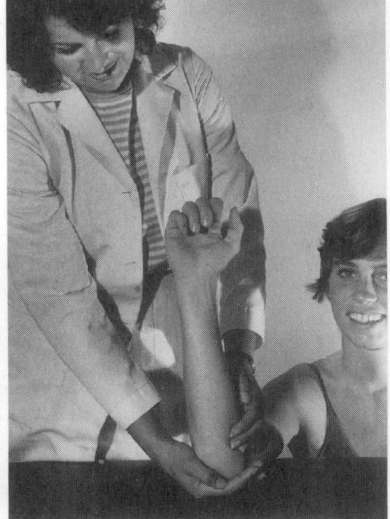

C

FIG. 22-17
Forearm pronation. **A,** Palpate and observe. **B,** Resist. **C,** Gravity-decreased position.

3. *Palpate:* The ECRL and ECRB tendons on the dorsal aspect of the wrist at the bases of the 2nd and 3rd metacarpals, respectively.[6,7,9] The tendon of the ECU may be palpated at the base of the 5th metacarpal, just distal to the head of the ulna (Fig. 22-18, *A*).[4,6,9,12]

4. *Observe:* S extend and radially deviate the wrist, lifting the hand from the supporting surface and simultaneously moving it medially (to the radial side). The movement should be performed without finger extension, which could substitute for the wrist motion (Fig. 22-18, *B*).[6,9,12]

5. *Resist:* Over the dorsum of the 2nd and 3rd metacarpals, toward flexion and ulnar deviation (Fig. 22-18, *C*).[6,9-11]

Procedure for Testing Grades P (2), T (1), and 0

1. *Position:* As described for the previous test, except that the forearm is resting in midposition on its ulnar border.[9,15]

2. *Stabilize:* At the ulnar border of the forearm, supported slightly above the table surface.[9]

3. *Palpate:* Radial wrist extensors as described for the previous test.

4. *Observe:* S extend the wrist, moving the hand away from the body (Fig. 22-18, *D*).

5. *Grade:* According to standard definitions of muscle grades.

Substitutions: Wrist extensors can substitute for one another. In the absence of the extensor carpi radialis muscles, the extensor carpi ulnaris will extend the wrist, but in an ulnar direction. The combined extension and radial deviation will not be possible. The extensor digitorum communis muscle and the extensor pollicis longus can initiate wrist extension, but finger or thumb extension will precede wrist extension.[6,7,10,12,15]

Motion

Wrist extension with ulnar deviation.

Muscles[9-1]	Innervation[10,11]
Extensor carpi ulnaris (ECU)	Radial nerve, C6-8
Extensor carpi radialis brevis (ECRB)	
Extensor carpi radialis longus (ECRL)	Radial nerve, C5-7

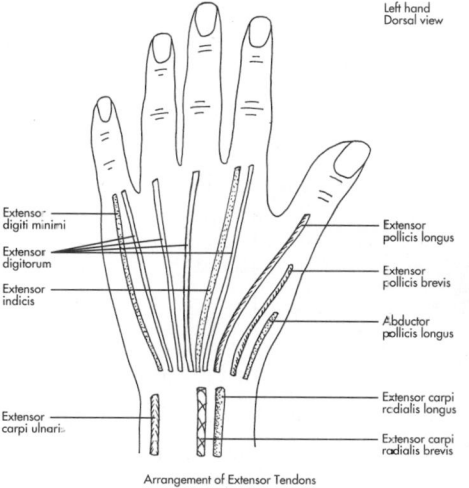

A

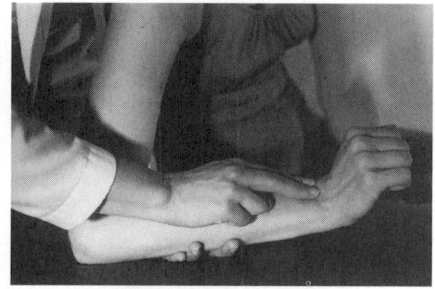

B

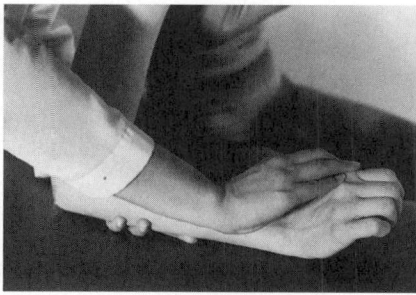

C

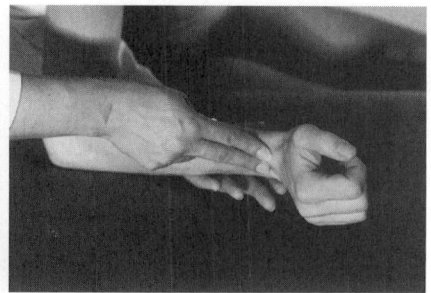

D

FIG. 22-18
A, Arrangement of extensor tendons at wrist. **B,** Wrist extension with radial deviation. Palpate and observe. **C,** Resist. **D,** Gravity-decreased position.

Procedure for Testing Grades N (5) to F (3)

1. *Position:* S seated, forearm pronated, wrist neutral, fingers and thumb relaxed, supported on a table. E sits opposite or next to S on the side to be tested.
2. *Stabilize:* Under the distal forearm.[9-11]
3. *Palpate:* ECU tendon at the base of the 5th metacarpal, just distal to the ulna styloid,[6] and the ECRL and ECRB tendons at the bases of the 2nd and 3rd metacarpals.
4. *Observe:* S extend the wrist and simultaneously move it laterally (to the ulnar side). E should observe that the movement is not preceded by thumb or finger extension (Fig. 22-19, A).[6,9,10,12]
5. *Resist:* Over the dorsal-lateral aspect of the 4th and 5th metacarpal toward flexion and radial deviation (Fig. 22-19, B).[6,9,11]

Procedure for Testing Grades P (2), T (1), and 0

1. *Position:* As described for the previous test, except that the forearm is in 45° of pronation and supported on a table. The wrist is flexed and radially deviated and the thumb and fingers are flexed.[6]
2. *Stabilize:* Under the distal forearm, supporting it slightly above the supporting surface.[9,11]
3. *Palpate:* Extensor tendons as described above.
4. *Observe:* S extend the wrist and move it ulnarly at the same time (Fig. 22-19, C).
5. *Grade:* According to standard definitions of muscle grades.

Substitutions: In the absence of the ECU muscle, the ECRL and ECRB muscles can extend the wrist but will do so in a radial direction. The ulnar deviation component of the test motion will not be possible. Long finger and thumb extensors can initiate wrist extension, but the movement will be preceded by finger or thumb extension.[6,7,10,12,15]

Motion

Wrist flexion with radial deviation.

Muscles[10,11]	Innervation[5,6,9]
Flexor carpi radialis (FCR)	Median nerve, C6-8
Flexor carpi ulnaris (FCU)	Ulnar nerve, C7-T1
Palmaris longus	Median nerve, C7-T1

Procedure for Testing Grades N (5) to F (3)

1. *Position:* S seated or supine, with the forearm resting in nearly full supination on the supporting surface, fingers and thumb relaxed.[7,10,12] E is seated next to S on the side to be tested.
2. *Stabilize:* Over the volar aspect of the midforearm.[6,9,11]
3. *Palpate:* The FCR tendon can be palpated over the wrist at the base of the second metacarpal bone. The palmaris longus tendon is at the center of the wrist at the base of the 3rd metacarpal, and the FCU tendon can be palpated at the ulnar side of the volar aspect of the wrist, at the base of the 5th metacarpal (Fig. 22-20, A).[4]
4. *Observe:* S flex and radially deviate the hand simultaneously. E should observe that the fingers remain relaxed during the movement[6] (Fig. 22-20, B).
5. *Resist:* In the palm at the radial side of the hand, over the 2nd and 3rd metacarpals toward extension and ulnar deviation (Fig. 22-20, C).[6]

Procedure for Testing Grades P (2), T (1), and 0

1. *Position:* S seated with the forearm in midposition with the ulnar border of the hand resting on the supporting surface.[9,15] E sits next to S on the side to be tested.
2. *Stabilize:* Under the ulnar border of the forearm, supporting the wrist slightly above the supporting surface.
3. *Palpate:* Wrist flexor tendons as described for the previous test.
4. *Observe:* S flex and radially deviate the wrist. Movement should not be initiated with finger flexion (Fig. 22-20, D).
5. *Grade:* According to standard definitions of muscle grades.

Substitutions: Wrist flexors can substitute for one another. If flexor carpi radialis is weak or nonfunctioning in this test, flexor carpi ulnaris will produce wrist flexion, but in an ulnar direction, and the radial deviation will not be possible. The finger flexors can assist wrist flexion, but finger flexion will occur before the wrist is flexed. The abductor pollicis longus, with the assistance of gravity, can initiate wrist flexion.[6,7,12]

Motion

Wrist flexion with ulnar deviation.

Muscles[9,10]	Innervation[5,9,10]
Flexor carpi ulnaris (FCU)	Ulnar nerve, C7-T1
Palmaris longus	Median nerve, C7-T1
Flexor carpi radialis (FCR)	Median nerve, C6-8

Procedure for Testing Grades N (5) to F (3)

1. *Position:* S seated or supine, with the forearm resting in nearly full supination on the supporting surface, fingers and thumb relaxed. E is seated opposite or next to S on the side to be tested.[9,11]
2. *Stabilize:* Over the volar aspect of the middle of the forearm.[9,11]
3. *Palpate:* Flexor tendons on the volar aspect of the wrist, the FCU at the base of the 5th metacarpal, the FCR at the base of the 2nd metacarpal, and the palmaris longus at the base of the 3rd metacarpal.[4]
4. *Observe:* S flex the wrist and simultaneously deviate it ulnarly (Fig. 22-21, A).

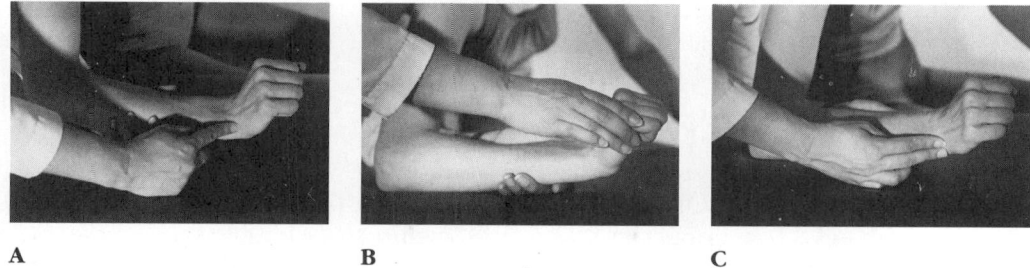

A   B   C

FIG. 22-19

Wrist extension with ulnar deviation. **A,** Palpate and observe. **B,** Resist. **C,** Gravity-decreased position.

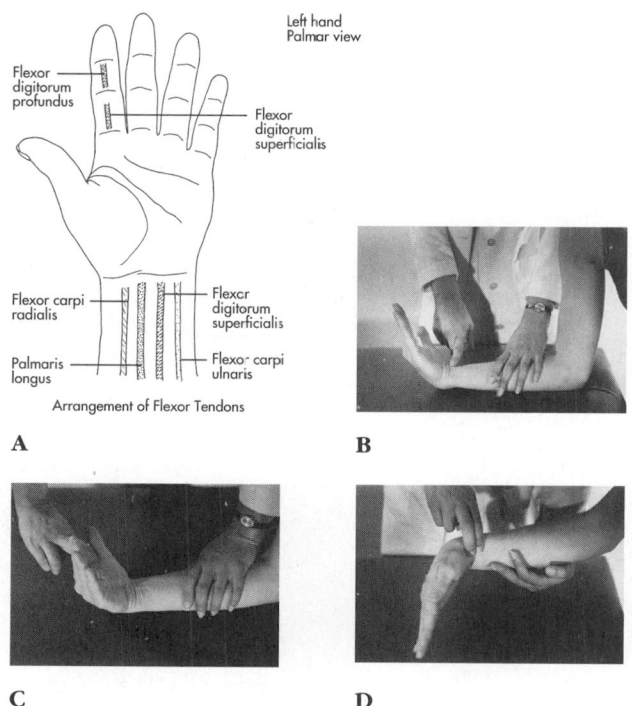

FIG. 22-20

A, Arrangement of flexor tendons at wrist. **B,** Wrist flexion with radial deviation. Palpate and observe. **C,** Resist. **D,** Gravity-decreased position.

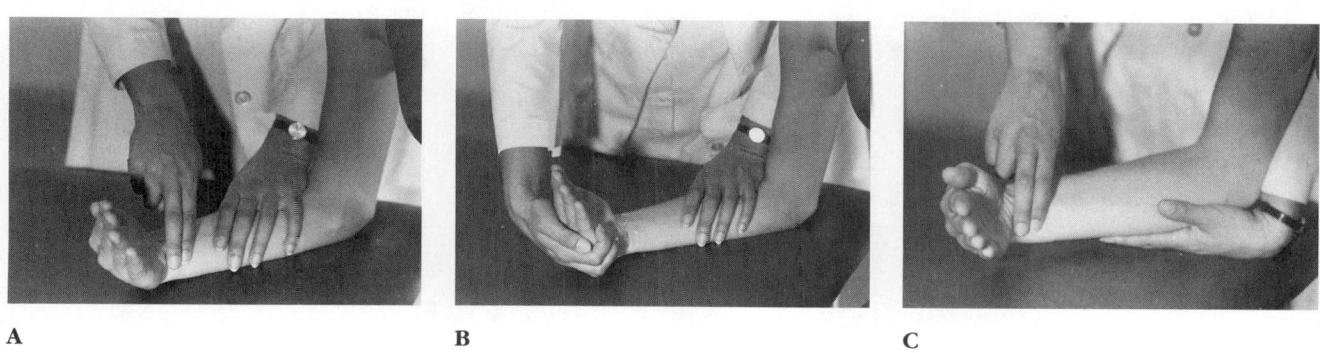

A   B   C

FIG. 22-21

Wrist flexion with ulnar deviation. **A,** Palpate and observe. **B,** Resist. **C,** Gravity-decreased position.

5. *Resist:* In the palm of the hand over the hypothenar eminence toward extension and radial deviation (Fig. 22-21, *B*).[6,7,11]

Procedure for Testing Grades P (2), T (1), and 0

1. *Position:* S seated, with the forearm in neutral rotation and resting in 45° of supination on the ulnar border of the arm and hand.[9] E sits opposite S or next to S on the side being tested.
2. *Stabilize:* S's arm can be supported slightly above the supporting surface and stabilized at the dorsal-medial aspect of the forearm to prevent elbow and forearm motion.
3. *Palpate:* Wrist flexor tendons as described for the previous test.
4. *Observe:* S simultaneously flex and deviate the wrist toward ulnar side (Fig. 22-21, *C*).
5. *Grade:* According to standard definitions of muscle grades.

Substitutions: Wrist flexors can substitute for one another. If FCU is weak or absent, FCR can produce wrist flexion in a radial direction and the ulnar deviation will not be possible. The finger flexors can also assist wrist flexion, but the motion will be preceded by flexion of the fingers.[6,12,15]

Motion

Metacarpophalangeal (MP) flexion with interphalangeal (IP) extension.

Muscles[1,4]	Innervation[9,10]
Lumbricals 1 and 2	Median nerve, C8,T1
Lumbricals 3 and 4	Ulnar nerve, C8,T1
Dorsal interossei	
Palmar interossei	

Procedure for Testing Grades N (5) to F (3)

1. *Position:* S seated, with forearm in supination, wrist at neutral, resting on the supporting surface.[8]

The MP joints are extended and the IP joints are flexed.[10,15] E sits next to S on the side being tested.

2. *Stabilize:* Over the metacarpals, proximal to the MP joints in the palm of the hand to prevent wrist motion.
3. *Palpate:* The first dorsal interosseous muscle just medial to the distal aspect of the 2nd metacarpal on the dorsum of the hand. The remainder of these muscles are not easily palpable because of their size and deep location in the hand.[12,15]
4. *Observe:* S flex the MP joints and extend the IP joints simultaneously (Fig. 22-22, *A*).[10,11]
5. *Resist:* Each finger separately by grasping the distal phalanx and pushing downward on the finger into the supporting surface toward MP extension and IP flexion, or apply pressure first against the dorsal surface of the middle and distal phalanges toward flexion, followed by application of pressure to the volar surface of the proximal phalanges toward extension (Fig. 22-22, *B*).[11]

Procedure for Testing Grades P (2), T (1), and 0

1. *Position:* S seated or supine, with the forearm and wrist in midposition and resting on the ulnar border on the supporting surface. MP joints are extended and IP joints are flexed.[9,10] E sits next to S on the side being tested.
2. *Stabilize:* The wrist and palm of the hand.
3. *Palpate:* As described for the previous test.
4. *Observe:* S flex the MP joints and extend the IP joints simultaneously (Fig. 22-22, *C*).
5. *Grade:* According to standard definitions of muscle grades.

Substitutions: Flexor digitorum profundus and superficialis may substitute for weak or absent lumbricals.[10] In this case, MP flexion will be preceded by flexion of the distal and proximal interphalangeal joints.[12,15]

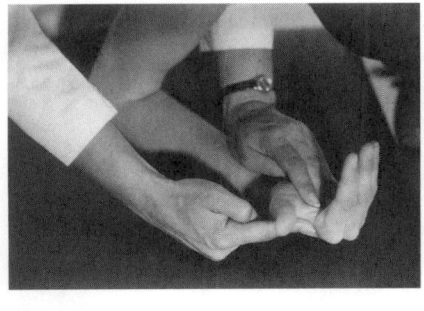 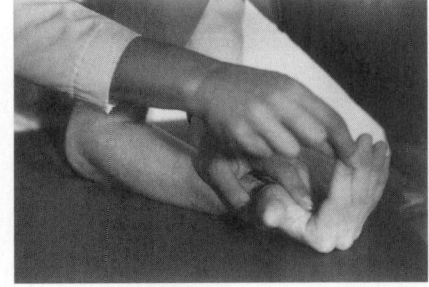 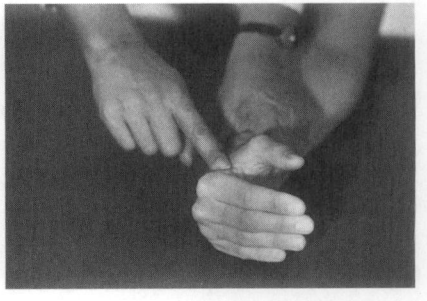

A   B   C

FIG. 22-22
Metacarpophalangeal flexion with interphalangeal extension. **A,** Palpate and observe. **B,** Resist. **C,** Gravity-decreased position.

Motion

MP extension.

<table>
<tr><td>Muscles[9,10]</td><td>Innervation[9,10]</td></tr>
<tr><td>Extensor digitorum communis (EDC)
Extensor indicis
Extensor digiti minimi (EDM)</td><td>Radial nerve, C7,8</td></tr>
</table>

Procedure for Testing Grades N (5) to F (3)

1. *Position:* S seated, with the forearm pronated and the wrist in the neutral position, MP and IP joints relaxed in partial flexion.[7,9,10] E sits opposite or next to S on the side to be tested.
2. *Stabilize:* The wrist and metacarpals slightly above the supporting surface.[9-11]
3. *Palpate:* The EDC tendons where they course over the dorsum of the hand.[6,7,9] In some individuals, the EDM tendon can be palpated or visualized just lateral to the EDC tendon to the 5th finger. The extensor indicis tendon can be palpated or visualized just medial to the EDC tendon to the first finger.[6]
4. *Observe:* S extend the MP joints, but maintaining the IP joints in some flexion (Fig. 22-23, A).[6,10]
5. *Resist:* Each finger individually on the dorsum of the proximal phalanx toward MP flexion (Fig. 22-23, B).[6,9,11]

Procedure for Testing Grades P (2), T (1), and 0

1. *Position:* The same as described for the previous test, except that S's forearm is in midposition and the hand and forearm are supported on the ulnar border.[9,10]
2. *Stabilize:* The same as described for the previous test.
3. *Palpate:* The same as described for the previous test.
4. *Observe:* S extend the MP joints while keeping the IP joints somewhat flexed (Fig. 22-23, C).
5. *Grade:* According to standard definitions of muscle grades.

Substitutions: With the wrist stabilized, no substitutions are possible. When the wrist is not stabilized, wrist flexion with tendon action can produce MP extension.[6,7,10,12,15]

Motion

PIP flexion, 2nd through 5th fingers.

<table>
<tr><td>Muscles[9,1?]</td><td>Innervation[6,9,10]</td></tr>
<tr><td>Flexor digitorum superficialis (FDS)</td><td>Median nerve, C7,8,T1</td></tr>
</table>

Procedure for Testing Grades N (5) to F (3)

1. *Position:* S seated, with the forearm supinated, wrist at neutral, fingers extended, and hand and forearm resting on the dorsal surface.[6,9,10] E sits opposite or next to S on the side being tested.
2. *Stabilize:* The MP joint and proximal phalanx of the finger being tested. (Fig. 22-24, A)[6,7,9,11] If it is difficult for S to isolate PIP flexion, hold all of the fingers not being tested in MP hyperextension and PIP extension. This maneuver inactivates the flexor digitorum profundus so that S cannot flex the distal joint (Fig. 22-24, B).[4,6,10,15] Most individuals cannot perform isolated action of the PIP joint of the 5th finger, even with this assistance.[12]
3. *Palpate:* The FDS tendon on the volar surface of the proximal phalanx.[6] A stabilizing finger may be used to palpate in this instance.[12] The tendon supplying the 4th finger may be palpated over the volar aspect of the wrist between the flexor carpi ulnaris and the palmaris longus tendons, if desired.[4,6]
4. *Observe:* S flex the PIP joint while maintaining DIP extension (Fig. 22-24, A).
5. *Resist:* With one finger at the volar aspect of the middle phalanx toward extension.[6,9,11] If E uses the index finger to apply resistance, the middle finger may be used to move the DIP joint to and fro to verify that the flexor digitorum profundus (FDP) is not substituting (Fig. 22-24, C).

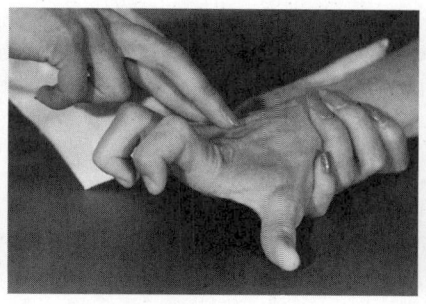 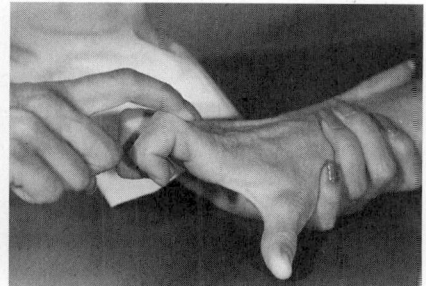 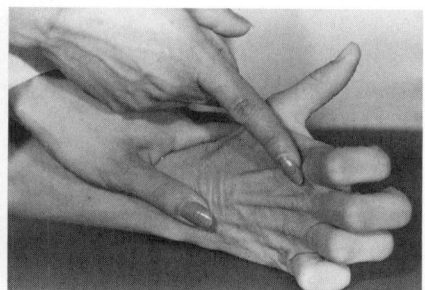

A   **B**   **C**

FIG. 22-23
Metacarpophalangeal extension. **A,** Palpate and observe. **B,** Resist. **C,** Gravity-decreased position.

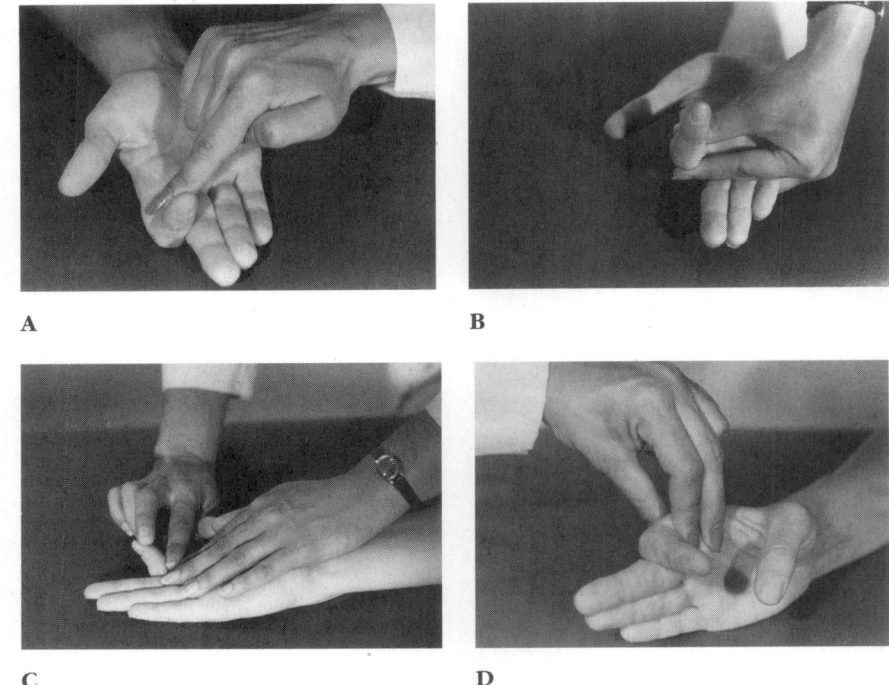

FIG. 22-24
Proximal interphalangeal flexion. **A,** Palpate and observe. **B,** Position to assist with isolation of proximal interphalangeal joint flexion. **C,** Resist. Therapist checks for substitution by flexor digitorum profundus. **D,** Gravity-decreased position.

Procedure for Testing Grades P (2), T (1), and 0

1. *Position:* S seated, with the forearm in midposition and the wrist at neutral, resting on the ulnar border.[10,15] E sits opposite or next to S on the side to be tested.
2. *Stabilize:* The MP joint and proximal phalanx of the finger.[9,11] If stabilization during the motion is difficult in this position, the forearm may be returned to full supination, because the effect of gravity on the fingers is not significant.
3. *Palpate and observe:* The same as described for the previous test, except that the movement is performed in the gravity-decreased position (Fig. 22-24, *D*).
4. *Grade:* According to standard definitions of muscle grades. If the test for grades poor and below is done with the forearm in full supination, partial ROM against gravity may be graded poor.[9]

Substitutions: The FDP may substitute for the FDS. DIP flexion will precede PIP flexion.[7,10,12,15] Tendon action of the long finger flexors accompanies wrist extension and can produce an apparent flexion of the fingers through partial ROM.[10,12,15]

Motion

DIP flexion, 2nd through 5th fingers.

Muscles[9,10]	Innervation[9,10]
Flexor digitorum profundus (FDP)	Median and ulnar nerves, C8, T1

Procedure for Testing Grades N (5) to F (3)

1. *Position:* S seated, with the forearm supinated, the wrist at neutral, and the fingers extended.[10] E sits opposite or next to S on the side being tested.[9]
2. *Stabilize:* The wrist at neutral and the PIP joint and middle phalanx of the finger being tested.[6,15]
3. *Palpate:* Use the finger stabilizing the middle phalanx to simultaneously palpate the FDP tendon over the volar surface of the middle phalanx.[6,9,12]
4. *Observe:* S flex the DIP joint (Fig. 22-25, *A*).
5. *Resist:* With one finger at the volar aspect of the distal phalanx toward extension (Fig. 22-25, *B*).[6,7,9,11]

Procedure for Testing Grades P (2), T (1), and 0

1. *Position:* S seated, with the forearm in midposition and with the wrist at neutral, resting on the ulnar border.[10,15] S may be positioned with the forearm supinated, if necessary.
2. *Stabilize:* The same as described for the previous test.
3. *Palpate:* The same as described for the previous test.
4. *Observe:* S flex the DIP joint (Fig. 22-25, *C*).
5. *Grade:* According to standard definitions of muscle grades, except that if the test for grades poor and below was done with the forearm in full supination, movement through partial ROM may be graded poor.[9]

Substitutions: None possible during the testing procedure if the wrist is well stabilized because the FDP is the only muscle that can act to flex the DIP joint when it

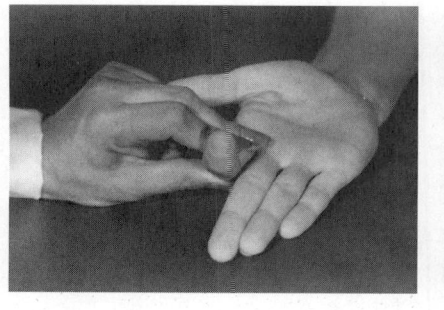 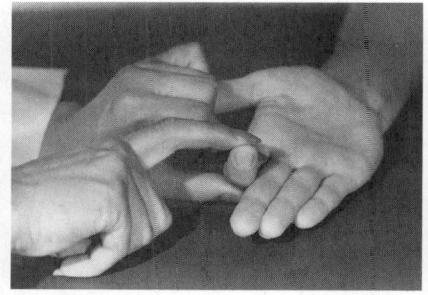 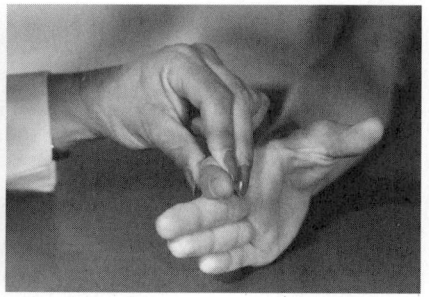

A   B   C

FIG. 22-25
Distal interphalangeal flexion. **A,** Palpate and observe. **B,** Resist. **C,** Gravity-decreased position.

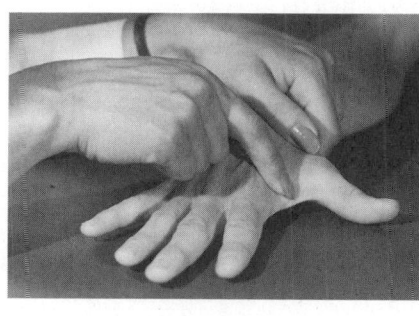 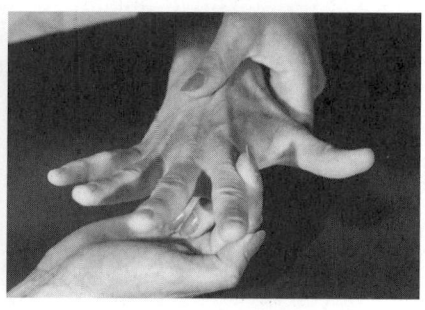

A   B

FIG. 22-26
Finger abduction. **A,** Palpate and observe. **B,** Resist.

is isolated. During normal hand function, however, wrist extension with tendon action of the finger flexors can produce partial flexion of the DIP joints.[10,12,15]

Motion

Finger abduction.

Muscles[9,10]	Innervation[9,10]
Dorsal interossei	Ulnar nerve, C8,T1
Abductor digiti minimi	

Procedure for Testing Grades N (5) to F (3)

1. *Position:* S seated or supine, with the forearm pronated, wrist at neutral, and fingers extended and adducted. E is seated opposite or next to S on the side to be tested.[9,10]
2. *Stabilize:* The wrist and metacarpals slightly above the supporting surface.
3. *Palpate:* The 1st dorsal interosseous muscle on the radial side of the second metacarpal or of the abductor digiti minimi on the ulnar border of the 5th metacarpal. The remaining interossei are not palpable.[6,7,9]
4. *Observe:* S spread the fingers; abduction of the little finger, the ring finger toward the little finger, the middle finger toward the ring finger, and the index finger toward the thumb. (Fig. 22-26, *A*).[10]

5. *Resist:* The first dorsal interosseus by applying pressure on the radial side of the proximal phalanx of the 2nd finger in an ulnar direction (Fig. 22-26, *B*); the 2nd dorsal interosseus on the radial side of the proximal phalanx of the middle finger in an ulnar direction; the 3rd dorsal interosseus on the ulnar side of the proximal phalanx of the middle finger in a radial direction; the 4th dorsal interosseus on the ulnar side of the proximal phalanx of the ring finger in a radial direction; the abductor digiti minimi on the ulnar side of the proximal phalanx of the little finger in a radial direction.[6,11] An alternative mode of resistance is to flick each finger toward adduction. If the finger rebounds, the grade is N (5).[10]

Procedure for Testing Grades P (2), T (1), and 0

The tests for these muscle grades are the same as described for the previous test.

1. *Grade:* Because the test motions were not performed against gravity, some judgment of the examiner must be used in grading. For example, partial ROM in gravity-decreased position may be graded poor and full ROM graded fair.[9,10]

Substitutions: EDC can assist weak or absent dorsal interossei, but abduction will be accompanied by MP extension.[6,12,15]

Motion

Finger adduction.

Muscles[9-11]	Innervation[9,10]
Palmar interossei, 1, 2, 3	Ulnar nerve, C8,T1

Procedure for Testing Grades N (5) to F (3)

1. *Position:* S seated, with forearm pronated, wrist in neutral, and fingers extended and abducted.[9,10]
2. *Stabilize:* The wrist and metacarpals slightly above the supporting surface.[6]
3. *Palpate:* Not palpable.[6]
4. *Observe:* S adduct the 1st, 4th, and 5th fingers toward the middle finger (Fig. 22-27, *A*).
5. *Resist:* The index finger at the proximal phalanx by pulling it in a radial direction, the ring finger at the proximal phalanx in an ulnar direction, and the little finger likewise (Fig. 22-27, *B*).[6,11] These muscles are very small, and resistance will have to be modified to accommodate their comparatively limited power. Fingers can also be grasped at the distal phalanx and flicked in the direction of abduction. If the finger snaps back to the adducted position, the grade is N (5).[10]

Procedure for Testing Grades P (2), T (1), and 0

The test for these muscle grades is the same as described for the previous test. The examiner's judgment must be used in determining the degree of weakness. Achievement of full ROM may be graded fair and partial ROM graded poor.[9,10]

Substitutions: FDP and FDS can substitute for weak palmar interossei, but IP flexion will occur with finger adduction.[10,12,15]

Motion

Thumb MP extension.

Muscles[9-11]	Innervation[9-11]
Extensor pollicis brevis (EPB)	Radial nerve, C6-8

Procedure for Testing Grades N (5) to F (3)

1. *Position:* S seated or supine, forearm in midposition, wrist at neutral, and hand and forearm resting on the ulnar border.[6,9,10] The thumb is flexed into the palm at the MP joint, and the IP joint is extended but relaxed. E sits opposite or next to S on the side to be tested.
2. *Stabilize:* The wrist and the thumb metacarpal.[6]
3. *Palpate:* The EPB tendon on the dorsoradial aspect of the base of the 1st metacarpal. It lies just medial to the abductor pollicis longus tendon on the radial side of the anatomical snuffbox, which is the hollow space created between the EPL and EPB tendons when the thumb is fully extended and radially abducted.[4,6,7]
4. *Observe:* S extend the MP joint. The IP joint remains relaxed (Fig. 22-28, *A*). It is difficult for many individuals to isolate this motion.
5. *Resist:* On the dorsal surface of the proximal phalanx toward MP flexion (Fig. 22-28, *B*).[6,9-11]

Procedure for Testing Grades (P), (T), and (0)

1. *Position and stabilize:* Positioning and stabilizing are the same as described for the previous test, except that the forearm is fully pronated and resting on the volar surface.[15] E may stabilize the 1st metacarpal, holding the hand slightly above the supporting surface. The test may also be performed in the same manner as for grades normal to fair, with modified grading.[9]
2. *Palpate and observe:* The same as described for the previous test. MP extension is performed in a plane parallel to the supporting surface (Fig. 22-28, *C*).
3. *Grade:* According to standard definitions of muscle grades. If midposition of the forearm was used, partial ROM is graded poor and full ROM is graded fair.[9,10]

Substitutions: Extensor pollicis longus may substitute for extensor pollicis brevis. IP extension will precede MP extension.[6,7,10.12,15]

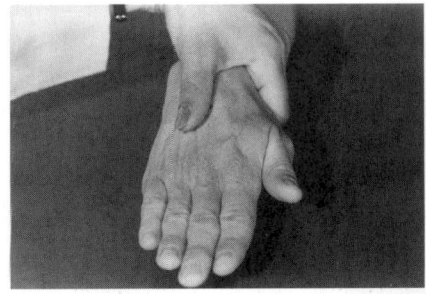
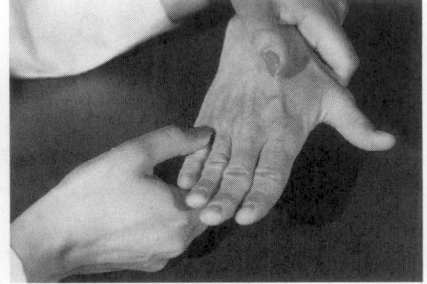

A   **B**

FIG. 22-27

Finger adduction. **A,** Therapist observes movement of fingers into adduction. Palpation of these muscles is not possible. **B,** Resist.

Motion

Thumb IP extension.

Muscles[9-11]	Innervation[9-11]
Extensor pollicis longus (EPL)	Radial nerve, C6-8

Procedure for Testing Grades N (5) to F (3)

1. *Position:* S seated or supine, forearm in midposition, wrist at neutral, and hand and forearm resting on the ulnar border.[6,9,10] The thumb is adducted, the MP joint is extended or slightly flexed, and the IP is flexed.[6] E sits opposite or next to S on the side being tested.
2. *Stabilize:* The wrist at neutral, 1st metacarpal, and the proximal phalanx of the thumb.[6]
3. *Palpate:* The EPL tendon on the dorsal surface of the hand medial to the EPB tendon, between the head of the 1st metacarpal and the base of the 2nd on the ulnar side of the anatomical snuff box.[4,6,9]
4. *Observe:* S extend the IP joint (Fig. 22-29, A).
5. *Resist:* On the dorsal surface of the distal phalanx, down toward IP flexion (Fig. 22-29, B).[6,9,11]

Procedure for Testing Grades P (2), T (1), and 0

1. *Position and stabilize:* Positioning and stabilizing are the same as described for the previous test, except that the forearm is fully pronated.[15] E may stabilize so that S's hand is held slightly above the supporting surface. The test may also be performed in the same position as for grades normal to fair with modification in grading.
2. *Palpate and observe:* The same as described for the previous test. IP extension is performed in the plane of the palm, parallel to the supporting surface (Fig. 22-29, C).
3. *Grade:* According to standard definitions of muscle grades. If the test was performed with the forearm in midposition, partial ROM is graded P (2).[9]

Substitutions: A quick contraction of the flexor pollicis longus followed by rapid release will cause the IP joint to rebound into extension.[6] IP flexion will precede IP extension.[7,12] The abductor pollicis brevis, flexor pollicis brevis, the oblique fibers of the adductor pollicis, and the 1st palmar interosseus can extend the IP joint because of their insertions into the extensor expansion of the thumb.[11,15]

Motion

Thumb MP flexion.

Muscles[9-11]	Innervation[9-11]
Flexor pollicis brevis (FPB)	Median and ulnar nerves, C8, T1

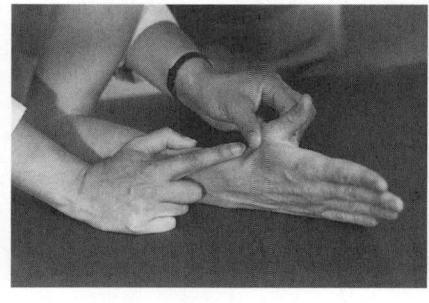
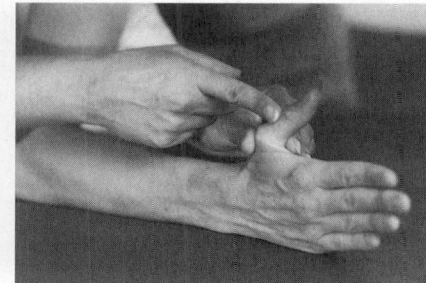
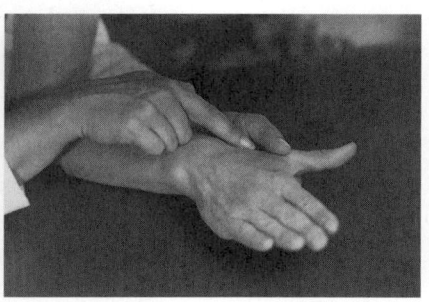

A   B   C

FIG. 22-28
Thumb metacarpophalangeal extension. **A,** Palpate and observe. **B,** Resist. **C,** Gravity-decreased position.

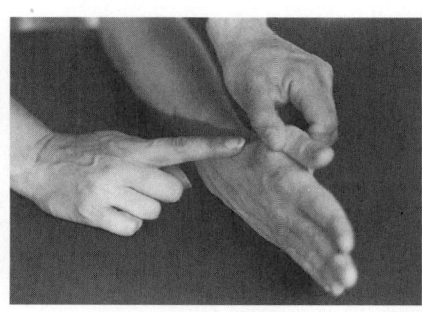
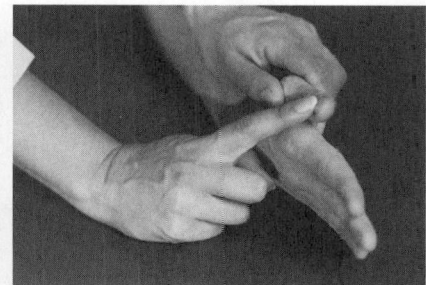
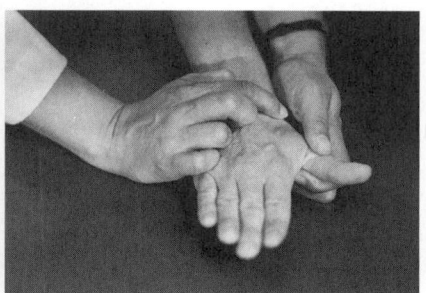

A   B   C

FIG. 22-29
Thumb IP extension. **A,** Palpate and observe. **B,** Resist. **C,** Gravity-decreased position.

Procedure for Testing Grades N (5) to F (3)

1. *Position:* S seated or supine, the forearm supinated, the wrist in the neutral position, and the thumb in extension and adduction.[6,10] E is seated next to or opposite S.[7,9,11]
2. *Stabilize:* The 1st metacarpal and the wrist.[10]
3. *Palpate:* Over the middle of the palmar surface of the thenar eminence just medial to the abductor pollicis brevis muscle.[6,9] The hand that is used to stabilize may also be used for palpation.
4. *Observe:* S flex the MP joint while maintaining extension of the IP joint (Fig. 22-30, *A*).[6] It may not be possible for some individuals to isolate flexion to the MP joint. In this instance, both MP and IP flexion may be tested together as a gross test for thumb flexion strength, and graded according to the examiner's judgment.
5. *Resist:* On the palmar surface of the first phalanx toward MP extension (Fig. 22-30, *B*).[6,7,9,11]

Procedure for Testing Grades P (2), T (1), and (0)

Positioning, stabilizing, and palpating are the same as described for the previous test.

1. *Observe:* S flex the MP joint so that the thumb moves over the palm of the hand.

2. *Grade:* Full ROM is graded fair; partial ROM is graded poor.[9,10]

   Substitutions: FPL can substitute for FPB. In this case, isolated MP flexion will not be possible and MP flexion will be preceded by IP flexion.[7,10,12,15]

Motion

Thumb IP flexion.

Muscles[6,9,10]	Innervation[9,10]
Flexor pollicis longus (FPL)	Median nerve, C7-T1

Procedure for Testing Grades N (5) to F (3)

1. *Position:* S seated, with the forearm fully supinated, wrist in neutral position, and thumb extended and adducted.[9,10] E is seated next to or opposite S.
2. *Stabilize:* The wrist, thumb metacarpal, and the proximal phalanx of the thumb in extension.[6,7,9,11]
3. *Palpate:* The FPL tendon on the palmar surface of the proximal phalanx.[6] In this instance the palpating finger may be the same one used for stabilizing the proximal phalanx.
4. *Observe:* S flex the IP joint in the plane of the palm (Fig. 22-31, *A*).[9,10]

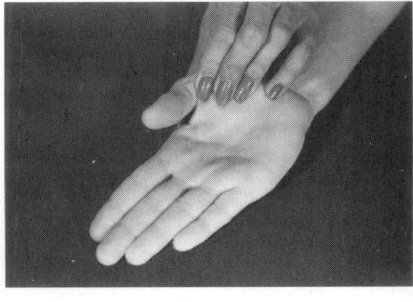
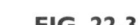
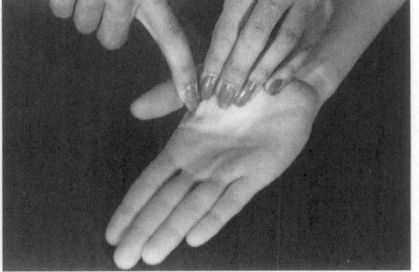

A   **B**

FIG. 22-30
Thumb metacarpophalangeal flexion. **A,** Palpate and observe. **B,** Resist.

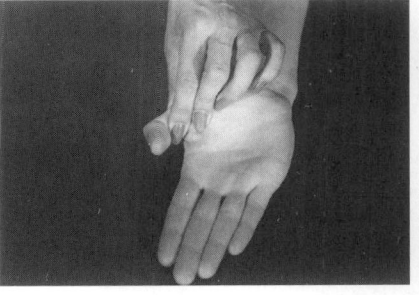
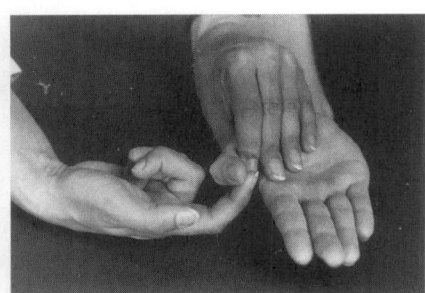

A   **B**

FIG. 22-31
Thumb interphalangeal flexion. **A,** Palpate and observe. **B,** Resist.

5. *Resist:* On the palmar surface of the distal phalanx, toward IP extension (Fig. 22-31, *B*).[6,9-11]

Procedure for Testing Grades P (2), T (1), and 0

The test for these muscle grades is the same as described for the previous test. The examiner's judgment must be used in determining the degree of weakness. Achievement of full ROM may be graded fair and partial ROM graded poor.[9,10]

Substitutions: A quick contraction and release of the EPL may cause an apparent flexion of the IP joint. E should observe for IP extension preceding IP flexion.[6,7,10,12,15]

Motion

Thumb palmar abduction.

Muscles[10,11]	Innervation[10,11]
Abductor pollicis brevis (APB)	Median nerve, C8,T1

Procedure for Testing Grades Fair (F) to Normal (N)

1. *Position:* S seated or supine, forearm in supination, wrist at neutral, thumb extended and adducted, and carpometacarpal (CMC) joint rotated so that the thumb is resting in a plane perpendicular to the palm. E sits opposite or next to S on the side to be tested.[6,7,9-11]
2. *Stabilize:* The metacarpals and wrist.
3. *Palpate:* The APB muscle on the lateral aspect of the thenar eminence, lateral to the flexor pollicis brevis muscle.[9]
4. *Observe:* S raise the thumb away from the palm in a plane perpendicular to the palm (Fig. 22-32, *A*).[6,11]
5. *Resist:* At the lateral aspect of the proximal phalanx, downward toward adduction (Fig. 22-32, *B*).[6,11]

Procedure for Testing Grades P (2), T (1), and 0

1. *Position:* As described for the previous test, except that the forearm and hand are supported on the ulnar border.[10,15]

2. *Stabilize:* The wrist and metacarpals.
3. *Palpate:* The APB muscle on the lateral aspect of the thenar eminence.
4. *Observe:* S move the thumb away from the palm in a plane at right angles to the palm of the hand and parallel to the supporting surface (Fig. 22-32, *C*).
5. *Grade:* According to standard definitions of muscle grades.

   Substitutions: APL can substitute for APB. Abduction will take place more in the plane of the palm, however, rather than perpendicular to it.[10,12,15]

Motion

Thumb radial abduction.

Muscles[10,11]	Innervation[10,11]
Abductor pollicis longus (APL)	Radial nerve, C6-8

Procedure for Testing Grades N (5) to F (3)

1. *Position.* S seated or supine, forearm in neutral rotation, wrist at neutral, thumb adducted and slightly flexed across the palm. Hand and forearm are resting on the ulnar border.[11] E sits opposite or next to S on the side being tested.
2. *Stabilize:* The wrist and metacarpals of the fingers.[9,11]
3. *Palpate:* The APL tendon on the lateral aspect of the base of the first metacarpal. It is the tendon immediately lateral (radial) to the EPB tendon.[4,6,9]
4. *Observe:* S move the thumb out of the palm of the hand, abducting away from the index finger at an angle of about 45° (Fig. 22-33, *A*).[6]
5. *Resist:* At the lateral aspect of the thumb metacarpal toward adduction (Fig. 22-33, *B*).[6,9,11]

Procedure for Testing Grades P (2), T (1), and 0

1. *Position:* As described for the previous test, except that the forearm is in supination.[9]
2. *Stabilize:* The wrist and palm of the hand.
3. *Palpate:* The same as described for the previous test.
4. *Observe:* S move the thumb out away from the palm of the hand in the plane of the palm (Fig. 22-33, *C*).

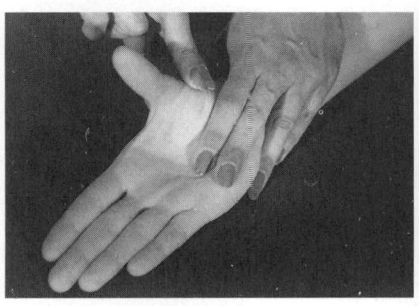
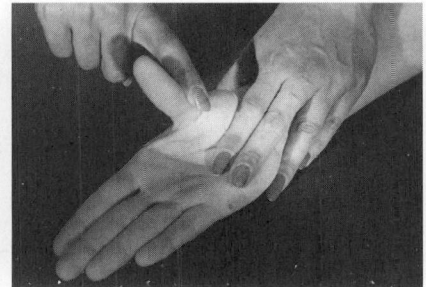
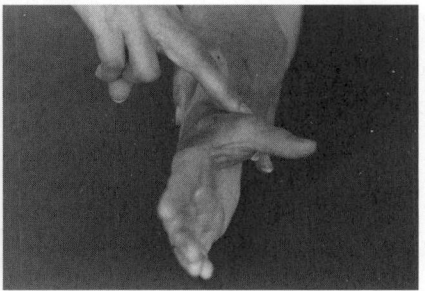

A   B   C

FIG. 22-32
Thumb palmar abduction. **A,** Palpate and observe. **B,** Resist. **C,** Gravity-decreased position.

5. *Grade:* According to standard definitions of muscle grades.

Substitutions: APB can substitute for APL. Abduction will not take place in the plane of the palm, but rather in a more ulnar direction.[12,15] EPB can substitute for APL. The movement will be more toward the dorsal surface of the forearm.[10]

Motion

Thumb adduction.

Muscles[9-11]	Innervation[9-11]
Adductor pollicis (AP)	Ulnar nerve, C8,T1

Procedure for Testing Grades N (5) to F (3)

1. *Position:* S seated or supine, forearm pronated, wrist at neutral, thumb is relaxed and in palmar abduction.[9,10,15] E is sitting opposite or next to S on the side to be tested.

2. *Stabilize:* The wrist and metacarpals by grasping the hand around the ulnar side and supporting it slightly above the resting surface.[9,10]
3. *Palpate:* AP on the palmar side of the thumb web space.[6,12]
4. *Observe:* S adduct the thumb to touch the palm (Fig. 22-34, A).[9,10] (The palm is turned up in the illustration to show the palpation point.)
5. *Resist:* By grasping the proximal phalanx of the thumb near the metacarpal head and pulling downward, toward abduction (Fig. 22-34, B).[9]

Procedure for Testing Grades P (2), T (1), and 0

1. *Position:* The same as described for the previous test, except that the forearm is in midposition and the forearm and hand are resting on the ulnar border.[15]
2. *Stabilize:* Over the wrist and palm of the hand.
3. *Palpate:* The same as described for the previous test.

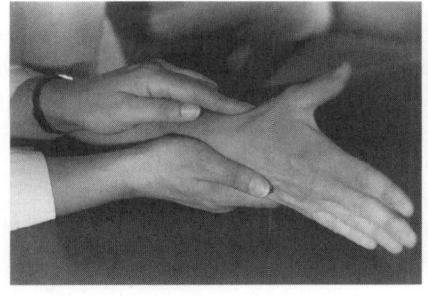 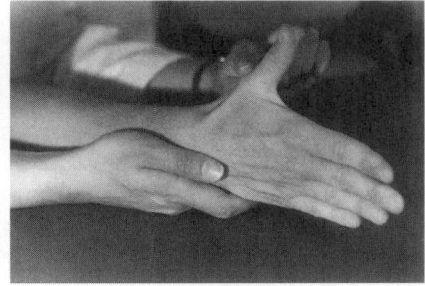 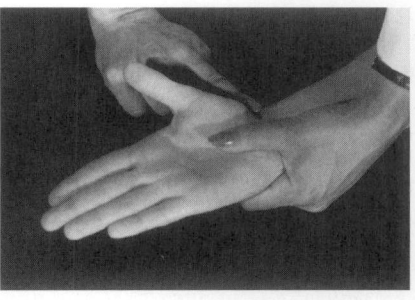

A   B   C

FIG. 22-33
Radial abduction. **A,** Palpate and observe. **B,** Resist. **C,** Gravity-decreased position.

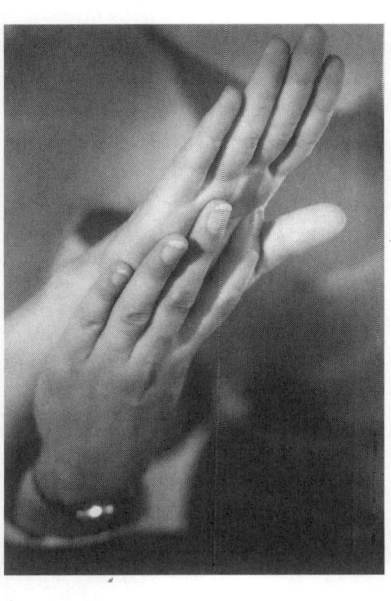 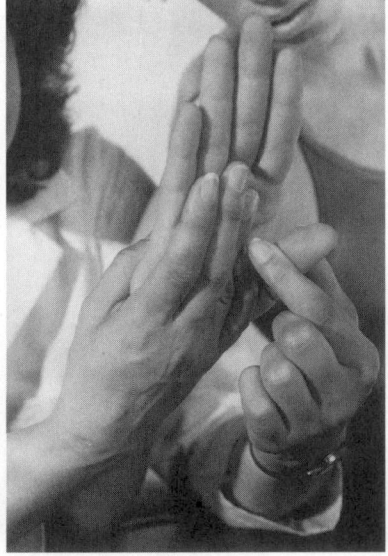 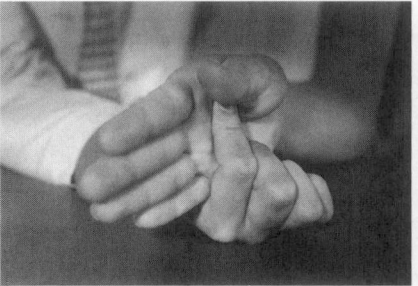

A   B   C

FIG. 22-34
Thumb adduction. **A,** Palpate and observe. **B,** Resist. **C,** Gravity-decreased position.

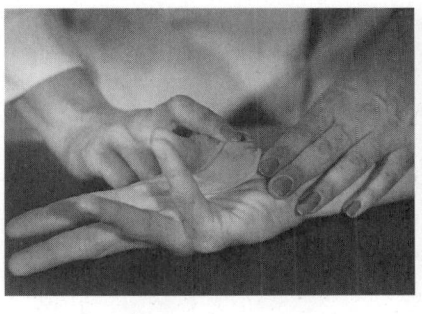 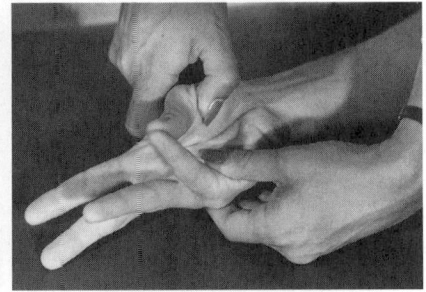

A   B

FIG. 22-35
Thumb opposition. **A,** Palpate and observe. **B,** Resist.

4. *Observe:* S adduct the thumb to touch the radial side of the palm of the hand or the 2nd metacarpal (Fig. 22-34, *C*).
5. *Grade:* According to standard definitions of muscle grades.

Substitutions: FPL or EPL may assist weak or absent AP. If one substitutes, adduction will be accompanied by thumb flexion or extension preceding adduction.[10,12,15]

Motion

Opposition of the thumb to the 5th finger.

Muscles[9,10]	Innervation[9,10]
Opponens pollicis	Median nerve, C8, T1
Opponens digiti minimi	Ulnar nerve, C8, T1

Procedure for Testing Grades N (5) to F (3)
1. *Position:* S seated or supine, with forearm supinated, wrist at neutral, thumb in palmar abduction, and 5th finger extended.[6,7,9,11] E sits opposite or next to S on the side to be tested.
2. *Stabilize:* The forearm and wrist.
3. *Palpate:* The opponens pollicis along the radial side of the shaft of the first metacarpal, lateral to the APB; the opponens digiti minimi on the shaft of the fifth metacarpal.[6,9,12]
4. *Observe:* S oppose the thumb to touch the thumb pad to the pad of the 5th finger, which flexes and rotates toward the thumb (Fig. 22-35, *A*).[6,7]
5. *Resist:* At the distal ends of the 1st and 5th metacarpals toward derotation of these bones and flattening of the palm of the hand (Fig. 22-35, *B*).[9,10]

Procedure for Testing Grades P (2), T (1), and 0
The procedure described for the previous test may be used for these grades, if grading is modified to compensate for the movement of the parts against gravity. For example, movement through full ROM would be graded fair and through partial ROM would be graded poor.[9,10]

Substitutions: APB will assist with opposition by flexing and medially rotating the CMC joint, but the IP joint will extend. The FPB will flex and medially rotate the CMC joint, but the thumb will not move away from the palm of the hand. The FPL will flex and slightly rotate the CMC joint, but the thumb will not move away from the palm and the IP joint will flex strongly.[12,15] The DIP joints of the thumb and little finger may flex to meet, giving the appearance of full opposition.[7,10]

MANUAL MUSCLE TESTING OF THE LOWER EXTREMITY
Motion

Hip flexion

Muscles[4,7,9]	Innervation[4,6,9]
Psoas major	Lumbar plexus, L1-3
Iliacus	Femoral nerve, L2,3
Rectus femoris	Femoral nerve, L2-4
Tensor fasciae latae	Superior gluteal nerve, L4,5,S1
Sartorius	Femoral nerve, L2-S1
Pectineus	Femoral nerve, L2,3

Procedure for Testing Grades N (5) to F (3)
1. *Position:* S seated, with knees flexed over the edge of the table and feet above the floor.[10] E stands next to S on the side being tested.[7]
2. *Stabilize:* The pelvis at the iliac crest on the side being tested. S may hold onto the edge of the table or fold arms across chest.[6,7,9-11]
3. *Palpate:* The psoas and iliacus are difficult to palpate.[6] The rectus femoris may be palpated on the middle anterior aspect of the thigh, just lateral to the sartorius muscle.[4,12]
4. *Observe:* S flex the hip so the femur rises above the table surface (Fig. 22-36, *A*).
5. *Resist:* Just proximal to the knee on the anterior surface of the thigh, down toward the table into hip extension (Fig. 22-36, *B*).[6,7,9-11]

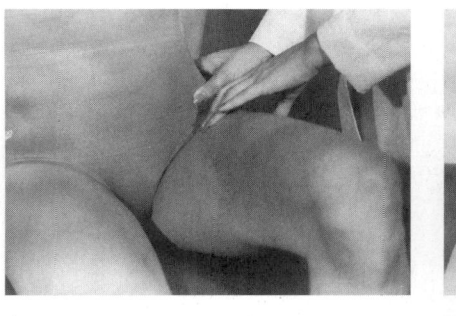
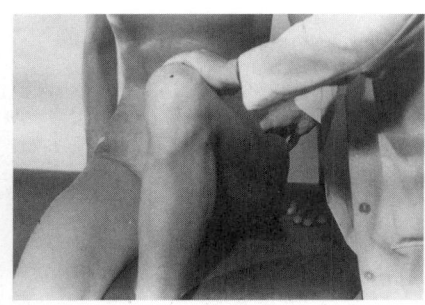
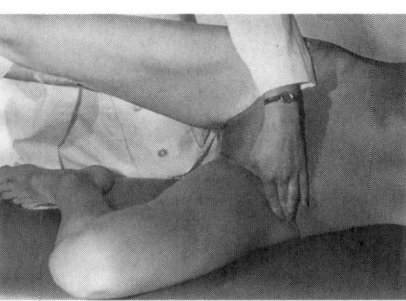

FIG. 22-36
Hip flexion. **A,** Palpate and observe. **B,** Resist. **C,** Gravity-decreased position.

Procedure for Testing Grades P (2), T (1), and 0

1. *Position:* S side-lying. E stands behind S, supporting the upper leg in neutral rotation and slight abduction, with the knee extended.[9,10] The lower leg (to be tested) is extended at the hip and knee.
2. *Stabilize:* The weight of the trunk may be adequate stabilization, or E may stabilize the pelvis.[9]
3. *Palpate:* The same as described for the previous test.
4. *Observe:* S bring the lower leg up toward the trunk, flexing the hip and knee (Fig. 22-36, C).[9]
5. *Grade:* According to standard definitions of muscle grades.

   Substitutions: Observe for internal rotation, external rotation, and abduction accompanying the flexion as signs of substitution or muscle imbalance in this muscle group.[6,7,10,11] The hip flexors can substitute for one another. If the iliacus and psoas major muscles are weak or absent, hip flexion will be accompanied by other movements: abduction and external rotation (sartorius), abduction and internal rotation (tensor fasciae latae), and adduction (pectineus).[9,12] If the anterior abdominal muscles do not stabilize the pelvis, it will flex on the thighs; the hip flexors may hold against resistance, but not at maximum ROM.[11]

Motion

Hip extension.

Muscles[6,10,11]	Innervation[9,10]
Gluteus maximus	Inferior gluteal nerve, L5-S2
Semitendinosus	Sciatic nerve, L5-S2
Semimembranosus	
Biceps femoris (long head)	Sciatic nerve, L5-S3

Procedure for Testing Grades N (5) to F (3)

1. *Position:* S lying prone, with the hip at neutral and the knee flexed to about 90°. This position is used to isolate the gluteus maximus.[6,10] S may also be positioned prone, with the knee extended.[10] E stands next to S on the opposite side.[11] Two pillows may be placed under the pelvis to flex the hips.[6,7]
2. *Stabilize:* Over the iliac crest on the side being tested.[9,10]
3. *Palpate:* The gluteus maximus on the middle posterior surface of the buttock.[12]
4. *Observe:* S extend the hip while keeping the knee flexed to minimize action of the hamstring muscles on the hip joint (Fig. 22-37, A).
5. *Resist:* At the distal end of the posterior aspect of the thigh, downward, toward flexion (Fig. 22-37, B).[9-11]

Procedure for Testing Grades P (2), T (1), and 0

1. *Position:* Side-lying. E stands in front of S, supporting the upper leg in extension and slight abduction.[9] The lower leg (to be tested) is flexed at the hip and knee.
2. *Stabilize:* The pelvis over the iliac crest.[9]
3. *Palpate:* The same as described for the previous test.

4. *Observe:* S extend the hip, bringing the lower leg backward, while maintaining flexion of the knee (Fig. 22-37, *C*).
5. *Grade:* According to standard definitions of muscle grades.

   Substitutions: Elevation of the pelvis and extension of the lumbar spine can produce some hip extension. In the supine position, gravity and eccentric contraction of the hip flexors can return the flexed hip to extension.[12] Hip external rotation, abduction, or adduction may be used to substitute.[7]

Motion

Hip abduction.

Muscles[6,9,10]	Innervation[9-11]
Gluteus medius	Superior gluteal nerve, L4-S1
Gluteus minimus	

Procedure for Testing Grades N (5) to F (3)

1. *Position:* S side lying, upper leg (to be tested) has the knee extended and hip extended slightly beyond the neutral position and slight forward rotation of the pelvis[10]; the lower leg is flexed at the hip and knee to provide a wide base of support.[7] E stands behind or in front of S.[6,7,9-11]

2. *Stabilize:* The pelvis over the iliac crest.[9,11]
3. *Palpate:* The gluteus medius on the lateral aspect of the ilium above the greater trochanter of the femur.[6,9]
4. *Observe:* S abduct the hip, lifting the leg upward (Fig. 22-38, *A*).
5. *Resist:* Just proximal to the knee in a downward direction, toward adduction (Fig. 22-38, *B*).[6,9,10]

Procedure for Testing Grades P (2), T (1), and 0

1. *Position:* S lying supine, with both legs extended and in neutral rotation. E stands next to S on the opposite side.[9] E may use one hand to support at the ankle and slightly lift the test leg off the surface, being careful to offer no resistance or assistance to the movement.[10]
2. *Stabilize:* The pelvis at the iliac crest on the side to be tested and the opposite limb at the lateral aspect of the calf.[9]
3. *Palpate:* Use the hand stabilizing over the pelvis to palpate the gluteus medius muscle simultaneously by adjusting the position of the hand so that the fingers are touching the lateral aspect of the ilium, above the greater trochanter, as described for the previous test.
4. *Observe:* S abduct the hip, moving the free leg sideward, while maintaining neutral rotation during this movement (Fig. 22-38, *C*).[9]

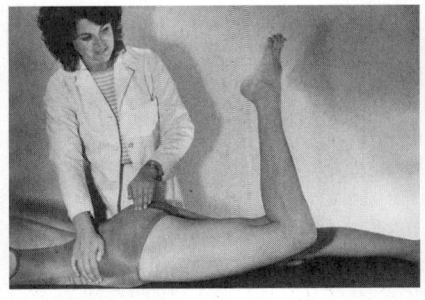
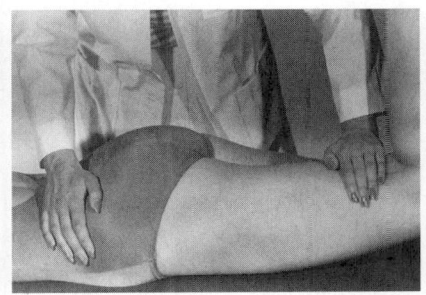
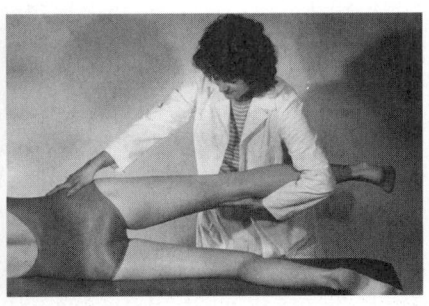

A   B   C

FIG. 22-37
Hip extension. **A,** Palpate and observe. **B,** Resist. **C,** Gravity-decreased position.

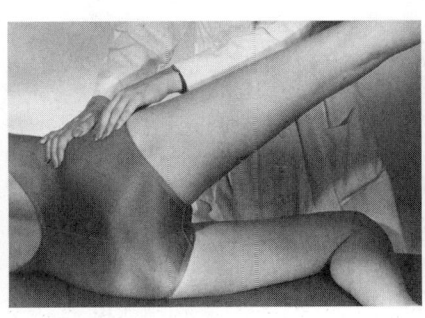
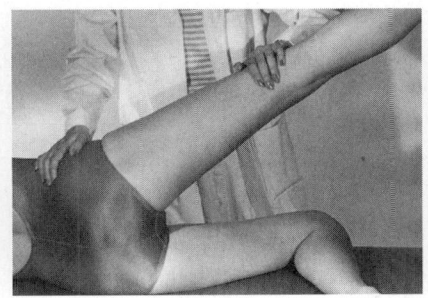
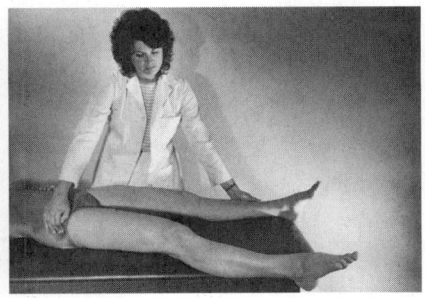

A   B   C

FIG. 22-38
Hip abduction. **A,** Palpate and observe. **B,** Resist. **C,** Gravity-decreased position.

5. *Grade:* According to standard definitions of muscle grades.

Substitutions: Lateral muscles of the trunk may contract to bring the pelvis toward the thorax, effecting partial abduction at the hip.[9] If the hip is externally rotated, the hip flexors may assist in abduction.[6,7,9,12]

Motion

Hip adduction.

Muscles[4,9,10]	Innervation[4,9,10]
Adductor magnus	Obturator L2-4
Adductor brevis	
Adductor longus	
Gracilis	
Pectineus	Femoral L2-4

Procedure for Testing Grades N (5) to F (3)

1. *Position:* S side lying, with the test limb lowermost; E supports the uppermost limb in 25° of abduction and stands behind S.[10] This test may also be done with S in the supine position.[6-9]
2. *Stabilize:* Support S's upper leg in partial abduction while S holds on to the supporting surface for stability.[5,6,9,11]
3. *Palpate:* Any of the adductor muscles as follows: adductor magnus at the middle of the medial surface of the thigh; adductor longus at the medial aspect of the groin; gracilis on the medial aspect of the posterior surface of the knee, just anterior to the semitendinosus tendon.[12]
4. *Observe:* S adduct the hip by raising the lower leg from the table until it meets the upper leg. Observe that there is no rotation, flexion, or extension of the hip or pelvic tilting (Fig. 22-39, *A*).[10,11]
5. *Resist:* Over the medial aspect of the leg, just proximal to the knee, downward toward abduction or outward if tested in supine position (Fig. 22-39, *B*).[6,7,9-11]

Procedure for Testing Grades P (2), T (1), and 0

1. *Position:* S supine; the limb to be tested is abducted to 45°. E stands next to S on the opposite side.
2. *Stabilize:* Over the iliac crest on the side to be tested.[9]
3. *Palpate:* The same as described for the previous test.
4. *Observe:* S adduct the leg toward midline (Fig. 22-39, *C*).
5. *Grade:* According to standard definitions of muscle grades.

Substitutions: Hip flexors may substitute for adductors. S will internally rotate the hip and tilt the pelvis backward. Hamstrings may be used to substitute for adduction. S will externally rotate the hip and tip the pelvis forward.[10-12]

Motion

Hip external rotation.

Muscles[9,10]	Innervation[9,10]
Quadratus femoris	Sacral plexus, L5, S1
Piriformis	Sacral plexus, S1,2
Obturator internus	Sacral plexus, L5-S2
Obturator externus	Obturator nerve, L3,4
Gemellus superior	Sacral plexus, L5-S2
Gemellus inferior	Sacral plexus, L4-S1

Procedure for Testing Grades N (5) to F (3)

1. *Position:* S seated, with knees flexed over the edge of the table. A small pad or folded towel is placed under the knee on the side to be tested. E stands in front of S toward the side to be tested.[6,9-11]
2. *Stabilize:* On the lateral aspect of the knee on the side to be tested. S may grasp the edge of the table to stabilize the trunk and pelvis.[6,9,11]
3. *Palpate:* These deep muscles are difficult or impossible to palpate.[6] Action of the external rotators may be detected by palpating deeply posterior to the greater trochanter of the femur.[9]

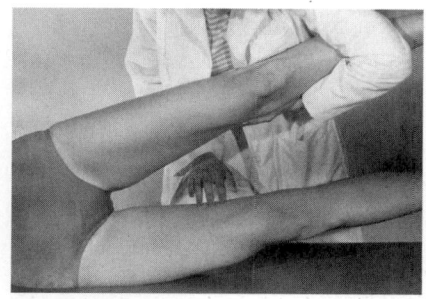
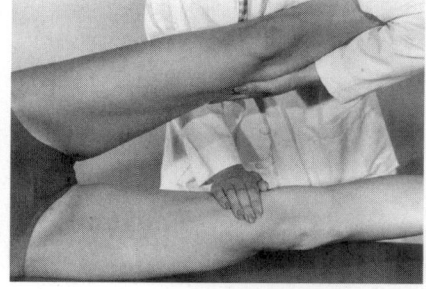
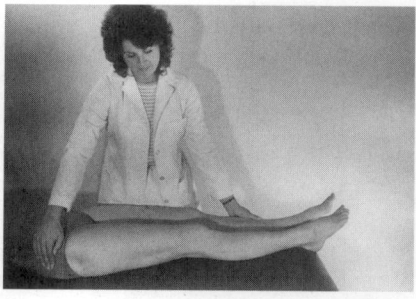

A   **B**   **C**

FIG. 22-39
Hip adduction. **A,** Palpate and observe. **B,** Resist. **C,** Gravity-decreased position.

4. *Observe:* S rotate the thigh outwardly, moving the foot medially (Fig. 22-40, *A*).

5. *Resist:* At the medial aspect of the lower leg, just proximal to the ankle in a lateral direction, toward internal rotation.[6,7,9-11] Resistance should be given carefully and gradually, because the use of the long lever arm can cause joint injury if sudden forceful resistance is given. Subjects with knee instability should be tested in supine position (Fig. 22-40, *B*).[7,9]

Procedure for Testing Grades P (2), T (1), and 0

1. *Position:* S lying supine, with hips and knees extended; the hip to be tested is internally rotated. E is standing next to S on the opposite side.[9,10]

2. *Stabilize:* The pelvis on the side to be tested.

3. *Palpate:* Action of the external rotators may be detected by palpating deeply posterior to the greater trochanter of the femur.[9]

4. *Observe:* S externally rotate the thigh (roll laterally). Gravity may assist this motion once S has passed the neutral position. E may use one hand to palpate and the other to offer slight resistance during the second half of the movement to compensate for the assistance of gravity. If the range can be completed with slight resistance, a grade of poor can be given (Fig. 22-40, *C*).[9]

5. *Grade:* According to standard definitions of muscle grades for fair to normal muscles. Muscles are graded poor if ROM in the gravity-decreased position can be achieved against slight resistance during the second half of the ROM. A grade of trace can be assigned if contraction of external rotators can be detected by the deep palpation, described for the previous test, when the movement is attempted in the gravity-decreased position.[9]

Substitutions: Gluteus maximus may substitute for the deep external rotators when the hip is in extension. Sartorius may substitute, but external rotation will be accompanied by hip flexion, abduction, and knee flexion.[7,12]

Motion

Hip internal rotation.

Muscles[4,9,11]	Innervation[9,11]
Gluteus minimus	Superior gluteal nerve, L4-S1
Gluteus medius	
Tensor fasciae latae	

Procedure for Testing Grades N (5) to F (3)

1. *Position:* S seated on a table, with the knees flexed over the edge and with a small pad placed under the knee. E stands in front of or next to S on the side to be tested.[6,9] (E is shown on the opposite side in the illustration so that the palpation and stabilization will be apparent.)

2. *Stabilize:* At the medial aspect of the knee. S may grasp the edge of the table to stabilize the pelvis and trunk.[6,9,11]

3. *Palpate:* The gluteus medius between the iliac crest and the greater trochanter.[4]

4. *Observe:* S internally rotate the thigh, moving the foot laterally. E should observe that S does not lift the pelvis on the side being tested (Fig. 22-41, *A*).[6,9,10]

5. *Resist:* At the lateral aspect of the lower leg, pushing the leg medially and, therefore, the thigh toward external rotation. The resistance is stressful to the knee joint. Subjects with knee instability should be tested in the supine position described for the next test (Fig. 22-41, *B*).[7,9,11]

Procedure for Testing Grades P (2), T (1), and 0

1. *Position:* S supine, with hips and knees extended; the hip to be tested in external rotation. E stands on the opposite side.[9,10]

2. *Stabilize:* Over the iliac crest on the side to be tested.[9]

3. *Palpate:* The same as described for the previous test.

4. *Observe:* S rotate the thigh inwardly or medially. As in external rotation, gravity may assist the motion once the neutral position is passed, but less than in the test for external rotation (Fig. 22-41, *C*).

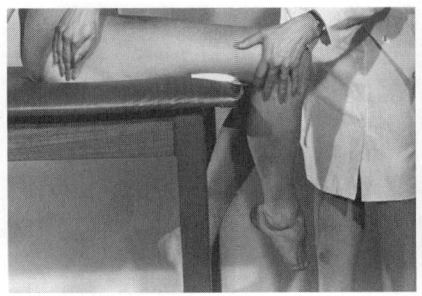
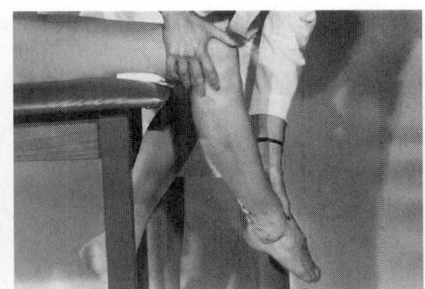
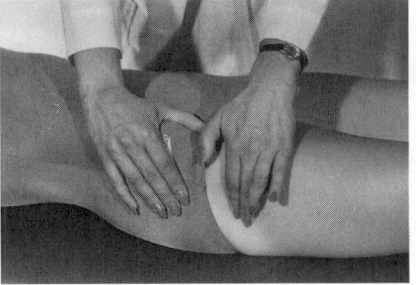

A   B   C

FIG. 22-40

Hip external rotation. **A,** Palpate and observe. **B,** Resist. **C,** Gravity-decreased position.

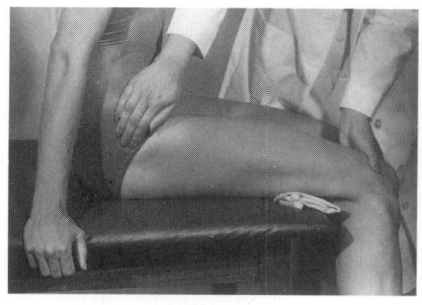 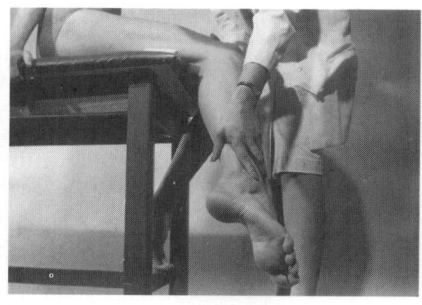 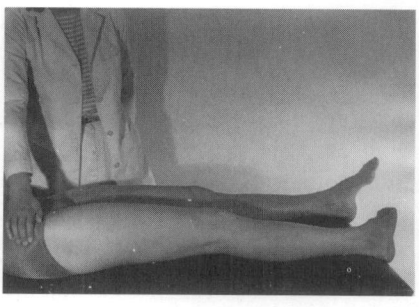

A   B   C

FIG. 22-41
Hip internal rotation. **A,** Palpate and observe. **B,** Resist. **C,** Gravity-decreased position.

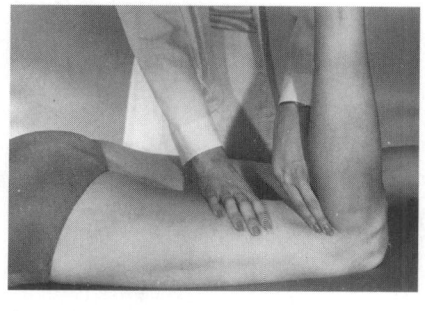 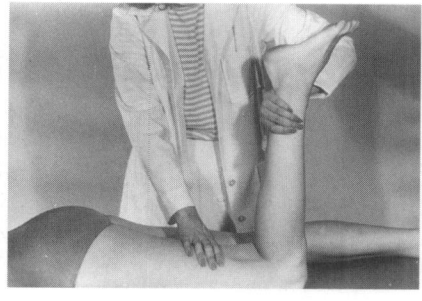 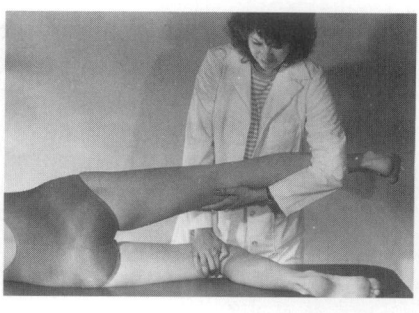

A   B   C

FIG. 22-42
Knee flexion. **A,** Palpate and observe. **B,** Resist. **C,** Gravity-decreased position.

5. *Grade:* According to standard definitions of muscle grades.

   Substitutions: Hip adduction and knee flexion; trunk medial rotation may also cause some internal rotation of the hip.[7,12]

Motion

Knee flexion.

Muscles[4,9,11]	Innervation[4,9,10]
Biceps femoris	Sciatic nerve, L5-S2
Semitendinosus	
Semimembranosus	
(Hamstrings)	

Procedure for Testing Grades N (5) to F (3)

1. *Position:* S lying prone, with knees and hips in extension and neutral rotation with the foot in midline and toes hanging over the end of the table.[5,7,9-11] E stands next to S on the opposite side, or the same side, toward the lower end of the supporting surface.[9]
2. *Stabilize:* Firmly over the posterior aspect of the thigh, above the tendinous insertion of the knee flexors.[6,9]
3. *Palpate:* For the biceps femoris tendon proximal to the knee joint, on the lateral aspect of the popliteal fossa; or for the semitendinosus tendon proximal to the knee joint, medial to the popliteal fossa.[4,6,12]

4. *Observe:* S flex the knee to slightly less than 90° (Fig. 22-42, A).[10,12]
5. *Resist:* Over the posterior aspect of the ankle downward toward knee extension.[6,9,10] Note that not as much resistance can be applied to knee flexion in this position as when tested in sitting position with the hip flexed (Fig. 22-42, B).[11]

Procedure for Testing Grades P (2), T (1), and 0

1. *Position:* S side lying, with knees and hips extended and in neutral rotation. E stands next to S and supports the upper leg in slight abduction to allow testing of the lower leg.[9]
2. *Stabilize:* Over the medial aspect of the thigh.
3. *Palpate:* The semitendinosus as described for the previous test.
4. *Observe:* S flex the knee of the lower leg (Fig. 22-42, C).
5. *Grade:* According to standard definitions of muscle grades.

   Substitutions: The sartorius may substitute or assist the hamstrings, but hip flexion and external rotation will occur simultaneously.[9,10,12] The gracilis may substitute, causing hip adduction with knee flexion.[10] The gastrocnemius may assist or substitute if strong plantar flexion of the ankle occurs during knee flexion.[9,10]

Motion

Knee extension.

Muscles[9]	Innervation[9]
The quadriceps group:	
Rectus femoris	Femoral nerve, L2-4
Vastus intermedius	
Vastus medialis	
Vastus lateralis	

Procedure for Testing Grades N (5) to F (3)

1. *Position:* S sitting, with knees flexed over the edge of the table and feet suspended off the floor. S may lean backward slightly to release tension on the hamstrings and grasp the edge of the table for stability.[6,9,10] E stands next to S on the side to be tested.[6,10]
2. *Stabilize:* The thigh by holding hand firmly over it, or place one hand under S's knee to cushion it from the edge of the table. S may grasp the edge of the table.[7,9-11]
3. *Palpate:* Any of the muscles in the quadriceps femoris group as follows: the rectus femoris on the anterior aspect of the midthigh; the vastus medialis on the medial aspect of the distal thigh; the vastus lateralis on the lateral aspect of the midthigh. The vastus intermedius cannot be palpated.[6,12]
4. *Observe:* S extend the knee to slightly less than full ROM. Observe for hip movements as evidence of substitutions (Fig. 22-43, A).
5. *Resist:* On the anterior surface of the leg, just above the ankle, with downward pressure toward knee flexion.[6,9,11] S should not be allowed to lock the knee joint at the end of the ROM when full extension is achieved.[7,9] Maintenance of a slight amount of knee flexion will prevent this condition. Resistance to a locked knee can cause joint injury (Fig. 22-43, B).[9]

Procedure for Testing Grades P (2), T (1), and 0

1. *Position:* S side lying on the side to be tested. The lower leg is positioned with the hip extended and the knee flexed to 90°. E stands behind S.

2. *Stabilize:* The upper leg in slight abduction with one hand, and with the other over the anterior aspect of the thigh on the leg to be tested.[9]
3. *Palpate:* Any of the muscles, as described for previous test, with the same hand used to stabilize S's thigh. Then ask S to straighten the leg, extending the knee. Observe for hip movements as signs of substitution (Fig. 22-43, C).
4. *Grade:* According to standard definitions of muscle grades.

Substitutions: Tensor fasciae latae may substitute for or assist weak quadriceps. In this case hip internal rotation will accompany knee extension.[6,9,11]

Motion

Ankle plantar flexion.

Muscles[4,9,11]	Innervation[11]
Gastrocnemius	Tibial nerve, S1,2
Soleus	Tibial nerve, L5-S2

Procedure for Testing Grades N (5) to F (3)

1. *Position:* S lying prone, with the hips and knees extended and the feet projecting beyond the edge of the table. E stands at the lower end of the table, facing S's feet.[6,7,10,11]
2. *Stabilize:* The weight of the leg is usually adequate stabilization. E may stabilize the leg proximal to the ankle.[6]
3. *Palpate:* The gastrocnemius on the posterior aspect of the calf of the leg, or the soleus, slightly lateral to and beneath the lateral head of the gastrocnemius.[12] The gastrocnemius tendon above the calcaneus may also be palpated.[9]
4. *Observe:* S plantar flex the ankle. Observe for flexion of the toes and forefoot before movement of the heel as evidence of substitutions (Fig. 22-44, A).[6,11,12]
5. *Resist:* On the posterior aspect of the calcaneus as if pulling downward and on the forefoot as if pushing forward.[10] If there is considerable weakness, pressure to the calcaneus may be sufficient (Fig. 22-44, B).[11]

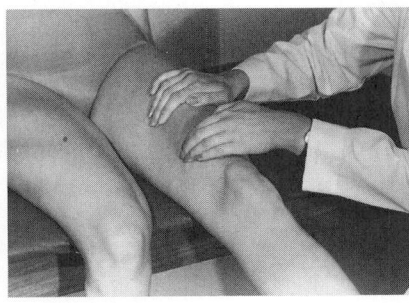
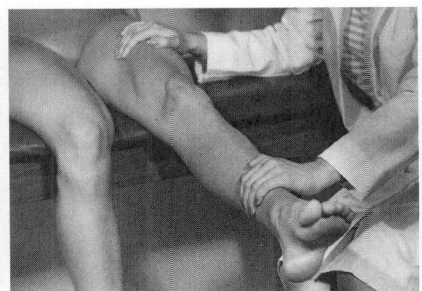
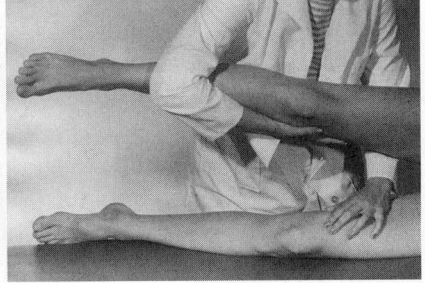

A   B   C

FIG. 22-43

Knee extension. **A,** Palpate and observe. **B,** Resist. **C,** Gravity-decreased position.

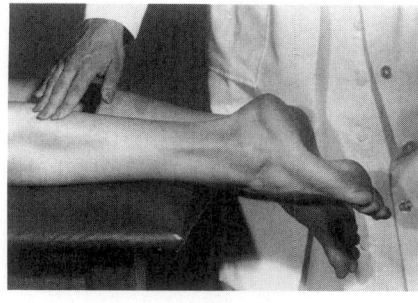 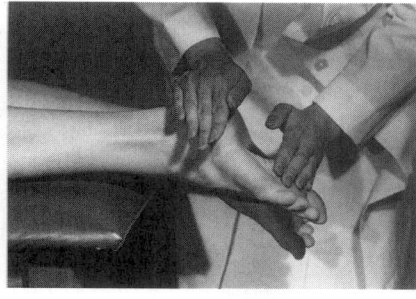 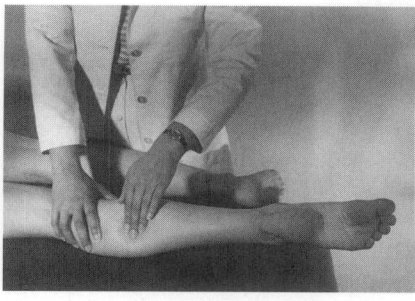

A   B   C

FIG. 22-44
Ankle plantar flexion. **A,** Palpate and observe. **B,** Resist. **C,** Gravity-decreased position.

Procedure for Testing Grades P(2), T (1), and 0

1. *Position:* S lying on the side to be tested; hip and knee of the lower limb are extended and the ankle is in midposition. The upper limb may be flexed at the knee to keep it out of the way. E stands at the lower end of the table.[6,9]
2. *Stabilize:* Over the posterior aspect of the calf.[9]
3. *Palpate:* As described for the previous test.
4. *Observe:* S pull the heel upward, pointing the toes down. Observe for toe flexion, inversion, or eversion of the foot as evidence of substitutions (Fig. 22-44, C).
5. *Grade:* According to standard definitions of muscle grades.

   Substitutions: The flexor digitorum longus and flexor hallucis longus can substitute for plantar flexors, producing toe flexion and flexion of the forefoot, with incomplete movement of the calcaneus. Substitution by the peroneus longus and brevis will cause foot eversion, and substitution by the tibialis posterior will cause foot inversion. Substitution by all three will effect plantar flexion of the forefoot, with limited movement of the calcaneus.[9,10,12]

Motion

Ankle dorsiflexion with inversion.

Muscles[6,9,10]	Innervation[6,9,11]
Tibialis anterior	Peroneal nerve, L4-S1

Procedure for Testing Grades N (5) to F (3)

1. *Position:* S seated, with the legs, flexed at the knees, over the edge of the table. E sits in front of S, slightly to the side to be tested.[6,9-11]
2. *Stabilize:* The leg just above the ankle. S's heel can rest in E's lap.[6,10]
3. *Palpate:* The tibialis anterior tendon on the anterior medial aspect of the ankle joint.[6,7,9] Muscle fibers may be palpated on the anterior surface of the leg, just lateral to the tibia.[12]

4. *Observe:* S dorsiflex and invert the foot, keeping the toes relaxed.[10] Watch for extension of the great toe preceding the ankle motion as a sign of muscle substitution (Fig. 22-45, A).[9,10]
5. *Resist:* On the medial dorsal aspect of the foot, toward plantar flexion and eversion (Fig. 22-45, B).[6,9,11]

Procedure for Testing Grades P (2), T (1), and 0

The same position and procedure described for the previous test may be used, with modified grading. The test may also be performed with S in side-lying or supine position.[7,9]

1. *Grade:* If the against-gravity position is used in the procedure for grades P to 0, clinical judgment of the examiner must be used to determine muscle grades. Partial ROM against gravity can be graded poor.[10] If the test is performed in the supine position for these grades, standard definitions of muscle grades may be used.[9]

   Substitutions: The extensor hallucis longus and extensor digitorum longus may assist or substitute. Movement will be preceded by extension of the great toe or by all of the toes.[7,9-12]

Motion

Foot inversion.

Muscles[9,11]	Innervation[7,8]
Tibialis posterior	Tibial nerve, L5, S1

Procedure for Testing Grades N (5) to F (3)

1. *Position:* S lying on the side to be tested, with the hip in neutral rotation, the knee slightly flexed, and the foot and ankle in a neutral position.[6] The upper leg may be flexed at the knee to keep it out of the way. E stands at the end of the table.
2. *Stabilize:* The leg to be tested above the ankle joint on the dorsal surface of the calf, being careful not to put pressure on the tibialis posterior muscle.[6,9]
3. *Palpate:* The tendon of the tibialis posterior muscle between the medial malleolus and navicular bone or above and just posterior to the medial malleolus.[6,7,9]

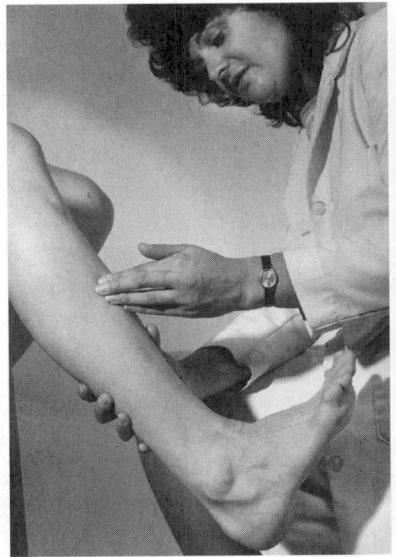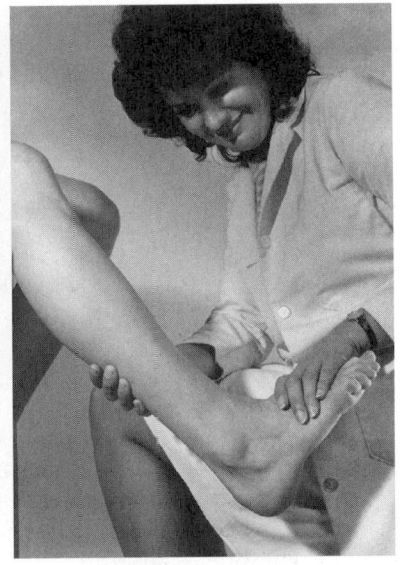

A   B

FIG. 22-45
Ankle dorsiflexion with inversion. **A,** Palpate and observe. **B,** Resist.

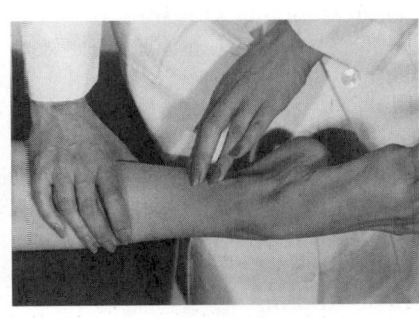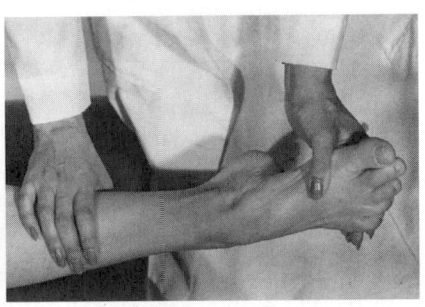

A   B

FIG. 22-46
Foot inversion. **A,** Palpate and observe. **B,** Resist.

4. *Observe:* S invert the foot, keeping the toes relaxed. There normally will be some plantar flexion as well (Fig. 22-46, A).[9,11]
5. *Resist:* On the medial border of the forefoot toward eversion (Fig. 22-46, B).[6,7,9,11]

Procedure for Testing Grades P (2), T (1), and 0
1. *Position:* S lying supine, with the hip extended and in neutral rotation, the knee extended, and the ankle in midposition.
2. *Stabilize:* The same as described for the previous test.
3. *Palpate:* The same as described for the previous test.
4. *Observe:* S move the foot inward (medially), inverting it while keeping the toes relaxed.
5. *Grade:* According to standard definitions of muscle grades.
   Substitutions: The flexor hallucis longus and flexor digitorum longus can substitute for the tibialis poste-

rior. Movement will be accompanied by toe flexion, or toes will flex when resistance is applied.[9-12]

Motion

Foot eversion.

Muscles[9,11]	Innervation[9,11]
Peroneus longus	Peroneal nerve, L4-S1
Peroneus brevis	

Procedure for Testing Grades Normal (N) and Fair (F)
1. *Position:* S side lying, with the lower leg flexed at the knee to keep it out of the way. The upper test leg is in hip extension with neutral rotation, knee extension, and ankle plantar flexion with foot inversion.[6]
2. *Stabilize:* Medially or laterally, above the ankle.[6]
3. *Palpate:* The peroneus longus over the upper half of the lateral aspect of the calf, just distal to the head

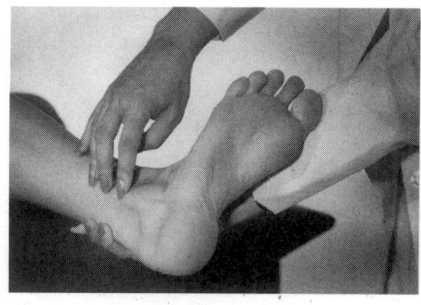
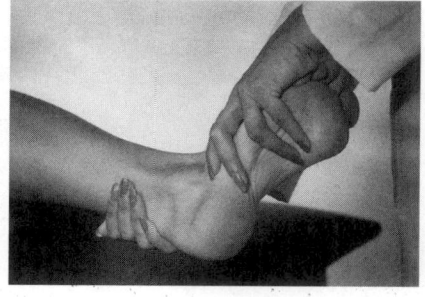
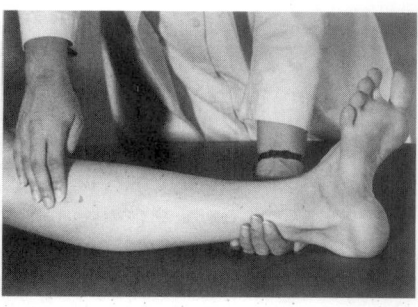

A   B   C

FIG. 22-47
Foot eversion. **A,** Palpate and observe. **B,** Resist. **C,** Gravity-decreased position.

of the fibula. Its tendon can be palpated on the lateral aspect of the ankle, above and behind the lateral malleolus. The peroneus brevis tendon may be palpated on the lateral border of the foot, proximal to the base of the 5th metatarsal.[6,9,12] Its muscle fibers can be found on the lower half of the lateral surface of the leg, over the fibula.[9]

4. *Observe:* S evert the foot. (Note that this movement is normally accompanied by some degree of plantar flexion.[11,12]) Observe for dorsiflexion or toe extension as evidence of substitutions (Fig. 22-47, *A*).

5. *Resist:* Against the lateral border and the plantar surface of the foot toward inversion and dorsiflexion (Fig. 22-47, *B*).[6,11]

Procedure for Testing Grades P (2), T (1), and 0

1. *Position:* S lying supine, hip extended and in neutral rotation.[9] The knee is extended, and the ankle is in midposition.

2. *Stabilize:* The leg under the calf.

3. *Palpate:* The same as described for the previous test.

4. *Observe:* S evert the foot (Fig. 22-47, *C*).

5. *Grade:* Grade according to standard definitions of muscle grades.

Substitutions: The peroneus tertius, while everting the foot, also dorsiflexes it. If it is substituting for the peroneus longus and peroneus brevis, dorsiflexion will accompany eversion. The extensor digitorum longus can also substitute for the peroneals, and toe extension will precede or accompany eversion.[7,12]

SUMMARY

Many diseases and injuries result in muscle weakness. Screening tests can be used to assess the general level of strength available for ADL and to determine which patients and which muscle groups might need the MMT.

Manual muscle testing evaluates the level of strength in a muscle or muscle group. It is used with patients who have motor unit (lower motor neuron) disorders

and orthopedic conditions. It does not measure muscle endurance or coordination, and it cannot be used accurately in upper motor neuron disorders when spasticity is present.

Accurate assessment of muscle strength depends on the knowledge, skill, and experience of the examiner. Although there are standard definitions of muscle grades, clinical judgment is important in accurate evaluation.

Muscle test results are used to plan treatment strategies to improve occupational performance, compensate for muscle weakness, and increase strength.

REVIEW QUESTIONS

1. List three general classifications of physical dysfunction in which muscle weakness is a primary symptom.

2. List at least three purposes for assessing muscle strength.

3. Discuss five considerations and their implications in treatment planning that are based on the results of the muscle strength assessment.

4. Define *endurance*.

5. How can muscle weakness be differentiated from joint limitation?

6. If there is joint limitation, can muscle strength be measured accurately? How is strength recorded when available ROM is less than normal?

7. What does the MMT measure?

8. What are the limitations of the MMT?

9. When is the MMT contraindicated?

10. What are the criteria for determining muscle grades?

11. In relation to the floor as a horizontal plane, describe or demonstrate what is meant by the terms "with gravity assisting," "with gravity decreased," "against gravity," and "against gravity and resistance."

12. List five factors that can influence the amount of resistance against which a muscle group can hold.

13. Define the muscle grades: N (5), F- (3-), F (3), P (2), P- (2-), T (1), and zero (0).

14. Explain what is meant by *substitution*.
15. How are substitutions most likely to be ruled out in the muscle testing procedure?
16. List the steps in the muscle testing procedure.
17. Is it always necessary to perform the MMT to determine level of strength? If not, what alternatives may be used to make a general assessment of strength?
18. List the purposes of screening tests.

REFERENCES

1. Basmajian JF: *Muscles alive*, ed 4, Baltimore, 1978, Williams & Wilkins.
2. Bobath B: *Adult hemiplegia: evaluation and treatment*, ed 2, London, 1978, William Heinemann Medical Books.
3. Brunnstrom S: *Movement therapy in hemiplegia*, New York, 1970, Harper & Row.
4. Brunnstrom S: *Clinical kinesiology*, Philadelphia, 1972, FA Davis.
5. Chusid J: *Correlative neuroanatomy and functional neurology*, ed 19, Los Altos, Calif, 1985, Lange Medical Publications.
6. Clarkson HM: *Musculoskeletal assessment*, ed 2, Philadelphia, 2000, Lippincott Williams & Wilkins.
7. Clarkson HM, Gilewich GB: *Musculoskeletal assessment*, Baltimore, 1989, Williams & Wilkins.
8. Cole JH, Furness AL, Twomey LT: *Muscles in action*, New York, 1988, Churchill Livingstone.
9. Daniels L. Worthingham C: *Muscle testing*, ed 5, Philadelphia, 1986, WB Saunders.
10. Hislop HJ, Montgomery J: *Daniels and Worthingham's muscle testing*, ed 6, Philadelphia, 1995, WB Saunders.
11. Kendall FP, McCreary EK: *Muscles: testing and function*, ed 2, Baltimore, 1983, Williams & Wilkins.
12. Killingsworth A: *Basic physical disability procedures*, San Jose, Calif, 1987, Maple Press.
13. Landen B, Amizich A: Functional muscle examination and gait analysis, *J Am Phys Ther Assoc* 43:39, 1963.
14. Pact V, Sirotkin-Roses M, Beatus J: *The muscle testing handbook*, Boston, 1984, Little, Brown.
15. Rancho Los Amigos Hospital, Department of Occupational Therapy: *Guide for muscle testing of the upper extremity*, Downey, Calif, 1973, Professional Staff Association of the Rancho Los Amigos Hospital.

CHAPTER 23

Motor Control

LINDA ANDERSON PRESTON

LEARNING OBJECTIVES

After studying this chapter the student or practitioner will be able to do the following:

1. Differentiate between upper and lower motor neuron pathological conditions.
2. List the components of motor control.
3. Differentiate between spasticity and hyperactive tonic stretch reflexes.
4. Recognize four types of rigidity.
5. Differentiate between spinal and cerebral hypertonus.
6. Identify all categories of the Ashworth Scale.
7. List standardized assessments designed for evaluating function after cerebrovascular accident.
8. Describe normal muscle tone.
9. List and describe at least four different abnormal tone states.
10. Describe how to assess muscle tone.
11. List the components of the postural mechanism.
12. List and describe at least four types of cerebellar disorders.
13. List and describe at least four extrapyramidal disorders.
14. Describe how to assess coordination.
15. Name several current medical and surgical treatment options for management of hypertonia.
16. List at least three conservative occupational therapy interventions for hypertonia.

Maureen (Mo) Johnson, OTR, BCN, and Jeffrey S. Hecht, MD, FAAPMR, are gratefully acknowledged for reviewing and assisting with this chapter.

Motor control is the ability to make dynamic postural adjustments and direct body and limb movement in purposeful activity.[83] Components necessary for motor control include normal muscle tone, normal postural tone and postural mechanisms, selective movement, and coordination. Complex neurological systems (i.e., the cerebral cortex, basal ganglia, and cerebellum) collaborate to make motor control possible. A neurological insult such as cerebrovascular accident (stroke or brain attack), brain injury, or a disease such as multiple sclerosis or Parkinson's disease affects motor control. Functional recovery depends on the initial amount of neurological damage, prompt access to medical treatment that limits the extent of neurological damage,[75] and therapeutic intervention that can facilitate motor recovery.

Plasticity is an important concept in neurological rehabilitation, because it helps explain why recovery is possible after brain injury or lesion. Plasticity is defined as "anatomical and electrophysiological changes in the central nervous system."[83] In some instances the central nervous system (CNS) is able to reorganize and adapt to functional demands after injury.[16] Motor relearning can occur through the use of existing neural pathways (unmasking) or through the development of new neural connections (sprouting).[68] In the case of unmasking, it is believed that seldom-used pathways become more active after the primary pathway has been injured. The adjacent nerves take over the function of the damaged nerves. In the case of sprouting, dendrites from one nerve form a new attachment or synapse with another (Fig. 23-1).[25] It is also believed that new axonal processes develop in sprouting.[68]

Observing for motor control dysfunction during occupational performance is a way to assess motor control. It is necessary to evaluate the specific components that underlie motor control. These components are muscle tone, postural tone and the postural mechanism, reflexes, selective movement, and coordination. A comprehensive assessment can help the patient and occupational therapist plan appropriate treatment intervention.

This chapter focuses on the functional effects of lesions in the upper motor neuron system (UMNS). The UMNS includes any nerve cell body or nerve fiber in the spinal cord (other than the anterior horn cells) and all superior structures. These structures include descending nerve tracts and brain cells of both gray and white matter that subserve motor function.

The lower motor neuron system includes the anterior horn cells of the spinal cord, the spinal nerves, the nuclei and axons of cranial nerves III through X, and the peripheral nerves. Lower motor neuron dysfunction results in diminished or absent deep tendon reflexes and muscle flaccidity. Figure 23-2 illustrates the influence of the upper motor neuron system over the lower motor neuron system.[65]

PERFORMANCE ASSESSMENTS

The occupational therapist has the challenge of maximizing the patient's ability to return to purposeful and meaningful occupation within his or her physical and social environment.[81] Therefore, evaluating functional performance is primary in helping patients to actualize realistic goals. The Canadian Occupational Performance Measure[60] is an assessment tool that ensures client-centered therapy. This tool helps prioritize the patient's

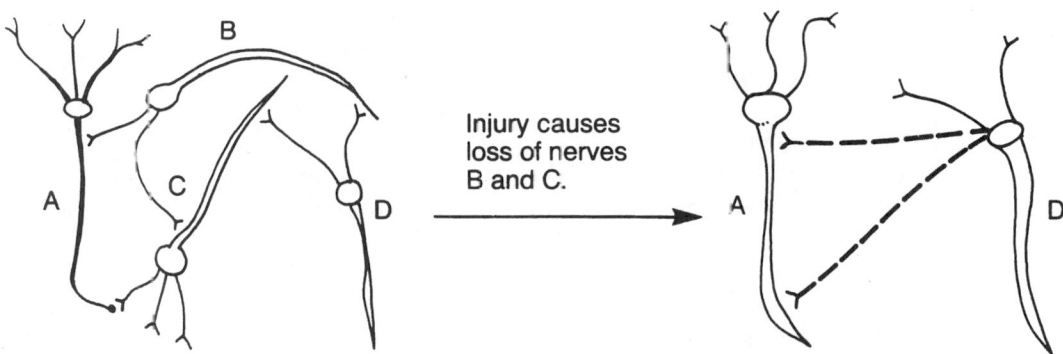

Injury causes loss of nerves B and C.

New dendrite connections "sprout" from nerve D to reestablish contact with nerve A.

FIG. 23-1

Sprouting theory of nerve cell replacement. Injury causes loss of nerves B and C. New dendrite connections "sprout" from nerve D to reestablish contact with nerve A. (From DeBoskey DS, Hecht JS, Calub CJ: *Educating families of the head injured*, Rockville, Md, 1991, Aspen Publishers.)

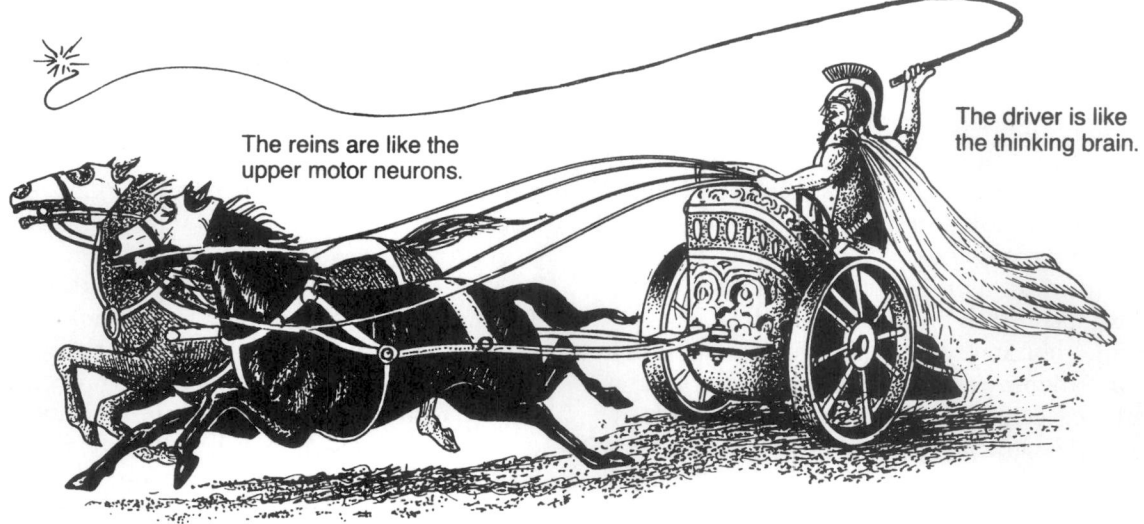

The reins are like the upper motor neurons.

The driver is like the thinking brain.

The horses are like lower motor neurons and muscles.

FIG. 23-2

Control of movement is comparable with a chariot driver with a team of horses. The upper motor neuron system facilitates or inhibits the lower motor neuron system. The driver is like the brain, the reins are like the descending nerve tracts, the horses are like lower motor neurons and muscles. (From DeBoskey DS, Hecht, JS, Calub CJ: *Educating families of the head injured*, Rockville, Md, 1991, Aspen Publishers).

functional activity goals in the areas of self-care, leisure, and productivity.[60]

The occupational therapist can observe the patient or client for motor control dysfunction during assessment of basic activities of daily living (BADL) and instrumental ADL (IADL), as well as of productive and leisure activities. The therapist must observe how problems in motor control affect motor performance. The therapist must also consider the patient's sensation, perception, cognition, and medical status. The following questions may be helpful to guide observation:

1. Is the patient having difficulty with sitting or standing balance?
2. Is the patient having difficulty making appropriate postural adjustments of the trunk and limbs to achieve the best position and motions needed to perform the activity?
3. Is there adequate trunk control to perform the activity?
4. Do changes in body and head position affect muscle tone?
5. Are primitive reflexes evoked during performance?
6. Is hypertonicity limiting movement or speed of movement?
7. Is there weakness that prohibits antigravity activity?
8. Are tremors, athetoid, or choreiform movements apparent?
9. Is there apparent incoordination (i.e., overshooting or undershooting the target)? Are there extraneous movements?
10. What is the spontaneous, functional use of involved extremities?

Many ADL tests are available to assess occupational performance and are also useful to observe motor control. The Test d'Evaluation des Membres Superieurs de Personnes Agees (TEMPA) is an upper extremity functional activity performance test for geriatric patients. The test was developed to help therapists distinguish between "normal and pathological aging in upper extremity performance."[28] Some of the test items are picking up and moving a jar, writing on an envelope, tying a scarf, and handling coins.[28]

Several assessments have been designed to assess function after cerebrovascular accident (CVA). These can be used to observe for motor control problems.

1. The Functional Test for the Hemiplegic/Paretic Upper Extremity[88] assesses the patient's ability to use the involved arm for purposeful tasks. This test provides objective documentation of functional improvement. The test includes tasks ranging from those that involve basic stabilization to more difficult tasks requiring fine manipulation and proximal stabilization. Examples include holding a pouch, stabilizing a jar, wringing a rag, hooking and zipping a zipper, folding a sheet, and putting in a light bulb overhead.[88]
2. The Fugl-Myer[53] is based on the natural progression of neurological recovery after CVA. Low scores on the Fugl-Myer have been closely correlated with the presence of severe spasticity.[53] Fugl-Meyer and associates developed a quantitative assessment of motor func-

tion following stroke, by using Brunnstrom's methods[14] and by measuring such parameters as range of motion (ROM), pain, sensation, and balance. The scores on the Fugl-Meyer assessment correlate with ADL performance.[32]

3. The Arm Motor Ability Test (AMAT)[55] is a functional assessment of upper extremity function. Cutting meat, making a sandwich, opening a jar, and putting on a T-shirt are some of the tasks included in this test. This test has high interrater reliability and test-retest reliability.[55]

4. The Motricity Index (MI)[21] is a valid and reliable test of motor impairment that can be performed quickly. The test assesses pinching a cube with the index finger and thumb, as well as elbow flexion, shoulder abduction, ankle dorsiflexion, knee extension, and hip flexion.[21]

5. The Assessment of Motor and Process Skills (AMPS)[6] is a standardized test that assesses motor and process skills in IADL. The test was created by occupational therapists. Although the test is not diagnosis specific, it has been widely used with patients who have had a CVA. Occupational therapy practitioners are eligible to become certified in the use of this test, through a five-day training course.[6]

After observing functional performance, the occupational therapist usually will find it necessary to assess the performance components that underlie motor control: muscle tone, the postural mechanism, reflexes, sensation, and coordination.

NORMAL MUSCLE TONE

Normal muscle tone, a component of the normal postural mechanism, is a continuous state of mild contraction, or a state of preparedness in the muscle.[76] It is dependent on the integrity of peripheral and CNS mechanisms and the properties of muscle. When normal muscle tone is present, a tension between the origin and insertion of a muscle is felt as resistance by the therapist when passively manipulating the limbs. The tension is determined partly by mechanical factors such as connective tissue and viscoelastic properties of muscle, and partly by the degree of motor unit activity.[31] When passively stretched, the normal muscle offers a small amount of involuntary resistance.

Normal muscle tone relies on normal function of the cerebellum, motor cortex, basal ganglia, midbrain, vestibular system, spinal cord functions, and neuromuscular system (including the mechanical-elastic features of the muscle and connective tissues)[52] and on a normally functioning stretch reflex.[10] The stretch reflex is mediated by the muscle spindle, a sophisticated sensory receptor continuously reporting sensory information from muscles to the CNS.

Normal muscle tone varies from one individual to another. Within the range that is considered normal, the degree of normal tone depends on such factors as age, sex, and occupation. Normal muscle tone is characterized by the following:

1. Effective coactivation (stabilization) at axial and proximal joints
2. Ability to move against gravity and resistance
3. Ability to maintain the position of the limb if it is placed passively by the examiner and then released[10]
4. Balanced tone between agonist and antagonistic muscles
5. Ease of ability to shift from stability to mobility and reverse as needed
6. Ability to use muscles in groups or selectively, if necessary[35]
7. Resilience or slight resistance in response to passive movement[26]

Hypertonicity (increased tone) interferes with performance of normal selective movement because it affects the timing and smoothness of agonist and antagonist muscles groups. Normalization of muscle tone and amelioration of **paresis** (slight or incomplete paralysis) are desirable when striving for selective motor control. Some function can be achieved even though tone may not be normal.

ABNORMAL MUSCLE TONE

Abnormal muscle tone is usually described with the following terms: *flaccidity, hypotonus, hypertonus, spasticity,* and *rigidity*. To plan appropriate treatment interventions the therapist must recognize the differences among these tone states and identify them during the clinical assessment, to plan the appropriate intervention.

Flaccidity

Flaccidity refers to the absence of tone. The patient will have the absence of deep tendon reflexes. Active movement is absent.[24,35] Flaccidity can result from spinal or cerebral shock immediately after a spinal or cerebral insult. In traumatic upper motor neuron lesions of cerebral or spinal origin, flaccidity is usually present initially and then changes to hypertonicity within a few weeks.[59]

Flaccidity also can result from lower motor neuron dysfunction, such as a peripheral nerve injury or a disruption of the reflex arc at the alpha motor neuron level. The muscles feel soft and offer no resistance to passive movement.[84] If the flaccid limb is moved passively, it will feel heavy. If moved to a given position and released, the limb will drop because the muscles are unable to resist gravity.

Hypotonus

Hypotonus is considered by many to be a decrease of normal muscle tone (i.e., low tone). Deep tendon reflexes are diminished or absent.[24,35] Van der Mech and Van der Gijn[86] suggested that hypotonus could be an erroneous clinical concept. They performed electromyography (EMG) analysis on the quadriceps muscles in "hypotonic" patients (e.g. peripheral neuropathy, cerebral infarction, and other diagnoses) and in relaxed normal subjects in a lower leg free-fall test. They concluded in their study that if a patient's limb feels hypotonic or flaccid, it is the result of weakness, not long-latency stretch reflexes.[85]

Hypertonus

Hypertonus is increased muscle tone. Hypertonicity can occur when there is a lesion in the premotor cortex, the basal ganglia, or descending pathways.[17] Damage to upper motor neuron systems increases stimulation of the lower motor neurons, with a resultant increased alpha motor activity.[37] Any neurological condition changing the upper motor neuron pathways that directly or indirectly facilitate alpha motor neuron activity may result in hypertonicity.

Hypertonicity often occurs in a synergistic neuromuscular pattern. Synergies are defined as "a fixed set of muscles contracting with a preset sequence of time and contraction."[89] A typical synergy seen in the upper extremity after CVA or traumatic brain injury is a flexion synergy.[14] For more details on synergies, refer to Chapter 34.

There is considerable energy cost in moving against hypertonicity. It takes a great deal of effort for patients with moderate to severe hypertonicity to move against this drawing force. Even patients with mild hypertonicity report frustration during functional activities. This frustration, coupled with the fatigue, decreased dexterity, and paresis associated with upper motor neuron syndrome, can influence therapy participation.[72] Furthermore, the architecture of hypertonic muscles changes over time. The muscles lose their ability to lengthen and shorten because of viscoelastic changes that result from the hypertonia.[16,52]

Hypertonicity can increase as a result of painful or noxious stimuli. These stimuli can often be reduced with good medical care. Stimuli that can increase tone are pressure sores, ingrown toenails, tight elastic straps on a urine collection leg bag, tight clothing, an obstructed catheter, urinary tract infections, constipation, and fecal impaction.[34,52] Other triggering factors include fear, anxiety, environmental temperature extremes, heterotopic ossification, and sensory overload.[37,41] These factors are true for both cerebral and spinal hypertonicity; however, they are more pronounced in spinal hypertonia. Therapeutic intervention should be designed to reduce, eliminate, or cope with these extrinsic factors.

Patients with hypertonicity often have difficulty initiating movement, especially rapid movement.[52] Although hypertonic muscles appear to be able to take a lot of resistance, they do not function as normal, strong muscles do. Through the mechanism of reciprocal inhibition, hypertonic muscles inhibit activity of their antagonists and thus can mask potentially good or normal function of antagonists.[72,83]

Cerebral Hypertonia

Cerebral hypertonia is caused by traumatic brain injury, stroke, anoxia, neoplasms (brain tumors), metabolic disorders, cerebral palsy, and diseases of the brain. In multiple sclerosis, hypertonia stems from both spinal and cerebral lesions.[72] Tone fluctuates continuously in response to extrinsic and intrinsic factors. Cerebral hypertonia usually occurs in definite patterns of flexion or extension, causing the limb to draw in one direction (Fig. 23-3).[10] Typically the patterns occur in the antigravity muscles of the upper and lower extremities (e.g., flexors of the upper extremities, extensors of the lower extremities).

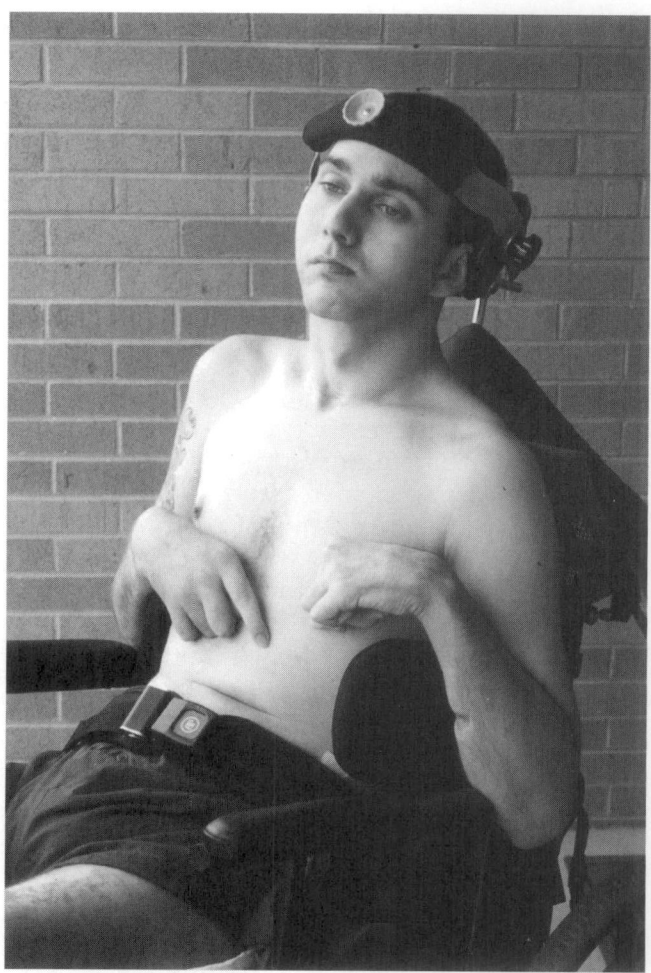

FIG. 23-3

A patient with upper extremity hypertonicity after traumatic brain injury.

The reemergence of primitive reflexes and associated reactions alters postural tone. When an individual is lying supine, muscle tone is less than when the individual is sitting or standing. The tone is at its highest during ambulation. Thus attention to postural tone is important when positioning a patient for splinting or casting. A cast or splint fabricated on a patient in a supine position may not fit when the patient is sitting up, because of the influence of gravity and posture on muscle tone.[72]

Spinal Hypertonia

Spinal hypertonia results from injuries and diseases of the spinal cord. In slow-onset spinal disease (e.g., spinal stenosis or tumor), there is no period of spinal shock. In traumatic spinal cord injury, spinal shock occurs and is characterized by flaccidity. With time (weeks or months) the flaccidity diminishes and hypertonus develops.[72] The affected extremities first develop flexor and adductor tone.[91] Over time, extensor tone develops and becomes predominant in the lower extremities. Spinal hypertonia can lead to muscle spasms severe enough to cause an individual to fall out of a wheelchair, off a gurney, or out of bed. The degree of hypertonicity in incomplete spinal lesions varies, depending on the degree and direction of remaining supraspinal influences.[77] The tone tends to be more severe in incomplete spinal cord lesions than in complete lesions.[72]

Spasticity

There has been much controversy in recent years about the difference between **spasticity** and hypertonia. Lance's[56] definition of spasticity is still accepted by many physicians and therapists. He defined spasticity as "a motor disorder characterized by a velocity-dependent increase in tonic stretch reflexes (muscle tone) with exaggerated tendon jerks resulting from hyperexcitability of the stretch reflex as one component of the upper motor neuron syndrome."[56]

Little, and Massagli[58,59] believe that pure spasticity is a subset of hypertonia. It is possible that Lance's definition does not adequately distinguish between the presence of phasic and tonic stretch reflexes, which present different clinical scenarios. This chapter attempts to clarify the differences using current physiatry literature.

Spasticity has three characteristics:

1. Hyperactivity of the muscle spindle's phasic stretch reflex with hyperactive firing of the IA afferent nerve
2. Velocity dependence, meaning the stretch reflex is only elicited by the examiner's rapid passive stretch[58,59]
3. The "clasp-knife" phenomenon. This means that when the examiner takes the extremity through a quick passive stretch, a sudden catch or resistance is felt, followed by a release of the resistance. What ac-

tually happens is that the initial high resistance of spasticity is suddenly inhibited.[52]

One of the main systems that has been affected when spasticity is present is the pyramidal system, which consists of the corticospinal and corticobulbar tracts. The corticospinal tract controls goal-directed, voluntary movement.[16]

Clonus

Clonus is a specific type of spasticity. This condition is often present in patients with moderate to severe spasticity. Clonus is characterized by repetitive contractions in the antagonistic muscles in response to rapid stretch. There are recurrent bursts of IA afferent activity, which result in a cyclical oscillation of phasic stretch reflexes.[52,59] Clonus is most commonly seen in the finger flexors and ankle plantar flexors.[59] The occurrence of clonus can interfere with participation in purposeful activity, transfers, and mobility. Therapists should educate the patient about how to bear weight actively, because this usually will stop the clonus. Therapists and physicians record clonus by counting the number of beats.[52] A three-beat clonus can be rated as mild and is less likely to interfere with ADL than clonus that is 10-beat or more. Clonus may be elicited during quick stretch tone evaluation or may become apparent during assessment of occupation (e.g., grasping or ambulation). If clonus greatly interferes with ADL, the patient may be a candidate for a referral to a physiatrist or neurologist for oral medication, Botox* injection, or a Phenol motor point block.[72]

Hypertonic Stretch Reflex

Therapists often confuse **hypertonic stretch reflexes** (HTSRs) with spasticity. These two conditions are similar in two ways:

1. HTSRs and spasticity both draw the limb into a unilateral direction.
2. HTSRs and spasticity are both types or subcategories of hypertonia.

HTSRs are different from spasticity in four ways:

1. HTSRs are typically not velocity dependent; that is, they are not evoked by rapid movement; rather, they are elicited by slow joint movement, and the hypertonus persists as long as the muscle stretch is maintained, because of the firing of group II muscle spindle afferents.[58,59]
2. HTSRs occur primarily in the flexor muscles in both upper and lower extremities, and often lead to contractures.[59]

---

*Allergan Pharmaceuticals, Inc., 2525 Dupont Drive, P.O. Box 19534, Irvine, CA 92713-9534

3. During passive movement, there is no catch felt with HTSR, as there is with the clasp-knife phenomenon of spasticity.
4. Most of the resistance with HTSRs is felt at the end of the ROM, and is objectively measurable by EMG.

Rigidity

Rigidity is an increase in muscle tone of agonist and antagonist muscles simultaneously (i.e., muscles on both sides of the joint). Both groups of muscles contract steadily, leading to increased resistance to passive movement in any direction and throughout the ROM.[27,63] Rigidity signals involvement of the extrapyramidal pathways in the circuitry of the basal ganglia, diencephalon, and brainstem. It occurs in isolated forms in disorders such as Parkinson's disease, traumatic brain injury, some degenerative diseases, encephalitis, tumors,[26] and certain toxins and after carbon monoxide poisoning. Rigidity is also seen in conjunction with spasticity in those with stroke and traumatic brain injury. Rigidity is not velocity dependent.[82]

Rigidity is evaluated during muscle tone evaluation (Fig. 23-4). Four types of rigidity are commonly seen:
1. Lead pipe rigidity
2. Cogwheel rigidity
3. Decorticate rigidity
4. Decerebrate rigidity

Both lead pipe and cogwheel rigidity can occur in Parkinson's disease. In *lead pipe rigidity*, constant resistance is felt throughout the ROM when the part is moved slowly and passively in any direction. The rigidity feels similar to the feeling of bending solder or a lead pipe, thus its name. In *cogwheel rigidity*, a rhythmic give occurs in the resistance throughout the ROM, much like the feeling of turning a cogwheel.[63] It is thought that cogwheel rigidity may be a rigidity superimposed on tremor, which results in the ratchety pattern.[48] It is crucial for the therapist to document the type of rigidity during initial assessment and how it affects the patient's performance. Deep tendon reflexes are normal or only mildly increased in Parkinson's rigidity.

Decerebrate and decorticate rigidity can occur after severe traumatic brain injury with diffuse cerebral damage or anoxia. These abnormal postures occur immediately after injury and can last a few days or weeks if recovery occurs, or persist indefinitely if there is little or no recovery.

Decerebrate rigidity results from lesions in the bilateral hemispheres of the diencephalon and midbrain. It appears as rigid extension posturing of all limbs and the neck. Bilateral cortical lesions can result in **decorticate rigidity,** which appears as flexion hypertonus in the upper extremities and as extension tone in the lower extremities. Supine positioning increases the abnormal tone, and with either type of rigidity it may be extremely difficult to position patients in a sitting position.[59]

MUSCLE TONE ASSESSMENT

Objective assessment of muscle tone in the patient with cerebral spasticity is difficult because the tone fluctuates continuously in response to extrinsic and intrinsic factors. The postural reflex mechanism, the position of the body and head in space, the position of the head in relation to the body, and stereotypical reflexes and associated reactions all influence the degree and distribution of abnormal muscle tone.[10,41]

Guidelines for Muscle Tone Assessment

The following steps describe the correct procedures for assessing muscle tone.
1. Record the test position of the patient because body and head position influence cerebral hypertonus. The patient's upper extremity muscle tone is usually evaluated with the patient sitting on a mat table when possible. Remember that the patient's posture (e.g., the seated patient bearing weight symmetrically versus slumped or leaning to one side) will affect the results of the tone evaluation.
2. Grasp the patient's limb proximal and distal to the joint to be tested and move the joint slowly through its range to determine the free and easy ROM available. Note the presence and location of pain.[8] If there is no active movement and the limb feels heavy, record that the limb is flaccid or "0" in strength. If the limb has some active movement and no evidence of increased tone, the affected muscle or muscle group may be labeled "paretic" instead of "hypotonic." The paretic antagonist muscle can then be graded in strength (usually the strength grade will fall between 1 and 4−). Grading the paretic antagonist muscles provides more objective clinical information than merely labeling the muscles as hypotonic. Strength grading antagonists can help the occupational therapist triage phenol block and Botox injection candidates who have potential to improve function; for example, a patient with triceps strength grade of 2− (in the presence of elbow flexor tone) would be a better block candidate than a patient with a triceps strength grade of 0.
3. Hold the limb on the lateral aspects to avoid giving tactile stimulation to the muscle belly of the muscle being tested. Note also if the limb feels light or heavy.[8]
4. Clinical assessment of tone involves holding the patient's limb as just described and moving it rapidly through its full range while the patient is relaxed. Label the tone "mild," "moderate," or "severe." (Refer to tone rating scales defined in the next section.)
5. Clinical assessment of rigidity and hyperactive tonic reflexes involves moving the limb slowly during the range, noting the location of first tone or resistance to movement in degrees, and labeling it "mild," "moderate," or "severe." Some physicians find gonio-

CRAIG HOSPITAL
TONE MANAGEMENT/ASSESSMENT FORM
OCCUPATIONAL/PHYSICAL THERAPY

Patient Name _____ Date _____

Unit # _____ DX _____

Date of Injury _____

Primary Physician _____

Therapist _____

1. Brief history of patient per team members:

2. Patient/caregiver chief complaints/concerns:
   Include results from Canadian Occupational Performance Measure©[1]:

3. Functional areas effected by spasticity/hypertonus:

   _____ skin   _____ transfers
   _____ positioning (w/c, bed) _____ ambulation
   _____ hygiene   _____ feeding
   _____ dressing   _____ other
   _____ mobility (w/c, bed)

4. Interventions tried and results:

Intervention	Date	Result
ROM program		
Splinting/types:		
Serial casting:		
Medicine/types:		
Blocks:		
Surgeries:		

---

[1] The Canadian Occupational Performance Measure is copyrighted. Published by CAOT Publications ACE.

FIG. 23-4

Occupational and Physical Therapy Tone Evaluation, Craig Hospital. (From Lori Daane, OTR, Occupational Therapy Department, Craig Hospital, Englewood, Colorado.) *Continued*

metric measuring of the location of the first tone helpful pre- and post long-acting nerve block.

6. Record findings for various muscle groups or movements (Fig. 23-4).

It is important to note the patient's overall posture during the evaluation of muscle tone. Is the patient's posture symmetrical, with equal weight bearing on both hips (if sitting) or on both feet (if standing)? Note how the patient moves in general. Is the head aligned or tilted to one side? Is one shoulder elevated? Is the trunk rotated or elongated on one side and shortened on the other? Such abnormalities will affect the patient's ability to move the limbs normally. Current intervention focuses heavily on quality of movement, achieving as normal movement as possible during occupation.

5. Describe spasticity/hypertonus: Assess using Scale A or B (not both)

   A. (Minimal = min., Moderate = mod., S = severe) (f = flexion or e = extension)
      (c = clonus) (r = rigidity)

      LUE: finger _____   wrist _____   elbow _____
               shoulder _____   scapula _____
      RUE: finger _____   wrist _____   elbow _____
               shoulder _____   scapula _____
      LLE: toes _____   ankle _____   knee _____   hip _____
      RLE: toes _____   ankle _____   knee _____   hip _____
      Neck: flexion _____   extension _____
               lateral flexion _____   rotation _____

      Note: Comment on flaccidity, paresis vs. paralysis.

   B. Ashworth Score involved muscle groups:

Motion	Date Initial L / R	Date Follow-up L / R	Date Follow-up L / R

   C. Spontaneous spasms:

	Date Initial	Date Follow-up	Date Follow-up
Grade:			

6. ROM measurements of involved joints:

Motion	Date Initial L / R	Date Follow-up L / R	Date Follow-up L / R

FIG. 23-4 cont'd
Occupational and Physical Therapy Tone Evaluation, Craig Hospital. (From Lori Daane, OTR, Occupational Therapy Department, Craig Hospital, Englewood, Colorado.)

Rating Scales for Spasticity and Hypertonicity

Ashworth Scale

The Ashworth Scale[2] and the Modified Ashworth Scale[11] were not designed to differentiate between pure spasticity and hyperactive tonic stretch reflexes. These scales are used to quantify the degree of the hypertonus.

Tone fluctuates from hour to hour and day to day because of the intrinsic and extrinsic factors that influence it. This fluctuation makes accurate measurement difficult, particularly for cerebral hypertonia. Rating tone is still worthwhile, especially in the managed care environment, in which objective measures of progress are needed to justify the continuation of therapy.

7. Team/occupational/physical therapy goals of spasticity/hypertonus management:

8. Recommendations:

9. Procedures completed

   A. Nerve/muscle Blocks

	Medication and Dose	Location	Administration by:
Local anesthesia (specify medication)			
Phenol			
Botox® (Botulinum toxin-type A)			
Other (specify medication)			

Joint/Muscle		Pretest Date	Post-test Date	Follow-up Date	Follow-up Date
	PROM				
	AROM				
	Ashworth				
	MMT				
	PROM				
	AROM				
	Ashworth				
	MMT				
	PROM				
	AROM				
	Ashworth				
	MMT				

FIG. 23-4 cont'd
Occupational and Physical Therapy Tone Evaluation, Craig Hospital. (From Lori Daane, OTR, Occupational Therapy Department, Craig Hospital, Englewood, Colorado.) *Continued*

Bobath proposed that specific assessment of hypertonus is not necessary. She believed that an assessment of the distribution of abnormal tone should be part of a comprehensive evaluation of the postural mechanism, including selective movement.[9,10]

Therapists familiar with the Ashworth Scale can help physicians evaluate candidates for neurosurgical proce-dures. For example, part of the selection criteria for the Synchromed* **Intrathecal Baclofen Pump** (ITB) implantation is based on the presence of a two-point reduction on the Ashworth Scale after the test dose of

*Medtronic, Inc., Neurological Division, 800 53rd Ave, NE, Minneapolis, Minn, 55421.

Casting/splinting post block:

Functional changes: (spasticity, isolated mvmt., positioning, pain, other)

B. Intrathecal baclofen
   Test dose protocol

Ashworth score

Muscle	Pre-test		1 hr.		2 hrs.		4 hrs.		6 hrs.	
	L	R	L	R	L	R	L	R	L	R
Iliopsoas										
Gluteals										
Hamstrings										
Quadriceps										
Adductors										
Gastroc/Soleus										
Pectoralis										
Triceps										
Biceps										
Wrist flexors										
Wrist extensors										

Spontaneous spasms

	Pre-test	1 hr.	2 hrs.	4 hrs.	6 hrs.
Grade					

Muscle grading (MMT, PROM, AROM) Comments:

Pre-test:

2 hr.

4 hr.

FIG. 23-4 cont'd
Occupational and Physical Therapy Tone Evaluation, Craig Hospital. (From Lori Daane, OTR , Occupational Therapy Department, Craig Hospital, Englewood, Colorado.)

medication is given.[72] Ashworth described the resistance encountered during passive muscle stretching as follows:
0 = normal muscle tone
1 = slight increase in muscle tone, "catch" when limb moved
2 = more marked increase in muscle tone, but limb easily flexed
3 = considerable increase in muscle tone
4 = limb rigid in flexion or extension[2]

Mild-Moderate-Severe Spasticity Scale
Some therapists and physicians find a mild-moderate-severe scale easier to use. The following two scales are suggested as a guide for estimating the degree of spasticity and hypertonicity:

Comments: (positioning, function, pt. responses)

Pre-test:

2 hr.

4 hr.

Ashworth Scale

1 –	No increase in tone.
2 –	Slight increase in tone, giving a "catch" when affected part(s) is moved in flexion or extension.
3 –	More marked increase in tone; passive movement difficult.
4 –	Considerable increase in tone; passive movement difficult.
5 –	Affected part(s) rigid in flexion or extension.

Spontaneous spasms

    The number of spontaneous sustained flexor and extensor muscle spasms per hour are to be recorded:

0 –	None.
1 –	No spontaneous spasms, vigorous sensory and motor stimulation results in spasms.
2 –	Occasional spontaneous spasms and easily induced spasms.
3 –	Greater than one, but less than 10 spontaneous spasms per hour.
4 –	Greater than 10 spontaneous spasms per hour.

FIG. 23-4 cont'd
Occupational and Physical Therapy Tone Evaluation, Craig Hospital. (From Lori Daane, OTR , Occupational Therapy Department, Craig Hospital, Englewood, Colorado.)   *Continued*

Mild: The stretch reflex (palpable catch) occurs at the muscle's end range (i.e., the muscle is in a lengthened position).

Moderate: The stretch reflex (palpable catch) occurs in midrange.

Severe: The stretch reflex (palpable catch) occurs when the muscle is in a shortened range.[35]

Preston's Three-Step Hypertonicity Scale

1 or Mild: First tone or resistance is felt when the muscle is in a lengthened position.

2 or Moderate: First tone or resistance is felt in the mid range of the muscle.

3 or Severe: First tone or resistance occurs when the muscle is in a shortened range.

Range of Motion Assessment in Tone Assessment

Passive ROM (PROM) assessment supplements and often correlates with tone assessment. For example, if a patient with acute CVA (1 month after onset) has a wrist ROM measurement of 20° extension (normal is 70°) and orthopedic etiology (e.g., arthritis or fixed contracture) has been ruled out, the therapist should assess the tone in the wrist flexors and extrinsic finger flexors. Hypertonicity of any of these muscles can prohibit full wrist extension. An assessment of PROM can reveal possible signs of joint changes (e.g., subluxation, dislocation, or contracture) that have occurred from chronic hypertonus, such as PIPs that measure −45° to 125° instead of 0° to 100°. Some physicians find PROM measurements useful in documenting the location of the first tone before and after nerve block and Botox injection.

Other Considerations in Tone Assessment

Changes in bone or other peripheral structures can lead to ROM limitations. For example, the presence of heterotopic ossification can limit joint ROM. Heterotopic ossification is the formation of new bone in soft tissue or joints, which can lead to joint anklyosis. Heterotopic ossification can occur in individuals with traumatic brain injury and spinal cord injury, along with severe spasticity, or in other types of severe injuries.[12,51,87] Conversely, the presence of fixed contractures may be incorrectly labeled as hypertonus. Physiatrists or other physician specialists can aid in the diagnosis of contractures with the use of diagnostic short-term nerve blocks or EMG.[72]

Assessing Movement and Control

Along with tone assessments previously described, the occupational therapist performs an assessment of upper extremity movement and control. The therapist identifies where and how much the patient's motor control is dominated by stereotypical patterns of movement, also known as synergies (Chapter 34), and where some isolated movement may be present. The degree to which abnormal tone interferes with selective control is identified. Also, determining in which direction of movement hypertonicity occurs and how it affects function helps determine the need for intervention.

Manual muscle testing usually is not appropriate for patients who exhibit moderate to severe hypertonicity or rigidity because the relative tone and strength of the muscles are not normal and movement is not voluntary or selective. Tone and strength are influenced by the position of the head and body in space, abnormal contraction, deficits in tactile and proprioceptive sensation, and failures in reciprocal innervation.[10] However, if hypertonia is mild and selective movements are possible, it may be helpful to grade the strength of the antagonists to measure progress objectively.[72]

Position change and labyrinthine and tonic neck reflexes influence muscle tone and motor control. Because the level and distribution of muscle tone changes as the position of the head in space and of the head in relation to the body change, tone cannot be assessed in isolation from postural mechanisms, motor function, synergies present, task specificity, and other factors related to motor control.[10]

Sensation

The following sensibility tests are recommended for patients with damage to the CNS: static two-point discrimination, kinesthesia, proprioception, pain, and light touch using the Semmes-Weinstein Monofilaments test.[3] The therapist can assess light touch more accurately with the Semmes-Weinstein monofilaments because they have better pressure control than a cotton ball. Chapters 25 and 44 provide descriptions of sensory tests.

Medical Assessment of Muscle Tone

Physiatrists, orthopedic surgeons, and neurologists are some of the physicians who may specialize in assessment of muscle tone. They may use static or dynamic surface or percutaneous (needle) EMG. Multiple channels are used in dynamic EMG to evaluate the hypertonicity of many contributing muscles.[58] EMG helps the physician determine abnormal, excessive electrical activity in muscles. EMG can help physiatrists and neurologists plan and implement short- and long-acting nerve blocks to treat hypertonia. Patients who show local muscle wasting, flaccidity, numbness, or unexplained paresis should receive EMG assessment to rule out peripheral neuropathy.[87]

NORMAL POSTURAL MECHANISM

The normal **postural mechanism** is composed of automatic movements that provide an appropriate level of stability and mobility.[17] These automatic reactions develop in the early years of life and allow for trunk control and mobility, head control, midline orientation of self, weight bearing and weight shifting in all directions, dynamic balance, and controlled voluntary limb movement. The components of the normal postural mechanism include normal postural tone and control, integration of primitive reflexes and mass movement patterns, righting reactions, equilibrium and protective reactions, and selective voluntary movement.[10,17]

In patients who have suffered UMNS damage, the normal postural mechanism is disrupted. Abnormal tone and mass patterns of movement dominate the patient's movements, and these patients lack balance and stability. Movements are slow and uncoordinated. Therapists must assess the extent of damage to the postural mechanism in patients with CNS trauma or disease.

Normal postural tone is tonus that is present in the postural muscles. It is high enough to resist gravity, yet low enough to allow movement.[10] It allows automatic and continuous adjustment to movement.[76] Postural control is the ability to control or regulate specific postural outputs.[61] This control provides the foundation for voluntary selective movements because normal selective movement cannot be superimposed on high degrees of hypertonicity.

It is important to assess the following automatic reactions, which are part of the postural mechanism, in patients with CNS trauma or disease.

Righting Reactions

Righting reactions are automatic reactions that maintain and restore the normal position of the head in space and the normal relationship of the head to the trunk, as well as the normal alignment of the trunk and limbs. Without effective righting reactions, the patient will have difficulty getting up from the floor, getting out of bed, sitting up, and kneeling.[10]

Equilibrium Reactions

Equilibrium reactions, elicited by stimulation of the labyrinths, are used to maintain and regain balance in all activities.[10,50] These reactions ensure sufficient postural alignment when the body's center of gravity is altered by a change in the supporting surface.[50] Without equilibrium reactions, the patient will have difficulty maintaining and recovering balance in all positions and activities.

Protective Reactions

Protective reactions are associated with equilibrium reactions and consist of protective extension of the arms and hands, which is used to protect the head and face when one is falling.[10,38] Without protective reactions the patient may fall or be reluctant to bear weight on the affected side during normal bilateral activities.

Assessment of Righting, Equilibrium, Protective Reactions, and Balance
Formal testing of these reactions may be difficult because of the cognitive and physical limitations of the patient or time constraints of the therapist. The therapist can evaluate righting reactions, however, during transfers and ADL. Equilibrium and protective reactions can be observed when the patient shifts farther out of

midline than necessary during functional activities, such as lower extremity dressing.

Balance depends on normal equilibrium and protective reactions. Balance is "the ability to maintain the center of gravity over the base of support, usually while in an upright position."[54] Balance involves a complex interaction between many systems, including the vestibular, proprioceptive, visual, and motor modulation from the cerebellum, basal ganglia, and cerebral cortex. Occupational and physical therapists must also observe the patient's ankle, hip, and step strategies and note areas of breakdown in the kinetic chain.[30,82]

When assessing a patient with CNS dysfunction, the therapist should assess the patient's static and dynamic balance before leaving the patient unattended on a mat table, in a wheelchair, or during ambulatory ADL. Dynamic balance involves maintaining balance while moving, and static balance involves maintaining equilibrium while stationary.

The Physical Performance Test assesses physical function during activity. Seven of the nine tested items involve static and dynamic balance.[86] The test only takes 10 minutes to complete.[74] Fig. 23-5 shows the test form and test protocol. Two other noteworthy balance assessments are the Tinetti Balance Test of the Performance-Oriented Assessment of Mobility Problems[80] and the Berg Balance Scale.[5]

Primitive Reflexes

The reemergence of primitive reflexes can interfere with the patient's occupational performance. Difficulties that may be encountered are described below. Observation of these motor behaviors is a way of evaluating for the presence of primitive reflexes.

Brainstem Level Reflexes
ASYMMETRICAL TONIC NECK REFLEX. The patient with asymmetrical tonic neck reflex may have difficulty maintaining the head in midline while moving the eyes toward or past midline.[9] The patient may be unable to (1) extend an arm without turning the head or (2) flex the arm without turning the head the other way.[9,24] The patient may be unable to move either or both arms to midline, especially when in the supine position, because movement of the arms is dependent on head positioning. This positioning causes asymmetry in the arms. Thus this reflex makes it difficult or impossible to bring an object to the mouth, hold an object in both hands, or grasp an object in front of the body while looking at it.

SYMMETRICAL TONIC NECK REFLEX. The patient with symmetrical tonic neck reflex will be unable to support the body weight on hands and knees, maintain balance in a quadruped position, or crawl normally without fixating the head.[10] The patient

PHYSICAL PERFORMANCE TEST SCORING SHEET

		Time*	Physical Performance Test Scoring	
	Score			
1.	Write a sentence (Whales live in the blue ocean.)	_____ sec	≤10 sec = 4 10.5-15 sec = 3 15.5-20 sec = 2 >20 sec = 1 unable = 0	_____
2.	Simulated eating	_____ sec	≤10 sec = 4 10.5-15 sec = 3 15.5-20 sec = 2 >20 sec = 1 unable = 0	_____
3.	Lift a book and put it on a shelf	_____ sec	≤2 sec = 4 2.5-4 sec = 3 4.5-6 sec = 2 >6 sec = 1 unable = 0	_____
4.	Put on and remove a jacket	_____ sec	≤10 sec = 4 10.5-15 sec = 3 15.5-20 sec = 2 >20 sec = 1 unable = 0	_____
5.	Pick up penny from floor	_____ sec	≤2 sec = 4 2.5-4 sec = 3 4.5-6 sec = 2 >6 sec = 1 unable = 0	_____
6.	Turn 360°	discontinuous steps continuous steps unsteady (grabs, staggers) steady	0 2 0 2	_____
7.	50-foot walk test	_____ sec	≤15 sec = 4 15.5-20 sec = 3 20.5-25 sec = 2 >25 sec = 1 unable = 0	_____
8.	Climb one flight of stairs	_____ sec	≤5 sec = 4 5.5-10 sec = 3 10.5-15 sec = 2 >15 sec = 1 unable = 0	_____
9.	Climb stairs†		Number of flights of stairs up and down (maximum 4)	_____

TOTAL SCORE (maximum 36 for nine-item, 28 for seven-item)

_____ nine-item
_____ seven-item

*For timed measurements, round to nearest 0.5 seconds.
†Omit for seven-item scoring.

FIG. 23-5

Physical performance test: scoring sheet and test protocol. (From Reuben DB, Siu AL: An objective measure of physical function of elderly outpatients—the physical performance test, *J Am Geriatr Soc* 38[10]:1111-1112, 1990.)

PHYSICAL PERFORMANCE TEST PROTOCOL

Administer the Physical Performance Test as outlined below. Subjects are given up to two chances to complete each item. Assistive devices are permitted for tasks 6 through 8.

1. Ask the subject, when given the command "go," to write the sentence, "Whales live in the blue ocean." Time from the word "go" until the pen is lifted from the page at the end of the sentence. All words must be included and legible. Period need not be included for task to be considered completed.

2. Five kidney beans are placed in a bowl, 5 inches from the edge of the desk in front of the patient. An empty coffee can is placed on the table at the patient's nondominant side. A teaspoon is placed in the patient's dominant hand. Ask the subject, on the command "go," to pick up the beans, one at a time, and place each in the coffee can. Time from the command "go" until the last bean is heard hitting the bottom of the can.

3. Place a *Physician's Desk Reference* or other heavy book on a table in front of the patient. Ask the patient, when given the command "go," to place the book on a shelf above shoulder level. Time from the command "go" to the time the book is resting on the shelf.

4. If the subject has a jacket or cardigan sweater, ask him or her to remove it. If not, give the subject a lab coat. Ask the subject, on the command "go" to put the coat on completely such that it is straight on his or her shoulders and then remove the garment completely. Time from the command "go" until the garment has been completely removed.

5. Place a penny approximately 1 foot from the patient's foot on the dominant side. Ask the patient, on the command "go," to pick up the penny from the floor and stand up. Time from the command "go" until the subject is standing erect with penny in hand.

6. With subject in a corridor or in an open room, ask the subject to turn 360°. Evaluate using scale on PPT scoring sheet.

7. Bring subject to start on 50-foot walk test course (25 feet out and 25 feet back) and ask the subject, on the command "go," to walk to 25-foot mark and back. Time from the command "go" until the starting line is crossed on the way back.

8. Bring subject to foot of stairs (9 to 12 steps) and ask subject, on the command "go" to begin climbing stairs until he or she feels tired and wishes to stop. Before beginning this task, alert the subject to possibility of developing chest pain or shortness of breath and inform the subject to tell you if any of these symptoms occur. Escort the subject up the stairs. Time from the command "go" until the subject's first foot reaches the top of the first flight of stairs. Record the number of flights (maximum is four) climbed (up and down in one flight).

FIG. 23-5 cont'd
Physical performance test: scoring sheet and test protocol. (From Reuben DB, Siu AL: An objective measure of physical function of elderly outpatients—the physical performance test, *J Am Geriatr Soc* 38[10]:1111-1112, 1990.)

will have difficulty moving from lying to sitting because when the head is lifted to initiate the task, increased hip extension resists the movement. As the patient struggles to sit up, increased leg extension can also interfere.[23] The patient will have difficulty with transfers from bed to wheelchair and wheelchair to bed because as the arms and neck are extended to initiate the transfer, one or both legs may show increased flexion, which may cause the patient to slide under the bed or wheelchair. Additionally, the affected leg may actually lift off the floor, causing an inability to bear weight on that extremity.[24]

TONIC LABYRINTHINE REFLEX. The patient exhibiting poorly integrated tonic labyrinthine reflex will be severely limited in the ability to move. A few examples of functional limitations are the inability to lift the head in the supine position, initiate flexion to sit up independently from the supine position, roll over, or sit in a wheelchair for long periods.[10,24] In attempting to move from a supine to sitting position, extensor tone will dominate until the patient is halfway up, when flexor tone begins to take over. Flexor tone continues until full sitting is reached, causing the head to fall forward, the spine to flex, and the patient to fall forward.[9] Sitting in a wheelchair for extended periods can lead to increased extensor tone as the patient hyperextends the head to view the environment. The knee is extended, the foot is pushed forward off the wheelchair foot rest, and eventually the patient may slip or remain in a half-lying asymmetrical position.[24]

POSITIVE SUPPORTING REACTION. The positive supporting reaction is caused by pressure on the ball of the foot. This stimulus elicits extension and internal rotation of the hip, knee extension, ankle plantar flexion, and foot inversion. The patient with a positive supporting reaction will have difficulty placing the heel on the ground for standing, putting the heel down first in walking, and having normal body weight transference in walking.[10,24] The patient will have difficulty getting up from a chair, sitting in a chair, or walking down steps, because the leg remains in rigid extension and it is not possible to move the joints while weight bearing. The rigid leg can carry the patient's body weight but is unable to contribute to any balance reactions. All balance reactions therefore are compensated for with other parts of the body.[9]

Spinal Level Reflexes

Spinal reflexes can occur after an upper motor neuron lesion. They appear because of a lack of inhibition from higher centers. Some examples of exaggerated spinal reflexes are hyperactive deep tendon reflexes, the Babinski sign, flexor withdrawal reflex, crossed extension, and grasp reflex.[52] Three spinal reflexes are reviewed.

CROSSED EXTENSION REFLEX. The crossed extension reflex causes increased extensor tone in one leg when the other leg is flexed. Therefore, if the patient with hemiplegia who is influenced by this reflex flexes the unaffected leg for walking, a strong extensor hypertonicity occurs in the affected leg and interferes with the normal pattern of ambulation. By the same token the patient can bridge (lift buttocks) in bed with the weight supported by both legs. If the unaffected leg is lifted (flexed), however, a total extension pattern occurs in the affected leg and the bridge cannot be maintained.[9,24]

FLEXOR WITHDRAWAL. The patient with flexor withdrawal will exhibit flexion of the ankle, knee, and hip when the sole of the foot is touched (swiped heel to ball of foot). This reflex clearly interferes with gait pattern and transfers.

GRASP REFLEX. The patient with a grasp reflex will not be able to release objects placed in the hand, even if active finger extension is present.[24] The reflexes just discussed are rarely seen in isolation.

Automatic Adaptation of Muscles to Changes in Posture

Normal muscles allow for smooth and well-controlled mobility against the force of gravity. A limb with normal muscles can be placed; that is, it can be moved by the examiner and will feel light because it follows the movement actively.[10] Otherwise, the limb will feel heavy and flop down if released by the examiner. The limb may also feel resistant to movement, which indicates that it does not have the ability to combat gravity appropriately for function.

If reflexes or stereotypical patterns are not integrated and righting, equilibrium, and protective reactions are impaired, patients will have difficulty using their limbs for function. These patients may not be able to place their limbs, stabilize an object, or manipulate an object. They may not be able to use their limbs to prevent a fall or maintain their balance.

Trunk Control Assessment

Collin and Wade[21] designed a quick and easily administered test of trunk control that is valid and reliable in patients with a diagnosis of CVA. It involves four timed tests: rolling to the weak side, rolling to the sound side, moving from supine to sitting, and sitting on the side of the bed with the feet off the floor for 30 seconds.[21]

To accurately assess trunk control, the therapist must evaluate strength and control in the following muscle groups: trunk flexors, extensors, lateral flexors, and rotators. The patient should be sitting upright on a mat table, with the feet supported for all tests. The patient should not be left unattended on the mat table until the therapist determines the patient has adequate trunk control and sitting balance. The procedures described in the following sections are condensed from Gillen and Burkhardt's *Stroke Rehabilitation: A Function-Based Approach*.[40]

Trunk Flexors

The examiner asks the patient to sit upright, slowly move his or her shoulders behind the hips, (eccentric control) and hold the end range posture (isometric control) (Fig. 23-6, *A*). The patient is then asked to

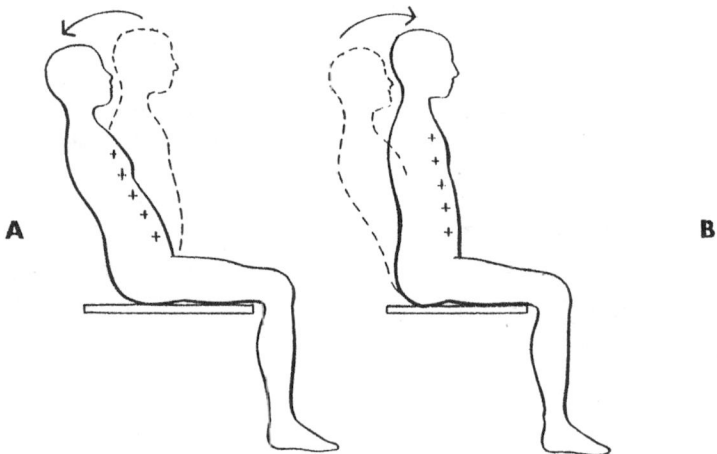

FIG. 23-6
Trunk flexor control. Dotted lines indicate trunk starting position, solid lines indicate trunk final position, arrows indicate movement direction, and plus symbols indicate muscle groups primarily responsible for control of pattern. (Skeletal muscle activity occurs on both sides of the trunk [reciprocal innervation].) (From Gillen G, Burkhardt A: *Stroke rehabilitation: a function-based approach*, St Louis, 1998, Mosby.)

move anteriorly (concentric control) to resume the initial upright posture (Fig. 23-6, *B*).

The examiner should observe for evidence of unilateral weakness, potential for falls, and symmetry of weight shift. A functional test for trunk flexor control is to observe the patient move from supine to sitting.

Trunk Extensors

TEST 1. The patient is sitting in a position of spinal flexion with a posterior pelvic tilt and moves into trunk extension while simultaneously moving the pelvis into neutral or into a slight anterior tilt. This test assesses concentric trunk extensor control, which is a prerequisite for lower extremity dressing and forward reach (Fig. 23-7, *A*).

TEST 2. The patient is seated in an upright posture. The examiner asks the patient to maintain an erect spine and lean forward. This test evaluates eccentric trunk extensor control (Fig. 23-7, *B*). For both trunk extensor tests the examiner should observe signs of unilateral weakness and note end-range control.

Lateral Flexors

The patient sits in an upright posture. The pelvis is stationary, and the upper trunk laterally flexes toward the mat table. Fig. 23-8, *A*, shows eccentric contraction of the left side and muscle shortening of the right side. The patient is then asked to return to the original test position (concentric control of the left side) (Fig. 23-8, *B*).

Fig. 23-8, *C*, shows assessment of trunk and pelvis lateral flexion, where the movement is initiated from the lower trunk and pelvis. The end position is one of trunk elongation on the weight-bearing side and shortening on the non-weight-bearing side, which involves concentric contraction of the right side.

Lateral flexion is needed for fall prevention when a patient is reaching to the side (e.g., shutting a car door).

Trunk Rotation

The primary muscles responsible for rotation are the obliques. When a person rotates the trunk to the left, the right external and the left internal obliques are recruited. Rotational control is a prerequisite for upper extremity dressing and reaching across the midline. The following three movement patterns are evaluated:

1. The patient sits upright, and the pelvis is in a neutral, stable position. The patient reaches with his or her right arm, across the body, in the direction of the floor. This motion helps assess concurrent flexion and rotation. The motion tests concentric control of the obliques and the back extensors (particularly the thoracic region). Both sides need to be tested.
2. The second movement pattern involves trunk extension with rotation. The upper trunk remains stable, and the lower trunk and pelvis move forward on one side (i.e., shifting forward). Again, both sides are tested.
3. The patient is positioned supine for the third movement. The patient initiates a "segmental roll by lifting the shoulders from the support surface and toward the opposite side of the body. This pattern is controlled by a concentric contraction of the abdominals (obliques)."[40]

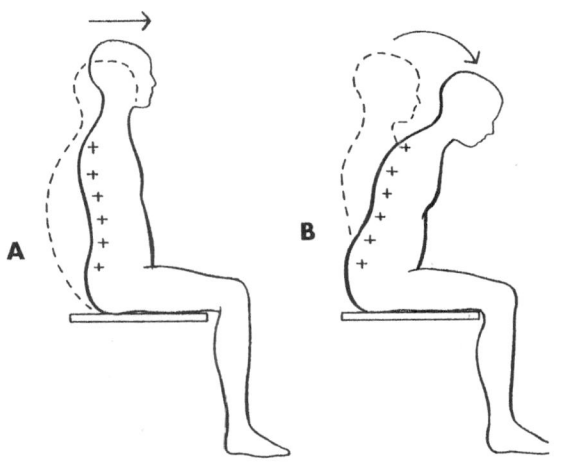

FIG. 23-7
Trunk extensor control. Dotted lines indicate trunk starting position, solid lines indicate trunk final position, arrows indicate movement direction, and plus symbols indicate muscle groups primarily responsible for control of pattern. (Skeletal muscle activity occurs on both sides of the trunk [reciprocal innervation].) (From Gillen G, Burkhardt A: *Stroke rehabilitation: a function-based approach*, St Louis, 1998, Mosby.)

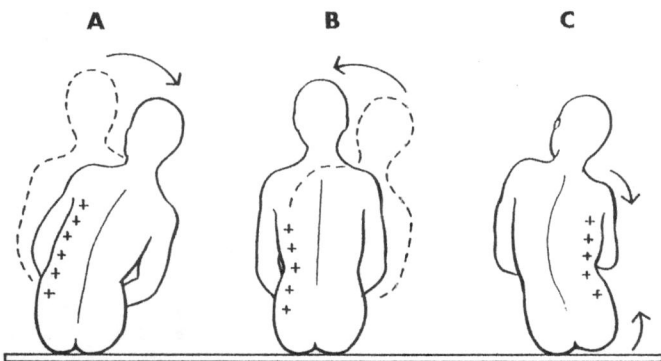

FIG. 23-8
Lateral flexor control. Dotted lines indicate trunk starting position, solid lines indicate trunk final position, arrows indicate movement direction, and plus symbols indicate muscle groups primarily responsible for control of pattern. (Skeletal muscle activity occurs on both sides of the trunk [reciprocal innervation].) (From Gillen G, Burkhardt A: *Stroke rehabilitation: a function-based approach*, 1998, St Louis, Mosby.)

COORDINATION

Coordination is the ability to produce accurate, controlled movement. Characteristics of coordinated movement are smoothness, rhythm, appropriate speed, refinement to the minimum number of muscle groups needed, and appropriate muscle tension, postural tone, and equilibrium. Coordination of muscle action is under the control of the cerebellum and influenced by the extrapyramidal system. Knowledge of the body

schema and body-to-space relationships is essential to the production of coordinated movement.

For coordinated movement, all of the elements of the neuromuscular mechanism must be intact. Coordinated movement depends on the contraction of the correct agonist muscles with simultaneous relaxation of the correct antagonist muscles, together with the contraction of the joint fixator and synergist muscles. In addition, proprioception, body schema, and the ability to judge space accurately and to direct body parts through space with correct timing to the desired target must be intact.[8]

INCOORDINATION

Many types of lesions can produce disturbances in coordination.[8] Disturbances of coordination often stem from cerebellar and extrapyramidal disorders. Noncerebellar causes include diseases and injuries of muscles and peripheral nerves, lesions of the posterior columns of the spinal cord, and lesions of the frontal and postcentral cerebral cortex. Paralysis of the limbs caused by a peripheral nervous system lesion prevents carrying out tests for coordination, even though CNS mechanisms are intact.[8,63]

Cerebellar Disorders

Cerebellar dysfunction can cause incoordination that can affect any body region and cause a variety of clinical symptoms. For example, the patient may have postural difficulties that include slouching or leaning positions (caused by bilateral lesions) or spinal curvature (caused by unilateral lesions) and wide-based standing. Eye movements, both voluntary and reflexive, may be affected, as well as the resting position of the eye. The following are common signs of cerebellar dysfunction that the therapist may encounter.[84]

Ataxia
Ataxia is manifested as delayed initiation of movement responses, errors in range and force of movement, and errors in the rate and regularity of movement. When a patient with ataxia reaches for an object, it is apparent that the shortest distance between the patient and object is not a straight line. Ataxia results in incoordination and irregularity of movement. The patient with ataxia has a staggering, wide-based gait with reduced or no arm swing. Step length may be uneven, and the patient may have a tendency to fall to the side of the lesion. Ataxia will result in a lack of postural stability, with patients tending to fixate to compensate for the instability.[20,39,62]

Adiadochokinesis
Adiadochokinesis is an inability to perform rapid alternating movements such as pronation and supination or elbow flexion and extension.[26]

Dysmetria

Dysmetria is an inability to estimate the ROM necessary to reach the target of the movement. Dysmetria is evident when an individual touches the finger to the nose or an object on a table, or when the individual places limbs in voluntary movement.[26]

Dyssynergia

Literally, dyssynergia is a "decomposition of movement" in which voluntary movements are broken up into their component parts and appear jerky. Dyssynergia can also cause problems in articulation and phonation.[26]

Rebound Phenomenon of Holmes

The rebound phenomenon of Holmes is the lack of a "check reflex"—that is, the inability to stop a motion quickly to avoid striking something. For example, if the patient's arm is flexed against the resistance of the examiner and the resistance is released suddenly, the patient's hand will hit the patient's face or body.[20,26]

Nystagmus

Nystagmus is an involuntary movement of the eyeballs in an up-and-down, back-and-forth, or rotating direction. It interferes with the head control and fine adjustments required for balance. Nystagmus can occur as a result of vestibular system, brainstem, or cerebellar lesions.[26]

Dysarthria

Dysarthria is explosive or slurred speech caused by an incoordination of the speech mechanism. The patient's speech may also vary in pitch, seem nasal and tremulous, or both.[20,26]

Extrapyramidal Disorders

Extrapyramidal disorders are characterized by hypokinesia or hyperkinesia. Parkinson's disease is characterized by hypokinesia (bradykinesia), cogwheel and lead pipe rigidity, a decrease or loss of postural mechanisms, and a resting, pill-rolling tremor.[29]

"Parkinson's Plus" is the name given to a group of movement disorders that have signs of Parkinson's disease with concomitant neurological deficits. Progressive supranuclear palsy is one such disease.[48] Affected persons have "loss of vertical ocular gaze, rigidity of the neck and trunk muscles, dementia, and parkinsonian signs,"[47] usually in the absence of tremor. Life expectancy is shorter than in Parkinson's disease. Death often occurs within 6 to 10 years.[47]

Chorea

Chorea is irregular, purposeless, involuntary, coarse, quick, jerky, and dysrhythmic movements of variable distribution. These movements may occur during sleep.[26] Two types of chorea are tardive dyskinesia and Huntington's disease. Tardive dyskinesia is a drug-induced disorder, often associated with neuroleptic drug use. Occupational therapists see tardive dyskinesia in psychiatric settings. Huntington's disease is an inherited, autosomal dominant disease. Patients with Huntington's disease have an ataxic gait with choreoathetoid movements. As the disease progresses, rigidity develops. Choreiform movements are faster than athetoid.[48]

Athetoid Movements

Athetoid movements are continuous, slow, wormlike, arrhythmic movements that primarily affect the distal portions of the extremities. These movements occur in the same patterns in the same subject and are not present during sleep.[26] Adult athetosis can occur after cerebral anoxia and Wilson's disease. Movement patterns include alternating "extension and flexion of the arm, supination and pronation of the forearm, and flexion and extension of the fingers."[48] Athetosis that occurs with chorea is termed "choreoathetosis."[48]

Dystonia

Dystonia results in persistent posturing of the extremities (e.g., in hyperextension or hyperflexion of the wrist and fingers) with concurrent torsion of the spine and associated twisting of the trunk.[1] Dystonic movements are writhing and often continuous and are often seen in conjunction with spasticity.[20] Dystonia can be primary or secondary, the latter occurring with other CNS disorders (e.g., hypoxic brain injury or tumor). Segmental dystonia involves two or more adjacent body parts. Generalized and multifocal dystonia also exist. Focal dystonia involves only one limb, as seen in writer's cramp, musician's cramp, and spasmodic torticollis.[47]

Ballism

Ballism is a rare symptom that is produced by continuous, abrupt contractions of the axial and proximal musculature of the extremity. Ballism causes the limb to fly out suddenly. It occurs on one side of the body (hemiballism) and is caused by lesions of the opposite subthalamic nucleus.[20,26]

Tremor

The following are three common types of tremor:

1. *Intention tremor*, associated with cerebellar disease, occurs during voluntary movement. It is intensified at the termination of the movement and is often seen in multiple sclerosis. The patient with intention tremor may have trouble performing tasks that require accuracy and precision of limb placement (e.g., drinking from a cup or inserting a key in a lock).
2. *Resting tremor* occurs at rest and subsides when voluntary movement is attempted. It occurs as a result of disease of the basal ganglia and is seen in Parkinson's disease.

3. *Essential familial tremor* is inherited as an autosomal dominant trait. It is most visible when the patient is carrying out a fine precision task.[47]

ASSESSMENT OF COORDINATION
Medical Assessment of Coordination

Incoordination consists of errors in rate, rhythm, range, direction, and force of movement.[39] Therefore observation is an important element of the clinical examination. The neurological examination for incoordination may include the nose-finger-nose test, the finger-nose test, the heel-knee test, the knee pat (pronation-supination) test, hand pat and foot pat tests, finger wiggling, and drawing a spiral.[8,63] Such tests can reveal dysmetria, dyssynergia, adiadochokinesis, tremors, and ataxia. Usually the neurologist or physiatrist performs these examinations. Magnetic resonance imaging and computerized tomography scans may also be ordered. Tremors are frequency rated with EMG, which helps the physician accurately diagnose tremor type.[47]

Occupational Therapy Assessment of Coordination

Selected activities and specific performance tests can reveal the effect of incoordination on function. The occupational therapist can observe for coordination difficulties during ADL assessment. The therapist can prepare simulated tasks that require coordinated muscle function, such as writing, opening containers, tossing and catching a bean-bag or ball, or playing a board game.[78] The therapist should observe for irregularity in the rate of movement and for sudden, corrective movements in an attempt to compensate for incoordination. Movement during the performance of various activities may appear irregular and jerky and overreach the mark.[63] The following general guidelines and questions can be used when evaluating incoordination:

1. Assess the muscle tone and joint mobility first.
2. Observe the patient in the sitting position and locate any overdeveloped muscle bulk.
3. Observe for ataxia, proximal to distal, during functional upper extremity movement. Are movements away from or toward the body more difficult for the patient? Where, within the ROM, is ataxia most prevalent?
4. Stabilize joints proximally to distally during the functional task and note differences in patient performance, as compared with performance without stabilization. (Stabilization can be by splinting or stabilizing the affected body part against a wall.) Weighted cuffs may be applied to the extremity during task performance to determine if weighting or resistance decreases the tremor (use caution). Note the amount of resistance provided. Observe whether the weights make the coordination worse. Sometimes the use of weights increases tremor.
5. Observe for tremor. Are the eyes and speech affected?
6. Does the patient's emotional status affect coordination?
7. How do the patient's ataxia or coordination problems affect coordination?
8. Perform an occupational history interview, asking about the patient's roles, routines, goals, and environment to determine which functions are important for the patient.

Several standardized tests of motor function and manual dexterity are available and can be used to evaluate coordination. Some of these tests are the Purdue Pegboard,[73] the Minnesota Rate of Manipulation Test,[66] the Lincoln-Oseretsky Motor Development Scale,[57] the Pennsylvania Bimanual Work Sample,[70] the Crawford Small Parts Dexterity Test,[22] and the Jebsen-Taylor Hand Function Test.[49] The standardized functional assessments for CVA and the TEMPA (geriatrics) mentioned earlier may also be useful for the geriatric population.[28]

RESULTS OF ASSESSMENT AS A BASIS FOR PLANNING INTERVENTION

Although the therapist bases intervention on the results of the patient's assessments, including cognition, vision, perception, sensation, psychological aspects, and occupational needs,[69] assessment of motor control suggests some directions for treatment. Several approaches to motor control management are described in Chapters 9 and 32 to 36. The sensorimotor approaches are often used to enhance CNS integration and improve the postural mechanism, muscle tone, and motor coordination and control.

Intervention for Hypertonicity and Spasticity

Hypertonicity is only one part of the UMNS. It is very important to treat other performance deficits of the UMNS such as paresis, fatigue, and decreased dexterity. These deficits can impede function more than hypertonia.[16]

Before treating hypertonus, the therapist and physician need to closely evaluate the function of the tone. Hypertonicity can have beneficial effects, such as aiding in standing and transfers, maintaining muscle bulk, and preventing deep vein thrombosis, osteoporosis, and edema. Intervention is necessary when spasticity interferes with ADL, gait, sleep, or wheelchair positioning or when it causes severe pain and limits hygiene (e.g., the patient is unable to wash hand or axilla) or leads to contractures or decubitus ulcers. Hypertonicity or spasticity may be treated with conservative therapeutic interventions, pharmacological agents, or surgery.

Conservative Treatment Approaches

For hypertonicity in the upper extremity, which is usually accompanied by synergy or patterned movement, treatment methods that use techniques of inhibition may be appropriate. This includes methods such as the sensorimotor approaches described in Chapters 32 through 36. The appropriateness of these methods depends on the disability, severity, and distribution of the hypertonicity and on concomitant problems. The goal of neurodevelopmental treatment is to balance the tone for more normal movement. Therefore intervention involving inhibition of the hypertonic muscles and facilitation of the antagonist muscles is implemented.[72]

Another OT objective is to have the patient manage muscle tone to accomplish essential daily living activities. Positioning and movement in patterns opposite to hypertonic or synergistic patterns are important in developing quality movement that is as close to normal as possible. At times it is appropriate to facilitate synergistic movements in the patient with chronic disease (or if the patient does not recover beyond Brunnstrom's[14] stage 3).[81] The synergy patterns can be facilitated to improve lateral pinch or elbow flexion function. The patient should be taught how to modulate the abnormal tone or how to instruct others to do so. The patient should also be taught how to incorporate the affected upper extremity as much as possible into all ADL.[14,33] ADL, crafts, games, and work activities can be used to teach incorporation of the extremities for a total approach to treatment.[8]

Even when motor control is adequate for some functions, the sensory and perceptual abilities of the patient may affect the achievement of functional goals. Perceptual dysfunction may alter the patient's abilities, requiring the therapist to focus on perceptual training as well.[6]

In some cases unilateral hypertonicity is severe enough to necessitate serial inhibitive casting or splinting (see Chapter 31). Casting in inhibitive postures has been shown to be effective in tone reduction.[24,43,67,90] The beneficial effect of casting on hypertonia and upper extremity contractures has also been well documented in the literature.[13,18,36]

Casting in inhibitive postures is effective because it provides neutral warmth, maintained pressure, and constant joint positioning with static lengthening of muscle.[46] **Serial casting** is most successful when a contracture has been present for less than 6 months. The cast may be bivalved (cut in half) and worn as a splint. This helps protect the skin and allows the therapist to work with the extremity out of the cast. However, many clinicians believe that a nonbivalved cast is more effective and actually causes less skin breakdown.[7] A dropout cast, which can be used as part of the serial casting process, includes a cut-out area, allowing movement of the joint in the desired direction. For example, for an elbow that has flexor hypertonicity, the dorsal upper arm portion of a long arm cast can be cut out to allow the triceps to be facilitated to extend the arm.

Serial casting should cease when desired position is achieved and tone is manageable with the last cast or splint. If there is no evidence of increased passive ROM after two to three casts are removed, serial casting must cease; however, the last cast should be kept, bivalved, and used as a splint to prevent further contracture.[72] Many innovations have occurred in commercially available spasticity reduction splints that are used to place the wrist and hand in inhibitive postures. The patient and family need to be educated in continuing to incorporate the extremity in occupation, and to bear weight on the extremity as much as possible to retain the ROM gains achieved during casting.

Physical agent modalities such as cold, superficial heat, ultrasound, and neuromuscular electrical stimulation can be used as preparation for or in conjunction with purposeful activity and muscle reeducation, provided the therapist has the appropriate training and can prove competency. Ultrasound can help inhibit or reduce hypertonicity temporarily and increase tendon and muscle extensibility. It is helpful to provide concurrent stretch during the ultrasound procedure.[72] Neuromuscular electrical stimulation has been shown to strengthen paretic muscles.[15,44]

Pharmacological Agents

Pharmacological agents prescribed and administered by physicians include oral medication, short-term nerve blocks, and long-term blocks.

Patients with severe hypertonicity accompanied by severe pain may need evaluation of the cause of the pain. Drug therapy and other pain management techniques may be part of the treatment approach. The four drugs most commonly used for spasticity of UMN origin are diazepam, baclofen, dantrolene sodium, and tizanidine. Dantrolene sodium acts at the skeletal muscle. Dantrolene sodium is preferred in cerebral spasticity because it is less apt to cause sedation. Dantrolene can cause weakness and liver damage.[72] Diazepam's side effects include drowsiness, fatigue, and possible addiction. Baclofen is more effective with spinal cord injuries than with cerebral injuries. Its potential side effects are confusion, drowsiness, and hallucinations. Neither diazepam nor baclofen can be discontinued suddenly because to do so may cause seizures. Tizanidine HCl is labeled for spasticity reduction in multiple sclerosis and spinal cord injury. Its side effects may include hypotension, sedation, and visual hallucinations. No matter which drug is used, it is crucial for the occupational therapist to communicate to the medical staff any noted side effects that interfere with the patient's overall function.[72]

Nerve blocks are injections of a chemical agent to diminish or obliterate tone. There are short and long-term nerve blocks. Short-term nerve blocks are injections of an anesthetic (e.g. bupivicaine) to temporarily reduce pain and muscle tone. These short-term blocks help the physician differentiate between hypertonus and contracture.[71] The short-term nerve blocks last from 1 to 7 hours, depending on which anesthetic is used.

Long-term blocks, usually injections of phenol or botulinum toxin-type A (Botox), generally last several months. Botox lasts for 3 to 5 months. Phenol blocks last from 2 to 8 months, depending on whether the motor points (2 to 3 months) or the motor branch (8 months) is injected. Phenol and Botox have different mechanisms of action. Botox exerts its effect via chemical denervation, and phenol works via motor point or motor branch neurolysis. Both blocks can be used to diminish or obliterate hypertonicity in the agonist. The blocks help to prevent contractures and render the hypertonic muscle weak or flaccid.[19,42,71] The effect and time interval of the long-term block provide therapists the opportunity to increase antagonistic strength and function. A combination of long-acting nerve blocks and casting or splinting is often used to treat hypertonicity. Long-term blocks in the upper extremities are commonly used in the subscapularis, brachioradialis, and flexor digitorum sublimis.

Surgical Methods

Surgery to control hypertonicity is also an option. Dynamic EMG can help orthopedic surgeons plan surgery. Orthopedic surgical intervention can improve function or release contractures. Examples of upper extremity functional surgery include lengthening of the biceps tendon to reduce elbow flexion and gain elbow extension, thumb-in-palm release, and transferral of the flexor carpi ulnaris tendon to the extensor carpi radialis longus or brevis tendons to decrease the deforming force of wrist flexion while simultaneously augmenting wrist extension.[72] An example of a contracture release procedure is the flexor digitorum superficialis to profundus transfer to gain length in the extrinsic finger flexors.[45]

A common neurosurgical procedure performed on adults with severe spasticity is **intrathecal baclofen pump** (ITB) implantation. This enables baclofen to enter the body at the spinal level and avoids the centrally mediated side effects of oral baclofen.[72] The ITB provides baclofen, a spasticity-reducing medication, directly into the intrathecal (subarachnoid) space via a catheter attached to a subcutaneous implantable pump in the abdomen. A patient must undergo a lumbar puncture test dose of intrathecal baclofen to determine candidacy before pump implantation.

ITB has been shown to be very effective in the reduction of severe spinal spasticity and spasticity associated with multiple sclerosis and is also effective for cerebral spasticity. For further details of medical and surgical

treatments and their relation to occupational therapy, the reader is referred to Preston and Hecht's *Spasticity Management: Rehabilitation Strategies*.[72]

Treatment of Rigidity

Decerebrate and decorticate rigidity can wax and wane. When the rigidity is waning, it is recommended that the patient be transferred to a wheelchair or reclining chair because the rigidity decreases in sitting. The rigidity is worse during episodes of agitation.[59] Parkinson's rigidity responds temporarily to heat, massage, stretching, and ROM exercises. Rocking back and forth before standing can aid in the transition. See Chapter 39 for additional treatment strategies for rigidity.[58]

Treatment of Flaccidity

Flaccidity stemming from upper motor neuron dysfunction (e.g., recovering from spinal or cerebral shock resulting from acute CNS insult) is treated with facilitation techniques such as weight bearing, high-frequency vibration, tapping, quick stretch, bed positioning with weight on the flaccid side the majority of the time, and functional neuromuscular electrical stimulation. Splinting the hand and wrist may be indicated for support. Therapists should closely supervise splinting, since contractures can result from excessive splint wear. Passive ROM exercises also are indicated.[72]

The arm can be positioned as normally as possible during ADL tasks to provide sensory and proprioceptive feedback. Patient education in proper positioning and joint protection is important to protect joint structures and prevent trauma.

Treatment of Incoordination

Admittedly, treatment of incoordination is difficult. Several approaches may be used. Incoordination arising from lesions of the corticospinal system may be improved using one of the sensorimotor approaches directed to the normalization of muscle tone and the development of more normal movement patterns. Specific sensory input is used to change muscle tone and evoke adaptive motor responses.

Activities graded on the basis of normal motor learning and control may be helpful for attaining proximal stability and then mobility. Therapy directed toward the modulation of reflexes and abnormal synergy patterns and the enhancement of postural control mechanisms, such as the righting and equilibrium reactions, can help to improve coordination. Weight bearing, joint approximation, placing and holding techniques, and fixed points of stability (tabletop) can be helpful.[17] The therapist should begin with small ranges of movement and gradually increase them as the patient progresses. Initially, work is done in the plane and direction of movement that are easiest for the patient, and the work progresses toward more difficult areas. Some of the involuntary movements of cerebellar or extrapyramidal origin, particularly primary movement disorders, are difficult to manage or change. Therapists have more influence over the movement disorders that are associated with traumatic brain injury and stroke.

Methods and devices to compensate for incoordination may be necessary to make ADL safer, more possible, and more satisfying. A thorough occupational history interview is necessary to make appropriate activity and equipment choices and determine adaptive strategies that the patient can carry over to the home environment. Some of these strategies are described in Chapter 13. The physician may employ pharmacological agents or surgical intervention in an effort to control tremors or other involuntary movements.

Surgical Intervention for Movement Disorders

Neurosurgical intervention for movement disorders may include stereotactic thalatomy for ballismus, chorea (Huntington's), Parkinson's disease, essential tremor, and athetosis. Surgical treatment for dystonia may include rhizotomy, neurectomy, cryothalotomy, or IBF implantation.[47] Deep brain stimulation has been effective in tremor reduction in essential tremor and Parkinson's disease.[4,79]

SUMMARY

Motor control is the ability to make postural adjustments in order to direct body and limb movement in purposeful activity. Motor control is the result of the interaction of complex neurological systems. Evaluation of motor control includes observation of motor performance and assessment of muscle tone, the postural mechanism, selective movement, and coordination. Associated reactions, stereotypic reflexes, and synergistic patterns are assessed.

The presence of abnormal elements of motor control affects the quality of movement and the ability to perform functional tasks. The occupational therapist assesses muscle tone, upper extremity recovery, and coordination, using standardized tests and observation of movement during occupational performance. The results of the motor control assessment can help the patient and therapist collaborate on appropriate intervention, such as one of the sensorimotor approaches or compensatory methods.

Because of the current managed care system, occupational therapists are receiving more referrals than ever before from primary care physicians. Occupational therapists who have a basic knowledge of the medical and surgical options in ameliorating motor control problems can play a triage role in suggesting referral to physician specialists.

REVIEW QUESTIONS

1. Define plasticity.
2. When would a physician recommend a long-term nerve block?
3. Describe the characteristics of rigidity.
4. Compare and contrast spasticity and HTSR.
5. Why should the assessment of muscle tone be performed in conjunction with the patient's overall motor function?
6. List the procedure for an upper extremity muscle tone evaluation.
7. What are the components of a normal postural mechanism?
8. Describe equilibrium reactions and the functional implications of their presence in motor control.
9. Describe functional difficulties encountered when the asymmetrical tonic neck reflex is present.
10. Compare and contrast chorea and athetosis.
11. Describe ataxia.
12. Compare and contrast the following tremors: essential familial, resting, and intention.

REFERENCES

1. Adams RD, Victor M, editors: Principles of neurology, ed 5, New York, 1993, McGraw-Hill.
2. Ashworth B: Preliminary trial of carisoprodol in multiple sclerosis, Practitioner 192:540-542, 1964.
3. Bell-Krotoski JA et al: Threshold detection and Semmes-Weinstein monofilaments, J Hand Ther 8(2):155-162, 1995.
4. Benabid AL et al: Chronic electrical stimulation of the ventralis intermedius nucleus of the thalamus as a treatment of movement disorders, J Neurosurg 84(2):203-214, 1996.
5. Berg KO et al: Measuring balance in the elderly: preliminary development of an instrument, Physiother Can 41:304-311, 1989.
6. Bernspang B, Fischer AG: Differences between persons with right or left CVA on the Assessment of Motor and Process Skills, Arch Phys Med Rehabil 76:1114, 1995.
7. Berrol S: The treatment of physical disorders following brain injury. In Wood RL, Eames P, editors: Models of brain injury rehabilitation, Baltimore, 1989, Johns Hopkins University Press.
8. Bickerstaff ER: Neurological examination in clinical practice, ed 3, 1973, Blackwell Scientific Publications.
9. Bobath B: Abnormal postural reflex activity caused by brain lesions, ed 2, London, 1975, William Heinemann Medical Books.
10. Bobath B: Adult hemiplegia: evaluation and treatment, ed 2, London, 1978, William Heinemann Medical Books.
11. Bohannon RW, Smith MB: Interrater reliability of a modified Ashworth scale of muscle spasticity, Phys Ther 67(2):206-207, 1987.
12. Bontke CF, Boake C: Principles of brain injury rehabilitation. In Braddom R, editor: Physical medicine and rehabilitation, Philadelphia, 1996, WB Saunders.
13. Booth BJ et al: Serial casting for the management of spasticity in the head injured adult, Phys Ther 63(2):1960-1966, 1983.
14. Brunnstrom S: Movement therapy in hemiplegia, New York, 1970, Harper & Row.

15. Carmick J: Clinical use of neuromuscular electrical stimulation for children with cerebral palsy. 2. Upper extremity, *Phys Ther* 73(8):514-527, 1993.

16. Carr JH, Shepherd RB: *Neurological rehabilitation: optimizing motor performance*, Oxford, 1998, Butterworth-Heinemann.

17. Charness A: *Stroke/head injury: a guide to functional outcomes in physical therapy management*, Rockville, Md, 1986, Aspen Publishers.

18. Cherry DB, Weigand GM: Plaster drop-out casts as a dynamic means to reduce muscle contracture, *Phys Ther* 61(11):1601-1603, 1981.

19. Chironna RL, Hecht JS: Subscapularis motor point block for the painful hemiplegic shoulder, *Arch Phys Med Rehabil* 71(6):428-429, 1990.

20. Chusid JG: *Correlative neuroanatomy and functional neurology*, ed 18, Los Altos, Calif, 1982, Lange Medical Publications.

21. Colin C, Wade D: Assessing motor impairment after a stroke: a pilot reliability study, *J Neurol Neurosurg Psychiatry* 53(7):576-579, 1990.

22. Crawford Small Parts Dexterity Test, New York, Psychological Corporation.

23. Cruickshank DA, O'Neill DL: Upper-extremity inhibitive casting in a boy with spastic quadriplegia, *Am J Occup Ther* 44(6):552-555, 1990.

24. Davies PM: *Steps to follow: a guide to treatment of adult hemiplegia*, New York, 1985, Springer Verlag.

25. DeBoskey DS, Hecht JS, Calub CJ: *Educating families of the head injured*, Gaithersburg, Md, 1991, Aspen Publishers.

26. deGroot J: *Correlative neuroanatomy*, ed 21, Norwalk, Conn, 1991, Appleton & Lange.

27. DeMyer W: *Technique of the neurologic examination: a programmed test*, ed 2, New York, 1974, McGraw-Hill.

28. Desrosiers J et al: Upper extremity performance test for the elderly (TEMPA): normative data and correlates with sensorimotor parameters, *Arch Phys Med Rehabil* 76(12):1125-1129, 1995.

29. Dombovy ML: Rehabilitation concerns in degenerative movement disorders of the central nervous system. In Braddom RL, editor: *Physical medicine and rehabilitation*, Philadelphia, 1996, WB Saunders.

30. Donato S, Pulaski KH: Overview of balance impairments: functional implications. In Gillen G, Burkhardt A: *Stroke rehabilitation: a function-based approach*, St Louis, 1998, Mosby.

31. Duncan PW, Badke MB: Determinants of abnormal motor control. In Duncan PW, Badke MB: *Stroke rehabilitation: the recovery of motor control*, Chicago, Ill, 1987, Year Book.

32. Duncan PW, Badke MB: Measurement of motor performance and functional abilities following stroke. In Duncan PW, Badke MB, editors: *Stroke rehabilitation: the recovery of motor control*, Chicago, 1987, Year Book.

33. Eggers O: *Occupational therapy in the treatment of adult hemiplegia*, London, 1984, William Heinemann Medical Books.

34. Eltorai I, Montroy R: Muscle release in the management of spasticity in spinal cord injury, *Paraplegia* 28(7):433-440, 1990.

35. Farber S: *Neurorehabilitation: a multisensory approach*, Philadelphia, 1982, WB Saunders.

36. Feldman PA: Upper extremity casting and splinting. In Glenn MB, White J, editors: *The practical management of spasticity in children and adults*, Philadelphia, 1990, Lea & Febiger.

37. Felten DL, Felten SY: A regional and systemic overview of functional neuroanatomy. In Farber S, editor: *Neurorehabilitation: a multisensory approach*, Philadelphia, 1982, WB Saunders.

38. Fiorentino M: *Normal and abnormal development: the influence of primitive reflexes on motor development*, Springfield, Ill, 1972, Charles C Thomas.

39. Ghez C: The cerebellum. In Kandel ER, Schwartz JH, Jessel TM, editors: *Principles of neural science*, ed 3, New York, 1991, Elsevier.

40. Gillen G: Trunk control: a prerequisite for functional independence. In Gillen G, Burkhardt A, editors: *Stroke rehabilitation: a function-based approach*, St Louis, 1998, Mosby.

41. Griffith ER: Spasticity. In Rosenthal M et al, editors: *Rehabilitation of the head injured adult*, Philadelphia, 1983, FA Davis.

42. Hecht JS: Subscapular nerve block in the painful hemiplegic shoulder, *Arch Phys Med Rehabil* 73(11):1036-1039, 1992.

43. Hill J: The effects of casting on upper extremity motor disorders after brain injury, *Am J Occup Ther* 48(3):219-224, 1994.

44. Hines AE et al: Functional electrical stimulation for the reduction of spasticity in the hemiplegic hand, *Biomed Sci Instrum* 29:259-266, 1993.

45. Hisey MS, Keenan MAE: Orthopedic management of upper extremity dysfunction following stroke or brain injury. In Green DP, Hotchkiss RN, Pederson WC, editors, *Operative hand surgery*, ed 4, New York, 1999, Churchill Livingstone.

46. Hylton N: Dynamic casting and orthotics. In Glenn MB, Whyte J, editors: *The practical management of spasticity in children and adults*, Philadelphia, 1990, Lea & Febiger.

47. Jain SS, Francisco GE: Parkinson's disease and other movement disorders. In DeLisa JA, Gans BM, editors: *Rehabilitation medicine: principles and practice*, ed 3, Philadelphia, 1998, Lippincott-Raven.

48. Jain SS, Kirshblum SC: Movement disorders, including tremors. In Delisa JA, editor: *Rehabilitation medicine: principles and practice*, ed 2, Philadelphia, 1993, JB Lippincott.

49. Jebsen RH et al: An objective and standardized test of hand function, *Arch Phys Med Rehabil* 50(6):311-319, 1969.

50. Jewell MJ: Overview of the structure and function of the central nervous system. In Umphred DA, editor: *Neurological rehabilitation*, ed 2, St Louis, 1990, Mosby.

51. Jordan CL, Allely RR: Burns and burn rehabilitation. In Pedretti LW, editor: *Occupational therapy: practice skills for physical dysfunction*, ed 4, St Louis, 1996, Mosby.

52. Katz RT: Management of spasticity. In Braddom RL, editor: *Physical medicine and rehabilitation*, Philadelphia, 1996, WB Saunders.

53. Katz RT et al: Objective quantification of spastic hypertonia: correlation with clinical findings, *Arch Phys Med Rehabil* 73(4):339-347, 1992.

54. Kisner C, Colby LA: *Therapeutic exercise foundations and techniques*, ed 3, Philadelphia, 1996, FA Davis.

55. Kopp B et al: The Arm Motor Ability Test: validity, and sensitivity to change of an instrument for assessing disabilities in activities of daily living, *Arch Phys Med Rehabil* 78(6):615-620, 1997.

56. Lance JW: Symposium synopsis. In Feldman, Young, Koella, editors: *Spasticity: disordered motor control*, Chicago, 1980, Year Book.

57. Lincoln-Oseretsky Motor Development Scale, Chicago, CH Stoelting Company.

58. Little JW, Massagli TL: Spasticity and associated abnormalities of muscle tone. In Delisa JB, editor: *Rehabilitation medicine: principles and practice*, ed 2, Philadelphia, 1993, JB Lippincott.

59. Little JW, Massagli TL: Spasticity and associated abnormalities of muscle tone. In Delisa JA, Gans BM, editors: *Rehabilitation medicine: principles and practice*, ed 3, Philadelphia, 1998, Lippincott Raven.

60. Law M et al: *Canadian Occupational Performance Measure*, ed 3, Ottawa, 1998, Canadian Association of Occupational Therapists.

61. Lee WA: A control systems framework for understanding normal and abnormal posture, *Am J Occup Ther* 439(5):291-301, 1989.

62. Marsden CD: The physiological basis of ataxia, *Physiotherapy* 61(11):326-328, 1975.

63. Mayo Clinic and Mayo Clinic Foundation: *Clinical examinations in neurology*, ed 5, Philadelphia, 1981, WB Saunders.

64. McCormack GL, Feuchter F: Neurophysiology for the sensorimotor approaches to treatment. In Pedretti LW, editor: *Occupational therapy practice skills for physical dysfunction*, ed 4, St Louis, 1996, Mosby.

65. McCormack G, Pedretti LW: Motor unit dysfunction. In Pedretti LW, editor: *Occupational therapy practice skills for physical dysfunction*, ed 4, St Louis, 1996, Mosby.

66. *Minnesota Rate of Manipulation Test*, Circle Pines, Minn, American Guidance Service.

67. Newton RA: Motor control. In Umphred DA, editor: *Neurological rehabilitation*, ed 2, St Louis, 1990, Mosby.

68. Nudo RJ et al: Neural substrates for the effects of rehabilitative training on motor recovery after ischemic infarct, *Science* 272(5269):1791-1794, 1996.

69. Pelland MJ: Occupational therapy and stroke rehabilitation. In Kaplan PE, Cerrillo LJ, editors: *Stroke rehabilitation*, Boston, 1986, Butterworth.

70. Pennsylvania Bi-Manual Work Sample: Educational Test Bureau, Circle Pines, Minn, American Guidance Service.

71. Preston LA: OT's role in enhancing nerve blocks for spasticity, *OT Practice* 3(10):28-35, 1998.

72. Preston LA, Hecht JS: *Spasticity management: rehabilitation strategies*, Bethesda, Md, 1999, American Occupational Therapy Association.

73. Purdue Pegboard: Science Research Associates, Inc, 259 East Erie Street, Chicago, Ill, 60611.

74. Reuben DB, Siu AL: An objective measure of physical function of elderly outpatients, *J Am Geriatr Soc* 38:1105-1112, 1990.

75. Roth EJ, Harvey RL: Rehabilitation of stroke syndromes. In Braddom RL, editor: *Physical medicine and rehabilitation*, Philadelphia, 1996, WB Saunders.

76. Ryerson S: Hemiplegia resulting from vascular insult or disease. In Umphred DA, editor: *Neurological rehabilitation*, ed 2, St Louis, 1990, Mosby.

77. Schneider F: Traumatic spinal cord injury. In Umphred DA, editor: *Neurological rehabilitation*, ed 2, St Louis, 1990, Mosby.

78. Smith HD: Occupational therapy assessment and treatment. In Hopkins HL, Smith HD, editors: *Willard & Spackman's occupational therapy*, ed 8, Philadelphia, 1997, JB Lippincott.

79. Tasker RR: Deep brain stimulation is preferable to thalamotomy for tremor suppression, *Surg Neurol* 49:145-154, 1998.

80. Tinetti ME: Performance oriented assessment of mobility problems in elderly patients, *J Am Geriatr Soc* 34:119-126, 1986.

81. Tomas ES et al: Nonsurgical management of upper extremity deformities after traumatic brain injury, *Phys Med Rehabil:* State of the art reviews, 7(3), October 1993.

82. Umphred DA: Classification of treatment techniques based on primary input systems. In Umphred DA, editor: *Neurological rehabilitation*, ed 3, St Louis, 1995, Mosby.

83. Umphred DA, editor: *Neurological rehabilitation*, ed 3, St Louis, 1995, Mosby.

84. Urbscheit NL: Cerebellar dysfunction. In Umphred DA, editor: *Neurological rehabilitation*, St Louis, 1990, Mosby.

85. Van der Meche F, Van der Gijn J: Hypotonia: an erroneous clinical concept? *Brain* 109(pt 6):1169-1178, 1986.

86. Whitney SL et al: A review of balance instruments for older adults, *Am J Occup Ther* 52(8):666-671, 1998.

87. Whyte J, Rosenthal M: Rehabilitation of the patient with traumatic brain injury. In DeLisa JA, editor: *Rehabilitation medicine: principles and practice*, ed 2, Philadelphia, 1993, JB Lippincott.

88. Wilson DJ, Baker LL, Craddock JA: *Functional test for the hemiplegic/paretic upper extremity*, Downey, Calif, 1984, Los Amigos Research and Education Institute.

89. Winkler PA: Head injury. In Umphred DA, editor: *Neurological rehabilitation*, ed 3, St Louis, 1995, Mosby.

90. Yasukawa A: Upper extremity casting: adjunct treatment for a child with cerebral palsy hemiplegia, *Am J Occup Ther* 44(9):840-846, 1990.

91. Young RR: Spasticity: a review, *Neurology* 44(suppl 9):S12-S20, 1994.

CHAPTER 24

Evaluation and Treatment of Visual Deficits

MARY WARREN

Visual perception
Visual perceptual hierarchy
Visual cognition
Visual memory
Pattern recognition
Visual scanning
Search
Visual attention
Oculomotor control
Visual fields
Visual acuity
Visual field deficit
Binocular vision
Sensory fusion
Diplopia
Paralytic strabismus
Convergence insufficiency
Hemi-inattention
Visual neglect

After studying this chapter the student or practitioner will be able to do the following:

1. Understand the role vision plays in enabling the person to adapt to the environment.
2. Understand how visual input is processed within the CNS to turn raw visual data into cognitive concepts of space and form through the process of visual perception.
3. Understand the concept of the visual perceptual hierarchy as a framework for evaluation and treatment of visual perceptual dysfunction.
4. Understand the purpose of evaluation completed by occupational therapy (OT) practitioners.
5. Understand how visual acuity, visual field, oculomotor control, visual attention, and visual scanning change following brain injury.
6. Understand how visual acuity, visual field, oculomotor control, visual attention, and visual scanning affect functional performance.
7. Understand how to assess and treat deficits in visual acuity, visual field, oculomotor control, visual attention, and visual scanning.

An understanding of visual perceptual dysfunction after cerebrovascular accident (CVA) and traumatic brain injury must be preceded by the realization that visual perception is a process used by the central nervous system (CNS) to adapt to the environment. Visual perception is not a series of discrete perceptual skills or the function of a single sensory modality, but rather a process that integrates vision with other sensory input for adaptation and survival.[54,83] The activities a person is required to complete in a day will dictate the visual perceptual processing needed. Whether a patient has a visual perceptual deficit after brain injury will depend on whether the ability to process visual information has been altered so that it prevents completion of a necessary activity of daily living.

ROLE OF VISION IN THE ADAPTATION PROCESS

According to Jean Ayres,[4] the overall function of the brain is to filter, organize, and integrate sensory information to make an adaptive response to the environment. The brain or CNS receives a variety of sensory information, including visual, proprioceptive, tactile, vestibular, and auditory information. Vision is used along with information from these other sensory systems to adapt to the environment—to act on it and to manipulate, mold, and improve it. In adapting to the environment, the CNS combines the isolated bits of sensory information it receives, integrating them to form a picture of the environment. This picture, created by sensory input, becomes the context of a situation, and an individual uses this context to make decisions and formulate plans to respond to various situations.

Successful adaptation to the environment depends on the ability to anticipate information. The key to survival is to stay one step ahead of circumstances, whether working with patients or navigating rush-hour traffic. Anticipation enables an individual to plan for situations, and planning allows manipulation of the environment. If a person was unable to plan for situations and able to react to them only once they occurred, the person might be able to survive the challenges of the environment but not to act on or change the environment. Anticipation and planning are driven by the sensory context of a person's circumstances: "It looks like rain. I'd better take an umbrella," or "It's dark in there. I'd better take a flashlight." How sensory information is perceived determines the plan formulated to respond to each situation.

Given the importance of sensory context, what role does vision, a basic sensory process, play in the adaptation process? Vision is our most far-reaching sensory system. It is the sensory system that takes us out into our environment, that is the first to alert us to danger (e.g., seeing a threatening storm approach), and that is the first to alert us to pleasure (e.g., seeing your pet in the yard as you drive up). Because of its far-reaching nature, visual input strongly dominates the construction of the environmental picture we use to adapt. We rely on vision to "size up" situations. We say to ourselves, "He looks harmless," or "That looks delicious." Our language is peppered with phrases that reflect the importance of vision in decision-making, such as, "I'll believe it when I see it," "I'll keep an eye out for it," or "I can see what you mean." Because visual input dominates the construction of sensory context, it plays a powerful role in the anticipatory process, and therefore in our ability to adapt to the environment. How a person "sees" a situation triggers the planning and decision-making processes.

The decision-making process guided by vision is not limited to manipulation of objects in the environment. Vision plays an important role in social communication, enabling a person to "read" and respond to the subtle gestural and facial expressions used to communicate emotional content in conversations. Vision also plays an important role in motor and postural accommodation by warning of upcoming challenges to postural control, such as the presence of a curb, stairs, a ramp, a banana peel, or obstacles in the travel path. The speed of visual processing enables the rapid intake of large amounts of detailed information. The person can instantly identify an object visually, whereas identifying the object tactilely would take longer. For example, a person groping for a bottle in the medicine cabinet late at night with the lights off knows that if a light is turned on, the bottle will be found instantly.

The speed at which vision is able to supply information about the environment is critical to the ability to negotiate dynamic environments safely. Dynamic environments are those in which objects and other persons are in motion independent of the individual in the environment. To be able to move safely through such an environment without colliding with other objects requires rapid information processing, which can be supplied only by vision. For example, it is possible to send a blindfolded person into an empty room to locate a chair to sit upon without that person's harshly colliding with other objects and possibly incurring injury. It will take only a few minutes longer to complete this task without vision than with vision. However, it is unlikely that the same person could be sent into a room full of people milling about and meet with the same success within the same time frame. The ADL most affected by visual impairment take place in dynamic, unpredictable environments such as those found in the community and workplaces. Reintegrating a person with a visual impairment into the stable environment of the home is a relatively easy process, but reintegrating a person into community environments is much more difficult.

Visual impairment can occur secondary to disease, trauma, and aging.[5,23,32,74] Often a combination of at least two of these causes is observed, especially in older patients. Visual impairment alters the quality and amount of visual input into the CNS or alters how the CNS is able to process and use incoming visual input. Either way, the result is a decrease in the ability to use vision to adapt to the environment. The therapist will be able to observe a decrease in the speed with which a patient can process information from the environment. This decrease in speed may prevent the patient from responding safely in dynamic environments. Changes in decision making may be observed in which the patient makes errors because not enough visual information was received or because the information received was faulty. The patient may even be unable to make decisions. Visual impairment has the potential to change the patient's interaction with all aspects of the environment and the persons and objects in it.

AN OVERVIEW OF VISUAL PROCESSING WITHIN THE CENTRAL NERVOUS SYSTEM

For vision to be used for adaptation, the raw material of vision (i.e., the pattern of light that falls on the retina) must be transformed into images of the surrounding environment. Those images must then be conveyed to the prefrontal areas of the brain, where decision making takes place.[54,64] The process begins as light enters the eye and passes through the cornea and lens to focus on the retina. The retina conveys this information over the optic nerve and tract to the lateral geniculate nucleus (LGN) of the thalamus. Because of the crossing of the retinal nasal fibers (of the optic nerve) at the optic chiasm, the LGN receives information from the retinal hemifields of both eyes. It integrates this information to provide binocular vision.[39,54] After synapsing in the LGN, visual information travels over the geniculocalcarine tracts to the visual cortex (found within the occipital lobe). Fig. 24-1 shows these pathways. The visual cortex sorts through the incoming visual information, sharpening and fine-tuning features such as orientation of line and color, then disperses this information for cortical processing.[39,90] From the visual cortex, visual information is processed by cortical circuitry and eventually sent to the prefrontal circuitry to be used in decision making. Before it can be used by the prefrontal areas, visual information must be combined (integrated) with other incoming sensory information to establish images and relationships between the body and the environmental surround.[54]

To integrate vision with other sensory input, visual information is sent from the visual cortex to the prefrontal area over two routes: a "northern" or superior route, which takes it through the posterior parietal circuitry, and a "southern" or inferior route through the posterior temporal circuitry.[30,53,54,63] This process is known as parallel-distributed sensory processing (Fig. 24-2). Visual information traveling the southern route through the posterior temporal circuitry is processed for visual object information and recognition.[53,54] The purpose of this processing is to identify objects and classify them. Neural processes in the posterior temporal lobe use precise visual input from the macular-foveal area of the retina to tune into the visual details of objects. Processing by posterior temporal circuitry is critical to the ability to distinguish discrete features of objects, such as the difference between the style of a can of diet Coke and regular Coke or particular facial features. This area of the CNS participates in directing attention to visual detail.[65]

Visual information taking the northern route to the prefrontal circuitry travels through the posterior parietal lobe. The parietal lobe is a synthesizer of sensory information, receiving input from all of the sensory systems and integrating the input to create internal sensory maps that are used to orient the body in space.[30,53,54,63] Visual information traveling through the parietal circuits is used to tune the CNS in to the presence of the objects surrounding the body and to determine the spatial relationship of the objects to the body and to

each other. Visual information must be integrated with other sensory information to provide this orientation. Tactile, proprioceptive, kinesthetic, vestibular, and auditory information is necessary, along with visual input, for people to accurately assess the relationship between them and the objects that surround them. The map created by information synthesized in the parietal circuitry is body centered and dynamic, changing in shape and content as the body moves through space.[30,52,54]

The posterior parietal circuitry in each hemisphere contains a map of the space on the contralateral side of the body. Thus the right hemisphere contains a map of the left side of the body and surrounding space, and the left hemisphere contains a map of the right side of the body and surroundings.[30] The map is not a detailed representation of space but provides a general impression of objects in space on that side of body. The CNS relies on visual information from the peripheral areas of the retinal fields to create and maintain these maps. This area of the brain participates in directing general attention to and awareness of space.[52,64]

The final destination for visual information traveling through the posterior temporal and parietal circuitry is the prefrontal area of the brain, where the information is used to make decisions and formulate plans. This area, along with the premotor circuitry and other areas, is responsible for planning skilled body movements, including eye movements.[29,30,54] The frontal eye fields are located in area eight of the prefrontal lobes and are responsible for voluntary visual search of the space on the contralateral side of the body[11,30]; that is, the frontal eye fields in the right hemisphere direct visual search toward the left visual space, and vice-versa. The frontal eye fields conduct visual search based on an expectation of where visual information will be found in the environment; the fields then direct the eyes to move toward that area.[50] For example, if you were looking for a light switch in a room, you would direct your visual search toward the walls, because that is where you expect to find a light switch. You would not waste time searching the floor or the ceiling. By directing visual search based on the expected location of crucial visual information, the CNS is able to process visual information quickly. This arrangement enables us to engage successfully in activities that require rapid visual processing, such as driving.

Not all visual information travels over the geniculocalcarine tracts for cortical processing. Many neural pathways leave the optic nerve and tract and travel to subcortical areas, including the hypothalamus and brainstem.[39,46,54] The brainstem contains important neural structures involved in visual processing. The superior colliculi, located in the midbrain of the brainstem, are primary brainstem processing centers. The superior colliculi are responsible for the detection of moving visual stimuli appearing in the peripheral visual

PARALLEL-DISTRIBUTED PROCESSING OF THE VISUAL SYSTEM-I

Schematic inferior view of a horizontal slice of the brain

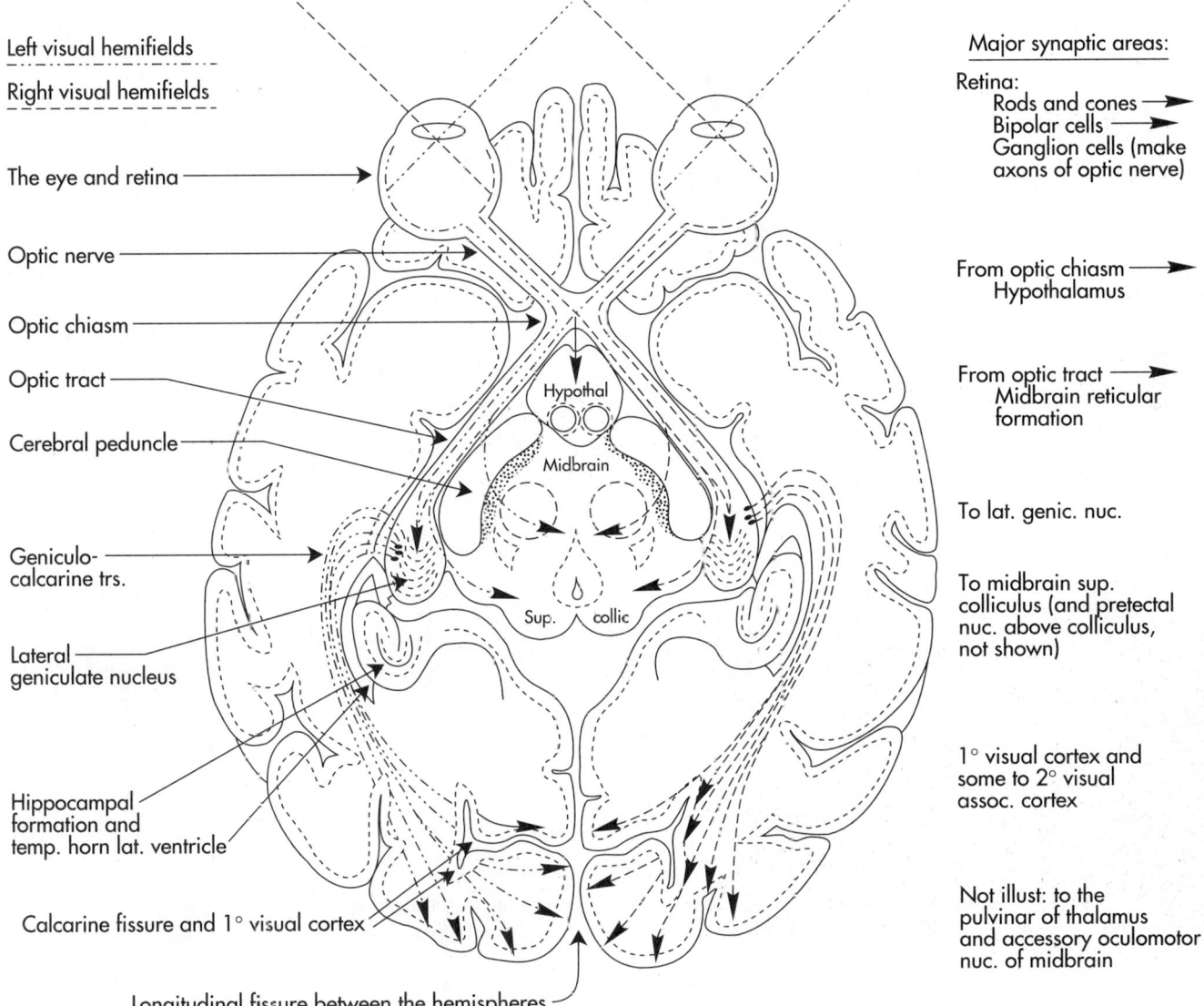

Left visual hemifields

Right visual hemifields

The eye and retina

Optic nerve

Optic chiasm

Optic tract

Cerebral peduncle

Geniculo-calcarine trs.

Lateral geniculate nucleus

Hippocampal formation and temp. horn lat. ventricle

Calcarine fissure and 1° visual cortex

Longitudinal fissure between the hemispheres

Hypothal

Midbrain

Sup. collic

Major synaptic areas:

Retina:
Rods and cones →
Bipolar cells →
Ganglion cells (make axons of optic nerve)

From optic chiasm →
Hypothalamus

From optic tract →
Midbrain reticular formation

To lat. genic. nuc.

To midbrain sup. colliculus (and pretectal nuc. above colliculus, not shown)

1° visual cortex and some to 2° visual assoc. cortex

Not illust: to the pulvinar of thalamus and accessory oculomotor nuc. of midbrain

The visual system is our most important sense in regard to:

A. Learning, memory, and recall including our ability to see color and fine details as well as the visual surround and global relationships.
B. Communication: use of symbolic language, speaking, and body language.
C. Spatiotemporal orientation in concert with vestibular-proprioceptive systems.
D. Early warning system to pleasure or danger, i.e., vision is our farthest reaching distance receptor and movement detector par excellence.
E. Visual-manual and visual-motor activities.

1°, Primary.
2°, Secondary.

FIG. 24-1
Pathways from retina to LGN to visual cortex. (Courtesy of Josephine C. Moore, PhD, OTR.)

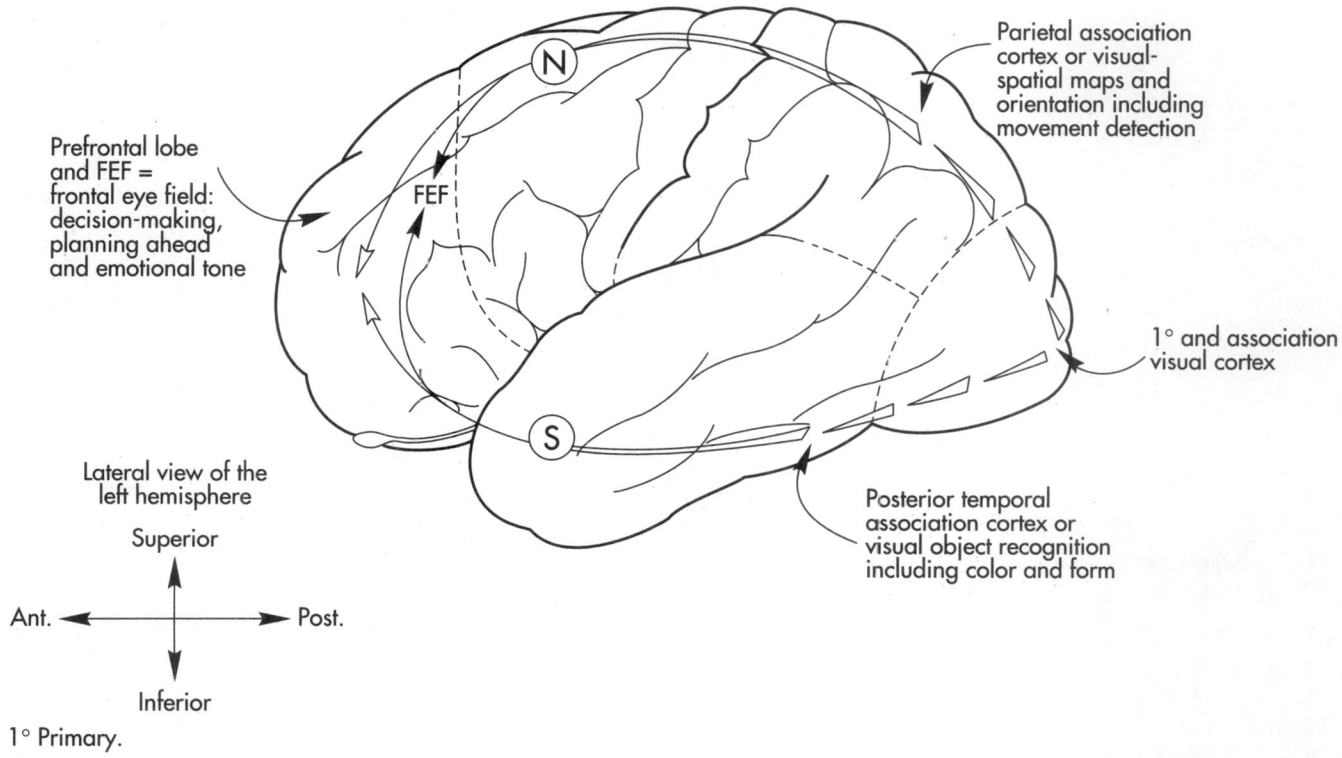

PARALLEL-DISTRIBUTED PROCESSING OF THE VISUAL SYSTEM

Two parallel routes carry visual information from the occipital lobe to the prefrontal lobe and frontal eye field (FEF). Fibers from these two routes distribute to many areas along each route (not illustrated) before terminating in the prefrontal cortex and FEF as illustrated.

(N) = "Northern" or superior route via parietal and frontal lobes.

(S) = "Southern" or inferior route via temporal and frontal lobes.

Prefrontal lobe and FEF = frontal eye field: decision-making, planning ahead and emotional tone

Parietal association cortex or visual-spatial maps and orientation including movement detection

1° and association visual cortex

Posterior temporal association cortex or visual object recognition including color and form

Lateral view of the left hemisphere

Superior

Ant. ← → Post.

Inferior

1° Primary.

FIG. 24-2
Visual input travels from the visual cortex through parietal and posterior temporal circuitry to the prefrontal lobe to complete cortical visual processing. (Courtesy of Josephine C. Moore, PhD, OTR.)

fields.[30,46,50,66] When motion is detected, the colliculi automatically initiate eye movement toward the direction of the detected motion. In performing this function, the colliculi serve as an early warning system to prevent the CNS from being "caught off-guard" by events occurring in the environment.[30,62] The brainstem also contains centers for the control of horizontal- and vertical-gaze eye movements. The nuclei of cranial nerves III, IV, and VI, which control the extraocular muscles of the eyes, are also located in the brainstem, along with basic visual functions such as the light (pupillary) reflex and the accommodation reflex.[28]

Various CNS areas are responsible for processing visual information, but all areas must work together for a person to make sense of what is seen and thus use visual information to adapt.[30,52,54,64] Millions of long and short neural fibers tie the various centers together within and between hemispheres to ensure effective and efficient visual processing. Like a car in which the fuel-injection system is as critical to performance as the spark plugs, the visual system will not run efficiently unless all of its components are working together. When brain injury or disease occurs, this communication system is disrupted and the organization of visual processing breaks down. Table 24-1 lists effects of various CNS lesions on different aspects of the visual system. In reviewing the table, remember that a patient will exhibit a functional limitation only in those ADL that require the type of visual processing compromised by the lesion. For example, a deficit in the ability to process visual detail caused by a lesion in the left posterior temporal lobe would significantly affect the ability of a proofreader to return to work but might have little effect on a piano tuner's ability to return to work.

TABLE 24-1

Summary of Cortical Hemispheric Functions for Visual Processing and Deficits Secondary to Lesion Site

Left Hemisphere Advantage		Right Hemisphere Advantage	
More detail-oriented in relation to persons, places, and things		More global or holistic	
Takes in minute details and compares and contrasts these details		Takes a general view of the environment	
Processes visual information sequentially in a systematic item-by-item, serial search strategy		Processes multiple visual inputs simultaneously, grouping them into meaningful categories	
Attends only to right visual fields		Attends globally to both left and right visual fields	
Parietal Lesion	**Post. Temp. Lesion**	**Parietal Lesion**	**Post. Temp. Lesion**
Biases attention to detail	Biases attention to global input	Biases attention to detail	Biases attention to global input
Biases brain to right hemisphere advantages	Biases brain to right hemisphere advantages	Biases brain to left hemisphere advantages	Biases brain to left hemisphere advantages
May have right inferior quadrant visual field loss	May have right superior quadrant visual field loss	May have neglect or hemi-inattention along with left inferior quadrant visual field loss	May have neglect or hemi-inattention along with left superior quadrant visual field loss

Modified with permission of Josephine C. Moore.

FRAMEWORK FOR EVALUATION AND TREATMENT OF VISUAL PERCEPTUAL DYSFUNCTION
A Hierarchical Model of Visual Perceptual Processing

The ability to use vision to adapt to the environment requires the integration of vision within the CNS to turn the raw data supplied by the retina into cognitive concepts of the perception of space and objects that can be manipulated and used for decision making. The process by which this occurs is known as **visual perception**. Visual perceptual function can be conceptualized as an organized hierarchy of processes that interact with and subserve each other.[83,86] Fig. 24-3 illustrates this hierarchy. Within the hierarchy, each process is supported by the one that precedes it and cannot properly function without the integration of the lower-level process. As Fig. 24-3 shows, the **visual perceptual hierarchy** consists of the processes of visual cognition (visuocognition), visual memory, pattern recognition, visual scanning, and visual attention. These perceptual processes are supported by three basic visual functions that form the foundation of the hierarchy: oculomotor control, visual fields, and visual acuity.

The ability to use visual perception to adapt to the environment is the result of the interaction of all of the processes in the hierarchy in a unified system. Each perceptual process is discussed individually in this section. The reader should remember that the ability to adapt

through vision is a result of the processes working in synergy. Although discrete perceptual processes can be identified, they do not operate independent of one another.

The highest-order visual perceptual process in the hierarchy is visual cognition. **Visual cognition** can be defined as the ability to manipulate visual information mentally and integrate it with other sensory information to gain knowledge, solve problems, formulate plans, and make decisions. Because visual cognition enables complex visual analysis, it serves as a foundation for all academic endeavors, including reading, writing, and mathematics, and many vocations, such as artist, engineer, surgeon, architect, and scientist.

Visual cognition cannot occur without the presence of **visual memory**, the next process level in the hierarchy. Mental manipulation of visual stimuli requires the ability to create and retain a picture of the object in the mind's eye while the visual analysis is being completed. In addition to being able to store visual images temporarily in short-term memory, a person must also be able to store and retrieve images from long-term memory. For example, to interpret the illustration in Fig. 24-4, one must be able to access visual memories of the shape of both a goose and a hawk. Adults and older children can easily resolve this illusion, but most toddlers cannot because they have not yet stored memories of the shapes of these birds.

Before a visual image can be stored in memory, an individual must recognize the pattern making up the

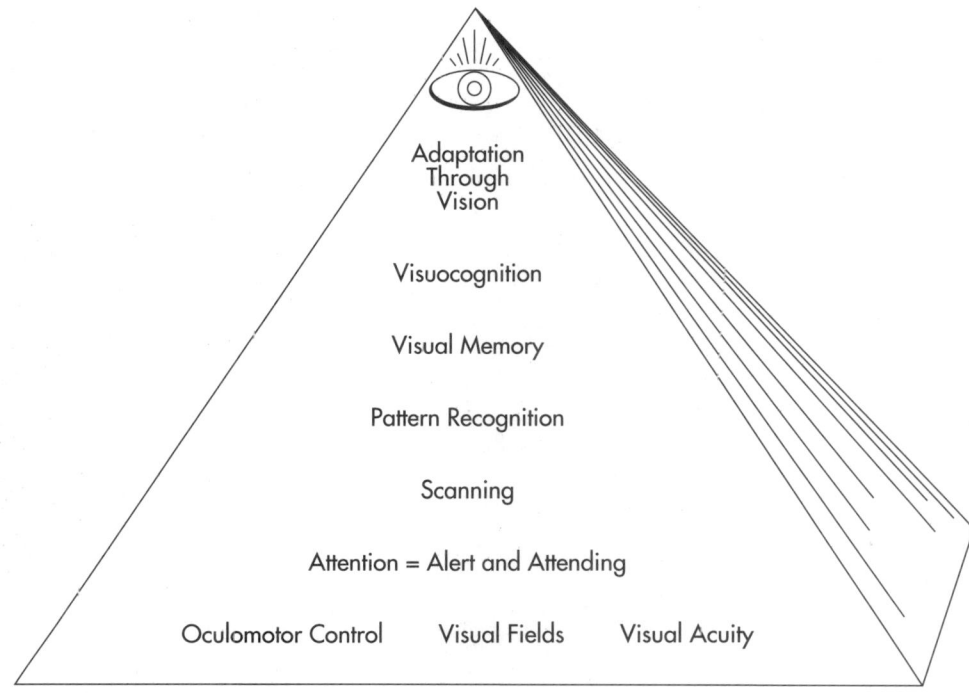

FIG. 24-3

Hierarchy of visual perceptual development in central nervous system. (Courtesy of Josephine C. Moore, PhD, OTR. From Warren M: A hierarchical model for evaluation and treatment of visual perceptual dysfunction in adult acquired brain injury, part I, *Am J Occup Ther* 47[1]:55-66, 1993.)

image. **Pattern recognition,** which subserves visual memory in the hierarchy, involves identifying the salient features of an object and using these features to distinguish the object from its surroundings.[37] A salient feature is a feature that distinguishes one object from another. For example, the salient feature that differentiates an "E" from an "F" is the lower horizontal line on the "E." Pattern recognition involves two abilities: the ability to identify the configural and holistic aspects of an object—to see its general shape, contour, and features—and the ability to identify specific features of an object, such as details of color, shading, and texture.[18] Both aspects of recognition must occur for accurate identification.[8]

Pattern recognition cannot be accomplished without the next process in the hierarchy: organized and thorough scanning of the visual scene. **Visual scanning** or **search** is accomplished through the use of saccadic eye movements. A saccade is a movement of the eye toward an object of interest in the environment. The purpose of a saccade is to focus on the object with the fovea, the area of the retina with the greatest ability to process detail.[28] In scanning a visual array, the eyes selectively focus on the elements that are critical for accurately interpreting the array.[22,56,68] The most important details are reexamined several times through a series of cyclic saccades to ensure that correct identification is made. Unessential elements in the scene are ignored.[68,93]

Visual scanning is actually a product of **visual attention.**[13,31,62] The saccadic eye movements observed in scanning reflect the engagement of visual attention as it is shifted from object to object. Visual search occurs on two levels: an automatic or reflexive level largely controlled by the brainstem and a voluntary level driven by the cortical processes of cognition.[52] On a reflexive level, visual attention (and therefore visual search) is automatically engaged by any novel object moving or suddenly appearing in the peripheral visual field, such as a flash of light.[50] This response serves to protect an individual from unexpected intrusions in the environment. Voluntary visual search, directed by the cortex, is completed for the explicit purpose of gathering information. Visual search is purposefully and often consciously driven by a desire to locate certain objects in the environment, such as a misplaced set of keys, or to obtain certain information, such as where an exit is located.[52]

Visual attention is a critical prerequisite for visual cognitive processing. If and how a person attends to an object or information determines if and how that visual input will be analyzed by the CNS, which becomes the basis for decision making. People who do not attend to visual information do not initiate a search for visual information, do not complete pattern recognition, do not lay down a visual memory, and cannot use this visual input for decision making. Likewise, those who attend

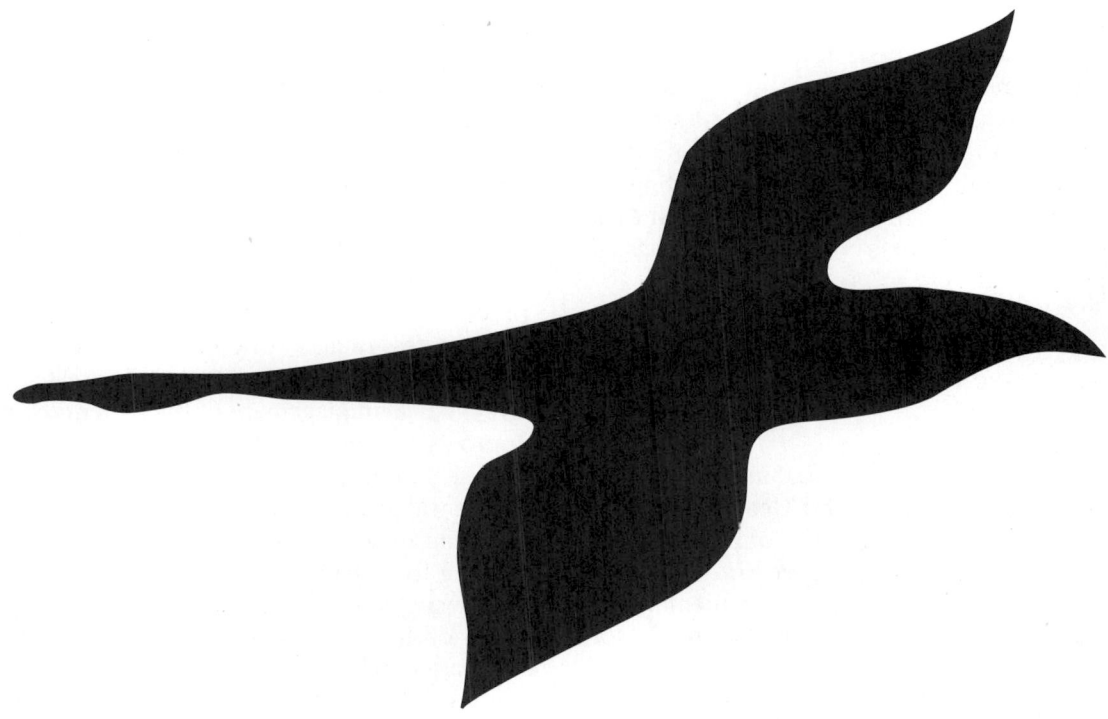

FIG. 24-4
Is this a goose or a hawk? (From Warren M: A hierarchical model for evaluation and treatment of visual perceptual dysfunction in adult acquired brain injury, part I, *Am J Occup Ther* 47[1]:55-66, 1993.)

to visual information in a random and incomplete way often do not have sufficient or accurate information on which to base a decision.

The type of visual attention engaged by the CNS depends on the type of visual analysis needed. For example, the type of attention needed for awareness that a chair is in the room is different from the type needed to identify the style of the chair. The first instance requires a *global* awareness of the environment and the location of objects within it; the second requires *selective* visual attention to the details of the chair to identify its features. Also, it is necessary to be able to employ more than one type of visual attention at the same time. When crossing a crowded room to talk to a friend, a person must be aware of the movement of people and the placement of obstacles in the room to avoid collision, while at the same time focusing on the friend (or target). The CNS employs several types of visual attention simultaneously and shifts constantly between types and levels of attention.[52] A large amount of neural processing is devoted to directing visual attention, causing visual attention to be disrupted easily by brain injury, but at the same time to be a highly resilient visual perceptual process.[52]

Engagement of visual attention and the other higher-level processes in the hierarchy cannot occur unless the CNS is receiving clear, concise visual information from the environment. Visual input is provided through the visual functions of oculomotor control, visual field, and visual acuity. **Oculomotor control** enables eye movements to be completed quickly and accurately and ensures perceptual stability. The **visual fields** register the visual scene and ensure that the CNS receives complete visual information. **Visual acuity** ensures that the visual information sent to the CNS is accurate. Without these prerequisite visual functions, an inadequate image is generated, preventing engagement of higher-level visual perceptual processing.

Brain injury or disease can disrupt visual processing at any level in the hierarchy. Because of the unity of the hierarchy, if brain injury disturbs a lower-level process or function, the processes above it will also be compromised. When this occurs, the patient may appear to have a deficit in a higher-level process, even though the deficit actually has occurred at a lower level in the hierarchy. For example, a patient who is unable to complete an embedded figures test appears to have a deficit in the visual cognitive process of figure-ground perception. In fact, this patient may be experiencing inaccurate pattern recognition, caused by an asymmetrical scanning pattern that results from visual inattention, compounded by a visual field deficit. Treatment of the higher-level process (figure-ground imperception) will not be successful unless the underlying deficits in visual attention and visual field are addressed first. This effect is similar to that observed in the motor system following brain injury. The high-level deficit observed is that the patient cannot use the hand to pick up an object.

The underlying deficits are reduced muscle tone and sensation and muscle weakness. Use of the hand for manipulation will not be possible until the deficits in muscle tone, strength, and sensation are addressed in treatment. Effective evaluation and treatment of visual perceptual dysfunction require an understanding of how brain injury affects the integration of vision at each process level and how the levels interact to enable visual perceptual processing.

MEDICAL FRAMEWORK FOR EVALUATION AND TREATMENT OF VISUAL IMPAIRMENT

Rehabilitation of the patient with visual impairment is a multidisciplinary process. The World Health Organization, in the International Classification of Diseases, Impairments, and Handicaps (ICDIH), established a four-step process for the management of permanent visual impairment. This process serves as the medical model for the rehabilitation of patients with visual impairment (Table 24-2).[16,17,91] The first step in the process is to identify the *visual disorder* or anatomical change causing the change in vision, such as damage to the geniculocalcarine tracts, retina, or prefrontal lobes of the brain. The second step is to identify the resulting *visual impairment*—the change in visual performance, such as the presence of a visual field deficit or a decrease in visual acuity, resulting from the anatomical change. An eye care specialist, either an ophthalmologist or an optometrist,

generally completes these first two steps. The two professions often collaborate with one another to complete this process and establish a diagnosis and prognosis of the visual condition. Steps three and four of the process consist of identifying the *visual disability*, which is the change in daily living performance that occurs as a result of the visual impairment, and the *visual handicap*, which is the socioeconomic consequence of having the disability, such as an inability to be gainfully employed. Occupational therapy (OT) practitioners and other rehabilitation professionals work collaboratively to complete these two steps of the evaluation process. Comprehensive medical management of the patient requires a team approach that integrates several disciplines to ensure that each step of the process is completed.

The value of rehabilitation is that it can alter the outcome in the last two categories of the process. According to Colenbrander,[16] rehabilitation is the art of influencing the links between the first and last categories of the process, "so that a given disorder results in the least possible handicap." Through treatment intervention it is possible to "optimize one's abilities in the presence of a given impairment."[17] OT intervention can facilitate this change because the relationship between impairment and ability is not rigidly fixed.[17] With treatment, it is possible to exploit a patient's capabilities while eliminating as many of the obstacles to success as possible, and in so doing to achieve better functional performance. Accomplishing this is the essence of treatment intervention.

OCCUPATIONAL THERAPY EVALUATION

To provide treatment intervention, the OT practitioner must link visual disability and handicap to the presence of a visual impairment. Establishing this relationship is the purpose of the assessment of visual performance completed by an occupational therapist. This process also is known as establishing "medical necessity," which is the prerequisite to receiving reimbursement for OT services. To achieve the link, the occupational therapist must be able to identify the functional limitation in performance of a daily activity and then connect it to the presence of a visual impairment. This often requires that the occupational therapist also complete assessments to identify visual impairment. However, whereas an ophthalmologist or optometrist evaluates visual impairment for the purpose of diagnosing a visual disorder, occupational therapists assess visual impairment to explain the presence of a functional limitation.

OT assessment has three purposes: to identify the functional impairment, to link the functional impairment to the presence of a visual impairment, and to determine appropriate treatment intervention based on the results of the assessment. In addressing evaluation and treatment, it is important to remember that a

TABLE 24-2
World Health Organization Aspects of Vision Loss

Visual Disorder	Visual Impairment	Visual Disability	Visual Handicap
← The Organ →		← The Person →	
Anatomical Changes	Functional Changes	Skills and Abilities	Social, Economic Consequences
Examples:			
Corneal opacity	Visual acuity	Reading skills	Need for extra effort
Cataract	Visual field	Writing skills	Loss of independence
Retinal scar	Color vision	ADL skills	Loss of earning potential
Optic atrophy	Night vision	Mobility skills	
Stroke	Ocular motility	Vocational skills	

From Colenbrander A, Fletcher DC: Basic concepts and terms for low vision rehabilitation, *Am J Occup Ther* 49(9):865-869, 1995.

patient's visual performance is significant not in terms of how it deviates from an established norm but in how it interferes with functional ability. A patient is considered to have a visual impairment that requires treatment if the impairment interferes with performance of a necessary ADL.

Several tests are available to occupational therapists to assess visual performance. Subtests from the Brain Injury Visual Assessment Battery for Adults (biVABA)* developed by the author are used in this chapter to describe assessment techniques.[82] The biVABA was designed specifically as a tool to help occupational therapists develop effective treatment plans and interventions for adults with visual impairment caused by brain injury. The biVABA consists of 17 subtests designed to measure visual processing ability. The assessments include evaluation tools used by ophthalmologists and optometrists to measure basic visual function, along with subtests designed specifically for occupational therapists.

OCCUPATIONAL THERAPY INTERVENTION

The focus of OT intervention is to change the outcome in the categories of visual disability and visual handicap. Three approaches are used in providing treatment. An *active* approach may be used, in which treatment attempts to change the patient's ability to complete visual processing by improving aspects of visual performance, such as increasing the efficiency of visual search or improving visual attention. A *passive* approach is also used, in which the emphasis of treatment is on changing the environment or task to enable the patient to use his or her current level of visual processing. These two approaches may be used alone or together to improve functional performance. The third approach that is always used in conjunction with the other two is *education* of the patient and family to increase their insight into how the patient's visual processing has changed and how it has affected functional performance. Education is a critical component of the treatment process because insight is crucial to the ability to learn compensatory strategies.[1]

OCCUPATIONAL THERAPY ASSESSMENT AND TREATMENT OF SPECIFIC VISUAL IMPAIRMENTS

The concept of a visual perceptual hierarchy provides the framework for the discussion of assessment and treatment. It is assumed that many changes in visual perceptual function after brain injury occur because of

*Brain Injury Visual Assessment Battery for Adults, visAbilities Rehab Services, Inc., 12008 W. 87th St., Suite 349, Lenexa, KS 66215; (888) 752-4364.

the alteration of the lower-level processes within the perceptual hierarchy, including visual acuity, visual field, oculomotor control, and visual attention and scanning. Deficits in these functions prevent the CNS from accurately completing complex visual processing and using vision for adaptation. Identification of deficiencies in these processes, followed by treatment to remediate the deficits, enables the CNS to process visual input more efficiently and facilitates adaptation. This section focuses on assessment and treatment of these processes within the visual perceptual hierarchy and examines how brain injury disrupts the functioning of each process, how the process is assessed, and how treatment intervention is provided.

Visual Acuity

Visual acuity is the ability to see small visual detail. Acuity contributes to the capability of the CNS to recognize objects. The dictionary defines acuity as "keenness or sharpness," and with regard to vision, acuity ensures that clear and precise visual information is provided to the CNS for processing.[2,39] The greater the quality of the visual input, the more precise the image created by CNS processing. The more precise the image, the faster and more accurate the ability of the CNS to recognize the object and discriminate it from other features in the environment. Good acuity therefore enables speed and accuracy of information processing and decision making.

Acuity occurs through a multistep process that begins with the focusing of light onto the retina. Light rays enter the eye through the pupil and are focused on the retina by the anterior structures of the eye: the cornea, lens, and optic media (Fig. 24-5).[27] The retina, acting like film in a camera, processes the light and records a "picture" that is relayed to the rest of the CNS by the optic nerve.[39] Although the concept is simple, the process is complex and involves many factors. These factors include the ability to focus light precisely onto the retina, the ability to maintain sharp focus over various focal distances, the ability to obtain sufficient illumination of the retina to capture a quality image, and the ability of the optic nerve to transmit the image through the CNS for perceptual processing.[27] Any compromise of the structures involved in this process will result in degradation of the image and reduced acuity.[27,74]

Visual acuity is most commonly measured by having the patient read progressively smaller optotypes on a chart. The optotypes may be letters, numbers, or symbols. The most common acuity measurement unit used in the United States is the Snellen fraction (20/20, 20/50, etc.).[17] The numerator of this fraction is the distance (in feet) from which the person views the chart, and the denominator is the distance at which a person with normal vision can identify a letter of a certain size.[74] A measurement of "20/20" means that standing

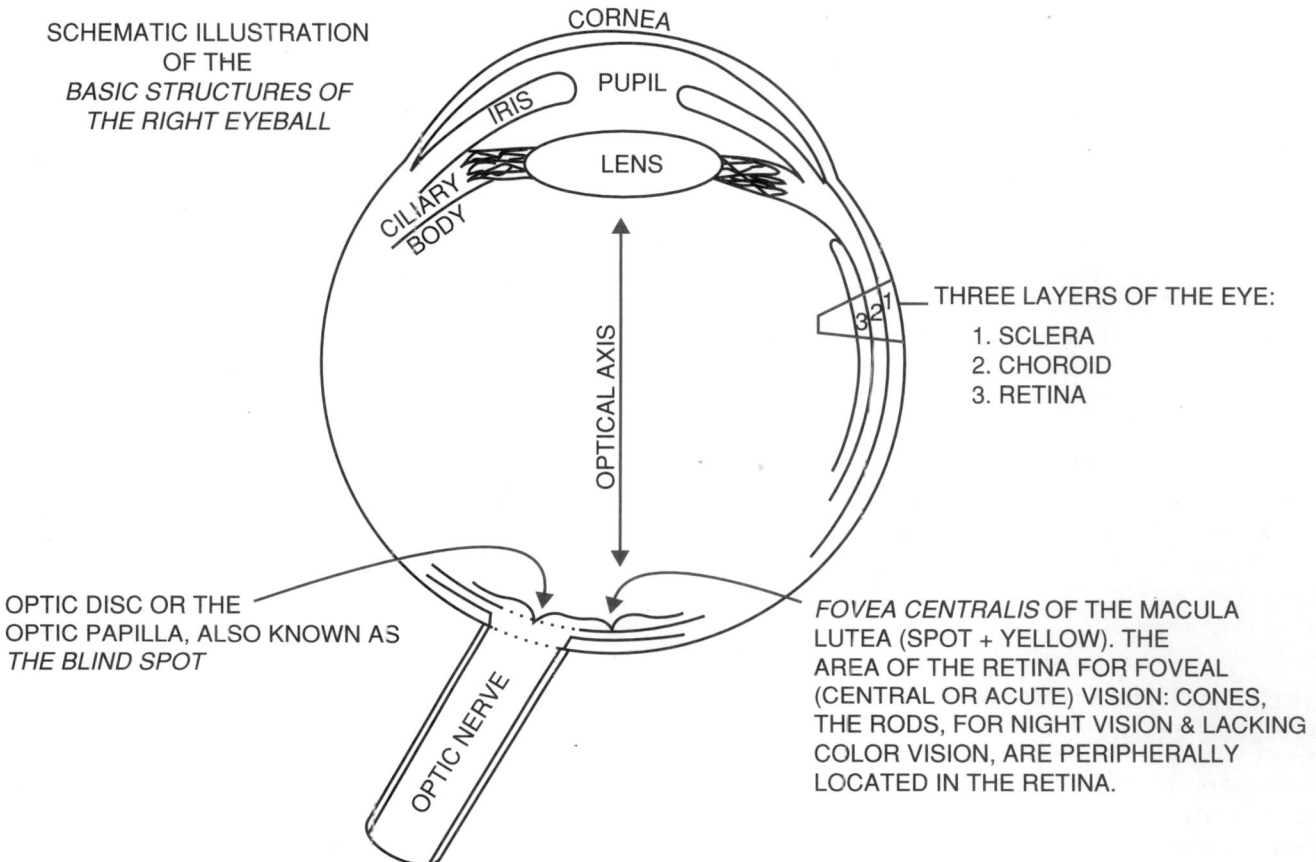

SCHEMATIC ILLUSTRATION
OF THE
*BASIC STRUCTURES OF
THE RIGHT EYEBALL*

CORNEA

PUPIL

IRIS

LENS

CILIARY BODY

OPTICAL AXIS

THREE LAYERS OF THE EYE:
1. SCLERA
2. CHOROID
3. RETINA

OPTIC DISC OR THE
OPTIC PAPILLA, ALSO KNOWN AS
THE BLIND SPOT

OPTIC NERVE

FOVEA CENTRALIS OF THE MACULA
LUTEA (SPOT + YELLOW). THE
AREA OF THE RETINA FOR FOVEAL
(CENTRAL OR ACUTE) VISION: CONES,
THE RODS, FOR NIGHT VISION & LACKING
COLOR VISION, ARE PERIPHERALLY
LOCATED IN THE RETINA.

FIG. 24-5
Anterior structures of the eyeball. Light passes through these transparent structures to focus on the receptor cells of the retina. (Courtesy of Josephine C. Moore, PhD, OTR.)

at a distance of 20 feet, the viewer can see the letter that a person with normal vision can see at 20 feet. Vision of 20/200 would indicate that a person standing at a distance of 20 feet can see a letter that a person with normal vision could identify at 200 feet.

Visual acuity typically is measured using a high-contrast, black-on-white test format. However, visual acuity actually represents a continuum of visual function ranging from the ability to detect high-contrast features on one end of the continuum to the ability to detect low-contrast features (such as beige on white) on the other end.[35] Low-contrast acuity, known as contrast sensitivity function (CSF), is the ability to detect the borders of objects reliably as they decrease in contrast (rather than size) from their backgrounds.[35] CSF makes it possible to distinguish and identify faint features of objects, such as the curve of a concrete curb or the protrusion of the nose on the face.[35] Because much of the environment is made up of low-contrast features (gradations of colors between objects rather than stark contrasts), CSF is a critical visual function for the ability to negotiate an environment safely.[9,35] For example, curbs and steps are routinely the same color throughout; without CSF, it would not be possible to see the depth in the curb or step. Carpets,

walls, doors, door frames, and furniture also are often monochromatic in design; without the ability to distinguish low-contrast features, it would not be possible to locate the door or avoid the chair jutting out into the pathway in such environments. One of the most common low-contrast objects is the human face. Human faces contain very little differentiation in contrast between the facial features. That is, the nose is the same color as the forehead, cheeks, and chin, and eye and hair color are designed to blend with skin tones. To see the unique features of a human face requires very good contrast sensitivity function. Although high- and low-contrast acuity represent opposite ends of a single continuum of visual acuity function, research has shown that CSF can be impaired in patients even when their high-contrast acuity is within normal limits.[9,12,34] Therefore both forms of acuity must be measured to obtain an accurate assessment of acuity function.

Besides high- and low-contrast acuity, two other measures of visual acuity are used: distance acuity and reading (near) acuity. Distance acuity is the ability to see objects at a distance. Near acuity is the ability to see objects clearly as they come closer to the eye. Near acuity is most accurately called "reading acuity" because reading is the primary function enabled by near acuity. Usually this form of acuity is measured by having the patient read sentences in progressively smaller sizes of print.

Reading acuity is dependent on the brainstem neural process of accommodation. Accommodation enables the eye to maintain clear focus on objects as they come closer.[27] As an object approaches the eye, its point of focus on the retina is pushed further back, eventually causing the image to go out of focus. The CNS adjusts for this situation through the three-step process of accommodation. As the object comes closer, (1) the eyes *converge* (turn inward) to ensure that the light rays entering the eye stay parallel and in focus, (2) the crystalline lens of the eye *thickens* to refract the light rays more strongly and shorten the focal distance, and (3) the pupil *constricts* to reduce scattering of the light rays. These three steps enable objects to stay in focus in the near vision range (distances between 3 and 16 inches from the eyes).[27]

Deficits in Visual Acuity

Until the fourth decade of life the accommodation process works efficiently to ensure equal acuity when an individual is viewing objects both up close and at a distance. As a person passes through the forties, the lens of the eye gradually becomes less flexible, reducing its ability to keep images in focus as they come closer. The condition created by this change is known as *presbyopia*.[72] Persons with this condition frequently complain of difficulty reading small print. Presbyopia is corrected either by using reading glasses to magnify print or, if the person already wears eyeglasses, by adding a magnifying lens or "reading ad" to the base of the lenses to create a bifocal.

In the normal eye, most deficiencies in visual acuity are caused by defects in the optical system (the cornea or lens or even the length of the eyeball), which cause images to be focused poorly on the retina.[27,72] The three most common optical defects reducing acuity are myopia (nearsightedness), hyperopia (farsightedness), and astigmatism. In *myopia* the image of an object is focused at a point in front of the retina and is therefore blurred when it reaches the retina. Myopia is corrected by placing a concave lens in front of the eye. In *hyperopia* the image comes into focus behind the retina, causing the image to remain out of focus on the retina. Hyperopia is corrected by placing a convex lens in front of the eye. Fig. 24-6 illustrates these defects. In *astigmatism* light is focused differently by two meridians 90° apart. This defect usually is caused by a cornea that is not totally spherical but shaped more like a spoon. The defect results in a blurring of the image because both meridians cannot be focused on the retina. Astigmatism is corrected by placing a cylindrical lens in front of the eye.

Visual acuity deficits primarily occur as a result of impairment in three areas of visual processing: disruption of the ability to focus light onto the retina, inability of the retina to accurately process the image, and inability of the optic nerve to transmit the information to the rest of the CNS for processing.[74] These impairments may be the direct result of a brain injury, a disease process, or a change in the eye occurring incidental to the injury. It is not possible to describe all of the conditions that can result in reduced acuity after brain injury, but the most common are described in the sections that follow.

DISRUPTION OF THE ABILITY TO FOCUS AN IMAGE ON THE RETINA. Sharp focusing of an image on the retina depends largely on the transparency of the intervening structures between the outside of the eye and the retina and on the ability of these structures to focus the light rays entering the eye. Light entering the eye passes through four transparent mediums: the cornea, aqueous humor, crystalline lens, and vitreous humor. An opacity or irregularity in these structures will prevent light from properly reaching the receptor cells in the retina.[27] Conditions that can occur in conjunction with head trauma include corneal scarring, trauma-induced cataract, and vitreous hemorrhage.[26] Corneal scarring may occur from direct trauma to the eye sustained during the assault to the head. The cornea is damaged and scars as it heals, creating an irregular surface that refracts the light unevenly. The person experiences blurred vision similar to that created by astigmatism. Trauma to the crystalline lens may cause displacement or result in the subsequent development of a cataract that clouds the lens and reduces acuity. Trauma to the eye also can result in bleeding into the vitreous humor. Because blood is an opaque medium, light cannot pass through it, and the patient experiences floaters, shadows, and episodes of darkness as the blood passes in front of the retina. Of these conditions, vitreal hemorrhage is the only one that is temporary and that usually will resolve on its own without treatment.

Impairment of accommodation is another condition that affects the focusing ability of the eye. This condition is associated with brainstem injury, either from head trauma or from stroke.[15,46,47,74] A brainstem injury can affect the functioning of one or all of the components of accommodation: convergence of the eyes, thickening of the lens, and pupillary constriction. When accommodation is impaired, the patient has difficulty achieving and sustaining focus during near-vision tasks. The most frequent complaint voiced by the patient is difficulty with maintaining focus during reading, which may cause the print to blur and swirl on the page.[15]

DISRUPTION OF THE ABILITY OF THE RETINA TO PROCESS THE IMAGE. The health and integrity of the retina also influence the quality of the image sent on to the CNS. The receptor cells of the retina can be damaged directly by injury or disease, preventing them

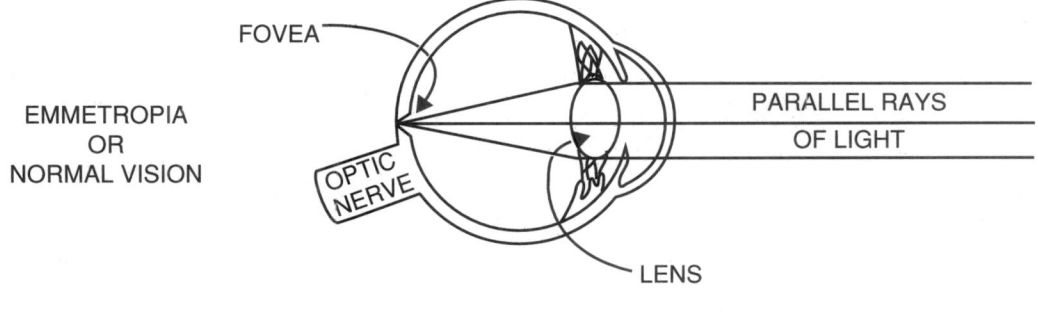

FOVEA

EMMETROPIA
OR
NORMAL VISION

PARALLEL RAYS
OF LIGHT

OPTIC NERVE

LENS

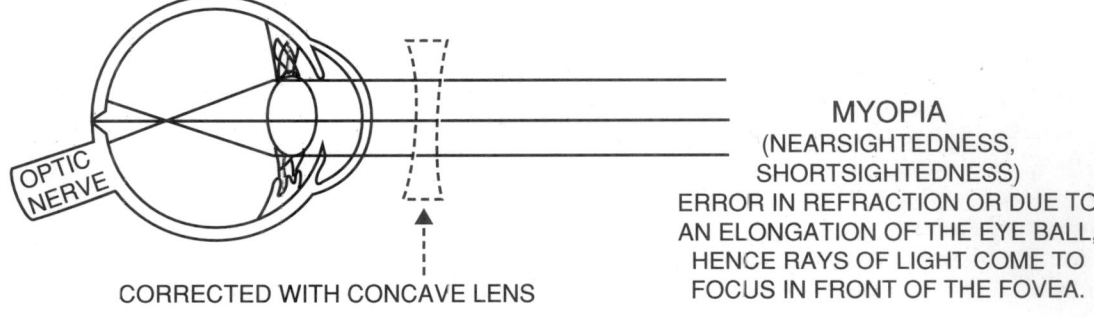

MYOPIA
(NEARSIGHTEDNESS,
SHORTSIGHTEDNESS)
ERROR IN REFRACTION OR DUE TO
AN ELONGATION OF THE EYE BALL,
HENCE RAYS OF LIGHT COME TO
FOCUS IN FRONT OF THE FOVEA.

OPTIC NERVE

CORRECTED WITH CONCAVE LENS

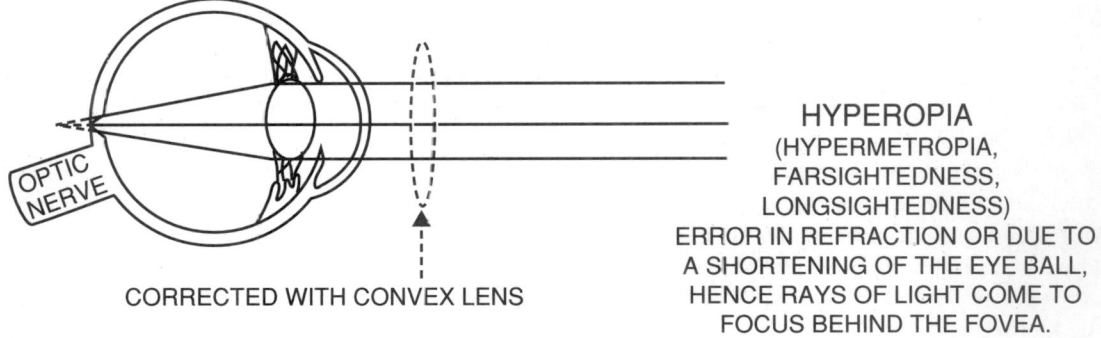

HYPEROPIA
(HYPERMETROPIA,
FARSIGHTEDNESS,
LONGSIGHTEDNESS)
ERROR IN REFRACTION OR DUE TO
A SHORTENING OF THE EYE BALL,
HENCE RAYS OF LIGHT COME TO
FOCUS BEHIND THE FOVEA.

OPTIC NERVE

CORRECTED WITH CONVEX LENS

FIG. 24-6
Normal, myopic, and hyperopic optical refraction of light coming into the eye and the type of lens used to correct myopic and hyperopic optical refractive errors. (Courtesy of Josephine C. Moore, PhD, OTR.)

from responding to light. Diseases that affect retinal function, such as macular degeneration and diabetic retinopathy, are associated with age and significantly increase in incidence in the seventh and eighth decades of life.[23] With damage to the retina (especially the macular area), both high- and low-contrast visual acuity are diminished, making accurate identification of features and objects difficult. It is estimated that approximately one in four persons over the age of 80 years has a visual impairment that affects the retina significantly enough to prevent the individual from reading standard print. It is not uncommon for an older adult who has been referred for treatment of a CVA (stroke) also to demonstrate reduced visual acuity secondary to eye disease. Too often the vision loss resulting from the disease is either overlooked or misdiagnosed as an attentional or cognitive impairment associated with the CVA.

DISRUPTION OF THE ABILITY OF THE OPTIC NERVE TO SEND THE RETINAL IMAGE. The most common cause of optic nerve damage in brain injury is trauma.[38] An injury can occur from a direct penetrating injury to the nerve, such as a missile wound to the head from a gunshot.[38] Indirect trauma can also occur from an optic canal fracture associated with facial or blunt forehead fractures. These fractures are most common in children and young adults and usually result in unilateral injuries.[38] Severe closed head injuries can cause stretching or tearing of the optic nerve, resulting in significant and usually bilateral damage to the nerves. Bilateral nerve injury can also result from compression of the nerves secondary to intracranial swelling or hematoma.[38]

Other common conditions that can cause optic nerve damage are glaucoma and multiple sclerosis. Glaucoma typically damages the optic nerve fibers carrying peripheral visual field input but can also affect the central visual field, reducing visual acuity. Multiple sclerosis can cause plaques to develop along the optic nerve, resulting in optic neuritis, reduced visual field acuity, and sensitivity to light.[74]

FUNCTIONAL DEFICITS CAUSED BY REDUCED VISUAL ACUITY. Reduced visual acuity can cause limitations in a significant number of ADL. The severity of the limitation depends on the extent of the acuity loss and whether there has been a loss of central acuity, peripheral acuity, or both. A loss of central acuity results in an inability to discriminate small visual details and to distinguish contrast and color. Activities dependent on reading, writing, and fine motor coordination (e.g., reading recipes and labels on foodstuffs, dialing a telephone, completing a check, paying a bill, applying makeup, shaving, identifying money, and shopping) will be affected. When peripheral acuity is reduced, as occurs with visual field deficit, mobility will be affected. The patient may be unable to identify landmarks, see obstacles in the path of travel, or accurately detect motion, which may impair his or her ability to ambulate safely and maintain orientation in the environment. This may reduce independence in driving, shopping, and participation in community activities.

Assessment

All evaluation begins with observation of the patient's performance in daily activities. Patients with deficits in visual acuity often complain of an inability to read print and may state that the print is too small or too faint to read. Complaints that print appears distorted, that parts of words are missing, or that words run together and swirl on the page are also common. Patients with CSF deficits may complain of an inability to see faces clearly. These patients also may be unable to distinguish between colors of similar hue, such as navy blue and black, or to detect low-contrast substances such as water on the floor.

If a decrease in visual acuity is suspected, a screening should be completed to determine how acuity has changed. To obtain a complete picture of the patient's visual acuity, both high- and low-contrast acuity are measured. High-contrast acuity testing generally is divided into two additional measurements: far acuity, measured with a test chart at a distance of 1 m or greater, and reading acuity, measured using a text card at 40 cm (16 inches).

Because brain injury can affect accommodative ability, it is important to measure both acuity distances.

When measuring visual acuity, the therapist must be sure that the chart is well illuminated and held at the specified distance from the patient. Adequate illumination is important because acuity shares a linear relationship with illumination; that is, as illumination decreases, so does acuity (no one can read a letter chart in the dark). Because acuity is depicted as a fraction of distance over letter size (e.g., 20/20 or 20/200), the measurement is not accurate unless the viewing distance is accurate. All test charts specify a distance at which they are to be used, and this should not be altered.

The patient's level of acuity is determined by the smallest line of optotypes (letters) he or she can read on the test chart. The patient is instructed to read the optotypes on the chart out loud, beginning with the largest line and continuing to lower lines until the print is too small to see. Patients with brain injury may have deficits in cognition, language, and perception, which interfere with the ability to provide an accurate and timely response in a testing situation. Extra time may be needed for this patient to locate the optotype on the chart, process the image, and respond. Slowness in responding therefore does not necessarily indicate that the patient lacks the acuity to identify the optotype. If the patient struggles with the identification of optotypes on each line but is accurate, the test should proceed until a line is reached on which the patient can no longer identify the majority of the optotypes.

The most useful chart for an occupational therapist is one that measures visual acuity as low as 20/1000 so that significant reductions in acuity can be measured. The standard charts used by doctors measure visual acuity only in the range that can be compensated for with eyeglasses, roughly to 20/100 Snellen acuity. When acuity is below that level, magnification must be used and the patient is referred to a low-vision specialist. Because some conditions such as optic nerve damage or macular diseases can result in profound vision loss (less than 20/400 acuity), it is important for a therapist to be able to measure acuity in the lower ranges so that appropriate referral and modifications can be made. The LeaNumbers Low Vision Test Chart* and the Warren Text card from the biVABA are examples of test charts that measure visual acuity in the low vision ranges.

Contrast sensitivity function also is assessed by viewing optotypes printed on a chart that is held at a specified distance from the patient. However, for this type of testing, the optotypes (which may be letters, numbers, symbols, or sine wave gratings) remain the same size but diminish in contrast as one proceeds down or across the chart. The patient is asked to identify as many optotypes as possible. There are many forms of

---

*LeaNumbers and LeaSymbols Low Contrast Tests, Precision Vision, 944 First St., LaSalle, IL 60301; (815)223-2022.

CSF tests on the market, from wall-mounted charts to tests such as the Optec 2000, which uses slides installed in vision testers. The least expensive and most portable test charts are those designed by Dr. Lea Hyvarinen, such as the LeaNumbers Low Contrast Screener included in the biVABA, the LeaSymbols Low Contrast Screener, and the LeaNumbers and LeaSymbols Low Contrast Tests available from Precision Vision.* When contrast sensitivity function is measured, the patient is asked to read down the chart as far as possible until the optotype is too faint to be identified. As with high-contrast acuity testing, the test chart must be held at a specific distance and must be well illuminated to obtain an accurate measurement.

In assessing visual acuity performance, the therapist does not have the job of diagnosing the cause of the deficiency, but rather linking the presence of the deficiency to a functional limitation the patient has. This is a subtle but important distinction that affects the assessment procedure. When a patient has reduced visual acuity, the ophthalmologist or optometrist uses the results of the assessment to determine the cause of the reduction (e.g., damage to the retina or cornea or the presence of a refractive error). With this information the eye care specialist determines how to manage the condition to restore optimum sight using optical devices (glasses or contact lenses), a surgical procedure, or the prescribing of medications. In contrast, when a therapist determines that a patient has reduced visual acuity, he or she uses this information to modify activities and the environment so that the patient can compensate for the loss and achieve optimal performance in daily activities. For example, if a patient cannot read the size of print on a medication label, the therapist determines whether the print can be enlarged to a size that the patient can read or determines another way for the patient to identify the medication bottle.

Treatment

If a significant reduction in visual acuity is noted, the patient should be referred to an ophthalmologist or optometrist to determine the nature and cause of the vision loss and whether vision can be restored. Referring patients to specialists can take days, weeks, and even months to complete. The patient's treatment program cannot be placed on hold while the referral is being processed; therefore the therapist uses the information obtained from the assessment to modify the environment and activities and enable the patient to use his or her remaining visual acuity. Examples of specific techniques used in this passive treatment approach are described in the following paragraphs.

*LeaNumbers and LeaSymbols Low Contrast Tests, Precision Vision, 944 First St., LaSalle, IL 60301; (815)223-2022.

INCREASING BACKGROUND CONTRAST. Increasing contrast by changing the background color to contrast with an object can help the patient see objects more clearly. The application of this technique can be as simple as using a black cup for milk and a white cup for coffee. In cases where background color cannot be changed readily, such as on carpeted steps, color can be applied to provide a marker. For example, a line of bright fluorescent tape can be applied to the end of each step riser on the carpeted stairs to distinguish between them.[21]

INCREASING ILLUMINATION. Increasing the intensity and amount of available light enables objects and environmental features to be seen more readily and reduces the need for high contrast between objects. For example, facial features can be identified more easily if a person's face is fully illuminated. The challenge in providing light is to increase illumination without increasing glare. Halogen, fluorescent, and full-spectrum lights provide the best sources of high illumination with minimum glare and are generally recommended over standard incandescent lighting for both room and task illumination. Lighting should be strategically placed to provide full, even illumination without areas of surface shadow. For example, if a 50-watt halogen lamp is used for reading, it should be positioned behind the patient's shoulder so that the page of print is fully illuminated without the light's shining directly in the patient's eyes.

REDUCTION IN BACKGROUND PATTERN. Patterned backgrounds have the effect of camouflaging the objects lying on them. The detrimental effect of patterns on object identification can be minimized by using solid colors for background surfaces such as bedspreads, place mats, dishes, countertops, rugs, towels, and furniture coverings. Objects in the environment also create background patterns. Cluttered environments with haphazardly placed objects challenge even a person with good acuity. If possible, the number of objects in the environment should be reduced and those remaining arranged in an orderly fashion. Closets, drawers, shelves, and countertops should be reorganized and simplified, as should such areas as sewing baskets, desks, refrigerators, and freezers.

ENLARGEMENT OF OBJECTS OR FEATURES THAT NEED TO BE SEEN. If possible, objects should be enlarged to make them more visible. Instructions can be reprinted in larger print, medications and other items relabeled, and calendars enlarged. The last line of print that is easily read on the reading acuity test card indicates the minimum size to which to enlarge print for the patient. Contrast should also be increased because it does little good to enlarge print if the print is faint. Black on white or white on black print is usually seen with greater ease than any other color combination. Many items now are manufactured with larger print, including calculators, clocks, watches, telephones, check registers, glucose monitors, scales, playing cards, games, and puzzles. These items can be purchased through specialty catalogs.

ORGANIZATION. Once closets and shelves are rearranged and simplified, every effort should be made to keep them organized. Putting items back where they belong and maintaining organization reduces frustration and facilitates independence. Establishing routines for activities such as filing nails and paying bills prevents daily tasks from becoming overwhelming. Steps that require visual monitoring should be eliminated as much as possible. For example, the patient should be advised to use prechopped and premeasured food ingredients, wrinkle-free clothing, electronic funds transfer, and voice-activated telephone dialing.

ACCESS TO COMMUNITY SERVICES. A variety of services are available to assist persons with vision loss. These services are generally free of charge and can be found in the resource section of the public library or by contacting an advocacy organization such as the American Foundation for the Blind or the Lighthouse Information and Resource Center. The following are some examples of available services:

1. The National Library Service for the Blind and Physically Handicapped, which offers books and magazines on cassette tape through its Talking Books program
2. The Bible Alliance in Bradenton, Florida, which provides a free Bible on tape
3. Local telephone companies, which may offer free directory assistance to persons with disabilities

Visual Field

The visual field is the visual surround that can be seen when a person looks straight ahead. It is analogous to the dimensions of a picture imprinted on the film in a camera (with the retina representing the film). The normal visual field extends approximately 60° superiorly, 75° inferiorly, 60° to the nasal side, and 100° to the temporal side.[3,74] As Fig. 24-7 shows, most of the visual

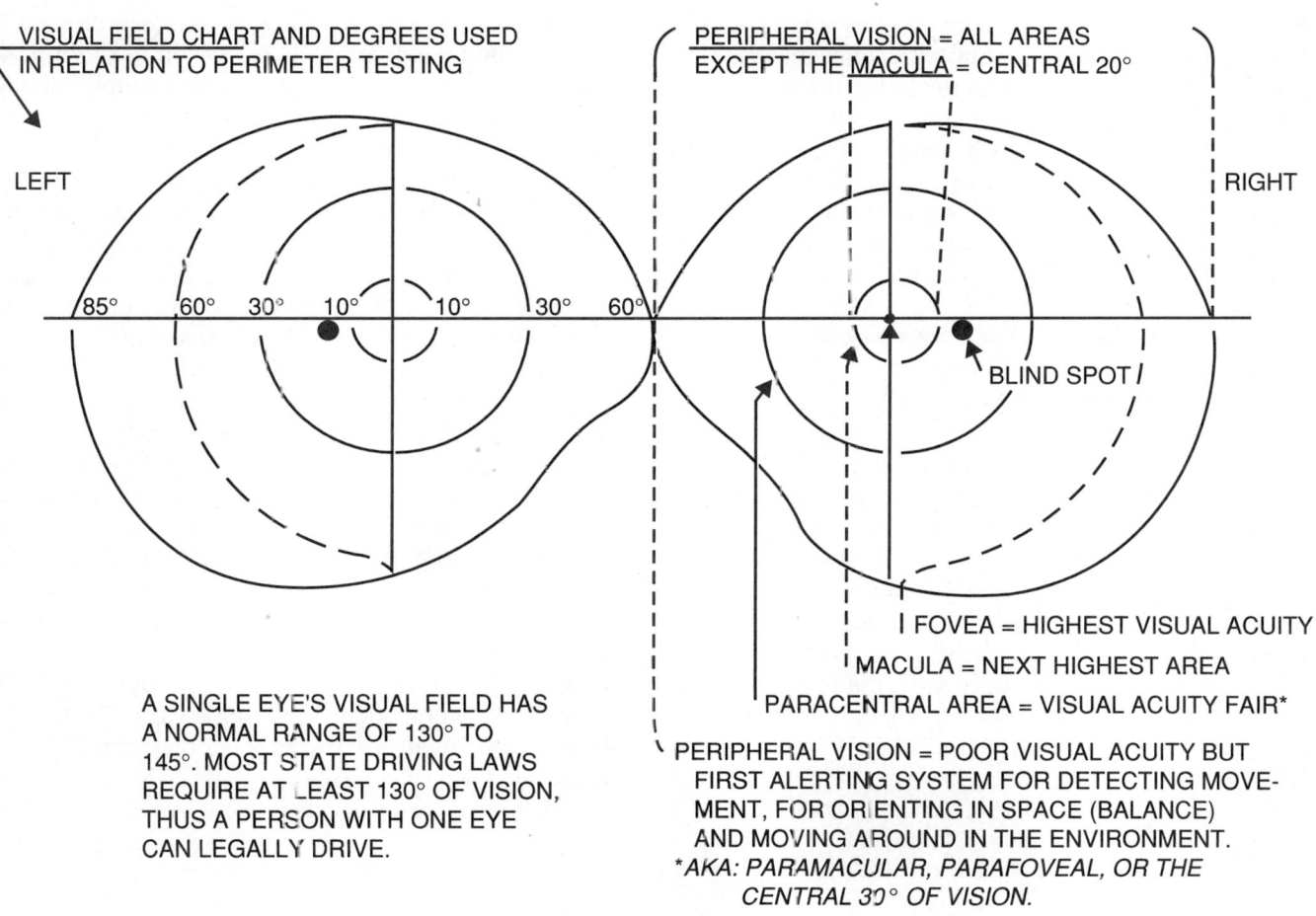

VISUAL FIELD CHART AND DEGREES USED IN RELATION TO PERIMETER TESTING

LEFT

85° 60° 30° 10° 10° 30° 60°

A SINGLE EYE'S VISUAL FIELD HAS A NORMAL RANGE OF 130° TO 145°. MOST STATE DRIVING LAWS REQUIRE AT LEAST 130° OF VISION, THUS A PERSON WITH ONE EYE CAN LEGALLY DRIVE.

PERIPHERAL VISION = ALL AREAS EXCEPT THE MACULA = CENTRAL 20°

RIGHT

BLIND SPOT

FOVEA = HIGHEST VISUAL ACUITY
MACULA = NEXT HIGHEST AREA
PARACENTRAL AREA = VISUAL ACUITY FAIR*
PERIPHERAL VISION = POOR VISUAL ACUITY BUT FIRST ALERTING SYSTEM FOR DETECTING MOVEMENT, FOR ORIENTING IN SPACE (BALANCE) AND MOVING AROUND IN THE ENVIRONMENT.
*AKA: PARAMACULAR, PARAFOVEAL, OR THE CENTRAL 30° OF VISION.

FIG. 24-7
Visual field chart illustrating the divisions of the visual field related to visual acuity. (Courtesy of Josephine C. Moore, PhD, OTR.)

field is binocular and is seen by both eyes. A small portion of the peripheral temporal field in each eye is monocular and can be seen only by one eye because the bridge of the nose occludes vision in the other eye. At the very center of the retinal visual field is the fovea, an area approximately 8° to 10° in diameter that records the visual details for object identification. Surrounding the fovea is the macular area of the field, also referred to as the central visual field (Fig. 24-8). This area is approximately 20° to 30° in diameter and is used for object identification.[39,54] The rest of the visual field is the peripheral field, which detects general shapes and movement in the environment. On the border between the central and peripheral visual fields on the temporal side is the blind spot, so called because the optic disc pierces the retina here and there are no sensory receptor cells.

Visual Field Deficits

Damage to the receptor cells in the retina or to the optic pathway that relays retinal information to the CNS for processing results in a **visual field deficit (VFD)**.[3,74] Fig. 24-1 illustrates this pathway as it changes from the optic nerve to the optic tract to the geniculocalcarine tracts. The location and extent of the visual field deficit depend on where damage occurs on the pathway. Although any type of visual field deficit is possible after brain injury, homonymous hemianopsia is the most common deficit observed.[96] Hemianopsia (hemi = half, anopsia = blindness) means that there has been a loss of vision in one half of the visual field in the eye. Homonymous means that the deficit is the same in both eyes. The patient may have either a left or a right hemianopsia, as well.

Functional Deficits Caused by Visual Field Deficits

Although VFD is often considered a mild impairment in comparison with the dramatic loss of use of the limbs, it can create changes in visual processing that significantly limit daily performance. The most important change occurs in the search pattern used by an individual to compensate for the blind portion of the visual field. Instead of spontaneously adopting a wider search strategy, turning the head farther to see around the blind field, patients tend to narrow their scope of scanning.[61,94] The patient typically turns the head very little

FIG. 24-8

Position of examiner and patient for completion of perimetry testing using the Damato 30-point Campimeter from the Brain Injury Visual Assessment Battery for Adults. (Courtesy of Precision Vision, LaSalle, Ill.)

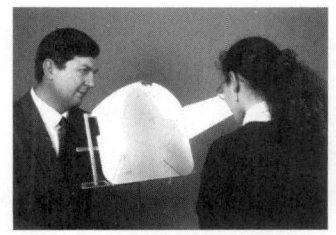

and limits visual search to areas immediately adjacent to the seeing side of the body. The reason for this odd strategy is the influence of a visual process known as "perceptual completion."[48,64,71,73] Perceptual completion is a process whereby the CNS fills in (or completes) absent visual information based on an expectation of the visual information to be found in the visual scene. The perceptual outcome of this process is that the viewer perceives that he or she is seeing a complete visual scene, even though part of the visual information in the scene is absent. The best known example of the effect of perceptual completion on the processing of visual field input is the lack of awareness of one's own physiological blind spot. The blind spot creates a 5° hole in the temporal visual field. Through perceptual completion, the CNS fills in the missing visual information in the field, causing the person to be unaware of this gap in vision.[73]

Perceptual completion provides speed in information processing by enabling an individual to infer a whole visual scene based on partial visual input. As such, it plays an important role in the person's ability to adapt to fast-paced and dynamic environments. However, in the case of significant visual field loss, the presence of perceptual completion makes it difficult for the patient to determine how his or her vision has changed.[48,71] Because of perceptual completion, the patient with a VFD is not immediately aware of the absence of vision after onset of the deficit.[48,71] He or she perceives the presence of a complete visual field—there are no gaps or black holes in the visual scene. However, the CNS cannot place objects in a visual scene that it does not actually see. Therefore the patient may not be aware of a chair, a plate of food, or other unanticipated objects on the blind side. As a result, the patient may run into a chair or other obstacles when navigating in the environment or may not be able to find items placed within the blind field. Until the patient becomes aware of the VFD, he or she will have the odd perception of a complete visual scene in which objects always seem to be appearing, disappearing, and reappearing, without warning, on the affected side. Uncertainty regarding the accuracy of visual input on the affected side causes the patient to adopt a protective strategy, which is tuned into input from the intact visual field.[61] This narrowed scope of scanning creates significant limitations in activities, such as driving a car or traversing a busy environment, that require monitoring of the full visual field.

In addition to resulting in a narrow scope of scanning, visual search into the blind field often is slow and delayed.[36,51,61] Again, the culprit is perceptual completion, which eliminates the presence of a marker to indicate the boundary between the seeing and nonseeing fields. Unable to determine the actual border of the seeing field or where a target might be within the nonseeing field, the patient naturally slows down when scanning toward the blind field. The slow visual search speed on the affected side increases the difficulties the patient has in moving and finding objects within the environment and also reduces reading speed.

If the VFD affects the macular portion of the visual field, especially the fovea, a patient may miss or misidentify visual details when viewing objects because part of the object falls into the blind area of the field. This can create significant challenges in reading.[10,95-97] Normal readers view words through a "window" or *perceptual span* that allows them to see approximately 18 characters (letters) with each fixation of the eye.[95] The reader typically moves from word to word using a series of successive saccadic eye movements to cross the line of print. Presence of a VFD can reduce the width of the perceptual window from 18 characters to as few as 3 to 4 characters. This may cause the patient to view only part of a word during a fixation and even skip over small words, often resulting in the transformation of words and sentences. For example, a patient with a left VFD may read the sentence, "She should not shake the juice" as "He should make juice," transforming "she" into "he" and "shake" into "make" and leaving out "not" and "the." Errors such as these cause the patient to have to stop and reread sentences, reducing reading speed and comprehension. Accuracy in reading numbers generally creates more challenge for the patient than reading words. Whereas context alerts the patient to an error when reading sentences (the sentence does not make sense), numbers appear without precise context, causing mistakes to go unnoticed. For example, a bill for $28.00 may be misread as $23.00 and the error missed until a notice of insufficient payment is received. Patients making these kinds of errors quickly lose confidence in their ability to pay bills and manage their checkbook and turn over these important ADL to someone else.

If the VFD has occurred on the same side as the dominant hand, the patient may have difficulty visually guiding the hand in fine motor activities. The most common functional change is a reduction of writing legibility. The patient often cannot visually locate and maintain fixation on the tip of the writing instrument as the hand moves into the blind visual field, causing handwriting to drift up and down on the line. Writing over something that was just written and improperly positioning handwriting on a form are also common mistakes. Quilting, hand sewing, pouring liquids, and other fine motor activities are also frequently impaired.

The behavioral changes described (narrow scope of scanning, slow scanning toward the blind side, missing or misidentification of visual detail, and reduced visual monitoring of the hand) contribute to a variety of functional limitations. The primary functional skills affected include mobility, reading, writing, and the ADL dependent on these skills. These activities include grooming, medication management, financial management, meal preparation, clothing selection and care, meal preparation, home management, telephone usage, and yard work. In general, the more dynamic the environment in which the ADL is completed and the wider the field of view required to complete the task, the greater the limitation. Therefore only minor limitations are generally experienced in self-care activities, compared with significant limitations in shopping and driving.

Persons with VFD commonly face significant emotional challenges in adapting to this considerable vision loss. For example, patients with VFD regularly report feeling a sense of anxiety when moving in unfamiliar environments. Sometimes the anxiety can be so severe that the patient has an autonomic nervous system reaction, becoming nauseated and short of breath and breaking out into a sweat in crowded environments. One individual with VFD described this sensation as "crowditis," reporting that he became physically ill if he had to go into a department store or other crowded environment.[86] This anxiety can become debilitating, leading to a withdrawal from community activities and to social isolation. Other patients report a tremendous loss of self-confidence because of the numerous mistakes they make during the course of a day, and many express that they experience depression because of their limitations, especially in the ability to drive a car and read accurately.

Assessment

The process of measuring the visual field is known as *perimetry*.[3] Several types of perimetry are available. These range from simple bedside assessments (such as the confrontation test), which give a gross indication of field loss, to the very precise imaging of a scanning laser ophthalmoscope (SLO).[3,73] The perimetry test selected depends on the availability and cost of the test and on the ability of the patient to participate in testing. For example, confrontation testing does not incur any expense and can be performed nearly anywhere, whereas SLO imaging must be completed by a specially trained technician in a center that has purchased the $120,000 instrument. In between these two extremes are the tangent screen, campimeter, manual bowl perimeters (the Goldmann), and automated bowl perimeters (the Humphrey), ranging in cost from $100 to $20,000. In general, the more expensive the apparatus, the more precise the measurement provided.

All perimetry testing involves three parameters: fixation on a central target by the patient while the testing is completed, presentation of a target of a specific size and luminosity in a designated area of the visual field, and acknowledgment of the target by the patient.[3] Testing is done with either static or kinetic presentation of the target. In static presentation the target appears in a specified area of the visual field without being shown moving to that location. In kinetic testing the target moves in from the periphery until it is identified.[3,72]

The most accurate perimetry test readily available clinically is computerized, automated perimetry.[3] In automated perimetry the person being tested places his or her chin on a chin rest and fixates on a central target inside a bowl-shaped device. As the person fixates on the central target, lights are displayed inside the bowl in varying locations and intensities. The person is asked to respond by pushing a small button each time he or she sees a light. The test is very thorough, presenting lights in over a hundred locations within the field and increasing the intensity of the light in a step threshold sequence if the target is not appreciated the first time. The result is an accurate measurement of the areas of absolute scotoma (total vision loss) and relative scotoma (decreased retinal sensitivity) within the field. To obtain an automated perimetry test, the patient must be referred to either an ophthalmologist or an optometrist.

For OT practitioners who want to screen for visual field deficit, an indication of visual field loss can be achieved using simpler perimetry testing in combination with careful observation of patient performance on ADL. Confrontation testing is a bedside examination that provides a crude indication of visual field loss.[72,78] To complete a static confrontation test, the examiner sits in front of the patient and has the patient fixate on a centrally placed target (often the examiner's eye or nose). The examiner then holds up a target in each of the four quadrants of the visual field (right upper, right lower, left upper, and left lower). The patient indicates whether he or she sees the target.[40,72,74] For a kinetic test the examiner stands behind the patient and moves a target (generally a penlight) in from the periphery while the patient fixates on a central target. The patient indicates as soon as he or she notices the target. Standardized versions of these tests are included in the biVABA. Therapists using confrontation testing to quantify visual field deficit must be careful to correlate their findings with observations of patient performance because confrontation testing has been shown to be unreliable in detecting all but gross defects.[78] The presence of a visual field deficit may be indicated if any of the following are observed: the patient changes head position when asked to view objects placed in a certain plane; the patient consistently bumps into objects on one side; the patient misplaces objects in one field; or the patient makes consistent errors in reading. If the confrontation test shows no deficit but the clinical observations suggest that a deficit is present, the clinical observations should carry the greater weight in deciding if a deficit exists.

Testing using perimetry devices such as the Damato 30-Point Multifixation Campimeter (biVABA) or a tangent screen enables therapists to obtain a more accurate measurement of central visual field function. The Damato campimeter shown in Fig. 24-8 is a portable test card that provides a precise measurement of the central 30° of the visual field. The test grid consists of 30 numbered targets that lead the patient's eye to move so as to place the test stimulus at known points in the visual field. The test stimulus is a 6-mm black circle that is shown in the center part of the card. The patient is instructed to fixate on one of the numbered targets. The test stimulus is then shown in the central window, and the patient indicates if and when he or she sees the circle. If the patient does not see the black circle, that point in the visual field is recorded as a loss. The test proceeds with the patient successively viewing the numbered targets until the entire field is mapped out.

The tangent screen consists of a black felt screen with a grid stitched into the felt in black thread so that the grid is visible only to the examiner.[3] The patient sits directly in front of the screen at a distance of 1 meter. The patient is instructed to fixate on the center of the screen as the examiner moves or places a white target attached to a black wand in a certain area of the screen. Without breaking fixation on the center of the screen, the patient indicates if and when he or she sees the target. If the patient does not see the target when it is presented, that point in the visual field is recorded as a loss. The examiner uses the grid to determine the location of the field deficit. Clinical observation of the patient's behavior is especially important to confirm the presence of VFD because of the limitations of perimetry testing.[72] Patients with fluctuating or limited attention, language, and cognition may give unreliable perimetry results. It also may be difficult to distinguish between VFD and a deficit in visual attention. However, the patient's performance of functional activities will strongly indicate the presence of a VFD.

The assessments previously described establish only whether a VFD is present and the size and location of the deficit. To determine whether treatment intervention is needed, the therapist must determine whether the patient is able to compensate for the VFD in performing functional activities, as well as the quality and consistency of that compensation. The presence of a VFD can cause significant limitations in ADL. The level of impairment in daily living skills will depend on whether the VFD occurs alone or in conjunction with visual inattention. An ADL assessment should be completed to evaluate patient performance in the primary ADL areas, including dressing, bathing, grooming, home management, and shopping. If the patient demonstrates difficulty completing an activity, the visual requirements of the activity should be analyzed to determine if the VFD is interfering with performance.

For example, if the patient is unable to locate a toothbrush during grooming, is it because the toothbrush is stored on the side of the patient's field deficit?

Reading is another functional task that may be affected by VFD. The *Visual Skills for Reading Test* (VSRT)* provides an effective way to measure the interference of the VFD on reading performance. The VSRT is designed to assess the influence of a scotoma (or field loss) in the macula on the visual components of reading, including visual word recognition and eye movement control.[87] The patient is asked to read single letters and words printed on a card. The words are not in context and are designed so that they can be misread and still make sense (e.g., "shot" can be mistakenly read as "hot"). The test measures reading accuracy and corrected reading rate and provides information on the prevalent types of reading errors made by the patient. The patient's performance on the letter and reading charts used to measure visual acuity also may indicate the influence of a VFD on reading performance. Because of the wider visual field, a patient with a VFD may have more difficulty reading the larger symbols and words on the chart and may be able to read faster and more accurately as the optotypes (and field) decrease in size. *Telephone Number Copy*, part of the biVABA, provides information about the patient's accuracy in reading numbers. In this test, the patient is required to copy down telephone numbers that include numbers easily misread by persons with VFD, such as 6, 8, 9, and 3.

To effectively compensate for the VFD, the patient must execute an organized and thorough search of the blind field, using the seeing portion of the visual field. This means that a patient with a left visual field deficit must use the right visual field to search both the left and right fields. Patients with VFD demonstrate difficulty searching both *peripersonal space* (the space immediately around the body) and *extrapersonal space* (the space extending from the body into the environment). Deficiencies in searching peripersonal space affect performance of self-care activities such as grooming, dressing, reading, and writing, as well as activities completed within a restricted visual field, such as meal preparation or leisure activities. Deficiencies in searching extrapersonal space have a pronounced impact on mobility and affect activities in outside and community environments, such as driving, shopping, and mowing the yard.

For mobility in dynamic community environments, the patient must use a wide scanning strategy that is initiated on the side of the deficit and executed quickly and efficiently. The patient also must be able to shift attention and visual search rapidly from the central visual field to the peripheral visual field. An objective assessment of the patient's ability to execute these strategies can be made with a Dynavision 2000,* an apparatus increasingly used in rehabilitation to assess and train visual motor performance (Fig. 24-9).[42-44] Therapists without access to a Dynavision can use a laser pointer to observe the patient's compensatory strategies. The beam of light from the pointer is projected onto various areas of a blank white wall, and the patient is instructed to locate and touch the projected red dot. The strategy used by the patient to locate the dot and the efficiency of the strategy are noted. Integration of visual scanning with ambulation is the final component of the assessment in this area and must be completed to determine whether the patient will be able to compensate for the deficit when moving in the environment. This is assessed by using such tests as the ScanCourse from the biVABA, to observe the patient search the environment while ambulating.

Treatment

Identifying the presence of VFD is not in itself justification for treatment unless the deficit affects the patient's independence in completing ADL. Safety and accuracy are the two aspects of performance most affected by VFD. The emphasis in treatment is on teaching the patient how to compensate for VFD in completion of ADL such as meal preparation, shopping, and financial management. Patients will have the greatest limitations in ADL that must be completed in dynamic environments, such as shopping, or activities that require monitoring of a wider visual field, such as meal preparation or yard work. Resumption of driving may or may not be a goal, depending on the state's driving statutes. Some states do not specify a minimum degree of visual field for licensure. In these states a patient may be able to safely resume driving if given the proper training. Reading and writing accurately may be addressed on the plan of care as specific goals but also may contribute to achievement of independent performance in other goals such as financial management and meal preparation.

The most important aspect of treatment is education of the patient regarding the nature of his or her vision loss and the resulting functional limitations. Compensation for VFD requires adopting a conscious, cognitive strategy of using head movement to broaden the visual field. Because the CNS exercises perceptual completion, the patient often lacks insight into the extent and boundaries of the field deficit. Successful compensation requires the patient to believe firmly that the deficit exists and that the visual input from the blind side cannot be trusted. The patient who is able to develop

---

*Visual Skills for Reading Test, Mattingly International, Low Vision Products, 938-K Andreasen Drive, Escondido, CA 92029; (800) 826-4200.

*Dynavision 2000, Performance Enterprises, 76 Major Buttons Drive, Markham, Ontario L3P3G7, Canada; (905) 472-9074.

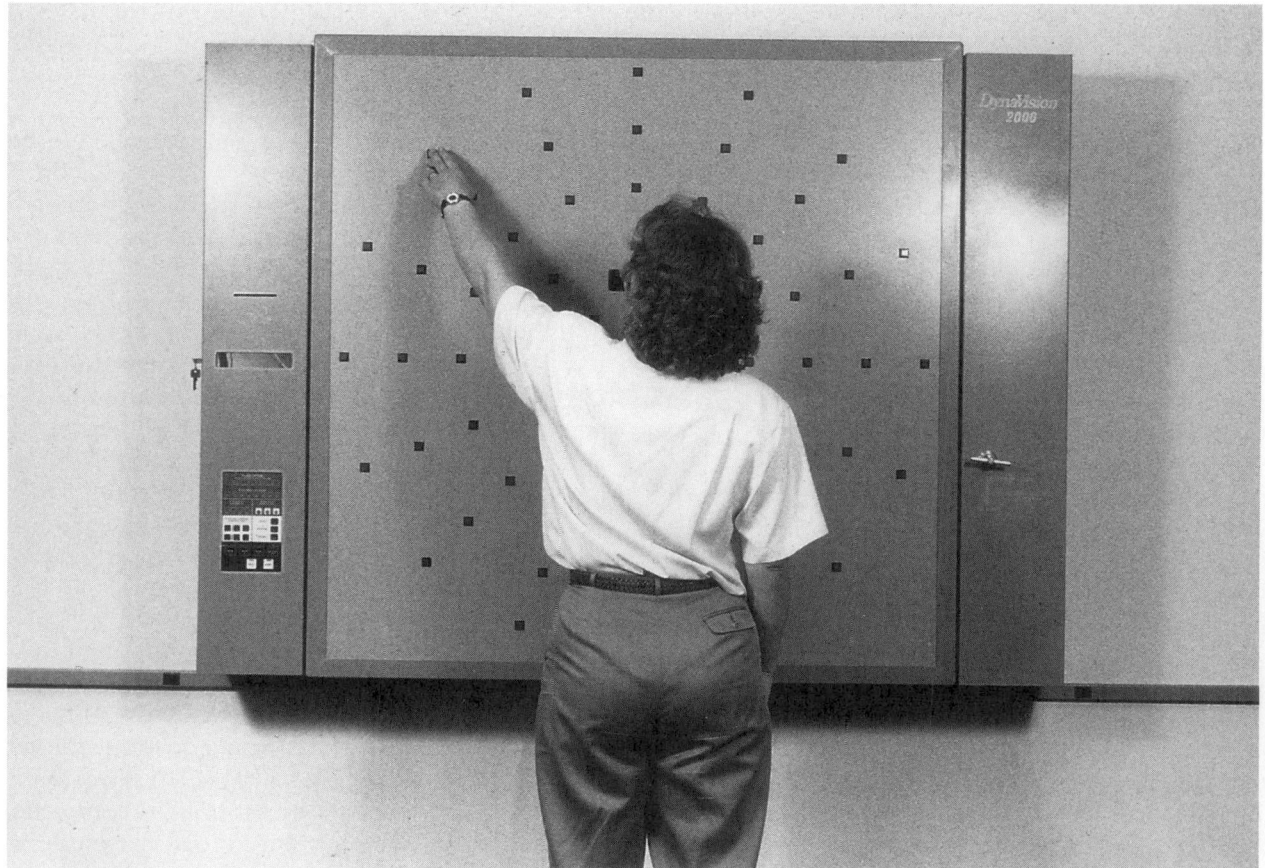

FIG. 24-9
Example of a visual search task using the Dynavision 2000. The lights on the board are illuminated one at a time in random patterns. The patient must locate the illuminated light and press it to turn it off. As light is pressed, another light is illuminated. The patient strikes as many lights as possible within a specified time. The activity can be used to teach and reinforce efficient search patterns to compensate for visual field deficits and visual inattention. (Dynavision 2000, manufactured by Performance Enterprises, Ontario, Canada.)

this level of insight will be able to learn to effectively compensate for the deficit. Every effort must be made through activities and educational materials to make the patient aware of the location and extent of the deficit.

In providing treatment, the therapist uses a combination of active and passive strategies. Active strategies focus on increasing the speed and width of the search pattern. The patient must learn to turn the head quickly to compensate for the restricted visual field. The therapist teaches the following components of an effective visual search strategy:

1. Initiation of a wide head turn towards the blind field
2. An increase in the number of head and eye movements toward the blind field
3. Faster completion of head and eye movement toward the blind field
4. Execution of an organized and efficient search pattern that begins on the blind side

5. Attention to and detection of visual detail on the blind side
6. Ability to quickly shift attention and search between the central visual field and the peripheral visual field on the blind side

The Dynavision 2000 apparatus has been shown to be effective in teaching the components of effective search patterns and is strongly recommended as a treatment tool.[43] The following are other therapeutic activities that facilitate head turning to compensate for VFD:

1. Ball games in which balls are passed quickly from player to player
2. Balloon batting
3. Projection of light from a laser pointer onto various locations on a white wall for the patient to search and find
4. Adhesive stick-on notes with numbers and letters printed on them, widely scattered over a wall for the patient to search and find

Use of the search strategy can be reinforced through the use of games such as concentration, solitaire, and checkers and in ADL such as walking on a crowded street, finding clothes in a closet, or locating items needed for meal preparation.

For patients who have limitations in functional mobility, practice in dynamic and in unfamiliar environments is beneficial. The patient is taught to watch out for features in the environment that could cause harm, such as steps, curb cuts, and other changes in the support surface. The patient also is taught to be more observant of landmarks such as a picture on a wall or a change in wall color to assist in maintaining orientation.

The patient's primary challenges in reading include locating and maintaining the correct line of print and accurately identifying words and numbers. Patients with left VFD often have difficulty accurately locating the next line of print on the left margin of the reading material and lose their place. Drawing a bold red line down the left margin provides the patient with a visual cue to use as an "anchor" to find the left margin.[88] The same technique used on the right margin helps the patient with right VFD who may be uncertain about the location of the end of the line of print. If the patient has difficulty staying on line or moving from line to line, a ruler or card can be used to underline the line of print and keep the patient's place. Accuracy in reading numbers, letters, and words is reestablished through practice. Prereading and prewriting exercises such as those designed by Warren[85]* or Wright and Watson,[92] and commercially available word and number searches† can be used to teach the patient to make the precise eye movements needed to see words completely.

Difficulty staying on line when writing is addressed by teaching the patient to monitor the pen tip and maintain fixation as the hand moves across the page and into the side of field loss. Activities that require the patient to trace lines towards the side of the VFD are effective in reestablishing eye-hand coordination. Practice in completing blank checks, envelopes, and check registers is also helpful.

Reading, writing, and ADL performance can be enhanced by modifying the visual environment of the patient. Adding color and contrast to the key structures in the environment needed for orientation (e.g., door frames and furniture) will help the patient locate these structures. Using black felt-tip pens can heighten the contrast in writing materials, and bold-lined paper can be used to help the patient monitor handwriting. The simple addition of more light often increases reading speed and reduces errors. Reducing pattern in the environment by reducing clutter and using solid-colored objects enhances the patient's ability to locate items.

Oculomotor Function

The purpose of oculomotor function is to achieve and maintain foveation of an object.[28] That is, oculomotor function ensures that the object the person wishes to view is focused on the fovea of both retinas (to ensure a clear image) and that focus is maintained as long as needed to accomplish the desired goal. This is a daunting task because human beings interact within dynamic, moving environments. An image focused on the fovea is always in danger of slipping off as the head or object is moved. Foveation is achieved and maintained by eye movements that keep the target stabilized on the retina during fixation, gaze shift, and head movement.[28,45,50]

Another function of oculomotor control is to provide **binocular vision.** Binocular vision ensures perception of a single image even though the CNS is receiving two separate visual images (one from each eye). The process of combining two visual images into one is called **sensory fusion.** For sensory fusion to occur, corresponding areas or points on the two retinas must be stimulated with the same image. If the retinas are thus stimulated, and if the images match in size and clarity, the CNS is able to fuse the two images perceptually into one. If the eyes do not align with each other or if there is a significant difference between the eyes in acuity, a double image **(diplopia)** may occur.[28,46,81]

Deficits in Oculomotor Function

Deficits in oculomotor control following brain injury generally result from either of two types of disruption: specific cranial nerve lesions causing paresis or paralysis of one or more of the extraocular muscles that control eye movements or disruption of central neural control of the extraocular muscles affecting the coordination of eye movements.[5,41,46,47,74] In the first case the message to the extraocular muscles through the cranial nerve is blocked; in the second case the message comes through but is scrambled. In both cases the functional result is decreased speed, control, and coordination of eye movements. Three pairs of cranial nerves (cn) control the extraocular muscles: the oculomotor nerve (cn III), the trochlear nerve (cn IV), and the abducens nerve (cn VI). Among them, these nerves are responsible for controlling seven pairs of striated muscles that surround and attach to the two eyeballs.

When a cranial nerve lesion occurs, the muscles controlled by that cranial nerve are weakened or paralyzed, a condition known as **paralytic strabismus.**[55,81] As a result, the eye is unable to move in the direction of the

---

*Warren Prereading and Writing Exercises for Persons with Macular Scotomas, Mattingly International, Low Vision Products, 938-K Andreasen Dr., Escondido, CA 92029; (800) 826-4200.
†Learn to Use Your Vision for Reading Workbook, Mattingly International, Low Vision Products, Escondido, CA 92029.

paretic muscles and may even be unable to maintain a central position in the eye socket (i.e., it drifts in or out). Because the eyes must always move in synergy and line up evenly to maintain a single visual image, an individual sees a double image when the movement of one eye is impeded or when the eye's position changes and does not match that of the other. This condition is known as diplopia or double vision and is the primary functional disruption observed with cranial nerve lesions.[55,81]

Functional Limitations Caused by Oculomotor Deficits

The presence of diplopia creates perceptual distortion, which may significantly affect eye-hand coordination, postural control, and binocular use of the eyes. The functional limitations this causes for the patient depend on where the diplopia occurs within the *focal range* (the range in which a person can keep objects in focus). Diplopia occurring within 20 inches of the face will disrupt reading and activities requiring eye-hand coordination, such as pouring liquids, writing, and grooming. Diplopia occurring at a distance (greater than 4 feet) will affect walking, driving, television viewing, and playing sports such as golf and tennis.

To eliminate the double image, the patient will often assume a head position that avoids the field of action of the paretic muscle.[5,47,54] For example, a patient with a left lateral rectus palsy (cn VI) will turn the head toward the left to avoid the need to abduct the eye. A patient with paralysis of the right superior oblique muscle (cn IV) will tilt the head to the right and downward to avoid the action of that muscle.[5] Unless oculomotor function is carefully assessed, these alterations in head position may be interpreted as resulting from changes in muscle tone in the neck rather than as a functional adaptation purposely assumed to stabilize vision.

Often it is not the cranial nerves that are damaged during brain injury, but the neural centers that coordinate their actions. These structures are scattered throughout the brainstem and communicate extensively with cortical, cerebellar, and subcortical areas of the CNS and the spinal cord.[50,74] In cases of traumatic brain injury, diffuse damage may take place throughout the brainstem, affecting these control centers. If the centers are damaged, the person will have difficulty executing eye movements even though the cranial nerves are intact.[70,72] Disconjugate eye movements may occur, causing the patient to have difficulty using the eyes together in a coordinated fashion. Dysmetric eye movement, in which the eye undershoots or overshoots a target, also may be observed.[74]

Damage to the pretectal nuclei in the brainstem can cause **convergence insufficiency,** a condition when the patient is unable to obtain or sustain convergence of the eyes.[15,47] Convergence is the muscle action of moving the eyes inward in adduction. It is one of the

three components of accommodation, the process that keeps objects in focus as they come into close view. When convergence insufficiency occurs, patients have difficulty obtaining or sustaining adequate focus during near vision tasks (tasks within 20 inches of the face). Patients with this condition often complain of fatigue, eye pain, or headache after a period of sustained viewing in near tasks such as reading. As the eye muscles fatigue from the exertion of sustaining convergence during reading, patients may begin to complain that the print is swirling and moving on the page. The condition often is overlooked in evaluation because cranial nerve function usually is intact and patients' complaints instead are attributed to inattention, lack of effort, or dyslexia.[15,47]

These disturbances in ocular motility can create a variety of functional deficits for the patient.[57,72] The speed and range of eye movement may be diminished. This will reduce the speed at which the patient is able to scan the environment and take in visual information, causing delays in responding to the environment. The patient may have difficulty maintaining a clear image and may experience doubling and blurring of visual images.[15,26,72] There may be difficulty focusing at different distances from the body. Depth perception may be diminished. These conditions will create significant visual stress for the patient, reducing concentration and endurance for activities. The patient may respond to this increased stress by becoming agitated and uncooperative in therapy sessions or complaining of headaches, eye strain, or neck strain.

Because a number of factors can disrupt the control of eye movements, much skill and expertise are needed to accurately diagnose the oculomotor deficit and design an appropriate treatment intervention. Therapists who treat this type of dysfunction should do so with the guidance of an optometrist or ophthalmologist who specializes in visual impairment caused by neurological conditions.[26,57]

Assessment

The purpose of an assessment completed by the OT practitioner is to determine whether the patient has functional limitations from dysfunction within the oculomotor system. It is *not* to determine whether the oculomotor dysfunction is the result of cranial nerve lesion, brainstem injury, or other conditions. Determining the etiology of the dysfunction is the responsibility of the ophthalmologist or optometrist. However, the occupational therapist is often one of the first members of the rehabilitation team to observe that the patient appears to have an oculomotor impairment affecting functional performance. This frequently places the occupational therapist in the position of requesting further evaluation by an eye care specialist. To make an appropriate referral, it is necessary to complete a screening to identify patterns of oculomotor dysfunction that may account for the functional limitations observed in the patient.

In assessing the patient, a "listen and look" approach is used, wherein the therapist *listens* to the complaints being voiced by the patient or the rehabilitation staff working with the patient and *looks* for deviations in oculomotor control that may contribute to these complaints. This approach is described in the biVABA, and the following steps in evaluation are from that assessment.

The first step in assessment is to obtain a visual history from the patient. The history is necessary because adults with childhood histories of oculomotor dysfunction or reduced acuity often display oculomotor abnormalities that do not affect functional performance. These individuals frequently wear eyeglasses to correct for the deficiencies; in this case the eyeglasses must be worn during the assessment to obtain accurate results. Areas addressed in this part of the evaluation include whether the patient had good vision before brain injury, whether the patient wears eyeglasses, and whether the patient has a history of conditions that may affect oculomotor control, such as congenital strabismus, lazy eye, or amblyopia.

Next, the patient is asked whether he or she is experiencing diplopia. If the response is affirmative, the patient should be questioned about the characteristics of the diplopia. Does the diplopia disappear when one eye is closed? This indicates impairment of the extraocular muscles. Do objects double side to side or on top of one another? Is the diplopia present at near distances or at far distances? Is there any area within the range of focus where the patient is able to achieve single vision? The answers to these questions may suggest which cranial nerve has been injured (Table 24-3). The therapist concludes the interview by identifying activities the patient has difficulty performing that could be caused by oculomotor dysfunction. The therapist should look for a pattern in the patient's response, such as difficulty with activities that require sustained focus in near space (reading, writing, and quilting). The therapist should pay attention to whether the patient's visual difficulty seems to change with the focal length of the task and whether the patient's levels of fatigue and concentration appear to be related to activities requiring sustained focusing.

The next part of the assessment is observing the patient's eyes and eye movements for deficiencies. First, the eyes are observed for asymmetries in pupil size, eyelid function, and eye position as the patient focuses on a distant object. Asymmetries such as a dilated pupil in one eye or a droopy eyelid may indicate cranial nerve involvement. Next, movement of the eyes is observed by asking the patient to track a moving object (such as a penlight) through the nine cardinal directions of gaze plus convergence.[59] This test can be thought of as an active ROM test of the eyes because the nine cardinal directions represent the directions through which the eyes move. The test is used to determine if there are deviations in strength and function of the extraocular muscles and is completed by observing the eyes move in a binocular test. During the test, the therapist observes the following: (1) the symmetry of the eye movement; (2) whether the eyes move the same distance in each direction; (3) whether the eyes are able to stay on target with a minimum of jerking movements; and (4) whether the patient is able to hold the eyes in a deviated position at the end of the range for 2 to 3 seconds. Restriction of eye movement in a specific direction or difficulty moving the eyes in a specific direction may indicate impaired oculomotor function.[55] Observing the eyes as they track an object moving toward the bridge of the nose tests convergence. Most adults can maintain focus and track an object to a distance of approximately 3 inches from the bridge of the nose. At that point one eye usually breaks fixation and moves outward. The point at which convergence is broken is known as the *near point of convergence*.[55]

Although the near point of convergence is 2 to 3 inches from the bridge of the nose, few adults ever view objects that closely. Therefore limitations in convergence are generally not *functionally* significant unless the patient is unable to converge the eyes and easily maintain convergence to a distance of 12 to 16 inches from the bridge of the nose. An inability to converge the eyes to this distance and maintain convergence for several seconds while focusing on an object may cause the patient to have difficulty performing tasks in near vision, especially those such as reading, which require a sustained focus. Observation of convergence insufficiency on testing should be correlated with complaints

TABLE 24-3

Summary of Oculomotor Deficits Associated with Cranial Nerve Lesions

Oculomotor Nerve 3	Trochlear Nerve 4	Abducens Nerve 6
Impaired vertical eye movements	Impaired downward and lateral eye movements	Impaired lateral eye movements
Lateral diplopia for near vision tasks	Vertical diplopia for near vision tasks	Lateral diplopia for far vision tasks
Dilation of pupil and impaired accommodation	With bilateral lesion assumes downward head tilt	
Ptosis of eyelid		

made by the patient regarding such tasks as reading, writing, quilting, or sewing.

The final component of the assessment is diplopia testing, which is completed only if the patient is complaining of diplopia.[74] Diplopia testing is used to determine the severity of the diplopia and whether it is caused by a tropia or a phoria. *Tropia* is the suffix applied when there is a noticeable deviation of the position of one eye in relation to the other when the patient is viewing an object.[74,81] *Phoria* is the suffix used when there is a deviation of the eye that is held in check by fusion and is therefore not noticeable when the patient is focusing on an object. These terms are used in conjunction with a prefix describing the direction of the deviation. Four prefixes are used: *eso-*, meaning a turning in of the eye; *exo-*, a turning out of the eye; *hypo-*, a turning downward of the eye; and *hyper-*, a turning upward of the eye. *Esotropia* therefore describes an observable, inward deviation of the eye commonly described as "crossed eyes," whereas *esophoria* indicates that the eye drifts inward when the patient is not focusing on an object but is held in check when the patient is focusing on an object.[72]

Diplopia testing is based on the principle that when an eye is required to fixate on an object, it will do so with the fovea. If an eye that is not fixating on a target is suddenly required to foveate, it will achieve foveation by making a saccade toward the target. By requiring the patient to fixate with both eyes on a target and then covering one of the patient's eyes during fixation, the examiner can determine whether both eyes are aligned in focusing on the target and, if not, which eye is the deviant (strabismic) eye.[59,80] Two tests are used: a cover/uncover test, which is completed when a tropia is suspected, and a cross or alternate-cover test, which is completed when a phoria is suspected.[59,80] If both eyes are aligned equally and fixating on the target, no movement of either eye will be observed when one is covered. If the eyes are not aligned, the deviating eye will move to take up fixation when the nonaffected eye is covered. Patients with tropias generally complain of constant diplopia when viewing objects and will need to have one eye occluded to eliminate the diplopia so that functional activities can be completed. Patients with phorias often complain of diplopia only intermittently, usually when fatigued or stressed by sustained viewing of a target. Although the phoric patient may complete most activities without diplopia, he or she may experience significant visual stress, which can manifest itself as headaches, eye strain, or decreased concentration.

The information gathered from the assessment should be compared with the patient's visual complaints and observations of his or her performance to determine if the oculomotor dysfunction is contributing to the patient's functional limitations. For example, the presence of convergence insufficiency may help explain the difficulty the patient is having in maintaining concentration when reading. As another example, the observation of downward movement of the left eye during the cover/uncover test may explain why the patient complains of feeling off balance and unsure when descending stairs. If oculomotor deficiencies are observed that appear to limit function, referral should be made to an ophthalmologist or optometrist for further evaluation to determine the cause of the deficiency, the prognosis for improvement, and treatment options.

Treatment

With the exception of reading and tasks requiring fine eye-hand coordination, the presence of oculomotor dysfunction usually does not prevent completion of most ADL; however, it does make completion of all ADL tedious and fatiguing. The patient may express reluctance to perform some activities, or even stop performing them, because of the constant visual stress. Motor and postural control also may be compromised, reducing safety in navigation of the environment. For these reasons oculomotor dysfunction must be addressed in treatment, although it is not specifically identified as a treatment goal. That is, the goal for therapy remains a functional goal such as safe and accurate completion of meal preparation, shopping, or bill paying, and management of the oculomotor dysfunction becomes one of the methods used to achieve the goal.

Treatment can be divided into four types of intervention: occlusion, application of prism, eye exercises, and surgery.[6,76,81] The last three interventions are used to reestablish fusion and binocularity. Most oculomotor dysfunction clears up without treatment intervention within 6 to 12 months after the brain injury.[81] Because of this, ophthalmologists generally do not believe that it is necessary to provide any treatment other than to eliminate the diplopia for the patient's comfort during the recuperation period. If the diplopia persists and becomes chronic, surgery can be used to reestablish fusion. Optometrists often choose a more active approach and prescribe eye exercises to reestablish binocularity, in addition to using occlusion and prism.[72] Brief descriptions of these treatment interventions follow. The treatment option selected for a patient depends on the prognosis for recovery, the patient's ability to participate in therapy, family and financial resources, and the eye specialist providing consultation.

OCCLUSION. The presence of diplopia causes perceptual distortion. This distortion creates confusion for the patient and limits participation in therapy. Therefore diplopia must be eliminated if the patient is to benefit fully from rehabilitation. Diplopia is eliminated by occluding the image presented to one eye. Occlusion can be achieved by assuming a head position or by covering one eye. Because assuming a deviant head position often affects motor and postural control, the preferred method is to cover one eye. Occlusion of the eye can be achieved through either full or partial occlusion.[6,72,76,81]

With full occlusion, vision is completely occluded in one eye by application of a "pirate patch," a clip-on occluder, or opaque tape. The challenge with full occlusion is that it eliminates peripheral visual input, disrupting normal CNS mechanisms for control of balance and orientation to space. This often causes the patient to feel off balance and disoriented and reduces depth perception. Another challenge is that the patient generally cannot tolerate long periods of occlusion of an eye, especially of the dominant eye. Therefore, for the comfort of the patient, the period of occlusion is alternated between the eyes every hour. Alternating occlusion between the eyes also reduces the likelihood of the development of secondary contracture of the muscles antagonistic to the paretic muscle.

For partial occlusion, a strip of opaque material (such as Transpore surgical tape) is applied to a portion of the eyeglass lens to block visual stimulation in the central visual field, while the peripheral visual field is left unoccluded (Fig. 24-10). The patient is instructed to view a target within the diplopic field. Tape is applied from the nasal rim toward the center of the lens until the patient reports that the diplopia is gone when viewing the target. The tape is applied to the nondominant eye for the greater comfort of the patient. The width of the tape is gradually reduced as the muscle paresis resolves. An advantage of partial occlusion is that the patient is more comfortable and therefore that compliance is increased. Another advantage is that peripheral vision is left intact and available for use in orientation to space and balance. The main disadvantage of this type of occlusion is that the patient must either wear prescription lenses or have tape applied to a pair of frames with plain, nonrefractive lenses. Either type of occlusion should be accompanied by daily ROM exercises. The unaffected eye is covered. The patient practices moving the strabismic eye toward the direction of the paresis, then repeats the ROM exercises binocularly (using the eyes together) in all directions of gaze to prevent contracture of the unaffected eye muscles.

PRISMS. Ophthalmologists and optometrists may use a prism to reestablish single vision in the primary directions of gaze: straight ahead and looking down. Application of a prism displaces the image, causing the disparate images created by the strabismus to fuse into a single image.[6,72] The prism can be ground into the eyeglass lenses worn by the patient or temporarily applied to the lens of the glasses using a plastic Fresnel press-on prism. A prism is used only as long as it is needed to maintain fusion. If the paresis is resolving, the patient is gradually weaned from the prism by reducing the dioptic strength of the prism over a period of time commensurate with the rate of recovery.

EYE EXERCISES. There has yet to be objective research unequivocally demonstrating that the use of eye exercises will restore binocular function following paretic strabismus. Eye exercises do not appear to adversely affect muscle function, however, and the use of eye exercises can empower the patient by increasing his

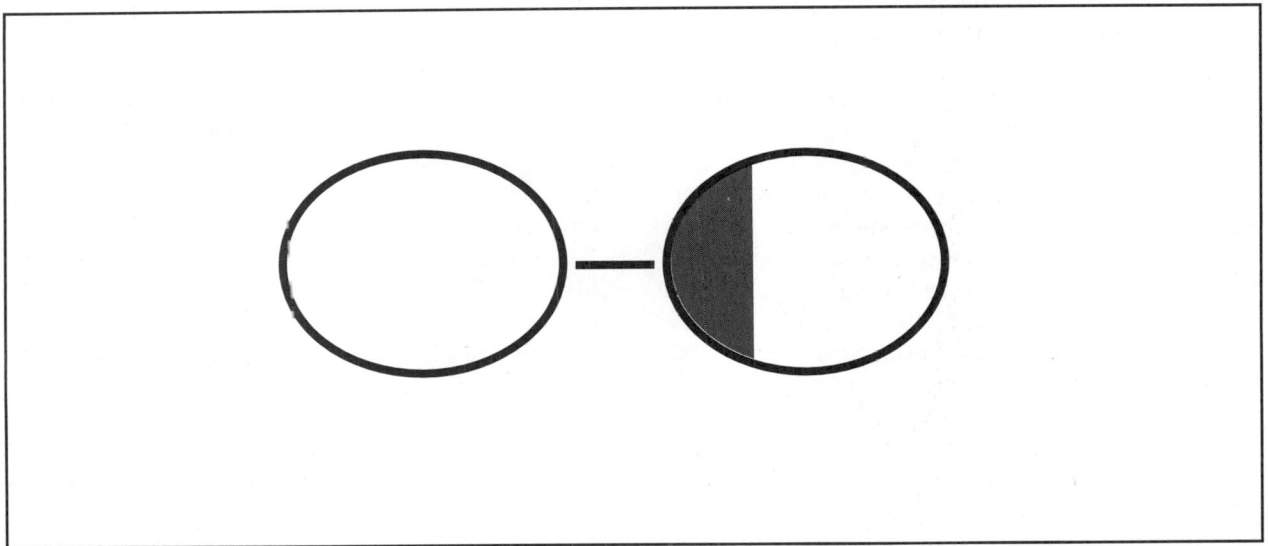

FIG. 24-10
Example of partial occlusion to eliminate diplopia. Translucent tape is applied to the nasal portion of the eyeglass lens on the side of the nondominant eye. (From Warren M: *Brain Injury Visual Assessment Battery for Adults Test Manual,* Lenexa, Kan, 1998, visAbilities Rehab Services)

or her participation in the recovery process. If eye exercises are undertaken, they should be directed toward correcting the deficiencies observed in binocular function. Recommended exercises are those that increase fusion and active ROM of the affected eye. An optometrist often directs the use of eye exercises in this aspect of the rehabilitation program.[72]

SURGERY. Surgery is recommended when the degree of strabismus is too large to be overcome consistently and easily by fusional effort, or when there is a significant strabismic condition that does not resolve in 12 to 18 months.[81] The general approach in surgery is to make the action of one of the extraocular muscles either weaker or stronger by changing the position of its attachment on the eyeball. The position of the eye in the socket is changed by the procedure, and the image is realigned. Surgery is completed by an ophthalmologist specially trained in strabismus surgery.

Visual Attention and Scanning

Visual attention is the ability to observe objects closely and carefully to discern information about their features and their relationship to oneself and other objects in the environment. It requires being able to ignore irrelevant sensory input and random thought processes and to focus over a period of several seconds to several minutes. Visual attention also entails being able to shift visual focus from object to object in an organized and efficient manner. Engagement of visual attention is accomplished through visual scanning or search (these two terms are used interchangeably). Although these two processes are separated within the visual perceptual hierarchy to assist in understanding them, they cannot be separated in function or in evaluation and treatment of the patient. Any change in visual attention will be observed in the patient as a change in the scanning pattern used for visual search.

Visual attention can be divided into two categories: focal, or selective, visual attention and ambient, or peripheral, visual attention.[37,67] Focal attention is used for object recognition and identification. Visual input from the macular area of the retina is used to complete this processing. Focal, or selective, attention enables an individual to accurately distinguish visual details such as differences between letters, numbers, and faces. Ambient, or peripheral, attention is concerned with the detection of events in the environment and their location in space and proximity to the person. It relies on input from the peripheral visual field. Peripheral attention ensures that a person is able to move safely through space and maintain orientation in space. Without peripheral attention, collisions with objects and disorientation when moving would be the norm. To have a fully operational and efficient visual system, these two modes of visual attention must work together. The contribution of each is equally important to perceptual processing.

In normal adults, visual search is completed using an organized, systematic, and efficient pattern.[13,25,62,84,89] The type of search pattern used depends on the demands of the task. In reading English, for example, a left-to-right and top-to-bottom linear strategy is used. In scanning an open array (such as a room), a circular, left-to-right strategy generally is used, following either a clockwise or a counterclockwise pattern.

Deficits in Visual Attention and Scanning

Studies have shown that disruption in the normal search strategy can occur after brain injury. The characteristics of the disruption vary, depending on which hemisphere was damaged. Visual search deficits associated with right hemisphere injury are characterized by avoidance in searching the left half of the visual space.[7,20,24,31,33,62,69] This condition is known as **hemi-inattention**. Instead of initiating the normal left-to-right visual search pattern, patients with right hemisphere injuries often begin and confine search to the right side of a visual array. This creates an asymmetrical rather than a symmetrical search pattern. The patient misses visual information on the left side and as a result may be deprived of information needed to make accurate identification and decisions.

Hemi-inattention is associated with only right hemisphere injuries and occurs because of a difference in the way the hemispheres are programmed to direct visual attention.[33,75] As illustrated in Fig. 24-11, the left hemisphere directs attention toward the right half of the visual space surrounding the body. In contrast, the right hemisphere directs visual attention toward *both* the right and left halves of the space surrounding the body. If a lesion occurs in the left hemisphere, visual attention and search toward the right side are diminished, but some attentional capability is still provided by the right hemisphere. A similar lesion in the right hemisphere may completely eliminate attentional capability toward the left because there is no other area directing attention toward the left side.

Hemi-inattention often is confused with the presence of left VFD in the patient. Although both conditions may cause the patient to miss visual information on the left side, they are distinctly different conditions and do not have the same effect on performance. When left VFD occurs, the patient attempts to compensate for the loss of vision by engaging visual attention.[36] The patient directs eye movements toward the blind left side in an attempt to gather visual information from that side. Because of the field deficit, however, the patient may not move the eyes far enough to acquire the needed visual information from the left side and as a result may appear inattentive. In contrast, the patient with hemi-inattention has lost the attentional mechanisms in the

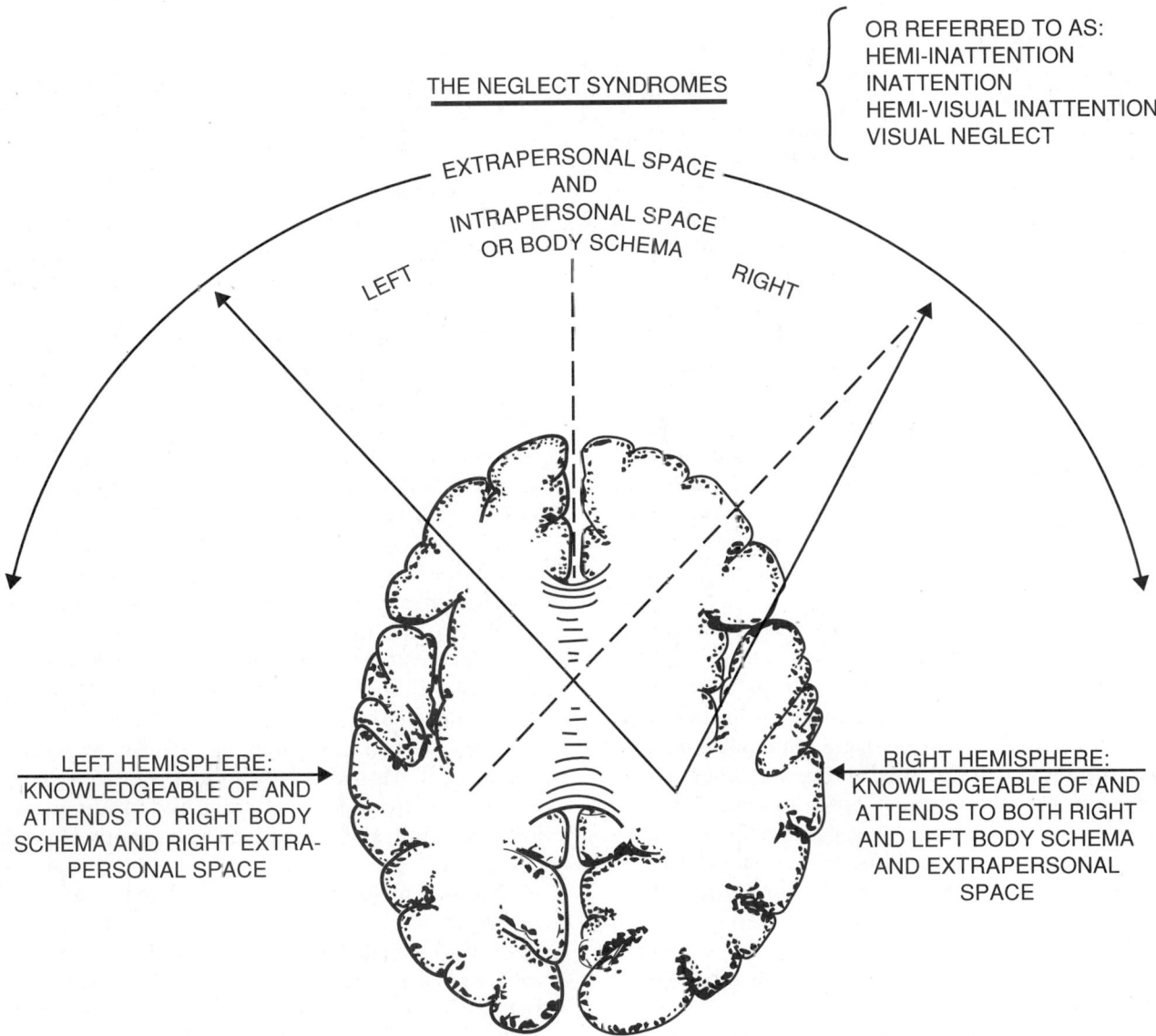

THE NEGLECT SYNDROMES

OR REFERRED TO AS:
HEMI-INATTENTION
INATTENTION
HEMI-VISUAL INATTENTION
VISUAL NEGLECT

EXTRAPERSONAL SPACE
AND
INTRAPERSONAL SPACE
OR BODY SCHEMA

LEFT   RIGHT

LEFT HEMISPHERE:
KNOWLEDGEABLE OF AND
ATTENDS TO RIGHT BODY
SCHEMA AND RIGHT EXTRA-
PERSONAL SPACE

RIGHT HEMISPHERE:
KNOWLEDGEABLE OF AND
ATTENDS TO BOTH RIGHT
AND LEFT BODY SCHEMA
AND EXTRAPERSONAL
SPACE

IN RELATION TO **MOVEMENT** AND **SENSORY PERCEPTIONS** SUCH AS <u>VISION</u> (VISUAL-SPATIAL AND VISUAL-OBJECT AWARENESS AND RECOGNITION), <u>AUDITORY</u> AND <u>SOMESTHETIC</u> (INCLUDING BODY IMAGE OR SCHEMA) COGNITION AND AWARENESS, IT APPEARS THAT THE LEFT HEMISPHERE PRIMARILY ATTENDS TO THE RIGHT EXTRAPERSONAL SPACE AND/OR BODY IMAGE PARAMETERS WHILE THE RIGHT HEMISPHERE ATTENDS TO BOTH RIGHT AND LEFT EXTRAPERSONAL SPACE AND BODY IMAGE. THUS **LEFT HEMISPHERE LESIONS** OF THE 1°, 2° OR 3° AREAS OF THE CEREBRAL CORTEX OR ASSOCIATED SUBCORTICAL FIBER TRACTS CONCERNED WITH <u>VISUAL</u>, <u>AUDITORY</u>, <u>SOMESTHETIC</u>, OR <u>MOTOR FUNCTIONS</u> RARELY RESULT IN A NEGLECT SYNDROME BECAUSE THE RIGHT HEMISPHERE CAN ATTEND TO AND COMPENSATE FOR THE LEFT HEMISPHERE DEFICIT. <u>HOWEVER</u> **RIGHT HEMISPHERE LESIONS** OF ONE OR MORE OF THESE FUNCTIONAL AREAS LEAVE THE BRAIN UNABLE TO ATTEND TO OR BE AWARE OF THE LEFT EXTRAPERSONAL SPACE AND BODY SCHEMA. VISUAL FIELD DEFICITS (ESPECIALLY LEFT HOMONYMOUS HEMIANOPSIA) ALWAYS COMPOUND THE NEGLECT SYNDROME

FIG. 24-11
Difference between the right and left hemispheres in the direction of visual attention and the relationship of hemisphere lesions to hemi-inattention and neglect syndrome. (Courtesy of Josephine C. Moore, PhD, OTR.)

CNS that drive the search for visual information on the left. No attempt will be made by the inattentive patient to search for information on the left side of the visual space, and no eye movements or head turning will be observed toward the left side.[36] The most significant change in visual search happens when the two conditions occur together in the patient. In this case the patient is not receiving visual input from the left side because of VFD and does not compensate for the loss of visual input by directing attention toward the left side. The combination of hemi-inattention and left VFD creates severe inattention, often called **visual neglect.** Patients with this condition show exaggerated inattention toward the left half of the visual space surrounding the body and often do not move the eyes past midline toward the left or turn the head toward the left side. Visual neglect may be compounded by neglect of the limbs on the left side of the body or neglect of auditory input from the left side.[19,20] The presence of neglect is associated consistently with poor rehabilitation outcomes.[14]

Another change in visual search associated with right hemisphere lesions is a tendency to fixate first on the most peripheral visual stimuli occurring in the right visual field.[20] If two visual stimuli simultaneously appear in the right visual field, the patient will attend first to the most peripheral stimulus. The patient with this tendency makes frequent head turns to attend to events occurring in the right peripheral field, giving the impression of being distractible. Yet another change in visual search is a reluctance to rescan for additional information once an area has been viewed, especially if the area is on the left side.[60,62] This may cause the patient to miss certain visual details when viewing complex visual arrays.

Although several distinct changes in visual search have been observed with right hemisphere lesions, only one has been observed following left hemisphere lesions. Patients with left hemisphere injury often show a symmetrical decrease in searching for detail when viewing a visual array.[7,31,79] These patients broadly scan the visual array for information but do not examine specific aspects of the visual scene to gather additional information. Because of this, they may miss visual details and often cannot accurately interpret or identify the objects around them. This may be because of a disruption in the selective item-by-item search strategy mediated by the left hemisphere.[58] Left hemisphere injury does not result in hemi-inattention or neglect.

In general, patients with injuries to either hemisphere are slower in scanning and show more erratic fixation patterns, compared with persons without brain injury.[49,89] They also have greater difficulty engaging selective attention and executing an organized and efficient visual search strategy. Research has shown that when persons with brain injuries are asked to search complex visual arrays for specific targets, they have difficulty maintaining attention on the salient features of the target and mistakenly select targets with similar features.[65,89] They also demonstrate an inability to superimpose an organized, efficient structure for visual scanning when asked to search an array with randomly displayed objects. For example, if asked to locate a certain individual seated among others on rows of benches (a structured visual array), the injured person would be able to accomplish the task. However, if asked to find the same individual standing in a jumbled crowd of persons (a random visual array), the injured person would display a random approach to searching the array and would likely miss the target.

Functional Deficits Caused by Visual Inattention

Disruption of visual attention creates asymmetry and gaps in the visual information gathered through visual search. The quality of an individual's adaptation to the environment decreases because the CNS is not receiving complete visual information in an organized fashion and therefore is unable to effectively use this information to make appropriate decisions. Reduction in visual attention will affect all aspects of the performance of ADL. However, the most affected activities will be those that require inspection and integration of significant amounts of visual detail and those completed in dynamic environments. Driving and reading are two diverse examples of tasks often significantly affected by inattention.

Because visual attention is modulated through an extensive neural network involving the entire CNS, some capacity for visual attention generally is retained even in cases of severe brain trauma.[54] On the other hand, changes in visual attention occur even with mild injuries. Whether a change in visual attention affects functional performance depends on the task to be completed. Tasks such as reading can require enormous amounts of selective visual attention if an individual is reading a highly technical textbook, and less selective attention if the individual is reading an advertisement. The task of driving requires continuous global attention to monitor the speed and position of other vehicles and objects, and sporadic selective attention to landmarks, street signs, and traffic lights. Whether a deficiency in visual attention manifests itself after brain injury depends on the circumstances and requirements of the tasks the patient is required to complete.

Assessment

As a process found at the intermediate level of the visual perceptual hierarchy, visual attention can be affected by deficits in lower-level visual functions (visual acuity, oculomotor function, and visual field). Therefore these functions should be assessed before visual attention is measured. The presence of aphasia and motor impairment can also affect performance on tests for visual attention. The criterion used in assessing visual search and attention is how efficiently and completely a person attends to and takes in visual information. That determines the ability to use the information for adaptation. Therefore, the emphasis in assessment is on observing how a patient initiates and carries out visual scanning to complete a task requiring visual search. During the assessment the therapist should answer the following questions: Does the patient initiate an organized search strategy? Can the patient carry out the search strategy in an organized and efficient manner? Does the patient obtain complete visual information from visual search? Is the patient able to identify visual detail correctly? Does the patient's ability to search for information decrease as the visual complexity of the task increases?

Research has shown that persons with good visual attention demonstrate specific characteristics of search patterns that make them effective in obtaining visual information.[13,84] These characteristics include strategies that are organized, symmetrical, thorough, resilient to challenge, and consistent. The use of these strategies usually results in good accuracy and speed in completion of visual search tasks. In contrast, persons with severe VFD or inattention often demonstrate ineffective search strategies. These individuals demonstrate incomplete or abbreviated patterns in which only a portion of the visual array is searched, usually in a random, unpredictable fashion.[7,13,14,18,25,36,37,49,65,89] The organization and accuracy of the pattern often break down when the person is challenged to search more complex visual arrays. Fig. 24-12 provides examples of some of the ineffective search strategies used on the visual search subtests of the biVABA by persons with brain injury. A patient who employs ineffective search strategies may not acquire sufficient visual information to complete perceptual processing accurately. He or she may acquire the information in such a way that it cannot be used to complete perceptual processing, or may not acquire the information rapidly enough to enable adaptation. The subsequent disruption of perceptual processing may cause errors in decision making and adversely affect performance of a variety of daily living activities.

When measuring visual attention, the therapist must be aware that visual search can be significantly affected by both the presence of a VFD and hemi-inattention. Because VFD and hemi-inattention are not the same condition, it is necessary to distinguish between the two conditions to establish an effective treatment plan. This can be difficult, both because similar errors are observed with the two conditions on search tasks and because the two can also occur together in the same patient. However, differentiation can be accomplished by observing the strategies used by the patient to complete visual search tasks such as those on the biVABA (Fig. 24-12). Although both VFD and hemi-inattention can

result in decreased accuracy in identifying targets on a visual search task, the characteristics of the search deficiencies are different.[36] For example, a patient with a left hemianopsia may demonstrate a left-to-right linear search pattern that is abbreviated on the blind side. The search pattern is organized but results in a number of errors on the left because the patient did not see that side of the array. In contrast, a patient with hemi-inattention may demonstrate an asymmetrical pattern, initiating and confining visual search to the right side using a disorganized and random search pattern. The pattern also results in a large number of errors on the left. Although accuracy on the search task may be similar for these two patients, the cause of the errors is different. By observing the strategy used by the patient to complete the search task, it is possible to distinguish between the two conditions. Table 24-4 compares the characteristics of search patterns used by persons with hemianopsia and persons with hemi-inattention. When the two conditions occur together, it is important to determine the severity of the inattention because this will determine whether the patient is able to learn the strategies needed to compensate for the VFD.

The visual search tests that have been described are pencil-and-paper tasks presented in a restricted and well-defined personal space. Determining how the patient applies a search strategy to broader extrapersonal space requires the use of a test such as the Scan-Board test described by Warren.[84] The test, part of the biVABA, consists of a large (20 inches by 30 inches) board with a series of 10 numbers displayed in an unstructured pattern. The board is placed at eye level and centered at the patient's midline. The patient is asked to scan the board and point out all of the numbers that he or she sees. The examiner records the pattern the patient follows in identifying the numbers. Research using this test has shown that adults with normal visual search employ an organized, sequential search pattern, beginning on the left side of the board and proceeding in either a clockwise or counterclockwise fashion until all of the numbers are identified. In contrast, adults with deficits in visual attention demonstrate disorganized, random, and often abbreviated search strategies, frequently missing numbers on one side of the board. Those with hemi-inattention often show an asymmetrical pattern, initiating and confining visual search to the right side of the board. Patients with VFD may miss numbers on the blind side but demonstrate an organized search strategy.

Treatment

Information gathered from observing the patient complete visual search tests should reveal specific deficiencies in the scanning pattern the patient uses to acquire visual information during completion of daily tasks. For example, it may be observed that the patient does not

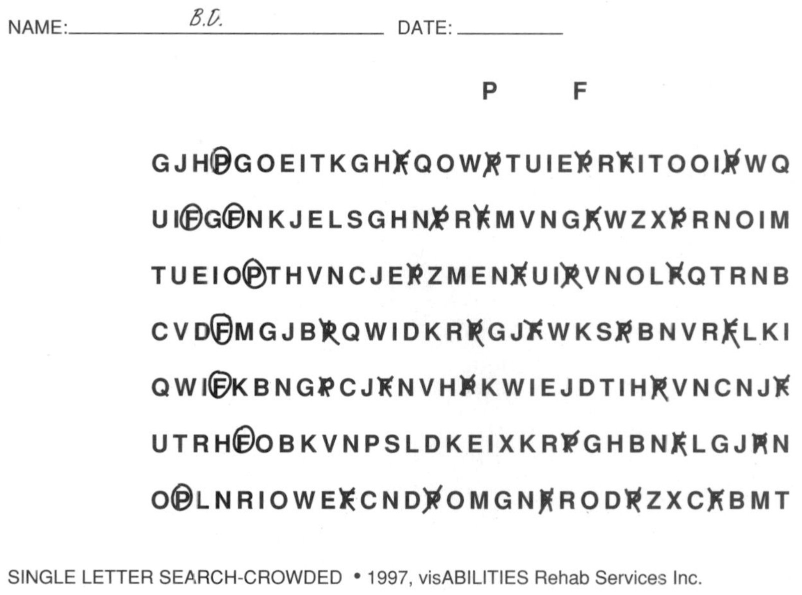

NAME: _____B.D._____ DATE: _____

P   F

GJH(P)GOEITKGHXQOWXTUIEXRXITOOIXWQ

UIF(G)NKJELSGHNXRXMVNGXWZXXRNOIM

TUEIO(P)THVNCJEXZMENXUIXVNOLXQTRNB

CVD(F)MGJBXQWIDKRXGJXWKSXBNVRXLKI

QWI(F)KBNGXCJXNVHXKWIEJDTIHXVNCNJX

UTRH(F)OBKVNPSLDKEIXKRXGHBNXLGJXN

O(P)LNRIOWEXCNDXOMGNXRODXZXCXBMT

SINGLE LETTER SEARCH-CROWDED • 1997, visABILITIES Rehab Services Inc.

A

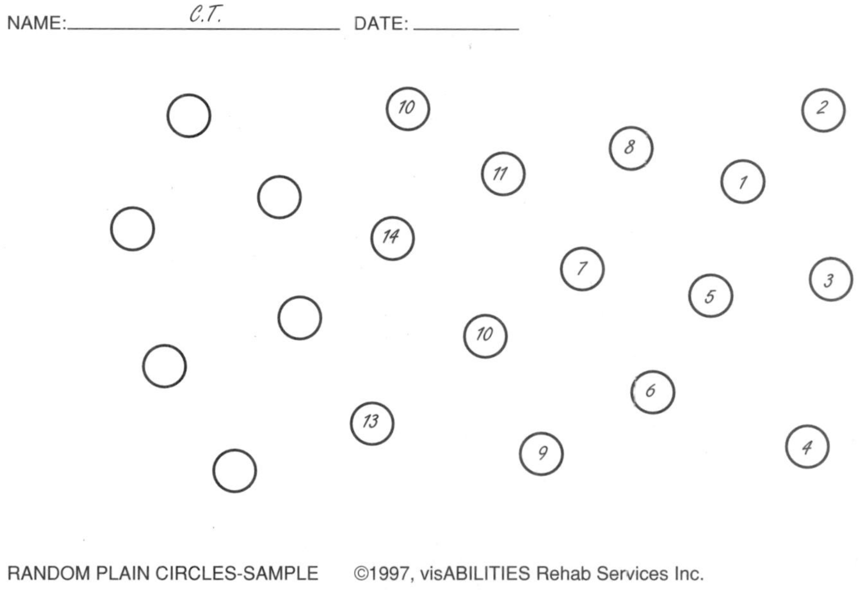

NAME: _____C.T._____ DATE: _____

RANDOM PLAIN CIRCLES-SAMPLE   ©1997, visABILITIES Rehab Services Inc.

B

FIG. 24-12

Examples of ineffective search patterns used by patients to complete two visual search subtests of the Brain Injury Visual Assessment Battery for Adults. **A,** An abbreviated search pattern used by a patient with left hemianopsia when crossing out the letters P and F on the subtest; the patient executed an organized left-to-right linear search pattern but failed to locate the beginning of the line on the left side, and as a result failed to cross out targets on that side (the circled letters). **B,** An asymmetrical and abbreviated search pattern executed by a patient with hemi-inattention and left hemianopsia. The patient was asked to number the circles consecutively, choosing any pattern desired. The patient began numbering the circles from the right rather than the left and failed to number circles on the left side of the array.

TABLE 24-4
Comparison of Search Patterns: Persons With Visual Field Deficit vs. Persons With Hemi-inattention

Visual Field Deficit	Hemi-inattention
Search pattern is abbreviated toward blind field	Search pattern is asymmetrical; initiated/confined to the right side
Attempts to direct search toward blind side	No attempt to direct search toward left side
Search pattern is organized and generally efficient	Search pattern is random and generally inefficient
Client rescans to check accuracy of performance	Client does not rescan to check accuracy of performance
Time spent on task is appropriate to level of difficulty	Client completes task quickly; level of effort applied is not consistent with difficulty of task

From Warren M: *Brain Injury Visual Assessment Battery for Adults Test Manual*, Lenexa, Kan, 1998, visAbilities Rehab Services.

search toward the left side of visual arrays. If this deficiency is significant, a similar performance should be observed when the patient completes a daily activity. This could be an inability to locate items placed to the left side of the sink in grooming or a tendency to begin reading a recipe in the middle of the line of print instead of at the left margin.

Depending on the severity of the deficit, some patients with inattention are able to complete simple and practiced daily activities and experience difficulty only on tasks that are unfamiliar or require search of a complex visual array. Others, especially those with neglect, may have difficulty with such a simple task as finding all the food on their plate. By combining information from visual search tests with that gained from observation of ADL performance, it is possible to determine if and how the patient's performance of daily activities has been affected by impairment of visual search. The treatment goals on the plan of care should be worded to reflect the specific daily activities compromised by the inattention. For example, the plan of care could include such treatments goals as, "The patient will be able to complete grooming independently" or, "The patient will be able to prepare a simple meal independently."

The goals established for independent ADL performance are achieved by ensuring that the patient learns to take in visual information in a consistent, systematic, and organized manner. Before a patient can learn to reorganize a visual search, he or she must understand how his or her visual search and attention have changed. To facilitate the development of this insight, the examiner should carefully review the results of the patient's performance on the visual search tests and show the patient how his or her search pattern differed from the norm and caused errors. If, after receiving this feedback, the patient wishes to retake one of the tests, he or she should be allowed to do so. If the patient's performance improves on the retest, this is an indication of capability to benefit from therapy intervention and serves as a jus-

tification for therapy services. Likewise, if the patient's performance does not improve, this helps to verify the significance of the deficit and also may indicate reduced rehabilitation potential.

The primary compensatory strategy taught to the patient with hemi-inattention is reorganizing the scanning pattern to begin visual search on the left side of a visual array and progress left to right.[88] The use of this pattern will counteract the patient's tendency to restrict all visual search to the right side and will increase the symmetry of the search pattern. Patients with left hemisphere injuries do not demonstrate asymmetry in visual search but often fail to notice details when searching visual arrays. These patients should be taught to initiate careful item-by-item search of visual arrays. Two scanning strategies are taught with all patients: a left-to-right *linear* pattern for reading and inspection of small visual detail, and a left-to-right *clockwise* or *counter-clockwise* pattern for viewing unstructured and extrapersonal visual arrays. Activities should be selected that encourage and reinforce the use of these patterns.

Compensatory strategies can be taught more effectively if treatment activities are designed using the following guidelines:

1. *Treatment activities should require the patient to scan as broad a visual space as possible.* Most daily activities require orientation to a broad visual space. To help the patient complete a wide visual search, the working field of the activity should be large enough to require the patient either to turn the head or to change body positions to accomplish the task. Many activities and games can be enlarged to require head turning for scanning. For example, a deck of playing cards can be laid out, facing up, in rows 2 to 3 feet wide. The patient is given another deck of playing cards and instructed to match the cards in hand to the cards on the table. The therapist ensures that the patient initiates a left-to-right, top-to-bottom, organized scanning pattern when searching for the matching cards to complete the task.

2. *Treatment activities will be more effective if the patient is required to interact physically with the target once it is located.* Research has shown that a stronger mental representation of a visual image is formed if what is seen is verified by tactual exploration.[4] Whenever possible, the treatment activity should be designed to be interactive. Games such as solitaire, dominoes, ball games, or activities such as putting together large puzzles are examples of treatment activities with interactive qualities.

3. *Treatment activities should emphasize conscious attention to visual detail and careful inspection and comparison of targets.* Because complex visual processing is dependent on initiation of the item-by-item search strategy of selective visual attention, it is important to include scanning activities that require discrimination of subtle details and matching. Patients should be taught consciously to study objects for their relevant features, with emphasis placed on attending to detail in the impaired space. Many games such as solitaire, double solitaire, concentration, Connect Four, checkers, Scrabble, and dominoes have these qualities. Large 300- to 500-piece puzzles, word or number searches, crossword puzzles, and needlecrafts such as latch hook also require these skills. Throughout performance of these tasks, patients should be encouraged to recheck their work to make sure that critical details are not missed.

4. *Practice the search strategy within context to ensure carryover of application to daily living activities.* Clinic activities provide a starting place to begin teaching the strategies needed for successful visual perceptual processing. Research has shown, however, that patients with brain injury often do not spontaneously transfer skills from one learning situation to the next. Toglia[77] suggests that having the patient apply the learned strategy in different contexts of daily living can facilitate transfer of learning. For example, the patient can be required to use a left-to-right search strategy when selecting clothes from a closet, searching for items in a refrigerator, or shopping for groceries. The more often the strategy is repeated under varied circumstances, the more the skill is generalized and transferred to new situations. There is no substitute in therapy for the practice of real-life situations to help the patient develop insight into abilities and compensation for limitations. Cafeterias, gift shops, and office areas within the hospital and fast food restaurants and shops surrounding the hospital can be used to expose the patient to more realistic and demanding visual environments.

Insight on the part of the patient into the nature of the visual deficit and how it has affected functional performance is critical to learning compensation. According to Toglia,[77] one of the reasons patients with brain injury do not spontaneously recognize their limitations and the need to compensate is that their concept of their capabilities is based on premorbid experiences. This causes these patients to overestimate their abilities after injury. Without a realistic understanding of his or her limitations, the patient may be unwilling to use compensatory strategies. To increase insight, Abreu and Toglia[1] advocate teaching a patient to monitor and control his or her performance by learning to recognize and correct for errors in performance. Giving the patient immediate feedback about the performance and pointing out deficiencies facilitate this process of error detection. The process can also be facilitated by teaching the patient to use self-monitoring techniques such as activity prediction, in which the patient predicts how successfully an activity will be performed and identifies the aspects of the activity in which errors are likely to occur. The patient then compares actual performance with predicted performance. This technique helps the patient develop anticipatory skills and increase awareness of how the deficit affects functional capabilities.

Some patients, because of the severity of their deficits, lack the cognition to benefit from training in compensatory strategies. Although treatment intervention is limited, such patients may benefit from a passive approach to treatment that emphasizes modification of the environment to help the patient use his or her limited attentional capabilities. The environment can be made more "user friendly" by reducing factors that place stress on visual processing. Suggested environmental modifications include the following:

1. *Reduce background pattern so that objects in the foreground can be seen more easily.* The more dense the background pattern, the greater the amount of selective attention needed to locate the desired object. Patients with severe brain injuries may not be able to sustain the effort needed to complete this level of processing and may view their environments as filled with "visual noise" rather than meaningful objects. Backgrounds can be simplified by eliminating patterned designs and using solid colors on support surfaces such as rugs, carpets, place mats, and bedspreads. Eliminating superfluous objects such as knickknacks and old magazines and organizing frequently used items on shelves and in containers also simplify the background. As a general rule, environments should be sparse and contain only the items needed by the patient for completion of daily activities. Items that contain a lot of pattern, such as reading materials, can be enlarged to decrease the density of the pattern.

2. *Ensure that room and task illumination is adequate.* Both too little and too much illumination can impair visual processing. However, environments usually contain too little rather than too much light. The type of lighting used should provide bright, even illumination without glare.

3. *Increase contrast between background and foreground objects to enhance the visibility of items in the environment that need to be noticed.* For example, the edge of a white plate placed on a black place mat is more visible than it would be if placed on a white place mat, and milk in a black cup is more visible than in a white cup. The use of glass or clear plastic items should be avoided because these items reduce contrast by absorbing whatever pattern or color is around them.

Complex Visual Processing

The processes of pattern recognition, visual memory, and visual cognition involve complex processing and integration of vision with other sensory information, past experiences, and cognitive function. To complete this sophisticated level of processing requires not only organized, high-quality sensory input, but also good cognitive ability such as the ability to categorize information and complete abstract reasoning. Complex visual processing, like other cognitive functioning, is elicited by the demands of a particular event. It is a learned skill, established by one's experiences in mastering the environment. With few exceptions, complex visual processing always is applied within context—used to solve a problem, formulate a plan, or make a decision regarding a specific situation. Because of the contextual nature of complex visual processing, the best way to assess it is not to ask the patient to complete some abstract, two-dimensional visual task, but rather to observe the patient complete daily tasks requiring this level of processing. For example, if the patient is an architect planning to return to work, his or her ability to design and execute building plans or other aspects of the job should be assessed, preferably at the patient's place of employment. If the patient wants to return to driving, his or her ability to handle complex traffic situations should be assessed with a behind-the-wheel assessment.

Visual input that is of poor quality or is incomplete or inaccurate will affect the ability to complete complex visual processing. Therefore visual acuity, visual field, oculomotor control, and visual attention and search should be assessed first to determine whether deficits exist that might contribute to deficiencies in complex processing. If deficits are identified, their effect on the patient's performance of ADL that require complex visual processing should be observed. For example, after having determined that a patient has left VFD and an incomplete search pattern indicative of hemi-inattention, the therapist should observe the patient complete an ADL requiring attending, planning, and decision making. The activity may be preparing a meal, sorting and completing laundry, shopping for groceries, measuring the oil level in the car, or completing a job-related task. In observing the patient, the therapist should make special note of how the patient's visual deficit affects his or her ability to process the more complex visual information needed to complete the task. If the patient has difficulty successfully completing the task and the visual deficit appears to be the cause, the therapist should determine if it is possible to improve the patient's performance with treatment of the visual deficit.

SUMMARY

The CNS relies on visual information to anticipate and plan adaptation to the environment. Brain injury or disease disrupts the processing of visual information, creating gaps in the visual input sent to the CNS. The quality of a person's adaptation to the environment decreases, because the CNS does not have sufficient or accurate visual information to make decisions. Whether a person's deficit in visual perceptual processing necessitates therapeutic intervention depends on the person's lifestyle and whether the visual deficit prevents successful completion of daily living activities. The framework for evaluation and treatment rests on the concept of a hierarchy of visual perceptual processing levels that interact with and subserve one another. Because of the unity of the hierarchy, a process cannot be disrupted at one level without an adverse effect on all perceptual processing. Evaluation must be directed at measuring function at all process levels, with particular emphasis on the foundation of visual functions and visual attention and scanning. Treatment focuses on increasing the accuracy and organization of visual input into the system through manipulation of the environment and by providing the patient with strategies to compensate for or minimize the effect of the deficit in ADL.

REVIEW QUESTIONS

1. What determines whether treatment intervention is needed for a patient with a visual impairment?
2. Describe the three purposes of the OT assessment.
3. What is the normal search pattern executed by most adults when viewing an unstructured visual array? A structured array?
4. What is the primary compensatory strategy taught to the patient with hemi-inattention?
5. What is the most crucial lower-level visual process contributing to the ability to complete visual cognitive processing?
6. What changes occur in the visual search pattern following right hemisphere injury?
7. What prevents a patient from automatically compensating for VFD by turning the head farther to see around the blind field?
8. What kind of protective behaviors do persons adopt following onset of visual field deficit? Why do they adopt these strategies?

9. Describe three of the treatment strategies for deficits in visual acuity. Give an example of how each could be applied in an activity of daily living.
10. Describe the assessments completed by the occupational therapist to assess the functional performance of the patient with VFD.
11. Give an example of an active treatment strategy that can be used to teach a patient to compensate for VFD.
12. Describe the assessment used to identify deficits in visual search and scanning.
13. Discuss some treatment strategies for visual scanning and visual inattention.
14. When would partial occlusion be used with the patient? Describe the technique used to apply partial occlusion.
15. How does convergence insufficiency affect functional performance?

REFERENCES

1. Abreu BC, Toglia JP: Cognitive rehabilitation: a model for occupational therapy, *Am J Occup Ther* 41:439-448, 1987.
2. *American Heritage dictionary of the English language*, New York, 1969, Houghton Mifflin.
3. Anderson BR: *Perimetry with and without automation*, ed 2, St Louis, 1987, Mosby.
4. Ayres AJ: *Sensory integration and learning disorders*, Los Angeles, 1972, Western Psychological Services.
5. Baker RS, Epstein AD: Ocular motor abnormalities from head trauma, *Surv Ophthalmol* 36:245-267, 1991.
6. Bedrossian EH: Non surgical management: acquired ocular muscle paralysis. In *The surgical and non surgical management of strabismus*, Springfield, Ill,1969, Charles C Thomas.
7. Belleza T et al: Visual scanning and matching dysfunction in brain damaged patients with drawing impairment, *Cortex* 15:19-36, 1979.
8. Bergen JR, Julesz B: Parallel vs serial processing in rapid pattern discrimination, *Nature* 303(5919):696-698, 1983.
9. Bodis-Wollner I, Diamond SP: The measurement of spatial contrast sensitivity in cases of blurred vision associated with cerebral lesions, *Brain* 99:695-710, 1976.
10. Brendler K, Trauzettel-Klosinski S, Sadowski B: Reading disability in hemianopic field defects: the significant of clinical parameters, *Invest Ophthalmol Vis Sci* 37:S1079, 1996.
11. Bruce CJ, Goldberg M: Physiology of the frontal eye fields, *Trends Neurosci* 7:436-441,1984.
12. Bulens C et al: Spatial contrast sensitivity in unilateral cerebral ischaemic lesion involving the posterior visual pathway, *Brain* 112:507-520, 1989.
13. Chedru F, Leblanc M, Lhermitte F: Visual searching in normal and brain damaged subjects, *Cortex* 9:94-111, 1973.
14. Chen Sea MJ, Henderson A, Cermak SA: Patterns of visual spatial inattention and their functional significance in stroke patients, *Arch Phys Med Rehabil* 74:355-60, 1993.
15. Cohen M et al: Convergence insufficiency in brain-injured patients, *Brain Injury* 2:187-191, 1989.
16. Colenbrander A: The functional vision score, a coordinated scoring system for visual impairments, disabilities and handicaps. In Kooijan AC et al, editors: *Low vision: research and new development in rehabilitation*, Amsterdam, 1994, IOS Press.
17. Colenbrander A, Fletcher DC: Basic concepts and terms for low vision rehabilitation, *Am J Occup Ther* 49(9):865-869,1995.
18. Delis DC, Robertson LC, Balliet R: The breakdown and rehabilitation of visuospatial dysfunction in brain injured patients, *Int Rehabil Med* 5:132-138, 1983.
19. DeRenzi E: *Disorders of space exploration and cognition*, New York, 1982, John Wiley & Sons.
20. DeRenzi E et al: Attentional shift towards the rightmost stimuli in patients with left visual neglect, *Cortex* 25:231-237, 1989.
21. Dickman IR: *Making life more livable*, New York, 1985, American Foundation for the Blind Press.
22. Festinger L: Eye movements and perception. In Bach Y, Rita P, Collins CC, editors: *The control of eye movements*, New York, 1971, Academic Press.
23. Fletcher D et al: Low vision rehabilitation: finding capable people behind damaged eyeballs, *West J Med* 154:554-556, 1991.
24. Gainotti G, Giustolisi L, Nocentini U: Contralateral and ipsilateral disorders of visual attention in patients with unilateral brain damage, *J Neurol Neurosurg Psychiatry* 53:422-426, 1990.
25. Gianutsos R, Matheson P: The rehabilitation of visual perceptual disorders attributable to brain injury. In Meier MJ, Benton AL, Diller L, editors: *Neuropsychological rehabilitation*, New York, 1987, Guilford Press.
26. Gianutsos R, Ramsey G, Perlin RR: Rehabilitative optometric services for survivors of acquired brain injury, *Arch Phys Med Rehabil* 69:573-578, 1988.
27. Gouras P: Physiological optics, accommodation, and stereopsis. In Kandel ER, Schwartz JH, editors: *Principles of neural science*, ed 2, New York, 1985, Elsevier.
28. Gouras P: Oculomotor system. In Kandel ER, Schwartz JH, editors: *Principles of neural science*, ed 2, New York, 1985, Elsevier.
29. Graziano MSA, Yap GS, Gross CG: Coding of visual space by premotor neurons, *Science* 266:1054-1057, 1994.
30. Gross CG, Graziano MSA: Multiple representations of space in the brain, *Neuroscientist* 1:40-50, 1995.
31. Halligan PW et al: Visuo-spatial neglect: qualitative difference and laterality of cerebral lesion, *J Neurol Neurosurg Psychiatry* 55:1060-1068, 1992.
32. Harrington DO: *The visual fields: a textbook and atlas of clinical perimetry*, ed 2, St Louis, 1964, Mosby.
33. Heilman K, Van Den Abel T: Right hemisphere dominance for attention: the mechanism underlying hemispheric asymmetries of inattention (neglect), *Neurology* 30:327-330, 1980.
34. Hess RF, Pointer JS: Spatial and temporal contrast sensitivity in hemianopia: a comparative study of the sighted and blind hemifields, *Brain* 112:871-894, 1989.
35. Hyvarinen L: *Vision testing manual*, Villa Park, Ill, 1996, Precision Vision.
36. Ishial S, Furukawa T, Tsukagoshi H: Eye fixation patterns in homonymous hemianopia and unilateral spatial neglect, *Neuropsychologia* 25:675-679, 1987.
37. Julesz B: Preconscious and conscious processing in vision, *Exp Brain Res* 3(suppl):333-359, 1985.
38. Kahn J: Blunt trauma to orbital soft tissues. In Shingleton BJ, editor: *Eye trauma*, St Louis, 1991, Mosby.
39. Kandel E: Processing of form and movement in the visual system. In Kandel ER, Schwartz JH, editors: *Principles of neural science*, ed 2, New York, 1985, Elsevier.
40. Kanski JJ: *Clinical ophthalmology*, Toronto, 1984, Mosby.
41. Keane JR: Fourth nerve palsy: historical review and study of 215 inpatients, *Neurology* 43:2439-2443, 1993.
42. Klavora P et al: The effects of dynavision rehabilitation on behind-the-wheel driving ability and selected psychomotor abilities of persons post-stroke, *Am J Occup Ther* 49:534-542, 1995.
43. Klavora P et al: Rehabilitation of visual skills using the dynavision: a single case experimental design, *Can J Occup Ther* 62:37-43, 1995.
44. Klavora P, Warren M: Rehabilitation of visuomotor skills in post-stroke patients using the dynavision apparatus, *Percept Motor Skills* 86:23-30, 1998.

45. Leigh RJ, Brandt T: A reevaluation of the vestibulo-ocular reflex: new ideas of its purpose, properties, neural substrate and disorders, *Neurology* 43:1283-1295, 1993.
46. Leigh RJ, Zee DS: *Neurology of eye movements*, ed 2, Philadelphia, 1991, FA Davis.
47. Lepore FE: Disorders of ocular motility following head trauma, *Arch Neurol* 52:924-926, 1995.
48. Levine DH: Unawareness of visual and sensorimotor deficits: a hypothesis, *Brain Cogn* 13:233-281,1990.
49. Locher PJ, Bigelow DL: Visual exploratory activity of hemiplegic patients viewing the motor-free visual perception test, *Percept Mot Skills* 57:91-100, 1983.
50. Marx P: Supratentorial structures controlling oculomotor functions and their involvement in cases of stroke, *Eur Arch Psychiatry Clin Neurosci* 239:3-8, 1989.
51. Meinenberg V et al: Saccadic eye movement strategies in patients with homonymous hemianopia, *Ann Neurol* 9:537-544, 1981.
52. Mesulam MM: A cortical network for directed attention and unilateral neglect, *Ann Neurol* 10:305-325, 1981.
53. Mishkin M, Ungerleider LG, Macko KA: Object vision and spatial vision: two cortical pathways, *Trends Neurosci* 6:414-417, 1983.
54. Moore JC: *The visual system*, Course syllabus for OT Australia national CPE program, Melbourne, 1997, Australian Occupational Therapy Association.
55. Neger RE: The evaluation of diplopia in head trauma, *J Head Trauma Rehabil* 4:27-34, 1989.
56. Noton D, Stark L: Scanpaths in eye movements during pattern perception, *Science* 171:308-311, 1971.
57. Padula WV: *A behavioral vision approach for persons with physical disabilities*, Santa Anna, Calif, 1988, Optometric Extension Program Foundation.
58. Palmer T, Tzeng OJL: Cerebral asymmetry in visual attention, *Brain Cogn* 13:46-58, 1990.
59. Park M: Eye movements and positions. In Duane TD, editor: *Clinical ophthalmology: strabismus, refraction, the lens*, Philadelphia, 1981, Harper & Row.
60. Petersen SF, Robinson DL, Currie JN: Influence of lesions of parietal cortex on visual spatial attention in humans, *Exp Brain Res* 76:267-280, 1989.
61. Pommerenke K, Markowitsch HJ: Rehabilitation training of homonymous visual field defects in patients with postgeniculate damage of the visual system, *Restorative Neurol Neurosci* 1:47-63, 1989.
62. Posner MI, Rafal RD: Cognitive theories of attention and the rehabilitation of attentional deficits. In Meier MJ, Benton AL, Diller L, editors: *Neuropsychological rehabilitation*, New York, 1987, Guilford Press.
63. Post RB, Leibowitz HW: Two modes of processing visual information: implications for assessing visual impairment, *Am J Optom Physiol Opt* 63:94-96, 1986.
64. Ramachandran VS, Blakeslee S: *Phantoms in the brain: probing the mysteries of the human mind*, New York,1998, William Morrow.
65. Rapesak SZ et al: Selective attention in hemispatial neglect, *Arch Neurol* 46:178-182, 1989.
66. Ratcliff G, Ross JE: Visual perception and perceptual disorder, *Br Med Bull* 37:181-186, 1981.
67. Reuter-Lorenz PA, Kinsbourne M: Hemispheric control of spatial attention, *Brain Cogn* 12:240-266, 1990.
68. Robinson DL, Petersen SE: The pulvinar and visual salience, *Trends Neurosci* 15:127-132, 1992.
69. Ron S, Gur S: Gaze and eye movement disorders, *Curr Opin Neurol Neurosurg* 5:711-715, 1992.
70. Ron S et al: Eye movements in brain damaged patients, *Scand J Rehabil Med* 10:39-44, 1978.
71. Safran AB, Landis T: Plasticity in the adult visual cortex: implications for the diagnosis of visual field defects and visual rehabilitation, *Curr Opin Ophthalmol* 7:53-64, 1996.
72. Scheiman M: *Understanding and managing vision deficits: a guide for occupational therapists*, Thorofare NJ, 1997, Slack.
73. Schuchard RA: Adaptation to macular scotomas in persons with low vision, *Am J Occup Ther* 49:870-876, 1995.
74. Simon RP, Aminoff MJ, Greenberg DA: Disturbances of vision. In *Clinical neurology*, Norwalk, Conn, 1989, Appleton & Lange.
75. Spier PA et al: Visual neglect during intracarotid amobarbital testing, *Neurology* 40:1600-1606, 1990.
76. Sterk CC: The conservative management of diplopia. In Sanders EACM, DeKeizer RJW, Zee DS, editors: *Eye movement disorders*, Boston, 1987, Martinus Nijhoff/Dr W Junk Publishers.
77. Toglia J: Generalization of treatment: a multicontext approach to cognitive perceptual impairment in adults with brain injury, *Am J Occup Ther* 45:505-516, 1991.
78. Trobe JD et al: Confrontation visual field techniques in the detection of anterior visual pathway lesions, *Ann Neurol* 10:28-34, 1981.
79. Tyler HR: Defective stimulus exploration in aphasic patients, *Neurology* 19:105-112, 1969.
80. Van Vliet AGM: Beside examination. In Sanders EACM, De Keizer RJW, Zee DS, editors: *Eye movement disorders*, Boston, 1987, Martinus Nijhoff/Dr W Junk Publishers.
81. Von Noorden GK: Paralytic strabismus. In *Binocular vision and ocular motility: theory and management of strabismus*, ed 3, St Louis, 1985, Mosby.
82. Warren M: *Brain injury visual assessment battery for adults test manual*, Lenexa, Kan, 1998, visAbilities Rehab Services.
83. Warren M: A hierarchical model for evaluation and treatment of visual perceptual dysfunction in adult acquired brain injury. I, II, *Am J Occup Ther* 47:42-66, 1993.
84. Warren M: Identification of visual scanning deficits in adults after cerebrovascular accident, *Am J Occup Ther* 44:391-399, 1990.
85. Warren M: *Prereading and writing exercises for persons with macular scotomas*, Lenexa, Kan, 1996, visAbilities Rehab Services.
86. Warren M: Visuospatial skills: assessment and intervention strategies. In Royeen CB, editor: *AOTA self study series: cognitive rehabilitation*, Rockville, Md, 1994, American Occupational Therapy Association.
87. Watson G, Baldesare J, Whittaker S: The validity and clinical uses of the Pepper Visual Skills for Reading Test, *J Visual Impair Blind* 84:119-123, 1990.
88. Weinberg J et al: Visual scanning training effect on reading-related tasks in acquired right brain damage, *Arch Phys Med Rehabil* 60(11):491-496, 1979.
89. Weintraub S, Mesulam MM: Visual hemispatial inattention: stimulus parameters and exploratory strategies, *J Neurol Neurosurg Psychiatry* 51:1481-1488, 1988.
90. Winckelgren I: How the brain "sees" borders where there are none, *Science* 256:1520-1521, 1992.
91. *World Health Organization: International classification of impairments, disabilities and handicaps*, Geneva, 1980, WHO.
92. Wright V, Watson G: *Learn to use your vision for reading workbook. LUV reading series*, Trooper, Pa, 1995, Homer Printing.
93. Yarbus AL: Eye movements during perception of complex objects. In Yarbus AL: *Eye movements and vision*, New York, 1967, Plenum Press.
94. Zangemeister WH et al: Eye head coordination in homonymous hemianopsia, *J Neurol* 226:243-254, 1982.
95. Zihl J: Eye movement patterns in hemianopic dyslexia, *Brain* 118:891-912, 1995.
96. Zihl J: Rehabilitation of visual impairments in patients with brain damage. In Kooijan Ac et al, editors: *Low vision: research and new development in rehabilitation*, Amsterdam, 1994, IOS Press.
97. Zihl J: Visual scanning behavior in patients with homonymous hemianopia, *Neuropsychologia* 33:287-303, 1995.

CHAPTER 25

Evaluation of Sensation and Treatment of Sensory Dysfunction

MEENAKSHI B. IYER
LORRAINE WILLIAMS PEDRETTI

KEY TERMS

Somatosensory systems
Sensory feedback
Feedforward control
Tactile (touch) sensation
Two-point discrimination
Sensation
Sensibility
Dermatome
Pressure sensation
Light touch sensation
Thermal sensation
Superficial pain sensation
Olfactory sensation
Hyposmia
Anosmia
Parosmia
Gustatory sensation
Proprioception
Kinesthesia
Anesthesia
Paresthesia
Hypesthesia
Hyperesthesia
Analgesia
Hypalgesia
Sensory reeducation
Compensatory treatment
Remedial treatment
Dysesthesia
Desensitization

LEARNING OBJECTIVES

After studying this chapter the student or practitioner will be able to do the following:
1. Define the keywords listed above.
2. Describe the normal function of sensation.
3. Describe the role of sensation in motor performance and the effects of sensory loss on motor performance.
4. Define the role of feedback and feedforward systems in motor performance.
5. Identify dysfunctions in which sensory assessment is indicated.
6. Describe the sensory modalities included in this chapter.
7. List the purposes of sensory assessment.
8. List three methods of occluding vision during the sensory test.
9. Describe the variability of normal responses in sensory testing.
10. Administer a sensory assessment using procedures described in this chapter.
11. Differentiate central nervous system disorders from peripheral nervous system sensory disorders.
12. Describe compensatory and remedial sensory reeducation programs.

This chapter is concerned with **somatosensory systems** of touch (tactile), deep pressure, pain, proprioception, and thermal sensation, and the special senses of taste and smell. Vision is discussed in Chapter 24.

Sensory systems allow us to enjoy life, warn us of danger, and cause discomfort in the form of pain. Sensory information from the environment is received by peripheral receptors and transmitted to the central nervous system (CNS) via the peripheral and spinal nerves. Almost all sensory information reaching the cerebral cortex is processed through the thalamus. The exception is olfaction, in which information is transmitted directly to the primitive cortex of the medial temporal lobe, *then* via the thalamus to the orbitofrontal cortex. Sensory information is used for sensory perception, cognitive processing, guidance of movement, and maintenance of arousal. Although sensation is a conscious experience, not all sensation is perceived (interpreted) before the production of a motor response. For example, the withdrawal of the hand from a hot object is driven by an automatic motor response before the perception that the object is hot occurs.[24] Diverse sensory systems have in common their ability to extract the same kinds of information from a sensory stimulus. That is, each system carries information about modality (e.g., touch, pain, or taste) and the intensity, duration, and location of the stimulus.[24]

SENSATION AND MOTOR PERFORMANCE

The external environment is represented internally through sensation. From this internal representation of the outside world, the information necessary to guide movement is derived (see Chapter 32).[17] Motor performance in purposeful activity is profoundly dependent on the continuous inflow of sensory information.[17,27] Sensory information is used to manage effective movement and to correct errors in movement through feedback and feedforward mechanisms.[17,26]

Feedback

Sensory feedback about the effectiveness of motor acts is received through the various sensory systems. Sensations derived from the ongoing movement are sent back to the CNS, where a comparison is made between intended action and what is actually happening. Most movements, such as dressing, eating, or bathing, depend on feedback from muscle spindles, joint receptors, and cutaneous receptors for sensory guidance. The

descending command for motor performance is compared with the incoming sensory information about the movements as they occur. When bathing, for example, if the soap slips from the hand, the individual makes immediate adjustments to grasp it tighter. Generally, sensory feedback is used during the performance of goal-directed movements for guiding the direction, force, and accuracy of movement. Knowledge of the outcome of actions can also serve as feedback. For example, if a wrong word or misspelling occurs when writing, visual feedback signals that an incorrect motor response has been made. This sensory information is then processed in the CNS, and a revision of the motor response is planned and executed. Feedback can be intrinsic (i.e., sensations arising from the body during movement) or extrinsic (e.g., information about effectiveness or outcome of motor performance from a therapist or teacher). Intrinsic feedback control is based on information from peripheral sense organs and is used primarily during postural adjustments and motor performance under sensory guidance because feedback processes operate relatively slowly.[17,26]

Feedforward

Feedforward control is used for rapid or ballistic movements that are planned in advance. Because of their ballistic nature, these movements cannot be altered by sensory feedback once initiated. It is not that the movement is performed without *any* sensory input. The movement was planned based on sensory information obtained before the movement was initiated.[17] For example, skiing is initiated with feedforward control. Anticipating the sensory experience is necessary to plan the motor act of descending the ski run. The slope of the ski run, the rate of speed of descent, potential obstacles, and the path to be taken must be considered before the descent is initiated. This anticipation results in assuming a specific posture, setting muscles, initiating the motion, making the appropriate balance responses, and directing movement along a given path toward the destination. As the motor act is being executed, the feedback system operates continuously to correct errors in the intended movement. The feedforward system operates intermittently to anticipate or reevaluate the required action and to plan movement responses.[17,26]

Effects of Sensory Loss on Movement

Proprioception and **tactile sensation** are essential for feedback and feedforward control systems. A schematic representation of the sensory distribution of major peripheral nerves and dermatomes corresponding to spinal segments is shown in Fig. 25-1. Patients with severe sensory loss as a result of peripheral neuropathies have major motor performance deficits because of the

Dr. A. Lee Dellon is gratefully acknowledged for reviewing this chapter.

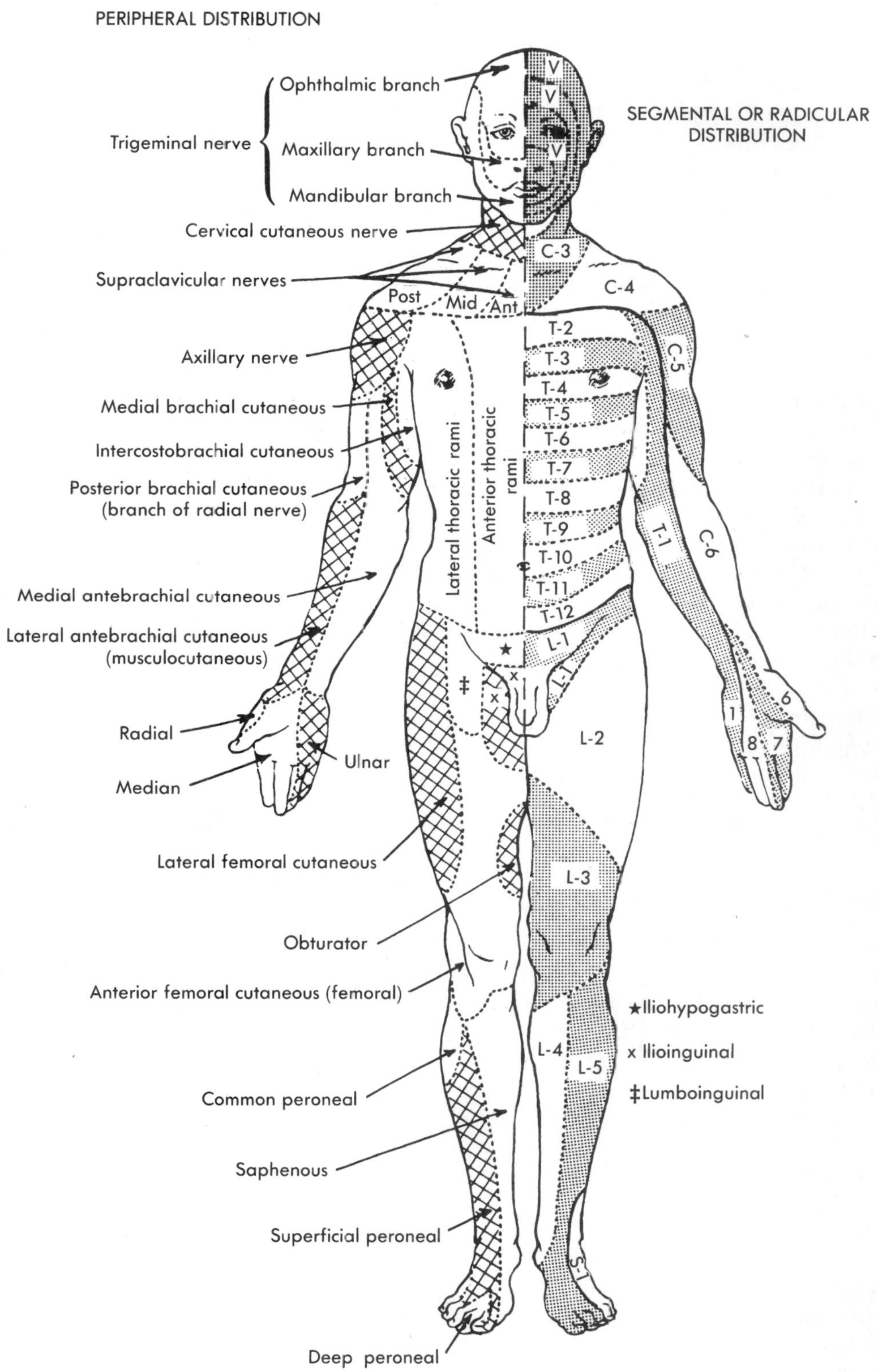
PERIPHERAL DISTRIBUTION
SEGMENTAL OR RADICULAR DISTRIBUTION
Trigeminal nerve
Ophthalmic branch
Maxillary branch
Mandibular branch
Cervical cutaneous nerve
Supraclavicular nerves
Post
Mid
Ant
Axillary nerve
Medial brachial cutaneous
Intercostobrachial cutaneous
Posterior brachial cutaneous (branch of radial nerve)
Medial antebrachial cutaneous
Lateral antebrachial cutaneous (musculocutaneous)
Radial
Median
Ulnar
Lateral thoracic rami
Anterior thoracic rami
Lateral femoral cutaneous
Obturator
Anterior femoral cutaneous (femoral)
Common peroneal
Saphenous
Superficial peroneal
Deep peroneal
V
V
V
C-3
C-4
C-5
C-6
T-1
T-2
T-3
T-4
T-5
T-6
T-7
T-8
T-9
T-10
T-11
T-12
L-1
L-2
L-3
L-4
L-5
S-1
1
6
7
8
★Iliohypogastric
x Ilioinguinal
‡Lumboinguinal

FIG. 25-1

A, Sensory distribution of major peripheral nerves and dermatomes corresponding to spinal cord segments, anterior view. (From Chusid JG: *Correlative neuroanatomy and functional neurology*, ed 19, Los Altos, Calif, 1985, Lange Medical Publications.)

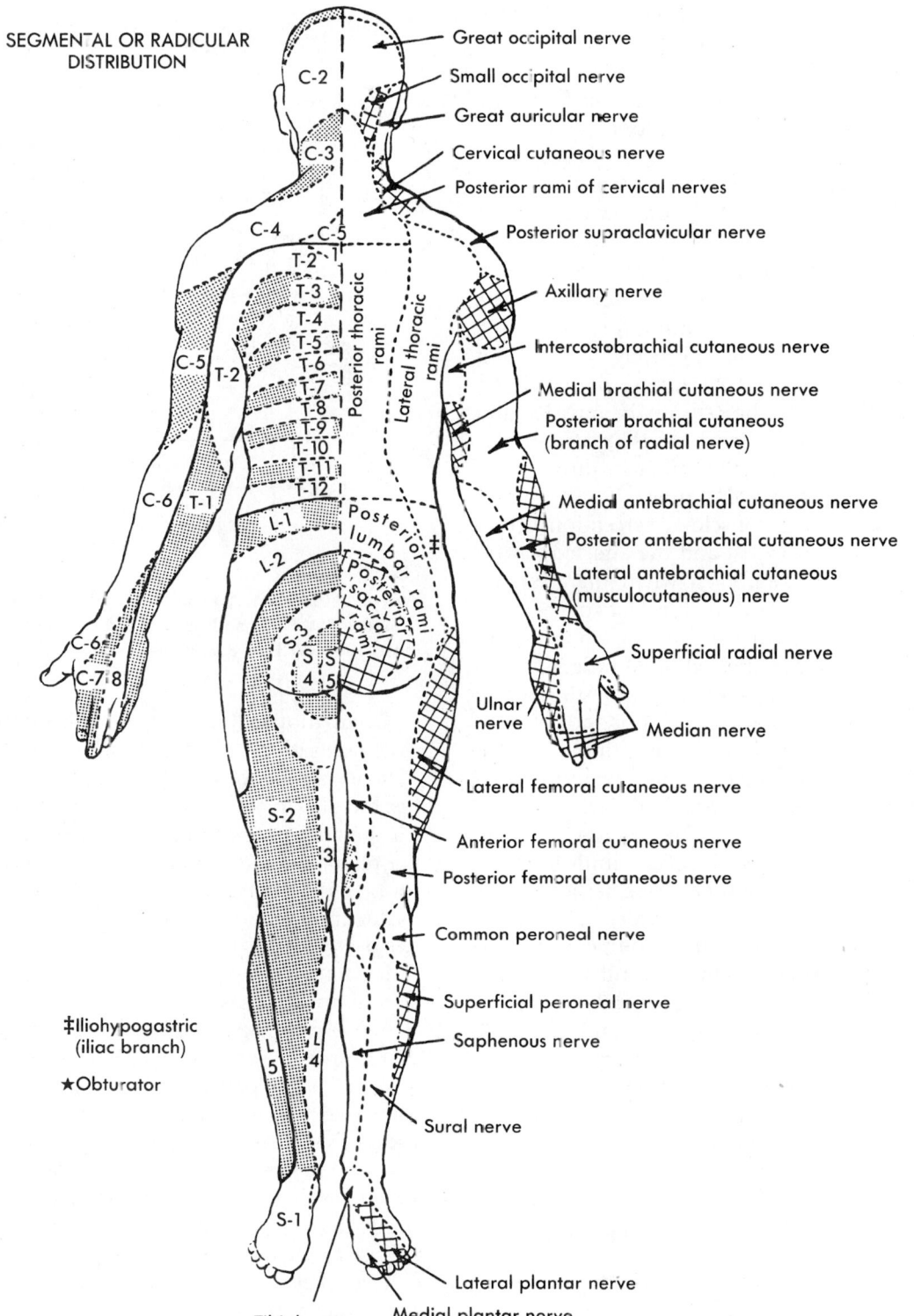

SEGMENTAL OR RADICULAR DISTRIBUTION

PERIPHERAL DISTRIBUTION

Great occipital nerve

Small occipital nerve

Great auricular nerve

Cervical cutaneous nerve

Posterior rami of cervical nerves

Posterior supraclavicular nerve

Axillary nerve

Intercostobrachial cutaneous nerve

Medial brachial cutaneous nerve

Posterior brachial cutaneous (branch of radial nerve)

Medial antebrachial cutaneous nerve

Posterior antebrachial cutaneous nerve

Lateral antebrachial cutaneous (musculocutaneous) nerve

Superficial radial nerve

Ulnar nerve

Median nerve

Lateral femoral cutaneous nerve

Anterior femoral cutaneous nerve

Posterior femoral cutaneous nerve

Common peroneal nerve

Superficial peroneal nerve

Saphenous nerve

‡Iliohypogastric (iliac branch)

★Obturator

Sural nerve

Lateral plantar nerve

Medial plantar nerve

Tibial nerve

FIG. 25-1 cont'd

B, Sensory distribution, posterior view.

425

absence of feedback control.[28] Those with tactile and proprioceptive dysfunction cannot sense the position and motion of joints or sense contact with objects, resulting in difficulties in the performance of the simplest activities of daily living (ADL). When patients who have sensory neuropathies with sensory loss but normal muscle strength are asked to move their fingers with their eyes closed, they can initially perform the movement in a feedforward mode. With time, however, their performance degrades because of the absence of sensory guidance. Vision can compensate for the loss of tactile and proprioceptive sensation, but the defects in feedback and feedforward control limit even the patient's ability to use vision effectively. The patient cannot sense the resistance of the surface on which the hand is moving or sense the tension in muscles and tendons. As a result, jerky movements occur because visual feedback is slow and the errors in direction of movement cannot be corrected in time.[17]

Without sensation the conscious perception of peripheral sensory stimuli is lost and the affected part(s) may be virtually paralyzed, even when there is adequate recovery of muscle function.[11] Patients with hemiplegia resulting from cerebrovascular accident (CVA) tend not to use the affected hand unless proprioception is intact and **two-point discrimination** at the fingertip is less than 1 cm apart, which is indicative of good discriminative sensation. The minimum distances for discrimination of two-point sensation vary from one part of the body to another (Fig. 25-2).[4] A test for two-point discrimination is described in Chapter 44. Even slight sensory deficits limit function of the affected hand because there are persistent problems in performing fine motor activities. The highly motivated patient may use visual compensation to engage the affected upper extremity in bilateral activities.[34] Adaptive motor behavior frequently occurs in response to external sensory stimuli, and adequate sensation is essential for effective movement. Therefore an understanding of the patient's sensory status is necessary to appreciate fully the causes of the apparent motor dysfunction and to plan appropriate treatment goals and methods.

PRINCIPLES OF SENSORY EVALUATION

The terms *sensation* and *sensibility* refer to the reception, transmission, and interpretation of sensory stimuli. These terms are sometimes used interchangeably, or they may be differentiated.[7,11,23] Callahan[7] defined **sensation** as the stimuli conveyed to the central interpretive centers by the afferent nerves and **sensibility** as the ability to perceive or interpret sensory stimuli.[7] For the purposes of this chapter, the term *sensation* will be used to refer to the ability to identify the sensory modality and its intensity and location.

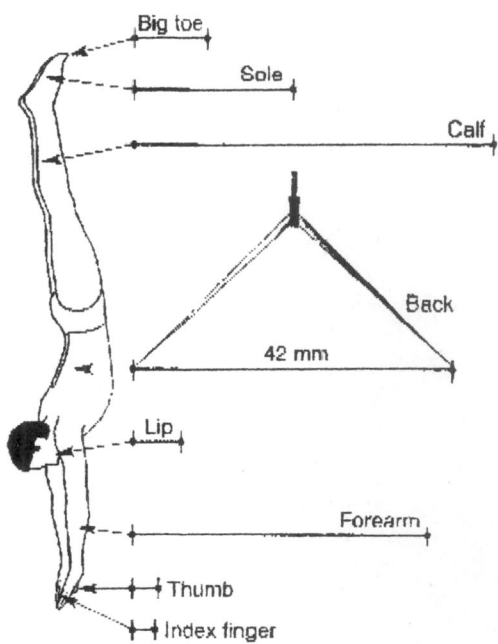

FIG. 25-2

Two-point discrimination on the body surface. (From Bear MS, Connors BW, Paradiso MA: *Neuroscience, exploring the brain,* Baltimore, 1996, Williams & Wilkins.)

Occupational therapy (OT) practitioners frequently assess sensation. It is important not only to assess the patient's ability to recognize a touch or pinprick stimulus, but also to determine whether sensation is adequate for the performance of ADL.[7] Any patient with CNS or peripheral nervous system (PNS) dysfunction should be routinely evaluated for sensory loss. Patients with CNS dysfunction tend to show loss of many sensory modalities over generalized areas, whereas those with PNS disorders tend to have loss of specific sensory modalities in circumscribed areas.

Sensory testing may also be indicated in (1) patients with burns, in whom sensory receptors in the skin are destroyed; (2) patients who have arthritis, in whom joint swelling may cause compression of a peripheral nerve; (3) patients with traumatic hand and upper extremity injuries, in whom skin, muscles, tendons, ligaments, and nerves may be involved; and (4) elderly individuals, who may show age-related changes in response to sensory stimuli.[1,19,21]

Examples of other diagnoses that require sensory testing are peripheral nerve injuries and diseases, spinal cord injuries and diseases, brain injuries and diseases, and fractures. With fractures, sensory testing may help to determine if there is peripheral nerve involvement.

Sensory Supply to Specific Areas

The sensory distribution of the major peripheral nerves of the body and limbs is shown in Fig. 25-1. In assessment of peripheral nerve dysfunction, it is important to test the area supplied by the nerve or nerves that are affected. The sensory distribution of the **dermatomes** that correspond to spinal cord segments is also shown in Fig. 25-1. A dermatome is the area of the skin supplied by one spinal dorsal root and its spinal nerve. Adjacent dermatomes overlap more for touch, pressure, and vibration than for pain and temperature. This means that assessment of pain and temperature will provide a better determination of spinal nerve injury. Testing of patients with spinal cord injury or disease according to this dermatomal distribution is important to determine the level or levels of spinal cord lesion and any sparing of spinal cord function.

Purposes of Testing

By performing a sensory test, the therapist can carefully outline areas of intact, impaired, or absent sensation. This information is sometimes of diagnostic or prognostic value to the physician and provides a baseline for progress. The sensory assessment can also be used to determine the need to teach the patient how to protect against injury, how to use compensatory techniques (such as visual guidance for movement during activities), and whether a sensory or sensorimotor retraining program is feasible. Sensory loss may affect the use of splints and braces because the patient may be unaware of pressure points during wear. Sensory loss may also affect controlled use of a dynamic splint, which requires good sensory feedback for effective operation. Consequently, the patient should be taught safety guidelines in the use of splints, particularly the need to check the insensitive body parts for early signs of injury.

Tests of sensory function do not always accurately predict functional use of the hand. Moberg, cited by Dellon,[11] studied patients with median nerve injury to determine whether a correlation existed between results of clinical sensory tests and hand function. He used a series of everyday activities that required several types of grip and prehension and a test of picking up small objects and placing them in a container (Moberg Picking Up Test) to evaluate hand function. Moberg concluded that tests of touch, pain, temperature, and vibration did not correlate with hand function. There was some correlation between two-point discrimination and hand function.[11] One of the reasons for the finding may be that the test did not include a test of proprioceptive function. Nevertheless, Moberg's work is important to OT because it underscores a primary purpose and principle of OT practice: to evaluate function or performance. Thus it is important for the occupational therapist not only to evaluate the sensory modalities, but also to evaluate function. The therapist can use one of several hand function tests to observe hand use under simulated conditions. More reliably still, the therapist

can observe for spontaneous use of the affected part(s) in bilateral ADL.

Occlusion of Vision During Testing

Almost all of the sensory tests described in this chapter require that the patient's vision be occluded so that the test stimuli cannot be seen. The use of a blindfold and keeping the eyes shut are the least desirable methods of occluding vision. A blindfold can be a source of sensory distraction and can provoke anxiety in patients with sensory, perceptual, and balance disturbances.[15] Additionally, many individuals with CNS dysfunction have difficulty maintaining eye closure because of apraxia and motor impersistence.

There are several alternative methods for occluding vision. As shown later with actual tests, a small screen made by suspending a curtain between two posts is convenient and effective. If such a device cannot be constructed, something similar can be made by folding in the sides of a corrugated box and draping a cloth over one side (Fig. 25-3, *A*), or a file folder can be held over the area being tested (Fig. 25-3, *B*). Sensory testing shields are also commercially available (Fig. 25-4).[32]

TESTS FOR SENSATION

The following tests are based on evaluation tools of clinical neurology and are designed to test gross sensation in adults with CNS or PNS dysfunction.[5,25] The reference list includes additional sensory tests and tests of discrete sensation.[7,11,36] Tests of moving touch, constant touch, vibration sense, and two-point discrimination are described in Chapter 44. Tests for discriminative tactile perception are described in Chapter 26.

General Procedure

Testing should take place in a quiet and nondistracting environment. Extraneous noises from the examiner or testing instruments should be minimized. Tests should always be administered to the analogous limb on the normal side if the patient has unilateral dysfunction, to establish a standard of accuracy for the individual patient and to assure that directions for test administration are understood. The parts to be tested should be exposed and positioned comfortably. In some instances, the examiner will have to support the part manually or with therapy putty, sandbags, or other cushioning material.[7] It is important for the examiner (E) to orient the subject (S) to the test procedures and to the rationale for administering the tests. E should be sure that S understands how to respond. S's vision can be occluded by shielding the parts being tested from view.

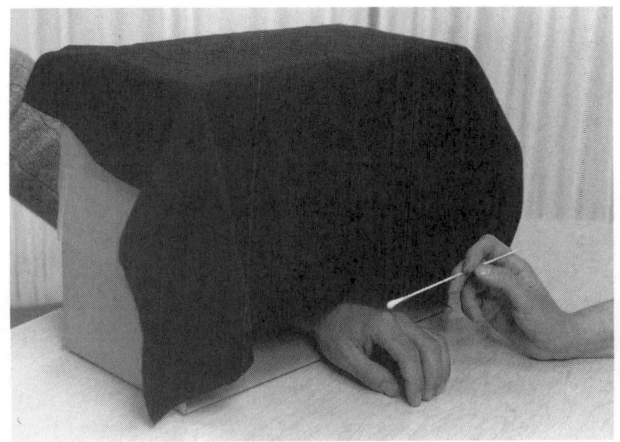

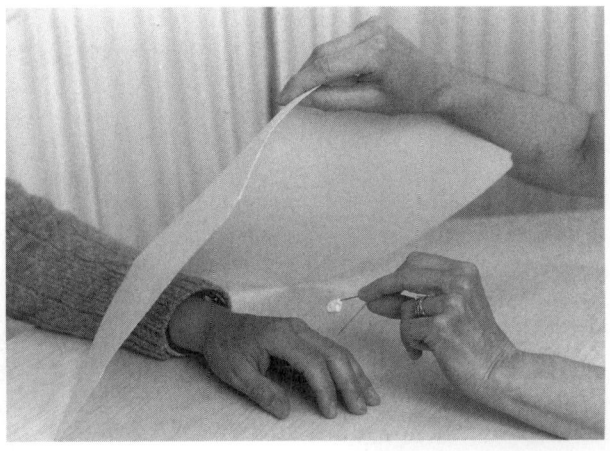

A

B

FIG. 25-3
A, Device for occluding vision during sensory testing: box with cloth drape. **B,** File folder used to occlude vision during sensory testing.

Light Touch and Pressure Sensation

Tactile sensitivity is critical to the performance of all ADL. For example, knowing an object is in the hand or feeling clothes on the body and knowing whether they are correctly adjusted is dependent on intact touch sensitivity. **Pressure sensation** is also important in ADL because it is continuously received in activities such as sitting, pushing drawers and doors, crossing the knees, wearing belts and collars, and a host of other activities that stimulate pressure receptors. It is possible for a patient to have intact pressure sensation if touch is impaired or absent because pressure receptors are in subcutaneous and deeper tissue and touch receptors are in the superficial layers of the skin. Touch sensation is necessary for fine discriminative activities, and pressure is a protective sensation because it warns of deep pressure or repetitive pressure that can lead to injury.[7] If touch sensation is impaired, pressure sensation can aid in performance of ADL and substitute for touch feedback in some activities.

Various tools have been used to apply stimuli for the light touch and pressure tests. These include a cotton ball, cotton swab, fingertip, or pencil eraser. All of these objects can provide a gross or cursory evaluation of **light touch sensation** and pressure sensation. More discrete and accurate testing of cutaneous pressure thresholds of light touch to deep pressure can be performed by using the Semmes-Weinstein Monofilaments described in Chapter 44[11,35] or the Pressure Specified Sensory Device.[12]

Test for Light Touch Sensation[5,7,18,24]

PURPOSE. To determine S's ability to recognize and localize light touch stimuli.

LIMITATIONS. Patients with receptive aphasia cannot be validly tested.

MATERIALS. A screen or manila folder to occlude vision; a cotton swab.

CONDITIONS. A nondistracting environment in which S is seated at a narrow table. The test may also be conducted at the bedside or in a wheelchair. The affected hand and forearm should be supported comfortably on the table. E sits opposite S.

METHOD. S's hand and forearm are hidden from S's view by placing them under the screen or by E holding a manila folder over them. The hand and forearm are touched lightly with a cotton swab at random locations, covering the area supplied by each peripheral nerve and each dermatome. A few trial stimuli should be administered while S is watching, to be sure that S understands the procedure and how to respond. The test should be administered on an uninvolved area first to establish a standard. If spasticity is a problem, E may support the hand on the dorsal surface and hold the thumb in radial abduction and extension to secure relaxation of the fingers for palmar testing (Fig. 25-5, which also shows the screen mentioned earlier).

RESPONSES. After each stimulus, E asks S if S was touched (recognition). S responds by nodding or saying yes or no. The screen is lifted or the folder is removed after each stimulus, and S is asked to point to the place where S was touched, using the unaffected hand if possible. Localization responses are more accurate if S is allowed to use vision.[4] If this cannot be done, S is asked to describe the location and E should select locations that are easy to name (e.g., "knuckle of middle finger").

SCORING. On the scoring chart E marks a "plus" (+) for the ability to recognize and localize touch

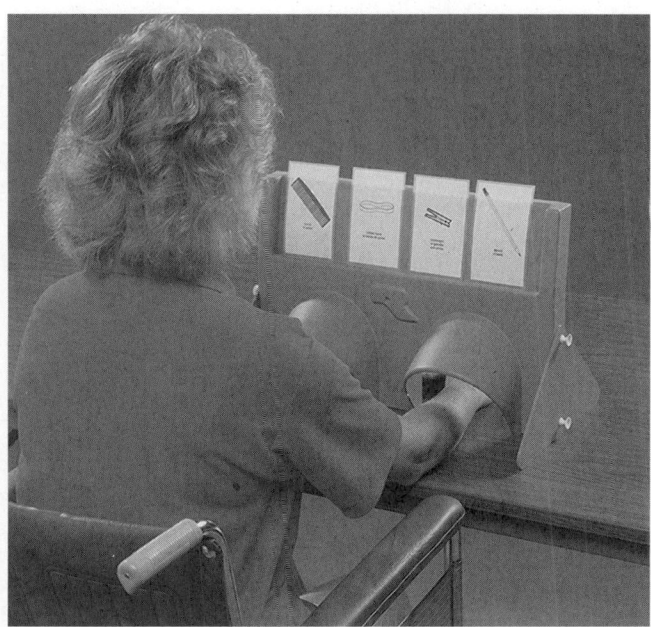

FIG. 25-4
Sensory testing shield. (From Smith & Nephew, Germantown, Wis.)

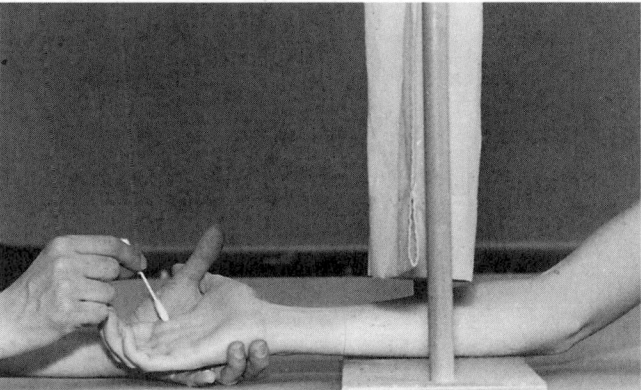

FIG. 25-5
Test for light touch and pressure sensation.

stimuli, a "minus" (−) for the ability to recognize only, and a "zero" (0) for an inability to recognize or localize a stimulus (Fig. 25-6).

INTERPRETATION OF RESULTS Deviations of $^3/_5$ to $1^1/_5$ inches (1.5 to 3 cm) from the point of application of the stimulus are normal for localization of stimuli, depending on the area of the hand or arm touched. Responses should be more accurate on the hand than on the forearm and more accurate on the forearm than on the upper arm. The ability to recognize and localize touch indicates intact sensation. The ability to recognize but not localize touch stimuli indicates sensory impairment, and an inability to recognize or localize touch stimuli means touch sensation is absent.

Test for Pressure Sensation

Pressure sensitivity may be tested as described for light touch, except that E should press hard enough with the cotton swab to dent and blanch the skin. If light touch sensitivity is severely impaired or absent, pressure sensitivity may be intact and may provide important sensory feedback, which can enhance function. Normally, pressure stimuli can be localized on the hand from 2.44 to 2.83 mg of pressure (Fig. 25-5).[35]

Thermal Sensation

Thermal sensation is another of the protective sensory modalities.[6] The ability to detect temperatures is essen-

tial for the prevention of injury in many ADL, such as bathing, cooking, and ironing. The ability to detect temperature also contributes to the enjoyment of food and to the detection of uncomfortable environmental temperatures. If the patient lacks accurate thermal discrimination, it will be necessary to teach precautions against injury and to structure ADL to prevent burns. As in the other sensory tests, the results can serve as a baseline for progress and changes in sensory status may be used to measure recovery or degeneration, depending on the diagnosis.

Techniques such as touching the skin with test tubes that are filled with hot and cold water, immersing the fingers or hand in hot or cold water, or touching small hot or cold compresses to the area being tested have been used in tests for thermal sensation. Another method is the Hot/Cold Discrimination Kit by Rolyan* (Fig. 25-7).[32] This kit includes two metal temperature probes with a thermometer at the head of each, two thermal cups, and a single-stem thermometer. One thermal cup is filled with ice and water, and the other is filled with hot tap water. The single thermometer is inserted into the thermal cup. When the desired temperature is reached, the probe is inserted into the thermal cup and allowed to reach the desired testing temperature. The metal probes, which look much like test tubes, are then put in contact with the skin surface to be tested. This kit makes it possible to control temperatures more precisely and to maintain constant temperature stimuli for the duration of the test.[32]

Test for Thermal Sensation[5,9,13,18]

PURPOSE. To determine S's ability to discriminate between extremes of hot and cold and to detect variations in temperature at four levels.

---

*Smith & Nephew, Inc., One Quality Drive, PO Box 1005, Germantown, Wis.

FORM FOR RECORDING SCORES ON TESTS OF SENSATION

Department of Occupational Therapy

Name_____ Age_____ Sex_____

Diagnosis_____ Disability_____

Date_____

TEST FOR LIGHT TOUCH SENSITIVITY	LEFT	RIGHT

Use a cotton swab and touch random locations on anterior and posterior surfaces.
Indicate on diagram:
  Intact: +
  Impaired: −
  Absent: 0
	Anterior
	
	Posterior
		Anterior
		
		Posterior

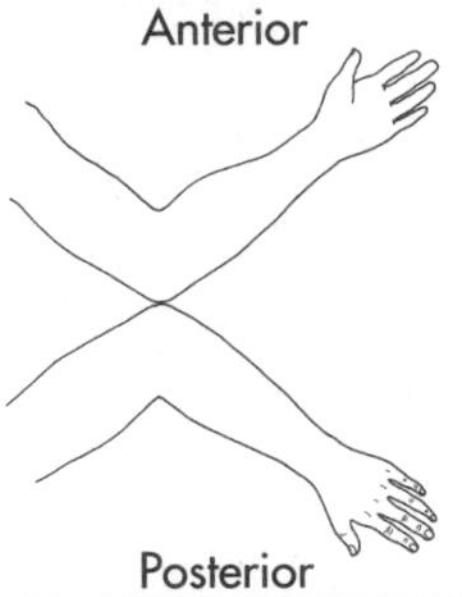

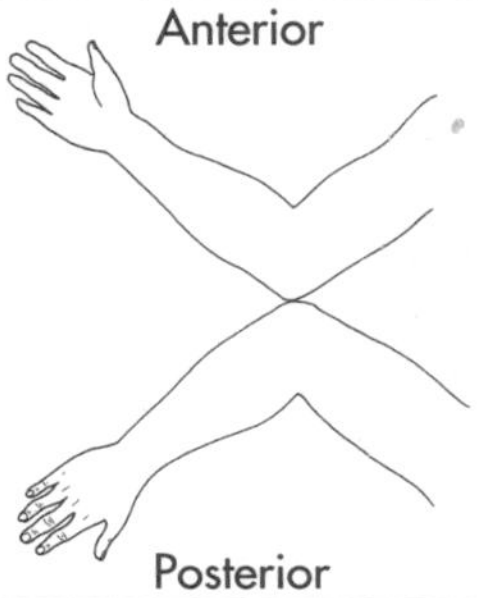

TEST FOR PRESSURE SENSITIVITY	LEFT	RIGHT

Use a cotton swab and press random locations on anterior and posterior surfaces.
Indicate on diagram:
  Intact: +
  Impaired: −
  Absent: 0
	Anterior
	
	Posterior
		Anterior
		
		Posterior

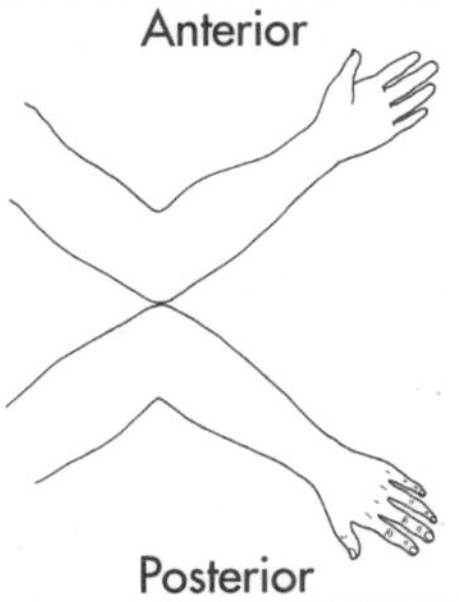

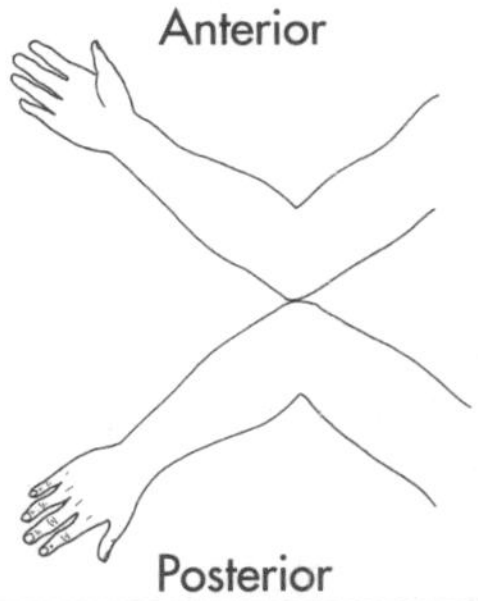

TEST FOR SUPERFICIAL PAIN	LEFT	RIGHT

Use a large safety pin and touch random locations with sharp and dull ends on anterior and posterior surfaces.
Indicate on diagram:
  Sharp:
    Correct response   +S
    Sharp reported dull   D
    No response   −S
  Dull:
    Correct response   +D
    Dull reported sharp   S
    No response   −D
	Anterior
	
	Posterior
		Anterior
		
		Posterior

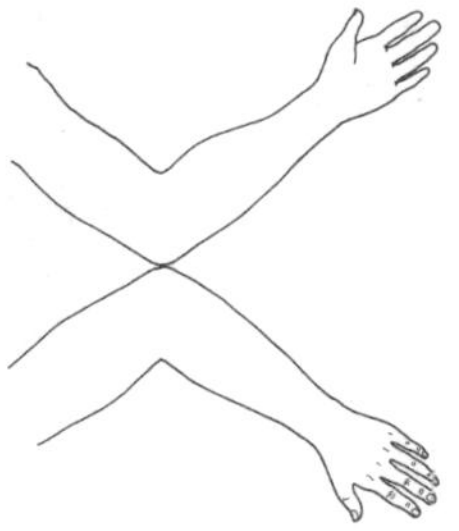

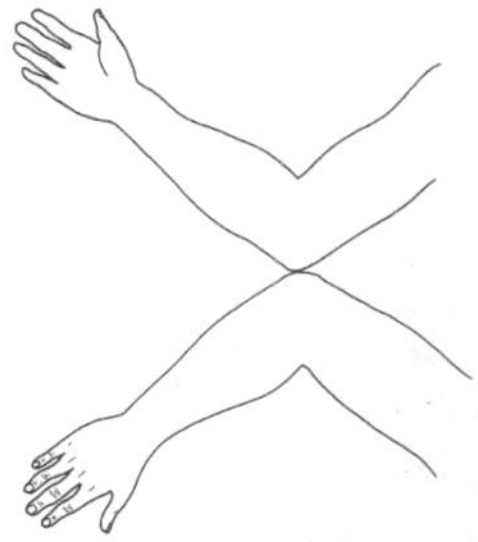

Remarks: _____

FIG. 25-6

Form for recording scores on tests of light touch, pressure, and superficial pain sensation.

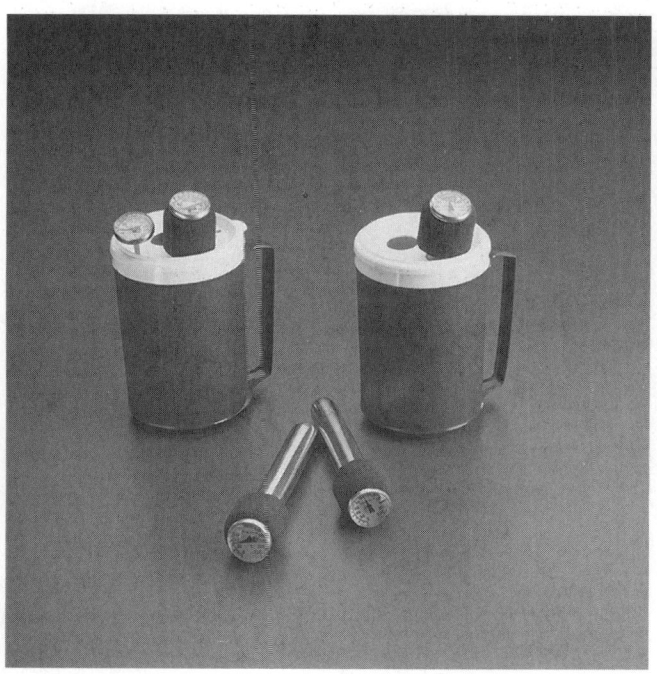

FIG. 25-7
Hot/cold discrimination kit. (From Smith & Nephew, Germantown, Wis.)

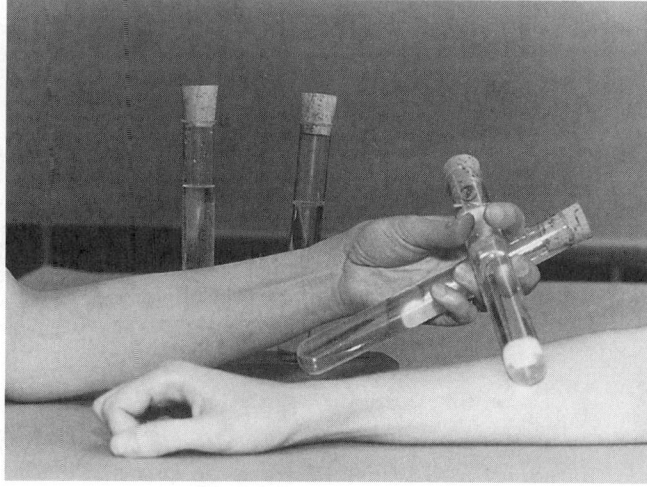

FIG. 25-8
Test for thermal sensation.

LIMITATIONS. Persons with receptive aphasia cannot be validly tested. It is difficult to control water temperature very accurately, and the temperature may change during the administration of the test. The results are subjective and may only detect ability to discriminate gross differences in temperature.

MATERIALS. Four test tubes (3/4-inch or 2-cm diameter) with stoppers; hot, warm, tepid, and cold water.

CONDITIONS. A nondistracting environment in which S is seated comfortably at a table with both the hand and forearm supported on a table, or alternative positioning described for previous tests.

METHOD
SUBTEST I. Two test tubes are used, one filled with cold water (45° F or 7° C) and one with hot water (110° F or 43° C). Extreme temperatures should not be used, because they can stimulate the pain receptors. Stoppers are placed in tubes. E touches the sides of the test tubes to the skin surfaces to be tested in random order and at random locations, being sure to cover the test area thoroughly (Fig. 25-8).
SUBTEST II. Four test tubes are used, one filled with cold water, one with tepid water, one with warm water, and one with hot water. E should color-code the stoppers as follows: yellow for hot, green for warm, orange for tepid, and red for cold. Place the stoppers in the tubes. E asks S to touch or hold test tubes with the affected

hand(s) in random order. If S is unable to hold the tubes, E may touch each one to S's palm and fingertips.

RESPONSES
SUBTEST I. S responds "hot" or "cold" in response to each stimulus. If S is aphasic, E should work out an alternative nonverbal response before beginning the tests.
SUBTEST II. S is asked to arrange the test tubes on a table from the hottest to the coldest, in order from left to right. E checks the correctness of the order by color-coded stoppers and feeling tubes.

SCORING
SUBTEST I. (Fig. 25-9) E marks a "plus" (+) if the temperature is correctly identified and marks a "zero" (0) if S cannot distinguish hot from cold. Subtest II is not administered if S succeeds at subtest I (Fig. 25-9).
SUBTEST II. E marks the appropriate blanks on the form with a check and the appropriate letter to indicate S's responses.

INTERPRETATION OF RESULTS. Adults in normal health should be able to complete all items on this test successfully. The normal hand can detect temperatures 1° to 5° C apart.[7]

Superficial Pain Sensation

Pain is one of the protective sensations that makes the detection of potentially harmful stimuli to the skin and subcutaneous tissue possible.[7] The ability to detect painful stimuli is critical to avoiding injury during the performance of daily activities and the prevention of skin breakdown while wearing splints and braces and using wheelchairs, crutches, and other adaptive devices. In normal circumstances pain sensa-

FORM FOR RECORDING SCORES ON
TESTS OF THERMAL SENSITIVITY

Department of Occupational Therapy

Name_____ Age _____ Sex _____

Diagnosis/Disability _____

Date of Onset_____ Date of Test _____
_____

TEST FOR THERMAL SENSITIVITY

SUBTEST I.

Touch sides of hot and cold test tubes to skin surfaces in random order and at random locations. Record scores on diagrams for tests of arms and hands or list site tested and record scores in columns.

Test site (fill in location tested)   Score (+, 0)

Dates			

Use diagram to record scores on test of arms and hands

LEFT

Anterior

Posterior

RIGHT

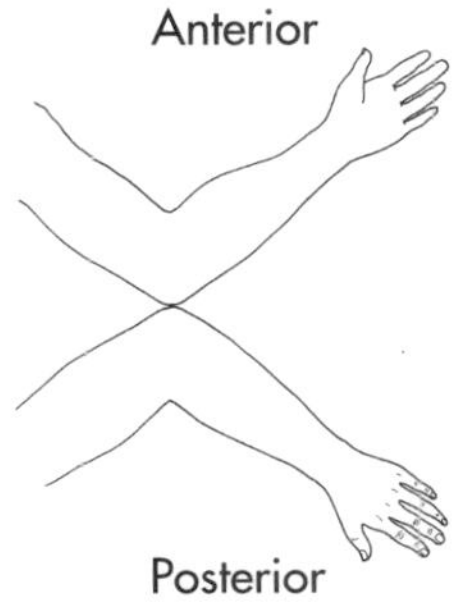

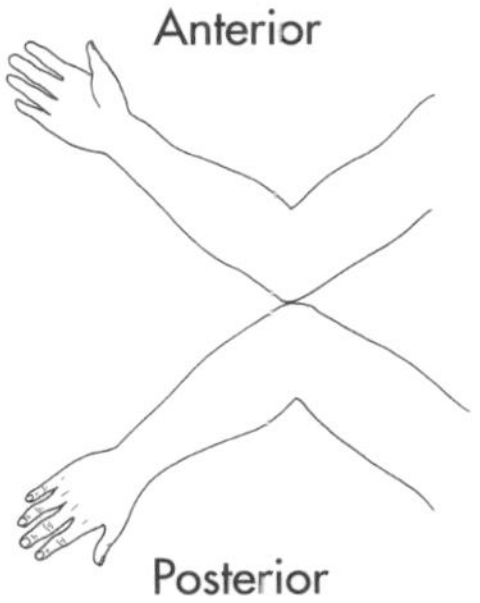

Anterior

Posterior

SUBTEST II.

Date _____   Date _____   Date _____

Arrange test tubes in correct order.   _____   _____   _____
Arrange test tubes in wrong order.   _____   _____   _____

Indicate arrangement of test tubes by filling in spaces below with H for hot, W for warm, T for tepid, and C for cold.

Date: _____   _____   _____   _____   _____

_____   _____   _____   _____   _____

_____   _____   _____   _____   _____

FIG. 25-9
Form for recording scores on the test for thermal sensation.

tion warns the individual to move quickly, as when withdrawing a finger from a hot surface. Pain sensation also signals the need to adjust the position of clothing that binds or to remove an offending article of apparel such as a shoe that is rubbing a blister on the foot. The patient who lacks the ability to detect such painful stimuli is more likely to be injured. If pain sensation is absent or impaired, it is important to teach sensory compensation and safety awareness in the treatment program.

The following test uses a safety pin to apply light pain stimuli. *A new safety pin should be used for each patient. The pin should be sterilized before testing and discarded after the test.* The examiner should be aware that atrophic skin is particularly susceptible to injury and that a pinprick stimulus, which would not break normal skin, could produce a tiny break in atrophic skin. Skin atrophy occurs after peripheral nerve injury. The interruption of nerve supply interferes with normal tissue nutrition and causes the atrophy.[7] If this possibility is a concern, the end of a straightened paper clip may be used for the test.

Test for Superficial Pain[5,18,25,27]

PURPOSE. To make a gross evaluation of superficial pain sensitivity.

LIMITATIONS. Persons with receptive aphasia cannot be validly tested. The pulp of the fingertips is relatively insensitive to a pinprick. Callused or toughened areas (e.g., the palms) are normally less sensitive to a pinprick than other areas. If S is fearful of a safety pin, the straightened paper clip may be used.

MATERIALS. The screen or a manila folder, to occlude S's vision; a large safety pin or straightened paper clip.

CONDITIONS. A nondistracting environment in which S is seated at a narrow table. The affected hand and forearm should be supported comfortably on the table. E sits opposite S on the other side of the table. If S cannot be positioned in this manner, the test may be administered while S is in bed or sitting in the wheelchair with his or her arms resting on a lap board.

METHOD. The hand and forearm to be tested are hidden from S's view by placing them under the screen or by E holding a manila folder over them. The affected hand and forearm are touched lightly at random locations, using sharp and dull stimuli in random order and at random speed. Each stimulus should be applied with the same degree of pressure (Fig. 25-10). It is important to apply stimuli to the area supplied by each peripheral nerve and each dermatome.[7] A few trial stimuli should be conducted with S watching, to be sure that S under-

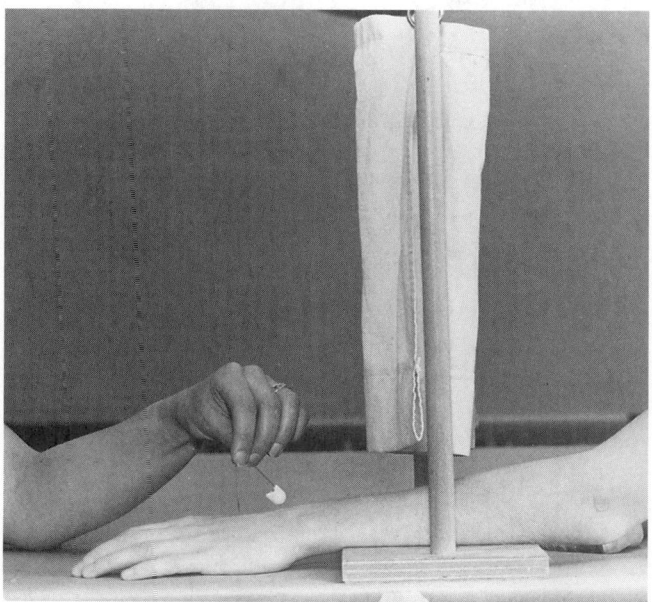

FIG. 25-10
Test for superficial pain sensation.

stands the test and knows how to respond. If spasticity is a problem, E may support the hand on the dorsal surface and hold the thumb in radial abduction and extension to secure relaxation for palmar testing as shown in Fig. 25-5.

RESPONSES. S should be asked to say "sharp" or "dull" in response to each stimulus. If S is aphasic or dysarthric, E should ask S to indicate a response by pointing to the appropriate side of an open safety pin in S's view.

SCORING. Callahan[7] recommended the following coding system for responses: E marks a "plus S" (+S) at the stimulus point on the scoring chart for a correct response to a sharp stimulus, a "minus S" (−S) for no response to a sharp stimulus, and a "D" if a sharp stimulus is reported as dull; a "plus D" (+D) for a correct response to a dull stimulus, a minus "D" (−D) for no response to a dull stimulus, and an S if a dull stimulus is reported as sharp.[7] A form for recording the results of the evaluation is shown in Fig. 25-6.

INTERPRETATION OF RESULTS. Correct responses to both sharp and dull indicate that protective sensation is intact. Incorrect responses to both sharp and dull are indicative of absent protective sensation. If dull stimuli are reported as sharp, the patient has hyperesthesia; if sharp stimuli are reported as dull, that patient has pressure sensation.[7] The computer-driven Automated Tactile Sensor may be used to record responses more accurately.[12]

Olfactory Sensation (Smell)

The sense of smell (**olfactory sensation**) is conveyed by receptors that lie deep within the nasal cavity. Normal individuals can detect thousands of odors at very low concentrations, making smell discrimination quite extraordinary. The sense of smell is important for detection of noxious and pleasant odors and is associated with the pleasure of taste. Smell is also connected to neuronal circuits that influence emotional states, and smell evokes certain memories. Olfactory acuity varies greatly among normal persons. Olfactory acuity normally declines with age.[14]

Hyposmia is a diminished sense of smell, whereas a loss of the sense of smell is known as **anosmia**. *Hyposmia* refers to impaired sensation of a general nature. It may occur in patients with cystic fibrosis of the pancreas, Parkinson's disease, and untreated adrenal insufficiency. Anosmia may be specific or general. *Specific anosmia* refers to lowered sensitivity to a specific odorant while perception of most other odors remains intact. *General anosmia* refers to absence of the sense of smell. Anosmia may result from local, chronic, or acute inflammatory nasal disease or from intracranial lesions that may be the result of CVA, head injury, tumors, and infections. In some disturbances the sense of smell is distorted. There may be perception of odors that do not exist, or pleasant odors may be distorted or perceived as noxious. This condition is known as **parosmia**.[5]

Anosmia interferes with function, as in the case of a patient who has an occupation in which the sense of smell is critical to safety, or for the detection of household gas, chemicals, smoke, car exhaust, and noxious environmental odors. The disturbance may interfere with the perception and enjoyment of food odors and taste because a decreased sense of smell affects the ability to taste. Therapists may also use olfactory stimulation in the treatment of certain neurological disorders.[16]

Test for Olfactory Sensation

PURPOSE. To determine if the sense of smell is intact, impaired, or lost and whether the loss is unilateral or bilateral.[5]

LIMITATIONS. Persons with receptive aphasia cannot be validly tested. Persons with expressive aphasia who cannot communicate using symbols such as pictures or words to indicate responses cannot be validly tested. The test is quite subjective, and E must rely on S's report.

MATERIALS Five small opaque or dark-colored bottles containing essences, powders, or crystalline material of familiar and natural odors; coffee, almond, chocolate, lemon oil, and peppermint are some that are suitable.[5] Vinegar, ammonia, or other irritating chemical odors should not be used in a test of olfaction because they stimulate all receptors of the mucous membranes and tend to be irritating.[13,16] If S cannot respond verbally, small cards with the word or a picture for each odor on them will be needed.

CONDITIONS. A nondistracting environment in which no strong odors are present, with S seated or semireclining.

METHOD. S is asked to compress one nostril, or this function may be provided by E. S is then asked to take a breath to demonstrate that the remaining nostril is open. If the substances can be recognized from their appearance, vision is occluded. The cork of the bottle or a cotton swab moistened with an essence is held under the open nostril. In the case of solid substances, the container may be held under S's nostril. S is asked to take two moderate sniffs. Each of the substances is tried, with a short delay between them, and the nostrils are tested alternately using the same and different substances.[5,9,25]

RESPONSES. E asks S if he or she can (1) detect an odor, (2) identify the odor, and (3) determine if the odors are the same or different to both nostrils.[5,25]

SCORING. E marks a "plus" (+) on the form if the odor is detected and correctly identified, a "minus" (−) if an odor is detected and incorrectly identified, and a "zero" (0) if no odor is detected (Fig. 25-11). Whether the same odors are perceived as the same by both nostrils and whether S can differentiate between dissimilar odors presented to each nostril should be noted on the form.

INTERPRETATION OF RESULTS. The ability to detect and identify odors quickly, the ability to detect an odor but not identify it, and the ability to detect and differentiate odors without identification may all be regarded as normal responses. Distortion of the odor (parosmia) and inability to detect odors (anosmia) are regarded as dysfunctional. If test responses are vague and variable, the results are unreliable and it is best to postpone the test to a more favorable time.[5]

Gustatory Sensation (Taste)

Taste receptor cells, located in the taste buds of the tongue, palate, pharynx, epiglottis, and esophagus, convey taste stimuli (**gustatory sensation**) to the brain via the facial, glossopharyngeal, and vagus nerves (cranial nerves VII, IX, and X). Generally, four basic tastes can be detected: sweet, sour, salty, and bitter. Detection of more complex taste sensations is thought to be a result of the activation of combinations of receptors for these four basic tastes.[14]

RECORDING SCORES OF OLFACTORY AND GUSTATORY SENSATION

Name:_____

Age:_____ Diagnosis:_____

Date:_____

Key: + = Can detect and identify odor
      − = Can detect odor, cannot identify odor
      0 = Cannot detect or identify odor
      S = Can detect same odors, both nostrils
      D = Can detect different odors, both nostrils

OLFACTORY SENSATION   Left nostril   Right nostril   Comparisons

Dates						
Coffee						
Almond						
Chocolate						
Lemon						
Peppermint						

GUSTATORY SENSATION

Key: + = Identifies taste correctly
      − = Cannot identify taste

Dates			Remarks
Sweet			
Salt			
Sour			
Bitter			

FIG. 25-11
Form for recording scores on olfactory and gustatory sensation.

Disturbances of taste may be caused by PNS or CNS lesions.[25] Smokers may demonstrate a decreased sense of taste with aging.[16] Taste is not only basic to the enjoyment of food, but also is one of the sensory stimuli that trigger salivation and swallowing.[31] Like smell, taste is connected to neural circuits that control emotional states and trigger specific memories.[14] Taste sensation may be of concern to the occupational therapist as part of a comprehensive evaluation of oral-motor mechanisms and for planning feeding training programs (Chapter 40).[31]

Test for Gustatory Sensation
PURPOSE. To determine if the sense of taste is intact, impaired, or absent.

LIMITATIONS. The same limitations as cited for the test of olfaction apply here. The most accurate method of administering the test requires that S keep the tongue extended.[5,8,31] Therefore S must respond by pointing to a word or picture. In instances where S has speech but cannot recognize words or pictures, a verbal response should be allowed. If S is aphasic, E should observe for aversive responses to the sour and bitter stimuli.[31] The appreciation of taste depends on an intact sense of smell.[5,16]

MATERIALS. A glass, pitcher of water, and small rinse basin; sugar or saccharin (sweet), salt or salt substitute (salty), lemon or vinegar (sour), and quinine (bitter) in small containers to test the four basic tastes[14]; cotton swabs; response cards with the word for the taste or a picture symbol of the taste on each.

CONDITIONS. A nondistracting environment in which S is seated or semireclining. E should sit directly in front of S. S's vision should be occluded. The oral cavity should be clean and free of residual food tastes.

METHOD. S is instructed to protrude the tongue, and a small amount of the test substance on the tip of a wet cotton swab is applied to the appropriate place on the tongue: sweet on the front or tip of the tongue, salty on the anterior lateral margins of the tongue, sour on the lateral middle margins of the tongue, and bitter on the posterior tongue margin.[9,14,16] Tastes are presented in that order because the bitter stimulus may evoke an aversive response.[16] If this technique is not effective, rubbing the substance along the side of the protruded tongue should be tried.[5,25] The tongue should be irrigated with plain water between each stimulus.[5,16,18]

RESPONSES. S is instructed to point to a response card before withdrawing the tongue and diffusing the taste to all areas of the tongue.[5,25]

SCORING. E should record a "plus" (+) if the taste is correctly identified and a "minus" (−) if the taste cannot be identified (Fig. 25-11).

INTERPRETATION OF RESULTS. Normal adults should be able to identify all tastes accurately.

Position and Motion Sense

Proprioception refers to the unconscious reception of information about joint position and motion that arises from receptors in the muscles, joints, ligaments, and bones. The conscious sense of motion may be referred to as **kinesthesia.** Equilibrium (balance) or vestibular sensation is part of proprioception.[2] These senses make it possible to detect joint motion and position of the body or any of its parts. Sensation that is evoked by movement is essential to being able to move effectively. Feedback and feedforward control mechanisms depend on proprioception.[17] These mechanisms provide information about the motion and position of the body and its parts. The mechanisms also help maintain erect posture, make postural adjustments, and localize action

of the limbs, trunk, and head at any moment. Proprioception, touch, and stereognosis make it possible to write without looking at the pencil, type without looking at the keys, and button clothes behind the back.

The awareness of motion and position is on a subcortical level and normally does not require conscious effort. To test position and motion sense, however, it is necessary to raise the sensation to a conscious level so that the patient can make the appropriate responses. A partial or complete loss of position and motion sense seriously impairs movement, even if muscle function is within normal limits. Therefore it is important for the occupational therapist to know if the patient has the sensory loss, so that the motor dysfunction can be more fully understood. The assessment will help to plan treatment by using compensatory methods or a sensory retraining program.

Test of Position and Motion Sense[5,10,18,20,22,27]
PURPOSE. To evaluate S's senses of motion and position.

LIMITATIONS. It is important that S comprehends instructions exactly. Thus patients with receptive aphasia may not be validly tested. Movements must be made slowly and carefully enough to be detected. Methods of responding must be well established and understood before beginning the test. The patient's concentration on motion and position is essential.[5]

MATERIALS. For testing hands and forearms, the screen or a manila folder used to occlude vision; for testing the elbow and shoulder, if space and equipment permit, a screen high and wide enough to conceal S's arm when held overhead or out in front when S is in a seated position. The curtain screen should be full, continuous, and attached only at the top. If such a screen is not available, an assistant can shield S's vision with a manila folder.

CONDITIONS. The test should be conducted in privacy in a nondistracting environment. When the fingers and wrist are being tested, S should be seated at a table with the screen in a position to accommodate the affected hand and forearm comfortably. E should sit opposite S on the other side of the screen and support S's hand for the test. When the elbow and shoulder are being tested, S should be seated away from the table, and the curtain screen should be draped over the affected shoulder so that S is unable to see the arm. If this position is not feasible, the test may be conducted with S seated or reclining in bed or seated in a wheelchair.

RESPONSES. To determine appreciation of direction of movement, S should be instructed to respond "up" (away from the floor) and "down" (toward the floor) or "out" (away from the body) and "in" (toward the body) as soon as he or she perceives direction of movement. Aphasic subjects may respond by pointing in the appropriate direction. If there is an unaffected extremity, as in hemiplegia, S should be asked to imitate the motion and final position with the unaffected extremity after E has ceased passive movement of the part being tested, to evaluate appreciation of motion and position.

METHOD

TEST OF FINGERS. Test positions are index finger flexion, middle finger extension, thumb extension, and little finger flexion, which should be presented in random order. No range of motion should be so extreme as to elicit pain or a stretch reflex. S's hand and forearm should be placed under the curtain, resting on the dorsal surface. When testing a right hand E should support S's hand with the left palm and hold the thumb out of the way with the left thumb if necessary. This position should induce relaxation of the fingers if S has flexor spasticity. With the right hand E should grasp the finger to be tested on each side at the distal phalanx to avoid giving pressure cues with E's thumb and index finger. The finger being tested should be separated from others and should be kept from touching the palm to avoid cues from contact. The position of E's hands is reversed when testing a left hand (Fig. 25-12).

TEST OF WRIST. Test positions are wrist flexion and extension. The ranges should not be so extreme as to elicit tendon action or a stretch reflex. E's and S's hands are positioned as for testing the fingers. E makes a somewhat firmer grasp at the sides of S's hand, but reducing contact between E's palm and the back of S's hand.

TEST OF ELBOW AND SHOULDER. The starting position

for all motions is with S's arm at the side, the shoulder supported in 20° to 30° of abduction, the elbow supported at 90° of flexion, and the wrist stabilized at neutral. Test positions are elbow extension, shoulder flexion, shoulder internal rotation, and shoulder scaption (halfway between 90° of flexion and 90° of abduction). Test positions should be presented in random order. Ranges should not be so extreme as to elicit a stretch reflex or cause pain if there is joint tightness. S should be seated away from the table. The curtain screen should be arranged at S's test side. E should stand at S's test side and guide the limb passively through the test positions. When a right arm is being tested, E's right hand should be placed along the ulnar border of S's hand and wrist, stabilizing the wrist at neutral. E's left hand should be placed on the dorsal surface of the upper arm, just proximal to the elbow. The position is reversed when testing the left arm. E may carry out all test positions for the elbow and shoulder without changing the position of the hands (Fig. 25-13).

SCORING. Appreciation of the direction of movement: E records "plus" (+) if the direction is correctly perceived or "zero" (0) if the direction is not perceived (Fig. 25-14).

APPRECIATION OF POSITION. E records "plus" (+) if the correct response is given, "minus" (−) if the response is delayed or nearly correct, and "zero" (0) if the response is obviously incorrect or if no response is given.

REMARKS. On the recording form, E comments on S's reactions, unusual statements, observations, and individual variations in test procedure adapted for specific dysfunctions.

INTERPRETATION OF RESULTS. Normal individuals can detect movements of 1 or 2 mm in a joint.[18] A grade of "intact" was given by Kent[22] if movement could be detected in the first 15° of the range of motion. It is possible for normal persons to duplicate the passive

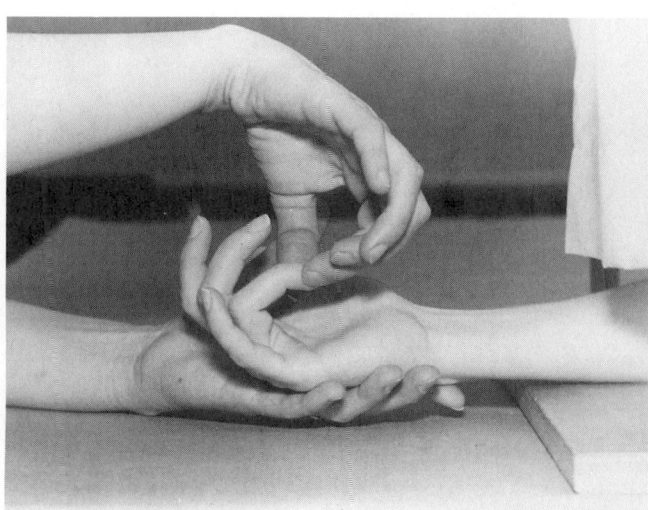

FIG. 25-12
Motion and position sense test of fingers.

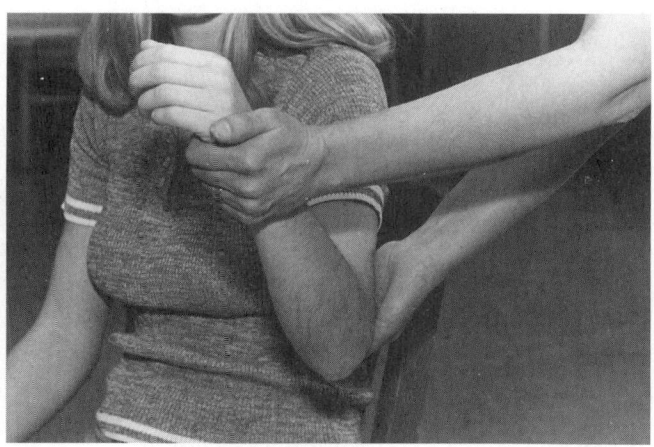

FIG. 25-13
Motion and position sense test of elbow and shoulder.

FORM FOR RECORDING TESTS OF POSITION/MOTION SENSE

Department of Occupational Therapy

Name_____ Age_____ Sex_____ Onset_____

Diagnosis/disability _____

Date_____

Directions:
  Fingers and Wrist: Grasp part laterally.
  Scoring: Direction of Movement
          + = Intact/correct response
          0 = Absent/incorrect response or no response

          Position Sense
          + = Intact/correct imitation of movement and position
          − = Impaired/delayed response, minor to moderate errors in response
          0 = Absent/significant errors or no response

  Elbow/Shoulder: Starting position for all movements is:
          Shoulder: 20° to 30° of abduction
          Elbow: 90° flexion
          Wrist: Stabilized at neutral
  Scoring: Same as above for fingers and wrist

Test of Motion/Position Sense	Shoulder flexion-abduction	Shoulder internal rotation	Shoulder flexion	Elbow extension	Wrist extension	Wrist flexion	Little finger flexion	Thumb extension	Middle finger extension	Index finger flexion
Appreciation of direction of movement										
Appreciation of position										
Remarks:										

FIG. 25-14
Form for recording the scores on tests of motion and position sense.

motion and position of the part being tested with the analogous uninvolved part quickly and with considerable accuracy.

SENSORY DYSFUNCTION

Sensory disturbances can result from CNS or PNS dysfunction or from cranial nerve disorders. In peripheral and cranial nerve lesions the sensory disturbance is localized to the area supplied by the affected nerve. Sensory disorders of nerve root origin are localized to the dermatome supplied by the affected nerve root. Sensory dysfunction of CNS origin is more generalized and affects the contralateral side of the body after stroke or head injury, resulting in hemiplegia. Some of the terms associated with sensory disturbances are **anesthesia** (complete loss of sensation), **paresthesia** (abnormal sensation such as tingling or crawling), **hypesthesia** (decreased sensation), **hyperesthesia** (increased tactile sensitivity), **analgesia** (complete loss of pain sensation), and **hypalgesia** (diminished pain sensation).[8]

Sensory loss may have a profound effect on the patient's ability to function in everyday activities. Therefore it is important to facilitate sensory recovery or reeducation to the extent possible or to teach compensatory techniques and safety precautions.

Treatment of Sensory Dysfunction

Before treatment of sensory dysfunction can be initiated, a sensory assessment and an assessment of functional use of the affected part should be completed. The therapist must have knowledge of the diagnosis, the cause of the sensory dysfunction, the prognosis for return of sensation, and the current progression of recovery. This information may help determine whether the treatment approach should be remedial, compensatory, or both. The patient who is to begin a **sensory reeducation** program should be motivated and able to concentrate. Cognitive ability should be adequate to understand the purpose of the training. Motivation to persevere in daily sessions and to make every effort to use the affected part in ADL is important.[6,15]

Central Nervous System Dysfunction

Effects of Sensory Loss

Following CVA and other CNS disorders such as head injury, sensory loss can be a considerable problem. Sensory loss inhibits movement even when there is good motor return. The inclination to move is based on sensory input and feedback. Persons with poor sensation have little urge to move. Attempted movement may be clumsy or uncoordinated. Sensory loss may contribute to, but is not the only cause of, the neglect of the affected extremity so often seen in patients with CVA. The possibility of injury is a serious concern, and the dependence on visual control negates carrying out many activities such as reaching into a purse or pocket to retrieve an item and fastening clothing at the side or back.[15]

Compensatory Treatment

A first concern of treatment is safety and ensuring that the patient is not injured by bumping, burning, or becoming snagged in furniture or equipment during the performance of ADL. If the loss of sensation is permanent, **compensatory treatment** will facilitate rehabilitation. The following are examples of compensation:

1. Using the less affected hand to perform such activities as cooking, eating, and ironing
2. Using vision to observe the motion and location of body parts; testing bath water with the less affected hand or a bath thermometer
3. Using adaptive devices such as the one-handed cutting board to avoid cutting the affected hand[33]

The patient with stroke (CVA) must be made aware of his or her sensory deficits. Safety factors during performance of everyday activities must be continuously brought to the patient's attention and reinforced. To compensate for sensory loss the patient can be trained to check the position of the limbs by looking at them. Patients must be evaluated for safety awareness and trained to consider safety in hazardous activities. The patient who wants to return to home management should demonstrate good judgment, safety awareness, and ability to use visual compensation for sensory loss.[29] Frequent repetition of instructions and cuing by the therapist are often necessary. Cognitive disturbances such as poor memory, perseveration, poor judgment, and inability to see cause-and-effect relationships make it difficult for some patients to learn and attend effectively to compensatory techniques. In such instances, supervision is required.

Remedial Treatment

Sensory bombardment involving as many of the senses as possible has been found to be useful for sensory retraining in some CVA patients. During regular therapeutic activities and handling, the therapist can touch or stroke the affected parts and encourage the patient to observe the movement and touch stimulation. Weight bearing on the legs, arms, and trunk increases proprioceptive feedback.[33]

Eggers[15] advocates integrating sensory retraining with motor retraining, with the neurodevelopmental approach as the basis for treatment (see Chapter 36). She described a sensory retraining program that focuses primarily on tactile and kinesthetic reeducation. A prerequisite to sensory retraining is having the therapist normalize the patient's muscle tone and find the optimal position for the sensory reeducation activities. The therapist must find ways to stimulate sensation without increasing spasticity. Sufficient time must be allowed for the patient to make responses because many patients exhibit delayed processing of sensory information. Other deficits, such as hemianopsia, aphasia, and visual perceptual deficits, must be considered when retraining for tactile-kinesthetic functions. Repetition and variation of sensory stimuli are necessary with CNS patients if they are to relearn sensation.[15]

Eggers[15] describes a graded treatment program for sensory deficits. Initially the patient is allowed to see and hear an object as it is being felt, for the benefit of intersensory facilitation. Then vision is occluded during the tactile exploration. Finally, a pad is placed on the tabletop so that both auditory and visual clues are eliminated and the patient relies on tactile-kinesthetic input alone. The program for tactile-kinesthetic reeducation begins with gross discrimination of objects that are very dissimilar—for example, smooth and rough textures or round and square shapes. Next the patient is asked to estimate quantities (such as the number of marbles in a box) through touch. Then the patient must discriminate between large and small objects hidden in sand, progressing to discriminate between two- and three-dimensional objects. Finally the patient is required to pick a specific small object from among several objects. The reader is referred to the original source for a detailed description of specific training activities.[15]

Peripheral Nervous System Dysfunction

Treatment of Hypersensitivity

Heightened, uncomfortable, or irritable responses to nonnoxious stimuli often occur after peripheral nerve injury.[3,30] Treatment of hypersensitivity, known as **dysesthesia,** is best done early and should precede a sensory reeducation program, provided that the patient does not have open wounds or infection.[30] Many patients with hypersensitivity tend to protect sensitive areas and avoid using the affected part in bilateral ADL. The therapist must reassure the patient that touching hypersensitive areas is beneficial.[3] **Desensitization** is most often done in hand rehabilitation and burn rehabilitation, which require advanced education and experience. Specific details of desensitization programs are beyond the scope of this chapter. Following is a summary of those details discussed by Barber[3] and Schutt and Opitz.[30]

Desensitization includes massage, tapping, or rolling with different textures over hypersensitive areas. Treatment begins at the patient's level of tolerance, and then textures are graded to coarser and rougher with increases in force, duration, and frequency of application. Vibration and immersion in materials such as soft Styrofoam balls, rice, beans, popcorn, buckshot, and plastic squares are also used. This method of treatment is based on increasing the pain threshold of the nerve.[3,30]

Compensatory Treatment

A compensatory approach for patients with PNS dysfunction is similar to that described previously for patients with CNS dysfunction. The patient must be made aware of the specific sensory deficits and taught safety awareness for ADL. It may be necessary to avoid use of the affected limb during bilateral activities that are potentially hazardous.

Callahan[6] proposed the following guidelines for patients with PNS dysfunction who lack protective sensation:

1. Avoid exposing the involved area to heat, cold, and sharp objects.
2. When gripping a tool or object, be conscious of not applying more force than necessary.
3. Be aware that the smaller the handle is, the less that pressure is distributed over gripping surfaces. Avoid small handles by building up the handle or using a different tool whenever possible.
4. Avoid tasks that require the use of one tool for long periods, especially if the hand is unable to adapt by changing the manner of grip.
5. Change tools frequently at work to rest tissue areas.
6. Observe the skin for signs of stress (e.g., redness, edema, and warmth) and for excessive force or repetitive pressure, and rest the hand if these signs occur.
7. If blisters, lacerations, or other wounds occur, treat them with the utmost care to avoid further injury to the skin and possible infection.
8. To keep skin soft and pliant, follow a daily routine of skin care, including soaking and oil massage to lock in moisture.[6]

The patient with PNS dysfunction may be more capable of learning and attending to the compensatory techniques than the patient with CNS dysfunction. The reason for this is that perceptual and cognitive skills are intact in patients with PNS dysfunction.

Remedial Treatment

Following nerve injury repair and recovery, the neural impulses received in the sensory cortex from sensory stimulation of the injured hand are altered. The new pattern of neural impulses may be so different as to preclude correct interpretation of the stimulus. Thus, although sensory information is received, it cannot be interpreted correctly. The purpose of sensory reeducation is to help the patient reinterpret the sensory impulses reaching his or her consciousness. The patient's potential for functional recovery following nerve repair will be enhanced by a sensory reeducation program.[11]

Dellon[11] described a sensory reeducation program that is divided into early and late phases. Progression of the program is based on the recovery process. The nerve recovery is determined by giving specific sensory tests. In the early phase of the program the focus is on reeducating moving touch, constant touch, pressure, and touch localization. For moving touch a pencil eraser or fingertip is moved up and down the area being treated. First, the patient observes the stimulus. Next, vision is occluded as the patient concentrates on the stimulus and then opens the eyes to verify what is happening. The patient verbalizes what is being felt by saying, for example, "I feel a soft object moving down the palm of my hand." A similar procedure is followed for constant touch. A pencil eraser is used to press down on one place on the finger or palm in an area where constant touch is recovered. The patient is encouraged to practice these reeducation techniques four times a day for at least 5 minutes each but is directed not to stimulate one hand with the other, because this action would send two sets of sensory stimuli to the brain.[6,11]

Late-phase sensory reeducation is initiated as soon as moving and constant touch are perceived at the fingertips and there is good localization, which is often 6 to 8 months after nerve repair at the wrist. The goal in this phase is to facilitate the recovery of tactile gnosis. The exercises involve a series of tactile discrimination tasks, which begin with the identification of large objects that are substantially different from one another and progress to objects with more subtle differences. Familiar household objects are used at the outset. The process is to grasp the object while looking at it, then to occlude the vision and concentrate on the perception, and, finally, to look again at the object for reinforcement. The next objects are those that differ in texture and then objects that are smaller and require more discrete discrimination. Manipulation of the training objects also contributes to motor recovery. Ultimately, the therapist can incorporate activities that simulate those of the patient's occupational roles.[6,11]

Wynn Parry[36] described a sensory retraining program for patients with PNS injuries affecting the hand. The rationale underlying the technique is that the patient can learn to "lay down a new code" in the CNS. It has been shown that in nerve regeneration following traumatic lesions, there is a marked disturbance of cortical representation of sensory nerve fibers in the hand. The training program works best with patients who are cooperative and well motivated and need to use their sensation for everyday activities.[36]

Wynn Parry's training program begins when the patient has sensation in the fingers, about 6 to 8 months after a nerve suture at the wrist. The program begins with the use of large wood blocks of different shapes. The patient's vision is occluded, and a block is placed in the affected hand. The patient is asked to feel the block, describe its shape, and compare its weight with a block placed in the unaffected hand. If an incorrect response is given, the patient is allowed to look at the blocks and repeat the manipulation, integrating visual and tactile information. The patient then compares the sensory experience in the affected hand with that of the normal hand. The procedure continues until various shaped blocks have been mastered. Then blocks are used with textures such as sandpaper or velvet on some surfaces. The patient is asked to differentiate textured surfaces from wood surfaces.[36]

In the next phase of training, the patient is asked to identify several textures such as sheepskin, leather, silk, canvas, rubber, plastic, wool, carpet, and sandpaper, all presented with the vision occluded. Finally, common objects are used in training, and the patient is asked to identify them without the aid of vision. If there are incorrect responses for texture and object identification, the patient is allowed to perform the manipulations while looking at the training objects and to relate what is felt to what is seen. Objects are graded from large to small. Training sessions may be varied by burying objects in a bowl of sand and asking the patient to retrieve a specific object, using a form board in which to place specific forms, or identifying wooden letters for spelling out words. Training is done in two to four 10-minute sessions a day.[36]

Wynn Parry[36] recommended the following procedure to train touch localization. Vision is occluded and the therapist touches several places on the volar surface of the hand. The patient is asked to locate each stimulus with the index finger of the unaffected hand. If the response is incorrect, the patient is directed to look at the place where the hand was touched and to relate where the touch was felt to where the stimulus was actually applied.[36]

Reevaluation is done at 1 month, 3 months, and 6 months after the initial examination to evaluate the effectiveness of training. The criteria used to evaluate treatment effectiveness are time to recognize objects, time to recognize textures, and time for correct localization. To avoid a training effect, the objects and some textures used in testing are different from those used in the training program.[36]

Turner[33] described a sensory reeducation program for patients with peripheral nerve lesions. Retraining is initiated when there is return of protective sensation with that (deep pressure and pinprick) and touch perception. The retraining activities consist of having the patient identify objects, shapes, and textures with the vision occluded. If the response is incorrect, the patient is allowed to look at the object and compare its sensation with that in the normal hand to allow the integration of tactile sensation and vision. Activities that may be helpful include using textured dominoes or checkers, handling cut-out shapes, and finding large to small common objects hidden in rice or lentils. Training with these objects is carried out three or four times a day for 45 minutes. The training periods are alternated with periods of general bilateral activity such as pottery, bread-kneading, weaving, and macramé. The patient is encouraged to use the affected hand in bilateral activities and to compare the feelings of the tools and materials in the affected hand with those in the unaffected hand.[33]

A program of sensory reeducation after nerve injury was described by La Croix and Helman.[23] The purpose of the program is to help the patient correctly interpret different sensory impulses. A series of graded stimuli is used in treatment, such as constant pressure, movement, light touch, and vibration. The least stressful stimuli are presented first. The patient does the training exercises several times a day for short periods. The exercises are done on the unaffected side and then on the affected side, first with the aid of vision and then with vision occluded. Areas of hypersensitivity are noted. Sensory stimulation such as stroking, deep pressure, rubbing, and maintained touch with different textures and shapes is used to reduce hypersensitivity.[23]

Sensory reeducation for PNS disorders focuses on applying graded stimuli according to the progression of nerve recovery. Sensory stimuli such as touch localization, moving touch, and constant touch are followed by exercises for tactile discrimination of shape, size, texture, and object identification. Intermodal reinforcement through visual, auditory, and tactile senses is an important part of the reeducation program.

SUMMARY

Exteroceptive receptors convey sensory information from the environment to the brain by way of peripheral and spinal nerves and the spinal cord. Almost all sensory stimuli are processed through the thalamus before reaching the cerebral cortex. Sensation presents the external environment to the brain and provides information necessary to guide purposeful and effective movement responses. Motor performance is dependent on sensory input, and significant motor deficits can result from dysfunction of sensory systems. Movement is guided by sensory feedback and feedforward control systems. Defects in sensation disrupt these systems.

Sensory testing should be part of the comprehensive OT evaluation of patients with upper and lower motor neuron disorders. Testing helps the therapist understand the complexity of the patient's motor dysfunction. Paralyzed muscles are not the sole cause of faulty or absent use of affected limbs. Rather, a sensory disturbance can be the primary or complementary cause of motor paralysis and movement disorders.

This chapter presents clinical screening tests for the senses of touch, pressure, superficial pain, thermal sensation, proprioception, smell, and taste. It provides information on setting up, administering, scoring, and interpreting results of these tests. Programs for the treatment of sensory dysfunction are reviewed.

REVIEW QUESTIONS

1. What is the role of normal sensation in movement?
2. What is the effect of sensory loss on motor performance?
3. Why is sensory evaluation necessary and important to occupational therapy?
4. What types of disabilities should be routinely given sensory evaluation?
5. What are the differences between sensory loss from CNS disorders and PNS disorders?
6. Do normal individuals all respond with the same accuracy on sensory tests?
7. How is vision occluded during the sensory assessment?
8. Describe how light touch sensitivity is assessed.
9. What are the alternatives for responses in the position sense test?
10. Why is it important to grasp the fingers and wrist laterally during the test for position sense?
11. Describe two methods for testing thermal sensation.
12. How are olfactory and gustatory sensations related?
13. Discuss two approaches to the treatment of sensory dysfunction and the purposes of each.
14. Describe the general principles for treatment of hypersensitivity.
15. With which disabilities is desensitization most likely to be used?
16. What is the neurophysiological principle on which sensory education for PNS dysfunction is based?

REFERENCES

1. Adams RD, Victor M: *Principles of neurology*, ed 5, New York, 1993, McGraw-Hill.
2. Ayres AJ: *Sensory integration and learning disorders*, Los Angeles, 1972, Western Psychological Services.
3. Barber LM: Desensitization of the traumatized hand. In Hunter JM et al, editors: *Rehabilitation of the hand*, St Louis, 1990, Mosby.
4. Bear MS, Connors BW, Paradiso MA: *Neuroscience, exploring the brain*, Baltimore, 1996, Williams & Wilkins.
5. Bickerstaff ER, Spillane JA: *Neurological examination in clinical practice*, ed 5, London, 1989, Blackwell Scientific Publications.
6. Callahan AD: Methods of compensation and reeducation for sensory dysfunction. In Hunter JM et al, editors: *Rehabilitation of the hand*, ed 3, St Louis, 1990, Mosby.
7. Callahan AD: Sensibility testing: clinical methods. In Hunter JM et al, editors: *Rehabilitation of the hand*, ed 3, St Louis, 1990, Mosby.
8. Chusid JG: *Correlative neuroanatomy and functional neurology*, ed 19, Los Altos, Calif, 1985, Lange Medical Publications.
9. deGroot J: *Correlative neuroanatomy*, Norwalk, Conn, 1991, Appleton & Lange.
10. De Jong R: *The neurologic examination*, New York, 1958, Paul B Hoeber.
11. Dellon AL: *Evaluation of sensibility and re-education of sensation in the hand*, Baltimore, 1981, Williams & Wilkins.
12. Dellon AL: *Somatosensory testing and rehabilitation*, Bethesda, Md, 1997, American Occupational Therapy Association.
13. De Myer W: *Technique of the neurologic examination: a programmed text*, ed 2, New York, 1974, McGraw-Hill.
14. Dodd J, Castellucci VF: Smell and taste: the chemical senses. In Kandel ER, Schwartz JH, Jessel TM, editors: *Principles of neural science*, New York, 1991, Elsevier Science Publishing.
15. Eggers O: *Occupational therapy in the treatment of adult hemiplegia*, Rockville, Md, 1984, Aspen Systems.
16. Farber SD: *Neurorehabilitation, a multisensory approach*, Philadelphia, 1982, WB Saunders.
17. Ghez C: The control of movement. In Kandel ER, Schwartz JH, Jessel TM, editors: *Principles of neural science*, New York, 1991, Elsevier Science Publishing.
18. Gilroy J, Meyer JS: *Medical neurology*, London, 1969, Macmillan.
19. Goldman J, Cote L: Aging of the brain: dementia of the Alzheimer's type. In Kandel ER, Schwartz JH, Jessel TM, editors: *Principles of neural science*, ed 3, New York, 1991, Elsevier.
20. Head H et al: *Studies in neurology*, London, 1920, Oxford University Press.
21. Jackson O: Brain function, aging, and dementia. In Umphred DA, editor: *Neurological rehabilitation*, St Louis, 1990, Mosby.
22. Kent BE: Sensory-motor testing: the upper limb of adult patients with hemiplegia, *Phys Ther J Am Phys Ther Assoc* 45:550, 1965.

23. La Croix E, Helman J: Upper extremity orthopedics. In Logigian MK, editor: *Adult rehabilitation: a team approach for therapists,* Boston, 1982, Little, Brown.

24. Martin JH: Coding and processing sensory information. In Kandel ER, Schwartz JH, Jessel TM, editors: *Principles of neural science,* New York, 1991, Elsevier Science Publishing.

25. Mayo Clinic and Mayo Foundation: *Clinical examinations in neurology,* Philadelphia, 1981, WB Saunders.

26. Montgomery PC: Perceptual issues in motor control. In *Contemporary management of motor control problems: proceedings of the II Step Conference,* Alexandria, Va, 1991, Foundation for Physical Therapy.

27. Occupational Therapy Department, Rancho Los Amigos Hospital: *Upper extremity sensory evaluation: a manual for occupational therapists,* Downey, Calif, 1985.

28. Rothwell JC. *Control of human voluntary movement,* ed 2, London, 1994, Chapman & Hall.

29. Ruskin A: Understanding stroke and its treatment. In Ruskin A, editor: *Current therapy in physiatry,* Philadelphia, 1984, WB Saunders.

30. Schutt AH, Opitz JL: Hand rehabilitation. In Goodgold J, editor: *Rehabilitation medicine,* St Louis, 1988, Mosby.

31. Silverman EH, Elfant IL: Dysphagia: an evaluation and treatment program for the adult, *Am J Occup Ther* 33(6):382-392, 1979.

32. Smith and Nephew: *Rehabilitative care catalog 1999,* Smith and Nephew, Inc, One Quality Drive, PO Box 1005, Germantown, Wis.

33. Turner A: *The practice of occupational therapy,* ed 2, New York, 1987, Churchill Livingstone.

34. Waters RL, Wilson DJ, Gowland C: Rehabilitation of the upper extremity after stroke. In Hunter JM et al, editors: *Rehabilitation of the hand,* St Louis, 1990, Mosby.

35. Werner JL, Omer GE: Evaluating cutaneous pressure sensation of the hand, *Am J Occup Ther* 24(5):347-356, 1970.

36. Wynn Parry CB: *Rehabilitation of the hand,* London, 1981, Butterworths.

CHAPTER 26

Evaluation and Treatment of Perceptual and Perceptual Motor Deficits

CAROL J. WHEATLEY

KEY TERMS

Perception
Adaptive approaches
Remedial approaches
Stereognosis
Graphesthesia
Body scheme
Finger agnosia
Right/left discrimination
Prosopagnosia
Agnosia
Gestalt
Form constancy
Position in space
Visual closure
Figure-ground discrimination
Spatial relations
Visuoconstructional skills
Praxis
Ideomotor apraxia
Ideational apraxia
Conceptual apraxia
Dressing apraxia

LEARNING OBJECTIVES

After studying this chapter the student or practitioner will be able to do the following:
1. Define perceptual motor function.
2. Identify the value of perceptual testing and functional assessment of perceptual motor skills.
3. Differentiate the two major approaches to treatment of perceptual motor dysfunction.
4. Define each of the perceptual motor skills cited.
5. Cite standardized assessment tools for each of the primary skill areas of perceptual motor function.
6. Describe specific treatment activities for targeted perceptual motor deficits.

Perception is the gateway to cognition[14]

Perception is the mechanism by which the brain interprets sensory information received from the environment. The perceived information is then further processed by the various cognitive functions (described in Chapter 27), and the individual may choose either to respond by a verbal expression or motor act, or to simply perceive and think about the observed stimuli. For example, when waiting in a check-out line in a grocery store, a person may observe the array of brightly wrapped candy lining the aisle, may remember the sweet taste of the chocolate, may remember a recent resolution to lose weight, and may choose to resist adding any candy bars to the grocery cart. The person may look over to the next aisle, recognize a neighbor, and begin a conversation. In a few minutes, the person may notice that another register has a shorter line and may choose to move over to that line to be able to complete grocery shopping in a shorter amount of time. Perception of the environment provides the information to enable these response options.

In early development, tactile, proprioceptive, vestibular, and visual perception provide an internalized sense of the body scheme, which is basic to all motor function.[6,57,88] Highly developed spatial skills are critical to an artist, architect, plumber, or designer.[33] The process of interpreting visual input is a learned skill, as evidenced by blind individuals who, when sight is restored later in life, have difficulty making sense of what they see.[75]

Acquired perceptual deficits are noted in persons with cerebrovascular accident (CVA), traumatic brain injury (TBI), and later stages of degenerative disorders, such as multiple sclerosis and Parkinson's disease.[54,65] Spatial disorders and apraxia of a progressive nature are also seen in Alzheimer's disease.[5,13]

Severe perceptual deficits, frequently combined with cognitive impairments, can affect every aspect of activities of daily living (ADL) and can present serious safety concerns. For example, the individual who cannot judge distance and the spatial relationship of his foot to the top step of his stairwell may be in danger of a serious fall. Another person who cannot judge the position of the dial on the stove when preparing a meal may cause a fire. It is often the occupational therapist's role to evaluate safe and independent functioning in everyday activities and to provide observations in real life of the skills assessed on standardized visual, perceptual, and cognitive testing.

This chapter describes higher-level tactile discriminative sensation, body scheme, spatial processing, praxis, and the deficits that result from impairment to these areas. Suggestions for standardized and functional testing are provided. General approaches to treatment are reviewed, and suggestions for specific treatment tasks are presented.

GENERAL PRINCIPLES OF EVALUATION

The optimal battery of standardized tests includes assessment tools that require a verbal response (e.g., naming a picture) or motor response (e.g., drawing) or have flexible response requirements of either mode (multiple choice indicated by verbalizing the number or letter or by pointing to the chosen item). With a variety of such tests, the therapist can gather information to discriminate between a deficit in the reception of information and a deficit in the verbal or motor output. This, in turn, influences the treatment approach. Observations of performance and analysis of the perceptual-motor demands of functional activities further complement standardized assessment tools and enable the determination of underlying causes of deficits in functional performance.

Arnadottir[2] recommends the use of ADL to assess neurobehavioral dysfunctions and their effect on the performance of tasks essential to functional independence. She maintains that it is preferable for occupational therapists to assess neurobehavioral deficits directly from the ADL evaluation. She developed the Arnadottir OT-ADL Neurobehavioral Evaluation (A-ONE), which provides information on neurobehavioral impairments and deficits in functional performance by assessing ADL skills.[2] The reader is referred to the original source for more information on this perspective and a detailed description of the A-ONE instrument.[2,3,4]

APPROACHES TO TREATMENT

An underlying assumption about perceptual-motor function is that perceptual deficits will adversely affect functional performance. Further, it is assumed that remediation of or compensation for perceptual deficits will improve functional performance.[60] In her critical analysis of approaches to treatment for perceptual deficits, Neistadt[60] described two general classifications of approaches: the adaptive and the remedial. **Adaptive approaches** provide training in daily living behaviors to facilitate adaptation to the environment for maximal functioning of the individual. In contrast, the **remedial approaches** seek to cause some change in central nervous system (CNS) functions.[60] The effectiveness of the various approaches to the remediation of perceptual deficits has not been well documented and requires scientific investigation.[28,60,73]

A therapist may use one approach or a combination of approaches in the treatment of perceptual deficits. The remedial and adaptive approaches can be used in a continuum, beginning with attempts to improve the basic skills and gradually incorporating compensatory techniques as the deficits persist.[48] The occupational therapy (OT) literature suggests many specific activities for treatment of perceptual deficits, but protocols for the use of such activities are lacking.[88] For measuring effectiveness of treatment, criteria are needed for successful performance, task grading, objective methods of evaluating performance, and guidelines for task modification.[59] In the absence of such objective criteria, the occupational therapist relies on empirical methods to measure and report improvement. The relationship between perceptual deficits and functional performance has been demonstrated in several studies.[7,27,79,81]

Remedial Approach

The **remedial,** or transfer of training, approach assumes that practice in a particular perceptual task carries over to performance of similar tasks or functional activities requiring the same perceptual skills.[60] For example, practice in reproducing pegboard designs for spatial relations training could carry over to dressing skills that require spatial judgment (such as matching blouse to body and discriminating between right and left shoes). The capacity for persons to improve their performance on perceptual tests following perceptual training has been documented.[39] However, reports conflict as to the effectiveness of such remediation in improving functional performance, and further research is needed to determine the benefits.[28,88]

Adaptive Approach

The **adaptive,** or functional, approach is characterized by the repetitive practice of particular tasks that help the person become more independent in the performance of ADL.[60] This approach is frequently used in clinics because current reimbursement for therapy services is based on functional outcome.[72] The therapist does not retrain specific perceptual skills. Rather, the person is made aware of the problem and taught methods of adapting to or compensating for the deficit during functional activities. For example, if the individual has difficulty with dressing because of a body scheme deficit, the therapist may set up a regular dressing routine and provide cues with repetitive practice. With these adaptations, the person may learn to dress. Adaptation of environment or materials is another way to compensate for a perceptual deficit. If an individual has difficulty discriminating a white shirt against the white sheets of the bed, the therapist may encourage the person to select a patterned shirt or may lay the white shirt on a colored towel or bedspread to provide a contrasting background.

ASSESSMENT AND TREATMENT OF SPECIFIC DEFICITS

Stereognosis

Stereognosis and graphesthesia are tactile discriminative skills of the parietal lobes. These skills require a higher level of synthesis than the basic tactile sensory functions of light touch and pressure described in Chapter 25.

Stereognosis, also known as tactile gnosis,[22] is the perceptual skill that enables an individual to identify common objects and geometric shapes through tactile perception without the aid of vision. It results from the integration of the senses of touch, pressure, position, motion, texture, weight, and temperature and is dependent on intact parietal cortical function.[37]

Stereognosis is essential to daily living because the ability to "see with the hands" is critical to many daily activities. It is the skill that makes it possible to reach into a handbag and find a pen and to find the light switch in a dark room. Along with proprioception, stereognosis enables the use of all hand tools and performance of hand activities without the need to concentrate visually on the implements being used. Examples are knitting while watching television, reaching into a pocket for house keys, and using a fork to eat while engaged in conversation. A deficit in stereognosis is called astereognosis. Persons who have astereognosis but retain much of their motor function must visually monitor their hands' activities. Thus they must be very slow and purposeful in their movements and tend to be generally less active.

Test for Stereognosis[11,21,41,50]

PURPOSE. To evaluate a person's ability to identify common objects and perceive their tactile properties.

MATERIALS. A means to occlude the person's vision is needed, such as a curtain or folder as described in Chapter 25. Typical objects that could be used for identification include a pencil, fountain pen, pair of sunglasses, key, nail, safety pin, paper clip, metal teaspoon, quarter, nickel, button, and small leather coin purse. Any common objects may be used, but it is important to consider the person's social and ethnic background to ensure that he or she has had previous experience with the objects. Three-dimensional geometric shapes (e.g., square, sphere, and pyramid) can also be used to test shape and form perception.

CONDITIONS. The test should be conducted in privacy in an environment with minimal distractions. The person should be seated at a table in a position that accommodates the affected hand and forearm comfortably. The therapist should sit opposite the person being tested. If the individual is unable to manipulate test objects because of motor weakness, the therapist should assist him or her to manipulate them in as near normal a manner as possible.

METHOD. The person's vision is occluded, with the dorsal surface of the hand resting on the table. Objects are presented in random order. Manipulation of objects is allowed and encouraged. The therapist assists with the manipulation of items if the person's hand function is impaired.

RESPONSES. The person should be asked to name the object, or, if he or she is unable to name the object, to describe its properties. Aphasic individuals may view a duplicate set of test objects after each trial and point to a choice.

SCORING. The person's response to each of the items presented is scored. The therapist notes if the object is identified quickly and correctly, if there is a long delay before the identification of the object, or if the individual can describe only properties (e.g., size, texture, material, and shape) of the object. The therapist also notes if the person cannot identify the object or describe its properties.

Test for Graphesthesia

An additional test of discriminative sensation that measures parietal lobe function is the test for **graphesthesia**, the ability to recognize numbers, letters, or forms written on the skin.[19,37,63] The loss of this ability is called agraphesthesia. To test graphesthesia, the examiner occludes the examiner's vision and traces letters, numbers, or geometric forms on the fingertips or palm with a dull-pointed pencil or similar instrument. The person tells the therapist which symbol was written.[63] If the person is aphasic, pictures of the symbols may be provided for the individual to indicate a response after each test stimulus.

Treatment of Astereognosis

A graded treatment program for sensory deficits is described by Eggers.[29] Initially, the person is allowed to see and hear an object while feeling it for the benefit of intersensory facilitation; then vision is occluded during the tactile exploration. Finally, a pad is placed on the tabletop so that both auditory and visual clues are eliminated and the person relies on tactile-kinesthetic input alone. The program for tactile-kinesthetic reeducation begins with gross discrimination of objects that are very dissimilar—for example, smooth and rough textures or round and square shapes. Next, the person is asked to estimate quantities (such as number of marbles in a box) through touch. Then the individual must discriminate between large and small objects hidden in sand and progress to discriminating between two- and three-dimensional objects. Finally, the person is required to pick a specific small object from among several objects. The reader is referred to the original source for a detailed description of specific training activities.[29]

Farber described a treatment approach to retrain stereognosis for adults and children with CNS dysfunction.[31] First, the person is allowed to examine the training object visually as it is rotated by the therapist. The person is then allowed to handle the object in the less affected hand while observing the hand. In the next step, the person is allowed to manipulate the object with both hands while looking. Then the object is placed in the affected hand and the person manipulates the object while looking at it. The individual may place the hand in a mirror-lined, three-sided box to increase visual input during these manipulations. This sequence is then repeated with the vision occluded. Once several objects can be identified consistently, two of the objects may be hidden in a tub of sand or rice. The person is then asked to reach into the tub and retrieve a specific object. If the sensation of the sand or rice is overstimulating or disturbing, the objects can be placed in a bag.[31]

Perceptual Processing

Body Scheme

Following a CVA or TBI, a person's sense of his or her body's shape, position, and capacity frequently is distorted. This is known as a disorder of **body scheme**, or autotopagnosia.[8] This can be noted in attempts to draw a human figure (Fig. 26-1) or in a person's unrealistic expectations of performance abilities.[54] For example, an individual with left hemiplegia after a traumatic brain injury expressed his intention to return to his previous manual labor job of installing garage doors. The disorder can affect egocentric perception of one's own body or allocentric orientation of another person's body.[62,65] A person may neglect one side of the body or demonstrate generally distorted impressions of the body's configuration. The person may confuse his or her body with that of another, such as the person who thought that her wedding ring had been stolen by the therapist, not realizing that the hand she was viewing was her own. **Finger agnosia**, or the inability to discriminate the fingers of the hand, can also be part of the disorder.[8] An individual may confuse the right and left side of his or her body, which is a deficit in **right-left discrimination**. An impaired body scheme will also affect self-care, since the individual may have difficulty with feeding, dressing, hygiene activities, or mobility.[73]

ASSESSMENT OF BODY SCHEME. Body scheme disorders can be assessed by asking the individual to draw a human figure (Fig. 26-1) or point to body parts on command. Finger agnosia is evaluated by occluding the person's vision and asking the person to name each finger as it is touched by the therapist. Assessment of right-left discrimination can be included in body part identification or finger agnosia testing.

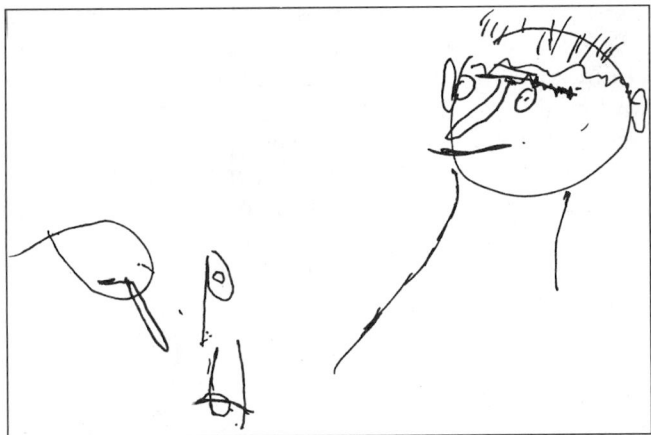

FIG. 26-1

Example of impaired body scheme. Drawing on left is the person's first attempt to draw a face. Therapist asked the person to try again. Second effort is drawing on right.

Facial Perception

Prosopagnosia refers to an inability to recognize faces.[15,45,74] The affected individual may have difficulty recognizing his or her own face, as well as the faces of family members and friends, or of famous individuals. When attempting to identify family members and acquaintances, the person tends to compensate by relying on auditory cues such as the sound of the family member's voice or a distinctive feature such as long, blond hair.

Brain damage can also impair the ability to interpret facial expressions, which can have significant social consequences.[17,86] For example, one individual tended to be very suspicious of others. He was observed to have difficulty describing the expressions of various persons depicted in photographs. Because he had emigrated to the United States from another country, it was considered that his difficulty could be a result of cultural differences. He was asked to bring in a newspaper that he regularly received from his native country. The captions of the photographs were occluded, and he was asked to describe the emotional expressions of the persons shown. He was then asked to translate the photo captions and became aware that he was unable to discriminate the emotions apparent on the faces.

ASSESSMENT OF FACIAL PERCEPTION. A standardized Test of Facial Recognition[12] is available, which presents a multiple-choice matching of faces presented in front view and side view and under various lighting conditions. A formal test of facial expression discrimination is not available,[54] but an informal assessment is possible using pictures and photographs.

Agnosia

Visual object recognition refers to the ability to identify objects via visual input. A deficit in this area is called **agnosia**.[45,54] The individual with agnosia demonstrates normal visual abilities, as indicated by the person's ability to ambulate around furniture through a room; further, the inability to name objects is not caused by a language deficit in naming the object, as noted in aphasic disorders. Rather, the person is unable to know an item using only visual means. If the person holds the object, he or she can identify it via tactile input, or by olfactory means if the object has a distinguishable odor, such as a flower.[74]

Testing is performed by informal means of asking the individual to identify various common objects by sight. Case studies describe compensatory methods of keeping frequently used objects, such as a hairbrush, in consistent locations, and teaching the individual to rely more heavily on stereognosis to seek and find desired items.[45] Efforts to retrain object recognition have met with limited success.[46]

Spatial Functions

Spatial abilities refers to the capacity to appreciate the spatial arrangement of one's body, objects in relationship to oneself, and relationships between objects in space. Various efforts have been made to subdivide spatial skills into components such as form recognition, figure-ground discrimination, and others, but recent writers acknowledge that spatial skills cannot be isolated easily from one another.[18] It is generally acknowledged that the right hemisphere, which controls spatial abilities, tends to function in the **gestalt** (whole), whereas the left hemisphere, which is responsible for linguistic operations, tends to focus on discrete details.[54]

Perception often occurs instantaneously, and it is because of this rapid processing of information that, when operating a motor vehicle, it is possible to react quickly to another driver's actions and so avoid a collision. An individual with mild perceptual impairment may need additional time to perform a task, but processes the information correctly, possibly by compensating with verbal analysis of the perceptual components. Severe impairment may result in the incorrect response despite additional time used in attempting to solve the problem.

Spatial skills are not limited to the visual domain.[53] Sounds can be localized in space, and the mobility and daily functions of blind individuals are heavily dependent on the tactile appreciation of the spatial arrangements of objects.[66] For example, a blind person's ability to navigate through a familiar room requires awareness of the layout of each piece of furniture in the area, and continual shifting of the individual's "cognitive map" while changing position in the room.

Spatial abilities are subdivided into the following skill areas[1]:

Form constancy is the recognition of various forms, shapes, and objects, regardless of their position, location, or size. For example, a person can perceive all of the pencils on a desk, in various sizes or in various positions in the pencil holder.

Position in space refers to the relative orientation of a shape or object to the self. It is this component of perception which allows a person to recognize that the tip of the pencil is pointed away from the individual, and so direct the hand to effectively grasp the pencil.

Objects may be partially occluded from view by other objects, and it is the skill of **visual closure** that allows an individual to recognize a pencil despite its partial concealment by a book.

Figure-ground discrimination allows the individual to perceive a particular pencil from the others in the pencil holder, thereby distinguishing the targeted object from the background.

As a pencil rolls across a desktop, it is the skill of **spatial relations** that enables a person to appreciate the

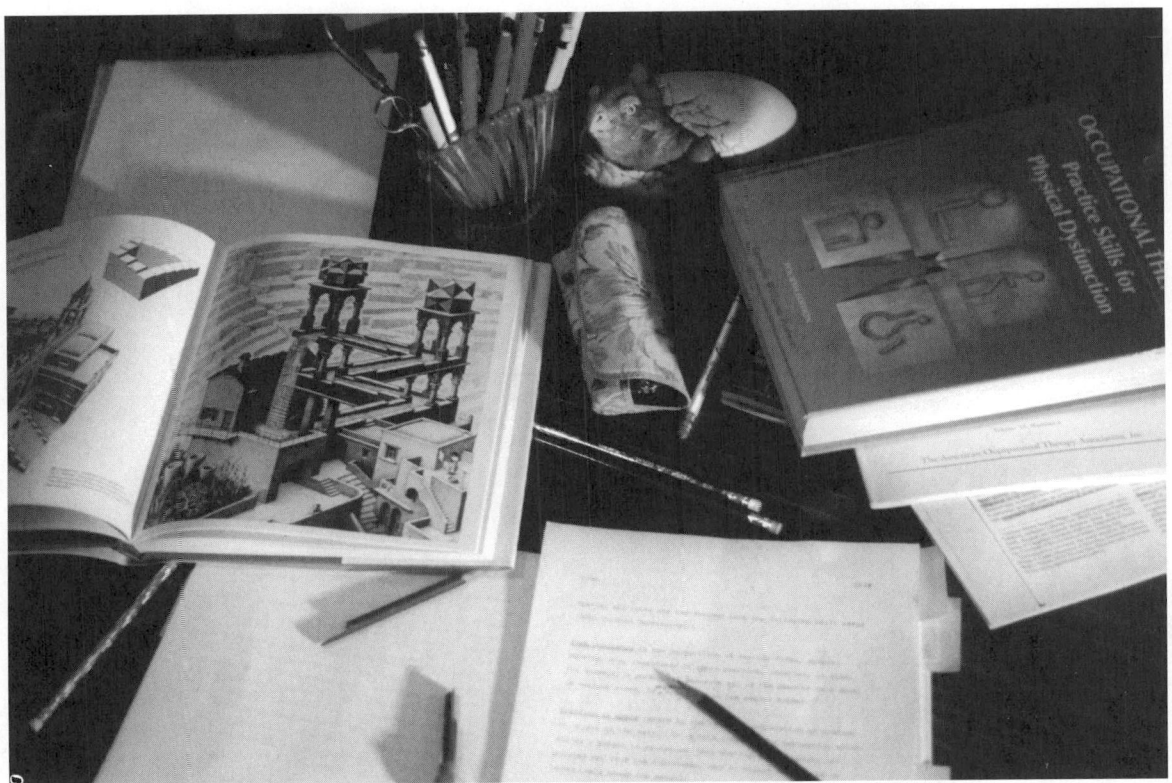

FIG. 26-2
Spatial functions in real life. Note that all components of spatial functions can be found in this scene.

relative orientation of the pencil to the table surface as the pencil nears the edge and is about to fall to the floor. Fig. 26-2 illustrates many of these spatial functions.

VISUOCONSTRUCTIONAL SKILLS. Many functional activities depend on **visuoconstructional skills,** or the ability to organize visual information into meaningful spatial representations. Constructional deficits refer to the inability to organize or assemble parts into a whole, as in putting together block designs (three-dimensional) or drawings (two-dimensional). Constructional deficits can result in significant dysfunction in activities that require constructional ability, such as dressing, following instructions for assembling a toy, and stacking a dishwasher.[61,79] Fig. 26-3, which shows evidence of left neglect, also demonstrates constructional deficits. An individual acts on his or her environment based on the information he or she perceives. Therefore, deficits in perception become more apparent when a person interacts with the environment in maladaptive ways.

ASSESSMENT OF PERCEPTUAL PROCESSING. Visual perceptual tests require either a verbal or simple motor (pointing) response to a multiple-choice selection or require a skilled motor response such as drawing or construction. This enables the therapist to assess visual perceptual function in a client with severe physi-

cal impairment or with significant limitations in communication ability. It is critical that an assessment of basic visual skills (see Chapter 24) be performed before visual perceptual assessment. For example, a deficit in visual acuity could be the underlying cause of poor performance on a test of visual perceptual function. The normal aging process also results in a decline in visual efficiency.[52] It is also possible that performance on visual perceptual tests may be affected by deficits in cognitive areas, such as attention, memory, or executive function (see Chapter 27). For example, an individual with severely limited attention and concentration is unlikely to perform well on any test, regardless of the modality or nature of the task.

Tsurumi and Todd[80] analyze the cognitive skills involved in the commonly used tests of visual perceptual functions and warn that individuals' performance using two-dimensional representations of visual stimuli may not be predictive of the person's performance in a three-dimensional world.[80] Tests that require three-dimensional object manipulation are available. (See the Tests of Constructional Functions section later in this chapter.)

The Loewenstein Occupational Therapy Cognitive Assessment (LOTCA)[47] and Rivermead Perceptual Assessment Battery[27,83] provide a comprehensive profile of visual perceptual and motor skills and involve both motor-free and constructional functions.

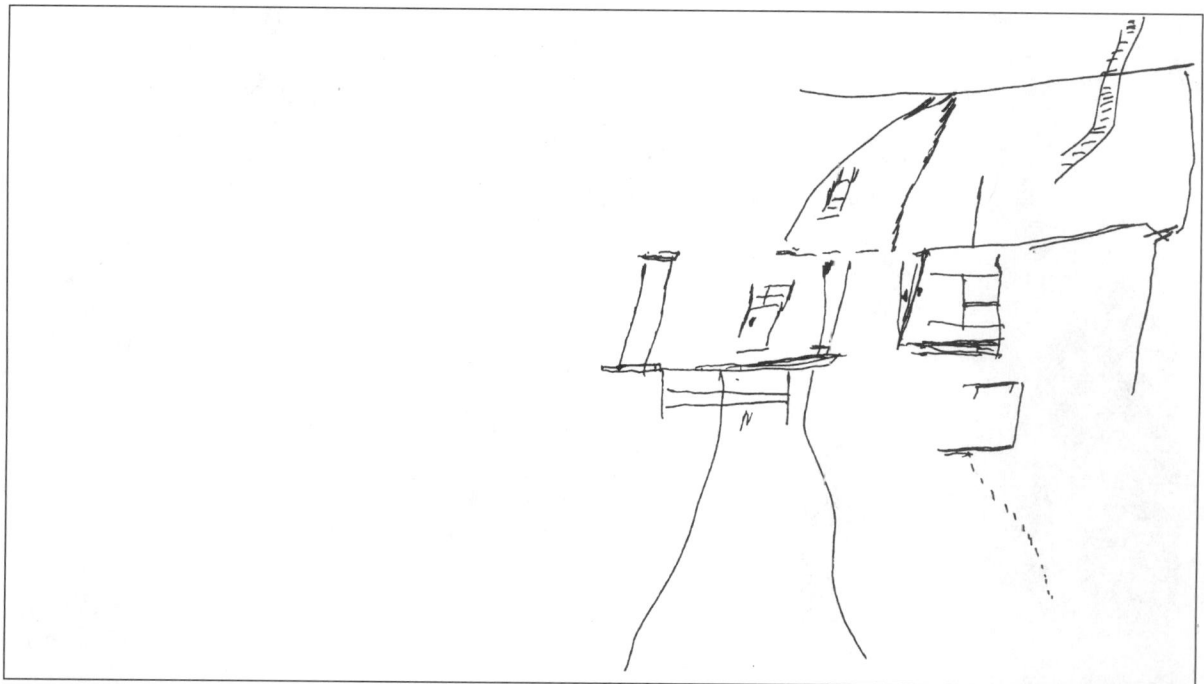

FIG. 26-3
Example of two-dimensional constructional disorder and left-sided inattention in a drawing of a house by a retired architect who had had a cerebrovascular accident (CVA) on the right side.

NON/LOW-MOTOR TESTING OF PERCEPTUAL SKILLS. A variety of assessment tools require either a verbal or a simple pointing response. The Motor-Free Visual Perceptual Test—Revised (MVPT-R)[20] assesses basic visual perceptual abilities. An alternative version of the test presents the multiple choices in a vertical format (MVPT-V) to reduce the interference of hemianopsia or inattention.[58] The Test of Visual Perceptual Skills—Upper Level (TVPS-UL)[35] also provides a multiple-choice format and has been normed for adults. Test items require a higher level of visual analysis compared with the MVPT, and the test is untimed. The Hooper Visual Organization Test[44] requires that the individual mentally assemble fragmented drawings of common objects. The Minnesota Paper Form Board Test[55] is a high-level assessment of visual organization, requiring mental rotation of fragmented geometric shapes.

TESTS OF CONSTRUCTIONAL SKILLS. Traditional tests of constructional abilities in a two-dimensional mode are the Test of Visual-Motor Skills,[34] the copy administration of the Benton Visual Retention Test,[76] and the Rey Complex Figure.[54] The latter two tests also are used to evaluate visual memory skills. Use of the Rey Complex Figure has been suggested for a quick screening of visual perceptual functions.[56] The Three-Dimensional Block Construction[10] involves the use of various blocks to copy a design from a three-dimensional model. Non-standardized tests that may be used are drawing, con-

structing matchstick designs, assembling block designs, or building a structure to match a model.[87] In daily living, tasks such as dressing or setting the table require constructional skills. To perform such tasks successfully, an individual must have integrated visual perception, motor planning, and motor execution.[10,38,59,82,88] Several studies have gathered data on the constructional skills of unimpaired subjects for use as a normative reference for persons with CVA and TBI.[30,59] In a study of constructional abilities in the well elderly, Fall[30] demonstrated that results are influenced by the type of test administration. Subjects tended to score higher on tests that used three-dimensional models as guides for construction than on those that used photographs or drawings. The implications of this finding for occupational therapists are that (1) the type of test administration affects scores, and (2) in teaching persons with constructional disorders, models or demonstrations of desired performance are likely to produce better results than would photographs or drawings.[30]

TREATMENT OF PERCEPTUAL AND CONSTRUCTIONAL DEFICITS. The remedial approach involves the use of perceptual tasks such as paper and pencil activities and puzzles to improve basic perceptual skills. The adaptive approach would include training for functional ADL tasks and developing compensatory approaches to the functional performance deficits. Many functional activities are suitable for perceptual motor treatment; folding towels, setting the dinner table, and weeding the garden are but a few examples. This is discussed further in the Approaches to Treatment section earlier in this chapter.

Praxis

Praxis is the ability to plan and perform purposeful movement. Apraxia has been classically defined as a deficit in "the execution of learned movement which cannot be accounted for by either weakness, incoordination, or sensory loss, or by incomprehension of or inattention to commands."[36] The disorder can result from damage to either side of the brain or to the corpus callosum[42,85] but is more frequently noted with left hemisphere damage.[43] Apraxia is often seen in persons with aphasia; however, not all aphasic persons are apraxic, nor are all apraxic persons aphasic.[40,42] This type of dysfunction may occur after CVA or TBI. Progressive apraxia is often noted with degenerative disorders such as Alzheimer's disease.[42,64] See also Chapters 37 to 39 in this text.

Apraxia has been strongly correlated with dependence in ADL.[77,81] For example, in a severe case of apraxia, an individual initially required full assistance with self-care. The individual was fully cognizant of ongoing events but could not even direct her arm and leg movements in a way that would assist the nursing staff during dressing. When asked to pick up a pencil, the individual walked around all four sides of the table in an attempt to position her hand correctly to grasp the object. She could describe the desired action in words ("I want to pick up the pencil between my thumb and index finger, with the lead point of the pencil close to the tips of my fingers") but reported after returning to her seat that her hand never "looked like it was in the right position" to take hold of the pencil.

The categories of apraxia are difficult to differentiate, and authors differ in their use of terms.[78] The principal types are ideomotor apraxia and ideational apraxia. Because the distinction between ideational and ideomotor apraxia is often perplexing, some authors recommend simply using the term *apraxia*.[51,54]

Ideomotor Apraxia

Ideomotor apraxia (IMA) is an inability to carry out a motor act on verbal command or imitation. However, the person with ideomotor apraxia is able to perform the act correctly when asked to use the actual object.[25, 42] For example, a person is unable to mime the action of brushing his teeth on request but is observed using a toothbrush correctly when he is performing grooming activities. Observation of the person in activity performance is critical to the identification of this deficit. The deficit is demonstrated only in the testing environment and appears to have little functional impact, as compared with ideational apraxia.[78]

Ideational Apraxia

Ideational apraxia (IA) is a conceptual deficit, seen as an inability to use real objects appropriately.[23,26,40] More recent authors suggest the use of the term **conceptual apraxia**.[43,64] The individual also may have difficulty sequencing acts in the proper order,[42] such as with folding a sheet of paper and inserting it into an envelope. The individual may use the wrong tool for the task or may associate the wrong tool with the object to be acted on, such as by attempting to write with a spoon.[42] This deficit has significant functional implications.

Another category seen in the literature is **dressing apraxia**. The classification of dressing impairment as a form of apraxia has been questioned in recent years because the difficulties in functional self-care are considered to be caused by perceptual or cognitive dysfunction[16,81,88] (if apraxia is not noted in other activities), or are seen as an extension of an ideational or ideomotor apraxic disorder.

The term *constructional disorder* is now favored over the previously used term of constructional apraxia since the deficit does not clearly fall within the definition of apraxia.[9,16,54] (See the Visuoconstructional Skills section of this chapter for further discussion.)

General Principles in the Assessment and Treatment of Apraxia

ASSESSMENT. It is important that assessments of sensory function, muscle strength, and dexterity are completed before the test of praxis because deficits in these areas would complicate any assessment of apraxia. If a person has a hemiplegia, the unaffected hand is used for testing. Input from the speech-language pathologist is important for establishing an individual's capacity for basic comprehension via words or gestures. Because of the frequent association of apraxia with aphasia and left hemisphere brain damage, an apraxia screening is included as a part of many aphasia batteries[78] used by speech-language pathologists.

The literature[16] offers several apraxia assessments used in research, such as the Florida Apraxia Screening Test (FAST),[70,71] the Movement Imitation Test,[24,25] and the Use of Objects Test.[24] The Loewenstein Occupational Therapy Cognitive Assessment (LOTCA)[47] includes a praxis subsection, as does the Rivermead Perceptual Assessment Battery,[83] both of which serve as screening tools for the disorder. The Santa Clara Valley Medical Center Praxis Test and the Solet Test for Apraxia are two additional evaluation tools developed by occupational therapists.[87]

A thorough assessment includes items presented, such as those shown in Table 26-1,[42] and involves both transitive movements (action involving both tool and use, such as writing with an imaginary pen), and intransitive movements (movements for communication,

TABLE 26-1

Elements of a Comprehensive Apraxia Assessment

Test Condition	Example
Gesture to command	"Show me how you would take off your hat." (transitive) "Show me how you would throw a kiss." (intransitive)
Gesture to imitation	"Copy what I do." *Therapist shrugs shoulders.* (intransitive) *Therapist flips an imaginary coin.* (transitive)
Gesture in response to seeing the tool	"Show me how you would use this object." *Therapist provides screwdriver for display.*
Gesture in response to seeing the object upon which the tool works	"Show me how you would use this object." *Therapist provides screwdriver and block of wood with screw partially inserted.*
Actual tool use	"Show me how you would use this object." *Therapist provides screwdriver for use.*
Imitation of the examiner using the tool	"Copy what I do." *Therapist makes stirring motion, using a spoon.*
Discrimination between correct and incorrect pantomimed movements	"Is this the correct way to blow out a match?" *Therapist pantomimes holding match in unsafe manner (e.g., match held upside down, with head of match near palm of hand).*
Gesture comprehension	"What object am I using?" *Therapist pantomimes shaving face with a razor.*
Serial acts	"Show me how you would open an imaginary can of soda, pour it into a glass, and take a drink."

From Heilman KM, Rothi LJG: Apraxia. In Heilman KM, Valenstein E, editors: *Clinical neuropsychology*, New York, 1993, Oxford University Press.

such as waving farewell). Lists of gestures used in assessment are noted in several studies.[16,42,68,70,84]

TREATMENT. The severely impaired individual who was described in the second paragraph of this section on praxis was treated first by practicing basic motor movements, then following a developmental sequence to more advanced functional motor activities. For example, following repetition of basic movement patterns, the person with apraxia progressed to coloring geometric shapes (felt-tip markers were initially placed in a vertical stand for easy grasp) and gradually to writing exercises. Independent telephone use was important to the individual, so a large calculator was used for keystroke practice. The individual gradually progressed to a disconnected telephone and then to a functional telephone. By the termination of the treatment program, the individual was independent in all aspects of self-care, although additional time was needed for each activity.

The clinical reasoning process was used in planning the treatment for an individual with apraxia, beginning with spoken instruction for each sequence in the task, written or pictorial instructions, and visual monitoring of her limbs throughout each aspect of the task.[16] Another case study of apraxia treatment involved conductive education—that is, breaking the task into smaller units and verbally guiding (conducting) the sequence.[67] The individual improved on targeted tasks, but minimal generalization was noted in everyday activities (see also the Generalization and Transfer section of Chapter 27).

The treatment of dressing impairment involves teaching a set pattern for dressing and giving cues that help the person distinguish right from left or front from back. A helpful method is to have the individual position the garment the same way each time—for example, positioning a shirt with the buttons face-up and pants with the zipper face-up. Labels, small buttons, or ribbons can be used as cues to differentiate the front from the back of the garment.[87,88]

BEHAVIORAL ASPECTS OF PERCEPTUAL MOTOR DYSFUNCTION

Some degree of accurate self-awareness and recognition of the effect of the disability on one's functioning is needed if the person is to invest energy in the therapy process.[32]

An individual who is unaware of perceptual deficits may be a serious safety risk and may attempt activities that are well beyond present physical abilities. Denial is often noted in early stages of recovery from CVA or TBI and may serve as a protective coping mechanism that allow the individual to gradually absorb the effect of the injury on his or her functioning. A person's innate trust of the accuracy of perceptions often is a basis for unrealistic self-confidence; demonstrating to the individual that his or her perceptions are now distorted and no longer trustworthy can profoundly affect the person's sense of self. A therapist needs to respect and be sensitive to the individual's sense of self and be prepared to aid the individual in understanding the changes in perceptual capacity and in reestablishing an accurate sense of self-awareness.

An individual who has some degree of awareness of the disability often is depressed, which seems an appropriate response to the gravity of the situation. The therapist needs to recognize and appreciate this emotional response and help the person achieve an emotional balance to reestablish quality of life through celebrating progress in therapy while acknowledging the impact of the disability.[32,69] (See also Chapter 28 on social and psychological aspects.)

Several questionnaires are available to assess an individual's self-awareness.[49] The questionnaires typically are issued to the person with deficits as well as to a family member or close acquaintance. The discrepancies in the two questionnaires are used as a measure of the accuracy of the individual's insight and serve as the basis for intervention.

The individual's behavior may also be the result of a disorder in executive function.[49] See Chapter 27 for additional discussion of this possibility.

SUMMARY

Deficits in perceptual and perceptual motor functioning can profoundly affect an individual's ability to perform daily activities. It is difficult to differentiate various perceptual motor skills, because the areas tend to overlap and complement each other. Perceptual motor functioning is optimally viewed in its *gestalt*, and treated in a holistic manner as well.

REVIEW QUESTIONS

1. Provide an example of the functional impact of a perceptual motor deficit.
2. Compare the advantages and disadvantages of perceptual testing and functional assessment.
3. Why are stereognosis and graphesthesia considered higher aspects of sensory function?
4. How would you adapt a stereognosis test for a person with aphasia?
5. Why is the speed of an individual's perceptual processing functionally important?
6. Define apraxia and describe the effect of apraxia on daily living skills.
7. How is ideomotor apraxia evaluated?
8. Describe the two approaches to treatment of perceptual deficits and give one example of a treatment activity for each.

REFERENCES

1. American Occupational Therapy Association: Uniform terminology for occupational therapy, ed 3, *Am J Occup Ther* 48:1047, 1994.
2. Arnadottir G: *The brain and behavior: assessing cortical dysfunction through activities of daily living,* St Louis, 1990, Mosby.
3. Arnadottir G: Impact of neurobehavioral deficits on activities of daily living. In Gillen G, Burkhardt A, editors: *Stroke rehabilitation: a function-based approach,* St Louis, 1998, Mosby.
4. Arnadottir G: Evaluation and intervention with complex perceptual impairment. In Unsworth C: *Cognitive and perceptual dysfunction: a clinical reasoning approach to evaluation and intervention,* Philadelphia, 1999, FA Davis.
5. Ashford JW, Schmitt F, Kumar V: Diagnosis of Alzheimer's disease. In Kumar V, Eisdorfer C, editors: *Advances in the diagnosis and treatment of Alzheimer's disease,* New York, 1998, Springer.
6. Ayres AJ: *Sensory integration and learning disorders,* Los Angeles, 1972, Western Psychological Services.
7. Baum B, Hall K: Relationship between constructional praxis and dressing in the head injured adult, *Am J Occup Ther* 35:438, 1981.
8. Benton A, Sivan AB: Disturbances of the body schema. In Heilman KM, Valenstein E: *Clinical neuropsychology,* New York, 1993, Oxford University Press.
9. Benton A, Tranel D: Visuoperceptual, visuospatial, and visuoconstructive disorders. In Heilman KM, Valenstein E, editors: *Clinical neuropsychology,* New York, 1993, Oxford University Press.
10. Benton AL, Fogel ML: Three-dimensional constructional praxis: a clinical test, *Arch Neurol* 7:347, 1962.
11. Benton AL, Schultz LM: Observations of tactile form perception (stereognosis) in pre-school children, *J Clin Psychol* 5:359, 1949.
12. Benton AL et al: *Contributions to neuropsychological assessment: a clinical manual,* Oxford, 1983, Oxford University Press.
13. Binetti G et al: Visual and spatial perceptions in the early phase of Alzheimer's disease, *Neuropsychology* 12:29, 1998.
14. Blakemore C, Movshon JA: Sensory system: introduction. In Gazzaniga MS, editor: *The cognitive neurosciences,* London, 1996, MIT Press.
15. Bruce V, Young A: *In the eye of the beholder: the science of face perception,* Oxford, 1998, Oxford University Press.
16. Butler JA: Evaluation and intervention with apraxia. In Unsworth C: *Cognitive and perceptual dysfunction: a clinical reasoning approach to evaluation and intervention,* Philadelphia, 1999, FA Davis.
17. Calder AJ et al: Facial emotion recognition after bilateral amygdala damage: differentially severe impairment of fear, *Cogn Neuropsychol* 13:699, 1996.
18. Caplan BM, Romans S: Assessment of spatial abilities. In Goldstein G, Nussbaum PD, Beers SR, editors: *Neuropsychology,* New York, 1998, Plenum Press.
19. Chusic JG: *Correlative neuroanatomy and functional neurology,* ed 19, Los Altos, Calif, 1985, Lange Medical Publications.
20. Colarusso RP, Hammill DD: *Motor-Free Visual Perception test—revised (MVPT-R),* Novato, Calif, 1996, Academic Therapy Publications.
21. DeJong R: *The neurologic examination,* New York, 1958, Paul B. Hoeber.
22. Dellon AL: *Evaluation of sensibility and re-education of sensation in the hand,* Baltimore, Md, 1981, Williams & Wilkins.
23. De Renzi E: Methods of limb apraxia examination and their bearing on the interpretation of the disorder. In Roy EA, editor: *Neuropsychological studies of apraxia and related disorders,* Amsterdam, 1985, North-Holland.
24. De Renzi E, Faglioni P, Sorgato P: Modality-specific and supramodal mechanisms of apraxia, *Brain* 105:301, 1982.

25. De Renzi E, Motti F, Nichelli P: Imitating gestures: a quantitative approach to ideomotor apraxia, *Arch Neurol* 37:6, 1980.

26. De Renzi E, Pieczuro A, Vignolo LA: Ideational apraxia: a quantitative study, *Neuropsychologia* 6:41, 1968.

27. Donnelly SM, Hextell D, Matthey S: The Rivermead Perceptual Assessment Battery: its relationship to selected functional activities, *Br J Occup Ther* 61:27, 1998.

28. Edmans JA, Lincoln NB: Treatment of visual perceptual deficits after stroke: single case studies on four patients with right hemiplegia, *Br J Occup Ther* 54:139, 1991.

29. Eggers O: *Occupational therapy in the treatment of adult hemiplegia*, Rockville, Md, 1984, Aspen Systems.

30. Fall CC: Comparing ways of measuring constructional praxis in the well elderly, *Am J Occup Ther* 41:500, 1987.

31. Farber SD: *Neurorehabiliation, a multisensory approach*, Philadelphia, 1982, WB Saunders.

32. Fleming J, Strong J: Self-awareness of deficits following acquired brain injury: considerations for rehabilitation, *Br J Occup Ther* 58:55, 1995.

33. Gardner H: *Frames of mind: the theory of multiple intelligences*, New York, 1983, Basic Books.

34. Gardner MF: *The Test of Visual-Motor Skills (TVMS)*, Burlingame, Calif, 1992, Psychological and Educational Publications.

35. Gardner MF: *The Test of Visual Perceptual Skills—revised (TVPS-R)*, Hydesville, Calif, 1997, Psychological and Educational Publications.

36. Geschwind N: The apraxias: neural mechanisms of disorders of learned movement, *Am Sci* 63:188, 1975.

37. Gilroy J, Meyer JS: *Medical neurology*, London, 1969, Macmillan.

38. Goodglass H, Kaplan E: *Assessment of aphasia and related disorders*, ed 2, Philadelphia, 1972, Thomas Publishers.

39. Gordon WA et al: Perceptual remediation in patients with right brain damage: a comprehensive program, *Arch Phys Med Rehabil* 66:353, 1985.

40. Haaland KY, Harrington DL: Neuropsychological assessment of motor skills In Goldstein G, Nussbaum PD, Beers SR, editors: *Neuropsychology*, New York, 1998, Plenum Press.

41. Head H et al: *Studies in neurology*, London, 1920, Oxford University Press.

42. Heilman KM, Rothi LJG: Apraxia. In Heilman KM, Valenstein E, editors: *Clinical neuropsychology*, New York, 1993, Oxford University Press.

43. Heilman KM et al: Conceptual apraxia from lateralized lesions, *Neurology* 49:457, 1997.

44. Hooper HE: *Hooper Visual Organization Test*, Los Angeles, 1983, Western Psychological Association.

45. Humphreys GW, Riddoch MJ: *To see but not to see: a case study of visual agnosia*, Hove, UK, 1987, Lawrence Erlbaum Associates.

46. Humphreys GW, Riddoch MJ: Visual object processing in normality and pathology: implications for rehabilitation. In Riddoch MJ, Humphreys GW, editors: *Cognitive neuropsychology and cognitive rehabilitation*, Hove, UK, 1994, Lawrence Erlbaum Associates.

47. Itzkovich M et al: *The Loewenstein Occupational Therapy Cognitive Assessment (LOTCA) manual*, Pequanock, NJ, 1990, Maddock.

48. Katz N, editor: *Cognition and occupation in rehabilitation: cognitive models for intervention in occupational therapy*, Bethesda, Md, 1998, American Occupational Therapy Association.

49. Katz N, Hartman-Maeir A: Metacognition: the relationships of awareness and executive functions to occupational performance. In Katz N, editor: *Cognition and occupation in rehabilitation: cognitive models for intervention in occupational therapy*, Bethesda, Md, 1998, American Occupational Therapy Association.

50. Kent BE: Sensory-motor testing: the upper limb of adult patients with hemiplegia, *Phys Ther J Am Phys Ther Assoc* 45:550, 1965.

51. Kimura D, Archibald Y: Motor functions of the left hemisphere, *Brain* 97:337, 1974.

52. Kline DW, Scialfa CT: Visual and auditory aging. In Birren JE, Schaie KW, editors: *Handbook of the psychology of aging*, ed 4, San Diego, 1996, Academic Press.

53. Kritchevsky M: The elementary spatial functions of the brain. In Stiles-Davis J, Kritchevsky M, Bellugi U, editors: *Spatial cognition: brain bases and development*, Hillsdale, NJ, 1988, Lawrence Erlbaum Associates.

54. Lezak MD: *Neuropsychological assessment*, New York, 1995, Oxford University Press.

55. Likert R, Quasha WH: *The revised Minnesota Paper Form Board Test*, New York, 1970, Psychological Corporation.

56. Lincoln NB et al: The Rey figure copy as a screening instrument for perceptual deficits after stroke, *Br J Occup Ther* 61:33, 1998.

57. MacDonald J: An investigation of body scheme in adults with cerebral vascular accident, *Am J Occup Ther* 14:72, 1960.

58. Mercier L et al: *Motor-free visual perception test—vertical(MVPT-V)*, Novato, Calif, 1997, Academic Therapy Publications.

59. Neistadt ME: Normal adult performance on constructional praxis training tasks, *Am J Occup Ther* 43:448, 1989.

60. Neistadt ME: A critical analysis of occupational therapy approaches for perceptual deficits in adults with brain injury, *Am J Occup Ther* 44:299, 1990.

61. Neistadt ME: The relationship between constructional and meal preparation skills, *Arch Phys Med Rehabil* 74:144, 1993.

62. Newcombe F, Ratcliff G: Disorders of visuospatial analysis. In Boller F, Grafman J, editors: *Handbook of neuropsychology*, vol 2, Amsterdam, 1989, Elsevier Science Publishers.

63. Occupational Therapy Department, Rancho Los Amigos Hospital: *Upper extremity sensory evaluation: a manual for occupational therapists*, Downey, Calif, 1985.

64. Ochipa C, Rothi LJG, Heilman KM: Conceptual apraxia in Alzheimer's disease, *Brain* 115:1061, 1992.

65. Ogden JA: Spatial abilities and deficits in aging and age-related disorders. In Boller F, Grafman J, editors: *Handbook of neuropsychology*, vol 4, Amsterdam, 1990, Elsevier Science Publishers.

66. Pick HL: Perception, locomotion, and orientation. In Welsh RL, Blasch BB, editors: *Foundations of orientation and mobility*, New York, 1980, American Foundation for the Blind.

67. Pilgrim E, Humphreys GW: Rehabilitation of a case of ideomotor apraxia. In Riddoch MJ, Humphreys GW: *Cognitive neuropsychology and cognitive rehabilitation*, Hove, UK, 1994, Lawrence Erlbaum Associates.

68. Poole JL et al: The mechanisms for adult-onset apraxia and developmental dyspraxia: an examination and comparison of error patterns, *Am J Occup Ther* 51:339, 1997.

69. Radomski MV: There is more to life than putting on your pants, *Am J Occup Ther* 49:487, 1995.

70. Rothi LJG, Heilman KM: Acquisition and retention of gestures by apraxic patients, *Brain Cogn* 3:426, 1984.

71. Rothi LJG, Heilman KM: Ideomotor apraxia: gestural discrimination, comprehension, and memory. In Roy EA, editor: *Neuropsychological studies of apraxia and related disorders*, Amsterdam, 1985, North-Holland.

72. Rubio KB: Treatment of neurobehavioral deficits: a function-based approach. In Gillen G, Burkhardt A, editors: *Stroke rehabilitation: a function-based approach*, St Louis, 1998, Mosby.

73. Rubio KB, Van Deusen J: Relation of perceptual and body image dysfunction to activities of daily living after stroke, *Am J Occup Ther* 49:551, 1995.

74. Sacks O: *The man who mistook his wife for a hat and other clinical tales*, New York, 1985, Summit Books.

75. Sacks O: *An anthropologist on Mars*, New York, 1995, Knopf.

76. Sivan AB: *The Benton Visual Retention Test*, San Antonio, Tex, 1992, Psychological Corporation.

77. Sundet K et al: Neuropsychological predictors in stroke rehabilitation, *J Clin Exp Neuropsychol* 10:363, 1988.

78. Tate RL, McDonald S: What is apraxia? The clinician's dilemma, *Neuropsychol Rehabil* 5:273, 1995.

79. Titus MND et al: Correlation of perceptual performance and activities of daily living in stroke patients, *Am J Occup Ther* 45:410, 1991.

80. Tsurumi K, Todd V: Theory and guidelines for visual task analysis and synthesis. In Scheiman M, editor: *Understanding and managing vision deficits: a guide for occupational therapists*, Thorofare, NJ, 1997, Slack.

81. Warren M: Relationship of constructional apraxia and body scheme disorders to dressing performance in adult CVA, *Am J Occup Ther* 35:431, 1981.

82. Warrington E, James M, Kinsborne M: Drawing ability in relation to laterality of lesion, *Brain* 89:53, 1966.

83. Whiting S et al: *RPAB—Rivermead Perceptual Assessment Battery*, Windsor, UK, 1985, NFER-Nelson Publishing Company.

84. Willis L et al: Ideomotor apraxia in early Alzheimer's disease: time and accuracy measures, *Brain Cogn* 38:220, 1998.

85. York CD, Cermack SA: Visual perception and praxis in adults after stroke, *Am J Occup Ther* 49:543, 1995.

86. Young AW et al: Face perception after brain injury, *Brain* 116:941, 1993.

87. Zoltan B: *Vision, perception, and cognition*, ed 3 (rev), Thorofare, NJ, 1996, Slack.

88. Zoltan B, Siev E, Freishtat B: *Perceptual and cognitive dysfunction in the adult stroke patient*, ed 2, Thorofare, NJ, 1986, Charles B Slack.

CHAPTER 27

Evaluation and Treatment of Cognitive Dysfunction

CAROL J. WHEATLEY

KEY TERMS

Cognition
Metacognition
Ecological validity
Orientation
Simultaneous multiple attention
Vigilance
Working memory
Declarative memory
Implicit memory
Explicit memory
Procedural memory
Everyday memory
Prospective memory
Confabulation
Learning style
Errorless learning
Domain-specific learning
Dyscalculia
Executive function
Anosognosia
Disinhibition
Stimulus-bound behavior
Perseveration

LEARNING OBJECTIVES

After studying this chapter the student or practitioner will be able to do the following:
1. Define cognition.
2. Explain the value of a team approach to cognitive rehabilitation.
3. Summarize the effects of environmental factors on a person's cognitive process.
4. Describe the effects of the aging process on cognitive skills.
5. Differentiate the major cognitive treatment approaches in the field of occupational therapy.
6. Provide examples of the use of assistive technology to compensate for cognitive dysfunction.
7. Cite standardized assessment tools for each of the primary skill areas of cognition.
8. Describe specific treatment efforts for targeted cognitive deficits.

Cognitive impairment can lead to profound functional limitations. Cognitive impairment often follows a cerebrovascular accident (CVA), traumatic brain injury (TBI), or acquired disease that results in brain damage, such as multiple sclerosis or Alzheimer's dementia. This chapter aims to increase the therapist's understanding of cognitive processes and to describe the principles of cognitive assessment and treatment.

Cognition is a series of complex thought processes by which we come to know and act on our environment, to benefit from past experiences, and to generate new ideas to advance our existence. Cognitive processing spans a wide range of activity and input. It can involve multiple sensory input from the external environment or can be carried on with only intrinsic material. For example, when driving a vehicle, an individual needs to process a continuous stream of information from the environment—the response of the automobile, the conditions of the road, traffic signs, and the movement of other vehicles or pedestrians in relationship to the vehicle being driven. In contrast, when a person is writing a term paper, much of the cognitive activity is internal, employing memories of information previously read, reasoning, analysis, and organization.

Metacognition, described as "knowing about knowing,"[21] is the ability to know and monitor the individual characteristics of cognitive skills. It is considered the bridge that links together all the various aspects of cognition and enables a person to choose memory strategies, problem-solving approaches, and reasoning methods that are uniquely beneficial to the completion of a cognitive activity.[43]

The assessment and remediation of cognitive deficits can be challenging and complex. Cognitive functions are discussed and evaluated in discrete subsections, but in practical reality, cognitive skills are employed together in every task to varying degrees. These functions include attention, memory, initiation, planning and organization, mental flexibility, abstraction, insight, reasoning, problem-solving, and judgment.

PRINCIPLES OF COGNITIVE ASSESSMENT
Team Approach to Evaluation

Many health care professionals from a variety of disciplines work together in the assessment and treatment of persons with cognitive dysfunction. Discussion of occupational therapy (OT) evaluation results with other members of the team increases the therapist's understanding of the person's capacity and the relationship of the deficits assessed to dysfunction in other skill areas. The OT approach to cognitive skills tends to emphasize the processing of visual, tactile, and spatial information, which is largely mediated by the right hemisphere of the brain. Consultation with the speech pathologist concerning the person's auditory, language, and linguistic and cognitive abilities is essential because these skills are processed mostly by the left brain hemisphere. Physical therapists can provide observations about the person's visual perceptual functioning during gross motor and ambulation tasks. The psychologist or neuropsychologist can provide information regarding the individual's intellectual range with an overview of the relative strengths and weakness of the various skills. In addition, the individual's family can provide the team with a description of the individual's functioning before the onset of the disability. Without prior knowledge of all these areas, interpretation of the OT cognitive assessment may be inaccurate. The therapist should always look at the total picture when interpreting an individual's behavior. Frequently the conclusions are the result of much team discussion.[40,63] The team may also

include the physician, therapeutic recreation specialist, and other disciplines, depending on the goals and resources of the facility.

Optimal Test Battery

The optimal test battery involves several tests, standardized and normed for the population, and a variety of functional activities that are relevant to the individual. Therapists need standardized tests to provide objective, quantifiable data, to measure the extent of the deficit compared to an established norm, to document progress, and to enable discharge planning. In addition, the common terminology, concepts, and testing conditions of standardized tests facilitate communication between practitioners. The **ecological validity** of a standardized test refers to the test's ability to predict functional performance based on test results—in other words, the extent to which a test predicts ability to function in important life tasks.[12,27]

Functional activities provide opportunities to observe the practical implications of deficits identified by standardized tests. Further, functional activities performed in the OT clinic allow the therapist to better predict an individual's functioning in the home environment.

The assessment process is similar to solving a puzzle in which a variety of tests and functional tasks are used to deduce the areas of strengths and weaknesses, to explain the person's behavior, and to identify potential treatment approaches.

Several test batteries are available that screen a range of cognitive skills, including the following: the Cognitive Assessment of Minnesota,[52] The Loewenstein Occupational Therapy Cognitive Assessment (LOTCA),[29] and the Neurobehavioral Cognitive Status Screening Examination (COGNISTAT).[31] The Arnadottir OT-ADL Neurobehavioral Evaluation (A-ONE) provides an analysis of functional activities to determine cognitive skill deficit areas.[4] The Cognitive Rehabilitation Workbook provides a pretest and posttest, as well as treatment exercises, for community living skills such as constructing a schedule and reading a map.[20]

Environmental Effects on Performance
Human performance is variable by nature. The testing environment can exert influence—sometimes strong, sometimes subtle—on the results of the cognitive assessment. The concept of environment includes not only the physical features and time of day, but also the amount of structure and feedback provided by the examiner. For example, the person's ability to attend to tasks may be very different early in the morning while lying in bed compared with taking a structured test, with cueing provided by the examiner, while seated in a wheelchair. The person's behavior in the foreign environment of the

hospital or rehabilitation facility may be quite different from performance in the familiar home setting. Health team members often disagree about the person's cognitive status when, in fact, discrepancies are merely the result of environmental differences in the administration and nature of testing. Instead of being alarmed by these differences in test results, the more constructive approach is to analyze and use the information in designing the most effective plan for remediation and compensation of deficits.

Therapist's Approach

When introducing a cognitive test to a person, the therapist should avoid a condescending attitude or a manner that is too bright or artificially positive. No matter what the level of functioning, the person must be approached in an age-appropriate manner.

It is important to avoid offering choices when there actually are none. Instead, choices should be offered, such as: "Would you prefer to perform coordination tests or cognitive tests first?" This suggests that all of the tests must be completed eventually. The therapist should not ask for cooperation as a personal favor ("I would like you to . . . ,") or imply that the test is a joint effort ("Let's do some testing today!"). Instead, recognize each person's responsibility, by such phrases as "I will be . . . , and your job is to . . . ."[34]

Avoid power struggles at all costs. Forcing a person to cooperate is not likely to produce valid assessment results.

It is also important that the therapist not provide cues to right or wrong responses; as an alternative, randomly reward the person's effort throughout the test by such comments as, "Good job" or "You put a lot of effort into that test."[34]

For a highly distractible individual, the therapist may model the desired behavior. The therapist who is gazing around the room during the test may serve as a distracting stimulus. In contrast, a therapist who is steadily gazing at the test items may cue the person to follow suit.

Test Administration

The therapist must adhere to the instructions that accompany standardized tests, or the results of the tests will be invalid. Later, when the test is repeated by a different therapist or different facility, variability in response may be difficult to explain. However, it is possible and sometimes clinically useful to test beyond the limits of a standardized assessment tool by following the rules as given until the assessment is completed and then exploring various modifications. It is important to document the adaptations and results.[34] For example, a person may perform poorly on a perceptual test because he has difficulty keeping the directions in working memory (see the Memory section) as he progresses through the items. After completion of the test, the therapist could return to earlier items, repeating the instructions for each item. A sharp improvement in performance may suggest a memory deficit rather than a perceptual deficit. Some of the newer testing instruments provide for the intervention of various cueing strategies, allowing for assessment of the effectiveness of the strategy, as well as of the skill area itself. An example is the Contextual Memory Test,[66] in which the therapist records the strategies used (e.g., imagery) and documents the effect of the strategy on the memory task. Frequently the therapist develops a repertoire of management strategies to support the optimum functioning of the person, but unless the strategies are documented, they will have to be rediscovered (or sometimes not) by other therapists who are working with that individual.

Relationship of Cognitive Deficits to Other Performance Components

As cognitive processes interrelate, the therapist must assess a broad spectrum of skill areas, from basic sensory functions to complex processing, and compare findings with those of other members of the team. A poor score on a test of complex cognitive function may be caused or complicated by a deficiency in a more basic skill. For example, a person with a left visual field loss may select a lightweight garment on a cold day, simply because he or she failed to scan the full contents of the closet to see the sweater hanging to the left. In addition, the individual who does not remember the selection of clothing brought to the rehabilitation facility will not search for the sweater among his or her belongings.

Intellectual Capacity Before Injury

The individual's family should be interviewed and existing records reviewed to determine the individual's level of functioning before the injury or CVA. For example, persons who were below average in intellectual level before injury cannot be expected to perform at a higher level on tests administered after the injury. Similarly, if a person has a previous learning disability affecting the ability to read and write, the therapist should recognize that the quality of the person's written responses on a given test may be the result of factors other than the CVA. Another example is the individual who functioned at a very high level before brain injury and who now scores in the average range. Although the person's functioning may be sufficient for daily activities, this is still a significant drop from previous capacity. The individual may need to learn new ways to cope with this change in functional level.

Impact of Substance Abuse

An individual with cognitive impairments caused by head trauma, CVA, or other causes may also have a history of substance abuse.[6] The long-term effects of use and abuse of illegal substances are widely recognized, but studies have been hindered by related factors of ongoing abuse, medical complications, and poor education.[34] It is important to know if a person has a history of alcoholism because prolonged use can lead to Korsakoff's syndrome, with significant loss of new learning capacity.[17]

Cognition and Aging

In the normal aging process, decline is noted in working memory, face recognition, speed of information processing, and spatial recall,[59] complicated by the decline in visual and auditory skills. This can have implications for everyday functioning, such as remembering a route, keeping to medication schedules, and facial recall of new acquaintances. An older adult's performance is relatively higher for familiar tasks in familiar settings than for unfamiliar tasks in unfamiliar settings.[28] Because the speed of information processing is slower for older persons, the therapist must match the pacing of the activity to the individual and allow for multiple repetitions and a longer response time.[32,73]

Some assessment tools, such as the Benton Visual Retention Test,[58] adjust the interpretation of scores based on age. The Mini-Mental State Examination frequently is used as a screening tool to assess the cognitive skills of the older population.[22,32]

An area of growing concern to geriatric therapists is that of the person with Alzheimer's dementia.[33] This disorder leads to progressive decline in behavior, attention, memory, visual perception, praxis, language, and executive functioning.[34,39] The goal of therapeutic intervention is to maximize the person's functional level, increase safety, minimize confusion, develop behavioral management strategies, and serve as a resource to families.[5,19,25] Rather than attempting to improve recall with drills or internal mnemonic strategies, the therapist makes changes to the environment to stimulate memory and orientation. Alzheimer's units in skilled nursing facilities may be designed to minimize residents' confusion. An example is placing a small display case next to a person's doorway, in which to store articles that have a strong personal meaning and thereby aid the person in recognizing which room is his or her own.[15,16]

APPROACHES TO TREATMENT
Models of Treatment

Table 27-1 summarizes various treatment approaches proposed in OT literature. The reader can consult the references for more in-depth discussions of each treatment approach.

Therapists may choose to follow a certain treatment philosophy or may adopt a more eclectic approach,

blending treatment models based on the response of the person.

The remedial and adaptive approaches were once viewed as incompatible but are now recognized as parts of a continuum. Acute care centers frequently find remedial intervention to be effective. Adaptive compensatory approaches are used in rehabilitation facilities as the period of rapid recovery diminishes.[30]

A treatment task can be analyzed and modified in several ways to improve performance.[68] This process is commonly known as providing *structure*. A treatment activity can be graded by changing the task parameters, which include the environment, familiarity with the task, directions for completing the task, number of items, spatial arrangement of items, number of response options, and response rate required.

Examples of task grading are the treatment of an inattentive individual in a quiet, uncluttered environment and the treatment of the person with poor memory in the same environment every day. Various environmental cues can be established in the person's work area to stimulate recall.

Cues are provided via systematic interpersonal interaction with the therapist or others and modified according to the client's response. Cues can direct attention to a particular aspect of a task, guide problem solving, and facilitate recall. Examples of cues are repetition ("Try again"), analysis ("What do these objects have in common?"), and direction of attention ("Look here on your left").[66] The client should be involved in the development of the cueing system whenever possible because the client will select the cues that are most meaningful.

The therapist's task is to identify the conditions that elicit the best performance from the client (e.g., styles of interaction with the client, cues to stimulate memory, or controls to elicit socially acceptable behavior). To challenge the client to expand his or her abilities, the therapist must achieve a delicate balance in presenting activities that are near, yet just beyond, the client's current capacity. One client described the OT program as "a moving target." Several resources offer a variety of treatment tasks and ideas.[18,20,69,84]

Technology in Cognitive Retraining

Recent advances in technology have provided additional options for remediation and compensation of cognitive deficits. Computers can be useful for rehabilitation, as a means by which to practice cognitive skills or strategies taught by the therapist.[26] In work-oriented tasks, the computer can be programmed to monitor, cue, and organize an individual's output.[47]

Miniaturization and the increased power of microprocessors have permitted the development of a number of electronic devices that can be used in compensation for cognitive and memory impairments.[44,45]

TABLE 27-1
Treatment Models

Model	Definition
Remedial, transfer of training approach	Uses practice with activities designed to target the deficit areas. Typically, tabletop pencil-and-paper tasks are used, involving skills that have been found by formal testing to be deficient.[84]
Adaptive approach	Focuses on the skills that are relatively intact, to develop compensatory methods for deficit areas. Treatment activities are functional, real-life tasks.[41,42]
Dynamic interactional approach	Resists labeling individual deficits (e.g., attention and memory). Instead, focuses on the processes used by the person as he or she performs various cognitive tasks; therapist teaches strategies to improve performance across the cognitive spectrum. The approach uses factors external to the patient (environmental context, nature of the task, and criteria of learning), as well as internal factors (metacognition, processing strategies, and the characteristics of the learner). A particular strategy is targeted and practiced in multiple environments to increase the likelihood of transfer, with a variety of tasks and movement demands.[60]
Quadraphonic approach	Integrates four theoretical approaches: information processing, learning theory, biomechanical, and neurodevelopmental, and emphasizes the need for the therapist to continuously adapt the treatment to the patient's changing status and the changing environment. Treatment guides the patient through the sequence of problem detection, discrimination and analysis, and hypothesis generation while performing therapeutic activities.[1]
Neurofunctional approach	Metacognitive training is combined with applied behavioral analysis to retrain for functional skills, using the behavioral approaches of shaping, fading, and reinforcement.[24]
Cognitive disabilities approach	Developed initially for chronic mental illness, this approach uses the Allen Cognitive Levels to determine a match between the patient's functioning and the environmental demands of the task, and to provide guidelines for caregivers.[2]

These include alarm watches; pocket-sized, computerized data storage units; electronic pillboxes; and telephones with phone number memory features. The therapist's role is to determine which device meets the client's need, to aid in the initial programming of the device, and to train the client and family to integrate the device into the client's daily routine.

ASSESSMENT AND TREATMENT OF SPECIFIC DEFICIT AREAS

Although cognitive processing relies on the complex integration of functions, isolation of various skills for close analysis is helpful. The therapist may find it useful to assess the client according to the following hierarchy of skills.

Orientation and Attention

Orientation refers to an individual's ongoing awareness of the situation, the environment, and the passage of time. From the point of a traumatic injury that results in cognitive impairment, an individual must develop an awareness of the events that preceded the accident and those occurring since that time. Frequently after a CVA the individual is initially disoriented. As the mental state clears, the individual becomes increasingly ori-

ented to his or her surroundings. A TBI can result in a period of coma, the length of which is indicative of the severity of injury. Chapters 37 and 38 provide further discussion on cerebrovascular accidents and traumatic head injury.

An unimpaired person is oriented to person ("Who am I?"), place ("Where am I?"), and time ("What year, month, day, or time of day is it?"). Orientation involves an individual's memory capacity, because a person must be able to remember past occurrences in order to place current events in their proper perspective. After a severe TBI or CVA, persons initially may be confused regarding their identity, indicating a disorientation to person. This deficit is more global than an inability to speak one's name, which may occur in the case of aphasia (difficulty with the verbal expression of any message). Some people may also confuse the identities of other individuals, such as by thinking that the therapist is a family member. *Orientation to place* refers to an individual's knowledge of the fact that he or she is in a hospital, for example, or the name of the immediate town, city, and state. Difficulty monitoring the passage of time can result in time disorientation. Persons often have difficulty beyond simply remembering the date; they may confuse the sequence of events in time. For example, a person may report that a certain family member visited the previous day, when the family member actually may have visited a week earlier. As with all aspects of cognition, discussion with other team members is critical to ensure a comprehensive understanding of the individual's deficit.

Topographical orientation describes an individual's awareness of his or her position in relation to the environment (e.g., the room, building, or town). Functional examples of this disorder are noted when an individual becomes confused while attempting to leave a room, locate another therapy department, or travel to the cafeteria. Such individuals frequently perform better in the familiar environment of the home and community, but deficits may still be apparent, particularly when there is a need to travel to a new environment.

Attention requires a fluid, ever-changing focus on relevant internal and environmental information. Attention involves the simultaneous engagement of alertness, selectivity, sustained effort, flexibility, and mental tracking.[64] An individual must be alert and awake and able to select a relevant focus of interest. The individual must be able to maintain focus for as long as needed, yet be able to shift focus if another event of interest or importance occurs. In addition, the individual must ignore information if it is not relevant and must be able to track multiple sequences of information simultaneously. Because these skills underlie all aspects of cognitive functioning, they are frequently affected by TBI or CVA, and deficits may hinder all higher skill levels. For example, a person who is unable to attend to a task for more than a few seconds cannot take in all the necessary information to perform a higher-level reasoning task.

Information processing can occur via well-established habits, referred to as *automatic processing*, or on a more conscious, *controlled processing* level.[81] A person undergoing rehabilitation often needs to use controlled processing to perform basic tasks that were handled automatically before the injury. A person who has difficulty with *divided attention*, or **simultaneous multiple attention**, may not be able to handle more than one task at a time. The person typically responds by reverting to focused attention. For example, during a physical therapy session, the person with hemiplegia who is asked a question while ambulating may stop walking in order to engage in conversation.

Concentration requires sustained attention, also referred to as **vigilance**. Persons may be highly distractible or very sensitive to events in the immediate environment, which pulls their focus away from the task at hand. It is important to note which types of stimuli (e.g., visual, auditory, tactile, or gustatory) distract the person easily. A low-stimulus environment or "quiet room" may be beneficial. Such a room is designed for minimal visual stimuli and for insulation from nearby noise and activity.

Some individuals have the opposite problem. That is, they can become very deeply focused on a given stimulus or activity and have difficulty maintaining a general awareness of events occurring around them. A family member once described his brother as tending to "get sucked into the computer," and a closer examination of the person's activity revealed that the person was not performing any useful work, only rearranging his computer files day after day. See the sections on executive function and behavior later in this chapter.

Either extreme is undesirable. Normal functioning requires that a person be able to focus, sustain a low level of awareness of peripheral events, and disengage, then reengage concentration as needed.

Assessment of Orientation and Attention

Orientation to person, time, and place can be assessed informally by asking the person basic questions about his or her identity, the date, time of day, and season of the year, and the name of the hospital, city, and state. Because levels of orientation can vary, it is best to ask these questions several times to determine the consistency of the person's awareness. Topographical orientation can be assessed informally by observing a person traveling from one site to another or by asking the person to draw a floor plan of his or her room, therapy area, or home, verifying the latter with the family. The therapist must also consider the influence of possible visuospatial deficits on this task. Orientation questions and route finding are also included as part of the Rivermead Behavioural Memory Test.[78]

Examples of standardized tests of attention include the Knox Cube Test[62] and, for divided attention, the Trail Making Test.[3] Additional information on these and other standardized tests of attention is given in sources referenced at the end of this chapter.[34,84] The occupational therapist's assessment of attention should include structured clinical observation and activity analysis during functional tasks.

Treatment of Deficits in Orientation and Attention

ORIENTATION. All staff and family members who come into contact with the person should make efforts to reestablish orientation as frequently as possible. External aids such as calendars, bulletin boards, and "orientation boards" with pertinent information (e.g., the name of the facility, the date, season, and current events) are often used in rehabilitation centers. An orientation group can be scheduled to meet at the start of each day to review the day's upcoming events and previous day's happenings.[36,83]

ATTENTION. The initial goal of treatment is to determine the optimal activities or environment that enables the person to focus for the longest time. As attention and concentration improve, the therapist can increase the duration, as well as the complexity, of the activity. Finally, the person should gradually be weaned from the low-stimulus environment as tolerance increases. Formalized attention-training models are available.[8,44,60]

MEMORY

Memory is the process by which all information is stored and retrieved in the cognitive system. It is a dynamic continuation of the attentional process that includes the factor of time. As an individual is able to maintain focus on a task, information becomes stored in the memory process. The memory process is summarized in Fig. 27-1.

The memory process can break down at any level. If a person is unable to maintain attention, the information may never enter the system. Some persons are able to process information in *short-term* or **working memory** but never encode the material into *long-term storage*. Others can store the information but have a deficit in the retrieval process. Strategic testing, comparing tests requiring free recall (open-ended questions) with recognition (multiple-choice responses), may help the therapist determine the breakdown in the memory process, which can then guide the treatment approach.

People with memory deficits, who need to expend additional effort to learn new material, may also have difficulty forgetting information when it is no longer needed. It is critical that the therapist be well prepared when planning to teach new information to a person, to avoid teaching incorrectly anything that the person will later need to unlearn.

The ability to recite or reproduce information is generally taken as an indication of recall and is referred to as **declarative memory**. Tests often require a person to repeat a word list or draw a set of geometric designs, or a therapist may quiz a person about events occurring earlier in the day. Declarative memory is divided into two categories. *Episodic memory* refers to an individual's recall of his or her personal history and lifetime of experiences. The general fund of knowledge shared by groups of people is called *semantic memory* and includes such information as language and rules of social behavior. Semantic memory is generally less affected than is episodic recall after an injury.[26]

Another distinction in memory function concerns the memory of the source of the information. Many memory-impaired individuals may recall the information but not the details of when, where, and from whom they learned it. This is labeled **implicit memory**.[53] In contrast, memory of the source of the information in addition to the information itself is called **explicit memory**. The difference can be seen in the example of a person who is informed by his nurse that there will be a cancellation for an appointment that day, because his therapist is not available. Later, another staff member observes the person in the recreation room during his regularly scheduled therapy time and admonishes the person for missing therapy. The person cannot explain the reason he is not in therapy because he lacks the explicit recall of the conversation with his nurse earlier that day. Nonetheless, he has acted on correct implicit memory for the change in schedule.

Some individuals have a considerable deficit in declarative memory, but less impaired **procedural memory**, memory for a skill or series of actions.[26] For example, a person may be unable to tell a therapist the steps in making a sandwich and a cup of coffee but may be able to perform the activity correctly. The process of obtaining a driver's license requires a written law test (declarative recall) followed by a behind-the-wheel test (procedural recall). It is procedural learning that enables a person to learn new self-care techniques despite severe memory deficits on standardized memory tests. This phenomenon underscores the need for integration between test performance and observations made during functional activities.

Everyday memory refers to a person's ability to remember information pertinent to daily life[79] (e.g., learning the names and faces of the doctors, nurses, and therapy staff who work regularly with the person in the hospital or rehabilitation facility). Learning a schedule of appointments or the locations of various departments may be difficult and further complicated by frequent changes. The hospital escort staff often assumes this responsibility for the person, which masks the deficit. Everyday memory also includes the ability to keep track of daily events in their proper sequence. **Prospective memory** refers to the ability to remember events that are set to occur at some future time, such as an appointment scheduled for later in the day.[79]

A person with memory deficits may tend toward **confabulation**,[14] or filling in the gaps in memory with imaginary material. This person is not aware of adding erroneous information to the factual data and so can become confused regarding past events or may insist on the accuracy of his memory, to the confusion of others around him. Some persons with memory deficits try to "fake it" to cover their embarrassment at the extent of their memory loss, but this practice is not considered confabulation.

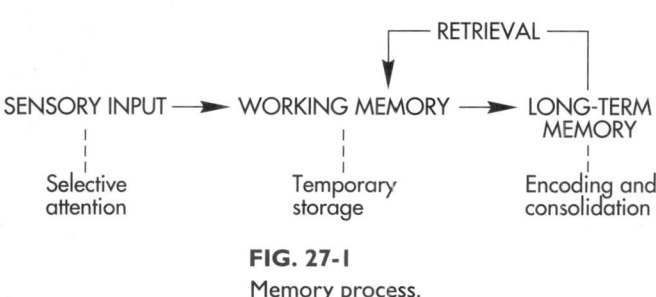

FIG. 27-1
Memory process.

Families frequently report that the individual recalls events from his or her life before the accident with great detail and accuracy but has very poor memory for events occurring in the immediate past. This phenomenon is called Ribot's Law.[50]

Just as is true for any individual, activities or topics of interest or of personal relevance tend to elicit the best performance. As a result, the family may minimize the deficit: "He can remember if he wants to." It is important to reinforce to the family that although the impairment may be less with certain types of material, the deficit remains.

Assessment of Memory Functions

One standardized test for the assessment of visual memory is the Benton Visual Retention Test,[58] which requires free recall of geometric figures and can also indicate an inattention deficit. Selected subtests of the Test of Visual Perceptual Skills assess recognition memory.[23] The Rey Complex Figure Test[34] provides a measure of incidental learning, since the test initially is presented to the person as a drawing task, with recall requested immediately after drawing a figure and then again 20 to 30 minutes later. The Learning Efficiency Test[71] provides a comparison of auditory versus visual recall. The Rivermead Behavioural Memory Test[78] is an evaluation of everyday memory skills and can immediately provide relevant information about the person's capacity to function safely in the home environment. The Contextual Memory Test[66] provides information on the awareness of the deficits, as well as the use and relative value of various strategies, thus offering important information to guide treatment.

A number of standardized memory questionnaires are available.[34] These can be filled out by both the person and a family member to determine the person's level of awareness of his or her memory deficits and the effect of the deficit on the person's everyday functioning.

Treatment of Memory Deficits

In concert with the psychologist, speech-language pathologist, and other team members, the occupational therapist can explore the person's optimal **learning style.**[48,74] Because flexibility in adapting to various teaching approaches is often lost or diminished in individuals with cognitive deficits, it becomes the responsibility of the therapist to present new information in the most efficient way for the person. If the deficit is one of *retrieval*, the team can explore the types of cues that most effectively facilitate the individual's recall. The therapist can identify a person's learning style by observing the response to instructions (oral, written, demonstrated, and diagrammatic) for standardized tests and functional activities, as well as by analyzing the data obtained from standardized memory tests. As

characteristics of optimal teaching methods become apparent, this information can be communicated to the team, the person's family, and the person, who can learn to request that new information be provided in the most effective manner.

The concept of **errorless learning** has been explored with memory-deficient individuals in recent years, with positive results in teaching everyday information and skills.[76,77] New information is taught to individuals in small increments, with many cues, feedback, and correct answers provided, so that the chance of failure is minimized. Over many learning trials, cues are gradually reduced. In contrast, the more common trial-and-error approach encourages the person to guess, sometimes resulting in incorrect responses. The person then must differentiate right from wrong responses in memory, which requires accurate explicit recall. The errorless technique maximizes the recall of the correct information and uses the implicit memory capacity of the person.[77]

A practical example of an errorful learning experience is the process of learning a new procedure on the computer. By attempting a variety of commands, the computer user eventually succeeds in performing the function, but may not recall the correct sequence when attempting to execute the function again. Errorless learning will occur when an experienced computer user teaches each step in sequence and observes the new user until he or she has learned all of the steps correctly.

Memory strategies can be divided into two groups: *internal,* referring to techniques carried out via mental effort by the person, and *external,* referring to methods used by the therapist or cues in the environment to trigger an individual's recall. Examples of external cues are oral reminders from the therapist, signs, cue cards, notebooks, written instructions, and electronic memory aids such as alarm watches and computer data storage units.[44,79] Internal mnemonic strategies include rehearsal, chunking, association, and imagery.[44,75] Table 27-2 lists some memory strategies.

Memory treatment techniques use several known characteristics of memory and cognitive functioning. Often the deficit is one of retrieval rather than recall, so many of the mnemonic techniques are designed to *cue* the memory system to elicit the information. An example is first-letter cueing for a list of words. It is also known that deeper processing of the information creates more retrieval possibilities, so mnemonic techniques can be a means to facilitate more complex examination of the information to be learned. Using association to remember a person's name requires that the individual generate an association between the name and the person; one client learned the author's name by visualizing a person singing holiday songs while standing in a wheat field. The use of environmental cues capitalizes on a person's tendency to be stimulus bound

TABLE 27-2
Memory Strategies

Functional Task	Internal Strategy	External Strategy
Names	Word mnemonic for association: **N**otice the person **A**sk the person to spell or pronounce his or her name **M**ention the name in conversation **E**xaggerate some facial feature	List of names with photographs in memory notebook
Schedule	Develop rhyme: *Breakfast pills are pink, two to help me think*	Alarm watch or hand-held computer data storage unit
Route	Develop series of landmarks to guide route	Map or building floor plan

Parente R, Herrmann D: *Retraining cognition: techniques and applications,* Gaithersburg, Md, 1996, Aspen.

(see the section on executive functions). One example of this is a brightly colored key rack located just inside the front door for the individual to store house keys.

The selection of mnemonic strategies depends on the characteristics of the learner. For example, an individual with relatively high spatial skills may profit from a visualization strategy, and a person who has limited attention and concentration may not be able to use internal mnemonics but may benefit from strategically placed environmental cues. If it has been determined that the individual has a deficit in storage of information but demonstrates good procedural recall, perhaps an electronic notebook would be useful. The therapist can assist the individual and family to set up the notebook, determine the critical information to be recorded, program the storage, and teach the individual to retrieve the information. The goal of therapy is to progress from the use of external cues designed by the therapist to internal and external cues established and maintained by the individual independently. A group approach, empowering individuals to guide the treatment process, has also been shown to be effective.[46]

The concepts of *generalization* and *transfer* are also critical to the learning of new skills. *Transfer of learning* refers to the application of information learned in one situation to another, similar situation. An example is the use of a clothes washer and dryer in the OT department to teach laundry skills; this training method requires that individuals transfer skills learned in the clinic laundry room to their homes. *Generalization* refers to the ability to apply knowledge and skills learned to a variety of similar but novel situations.[44] A person who can generalize could perform clothes cleaning tasks in any laundry setting. Individuals with cognitive deficits frequently have difficulty with transfer of learning and may be unable to generalize skills to novel situations. Transfer of new skills must be built into treatment planning, because the person may not be able to transfer skills independently.

The principle of **domain-specific learning** is based on the assumption that generalization is not likely to be achieved by severely memory-impaired individuals. However, a person may be able to learn specific skills relative to a particular situation and to continue to apply these skills in that specific environment.[54] Teaching one-handed cooking skills in the OT department kitchen may be ineffective if the person is unable to generalize those skills to the kitchen at home. This person may be better served if the instruction is provided in the home environment by the home health therapist.[55] Job coaching, a type of supported employment, also is based on this premise. The skills needed for the job are taught on the job site rather than being taught in advance in a setting other than the job site.[72]

REASONING AND PROBLEM-SOLVING SKILLS

Abstract thinking enables a person to see relationships between objects, events, or ideas, to discriminate relevant from irrelevant detail, and to recognize absurdities.[34] Cognitive deficits in this area and resultant behaviors create difficulty in transfer of knowledge to new situations and in problem solving.[84] Persons with frontal lobe damage commonly lose abstract thinking ability and think only in the most concrete, literal manner. This literal thinking is often paired with mental inflexibility.

The following is an example of *concrete thinking*. A person is asked the interview question, "What brought you to this hospital?" The person responds, "My parent's car." The person is interpreting the question literally, rather than understanding it as a reference to the accident that resulted in brain injury.

Problem solving is a complex process involving many cognitive skills. Problem solving can take the form of *convergent thinking*, which enables a person to arrive at a central idea, and *divergent thinking*, which is aimed at generating alternatives.[82] The process of grocery shopping provides an example of both types of thinking. An individual knows that milk, eggs, and butter are needed and by convergent thinking identifies them as dairy products. Divergent thinking is used to arrive at a list of stores that carry these items.

Various types of reasoning can be used in the problem-solving process. *Deductive reasoning* refers to the ability to arrive at conclusions. For example, a person notices that items grasped in the affected right hand tend to drop to the floor and concludes that the hand is not reliable for grasping and holding. *Inductive reasoning* enables a person to draw generalizations from specific experiences. For example, after a period of persistent right-hand incoordination, the person realizes that the ability to return to a previous occupation involving bilateral manual skills (such as assembly-line work) is now questionable.[9,82]

Reasoning deficits can be noted in a person's inability to recognize the long-term consequences of an action and focus instead on the immediate effect. Persons with deficits in reasoning may have difficulty establishing priorities when faced with a number of tasks to be accomplished.

Dyscalculia is a deficit in the reasoning ability used to perform simple calculations. This deficit can have important implications for an individual's independent functioning in the community. Various types of calculation disorders have been identified.[37] A person may have difficulty reading (alexia) or writing (agraphia) numbers, and consultation should be sought with the speech-language pathologist or psychologist on the team.

Spatial dyscalculia refers to a deficit in the spatial arrangement of numbers (Fig. 27-2). *Anarithmetria* is an inability to perform calculations in someone who has no deficits in reading and writing numbers or spatially arranging the numbers in the calculation and who had a satisfactory educational background and academic skills before the injury.[37]

Assessment of Reasoning and Problem Solving

Abstract conceptual thinking can be assessed in a number of ways. The Test of Nonverbal Intelligence (TONI),[11] the Space Visualization subtest of the Employee Aptitude Series,[55] and the Minnesota Paper Form Board Test[35] all assess complex spatial reasoning skills. The Toglia Category Assessment can test a person's ability to organize and group objects and to change

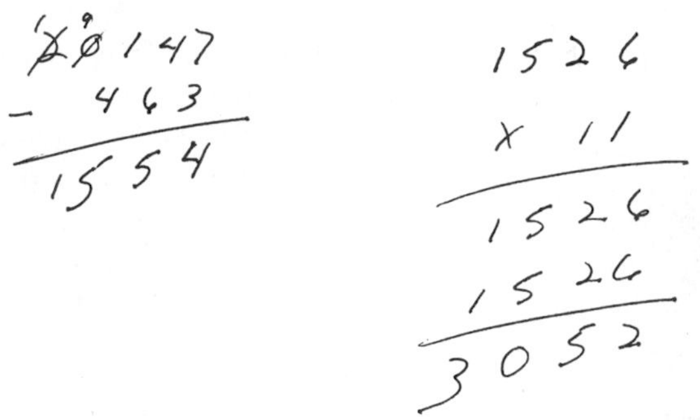

FIG. 27-2
Examples of spatial dyscalculia.

groupings from one category to another.[67] Assessment of reasoning skills during functional task performance can provide predictions of a person's safety and readiness to return home from the rehabilitation facility.

An assessment of calculation abilities should include number recognition and simple to complex mathematical problems, as well as functionally oriented items such as calculating change, recognizing coins, and budgeting. The Cognitive Rehabilitation Workbook[20] includes everyday calculation tasks, providing pretest and posttest measures and training exercises.

Treatment of Reasoning and Problem-Solving Deficits

The steps that comprise the problem-solving process have been organized into the acronym SOLVE[45] for easy recall:

Specify the problem	Frequently, persons have difficulty defining the problem and so tend to generate misdirected solutions
Options	For those who focus narrowly on one solution, developing several possible solutions increases the likelihood of success
Listen to other's advice	This encourages the person to fully explore the problem to avoid missing some critical element.
Vary the solution	This encourages expanded mental flexibility.
Evaluate	Individuals are encouraged to assess what worked and what did not and use the new information for future situations.

This sequence can be taught to the individual, with instructions to use the steps when a problem is encountered in therapy or in functional tasks.[9,82] The therapist assists the individual in transferring this technique to a variety of functional situations.[70]

Executive Functions

Deficits in executive skills are generally the result of damage to the frontal lobes of the brain. The *dysexecutive syndrome*[12] is composed of deficits in the following areas: goal formation and follow-through, memory, disinhibition, and behavior and personality changes. Memory and behavior are discussed in separate sections of this chapter.

GOAL FORMATION AND FOLLOW THROUGH.
An example of a deficit in goal formation is the person who does not generate an idea for activity, but who responds well to an established routine. The structured

schedule of a hospital or rehabilitation facility may mask deficits in this area. These deficits become apparent once the person is discharged to his or her home, where the routine is less formalized. Some persons are able to verbalize an intended goal and plan a course of action but are unable to carry it out. The problem may be one of initiation of the activity or of sequencing the steps of the plan in a profitable manner. Individuals with this deficit often seem far more capable than their behavior demonstrates. Effective performance requires that the individual continually monitor and adjust performance throughout the execution of a task. Some people demonstrate an inability to perceive errors, while others may recognize an error but make no effort to correct it.

When trying to carry out the plan, a person may demonstrate poor mental flexibility or may have difficulty changing mental set. For example, a person is attempting to solve a problem using a selected solution. The solution proves ineffective, but the person continues the effort unabated. The therapist may guide the person's awareness to acknowledge the lack of success, but the person may persist in trying the same solution.

Assessment of Executive Functions
Family members are frequently the best source of information about the person's **executive functioning.** The Dysexecutive Questionnaire[13] is designed to be completed by both the person and the family, thus providing a comparison with which to determine the person's insight into his or her own deficits.

Standardized assessments include the Behavioural Assessment of the Dysexecutive Syndrome,[80] as well as formal assessments of everyday tasks such as route finding[10] and errand planning.[56] The therapist should also assess these skills through close clinical observation. A homemaking assessment that includes planning and simultaneous preparation of a variety of dishes for a meal may be useful. Perseverative or stimulus-bound behavior should be noted, as related to both a specific environment and particular tasks. The therapist must remember that similar behaviors may be related to other clinical deficits such as poor comprehension or apraxia or may be a sign of depression. Ongoing close observation, assessment, and consultation with other team members increase the likelihood of correct interpretation and management of behavior.

Treatment of Deficits in Executive Functions
An individual's level of awareness of the executive deficits will determine the treatment approach.[61] A person with relatively good metacognitive skills, one who can recognize, comprehend, and appreciate the implications of inactivity, may be responsive to self-monitoring strategies or environmental cues. A more severely impaired individual, one who cannot acknowl-edge or tends to devalue the deficit, may require supervision by another individual. A family member or significant other may be trained to set up a daily routine, provide the verbal prompts needed, and maintain the system of environmental cues established.

BEHAVIORAL DEFICITS

A variety of behavioral deficits can be the result of cognitive dysfunction or may also develop in response to the frustration and outrage at the disability and the profound changes in a person's life and sense of self.

IMPAIRED AWARENESS. In the immediate postinjury stage, persons frequently attempt activities that are beyond their physical or mental capacity, demonstrating a deficit in the awareness of their limitations. People may be operating on old intrinsic knowledge of their capacities and may not have incorporated their limitations into their sense of self since the injury.[24] Years later, an individual may tell stories of gradual realization of deficits: "I didn't realize that my left side was paralyzed until I tried to get out of bed." With individuals whose awareness is impaired, the rehabilitation effort may become a power struggle, since the person may see no reason to have therapy.[38] A person's insight frequently increases as the body scheme is modified in response to changes imposed by the disability—a long and complex process.

Memory deficits may also complicate a person's awareness of the frequency with which a problem occurs. For example, the person who acknowledges difficulty recalling a nurse's name only two or three times a day may consider the memory problem minimal, although the incidence is actually closer to 12 to 15 times a day and extends to the entire staff. Sometimes the use of a frequency check sheet, recorded by the person under the supervision of the therapist, may help the person more fully understand the extent of the problem.

ANOSOGNOSIA. Anosognosia is a total inability, exceeding common denial, to recognize deficits.[49] Use of the normal coping strategy of denial implies that the individual appreciates the problem on some level; the anosognosic person is completely unable to acknowledge the impaired function. A team approach is needed to distinguish between neurological and psychological types of awareness deficits.[7] An example is a person (with intact basic perceptual and language abilities) who cannot recognize her own handwriting on a task performed earlier in the day and accuses the therapist of falsifying the work.

INAPPROPRIATE EMOTIONAL RESPONSE. A person may laugh, cry, or express other emotions that have no relation to the actual emotional context of a situation. Other individuals may respond with the correct category of emotion, such as laughing at a humorous situation, but the extent and forcefulness of their laughter may be inappropriately exaggerated. People cope with this trait in various ways. Some avoid social contact, and others learn to mask this trait or even use it to their advantage. One person developed a repertoire of jokes to tell; another person realized that people enjoyed socializing with him, since he smiled all the time and appeared to have a lighthearted approach to life. In more serious relationships, this person would explain the deficit to his friends so they could learn to read his emotions more accurately.

DISINHIBITION. Some people with executive dysfunction demonstrate **disinhibition,** or impulsive behavior.[12] These people may continuously generate ideas for activity but cannot delay or resist the need to act on the thought immediately. A person may greet a newcomer and announce his first impression: "You have a stain on your shirt." Other people are able to recognize and discuss their inappropriate behavior but may still be unable to control it An individual may demonstrate **stimulus-bound behavior** as he or she impulsively begins the task before being instructed or cannot draw attention away from a task when necessary. One person, when presented with the first item of a multiple-choice visual closure test (the Motor-Free Visual Perception Test), immediately began drawing on the test booklet to complete the partially drawn items. **Perseveration,** which refers to the rapid continuation or repetition of an action beyond its purpose, can be seen in motor acts, verbalizations, or thought processes. Fig. 27-3 provides an illustration of writing perseveration.

PERSONALITY AND EMOTIONAL FACTORS. The person may demonstrate apathy, indifference, or decreased spontaneity. The person may also exhibit a slowness of response or absence of initiative unless specifically instructed to perform the task. Other individuals may be inappropriately happy or euphoric and in conversation may minimize the effect that their deficits have had on their lives and families.[49] An additional factor is the person's emotional response to the effects of the disability on his or her life; a person with cognitive deficits will still pass through the stages of emotional adjustment to disability that can be expected of anyone undergoing the rehabilitation process.

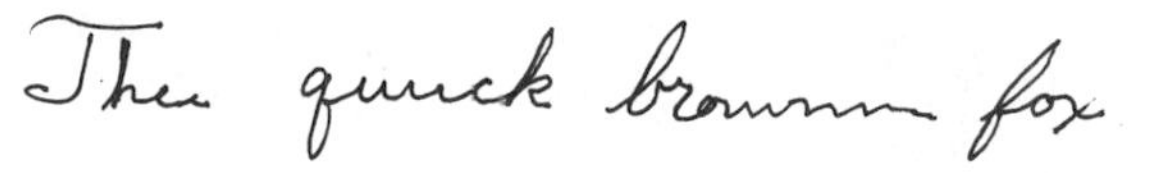

FIG. 27-3
Example of writing perseveration.

Assessment of Behavioral Deficits

Assessment of these behavioral deficits is made by behavioral observation and interviews with the family. Subjective questionnaires[12] can be completed by both the person and a family member, and the results can be compared and discussed with both parties. The behavior must be considered in relation to the social and cultural background of the person and his or her personality characteristics before the onset of the disability.

Treatment of Behavioral Deficits

Awareness can be further addressed in treatment using several approaches.[65] Self-estimation can be encouraged by asking questions requiring an individual to predict performance on a certain task. Role reversal can be used between the therapist and the individual. Self-questioning during an activity and self-evaluation after completion of the task can also be important tools for increasing awareness.[57]

Behavioral management strategies can be developed to impose restrictions on an individual's behavior. Specific, direct feedback regarding the inappropriateness of a behavior should be given to the person. If the person's level of insight and control warrants, internal strategies can be taught, such as "time out," in which the person voluntarily leaves the situation. If this approach fails, external controls may be used and a staff person may escort the person to a quiet area until behavioral control is reestablished. It is critical that the staff person remain calm because a strong emotional response from staff can further exacerbate the situation.[24]

A group approach can also be useful for providing feedback from peers.[36,70] Videotaping can provide a visual record of behavior that can be discussed with the person.

SUMMARY

As a reader, you have been using your own metacognitive skills in processing the preceding material. This chapter has provided a description of basic cognitive processing, the principles of cognitive assessment, and suggested methods of remediation and compensation. The field of cognitive neuroscience is ever changing, as new mechanisms are developed to explore, image, and understand the complexity of the brain. Students and therapists are encouraged to continue to stay abreast of new developments to provide the optimal benefit to patients and clients.

REVIEW QUESTIONS

1. Discuss the difference between cognition and metacognition.
2. List the areas of cognition that the occupational therapist should assess.

3. What are the related factors of performance that the therapist should consider when evaluating cognitive function?

4. Describe and compare the various theoretical approaches to treatment of cognitive dysfunction.

5. What is environmental feedback, or cueing?

6. What are the implications of a deficit in attention and concentration for an individual's functioning in everyday activities?

7. Describe the various types of memory functioning.

8. What considerations are important in choosing a memory strategy for a particular person?

9. What are some behavioral manifestations of poor initiation?

10. What behaviors does the person with poor mental flexibility display?

11. What are the five steps to problem solving?

12. What are the social implications of behavioral deficits?

REFERENCES

1. Abreu BC: The quadraphonic approach: holistic rehabilitation for brain injury. In Katz N, editor: *Cognition and occupation in rehabilitation: cognitive models for intervention in occupational therapy*, Bethesda, Md, 1998, American Occupational Therapy Association.

2. Allen CK, Blue T: Cognitive disabilities model: how to make clinical judgments. In Katz N, editor: *Cognition and occupation in rehabilitation: cognitive models for intervention in occupational therapy*, Bethesda, Md, 1998, American Occupational Therapy Association.

3. *Army individual test battery: manual of directions and scoring*, Washington, DC, 1944, War Department, Adjutant General's Office.

4. Arnadottir G: *The brain and behavior: assessing cortical dysfunction through activities of daily living*, St Louis, 1990, Mosby.

5. Aronson MK: Caring for the dementia patient. In Aronson MK, editor: *Understanding Alzheimer's disease*, New York, 1988, Charles Scribner's Sons.

6. Babor TF: Substance use disorders and persons with physical disabilities: nature, diagnosis and clinical subtypes. In Heinemann AW, editor: *Substance abuse and physical disability*, New York, 1993, Hayworth Press.

7. Barco PP et al: Training awareness and compensation in postacute head injury rehabilitation. In Kreutzer JS, Wehman PH, editors: *Cognitive rehabilitation for persons with traumatic brain injury*, Baltimore, 1991, Paul H Brookes Publishing.

8. Ben-Yishay Y, Piasetsky EB, Rattock J: A systematic method for ameliorating disorders in basic attention. In Meier MJ, Benton AL, Diller L, editors: *Neuropsychological rehabilitation*, New York, 1980, Guilford Press.

9. Beyer BK: *Practical strategies for the teaching of thinking*, Boston, 1987, Allyn & Bacon.

10. Boyd TH, Sautter SW: Route-finding: a measure of everyday executive functioning in the head-injured adult, *Appl Cogn Psychol* 7:171, 1993.

11. Brown L, Sherbenou RJ, Johnsen SK: *The Test of Nonverbal Intelligence (TONI)*, Austin, Tex, 1982, Pro-Ed.

12. Burgess PW et al: Ecological validity of tests of executive function, *J Int Neuropsychol Soc* 4:547, 1998.

13. Burgess PW et al: The dysexecutive questionnaire. In Wilson BA et al: *Behavioural Assessment of the Dysexecutive Syndrome*, Bury St Edmunds, UK, 1996, Thames Valley Test.

14. Burgess PW, Shallice T: Confabulation and the control of recollection, *Memory* 4:359, 1996.

15. Calkins MP: Designing special care units: a systematic approach, *Am J Alzheimer's Care Res* March/April:16, 1987.

16. Calkins MP: Designing special care units: a systematic approach. Part II, *Am J Alzheimer's Care Res* May/June:16, 1987.

17. Cermack LS: Models of memory loss in Korsakoff and alcoholic patients. In Parsons OA, Butters N, Nathan PE, editors: *Neuropsychology of alcoholism*, London, 1987, Guilford Press.

18. Craine JF, Gudeman HE: *The rehabilitation of brain functions: principles, procedures and techniques of neurotraining*, Springfield, Ill, 1981, Charles C Thomas.

19. Davis CM: The role of the physical and occupational therapist in caring for the victim of Alzheimer's disease. In Taira ED: *Therapeutic interventions for the person with dementia*, New York, 1986, Hayworth Press.

20. Doughterty PM, Radomski MV: *The cognitive rehabilitation workbook*, Rockville, Md, 1993, Aspen.

21. Flavell JH: *Cognitive development*, Englewood Cliffs, NJ, 1985, Prentice-Hall.

22. Folstein MF, Folstein SE, McHugh PR: Mini-mental state: a practical method for grading the cognitive state of patients for the clinician, *J Psychiatr Res* 12:189, 1975.

23. Gardner MF: *The Test of Visual Perceptual Skills, upper Level, revised (TVPS [UL]-R)*, Hydesville, Calif, 1997, Psychological and Educational Publications.

24. Giles GM: A neurofunctional approach to rehabilitation following severe brain injury. In Katz N, editor: *Cognition and occupation in rehabilitation: cognitive models for intervention in occupational therapy*, Bethesda, Md, 1998, American Occupational Therapy Association.

25. Glickstein JK: *Therapeutic interventions in Alzheimer's disease*, Rockville, Md, 1988, Aspen.

26. Harrell M et al: *Cognitive rehabilitation of memory: a practical guide*, Gaithersburg, Md, 1992, Aspen.

27. Hart T, Hayden ME: The ecological validity of neuropsychological assessment and remediation. In Uzzell BP, Gross Y, editors: *Clinical neuropsychology of intervention*, Boston, 1986, Martinus Nijihoff.

28. Hess TM, Pullen SM: Memory in context. In Blanchard-Fields F, Hess TM: *Perspectives on cognitive change in adulthood and aging*, New York, 1996, McGraw-Hill.

29. Itzkovich M et al: *LOTCA manual*, Pequannock, NJ, 1990, Maddock.

30. Katz N: *Cognition and occupation in rehabilitation: cognitive models for intervention in occupational therapy*, Bethesda, Md, 1998, American Occupational Therapy Association.

31. Kiernan RJ et al: The neurobehavioral cognitive status examination, *Ann Intern Med* 107(4):481-485, 1987.

32. Levy LL: Cognitive changes in later life: rehabilitation implications. In Katz N, editor: *Cognition and occupation in rehabilitation: cognitive models for intervention in occupational therapy*, Bethesda, Md, 1998, American Occupational Therapy Association.

33. Levy LL: The cognitive disabilities model in rehabilitation of older adults with dementia. In Katz N, editor: *Cognition and occupation in rehabilitation: cognitive models for intervention in occupational therapy*, Bethesda, Md, 1998, American Occupational Therapy Association.

34. Lezak MD: *Neuropsychological assessment*, New York, 1995, Oxford University Press.

35. Likert R, Quasha WH: *The revised Minnesota Paper Formboard Test*, New York, 1970, Psychological Corporation.

36. Lundgren CC, Persechino EL: Cognitive group: a treatment program for head injured adults, *Am J Occup Ther* 40:397, 1986.

37. McCarthy RA, Warrington EK: *Cognitive neuropsychology: a clinical introduction*, San Diego, 1990, Academic Press.

38. McGlynn SM, Schacter DL: Unawareness of deficits in neurological syndromes, *J Clin Exp Neuropsychol* 11:143, 1989.

39. McGowin DF: *Living in the labyrinth: a personal journey through the maze of Alzheimer's*, New York, 1993, Delacorte Press.
40. Morse PA, Morse AR: Functional living skills: promoting the interaction between neuropsychology and occupational therapy, *J Head Trauma Rehabil* 3:33, 1988.
41. Neistadt ME: Occupational therapy for adults with perceptual deficits, *Am J Occup Ther* 42:434, 1988.
42. Neistadt ME: A critical analysis of occupational therapy approaches for perceptual deficits in adults with brain injury, *Am J Occup Ther* 44:299, 1990.
43. Nelson TO, Narens L: Why investigate metacognition? In Metcalfe J, Shimamura AP, editors: *Metacognition: knowing about knowing*, Cambridge, Mass, 1994, MIT Press.
44. Parente R, Anderson-Parente J: *Retraining memory: techniques and applications*, Houston, 1991, CSY Publishing.
45. Parente R, Herrmann D: *Retraining cognition: techniques and applications*, Gaithersburg, Md, 1996, Aspen.
46. Parente R, Stapleton M: An empowerment model of memory training, *Appl Cogn Psychol* 7:585, 1993.
47. Parente R, Stapleton M: Vocational evaluation, training, and job placement after traumatic brain injury: problems and solutions, *J Voc Rehabil* 7:181, 1996.
48. Parente R, Stapleton MC, Wheatley CJ: Practical strategies for vocational reentry after traumatic brain injury, *J Head Trauma Rehabil* 6:35, 1991.
49. Prigatano GP: *Neuropsychological rehabilitation after brain injury*, Baltimore, 1986, Johns Hopkins University Press.
50. Ribot T: *Diseases of memory*, New York, 1882, Appleton-Century-Crofts. Cited in Schacter DL: *Searching for memory: the brain, the mind, and the past*, New York, 1996, Basic Books.
51. Ruch FL, Ruch M: *Employee aptitude survey*, San Diego, 1963, Educational & Industrial Testing Service.
52. Rustad RA et al: *The Cognitive Assessment of Minnesota*, Tucson, Ariz, 1993, Therapy Skill Builders.
53. Schacter DL: *Searching for memory: the brain, the mind, and the past*, New York, 1996, BasicBooks.
54. Schacter DL, Glisky EL: Memory remediation: restoration, alleviation, and the acquisition of domain-specific knowledge. In Uzzell BP, Gross Y, editors: *Clinical neuropsychology of intervention*, Boston, 1986, Martinus Nijihoff.
55. Schwartz SM: Adults with traumatic brain injury: three case studies of cognitive rehabilitation in the home setting, *Am J Occup Ther* 49:655, 1995.
56. Shallice T, Burgess PW: Deficits in strategy application following frontal lobe damage in man, *Brain* 114:727, 1991.
57. Sherer M et al: The awareness questionnaire: factor structure and internal consistency, *Brain Injury* 12:63, 1998.
58. Sivan AB: *The Benton Visual Retention Test*, San Antonio, Tex, 1992, Psychological Corporation.
59. Smith AD: Memory. In Birren J, Schaie KW, editors: *Handbook of the psychology of aging*, ed 4, San Diego, 1996, Academic Press.
60. Sohlberg MM, Mateer CA: *Attention process training*, Puyallup, Wash, 1986, Association for Neuropsychological Research & Development.
61. Sohlberg MM, Mateer CA, Stuss DT: Contemporary approaches to the management of executive control dysfunction, *J Head Trauma Rehabil* 8:45, 1993.
62. Stone MH, Wright BD: *Knox's Cube Test*, Wood Dale, Ill, 1980, Stoelting.
63. Tankle RS: Application of neuropsychological test results to interdisciplinary cognitive rehabilitation with head injured adults, *J Head Trauma Rehabil* 3:24, 1988.
64. Toglia J: Attention and memory. In Royeen CB, editor: *AOTA self study series: cognitive rehabilitation*, Rockville, M, 1993, American Occupational Therapy Association.
65. Toglia JP: Generalization of treatment: a multicontext approach to cognitive perceptual impairment in adults with brain injury, *Am J Occup Ther* 45:505, 1991.
66. Toglia JP: *The Contextual Memory Test manual*, Tucson, Ariz, 1993, Therapy Skill Builders.
67. Toglia JP: *Dynamic assessment of categorization skills: the Toglia Category Assessment*, Pequannock, NJ, 1994, Maddock.
68. Toglia JP: A dynamic interactional model to cognitive rehabilitation. In Katz N: *Cognition and occupation in rehabilitation*, Rockville, Md, 1998, American Occupational Therapy Association.
69. Toglia JP, Golisz K: *Cognitive rehabilitation: group games and activities*, Tucson, Ariz, 1990, Therapy Skill Builders.
70. Von Cramon DY, Matthes-von Cramon G: Reflections in the treatment of brain-injured patients suffering from problem-solving disorders, *Neuropsychol Rehabil* 2:207, 1992.
71. Webster RE: *The Learning Efficiency Test*, ed 2, Novato, Calif, 1992, Academic Therapy Publications.
72. Wehman PH: Cognitive rehabilitation in the workplace. In Kreutzer JS, Wehman PH, editors: *Cognitive rehabilitation for persons with traumatic brain injury: a functional approach*, Baltimore, Md, 1991, Paul H Brookes Publishing.
73. West RL: Compensatory strategies for age-associated memory impairment. In Baddeley AD, Wilson BA, Watts FN, editors: *Handbook of memory disorders*, Chichester, UK, 1995, John Wiley & Sons Ltd.
74. Wheatley CJ, Rein JJ: Intervention in traumatic head injury: learning style assessment. In Hertfelder S, Gwin C, editors: *Work in progress: occupational therapy in work programs*, Rockville, Md, 1989, American Occupational Therapy Association.
75. Wilson BA: *Rehabilitation of memory*, New York, 1987, Guilford Press.
76. Wilson BA: Management and remediation of memory problems in brain-injured adults. In Baddeley AD, Wilson BA, Watts FN, editors: *Handbook of memory disorders*, Chichester, UK, 1995, John Wiley & Sons.
77. Wilson BA, Baddeley A, Evans J: Errorless learning in the rehabilitation of memory impaired people, *Neuropsychol Rehabil* 4:307, 1994.
78. Wilson B, Cockburn J, Baddeley A: *The Rivermead Behavioural Memory Test*, Suffolk, UK, 1985, Thames Valley Test.
79. Wilson BA, Moffat N, editors: *Clinical management of memory problems*, Rockville, Md, 1984, Aspen Publishers.
80. Wilson BA et al: *Behavioural Assessment of the Dysexecutive Syndrome*, Bury St Edmunds, UK, 1996, Thames Valley Test Company.
81. Wood RL: Management of attention disorders following brain injury. In Wilson BA, Moffat N, editors: *Clinical management of memory problems*, Rockville, Md, 1984, Aspen Publishers.
82. Ylvisaker M et al: Topics in cognitive rehabilitation therapy. In Ylvisaker M, Gobble EM: *Community re-entry for head injured adults*, Boston, 1987, Little, Brown.
83. Zencius AH, Wesolowski MD, Rodriguez IM: Improving orientation in head injured adults by repeated practice, multi-sensory input and peer participation, *Brain Injury* 12:53, 1998.
84. Zoltan B: *Vision, perception and cognition*, ed 3, Thorofare, NJ, 1996, Charles B Slack.

CHAPTER 28

The Social and Psychological Experience of Having a Disability: Implications for Occupational Therapists

ELIZABETH JUNE YERXA

KEY TERMS

Values
Spread
Stigma
Liminality
Stereotypy
People with disabilities
Patient-agent
Americans with Disabilities Act
Equality of capability
Occupation as therapy
Adaptation with disability
Mutual cooperation
Comanagement
Independent living movement

LEARNING OBJECTIVES

After studying this chapter the student or practitioner will be able to do the following:

1. Compare and contrast the values of occupational therapy with those of traditional medicine, showing how these translate into complementary goals for the two professions.
2. Discuss several implications of the use of the term *patient-agent* for the recipient of occupational therapy services.
3. Visualize new models of practice employing occupation as therapy.
4. Name three positive outcomes of the patient-agent's engagement in occupation.
5. Discuss a new, alternative view of health that includes rather than excludes people with disabilities.
6. Identify two provisions of the *Americans With Disabilities Act*.
7. Discuss how practicing occupational therapists might use people's experiences of having disabilities to improve service.
8. List three characteristics of a constructive parent-professional relationship.

I was quite literally separated from the earth, for while I spent my time in an iron lung, in a bed, or in a wheelchair, my feet almost never touched the ground.

But more important, I believe, was being separated from so many of the elemental routines that occupy people. I felt no longer connected with the familiar roles I had known in family, work, sports. My place in the culture was gone.

Many years ago I met "Jeff," a patient undergoing rehabilitation at a large hospital in which I worked as an occupational therapist. My encounter with Jeff created a turning point in my thinking about people with disabilities and influenced the direction of my entire subsequent career.

One day Jeff wheeled into my office. I could see that he was very excited about something. "Betty, if you have a minute, I want to show you something," he exclaimed, his eyes bright with anticipation.

"Sure, Jeff," I replied. "What is it?" He handed me a manuscript. As I examined it, I realized that it was a scholarly paper. It was titled something like this: "The Social Status of People with Disabilities as a Maligned Minority Group." Because it was the early 1960s, Jeff's paper conveyed a new idea to me.

"I've written it for a sociology class I'm taking at UCLA. I thought you might like to read it." His tone of voice conveyed both a question and a hope.

"I'd love to read it," I replied, full of curiosity by now. "Could I borrow it for a few days?" He nodded, left his paper, and told me he would return by the end of the week.

I took Jeff's paper home that night and read it with increasing interest. He proposed and supported, with many references, the idea that people with disabilities were treated as second-class citizens in American society and were the recipients of pervasive prejudice that limited their life opportunities. I saw images in my mind of events that had occurred at our rehabilitation center, events that had bothered me. For example, I remembered patients being talked about as though they were invisible in conferences at which they were present. I saw patients segregated from professional staff members into separate eating areas and rest rooms clearly labeled "patients" versus "staff." References to some patients were in such terms as "uncooperative" or "has not accepted his or her disability." Such labels were the kiss of death, since these patients were discharged as soon as possible, often in an atmosphere of contempt and hostility.

With these pictures racing through my mind and the increasing conviction that Jeff was onto something important, I showed his paper to a colleague the next day.

"Take a look at this," I exclaimed. My coworker quickly scanned Jeff's paper. Then she turned to me with a slight smile and in a tone of incredulity, as though I had been taken in, said, "Betty, remember this. Jeff has brain damage!"

Both Jeff's paper and the rejection of his experiences by this professional colleague created a new impetus for me to explore what it is like to have a disability. I hoped that such a quest would enable me to do a better job as an occupational therapist.

I am indebted to Carol Stein, MA, OTR, for helpful suggestions that strengthened this work, to the Occupational Therapy Department at the University of Southern California for their support in preparing the manuscript, and to Marian Karsjens who processed the words so competently.

QUESTIONS

This chapter explores several questions that are central to occupational therapists who work with people with disabilities. These queries permeate our practice regardless of the technology we employ, the theories that guide us, or the particular type of disability with which the patient must live. The four major themes of this chapter are as follows:

1. Through what "pair of glasses" do occupational therapists view the recipients of their services?
2. What is it like to have a disability?[6]
3. What, if anything, does our society need to do for people with disabilities?
4. (The bottom-line question) How can occupational therapists help improve life opportunities for people with disabilities?

THE "PAIR OF GLASSES" THROUGH WHICH OCCUPATIONAL THERAPISTS VIEW THEIR PATIENTS

Before we examine these important questions, let me identify some of my assumptions. The first assumption is that all professionals, including occupational therapists, wear a particular "pair of glasses" through which we view the people who receive our services. These glasses are constructed of the beliefs, values, and traditions of the profession and are transmitted via education, including clinical socialization.[30] I assume that the lenses worn by occupational therapists are different from those worn by physicians and other medical personnel, even though occupational therapists often practice within a medical or rehabilitation milieu.[71]

Table 28-1 summarizes key **values** and beliefs of occupational therapists, derived from our history and literature. Occupational therapists' values seem to center on a humanistic concern for the individual who may have a chronic, severe, and lifelong disability and who will never be cured.[71] The occupational therapists' lenses see the essential humanity of each person, including the need to maximize his or her capacity or capability. Rather than eradicating disease, occupational therapists identify and strengthen the healthy aspects or potential of the person. Self-directedness and self-responsibility of the person are emphasized rather than compliance or adherence to orders. A generalist, integrated view of the person as one who interacts with his or her environment guides occupational therapy (OT) practice, rather than a specialist, reductive perspective. This integration is required by our emphasis on patients' daily life activities and their engagement in the occupations expected by their culture. In OT, therapeutic relationships are based upon a model of **mutual cooperation**[57] with the

TABLE 28-1

Comparison of Traditional Values Supporting Practice of Occupational Therapy With Those of Medicine

Occupational Therapy	Medicine
Essential humanity of patient-agent; obligation to seek life satisfaction for people with severe disability	Freedom from threat of death; responsibility limited to illness
Maintain and enhance health; support healthy aspects of patient-agent	Eradicate disease, pathological conditions; confer the sick role
Self-directedness and responsibility of patient-agent	Patient compliance to orders; moral authority
Generalist, integrated view of patient-agent	Specialist, reductionistic emphasis on organ systems
Therapeutic relationship of mutual cooperation with patient-agent; shared authority	Therapeutic relationship of activity of physician, passivity of patient; Aesculapian and sapient authority of physician
Patient-agent acts on environment rather than being determined by it	Patient as determined by environment and "body machine"
Faith in patient-agent's potential	Faith in science and healer's competence and charismatic authority
Patient-agent productivity and participation	Patient relieved of all responsibilities except getting well
Play, leisure activities as essential components of balanced life	Recovery from illness, freedom from disease as major concern
Understanding of subjective perspectives of patient-agent	Emphasis on objectivity, analysis, observation, and diagnosis

Modified from Yerxa EJ: Audacious values: the energy source for occupational therapy practice. In Kielhofner G, editor: *Health through occupation*, Philadelphia, 1983, FA Davis.

patient rather than a model of an active therapist and passive patient. The patient is viewed as an agent or actor with goals, interests, and motives and not as one whose behavior is determined by physical laws.[33] The occupational therapist seems to possess faith in the patient's potential ability, which is actualized by engagement in activity.

Therapeutic intervention emphasizes the recipient's productivity and participation rather than relief from responsibility. Occupational therapists seek to facilitate a balance among work, rest, play, and sleep in the patient's daily life rather than only recovery from illness.

Finally, the occupational therapist seeks to understand the patient's experience and point of view instead of relying solely on observation as the only credible source of information. The patient's view is essential to our understanding of people's motivation to engage in the activities of daily life.

By way of contrast, in their classic work, Siegler and Osmond[58] identified important values supporting the traditional practice of medicine. These values constitute the glasses through which physicians have historically viewed their patients. The values are based on Aesculapian authority, conferred by society, which defines the physician-patient relationship. The physician has the power to confer the sick role upon the patient. This role requires that the patient admit to being ill, submit to treatment, and curtail his or her usual activities while being exempted from normal responsibilities. The patient's job is to get well by complying with orders.

A physician's authority ends when the illness ends. It does not deal with the state of impairment that results when the person recovers from the illness but still has a disability.

The values supporting the traditional practice and science of medicine include freeing the patient from the threat of death; eradicating disease while conferring the sick role; expecting patient compliance; employing a specialist approach in order to possess superior, precise knowledge; promoting a physician-patient relationship in which the physician is active and the patient is passive; perceiving the patient as more or less of a body machine determined by physical laws; placing faith in natural science and the competence of the physician-healer; relieving the patient of everyday responsibilities; focusing on recovery from illness rather than engagement in daily activities; and relying on an objective, observable assessment of the patient's symptoms to produce a diagnosis and to indicate a course of treatment, which usually employs technology such as drugs or surgery.

Throughout this chapter I will assume that occupational therapists focus on improving life opportunities for people who often do not recover but must live with the impact of having a chronic condition. According to the American Occupational Therapy Association, the majority of occupational therapists work with people who have chronic and often severe disabling conditions.[1] Thus, although occupational therapists may provide services in a medical milieu, we view the patient in a way different from the traditional medical perspective of diagnosis, cure, and recovery, and we follow a different thought process. I also assume that our concern for people's capacity to engage in their rounds of daily life activities means that our scope of practice includes not only the hospital, but also the patient's home and community. Thus occupational therapists practice both within and outside of the medical milieu, often helping patients to become agents. In this sense OT practice bridges the sometimes alien world of acute medical care with the familiar world of home, family, and culture.

WHAT IS IT LIKE TO HAVE A DISABILITY?

Bickenbach,[6] a philosopher, suggested that society has not yet answered in a satisfactory manner the "straightforward" and "childishly simple" query, "What does it mean to have a disability?" As with the contrasting glasses worn by physicians and occupational therapists, the answer depends on one's perception or point of view.

World Health Organization Classification

In 1980 the World Health Organization (WHO),[67] to assess the effectiveness of health care systems, adopted a classification of the outcomes of the physical event of a disability ("Definition" column of Table 28-2). This classification system is used internationally to provide consistent terminology, formulate research questions, and influence public policy.

Impairment means an abnormality of a physiological structure or deviation from a biomedical norm.[6] For example, a fracture-dislocation of the cervical vertebra at the level of C5,6 is an impairment.

A disability is a limitation resulting from the impairment. It may be an inability to perform any activity considered normal or required for some recognized social role or occupation.[6] For example, an inability to dress oneself because of the loss of hand function caused by the impairment of the cervical fracture with resultant spinal cord injury constitutes a disability.

A handicap is any disability-related social disadvantage for an individual that limits the fulfillment of a normal role or occupation.[6] For example, for a person with quadriplegia, the lack of accessibility to a job site caused by architectural or social barriers constitutes a handicap.

TABLE 28-2
Three Models of Disability

Definition	Model	Problem	Power
Impairment	Biomedical	Body	Medicine
Disability	Economic	Individual's contribution to economy	Marketplace/state
Handicap	Sociopolitical	Social Environment	Self-advocacy

Modified from Bickenbach JE: *Physical disability and social policy,* Toronto, 1993, University of Toronto Press.

Table 28-2 presents the WHO classification as three models of disability. To include some important implications of the separate perspectives, I have expanded these to include the columns labeled "Problem" and "Power." Each of the three classifications—impairment, disability, and handicap—represents a different view of what it is like to have a disability.[6] Because impairment emphasizes pathological structures, it reflects the traditional biomedical model of disability. In this view the problem of having a disability resides in the body, which needs to be cured or modified in some way (for example, through surgery or technology). The power to accomplish a solution to the problem therefore rests in the medical profession by virtue of its superior knowledge and authority.

A disability presents a contrasting economic model. The problem resides in those who are unable to contribute to society by fulfilling an occupational or social role as a result of their limitations. The beginning of the rehabilitation movement in the United States was marked by efforts to restore people with disabilities to gainful employment so that they would contribute to the economic well-being of the country rather than deplete its resources.[6] The power in this model rests in the marketplace or state, which assesses the value of the individual according to his or her capacity to be a productive contributor to society. The state may intervene by providing vocational rehabilitation services to increase productivity.

The handicap model adopts a sociopolitical pair of glasses. In this view, the problem does not reside in the body or in the individual's ability to contribute to society's productivity; rather, it resides in the social environment in which the person with a disability goes about daily life. Thus, to have a handicap means to experience a social disadvantage or injustice because of social stigma, prejudice, or other environmental constraints.[6] Therefore, the power and solution rest in self-advocacy, in which people with disability work to bring about social change to achieve equality of opportunity and justice. An example of such self-advocacy is the political organization by and for people with disability to influence legislation designed to remove barriers to their full participation in society.[54]

Each of these models represents a different perception of what it means to have a disability. According to Bickenbach,[6] none is complete or integrated; rather, each model represents only a partial and selective viewpoint. He urges society to develop an integrated, comprehensive model of disability rather than focusing on these partial and conflicting views.

Perhaps in recognition of these significant issues,[46] the WHO is currently considering revising its classification of people's health status.[68] The three proposed dimensions of function are body level, person level, and society level. The categories are named "(B) Body functions and structures," "(A) Activities," and "(P) Participation." All dimensions interact in an environmental context. I see three implications of this proposed revision. It refers to "all people," integrating those with disabilities into the mainstream. It avoids such pejorative terms as *disability* and *handicap* by emphasizing ability to function. It reflects a dynamic, interactive systems view (biopsychosocial) of human beings. All occupational therapists will want to be alert to whether this new classification is adopted, because it appears more integrated and congruent with our perspectives.

Need for an Integrated Model

The biomedical and economic models necessarily emphasize what is wrong with the person who has disability as seen by an outside observer (the physician or potential employer). In contrast, the sociopolitical model emphasizes what is wrong with the social environment as seen by the person who has the disability, and in this sense provides an insider's view. Occupational therapists working with individuals who have lifelong disability need an integrating model of what it means to have a disability, a model that reflects our ethical values and seeks to understand both the outsider's and insider's view of disability. Although we often provide our services in a medically oriented environment, we know that OT cannot be limited to concern with the body. It must also focus on people's ability to connect with the daily routines of their culture[3] in their own physical and social environments.

One of the insights of the occupational behavior frame of reference,[51] the model of human occupation,[27] and of the newly emerging discipline of occupational science[73] is the recognition of the complexity of the people served by occupational therapists. In these conceptual frameworks a person is viewed as a multilevel, open system interacting with his or her environment. Thus all people, with or without disabilities, have biological, psychological, sociocultural, and spiritual or transcendental levels of existence, open to a multitude of inputs from the outside world.

In the sciences each level also represents a pair of glasses through which outsiders may perceive a human being. Many respected and powerful academic disciplines tend to focus on only one level, ignoring the others or reducing them to lower levels. For example, medical knowledge, emanating from the natural sciences, may focus primarily on the microbiological level, emphasizing the integrity of body structures. Sociologists may focus on the level of society and culture. Although these are legitimate disciplines, their partial views may fail to address significant aspects of human life and their tools for helping people may be limited or even distorting. In the realm of people with disability, medicine emphasizes impairment, whereas sociology emphasizes handicap.

Because of OT's values and its emphasis on what people want and need to do in daily life, many of our theorists seek to integrate and address all of these levels, as well as the environments in which people actually live. Although different levels present valid perspectives, these perspectives must be integrated to provide a complete picture, supplemented by the insider's experiences of daily life (i.e., experiences of the person with the disability) and the characteristics of the environment.

The scientists and practitioners of OT need to develop new approaches to augment the strengths and potential of people beyond current models and integrating perspectives. The remainder of this chapter describes a systems view of what it is like to have a disability, emphasizing the complexity and uniqueness of interactions between the individual and the environment.

Social Attitudes Toward People With Disabilities

OT students at Boston University participated in a class designed to provide a first-person experience of architectural barriers. Students spent most of the day in wheelchairs going about their daily routines as students, visiting classrooms, libraries, and cafeterias. At the end of the day they returned to the classroom for discussion.

Although the students discovered architectural barriers, many were much more impressed with the behaviors of able-bodied people they encountered. Students were the recipients of stares, averted eye contact, obvious social discomfort, and conversations directed to their wheelchair pushers rather than to them. (Most people didn't know these students were able bodied.) One student put it this way: "I couldn't wait until 4:00 PM when I could get out of that damned wheelchair. What must it be like for people who really have a disability and cannot walk away?"

Outsiders' Views

How society views people with disability, an outsider's view, is sometimes categorized as *social attitude*. Wright,[69] a social psychologist, has studied society's reactions to people with disability for many years. She used the term **spread** to describe how the presence of disability or an atypical physique serves as a stimulus to inferences, assumptions, or expectations about the person who has disability. For example, a person who is blind may be shouted at, as though lack of vision indicates impaired hearing as well, or a person with cerebral palsy may be assumed to be mentally retarded.

One extreme manifestation of spread is the belief that an individual's life must be a tragedy because of having a disability. This attitude may be expressed in such statements as, "I would rather be dead than have multiple sclerosis." The assumption of a life sentence to a tragic existence denies that satisfaction and happiness may ever be obtained in the presence of a disabling condition. This attitude is of particular ethical concern today, when genetic counseling and euthanasia may provide a socially acceptable means of exterminating people with disability.[61] If life is seen as tragic or not worth living, it is a fairly easy step to argue that it would be better for everyone if people with disability ceased to exist.[48]

Goffman's classic work[23] used the term **stigma** to describe the social discrediting process that reduces the life chances of people with disability or other differences. An obvious impairment is translated into "something bad about the moral status of the signifier."[23] The individual with stigma is seen as not quite human. Society tends to impute a wide range of imperfections on the basis of the original stimulus (impairment) and at the same time project some positive (but undesired) attributes such as heroism or a sixth sense.

Stigma often is a societal reaction to fear of the unknown. Despite mainstreaming in education and the removal of many environmental barriers, the general public has little social contact with people who have disability and does not know what to expect of them in daily life. As a result, people with disability are often categorized as different from other people. This treatment may be complicated by the just-world hypothesis.[32] If the world is just and having a disability is a tragedy, then the person or the family must have done something morally reprehensible to be the recipients of such a fate. Such thinking leads easily to stigmatization and social distancing. Liachowitz[34] argued that, historically, people who were physically different were often the recipients of philanthropy that inadvertently reinforced negative beliefs of helplessness and dependency by society at large. One current example is the approach used in telethons or other fund-raising ventures, in which people with disabilities may be portrayed as victims, reinforcing negative attitudes and stigmas. In contrast, some network television programs and commercials include people with disabilities as regular participants in daily life, as workers or family members.

Echoing the WHO classification of handicap, Wright[69] posited that outside observers may attribute the behavior of people with disability to the disability rather than the environmental situation, which is often the real culprit. For example, a child's inattentiveness may be accounted for in terms of presumed hyperactivity or mental retardation, disregarding possible environmental contributions to the observed behavior. People with disabilities may be blamed for being unemployed, when in fact environmental factors such as employer attitudes, transportation and architectural barriers, community unemployment levels, or family obstacles are the cause, rather than personal attributes. Dawes,[15] a research psychologist, pointed out that in general people

are likely to attribute their own failures to environmental conditions but other people's failures to personality factors. This observation seems to describe how society views people with disability, except that failures are blamed on the disability.

Attitudes are often reflected in research approaches. Twenty-five years ago I conducted a small study comparing the self-esteem of children with and without disability. I expected to find lower self-esteem in the children with disability, but I did not. I know now that my expectation was based on the erroneous assumption that to have disability meant to have a more negative self-concept. My previous view was recently echoed by another researcher's perspective.[21] Having found that the self-esteem of college students with disability was similar to that of nondisabled students, the authors asked, "Why then do people with disabilities have positive self-images?" This question reflects an unstated assumption that such people should have negative self-images. This study also was based on the unstated assumption that disability is such a powerful, salient stimulus that it overrides every other aspect of the person and his or her environment—a questionable assumption, to say the least. When reading research about people with disability, it is useful to determine what assumptions are embedded in the study and what sort of attitudes they reflect.

Siller,[59] a social psychologist, has studied attitudes toward people with disability for over 30 years. In a wide-ranging review of the extant research he concluded, "Any inclination to consider disability outside of the larger social context and as something that resides only in the disabled person is destructively wrong" (p. 280).

Cultural Influences

Edgerton,[18] an anthropologist, discussed social reactions to disability within the context of the social rules of culture. "Rules are a shared understanding of how people ought to behave and what should be done if someone behaves in a way that conflicts with that understanding" (p. 24).

Cultural rules influence the treatment of people with disability. Societies differ in the extent to which they relieve their sick members of responsibilities. Often, the rules are different when someone is sick. For example, the Chinese in Taiwan are more willing than those in America to exempt sick people from their responsibilities. In some societies, people with severe mental retardation may receive almost total exemption from responsibility to follow the rules, whereas in other societies (e.g., that of the Northern Salteaux Indians), such people could be burned alive as children. Some societies do not indulge their ill members. For example, it is inexcusable for married females to be sick among the Sarakatsani shepherds of Greece, and anyone too ill to travel was left to die in the Siriond culture of the tropical forests of Bolivia.

Many impairments are culturally recognized as brief periods during which the temporarily ill person is expected to behave in ways that normally would be prohibited. Culture also dictates great differences in a person's responses to pain. For example, Jews and Italians are encouraged to respond to pain as an expression of their feelings and emotions, whereas other cultures disapprove of such expression.[18] Culture and its rules create profound differences in both the expectations and opportunities for people with disability.

Attitudes of Rehabilitation Workers

Many people with disability encounter the health care system, but what is known about the attitudes of those providing services? Siller[59] described an array of studies about rehabilitation personnel. First, he observed that certain conditions have less appeal to medical students than do others. Patients who are elderly, have mental retardation, are dying, or have a chronic disability seem to have less appeal than patients who are seen as most like the medical students or are perceived as more capable of being helped.

The expectations of the teacher influence the performance of students. This is referred to as the "Pygmalion effect." For example, higher expectations are correlated with better school performance. Several studies in rehabilitation settings support this theory for professionals (who have higher status) and their patients (who have lower status). For example, a correlation was found between the expectations of house parents and the performance of institutionalized adolescents. Siller[59] concluded that such findings about expectations probably can be generalized to all disability conditions and all rehabilitation professions. Lower expectations may lead to lower performance, and higher expectations produce better performance.

Having relatives with a particular type of disability and knowing more about a certain disability are correlated with a professional's preference to work in that area.[59] In another study, counselors who rated people with disability similarly to people without disability were judged by their superiors as more effective than counselors who rated the two groups differently.[59]

Siller[59] observed that medical personnel, particularly physicians, may see themselves as healers. They have often been trained within an acute medical care frame of reference in which passivity on the part of the patient is encouraged or insisted upon. Some rehabilitation professionals may need to emphasize the negative aspects of disability to reassure themselves of the importance of their services. Siller concluded, "One cannot overly stress the crucial importance for those with chronic disabling conditions to be self-sufficient and active in their own behalf."[59]

What sorts of attitudes are displayed by OT students? Lyons[35] studied the attitudes of Australian students. He found that the attitudes of first-year OT students did not differ significantly from those of business majors. The OT students' attitudes did not vary with the years of undergraduate education completed. However, those students who had valued social role contact with people with disability (e.g., a friend, family, or coworker, rather than a patient) had significantly more positive attitudes than those without such contact. He recommended that educational programs in OT facilitate such valued social role contact. In another study of social distance, Lyons[36] found that undergraduate OT students most preferred to work with people who had less visible types of disabilities and least preferred to work with those who had disorders of the mind—namely, people with cerebral palsy, mental retardation, mental illness, or alcoholism or those with a criminal record.

Other studies of occupational therapists[4,20] yielded conflicting results, some finding more positive attitudes than those reported by Lyons. Westbrook and Adamson[64] concluded that "occupational therapy students tend to underestimate the normalcy of lives that handicapped people are managing to live in a relatively prejudiced society."

Vash,[62] a psychologist who also has disability, recounted a rehabilitation conference held in 1974. A psychiatrist addressed the audience, alternately standing up and sitting in a wheelchair, all the while challenging observers to deny that their perceptions of his competence fluctuated as he stood and sat, over and over. Vash reported that much discussion followed and that virtually all in attendance acknowledged that their views of his competence had changed; the psychiatrist appeared more credible and more worthy of attention when he stood. The experience was emotionally draining for many because it forced them to confront the prejudice they had denied or ignored previously. A wheelchair can be a powerful social symbol, conveying devaluation of the person in it.

Vash[62] introduced her work on the psychology of disability with this bit of wisdom: some dangers inhere in even acknowledging the validity of the concept "the psychology of disability," since in the past it has led to unhelpful exaggerations of the perceived differences between people with disabilities and those without. The fact is, human beings are more alike than different, regardless of variances in their physical bodies, sensory capacities, or intellectual abilities.

How Different Are People With Disabilities?

What is actually known about the similarities and differences between people with and people without disability? Siller[59] reported mixed results. He inferred that, "As soon as one departs from the direct fact of disability, evidence can be provided to demonstrate that persons with disabilities do or do not have different developmental tracks, social skills and precepts, defensive orientations, empathetic potential, etc. The data suggest that if the disabled* do present themselves as 'different' this is often a secondary consequence of the social climate rather than inherent disability-specific phenomena" (p. 142).

Weinberg[63] reported that a group of people with disability showed no differences in life satisfaction, frustration, or happiness, compared with a group without disability. The only difference found was on ratings of the difficulty of life. People with disability judged their lives to be more difficult and more likely to remain so. She reported another study in which people with chronic, but not fatal, health problems not only seemed to be quite happy, but also derived some happiness from their ability to cope with their difficulty. She concluded that, "we need to question the assumption that physical limitations are directly related to happiness. Instead, it may be that many people with disabilities find happiness despite their disabilities, even though the able-bodied public would not always expect this."[63]

Studies in Sweden showed that among community-based people who had had strokes, life satisfaction was not correlated with the degree of physical impairment. Rather, it was related to people's ability to achieve their own valued goals.[5]

Another longitudinal study found that although adolescent girls with cerebral palsy scored significantly lower on physical, social, and personal self-esteem, as adults they no longer scored significantly differently from other able-bodied groups.[38] The authors speculated that factors in their subjects' changed self-esteem might have been a greater choice of environments in which to interact, better social relationships, or a wider range of experiences in education, work, and commerce.

A study of adolescents with disability (e.g., cerebral palsy, orofacial clefts, and spina bifida) found that the subjects' self-evaluations of global self-worth did not differ from those of an able-bodied comparison group. Speaking to occupational therapists, the authors of this study concluded that, "clinicians should not assume that adolescents with physical disabilities will have problems in self-esteem."[28]

Social attitudes toward people with disability are often stigmatizing and devaluing, increasing the degree of handicap and decreasing life opportunities. Such attitudes may be found among professional rehabilitation workers, including occupational therapists. Positive attitudes are associated with valued social role contact as friends, family, or coworkers. Much research supports the finding that people with disability are more like their nondisabled peers than they are different from them in life satisfaction, happiness, and self-esteem. Apparently, when we know only that a person has an impairment or disability, we cannot assume anything about his or her social or psychological status.

Insider's Views of Having a Disability

How do people with disabilities perceive themselves? A growing body of literature provides us with the insiders' viewpoint of what it is like to have disability.

Zola,[74] a sociologist who has disability, observed that, at its worst, society denigrates, stigmatizes, and distances itself from people with chronic conditions. He experienced little encouragement to integrate his "disabled self into the rest of his life" because this integration would be interpreted as "giving up the struggle to be normal." In letting his disability surface as a real and not necessarily bad part of himself, he was able to shed his super strong, "I can do it myself" attitudes and be more demanding for what he needed. Only later did he come to believe that he had the right to ask for or demand certain accommodations. He began to refuse invitations for speaking engagements unless they were held in a fully accessible facility (not only for him as the speaker, but also for the audience).

Vash[62] reported that at the age of 19, about 3 years after the onset of poliomyelitis, she was rejected for service by the state-funded vocational rehabilitation program. The reason given was that she refused to abandon her "unrealistic" goal of becoming a psychologist for the practical goal of becoming a secretary. She has subsequently had a productive career as a psychologist, professor, and writer who still cannot type.

In one of her books, Vash[62] described the impact of disability from her unique insider-outsider perspective as a person with disability and as a psychologist. She observed that an individual's reactions to having disability are influenced not only by the type of disability, but also by its severity and stability, as well as the person's gender, inner resources, temperament, self-image, family support, income, technology, and even government funding trends.

The stage of life at which disability occurs influences a person's reaction because it affects the way the person is perceived and the developmental tasks that might be interrupted. The person who is born with disability or acquires disability in infancy or childhood may experience isolation or separation from the mainstream in family life, play, and education. A person who acquires disability later in life may face different issues, such as the need to change vocations, find a marital partner, or remain a part of his or her culture via the routines of daily life.[3,62]

In terms of functions impaired, Vash[62] believed that different disabilities (such as blindness or paralysis) generate different reactions because each creates different problems or challenges. She observed, however, that the insider-outsider perspective also applies to people

---

* "The disabled" is Siller's terminology.

with disability. Thus the person with disability may feel that his or her condition is not as difficult as that of others; for example, a person who is blind may feel that it would be worse to be deaf. Reactions are also tempered by the impact of the disability on the valued skills and capacities the person has lost. For example, a person who loves music more than the visual arts may have a stronger reaction to loss of hearing than a visual person with the opposite pattern. (Note the use of the word "may" throughout this paragraph, indicating that reactions are individualized and unpredictable.)

The severity of disability does not have a direct, one-to-one relationship with the person's reaction to it. Vash[62] stated, "One person can assimilate total paralysis with fair equanimity, while another is devastated by the loss of a finger."

The visibility or invisibility of impairment may influence a person's response to his or her disability because of social reactions.[62] For example, invisible disabilities such as pain may create difficulties because other people expect the person to perform in impossible ways. One woman with arthritis indicated that it was easier for her to go grocery shopping when she wore her hand splints because then her disability was visible and people would carry her packages for her without her having to ask.

The stability of the disability or the extent to which it changes over time may influence reactions.[62] In some progressive disabilities the individual faces uncertainty as to the degree of limitations, as well as (in some cases) a hastened death. Reactions to such disabilities are shaped by these realities and by what the affected people tell themselves about their projected futures. When hope for neither containment nor cure is substantiated, the person may experience a new round of disappointment, fear, or anger.

Pain tends to usurp consciousness whenever it is present. As Vash[62] observed, "It is hard to be jolly, creative or maybe even civil when you hurt—but some [people] can learn to do so." Reactions to pain are highly individualized and influenced by culture.[18]

In discussing reactions to disability, Vash[62] observed that they depend not only on the disability, but also on the people who become disabled. She observed that we need to ask, "What remaining resources do they have for developing effective and gratifying lifestyles?" This question seems particularly important for occupational therapists because of our concern for what people can do and how their own occupations influence their health and quality of life. Vash raised other questions relevant to occupational therapists: "What activities and behavior patterns are interrupted by disablement, and how central are these to their happiness? What is the spiritual or philosophical base of their lives?"

Gender influences a person's reactions. Certain societal expectations that people fulfill their social and sexual roles and live up to social ideals may influence men's and women's reactions differently. For example, the need for women to be "physically perfect specimens"[62] or to carry the major responsibility for managing the home and caring for children may create a different impact for women.

Vash[62] gave great importance to the activities affected by disablement. In fact, she stated that, "The impact of disablement is largely contingent on the extent to which it interferes with what you are doing." It is not only actual activities that influence a person's reactions, but also the potential activities that are held as goals for the future.

Interests, values, and goals influence a person's reaction to disablement. The individual with a limited range of interests may react more negatively to a disability that prevents their expression, whereas an individual with a wide range of interests and goals may adapt more readily. Vash[62] observed that people may not be aware of their interests, values, and goals and therefore may not be conscious of those that have the potential to lead to satisfaction after acquiring a disability. She emphasized the importance of interests: "The more varied this potential, the more protected is the individual from frustration and dejection over being disabled."*

Vash[62] proposed that the resources the individual possesses for coping with and enjoying life are assets that may counterbalance the devastation of loss of function. Some of these, such as social skills and persistence, may be developed to a level enabling paid employment, whereas others, such as artistic talent or leisure skills, may contribute to a more satisfying life.

Vash[62] is one of the few authors who emphasized the importance of spiritual and philosophical beliefs to a person's reactions to disablement. She separated spirituality from religiosity, with the observation that people who acknowledge a spiritual dimension of life and who have a philosophy of life into which disablement can be integrated in a meaningful, nondestructive way may be better able to deal with having a disability. Specific religious beliefs may or may not be helpful. The person who views having a disability as punishment for past sins will respond differently from one who views the disability as a test or opportunity for spiritual development.

Finally, Vash[62] acknowledged the importance of the person's environment in influencing his or her reactions to having disability. Immediate environmental qualities such as family support and acceptance, income, community resources, and loyal friends are powerful contributors. The institutional environment if one is hospitalized also has a profound effect, especially the attitudes and behaviors of the staff members. The culture and its support (or lack thereof) for resolving

---

*"Being disabled" is Vash's term.

functional problems or protecting the civil rights of people with disability is another significant influence.

Vash[62] provided a broad and complex picture of people's reactions to having a disability. In her portrayal of the impact of impairment and disability on the biological, psychological, social, and spiritual levels of the human, she recognized the need to discover resources at all of these levels and stressed the importance of the person's interaction with his or her environment, especially in being able to do something, to act. Vash's work supported both OT's values and its open-systems view of human beings.

A growing body of literature provides insight into the experiences of having disability.[2,3,17,22,24,42,43,65] These works provide occupational therapists with a much needed insider's view.

Beisser[3] had just completed medical school at age 23 when he acquired poliomyelitis, which left him totally paralyzed and unable to breathe without a respirator. He spent a year in the hospital, occupying the same room. Later, he was able to articulate his experiences with a clarity and sensitivity that enable us, almost, to share them. Some of his experiences in the hospital are noteworthy.

Beisser frequently felt that those who attended to his body were more the owners of it than he was. Although he was often cold because his paralysis prevented his muscles from generating heat, the nurse doubted his judgment. She would feel his leg and say, "Oh, it's all right, you're not cold." These experiences happened over and over. Beisser[3] observed, "They thought they knew how I felt better than I did. I was not even acknowledged as a separate person." Although enraged by his imposed powerlessness, he learned that you "cannot get mad in hospitals" because "angry patients come last" (i.e., have their needs attended to last). He compared his experience of hospitalization to being a prisoner of war, except that, although he depended upon his captor's feelings and behaviors for his self-esteem, he could never become one of them no matter how hard he tried to be a good patient.

Depersonalization was common. Some of the employees on whom Beisser depended made it clear that it was just a job to them. In one hospital the first hour of the nurses' shift was spent deciding about coffee breaks. Patient needs were secondary. Sometimes workers even left him in midair in a lift to go on a coffee break. "One of the worst times was at 'change of shift' because then there was absolutely no chance of getting anyone to help even if the problem was urgent." Beisser[3] observed, "To me, what they did or did not do was not 'just a job' but a matter of survival, of both my physical body and my sense of myself as a person."

Fortunately, he sometimes had other sorts of helpers who helped willingly with interest and compassion, whose primary goal was the comfort of patients. When one of them came to a ward of patients, the room brightened and the patients' fears and tensions lessened considerably.

Beisser[3] discussed his reactions to acquiring disability. First he had to give up the "old and obsolete, preparing the ground for something new." Then he had to find something positive, available for a new commitment. The first step in giving up the old was a grieving process, which involved a gradual reduction in the energy invested in what had been lost. He described passing through stages of denial (he had not really lost anything of value), blaming (whose fault is this?), and bargaining (with physicians, God, and the universe) that if he did X, he would get back what he had lost. When he discovered that there was no one to blame or bargain with or rage against, despair and depression appeared. Although this stage is supposed to lead to acceptance, Beisser[3] asked, "Acceptance of what?" Why would a person accept the loss of something valued unless there was something new of value to take its place? There had to be a positive replacement. In his case he had to find a new way of being, involving his old enthusiasms. The first was sports, then people in his life, and finally work, but these discoveries took a long time.

Although he couldn't become a surgeon, he did become a psychiatrist; although he could no longer play tennis, he could become an enthusiastic sports fan (he later wrote a book about sports). The stages of acceptance, which needed to occur simultaneously with grief, were the following: "Rejection of unfamiliar options; looking for something new; a grudging acceptance of something new; behaving 'as if' you accept it; discovering some of the same satisfaction in the new that you had with the obsolete."

Another insider's view of disability is provided by Robert Murphy,[42] a professor of anthropology who developed a progressive spinal cord tumor that moved from "a little muscle spasm in 1972 to quadriplegia in 1986," the year he wrote his book.

Murphy[42] described his initial reaction to having disability: "But what depressed me above all else was the realization that I had lost my freedom, that I was to be an occasional prisoner of hospitals for some time to come, that my future was under the control of the medical establishment." This feeling was like falling into a vast web, a trap from which he might never escape.

Murphy's view of hospitalization was similar to Beisser's.[3] He described the key rules for a sick person as (1) don't complain, and (2) maintain a cheery exterior. Doctors and nurses appreciate patients who can follow these rules.

The hospital patient must conform to the routine imposed by the establishment. For example, Murphy spent 5 weeks on one ward where he was bathed at 5:30 every morning because the day shift nurses were too busy to do it. The chain of authority from physicians on down creates a bureaucratic structure that breeds and feeds on impersonality.[42] The totality (social isolation) of such institutions is greater in long-term care facilities, such as mental hospitals and rehabilitation centers. A closed-off, total institution generally attempts to erase prior identity and make the person assume a new one, imposed by authority. The hospital requires that the inmates think of themselves primarily as patients, a condition of "conformity and subservience."

In relation to his social world, Murphy[42] experienced an increase in social isolation because some of his friends avoided him. He often encountered physical barriers in his environment. He was surprised to discover that in attending meetings of organizations of people with disability, often more attention was paid to the opinions of outside experts who were able bodied than to his views (in spite of his having disability and being a professor of anthropology). He observed that people with disability fit into a mold of **liminality** (invisibility); as their bodies are impaired, so is their social standing. "Their persons are regarded as contaminated; eyes are averted and people take care not to approach wheelchairs too closely."[42] One of his colleagues viewed wheelchairs as portable seclusion huts or isolation chambers. Even so, Murphy[42] expressed a sense of wonder that so many people with disability manage to break out into the world.

A great deal of Murphy's book[42] recounts his struggle for autonomy. Because of changes in his physical condition, he decided to have his wife, Yolanda, do the driving. Later he realized that this change was a mistake because it resulted in the loss of his sense of mastery and power. Driving an automobile meant not only mobility, but also spontaneity and free will. Having to rely on other people and the planning necessary to go anywhere because of his increasing paralysis "invaded my entire assessment of time." He observed that not only he, but all people with paraplegia and quadriplegia, have problems of planning activities and often have to conform to the timetables of family members, aides, and service providers.

A major contributor to Murphy's sense of mastery was his work as a professor, which he continued as long as possible. But even with his status as an internationally recognized anthropologist and researcher, hospital personnel often saw him as an anomaly. A social worker asked him, "What was your occupation?" even though he was working full time and doing research in areas related to medical expertise. With their mindset, hospital workers seemed unable to place him in the mainstream of society. Murphy[42] concluded that people with disability must make extra efforts to establish themselves as autonomous, worthy individuals. His book ended with this observation: "But the essence of the well-lived life is the defiance of negativity, inertia

and death. Life has a liturgy which must be constantly celebrated and renewed; it is a feast whose sacrament is consummated in the paralytic's breaking out from his prison of flesh and bone, and in his quest for autonomy."

Williams' autobiography[65] provides a glimpse into the experiences of a woman with diagnosed autism. The book provides a rich portrait of one person's experience of growing up in an alien world. When she was a child, her mother and brother often joined together to put her down. "To them, I was a nut, a retard, a spastic. I threw mentals and couldn't act normal." She sought safety in hanging on to an insular little world in which communication via objects was comfortable but any physical contact with people was anxiety ridden. "I felt that all touching was pain, and I was frightened" (at the prospect of hugging or being hugged).

Fortunately, Williams' father was sensitive to her needs. "He simply sat within my presence, letting me show him how I felt in the only way I could—via objects. I eventually had the courage to show him some of the secret pictures I'd drawn and the poems I'd written."[65]

Williams' existence became one of her own construction as she tried to resist intrusion from the outside world of fragments and incoherence. For example, although she could read novels fluently, she was unable to understand what books were about. The meaning got lost in "the jumble of trivial words."[65] Concentration was difficult, especially for imposed tasks. Unless the activity was one she had chosen, she would drift off, no matter how hard she tried. "Anything I tried to learn, unless it was something I sought and taught myself, closed me out and became hard to comprehend, just like any other intrusion from 'the world.'"

At the end of her odyssey, often similar to that of being on a strange planet, Williams[65] recounted those experiences that had been helpful:

Allowing me my privacy and space was the most beneficial thing I ever got. As much as many of the things I did were dangerous and as much as people could sense my isolation, this isolation was not from being left to my own devices. It stemmed from the isolation of my inner world, and only the unthreatening nature of privacy and space would inspire the courage to explore the world and get out of my world under glass step by step.

Williams' book conveys the experiential basis of her behavior, which often might otherwise appear bizarre and incomprehensible to an outside observer. The book also offers support for the importance of choices, a safe space for exploration, and intrinsic motivation for engagement in activities.

Dubus,[17] an accomplished novelist, acquired a severe disability when he was hit by an automobile after he had stopped to help a couple whose car had broken down on a busy highway. He was suddenly transformed into a "disabled man" with one leg amputated and the other so badly shattered that he needed to use a wheelchair as a permanent mode of transportation. He gradually moved from initial despair toward surrender and acceptance. Along the way he told of changes in how he perceived his environment:

The world is a different place when seen from a wheelchair. It's a landscape made up of obstacles and traps. How to get a glass of water the nurse has put out of reach? How to get in and out of a car? How to shave, how to shower? How to reach the dials on the stove? What do you do if your car breaks down? How do you ask for things without making every request a statement of disability?

Dubus' solution to the last question in his list was, "I say things like 'I wonder if there's any cheese?' or 'Does anyone want hot chocolate?'"[17]

Like Murphy[42] and Beisser,[3] Dubus[17] had a profound change in his sense of time. Everything took him three times as long to do as it had previously. As a result, time seemed to move "three times as fast as the action that once used a third of it." Dubus' experiences underline his need to develop extraordinary new skills to manage his space, time, and social relationships as a person with disability.

Osborn[43] is a physician who received a traumatic head injury as a result of a bicycle-automobile accident. Her book is one of the few memoirs written by someone who is both a physician and a person who needed to learn how to live with the effects of a brain injury. Although she completed two 5-month stints of cognitive rehabilitation at an internationally recognized center, little or no help was available to enable her to function in her daily routines in her own environments. She reported that while living alone in New York City (so that she could attend the rehabilitation program), she had extreme problems in performing daily occupations such as organizing her time and space, using public transportation, and completing the tasks of daily living. For example, she often went to bed hungry because she forgot to shop or because she botched shopping: "I couldn't decide what to put on my list. I didn't know where to go or what to buy."

As she engaged in the lengthy process of recovery and adaptation to her changed status, Osborn discovered the joys of painting and writing. "If I could not speak what I felt, I would draw and write it." She began to value the fledgling part of the new individual she was becoming, while recognizing the loss of the old. "I would love to be that woman again, but she died in 1988. While I shall always miss her, I do not idealize her. She wasn't much fun. She steeped herself in her work and was often unavailable to her friends and family; she was so attentive to her patients' needs that there was not much left for herself. She could not paint and she wrote nothing that was not medical."

Osborn's story is an honest portrait of a woman struggling to survive, contribute, find something worth doing, and forge a new identity. As I read it, I was struck with her unmet needs for (1) engagement in occupation and (2) the discovery, via occupations, of her nascent capabilities.

These articulate people help us understand the experience of having disability from an insider's point of view. An increasing amount of literature provides new insights into experiences such as encounters with social stigma, reactions to the medical system, and the need to have a supportive environment. Of particular relevance to occupational therapists are these insiders' quests for autonomy and a sense of mastery over their daily lives, their needs to discover substitute interests for those lost, and the essential strength of their unique resources and their embeddedness in the mainstream of humanity. Reading these and other[2,22,24,25,29,49] original sources may provide occupational therapists with new understanding of how to make their services better fit the needs of people—needs identified by the people themselves. These sources cast light on how people adapt to the challenges of their environments in the presence of a disabling condition by discovering, enhancing, and using their strengths and resources. This process can be profoundly affected by OT.

WHAT, IF ANYTHING, DOES SOCIETY NEED TO DO FOR PEOPLE WITH DISABILITIES?

This section explores the social context of having a disability. The first issue is current trends in terminology, followed by changes in health care affecting life opportunities for people with disability. Finally, some current social policies regarding the civil rights of people with disability and attempts to reduce social handicapping[6] are presented.

Terminology

The language used to communicate ideas about people with disability is important because it conveys images about the people that may or may not diminish their status as human beings. For example, in the jargon of the medical environment people may be called "quads," "paras," "CPs" or "that stroke down the hall." This categorization easily leads to viewing individuals as categories (stereotypy), and also as being "engulfed"[6] by their impairments. Additionally, referring to such people as "the disabled" or "a disabled person" seems to make the disability swallow up their entire identity, leaving them outside the mainstream of humanity. How, then, might one talk about them in a spirit of dignity?

Many years ago, Vash[62] edited a chapter I had written for one of her books. In the margin she wrote, "Why not refer to 'people with disabilities' rather than 'the disabled'?" This was her way of emphasizing that each individual was a person first, with all of the uniqueness and the similarity to everyone else that personhood conveys. I have used that terminology throughout this chapter with the intention that disability be defined in the broadest sense to include any condition (internal or external) that may interfere with the accomplishment of goals and intentions. **People with disabilities** is increasingly being used by other writers in this field.[6,62,69]

Another issue is that of what to call the recipient of OT: "patient," "client," or even "patient-client." In a medical setting, "patient" may convey both a sense of ethical responsibility[52] toward, and a state of passivity and dependence[42] of, people receiving care. "Client," on the other hand, conveys an economic relationship,[56] as does "consumer." What these latter terms may gain in autonomy, they seem to lose in beneficence. Most people do not choose to need health care and are especially vulnerable to professional practices because of the traumatic nature of illness and disability. Therefore I suggest that the term **patient-agent** be used in a medical setting, to convey both the ethical responsibility of care givers and the goal of enabling patients to become agents (an agent is one who acts, has power, and is capable of producing an effect).

In a community or nonmedical setting it may be appropriate to use such terms as "students" (in an educational program) or the more generic "service recipient." I prefer the latter term because it conveys the important point that OT is a service and not a commodity to be consumed. Service conveys benefits, help, and usefulness rather than a business (client) relationship in which the buyer may need to beware that the goal of the provider is to maximize his or her profits.

The WHO terminology of "impairment," "disability," and "handicap"[67] also may be useful in separating the biomedical, economic, and social perspectives of disability. The terminology is used widely in the international community. Whatever terminology is selected needs to be chosen with care and thoughtfulness to ensure that it conveys respect, dignity, and a sense of ethical responsibility toward those who receive OT.

Changes in Health Care

Changes in the health care system are resulting from the increased population of people with chronic conditions and the increased knowledge and activism of those receiving care, especially long-term care such as rehabilitation. These changes will certainly affect the way society provides opportunities for people with disability.

Robinson,[53] a British social scientist who has written about the experience of having multiple sclerosis, urged that major changes be made in the organization of rehabilitative care. Such changes are needed to support the patient's active and involved commitment to the process of rehabilitation, to achieve a good quality of life, and to restore viable social functioning.

Because rehabilitation is often based on a model of acute medical care, Robinson recommended that the traditional goals of short-term, acute medical care be radically changed to goals appropriate to the rehabilitation of people with long-term disability. The aim of rehabilitation would thus change from cure to alleviation, its focus from impairment to handicap,[6] and its style from technique centered to patient centered. He recommended that the physician's role change from controller to coordinator and that therapists change from medical agents (carrying out medical orders) to autonomous contractors (who can deal with the long-term complex relationships among impairment, disability, and handicap).[53] The patient's role would change from that of passive complier with preset goals to active definer of rehabilitation goals. The site of service provision would change from the hospital to the community.[53]

Interestingly, Robinson[53] observed that of the health professionals involved in rehabilitation, occupational therapists were most likely to adapt to these needed changes because of their traditional involvement with long-term impairments and "the very adaptability and diversity of occupational therapy, centered around ideas of occupation and activity." As more and more people live with disability in an increasingly complex environment,[72] such changes in rehabilitation will be urgently needed to improve the life opportunities of people with disability and to ensure that they can achieve their goals and purposes in real-life environments.

Legislation

Legislation is another way for society to improve life by decreasing the handicap of people with disability. After decades of work by people with disability and their advocates, the *Rehabilitation Act of 1973* was passed as a first step toward full recognition of the rights of such people. It prohibited discrimination on the basis of disability in all federally funded programs and activities and required that federal contractors use affirmative action in hiring and promoting qualified people with disability.[6]

In 1990, the **Americans With Disabilities Act**[66] was passed, reflecting further progress in achieving civil rights. At the time the act was passed, 67% of the estimated 43 million people with disability residing in the USA were unemployed. The act consists of 5 sections (called *titles*) designed to prevent employers and businesses from discriminating on the basis of physical or mental disability. It broadens the scope of the Rehabilitation Act of 1973 to prohibit discrimination by all businesses (not just federally funded businesses). The act prohibits discrimination on the basis of physical or mental disability. Disability is defined as an impairment that substantially limits a major life activity such as caring for oneself, performing manual tasks, walking, learning, and working.[66] Major provisions include prohibition of discrimination in employment of those with disability who are qualified to perform the job, with or without accommodations at the work site; accessibility to all state and local government services without discrimination against individuals with disability; and accessibility to public goods and services (e.g., restaurants and inns, hospitals, universities, zoos, amusement parks, and homeless shelters). Such accessibility may be achieved through removal of architectural barriers and by changes in company policies and practices. Telephone systems must make public accommodations more accessible to hearing-impaired and speech-impaired persons. Finally, the act prohibits retaliation or coercion against people who seek the rights granted by the act. (See also Chapter 17.)

Any legislation is only as effective as its enforcement. According to public television,[37] complying with the act has not resulted in the huge expenditure predicted by many business owners. But although progress is being made, many medium-sized and smaller businesses are still not in compliance, as is true of many universities. As a result, more people with disability are filing lawsuits to achieve their rights by bringing about needed changes in their social and physical environments. Occupational therapists may help achieve the goals of the act by serving as both advocates and sources of information for people with disability about their rights.

Public Policy

A final point about society's responsibility to people with disability concerns public policy. Bickenbach's entire book[6] deals with the issue of how the decisions made by social entities such as governments affect the lives of individuals with disability. He pointed out that such policies ultimately affect almost everyone because those without disability are really TABs (temporarily able bodied), whose status may change because of aging, acute conditions such as fractures, or pregnancy.

Bickenbach[6] concluded that policies should promote the goals of respect for, social participation of, and accommodation for people with disability. He viewed disablement as a condition of social, structural inequality. He then raised the question of what equality might mean, asking "Equality of what?" For example, it might be defined as equality of respect, antidiscrimination, opportunity, or equality of result (such as political and economic power). After exploring each of these ideas, he concluded that **equality of capability** is the most just and encompassing goal.

Equality of capability seems relevant to OT and is reminiscent of Reilly's goal[51] of reduction of incapacity

as central to OT practice. In Bickenbach's[6] view, capability is a "set of functionings, over which a person has a choice, so that the set of a person's capabilities constitute his or her actual freedom of choice over alternative lives he or she can lead." The value of this freedom is in its positivity, range of options, and functionings (things people can do or become or have a realistic choice about). For example, equality of capability for a man with blindness might mean a world in which he could rise in the morning, help get the children off to school, bid his wife good-bye, and proceed along the street to his daily work without dog, cane, or guide (if he so desired), proceeding with assurance and knowing that he is a member of the public for whom the streets are maintained with the help of his taxes and that he shares a world in which he also has a right to live.[6] Equality of capability respects people as agents and emphasizes not what they do choose but what they can and might choose.

In answer to the question of society's responsibilities to people with disability, several directions are now apparent. The words used to refer to people with disability need to be chosen carefully so that they convey dignity and reflect individual personhood rather than stereotypy. Changes are needed in the health care system so that the current paradigm of acute medical care is replaced with a model of long-term commitment to improving life opportunities for people with disability, leading to more autonomy for both patient-agents and the occupational therapists who serve them. Legislation to protect the civil rights of people with disability needs to be passed, widely publicized, and enforced so that handicap is no longer a social barrier. People with disability need to know about their rights to participate fully in life. Finally, society needs to understand and support the goal of equality of capability so that people with disability can enjoy their agency and have full participation in the routines of their culture, to the degree that they so desire.

HOW MAY OCCUPATIONAL THERAPISTS HELP IMPROVE THE LIFE OPPORTUNITIES OF PEOPLE WITH DISABILITIES?
Mind-Body Split

Several years ago, a patient in a large rehabilitation center attempted suicide. The administrators tried to transfer him to a psychiatric facility. However, that hospital would not accept him because he had a spinal cord injury. This incident emphasizes the mind-body split[14,31] in categorization that forces whole people into medically defined, diagnostic boxes. It is often assumed that a person with physical disability has a physical impairment that can be fixed via technology and therapy.

If such a person displays so-called psychosocial problems, these are viewed as adjustment or behavioral deficits requiring counseling or psychotherapy. Because occupational therapists are educated to provide services for people with diagnoses of both physical and psychiatric disability, therapists might similarly dichotomize their patients and approach those with physical impairments by providing technical solutions, including devices and physical modalities. If these patients display emotional reactions such as depression, the occupational therapists might supplement their techniques with counseling or talk therapy. But note that the patient-agent is fragmented and the approach is one of "doing to" a patient by a professional. The majority of people seen by occupational therapists have lifelong conditions that cannot be cured,[1] so the fixing is only partially successful and the cost of what is neglected may be high in terms of loss of the patient-agent's autonomy and future quality of life.

Occupation as Therapy

In contrast to the previously described approach, the occupational therapist might employ **occupation as therapy,** engaging the recipient of services in self-initiated, self-directed, purposeful (to the patient-agent) activity. Here I do not mean only self-care, but rather the whole gamut of playful, creative, and productive human activity that is recognized as meaningful by both the individual and his or her culture. Such occupation helps to put the patient-agent back together again because it is not exclusively physical or mental but, as Reilly[50] said, is energized by mind and will. The use of occupation performed by the recipient of OT services has several implications relevant to the social and psychological experience of having disability. First, it enables the expression of the unique pattern of interests each individual possesses. Pursuing old interests and developing new ones are vital ingredients in enabling people to adapt to their environments in the presence of disabling conditions.[3,39,43,62,65] The activation of interests through occupation also is a way of tapping into the intrinsic motivation[8,13] that will energize the person—not only for the short term, but also for life in the real world of home and community.

Engagement in occupation involves the whole human being in the development of skill, which he or she will possess as a resource. Occupation requires such subroutines as planning, problem solving, application of work habits, knowing and following rules, and identifying and correcting mistakes, all of which contribute to the ability of the eye, hand, and mind[7] to function cooperatively in producing an effect on the environment.

Because occupation enables the actor to produce an effect, it contributes to a sense of mastery. The need to achieve mastery, efficacy, and autonomy is identified by many authors with disability as an important contributor to the quality of their lives and their sense of well-being.[3,22,24,42,43,62] Humans possess an innate need to exercise control over their environment, a need that rarely seems to be recognized in the traditional medical milieu and therefore compounds the impact of the disability. Instead of learned helplessness,[55] in which people see themselves as the victims of overwhelming forces in their environment, the ability to do[62] something the person really wants to do contributes to a sense of efficacy. Dawes[15] wrote that self-esteem frequently results from achievement and effort rather than being their precursor. He also cited research supporting the idea that mild depression is often alleviated by simply encouraging and enabling people to engage in the activities they enjoy. Engagement in occupation may contribute to self-esteem and mitigate depressive emotions.

Occupation as therapy enables people to learn those skills they need to fulfill their social roles.[51] For example, Beisser[3] needed to learn how to pursue his interest in sports in a new way (by writing a book) and how to work as a physician (as a psychiatrist rather than a surgeon). These are examples of how occupations enabled him to be reconnected with his culture and to find his place in society.

The use of occupation as therapy demands a systems perspective of the recipient, rather than a perspective limited to impairment, disability, or handicap alone. Occupation involves all levels of the human system (biological, psychological, sociocultural, and spiritual) in interaction with that person's real environment. The activity is the integrator of these levels, producing an output such as competence or skill.

The occupational therapist has a significant, complex, and sensitive part to play in the use of occupation as therapy. He or she creates an environment in which the patient-agent can make an adaptive response. This role requires setting the stage at the right level of challenge—neither too difficult nor too easy—for each individual. It also requires suggesting activities that are consonant with the individual's interests and that may need to be adapted so that the individual can perform them. One of my colleagues had a serious traumatic head injury when her children were still young. Her occupational therapist helped her learn how to resume her responsibilities as a mother by performing a task analysis of subroutines. The therapist broke these occupations into small, achievable units. When accomplished, these units were synthesized to enable my colleague to achieve the global skills of child care. The ability to resume her role of mother was a powerful contributor to her sense of competence and the reuniting of her family.

Using occupation as therapy requires discovering the resources each individual possesses. This process is grounded in an optimistic view of human nature[50] in which all persons are seen as having resources that can be reclaimed,[41] regardless of the degree of impairment. Much of the literature[6,59,62,70] supports the validity of viewing people with disability not according to what is wrong with them but according to what is right about them. For example, psychologists Wright and Fletcher[70] claimed that a professional preoccupation with the negative leads rehabilitation workers to underestimate people's abilities. They recommended that more attention be given in assessment procedures to the environments in which the patient-agent will live (e.g., school, workplace, community). They also urged that evaluators pay as much attention to describing the strengths and resources of the individual (and his or her environments) as to exposing deficiencies and problems.

A study by Burnett and Yerxa[10] of the self-identified needs of community-based people with disabilities demonstrated many unmet needs. Our subjects reported lower confidence levels than a sample of people without disabilities in performing problem-solving, social, recreational, school, vocational, and home skills, as well as in community mobility. Basic activities of daily living was the only area of similar confidence. Many of these people had received previous hospital-based rehabilitation services including OT, yet pervasive needs for the skills required to live in the community persisted. As a result, a new program was established by the authors at a community college. It is directed by Burnett,[9] an occupational therapist. The program includes not only skill development for independent living in the community, but also training in self-advocacy (to reduce or eliminate handicap).

The use of occupation as therapy reveals the occupational therapist's role as coach (a term suggested by Mary Reilly). Rather than doing to or for the patient, the occupational therapist has the role of fostering the patient-agent's adaptive response, often by making it possible for the patient to use existing strengths and capabilities or to develop new ones. This approach takes sensitivity, skill, and an understanding of intrinsic motivation[7] far beyond that required for the "laying on of hands." Just as an athlete needs coaching to achieve the highest level of performance, the recipients of our services need coaching from occupational therapists to reach a level of competence that enables them to achieve their goals in their own environments. This is the process by which patients may be transmuted to agents. We need to study and learn much more about this process, a process that is consonant with needed changes in the health care system.[53]

Finally, the use of occupation as therapy requires that patient-agents learn to organize their lives to reduce the interference of the disability. This aspect requires a knowledge of how people may organize their time, space, resources, and daily routines to achieve their goals. Almost all of the people who wrote about their experiences of having a disability mentioned problems and frustrations with time, space, and daily routines.[17,22,24,42,43,49] Such organization is becoming more overwhelming as society increases in technological complexity. Some patient-agents never may have learned how to plan and might need help in determining their goals. This possibility is especially likely if, instead, they have learned helplessness. Occupational therapists with a knowledge of organization can help patient-agents organize their lives for maximum satisfaction and participation, contributing to their equality of capability.[6]

Mourning and Value Changes

Wright[69] discussed the common experience of people who acquire disability as feelings of shame and inferiority along with avoidance of being identified as a person with disability. She urged that caregivers conceptualize acceptance of disability in a new way. Rather than resignation or preference of one's state over another, she recommended the goal of acceptance of one's disability as nondevaluing. The disability may still be seen as inconvenient and limiting, requiring work to improve certain facets of life, but the person will not feel debased or need to hide in shame. Almost all of the people whose experiences were described earlier talked at length about the devaluation they experienced.[2,22,24,42,43,62,65,74]

The crisis of suddenly having disability may produce a gamut of emotions and thoughts, including disbelief and denial, anger, panic, self-devaluation, and guilt, fluctuating with hope and encouragement, feelings of being comforted, relief, and exaltation. These rapidly occurring cycles are highly individual and may become less acute as the person begins to acknowledge reality.[69]

How might health care workers help people through such crises toward nondevaluing acceptance of loss? Wright[69] suggested that changes are needed in people's value systems. These changes include "(1) enlarging the scope of values, (2) subordinating physique relative to other values, (3) containing disability effects, and (4) transforming comparative-status values into asset values." Note that these changes apply both to the person with disability and to outsiders such as occupational therapists and the patient-agent's family members. The value changes are discussed in the paragraphs that follow.

In enlarging the scope of values, the person with disability may initially be preoccupied with loss, going through a period of mourning. Wright[69] viewed this process as unique to the individual in length and depth. She observed that caregivers who are outsiders may overestimate the degree of depression, whereas the insider, because his or her life depends on it, may have a strong need to cope and to discover and hold onto hope and positive aspects of the situation. Some forces that may keep the person in a mourning state are a need to hold on to the preferred state that was, the need for time to absorb the changes, and perceptual emphasis on the difference of disability, rather than on commonalities and continuity with the past. In contrast, the scope of values may be enlarged by the comparison of one's state with other states (e.g., death or having other disabilities); arousal of dominant values such as awakened pride or the need to deal with the problems at hand; the satiation factor, whereby the emotions devoted to mourning are worn out and the person feels wrung out and becomes ready for something new; and, finally, involvement in the necessities of daily living.

Mourning may not always be protracted or intense, but it needs to be recognized as a healing period during which the wound is first anesthetized and then closed gradually with some scarring. Wright[69] observed that as depression lifts, the sheer necessities of living contribute to needed changes in values. Bodily needs prod the person with paraplegia; for example, trying to move or sit up represents a "here and now" challenge. Mastering the activities of daily living (ADL) helps enlarge the scope of values, although as Wright observed, "Mastering ADL is surely not sufficient for enjoying a new lease on life." Seeing films of other patient-agents who can manage the ordinary affairs of daily life may also provide valuable support for the person who has recently acquired disability.[69] The occupational therapist's regulated optimism regarding the patient-agent's potential may contribute to a sense of the possible.

As mourning subsides after sufficient time has elapsed for its expression and the opportunity to engage in activity, physique may still hold a potent value. Value changes may eventually override this potency through a shift in emphasis from appearance to personality or capability, reducing the effects of spread.

Containing disability effects involves understanding that although a physical impairment is a fact that may affect aspects of life, it does not affect all of life, and its effects are not necessarily negative. Instead, "It involves certain limitations in certain situations. The source of limitation is due to barriers imposed by society and not only to personal incapacity."[69]

Finally, transforming comparative-status values into asset values is an important shift. Status values or judgments of the worthiness of a person can be replaced by asset values. Asset values are attributes that, rather than being competitive or judgmental, are seen as useful or intrinsically worthwhile. For example, being able to get around in one's community while using a wheelchair may constitute an asset value without comparison with how other people do it or even how the person with disability used to do it. Occupational therapists who enable people to achieve their personal goals by discovering and using their strengths and resources may help people with disability to enlarge their scope of values so

that physique is less important than what one can do and be[62] and so that new possibilities are discovered as asset values.

Although psychologists such as Wright[69] and Siller[59] emphasize adjustment to disability, I prefer the broader concept of **adaptation with disability**.[40] This goal suggests that the disability or handicap constitutes only one class of challenges among many others with which all human beings must deal to achieve a good fit with their environment. Adaptation places the person with disability within the mainstream of humanity and acknowledges his or her resources gained by evolution. It places proper attention on the social barriers of handicap, rather than putting the entire responsibility on the person with disability.

Relationship Between Occupational Therapist and Patient-Agent

Occupational therapists are said to value a model of **mutual cooperation**[57,71] as the ideal relationship with the patient-agent. This collaborative relationship is different in style and substance from the traditional physician-patient relationship in which the professional is active and the patient is passive. What are some characteristics of the occupational therapist/patient-agent relationship?

Peloquin[44] urged that occupational therapists be not only competent but also caring. She observed that the profit-driven nature of health care provision often leads to treatment of patients as mere customers and results in a budgeting of caring actions. Many patients complain about the impersonality and overreliance on technical methods they experience in the hospital or clinic. The system values competence over caring because of three social trends: "(1) emphasis on rational fixing of health care problems, (2) overreliance on methods and protocols, and (3) a health care system driven by business, efficiency, and profits." Peloquin challenged occupational therapists to recognize the extent to which such social forces shape the manner in which they relate to patients.

Despite the influence of the profit-driven nature of health care provision, Peloquin[44] observed that occupational therapists can be both competent and caring. This goal may be accomplished by getting to know each patient as a person, gaining more power in the system (in order to change it), tempering that power with care, seeking to understand patients' feelings about their illness, and, rather than acting as an authoritarian parent or technician, providing patients with opportunities for control over their own lives. These recommendations seem congruent with valuing mutual cooperation in planning and implementing OT. For example, if the occupational therapist wishes to elicit the patient's interests and goals, he or she must get to know each patient as an individual. Providing opportunities for control and self-direction is congruent with the ultimate goal of independent living in the community, whereas expecting compliance with professional orders may seem more efficient but may subvert the learning of habits of independence and self-sufficiency.

Schlaff,[54] an occupational therapist, proposed that occupational therapists help redefine disability. This redefinition would include working for changes in social attitudes and practices so that society would recognize the dignity and worth of people with disability, granting their rights to self-definition and self-direction. The occupational therapist would strive to work in an independent living paradigm as a consultant, helper, and advocate, rather than as a diagnostician or a prescriber and manager of treatment. "The consumer is or becomes self-directed, and both the consumer and occupational therapist work to remove community barriers and disincentives" for economic independence.[12,54]

Wright's perspective[69] of the client as comanager in rehabilitation echoes the valuing of mutual cooperation by OT. She observed that if the goal of rehabilitation is independence and self-directedness, these must be nurtured during rehabilitation. She proposed that **comanagement** could result in increased self-esteem, intrinsic motivation, and better potential for learning because the patient-agent is actively involved. Besides, health care professionals need the knowledge that only the patient-agent can provide to recommend the best course of action. Vash[62] obviously knew herself better than her vocational counselor did when she decided to become a psychologist rather than a secretary. If mutual cooperation is actualized by comanagement, what might impede this cooperation?

Wright[69] observed that the helping relationship itself might get in the way because it conveys subservience and less power for the person being helped, reinforcing the view that the expert has (or should have) the answers. The patient-agent might expect and want the professional to take complete charge. In some circumstances, such as acute illness, this approach is necessary and commendable. However, the shifting of responsibility to the therapist can interfere substantially with the goals of rehabilitation and OT, especially those of eventual unsupervised and independent living. Wright[69] therefore asserted that "It is essential that the client be brought into a directorship role as soon as feasible."

Wright[69] also acknowledged that helpers may have needs that interfere with comanagement. They might need to assert themselves, display their knowledge, gain power, or achieve satisfaction in an authoritative role. Wright also cited the increasing pressure for efficiency and cost containment in the system as a stumbling block because comanagement may require more time and effort than would professional prescriptions. Her advice was, "Don't get stuck with the problem; move on

to the solution" to prod constructive thinking. For example, why not employ more people with disability to work in OT departments, to pave the way for real participation on the part of patient-agents?

Some other suggestions for comanagement are that patient-agents be given more active roles and responsibilities in the day-to-day activities of the hospital, such as administrative problem solving that planning the rehabilitation program be a joint effort of patient-agents and staff; that patient-agents be encouraged to make decisions and evaluate options (at every stage of the therapeutic process); and that professionals be given training in encouraging participants to become comanagers.[69] I would add that patient-agents, too, may need training in how to be comanagers and that OT, with its emphasis on self-directed occupations, is a likely learning laboratory for the development of such skills.

Wright[69] cited research that supported the findings about long-term effects of comanagement. A group of 100 patients with severe disability underwent rehabilitation in a hospital that encouraged their maximum involvement and participation. One year after discharge, their status was compared with that of a control group who had completed a conventional rehabilitation program at the same hospital. The experimental group showed a greater degree of sustained improvement in self-care and ambulation and a lower mortality rate.[69]

Wright[69] concluded with the conviction that whenever feasible, comanagement on the part of the client should be promoted. The therapist should support this belief by showing that he or she likes the patient-agent, by being friendly and caring, and by showing concern about the patient-agent's welfare. Basic civilities such as introducing oneself and addressing the recipient of services by name are also important. The professional person needs "to question at all times whether the client is at the helm" or whether the person is being "paternalistically directed."[69] This last test is especially important for occupational therapists who may work in an environment in which professional authoritarianism is the norm.

The therapeutic relationship of mutual cooperation and comanagement extends to the interaction between the occupational therapist and parent when providing services to a child with disability. Parents need to learn the skills of relating to a wide range of professionals to obtain needed services, often in an atmosphere that fosters an uneven distribution of power. Parents deal with the diagnosis of a lifelong disability in highly individual ways, attempting a resolution between professionally provided definitions and their everyday experiences of living with a child who is not a clinical category but a real person with both resources and problems.[60]

Wright[69] viewed the parent as a key participant in the rehabilitation process. Parents offer knowledge about their children, and their cooperation is essential. They also may need help and support in accepting the child's disability as nondevaluing and in learning to cope with the challenges awaiting them.

Wright cited three characteristics of a constructive professional-parent relationship: parents need to feel that the professional is not working against them and that together they are seeking solutions; they need to believe that the professional likes their child and sees him or her as a special individual; and they need to feel that the professional appreciates their struggle to do the best they can for their child and that although they may have shortcomings, they also have strengths and ideas.[69]

Wright[69] proposed that rather than an exaggerated valuing of independence, the goal of balancing independence, dependence, and interdependence is more helpful. Finding this balance is a necessity in all human relationships, and it is likely to ensure the proper emphasis on warmth, love, and caring, which every child needs. Independence often means making choices and calling the shots while still depending on others for some things. For example, a person might be independent in hiring or firing an attendant for some personal care but dependent in needing a person to perform such services.

There are many ways to achieve the balance among independence, dependence, and interdependence. For example, the balance might be enhanced by opportunities for parents to observe other children with the same disability as that of their own child; parent discussion groups, including brainstorming for problem solving; special techniques that make life easier at home; creation of opportunities for specific experiences such as play and leisure activities; the judicious use of reading material to impart factual information and constructive attitudes; and opportunity for the child to assume increasing responsibility for his or her own self-help behavior and activities involving other people[69] (such as doing chores at home).

Occupational therapists can contribute to achieving balance by working in partnership with the families of children who have disability.[19] For example, therapists can assist family members in setting aside space and time for play, leisure, and social activities in the home, as well as personal time and space for the primary caregiver, who is often the mother.[19] (Housework, child care, lack of financial resources, and fatigue often make such time out essential.) Other ways occupational therapists can help are by reducing environmental barriers to the child's participation in daily life; determining the child's strengths and resources (reducing negative spread); enlarging the child's scope of activities by providing the necessary time, patience, and opportunity for learning; and helping the family organize its time and resources to avoid frustrations and fatigue and to ensure participation in satisfying family activities.

A study of mothers of children with cerebral palsy[11] uncovered frustration at the fact that their input was sometimes disregarded by professionals and at the high rate of turnover of therapists and resulting lack of continuity in the care of their children. These mothers viewed occupational therapists as agents of change, sources of information, and sources of support. Recommendations for occupational therapists working with such children included the following: developing active, respectful listening skills; establishing a priority of therapist continuity; increasing mothers' trust and confidence; providing expressions of optimism; and enabling children to receive as much therapy as possible.

The relationship between the patient-agent and the occupational therapist is both complex and sensitive. It emphasizes the model of mutual cooperation and the full participation of the service recipient in identifying goals. It provides a safe space for growth and the learning of skills, as well as the discovery and nurturing of the patient-agent's resources for adaptation and competence.

New Models of Practice

The literature provides several examples of new models of OT practice with patient-agents who have physical disability. These examples have been selected because they appear congruent with both the values of the profession and the experiences of people with disability; they foster positive attitudes and emphasize the strengths and resources of the individual (such as adaptive capacities) and employ occupation as therapy.

Montgomery[41] described the OT hospital-based clinic as a resource reclamation center. The occupational therapist discovers and augments the patient's potential strengths, which have developed over the three time spans of evolution, development, and learning. As these resources are enhanced through activity, the patient-agent is helped to resume daily living in the real world of home and community—not as a disabled person, but as a person who is part of the mainstream of humanity with the same needs and resources as anyone else.

In a classic article, Burke[8] explored the complex issue of intrinsic motivation that cuts across all dimensions of OT practice. Her paper provides occupational therapists with useful information on coaching patient-agents to engage in occupations and become self-directed originators rather than pawns. It addresses creation of a just-right challenge from the environment so that patient-agents may make their own adaptive response.

Several models of OT practice are devoted to the development of independent living skills for community living. Pendleton[45] found that occupational therapists working in rehabilitation centers frequently place much more emphasis on technical goals (such as range of motion and muscle strengthening) than on the skills needed for independent living. She urged occupational therapists to devote more time and energy to preparing patient-agents for the capacity to function in their own communities.

The **independent living movement**[16] arose to increase the self-direction and ensure the civil rights of people with disability. The movement is based on the idea that people with disability are the best judges of their own needs. It emphasizes the goals not only of self-care, but also of mobility, employment, accessible living arrangements, out-of-home activity (to enlarge the environment), and consumer assertiveness. This movement appears compatible with the goals and values of OT in its pursuit of equality of capability, enabling people to manage their own environments, including their time, space, and energy. In some respects it addresses the shortcomings of the medical and rehabilitation system, which may foster paternalistic dependence on professionals. For example, one of the movement's goals is to enable people with disability to take risks. "Without the possibility of failure, the disabled person* lacks true independence and the ultimate mark of humanity, the right to choose for good or evil."[16]

Some models of OT practice reflect an emphasis on autonomy, choice, and the skills needed to increase people's capacity for daily living. Several models are based in community settings such as schools and independent living centers rather than in hospitals. Community-based OT practice is likely to become more common in the 21st century because of the high cost of hospital care and the need for long-term services for those with chronic conditions.

Cole (now Cole-Spencer),[12] an anthropologist and occupational therapist, described a program for teaching independent living skills. She observed that such skills must include planning and management and the skills for self-direction rather than task-oriented behavioral capabilities (such as basic self-care). Some skills her program emphasized were communicating effectively to have one's needs met; identifying and using resources; identifying and comparing choices; making decisions and setting priorities; committing oneself to long-term goals and persisting until they are attained; developing sequential plans so that efforts produce a cumulative effect and outcome; assessing risks and developing judgment about risk taking; managing crises such as medical or financial emergencies; and solving problems. These skills are needed by every human being and are not limited to people with disability. (They are even useful for students studying OT!) Such skills are developed through engagement in self-directed activity rather than doing to or for the recipients of service.

Burnett (now Burnett-Beaulieu)[9] developed a nontraditional OT program for community college students with disability. The goals of the program are similar to those described by Cole,[12] with a primary emphasis upon enabling students with disability to function successfully in their roles as college students. She reported that this program often serves as a bridge between medical rehabilitation and life in the mainstream. It includes three levels of skills: self-care, home management, and community mobility; social-recreational, cognitive, and classroom skills; and consumer rights skills. Burnett-Beaulieu[9] posited that these skills can be grouped into a hierarchy, with the first level basic to the achievement of the other two levels.

Another OT program was developed by Jackson[26] and colleagues. It was designed for adolescents with developmental disability. This Options program is provided at a nonmainstreamed high school campus. The goal of the program is to enable students to make a successful transition from school to community living through exploring and broadening their choices about employment, living arrangements, and social activities. It focuses not only on the skills and resources of the students, but also on the characteristics of their environments. Parents and family members are included as advocates. An important feature of the program is the learning of employment skills in a supported work environment.

The programs described in the preceding paragraphs may stimulate occupational therapists to think about and develop new models of community-based practice as a needed alternative to traditional hospital-based practice. This alternative is made more urgent by revolutionary changes in the health care system,[53] the needs and experiences of people with disability,[42,62,74] and the values and traditions of OT.[71] We need many more such models to achieve our potential contribution as a profession, to improve life opportunities for people with disability, and to influence public attitudes toward people with disability in a positive way by emphasizing the skills of such people and their similarities rather than their differences as human beings.

SUMMARY

This chapter explores important questions about the social and psychological experiences of having disability and what implications these experiences hold for OT practice. I have suggested that the experiences of people with disability are important resources for occupational therapists in enabling us to broaden our vision and potential contribution to the quality of life of the recipients of our services. In widening our scope, we need to take a systems view of each individual as one who interacts with a unique environment by engaging in a unique pattern of occupations, dictated by both culture and unique interests.

---

*"The disabled person" is De Jong's terminology.

TABLE 28-3
Model of Occupational Therapy

Definition	Model	Problem	Power
Capability	Occupational therapy	Discover/ nurture potential for agency	Human system acting on the environment with a repertoire of skills

When Reilly[50] proposed her great hypothesis that humans could influence the state of their own health through the use of hands, mind, and will, she was conveying not only the essence of OT, but also perhaps a much needed new view of health. Occupational therapists work primarily with people having chronic conditions who will never get well. Therefore we need to help society redefine health, not as the absence of impairment or disease, but as the possession of a repertoire of skills[47] that enable a person to achieve his or her valued goals. Thus people with irremediable impairments can still look forward to a healthy life.

Returning to Bickenbach's[6] three models of disability (Table 28-2), we can now add a fourth model, that of OT (Table 28-3). In this model the problem is the need to discover and nurture the individual's potential for agency. The definition is human capability, which emphasizes people's abilities to do what they want and need to do and their opportunities to make choices. Although it may be threatened or diminished by impairment, disability, or handicap, capability is the desired outcome of the physical event of a disability. The power rests in the human system itself, which acts on the environment through occupation, possessing a repertoire of skills. This model of OT assumes that people have or can develop the strengths and resources to achieve their own goals by engagement in occupation. The model integrates people with disability into their own environments and welcomes them into the mainstream of society. The model of OT provides new hope for attaining equality of capability[6] and influencing health.[50]

REVIEW QUESTIONS

1. Compare and contrast the values of occupational therapy with those of traditional medicine.
2. How do these differences in values translate into different, complementary goals for each profession?
3. Describe a systems view of human beings and apply it to occupational therapy for people with physical disabilities.

4. Define *stigma* as described by Goffman.
5. Why is it essential for occupational therapists and other health professionals to consider the environment and social context of the person with disability?
6. To what extent is it valid to predict that a person with disability will have low self-esteem?
7. How do a person's interests, values, and goals influence his or her reactions to acquiring disability?
8. Which aspects of Murphy's daily life contributed to his sense of autonomy and which diminished it?
9. What needs that could be met by occupational therapy were revealed in the autobiographies of people with disabilities?
10. What unmet needs for community living skills were identified in Burnett and Yerxa's study?
11. Differentiate between the terms "adjustment to disability" and "adaptation with disability."
12. Discuss a new view of health as it applies to people with chronic conditions.

EXERCISE

1. Please read the following description: "James, an adolescent of fourteen, has spastic cerebral palsy, frequently relates to his siblings and peers aggressively, is 2 years below grade level in reading and arithmetic, and has parents who are rarely present at home."[70] Stop here. What is your impression of James?
2. Now add this: "James does an outstanding job on his paper route, likes to write poetry and fantasy stories, has a close relationship with his uncle and aunt who live nearby, and is making steady progress in physical therapy." What is your impression of James?
3. Relate this exercise to how occupational therapists assess or evaluate their patient-agents.

REFERENCES

1. American Occupational Therapy Association: *Summary report: 1990 member data survey*, Rockville, Md, 1990, The Association.
2. Bauby JD: *The diving bell and the butterfly*, London, 1997, Fourth Estate.
3. Beisser A: *Flying without wings: personal reflections on being disabled*, New York, 1989, Doubleday.
4. Benham P: Attitudes of occupational therapy personnel toward persons with disabilities, *Am J Occup Ther* 42(5):305-311, 1988.
5. Bernspång B: *Consequences of stroke: aspects of impairments, disabilities and life satisfaction with special emphasis on perception and occupational therapy*, Umeå, Sweden, 1987, Umea University Printing Office.
6. Bickenbach JE: *Physical disability and social policy*, Toronto, 1993, University of Toronto Press.
7. Bruner JS: Eye, hand, and mind. In Bruner JS, editor: *Beyond the information given: studies in the psychology of knowing*, New York, 1973, WW Norton.
8. Burke JP: A clinical perspective on motivation: pawn versus origin, *Am J Occup Ther* 31(4):254-258, 1977.
9. Burnett SE: *Seven modules for independent living skills: instruction for physically disabled college students*, Santa Monica, Calif, 1982, Disabled Students Center, Santa Monica College.
10. Burnett SE, Yerxa EJ: Community based and college based needs assessment of physically disabled persons, *Am J Occup Ther* 34(3):201-207, 1980.

11. Case-Smith J, Nastro MA: The effect of occupational therapy intervention on mothers of children with cerebral palsy, *Am J Occup Ther* 47(9):811-817, 1993.

12. Cole JA: Skills training. In Crewe NM, Zola IK, editors: *Independent living for physically disabled people: developing, implementing and evaluating self-help rehabilitation programs*, San Francisco, 1983, Jossey-Bass.

13. Csikszentmihalyi M: *Beyond boredom and anxiety: the experience of play in work and games*, San Francisco, 1975, Jossey-Bass.

14. Damasio A: *Descartes' error: emotion, reason and the human brain*, New York, 1994, Avon Books.

15. Dawes RM: *House of cards: psychology and psychotherapy built on myth*, New York, 1994, Free Press.

16. De Jong G: Defining and implementing the independent living concept. In Crewe NM, Zola IK, editors: *Independent living for physically disabled people: developing, implementing and evaluating self-help rehabilitation programs*, San Francisco, 1983, Jossey-Bass.

17. Dubus A: *Broken vessels*, Boston, 1991, David R Godine.

18. Edgerton RB: *Rules, exceptions and social order*, Berkeley, 1985, University of California Press.

19. Esdaile SA: A focus on mothers, their children with special needs and other caregivers, *Aust Occup Ther J* 41:3, 1994.

20. Estes J et al: Influences of occupational therapy curricula on students' attitudes toward persons with disabilities, *Am J Occup Ther* 45(2):156-159, 1991.

21. Fichten CS et al: College students with physical disabilities: myths and realities. In Eisenberg MG, Glueckauf RL, editors: *Empirical approaches to the psychosocial aspects of disability*, New York, 1991, Springer.

22. Fiffer S: *Three quarters, two dimes, and a nickel, a memoir of becoming whole*, New York, 1999, Free Press.

23. Goffman E: *Stigma: notes on the management of spoiled identity*, Englewood Cliffs, NJ, 1963, Prentice-Hall.

24. Hockenberry J: *Moving violations, a memoir*, New York, 1995, Hyperion.

25. Hodgins E: Whatever became of the healing art? *Ann New York Acad Sci* 164:838, 1964.

26. Jackson J: En route to adulthood: a high school transition program for adolescents with disabilities. In Johnson JA, Yerxa EJ, editors: *Occupational science: the foundation for new models of practice*, New York, 1990, Haworth Press.

27. Kielhofner G: *A model of human occupation: theory and application*, Baltimore, 1985, Williams & Wilkins.

28. King GA et al: Self-evaluation and self-concept of adolescents with physical disabilities, *Am J Occup Ther* 47(2):132-140, 1993.

29. Kisor H: *What's that pig outdoors? A memoir of deafness*, New York, 1990, Penguin.

30. Konner M: *Becoming a doctor: a journey of initiation in medical school*, New York, 1987, Viking.

31. Lakoff G, Johnson M: *Philosophy in the flesh: the embodied mind and its challenge to Western thought*, New York, 1999, BasicBooks.

32. Lerner MJ, Miller DT: Just world research and the attribution process: looking back and ahead, *Psychol Bull* 85:1030, 1978.

33. Lewontin RC: *Biology as ideology*, New York, 1991, Harper Collins.

34. Liachowitz CH: *Disability as a social construct: legislative roots*, Philadelphia, 1988, University of Pennsylvania.

35. Lyons M: Enabling or disabling? Students' attitudes toward persons with disabilities, *Am J Occup Ther* 45(4):311-316, 1991.

36. Lyons M, Hayes R: Student perceptions of persons with psychiatric and other disorders, *Am J Occup Ther* 47(6):541-548, 1993.

37. *The MacNeil/Lehrer NewsHour*, Public Broadcasting System, April 4, 1994.

38. Magill-Evans JE, Restall G: Self-esteem of persons with cerebral palsy: from adolescence to adulthood, *Am J Occup Ther* 45(9):819-825, 1991.

39. Matsutsuyu JS: The interest checklist, *Am J Occup Ther* 23(4):323-328, 1969.

40. McCuaig M, Frank G: The able self: adaptive patterns and choices in independent living for a person with cerebral palsy, *Am J Occup Ther* 45(3):224-234, 1991.

41. Montgomery MA: Resources of adaptation for daily living: a classification with therapeutic implications for occupational therapy, *Occup Ther Health Care* 1:9, 1984.

42. Murphy RF: *The body silent*, New York, 1990, WW Norton.

43. Osborn CL: *Over my head, a doctor's own story of head injury from the inside looking out*, Kansas City, 1998, Andrews McMeel.

44. Peloquin SM: The patient-therapist relationship: beliefs that shape care, *Am J Occup Ther* 47(10):935-942, 1993.

45. Pendleton HM: Occupational therapists' current use of independent living skills training for adult inpatients who are physically disabled, *Occup Ther Health Care* 6:93, 1989.

46. Pfeiffer D: The categorization and control of people with disabilities, *Disabil Rehabil* 21(3):106-107, 1999.

47. Pörn I: Health and adaptedness, *Theor Med* 14(4):295-303, 1993.

48. Proctor RN: *Racial hygiene: medicine under the Nazis*, Cambridge, Mass, 1988, Harvard University Press.

49. Puller LB: *Fortunate son: the autobiography of Lewis B Puller, Jr*, New York, 1991, Grove Weidenfeld.

50. Reilly M: Occupational therapy can be one of the great ideas of 20th century medicine, *Am J Occup Ther* 16:300, 1962.

51. Reilly M: The educational process, *Am J Occup Ther* 23(4):299-307, 1969.

52. Reilly M: The importance of the client versus patient issue for occupational therapy, *Am J Occup Ther* 38(6):404-406, 1984.

53. Robinson I: The rehabilitation of patients with long term physical impairments: the social context of professional roles, *Clin Rehab* 2:339, 1988.

54. Schlaff C: Health policy from dependency to self-advocacy: redefining disability, *Am J Occup Ther* 47(10):943-948, 1993.

55. Seligman MEP: *Helplessness*, New York, 1975, WH Freeman.

56. Sharrott GW, Yerxa EJ: Promises to keep: implications of the referent "patient" versus "client" for those served by occupational therapy, *Am J Occup Ther* 39(6):401-405, 1985.

57. Shortell SM: Occupational prestige differences within the medical and allied health professions, *Soc Sci Med* 8(1):1-9, 1974.

58. Siegler M, Osmond H: *Models of madness, models of medicine*, New York, 1975, Macmillan.

59. Siller J: The measurement of attitudes toward physically disabled persons. In Herman CP, Zanna MP, Higgins ET: editors: Ontario symposium on personality and social psychology, vol 3, *Physical appearance, stigma and social behavior*, Hillsdale, NJ, 1986, Lawrence Erlbaum.

60. Thomas D: *The experience of handicap*, New York, 1982, Methuen.

61. Turner C: Death of Canada "right to die" advocate triggers new debate, *Los Angeles Times*, p A5, April 8, 1994.

62. Vash CL: *The psychology of disability, Springer series on rehabilitation*, vol 1, New York, 1981, Springer.

63. Weinberg N: Another perspective: attitudes of people with disabilities. In Yuker E, editor: *Attitudes toward persons with disabilities*, New York, 1988, Springer.

64. Westbrook M, Adamson B: Knowledge and attitudes: aspects of occupational therapy students' perceptions of the handicapped, *Aust Occup Ther J* 36:120, 1989.

65. Williams D: *Nobody nowhere: the extraordinary autobiography of an autistic*, New York, 1992, Avon.

66. Williams MR, Russell ML: *ADA handbook: employment and construction issues affecting your business*, Chicago, 1993, Dearborn Financial Publications.

67. World Health Organization: *International classification of impairments, disabilities and handicaps: a manual of classification relating to the consequences of disease*, Geneva, 1980, The Organization.

68. World Health Organization: *I C I DH-2, Beta 2 Draft*, Introduction, Geneva, April 1999, The Organization.

69. Wright B: *Physical disability: a psychosocial approach*, ed 2, New York, 1983, Harper & Row.

70. Wright B, Fletcher BL: Uncovering hidden resources: a challenge in assessment, *Prof Psychol* 13:229, 1982.

71. Yerxa EJ: Audacious values: the energy source for occupational therapy practice. In Kielhofner G, editor: *Health through occupation,* Philadelphia, 1983, FA Davis.

72. Yerxa EJ: Dreams, dilemmas and decisions for occupational therapy practice in a new millenium: an American perspective, *Am J Occup Ther* 48:586, 1994.

73. Yerxa EJ et al: An introduction to occupational science, a foundation for occupational therapy in the 21st century, *Occup Ther Health Care* 6:1, 1989.

74. Zola IK: *Missing pieces: a chronicle of living with disability,* Philadelphia, 1982, Temple University Press.

CHAPTER 29

Pain Management

JOYCE M. ENGEL

Acute pain
Chronic pain
Gate control theory
Pain behavior
Pain assessment
Pain intervention

After studying this chapter the student or practitioner will be able to do the following:
1. Discuss the differences between acute and chronic pain.
2. Explain the gate control theory of pain transmission.
3. Identify two pain syndromes.
4. Summarize two approaches to pain assessment.
5. Describe three approaches to pain intervention.

Despite advances in medicine, rehabilitation, and technology, pain often affects an individual's occupational performance and quality of life. Pain may coexist with a medical condition (e.g., arthritis) or rehabilitation procedure (e.g., stretching) or be the primary complaint (e.g., low back pain). Occupational therapists may suspect that pain is impeding the patient's progress but feel unsure about how to approach evaluation and intervention. This chapter defines pain, discusses pain transmission, describes common pain syndromes, outlines evaluation procedures, and proposes intervention strategies.

DEFINITION OF PAIN

Pain is an unpleasant sensory and emotional experience associated with actual or potential tissue damage or described in terms of such damage.[18] This definition conveys that pain is a subjective experience and multidimensional. Individual variables such as mood, attention, prior pain experiences, and culture are known to affect one's experience of pain.[25]

Most investigators agree in differentiating acute from chronic pain, which is critical for selecting appropriate assessment and intervention strategies.[20] **Acute pain** has a well-defined pain onset. It is associated with sympathetic nervous system arousal (e.g., increases in muscle tone). Acute pain serves a biological purpose, directing attention to injury, irritation, or disease and signaling the need for immobilization and protection of a body part.[20] Fortunately, acute pain usually responds to medication, management, and treatment of the underlying cause of pain.[16]

In contrast, **chronic pain** may begin as acute pain or may be more insidious and endure beyond the point at which an underlying pathological condition can be identified. Increased sympathetic nervous system activity does not continue. Chronic pain does not appear to serve a biological purpose. Chronic pain often produces significant changes in personality, lifestyle, and functional ability.[16]

PAIN TRANSMISSION

Multiple theories of pain transmission have been proposed. To date, the **gate control theory**[26] represents the single most important theoretical contribution to our understanding of pain. Melzack and Wall[26] offered a variation of the previously accepted specificity and pattern theories to explain pain transmission. They suggested that pain is modulated by a "gating" mechanism in the spinal cord that can increase or decrease the flow of nerve impulses to the brain. Sensory impulses travel to the dorsal horn along large- and small-diameter nerves associated with pain impulses. At the dorsal horn, these impulses encounter a gate believed to be composed of substantia gelatinosa cells. This gate, which may be presynaptic, postsynaptic, or a combination of both, can be closed, partially open, or open. If the gate is closed, pain impulses cannot proceed. If the gate is at least partially open, pain impulses stimulate transmission or trigger cells in the dorsal horn which then ascend the spinal cord to the brain and result in pain perception. Once the pain impulses are perceived, higher central nervous system structures (brain stem, thalamus, cerebral cortex) can modify pain by influencing T-cell activity. These structures can alter such factors as attention, memory, and affect, contributing to an individual's unique pain perception. Pain management therefore focuses on "closing the gate" through a combination of interventions.[1,8,9]

Fordyce[12] proposed a different perspective of pain transmission based on learning theory. **Pain behaviors** communicate to others that pain is being experienced. According to Fordyce, pain behavior can be classified as *respondent* if its onset was caused by antecedent tissue irritation or damage. Respondent pain may be reduced by medication, avoidance of specific activities, and certain body postures. As individuals in the patient's environment respond to these pain behaviors (e.g., moaning, grimacing, limping, and taking medications), the behaviors may be reinforced. This contingent relationship may continue after initial tissue irritation or damage has subsided and may result in operant pain, with the patient taking on a "sick role." Intervention for operant pain requires that reinforcement of operant pain behaviors be removed, so as to increase the occurrence of healthy behaviors (e.g., functional activity).

The above theories help to explain the variation in pain perception and expression. These theories guide the occupational therapist in multidimensional pain assessment and intervention.

PAIN SYNDROMES

Pain is a primary reason for seeking health care. The evaluation and treatment of pain resulting from trauma, disease, or unknown etiology are a significant health care concerns. The following sections provide descriptions of common pain syndromes.

Headache Pain

Recurrent headaches are one of the most common pain problems, affecting over 40% of the U.S. population. Over half of the population of persons with head-aches do not seek treatment because they perceive the problem as too trivial, have concerns about medication side effects, and believe no adequate treatment is available.[23]

Migraines affect 17.6% of women and 5.7% of men.[23] A strong genetic predisposition exists for migraines. These headaches are characterized by recurrent pain episodes varying in frequency, duration, and intensity. The pain is typically unilateral and pulsatile and may be accompanied by anorexia, nausea, vomiting, neurological symptoms (e.g., photosensitivity and photophobia), and mood changes (e.g., irritability).[23]

Tension-type headaches are the most common headache disorder. Approximately 73% of adult Americans experience one or more headaches in a year.[5] These headaches are typically of mild to moderate intensity. The pain is bilateral and of a pressing character and does not have associated symptoms. Precipitating headache factors include situational stress, missed meals, sleep deprivation, and noxious stimuli (e.g., heat exposure).[23]

Low Back Pain

Low back pain (LBP) is the second most common pain complaint among the adult population. Eighty percent of workers with LBP are absent from their jobs as a result of the pain.[30] The incidence of LBP is influenced by occupation; individuals employed in jobs that involve heavy physical work and lifting are more susceptible to LBP than others.[16]

The most common causes of LBP are injury and stress, resulting in musculoskeletal and neurological disorders (e.g., muscle spasm and sciatica). Back pain also may result from infections, degenerative diseases (e.g., osteoarthritis), rheumatoid arthritis, spinal stenosis, tumors, and congenital disorders.[30] Once significant back pain has lasted for 6 months, the chance of return to work is only 50%.[7]

Arthritis

Bonica[2] estimated that 24 million Americans experience painful arthritis and 11.5 million are at least partially disabled. Osteoarthritis is characterized by a progressive, dull ache and swelling, typically affecting the fingers, elbows, hips, knees, and ankles. Osteoarthritis may be exacerbated by movement. Degeneration of the articular cartilage and swelling occur, typically affecting weight-bearing joints.[34]

Rheumatoid arthritis usually has a slow insidious onset, characterized by aches, pains, swelling, and stiffness. Any joint may be involved, but usually there is a symmetrical pattern affecting the fingers, wrists, knees, ankles, and cervical spine.[16] This systemic disease involves remissions and exacerbations of destructive inflammation of connective tissue, especially in the synovial joints.[34] See Chapter 43 for more information on arthritis.

Reflex Sympathetic Dystrophy Pain

Reflex sympathetic dystrophy (RSD) pain is continuous burning pain that results from trauma, postsurgical inflammation, infection, or laceration to an extremity, causing a cycle of vasospasm and vasodilatation. Pain, edema, shiny skin, and coolness of the hand occur. An individual experiencing RSD pain may also have excessive sweating or dryness. Exacerbating pain factors include movement, cutaneous stimulation, and stress.[19]

Myofascial Pain

Myofascial pain is a common pain syndrome defined by the presence of "trigger points" (localized areas of deep muscle tenderness). Pressure on the trigger point elicits pain to a well-defined distal area. Myofascial pain may result from sustained muscle contraction or from trauma to the head, neck, shoulder, or lower back regions.[15]

Cancer Pain

Patients with cancer often have multiple pain problems that are frequently undertreated. Cancer pain is often chronic. In the initial and intermediate stages 30% to 45% of patients experience moderate to severe pain. About 75% of patients with advanced cancer have pain. Cancer pain may result from tumor progression, interventions (e.g., surgery, chemotherapy, and radiation), infection, or muscle aches when patients decrease their activity.[37]

Referred Pain

Referred pain is a common feature of low back and myofascial pain. Referred pain is experienced within the same dermatome as the tissue damage, in a distant area supplied by the same nerve, or in areas with no anatomical correlation.[15]

EVALUATION

A referral for occupational therapy (OT) evaluation is made when pain interferes with the patient's performance of activities of daily living (ADL), work and other productive activities, or leisure. Occupational therapists focus evaluation on psychosocial and environmental factors that contribute to the patient's pain perception and on the effects of pain on functional performance. Before interventions are implemented, objective measures of occupational performance should be obtained to assess the status of the patient and the value of those activities. Factors that may contribute to pain perception and decreased functional performance should be identified.

The occupational therapist performs a **pain assessment**, viewing pain as a complex phenomenon involving psychological arousal, sensations of noxious stimulation, tissue damage or irritation, behavioral avoidance, and complaints of subjective distress. Pain is conceptualized as an interacting cluster of overt and covert behaviors. Overt behaviors, or observable pain behaviors, are commonly targeted in evaluation. Such pain behaviors include guarded movement, bracing, posturing, limping, rubbing, and facial grimacing, all of which suggest discomfort.[21] The University of Alabama Pain Behavior Scale[29] is an example of a standardized rating scale that is reliable, valid, and an easy method for documenting overt behaviors. Analysis of the patient's overt behaviors before, during, and after intervention can provide valuable information about the role of situational and learned factors in the individual's pain perception, as well as responses to treatment procedures. Merskey[27] cautions practitioners not to provide treatment for reducing pain behaviors in lieu of attempts at alleviating the pain. Evaluation that focuses solely on pain behavior may lead to the inaccurate conclusion that pain behavior suggests malingering, lack of motivation, or hypochondriasis.

Covert behaviors or self-reports of pain are also assessed because pain is considered to be primarily a subjective phenomenon. The clinical interview focuses on the patient's identification of pain location, frequency, duration, intensity, onset, exacerbating and relieving pain factors, past and present pain treatments, affect, and functional performance. The single most reliable indicator of the existence and intensity of pain, and any resultant affective discomfort, is the patient's self-report.[37] A Simple Descriptive Pain Intensity Scale, 0-10 Numeric Pain Intensity Scale, or Visual Analog Scale (Box 29-1) may be used in assessing self-reports of pain intensity.[37] These instruments are easy to use and can be adapted to the patient's vocabulary.

Activity performance is the primary focus of the occupational therapist. The patient may complete daily activity diaries as an assessment technique and outcome measure. With this technique, hourly entries of time spent in sitting, standing, reclining, and other productive activities are recorded by the patient and may be corroborated by trained staff.[10] The Brief Pain Inventory[6] is a reliable and valid instrument that may also be used to measure pain interference. Patients rate on an ordinal scale how much their pain has interfered with general activity, mood, mobility, work, interpersonal relationships, sleep, enjoyment of life, self-care, and recreation (Box 29-2). This information may be helpful in determining baseline tolerance levels for specific functional tasks that may be addressed in treatment.

BOX 29-1

Examples of Pain Intensity Scales

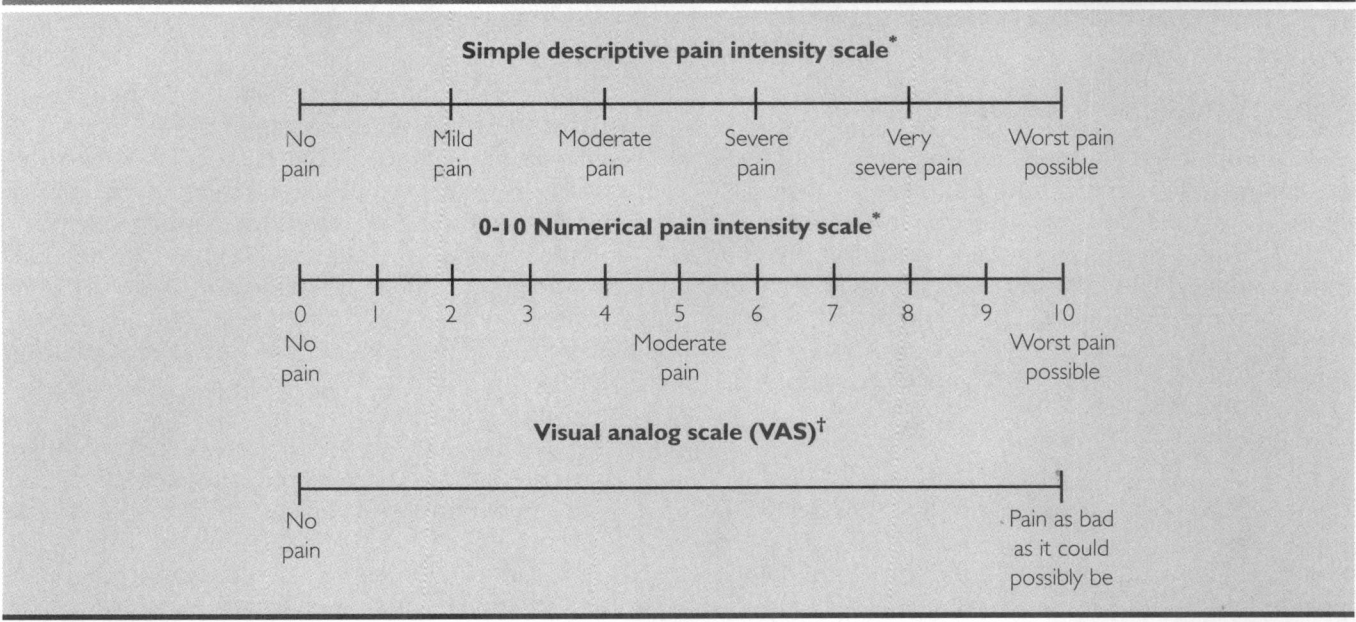

Simple descriptive pain intensity scale*＊

| No pain | Mild pain | Moderate pain | Severe pain | Very severe pain | Worst pain possible |

0-10 Numerical pain intensity scale*＊

0 1 2 3 4 5 6 7 8 9 10

No pain · Moderate pain · Worst pain possible

Visual analog scale (VAS)†

No pain · Pain as bad as it could possibly be

From US Department of Health and Human Services, Acute Pain Management Guideline Panel: *Acute pain management in adults: operative procedures. Quick reference guide for clinicians*, AHCPR Pub No. 92-0019, Rockville, Md, 1995, US Government Printing Office.
*If used as a graphic rating scale, a 10-cm baseline is recommended.
†A 10-cm baseline is recommended for VAS scales.

BOX 29-2

Pain Interference Scales

A. *In the past week,* how much has pain interfered with your daily activities?

0-10 Numerical pain intensity scale

0 1 2 3 4 5 6 7 8 9 10

No interference · Unable to carry out any activities

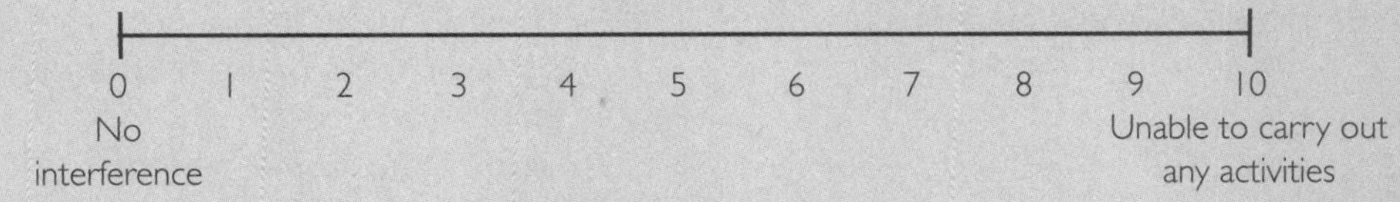

B. *In the past week,* how much has pain interfered with your ability to take part in recreational, social, and family activities?

0-10 Numerical pain intensity scale

0 1 2 3 4 5 6 7 8 9 10

No interference · Unable to carry out any activities

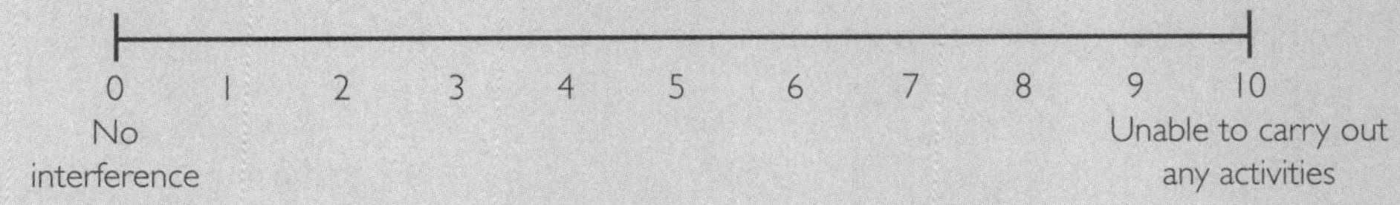

C. *In the past week,* how much has pain interfered with your ability to work (including housework)?

0-10 Numerical pain intensity scale

0 1 2 3 4 5 6 7 8 9 10

No interference · Unable to carry out any activities

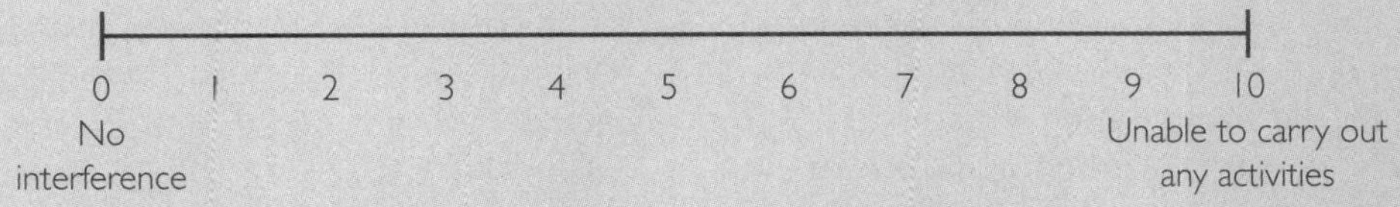

From National Institutes of Health, National Institute of Child Health and Human Development, National Institute of Neurological Disorders and Stroke: Ongoing research, (Grant No. 1 PO1 HD/NS33988).

INTERVENTION

The obligation to manage pain and relieve a patient's suffering is fundamental. Occupational therapy interventions focus on increasing physical capacities, productive and satisfying performance of life tasks and roles, mastery of self and environment through activities, and education.[17] As the causes of pain are multifactorial, so are the approaches to treatment. Typical **pain interventions** may include the following.

Medication

Medications are generally the treatment of choice for individuals experiencing acute pain. Occupational therapists need to observe patients for possible drug reactions. To reduce possible discomfort from rehabilitative procedures, practitioners should check that patients are adequately medicated. Aspirin and acetaminophen are frequently used in the treatment of mild pain (e.g., headache) because of their high level of effectiveness, low level of toxicity, and limited abuse potential. Nonsteroidal antiinflammatory agents have been used in the treatment of arthritis and inflammation of a musculoskeletal origin. Codeine is often used for moderate-intensity pain that has not responded adequately to aspirin or acetaminophen. Morphine is the standard medication used in the relief of severe pain. The use of opioid analgesics (a newer term for narcotics) in chronic nonmalignant pain has been controversial because of concerns about addiction.[16]

Activity Tolerance

Although a few days of rest may be indicated for acute pain, therapeutic activity is important for the treatment of any underlying impairment. Activity levels are increased on a gradual basis, with the patient working to "tolerance" (gradual increase in task demands such as duration, mobility, strength, and endurance), as opposed to "pain," before a scheduled rest period. The patient should not initiate rest at the time of the pain onset or exacerbation because this may reinforce pain behaviors.[12] A gradual increase in activity also lessens the likelihood of an exacerbation of pain. Fordyce[12] provides guidelines for the use of quota programs for patients with chronic pain. Modalities (e.g., heat or cold) may be applied before activity as a means of enhancing functional performance. Patients are also most likely to adhere to functional tasks that they find interesting.[31,35]

Therapeutic Modalities

Physical agent modalities (PAM) may be used by occupational therapists as adjuncts to or preparation for purposeful activities. Appropriate postprofessional education is needed to ensure that the practitioner is competent in the use of these modalities.[28] Both heat and ice are useful in reducing pain and muscle spasm of musculoskeletal and neurological pathologies. Superficial heat includes hot packs, heating pads, paraffin wax, fluidotherapy, hydrotherapy, Hubbard tank, whirlpool, and heat lamps. The application of heat results in an increase in local metabolism and circulation. Vasoconstriction occurs initially, followed by vasodilatation resulting in muscle relaxation. The use of heat is indicated in the treatment of subacute and chronic traumatic and inflammatory conditions such as muscle spasms, arthritis of the small joints of the hands and feet,[11,22] tendonitis, and bursitis.

The use of heat is contraindicated in several instances. Heat is not to be used for patients who have acute inflammatory conditions, cardiac insufficiency, malignancies, or peripheral vascular disease. Preexisting edema may be aggravated. Heat may cause malignancies to spread. Paraffin therapy produces increased skin tissue temperature while decreasing the temperature of subcutaneous tissue.

Cold can improve pain control by elevating the pain threshold (i.e., the minimal level of noxious stimulation at which the patient first reports pain). Local vasoconstriction occurs in direct response to cold therapy (cryotherapy). When the area is subsequently exposed to air, vasodilatation occurs. Cold applications also result in decreased local metabolism, slowing of nerve conduction velocity, diminished muscle spasm secondary to joint or skeletal pathological conditions and spasticity, decreased edema, and lessened tissue damage. Cold can be applied via packs, sprays, or a massage stick.[22]

There are several contraindications in the use of cryotherapy. Patients who are extremely sensitive may not be able to tolerate cold. If a patient has a history of frostbite in the area to be treated, another modality must be used. If a patient has Raynaud's disease, severe pain may occur in the treated area. Cryotherapy is contraindicated in the very young and elderly because their thermoregulatory responses may not function sufficiently.[11]

Transcutaneous Electrical Nerve Stimulation

Transcutaneous electrical nerve stimulation (TENS) is a noninvasive pain relief measure that uses cutaneous stimulation. A TENS unit consists of a battery-powered generator that sends a mild electrical current through electrodes placed on the skin at or near the pain site, stimulating A fibers. Some success has been demonstrated with using TENS to relieve acute and chronic painful conditions caused by disease or injury of nervous system structures or the skeleton, muscle pain of ischemic origin in the extremities, and angina pectoris.[32]

Body Mechanics and Posture Training

Instruction in and rehearsal of proper body mechanics and postures that will not increase the risk of low back injury or strain are essential for patients experiencing both acute and chronic LBP.[24] Practice in using the body safely and to maximum performance during routine tasks in natural (i.e., home, work, or leisure) environment is particularly important.[35] The patient should be taught to avoid tasks or positions that do not allow balanced posture. For detailed guidelines on proper posture and body mechanic principles, please refer to Chapter 46. For patients in wheelchairs, the information on positioning in Chapter 14 is also important.

Energy Conservation, Pacing, and Joint Protection

Instruction in energy conservation, pacing, and joint protection may be beneficial for achieving recommended amounts of rest during task completion, time spent physically active, and balance between rest and physical activity. Patients, especially those with rheumatoid arthritis, are taught to use these strategies before they experience pain and fatigue so that occupational performance can continue as long as possible without pain and fatigue.[13]

Splinting

Splinting of the upper extremity may be necessary if contractures or muscle imbalances occur. In RSD static resting splints may provide pain relief. Splint use is alternated with tasks that require joints to be taken through range of motion, since total immobilization could lead to increased pain and dysfunction. Static resting splints maintain joint alignment, reducing inflammation and pain during flare-ups of rheumatoid arthritis. Splints that support the wrist in a functional position throughout the day and night may be necessary for 4 to 6 weeks.[3] People with compromised proximal joint mobility should use caution because orthoses may add to the stress on proximal joints when the wrist is confined.[4]

Adaptive Equipment

Patients with acute LBP may use a back support for stabilization of the lumbar area and increased abdominal pressure to improve postural alignment. This can result in decreased muscle spasm, reduced pain, and improved ability to engage in occupations.[3,36]

Relaxation

Relaxation training can be used to decrease muscle tension, which is believed to precipitate or exacerbate pain. Progressive muscle relaxation involves the systematic tensing of major musculoskeletal groups for several seconds, passive focusing of attention on how the tensed muscles feel, and release of the muscles and passive focusing on the sensations of relaxation. As the patient learns to recognize muscle tension, he or she can direct attention to inducing relaxation.

Autogenic training is another means to inducing relaxation. This approach involves the silent repetition of self-directed formulas that describe the psychophysiological aspects of relaxation (e.g., "My arms and legs are warm"). The patient passively concentrates on these phrases while assuming a relaxed body posture, with eyes closed, in a quiet setting. Relaxation training has been used successfully to modify a variety of chronic pain complaints, including headache, LBP, myofascial pain, arthritis, and cancer pain.[14]

Biofeedback

Biofeedback is the use of instrumentation to provide visual or auditory signals that indicate some change in a biological process, such as skin temperature, as it occurs. The signals are used to increase the patient's awareness of these changes so that the changes may come under voluntary control. Biofeedback is based on the assumption that a maladaptive psychophysiological response results in chronic pain. Despite the questionable validity of this assumption, data do exist to support the use of biofeedback for the treatment of headache disorders, LBP, arthritis, myofascial pain, and RSD.[14]

SUMMARY

Pain is a complex phenomenon. Occupational therapists bring their understanding of anatomy, physiology, kinesiology, psychology, and function to the comprehensive evaluation and treatment of the patient with pain. Interventions focus on relieving pain, improving functional levels, and developing coping strategies. Data are needed to support the use of the OT interventions described in this chapter.

BOX 29-3 Glossary

Gating Mechanism: A neural mechanism in the spinal cord that acts like a gate to facilitate or inhibit the flow of nerve impulses from peripheral fibers to the central nervous system.

Operant Pain: Pain behaviors that occur as responses to cues in the environment.

Pain: An unpleasant sensory *and* emotional experience associated with actual or *potential* tissue damage.

Pain Behavior: Observable and measurable behaviors used by the patient to communicate the experience of pain to others.

Pain Contingent Rest: Breaks taken when the patient experiences an aversive task.

CASE STUDY 29-1

CASE STUDY—C.A.

C.A., a 34-year-old woman, was injured 5 months ago when catching a heavy weight while employed as an electrician. She sustained a lumbar strain. C.A. was initially treated at an emergency room, where narcotics, muscle relaxants, heat application, and bed rest were prescribed. After persistent pain complaints, she was given pelvic traction and TENS. C.A. has not returned to work since her injury and described her current lifestyle as sedentary. She described her pain as severe (a "9" or "10" on an 10-point numerical scale, with "0" = "no pain" and "10" = "pain as bad as could be") and almost constant. She identified prolonged sitting, standing, and ambulation as exacerbating pain factors. C.A. described occasional mild pain relief with ibuprofen use and bed rest. Her self-report on the Brief Pain Inventory revealed moderate to high pain interference with IADL and recreational, social, and work activities. C.A. described using pain-contingent rest and asking for assistance as the means of coping with her pain.

During evaluation, C.A. was found to have decreased active right shoulder range of motion and strength, decreased left lower extremity strength, and muscle spasms throughout the left lumbar paraspinal muscles and into the left buttocks. She demonstrated poor body mechanics, poor posture, and mild shortness of breath. C.A. offered numerous verbal complaints of pain and expressed fear that the pain would never go away.

Physical retraining and cognitive behavioral techniques were emphasized in intervention. C.A. participated in generalized mobility, strengthening, and cardiovascular endurance exercises as a means of increasing her occupational performance, minimizing fatigue, and increasing feelings of well-being. Functional tasks were incorporated into treatment. C.A. was instructed in how to monitor her daily routine (e.g., balance of rest, relaxation, and activity) and modify faulty thinking (e.g., catastrophizing, such as thinking there is nothing that can stop the pain). Her daily routine included progressive relaxation rehearsal.

C.A. made fair progress in her 4-week treatment program. She demonstrated normal mobility, strength, and endurance. Bed rest during the day was eliminated. C.A. was taught proper posture and body mechanics and was observed to use them in her routine activities. Her verbal complaints of pain remained unchanged, but she stated that she no longer felt the pain was controlling her. C.A. was now ready to progress to a work-hardening program.

REVIEW QUESTIONS

1. Contrast acute pain and chronic pain.
2. Contrast the gate control theory of pain with the learning theory model of Fordyce.
3. List and describe seven different pain syndromes that may be present in persons referred for occupational therapy.
4. Identify the essential elements of a pain assessment.
5. Identify at least eight interventions used in the treatment of pain.
6. Describe the role and define the scope of occupational therapy in the evaluation and treatment of pain.

REFERENCES

1. Bockrath M: Fundamentals. In Carey KW et al, editors: *Pain*, Springhouse, Penn, 1985, Springhouse.
2. Bonica JJ: General considerations of chronic pain. In Bonica JJ, editor: *The management of pain*, ed 2, Philadelphia, 1990, Lea & Febiger.
3. Borrelli EF, Warfield CA: Occupational therapy for pain, *Hosp Pract*, August 15, 1986.
4. Bulthaup S, Cipriani D, Thomas JJ: An electromyography study of wrist extension orthoses and upper-extremity function, *Am J Occup Ther* 53(5):434-440, 1999.
5. Cailliet R: *Headache and face pain syndromes*, Philadelphia, 1992, FA Davis.
6. Cleeland CS: Research in cancer pain: what we know and what we need to know, *Cancer* 67:823, 1991.
7. Ellis RM: Back pain, *BMJ* 310(6989):1220, 1995.
8. Engel JM: *Pediatric pain*, Athens, Ga, 1988, Elliott & Fitzpatrick.
9. Engel JM: Pain management. In Hopkins HL, Smith HD, editors: *Willard and Spackman's occupational therapy*, ed 8, Philadelphia, 1993, JB Lippincott.
10. Follick MJ, Ahern DK, Laser-Wolston N: Evaluation of a daily activity diary for chronic pain patients, *Pain* 19(4):373-382, 1984.
11. Fond D, Hecox B: Superficial heat modalities. In Hecox B, Mehreteab TA, Weisberg J, editors: *Physical agents: a comprehensive text for physical therapists*, Norwalk, Conn, 1994, Appleton & Lange.
12. Fordyce WE: *Behavioral methods for chronic pain and illness*, St Louis, 1976, Mosby.
13. Furst GP et al: A program for improving energy conservation behaviors in adults with rheumatoid arthritis, *Am J Occup Ther* 41(2):102-111, 1987.
14. Gaupp LA, Flinn DE, Weddige RL: Adjunctive treatment techniques. In Tollison CD, Satterthwaite JR, Tollison JW, editors: *Handbook of pain management*, ed 2, Baltimore, 1994, Williams & Wilkins.
15. Goldberg DL: Controversies in fibromyalgia and myofascial pain syndromes. In Arnoff GM, editor: *Evaluation and management of chronic pain*, ed 3, Baltimore, 1998, Williams & Wilkins.
16. Hawthorn J, Redmond K: *Pain: causes and management*, Malden, Mass, 1998, Blackwell Science.
17. International Association for the Study of Pain, ad hoc Subcommittee for Occupational Therapy/Physical Therapy Curriculum: Pain curriculum for students in occupational therapy or physical therapy, *IASP Newsletter* November/December, 1994, The Association.
18. International Association for the Study of Pain, Subcommittee on Taxonomy: Pain terms: a list with definitions and notes on usage, *Pain* 6(3):, 249, 1979.
19. Kasch MC: Hand injuries. In Pedretti LW, editor: *Occupational therapy: practice skills for physical dysfunction*, ed 4, St Louis, 1996, Mosby.

20. Katz ER, Varni JW, Jay SM: Behavioral assessment and management of pediatric pain. In Hersen M, Eisler RM, Miller PM, editors: *Progress in behavior modification*, vol 18, Orlando, Fla, 1984, Academic Press.

21. Keefe FJ, Block AR: Development of an observation method for assessing pain behavior in chronic low back pain patients, *Behav Ther* 13:363, 1982.

22. Lee MHM et al: Physical therapy and rehabilitation medicine, In Bonica JJ, editor: *The management of pain*, ed 2, Philadelphia, 1990, Lea & Febiger.

23. Mauskop A: Head pain. In Ashburn MA, Rice LJ, editors: *The management of pain*, New York, 1998, Churchill Livingstone.

24. McCauley M: The effects of body mechanics instruction on work performance among young workers, *Am J Occup Ther* 44(5):402-407, 1990.

25. Melzack R: *The puzzle of pain*, New York, 1973, BasicBooks.

26. Melzack R, Wall PD: Pain mechanisms: a new theory, *Science* 150(699):971-979, 1965.

27. Merskey H: Limitations of pain behavior, *APS* 1:101-104, 1992.

28. Pedretti LW, Wade IE: Therapeutic modalities, In Pedretti LW, editor: *Occupational therapy: practice skills for physical dysfunction*, ed 4, St Louis, 1996, Mosby.

29. Richards JS et al: Assessing pain behavior: the UAB Pain Behavior Scale, *Pain* 14:393, 1982.

30. Rowlingson JC, Keifer RB: Low back pain. In Ashburn MA, Rice LJ, editors: *The management of pain*, New York, 1998, Churchill Livingstone.

31. Sakamoto BJ, Warner K: The role of occupational therapy in the treatment of chronic pain. In Crue BL, editor: *Chronic pain*, New York, 1979, SP Medical & Scientific Books.

32. Sjolund BH, Eriksson M, Loeser JD: Transcutaneous and implanted electrical stimulation of peripheral nerves. In Bonica JJ, editor: *The management of pain*, ed 2, Philadelphia, 1990, Lea & Febiger.

33. Smithline J: Low back pain. In Pedretti LW, editor: *Occupational therapy: practice skills for physical dysfunction*, ed 4, St Louis, 1996, Mosby.

34. Spencer EA: Orthopedic and musculoskeletal dysfunction in adults. In Neistadt ME, Crepeau EB, editors: *Willard & Spackman's occupational therapy*, ed 9, Philadelphia, 1998, Lippincott.

35. Strong J: *Chronic pain: the occupational therapist's perspective*, New York, 1996, Churchill Livingstone.

36. Tyson R, Strong J: Adaptive equipment: its effectiveness for people with chronic lower back pain, *Occup Ther J Res* 10:111, 1990.

37. U.S. Department of Health and Human Services: *Management of cancer pain*, Rockville, Md, 1994, AHCPR.

PART FIVE

OCCUPATIONAL THERAPY INTERVENTIONS

CHAPTER 30

Therapeutic Occupations and Modalities

ESTELLE B. BREINES

KEY TERMS

Active occupation
Egocentric realm
Exocentric realm
Consensual realm
Occupational genesis
Physical agent modalities
Purposeful occupation and activity
Grading activity
Resistive exercise
Simulated or enabling activity
Adjunctive modalities
Isotonic exercise
Isometric exercise
Active exercise
Passive exercise

LEARNING OBJECTIVES

After studying this chapter the student or practitioner will be able to do the following:

1. Recognize the organizing concepts of occupational genesis as they relate to active occupation.
2. Discuss the role of activity analysis in the selection of therapeutic activity.
3. Understand the similarities and distinctions between therapeutic activity and therapeutic exercise.
4. Identify the role of physical agent modalities in occupational therapy (OT) practice.
5. Describe how grading activity heightens functional performance.
6. Differentiate between the various types of therapeutic exercise.
7. Describe how and why simulated and enabling activities are used in practice.
8. Describe how and why adjunctive modalities are used in OT practice.
9. Identify the requirements established by the American Occupational Therapy Association for the use of adjunctive modalities in OT practice.
10. Perform an activity analysis appropriate for physical dysfunction.

ACTIVE OCCUPATION

Active occupations are the foundation of occupational therapy (OT) practice. Active occupations are those activities in which people engage as part of their life's roles. These include personal care, the constructional tasks that involve the use of hand and mechanical tools, technological activities involving such tools as calculators, computers, and electronics, games of various sorts, and vocational skills. They function together in a complex process, stimulating growth and health throughout the life span.

When physical disability strikes and the ability to perform occupational roles and activities becomes impaired, the occupational therapist helps patients regain their skills using active occupations as therapeutic tools to stimulate performance.

Active occupation is the primary therapeutic modality of OT, designed both to stimulate function and to lead to improved function.

Engagement in activity enhances performance beyond the given task. Learning to perform one activity skillfully leads to skillful performance in other activities. Therefore active occupations are both the objectives and the tools of practice. Activities are the means and the end to heightened performance. Whether related to personal care, work, or leisure, active occupations constitute an effective and substantial portion of any OT program.

The needs and interests of patients guide the selection of occupations used for therapy. These needs are governed by the roles patients play in their worlds. As members of society, patients represent the societies in which they perform activities, and the activities in which they engage reflect their worlds. Patients' needs and interests are tied to the societies in which they live.

Patients must assume their personal and social obligations to become effective members of society. To assume these responsibilities, patients must acquire the skills needed to perform their occupational roles. The roles people assume reflect their participation. For persons with disabilities, participation may require relearning skills or learning to perform in new ways. Therefore the occupational therapist must be prepared with a broad knowledge of activities and techniques that may then be used as tools of therapy in a patient-centered approach. Occupational therapists must understand the roles and activities in which people engage to perform their life's tasks. As a consequence, occupational therapists must be prepared to meet the challenges that ordinarily occur as people and societies evolve and change.

Just as society changes and adapts with the invention of new objects and methods, so do the activities patients use in their lives. Nowhere is this more readily observed than by examining the OT treatment environment. Just as the nature of activity has changed over time as societies have evolved and adapted, the scope of OT's treatment methods and modalities has changed and broadened considerably over the years.

When the field of OT became formalized in the early 1900s, the nature of human occupation was limited to the scope of activities that had been developed up to that time. Consequently, the use of handicrafts and early industrial tasks guided activity at the outset of the profession. Although commonly described as crafts, these activities can be viewed from an anthropological perspective, representing the times in which they were developed and in which they met people's personal and social needs. But times changed, and along with these changes society developed new and different occupations, requiring occupational therapists to expand their skills to incorporate activities and techniques of the modern era.

Today's occupational therapists are qualified and competent in the use of a wide variety of therapeutic occupations and modalities, both traditional and modern.[1] Their competence is derived from entry-level through graduate education, specialty certification, continuing education, and work experience. The scope of practice is broad and addresses the continuum of treatment from acute care through advanced rehabilitation. Therefore OT offers comprehensive services and challenges the OT practitioner to keep pace with new developments in society and in practice.

PHILOSOPHICAL FOUNDATIONS

Occupational therapists organize treatment by integrating a comprehensive knowledge of the patient's mind and body (the **egocentric realm**) with knowledge of the tangible world (the **exocentric realm**) and the social influences (the **consensual realm**) that contribute to function. The relationships among these three interactive forces are in constant flux in a lifelong developmental process that is stimulated by active occupation.

These ideas stem from the work of John Dewey[18] and the other American philosophers of pragmatism whose work influenced the mental hygiene movement, which in turn influenced the founders of the profession.[12] Dewey's use of the terms *purposive activity* and *active occupation*, along with his renowned concept of learning through doing, are found in his text *Democracy and Education*,[18] published in 1916 in Chicago, a year before the establishment of the National Society for the Promotion of Occupational Therapy.

Egocentric Realm

Intensive training in the motor, neurological, and perceptual-cognitive components of performance prepares the occupational therapist with a refined knowledge of what contributes to a patient's performance in all aspects of the mind and body. Mind and body are seen as interactive and together govern performance.

Exocentric Realm

Occupational therapists have an equally refined understanding of the material world in which people live, act, and react. Textures, weights, direction, location, time, and other objective means regulate performance in the world. A person functions within a real world filled with objects and environments that must be manipulated in one manner or another. Occupational therapists are expert in adapting the tangible and durable elements of the world to enhance function.

Consensual Realm

Occupational therapists also bring their knowledge of the effect of society on individual and group performance. This knowledge is used to enhance patients' function by effectuating the roles they play in their social worlds. Recognizing and valuing the sociocultural aspects of occupation and their implications for patient performance contribute to the occupational therapist's knowledge base.

Relationships Among Realms

The three major aspects of OT's knowledge base, the egocentric (mind and body), exocentric (time and space), and consensual (society) realms, are thoroughly integrated in active performance, regardless of interest, purpose, environment, or era.[11,12] Occupational therapists use one or more of these realms to influence or heighten performance in impaired aspects (Fig. 30-1). For example, a splint (exocentric) can be used to stabilize a wrist to reduce pain (egocentric), enabling the patient to prepare a meal for the family (consensual). A walker can be adapted so a patient can carry her knitting (exocentric), allowing her to prepare gifts for her grandchild (consensual) and heighten her feelings of efficacy (egocentric).

Development and Evolution

The interaction among these three realms represents a developmental continuum. They influence one another throughout the life span in a process defined as **occupational genesis**.[10] Interactions among physical and mental capacities, the tangible world, and the roles people play in their worlds are reflected and governed by the activities in which people engage throughout their lives.

Intensive preparation in these three realms and their interaction constitute the education and preparation of the OT practitioner and guide the therapist in treatment. With this comprehensive foundation, occupational therapists use various modalities to integrate these three realms, thus enhancing patient performance and enabling patients to meet life needs.

EVOLVING PRACTICE

Just as society and its occupations have evolved and continue to evolve, occupational therapy practice has evolved. New media and modalities have emerged to enable patients to become skilled in functional performance. In addition to therapeutic exercise and activity and the facilitation and inhibition techniques associated with the sensorimotor approaches to treatment, therapists have added adjunctive therapies to their repertoires, all designed to enhance patients' performance in purposeful occupation.

Although use of adjunctive therapies such as **physical agent modalities** is not considered to be an entry level skill,[3-4] some therapists have become increasingly skilled in the application of these therapies. These modalities traditionally belonged to the field of physical therapy but have since entered the realm of OT practice. They are used by trained occupational therapists to enhance the development of the individual's ability to perform purposeful occupation, the primary objective of OT. Their use by occupational therapists should be limited to the role of an adjunct to purposeful active occupation.

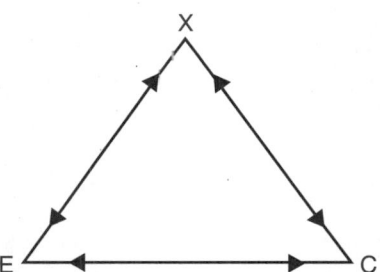

FIG. 30-1
The egocentric (E), exocentric (X), and consensual (C) realms of occupational therapy's knowledge base are related. (From Breines EB: *Occupational therapy from clay to computers: theory & practice,* Philadelphia, 1995, FA Davis.)

BOX 30-1
Occupational Therapy Modalities

Modality: The employment of, or method of employment of, a therapeutic agent (Webster's New World College Dictionary, edition 2).[1] Traditionally, the modalities of occupational therapy were its crafts. The term has grown to be understood more broadly and defines active occupation as the primary therapeutic modality of occupational therapy. The term "modality" also includes both media and methods.[42] Media are the means by which therapeutic effects are transmitted. For example, media can include a variety of objects such as an article of clothing, a vestibular ball, or an adapted tool. Methods are the steps, sequence, or approaches used to activate the therapeutic effect of a medium, such as the movements required in the creation of a macramé plant hanger to heighten shoulder flexion or reduce edema, or the movements used with the vestibular ball to effect the desired motor responses. The modalities, media, and methods of occupational therapy are variable in their application and require considerable expertise to select, modify, adapt, and apply to elicit therapeutic effects.

PURPOSEFUL OCCUPATION AND ACTIVITY

One of the first principles of OT, stated by Dunton in 1918, is that there must be some useful end to occupation for it to be effective in the treatment of mental and physical disability.[48] This principle implies that occupation has a purpose and that purposeful activity has an autonomous or inherent goal beyond the motor function required to perform the task.[8] An individual engaged in purposeful activity focuses attention on the goal rather than the processes required to reach the goal.[2,5]

Conversely, nonpurposeful activity has been defined as activity that has no inherent goal other than the motor function used to perform the activity.[48] The person performing a nonpurposeful activity is likely to be focused on the activity process or movements rather than a functional or meaningful goal. Therapeutic exercise and enabling activities such as moving cones and stacking blocks cannot be considered purposeful activity when they have no purpose for the patient. This statement does not imply that such media have no place in the treatment continuum. Yet treatment must consider the inherent occupational objectives of the patient as both tools of treatment and skills to be acquired, for these are more readily tied to purpose, meaning, and therapeutic value and constitute the occupational nature of therapy.

Purposeful activity is the cornerstone of OT, and is its primary treatment modality.[48,50] In a position paper on purposeful activity, the American Occupational Therapy Association (AOTA) defined the term as "goal-directed behaviors or tasks that comprise occupations. An activity is purposeful if the individual is an active, voluntary participant and if the activity is directed toward a goal that the individual considers meaningful."[5] The uniqueness of OT lies in its emphasis on the extensive use of purposeful or meaningful activity. This emphasis gives OT the theoretical foundation for its broad application to psychosocial, physical, and developmental dysfunction, as well as to health maintenance.[2]

Purposeful activity has both inherent and therapeutic goals. For example, sawing wood (Fig. 30-2) may have the inherent goal of securing parts for construction of a bookshelf, whereas the therapeutic objectives may be to strengthen shoulder and elbow musculature. The conscious effort of the patient is focused on the ultimate outcome of the project and not on the movement itself.[8] The patient directs and is in control of the movement, yet that control is ordinarily outside of conscious awareness as the patient focuses on the goal aspects of performance. In fact, performance outside of conscious awareness distinguishes OT's therapeutic effectiveness. Performance that is deliberate is not effective in producing enhanced levels of skill. To enhance skill building, performance must become automatic.[12] Automatic performance serves as a subskill for more advanced performance. For example, Huss[23] suggested that the child who must attend to sitting is unable to focus on the task performance that automatic sitting would ordinarily enable. Consequently, the child cannot engage in active occupations essential to growth and the development of social roles.

The importance of purposeful activity is readily observed in goal-directed performance. As the patient becomes absorbed in the performance of any given activity, affected parts are used more naturally and with less fatigue.[47] Concentration on motion has a detrimental effect on that motion, and muscles controlled by conscious attention and focused effort fatigue rapidly. The value of goal-oriented effort in purposeful tasks is clear. It is of greater therapeutic value to focus attention on an activity of interest to the patient and its inherent goal than on the muscles or motions being used to accomplish the activity.[8]

A number of studies have shown the efficacy of purposeful activity.[38] Steinbeck[48] demonstrated that patients performing purposeful activity perform for a longer period than when they are performing nonpurposeful activity. A study of motivation for product-oriented versus non-product-oriented activity by Thibodeaux and Ludwig[50] indicated the need to determine the patient's level of interest in the process and the product and to incorporate his or her image of the activity in treatment planning. Rocker and Nelson[44] found that not being allowed to keep an activity product can elicit hostile feelings in normal subjects, demonstrating the importance of tangible productivity for sustaining people's interest. Yoder, Nelson, and Smith[54] studied the effects of added-purpose versus rote exercise in female nursing home residents. The added-purpose exercise resulted in significantly more movement repetitions than did rote exercise.[54] These studies suggest that goal-directed, purposeful activity increases motivation for participation in sustained activity and can therefore be assumed to heighten the willingness of patients to engage in therapeutic activity.

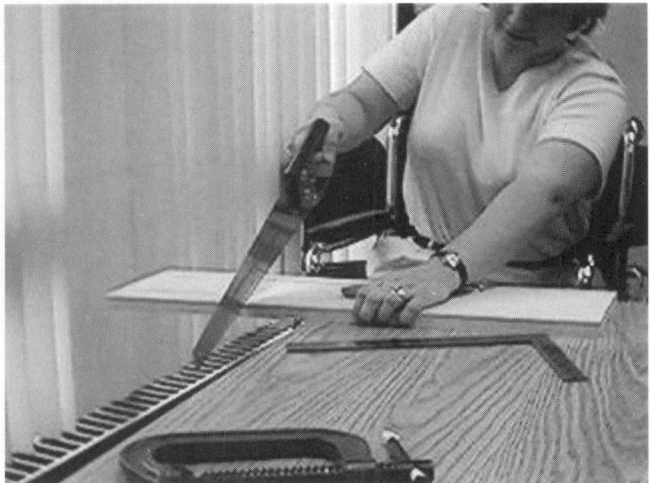

FIG. 30-2
Sawing wood to strengthen shoulder and elbow musculature.

When a treatment plan is being developed, the inherent goals of the activity, the patient's level of interest in the activity, and the meaning of the activity and its product are important considerations in the ultimate effectiveness of the media and methods selected for treatment. Purposeful activities are used, or adapted for use, to meet one or more of the following therapeutic objectives: to develop or maintain strength, endurance, work tolerance, range of motion (ROM), and coordination; to practice and use voluntary, automatic movement in goal-directed tasks; to provide for purposeful use of and general exercise to affected parts; to explore vocational potential or train in work skills; to improve sensation, perception, and cognition; to improve socialization skills and enhance emotional growth and development; and to increase independence in occupational role performance. It is recognized that some of these objectives alone might not be considered purposeful unless they relate to function. Arts, crafts, games, sports, leisure, self-care, home management, purposive mobility, and work-related activities are considered purposeful activities.

OCCUPATION AND HEALTH

OT was founded on the concept that human beings have an occupational nature. That is, it is natural for humans to be engaged in activity, and the process of being occupied contributes to the health and well-being of the organism.[8,11,16,24] Activity is valuable for the maintenance of health in the healthy person and for the restoration of health after illness and disability. When the patient engages in relevant, meaningful, and purposeful activity, change is possible and dysfunction is reversible.[16] The occupational therapist acts as facilitator of the change process.[15] Therefore physical dysfunction can be ameliorated when the patient participates in goal-directed (purposeful) and thus therapeutic activity.[8]

The value of purposeful activity lies in the patient's simultaneous mental and physical involvement. Activity provides the exercise needed to help develop the use of affected parts and also provides an opportunity to meet emotional, social, and personal gratification needs.[8,47] Cynkin and Robinson[16] pointed out that, for the attainment of optimal function and health, the human being must be consciously involved in problem-solving and creative activity, processes that are linked with the use of the hands.[16]

Virtually all occupational performance involves the hands or requires the substitution of methods that simulate the use of hands. One example of an activity ordinarily performed by the hands is the use of a computer-driven environmental control unit operated by a puff-and-sip mechanism.

The activities that form the pattern of a person's life, that are performed routinely and automatically, are taken for granted until some dysfunction disrupts their performance. It is the role of the occupational therapist to adapt activity so that patients can resume their ability to perform life's tasks. OT is founded on the notion that dysfunction can be modified, altered, or reversed toward function through engagement in activities of real life. Cynkin and Robinson[16] make several assumptions about activities that are summarized as follows:

1. A wide variety of activities are important to the individual. Activities fulfill many of a person's needs and wants, and they are essential to physical and psychosocial growth and development and the attainment of mastery and competence.
2. Activities are socioculturally regulated by the values and beliefs of the culture that defines acceptable behavior for groups of people in the culture. Whether a society is rigid or flexible in its interpretation of acceptable behaviors for various groups, at some point deviations in behavior or activity patterns are deemed unacceptable.
3. Activity-related behavior can change from dysfunctional toward more functional. Persons can change and desire change.
4. Changes in activity-related behavior take place through motor, cognitive, and social learning.[16]

Assessment of Occupational Role Performance

The therapist should establish the patient's occupational goals and needs, as described in Chapter 12. A top-down, client-centered approach is recommended. Identifying appropriate and meaningful therapeutic activities should begin with obtaining and analyzing the patient's occupational history and interests.[50]

The Canadian Occupational Performance Measure[29] and the Activity Configuration[15] are two examples of occupational performance assessments. See Chapter 12 for more information about assessing occupational performance.

ACTIVITY ANALYSIS

Careful activity analysis is essential to the selection of appropriate treatment activities. It should yield information about various activities as intervention strategies for physical dysfunction and health maintenance. Activities should be analyzed from three perspectives: the contributions of the person or actor, the effects of the physical environment, and the implications of the social environment. The therapist should recognize that these three elements are inextricable and form the context for treatment. The importance of context in treatment is widely recognized throughout the profession.[6]

Comprehensive guides to activity analysis have been developed by a number of theorists[11,30,51] and can serve as useful resources. A guide to activity analysis specifically relevant to practice in physical dysfunction follows on page 526.

Principles of Activity Analysis

Activities selected for therapeutic purposes should be goal directed; have some meaning to the patient to meet individual needs in relation to social roles; require the mental or physical participation of the patient; be designed to prevent or reverse dysfunction; develop skills to enhance performance in life roles; relate to the patient's interests; be adaptable, gradable, and age appropriate; and be selected through knowledge and professional judgment of the occupational therapist in concert with the patient.[21] A comprehensive activity analysis includes all aspects of performance that are potentially elicited by specific activities and serves to reveal their potential for therapeutic application.

THERAPEUTIC APPROACHES

A variety of therapeutic approaches are available to occupational therapists. Although these approaches differ in their emphasis, all are consistent with an occupational approach to treatment. Aspects of activity analysis relevant to various therapeutic approaches are listed below.

Biomechanical Approach

The biomechanical approach to treatment is likely to be used in the treatment of lower motor neuron and orthopedic dysfunctions. Improvements in strength, ROM, and muscle endurance are the goals of OT for such dysfunctions. Thus the emphasis of activity analysis is on muscles, joints, and motor patterns required to perform the activity. Steps of the activity must be identified and broken down into the motions required to perform each step. ROM, degree of muscle strength, and type of muscle contraction to perform each step should be identified. The activity analysis format at the end of this chapter is based on the biomechanical approach.

Sensorimotor Approach

Sensorimotor approaches to treatment are likely to be used for upper motor neuron disorders such as cerebral palsy, stroke, and head injury. Activity analysis for these dysfunctions should focus on the sensory perception of the patient and the movement patterns required in the particular treatment approach. The therapist must also consider the effect of the activity on balance, posture, muscle tone, and the facilitation or inhibition of abnormal reflexes and movements. For example, if the therapist is using the proprioceptive neuromuscular facilitation

(PNF) approach, it is important to incorporate PNF patterns in the activity or to select activities that use these patterns naturally. For the neurodevelopmental (Bobath) approach, postures and movements that inhibit abnormal reflexes, reactions, and tone are important. These and other sensorimotor approaches and their applications to activity are discussed in Chapters 32 through 36.

Analysis of the perceptual and cognitive requirements of the activity is particularly important for patients with upper motor neuron disorders because these functions are often disturbed. It is important for the therapist to select activities that not only meet the requirements for motor performance but also can be performed with some success.

Regardless of diagnosis or therapeutic approach, activity analysis should include the contextual aspects of performance. The tangible environment and the social environment dictate occupational performance to the same extent that physical and mental capacities do, and they must be considered in developing a treatment plan.

ADAPTING AND GRADING ACTIVITY
Adaptation of Activity

It may be necessary to adapt activities to suit the special needs of the patient or the environment. An activity may need to be performed in a special way to accommodate the patient's residual abilities—for example, eating using a special splint with a utensil holder fitted to the hand (Fig. 30-3). An activity may need to be adapted to the positioning of the patient or to the environment—for instance, by setting up a special reading stand and providing prism glasses to enable a patient to read while supine in bed. The

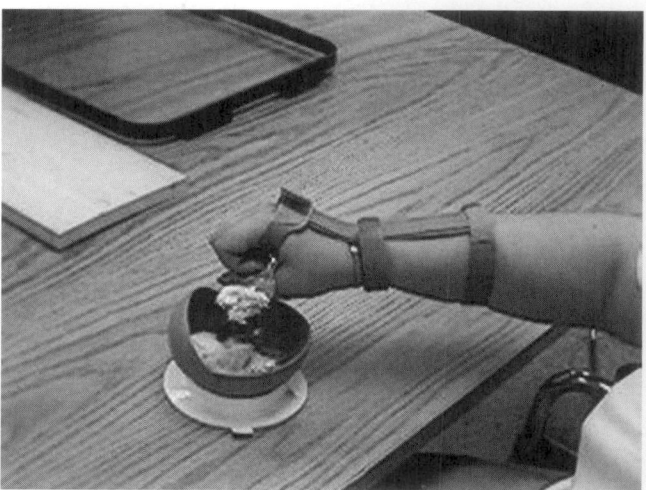

FIG. 30-3
Eating using a special splint with a utensil holder fitted to the hand.

problem-solving ability, creativity, and ingenuity of occupational therapists in making adaptations are some of their unique skills.

The therapist should remember that for adaptations to be effective, the patient must be able to use them in a comfortable position. The patient must understand the need and purpose of the activity and the adaptations and be willing to perform the activity with the simple modifications. Peculiar and complicated adaptations that require frequent adjustment and modification should be avoided.[41,47]

Grading of Activity

Grading an activity means pacing it appropriately and modifying it for the patient's maximal performance. If movement patterns or degree of resistance cannot be attained when the activity is performed in the usual manner, simple modifications may be made. The patient usually accepts changes if they are not complex and do not require strained and unnatural motions. The novice is cautioned that the value of the activity may be diminished if it is designed to be performed with artificial movements or excessive resistance. Such methods discourage participation and interfere with the development of coordination.[26,47] They also require that the patient focus on movements rather than on the goal of the activity, which reduces satisfaction and defeats the primary purpose of purposeful activity as described earlier. The skilled occupational therapist adapts and grades activities so that they are easily accepted by the patient and provide the "just right" demand upon performance.

Activities may be graded in many ways to suit the patient's needs and the treatment objectives. Activities can be graded for increasing strength, ROM, endurance and tolerance, coordination, and perceptual, cognitive, and social skills.

Strength

Strength may be graded by increasing resistance. Methods include changing the plane of movement from gravity eliminated to against-gravity, by adding weights to the equipment or to the patient, using tools of increasing weights, grading the texture of the materials from soft to hard or fine to rough, or changing to another more or less resistive activity.

For example, a weight attached to the wrist by a strap increases resistance to arm movements during needle or leatherwork (Figure 30-4). A pulley-and-weight system can be attached to an inclined plane sanding board to increase resistance to the biceps when the sanding block is pulled downward, as the patient sands a cutting board for use in one-handed cutting. Springs may be used to increase resistance on a block printing press. When grasp strength is inadequate, grasp mitts may be used to

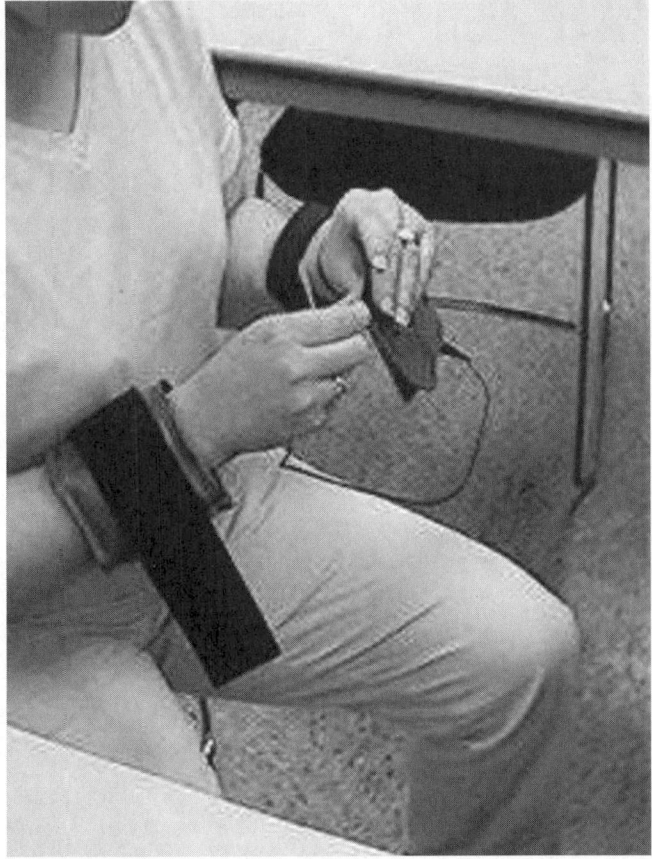

FIG. 30-4
Weight attached to the wrist increases resistance during needlework or leatherwork.

fasten the hand to a tool or equipment handle to assist grip strength and allow arm motion.

Range of Motion

Activities for increasing or maintaining joint ROM may be graded by positioning materials and equipment to demand greater reach or excursion of joints or by adapting equipment with lengthened handles to facilitate active stretching.

An example of a simple adaptation is positioning a weaving project in a vertical position to achieve the desired range of shoulder flexion while working. As the work progresses, the activity itself establishes increased demands on active range. Positioning objects, such as tiles used in a mosaic tile project, at increasing or decreasing distances from the patient changes the range needed to reach the materials (Fig. 30-5). Tool handles such as those used in woodworking may be increased in size by using a larger dowel or by padding the handle with foam rubber to accommodate limited ROM or to facilitate grasp (Fig. 30-6). Reducing the amount of padding as range increases can effect grading.

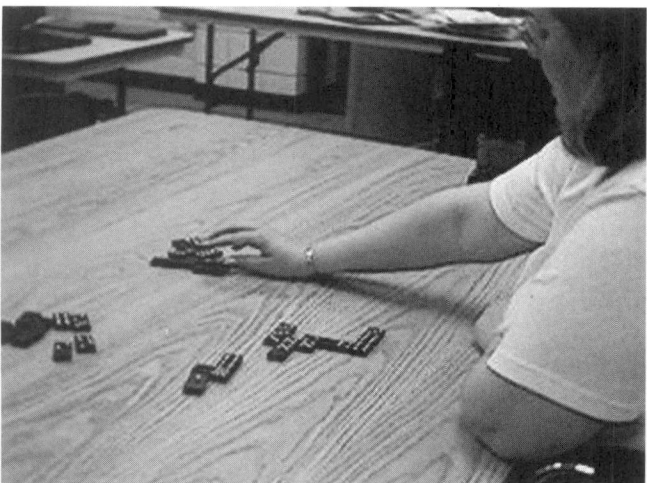

Fig. 30-5
Placing objects at alternate distances changes the range needed to reach materials.

Endurance and Tolerance

Endurance may be graded by moving from light to heavy work and increasing the duration of the work period. For example, an initial household task of folding paper napkins can be graded to sorting heavier and heavier objects, such as the task of sitting to sort kitchen utensils, and then grading to a standing position to organize tools on a pegboard. Standing and walking tolerance may be graded by increasing the time spent standing to work, perhaps at first at a stand-up table (Fig. 30-7), and increasing the time and distance spent in activities requiring walking, perhaps including home management and workshop activities.

Conditions that are progressively degenerative, such as muscular dystrophy, multiple sclerosis, or Parkinson's disease, may require grading endurance in a negative direction to accommodate a diminishing physical condition. In such cases it is advisable to change the activity to one that requires less effort rather than reducing the demand of an existing project. The latter can have a negative psychological effect if the patient readily recognizes the reduction in performance capacity.

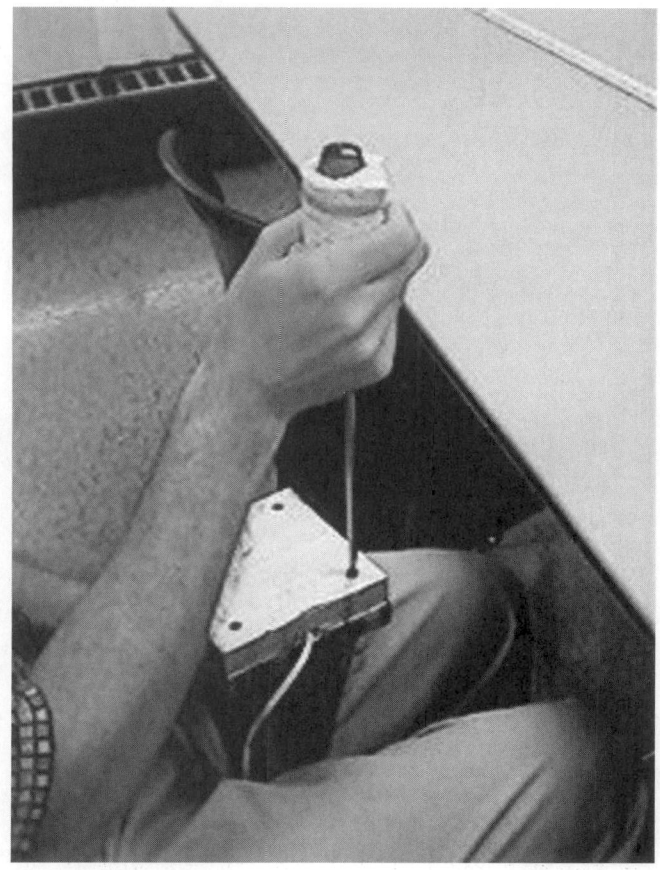

FIG. 30-6
The size of tool handles may be increased by padding the handle with foam rubber.

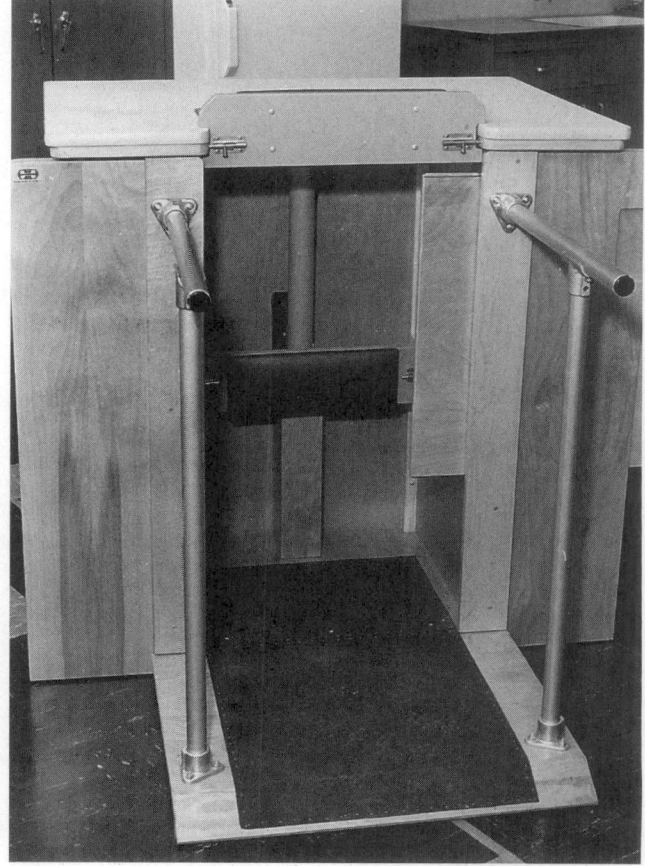

FIG. 30-7
Stand-up table with sliding door, padded knee supports, and backrest.

Coordination

Coordination and muscle control may be graded by decreasing the gross resistive movements and increasing the fine controlled movements required. An example is progressing from sawing wood with a crosscut saw to using a coping saw to using a jeweler's saw. Dexterity and speed of movement may be graded by practice at increasing speeds once movement patterns have been mastered through coordination training and neuromuscular education.

Perceptual, Cognitive, and Social Skills

In grading cognitive skills, the therapist can begin the treatment program with simple one- or two-step activities that require little judgment, decision making, or problem solving, and progress to activities with several steps that require some judgment or problem-solving processes. A patient in a lunch preparation group may butter bread that has already been lined up on the work surface. This task could be graded to lining up the bread, then buttering it and placing a slice of lunch meat on it, and, ultimately, to making sandwiches.

For grading social interaction, the same treatment may begin with an activity that demands interaction only with the therapist. The patient can progress to activities requiring dyadic interaction with another patient and, ultimately, to small group activities. The therapist can facilitate the patient's progression from the role of observer to that of participant and then to leader. Concomitantly, the therapist decreases his or her supervision, guidance, and assistance to facilitate more independent functioning in the patient.

SELECTION OF ACTIVITY

In the treatment of physical dysfunction, activities are usually selected for their potential to improve both sensorimotor and psychosocial components in order to ensure that patients' motivation to engage in activity is sustained. Activities selected for the improvement of physical performance should provide desired exercise or purposeful use of affected parts. They should enable the patient to transfer the motion, strength, and coordination gained in adjunctive and enabling modalities to useful, normal daily activities. If activities are to be used for physical restoration, they should have certain characteristics, as follows:

1. Activities should provide action rather than merely the position of involved joints and muscles; that is, they should allow alternate contraction and relaxation of the muscles being exercised and allow patients to course through their available ROM.
2. Activities should provide repetition of motion. That is, activities should allow for a considerable number of repetitions of movement patterns sufficient to be of benefit to the patient

3. Activities should allow for one or more kind of grading, such as for resistance, range, coordination, endurance, or complexity.[21,47]

The type of exercise that is needed must be considered when choosing an activity. Active and **resistive exercises** are most often used in the performance of purposeful activity.[47] Requirements for passive and active assisted exercise are harder (although not impossible) to apply to purposeful activities, for example, bilateral sanding or bilateral sponge wiping. Other important considerations in the selection of activity are the objects and environment required to perform the activity; safety factors; preparation and completion time; complexity, type of instruction, and supervision required; structure and controls in the activity; learning requirements; independence, decision making, and problem solving required; social interaction potential and communication skills required; and potential gratification to the person.

If an activity is selected in which the patient has an interest, the patient is more likely to experience sufficient satisfaction to sustain performance. The therapist's job is to guide the patient to suitable therapeutic activities at just the right level of challenge so that the patient will achieve satisfaction by engaging in the activity. This satisfaction is an important characteristic of intrinsic motivation. Thus purposeful activities both meet the requirements for motor performance and can be performed with success.

SIMULATED OR ENABLING ACTIVITY

The clinical environment may not be fully equipped to meet the exact occupational needs of all patients. When this is the case, it may be necessary to simulate appropriate active occupation by adapting the environment or activity to meet the patient's needs and retain his or her interest.

Occupational therapists have developed a variety of methods to simulate active occupation. A number of these activities were devised initially from equipment and found materials used in other activities. For example, a common item found in every OT clinic in its earliest days was empty cones that had held the thread that was used to warp looms. Because of their availability, these cones were adapted for many uses in the clinic. Some activities that were devised are moving a series of cones from one side of a tabletop to the other, or stacking them, to increase ROM in the shoulder along with grasp. Cones can also be used to train gross coordination and a combined (out of synergy) movement pattern in the Brunnstrom approach, discussed in Chapter 34.

Another devised activity is the simulated inclined sanding board (Fig. 30-8). The sanding board was designed to incline wood while the wood was being

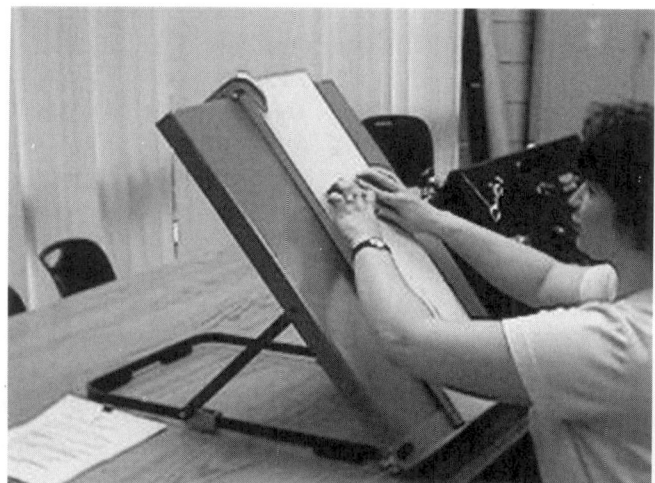

FIG. 30-8
Inclined sanding board used to sand wood.

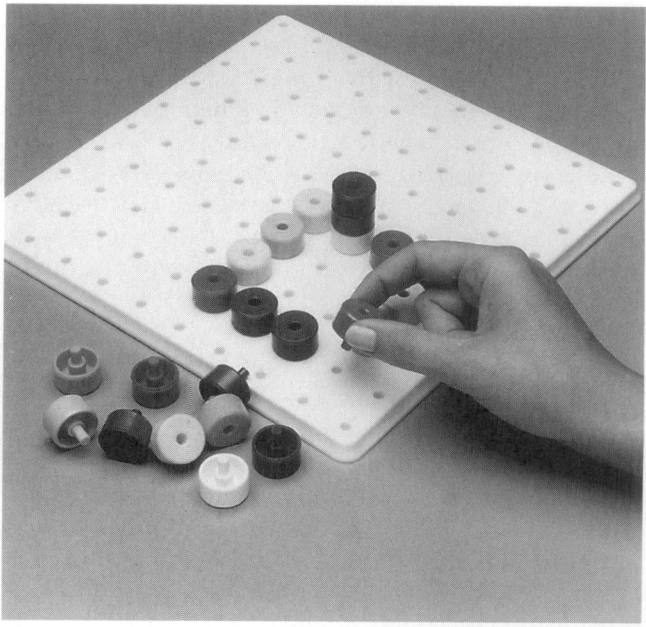

Fig. 30-9
Puzzles and other perceptual and cognitive training media are used on the tabletop. (Courtesy of North Coast Medical, Morgan Hill, Calif.)

sanded. Therapists began using the board, without the wood, to exercise muscles of the elbow and shoulder. Without the wood there is no end product and thus no inherent purposefulness. However, incorporating wood for a project can turn this activity from a simulated to a meaningful one.

Puzzles and other perceptual and cognitive training media are used to train patients in visual perceptual functions, motor planning skills, memory, sequencing, and problem solving, among other skills (Fig. 30-9). Clothing fastener boards and household hardware boards may provide practice in the manipulation of everyday objects before the patient is confronted with the real task (Fig. 30-10). At a higher level of technological sophistication, commercial work simulators (see Chapter 16) and computer programs are used to train patients in physical and cognitive skills.

Although many of these items are readily available in clinics, the nature and purpose of occupational therapy are best met when the patient can be engaged in an activity in which he or she finds purpose and meaning. The therapist should take into consideration the needs and interests of the patient in selecting activities, rather than relying on available objects that meet only physical needs.

Enabling activities are considered nonpurposeful and generally do not have an inherent goal, but they may engage the mental and physical participation of the patient. The purposes of engaging in enabling activities are to practice specific motor patterns, to train in perceptual and cognitive skills, and to practice sensorimotor skills necessary for function in the home and community. Indeed, many enabling modalities used in OT practice facilitate perceptual, cognitive, and motor learning. Such activities may be appropriate for the skill acquisition stage of learning, when the patient

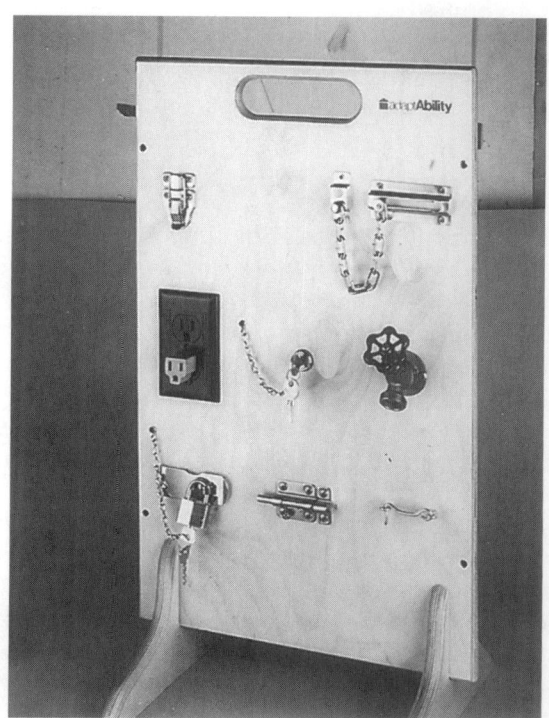

FIG. 30-10
Boards built with household fasteners are simulations used for practicing manipulation and management of common household hardware. (Reprinted with permission, S & S Worldwide, adaptAbility, 1995.)

is getting the idea of the movement and practicing problem solving. Practice should be daily or frequent and feedback given often so that errors are decreased and skills refined to prepare for performance of real-life purposeful activity. These activities should be used judiciously, and their place in the sequence of treatment and motor learning should be well planned. They may be used along with **adjunctive modalities** and purposeful activities as part of a comprehensive treatment program.

ADJUNCTIVE MODALITIES

Adjunctive modalities may be used as a preliminary to purposeful activity. When used by the occupational therapist they are meant to prepare the patient for occupational performance. Examples of adjunctive modalities are exercise, orthotics, sensory stimulation, and physical agent modalities.[39] Therapeutic exercise and physical agent modalities are described below. Many of the principles of therapeutic exercise are readily and customarily incorporated into therapeutic activity and consequently are inherent aspects of OT practice.

THERAPEUTIC EXERCISE AND ACTIVITY

From the earliest history of OT it was recognized that the mind and body are inextricably united in performance. Both the psychological and physical effects of purposeful activity were recognized in the treatment of individuals with mental conditions, as well as in the treatment of persons with physical dysfunction.[9,12,19,24] Because it was recognized that physical benefits accrued from the performance of activity, kinesiological considerations were applied in the selection of appropriate therapeutic activities. To apply kinesiologic considerations to purposeful activity, it was necessary to understand the principles of therapeutic exercise.

As treatment methods evolved, occupational therapists began to use therapeutic exercise alone to prepare patients for purposeful activity and to expedite treatment in a health care system constrained by budget and time. The treatment of patients in acute stages of illness and disability imposed new demands and role responsibilities on occupational therapists. Short treatment sessions in acute care settings, the extent of the patient's physical incapacities, and shortened length of stay in hospital and rehabilitation facilities caused occupational therapists to expand the range of modalities used in treatment.

The use of therapeutic exercise as an isolated modality raised considerable controversy.[20] It was feared that if occupational therapists used exercise or other preparatory modalities, purpose would be forgotten. Exercise and activity tended to be seen by some as mutually exclusive, yet the principles of exercise had been applied to purposeful activity from early in the history of OT. Exercise and activity are complementary in the treatment continuum, and both may be used in a single treatment plan. However, if only pure exercise is used, the patient has not received OT.[20]

When used by occupational therapists, therapeutic exercise should be used to remediate sensory and motor dysfunction, augment purposeful activity, and prepare the patient for performing a functional occupation.

A comprehensive understanding of the principles of exercise is basic to the application of therapeutic activity. Therapeutic exercise is defined as any body movement or muscle contraction to prevent or correct a physical impairment, improve musculoskeletal function, and maintain a state of well-being.[14,27] A wide variety of exercise options are available; each should be tailored to meet the goals of treatment and the specific capacities and precautions relative to the patient's physical condition.

Exercise can be used to increase ROM and flexibility, strength, coordination, endurance, and cardiovascular fitness.[27] Specific exercise protocols may be used to achieve specific goals. However, exercise without activity is apt to place the exercise in the realm of deliberate rather than automatic performance, therefore violating essential principles of OT discussed earlier. Although judicious application of therapeutic exercise may have a limited place in the therapeutic program, the occupational therapist should structure treatment so that the patient is primarily engaged in activity to take advantage of the automaticity generated by purposeful goal-directed therapeutic activity.

Purposes

The general purposes of therapeutic exercise, as with therapeutic activity, are as follows:

1. To develop awareness of normal movement patterns and improve voluntary, automatic movement responses
2. To develop strength and endurance in patterns of movement that are acceptable and necessary and do not produce deformity
3. To improve coordination, regardless of strength
4. To increase the power of specific isolated muscles or muscle groups
5. To aid in overcoming ROM deficits
6. To increase the strength of muscles that will power hand splints, mobile arm supports, and other devices
7. To increase work tolerance and physical endurance through increased strength
8. To prevent or eliminate contractures developing as a result of imbalanced muscle power by strengthening the antagonistic muscles[41]

Indications for Use

Therapeutic exercise is most effective in the treatment of orthopedic disorders (such as contractures and arthritis) and lower motor neuron disorders that produce weakness and flaccidity. Examples of the latter are peripheral nerve injuries and diseases, poliomyelitis, Guillain-Barré syndrome, infectious neuronitis, and spinal cord injuries and diseases.

The candidate for therapeutic exercise must be medically able to participate in the exercise regimen, able to understand the directions and purposes, and interested and motivated to perform. The patient must have available motor pathways and the potential for recovery or improvement of strength, ROM, coordination, or movement patterns, as applicable. It is important that some sensory feedback be available to the patient; that is, sensation must be at least partially intact so the patient can perceive motion and the position of the exercised part and sense superficial and deep pain. Muscles and tendons must be intact, stable, and free to move. Joints must be able to move through an effective ROM for those types of exercise that use joint motion. The patient should be relatively free of pain during motion and should be able to perform isolated, coordinated movement. If the patient has any dyskinetic movement, he or she should be able to control it so that the procedure can be performed as prescribed.[40] The type of exercise selected depends on muscle grade, muscle endurance, joint mobility, diagnosis and physical condition, treatment goals, position of the patient, and desirable plane of movement. Each of these requirements is also applicable to the use of exercise-focused therapeutic activity, and should underlie its selection as a therapeutic tool.

Contraindications

Therapeutic exercise and exercise-focused therapeutic activity are contraindicated for patients who have poor general health or inflamed joints or who have had recent surgery.[40] They may not be useful where joint ROM is severely limited as the result of well-established, permanent contractures. As defined and described here, they cannot be used effectively for those who have spasticity and lack voluntary control of isolated motion or those who cannot control dyskinetic movement. The latter conditions are likely to occur in upper motor neuron disorders, which are more amenable to exercise regimens of the sensorimotor approaches to treatment (see Chapters 32 to 36).

Exercise Programs

Muscle Strengthening

Active-assisted, active, and resistive **isotonic** and **isometric exercises** are used to increase strength. After partial or complete denervation of muscle and during inactivity or disuse, muscle strength decreases. When strength is inadequate, substitution patterns or "trick" movements are likely to develop.[53] A substitution is the attempt to achieve a functional goal by using muscle groups and patterns of motion not ordinarily used. Substitution is used when there is loss or weakness of the muscles normally used to perform the movements or restrictions in ROM because of structural dysfunction. An example is using shoulder abduction to achieve a hand-to-mouth movement if elbow flexors cannot perform against gravity (Fig. 30-11). When muscle loss is permanent, some substitution patterns may be desirable as a compensatory measure to improve performance of functional activities, such as the use of tenodesis to permit grasp that will enable self-feeding. Many substitute movements are not desirable, however, and it is often the aim of therapeutic exercise to prevent or correct substitution patterns.[53]

A muscle must contract at or near its maximal capacity and for enough repetitions and time to increase strength. Strengthening programs generally are based on having the muscle contract against a large resistance for a few repetitions. Strengthening exercises are not effective if the contraction is insufficient.[14,28] Excess strengthening, however, may result in muscle fatigue, pain, and temporary reduction of strength. If a muscle is overworked, it becomes fatigued and is unable to contract. The type of exercise must suit the muscle grade and the patient's fatigue tolerance level. Fatigue level varies from individual to individual, and the threshold for muscle fatigue decreases in pathological states.[28] Many patients may not be sensitive to fatigue or may push themselves beyond tolerance in the belief that this approach hastens recovery. Therefore the therapist must carefully assess the patient's muscle power and capacity for performance. The therapist must also supervise the

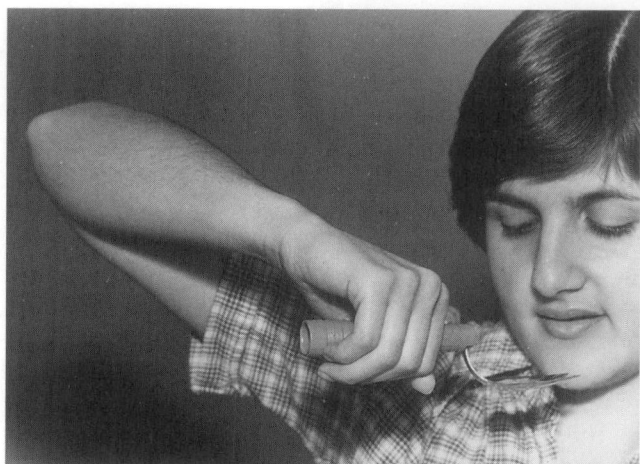

FIG. 30-11

Using shoulder abduction as compensation to achieve hand-to-mouth movement.

patient closely and observe for signs of fatigue. These signs may be slowed performance, distraction, perspiration, increase in rate of respiration, performance of exercise pattern through a decreased ROM, and inability to complete the prescribed number of repetitions.

Increasing Muscle Endurance

Endurance is the ability of the muscle to work for prolonged periods and resist fatigue. Although a high-load, low-repetition regimen is effective for muscle strengthening, a low-load and high-repetition exercise program is more effective for building endurance.[14,17] Having determined the patient's maximum capacity for a strengthening program, the therapist can reduce the maximum resistance load and increase the number of repetitions to build endurance in specific muscles or muscle groups. The strength versus endurance training may be seen as a continuum. Resistance and the number of repetitions can be modulated so that gains in strength and endurance accrue.[14]

Physical Conditioning and Cardiovascular Fitness

Improving general physical endurance and cardiovascular fitness requires the use of large muscle groups in sustained, rhythmic aerobic exercise or activity. Examples are swimming, walking, bicycling, jogging, and some games and sports. This type of activity is often used in cardiac rehabilitation programs in which the parameters of the patient's physical capacities and tolerance for exercise should be well defined and medically supervised. To improve cardiovascular fitness, exercise should be done 3 to 5 days per week at 60% to 90% of maximum heart rate or 50% to 85% of maximum oxygen uptake. Fifteen to 60 minutes of exercise or rhythmic activities using large muscle groups is desirable.[14]

Range of Motion and Joint Flexibility

Active and passive ROM are used to maintain joint motion and flexibility. **Active exercise** is that performed solely by the performer. An outside force such as the therapist or a device can be used for performing **passive exercise.** The continuous passive motion machine, a device that can be preset to provide continuous passive motion throughout the joint range, is an example. Application of any mechanical device requires caution and careful monitoring to prevent mishaps and possible deleterious effects.[14]

Stretching or forced exercise may be necessary to increase ROM. Some type of force is applied to the part when soft tissue (muscles, tendons, and ligaments) is at or near its available length. The use of a low-resistance stretch of sustained duration is preferred to high resistance and repetitive, quick, bouncing movements. The former method is less likely to produce tissue tearing, trauma, and activation of stretch reflexes in hypertonic muscles. The use of thermal agents or neuromuscular facilitation techniques may enhance static stretching.[14]

Coordination and Neuromuscular Control

Coordination is the combined activity of many muscles into smooth patterns and sequences of motion. Coordination is an automatic response monitored primarily through proprioceptive sensory feedback. Kottke[26] differentiated between neuromuscular control and coordination. He defined control as "the conscious activation of an individual muscle or the conscious initiation of a pre-programmed engram." Control involves conscious attention to and guidance of an activity. Conscious attention to activity may limit the achievement of further skill.

A preprogrammed pattern of muscular activity represented in the central nervous system (CNS) has been described as an *engram*. An engram is formed only if there are many repetitions of a specific motion or activity. With repetition, conscious effort of the patient is decreased and the motion becomes more and more automatic. Ultimately the motion can be carried out with little conscious attention. It has been hypothesized that when an engram is excited, the same pattern of movement is produced automatically. Neuromuscular education or control training involves teaching the patient to control individual muscles or motions through conscious attention. Coordination training is used to develop preprogrammed multimuscular patterns or engrams.[26]

Types of Muscle Contraction

Isometric or Static Contraction

During an isometric contraction no joint motion occurs, and the muscle length remains the same. The limb is set or held taut as agonist and antagonist muscles are contracted at a point in the ROM to stabilize a joint. This action may be without resistance or against some outside resistance, such as the therapist's hand or a fixed object. An example of isometric exercise of the triceps against resistance is pressing down against a tabletop with the ulnar border of the forearm while the elbow remains at 90° flexion. An example of an activity that requires isometric contraction is stabilizing the arm in a locked position when carrying a shopping bag slung over the forearm.[22,28]

Isotonic or Concentric Contraction

During an isotonic contraction there is joint motion and the muscle shortens. This contraction may be done with or without resistance. Isotonic contractions may be performed in positions with gravity decreased or against gravity, according to the patient's muscle grade and the goal of the exercise or activity. An isotonic contraction of the biceps is used to lift a fork to the mouth for eating.[22,28]

Eccentric Contraction

When muscles contract eccentrically, the tension in the muscle increases or remains constant, while the muscle lengthens. This contraction may be performed with or without resistance. An example of an eccentric contraction performed without resistance is the lowering of the arm to the table when placing a napkin next to a plate. The biceps contracts eccentrically in this instance. An example of eccentric contraction against resistance is the controlled return of a pail of sand lifted from the ground. In this example the biceps is contracting eccentrically to control the rate and coordination of the elbow extension in setting the pail on the ground.[22,28]

Exercise and Activity Classifications

Isotonic Resistive Exercise

Resistive exercise uses isotonic muscle contraction against a specific amount of weight to move the load through a certain ROM.[14,22,28] It is also possible to use eccentric contraction against resistance. Resistive exercise is used primarily for increasing the strength of fair plus to normal muscles but may also be helpful for producing relaxation of the antagonists to the contracting muscles. This latter purpose can be useful if increased range is desired for stretching or relaxing hypertonic antagonists.

The patient performs muscle contraction against resistance and moves the part through the available ROM. The resistance applied should be the maximum against which the muscle is capable of contracting. Resistance may be applied manually or by weights, springs, elastic bands, sandbags, or special devices. The source of resistance depends on the activity, and resistance is graded progressively with an increasing amount of resistance.[14,22,28] The number of possible repetitions depends on the patient's general physical endurance and the endurance of the specific muscle.

There are many types of strength training programs, most based on the principle that to increase strength, the muscle must contract against its maximal resistance. The number of repetitions, rest intervals, frequency of training, and speed of movement vary with the particular approach and with the patient's ability to accommodate to the exercise or activity regimen.[9] One specialized type of resistive exercise is the DeLorme method of progressive resistive exercise (PRE).[17,46] PRE is based on the overload principle: muscles perform more efficiently if given a warmup period and must be taxed beyond usual daily activity to improve in performance and strength.[17] During the exercise procedure small loads are used initially and increased gradually after each set of 10 repetitions. The muscle is thus warmed up to prepare to exert its maximal power for the final 10 repetitions. The exercise procedure consists of three sets of 10 repetitions each, with resistance applied as follows: first set, 10 repetitions at 50% of maximal resistance; second set, 10 repetitions at 75% of maximal resistance; third set, 10 repetitions at maximal resistance.[14,17,46] The load must be sufficient so that the patient can perform 10 repetitions. As strength improves, resistance is increased so that 10 repetitions can always be performed.[9] The patient is instructed to inhale during the shortening contraction and exhale during the relaxation or eccentric contraction.[17,46]

An example of a PRE is a triceps, capable of 12 pounds maximal resistance, extending the elbow, first against 6 pounds, then against 9 pounds, and the final 10 repetitions against 12 pounds. Maximal resistance, the amount of resistance the muscle can lift through the ROM 10 times, is determined by contracting the muscle and moving the part through the full ROM against progressively increasing loads for sets of 10 repetitions, until the maximal load that can be lifted 10 times is reached.

At the beginning of the treatment program it is often difficult for the therapist to determine the patient's maximal resistance. Reasons may be that the patient may not know how to exert maximal effort, may be reluctant to exercise strenuously for fear of pain or reinjury, may be unwilling or unable to endure discomfort, and may have difficulty with the timing of exercises.

The experience of the therapist and trial and error aid in determining maximal resistance. The therapist should estimate the amount of resistance the patient can take based on the muscle test results, and add or subtract resistance (weight or tension) until the patient can perform the sets of repetitions adequately.

The exercises should be performed once daily, four or five times a week, and rest periods of 2 to 4 minutes should be allowed between each set of 10 repetitions. The exercise procedure may be modified to suit individual needs. Some possibilities are 10 repetitions at 25% of maximal resistance, 10 repetitions at 50%, 10 repetitions at 75%, and 10 repetitions at maximal resistance. Another possibility is five repetitions at 50% and 10 repetitions at maximal resistance. Still another possibility is to omit the second set of exercises. Adjustments in the first two sets of exercises may be made to suit the capacity of the individual.[17]

Another approach is the Oxford technique, essentially a reverse of the DeLorme method. The exercise sequence begins with 100% resistance and decreases to 75%, and then to 50% on subsequent sets of 10 repetitions each.[17,46] The greatest gains may be made in the early weeks of the treatment program, with smaller increases occurring at a slower pace in the subsequent weeks or months. During performance of the exercise, the therapist should be aware of joint alignment of the exercise device; proper fit and adjustment of the device; ruling out of substitute movements; and clear instruction of speed, ROM, and proper breathing.[17,41]

APPLICATION TO ACTIVITY. Many purposeful activities lend themselves well to resistive exercise. For instance, leather lacing can offer slight resistance to the anterior deltoid if the lace is pushed in an upward direction. Sanding wood with a weighted sand block can offer substantial resistance to the anterior deltoid and triceps if done on an inclined plane. Activities such as sawing and hammering offer resistance to upper extremity musculature. Kneading dough and forming clay objects offer resistance to muscles of the hands and arms.

Isotonic Active Exercise

Isotonic muscle contraction is used in active exercise. Eccentric contraction may also be used. Active exercise is performed when the patient moves the joint through its available ROM against no outside resistance. Active motion through the complete ROM with gravity decreased or against gravity may be used for poor to fair muscles to improve strength, with the added benefit of maintaining ROM. It may be used with higher muscle grades for the maintenance of strength and ROM when resistance is contraindicated. Active exercise is not used to increase ROM because this purpose requires added force not present in active exercise.

In active exercise the patient moves the part through the complete ROM independently. If the exercise is performed in a gravity-decreased plane, a powdered surface, skateboard, deltoid aid, or free-moving suspension sling may be used to reduce the resistance produced by friction. The exercise is graded by a change to resistive exercise as strength improves.[22,28]

APPLICATION TO ACTIVITY. Activities that offer little or no resistance can be used as active exercise. A needlework activity performed in the gravity-decreased plane provides active exercise to the wrist extensors. When a grade of fair or 3 is reached, the activity can be repositioned to move against gravity, as in latch hooking (Fig. 30-12).

Active-Assisted Exercise

Isotonic muscle contraction is used in active-assisted exercise. The patient moves the joint through partial ROM, and the therapist or a mechanical device completes the range. Slings, pulleys, weights, springs, or elastic bands may be used to provide mechanical assistance.[46] The goal of active-assisted exercise is to increase strength of trace, poor minus, and fair minus muscles while maintaining ROM. In the case of trace muscles the patient may contract the muscle, and the therapist completes the entire ROM. This exercise is graded by decreasing the amount of assistance until the patient can perform active exercises.[22,28]

APPLICATION TO ACTIVITY. If assistance is required to complete the movement, an activity must be

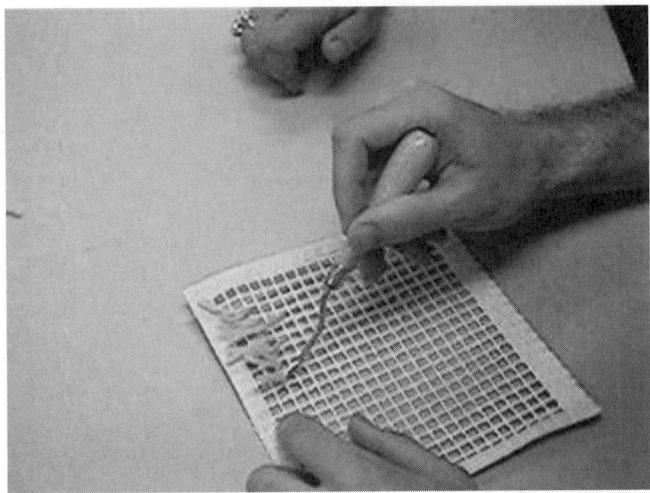

Fig. 30-12
Latch hooking to provide active resistive exercise to the wrist extensors.

structured so that assistance can be offered by the therapist, the patient's other arm or leg, or a mechanical device. Various bilateral activities lend themselves well to active-assisted exercise. Bilateral sanding, bilateral sponge wiping, using a sweeper, and sawing are some examples. In bilateral activities the unaffected arm or leg can perform a major share of the work, and the affected arm or leg can assist to the extent possible.

Passive Exercise

In passive exercise there is *no* muscle contraction. Therefore passive exercise is not used to increase strength because no force is applied. The purpose of passive exercise is to maintain ROM, thereby preventing contractures, adhesions, and deformity. To achieve this goal, the person should perform exercise for at least three repetitions, twice daily.[27] It is used when absent or minimal muscle strength (grades 0 to 1) precludes the active motion or when active exercise is contraindicated because of the patient's physical condition. During the exercise procedure the joint or joints to be exercised are moved through their normal ranges manually by the therapist or patient, or mechanically by an external device such as a pulley or counterbalance sling. The joint proximal to the joint being exercised should be stabilized during the exercise procedure (Fig. 30-13).[22]

APPLICATION TO ACTIVITY. It is often possible to include a passive limb in a bilateral activity if the contralateral limb is unaffected. Several of the activities described previously for active-assisted exercise can also be used for passive exercise.

Passive Stretch

For passive stretching, the therapist moves the joint through the available ROM and holds momentarily,

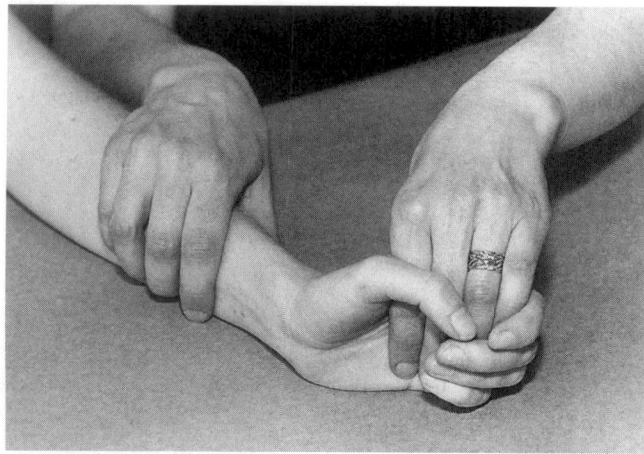

FIG. 30-13
Passive exercise of the wrist with stabilization of the joint proximal to the one being exercised.

applying a gentle but firm force or stretch at the end of the ROM. There should be no residual pain when the stretching is discontinued. Passive stretch or forced exercise is meant to increase ROM. It is used when there is a loss of joint ROM and stretching is not contraindicated. If muscle grades are adequate, the patient can move the part actively through the available ROM and the therapist can take it a little farther, thus forcing or stretching the soft-tissue structures around the joint.

Passive stretching requires a good understanding of joint anatomy and muscle function. It should be carried out cautiously under good medical supervision and with medical approval. Muscles to be stretched should be in a relaxed state.[28] The therapist should never force muscles when pain is present, unless ordered by the physician to work through pain. Gentle, firm stretching held for a few seconds is more effective and less hazardous than quick, short stretching. The parts around the area being stretched should be stabilized, and compensatory movements should be prevented. Incorrect stretching procedures can produce muscle tearing, joint fracture, and inflammatory edema.[27]

APPLICATION TO ACTIVITY. Passive stretching may be incorporated into an activity if an unaffected part guides the movement of the affected part and forces it slightly beyond the available ROM. One example is the passive stretch of wrist flexors during a block printing activity if the block is pressed down to stabilize the block with an open hand while the patient is standing.

Active Stretch

The purpose of active stretch is the same as for passive stretch: to increase joint ROM. In active stretching, the patient uses the force of the agonist muscle to increase the length of the antagonist. This requires good to normal strength of the antagonist, good coordination,

and motivation of the patient. For example, forceful contraction of the triceps to stretch the biceps muscle can be performed. Because the exercise may produce discomfort, there is a natural tendency for the patient to avoid the stretching component of the movement. Therefore supervision and frequent evaluation of its effectiveness are necessary.

APPLICATION TO ACTIVITY. Many activities can be used to incorporate active stretching. For example, slowly sawing wood requires a forceful contraction of the triceps with a concomitant stretch of the biceps.

Isometric Exercise Without Resistance

Isometric exercise uses isometric contractions of a specific muscle or muscle group. In isometric exercises a muscle or group of muscles is actively contracted and relaxed without producing motion of the joint that it ordinarily mobilizes. The purpose of isometric exercise without resistance is to maintain muscle strength when active motion is not possible or is contraindicated. It may be used with any muscle grade above trace. It is especially useful for patients in casts, after surgery, and with arthritis or burns.[14]

The patient is taught to set or contract the muscles voluntarily and to hold the contraction for 5 or 6 seconds. Without offering resistance, the therapist's fingers provide a kinesthetic image of resistance and help the patient learn to set the muscle. If needed, the therapist's fingers may be placed distal to the joint on which the muscles act. If passive motion is allowed, the therapist may move the joint to the desired point in the ROM and ask the patient to hold the position.

Isometric exercise affects the cardiovascular system, which may be a contraindication for some patients. It may cause a rapid and sudden increase in blood pressure, depending on the age of the patient, the intensity of contraction, and muscle mass being contracted. Therefore it should be used with caution.[14]

Isometric Exercise With Resistance

Isometric exercise with applied resistance uses isometric muscle contraction performed against some outside resistance. Its purpose is to increase muscle strength in muscles graded fair+ or 3+ to normal or 5. The patient sets the muscle or muscle group while resistance is applied, and holds the contraction for 5 or 6 seconds. Isometric exercises should be performed for one exercise session per day, 5 days a week. In addition to manual resistance, the patient may hold a weight or resist against a solid surface, depending on the muscle group being exercised. A small weight held in the hand while the wrist is stabilized at neutral requires isometric contractions of the wrist flexors and extensors.

Exercise is graded by increasing the amount of resistance or the degree of force the patient holds against. A tension gauge should be used to monitor accurately the amount of resistance applied. Isometric exercises are effective for increasing strength, but isotonic exercise is the method of choice. Isometric exercise has several specific applications, as in arthritis, when joint motion may be contraindicated but muscle strength must be increased or maintained.[22,41] The cardiovascular precautions stated previously are particularly important with isometric resistive exercise.

APPLICATION TO ACTIVITY. Any activity that requires holding or static posture incorporates isometric exercise. Holding tool handles and holding the arm in elevation while painting are examples. This type of exercise, if contraction is sustained, can be very fatiguing.

Neuromuscular Control and Coordination

Procedures for the development of neuromuscular control and neuromuscular coordination are briefly outlined in the following paragraphs. The reader is referred to original sources for a full discussion of the neurophysiological mechanisms underlying these exercises. Neuromuscular education or control training involves teaching the patient to control individual muscles or motions through conscious attention. Coordination training is used to develop preprogrammed multimuscular patterns or engrams.[26]

NEUROMUSCULAR CONTROL. It may be desirable to teach control of individual muscles when they are so weak that they cannot be used normally. The purpose is to improve muscle strength and muscle coordination to new patterns. To achieve these ends, the person must learn precise control of the muscle, an essential step in the development of optimal coordination for persons with neuromuscular disease.

To participate successfully the patient must be able to learn and follow instructions, cooperate, and concentrate on the muscular retraining. Before beginning, the patient should be comfortable and securely supported. The exercises should be carried out in a nondistracting environment. The patient must be alert, calm, and rested. He or she should have an adequate pain-free arc of motion of the joint on which the muscle acts, as well as good proprioception. Visual and tactile sensory feedback may be used to compensate or substitute for limited proprioception, but the coordination achieved will never be as great as when proprioception is intact.[26]

The patient's awareness of the desired motion and the muscles that effect it is first increased by passive motion to stimulate the proprioceptive stretch reflex. This passive movement may be repeated several times. The patient's awareness may be enhanced if the therapist also demonstrates the desired movement and if the movement is performed by the analogous unaffected

part. The skin over the muscle belly and tendon insertion may be stimulated to enhance the effect of the stretch reflex. Stroking and tapping over the muscle belly may be used to facilitate muscle action.[26]

The therapist should explain the location and function of the muscle, its origin and insertion, line of pull, and action on the joint. The therapist should then demonstrate the motion and instruct the patient to think of the pull of the muscle from insertion to origin. The skin over muscle insertion can be stroked in the direction of pull while the patient concentrates on the sensation of the motion during the passive movement performed by the therapist.

The exercise sequence begins with instructions to the patient to think about the motion, while the therapist carries it out passively and strokes the skin over the insertion in the direction of the motion. The patient is then instructed to assist by contracting the muscle while the therapist performs passive motion and stimulates the skin as before. Next the patient moves the part through ROM with assistance and cutaneous stimulation, while the therapist emphasizes contraction of the prime mover only. Finally the patient carries out the movement independently, using the prime mover.

The exercises must be initiated against minimal resistance if activity is to be isolated to prime movers. If the muscle is very weak (trace to poor), the procedure may be carried out entirely in an active-assisted manner so that the muscle contracts against no resistance and can function without activating synergists. Progression from one step to the next depends on successful performance of the steps without substitutions. Each step is carried out three to five times per session for each muscle, depending on the patient's tolerance.

COORDINATION TRAINING. The goal of coordination training is to develop the ability to perform multimuscular motor patterns that are faster, more precise, and stronger than those performed when control of individual muscles is used. The development of coordination depends on repetition. Initially in training, the movement must be simple and slow so that the patient can be consciously aware of the activity and its components. Good coordination does not develop until repeated practice results in a well-developed activity pattern that no longer requires conscious effort and attention.

Training should take place in an environment in which the patient can concentrate. The exercise is divided into components that the patient can perform correctly. Kottke calls this approach desynthesis.[26] The level of effort required should be kept low, by reducing speed and resistance, to prevent the spread of excitation to muscles that are not part of the desired movement pattern. Other theorists offer contrary advice, emphasizing the integration of movements that customarily occurs during activity. The therapist's experience and judgment are important in determining which method to use.

When the motor pattern is divided into units that the patient can perform successfully, each unit is trained by practice under voluntary control, as described previously for training of control. The therapist instructs the patient in the desired movement and uses sensory stimulation and passive movement. The patient must observe and voluntarily modify the motion. Slow practice is imperative to make this monitoring possible. The therapist offers enough assistance to ensure precise movement while allowing the patient to concentrate on the sensations produced by the movements. When the patient concentrates on movement, fatigue occurs rapidly and the patient should be given frequent, short rests. As the patient masters the components of the pattern and performs them precisely and independently, the sequence is graded to subtasks or several components that are practiced repetitively. As the subtasks are perfected, they are linked progressively until the movement pattern can be performed.

The protocol can be graded for speed, force, or complexity, but the therapist must be aware that the increased effort put forth by the patient may result in incoordinated movement. Therefore the grading must remain within the patient's capacity to perform the precise movement pattern. The motor pattern must be performed correctly to prevent the development of faulty patterns.

If CNS impulses irradiate improperly to muscles that should not be involved in the movement pattern, incoordinated motion results. Constant repetition of an incoordinated pattern reinforces the pattern, resulting in a persistent incoordination. Factors that increase incoordination are fear, poor balance, too much resistance, pain, fatigue, strong emotions, prolonged inactivity,[26] and excessively prolonged activity.

APPLICATION TO ACTIVITY. OT can be used to develop coordination, strength, and endurance. Active occupations have the advantage of engaging the patient's attention and interest. Activities should be structured to enable the patient to use the precise movement pattern and to work at speeds consistent with the maintenance of precision.

Therapists may initiate coordination training with neuromuscular education and progress to repetitious activities requiring desired coordinated movement patterns. Placing small blocks, marbles, cones, paper cups, or pegs is an enabling activity that demands repetitious patterns of nonresistive movement. Purposeful activities such as leather lacing, mosaic tile work, needlecrafts, and household tasks such as wiping, sweeping, and dusting also provide such repetitive movements.

PHYSICAL AGENT MODALITIES*

The introduction of **physical agent modalities** (PAMs) into OT practice generated considerable controversy.[49,52] The use of such modalities was initiated by occupational therapists specializing in hand rehabilitation in which inclusion of physical agents in a comprehensive treatment program became expedient.[43,45] After much study and discussion, the AOTA published a position paper on physical agent modalities.[3,4] In this official document, physical agents were defined and their use as adjuncts to or preparation for purposeful activity was specified. "The exclusive use of physical agent modalities as a treatment method during a treatment session without application to a functional outcome is not considered occupational therapy."[4] Further, the use of PAMs is not considered entry-level practice: rather, appropriate postprofessional education is required to ensure competence of the OT practitioners using these modalities.[4] The AOTA stipulated that the practitioner must have documented evidence of the theoretical background and technical skills to apply the modality and integrate it into an OT intervention plan.[3,4] Generating from these notions, several states have required in their licensure laws that occupational therapists have advanced training in order to use PAMs in treatment.

Physical agent modalities are used before or during functional activities to enhance the effects of treatment. This section introduces the reader to basic techniques and when and why they might be applied. Examples of the treatment of upper extremity injuries are presented because modalities are most commonly used by occupational therapists for treatment of hand injuries and diseases. The use of the techniques described is not limited to the treatment of hands, however.

Thermal Modalities

In a clinical setting heat is used to increase motion, decrease joint stiffness, relieve muscle spasms, increase blood flow, decrease pain, and aid in the reabsorption of exudates and edema in a chronic condition.[31] Collagen fibers have an elastic component and when stretched will return to their original length. Applying heat before a prolonged stretch, as in dynamic splinting, allows the permanent elongation of these fibers. The blood flow maintains a person's core temperature at 98.6° F. To obtain maximum benefits from heat, tissue temperature must be raised to 105° to 113° F. Precautions must be taken with temperatures above this range to prevent tissue destruction.

Contraindications to the use of heat include acute conditions, sensory losses, impaired vascular structures,

*Ingrid E. Wade, OTR, is gratefully acknowledged for her contribution of this topic in the fourth edition of this book.

malignancies, and application to the very young or very old. The use of heat may substantially enhance the effects of splinting and therapeutic activities that attempt to increase range of motion and functional abilities.

Conduction

Conduction is the transfer of heat from one object to another through direct contact. Paraffin and hot packs provide heat by conduction. Paraffin is stored in a tub that maintains a temperature between 125° and 130° F. The client repeatedly dips his or her hand into the tub until a thick, insulating layer of paraffin is applied to the extremity. The hand is then wrapped in a plastic bag and towel for 10 to 20 minutes.[31] This technique provides an excellent conforming characteristic, so it is ideal for use in hands and digits. Partial hand coverage is possible. The paraffin transfers its heat to the hand, and the bag and towel act as an insulator against dissipation of heat to the air.

Care must be taken to protect insensate parts from burns. To prevent excessive vasodilation, paraffin should not be applied when moderate to severe edema is present. It cannot be used if open wounds are present. Paraffin can be used in the clinic or incorporated into a home program. The tubs are small, and the technique is safe and easy to use in the home. It is an excellent adjunct to home programs that include dynamic splinting, exercises, or general ADL. It may be used in the clinic before therapeutic exercises and functional activities.

Hot packs contain either a silicate gel or a bentonite clay wrapped in a cotton bag and submerged in a hydrocollator, a water tank that maintains the temperature of the packs at 160° to 175° F.[31] Because tissue damage may occur at these temperatures, the packs are separated from the skin by layers of towels. As with paraffin, precautions should be taken when applying hot packs to insensate tissue that has sustained vascular damage. Hot packs are commonly used for myofascial pain, before soft-tissue mobilization, and before any activities aimed at elongating contracted tissue.[13] For a client with a hand injury the packs may be applied to the extrinsic musculature to decrease muscle tone caused by guarding, without also heating the hand. Unless contraindicated, hot packs can be used (with precautions) when open wounds are present.

Convection

Convection supplies heat to the tissues by fluid motion around the tissues. Examples of convection are whirlpool and fluidotherapy. Whirlpool is used more commonly for wound management than for heat application. Fluidotherapy involves a machine that agitates finely ground cornhusk particles by blowing warm air through them. This device is similar to the whirlpool, but corn particles are used instead of water. The temper-

ature is thermostatically maintained, with the therapeutic range extending to 125° F. Studies have shown this technique to be excellent for raising tissue temperature in the hands and feet.[13] An additional benefit is its effect on desensitization. The agitator can be adjusted to decrease or increase the flow of the corn particles, thus controlling the amount of stimulation to the skin. Because an extremity can be heated generally, this technique is effective as a warmup before exercises, dexterity tasks, functional activities, and work simulation tasks.

Conversion

Conversion occurs when heat is generated internally by friction, for example, by means of ultrasound. The sound waves penetrate the tissues, causing vibration of the molecules, and the resulting friction generates heat. The energy of sound waves is thus converted to heat energy. The sound waves are applied with a transducer, which glides across the skin in slow, continuous motions. Gel is used to improve the transmission of the sound to the tissues. Ultrasound is considered a deep heating agent. At 1 MHz (1 million cycles per second), it can heat tissues to a depth of 5 cm. The previous methods produce heating to 1 cm.[35] Many therapeutic ultrasound machines provide a 3-MHz option for treatment of more superficial structures, with the corresponding heating depth reduced to 3 cm. Ultrasound at frequencies higher than recommended standards can destroy tissue. In addition, precautions must be taken to avoid growth plates in the bones of children, an unprotected spinal cord, and freshly repaired structures such as tendons and nerves. Because of its ability to heat deeper tissues, ultrasound is excellent for treating problems associated with joint contractures, scarring with its associated adhesions, and muscle spasms. When applying the ultrasound, the therapist should apply a stretch to the tissues while they are being heated, followed by activities, exercises, and splints to maintain the stretch.

Ultrasound may also be used in a nonthermal application in which the ultrasound waves are used to drive antiinflammatory medications into tissues. This process is called phonophoresis. Ultrasound is thought to increase membrane permeability for greater symptom relief, and may also be used after corticosteroid injections.

Cryotherapy, the use of cold in therapy, is often used in the treatment of edema, pain, and inflammation. The cold produces a vasoconstriction, which decreases the amount of blood flow into the injured tissue. Cold decreases muscle spasms by decreasing the amount of firing from the afferent muscle spindles. Cryotherapy is contraindicated for clients with cold intolerance or vascular repairs. The use of cryotherapy may be incorporated into clinical treatment; however, it is particularly useful in a home program.

Cold packs can be applied in a number of ways. There are many commercial packs, ranging in size and cost. An alternative to purchasing a cold pack is to use a bag of frozen vegetables or to combine crushed ice and alcohol in a plastic bag to make a reusable slush bag. Ice packs should be covered with a moist towel to prevent tissue injury. The benefit of commercial packs is that they are easy to use, especially if the client must use them frequently during the day. When clients are working, it is recommended that they keep cold packs at home and at work, to increase the ease of use. The optimum temperature for storing a cold pack is 45° F.

Other forms of cryotherapy include ice massage and cooling machines. Ice massage is used when the area to be cooled is small and very specific—for example, inflammation of a tendon specifically at its insertion or origin. The procedure entails using a large piece of ice (water frozen in a paper cup) and massaging the area with circular motions until the skin is numb, usually for 4 to 5 minutes. Cooling devices, which circulate cold water through tubes in a pack, are available through vendors. These devices maintain their cold temperatures for a long time, but they are expensive to rent or purchase. They are effective in reducing edema immediately after surgery or injury, during the inflammatory phase of wound healing.

Contrast baths combine the use of heat and cold. The physical response is alternating vasoconstriction and vasodilation of the blood vessels. The client is asked to submerge the arm, for example, alternating between two tubs of water. One contains cold water (59° to 68°F), and the other contains warm water (96° to 105°F). The purpose is to increase collateral circulation, which effectively reduces pain and edema. As with the use of cold packs, contrast baths are a beneficial addition to a home therapy program. This technique is contraindicated for clients with vascular disorders or injuries.

Electrical Modalities

Electrical modalities are used to decrease pain, decrease edema, increase motion, and reeducate muscles. As with all PAMs, occupational therapists use these modalities to increase a client's functional abilities. Many techniques are available; those most commonly used are presented here. Electrical modalities should not be used with clients with pacemakers or cardiac conditions.

Transcutaneous Electrical Nerve Stimulation (TENS)

TENS employs electrical current to decrease pain. Pain is classified in three categories: physical, physiological, and psychological. When trauma occurs, an individual responds to the initial pain by guarding the painful body part. This guarding may result in muscle spasms and fatigue of the muscle fibers, especially after prolonged guarding. The supply of blood and oxygen to the affected area decreases, and resultant soft-tissue and joint dysfunction occurs.[34] These reactions magnify and compound the problems associated with the initial pain response. The therapist's goal after an acute injury is to prevent this cycle. In the case of chronic pain the goal is to stop the cycle that has been established. TENS is an effective technique for controlling pain without the side effects of medications. Pain medications are frequently used in conjunction with TENS, which often reduces the duration of their use. TENS is safe to use, and clients can be educated in independent home use.

TENS provides constant electrical stimulation with a modulated current and is directed to the peripheral nerves through electrode placement. The therapist can control several attributes of the modulation waveform such as the frequency, amplitude, and the pulse width. When TENS is applied at a low-fire setting, endogenous opiates are released. Endorphins, naturally occurring substances, reduce the sensation of pain. The effects of high-frequency TENS are based on the gate control theory originally proposed by Melzack and Wall in 1965. This theory describes how the electrical current from TENS, applied to the peripheral nerves, blocks the perception of pain in the brain. Nociceptors (pain receptors) transmit information to the CNS through the A, delta, and C fibers. A fibers transmit information about pressure and touch. It is thought that TENS stimulates the A fibers, effectively saturating the gate to pain perception, and the transmission of pain signals via the A, delta, and C fibers are blocked at the level of the spinal cord.[34] TENS can be applied for acute or chronic pain. TENS is frequently used postsurgically, when it is mandatory that motion be initiated within 72 hours such as in tenolysis and capsulotomy surgeries or when is important to maintain tendon gliding through the injured area after fractures. TENS can be especially helpful with clients who have a low threshold to pain, making exercising easier. TENS is also useful in treating clients with reflex sympathetic dystrophy because continued active motion is crucial.

TENS can be used to decrease pain from an inflammatory condition such as tendonitis or a nerve impingement; however, it is mandatory that the client be educated in tendon and nerve protection and rest, with a proper home program of symptom management, positioning, and ADL and work modification. Without the sensation of pain, it is possible for the client to overdo and stress the tissues. It is recommended that other techniques be tried first to decrease pain for these clients. TENS is also used for treating trigger points, with direct electrode application to the trigger point to decrease its irritability.[36]

Neuromuscular Electrical Stimulation

Neuromuscular electrical stimulation (NMES) provides a continuous interrupted current. It is applied through an electrode to the motor point of innervated muscles to provide a muscle contraction. The current is interrupted to enable the muscle to relax between contractions, and the durations of the on and off times can be adjusted by the therapist. Adjustments can also be made to control the rate of the increase in current (ramp) and intensity of the contraction.

NMES is used to increase ROM, facilitate muscle contractions, and strengthen muscles.[37] It may be used postsurgically to provide a stronger contraction for released tendon gliding—for example, after a tenolysis. It also may be used later in the tendon repair protocol, once the tendon has healed sufficiently to tolerate stress, usually at a minimum of 6 weeks. NMES may be used to lengthen a muscle that has become weakened because of disuse. During the reinnervation phase after a nerve injury, this technique may be used to help stimulate and strengthen a newly innervated muscle. Care must be taken not to over-fatigue the muscle. NMES can be applied during a dexterity or functional activity, which allows the muscle to be retrained in the purpose of its contraction. As with TENS, NMES may be incorporated into a home program with proper client education and follow-through.

Other techniques that use an electrical current include high-voltage galvanic stimulation (HVGS) and inferential electrical stimulation. These techniques are applied to treat pain and edema.[37] Electrical stimulation may be applied in conjunction with ultrasound through a single transducer to provide heat simultaneously with current. This approach is beneficial in treating trigger points and myofascial pain. Iontophoresis uses a current to drive ionized medication into inflamed tissue and scar tissue. The technique uses an electrode filled with the medication of choice. The medicine is transferred by applying an electric field that repels the ions into the tissues.

SELECTION OF APPROPRIATE MODALITIES IN THE CONTINUUM OF CARE

Many years ago treatment roles and responsibilities were more specifically delineated. Occupational therapists treated patients only after the patients were capable, at least to some degree, of performing purposeful activity.[20] Evolution of treatment methods, trends in health care (Chapter 2), and medical technology have significantly altered the role of the respective therapists and expanded the repertoire of treatment modalities that therapists are competent to practice.

Patients are now referred to OT long before they are capable of performing purposeful activity. Therapists are treating patients in the very acute stages of illness and disability. Treatment is directed toward preparing the patient for the time when purposeful activity is possible. This approach may mean that the occupational therapist applies a positioning splint to a patient immediately after hand surgery, considering how the hand will be used later in treatment and in real life. It means the therapist may use sensory stimulation on the comatose patient because arousal and a return to interacting with persons and objects in the environment will make performance of purposeful activity possible in the future. It means the therapist may apply paraffin to decrease joint stiffness and increase mobility of finger joints before performance of a macrame project. It also may mean preparing the patient and family to plan for the future, when life skills may need to be performed in ways new to them, such as modified sexual positioning for arthritic or spinal cord patients or learning self-care of the colostomy. The unique perspective of the occupational therapist is seeing the potential for performance and using modalities that lead incrementally to performance relevant to the lives patients wish to lead.

SUMMARY

Active occupation is the primary tool and objective of OT practice. Occupational therapists use purposeful activity, activity analysis, adaptation, grading of activities, therapeutic exercise, simulated or enabling activities, and adjunctive modalities in the continuum of treatment, and they may use these methods simultaneously toward these ends. Through this breadth of practice skills, based on the patient's personal and social needs, the occupational therapist helps the patient apply newly gained strength, ROM, and coordination during the performance of purposeful activity, preparing the patient to assume or reassume life roles. Appropriate therapeutic activity is individualized and designed to be meaningful and interesting to the patient, while meeting therapeutic objectives.

Therapeutic activity may be adapted to meet special needs of the patient or the environment. It may be graded for physical, perceptual, cognitive, and social purposes to keep the patient functioning at maximal potential at any point in the treatment program. The uniqueness of OT lies in its extensive use of goal-directed purposeful activities as treatment modalities, making use of the mind-body continuum within the tangible and social context. Purposeful activity is the core of OT practice.

In practice, therapists' roles may not be sharply defined because they are subject to variations in expectations that stem from regional differences, health care developments, legislation, institutional philosophy, and the roles and responsibilities assigned by the treatment facility. In all instances, therapists must be well trained and well qualified to deliver all aspects of practice. They should not hesitate to refer patients to experts for treatment whenever appropriate.

REVIEW QUESTIONS

1. Identify the three realms of occupational genesis and their relation to the concept of development.
2. Define modality.
3. What is required for an activity to be considered purposeful?
4. Name two reasons that activity is valuable.
5. List the six elements of an activity configuration.
6. Name a client-centered tool used to identify patients' goals, objectives, and lifestyles.
7. Name the three perspectives of activity analysis.
8. What term bests describes how activities and environments are modified to meet the individualized needs of patients?
9. What is used to create the "just right" challenge in performance?
10. What is the term that refers to activities that are contrived to elicit movements but are considered non-purposeful?
11. When are adjunctive modalities appropriately used by occupational therapists?
12. For which types of disabilities would therapeutic exercise (as defined in this chapter) be inappropriate?
13. List and define three types of muscle contraction.
14. Identify an activity that can be used to provide resistive exercise, and describe how it could be done.
15. List four general categories of physical agent modalities.
16. What kinds of symptoms are treated with cryotherapy?

REFERENCES

1. American Occupational Therapy Association: Association policy: occupational therapists and modalities (Representative Assembly, April, 1983), *Am J Occup Ther* 37(12):816, 1983.
2. American Occupational Therapy Association: Position paper on purposeful activities, *Am J Occup Ther* 37(12):805-806, 1983.
3. American Occupational Therapy Association: Official AOTA statement on physical agent modalites, *Am J Occup Ther* 45(12):1075, 1991.
4. American Occupational Therapy Association: Position paper: physical agent modalities, *Am J Occup Ther* 46(12):1090, 1992.
5. American Occupational Therapy Association: Position paper: physical agent modalities, *Am J Occup Ther* 47(12):1081-1082, 1993.
6. American Occupational Therapy Association: Uniform terminology for occupational therapy, ed 3, *Am J Occup Ther* 35(12):499-518, 1994.
7. Ayres AJ: Basic concepts of clinical practice in physical disabilities, *Am J Occup Ther* 12(8):300-302, 1958.
8. Ayres AJ: Occupational therapy for motor disorders resulting from impairment of the central nervous system, *Rehabil Lit* 21:302, 1960.
9. Barton G: *Teaching the sick: a manual of occupational therapy and reeducation*, Philadelphia, 1919, WB Saunders.
10. Breines EB: Genesis of occupation: a philosophical model for therapy and theory, *Aust Occup Ther J* 37:45-49, 1990.
11. Brienes EB: *Occupational therapy from clay to computers: theory & practice*, Philadelphia, 1995, FA Davis.
12. Breines EB: *Origins and adaptations: a philosophy of practice*, Lebanon, NJ, 1986, Geri-Rehab.
13. Cannon NM, Mullins PT: *Manual on management of specific hand problems*, Pittsburgh, 1984, American Rehabilitation Educational Network.
14. Ciccone CD, Alexander J: Physiology and therapeutics of exercise. In Goodgold J, editor: *Rehabilitation medicine*, St Louis, 1988, Mosby.
15. Cynkin S: *Occupational therapy: toward health through activities*, Boston, 1979, Little, Brown.
16. Cynkin C, Robinson AM: *Occupational therapy: toward health through activities*, Boston, 1990, Little, Brown.
17. DeLateur BJ, Lehmann J: Therapeutic exercise to develop strength and endurance. In Kottke FJ, Stillwell GK, Lehmann JF, editors: *Krusen's handbook of physical medicine and rehabilitation*, ed 4, Philadelphia, 1990, WB Saunders.
18. Dewey J: *Democracy and education: an introduction to the philosophy of education*, Toronto, 1916, Collier-Macmillan.
19. Dunton WR: *Prescribing occupational therapy*, Springfield, Ill, 1928, Charles C Thomas.
20. Dutton R: Guidelines for using both activity and exercise, *Am J Occup Ther* 43(9):573-580, 1989.
21. Hopkins HL, Smith HD, Tiffany EG: The activity process. In Hopkins HL, Smith HD, editors: *Willard & Spackman's occupational therapy*, ed 7, Philadelphia, 1988, JB Lippincott.
22. Huddleston OL: *Therapeutic exercises*, Philadelphia, 1961, FA Davis.
23. Huss AJ: From kinesiology to adaptation, *Am J Occup Ther* 35(9):574-580, 1981.
24. Kielhofner G: A heritage of activity: development of theory, *Am J Occup Ther* 36(11):723-730, 1982.
25. Killingsworth A: *Activity module for OCTH 120, functional kinesiology*, 1989, San Jose State University, San Jose, California (unpublished).
26. Kottke FJ: Therapeutic exercises to develop neuromuscular coordination. In Kottke FJ, Stillwell GK, Lehmann JF, editors: *Krusen's handbook of physical medicine and rehabilitation*, ed 4, Philadelphia, 1990, WB Saunders.
27. Kottke FJ: Therapeutic exercise to maintain mobility. In Kottke FJ, Stillwell GK, Lehmann JF, editors: *Krusen's handbook of physical medicine and rehabilitation*, ed 4, Philadelphia, 1990, WB Saunders.
28. Kraus H: *Therapeutic exercise*, Springfield, Ill, 1963, Charles C Thomas.
29. Law M, Baptiste S, Carswell A, et al: *Canadian occupational performance measure*, ed 3, Ottowa, Canada, 1998, Canadian Association of Occupational Therapists.
30. Lamport NK, Coffey MS, Hersch GI: *Activity analysis & application: building blocks of treatment*, Thorofare, NJ, 1996, Slack.
31. Lehmann JF: *Therapeutic heat and cold*, ed 3, Baltimore, 1982, Williams & Wilkins.
32. Llorens LA: Activity analysis: agreement among factors in a sensory processing model, *Am J Occup Ther* 40(2):103-110, 1986.
33. Llorens L: *Activity analysis for sensory integration (CPM) dysfunction*, 1978 (unpublished).
34. Mannheimer JS, Lampe GN: *Clinical transcutaneous electrical nerve stimulation*, Philadelphia, 1990, FA Davis.
35. Michlovitz SL: *Thermal agents in rehabilitation*, ed 2, Philadelphia, 1990, FA Davis.
36. Moran CA, Saunders SR, Tribuzi SM: Myofascial pain in the upper extremity. In Hunter JM et al, editors: *Rehabilitation of the hand*, ed 3, St Louis, 1990, Mosby.
37. Mullins PT: Use of therapeutic modalities in upper extremity rehabilitation. In Hunter JM et al, editors: *Rehabilitation of the hand*, ed 3, St Louis, 1990, Mosby.
38. Nelson D et al: The effects of occupationally embedded exercise on bilaterally assisted supination in persons with hemiplegia, *Am J Occup Ther* 50(8):639-646.

39. Pedretti LW, Smith RO, Hammel J, et al: Use of adjunctive modalities in occupational therapy, *Am J Occup Ther* 46(12):1075-1081, 1992.

40. Rancho Los Amigos Hospital: *Muscle reeducation* (unpublished), Downey, Calif, 1963, the Hospital.

41. Rancho Los Amigos Hospital: *Progressive resistive and static exercise: principles and techniques* (unpublished), Downey, Calif, the Hospital.

42. Reed KL: Tools of practice: heritage or baggage? *Am J Occup Ther* 40(9):597-605, 1986.

43. Reynolds C: OTs and PAMs: a physical therapist's perspective, *OT Week* 8(37):17, Bethesda, Md, 1994, American Occupational Therapy Association.

44. Rocker JD, Nelson DL: Affective responses to keeping and not keeping an activity product, *Am J Occup Ther* 41(3):152-157.

45. Rose H: Physical agent modalities: OT's contribution, *OT Week* 8(37):16-17, Bethesda, Md, 1994, American Occupational Therapy Association.

46. Schram DA: Resistance exercise. In Basmajian JV, editor: *Therapeutic exercise*, ed 4, Baltimore, 1984, Williams & Wilkins.

47. Spackman CS: Occupational therapy for the restoration of physical function. In Willard HS, and Spackman CS, editors: *Occupational therapy*, ed 4, Philadelphia, 1974, JB Lippincott.

48. Steinbeck TM: Purposeful activity and performance, *Am J Occup Ther* 40(8):529-534, 1986.

49. Taylor E, Humphrey R: Survey of physical agent modality use, *Am J Occup Ther* 45(10):924-931, 1991.

50. Thibodeaux CS, Ludwig FM: Intrinsic motivation in product-oriented and non-product-oriented activities, *Am J Occup Ther* 42(3):169-175, 1988.

51. Watson DE. Llorens LA: *Task analysis: an occupational performance approach*, Bethesda, Md, 1997, American Occupational Therapy Association

52. West WL, Weimer RB: This issue is: should the representative assembly have voted as it did, on occupational therapist's use of physical agent modalities? *Am J Occup Ther* 45(12)1143-1147, 1991.

53. Wynn-Parry CB: Vicarious motions. In Basmajian JV, editor: *Therapeutic exercise*, ed 3, Baltimore, 1982, Williams & Wilkins.

54. Yoder RM, Nelson DL, Smith DA: Added-purpose versus rote exercise in female nursing home residents, *Am J Occup Ther* 43(9):581-586, 1989.

APPENDIX
Activity Analysis Model

The activity analysis offers the reader one systematic approach for looking at the therapeutic potential of activities. This model includes some factors that must be considered about the performer, the environmental context, and the activity in the selection of purposeful, therapeutic activity. In the model, just two steps of a multistep activity are analyzed for the sake of space and simplicity. The reader is encouraged to complete the motor analysis by considering movements of the shoulder, forearm, and wrist that accompany the pinch and release pattern analyzed.

I. Preliminary information
   1. Name of activity: Pinch pottery
   2. Components of the task
      a. Roll some clay into a ball, 3 to 4 inches in diameter.
      b. Place the ball centered on the work table in front of the performer.
      c. Make a hole in the center of the ball with the right or left thumb (Fig. 30-14).
      d. With the thumb and first two fingers of both hands, pinch around and around the hole from base to top of the ball.
         i. Pinch by pressing thumb against index and middle fingers.
         ii. Release pinch by extending thumb and index and middle fingers slightly.
      e. Continue pinching in this way, gradually spreading the walls of the clay until a small bowl of the desired size is formed.
   3. Steps of activity being analyzed
      a. Pinch
      b. Release

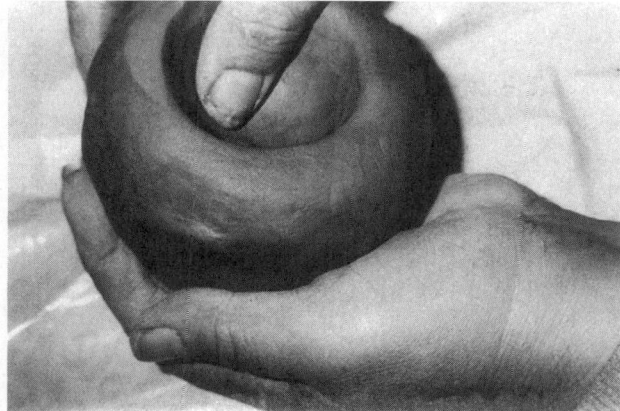

FIG. 30-14

Opening pinch pot with thumb. (From Breines EB: *Occupational therapy from clay to computers: theory & practice*, Philadelphia, 1995, FA Davis.)

4. Equipment and supplies necessary
   a. Ball of soft ceramic clay
   b. Wooden table 30 to 32 inches high or a wooden work surface fastened to a table with C clamps
   c. Chair at the work table
   d. Sponge and bowl of water
   e. Ceramic smoothing tool
5. Environmental context[15,16]: Occupational therapy workshop or craft activity room. A sink and damp storage area should be available in the work area. There should be ample room around the work table so that the performer is not crowded and can move freely between the table and the sink and damp storage closet. Lighting should be adequate for clear visualization of clay object and work area.
6. Position of the performer in relation to the work surface and equipment: The performer is seated in the chair at the table, at a comfortable distance for reaching and manipulating the clay and tools. The clay is centered in front of the performer, and the tool, sponge, and water bowl are to the right and near the top of the work area.
7. Starting position of the performer: Sitting erect with feet flat on the floor; shoulders are slightly abducted and in slight internal rotation, bringing both hands to the center work surface; elbows are flexed to about 90°; forearms are pronated about 45°; wrists are slightly extended and in ulnar deviation, thumbs are opposed to index and middle fingers, ready to pinch the posterior surface of the opened clay ball.
8. Movement pattern used to perform the steps under analysis: Flexion of the MP and IP joints of index and middle fingers; opposition and flexion of the thumb (pinch) followed by extension of the MP and IP joints index and middle fingers and extension and palmar abduction of the thumb (release). Repeat the pattern around ball of clay until a small bowl of desired size and thickness is formed.

II. Motor analysis[25]
   1. Joint and Muscle activity: List the joint motions for all movements used during performance of the activity. For each, indicate amount of ROM used (minimal, moderate, or full), muscle group used to perform the motion, strength required (minimal [P+ to F], moderate [F+ to G], and full [G+ to N]), and type of muscle contraction (isotonic, isometric, eccentric) (Table 30-1).
   2. Grading: Grade this activity for one or more of the following factors:
      a. ROM: Cannot be graded for ROM.
      b. Strength: Grade for strength by increasing the consistency of the clay.

TABLE 30-1
Motions For Pinch

Joint Motion	Range of Motion	Muscle Group	Strength	Type of Muscle Contraction
Index and Middle Fingers				
MP flexion	Minimal	FDP, FDS lumbricales	Moderate	Isotonic
PIP flexion	Minimal	FDP, FDS	Moderate	Isotonic
DIP flexion	Minimal	FDP	Moderate	Isotonic
Finger adduction	Maximal	Palmar interossei	Moderate	Isometric
Thumb				
Opposition	Full	Opponens pollicis, FPl, FPB	Moderate	Isotonic
Motions for Release Index and Middle Fingers				
MP extension	Minimal	EDC, EIP	Minimal	Isotonic
PIP and DIP extension	Minimal	EDC, EIP	Minimal	Isotonic
Finger adduction	Maximal	Palmar interossei	Moderate	Isometric
Thumb				
Radial abduction	Moderate	APL, APB	Minimal	Isotonic
MP, IP extension	Full	EPL, EPB	Minimal	Isotonic

Adapted from Killingsworth A: *OT120 activity module,* San Jose, Calif, 1989, San Jose State University.
APB, Abductor pollicis brevis; *APL,* abductor pollicis longus; *DIP,* distal interphalangeal; *EDC,* extensor digitorum communis; *EIP,* extensor indicis proprius; *EPB,* extensor pollicis brevis; *EPL,* extensor pollicis longus; *FDP,* flexor digitorum profundus; *FDS,* flexor digitorum superficialis; *FPB,* flexor pollicis brevis; *FPL,* flexor pollicis longus; *IP,* interphalangeal; *MP,* metacarpophalangeal; *PIP,* proximal interphalangeal.

c. Endurance: Grade for sitting tolerance by increasing the length of activity sessions.

d. Grade for sitting balance by decreasing sitting support.

e. Coordination: Requires fine coordination as performed; grade coordination by adding scored or painted designs to surface; grade to sculpture of small clay figures.

3. Criteria for activity as exercise

a. Action of joints: Movement localized to flexion and extension of MP and IP joints of index and middle fingers; CMC, MP, and IP joint of thumb.

b. Repetition of motion: The pinch and release sequence is repeated until the bowl has reached the desired height and thickness.

c. Gradable: The activity is gradable for strength and endurance.

III. Sensory analysis[32,33]

1. Check the sensory stimuli received by the person performing the activity. Include any sensory experience obtained from position, motion, materials, or equipment. Describe how sensation is received (Table 30-2).

TABLE 30-2
Sensory Analysis

Sensory Modality		How Received
Tactile	X	Touching clay and tools
Proprioceptive (joint motion and position sense)	X	Being aware of joint position and motion during pinch/release
Vestibular (balance, sense of body, head motion)	X	Maintaining posture in chair while performing activity
Visual	X	Seeing clay object, environment
Olfactory (smell)	X	Smelling a slight odor of damp clay
Pain	O	
Thermal (temperature)	X	Hands sensing coldness of clay
Pressure	X	Fingertips and thumb tips pressing against walls of clay bowl
Auditory (hearing)	O	
Other		

O, Sensory stimuli not received; *X,* sensory stimuli received.

TABLE 30-3
Cognitive Analysis

Cognitive Skill		Justification
Memory	X	Remembers instruction
Sequencing (steps in order)	X	Performs steps in order
Problem-solving skills	X	Knows what to do if clay is too wet or too dry, if walls of bowl are too thin or too thick
Following Instructions		
Spoken	X	Is able to comprehend and follow spoken instructions
Demonstrated	X	Is able to comprehend and follow demonstrated instructions
Written	O	
Concentration and attention required	X	Moderate: focuses on bowl and knows when its walls are thin enough and high enough

O, Cognitive skill note used; X, cognitive skill required in activity.

IV. Cognitive analysis[32]: Check all that apply and justify your answer (Table 30-3).

V. Safety factors: What are the potential hazards of this activity? Describe safety precautions necessary for this activity. There are few hazards in this activity. Ingesting clay or using the smoothing tool inappropriately is possible. Also, sitting balance must be adequate to maintain upright posture to perform the activity. Precautions must be taken: Adequate supervision should be provided to ensure appropriate use of clay and tool, and the task should be performed from a wheelchair with supports if sitting balance is impaired.

VI. Interpersonal aspects of activity
1. Solitary activity: May be done alone.
2. Potential for dyadic interaction: May be done in parallel with one other person but does not require interaction.
3. Potential for group interaction: May be done in a group but does not require interaction.

VII. Psychological and psychosocial factors
1. Symbolism in performer's culture[15]: May be seen as more feminine than masculine in mainstream American culture; may be associated with the artistic, liberal, naturalist groups of people in American society.
2. Symbolic meaning of activity to performer: May be seen as leisure skill rather than work: may be regarded as child's play by some persons.
3. Feelings or reactions evoked in performer during performance of activity[32]: The soft, moist, pliable, and plastic properties of the clay may evoke soothing feelings in many persons. Others may regard it as messy or dirty. Potential for personal gratification is good because attractive end product is easy to achieve; activity is creative, individualistic, and useful.

VIII. Therapeutic use of activity
1. List the autonomous goal of the activity: To make a small clay bowl.
2. List possible therapeutic objective(s) for the activity
   a. To increase pinch strength
   b. To improve coordination of opposition
   c. To increase sitting tolerance

CHAPTER 31

Orthotics

JULIE BELKIN
LYNN YASUDA

KEY TERMS

LEARNING OBJECTIVES

After studying *Section 1* the student or practitioner will be able to do the following:
1. Identify basic hand anatomy.
2. Describe the difference between single-axis and multiaxis joints, and explain how they relate to splinting.
3. Define torque, and describe how a splint produces torque.
4. Discuss the relationship of angle of approach to dynamic splinting.
5. Describe the three major purposes of splints.
6. Demonstrate an understanding of the principles of making a splint pattern.
7. Identify three characteristics of low-temperature thermoplastic material.
8. Discuss two ways in which splints may apply force.
9. Demonstrate how to determine the proper length of a forearm-based splint.

After studying *Section 2* the student or practitioner will be able to do the following:
1. List the purposes of suspension arm devices.
2. List physical disabilities with which suspension arm devices are used.
3. List the elements of adjustment and the training program for suspension arm devices.
4. Briefly describe the evolution of the mobile arm support (MAS) and name its parts.
5. List the benefits of the MAS to persons with severe upper extremity weakness.
6. List the criteria for use of the MAS and describe how it works.
7. List two special parts of the MAS.
8. Name the flexible, low-profile device that facilitates passage through doorways.

According to *Mosby's Medical, Nursing, & Allied Health Dictionary,*[1] orthotics is "the design and use of external appliances to support a paralyzed muscle, promote a specific motion, or correct musculoskeletal deformities;" an **orthosis** is "a force system designed to control, correct, or compensate for a bone deformity, deforming forces, or forces absent from the body . . . [and] often involves the use of special braces;" and a splint is "an orthopedic device for immobilization, restraint, or support of any part of the body." Both splints and suspension arm devices can be considered orthoses. Occupational therapists often design and contruct splints. An orthotist usually designs and constructs suspension arm devices, and occupational therapists adjust them and train patients to use them. In practice, the term *orthosis* is more frequently used to refer to suspension arm devices than splints. Hand splinting is the topic of Section 1 of this chapter and suspension arm devices are described in Section 2.

Section 1
Hand Splinting; Principles, Practice, and Decision Making

JULIE BELKIN

The human hand is the brain's most important instrument with which to explore and master the world. It is the only body part that can substitute for other senses. We read with our hands if we suffer a loss of vision; we communicate with our hands in the absence of speech or hearing. Our hands give us expression and console us. We first explore our hands and explore with our hands as infants. The wonder of the human hand is the precision with which it functions and the extremes of abuse it tolerates. We can and do take our hands for granted because they seem to function effortlessly— that is, until we experience some level of impairment or dysfunction.

The hand does not function independent of the whole human organism. It is connected to the brain via a complex tangle of nerves and is dependent on precise synaptic connections. The hand does not function independent of the upper extremity (UE); stability and control of the shoulder, elbow, and wrist are needed to position the hand in space. Dysfunction anywhere from the brain to the fingertips may cause impaired function of the hand.

Humans achieve mastery and independence over their environment because of the superiority of the human brain and the dexterity of the hand. Tying a knot, opening a necklace clasp, wielding a hammer, and throwing a ball are all abilities unique to the human hand. That we can close a necklace with our vision occluded is testament to the sensibility of the hand. That we can wield a hammer to drive a nail is testament to the integrity of the skin and the strength of the muscles that power the hand. That we can speak volumes with a sweep of our hands or a caressing touch is testament to the aesthetics of the hand. It is a remarkable instrument indeed.

Occupational therapists deal with the human being as a whole, not as just a hand, a toe, or a shoulder. With the human hand, even the smallest impairment may affect function. Loss of placement of the hand may mean an inability to achieve a hand-to-mouth pattern, making independent feeding impossible. Pain and fear can and do accompany injury, and when independence or livelihood is threatened by hand dysfunction, the outcomes are often dramatic. The hand is perhaps most valued only when it ceases to function and we must pay it attention.

A splint is one of the most important tools therapists use to minimize or correct impairment and to restore or augment function. Little else so readily calls attention to the hand as a splint. An individual may not receive comments on a new ring or a recent manicure, but put a splint on the hand and all will take notice. The decision to provide or fabricate a splint requires an in-depth understanding of the pathological condition to be affected and of the many splinting choices available.

Section 1 of this chapter serves as an introduction to the anatomical and biomechanical principles necessary to the understanding of the basic concepts and models of splinting. This section briefly reviews the anatomy of the hand and its relationship to principles of splinting, introduces the biomechanical principles involved in splint design and fabrication, and introduces a five-step splint fabrication process. This process involves instruction in pattern making, material choices, types of traction, and techniques of fabrication.

ROLE OF THE OCCUPATIONAL THERAPIST

The education an occupational therapist receives in the analysis of activity and the assessment of human occupation and function leads naturally to the use of splinting as one therapeutic tool in the treatment regimen. Occupational therapists most commonly fabricate splints for the hand and UE, but they also may be called on to design and fabricate splints for the lower extremity (LE) and even for the back or spine. The basic principles of splinting apply regardless of which part is being splinted.

Involvement of the occupational therapist in all phases of splint fabrication is recommended from the initial assessment of need, through the design phase, the fabrication, and the training and follow-up necessary to ensure proper use and fit of the splint. This involvement requires an understanding of the anatomy and biomechanics of the normal, unimpaired hand and of the pathology of the impaired hand. Many excellent texts describe both hand anatomy and biomechanics in extensive detail and should be included in the library of any occupational therapist treating the hand. This chapter briefly reviews the anatomy and biomechanics of the hand most pertinent to splinting. The lists of references and suggested readings at the end of this chapter provide several excellent selections for further study.

One reference of note that should be included in every therapist's library is *Clinical Mechanics of the Hand*,[3] third edition, by Paul W. Brand and Anne Hollister. This text is an excellent source for a straightforward explanation of the mechanics of muscles, joints, and skeletal structures and how they contribute to the remarkable dexterity and strength of the hand. Brand and Hollister also discuss clinical approaches and how they affect the natural biomechanics of the hand.

ANATOMICAL STRUCTURES OF THE HAND
Wrist

The hand and wrist are composed of an arrangement of 27 bones that contribute to mobility and adaptability. The wrist is a complex consisting of the distal ulna and radius and the eight carpal bones arranged in two rows. The carpal bones form the concave transverse arch and, with the configuration of the distal radius, contribute substantially to the conformability of the hand.[8] The distal ulna does not articulate with any carpal bone and its contribution to wrist stability is through the attachments of the ulnar collateral ligament, which places a check on radial deviation (Fig. 31-1).

The wrist complex allows a greater arc of motion than any other joint complex except the ankle. This mobility is a result of a unique skeletal configuration and an involved ligamentous system. All motion at the wrist is component motion occurring in more than one anatomical plane; there are no pure or isolated motions. This concept is key in any treatment directed at the wrist. Extension occurs with a degree of radial deviation and supination. Wrist flexion includes both ulnar deviation and pronation. The wrist is contiguous and continuous with the hand. The distal carpal row (the trapezium, trapezoid, capitate, and hamate) articulates firmly with the metacarpals. Motion is produced across these articulations by muscles that cross the carpals and attach to the metacarpals. The proximal carpal row (the scaphoid, lunate, and triquetrum) articulates distally with the distal carpal row and proximally with the radius and the triangular cartilage. Gliding motions occur between the carpal rows during

flexion, extension, and deviation, with excessive motion checked by the carpal ligaments.

Placement of the hand for functional tasks is reliant on the stability, mobility, and precision of placement permitted by the wrist complex. Any mechanism of injury or disease that alters this complex system translates into some level of dysfunction. Even the simplest splint that crosses the wrist will in some way alter the functional abilities of the hand. Splint designs that attempt to augment or substitute for wrist motion are likely to limit component motions or be too complex to fabricate or wear.

When static positioning of the wrist is required, the optimal degree of flexion or extension and ulnar or radial deviation will vary with the task and with the patient's preference.

Wrist Tenodesis

Tenodesis is the reciprocal motion of the wrist and fingers that occurs during active or passive wrist flexion and extension. Tenodesis is the action of wrist extension producing finger flexion and wrist flexion producing finger extension. It is caused by the lack of change in length of the long finger muscles during wrist flexion or extension (Fig. 31-2). The extrinsic finger muscle tendon units have a fixed resting length, and because they cross multiple joints before inserting onto the phalanges, they can affect the position of several joints without any contraction or length change required of the muscles. This concept is crucial to understanding

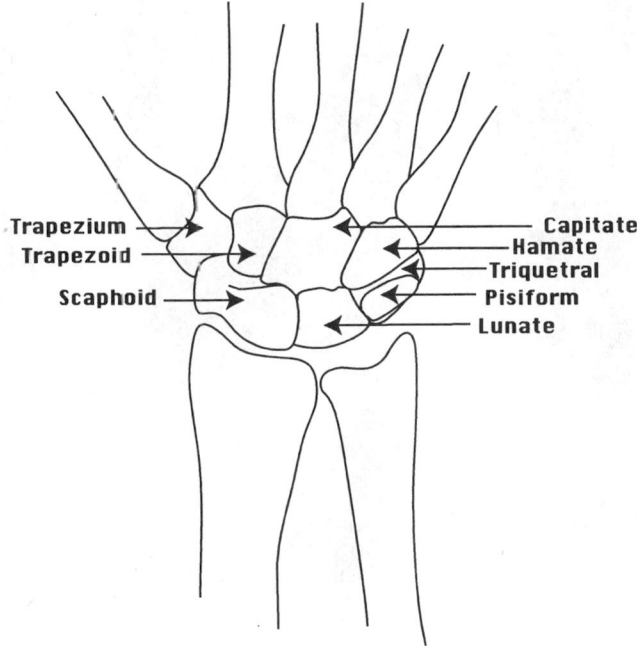

FIG. 31-1
Skeletal structures of the wrist, dorsal view.

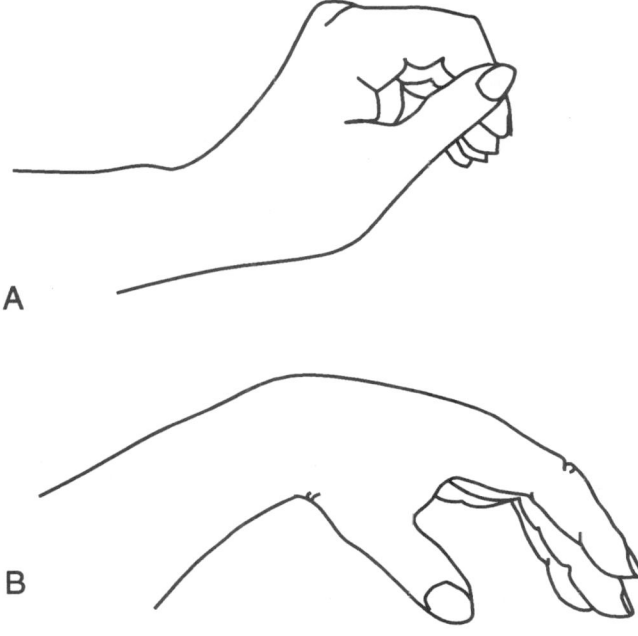

FIG. 31-2

Tenodesis. **A,** Active wrist extension results in passive finger flexion. **B,** Active wrist flexion results in passive finger extension.

how passive positioning of the wrist affects the resting position of the digits. In the nerve-injured hand, tenodesis is often harnessed by splints to provide function. The patient with spinal cord injury with sparing of a wrist extensor (C6, 7 level) gains considerable function from a tenodesis splint. In a **dynamic splint,** the effect that tenodesis has on tendon length will in part dictate the wrist position that will optimize forces directed at the digits.

Metacarpal Joints

The metacarpals articulate with the carpal bones proximally and with the phalanges distally. The first metacarpal, the thumb, articulates with the saddle-shaped trapezium and is considered separately. The second metacarpal fits into the central ridge of the trapezoid, and the third articulates firmly with the facets of the capitate. These articulations form the immobile central segment of the hand around which the other metacarpals rotate. The fourth and fifth metacarpals articulate with the concave distal surface of the hamate. The shorter length of the ulnar two metacarpals and their greater mobility form the flexible arches of the hand, allowing it to conform and fold around objects of various shapes.

The distal transverse arch of the hand lies obliquely across the metacarpal heads. This obliquity is critical to the hand's ability to adapt its shape to objects. The

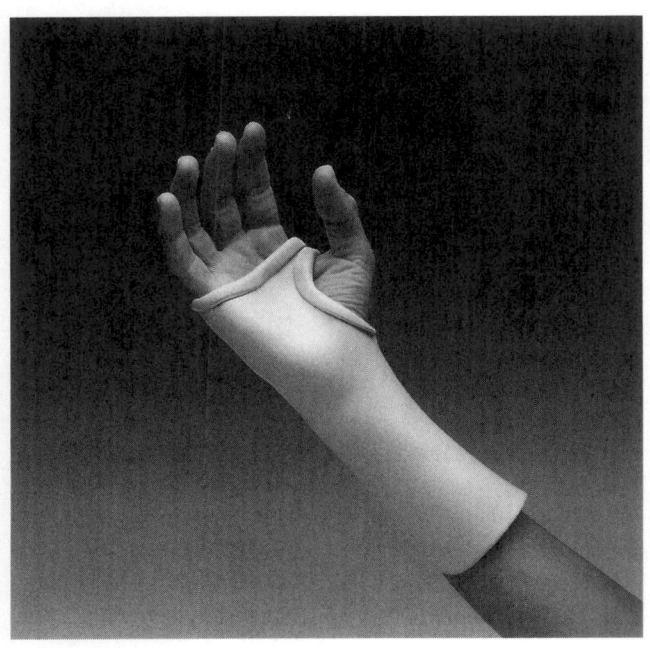

A

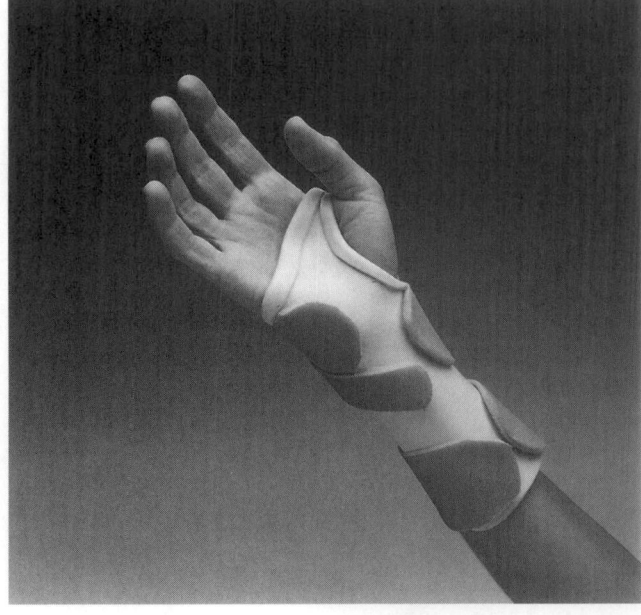

B

FIG. 31-3

A, Trim lines of splint extend distal to metacarpophalangeal creases and limit finger flexion. **B,** Splint's distal trim lines fall proximal to metacarpophalangeal creases and permit full finger flexion.

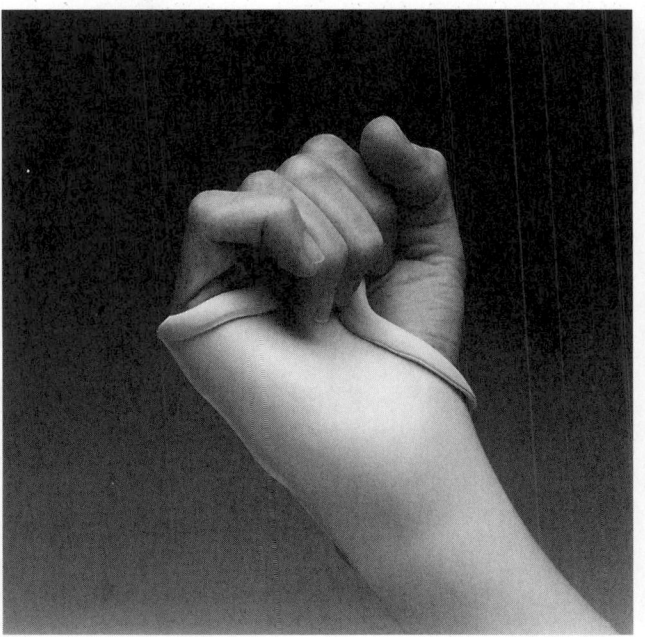
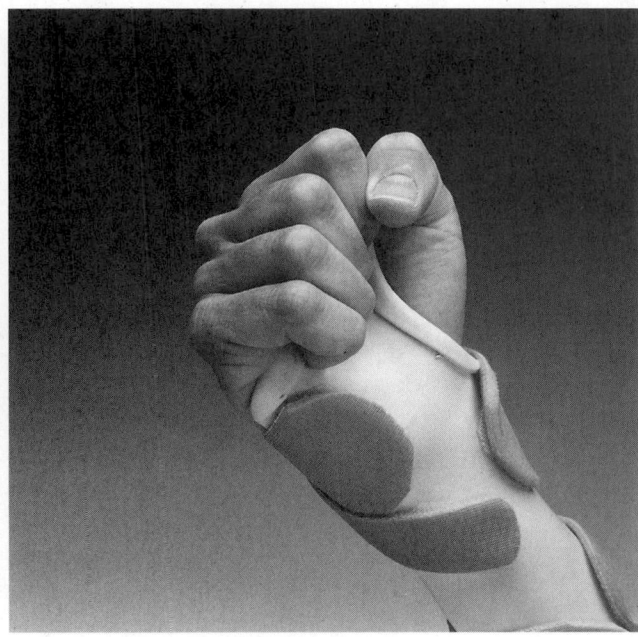

A

B

FIG. 31-4
A, Fourth and fifth digits are prevented from full flexion. **B,** Full finger flexion is possible with proper trim lines.

hand does not form a cylinder as it closes but instead assumes the position of a cone. In making a fist, the ulnar two digits of the hand contact the palm first, and the radial two digits follow. This cascade of the fingers is a direct result of the oblique angle formed at the metacarpal heads. This concept is most important in splinting in determining the distal trim lines for a wrist support when full metacarpophalangeal (MP) flexion is desired. The splint in Fig. 31-3, *A,* is improperly trimmed distal to the MP creases. Distal trim lines should be established proximal to the MP creases, as in Fig. 31-3, *B*.

Metacarpophalangeal Joints

The distal heads of the metacarpals articulate with the proximal phalanges to form the MP joints. Active motion is possible along an axis of flexion and extension and along an axis of abduction and adduction. Additionally, a small degree of rotation is present at the MP joints. These axes of motion allow for expansion or spreading of the hand and contribute to the ability of the hand to conform to different shapes and sizes of objects. An attempt to hold a softball without abducting the fingers shows the importance of this motion. A splint with trim lines along the ulnar border of the hand that extend too far distally limits both flexion and abduction of the fourth and fifth digits. As a result, the hand will have a limited ability to grasp large objects, and function will be restricted (Fig. 31-4, *A*).

Distal trim lines that fall proximal to the MP creases will allow for full MP flexion (Fig. 31-4, *B*).

Thumb

The base of the first metacarpal articulates with the trapezium to form a highly mobile joint that is often compared to the shape of a saddle. The base of the first metacarpal is concave in the anteroposterior plane and convex in the lateral plane. This surface is met by reciprocal surfaces on the trapezium. This configuration allows for a wide arc of motion, with the thumb able to rotate not only for pad-to-pad opposition but also for full extension and abduction to move away from the palm.[8] Both motions are important to function. That is, a thumb posted in permanent opposition may make grasp possible but release of objects impossible. This concept is crucial to the understanding of splints that augment the tenodesis action of the hand by posting the thumb in opposition to the index and long fingers. With such splints the therapist must carefully consider the degree of abduction and opposition in which the thumb is posted, to maximize both grasp and release.

Interphalangeal Joints

The proximal interphalangeal (PIP) and distal interphalangeal (DIP) joints are true hinge joints, with motion in only one plane. This limitation of motion ensures

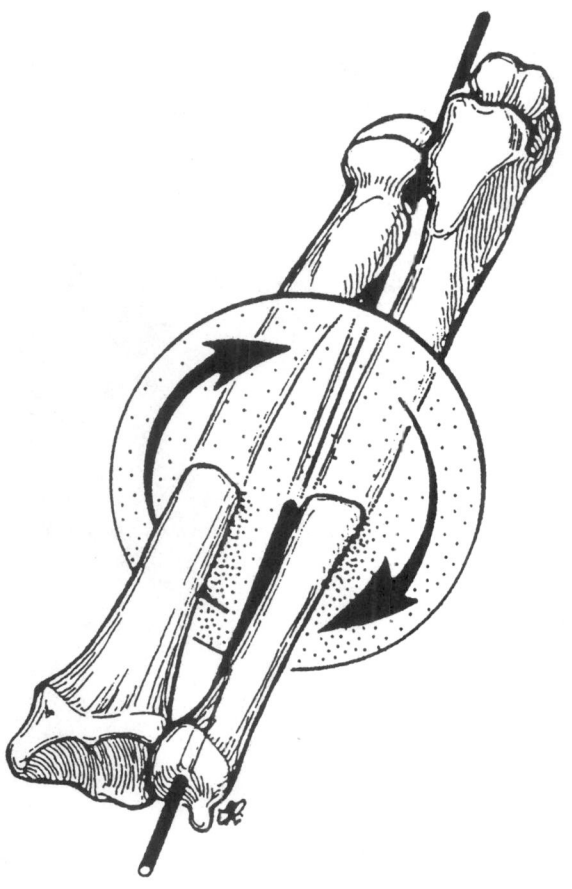

FIG. 31-5
The axis of motion for supination and pronation extends the length of the forearm and is centered through the radial head and capitulum and the distal ulnar styloid. (From Colello-Abraham K: *Rehabilitation of the hand*, ed 3, St Louis, 1990, Mosby).

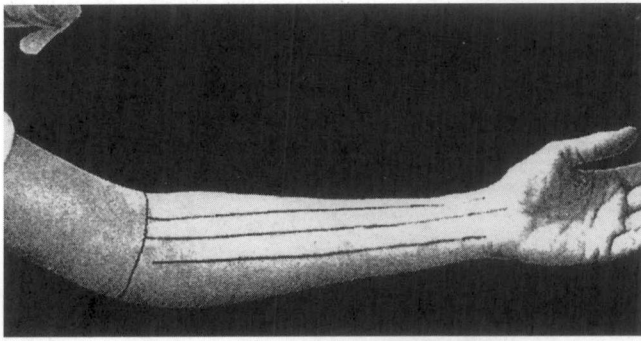

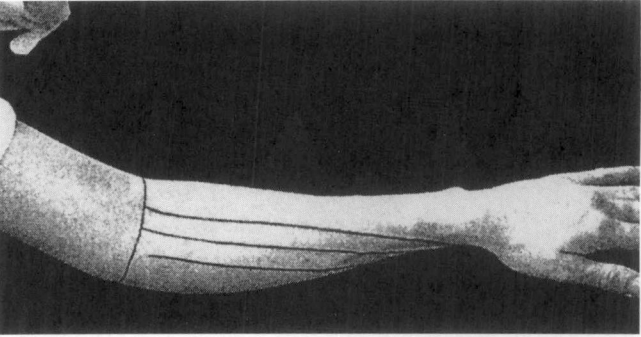

FIG. 31-6
The shape of the forearm is altered as it moves from supination to pronation. Forearm-based splints must be repositioned to accommodate this if the forearm is rotated during the fabrication process. (From Wilton JC: *Hand splinting, principles of design and fabrication*, Philadelphia, 1997, WB Saunders.)

greater stability in these joints, which contributes to their ability to resist palmar and lateral stresses and so impart strength and precision to functional tasks.

Forearm Rotation

Close consideration of forearm rotation (i.e., supination and pronation) is necessary because of the importance of these motions to function and to the fitting of splints. Forearm rotation occurs at the elbow and at the distal forearm, with axes of rotation through the center of the radial head and capitulum and along a line extending through the base of the ulnar styloid (Fig. 31-5). During pronation the ulnar styloid moves laterally as the radial styloid travels medially. During supination the opposite occurs, with the ulnar styloid moving medially. This movement results in a displacement of the styloids, which in turn alters the architecture of the forearm in supination as compared with pronation.

The way in which this change in dimensions affects splint trim lines is shown in Fig. 31-6. Lines drawn at midline along the supinated forearm shift dramatically upon pronation. Splints are generally used for function with the forearm in pronation, but they are easier to fabricate with the forearm in supination. If the forearm is not pronated before the splint material is set, the trim lines will be high on the radial border and low on the ulnar border.

One final active demonstration highlights the importance of forearm position on hand function. Place a coin of any size on a tabletop, and, holding the forearm in neutral (thumb straight up), attempt to pick up the coin. It becomes rapidly apparent that the ability to position the hand for function relies in great part on the more proximal joints of the forearm.

Ligaments of Wrist and Hand

The ligamentous structures of the hand act as checkreins for the hand and wrist, limiting extremes of motion and providing stability. The complex motions of the wrist are dependent in large part on the ligaments that restrain them, rather than on the contact surfaces between the carpals and metacarpals. Three groups of ligaments are discussed briefly to highlight their contribution to wrist stability and mobility.

The palmar ligaments include the radioscapho-capitate ligament, which contributes support to the scaphoid; the radiolunate, which supports the lunate; and the radioscapholunate ligament, which connects the scapholunate articulation with the palmar surface of the distal radius. The stability and mobility of the thumb and radial carpus depend on the integrity of these ligaments. Disruption of the ligaments results not only in instability and pain at the wrist, but also in significant dysfunction of the thumb. Splinting is frequently the treatment of choice to supply stability for pain reduction.

The radial and ulnar collateral ligaments provide dorsal stability. These capsular ligaments, along with the radiocarpal and dorsal carpal ligaments, provide carpal stability and permit range of motion (ROM). Disruption of any of these ligaments may result in pain, loss of strength, and functional impairment.

The triangular fibrocartilage complex (TFCC) includes the ligaments and the cartilaginous structures that suspend the distal radius from the distal ulna and the proximal carpus. Tears or strains in this complex are evidenced by pain and weakness with resultant loss of function in resistive tasks. The advent of new imaging techniques has made the diagnosis of TFCC tears more common, and splinting is often ordered for support and pain relief.

Metacarpophalangeal Joints

The soft-tissue structures that surround the MP joints include the joint capsule, collateral ligaments, and an anterior fibrocartilage or volar plate. The capsule covers the head of the metacarpal and is reinforced by the collateral ligaments. The collateral ligaments are configured to allow side-to-side motion when the MP is in extension and to tighten as the MP is flexed. The volar plate is attached to the base of the proximal phalanx and loosely attached to the base of the neck of the metacarpal through the joint capsule. This configuration allows for sliding of the plate proximally during MP flexion. The plate returns to its lengthened state with the MP in extension and acts as a checkrein to volar displacement of the MP joint when it is extended.

When the MPs are immobilized in extension, there is a strong tendency for secondary shortening of the lax collateral ligaments, as well as contraction and adherence of the volar plate, resulting in limited MP flexion and loss of functional grasp patterns. The commonly accepted resting position splint, which places the wrist in 25° to 35° of extension, the MP joints at 60° to 70° of flexion, and the PIP and DIP at 10° to 35° of flexion, is designed to prevent shortening and maintain the joints in midrange for optimal function. An important consideration is to ensure that the mobile fourth and

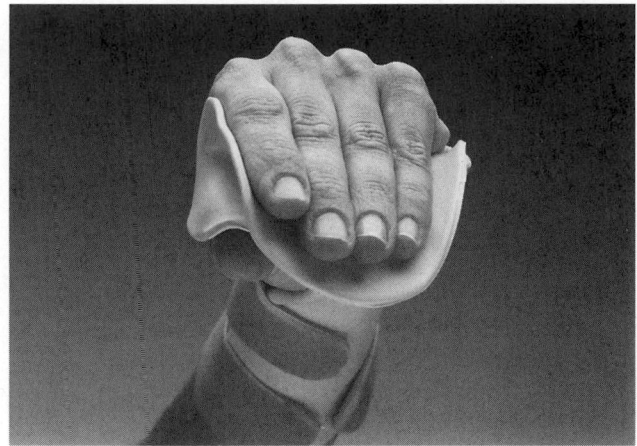

FIG. 31-7
Oblique angle of transverse arch at metacarpophalangeal joints must be accommodated to ensure maintenance of more mobile fourth and fifth digits.

fifth digits are positioned in the splint to accommodate their additional degree of mobility by allowing somewhat greater flexion at their MP joints (Fig. 31-7).

Proximal Interphalangeal Joints

The PIP joint capsule and ligaments provide stability and allow mobility in one plane only. Collateral ligaments on each side of the joint run in a dorsal-to-palmar direction, inserting into the fibrocartilage plate of the PIP. These ligaments and plate are lax with the PIP joint in flexion and taut with it in extension. The seemingly simple joint is made more complex by the inclusion of the extensor mechanism passing through the capsule dorsally and contributing slips to the system of ligaments affecting this joint. The potential for disruption of the extensor mechanism is high. Many of the most commonly fabricated finger splints are used to correct the PIP boutonniere (Fig. 31-8, A), and swan neck (Fig. 31-8, B) deformities.

Distal Interphalangeal Joints

The DIP joint capsule and ligaments are similar to the PIP joint, but with less structural strength to the terminal insertions of its palmar plate and collateral ligaments. As the structures become smaller, they lose integrity and strength. It is no wonder that one of the most frequent injuries to the digits is the disruption of the terminal end of the extensor tendon, resulting in a mallet or "baseball" finger (Fig. 31-8, C).

Muscles and Tendons of Forearm, Wrist, and Hand

Balance in the hand must be considered when the hand is assessed for a splint. Two groups of muscles act on the wrist and hand: the extrinsic muscles that arise from the

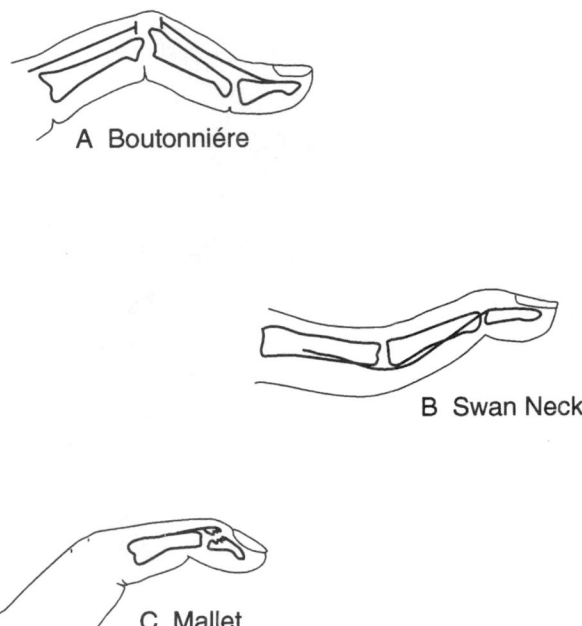

FIG. 31-8

A, Boutonniere deformity characterized by proximal interphalangeal joint flexion and distal interphalangeal joint hyperextension. **B**, Swan neck deformity with proximal interphalangeal joint hyperextension and distal interphalangeal joint flexion. **C**, Mallet deformity with distal interphalangeal joint flexion and loss of active extension.

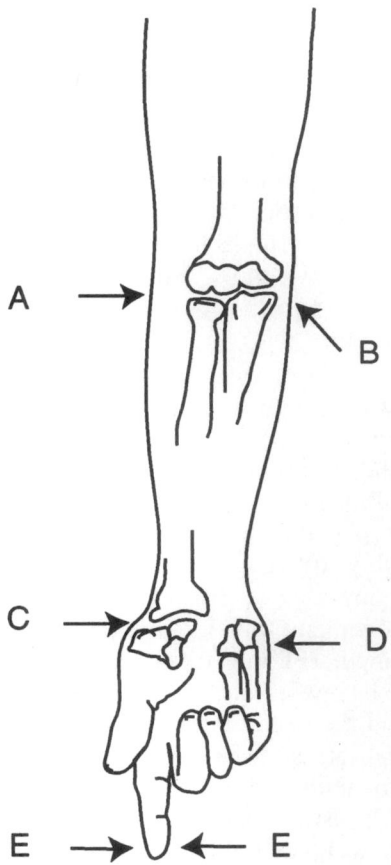

FIG. 31-9

Potential sites for nerve compression from improperly fitted splints. **A**, Radial nerve. **B**, Ulnar nerve. **C**, Radial digital nerve in anatomical snuffbox. **D**, Ulnar nerve in Guyon's canal. **E**, Digital nerves.

elbow and the proximal half of the midforearm, and the intrinsic muscles with origins and insertions entirely in the hand. The extrinsic muscles include both a flexor and extensor group acting on the wrist and on the digits. The intrinsics include the lumbricals, the dorsal and palmar interossei, and the thenar and hypothenar groups. Smooth, coordinated motions of the hand depend on a well-integrated balance between and within these two muscle groups. Many of the contractures occupational therapists are called on to correct with splinting are caused by neurological dysfunction (central or peripheral), which results in imbalance of muscle tone or innervation.

Nerve Supply

In a discussion of the nerve supply to the hand it is important to mention the continuity of the brachial plexus from its origins in the spinal cord to its terminal innervations in the hand. Injuries or compressions occurring anywhere along this continuum may result in motor or sensory dysfunction. When splinting the UE, the therapist must give attention to the pathways of the nerves supplying the UE and to the potential sites for entrapment. In the fabrication of splints, care must be taken to avoid applying pressure over sites

where the nerves are superficial and prone to compression. These sites include the ulnar nerve at the elbow and in the Guyon canal in the palm, the radial nerve at the elbow and in the thenar snuffbox, and the digital nerves along the medial and lateral borders of the digits (Fig. 31-9).

Three peripheral nerves supply the motor and sensory function to the hand (Fig. 31-10). The radial nerve is the primary motor supplier to the extensor and supinator muscles. The sensory fibers of the radial nerve supply the dorsum and radial border of the hand. The median nerve provides motor supply to the flexor-pronator group, including most of the long flexors and the muscles of the thenar eminence. The sensory distribution of the median nerve is functionally the most important because it includes the palmar surface of the thumb, index, and long fingers and the radial half of the ring finger. The ulnar nerve supplies most of the intrinsic muscles, the hypothenar muscles, the ulnarmost profundi, and the adductor pollicis brevis. The sensory supply of the ulnar nerve includes the palmar surface of

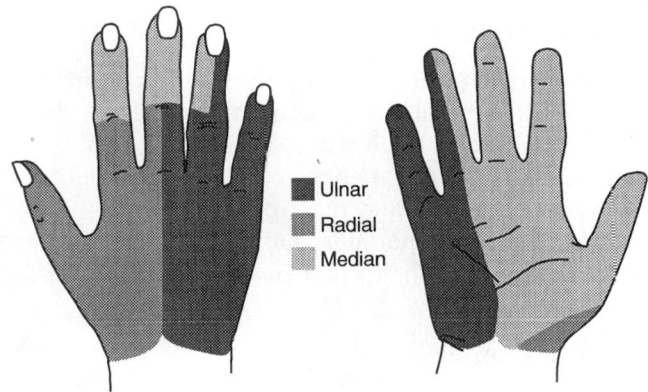

FIG. 31-10
Sensory distribution in hand. Median nerve distribution includes most of the prehensile surface of the palm.

Ulnar
Radial
Median

the ulnar half of the ring finger, the little finger, and the ulnar half of the palm.

Nerve dysfunction presents a challenge to the splint maker. Muscle imbalance leads to dysfunctional posturing of the hand and muscle atrophy that reduces the natural padding of the hand. Abrasions or ulcerations may occur in persons who do not remove their splints because they do not feel pain caused by shearing forces or pressure areas inside the splint. Finally, skin with marked sensory impairment lacks natural oils and perspiration, leading to dry skin that abrades easily. These factors must be assessed and considered carefully when splints are being fitted on persons with sensory impairment.

Splinting the neurologically impaired hand is directed at prevention of joint and soft-tissue contractures and at restoration of functional positioning. Splinting cannot restore sensibility, and care must be taken to prevent damage to sensory-impaired skin and to limit further reduction of sensory feedback by covering sensate surfaces.

Blood Supply

Blood supply to the hand is carried by the radial and ulnar arteries. The ulnar artery lies just lateral to the flexor carpi ulnaris tendon, where it divides into a large branch that forms the superficial arterial arch and a small branch that forms the lesser part of the deep palmar arch. The ulnar artery is vulnerable to trauma where it passes between the pisiform and the hamate (the canal of Guyon). The radial artery divides at the proximal wrist crease into a small, superficial branch and a larger, deep radial branch. The superficial arterial arch further divides into common digital branches and then into proper digital branches.

Venous drainage of the hand is accomplished by two sets of veins: a superficial and a deep group. Therapists are more likely to be concerned with the superficial venous system because it lies superficially in the dorsum of the hand. Disruption of this superficial system may result in extensive fluid edema in the dorsum of the hand, that requires the therapist's intervention.

Skin

The mobility of the hand is directly related to the type and condition of the skin. Anyone who has put on a ring that is slightly too small, only to be unable to remove it, has experienced the redundancy of the skin on the dorsum of the hand. The skin on the dorsum of the hand is loosely anchored to underlying structures and moves easily to allow flexion and extension of the digits. The ring "problem" occurs because of a greater degree of elasticity in the dorsal skin when it is pulled distally, as opposed to when it is pulled proximally. This fact should be considered when the use of finger splints is contemplated.

The palmar skin, by contrast, is thicker and relatively inelastic. It is firmly connected to the underlying palmar aponeurosis for stability and protection during **prehension** activities. Furthermore, the underlying fascia of the palmar skin is thicker and protects the nerve endings, while acting to supply adequate moisture and oils to the skin surface.

Superficial Anatomy and Landmarks

When fabricating a splint, therapists must consider where to apply **force** without causing further trauma. Despite its deftness and power, the hand's lack of protective fascia means that it tolerates external pressures poorly and shearing stresses not at all. The prominent ulnar styloid, the distal head of the radius at the ulnar snuffbox, and the thumb carpometacarpal joint are common sites for pressure. A truism that will always hold in splinting is that padding adds pressure. The softest padding added to a too-tight splint will only add pressure. Pressure is relieved by creation of a relief in the splint or by application of padding and material molded over the pad to make it an integral part of the splint (Fig. 31-11). Added padding to relieve pressure after the splint is formed, should be avoided.

PREHENSION AND GRASP PATTERNS

The ability of the human hand to assume myriad positions and to apply only the precise amount of pressure necessary to hold an object is a result of the mobility and stability supplied by the skeleton, the power of the muscles, and the remarkable degree of sensory feedback from the nerves. This sensory feedback is used to assess the size, shape, texture, and weight of an object. The brain then determines which type of prehension to use.

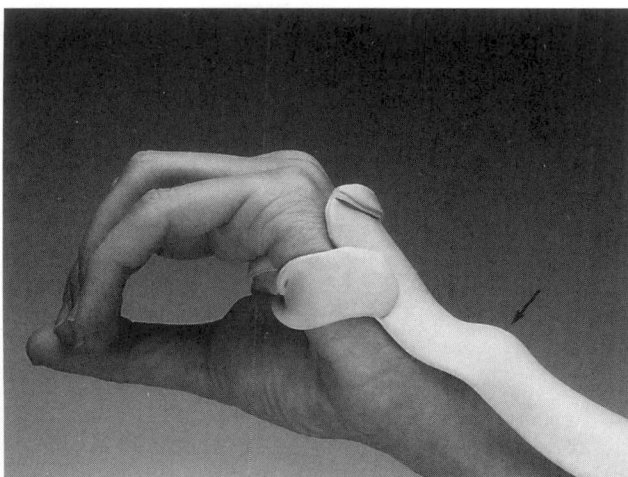

FIG. 31-11
Relief "bubbled" over the ulnar styloid accomplished by molding plastic over a pad placed on the styloid.

The feedback used in the grasping and lifting of an object is dependent both on the brain's interpreting correctly what is seen and on the hand's responding appropriately. Once an object is in the hand, further adaptation in prehension will occur if the initial visual assessment was faulty.

Splints can maximize functional prehension. In achieving this goal the therapist must be aware of what a splint can and cannot do; a splint can stabilize an unstable part, position a thumb in opposition, and even assist or substitute for lost motion. The splint maker must be aware that a splint may also limit mobility at uninvolved joints, reduce sensory feedback, add bulk to the hand, and transfer stresses to unsplinted joints proximal or distal to the part being splinted.

The prehension patterns the hand is able to achieve are as exhaustive as the objects that are available to grasp or pinch. Several authors have contributed to classifications of normal prehension, and the presentation by Flatt[5] is recommended for further study of the subject. It is possible to reduce the many patterns to two basic classifications, prehension and grasp, from which other patterns may be derived. Prehension is defined as a position of the hand that allows finger and thumb contact and facilitates manipulation of objects. Grasp is defined as a position of the hand that facilitates contact of an object against the palm and the palmar surface of the partially flexed digits.

The thumb is involved in all but one type of grip, that of hook grasp. Carpometacarpal and MP rotation is crucial to prehension and cannot be overstressed in its importance in splinting to achieve function. This rotation allows for full contact of the thumb in pad-to-pad prehension.

Lateral Prehension

In lateral prehension the pad of the thumb is positioned to contact the radial side of either the middle or distal phalanx of the index finger (Fig. 31-12). Most commonly this pattern of prehension is used in holding a pen or eating utensil and in holding and turning a key. The short or long opponens splint is used to stabilize the thumb to achieve this prehension pattern.

Palmar Prehension

Palmar prehension is also called three-jaw chuck pinch. The thumb is positioned in opposition to the index and long fingers (Fig. 31-13). The important component of motion in this pattern is thumb rotation, which allows for pad-to-pad opposition. This prehension pattern is used in lifting objects from a flat surface, in holding

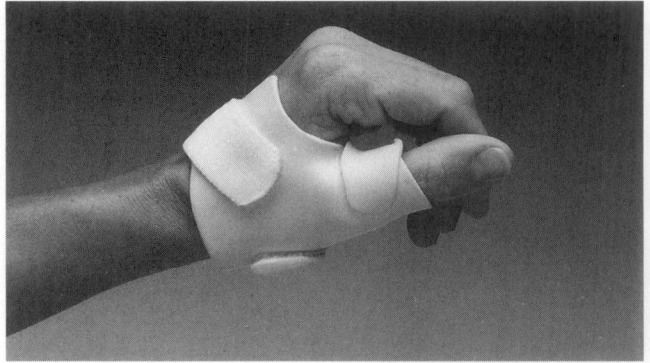

FIG. 31-12
Lateral prehension or key pinch in short opponens splint that positions thumb in lateral opposition to index finger.

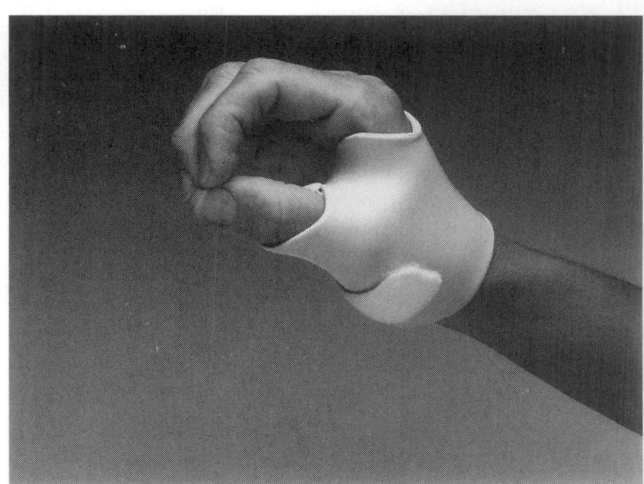

FIG. 31-13
Palmar prehension or three-jaw chuck pinch in short opponens that positions thumb in opposition to index and long fingers.

small objects, and in tying a shoe or bow. The short and long opponens splints may also be fabricated to position the thumb in palmar prehension.

Tip Prehension

In tip prehension the IP joint of the thumb and the DIP and PIP joints of the finger are flexed to facilitate tip-to-tip prehension (Fig. 31-14). These motions are necessary to pick up a pin or a coin. It is difficult to substitute for tip prehension because it is rarely a static holding posture. Once a pin is in the hand, tip prehension will convert to palmar prehension to provide more skin surface area to retain a small object. A thumb IP hyper-

extension block is useful to limit IP hyperextension and to facilitate the IP flexion required for tip prehension.

Cylindrical Grasp

Cylindrical grasp, the most common static grasp pattern, is used to stabilize objects against the palm and the fingers, with the thumb acting as an opposing force (Fig. 31-15). This pattern is assumed for grasping a hammer, pot handle, drinking glass, or the handhold on a walker or crutch. Splinting offers little to restore this grasp directly, although positioning the wrist in extension offers greater stability to the hand as it assumes this grasp pattern. A dorsal wrist stabilizer offers stability while minimizing palm coverage.

Spherical Grasp

Also called ball grasp, this pattern is assumed for holding a round object such as a ball or apple. It differs from cylindrical grasp primarily in the positioning of the fourth and fifth digits. In cylindrical grasp the two ulnar metacarpals are held in greater flexion. In spherical grasp the two ulnar digits are supported in greater extension to allow a more open hand posture (Fig. 31-16). In splinting, to facilitate or support this pattern of grasp, the wrist-stabilizing splint must be proximal to the distal palmar crease and contoured to allow for the obliquity at the fourth and fifth metacarpal heads.

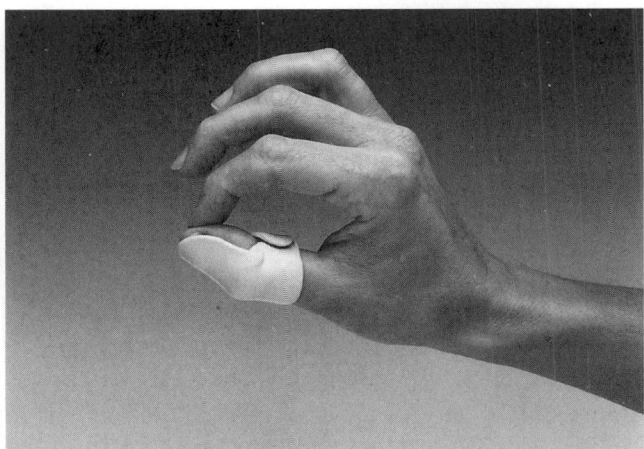

FIG. 31-14
Tip prehension with thumb and index finger in interphalangeal blocker that secures interphalangeal joint in slight flexion to assist tip prehension.

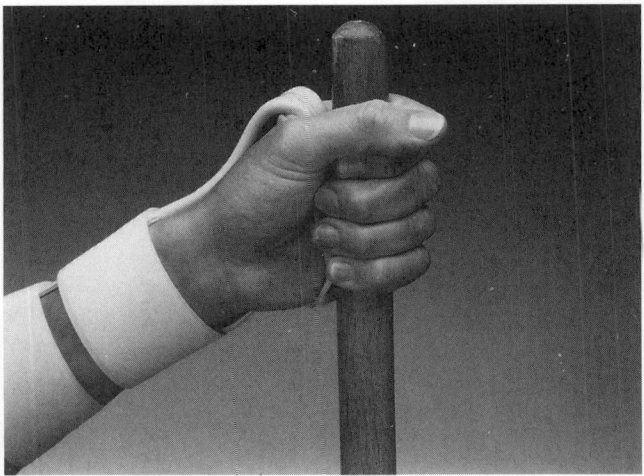

FIG. 31-15
Cylindrical grasp in dorsal splint that stabilizes wrist to increase grip force and minimizes palm covering.

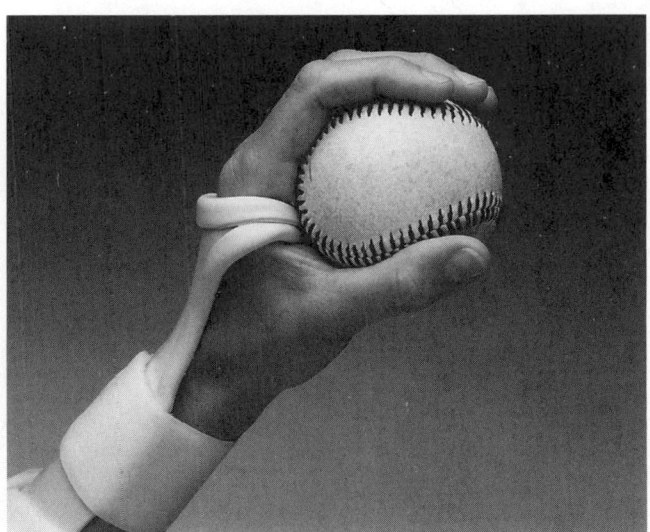

FIG. 31-16
Spherical grasp in dorsal splint. Splint stabilizes wrist to increase grip force and permits metacarpal mobility required for spherical grasp.

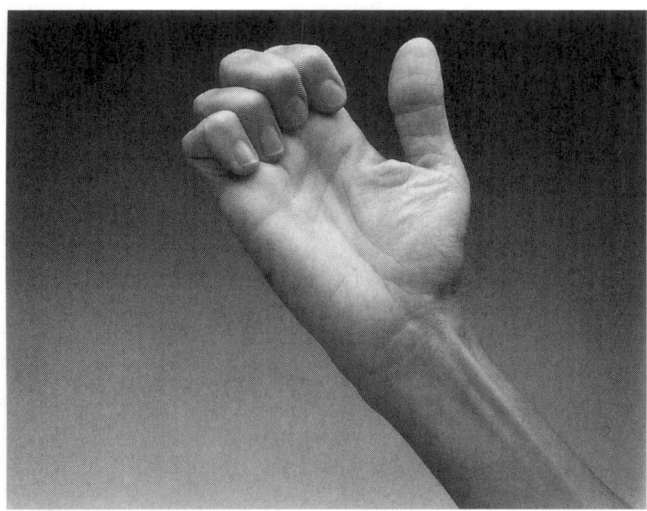

FIG. 31-17
Hook grasp does not involve thumb. Grasp pattern is seen in median and ulnar neuropathy; splinting is aimed at correcting rather than augmenting grasp.

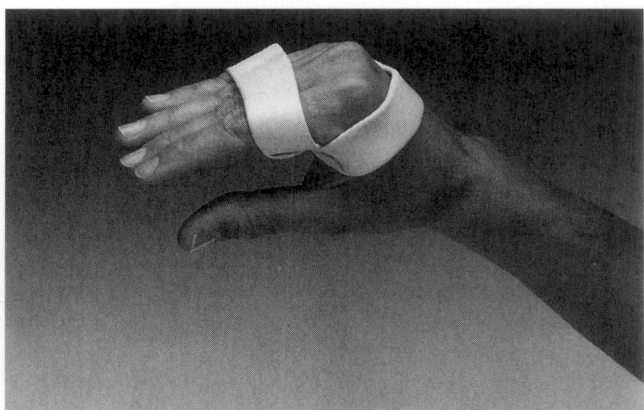

FIG. 31-18
Figure-eight splint substitutes for loss of intrinsic function with median and ulnar neuropathy.

Hook Grasp

Hook grasp is the only prehension pattern that does not include the thumb to supply opposition. The MPs are held in extension, and the DIP and PIP joints are held in flexion (Fig. 31-17). This is the attitude the hand assumes when holding the handle of a shopping bag, a pail, or a briefcase. In the nerve-injured hand, splinting is more commonly directed at correcting this posture than at facilitating it.

Intrinsic Plus Grasp

Intrinsic plus grasp is characterized by the positioning of all the MPs of the fingers in flexion, the DIP and PIP joints in full extension, and the thumb in opposition to the third and fourth fingers (Fig. 31-18). This pattern is used in grasping and holding large, flat objects such as books or plates. Intrinsic plus grasp is often lost in the presence of median or ulnar nerve dysfunction, and a figure-eight or dynamic MP flexion splint is used for substitution.

MECHANICS OF THE HAND AND PRINCIPLES OF SPLINTING

McCollough and Sarrafian[7] stated that the three basic motor functions of the upper limb are "prehension and release, transfer of objects in space, and manipulation of objects within the grasp."[9] These functions depend on the structural integrity of the skeleton, the muscles that provide power, and feedback to which the brain responds when enabling the limb to meet functional demands. The task of restoring any one of these basic

functions through the application of a splint is complex and relies on an understanding of the biomechanics of the hand and the mechanics involved in splinting. It is beyond the scope of this chapter to present this topic in depth. Presented here is an introduction to those tenets of clinical mechanics deemed necessary for the beginning splint maker.

Mechanics deals with the application of force, and biomechanics may be viewed as the body's response to those forces. In the hand the force required for producing motion is supplied by muscles. The force is then transmitted by the tendons to the bones and joints, with control supplied by the skin and pulp of the fingers and palm.[6] How the application of a splint affects the transmission of force to produce motion depends on the relationship between the axis of rotation of joints and anatomical planes and the forces imposed on the hand.

Axis of Motion

Hollister and Giurintano[6] define **axis of motion** as a stable line that does not move when the bones of a joint move in relation to each other (Fig. 31-19). This stable line is illustrated by Fig. 31-19, *B*, which shows a tire perfectly balanced around its axis of motion. When a tire is perfectly balanced, it does not wobble; it has pure motion around a single point.

In a single-axis joint, motion occurs in only one plane. The PIP joint is an example of a single-axis joint in alignment with an anatomical plane. It moves only in the plane of flexion and extension.

Joints that have more than one axis of motion may move in more than one plane at a time. For example, the wrist complex has two axes of motion: flexion-extension and radial-ulnar deviation. A joint with multiple axes has conjoint motions that occur in addition to the primary motions described by the joint. Wrist flexion occurs with a moment of ulnar deviation and with a small degree of pronation. Wrist extension occurs with radial deviation and slight supination. These conjunct motions are what make circumduction of the wrist possible. They are also what makes splinting the wrist with hinged joints a challenge.

A splint with a movable hinge or coil has a single axis. When used to splint a single-axis joint such as a PIP joint, a hinge can and should be properly aligned to avoid binding that will limit motion. If a single-axis hinge or coil is used to reproduce motion in a multiaxis joint, there will always be some binding or **friction**, no matter how well aligned, because the hinge or coil does not allow for, or reproduce, the conjunct motions available in the unsplinted joint.

Force

It is crucial to understand basic principles of force and apply them correctly in splinting. An understanding of the forces applied by levers and the stresses that occur between opposing surfaces can help explain what

A

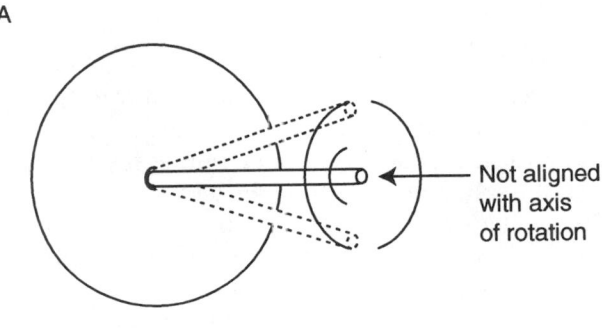

Not aligned with axis of rotation

B

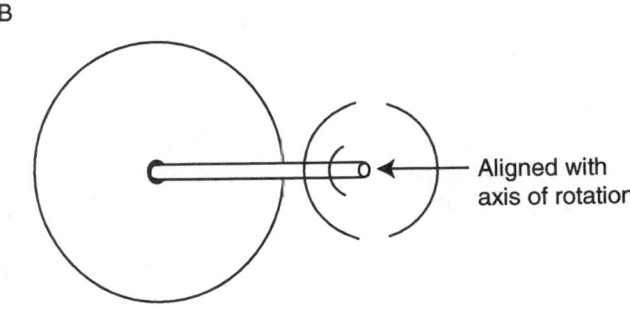

Aligned with axis of rotation

FIG. 31-19

A, If a tire is not balanced around its axis, it wobbles. If a splint hinge is not aligned with joint axis, wobble is seen as binding of joint. **B,** Proper alignment of a tire or of a hinge with anatomical joint results in smooth, unimpeded motion.

happens as forces are applied within the body by muscles and externally by splints.

Definitions

The use of the term **force**, as it relates to splinting, describes the effect materials and dynamic components have on bone and tissue. Force is a measure of stress, friction, or **torque**. Stress is resistance to any force that strains or deforms tissue. Shear stress occurs when force is applied to tissues at an angle or in opposing directions. Pinching skin between the surface of a splint and the underlying bony structures causes shear stress.

Friction occurs when one surface impedes or prevents gliding of a surface on another. Friction is produced in the stiff or contracted joint when soft-tissue restriction prevents gliding of the bones. Splints may contribute to friction if they are misaligned in relation to a joint axis. For example, a hinged splint that is not properly aligned with the axis of rotation will limit motion by producing friction as the joint attempts to move.

Torque is a measure of the force that results in rotation of a lever around an axis. The torque created when a lever rotates depends on the force used and the length of the lever employed. In the body, muscles are the levers that create torque when they act to move a joint. Externally, splints may act as levers to apply the force necessary to move a bone around its axis. The measure of torque is given by the formula:

Torque = (amount of) Force × (length of) Lever arm

Internally, the length of the lever arm is measured as the perpendicular distance from the axis of the joint to the tendon. Externally, the length of the lever arm is measured as the estimated distance from the joint axis to the attachment of force. In splinting, the attachment point of the force is usually a soft or molded cuff. If the splint includes an outrigger with a finger cuff, as shown in Fig. 31-20, the lever arm is the distance from the axis of the joint to the finger cuff, as indicated in line M.

It can be seen in the illustration in Fig. 31-20 that the angle of approach of the force to the finger also affects the length of the lever arm and ultimately the torque applied. The angle of approach is the angle that the line of traction makes as it meets the part being splinted. When the angle of approach is at a right angle (90°) to the long axis of the phalanx, the lever arm is M. When the cuff is at less than 90° to the long axis of the phalanx, the lever arm is shortened to M1. This shorter lever arm will produce less torque and therefore less rotation unless greater force is applied.

Given an equal amount of resistance or load, a 2-foot lever will require half as much force to create motion around an axis as will a 1-foot lever. The important principle for splint makers is that the greater the distance between the attachment of the cuff or strap to the joint axis, the less the force required to achieve motion.

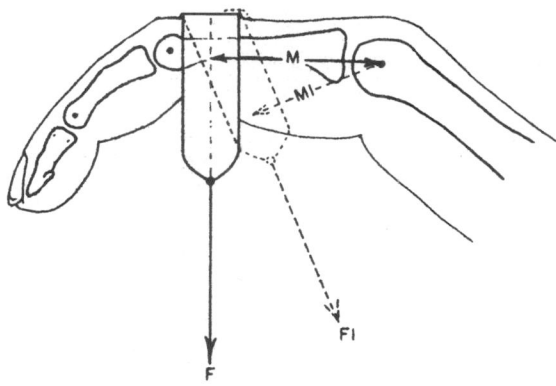

FIG. 31-20
Tension *F* on the phalanx has a moment arm of *M* acting on the joint. Tension *F1* has a smaller moment arm, *M1*, (with less resulting torque) when the angle of approach is not 90°. (From Brand PW, Hollister A: *Clinical mechanics of the hand*, ed 2, St Louis, 1993, Mosby).

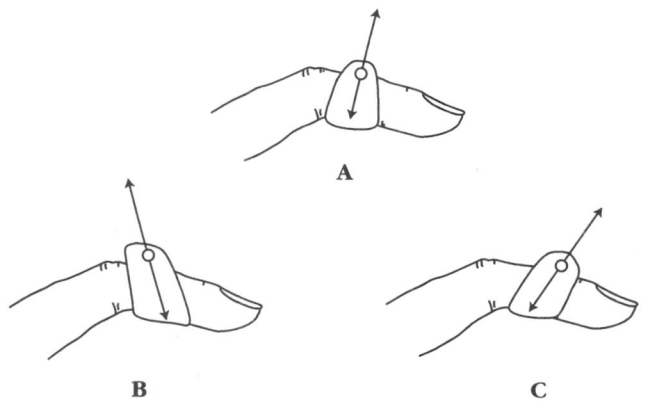

FIG. 31-21
A, Angle of approach is 90° to middle phalanx, ensuring force pulling proximal interphalangeal joint in to extension is not dissipated. **B**, Angle of approach less than 90° to middle phalanx causes joint compression. **C**, Angle of approach greater than 90° distracts joint.

Translational Forces

In addition to the angle of approach affecting the length of the lever arm, an approach of less than or greater than 90° results in **translational forces**. The outrigger splint in Fig. 31-21, *A*, shows a 90° angle of approach between the nylon line and the phalanx, producing only rotation around the axis of the joint.

When force is applied at any angle other than 90°, translational forces are created. This alteration of the angle of approach translates some of the rotational force away from producing joint extension and directs the force into joint compression or joint distraction (Fig. 31-21, *B* and *C*). The greater the deviation from 90°, the greater the translational force. Depending on the type of splint and the condition of the joint, the

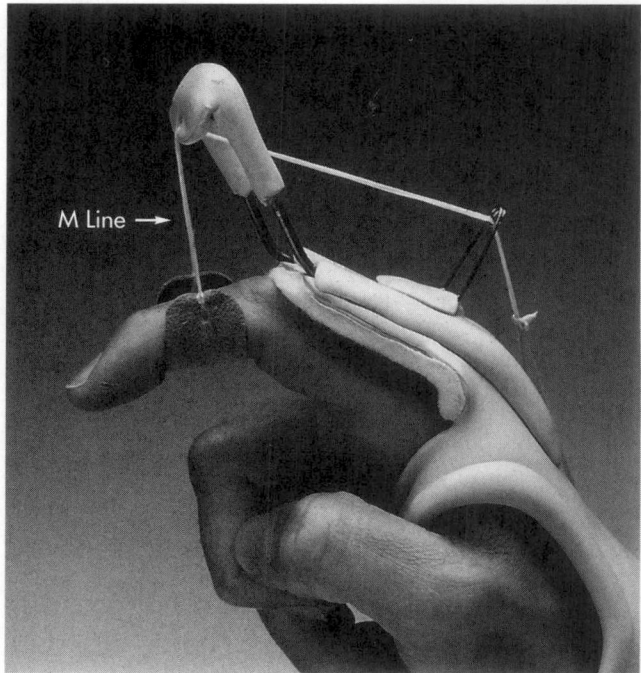

FIG. 31-22
As dynamic traction acts on range of motion at the proximal interphalangeal joint, splint must be adjusted to maintain 90° angle of approach.

joint compression or distraction may lead to mere discomfort or to actual joint damage. Translational force also is undesirable because it undermines the effectiveness of the splint by shortening the lever arm.[3]

The challenge in splinting with an outrigger is to position the splint so there is a 90° angle of approach. In the outrigger in Fig. 31-22, as long as the finger does not move, the 90° angle will remain. As soon as the finger moves, however, the 90° angle changes. Since few outriggers allow for this automatic readjustment in position, it is important to adjust the outrigger as the contracture lessens in order to maintain the 90° angle of approach.

SPLINT CLASSIFICATIONS

Splints may be described in a number of ways. Terminology varies, and it is useful to understand some of the ways splints may be described. For purposes of clarity, splint classifications are described here according to type, purpose, and design.

One reference to be considered when discussing classification is the *Splint Classification System* (SCS)[1] published by The American Society of Hand Therapists (ASHT). The SCS describes splint nomenclature based on the functional requirement of a splint, as well as on the anatomy affected. This nomenclature is quite inclusive of the broad variety of UE splints fabricated by occupational therapists and is suggested for study.

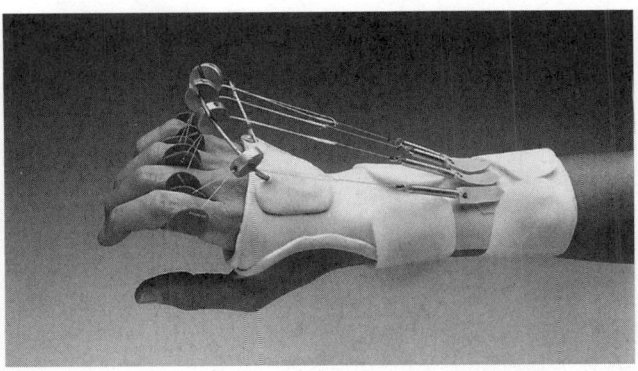

FIG. 31-23
Forearm-based four-digit outrigger with dynamic extension assist supplied by springs.

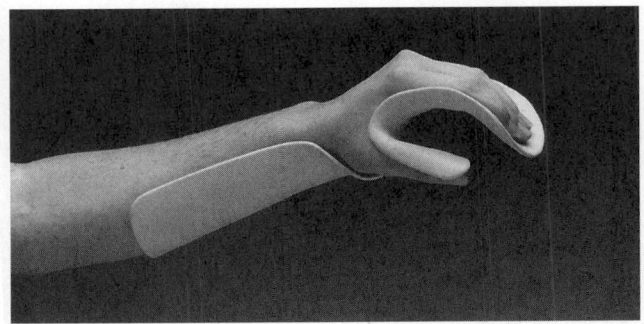

FIG. 31-24
Single-surface static resting splint positions hand in 20° to 30° wrist extension, 45° to 60° metacarpophalangeal flexion, and 15° to 30° proximal interphalangeal and distal interphalangeal flexion.

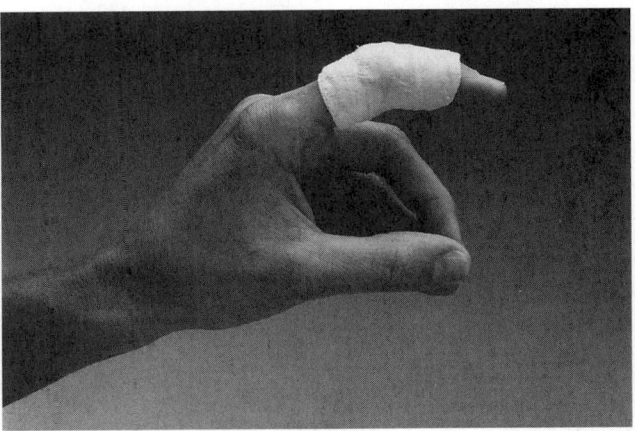

FIG. 31-25
A series of cylindrical plaster casts is made to reduce flexion contracture at proximal interphalangeal joint.

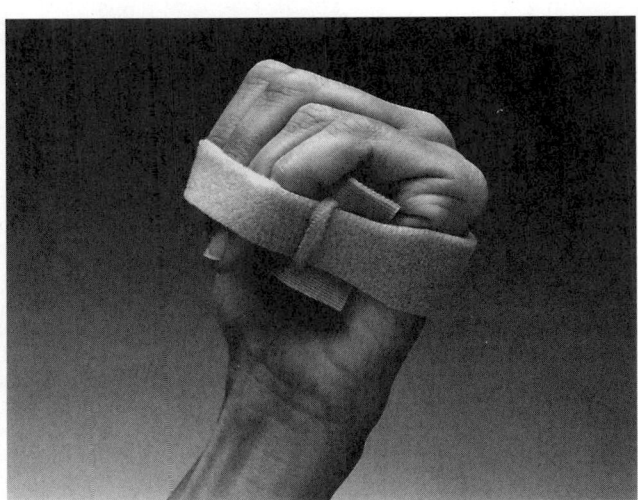

FIG. 31-26
Static progressive web strap adjusts with hook closure. Patient is taught to adjust strap as tolerance permits.

Splints Classified by Type

Dynamic splints include one or more resilient components (elastics, rubber bands, or springs) that produce motion. The force applied from the resilient component is constant even when tissues have reached end range. Dynamic splints are designed to increase passive motion, to augment active motion by assisting a joint through its range, or to substitute for lost motion. Dynamic splints generally include a static base on which to attach the movable, resilient components (Fig. 31-23).

A *static splint* has no movable components and immobilizes a joint or part. Static splints are fabricated to rest or protect, to reduce pain, or to prevent muscle shortening or contracture. An example of a static splint is a resting pan splint that maintains the hand in a functional or resting position (Fig. 31-24).

A **serial static** splint achieves a slow, progressive increase in ROM by repeated remolding of the splint or cast. The serial static splint has no movable or resilient components, but rather is a static splint whose design and material allow repeated remoldings. Each adjust-

ment repositions the part at the end of the available range to progressively gain passive motion. A cylindrical cast designed to reduce a PIP joint flexion contracture through frequent removal and recasting is a classic example of a serial static splint (Fig. 31-25).

Static progressive splints include a static mechanism that adjusts the amount or angle of traction acting on a part. This mechanism may be a turnbuckle, cloth strap, nylon line, or buckle. The static progressive splint is distinguished from the dynamic splint by its lack of a resilient force. It is distinguished from a serial static splint in having a built-in adjustment mechanism so that the part can be repositioned at end range without the need to remold the splint. Generally the static progressive mechanism can be adjusted by the patient as prescribed or as tolerated (Fig. 31-26).

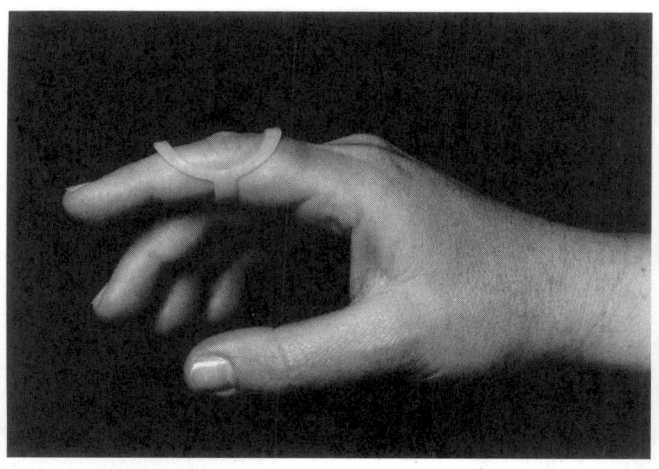

A

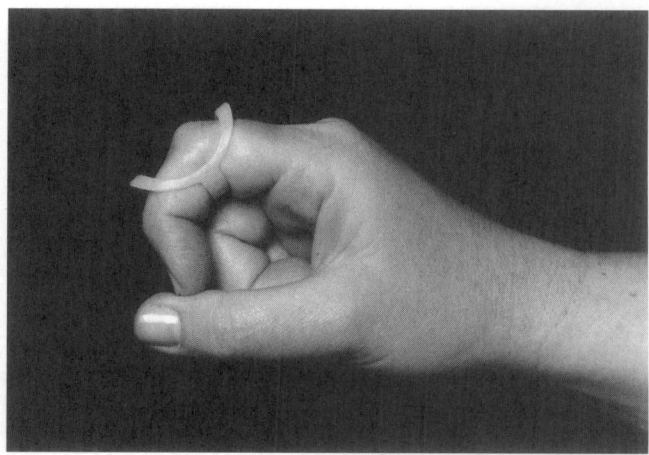

B

FIG. 31-27
Oval-8 ring splints. **A**, Ring splint restricts proximal interphalangeal joint hyperextension. **B**, Ring splint allows full flexion.

Splints Classified by Purpose

Though nomenclatures may vary, the categories presented in the splint classification system (SCS) describe splints in functional rather than in design terms.[1] The SCS describes three overriding purposes of splints: restriction, immobilization, and mobilization. The publication also lists many functions of splints, each of which is placed in one of three categories. Splints may fulfill more than one function or purpose, depending on the method of fabrication and the problems they address.

Restrictive Splints

Restrictive splints limit joint ROM but do not completely stop joint motion. One example is the splint in Fig. 31-27 that blocks PIP joint hyperextension while allowing unlimited PIP joint flexion. Semiflexible splints are available that limit motion at the extremes of range but allow motion in the middle of range. Although the splint may be restrictive, the goal or function of the splint may vary.

Immobilizing Splints

Immobilizing splints may be fit for protection to prevent injury, for rest to reduce inflammation or pain, or for positioning to facilitate proper healing after surgery. The classic example is the resting pan splint (see Fig. 31-24) that serves two of the three functions. A resting splint fit for a patient after a cerebrovascular accident (CVA) positions the wrist and digits to prevent contractures and can protect the desensate hand against damage.

Mobilizing Splints

Mobilizing splints are designed to increase limited ROM or to restore or augment function. A mobilizing splint may assist a weak muscle or substitute for motion

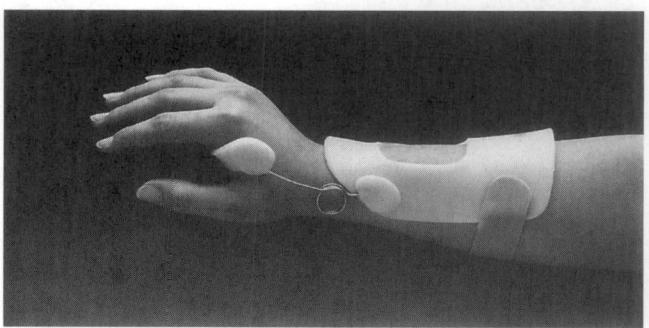

FIG. 31-28
Spring coil splint substitutes for absent wrist extension in radial nerve injury.

lost because of nerve injury or muscle dysfunction (Fig. 31-28). The splint may attempt to balance the pull of unopposed spastic muscles to prevent deformity, as well as to assist function. A splint may resist a weak muscle to improve its strength or to facilitate tendon gliding after tendon surgery. Frequently, a mobilizing splint is used to increase the ROM of a contracted joint.

Splints Classified by Design

After the purpose of the splint has been determined, the next decision relates to its design. Each of the types of splints described earlier (static, dynamic, serial static, and static progressive) may be fabricated as a single surface design, a circumferential design, or a three-point design. A final category, the loop design, is generally limited to acting on finger IP joints by providing a loop of material that wraps around the joints to restore the final degrees of joint flexion.

All splints are designed to provide some degree of force. That force may be distributed as a continuous

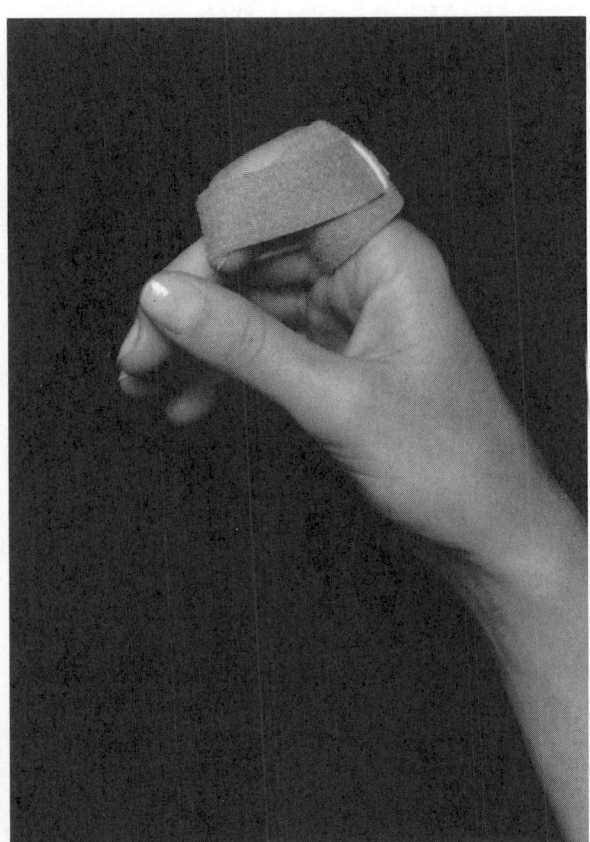

FIG. 31-29
Final flexion strap designed to restore full interphalangeal joint flexion provides equal force on all surfaces of the digit.

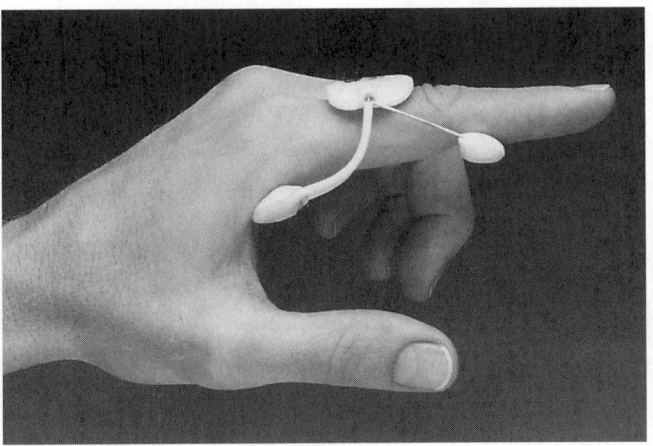

FIG. 31-30
Three-point pressure splint with spring wire reduces proximal interphalangeal joint flexion contractures of 35° or less.

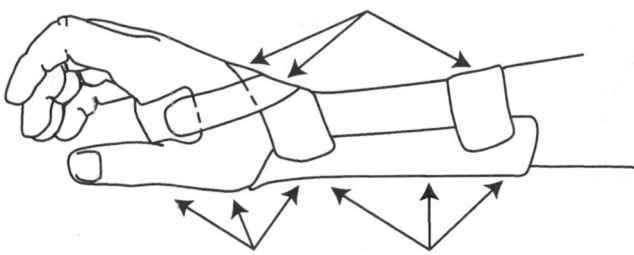

FIG. 31-31
Single-surface splint requires properly placed straps to create three-point pressure systems to secure splint and ensure distribution of pressure.

loop, with equal and opposing forces wrapping around two or more joints (Fig. 31-29). More commonly the force is applied through three points of pressure (Fig. 31-30). Although the loop design is generally used only on finger IP joints, some variation of the three-point pressure design is used in all other splints.

Three-point finger splints that incorporate springs, spring wire, or elastics are often used to correct DIP and PIP joint flexion contractures. A flexion contracture exists when a joint will not move passively out of a closed position into extension. These designs include two points of pressure, one proximal to the joint and one distal, and the third or central opposing force acting directly over or close to the joint, as in Fig. 31-30. In a three-point finger splint the force of the central point is equal to the sum of the two forces of the correcting points. This fact is clinically important because tissue tolerance under this central point may be insufficient and may react with pain and inflammation. This problem is seen frequently at the PIP joint where there is limited surface area over which to distribute pressure. It is important to distribute pressure with contoured surfaces that are as broad as possible and to adjust the spring or elastic force and the wearing time to tolerance. Proper padding incorporated into the splint can also aid in distributing pressure.

The dynamic finger-based three-point splint just described is a unique design that does not adhere to the 90° rule. That is, when the splint is applied to a joint with a flexion contracture, the angle of approach of the line of traction is never 90°. The more severe the contracture, the more translational force is present; therefore it is less effective than a properly contoured outrigger splint that adheres to the 90° rule. This design should be fitted only in the presence of IP joint flexion contractures of 35° or less. For finger contractures in excess of 35° a hand- or forearm-based outrigger splint is recommended because it can be positioned to apply force at a 90° angle of attack. Alternatively, a conforming, serial static splint can be used, as described in the section on traction.

Single-Surface or Circumferential Design

If a molded splint is to be fabricated, the next decision is whether to use a circumferential or single-surface design. Single-surface splints are fabricated to cover only one surface, either the palmar or dorsal surface of a limb or the ulnar or radial half of the hand or forearm. Straps are added to create the three points of pressure necessary to secure the splint (Fig. 31-31).

Circumferential splints wrap around a part, covering all surfaces with equal amounts of pressure (Fig. 31-32). Straps are used solely to close the splint or to create an overlap. Thinner materials can be employed in molding a circumferential splint, since the increased contours in the material add to the splint's rigidity. That contours add strength to materials is clearly seen when corrugations that create contours are added to paper to increase strength. Circumferential splints then can be made lighter and out of highly perforated materials for air circulation without a sacrifice of control.

Indications for Single-Surface Splinting

Single-surface splinting is effective for supporting joints surrounded by weak or flaccid muscles, such as following a CVA or peripheral nerve injury. Because little or no active motion is available, the extra control given by circumferential splinting is not needed, and donning and doffing the splint will be easier. A single-surface splint is also effective as the base for attaching outriggers in dynamic splinting and for postoperative splints in which the fabrication of a circumferential splint may damage repaired structures.

Indications for Circumferential Splinting

Circumferential splinting is effective for immobilizing painful joints or for protecting soft tissue (Fig. 31-32). Because the circumferential design gives comfortable, complete control, it is particularly helpful when the patient has active motion and will be wearing the splint during activity, when shear forces can be a problem. This comfortable, complete control also makes a circumferential design useful for serial **static splints** used to reduce contractures. The control a circumferential design supplies also makes it a good design for stabilizing proximal joints when outriggers are applied to act on more distal joints.

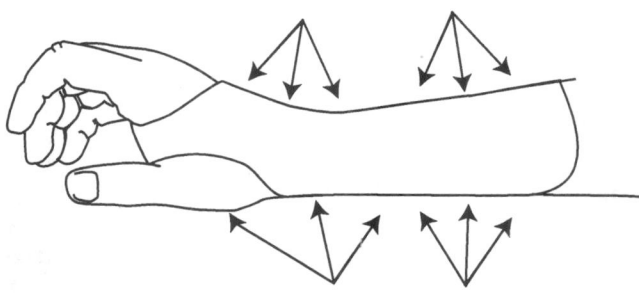

FIG. 31-32
Circumferential splints create multiple three-point pressure systems to secure splint for immobilization.

WHEN TO SPLINT AND WHEN NOT TO SPLINT

A first step in deciding which splint style and design to choose is determining if the patient is a good candidate for wearing a splint. Several issues should be examined in this regard.

Compliance Issues

First, the therapist must consider whether the patient is likely to comply with the splinting program. The splint may have a negative effect on the patient's ability to be independent in self-care or to function at work. Some patients are extremely sensitive about their appearance and refuse to wear a splint if it offends their aesthetic sense. Compliance with a splinting program may be poor if the patient's general level of motivation to get better is low. On the other hand, some patients are so highly motivated that they will overdo the splinting program and cause themselves damage. Finally, the patient's cognitive and perceptual ability to follow a splinting program should be considered, especially if there is no responsible caretaker.

Ability to Don and Doff a Splint

Even if compliance is not an issue, there may be problems with the patient's donning and doffing (putting on and removing) the splint. For example, the patient may have no one at home to assist in donning and doffing a difficult splint. The hospitalized patient may not have adequate staff for help with following the wearing schedule or applying the splint correctly.

Skin Tolerance and Hypersensitivity

The therapist must assess the skin condition of the patient before deciding to fit a splint. If the patient suffers from brain or spinal cord damage, he or she may be diaphoretic and produce excessive perspiration, that can lead to rapid skin maceration. Some patients are intolerant of any pressure because of extremely thin and fragile skin. Patients with sensory dysfunction may be hypersensitive and unable to tolerate many hard or even soft splints. If any of these issues exist and cannot be ameliorated, safe alternative therapeutic interventions must be substituted for the splint.

Wearing Schedule

If none of the preceding issues prevents the patient from being a candidate for splinting, the therapist must decide on the best wearing schedule for the splint. Nighttime may be the optimal time for the patient to wear a static splint designed to change ROM. It is also the time when patients need resting splints to prevent them from sleeping in positions that damage the hand. During the daytime the patient may wear a dynamic splint or a splint designed to assist function. It is often best to minimize splinting during the day if possible, so that the patient can use his or her hand as normally as possible.

SPLINT FABRICATION PROCESS
Step One—Creating A Pattern

Once the decision has been reached to fabricate a splint, arguably the most important step in the fabrication process is deciding on and creating a pattern. Although it may seem elementary even to the novice splint maker, this step can determine the success of the splint in terms of both fit and function. Allowing the time to make a well-thought-out and properly fitted pattern gives the splint maker the chance to deal with such issues as what he or she is trying to accomplish with the splint, why the splint is being made, and how and where that splint is going to fit. Ultimately a properly fitted pattern will make the entire fabrication process easier and faster and will increase the chance of success.

The process of making a pattern involves an understanding of the geometry of the hand and the materials to be used, as well as a bit of old-fashioned dressmaking. Understanding how positional changes alter length and how depth and width relate to the pattern is paramount to success.

The common technique of making a pattern starts with a tracing or outline of the hand. This is generally taken with the hand lying flat when possible, or by tracing the uninvolved hand if necessary. An amount is added to this outline to approximate the width and length needed for the splint. A common error in this technique is not taking into account the position in which the hand (or other body part) will ultimately be held in the splint.

Fig. 31-33, *A* and *B*, shows a pattern taken with the hand lying flat, without adding any length to the pattern. In Fig. 31-34, when the pattern is fit on the volar surface of the hand with the hand in functional position (the wrist in 35° of extension, the MP joints at 70° of flexion, and the IP joints in 10° to 20° of flexion), the pattern extends beyond the fingertips and is in fact too long. The same pattern on the dorsum of the hand (Fig. 31-35) with the wrist now in flexion illustrates that the pattern is now too short. Going from the volar surface of the hand to the dorsal surface is akin to driving around the inside of a curve as opposed to the outside of a curve. As any race car driver knows, the inside of a curve is the shorter distance. Altering the position of the hand and altering the surface to which the splint will be fit alters the length of the pattern. The splint maker must accommodate for this

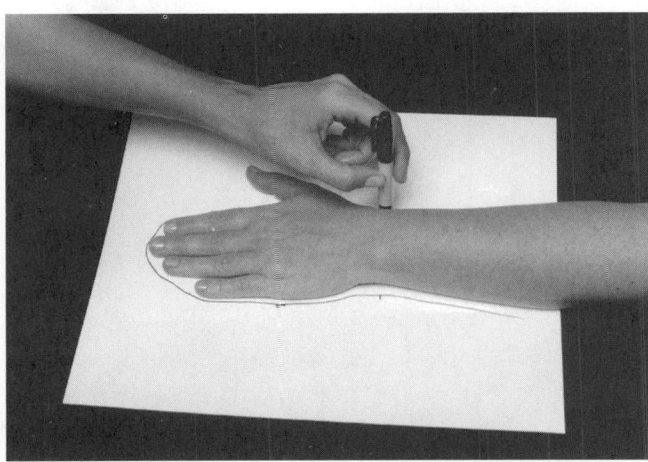

A

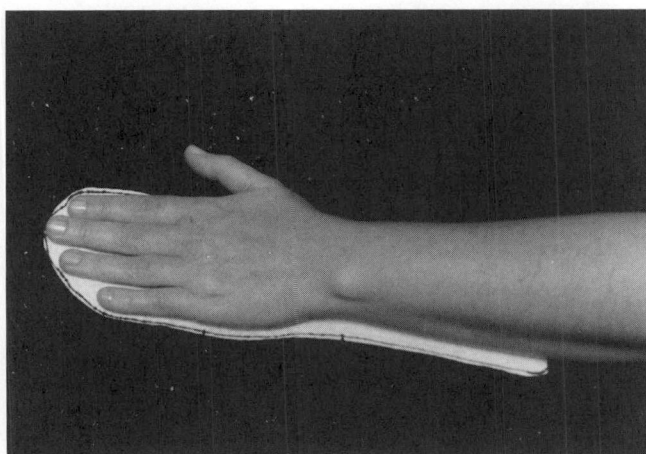

B

FIG. 31-33
A, Tracing with pencil perpendicular to arm creates a true size pattern. **B,** Pattern is full length with hand flat.

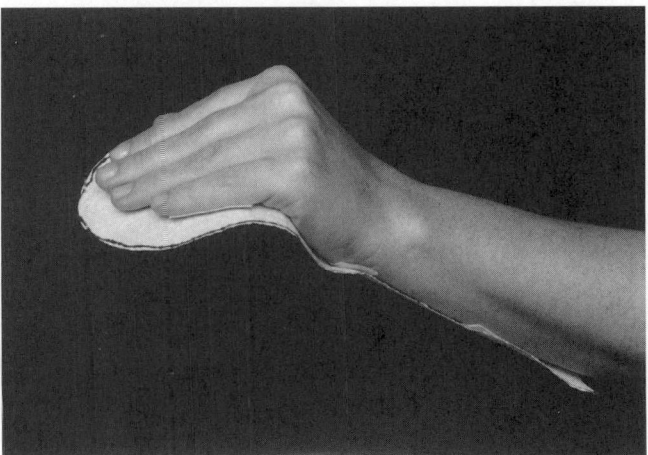

FIG. 31-34
Pattern is too long when fit on the volar surface with hand in resting position.

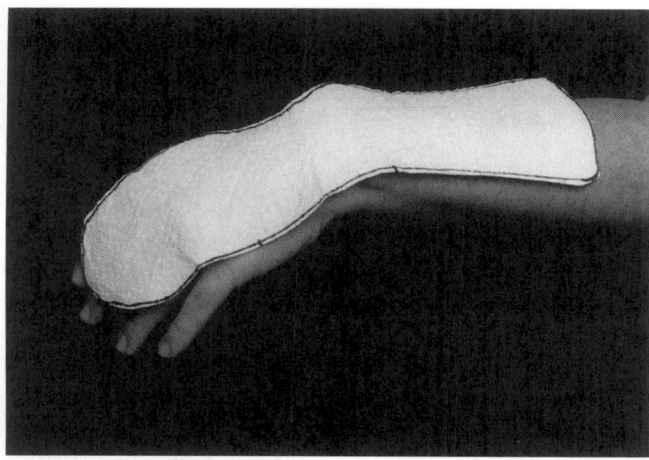

FIG. 31-35
Pattern is too short when fit on dorsum of hand with wrist and fingers in flexion.

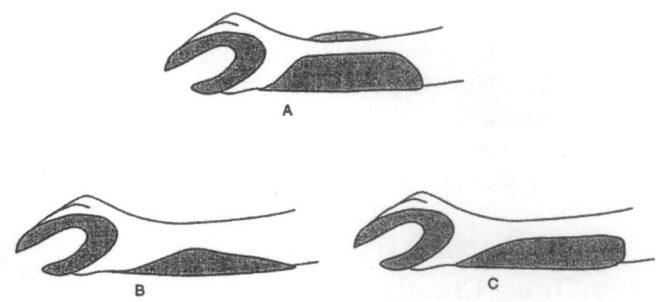

FIG. 31-36
Forearm trim lines. **A**, Trim lines are too high, extending above forearm. Straps will bridge arm and be ineffective. **B**, Trim lines too low. Straps cannot substitute for too-low trim lines without applying excessive pressure. **C**, Midline trim lines ensure straps properly secure splint on arm and hand.

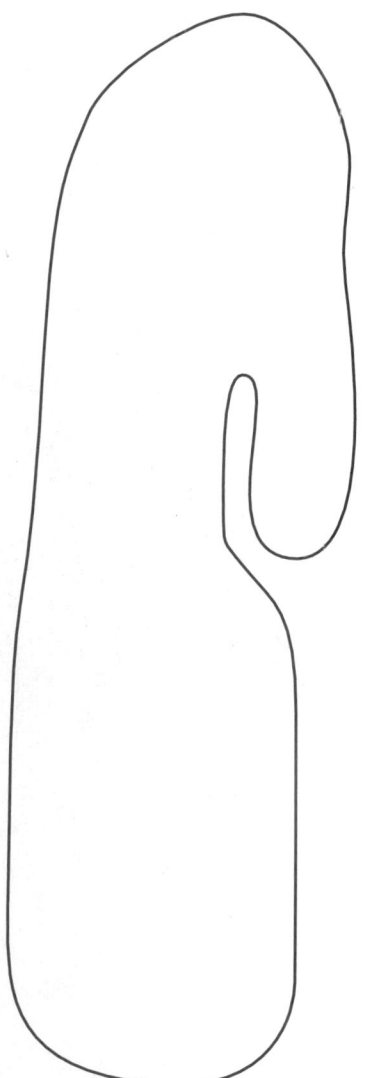

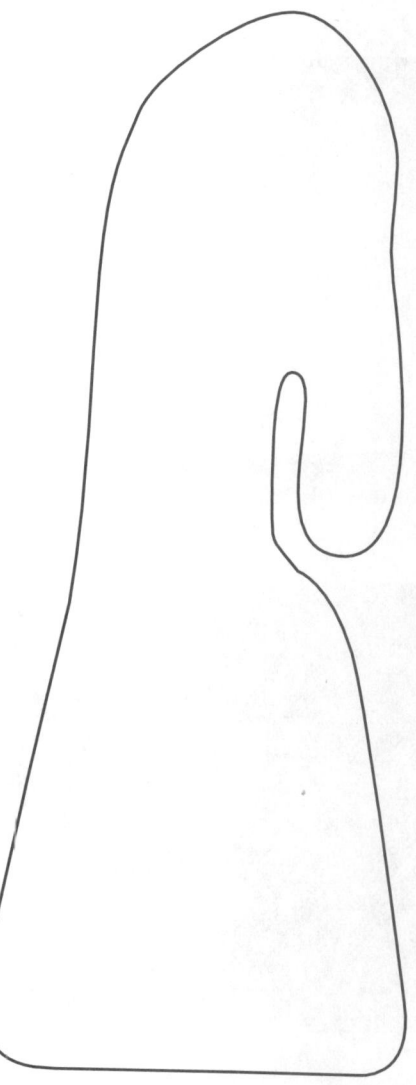

FIG. 31-37
A, Narrowing the proximal pattern will cause trim lines to drop below midline. **B**, Flaring the proximal border of the splint maintains trim lines at midline.

by checking the splint pattern on the hand in the position in which the hand will be splinted.

Depth is the second dimension that needs to be considered when a pattern is made. The ideal trim lines of a single-surface splint will fall at midline along the arm, hand, leg, or foot. A splint trimmed at midline will provide optimal support and will allow for proper strapping to help secure the splint in place (Fig. 31-36).

To determine how much to add to the outline to achieve midline trim lines, the maker must observe the width and depth of the arm or hand. The forearm is a cone shape, not a straight cylinder, and it graduates in depth over the forearm muscle. Even the thinnest forearm graduates in width and depth proximally. Persons with significant muscle bulk may have graduation at quite an acute angle from the wrist to the proximal forearm. Determination of how much to add to a forearm trough must consider how much the splint must come out, around, and up the forearm to reach midline. The depth of the hand, particularly the depth of the hypothenar eminence, must be known to create the proper trimlines for a hand platform.

It is important in the fit of any forearm-based splint that the proximal trimlines take advantage of the soft muscle bellies that protect the radius and ulna. The proximal borders of the splint should be flared so that the trimline remains at midline to help secure the splint in place on the arm (Fig. 31-37).

A forearm-based splint should extend approximately two thirds of the length of the forearm, as measured from the wrist proximally. A good rule to remember is to bend the patient's elbow fully and mark where the forearm and the biceps muscle meet. The splint should be trimmed ¼ inch below this point to avoid limiting elbow flexion and to prevent the splint from being pushed distally when the elbow is flexed (Fig. 31-38).

Most low-temperature thermoplastics used to make splints will stretch to conform around angles and contours. When a pattern is created that will go around an acute angle, such as a 90° angle around a flexed elbow or wrist, the pattern should include a dart where the material can be overlapped without causing undue bulk (Fig. 31-39). The pattern may also be angled where necessary to accommodate acute angles. A well-fit and thought out pattern translates to less material wasted, less expense, and shorter fabrication time.

Step Two—Choosing Appropriate Material

The materials commonly used for custom fabricated splints are those in a family of plastic polymers that become pliable at a temperature low enough for the material to be molded directly on the skin. The **low-temperature thermoplastics** (LTTs) available today

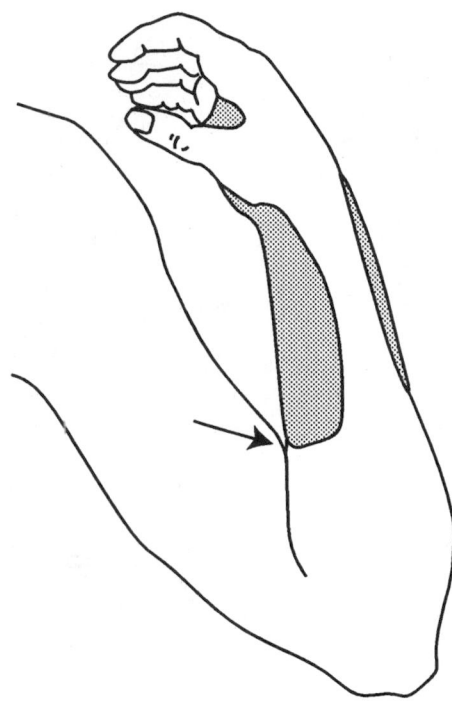

FIG. 31-38
Length of forearm-based splint is checked by flexing elbow and noting where biceps meets forearm. Splint is trimmed ¼ to ½ inch distal to point of contact.

have certain characteristics that can be defined according to how a material reacts or handles when warm and how it reacts once molded.

Choosing the optimal material for a given splint application can make the difference between a quick and easy splint-making process or one that requires extensive adjustments and reheating. It behooves every splint maker, novice to advanced, to sample a variety of materials and test for the handling characteristics so no surprises occur when a material is heated and ready to be cut and fitted to a patient.

Characteristics of Splint Materials

Each LTT has some handling characteristics that apply when the materials are warm and pliable and some that apply when they are cold or molded. The following is a list of the most common characteristics and how they contribute to the choice of a material for a specific application.

RESISTANCE TO STRETCH. Resistance to stretch describes the extent to which a material resists pulling or stretching. The greater the resistance, the greater the degree of control the splint maker will have over the material. Materials that resist stretch tend to hold their shape and thickness while warm and can be handled more aggressively without thinning. The more resistive

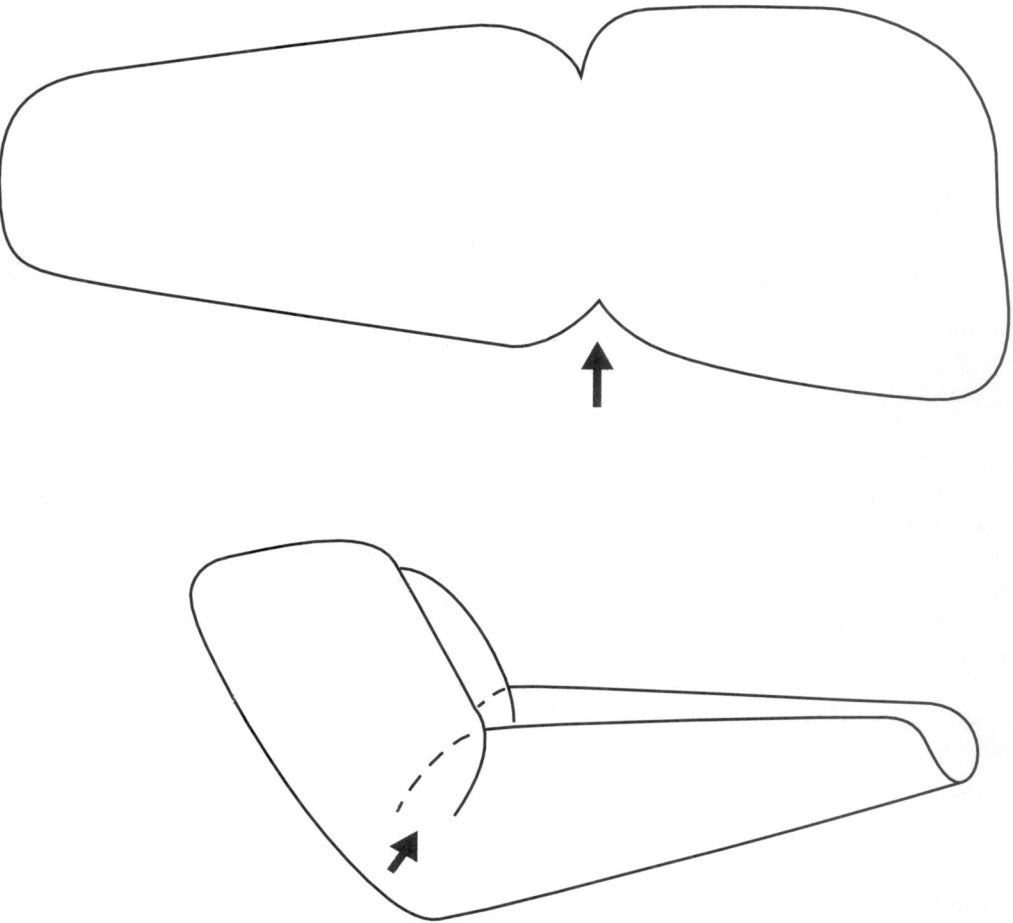

FIG. 31-39
Drawing darts in elbow pattern allows material to be overlapped and contoured without excess material.

materials are recommended for large splints and for splints made for persons who are unable to cooperate in the fabrication process. In contrast, the less resistance to stretch a material has, the more the material is likely to thin during the fabrication process and the more delicately it must be handled. The advantage of stretch is seen in the greater degree of conformability obtained with less effort on the splint maker's part.

CONFORMABILITY OR DRAPE. Resistance to stretch and conformability or drape describe nearly the same characteristic; that is, if a material stretches easily, it will have better drape and conformability. The great advantage of materials with a high degree of drape or conformability is that with a light, controlled touch or simply the pull of gravity, they readily conform around a part for a precise fit, with minimal effort on the splint maker's part. The disadvantage of materials with a high degree of drape (and generally also low resistance to stretch) is that they tolerate only minimal handling, and care must be taken to prevent

overstretching and fingerprints in the material. Materials with a high degree of drape are not recommended for large splints or for uncooperative patients. They are ideal, however, for splinting postoperative patients when minimal pressure is desired and for dynamic splint bases where conformability secures the splint against migration (movement distally) when components are attached. Materials with a low degree of drape must be handled continuously until the materials are fully cooled to achieve a contoured fit and often will not conform intimately around small parts such as the fingers.

MEMORY. Memory is the ability of a material, when reheated, to return to its original, flat shape after it has been stretched and molded. The advantage of high memory in a material is that the splint can be remolded repeatedly without the material thinning and losing strength. Materials with memory require handling throughout the splint-making process because until they are fully cooled and molded, they tend to return to a flat shape. This and the slightly longer cooling time of materials with high memory can be used to advantage with patients who require more aggressive handling to achieve the desired position. Disadvantages of materials with excellent memory are their tendency to return to a flat sheet state when an area is spot heated for adjustment and their need for longer handling to ensure that they maintain their molded shape until fully cooled.

RIGIDITY VERSUS FLEXIBILITY. Rigidity and flexibility in cold splint material are terms describing the amount of resistance a material gives when force is applied to it. A highly rigid material is very resistive to applied force and may, with enough force, break. A highly flexible material bends easily when even small force is applied to it, and it is not apt to break under high stress. Materials are available that fall all along this continuum.

Generally, the thicker a thermoplastic and the more plastic its formula contains, the more rigid the material will be. Thermoplastics come in thicknesses from 1/8 inch (3.2 mm) to as thin as 1/16 inch (1.6 mm). The thinner materials and the thermoplastics that contain rubberlike polymers in their formula tend to have greater flexibility in their molded state. Flexibility in a material allows for easier donning and doffing of circumferential splints and may be desirable for patients unable to tolerate the more unforgiving rigid materials. Rigidity is also a factor of the number and depth of the contours included in the design. A material may yield a semiflexible splint when used to make a single-surface splint with shallow contours, and rigid when used to make a tightly fit circumferential splint.

BONDING. Bonding is the ability of a material to adhere to itself when warmed and pressed together. Many materials are coated to resist accidental bonding and require solvents or surface scraping to remove the coating in order to bond. Uncoated materials, which require no solvents or scraping, have very strong bonding properties when two warm pieces are pressed together. Self-bonding is helpful when outriggers or overlapping corners are applied to form acute angles but can be a problem if two pieces adhere accidentally.

SELF-SEALING EDGES. Self-sealing edges are edges that round and seal themselves when heated material is cut. This characteristic produces smooth edges that require no additional finishing, which adds time to the fabrication process. Materials with little or no memory and high conformability generally produce smooth, sealed edges when cut while warm. Materials with memory, or those that have a high resistance to stretch, resist sealing and require additional finishing.

SOFT SPLINT MATERIALS. Soft, flexible materials such as cotton duck, neoprene, knit elastics, and plastic-impregnated materials may be used alone or in combination with metal or plastic stays to fabricate semiflexible splints. These materials allow fabrication of splints that permit partial motion around a joint, yet still limit or protect the part. Semiflexible splints are sometimes used during sporting activities and to assist patients with chronic pain in returning to functional activity. Semiflexible splints are also used for geriatric patients and patients with arthritis who often cannot tolerate rigid splints.

Neoprene splints can be fabricated with use of a sealing glue or iron-on tapes. Careful attention must be given to the patterns for soft splints because the support they offer relies primarily on achieving a secure fit without gapping or excess material. Most other soft materials require sewing, and the fully equipped OT department should include a sewing machine. A sewing machine is useful for adapting and adjusting prefabricated soft splints to ensure that each splint that leaves the clinic is indeed custom fit, if not custom fabricated.

Choosing the Best Category of Material for the Splint

Although an experienced splint maker can make many types of splints from the same material, it is better to choose a material with the appropriate handling characteristics for the type of splint being made. The following list can be used as a guideline from which to start choosing materials for different applications. The availability of materials and the experience level of the therapist will further determine the most appropriate material.

FOREARM- AND HAND-BASED SPLINTS. Splints need close conformability around a part when they serve as a base for a dynamic splint, stabilize a part of the body, reduce contractures, remodel scar tissue, or immobilize to facilitate healing of an acute condition. Such splints should be made from a material with a high degree of conformability to achieve a conforming fit. When conformability is not crucial, the splint can be made from a material with high resistance to stretch and low to moderate drape. Splints fabricated for burns and other acute trauma do not require as conforming a fit and can be made from low-drape materials. Materials that resist stretch and tolerate aggressive handling are also recommended for positioning of a spastic body part, since such a material will not stretch and thin during the splint-making process.

LARGE UPPER AND LOWER EXTREMITY SPLINTS. Long splints fabricated for the elbow, shoulder, knee, or ankle should generally be made of materials that have high resistance to stretch to provide the control necessary for dealing with large pieces of material. Such splints generally do not need to be highly conforming because they are molded over broad expanses of soft tissue. Care must be taken to provide relief for bony prominences or to provide padding to distribute pressure.

CIRCUMFERENTIAL SPLINTS. A splint designed to wrap all the way around the part should be fabricated from materials that have a high degree of memory and that tolerate stretching without forming thin spots. The materials should be highly perforated, thin, or able to be stretched evenly. After being stretched, these materials will cinch in around the body part but still allow sufficient flexibility for easy donning and doffing. These materials work very well for fracture bracing and for circumferential splints that are used for contracture reduction and for stabilizing or immobilizing joints. Another choice for making less restrictive circumferential splints is the use of semiflexible materials, which facilitate easy donning and doffing and allow limited motion within the available arc of motion.

SERIAL SPLINTS. Serial splints that require frequent remolding to accommodate increases in joint range of motion should be made from a material that has considerable memory or is highly resistant to stretch to avoid thinning with repeated remolding. The chosen material should have moderate to high rigidity when molded to resist forces from contracted joints or from spastic muscle tone.

Step Three—Choosing the Type of Traction

All splints provide some form of traction to move or stabilize a joint or joints. The traction mechanism may be dynamic, using a spring, hinge, or elastic. Traction may also be static, employing straps or turnbuckles or involving remolding of the splint base itself. If the mechanism moves or is resilient, the splint is called a dynamic splint, and if it does not move, the splint is called a static splint. The following section describes the various options for applying traction and discusses the appropriate uses of each option.

Dynamic Traction
The purpose of dynamic splints is the mobilization of a joint through the use of a resilient force attached to an outrigger or through the use of a spring coil. Each mechanism of force has advantages and disadvantages that make it suited for some uses and ill suited to others. The construction techniques differ substantially when spring coils are used, versus outriggers with elastic components. Thus the indications for each style of splint vary.

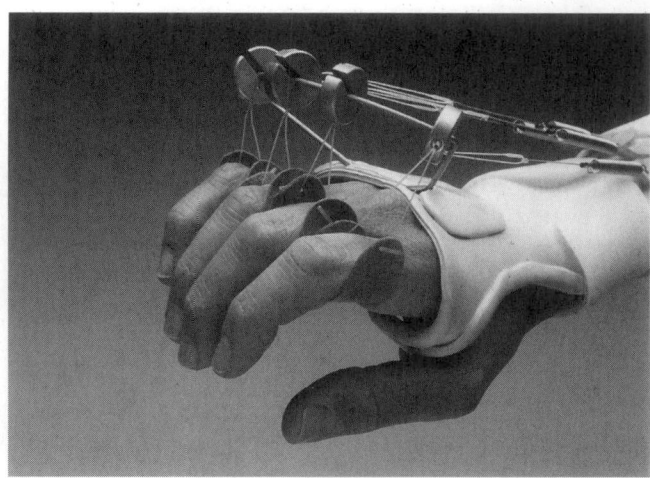

FIG. 31-40
Easily adjustable Phoenix outrigger with slotted pulleys allows frequent changes in angle of approach.

Spring coils are best suited to assist weak muscles or substitute for paralyzed muscles (Fig. 31-28). Patients with weak or paralyzed muscles will likely require the splint for a long time and will wear it while working or performing their ADL. The low-profile, lightweight construction of a coil splint is recommended because it is less likely to interfere with hand function. Spring coils retain their force and alignment over time, rarely require adjustment, and are ideal for long-term conditions.

Splints with outriggers are the optimal choice for splinting postoperative patients (Fig. 31-40). These splints allow frequent adjustments to maintain correct positioning and to accommodate changes in bandage thickness and edema as the healing and rehabilitation progresses. The postoperative patient will likely use the splint for only a short time, generally 4 to 6 weeks. Such a patient will not be returning to normal functional activities with the affected hand during that time. Thus the bulkiness and limitation of function with an outrigger splint are relatively unimportant.

Splints with outriggers are also used for contracture reduction. For this purpose they are generally most effective when used during the early stages of healing when the contracture feels soft and is easy to reduce.[4] Frequently patients at this stage still have pain and inflammation. They cannot tolerate a rigid, static splint, but they will tolerate a light force provided by an outrigger.

Static Traction
The overall purpose of static splints is to apply traction to immobilize or restrict motion. When static splints immobilize, they are protecting, resting, or positioning. When they restrict, they are blocking motion, aligning joints, or limiting motion. When static splints are used to mobilize, they are used in either a serial static or static

progressive fashion to reduce contractures and remodel scar.

Serial Static Traction

A serial static splint is fabricated by repeated adjustments that position a joint at its end range of motion each time to achieve slow, progressive increases in ROM. For example, a cylindrical cast made for gaining PIP extension must be remade after a time (usually 1 to 3 days) to reposition the joint at the end of its range of motion (Fig. 31-25).

Static Progressive Traction

A static progressive splint requires a built-in mechanism for adjusting the traction. Choosing which mechanism to use, be it a turnbuckle, Velcro strap, or buckle, depends on availability, the therapist's experience, and the patient's ability to manage the mechanism. A good rule to follow is to choose the simplest component that will achieve the desired goal.

Serial static splints and static progressive splints each have certain advantages and disadvantages. Serial static splints are useful for difficult patients who have high muscle tone or who are cognitively impaired and would have problems with the adjustment mechanisms. Also, the therapist has the control necessary for patients who are noncompliant or who would be overly zealous and apply too much force. The disadvantages are that the splint requires more therapist time because it must be remolded many times and that if the patient does not remove it for several days, some ROM may be lost in the direction opposite to that in which the splint is applying force.

The advantages of a static progressive splint are that the therapist has to make only one splint and that reliable patients with normal muscle tone may make more rapid progress because they can tailor the adjustment to their own pace and tolerance. The disadvantage of a static progressive splint is that it cannot be used on the patient who has abnormal tone or who is unreliable.

IMPLICATIONS OF APPLICATION OF FORCE. All splints, whether static or dynamic, apply force and to some degree stress on the structures they contact. The unimpaired hand tolerates a wide range of stresses by adaptation when possible and by avoidance when not. The patient with sensory or cognitive impairment may lack the protective responses necessary to reposition the hand away from the stresses applied by splints.

Pressure causes ischemia (localized anemia caused by obstruction of blood supply to tissues), and pressure increases when splints are contoured too sharply, when they do not conform uniformly, or when they do not cover a broad enough area of soft tissue. Splints that migrate or move on the hand because of insufficient strapping or contouring may actually apply pressure in areas that the splint was designed to relieve.

AMOUNT OF FORCE TO APPLY. How much force can be applied safely? There are no absolute rules about the amount of force that can be applied for immobilization or to a restricted joint to produce motion. The splint maker must apply sufficient force to create motion, but not so much as to cause ischemia. Much depends on the degree of the contracture, how long the restriction has existed, the age of the patient, and the location of the restriction. This leaves the therapist with several options when choosing which force and how much force to apply.

For example, external force in dynamic splints is generally applied through the addition of rubber bands, elastic, or springs. Neither option is ideal, and both require careful selection and frequent adjustment. The amount of force supplied by rubber bands and springs depends on both their thickness and their length. The thickness of the band or spring determines its potential force, whereas the length of the band or spring (or the number of coils in the spring) determines the ROM through which the force can be applied. When either bands or springs are used, it is desirable to use the optimal force (i.e., the greatest tolerable force over the longest wearing time) that does not produce ischemia. To accomplish this, the midrange of the bands or springs should be used, rather than their end ranges, which are either too slack or too strong. A gauge is available for measuring the applied force of elastic, which should generally be between 100 and 300 grams.

Techniques are available for avoiding pressure areas and shear forces in a dynamic splint, particularly where traction is applied to mobilize a finger joint. First, it is important to stabilize the joint(s) proximal to the finger joint being splinted. For instance, to mobilize a PIP joint with an outrigger and cuff, the MP joint must be held securely so that no movement occurs to cause the splint to produce pressure points elsewhere on the hand or digits. Care must be taken in the contouring of the splint around the proximal phalanx to distribute pressure and prevent motion that could cause shearing over the dorsum of the finger. In this case, padding may be necessary to help distribute pressure over the small and thinly padded phalanx (Fig. 31-41).

DURATION OF TRACTION. Basic to answering the question, "How long should traction be applied?" is an understanding of theories of tissue stretching versus tissue growth. Three key concepts aid in the understanding of these two different tissue responses. First, all materials, including human tissue, respond to applied stress. If stress is applied over time and then relaxed, the tissue will no longer return to its original

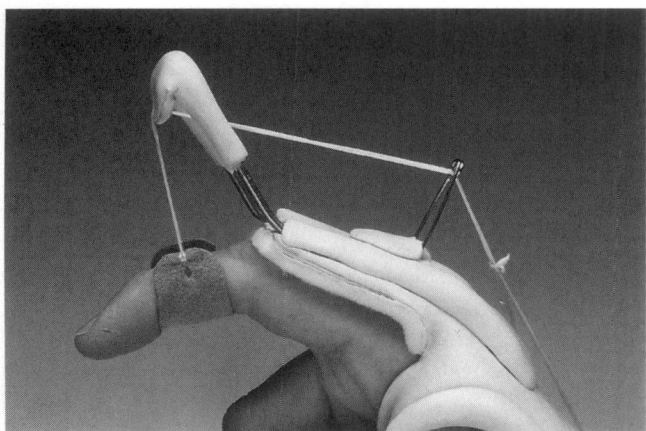

FIG. 31-41
Felt padding distributes pressure over bony proximal phalanx.

shape but will adapt to the new shape. This stretching phenomenon in skin is a result of its plastic behavior and is known as creep. The lengthening that occurs with creep is found to be the result of "a slippage of short collagen fibers on one another within the tissue. Some fibers may rupture while others just slide on each other."[3]

The second concept is that of the elastic limit of tissue. Think of pulling on a rubber band. As the band is pulled, tension increases until the elastic limit is reached. If pulled beyond its elastic limit, the rubber band will break. In clinical terms the end of the elastic limit is the point of tissue elongation at which pain will be felt and tissue damage may occur. Stretching tissue beyond its elastic limit does not lead to permanent lengthening, but instead to unwanted tearing and probable further tissue contracture.[3]

For creep to occur in living tissue, traction must hold the skin with sufficient force to exceed the skin's elastic limit. This may cause tearing of small fibers and possible hemorrhaging, leading to inflammation and additional scarring caused by fibrogen deposits.

The third concept is tissue growth. True growth occurs when "living cells will sense strain and collagen fibers will be actively and progressively absorbed and laid down again with modified bonding patterns with no creep and no inflammation."[3] This is the aim of splinting when the goal is contracture reduction or lengthening of restricted soft tissue.

There are two approaches to the application of traction to lengthen soft tissue and reduce contractures. One approach is to position the tissue at the end range of its elastic limits and hold it statically for short periods, and then to relax and reposition it frequently. This approach is termed stress relaxation.[2] The second approach is to apply force within the elastic limits of the tissue, hold it for a long period, and then reposition it.

The difference in these two approaches is one of time and of being able to judge the elastic limits of tissue. The first approach relies on principles of stress relaxation, which theorizes that tissues reach their elastic limit over a shorter period with frequent repositioning and will retain this newly set limit over time.[2] The second and more commonly used approach relies on the application of a low load over a long time to allow tissue growth to occur. Both approaches have merit, and it is up to the therapist and prescribing physician to determine the appropriate approach in each instance.

Step Four—Choosing a Splint Design for a Given Purpose

Mobilizing Splints to Remodel Scar Tissue and Reduce Contractures

Scar tissue is one of the major contributors to deformity. Anytime there is an insult to tissue, as occurs after an open injury or after surgery, scar tissue is produced by the body to heal the wound. The scar may be subcutaneous, superficial, or both. When it is subcutaneous, it often results in loss of motion because it acts like glue, keeping tissue planes from gliding. Scar also contracts, and when that contracture occurs over a joint, loss of joint motion results. To restore motion, scar tissue must be remodeled; that is, it must be softened and lengthened. If the contracture is caused by shortened soft tissue that is not scar, that soft tissue must also be lengthened. The process is the same for scar or soft tissue.

The effectiveness of splinting for remodeling scar and reducing contractures can be increased greatly by applying a deep heat modality, such as paraffin or moist heat, before applying the splint. When tissue is unheated it is less elastic, meaning it has a great deal of tension and is difficult to elongate. With the application of heat, tissue becomes temporarily more elastic, meaning that the tension in the tissue is reduced and the tissue is much easier to elongate.

There are many approaches to splinting for remodeling scar and reducing contractures. Three-point splints can be used for flexion contractures, loop splints for IP joint extension contractures, and outriggers for MCP extension contractures. Dynamic outriggers can be used for reducing early, soft contractures, particularly when the patient cannot tolerate a static splint. Static progressive splints or static splints can be used in a serial fashion.

Immobilizing and Restrictive Splints for Pain Reduction

Of the many uses of splints, perhaps the most common is to limit or reduce pain by providing rest and support. The most common splint prescriptions are written for splints to reduce the pain caused by the inflammatory processes of tendinitis or following sprain or strain injuries.

Several questions help determine which splint will best serve the patient's need. First, if the injury is caused by an acute sprain, the choice may be for an immobilizing splint until pain and edema have subsided. If the pain is chronic in nature and caused by the performance of a particular activity, a semiflexible splint may serve best. A semiflexible restrictive splint may sufficiently reduce pain by limiting ROM, yet still allow function without increasing stress on unaffected joints or tissue (Fig. 31-42).

A second question concerns the need for full-time splinting versus intermittent wear. In the presence of an acute injury with orthopedic involvement or tissue damage, the splint may not only need to immobilize, but also to protect the part from further damage. Here, patient tolerance and compliance will in part determine material and design choice. The therapist may also need to consider the integrity of tissue and the need to accommodate bandages and bandage changes. If the splint is indicated only for intermittent wear, the design choice may depend more on the patient's ability to readily don and doff the splint. The choice of materials may be dictated by the functional needs of the patient. For intermittent splints used for vocational activities, lightweight, well-aerated materials may be indicated. For intermittent splints used for positioning, such as a resting splint designed to maintain functional position between exercise sessions, stronger materials may be indicated and perforations may not be necessary.

A third important question in deciding on a splint design is, "What structures need to be immobilized or supported, and which should be left free?" When protective or pain-reducing splints are provided, care must be taken to splint only the involved structures and not

impede motion elsewhere. If the purpose of the splint is to rest the tendons at the wrist to reduce inflammation, the splint must not limit CMC or MP joint motion if these structures are not symptomatic. If used during the performance of ADL, splints that fully immobilize a joint may transfer stress to joints proximal or distal to the immobilized joint. For this reason semiflexible splints that restrict only end ranges of motion may be indicated during activity, whereas an immobilizing splint may be indicated for total rest at night.

Immobilizing Splints For Positioning

One of the splints most frequently fabricated by occupational therapists is the resting pan (also known as the resting hand or functional position splint), used to maintain the hand in a functional position (Fig. 31-24). The purpose of this positioning splint is to keep the soft tissues of the hand in midrange in order to maintain optimal mobility and prevent shortening of the soft tissue structures around the joints. Occasionally, positioning splints are prescribed to position joints at end range to prevent contractures in the presence of severe tissue damage. Resting splints fitted on persons with burns are the prime example of this splint because the MP joints are positioned in full available flexion. The important decision in this case is determination of the optimal position for the most functional outcome.

Positioning splints may be fabricated for temporary use after surgery and may require frequent adjustment to accommodate changes in edema and bandages. The materials chosen for these splints should have memory to allow for remolding while keeping its thickness and strength. Resting splints fabricated for patients after a CVA will likely require only minimal adjustment, so more conforming plastic materials with little or no memory can be used. Further choices of a dorsal- versus a volar-based splint and a single-surface versus a circumferential splint will depend on surgical and wound sites, need for ease of donning and doffing, and therapist and physician preference and experience.

Step Five—Fabrication

The fabrication processes for single-surface and circumferential splints differ significantly. They do have a starting point in common: the pattern from which the splint will be made. Starting with a paper pattern is recommended, particularly for the novice splint maker. One very basic rule of splinting is to get the pattern right before beginning to work with plastic. It is far less expensive to discard a few pieces of paper than even a small piece of LTT. Pattern making is discussed in detail earlier in this chapter and should be reviewed before creating the pattern as step one in the fabrication process.

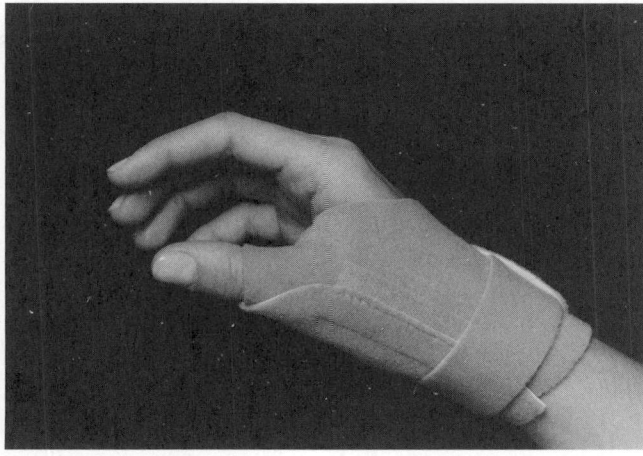

FIG. 31-42
Flexible thumb splint provides support yet allows midrange movement.

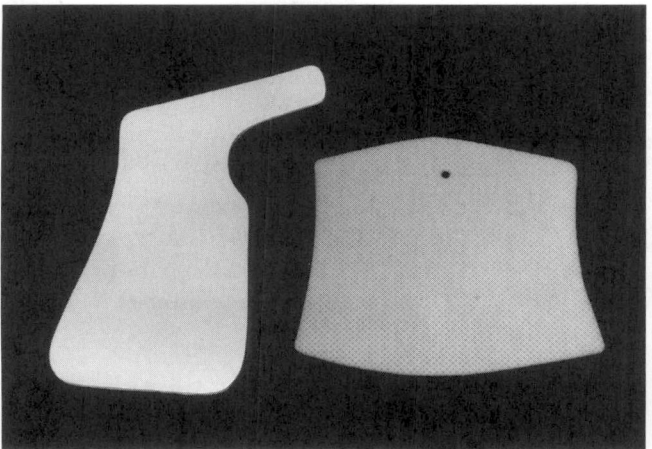

FIG. 31-43
Pattern for single-surface cock-up splint on left requires precision for a proper fit. Pattern on right for circumferential splint does not need precise fit because material stretches and overlaps to achieve proper size.

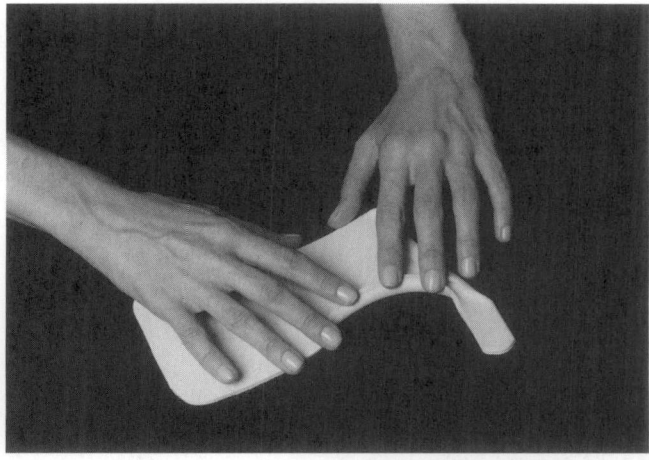

FIG. 31-45
Fold edges of material and gently press flat to create thin, smooth edges that distribute pressure better.

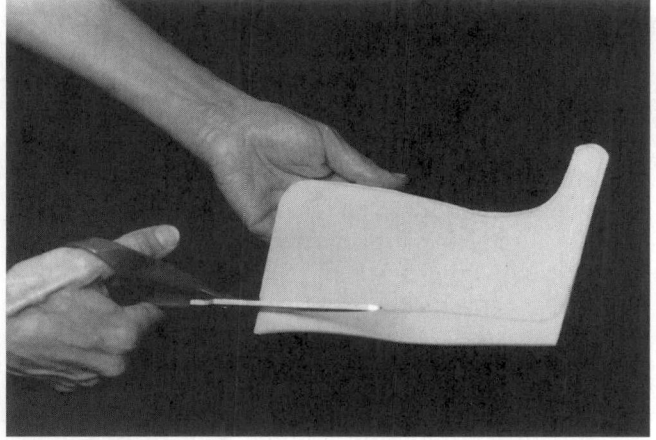

FIG. 31-44
Support material on table to prevent stretching and cut with long strokes of scissors.

Fabrication Techniques for Single-Surface Splinting

Single-surface splints cover the volar surface, the dorsal surface, the ulnar half, or the radial half of the arm and hand. Generally, single-surface splints have gentle contours and cover as broad an area of tissue as is feasible to distribute pressure. The following steps should be used as a guideline in the process of creating a single-surface splint. For the sake of demonstration, the single-surface and the circumferential splints described and pictured are wrist extension (cock-up) splints (Fig. 31-43).

1. Except for the fingers, ⅛-inch-thick material is recommended to obtain sufficient rigidity to hold the joint firmly in position. The broad contours of single-surface splints require thicker materials to provide sufficient support.
2. Etch the pattern onto the cold thermoplastic material with a scratch awl or wax pencil before placing the material in a hot water bath. The water temperature for most materials to soften properly is approximately 160° F. Temperature and time will vary, depending on the material and its thickness. Most materials heat to the pliable stage in 2 to 3 minutes.
3. Carefully remove the material from the hot water bath and lay it flat on the table to cut. To prevent stretching, avoid holding material unsupported while cutting (Fig. 31-44).
4. Starting in the neck of the scissors, cut with long, even strokes to prevent jagged edges.
5. Reheat the material if it has cooled too much to be formed. Place the material on the forearm and hand with the forearm in supination so that gravity can assist the initial molding. Check that the trim lines fall at midline. If they do not, mark where excess material needs to be removed. Trim the material before it cools. Note areas that will need to be folded for clearance and to create smooth edges. Fold and secure the edges firmly in place (Fig. 31-45).
6. Reposition the splint on the forearm. Maintaining control on the wrist and forearm sections, carefully pronate the forearm. Maintain the wrist in extension at all times. The tendency for the wrist to drop into flexion when the forearm is pronated is universal. Controlling the wrist will ensure that the desired wrist position is maintained at all times (Fig. 31-46). If necessary, rotate the forearm section to ensure that the trim lines are at midline. Refer to

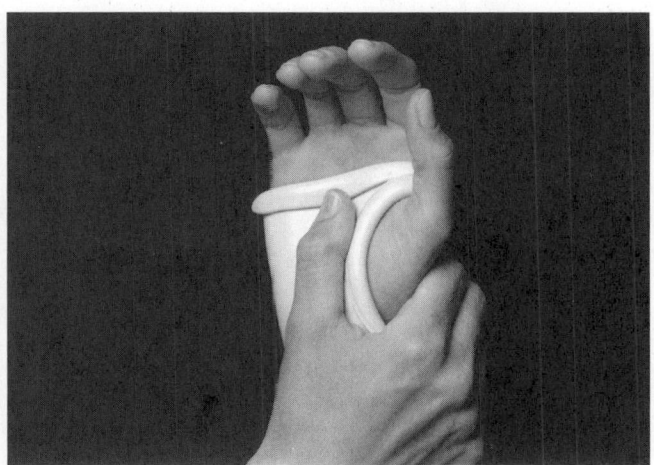

FIG. 31-46
Gently support the wrist at all times to achieve proper fit.

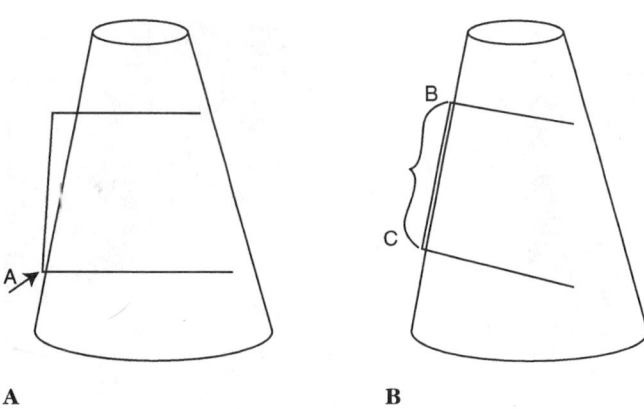

A   B

FIG. 31-47
Forearm is cone shaped, gradually widening from wrist to elbow. **A,** Strap laced straight across broader proximal forearm contacts skin only at point A and does not secure splint. **B,** Strap placed at angle applies even pressure along line BC to secure splint.

Fig. 31-6 to review the importance of the changing shape of the forearm from a supinated to a pronated position.

7. Allow the splint to cool until it holds its shape. It does not have to be held in place until completely cold. Remove the splint. Heat and smooth any rough edges as needed and apply the straps.

8. Strapping is critical to secure the splinted part in the splint and diminish both shear forces and the possibility of pressure areas developing. The splint may require several straps, and wide or crossed straps are suggested to obtain the necessary control. Because the forearm is cone shaped, straps placed straight across the forearm will contact the skin effectively only on their proximal surface (Fig. 31-47). To have the forearm straps apply effective and well-distributed pressure, place them at an angle.

9. Single-surface splints rely on strapping to hold them in place and create one or more three-point pressure systems to securely hold the joint or joints being splinted (Fig. 31-30). To ensure that straps function properly, trim lines must fall midline along the arm and hand. If the trim lines are left too high, making the trough too deep for the part, the straps will bridge the part and sit up on the edge of the splint, where they are ineffective. The most effective way to secure a splint in place on the forearm is to apply pressure through the splint onto the soft tissue of the forearm muscle bellies. If the forearm trim lines angle below the muscle bellies, the splint will no longer be secured on the muscle bellies.

10. Instruct the wearer in the wearing schedule and in the proper care of the splint. To prevent ischemia and shear forces, check the fit of the splint regularly.

Fabrication Techniques for Circumferential Splints

1. Use a thin or highly perforated elastic material or flexible rubber material that has some memory. For hand and forearm-based splints, thin elastic materials ($\frac{1}{16}$-, $\frac{1}{12}$-, or $\frac{3}{32}$-inch) provide sufficient strength because of the rigidity provided by the curves of the splint. For splints covering larger areas, a highly perforated $\frac{1}{8}$-inch material is recommended. Materials for circumferential splints should be coated to prevent permanent adherence when warm or should be able to be pulled apart once cooled.

2. Etch the pattern onto the material. Because the materials for circumferential splints are generally stretched to contour around the arm, the pattern does not need to be as precise as for a single-surface splint. It is important to know how much the material will be pulled and if it will be overlapped or finished edge to edge so that a piece of sufficient size is cut (Fig. 31-48).

3. Wrap the material all the way around the part being splinted. Two techniques can be used in creating a closure for a circumferential splint. The first is to pull the material around the part and pinch the remaining material together to create a seam. Gently tug on the seam to conform the material. When the material is cool, open the seam and trim the splint. The second technique is to overlap the two ends to form a flap (Fig. 31-49). To prevent the flap from adhering (this may happen when the coating is thinned as the material is stretched), wait until it has cooled slightly before overlapping.

4. Smooth edges as necessary. The circumferential splint creates multiple three-point pressure systems

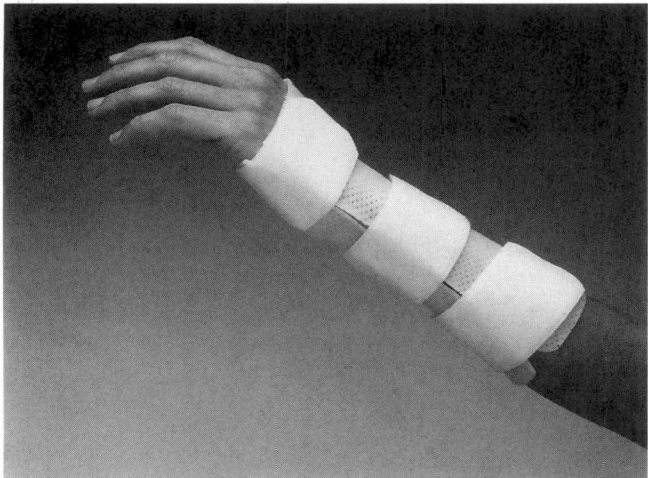

FIG. 31-48
Circumferential splint trimmed to close edge to edge.

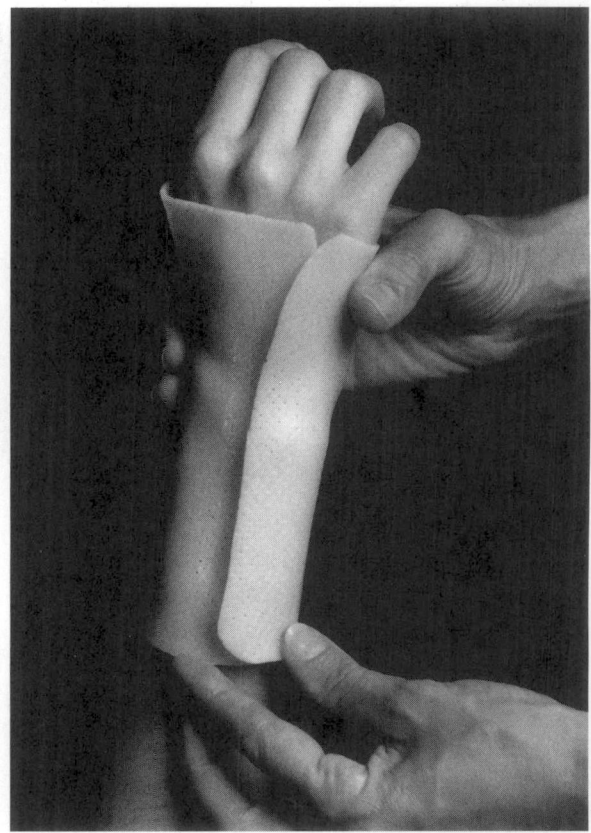

FIG. 31-49
Circumferential splint made from flexible material with overlap for easy donning and doffing.

by virtue of its design, and strapping is used only to hold the splint firmly closed.

Fabrication and Fitting of Semiflexible Splints and Prefabricated Splints

Materials used in the fabrication of semiflexible splints include neoprene, cotton duck, woven elastics, and thermoplastic-impregnated materials. Neoprene splints are generally fabricated using a special glue that adheres pieces together at the edges. The patterns for neoprene splints must be very precise to achieve a conforming fit. Cotton duck and other woven materials require sewing and considerable skill in pattern creation and the addition of darts to assure a good fit. Very thin thermoplastic materials can be used to create semiflexible splints, and certain patterns can be adapted to allow for partial range of motion within a splint.

Many of the commercially prefabricated splints are made from woven materials, because they present the broadest range of size adjustability and are less likely to require custom fabrication. It is highly recommended that even a prefabricated splint be custom fit by a therapist to ensure proper fit and adherence to an appropriate wearing schedule. A well-supplied splint department should include a sewing machine to custom fit all splints. Remember when fitting prefabricated supports that if a patient comes to see a therapist with a prescription for a splint, it is the therapist's responsibility to take the time and develop the skills to be certain that even prefabricated splints fit as if they were custom made.

SUMMARY

Section 1 of this chapter introduces the basic concepts of splint design and problem solving that must precede the

fabrication of a splint. The anatomy and biomechanics of the hand and types of grasp and prehension are reviewed. Splint classification and the purposes of splinting are described. The section presents a variety of splinting materials and their appropriate uses for different types of splints. Principles of safe and effective splinting and basic fabrication techniques are also described.

The occupational therapist must bring to the splinting process a knowledge of anatomy and biomechanics, skills in assessing function, and the ability to determine the optimal intervention for each patient, whether it includes a splint or not.

SECTION 2
Suspension Arm Devices and Mobile Arm Supports

LYNN YASUDA

Suspension arm devices and **mobile arm supports** are commonly used and can fulfill several treatment objectives for the person with severe physical disability. These devices can support the shoulder and forearm, encourage motion of weakened proximal musculature, prevent loss of ROM, provide pain relief, provide proximal support for distal function, and enable occupational performance.

SUSPENSION ARM DEVICES

Suspension arm devices are suspended from above the head, generally on an overhead **suspension rod** that is most often attached to a wheelchair. They can also be attached to regular chairs, a child's highchair, a body jacket, and even an overhead track used for walking patients.[3] Without the **overhead rod,** they are also attached to over-bed frames to allow the patient to use the device while in bed. These suspension arm devices were found in OT clinics as early as the 1940s. The ease of management, low cost, and ability to support proximal weakness of the upper limb contributed to their early popularity,[6] and they continue to be used for selected purposes.

Purposes

Suspension arm devices may be used to meet some of the following objectives:

- To position the shoulder girdle musculature to allow distal muscles to engage in functional activities
- To assist and support below fair-grade (F or 3) shoulder girdle musculature
- To allow gravity-eliminated exercise for weak shoulder girdle musculature
- To encourage use of increased ROM through repetitive activities[6]
- To prepare patients to use the mobile arm supports (MAS) by encouraging weak proximal musculature to move
- To support a painful shoulder
- To position an edematous hand away from a dependent position
- To prevent loss of shoulder ROM

Suspension arm devices are generally more effective for positioning and exercise than for function because of the mechanical principles on which they operate. The upper limb swings as a pendulum from straps attached to the suspension rod, thus making it difficult for fine adjustments in movement.[6]

Variations in Suspension Arm Devices

There are several variations of suspension arm devices. The overhead rod may be the same, but the attachments to the rod identify the variation. The variations listed here are commercially available and are in current use.

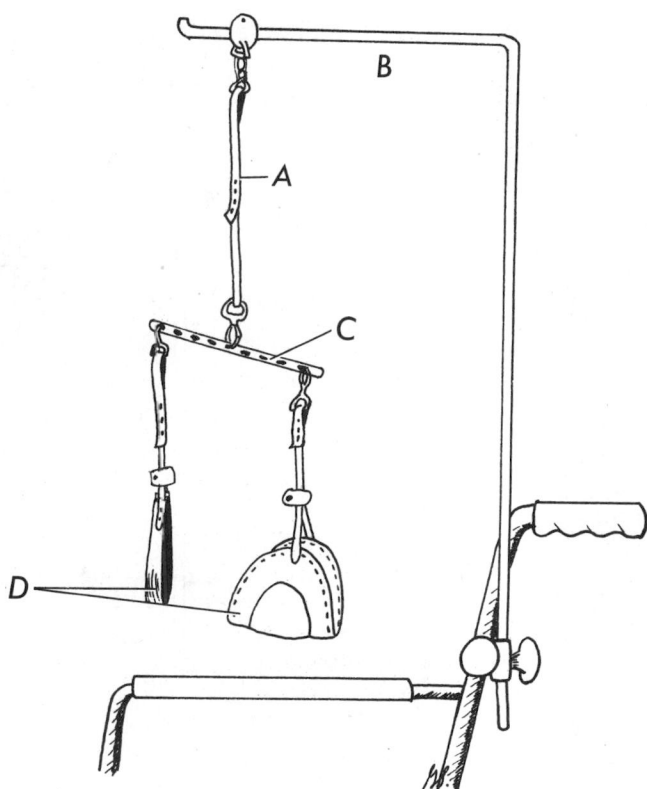

FIG. 31-50

Suspension sling. (Modified with permission from Occupational Therapy Department, Rancho Los Amigos Hospital, Downey, Calif.)

Suspension Sling

The **suspension sling** (Fig. 31-50) has a single strap (A) suspended from the overhead bar (B). A horizontal bar (adjustable balance bar, JAECO[5]) with holes for adjustment of the fulcrum (C), supports the two vertical straps (D). These straps provide support for the wrist and elbow separately.

Suspension Arm Support

The **suspension arm support** (offset suspension arm positioner, JAECO[5]) (Fig. 31-51) has a forearm trough that is the same as that used in the mobile arm support. It is suspended from a single point on the overhead bar. This device can be used as an initial step for the patient who can benefit from a MAS and is easily applied to the wheelchair. It can be easily attached and adjusted to over-bed frames to allow patients who are confined to bed to perform tabletop activities, as well as hand-to-face activities with this device (Fig. 31-52). However, it does not have the fine adjustment capabilities of the MAS, which extremely weak patients need. With a special bracket (Fig. 31-53), the suspension arm support is easily adaptable to the

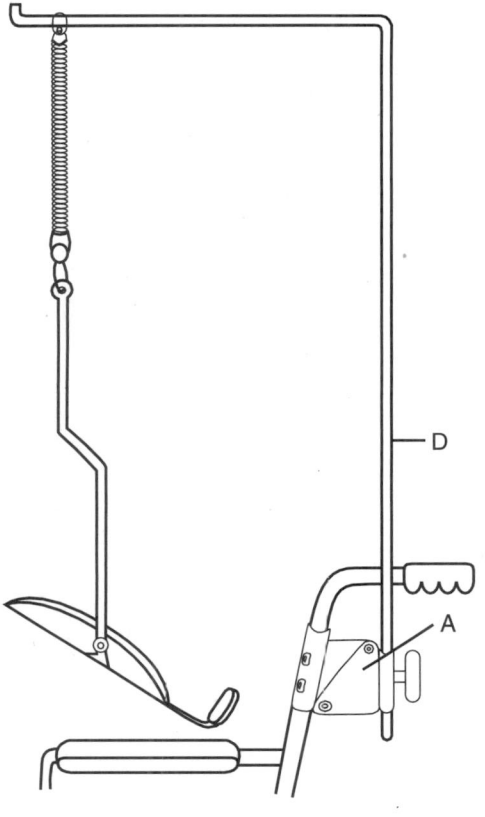

FIG. 31-51
Suspension arm support.

reclining wheelchair. This feature makes it useful during the rehabilitation of patients who cannot yet sit upright.

Adjustment of Suspension Arm Devices

Straps

The strap that connects the overhead rod to the limb directly or by the horizontal bar or forearm trough rocker attachment may be adjusted for length. This provides elevation control for the entire limb or for the wrist and elbow separately when separate supports are provided. Adjustments for height relative to the work surface or to the face are similar to those discussed in the later section on mobile arm supports.

Overhead Rod

HEIGHT. The overhead rod can be adjusted on the wheelchair **sling bracket.** The higher the overhead rod, the flatter the arc of pendulum swing when the arm is in motion. Usually the bar is kept as high as is possible while still allowing the wheelchair to pass through doorways. Lowering the bar shortens the pendulum arc

and causes the upper limb to move uphill at each extreme of the arc. Lowering the overhead rod can thus add undesirable resistance to a group of muscles during functional performance.

ROTATION. The shoulder can be placed in horizontal abduction and external rotation as the suspension rod is rotated outward, or in horizontal adduction and internal rotation if the suspension rod is rotated inward. This gives mechanical advantage to those muscles that are held in shortened range and offers resistance to the opposing muscles.[2,6]

SPRINGS. Springs of various tensions may be inserted in the straps supporting the upper limb. In early muscle reeducation, these springs allow the very weak patient to produce and visualize some slight bouncing movement while upright by contracting available muscles, a motion not as easily possible with straps alone.

HORIZONTAL BAR. Moving the strap on the holes on the horizontal bar (also called adjustable balance bar, made by JAECO[5]) will position the elbow in greater or lesser degrees of flexion. The bar is often positioned for the comfort of the patient, or, if edema is present, the hand is held higher than the elbow.

ROCKER TROUGH. The **rocker trough** (also called forearm trough, made by JAECO[5]) is the same one used in the MAS. However, this trough has a vertical metal rod attached to the rocker arm. The rocker arm can be moved on the trough, permitting greater directional assistance for **vertical motion,** up or down, depending on the patient's specific weakness in shoulder rotator or elbow musculature.

FULLY RECLINING SLING BRACKET. For all suspension devices, the overhead rod may be supported by a reclining bracket that permits the suspension to be perpendicular to the floor when the patient is reclined in the wheelchair.

Training in the Use of Suspension Arm Devices

Suspension arm supports can be used as training for or as an interim device before using the MAS. Training can include exercises for the shoulder and elbow, including scapular protraction and adduction, shoulder flexion and extension, elbow flexion and extension, and shoulder internal and external rotation (especially with the use of the forearm trough and rocker arm). Because the forearm trough is easily attached to over-bed frames, functional activities can be practiced using a table surface and any distal orthoses and adapted equipment that are needed[6] before the patient is able to be upright in a wheelchair.

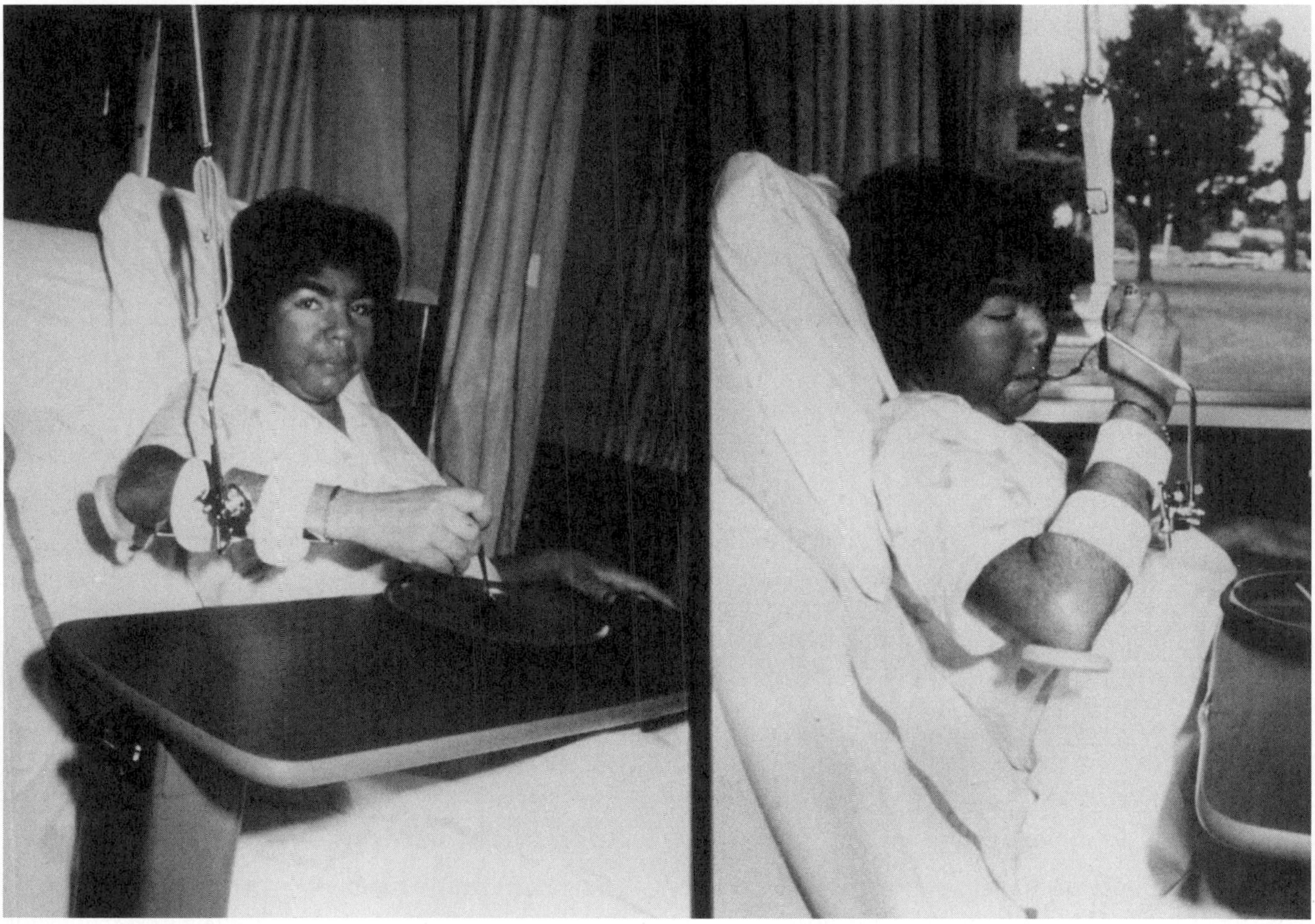

FIG. 31-52
Suspension arm support attached to bed. (From ARHP Arthritis Teaching Slide Collection, American College of Rheumatology.)

MOBILE ARM SUPPORTS

Mobile arm supports are mechanical devices that support the weight of the arm and provide assistance to shoulder and elbow motions through a linkage of ball-bearing joints. They are used for persons with weakness of the shoulder and elbow that affects their ability to position the hand. Mobile arm supports are or have been known by other names. Among these are MASs, ball-bearing feeder, ball-bearing arm support, balanced forearm orthosis (BFO), and arm positioner.

The MAS in current use (Fig. 31-54) has not changed significantly in design since 1952.[1] Earlier prototypes were reported as long ago as 1936, when a patient at the Georgia Warm Springs Foundation was given a Barker feeder, a device that was bolted to the lap board of a wheelchair and that required shoulder depression to bring the hands toward the head. Several other models were subsequently reported in the literature, until the design of the 1952 segmented arm feeder, which has close similarities to that seen today.[1,10]

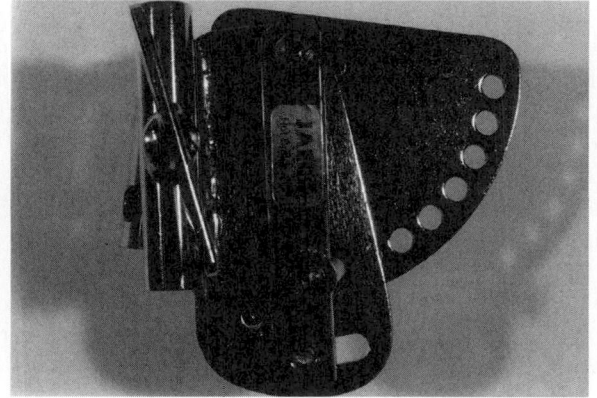

FIG. 31-53
Reclining suspension arm support bracket. (Courtesy of Paul Weinreich, Rancho Los Amigos National Rehabilitation Center.)

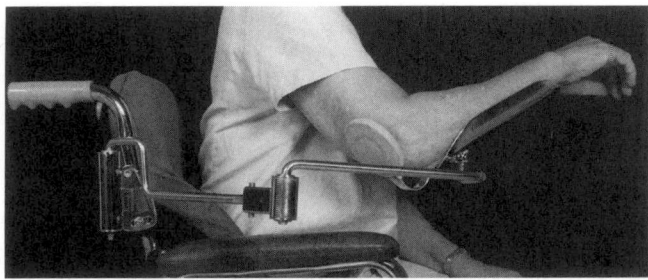

FIG. 31-54
Patient in standard mobile arm support set up on a wheelchair. (Courtesy of Paul Weinreich, Rancho Los Amigos National Rehabilitation Center.)

Mobile arm supports have increased UE function for persons with severe arm paralysis caused by such disabilities as cervical spinal cord injury, muscular dystrophy, Guillain-Barré syndrome, amyotrophic lateral sclerosis, poliomyelitis, and polymyositis.[4,11] The MAS has also been used for pain relief in the upper arm during function for patients with arthritis and other painful conditions.

How Mobile Arm Supports Work

Mobile arm supports compensate for proximal weakness in the UE in three ways. They provide arm motion, which allows for active ROM in the shoulder and elbow, they allow weak muscles that are below functional level to be used for movement; and they enable hand placement for activity in a variety of positions.

The purposes of mobile arm supports can be functional (i.e., allowing the weak arm to perform tabletop and hand-to-face activities, which otherwise are impossible or difficult) and therapeutic (i.e., improving ROM, strength, and endurance). The devices can be temporary or permanent.[8]

The mechanical principles of mobile arm supports are threefold. The MAS uses gravity to assist weak muscles, supports a weak arm to reduce the load of weak muscles, and reduces friction by using ball-bearing joints.[8]

Criteria for Use

Functional Need
The person must have a need to perform specific activities that cannot otherwise be accomplished because of weak shoulder and elbow musculature.

Adequate Source of Power
The source of power can be the muscles of the neck, trunk, shoulder, shoulder girdle, and elbow.

Adequate Motor Control
The person must be able to contract and relax functioning muscles. People with such conditions as cerebral palsy or significant elbow flexor tone are not usually good candidates for the mobile arm supports.

Sufficient Range of Motion
The preferred ROM for joints to use the MAS well is shoulder flexion and abduction (90°), shoulder external rotation (30°), shoulder internal rotation (normal), elbow flexion (normal), forearm pronation (80°), and hip flexion (100°).

Stable Trunk Positioning
An upright sitting posture is ideal. Good head and neck positioning is important.

Patient Motivation
The patient must want to use the device and have sufficient motivation for training to use it proficiently.

Supportive Environment
Generally, people who use this device cannot put it on themselves and will need support to help with the use of the device.[8]

Adjustment of Mobile Arm Supports

The adjustment of mobile arm supports generally requires postgraduate practical training. However, having some knowledge of adjustment will give the reader a greater appreciation for the need to have additional training to learn how to make fine adjustments. One study has shown that even when the MAS is not adjusted correctly, a person with sufficient muscle power can overcome the lack of fine adjustment.[12] This does not negate the need for therapists to be trained to ensure the best possible adjustment and mechanical advantage possible for the patient using the MAS.

Even with practical training, there are additional parts beyond the basic pieces that enhance the effectiveness of the device. The training needed to use these additional parts comes with practice, experience, and consultation with therapists familiar with the use of special parts.

Adjustment of Basic Parts
(Fig. 31-55)

FOREARM TROUGH. (Fig. 31-55, *D*). The forearm trough is initially fitted by bending the dial to accommodate the left or right elbow.

ROCKER ARM. The rocker arm is attached to the trough. The standard rocker arm is attached to the first and third holes closest to the elbow.

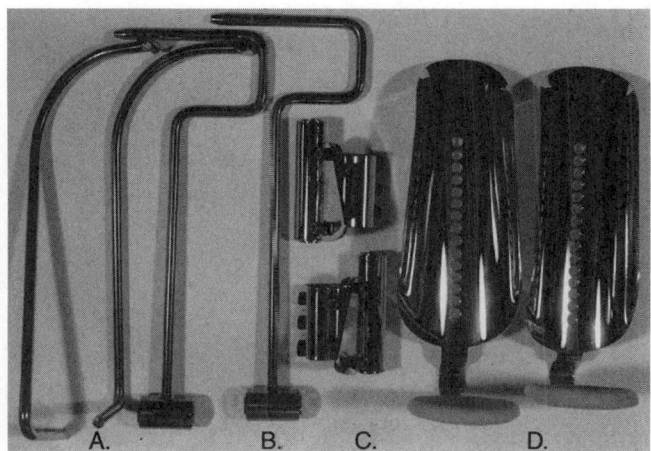

FIG. 31-55

Parts of standard mobile arm support. *A,* Distal arms, right and left; *B,* proximal arms; *C,* semireclining brackets, right and left; *D,* forearm troughs.

SEMIRECLINING BRACKET, PROXIMAL ARM, DISTAL ARM, AND FOREARM TROUGH. The bracket (Fig. 31-55, *C*) is attached to the wheelchair, the **proximal arm** (Fig. 31-55, *B*) is placed in the bracket, the **distal arm** (Fig. 31-55, *A*) is placed in the proximal arm, and the forearm trough is placed in the distal arm.

BALANCING THE MOBILE ARM SUPPORT AT NEUTRAL. The bracket is adjusted so that the ball bearings are parallel to the floor.

CHECKING THE BRACKET HEIGHT. The patient is placed in the MAS, and the therapist passively moves the hand to the mouth. If the shoulder is elevated or depressed, the height of the bracket should be adjusted.

ASSESSING TROUGH FOR FIT AND ADAPTATIONS. The trough is observed for forearm comfort and allowance of wrist flexion (if patient has active motion). Measurements are taken to have the trough cut if necessary to prevent discomfort and nonconformity to the size and shape of the forearm.

ADJUSTING FOR HORIZONTAL MOTION. The bracket is rolled to assist horizontal abduction or adduction. The pitch of the bracket or the distal bearing is adjusted to achieve maximum **horizontal motion** in front of the patient.

ADJUSTING FOR VERTICAL MOTION. The rocker arm is moved on the trough if up or down motion is difficult.

READJUSTING FOR FINE BALANCE. The therapist reviews all the adjustments to ensure maximum motion.

CHECKING FIT DURING OCCUPATIONAL PERFORMANCE. Further adjustments may be needed with the weight of objects in the hand.[8]

Training

Training proceeds using all activities that interest the patient and that need to be performed. Any of these activities may require various adjustments until the final settings are achieved. If strength or ROM increases during the training period, further adjustments may be needed. Adapted equipment can be used in conjunction with the MAS. A wrist-hand orthosis may be required or adjusted for use with the MAS.[8]

Follow-up with patients is indicated, especially for a growing child. Mobile arm supports can come out of adjustment over time. The questions in Box 31-1 are from a mobile arm support appraisal form that was

---

BOX 31-1

Mobile Arm Support Appraisal

1. Are the patient's hips set back in the chair?
2. Is the spine in good vertical alignment?
3. Is there good lateral trunk stability?
4. Is the chair seat and back adequate for comfort and stability?
5. Is the patient able to sit upright?
6. If the patient wears hand splints, are they on?
7. Does the patient have adequate passive range of motion?
8. Is the bracket tight on the wheelchair and positioned perpendicular to the floor?
9. Is the bracket at the proper height, so that the shoulders are not forced into elevation?
10. Is the proximal arm all the way down in the bracket?
11. Does the elbow dial clear the lap surface when the trough is in the "up" position?
12. When the trough is in the "up" position, is the patient's hand as close to the mouth as possible?
13. Can the patient obtain maximal active reach?
14. Is the trough the correct length? Does the distal end of the trough stop at the wrist joint?
15. Are the trough edges rolled so that they do not contact the forearm?
16. Is the elbow secure and comfortable in the elbow support?
17. Is the trough balanced correctly?
18. In vertical motion, is the dial free of the distal arm?
19. Can the patient control motion of the proximal arm from either extreme?
20. Can the patient control motion of the distal arm from either extreme?
21. Can the patient control vertical motion of the trough from either extreme?
22. Have stops been applied to limit range, if necessary?
23. Can the patient lift a sufficient amount of weight to perform appropriate functional tasks?

developed at Rancho Los Amigos National Rehabilitation Center in the polio era.[7] It can be a useful tool to check the adequacy of the fit of the MAS when the patient returns to the clinic for follow-up visits.

Special Parts of the Mobile Arm Support

Some commonly used special parts include the **outside rocker assembly** (also known as an offset swivel) and the **elevating proximal arm** (Fig. 31-56). The outside rocker assembly has a ball-bearing joint that allows greater freedom in vertical motion. The elevating proximal arm is useful for the person who has deltoid muscles that are between fair (F or 3) and poor (P or

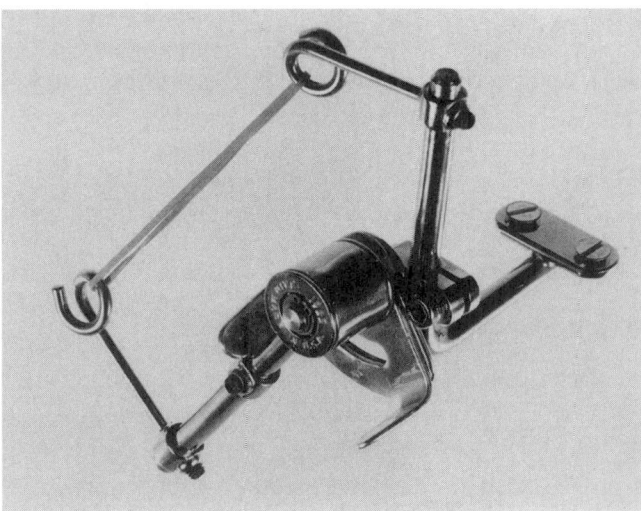

A

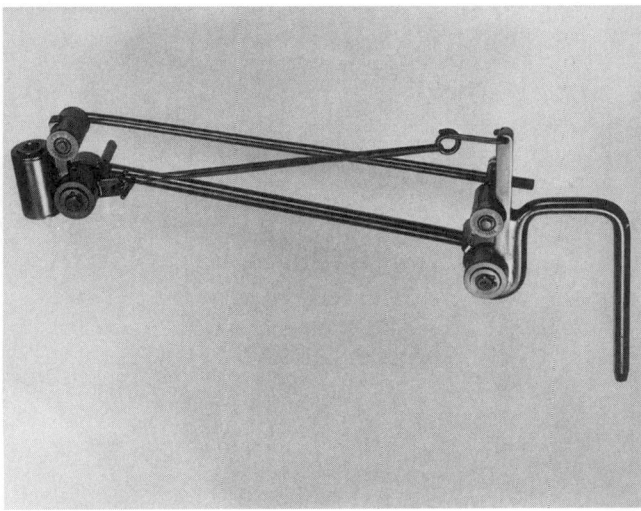

B

FIG. 31-56
A, Offset swivel with up and down stops and humeral rotation assist (outside rocker arm with rocker band assist). **B,** Elevating proximal arm. (Courtesy of JAECO Orthopedic Specialities, Hot Springs, Ark.)

2).[5] The patient initiates the elevating motion, and rubber band assists allow the patient to flex and abduct the humerus to a higher level.

Many other useful, but not commonly used, special parts are commercially available for patients with special problems. Understanding the use and adjustment of these special parts generally requires training.[8] With the advent of new designs for wheelchairs, it is sometimes necessary to adapt the MAS bracket to attach to the newer wheelchairs. Some wheelchair manufacturers can assist with providing solutions to these problems, and some centers have developed common solutions.[8]

FUTURE RESEARCH

Problems with the standard MAS have included difficulty mounting to wheelchairs, difficulty with learning adjustment strategies, and difficulty going through common doorways. As a part of a research grant funded by the National Institute on Disability and Rehabilitation Research (NIDRR), U.S. Department of Education for Rehabilitation Engineering Research Center on Technology for Children, a **multilink articulated arm** for the MAS that shows promise was developed at Rancho Los Amigos National Rehabilitation Center (Fig. 31-57).

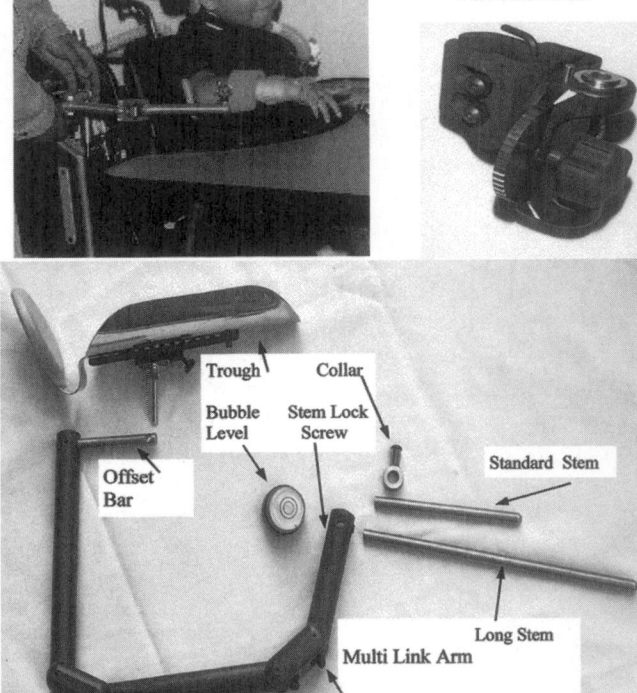

FIG. 31-57
New multilinked mobile arm support. (From Rancho Los Amigos National Rehabilitation Center, Rehabilitation Engineering Center, Downey, Calif.)

The multilink articulated arm for the MAS is low profile and flexible to facilitate passage through doorways. Children who tested the arm were pleased with the appearance and operation of the multilink design. It is not intended to replace the current MAS design but may offer a simpler option for users who do not have complex fitting problems.[9] At the time of this writing, the research is in its pilot phase of trial use with patients throughout the United States.

SUMMARY

Suspension arm devices and mobile arm supports can support the shoulder and forearm and afford increased occupational performance for persons with severe UE weakness. The MAS has been used for over 40 years. Adjustment of the device and training patients in its use require postgraduate training and experience.

Patients have been known to have the device originally ordered for at least 10 years, and probably beyond this. When fitted correctly the MAS enhances increased occupational performance and can facilitate remediation of performance components. For some patients the device is useful for life. For other patients the mobile support is a temporary device that allows function and enables exercise until musculature is strong enough to perform purposeful activities without them.

REVIEW QUESTIONS

SECTION 1

1. Describe the role of the occupational therapist in the splint-making process.
2. What is wrist tenodesis, and how can it be used functionally?
3. Describe the axis of motion of forearm rotation, and discuss how it affects the fit of a splint.
4. Name the three major nerves supplying the hand, and describe their sensory innervation patterns.
5. Why is tip prehension considered to be a dynamic prehension pattern rather than static?
6. What is the one grasp pattern that does not include the thumb?
7. Define the terms "friction," "torque," and "stress."
8. How is shear stress created, and how can it best be avoided?
9. Why do translational forces minimize the effectiveness of a splint?
10. Describe the difference between a dynamic and a static splint.
11. How might a splint pattern vary if it is to be fitted on the dorsum of the hand, as compared with the volar surface?

12. How does the amount of drape in a low-temperature thermoplastic material affect the making of a splint?
13. What is the recommended type of material for small finger splints? Why?
14. What is the recommended type of material for large elbow and lower extremity splints? Why?
15. What is the importance of straps on a single-surface splint?

SECTION 2

1. What are the purposes of suspension arm devices?
2. Where are suspension arm devices attached?
3. What are the limitations of suspension arm devices?
4. What is the difference between a suspension arm sling and a suspension arm support?
5. Which types of patients are good candidates for suspension arm devices? Which are not good candidates?
6. How are suspension arm devices adjusted?
7. When were mobile arm supports first used?
8. Name the parts of the MAS.
9. What are the benefits of the MAS?
10. How does the MAS work?
11. What are the criteria necessary to use the MAS?
12. How is the MAS adjusted for each patient?
13. What is the multilink articulated arm?

REFERENCES

1. Anderson KN, Anderson LE, Glanze WD, editors: *Mosby's medical, nursing, and allied health dictionary*, ed 4, St Louis, 1994, Mosby.

SECTION 1

1. American Society of Hand Therapists: *Splint classification system*, Chicago, 1992, The Society.
2. Bonutti PM, Windau JE, Ables BA, et al: Static progressive stretch to reestablish elbow range of motion, *Clin Orthop* June(303):128-134, 1994.
3. Brand PW, Hollister A: *Clinical mechanics of the hand*, ed 3, St Louis, 1999, Mosby.
4. Colditz J: Dynamic splinting of the stiff hand. In Hunter J, Schneider L, Mackin E, et al: *Rehabilitation of the hand: surgery and therapy*, ed 3, St Louis, 1990, Mosby.
5. Flatt AE: *Care of the arthritic hand*, St Louis, 1983, Mosby.
6. Hollister A, Giurintano D: How joints move. In Brand PW, Hollister A: *Clinical mechanics of the hand*, ed 3, St Louis, 1999, Mosby.
7. McCollough N, Sarrafian S: Biomechanical analysis system. In *Atlas of orthotics, biomechanical principles and application*, St Louis, 1975, Mosby.
8. Strickland JW: Anatomy and kinesiology of the hand. In Fess E, Philips C: *Hand splinting: principles and methods*, St Louis, 1987, Mosby.

SECTION 2

1. Bennett RL: The evolution of the Georgia Warm Springs Foundation Feeder. *Artif Limb* 10(1):5-9, 1966.

2. Bennett RL: Orthotics for function. I. Prescription, *Phys Ther Rev* 36(11):1-25, 1956.
3. Bennett RL, Stephens HR: Care of severely paralyzed upper extremities, *JAMA* 149(2):105-109, 1952.
4. Haworth R, Dunscombe S, Nichols PJR: Mobile arm supports: an evaluation, *Rheumatol Rehabil* 17(4):240-244, 1978.
5. *JAECO Orthopedic Specialties catalog*, Hot Springs, Ark (undated).
6. Long C: Upper limb bracing. In Licth S, editor: *Orthotics etcetera*, Baltimore, 1966, Waverly Press.
7. Rancho Los Amigos Medical Center, Occupational Therapy Department: *Mobile arm support appraisal*, Downey, Calif, 1969, the Center (unpublished).
8. Rancho Los Amigos National Rehabilitation Center, Occupational Therapy Department: *Mobile arm support workshop manual*, Downey, Calif, 1998, the Center.
9. Rehabilitation Engineering Program: *Annual report, 1997, RERC on Technology for Children*, Downey, Calif, 1997, Rancho Los Amigos Medical Center Research and Education Institute.
10. Snelson R, Conry J: Recent advancements in functional arm bracing correlated with orthopedic surgery for the severely paralyzed upper extremity, *Orthop Prosthet Appliance J*, 41-49, 1958.
11. Wilson DJ, McKenzie MW, Barber LM: *Spinal cord injury: a treatment guide for occupational therapists*, rev ed, Thorofare, NJ, 1984, Slack.
12. Yasuda, YL, Bowman K, Hsu JD: Mobile arm supports: criteria for successful use in muscle disease patients, *Arch Phys Med Rehabil* 67(4):253-256, 1986.

PATRICIA ANN GENTILE
MEENAKSHI B. IYER

CHAPTER

32

Traditional Sensorimotor Approaches to Treatment: An Overview

KEY TERMS

Lower motor neurons
Upper motor neurons
Information flow
Motivational urge
Ideation
Movement strategy
Motor program
Execution level
Sensorimotor system
Reflex and hierarchical models
Top-down orientation
Sensory stimulation
Evolution in reverse
Mass movement patterns

LEARNING OBJECTIVES

After studying this chapter the student or practitioner will be able to do the following:

1. Name the structures that constitute the upper motor neurons.
2. Describe the four general processes of information flow related to control of movement.
3. Define *motivational urge,* and name the locus of this function in the brain.
4. Describe where in the brain *motivational urge* is transformed to ideas for purposeful movement.
5. Trace the flow of information in the central and peripheral nervous systems that leads to purposeful movement.
6. Define *sensorimotor system* and give its locus in the brain.
7. Describe where movement planning takes place in the brain.
8. List the structures that constitute the higher, middle, and lower levels of the central nervous system components for movement.
9. Name the four traditional sensorimotor approaches to treatment and the theorist responsible for each.
10. Name the two models of motor control that form the basis for the sensorimotor approaches to treatment.
11. Briefly describe each of the four traditional sensorimotor approaches to treatment; compare and contrast their similarities and their differences.

ccupational therapists working with patients who have sustained damage to the central nervous system (CNS) are concerned with enhancing functional movement and promoting independence in occupational performance. To achieve this objective, a variety of treatment approaches are available from which the therapist may choose. This chapter reviews the neurological considerations for these approaches and presents a brief description of each. More detailed explanations of the approaches can be found in Chapters 33 to 36.

NEUROLOGICAL CONSIDERATIONS FOR THE TRADITIONAL SENSORIMOTOR APPROACHES TO TREATMENT

Occupation presupposes voluntary movement that is controlled and monitored by the nervous system. This control is precise and all encompassing, whether the movement is to maintain a posture, carry a load, or play the piano. The nervous system determines both the muscles to be activated and the extent of their activation. If a movement is poorly performed, learning occurs through feedback and the commands to the muscles are updated so that accuracy of movement is achieved. This requires the coordinated activity of many brain regions. Knowledge of the intricate working of the nervous system is of special importance to the occupational therapist concerned with refining and improving the motor performance of patients with neurological conditions. A brief overview of the flow of information associated with the control of movement is described in the following sections.

Brain Control of Movement

The firing of motor neurons located in the spinal cord produces all movements.[17] These neurons directly innervate the skeletal muscles. The activity of the spinal or **lower motor neurons** can be modulated by local segmental spinal circuitry and by the descending drive from the motor neurons located in the motor cortex and brainstem. Two other structures, the basal ganglia and the cerebellum, and their associated pathways are intimately involved with motor control. Thus there are three structures or **upper motor neurons** involved in movement production. Lesions of each of these structures are associated with characteristic weaknesses. The unmodified term *upper motor neuron* can be confusing and inappropriate, since the upper motor neuron is composed of three structures.

Movement production does not begin and end with the motor system. Many CNS structures contribute to the development of the signals that activate muscles. Although there is much about the control of movement that is still unknown, both animal and human research suggest that there are four general processes related to the control of movement. The four general processes of **information flow** are motivation, ideation, programming, and execution.[2,3] A schematic diagram indicating the main direction of information flow and connecting the various motor centers appears in Fig. 32-1.

The motivation or emotive component of the movement is a function of the limbic system.[2,14] The **motivational urge** or *impulse to act* of the limbic system is transformed to ideas by the cortical association areas. The association areas of the frontal, parietal, temporal, and occipital lobes are concerned with **ideation,** or the goal of the movement, and the programming or **movement strategy** (plan) that best achieves the goal. Programming also involves the premotor areas, the basal ganglia, and the cerebellum. The **motor program** is the procedure or the spatiotemporal order of muscle activation that is needed for smooth and accurate motor performance. The **execution level,** represented by the motor cortex, the cerebellum, and the spinal cord, is concerned with the activation of the spinal motor neurons and interneurons that generate the goal-directed movement and the necessary postural adjustments.

To appreciate the flow of information leading to purposeful movement, consider the actions of a person who is thirsty and who is reaching out for a glass of water (Fig. 32-2). The limbic system, which connects with the areas of the midbrain and brainstem that control vital functions such as hunger and thirst, has registered the need for water.[6] This need for drinking water has been conveyed to the cortical association areas, which have information based on vision, audition, somatic sensation, and proprioception about precisely where the body is in space and where the glass of water is relative to the body. This sensory information is needed before the movement is initiated. Strategies or motor plans are formulated to move the arm and hand from their immediate location in space to one in which the glass of water is picked up and moved to the mouth. Motor programs are generated by the association cortex in conjunction with the basal ganglia, lateral cerebellum, and premotor cortex. Once strategy is determined, the motor cortex is activated. The motor cortex, in turn, conveys the action plan to reach and lift the glass in a particular manner to the brainstem and spinal cord. Activation of the cervical spinal neurons generates a coordinated and precise movement of the shoulder, elbow, wrist, and fingers. Input from the brainstem ensures that the necessary postural adjustments are made by the axial musculature. Sensory information during the movement is necessary not only to ensure the smooth performance of the ongoing movement, but also to improve subsequent similar movements. Since the motor areas rely so heavily on sensory information, provided

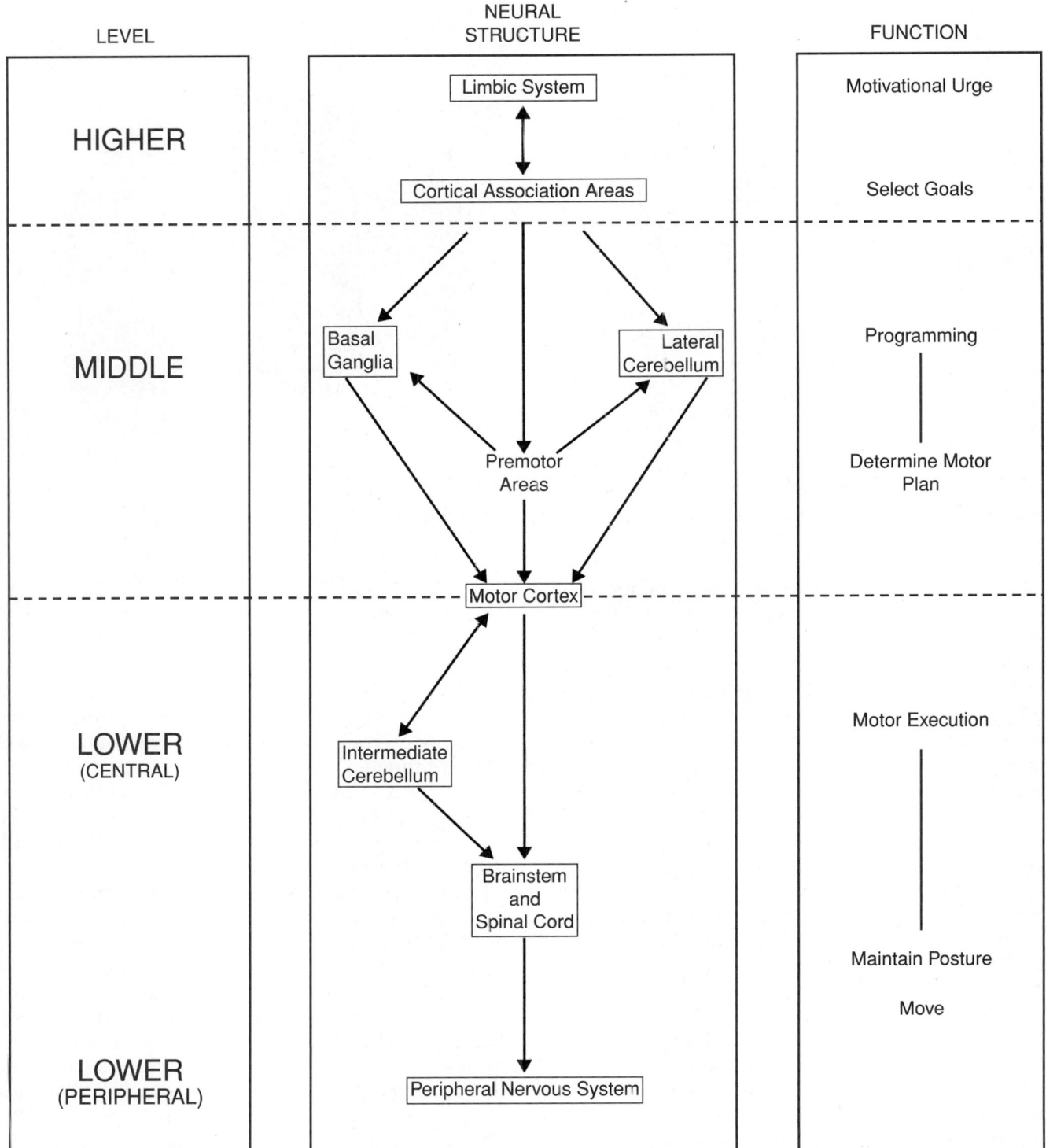

FIG. 32-1
Schematic representation of the hierarchy of the neural structures involved in motor control. The left column indicates the hierarchical level and the right column the major function of the neural structures shown in the center column during motor performance. (Adapted from Cheney PD: Role of cerebral cortex in voluntary movements: a review, *Phys Ther* 65[5]:624-635, 1985.)

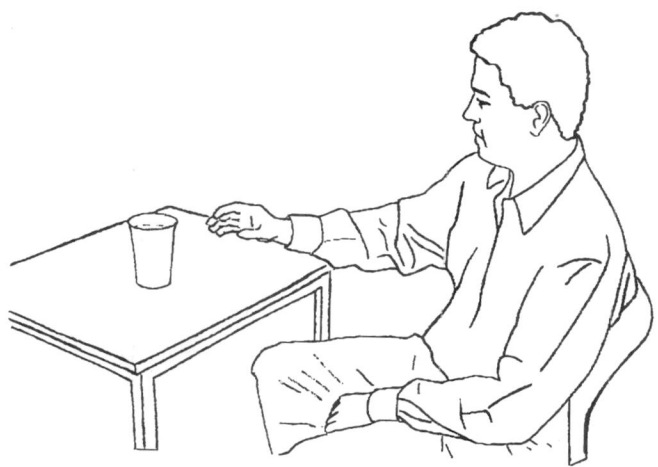

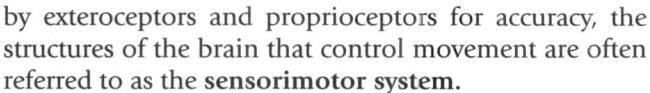

FIG. 32-2
A person reaching out for a glass of water.

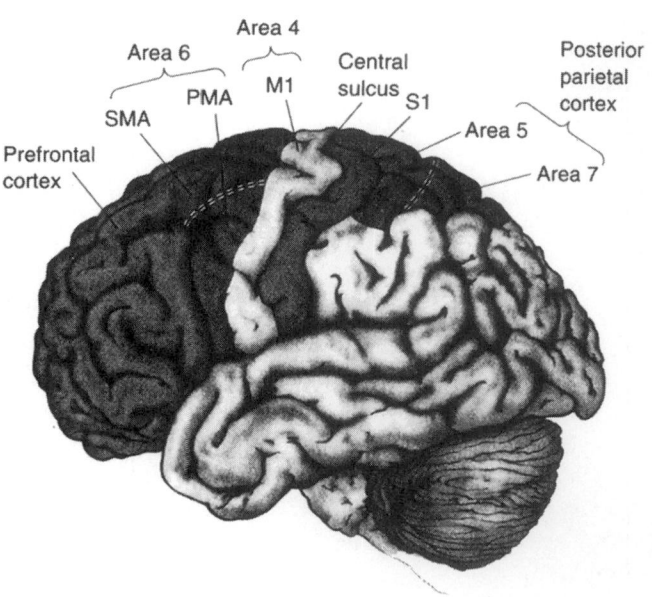

FIG. 32-3
Areas of the neocortex intimately involved in planning and instruction of voluntary movement. Areas 4 and 6 constitute motor cortex. (From Bear MF, Connors BW, Paradiso MA: *Neuroscience: exploring the brain*, Baltimore, 1996, Williams & Wilkins.)

by exteroceptors and proprioceptors for accuracy, the structures of the brain that control movement are often referred to as the **sensorimotor system.**

Given the motivation-ideation-programming-execution scheme of organization of information through the nervous system, it is obvious that control of voluntary movement involves almost all of the neocortex. Voluntary movement depends on knowledge of where the body is in space, where the body intends to go with respect to this external space, the internal and external loads that must be overcome, and formulation of a strategy or plan to perform the movement. Once a strategy or plan has been formulated, it must be held in memory until execution, at which point appropriate instructions are sent to the spinal motor neurons. The major functional aspects of some of the sensorimotor areas involved in motor control are examined below. References 2, 10, and 14 provide more details on this topic.

Sensorimotor Cortex

The sensorimotor cortex is the major integrating center of sensory input and motor output. It is composed of cortical areas located immediately anterior and posterior to the central sulcus (Fig. 32-3). The three principal motor regions located in the frontal lobe are the primary motor area, the supplementary motor area, and the premotor area. The two principal sensory regions located in the parietal lobe are the primary somatosensory cortex and the posterior parietal cortex. Both anterior and posterior regions contribute to the descending corticospinal tract, which influences the activity of the motor neurons located in the ventral spinal cord. The output from the sensory cortical areas goes to the dorsal spinal cord and modulates peripheral sensory input, ev-

idenced by the presence of the long latency stretch reflex.[15] In addition, there are other networks of descending, ascending, and cortico-cortical connections of the sensorimotor cortex.[5,7,9]

Each area of the sensorimotor cortex (primary motor cortex, primary somatosensory cortex, posterior parietal cortex, supplementary motor area, and premotor cortex) is arranged in a manner that provides a topographical representation of the contralateral body segments.[10,12] Each of these areas is principally responsible for certain aspects of movement generation. In the case of the previous example of reaching out for the glass of water, the mental image of the body and its relation to the surrounding space depends on somatosensory, proprioceptive, and visual inputs to the posterior parietal cortex. Patients with a lesion in this area demonstrate impairment of body image and its relation to extrapersonal space, and in the extreme situation a neglect of the contralateral body segments.

The posterior parietal cortex integrates and translates sensory information so that the ensuing movements are directed appropriately in extrapersonal space. It is extensively interconnected with the association areas of the frontal lobe that are considered to be involved in determining the consequences of movement strategies such as moving the arm forward, curling the fingers around the plastic cup, and lifting the cup to the mouth. The fingers begin to curl appropriately before there is any contact with the cup; therefore the size and shape of the cup must be recognized before grasping. Both the prefrontal association areas and the posterior parietal cortex project to the premotor area, which is thought to be concerned with orientation of body segments before initiation of movement. The input of the posterior parietal cortex to the premotor area may be important in the somatosensory guidance of movement.[3] Lesions of the premotor area or posterior parietal cortex have been demonstrated to result in the generation of inappropriate movement strategy.[8]

Planning of movement is considered to be the function of the supplementary motor area. Electrophysiological recordings of the cells in this area in behaving animals indicate that the cells typically increase discharge rates about a second before the execution of movement of either hand.[18] The same findings have been corroborated in humans, using imaging studies to study patterns of cortical activation. Imaging studies using positron emission tomography (PET) monitor changes in local blood flow, since an increase in the local cerebral blood flow is associated with increased neuronal activity. Under these conditions, when subjects were asked to imagine a movement without actually moving the finger, the blood flow to the supplementary motor cortex increased and no similar increase in blood flow was seen in the primary motor area.[13] When subjects were asked to perform a series of finger movements from memory, blood flow to the supplementary motor cortex increased in advance of the movement, but not during the performance of the movement. Unilateral lesions of the supplementary motor area result in apraxia (the loss of the ability to perform movement in the absence of motor or sensory impairments). Another effect of such lesions is the inability to produce the correct sequence of muscle activation for complex motor activities such as speaking, writing, buttoning, typing, sewing, and playing the piano.

The primary somatosensory cortex projection to the primary motor cortex and association areas provides the sensory input needed for motor planning, movement initiation, and regulation of ongoing movement.[4] The primary motor cortex integrates the information it receives from other areas of the brain and generates the descending command for the execution of movement. Not only is this descending command sent to the brainstem and spinal cord, but a copy of it is also sent to the basal ganglia and cerebellum. The descending command specifies the muscles to be activated and the direction, speed, and required force.[3] Lesions of the primary somatosensory cortex typically result in contralateral sensory loss. Movements are uncoordinated because of an inability to register sensory feedback during and after the movement. Damage to the primary motor area results in execution deficits. The patient presents the classic picture of muscle weakness, spasticity, and decreased fractionation of movement with corresponding loss of function.

Relation to Sensorimotor Treatment Approaches

The CNS components for movement can be grouped functionally into higher, middle, and lower levels. The higher level consists of the limbic system and association areas. The sensorimotor areas, along with the basal ganglia and cerebellum, form the middle level, and the lower level consists of the nuclei in the brainstem and spinal cord. Under normal circumstances the repertoire of muscle activity is quite large. Following damage to higher centers there is a loss of descending excitatory input. The possible levels of modulation of spinal motor neurons become quite limited, and the muscle response may be limited or stereotyped. Traditional sensorimotor approaches to treatment (described in the subsequent chapters) can be viewed as targeting the middle sensorimotor level, the motor planning–strategy formulation process, and the lower-level execution process, with the aim of reintegrating, as far as possible, a complete motor control hierarchy. It easily can be seen that the motor relearning program should be cognitively oriented and targeted toward achieving a goal or "occupational" task.

Patients need to be taught motor strategies or compensatory mechanisms to adapt to the deficits produced by a lesion. Compensatory mechanisms and the shaping of motor programs are brought about by the use of sensory inputs. The sensorimotor approaches use sensory stimulation to elicit specific movement patterns. Early in the treatment phase, the emphasis is on the use of external sensory stimuli. Once a movement response is obtained, in order to reinforce and strengthen the response, the focus shifts to the use of intrinsic sensory information, thereby encouraging voluntary motor control.

The four traditional sensorimotor treatment approaches historically used by occupational therapy (OT) practitioners are the Rood approach, the Brunnstrom (movement therapy) approach, the proprioceptive neuromuscular approach (PNF), and the neurodevelopmental (Bobath) approach. These approaches, developed in the 1950s and 1960s, all have their theoretical basis in the **reflex and hierarchical models** of motor control. Although more contemporary models are currently being used to guide treatment with patients who demonstrate CNS dysfunction, an understanding of these traditional approaches is warranted to appreciate their contributions to clinical practice and to recognize the appropriate application of these approaches in selected patient populations.

Reflex and Hierarchical Models of Motor Control

Both reflex and hierarchical models of motor control view movement developmentally. There are two major fundamental assumptions underlying the reflex and hierarchical models:

1. *The basic units of motor control are reflexes.* Reflexes are motor responses that occur in response to specific sensory stimuli. Reflexes are automatic, predictable, and stereotypical; they are normal responses that are seen from early infancy. As the CNS matures, reflexes become integrated and are believed to form the foundation for volitional motor control. Volitional (purposeful) movement is the summation and integration of reflexive movement. When damage to the CNS occurs, there is a resurgence of reflexive motor activity and an inability to modulate these reflexive movements.

2. *Motor control is hierarchically arranged.* In a hierarchical model of motor control, it is believed that the CNS has a specific organizational structure and motor development and function are dependent upon that structure. This organization is in a **top-down orientation;** that is, the higher centers of the brain regulate and exert control over lower centers of the CNS. The higher centers, specifically the cortical and subcortical areas, are responsible for regulating and controlling volitional, conscious movement. The lower levels regulate and control reflexive, automatic, and responsive movement. Based on this conceptual-

TABLE 32-1

Comparison of Key Treatment Strategies Used in the Traditional Sensorimotor Approaches to Treatment

Key Treatment Strategies	Rood Approach	Brunnstrom Approach (Movement Therapy)	Proprioceptive Neuromuscular Approach	Neurodevelopmental Treatment
Sensory stimulation used to evoke a motor response	YES (Uses direct application of sensory stimuli to muscles and joints)	YES (Movement occurs in response to sensory stimuli)	YES (Tactile, auditory, visual sensory stimuli promote motor responses)	YES (Abnormal muscle tone occurs, in part, because of abnormal sensory experiences)
Reflexive movement used as a precursor for volitional movement	YES (Reflexive movement achieved initially through the application of sensory stimuli)	YES (Move patient along a continuum of reflexive to volitional movement patterns)	YES (Volitional movements can be assisted by reflexive supported postures)	NO
Treatment directed toward influencing muscle tone	YES (Sensory stimuli used to inhibit or facilitate tone)	YES (Postures, sensory stimuli used to inhibit or facilitate tone)	YES (Movement patterns used to normalize tone)	YES (Handling techniques and postures can inhibit or facilitate muscle tone)
Developmental patterns/sequences used for the development of motor skills	YES (Ontogenic motor patterns used to develop motor skills)	YES (Flexion and extension synergies; proximal to distal return)	YES (Patterns used to facilitate proximal to distal motor control)	NO
Conscious attention is directed toward movement	NO	YES	YES	NO
Treatment directly emphasizes development of skilled movements for task performance	NO	NO	NO	NO

ization , when damage occurs to the CNS, it is believed that the damaged area can no longer regulate and exert control over the underlying areas. Motor control, according to this belief, becomes a function of the next lower functioning level of the CNS. Typically this means a return to more reflexive and primitive movement patterns.

The four traditional sensorimotor treatment strategies rely heavily on these basic assumptions about motor development and motor control. Consequently, treatment strategies used in these approaches frequently involve the application of sensory stimulation to muscles and joints to evoke specific motor responses, handling and positioning techniques to effect changes in muscle tone, and the use of developmental postures to enhance the ability to initiate and carry out movements. Table 32-1 presents a comparison and summary of key treatment strategies used in each of the four traditional sensorimotor approaches.

OVERVIEW: THE TRADITIONAL SENSORIMOTOR TREATMENT APPROACHES
Rood Approach

Margaret Rood drew heavily from both the reflex and the hierarchical models in designing her treatment approach. Key components of the Rood approach are the use of **sensory stimulation** to evoke a motor response and the use of developmental postures to promote changes in muscle tone.[11] Sensory stimulation is applied to muscles and joints to elicit a specific motor response. Stimulation has the potential to have either an inhibitory or a facilitatory effect on muscle tone. Types of sensory stimulation described by Rood include the use of slow rolling, neutral warmth, deep pressure, tapping, and prolonged stretch. Examples of how this stimulation may be applied include tapping over a muscle belly to facilitate (increase) muscle tone and applying deep pressure to a muscle's tendinous insertion to elicit an inhibitory (decreased) effect. Rood also described the use of specific developmental sequences believed to promote motor responses. These sequences were proximal to distal and cephalocaudal. Treatment strategies move patients through these developmental sequences.

In current clinical practice, practitioners may use selected principles from Rood's work as adjunctive or preliminary interventions in order to prepare a patient to engage in a purposeful activity—for example, the application of quick stretch over the triceps before instructing a patient to reach for a cup. A patient may be instructed in ways to apply his or her own sensory stimulation in order to enhance ADL performance. For example, during upper extremity dressing, a patient might perform a prolonged stretch to the biceps, resulting in a

reduction of muscle tone, which may increase the ease in which the arm is moved through the sleeve of a shirt.

Limitations in the use of Rood's approach are numerous and include the passive nature of the sensory stimulation (it is applied "to" a patient) and the short-lasting and unpredictable effect of some of the sensory stimulation.

The Brunnstrom (Movement Therapy) Approach

Signe Brunnstrom, a physical therapist, developed a treatment approach specifically for patients who had sustained a cerebrovascular accident (CVA). The approach she designed draws strongly from both the reflex and hierarchical models of motor control. Brunnstrom conceptualized patients who had sustained a CVA as going through an **"evolution in reverse"**; within this concept the early reflexive movement that may be present is seen as a normal process of this evolution. Spastic or flaccid muscle tone and the presence of reflexive movements that might be evident after a CVA are considered a normal process of recovery; they are viewed as necessary intermediate steps in regaining volitional movement.[16] Brunnstrom clearly detailed stages of motor recovery following a CVA. These stages include the description of flexor synergy patterns and extensor synergy patterns for the upper and lower limbs.

In the Brunnstrom approach emphasis is on facilitating the progress of patients by promoting movement, from reflexive to volitional. In the early stages of recovery this may include the incorporation of reflexes and associated reactions to affect tone and achieve movement. For example, to generate reflexive movement in the upper limb, resistance may be applied to one side of the body in order to increase muscle tone on the opposite side. This technique is applied until the patient demonstrates volitional control over the movement pattern.

In current clinical practice most OT practitioners do not use Brunnstrom's treatment strategies for fear of increasing and encouraging the development of abnormal movement patterns, which may be difficult to undo later on. However, the stages of recovery are used in some rehabilitation settings to describe motor recovery.

Proprioceptive Neuromuscular Facilitation Approach

The proprioceptive neuromuscular facilitation (PNF) approach is grounded in both the reflex and hierarchical models of motor control. Major emphasis in this approach is on the developmental sequencing of movement and the balanced interplay between agonist and antagonist in producing volitional movement.[19] PNF describes **mass movement patterns**, which are diagonal in nature, for the limbs and trunk. Treatment strategies use these patterns to promote movement. The use of sensory stimulation, including tactile, auditory, and visual inputs, is also actively incorporated into treatment to promote a motor response.

In OT clinical practice the inclusion of PNF patterns often can be seen in the way functional activities are designed, especially in the placement of objects during purposeful activities. Asking a patient to reach into a shopping bag placed on his left side in order to retrieve objects that will then be placed into a cabinet on the right side is an example of this.

Neurodevelopmental Treatment Approach

Neurodevelopmental treatment, also known as the Bobath treatment approach, is based on normal development and movement. It draws from the hierarchical model of motor control. The primary objectives of neurodevelopmental treatment are to normalize muscle tone, inhibit primitive reflexes, and facilitate normal postural reactions.[1] Improving the quality of movement and helping patients relearn normal movement patterns are key objectives of treatment. To achieve these objectives, therapists employ numerous techniques, including handling techniques, weight bearing over the affected limb, the use of positions that encourage the use of both sides of the body, and the avoidance of any sensory input that might adversely affect muscle tone. In clinical practice today, many of these techniques and strategies are used in treatment within the context of purposeful activities.

SUMMARY

Movement takes place within an occupational context. Emotional needs influence motor strategies. The spinal cord or brainstem can mediate reflexive responses, but interpretation and transformation of sensory signals by all areas of the sensorimotor system are essential for voluntary movement to occur with precision. The primary somatosensory cortex and posterior parietal cortex are primarily responsible for processing sensory information. The premotor area uses sensory information for the planning of movements, the supplementary motor area is important for bimanual coordination, and the motor cortex is important for execution.

The traditional sensorimotor treatment approaches have their theoretical basis in reflex and hierarchical models of motor control. These approaches offer a valuable link between neurophysiological principles and the rehabilitation treatment of patients with CNS dysfunction. In contemporary practice many of the techniques described in these approaches are used as adjunctive or preliminary techniques or are incorporated into more task-directed treatment activities.

REVIEW QUESTIONS

1. Which structures constitute the upper motor neurons?
2. What are the four general processes of information flow related to control of movement?
3. Define *motivational urge* and name the locus of this function in the brain.
4. Where in the brain is *motivational urge* transformed to ideas?
5. Define *motor program*.
6. Trace the flow of information in the central and peripheral nervous systems that leads to purposeful movement.
7. What is the sensorimotor system?
8. List the areas of the sensorimotor cortex.
9. Where does movement planning take place?
10. List the structures that constitute the higher, middle, and lower levels of the central nervous system components for movement.
11. Name the four traditional sensorimotor approaches to treatment and the theorist responsible for each.
12. Which two models of motor control form the basis for the sensorimotor approaches to treatment?
13. Briefly describe each of the four traditional sensorimotor approaches to treatment. Compare and contrast their similarities and their differences.
14. List some techniques used by therapists to influence or modify motor responses in each of the traditional sensorimotor approaches.
15. How are the sensorimotor approaches used in current clinical practice?

REFERENCES

1. Bobath B: *Adult hemiplegia: evaluation and treatment,* ed 3, London, 1991, Heinemann Medical Books.
2. Brooks VB: *The neural basis of motor control,* New York, 1986, Oxford University Press.
3. Cheney PD: Role of cerebral cortex in voluntary movements: a review, *Phys Ther* 65(5):624-635, 1985.
4. Fromm C, Wise SP, Evarts EV: Sensory response properties of pyramidal tract neurons in the precentral motor cortex and postcentral gyrus of the rhesus monkey, *Exp Brain Res* 54(1):177-185, 1984.
5. Georgopoulus AP et al: The motor cortex and the coding of force, *Science* 256(5064):1692-1695, 1992.
6. Holstege G: The emotional motor system, *Eur J Morphol* 30(1):67-79, 1992.
7. Houk JC, Keifer J, Barto AG: Distributed motor commands in the limb premotor network, *Trend Neurosci* 16(1):27-33, 1993.
8. Jeannerod M: *The neural and behavioral organization of goal-directed movements,* Oxford, 1988, Clarendon Press.
9. Kalaska JF, Crammond DJ: Cerebral cortical mechanisms of reaching movements, *Science* 255(5051):1517-1523, 1992.
10. Kandel ER, Schwartz JH, Jesell TM, editors: *Principles of neural science,* ed 3, New York, 1991, Elsevier.
11. McCormack G: The Rood approach to treatment of neuromuscular dysfunction. In Pedretti LW, editor: *Occupational therapy: practice skills for physical dysfunction,* ed 4, St Louis, 1996, Mosby.

12. Penfield W: *The excitable cortex in conscious man*, Liverpool, 1958, Liverpool University Press.
13. Roland P et al: Supplementary motor area and other cortical areas in organization of voluntary movements in man, *J Neurophysiol* 43(1):118-136, 1980.
14. Rothwell JC: *Control of human voluntary movement*, ed 2, London, 1994, Chapman & Hall.
15. Rothwell JC et al: Physiological studies in a patient with mirror movements and agenesis of the corpus collosum, *J Physiol* 438:34P, 1991.
16. Sawner K, LaVigne J: *Brunnstrom's movement therapy in hemiplegia: a neurophysiological approach*, ed 2, Philadelphia, 1992, JB Lippincott.
17. Sherrington C: *The integrative action of the nervous system*, ed 2, New Haven, Conn, 1947, Yale University Press.
18. Tanji J, Taniguchi K, Saga T: Supplementary motor area: neuronal response to motor instructions, *J Neurophysiol* 43(1):60-68, 1980.
19. Voss DE, Ionta MK, Myers BJ: *Proprioceptive neuromuscular facilitation*, ed 3, Philadelphia, 1985, Harper & Row.

CHAPTER 33

The Rood Approach: A Reconstruction

CHARLOTTE BRASIC ROYEEN
MAUREEN DUNCAN
GUY McCORMACK

KEY TERMS

Chaos theory
Dynamic systems
Coeffect
Nonlinear
Generalizability
Somatic marker
Meta-emotion
Reciprocal inhibition
Cocontraction
Heavy work
Skill
Supine withdrawal
Rollover
Pivot prone
Neck cocontraction
Ontogenetic patterns
Proprioceptive neuromuscular techniques
Vestibular stimulation
Inversion
Inhibitory techniques

LEARNING OBJECTIVES

After studying this chapter the student or practitioner will be able to do the following:
1. Identify the importance of Margaret Rood's work.
2. Define key concepts first proposed by Margaret Rood.
3. Delineate how Rood's concepts have been redefined in light of current understanding of neuroscience.
4. Recognize the four components of motor control emphasized by Rood.
5. Describe the major motor patterns of development identified by Rood.
6. Delineate examples of how Rood's major motor patterns are used during occupation.
7. State reasons for caution when employing Rood's treatment techniques.
8. Give two examples of Rood techniques still used today.
9. Contrast the traditional Rood approach and the Rood approach reconstructed for occupation-based practice.

Margaret S. Rood was formally educated in both occupational and physical therapy. She originated her theory in the 1940s and revised it many times. Rood did not write extensively; she seemed to prefer clinical teaching for the dissemination of her ideas. Most of the literature that describes the Rood approach is based on interpretations by accomplished occupational and physical therapists such as Ayres,[1] Farber,[8,9] Heininger,[12] Randolph,[20] Huss,[13] and Stockmeyer.[26]

Theories and related frames of reference exist within the context of the time and level of knowledge from which they originate. Many would say that the work of Margaret Rood is out of date and thus not worthy of study. Many of the particular techniques and some of the hypotheses posed by Rood have never been adequately tested or researched. Nonetheless, to discount Rood's work as out of date is to discount an important historical perspective of occupational therapy (OT) and to dismiss

The first author wishes to acknowledge the inspirational leadership of Virginia Scardina in promoting the work of Margaret Rood.

the possibility of incorporating elements of her work into more recent understanding of central nervous system (CNS) processing linked to therapeutic intervention. Thus the purpose of this chapter is to offer a reconstruction of Rood's work based on current understanding of CNS processing and occupation-based intervention.

A measure of the contribution of a scholar to a field is not whether he or she is ultimately determined to be right or wrong, but how much research and deliberation the person's work engendered. Rood's work continues to be valuable to OT in terms of orientation to the interaction of the nervous system with behavior, function, and, most significantly, occupation. For all of these reasons, the work of Margaret Rood is important for therapists to study.

The work of Margaret Rood was set in the context of the developmental and neurophysiological literature of the 1930s through the 1970s. At that time the neuroscience literature was based on assumptions of the hierarchical nature of the nervous system that have subsequently been revised. In light of current understanding of the heterarchial (flattened hierarchy) nature of nervous system functioning, a reconstruction of Rood's work is executed based in part on current understanding of **chaos theory** and **dynamic systems**. Rood's main contribution has been to highlight the importance of interactions that occur between the nervous system and occupation (i.e., that the nervous system and occupation **coeffect** one another in a dynamic, **nonlinear** manner). Coeffect refers to the interaction of one or more forces upon the other force(s), suggesting a state or condition of active interdependence.

Specifically, Rood identified (1) that the feedback loop of motor and sensory signals coeffect each other, (2) that patterns of sensory-motor behaviors emerge over time, and (3) that the psychic, somatic, and autonomic functions operate within a system of coeffects or interrelationships.

RECONSTRUCTION OF ROOD'S THEORY FOR OCCUPATION-BASED PRACTICE

Rood's work has been synthesized into the essential concepts presented in Table 33-1, which provides a historical view with a reinterpretation of concepts that still apply.

As delineated in Table 33-1, six key concepts of Rood have been reconstructed (right column) from the traditional view, (left column), in light of current knowledge and understanding pertaining to the areas. Each of these reconstructed concepts is briefly discussed in the following paragraphs.

"Muscle tone and motor control coeffect each other" refers to the relationship that exists between the tone of the muscles and the execution of the motor act. These are but two parameters among a myriad of variables

TABLE 33-1
Summary of Main Concepts of Rood's Work

Traditional Rood	Reconstruction of Rood
Normalization of muscle tone is a prerequisite for movement.	Muscle tone and motor control coeffect each other.
Treatment begins at the developmental level of functioning.	Flexion and extension patterns coeffect each other.
Reeducation of muscular responses occurs through repetition.	Repetition of muscular responses creates movement patterns.
Movement is directed toward functional goals.	Intention or goal direction coeffects movement.
Approximation of real life context increases treatment effectiveness and generalizability.*	Approximation of real life context increases treatment effectiveness and generalizability.
Therapeutic use of self should match client needs.*	Therapists use somatic markers to select interaction methods with clients.†

*This was a basic Rood premise taught to the first author by Margaret Rood during a 2-week training course in Cincinnati in the 1970s.
†See Chapter 8, "The Somatic Marker Hypothesis," in Damasio AR: *Descartes' error: emotion, reason and the human brain*, New York, 1994, Avon Books.

that affect movement. Yet they are singled out for this special emphasis because Rood was the person who called for therapists to look at muscle tone as a contributor to movement. It is now known that muscle tone is not the only prerequisite for motor control and that relative degrees of motor control can, in fact, exist in spite of poor or inadequate muscle tone.

"Flexion and extension patterns coeffect each other" refers to the dynamic relationship between flexion patterns experienced through everyday occupations and extension patterns also experienced through everyday occupations (e.g., sitting in a flexion pattern while reading this text!). It is hypothesized that the total balance or imbalance between flexion and extension patterns affects both in a dynamic system of postural patterns.

"Repetition of muscular response creates movement patterns" refers to the learning that occurs through repeated neuromuscular actions that lay down the engrams for the repertoire of motor behavior available to a given individual.

"Intention or goal direction coeffects movement" refers to the developing research base that shows that intent of a motor action influences the nature and quality of motor action.

"Activities which provide approximation of real life context increase treatment effectiveness and **generaliz-**

ability" refers to the supposition that performance in real life or simulated contexts increases the effectiveness of "practice" and indeed of therapy itself.

"Therapists use somatic markers to select interaction methods with clients" refers to a working hypothesis that master clinicians intuitively and automatically "fit" their demeanor and emotional state to those of the client being served. **Somatic marker**, a term coined by Damasio,[5] is used here to refer to the collection of feelings or emotional tone of a person at any given time, in a learned response to a given situation. Somatic marker is a concept related to the larger conceptualization of meta-emotion. The term **meta-emotion** is used here to refer to the conceptualization and study of the interactions or coeffects between emotions, the body, and occupation (i.e., "feeling while doing").

ROOD'S FOUR COMPONENTS OF MOTOR CONTROL

Table 33-1 reveals that Margaret Rood's concepts pertaining to motor function were far ranging. An important contribution of her work is the emphasis she placed on components of motor control. She was a forerunner of current motor control theories in that she was among the first to identify and articulate the importance of components of motor control in the therapeutic context. Therapists can apply these same concepts today in occupation-based practice. Accordingly, the four components of motor control Rood emphasized are summarized below.

Reciprocal Inhibition (Innervation)

Reciprocal inhibition is an early mobility pattern that serves a protective function. It is a phasic (quick) type of movement that requires contraction of the agonist muscle as the antagonist muscle relaxes. This basic movement pattern is primarily a reflex governed by spinal and supraspinal centers. It is, in fact, the underpinning for movement needed to engage in occupation.

Cocontraction (Coinnervation)

Cocontraction or coinnervation provides stability and is considered a tonic (static) muscle pattern. This muscle pattern provides the ability to hold a position or an object for a longer duration. Cocontraction is the simultaneous contraction of the agonist muscle and antagonist muscle, with the antagonist supreme. It is the foundation of postural control, which provides the stability needed for engaging in occupation.

Heavy Work

Heavy work is described by Stockmeyer as "mobility superimposed on stability."[26] In this postural pattern the proximal muscles contract and move, whereas the distal segment is fixed. A good example of heavy work is creeping. In the quadruped position, the distal segments, wrists, and ankles are in a fixed position. The proximal joints, such as the neck and thorax, are stable, whereas the shoulder and hip girdles are free to move. Heavy work patterns may be associated with many of the occupations typically involved with agriculture and industry, such as lifting, moving, or pulling. It is hypothesized that modern society (Western civilization) lacks "heavy work" patterns, resulting in a functionally deficient neurophysiological state for members of this society.

Skill

Skill is the highest level of motor control and combines the effort of mobility and stability.[11,22] In the execution of a skilled pattern the proximal segment is stabilized while the distal segment moves freely. The art of oil painting demonstrates this pattern. The artist stands back from the canvas, holds his or her arm at full length, and manipulates the brush freely in the hand. Skill is associated with many of the functions needed in the information age, such as typing and fine eye-hand coordination for computer work. It is further hypothesized that modern society has an excessive preponderance of skill demands, to the exclusion of heavy work patterns, with a resultant imbalance.

MOTOR PATTERNS

In this section the major motor patterns of development that Rood emphasized are reviewed. For each motor pattern photographs of humans engaged in the postural pattern as an activity or an occupation are shown.

Supine Withdrawal (Supine Flexion)

Supine withdrawal is a total flexion response toward the vertebral level of T10. This position is protective because the flexion of the neck and the crossing of the arms and legs protect the anterior surface of the body. This position is a mobility posture requiring reciprocal innervation, yet it also requires heavy work of the proximal muscles and the muscles of the trunk.[22] Therapeutically, supine withdrawal aids in the integration of the tonic labyrinthine reflex. Rood recommended this pattern for patients who lacked reciprocal flexion pattern and for individuals dominated by extensor tone (Fig. 33-1).

Rollover (Toward Side Lying)

When an individual is rolling over, the arm and leg flex on the same side of the body. This movement, **rollover**, is a mobility pattern for the extremities and activates the lateral trunk musculature.[26] Rollover is encouraged for individuals who are dominated by tonic reflex patterns in

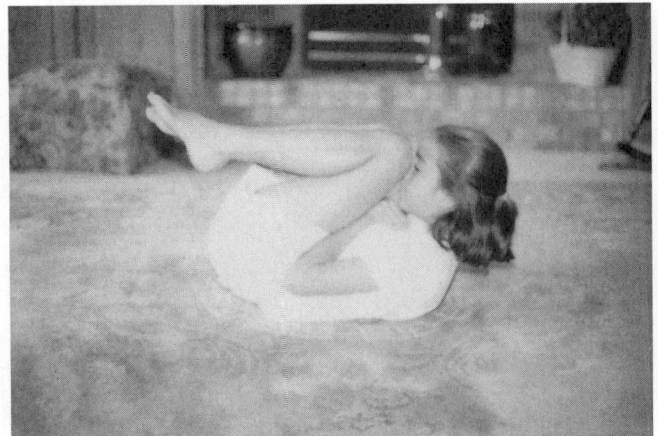

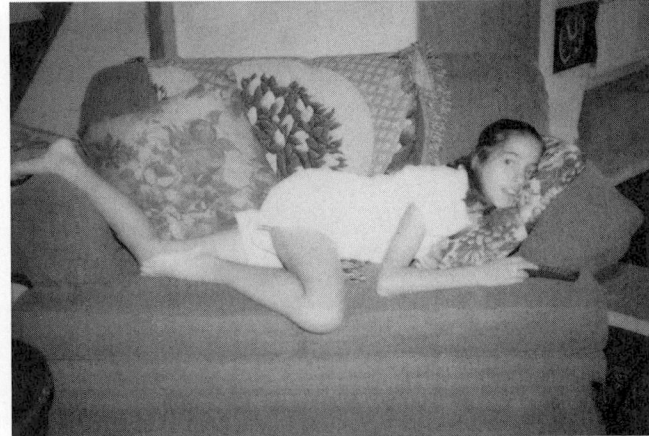

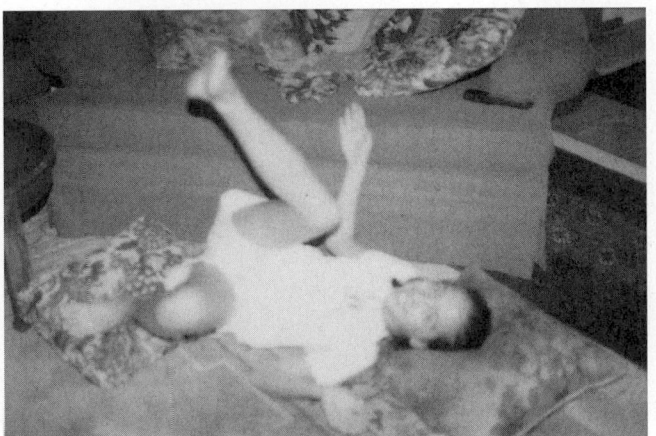

FIG. 33-2
Rollover toward side lying.

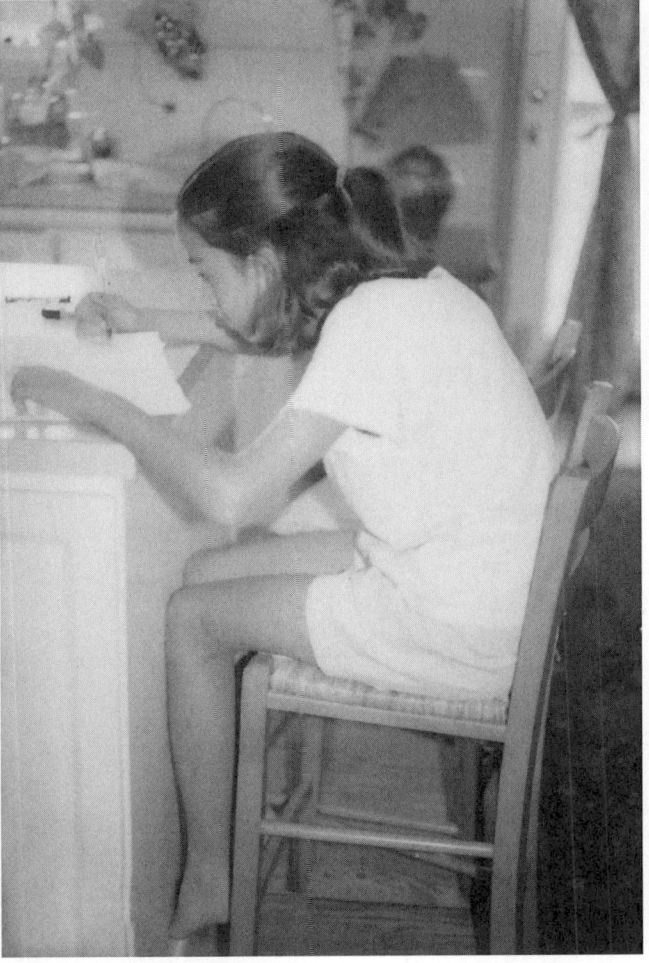

FIG. 33-1
Supine withdrawal or supine flexion.

the supine position. The rolling action also stimulates the semicircular canals of the vestibular system, which in turn activate the neck and extraocular muscles (Fig. 33-2).

Pivot Prone (Prone Extension)

The **pivot-prone** position demands a full range of extension of the neck, shoulders, trunk, and lower extrem-

ities. This pattern has been called both a mobility pattern and a stability pattern. The position is difficult to assume and hold against gravity. Therefore the pivot-prone position plays an important role in preparation for stability of the extensor muscles in the upright position. The pivot-prone position has been associated with the labyrinthine righting reaction of the head. The ability to maintain the position indicates integration of the symmetric tonic neck reflexes and the tonic labyrinthine reflexes (Fig. 33-3).

Neck Cocontraction (Coinnervation)

Neck cocontraction is the first genuine stability pattern. In keeping with the cephalo-caudal and cephalo-rostral rules, cocontraction of the neck precedes cocontraction of the trunk and extremities. As the head bobs up and down, the extensors and rotators are stretched. This action is thought to activate both flexors and deep tonic extensors of the neck.[22] It is important to make sure the neck flexors are well established, however, before the prone position is assumed. To raise the head against gravity, the patient needs to have good cocontraction of the flexors and extensors of

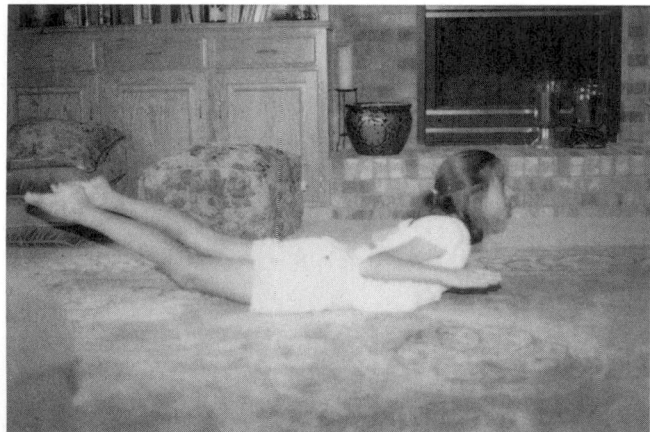
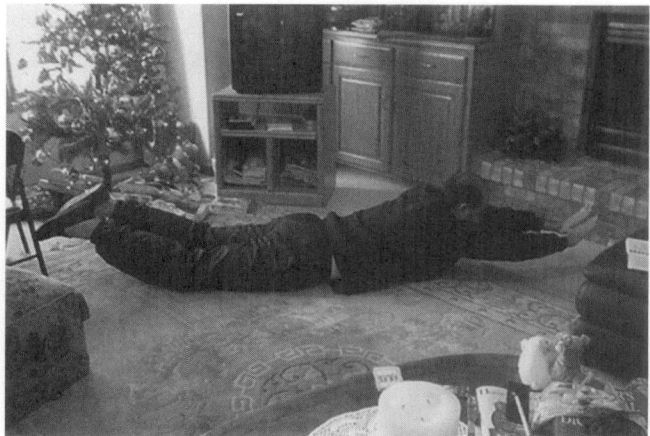

FIG. 33-3
Pivot prone or prone extension.

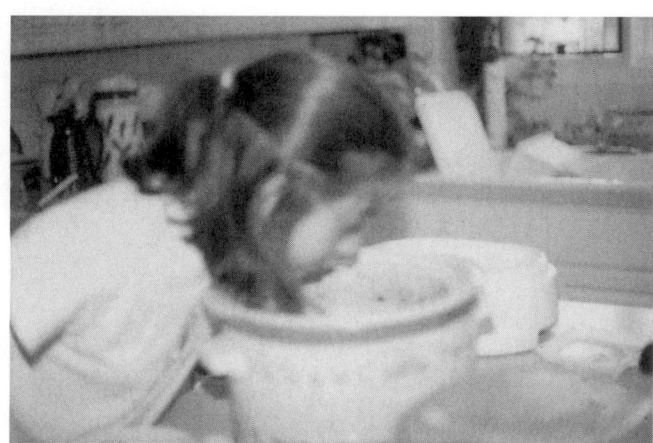
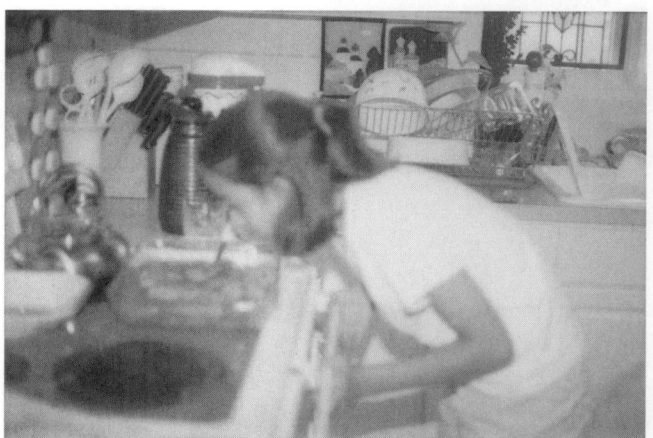

FIG. 33-4
Neck cocontraction or coinnervation.

the neck.[8] Neurologically this pattern elicits the tonic labyrinthine righting reaction when the face is perpendicular to the floor. As the head flexes, it stretches the proprioceptors in the neck and upper trapezius, causing them to contract against the forces of gravity.[19,21,23] This position also promotes neck stability and extraocular control (Fig. 33-4).

ONTOGENETIC DEVELOPMENT PATTERNS

Ontogenetic development patterns observed in normal development are outlined in the following sections. In the past these patterns were used as a basis for therapy. It was assumed that motor control could be inhibited or facilitated by positioning in the patterns. It may be the case that these patterns have beneficial effects when combined with occupational engagement, but that these effects are not necessarily or exclusively on motor control. Future research will shed more light on these assumptions.

On Elbows (Prone on Elbows)

After cocontraction of the neck and prone extension, weight bearing on the elbows is the next pattern to be achieved. Bearing weight on the elbows stretches the upper trunk musculature to influence stability of the scapular and glenohumeral regions. This position gives the patient better visibility of the environment and an opportunity to shift weight from side to side. It is also inhibitory to the symmetrical tonic neck reflex (Fig. 33-5).

All Fours (Quadruped Position)

The quadruped position follows stability of the neck and shoulders. The lower trunk and lower extremities are brought into a cocontraction pattern. Initially the position is static and the abdomen may sag at the T10 level, causing stretching of the trunk and limb girdles. This stretching develops cocontraction of the trunk flexors and extensors. Eventually shifting weight

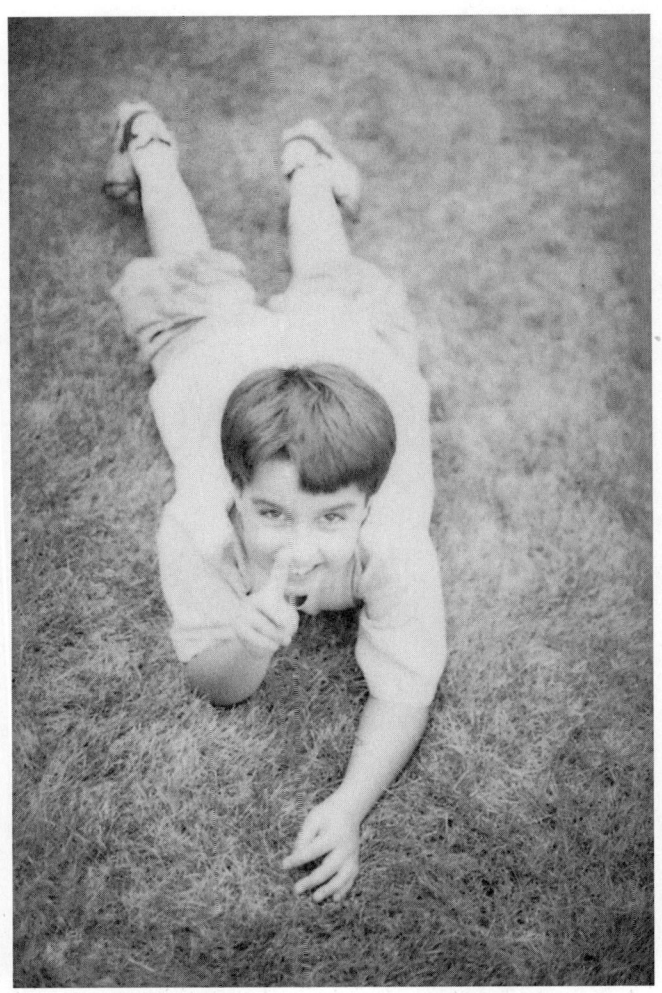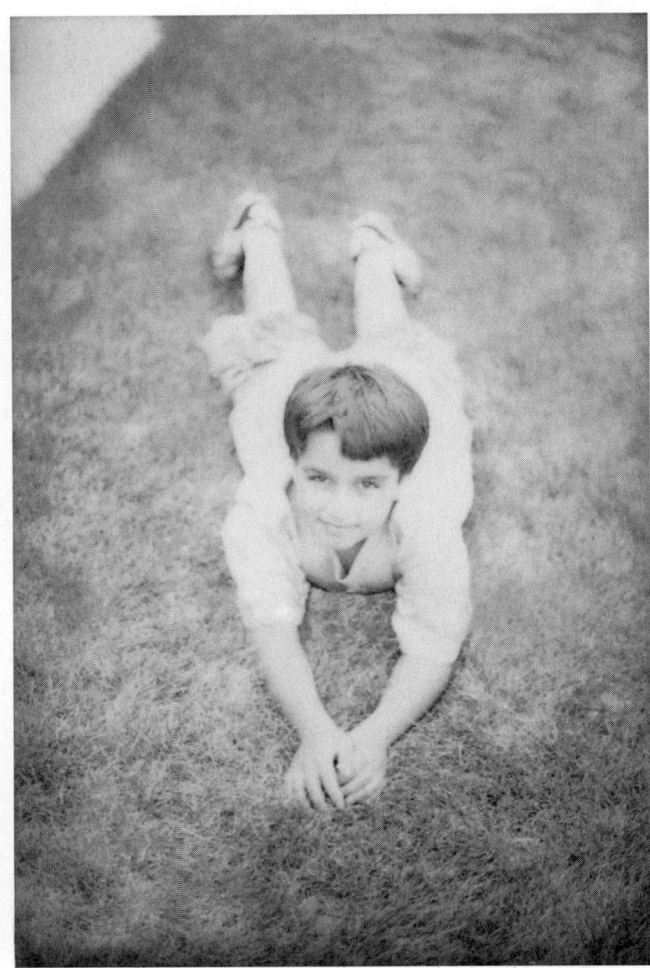

FIG. 33-5
Prone on elbows.

forward, backward, side to side, and diagonally provides a mobility superimposed on the stability phase. The weight shifting may be preparatory to equilibrium responses (Fig. 33-6).

Static Standing

Assuming the upright bipedal position, static standing is thought to be a skill of the upper trunk because it frees the upper extremities for prehension and manipulation.[26] Weight is first equally distributed on both legs, and then weight shifting begins. This position brings into play higher level neurological integration, such as righting reactions and equilibrium reactions (Fig. 33-7).

Walking

The gait pattern unites skill, mobility, and stability. According to Murray,[18] normal locomotion entails the ability to support the body weight, maintain balance, and execute the stepping motion. Walking includes a stance phase, push off, swing, heel strike, and stride length.[26] Walking is a sophisticated process requiring coordinated movement patterns of various parts of the body, including weight shifting (Fig. 33-8).

In addition to the theoretical emphasis Rood placed upon the previously discussed motor patterns, she developed many innovative treatment strategies and techniques, as described in the following section.

TRADITIONAL ROOD TREATMENT TECHNIQUES FOR OCCUPATION-BASED PRACTICE

The reader is likely to encounter Rood techniques in practice. However, these techniques lack empirical study to determine their effectiveness, and knowledge of advanced neuroscience is needed to even consider the use of these techniques in practice. Table 33-2 presents a summary of traditional treatment techniques employed by Rood.

Caution is urged in adopting any or all of these techniques in current occupation-based practice because these interventions are designed to specifically influence

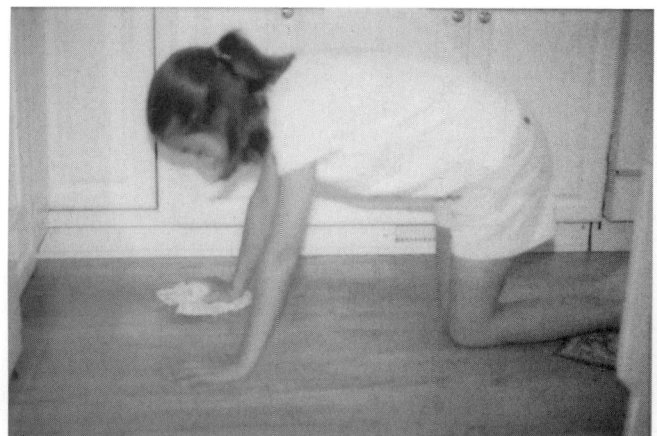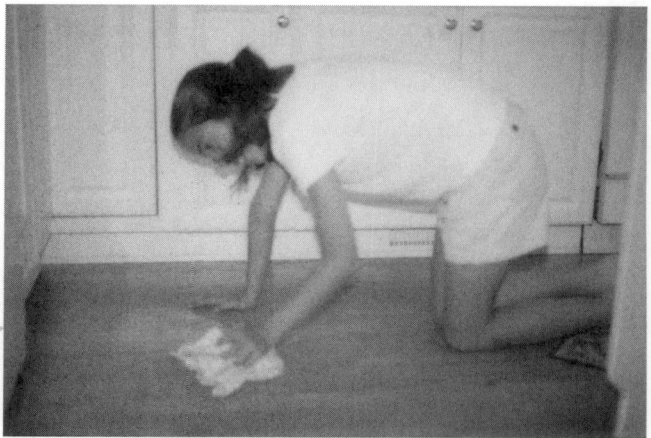

FIG. 33-6
Quadruped (all fours).

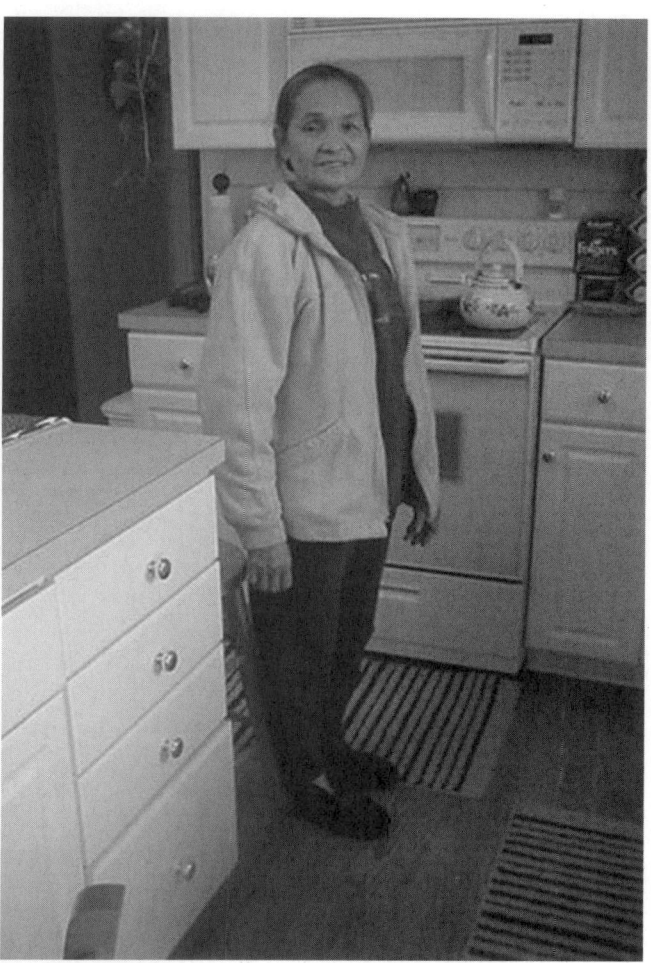

FIG. 33-7
Static standing.

TABLE 33-2

Summary of Rood Facilitatory and Inhibitory Techniques

Cutaneous Facilitation Techniques	Proprioceptive Facilitation Techniques	Inhibitory Techniques
Light moving touch*	Heavy joint compression	Neutral warmth
Fast brushing*	Resistance	Joint approximation
Icing*	Vestibular stimulation	Slow stroking
	Inversion	Rocking
	Stretch pressure*	Gentle shaking or rocking*
	Stretch*	Tendinous pressure*
	Intrinsic stretch*	Maintained stretch*
	Secondary ending stretch*	Slow rolling*
	Tapping*	
	Therapeutic vibration*	
	Osteopressure*	

*These techniques are well beyond the scope of entry-level practice and are therefore not dealt with in this chapter.

performance components and not occupation per se. Thus, occupation-based practice would never include the provision of any of these treatment techniques isolated from an occupation. Also, these interventions unduly address motor function as isolated from the dynamical system of engagement in occupation.

Of the previously identified Rood intervention techniques, those most relevant to today's practice and those consistent with the current understanding of neuroscience were selected for summary presentation in this

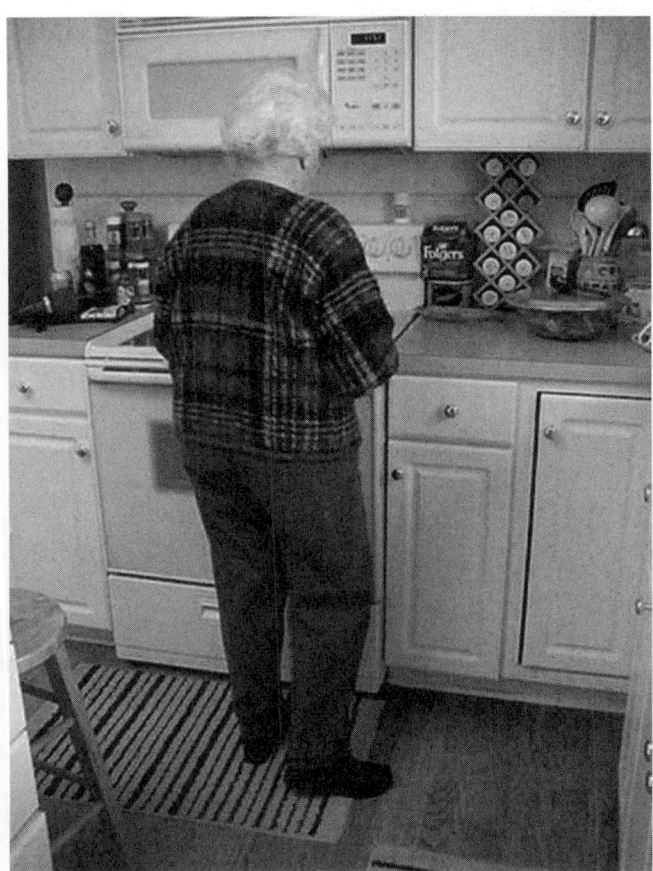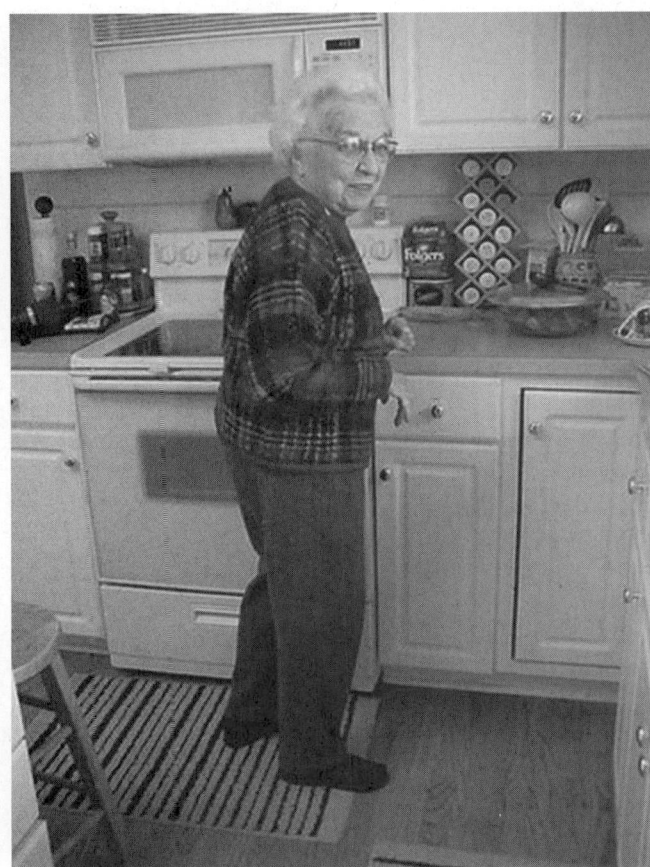

FIG. 33-8
Weight shifting.

section. Further, only interventions appropriate for entry-level practice are discussed.

Proprioceptive Facilitatory Techniques

Proprioceptive stimulation refers to the facilitation of muscle spindles, Golgi tendon organs, joint receptors, and the vestibular apparatus.[15,17,29] In general, proprioceptive stimulation gives the therapist and the client more control over the motor response. Proprioceptors adapt more slowly than exteroceptors and can produce sustained postural patterns.[3] There is little or no neuronal recruitment in the proprioceptive system. Therefore the motor response is thought to last as long as the stimulus is applied.[7,25] Four types of proprioceptive facilitatory techniques are described in the following paragraphs: heavy joint compression, resistance, vestibular stimulation, and inversion.

Heavy Joint Compression

Heavy joint compression is joint compression greater than body weight applied through the longitudinal axis of the bone.[1] The amount of force in heavy joint compression is more than that of the normal body weight

above the supporting joint.[9,12] Heavy joint compression is used to facilitate cocontraction at the joint undergoing compression. This approach can be combined with developmental patterns, such as prone on elbows, quadruped, sitting, and standing positions. The joint compression may be done manually by the therapist or with weighted wrist cuffs or sandbags. Clinically, joint compression is most effective when applied through the longitudinal axis of long bones such as the humerus (glenohumeral joint) and the femur (acetabulum).

Resistance

Rood used heavy resistance to stimulate both primary and secondary nerve endings of the muscle spindle. Resistance is used in an isotonic fashion in developmental patterns to influence the stabilizer muscles. According to Stockmeyer,[26] resistance to contraction of muscles in the shortened range facilitates muscle spindle afferents in the deeper, tonic postural muscles. Fast brushing is used over the stabilizers before resistance is applied, to maximize the response. Farber[9] used quick stretch before resistance to increase the responsiveness of the muscle spindle. In addition, when a muscle contracts against resistance, it assumes a shortened length that causes the muscle spindles to contract to readjust to the shorter length. This is the process of biasing the muscle spindle so it is more sensitive to stretch. Intermittent resistance graded to the desired motion is better than manual stretching for alleviating tight muscles.[15,16,22]

Vestibular Stimulation

Vestibular stimulation is a powerful proprioceptive input.[6] The static labyrinthine system can be used to promote extensor patterns of the neck, trunk, and extremities.[30] The kinetic labyrinth can be used to elicit phasic subcortical responses such as protective extension.[10] Jones and Watt[14] studied muscular responses to unexpected falls in human subjects. Their findings demonstrate that the vestibular system activates the antigravity muscles and their antagonists before the stretch reflex of the muscle spindles. The vestibular system is a divergent system that affects tone, balance, directionality, protective responses, cranial nerve function, bilateral integration, auditory language development, and eye pursuits.[4,12,30] The vestibular system is stimulated during linear acceleration and deceleration in horizontal and vertical planes and during angular acceleration and deceleration, such as spinning, rolling, and swinging. Vestibular stimulation can be either facilitatory or inhibitory, depending on the rate of stimulation. Fast rocking tends to stimulate, whereas slow, rhythmic rocking tends to cause a generalized relaxation response.[1,2]

Inversion

Rood encouraged the use of the inverted position (**inversion**) to alter muscle tone in selected muscles. In the inverted position the static vestibular system produces increased tonicity of the muscles of the neck, midline trunk extensors, and selected extensors in the limbs.[12] Tokizane[27] used human subjects to study the effects of head position on selected skeletal muscles. His findings indicate that extensor tone is maximized in certain muscles in the head-down position, whereas extensor tone is minimized in those muscles in the upright position. For best results, the head must be in normal alignment with the neck. If the neck is flexed or extended, the tonic neck reflex interferes with the response.[21,27] Inversion should be used with extreme care for individuals with cardiovascular disease. As the head approaches a point below the level of the shoulders, baroreceptors in the carotid sinus are stimulated by blood pressure changes. This positioning produces a physiological response through the parasympathetic nervous system, reducing blood pressure, decreasing muscle tone, and promoting generalized relaxation. Inversion techniques can be combined with vibration or neck compression to change tone in selected muscles.[9,12]

Inhibitory Techniques

Four **inhibitory techniques** are neutral warmth, slow stroking, light joint compression, and rocking in developmental patterns.

Neutral Warmth

The neutral warmth technique most likely affects the temperature receptors of the hypothalamus and stimulates the parasympathetic nervous system.[25] Neutral warmth can be used for individuals with hypertonia, particularly those with spasticity and rigidity. It may also be helpful for children with attention deficit disorders.[9] The provision of neutral warmth can be accomplished by having the individual assume a recumbent position while the entire body is wrapped in a cotton blanket or comforter for approximately 5 to 10 minutes. Neutral warmth provides a moderate amount of heat that is homeostatically compatible with the receptors of the hypothalamus. The individual usually feels relaxed, and muscle tone is decreased.[8,13]

Slow Stroking

Slow stroking has been described as an inhibitory technique. The individual lies in the prone position while the therapist provides rhythmic, moving, deep pressure over the dorsal distribution of the primary posterior rami of the spine. The therapist applies fingertip pressure on both sides of the spinous process to affect the nerve endings and the sympathetic outflow of the autonomic nervous system. The stroking action is done slowly and continuously from the occiput to the coccyx. The hands are alternated so that as one hand reaches the bottom of the spine, the other is starting downward from the top.[9,12,13] Inhibition techniques have been found to be clinically beneficial when accompanied by soft music. Music also has been used as a closure technique following sensory integrative therapy to calm children after vestibular and proprioceptive facilitation. Slow stroking should not exceed 3 minutes because it may cause a rebound phenomenon, resulting in excitation of the sympathetic branch of the autonomic nervous system.[26]

Light Joint Compression (Approximation)

Joint compression of body weight or less than body weight can be used to inhibit spastic muscles around a joint.[24] This technique may be used with individuals who have hemiplegia, to alleviate pain and temporarily offset the muscle imbalance around the shoulder joint.[9] The individual can be sitting or lying in the supine position. The therapist places one hand over the individual's shoulder and the other hand under the flexed elbow joint. The arm is abducted 35° to 45°, and a compression force of body weight or less is applied through the longitudinal axis of the humerus.[1] This procedure compresses both the glenohumeral joint and the articulation between the humerus and ulna. Moreover, if applied properly, this technique compresses two joints but has the most dramatic effect on the shoulder. Once the muscles begin to relax, the therapist can slowly and gently circumduct the humerus in small circles to reduce pain and stiffness in the shoulder joint.[9] Joint compression of the shoulder and elbow joints can also be achieved when the patient is in the on-elbows position.[26] Light joint compression is also beneficial when applied through the longitudinal axis of the wrist and elbow joints.[9] The therapist places one hand behind the elbow and places the individual's forearm in midposition; the wrist joint is extended, and compression is applied through the heel of the patient's hand. Joint compression has its greatest effect during the time that the stimulus is applied.[28]

Rocking in Developmental Patterns

In keeping with the developmental sequence and Rood's concept of mobility superimposed on stability, Rood encouraged movement as the individual gained mastery of the static position.[26] Developmentally, the individual first must assume and be able to achieve a static position and then integrate coordinated movements while maintaining the posture. Rood referred to this process as the development of "skill." For example, in the quadruped position, the patient shifts weight to a three-point stance so that one hand is free to reach forward to grasp and explore the immediate environment. Movement may begin by shifting the weight forward and backward. The shifting may progress to side-to-side and diagonal patterns as the patient becomes comfortable with the rhythmic movements.[9] In the quadruped position, individuals with hemiplegia are assisted by achieving stability of the involved elbow when the therapist applies pressure and stretch to the triceps brachii and anconeus. As the therapist applies compression that is greater than body weight to facilitate cocontraction, the pressure exerted on the extended wrist and heel of the hand inhibits the wrist flexors. Light, moving touch over the dorsum of the hand is performed to promote finger extension.[24] Rocking in the quadruped position should first be performed with the neck in a straight, normal relationship to the body so that the proprioceptors of the neck do not influence the tonicity of the limbs.[7] As the individual moves in an anteroposterior plane, the shoulder and pelvic girdles are mobilized. Later in treatment, the therapist may want to incorporate flexion, extension, and rotation of the neck as a reflex inhibition measure.[19]

RECONSTRUCTION OF THE ROOD APPROACH FOR OCCUPATION-BASED PRACTICE

Traditionally, occupational therapists used the previously described techniques primarily to prepare an individual for purposeful activities. Hence, a basic tenet of the Rood approach is that activity should be purposeful—that is, occupation based. The introduction of purposeful activities leading to occupation adds meaning and relevance to the endeavor. Rood's methods are most useful in preparation for engagement in occupation. Reconceptualization of her work in light of current research and knowledge is most useful in understanding and thinking about occupational performance in context. Specifically, Rood's conceptual framework is reconstructed in the next section.

ROOD'S CONCEPTUAL FRAMEWORK: A RECONSTRUCTION

Five key assumptions underlie thinking about occupation-based practice in context (Fig. 33-9). These functions are adapted from Stockmeyer,[26] who presented Rood's initial work.

Assumption 1: Neuromuscular function related to occupation is a chaotic system of multiple networks interacting and changing, based upon coeffects and sensitivity to initial conditions.

Assumption 2: As a chaotic system, neuromuscular function unfolds in a dynamic process.

Assumption 3: Key control parameters influencing the neuromuscular system are the somatic, autonomic, emotional, and cognitive or motivational variables.

Assumption 4: Motor and sensory systems coeffect each other.

Assumption 5: Occupation shapes function.

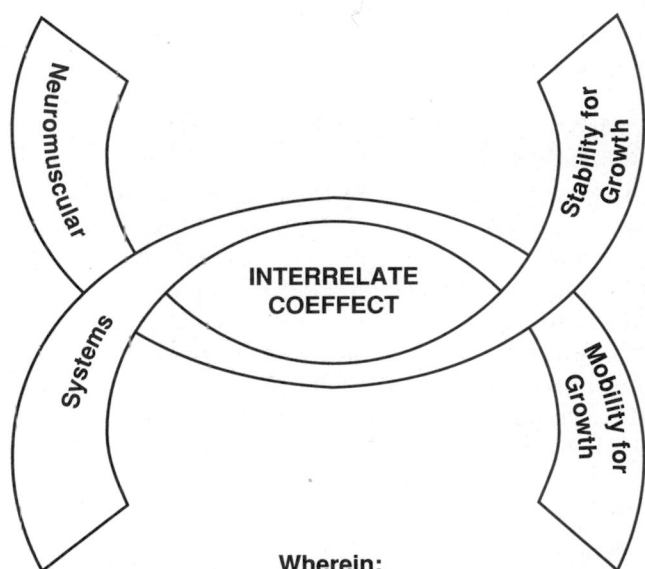

Wherein:
Stability based upon structural and functional design
Mobility for survival through protection and movement

FIG. 33-9

A reconstruction of Rood's conceptual framework. (Figure designed by Rene Padilla OTR-L.)

TABLE 33-3
Heuristic of Rood Reconstructed

Neuro-Muscular Network	Function	Key Control Parameter	Associated Outcome
Network I	Inspiration Suck Swallow Flexion	Cranial nerve V Medial longitudinal fasciculus (MLF)	Supine flexion: body functions
Network II	Extension	Vestibulospinal tract (VST)	Pivot prone: antigravity
Network III	Cocontraction	Muscle spindle	Joint stability: posture
Network IV	Mobility	Corticospinal tract (CST)	Movement through space: skill
Network V	Motivation	Limbic system Frontal lobe Cognition Emotions	Engagement in occupation

In the future, it is likely that others will elaborate on these key assumptions based on the work of Rood.

Finally, as a way to think about the networks that subserve motor function as a foundation for occupation, Table 33-3 is provided as an heuristic. Note that this heuristic links networks to function, control parameters, and associated outcomes and reflects the essence of Rood's thinking as updated with current neuroscientific knowledge and understanding.

SUMMARY

This chapter offers a reconstruction of Margaret Rood's work based on current understanding of CNS processing and therapeutic intervention. Chaos theory and dynamic systems theory are used to help reconstruct her theory for occupation-based practice. Rood's original components of motor control in therapeutic intervention provide the basis for engagement in occupation. Major motor patterns of development originally developed by Rood and their purpose in occupations are delineated. Traditional Rood treatment techniques for entry-level practice and the application of these techniques to occupation-based practice are summarized, based on current findings in neuroscience. In conjunction with Rood's tenet that activity should be purposeful, the context of occupational performance is emphasized. A conceptual framework is proposed based on Rood's important concepts, which provided five key assumptions in occupation-based practice in context. Finally, a

heuristic is provided to identify the networks that subserve motor function as a foundation for occupation.

REVIEW QUESTIONS

1. Why is it important to study Margaret Rood's work?
2. How have key concepts identified by Rood been redefined today?
3. What were the four components of motor control emphasized by Rood?
4. What were the major motor patterns of development described by Rood?
5. Give examples of how Rood's major motor patterns are used during occupation.
6. It was stated that caution is needed when using traditional Rood treatment techniques in current occupation-based practice. What reasons are given for this caution?
7. List which Rood techniques are used today and why. Give examples of two techniques.
8. What are the similarities and differences of the traditional Rood approach and the Rood approach in occupation-based practice?
9. Name the five key assumptions underpinning the reconstruction of Rood.

REFERENCES

1. Ayres J: *The development of sensory integrative theory and practice,* Dubuque, Iowa, 1974, Kendall/Hunt.
2. Ayres J: *Sensory integration and learning disorders,* Los Angeles, 1972, Western Psychological Services.
3. Buchwald J: Exteroceptive reflexes and movement, *Am J Phys Med* 46(1):141-150, 1967.
4. Clark B: The vestibular system. In Mussen PH, Rosenzweig MR, editors: *Annual review of psychology,* New York, 1970, Harper & Row.
5. Damasio AR: *Descartes' error: emotion, reason and the human brain,* New York, 1994, Avon Books.
6. DeQuiros JB: Diagnosis of vestibular disorders in the learning disabled, *Learning Disabilities* 9:50, 1974.
7. Eldred E: Peripheral receptors: their excitation and relation to reflex patterns, *Am J Phys Med* 46(1):69-87, 1967.
8. Farber S: *Sensorimotor evaluation and treatment procedures for allied health personnel,* Indianapolis, 1974, Indiana University and Purdue University Medical Center.
9. Faber S: *Neurorehabilitation: a multisensory approach,* Philadelphia, 1982, WB Saunders.
10. Fukuda T: Studies on human dynamic postures from the viewpoint of postural reflexes, *Acta Otolaryngol* 161(suppl):8, 1961.
11. Gardner E: *Fundametals of neurology,* ed 6, Philadelphia, 1975, WB Saunders.
12. Heininger M, Randolph S: *Neurophysiological concepts in human behavior,* St Louis, 1981, Mosby.
13. Huss AJ: Sensorimotor approaches. In Hopkins H, Smith H, editors: *Willard and Spackman's occupational therapy,* Philadelphia, 1978, JB Lippincott.
14. Jones GM, Watt D: Muscular control of landing from unexpected falls in man, *J Physiol* 219(3):729-737, 1971.
15. Loeb GE, Hoffer JA: *Muscle spindle function: in muscle receptors in movement control,* London, 1981, Macmillan.
16. Matthews PBC: Muscle spindles and their motor control, *Physiol Rev* 44:219, 1964.

17. McCloskey DI: Kinesthetic sensibility, *Physiol Rev* 58:763, 1978.

18. Murray MP: Gait as a total pattern of movement, *Am J Phys Med* 46(1)290-333, 1967.

19. Payton R et al, editors: *Scientific basis for neurophysiologic approaches to therapeutic exercise: an anthology,* ed 2, Philadelphia, 1978, FA Davis.

20. Randolph G: Therapeutic and physical touch: physiological response to stressful stimuli, *Nurs Res* 33(1):33-136, 1984.

21. Roberts T: *Neurophysiology of postural mechanisms,* New York, 1976, Plenum.

22. Rood M: Neurophysiological mechanisms utilized in the treatment of neuromuscular dysfunction, *Am J Occup Ther* 10:4, 1956.

23. Rood M: Occupational therapy in the treatment of the cerebral palsied, *Phys Ther Rev* 32:220, 1952.

24. Rood M: The use of sensory receptors to activate, facilitate and inhibit motor response, automatic and somatic, in developmental sequence. In Sattely C, editor: *Approaches to the treatment of patients with neuromuscular dysfunction,* Dubuque, Iowa, 1962, William C Brown.

25. Schmidt R: *Fundamentals of sensory physiology,* New York, 1978, Springer-Verlag.

26. Stockmeyer S: An interpretation of the approach of Rood to the treatment of neuromuscular dysfunction, NUSTEP proceedings, *Am J Phys Med* 46(1):900-961, 1967.

27. Tokizane T et al: Electromyographic studies on tonic neck, lumbar and labyrinthine reflexes in normal persons, *Jpn J Physiol* 2:30, 1951.

28. Vallbo A et al: Somatosensory proprioceptive and sympathetic activity in human peripheral nerves, *Physiol Rev* 59(4):919-957, 1979.

29. Werner J: *Neuroscience: a clinical perspective,* Philadelphia, 1980, WB Saunders.

30. Wilson VJ, Paterson BW: The role of the vestibular system in posture and movement. In Mountcastle V, editor: *Medical physiology,* St Louis, 1979, Mosby.

Movement Therapy: The Brunnstrom Approach to Treatment of Hemiplegia

LORRAINE WILLIAMS PEDRETTI

KEY TERMS

Associated reactions
Proximal traction response
Limb synergies
Flexor synergy (upper and lower limbs)
Extensor synergy (upper and lower limbs)
Resting posture (upper extremity)
Homolateral limb synkinesis
Grasp reflex
Instinctive grasp reaction
Instinctive avoiding reaction
Souques' finger phenomenon
Glenohumeral subluxation
Wrist fixation for grasp

LEARNING OBJECTIVES

After studying this chapter the student or practitioner will be able to do the following:
1. Describe the theoretical foundations for movement therapy.
2. Describe the evaluation procedure for the upper limb.
3. List the goal of treatment for each recovery stage of the upper limb.
4. Describe facilitation techniques used in this approach.
5. List the sequential stages of motor recovery for arm, hand, and leg.
6. Define terms associated with this approach.
7. Identify the synergy patterns of the arm and leg.
8. Identify characteristic movements for each stage of recovery of arm function.
9. Describe applications of movement patterns available in stages three to six to purposeful activities.

PROFILE

Signe Brunnstrom was a physical therapist from Sweden. Her practice, teaching, and theory development in the United States extended from the World War II years through the 1970s. Her clinical observation and research at major treatment and educational institutions, primarily in the Northeast, led to the development of the treatment approach called *movement therapy*. It was the first systematic approach to the treatment of motor dysfunction after cerebrovascular accident (CVA). The last of the three major works Brunnstrom published in the United States was *Movement Therapy in Hemiplegia* (1970).[3] Signe Brunnstrom died in February 1988.[10]

The theoretical foundations, therapeutic goals, and intervention techniques described in this chapter are an overview of and introduction to some of the procedures that constitute movement therapy. This treatment approach is valuable for its historical significance, its description of the recovery process, its approach to motor assessment, and the effectiveness of selected intervention strategies. To learn the details of the treatment approach, the reader is referred to the original source.[3]

THEORETICAL FOUNDATIONS

Brunnstrom developed her treatment approach on the basis of an extensive review of the literature in neurophysiology, central nervous system (CNS) mechanisms, effects of CNS damage, sensory systems, and related topics, as well as clinical observation and application of training procedures.[3]

The work of several major theorists, such as Gellhorn, Denny-Brown, Hagbarth, Jackson, Magnus and Sherrington, and Twitchell, served as the foundation for the treatment approach. Sherrington, whose work dates to the late 1800s, stated that afferent-efferent (sensory-motor) mechanisms in phylogenesis are retained in humans, and that these mechanisms serve as the basis for the evolutionary process that result in human movements being more voluntary than automatic. Sherrington postulated that sensory denervation abolished all voluntary movement and that sensation is necessary for effective movement.[3]

In the early 1900s Magnus stated that peripheral influences continuously affect the CNS and may work together to facilitate a movement or exert opposite influences that compete with each other. Magnus demonstrated in experimental animals that the same stimulus can evoke opposite motor responses, depending on the position of the responding part.[3] The studies of Magnus support the hypothesis that sensory stimuli and positioning can be used to influence motor behavior.

In the late 1800s Hughlings Jackson described the successive levels of CNS integration. He postulated that the spinal cord and cranial nerve nuclei are located at the lowest motor centers and that muscles in all parts of the body are represented at this level, but few movement combinations are possible. Movements are simple and more automatic than voluntary at this level. Jackson described the middle motor centers in the Rolandic region of the brain. All the muscles represented at the lowest motor centers also are represented here. More complex movements are possible, however, but movement is still more automatic than voluntary at the middle motor centers. Jackson stated that the frontal lobes contain the highest motor centers, along with corresponding sensory centers. The body parts represented at the middle and lowest motor centers are represented here in a still more complex manner than before. This level subserves complex voluntary movement.[11]

Jackson hypothesized that the damaged CNS has undergone an "evolution in reverse." The same reflexes present in earlier phylogenesis and ontogenesis are present once again after CNS damage. Therefore these reflexes were considered normal for the regressed CNS. Jackson also stated that reflexes are precursors of purposeful movement and that they support purposeful movement.[3] Brunnstrom's treatment approach was based on Jackson's hypotheses. In recent years these hypotheses have been challenged and are being modified by newer concepts in neurophysiology.[6,7]

The successive levels of CNS integration, and the reflexes and reactions thought to be integrated at each level, are summarized as follows:

1. *Spinal level (apedal):* flexor withdrawal, extensor thrust, crossed extension
2. *Brainstem level (apedal):* tonic neck reflexes (TNRs), tonic labyrinthine reflex (TLR), **associated reactions,** positive and negative supporting reactions
3. *Midbrain level (quadrupedal):* neck righting, body righting, labyrinthine righting, optical righting, amphibian reaction, Moro reflex
4. *Cortical level (bipedal):* equilibrium reactions[5]

Twitchell[12] described a sequence of motor recovery after CVA. He hypothesized that recovery after CVA constitutes a reversal of the regression of CNS function. He stated that primitive responses are the bases for the evolution of more elaborate motor responses. Twitchell also postulated that all proprioceptive responses are influenced by neck- and body-righting reactions, reflexes, and tactile stimulation. He replicated Sherrington's study and concluded that (1) sensation is critical to movement, (2) a limb is essentially useless without sensation, (3) preservation of cutaneous sensation in the hand is indispensable for motor function of the upper limb, and (4) movements of the upper limb, particularly grasp function, are directed by contactual stimuli. The recovery process after CVA described by Twitchell is summarized sequentially as follows:

1. Flaccidity
2. Stretch reflexes
3. Complex proprioceptive reactions such as the **proximal traction response**
4. **Limb synergies** with ability to use these movement patterns
5. Decline in spasticity
6. Improvement of willed movement and ability to be influenced by tactile stimuli[12]

Brunnstrom subscribed to the concept that the damaged CNS has undergone an evolution in reverse and regressed to phylogenetically older patterns of movement. These include the limb synergies, gross patterns of limb flexion and extension that are primitive spinal cord patterns, and primitive reflexes.[2,3] These primitive movement patterns are modified in humans during development through the influence of higher centers of nervous system control. After CVA they return to their primitive, stereotyped character. Thus, when the influence of higher centers is disturbed or destroyed, reflexes present in early life (e.g., TNRs, tonic lumbar reflex, and TLR) reappear and normal deep tendon reflexes (DTR) become exaggerated. In this approach the TNRs, TLR, and tonic lumbar reflex are considered "normal" when the central nervous system (CNS) has regressed to an earlier developmental stage, as in hemiplegia.[3]

Movement therapy is based on the use of motor patterns available to the patient at any point in the recovery process. Its goal is to enhance progress through the stages of recovery toward more normal and complex movement patterns. Brunnstrom saw synergies, reflexes, and other abnormal movement patterns as a normal part of the process that the patient has to go through before normal voluntary movement could occur.

Brunnstrom believed that the synergies constituted a necessary intermediate stage for further recovery. Accordingly, gross movement synergies of flexion and extension always precede the restoration of advanced motor functioning after hemiplegia.[3] Therefore, during the early stages of recovery (stages one to three) the patient is aided to gain control of the limb synergies. Selected afferent stimuli (TNRs, TLR, cutaneous and stretch stimuli, positioning, and associated reactions) are used to help the patient initiate and gain control of movement. Once the synergies can be performed voluntarily with some ease, they are modified and simple to complex movement combinations are initiated (stages four and five). These combined movements deviate from the stereotypical synergy patterns of flexion and extension.[3] Synergistic movements are used by normal persons all of the time, but they are controlled, occur in a wide variety of patterns, and can be modified or stopped at will.

The advisability of using reflexes, synergies, and associated reactions to effect motion was challenged by Bobath.[1] It was argued that no pathological responses should be used in training because by repeated use the efferent pathways may become too readily available for use at the expense of normal pathways.[2,3] Brunnstrom, however, concluded that the opposite was true. She believed that during the early stages of recovery the development of the synergies should be facilitated and that the use of selected exteroceptive and proprioceptive stimuli was justified for this purpose.[2,3] Both Bobath and Brunnstrom based their hypotheses on neurophysiology. Brunnstrom proposed that the approaches may not be as opposed as they appear. She stated that in the early recovery stage, only reflex movement is available, whereas at later stages of recovery, reflex activity is inhibited and more normal movement is possible. Brunnstrom proposed that both approaches can be useful if applied to a specific patient at a specific time.[3]

Limb Synergies

A limb synergy of flexion or extension is a pattern of movement acting as a bound unit in a primitive and stereotypical manner.[3] The muscles in the pattern are neurophysiologically linked and cannot act alone or perform all of their functions. If one muscle in the synergy is activated, each muscle in the synergy responds partially or completely. The patient thus cannot

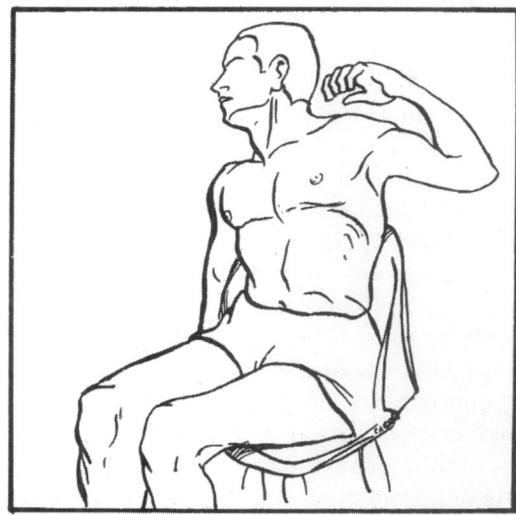

FIG. 34-1

Flexor synergy of upper limb in hemiplegia. The flexor synergy is being performed voluntarily and is facilitated by the tonic neck reflex. (From Brunnstrom S: *Movement therapy in hemiplegia*, New York, 1970, Harper & Row. Used by permission, Lippincott Williams & Wilkins).

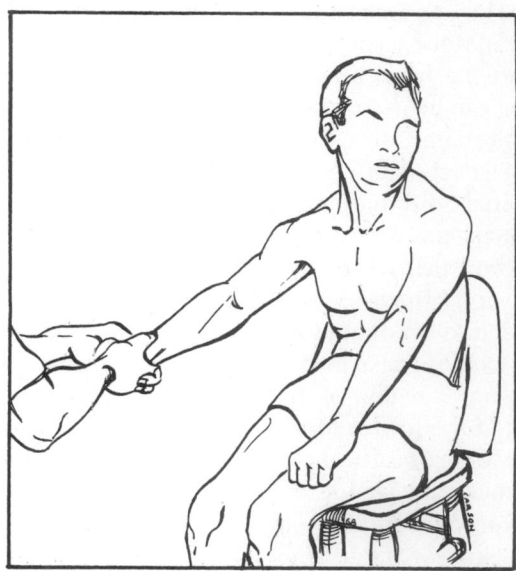

FIG. 34-2

Extensor synergy of the upper limb in hemiplegia. This semivoluntary performance of the extensor synergy is being facilitated by stabilization of the unaffected arm and rotation of the head to the affected side for facilitation through the ATNR. (From Brunnstrom S: *Movement therapy in hemiplegia*, New York, 1970, Harper & Row.)

perform isolated movements when bound by these synergies.

The **flexor synergy** of the upper limb consists of scapular adduction and elevation, shoulder abduction and external rotation, elbow flexion, forearm supination, wrist flexion, and finger flexion. Hypertonicity (spasticity) is usually greatest in the elbow flexion component and least in shoulder abduction and external rotation (Fig. 34-1). The **extensor synergy** consists of scapula abduction and depression, shoulder adduction and internal rotation, elbow extension, forearm pronation, and wrist and finger flexion or extension. Shoulder adduction and internal rotation are usually the most hypertonic components of the extensor synergy, with much less tone in the elbow extension component (Fig. 34-2).

In the lower limb the flexor synergy consists of hip flexion and abduction and external rotation, knee flexion, ankle dorsiflexion and inversion, and toe extension (Fig. 34-3). Hip flexion is usually the component with the highest tone, and hip abduction and external rotation are the components with the least tone. The extensor synergy is composed of hip adduction, extension,

and internal rotation; knee extension; ankle plantar flexion and inversion; and toe flexion (Fig. 34-4). Hip adduction, knee extension, and ankle plantar flexion are usually the most hypertonic components, whereas hip extension and internal rotation are usually less so.

Characteristics of Synergistic Movement

The flexor synergy dominates in the arm, and the extensor synergy dominates in the leg. Performance of synergistic movement, either reflexively or voluntarily, may be influenced by the postural mechanism. When the patient performs the synergy, the components with the greatest degree of hypertonicity are often most apparent, rather than the entire classic patterns described previously (Fig. 34-5). With facilitation or voluntary effort, however, the more classic synergy pattern can usually be

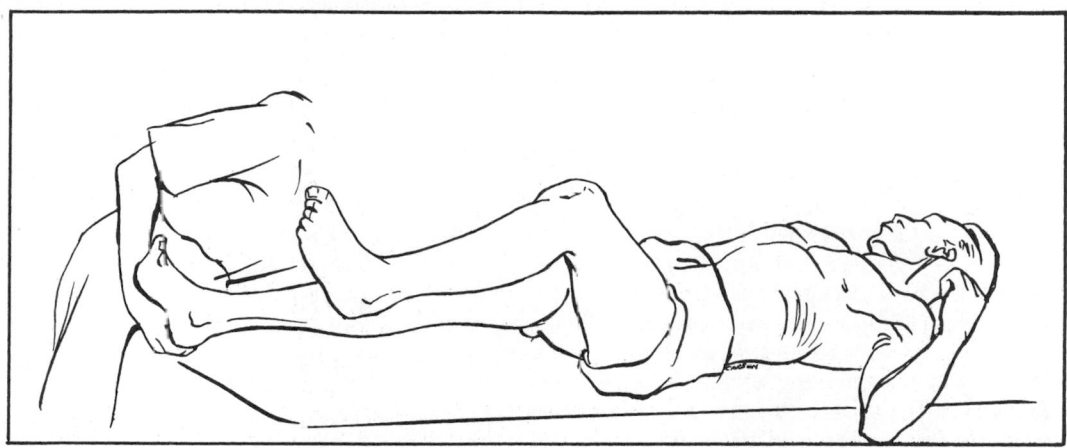

FIG. 34-3
Flexor synergy of the lower limb is evoked as an associated reaction by giving resistance to ankle plantar flexion on the unaffected side. (From Brunnstrom S: *Movement therapy in hemiplegia*, New York, 1970, Harper & Row.)

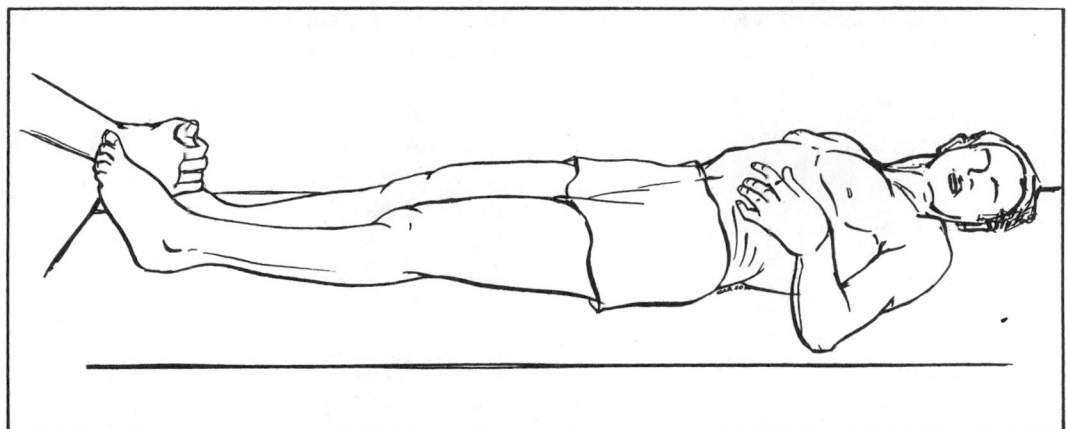

FIG. 34-4
Extensor synergy of the lower limb is evoked as an associated reaction by giving resistance to ankle dorsiflexion on the unaffected side. (From Brunnstrom S: *Movement therapy in hemiplegia*, New York, 1970, Harper & Row.)

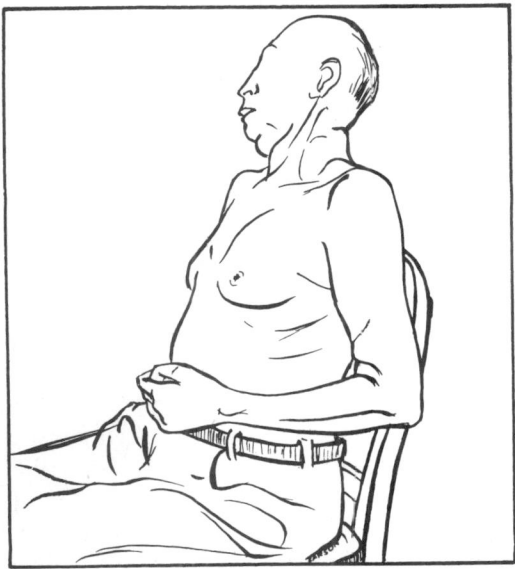

FIG. 34-5
Flexor synergy of the upper limb, alternate pattern with hyperextension at the shoulder and half-range forearm supination. (From Brunnstrom S: *Movement therapy in hemiplegia,* New York, 1970, Harper & Row.)

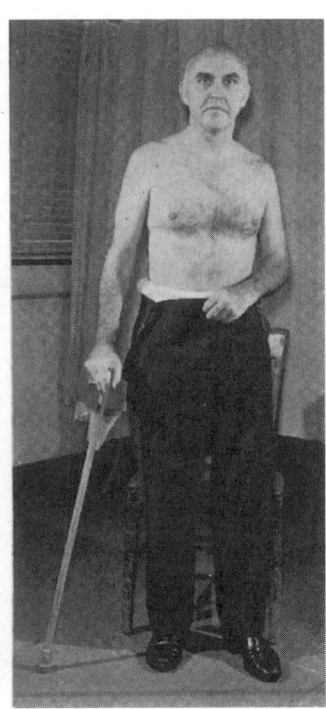

FIG. 34-6
Typical resting posture of the upper limb in standing. Shoulder adduction, elbow flexion, forearm pronation, and wrist and finger flexion. (Adapted from Brunnstrom S: *Movement therapy in hemiplegia,* New York, 1970, Harper & Row.)

evoked.[3] The **resting posture** of the limb, particularly the arm, is characterized by a position that represents the most hypertonic components of both flexor and extensor synergies-that is, shoulder adduction, elbow flexion, forearm pronation, and wrist and finger flexion (Fig. 34-6).

Motor Recovery Process

Brunnstrom observed that after a CVA resulting in hemiplegia, the patient progresses through a series of recovery steps or stages in a fairly stereotypical fashion (Table 34-1). The progress through these stages may be rapid or slow.

Spontaneous motor recovery follows an ontogenetic process, usually proximal to distal, so that shoulder movement can be expected before hand movement. Flexor patterns occur before extensor patterns, reflex motion occurs before voluntary movement, and gross movement patterns can be performed before isolated, selective movement.[3]

Recovery may cease at any stage and is influenced by such factors as sensation, perception, cognition, motivation, affective states, and concomitant medical problems. Few patients make a very good recovery of arm function, and the greatest loss is usually in the wrist and hand.

No two patients are exactly alike. There is much individual variation in the characteristic motor disturbances and the recovery process among patients. The motor behavior and recovery process described represent common characteristics that may be observed in most persons after CVA occurs.[3]

DEFINITION OF TERMS

A definition of terms is necessary before the discussion of treatment principles that follows. *Associated reactions* are movements on the affected side in response to voluntary, forceful movements in other parts of the body.[3] Resistance to flexion movements of the normal upper extremity (UE) usually evokes a flexor synergy or some of its components in the affected UE. Resistance to extension on the sound side evokes the extensor synergy on the affected side. In the lower extremities the responses are reversed. Resisted flexion of the normal limb evokes extension of the affected limb, and vice versa.[9]

Homolateral limb synkinesis is a mutual dependency between the synergies of the affected upper and lower limbs. The same or similar motion occurs in the limb on the same side of the body. For example, efforts at flexion of the affected UE evoke flexion of the lower extremity (LE).[3,9] The mirroring of movements attempted or performed on the affected side by the unaffected side, perhaps in an effort to facilitate the movement, is called *imitation synkinesis.*[3]

Several specialized reactions can be noted in the hemiplegic hand. The *proximal traction response* is elicited by a stretch to the flexor muscles of one joint of the upper limb, which evokes contraction of all flexors of that limb, including the fingers. This response may

TABLE 34-1

Motor Recovery After Cerebrovascular Accident*

Stage	Characteristics		
	Leg	**Arm**	**Hand**
1	Flaccidity	Flaccidity; inability to perform any movements	No hand function
2	Spasticity develops; minimal voluntary movements	Beginning development of spasticity; limb synergies or some of their components begin to appear as associated reactions	Gross grasp beginning; minimal finger flexion possible
3	Spasticity peaks; flexion and extension synergy present; hip-knee-ankle flexion in sitting and standing	Spasticity increasing; synergy patterns or some of their components can be performed voluntarily	Gross grasp, hook grasp possible; no release
4	Knee flexion past 90° in sitting, with foot sliding backward on floor; dorsiflexion with heel on floor and knee flexed to 90°	Spasticity declining; movement combinations deviating from synergies are now possible	Gross grasp present; lateral prehension developing; small amount of finger extension and some thumb movement possible
5	Knee flexion with hip extended in standing; ankle dorsiflexion with hip and knee extended	Synergies no longer dominant; more movement combinations deviating from synergies performed with greater ease	Palmar prehension, spherical and cylindrical grasp and release possible
6	Hip abduction in sitting or standing; reciprocal internal and external rotation of hip combined with inversion and eversion of ankle in sitting	Spasticity absent except when performing rapid movements; isolated joint movements performed with ease	All types of prehension, individual finger motion, and full range of voluntary extension possible

From Brunnstrom S: *Movement therapy in hemiplegia*, New York, 1970, Harper & Row.
*Recovery of hand function is variable and may not parallel the six recovery stages of the arm.

therefore be used to elicit the flexor synergy. To elicit the **grasp reflex,** the examiner applies deep pressure to the palm and moves the pressure distally over the hand and fingers, mostly on the radial side. The responses are complex, but in general, adduction and flexion of the digits are present. The **instinctive grasp reaction** was differentiated by Brunnstrom from the grasp reflex. It is a closure of the hand in response to contact of a stationary object with the palm of the hand. The person is unable to release the object-stimulus once the fist has been closed.

A hyperextension reaction of the fingers and thumb in response to forward-upward elevation of the arm is the **instinctive avoiding reaction.** Brunnstrom reported that with the arm in this position, stroking distally over the palm and attempting to reach out and grasp an object resulted in an exaggeration of the reaction. The automatic extension of the fingers when the shoulder is flexed is known as the **Souques' finger phenomenon,** and can be observed in some, but not all, patients with

hemiplegia. Brunnstrom found that although this phenomenon may not be exhibited, the elevated position of the affected arm is favorable for the facilitation of finger extension.[3]

MOTOR ASSESSMENT OF THE PATIENT WITH HEMIPLEGIA

Brunnstrom in *Movement Therapy in Hemiplegia* described an assessment procedure that measures muscle tone, stage of recovery, movement patterns, motor speed, and prehension patterns of the UE.[3] The assessment is based on the recovery stages after the onset of hemiplegia. In this test the patient performs motor acts that are graduated in complexity and require increasingly finer neuromuscular control.

Progress through the recovery stages is gradual, and signs of two stages may be apparent at any given time in the patient's recovery. Because it is not possible to establish an absolute point between one recovery stage and the next, the patient may be classified as being at stages two and three or three and four, for example. This rating indicates progression from one stage to the next. The Hemiplegia Classification and Progress Record is presented in Fig. 34-7. The reader should refer to this form while reading the directions for test administration, which have been summarized from *Movement Therapy in Hemiplegia*.[3]

Gross Sensory Testing

Sensory testing precedes motor assessment and includes assessment of passive motion sense and touch localization in the hand. Tests of passive motion sense of the shoulder, elbow, forearm, wrist, and fingers are carried out by procedures similar to those described in Chapter 25. Results are recorded on the first and second pages of the form (shown in Fig. 34-7, *A* and *B*).

HEMIPLEGIA CLASSIFICATION AND PROGRESS RECORD

Upper limb-test sitting

Name _____ Age _____ Date of onset _____ Side affected _____

Date _____

___ Passive motion sense: Shoulder _____ Elbow _____

___ Pronation-supination _____ Wrist flexion-extension _____

___ 1. NO MOVEMENT INITIATED OR ELICITED _____

___ 2. SYNERGIES OR COMPONENTS FIRST APPEARING. Spasticity developing _____

___   Flexor synergy _____

___   Extensor synergy _____

___ 3. SYNERGIES OR COMPONENTS INITIATED VOLUNTARILY. Spasticity marked _____

FLEXOR SYNERGY		ACTIVE JOINT RANGE	REMARKS
___ Shoulder girdle	Elevation		
	Retraction		
___ Shoulder joint	Hyperextension Abduction		
	External rotation		
___ Elbow	Flexion		
___ Forearm	Pronation		
EXTENSOR SYNERGY			
___ Shoulder	Pectoralis major		
___ Elbow	Extension		
___ Forearm	Pronation		
4. MOVEMENTS DEVIATING FROM BASIC SYNERGIES. Spasticity decreasing	Hand to sacral region		
___	Raise arm forward-horizontally		
___	Pronate-supinate elbow at 90 degrees		
5. RELATIVE IN-DEPENDENCE OF BASIC SYNERGIES. Spasticity waning	Raise arm sideways-horizontally		
___	Raise arm over head		
___	Pronate-supinate elbow extended		
6. MOVEMENT COORDINATION NEAR NORMAL. Spasticity minimal			

A

FIG. 34-7
Hemiplegia classification and progress record. (From Brunnstrom S: *Movement therapy in hemiplegia,* New York, 1970, Harper & Row.)

Fingertip recognition is tested by asking the patient to localize touch stimuli to specific fingers. The patient is seated, with forearms pronated and resting on a pillow in the lap. The test is given with the vision occluded after a rehearsal in full view. The palmar surface of the fingertips is lightly touched with a pencil eraser in a random sequence. The patient must indicate which finger is being touched. Results are recorded on the second page of the form (Fig. 34-7, B).

Motor Tests of Upper Extremity

The patient is classified as being in recovery stage one when no voluntary movement of the affected arm can be initiated.[3] The examiner should move the limb passively through the synergy patterns and assess the degree of resistance to passive movement. The patient should be asked to attempt movement during these maneuvers. During recovery stage one the limb is predominantly flaccid and feels heavy, there is little or no resistance to passive movement, and the patient is unable to initiate or effect any movement voluntarily.

During recovery stage two, tone begins to increase and the limb synergies or some of their components may be evoked on voluntary effort or as associated reactions. The flexor synergy usually appears first.[3] The therapist may again move the limb passively, alternating between flexor and extensor synergy patterns. The

---

HEMIPLEGIA CLASSIFICATION AND PROGRESS RECORD

Upper limb-test sitting cont'd

Name _____

Date _____

SPEED TESTS FOR Classes 4, 5, 6		Strokes per 5 seconds		
Hand from lap to chin	Normal Affected			
Hand from lap to opposite knee	Normal Affected			

____ Passive motion sense, digits_____

____ Fingertip recognition_____

____ Wrist stabilization for grasp   1. Elbow extended_____

                                      2. Elbow flexed_____

____ Wrist flexion and extension   1. Elbow extended_____

____ Fist closed   2. Elbow flexed_____

____ Wrist circumduction_____

DIGITS

____ Mass grasp_____ Dynamometer test   Normal_____lb.
                                                    Affected_____lb.

____ Mass extension _____

____ Hook grasp (handbag, 2 lb.)_____

____ Lateral prehension (card)_____

____ Palmar prehension (pencil)_____

____ Cylindrical grasp (small jar)_____

____ Spherical grasp (ball)_____ Catch_____ Throw_____

Indiv. thumb movements, hands in lap ulnar side   1. Vertical movements_____

____ down   2. Horizontal movements_____

____ Individual finger movements_____

____ Button and   Using both hands_____

____ unbutton shirt   Using affected hand only_____

____ Other skilled activities_____

B

FIG. 34-7 cont'd

Hemiplegia classification and progress record. (From Brunnstrom S: *Movement therapy in hemiplegia,* New York, 1970, Harper & Row.)

Continued

HEMIPLEGIA CLASSIFICATION AND PROGRESS RECORD

Trunk and lower limb

Name _____   Evaluation date _____

SUPINE

Passive
motion
sense

Hip _____   Knee _____

Ankle _____   Big toe _____

Flexor synergy _____

Extensor synergy _____

Hip: Abduction _____   Adduction _____

SITTING ON CHAIR		STANDING	
Trunk balance (no back support)		With _____ without _____ support Balance, normal limb sec.	
Sole sensation (no. of answers)	Correct Incorrect	Double scale reading†	(a) _____ (b) _____
Hip-knee-ankle flexion		Hip-knee-ankle flexion	
Knee flexion-extension small range		Knee flexion-extension small range	
Knee flexion beyond 90°		Knee flexion hip extended	
Ankle, isolated dorsiflexion		Ankle, isolated dorsiflexion	
Reciprocal hamstring action*		Hip abduction knee extended	

AMBULATION   Evaluation date _____

Brace? _____   Cane? _____   In parallel bars _____

Supported _____   Escorted _____   Alone _____

Arm in sling _____   Arm swings loosely _____   Elbow held flexed _____

Arm swings near normal _____

GAIT ANALYSIS   Evaluation date _____

STANCE PHASE   SWING PHASE

Ankle _____   _____

Knee _____   _____

Hip _____   _____

Walking cadence: Steps per min.   Speed: Feet per min.

*Inward and outward rotation at knee with inversion-eversion at ankle.
†Recorded as normal/affected; (a) preferred stance, (b) weight shift on affected limb.

C

FIG. 34-7 cont'd

Hemiplegia classification and progress record. (From Brunnstrom S: *Movement therapy in hemiplegia,* New York, 1970, Harper & Row.)

therapist should ask the patient to help in the movements. Thus it is possible to assess the degree of hypertonicity and to assess whether the subject's voluntary efforts are evoking any movement responses.

During recovery stage three, hypertonicity is increased and may be marked. The limb synergies or some of their components are performed voluntarily, although with much effort and cognitive control. The patient may remain at this stage for a long time, and se-

verely involved patients may never progress beyond it. The pectoralis major, pronators, and wrist and finger flexors may be very hypertonic, causing limited performance of their antagonists.

The patient is seated, and the therapist demonstrates the complete flexor synergy. The patient is asked to perform the movement pattern with the unaffected side to demonstrate that the directions are understood. The patient is then asked to perform the movement pattern with the affected side after a command such as "touch your ear" or "touch your mouth," which gives purpose and direction to the effort. A similar procedure is used to assess performance of the extensor synergy. The patient is asked to reach forward and downward to touch the therapist's hand, which is held between the patient's knees. The responses may be influenced by the predominant hypertonicity seen in components of each of the synergies. For instance, the very spastic pectoralis major and elbow flexors may predominate during the patient's efforts and result in the patient reaching across the thorax to touch the opposite shoulder. The status of the synergies is recorded on the evaluation form in terms of the active joint range achieved for each motion in the pattern. The joint ranges are estimated and recorded as 0, ¼, ½, ¾, or full range.

When the patient has reached recovery stage four, there is a decrease in spasticity and the patient is capable of performing gross movement combinations that deviate from the limb synergies. Brunnstrom chose three movements to represent stage four. These are (1) placing the hand behind the body to touch the sacral region, (2) raising the arm forward to 90° of shoulder flexion with elbow extended, and (3) pronating and supinating the forearm with the elbow flexed to 90° and stabilized close to the side of the body. The patient performs all of the movements while seated, and as in all test items, no facilitation is allowed. During the test for pronation-supination, bilateral performance is allowed so that the therapist can compare the two sides.

Further decrease of hypertonicity and ability to perform more complex combinations of movement characterize recovery stage five. The patient is relatively free of the influence of the limb synergies and performs the stage four movements with greater ease. Three movements chosen to represent stage five are (1) raising the arm to 90° of shoulder abduction with the elbow extended and forearm pronated, (2) raising the arm forward, as in stage four, but above 90° of shoulder flexion, and (3) pronating and supinating the forearm with the elbow extended. The third movement is performed with the arm in the forward or side horizontal position and is not isolated from shoulder internal and external rotation.

Persons who progress to recovery stage six are able to perform isolated joint motions and demonstrate coordination that is comparable or nearly comparable to that of the unaffected side. On close inspection the trained observer may detect some awkwardness of movement, and there may be some incoordination when rapid movement is attempted. The patient may be assessed while performing a variety of daily living tasks, provided that recovery of hand function has kept pace with recovery of arm function.

The tests of motor speed on the second page of the evaluation form (Fig. 34-7, *B*) may be used to assess hy-

pertonicity during any recovery stage, provided that the patient has enough range of active motion to perform the necessary movement. The tests are especially useful in stages four, five, and six. The normal side is tested first for comparison, then the affected side is tested. The two movements that are tested are (1) hand to chin and (2) hand to opposite knee. The patient is seated in a sturdy chair without armrests. The trunk should be stabilized against the back of the chair, and the head should be erect. The hand is closed, but not tightly, and rests in the lap. For the hand-to-chin test, the forearm is at 0° neutral between pronation and supination. The therapist asks the patient to bring the hand from lap to chin as rapidly as possible, first with the unaffected side and then with the affected side, and records the number of full back-and-forth movements accomplished in 5 seconds. If speed is slow because of marked spasticity, half movements may be counted. The same procedure is followed for the hand-to-opposite knee test, except that the forearm is positioned in full pronation on the lap. The hand is moved from the lap to the opposite knee, using full range of elbow extension. These two tests measure the hypertonicity of elbow flexors and extensors.

Wrist stabilization, which is automatic during normal grasp, is often lacking after a stroke. Therefore it is important to evaluate wrist stabilization during fist closure. This test is performed with the elbow both flexed and extended. During the recovery stages when the synergies are dominant, the wrist tends to flex when the elbow flexes. The patient is asked to make a fist while the elbow is extended across the front of the body. The patient is then asked to make a fist while the elbow is flexed at the side of the body. Whether the wrist remains stabilized in the neutral position or extends slightly is observed. This test is followed by a request for wrist flexion and extension with the fist closed. The patient holds an object such as a wide dowel rod and extends and flexes the wrist. This is done in the elbow-extended and elbow-flexed positions as on the previous test. Circumduction of the wrist indicates significant recovery to the advanced stages. When evaluating the ability to perform this movement, the therapist should stabilize the forearm in pronation. The upper arm should be stabilized against the trunk.

Mass grasp is tested with a dynamometer, which measures pounds of pressure of grasp strength. The normal side is tested first, then the affected side, and the results are recorded for comparison. Mass extension is evaluated by asking the patient to release and actively extend the fingers to the degree possible. Whether active extension is accomplished and the approximate amount of range achieved should be noted on the form. Active release to full range of extension is very difficult for many persons with CVA.

All types of prehension are evaluated in order of their difficulty. Everyday tasks that require the particular prehension pattern are used. Hook grasp may be assessed by asking the patient to hold a bag by its handle. Holding a card demands lateral prehension. Palmar prehension is required for grasping a pencil. Cylindrical grasp may be assessed by asking the patient to hold a small, narrow jar. Grasping a ball requires spherical grasp. The patient's ability to catch and throw the ball may be observed. These activities are difficult for persons with hemiplegia because they require rapid grasp and release, coordination of the entire limb, and time-space judgment. In all the prehension tests the normal side should be observed first for purposes of comparison.

Individual thumb movements are assessed with the patient's hand resting in the lap, ulnar side down. The normal side is observed first, then the affected side. The patient is asked to move the thumb up and down (flexion-extension) and side to side (adduction-abduction).

The therapist tests individual finger movements by asking the patient to tap the index and middle fingers on the tabletop or on a pillow held in the lap. Isolated control of metacarpophalangeal (MP) flexion and extension is assessed and noted on the evaluation form.

Fine, coordinated use of the affected hand and arm and of both hands together usually is indicative of advanced recovery. Patients who have succeeded well at the prehension tests may be asked to button and unbutton a shirt, first using both hands, then using the affected hand only. Other skilled activities, such as writing, threading a needle, removing a small bottle cap, and picking up and placing small objects such as mosaic tiles or coins, may be used to further test skilled hand use.

Motor Tests of Trunk and Lower Extremity

To assess trunk and LE function, the patient is tested first in the supine position, then in the sitting position, and then in the standing position. If the patient is ambulatory, a gait analysis is made (Fig. 34-7, C). Tests in the supine position include tests of passive motion sense, flexor and extensor synergies, and hip abduction and adduction. In the sitting position trunk balance, sole sensation, and specific movements of the lower limb are tested. These tests include hip-knee-ankle flexion, knee flexion and extension in small range, knee flexion beyond 90°, isolated ankle dorsiflexion, and reciprocal hamstring action (inward and outward rotation at the knee with inversion-eversion at the ankle). In the standing position balance and selected movements are assessed. These tests are hip-knee-ankle flexion, knee flexion-extension in small range, knee flexion with the hip extended, isolated ankle dorsiflexion, and hip abduction with the knee extended. The LE assessment concludes with a gait analysis, including timed walking

cadence.[3] The physical and occupational therapists perform the motor assessment cooperatively and use an integrated approach in treatment, which incorporates upper limb, trunk, and lower limb function, according to prescribed treatment goals.

TREATMENT GOALS AND METHODS

Before the initiation of any intervention strategies, the occupational and physical therapists make a thorough evaluation of the motor, sensory, perceptual, and cognitive functions of the patient. The motor assessment yields information about stage of recovery, muscle tone, passive motion sense, hand function, sitting and standing balance, leg function, and ambulation.

The goal of Brunnstrom's movement therapy is to facilitate the patient's progress through the recovery stages that occur after onset of hemiplegia (Table 34-1). Use of the available afferent-efferent mechanisms of control is the means for attainment of this goal. Postural and attitudinal reflexes are used as means to increase or decrease tone in specific muscles.[9] For instance, changes in head and body position can influence muscle tone by evoking the tonic reflexes, such as the TNRs, tonic lumbar reflex, TLR, and equilibrium and protective reactions. Associated reactions can be used to initiate or elicit synergies in the early stages of recovery by giving resistance to the contralateral muscle group on the normal side. Through homolateral limb synkinesis, efforts at flexion synergy of the affected leg are used to elicit a flexor synergy of the arm.

Stimulating the skin over a muscle by rubbing with the fingertips produces contraction of that muscle and facilitation of the synergy to which the muscle belongs. An example is brisk stimulation of the triceps muscle during other efforts at performance of the extensor synergy, which enhances elbow extension and amplifies the synergy pattern. Muscle contraction is facilitated when muscles are placed in their lengthened position, and the quick stretch of a muscle facilitates its contraction and inhibits its antagonist. Resistance facilitates the contraction of muscles resisted. Synergistic movement is augmented by the voluntary effort of the patient. Visual stimulation through the use of mirrors, videotape, and movement of parts facilitates motion in some patients. Loud and repetitive commands to perform the desired movement can also be used as facilitation.

The strongest component of a synergy pattern inhibits its antagonist through reciprocal innervation. It follows that if relaxation of the stronger or hypertonic muscle can be effected, it may be possible to evoke some activity in the weaker antagonist, which may appear to be functionless because of its inability to overcome the very hypertonic agonist.[2,9]

Some treatment goals and methods are summarized below. The point at which the therapist initiates treatment depends on the stage of recovery, muscle tone, and sensory status of the individual patient.

Bed Positioning

Proper bed positioning begins immediately after the onset of the stroke, when the patient is in the flaccid stage.[3] During this period the limbs can be placed in the most favorable positions without interference from hypertonic muscles. Correct bed positioning is often the responsibility of the nurse; therefore it is essential that the physical therapist or occupational therapist provide information about the influence of the limb synergies on bed postures.

If left unsupervised, the lower limb tends to assume a position of hip external rotation and abduction and knee flexion. This posture is partly a result of mechanical influences on the flaccid limb; that is, the weight of the part tends to pull the hip into external rotation. Neurologically, this position mimics the flexor synergy of the LE. The advent of muscular tension in the flexor and abductor muscle groups of the hip and the flexor group of the knee contributes to the posture of the LE as described previously.

If the extensor synergy is developed in the LE, the leg may assume a different position. Hypertonicity of the extensor muscles usually exceeds that of the flexor muscles in the lower limb. In this case, hip extension and adduction, knee extension, and ankle plantar flexion characterize the posture of the leg. If adductor hypertonicity is severe, the patient may habitually place the unaffected leg under the affected leg, which allows the affected limb to adduct even more and results in a crossed-limb posture.

If the extensor synergy dominates in the lower limb, the recommended bed position in supine is slight flexion of the hip and knee maintained by a small pillow under the knee. Lateral support of the leg at the knee with pillows or a rolled blanket or bolster should be provided to prevent abduction and external rotation. The bed covers should be supported to prevent them from resting on the foot. This helps to prevent excessive ankle plantar flexion. The position of slight flexion at the hip and knee is beneficial because it has an inhibitory effect on the extensor muscles of the knee and ankle, counteracting the development of severe hypertonicity in these muscles, which hinders ambulation.

If the flexor synergy dominates in the lower limb, the knee must be maintained in extension. Hip external rotation can be prevented with supports as described previously. The choice of bed position is determined on an individual basis. The position selected is opposite the pattern of the greatest amount of muscle tone to effect the inhibition of excessive hypertonicity.

The affected UE is supported on a pillow, in a position comfortable for the patient. Abduction of the humerus in relation to the scapula is prevented because in this position the stabilizing action of the lower portion of the glenoid fossa on the humeral head is reduced and the superior portion of the joint capsule is slackened. This position can predispose the humeral head to downward subluxation. When the patient is being handled, traction on the affected UE is avoided. The patient is instructed to use the unaffected hand to support the affected arm when moving about in bed.

Bed Mobility

Turning toward the affected side is easier than turning toward the unaffected side because it requires little activity of the affected limb(s). The affected arm is placed close to the body, and the patient rolls over the affected arm when turning. Turning toward the unaffected side requires muscular effort of the affected limbs. The unaffected arm is used to elevate the affected arm to a vertical position over the face, with the shoulder in 80° or 90° of flexion and the elbow fully extended. The affected LE is positioned in partial flexion at the knee and hip and could be stabilized in this position momentarily by the therapist. The patient turns by swinging the arms and the affected knee across the body toward the unaffected side. The movements of the limbs assist in the turn of the upper body and pelvis. When control improves, the patient carries out the maneuver independently, in one smooth, continuous movement, to turn from the supine position to the side-lying position on the unaffected side.

Trunk Movement and Balance

One of the early goals in treatment is for the patient to achieve good trunk or sitting balance. Most persons with hemiplegia lean to the affected side, which may cause a fall when the appropriate equilibrium responses do not occur. To evoke balance responses the therapist deliberately disturbs the patient's erect sitting posture in forward-backward and side-to-side directions while the patient sits on a chair, edge of a bed, or mat table. The patient is prepared for the procedure with an explanation, and is pushed, at first gently and then more vigorously. The patient may support the affected arm by cradling it to protect the shoulder. This prevents the patient from grasping the supporting surface during the procedure. Later, the therapist initiates and assists the patient with bending the trunk directly forward and obliquely forward. The patient sits and supports the affected arm as previously described. The therapist's hands are held under the patient's elbows. The therapist can use his or her knees to stabilize the patient's knees if balance is poor. In this position the therapist guides the patient while inclining the trunk forward and obliquely and obtains some passive glenohumeral and scapular motion at the same time.

Trunk rotation is encouraged in a similar manner, with the therapist sitting in front of the patient or standing behind and supporting the patient's arms as before. Trunk rotation is first performed through a limited range and is gently guided by the therapist. The range is gradually increased. Some neck mobilization can be obtained almost automatically during these maneuvers. As the trunk rotates, the patient cradles the affected arm and moves the arms rhythmically from side to side to achieve shoulder abduction and adduction alternately. The shoulder components of the flexor and extensor synergies may be evoked during these procedures through the TNR and tonic lumbar reflexes.[3]

Shoulder Range of Motion

A second important early goal in treatment is maintaining or achieving pain-free range of motion (ROM) at the glenohumeral joint. There appears to be a relationship between the shoulder pain common in patients with hemiplegia and the stretching of hypertonic muscles around the shoulder joint. Traditional forced passive exercise procedures may actually produce this stretching and contribute to the development of pain. Such exercise is harmful and contraindicated. Once the patient has felt the pain, the anticipation of pain increases the muscular tension which in turn decreases the joint mobility and increases the pain experienced on passive motion. Therefore the shoulder joint is mobilized through guided trunk motion, without forceful stretching of hypertonic musculature about the shoulder and shoulder girdle.

The patient sits erect, cradling the affected arm. The therapist supports the arms under the elbows while the patient leans forward. The more the patient leans, the greater the range of shoulder flexion that can be attained. The therapist guides the arms gently and passively into shoulder flexion while the patient's attention is focused on the trunk motion. In a similar fashion the therapist guides the arms into abduction and adduction while the patient rotates the trunk from side to side. The asymmetrical tonic neck reflex (ATNR) and tonic lumbar reflex facilitate relaxation of muscles during this maneuver. When the patient is confident that the shoulder can be moved painlessly, active-assisted movements of the arm in relation to the trunk are begun. First, the patient moves both shoulders into elevation and depression and scapula adduction and abduction. These movements are then combined with glenohumeral movements. The therapist supports the arm from behind, with the shoulder between forward flexion and abduction and the elbow flexed less than 90°, and supports the wrist in slight extension. The therapist asks the patient to elevate the shoulders, while tapping the upper trapezius with the fingertips. At the same time the therapist assists the patient to elevate the arm. Active shoulder elevation tends to elicit other components of the flexor synergy. That, in turn, tends to inhibit the very hypertonic adduction component of the extensor synergy (pectoralis major). This allows the therapist to elevate the arm into abduction by small degrees each time the patient repeats the active shoulder girdle elevation. The procedure is repeated, and the therapist gives the appropriate verbal commands "Pull up" and "Let go."

The abduction movement is at an oblique angle between forward flexion and full abduction. Sideward abduction with the arm in the same plane as the trunk is likely to be painful and should be avoided. Alternate pronation and supination of the forearm by the therapist accompany the elevation and lowering of the arm throughout the procedure. The forearm is supinated when the shoulder is elevated and pronated when the arm is lowered. Head rotation to the normal side inhibits activity in the pectoralis major muscle through the ATNR. When abduction movement above the horizontal is accomplished without pain, the patient is directed to reach overhead and straighten out the elbow if there has been sufficient recovery to do so. The patient is directed to rotate the head to the affected side to facilitate the elbow extension, while observing the movement of the arm.

These techniques result in increased ROM at the shoulder and also help the development of the flexor synergy. A small ROM in the path of the extensor synergy is performed between the patient's efforts at flexion so that both synergies are developed. As training progresses, greater emphasis is placed on the development of the extensor synergy.

Shoulder Subluxation

Brunnstrom believed that **glenohumeral subluxation** resulted from dysfunction of the rotator cuff muscles (supraspinatus, infraspinatus, teres minor, and subscapularis). Activation of these muscles in treatment is necessary if subluxation is to be minimized or prevented. Function of the supraspinatus muscle is particularly important for the prevention of subluxation. Slings were used in an effort to hold the humeral head in the glenoid fossa. However, slings do not in any way activate the muscles needed to protect the integrity of the shoulder joint.[3] The use of slings has been found to be of little value and may actually be harmful.[4] A more complete discussion of shoulder problems and slings appears in Chapter 36.

Upper Limb Training

The training procedures for improving arm function are geared to the patient's recovery stage. During stages one and two, when the arm is essentially flaccid or some components of the synergy patterns are beginning to appear, the aim is to elicit muscle tone and the synergy patterns on a reflex basis. This improvement is accomplished through a variety of facilitation procedures. Associated reactions and tonic reflexes are employed to influence tone and evoke reflexive movement. The proximal traction response is used to activate the flexor synergy. Tapping over the upper and middle trapezius, rhomboids, and biceps is used to elicit components of the flexor synergy. Tapping over the triceps and stretching of the serratus anterior is used to activate components of the extensor synergy. Quick stretch and surface stroking of the skin are also used to activate muscles. Passive movement alternately through each of the synergy patterns is not only an excellent means for maintaining ROM of several joints, but also provides the patient with proprioceptive and visual feedback for the desired patterns of early movement.

The methods are not employed in any set order or routine but are selected to suit the particular responses of each individual patient. Because the flexor synergy usually appears first, it is useful to begin trying to elicit the flexor patterns. This attempt is followed immediately with facilitation of the extensor synergy components, which tend to be weaker and more difficult to perform in later stages of recovery.[3,8]

When the patient has recovered to stages two and three, the synergies or their components are present and sometimes can be performed voluntarily. Hypertonicity is developing and reaches its peak in stage three. During this period the aim is for the patient to achieve voluntary control of the synergy patterns. This goal is reached by repetitious, alternating performance of the synergy patterns, first with the assistance and facilitation of the therapist. Facilitation is provided through resistance to voluntary motion, verbal commands, tapping, and cutaneous stimulation. This step is followed by voluntary repetition of the synergy patterns without the facilitation and, finally, concentration on the components of the synergies from proximal to distal, first with facilitation and then without.

Bilateral rowing movements with the therapist holding the patient's hands are used for reciprocal motion of the synergies and are started during this time. Bearing weight on the affected arm is employed to reinforce elbow extension. The patient uses the normal hand to guide the affected hand, fist clenched, to a low stool positioned in front of him or her. A sandbag or cushion is placed on the stool, and a concavity is made in it to accommodate the fist. The patient's body weight is shifted to the affected arm to facilitate the elbow extensors through weight bearing.[3,8]

The treatment aim during stages four and five is to break away from the synergies by mixing components

from antagonistic synergies to perform new and increasingly complex patterns of movement. One means for accomplishing this goal is to use exercises in arcs of movement to get elbow flexion, combined with shoulder horizontal adduction and forearm pronation, and alternating with shoulder horizontal abduction and elbow extension with forearm supination, such as with a skateboard or powder board. Later the patient might be able to perform the more complex figure-eight pattern. In the final recovery, stages five and six, increasingly complex movement combinations and isolated motions are possible. The aims in treatment are to achieve ease in performance of movement combinations and isolated motion, and to increase speed of movement.

Although the hemiplegic UE seldom makes a full recovery, the patient should be trained to use the limb to assist the unaffected arm to whatever extent possible in bilateral activities.

Hand Training

Because recovery of hand function does not always coincide with arm recovery, methods for retraining hand function are addressed separately. Hand retraining commensurate with the recovery status of the patient should be carried out continuously.

The first goal of hand retraining is to achieve mass grasp. The proximal traction response and grasp reflex are used to elicit early grasp movement on a reflex level. During the proximal traction response maneuver, the therapist maintains the patient's wrist in extension and gives the command "Squeeze."

Because the normal association between wrist extension and grasp is disturbed, the second goal is to achieve **wrist fixation for grasp.** Wrist extension often accompanies the extensor synergy. Wrist extension can be evoked if the therapist applies resistance to the proximal palm or fist while supporting the arm in the position described earlier for elevation of the arm into abduction. Percussion of the wrist extensors with the elbow in extension and arm elevated and supported by the therapist can activate wrist extension. The proximal portions of the extensors are tapped, and the therapist directs the patient to squeeze simultaneously. The commands to squeeze and stop squeezing are given at appropriate points in the facilitation procedures.

During the wrist extension and fist closure the therapist carries the elbow forward into extension. During the wrist and finger relaxation the therapist carries the elbow back into flexion. While the patient maintains fist closure, the therapist can withdraw the wrist support and give the command "Hold." The therapist may continue tapping the wrist extensors while the patient attempts to hold the posture. The goal is to synchronize the muscles for fist closure with wrist extension.

This procedure is alternated with the command "Stop squeezing," and the wrist is allowed to drop and fingers to open while the elbow is moved into flexion. These steps are alternated, and the wrist extension-fist closure is performed gradually, with increasing amounts of elbow flexion, so that the patient can learn to grasp with wrist stabilization when the arm is in a variety of positions.

A third objective in hand retraining is to achieve active release of grasp. This movement is difficult because there is usually a considerable degree of hypertonicity in the flexor muscles of the hand. A release of tension in the finger flexors, then, is primary to the achievement of any active finger extension. Active grasp is alternated with manipulations to release tension in the flexors. The therapist sits facing the patient and pulls the thumb out of the palm by gripping the thenar eminence. The forearm is supinated. The wrist is allowed to remain in slight flexion. The therapist maintains the grasp around the thumb and alternately pronates and supinates the forearm, with emphasis on supination. Pressure on the thumb is decreased during pronation and increased during supination. Cutaneous stimulation is given to the dorsum of the hand and wrist when the forearm is supinated. This manipulation facilitates some tension in the finger extensors, and the fingers are extended. The patient could actually participate in opening the hand when the forearm is supinated. Strong efforts on the part of the patient may evoke flexion instead, however, and are to be avoided.

If the manipulation is inadequate, stretch of the finger extensors can be used. With the therapist and patient positioned and the hand manipulated as just described, the therapist uses the free hand for distally directed, rapid stroking movements over the proximal phalanges of the affected hand. This action causes momentary flexion of the MP joints, which then bounce back into partial extension. The stroking movement is performed so that the proximal, then distal interphalangeal (IP) joints are included. The movement is performed rapidly and continuously, causing rapid flexion and then bounce back of MP and IP joints. The fingers become extended, and the finger flexors are relaxed because they are reciprocally inhibited by the stretch reflex response in the extensors. If the flexors are stretched or stroking is performed over the palmar surface of the fingers, the spasticity returns to the finger flexors and they act to close the hand.[3] For this reason the fingers should not be pulled into extension.

Active finger extension may be further facilitated by the use of a finger extension exercise glove with rubber bands, which the patient uses while the hand is manipulated into supination with the thumb pulled out of the palm as described earlier (Fig. 34-8).

Elevation above the horizontal position evokes the extensor reflexes of the fingers. After flexor spasticity is

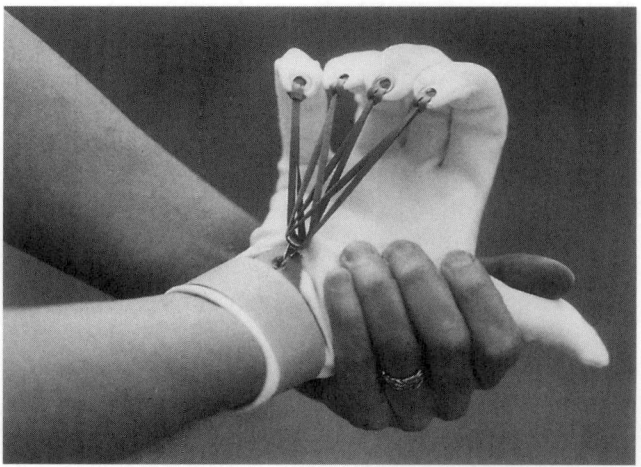

FIG. 34-8
Finger extension exercise glove.

decreased by the maneuvers just described, the therapist stands on the affected side and maintains the thumb in abduction and extension and the forearm in pronation. The fingers are kept in extension by pressure over the IP joints and stabilization of the fingertips. The grip on the thumb is released, and the arm is raised above the horizontal position.

The therapist strokes distally over the IP joints with the heel of the hand. The fingers extend or hyperextend, and the therapist gradually discontinues contact with the patient's hand. If the patient is ready, slight voluntary mental effort can be superimposed on the reflex extension, which might bring about additional extension of the fingers. If the forearm is supinated while the arm is elevated, thumb extension is enhanced. The hand is positioned overhead for this maneuver. To facilitate extension of the fourth and fifth fingers, the forearm is pronated as the arm is elevated and friction is applied over the ulnar side of the dorsum of the forearm.

When reflex extension of the fingers is well established, alternate fist opening and closing begins. The arm is lowered passively, and the elbow is flexed. The forearm and wrist are supported, and the patient is asked to squeeze, then stop squeezing. As soon as the fingers relax, the manipulations to facilitate finger extension are carried out. These two steps are alternated, and the patient's voluntary efforts are superimposed on the reflex activity so that the movements begin to assume a semivoluntary character. Semivoluntary finger extension is influenced by the position of the limb and appears to be linked to gross movements other than the synergy patterns. Voluntary movements of the thumb appear when semivoluntary mass extension becomes possible.

Once the flexor muscles are relaxed, the hand is placed in the patient's lap, ulnar side down, and the patient attempts to move the thumb away from the first finger, a preliminary for lateral prehension. The therapist can stimulate the tendons of the abductor pollicis and the extensor pollicis brevis by tapping or friction at the point where they pass over the wrist, to enhance the patient's effort. The patient can learn to twiddle the thumbs to attain further control of thumb motion. The patient folds the hands, with wrists slightly flexed, and moved the thumbs around each other. Initially the normal thumb could push the other around, but the involved thumb may begin to participate actively. The willed effort, visual input, and sensory feedback from affected and unaffected sides contribute to the development of this movement.

During treatment sessions the patient has to be comfortable and relaxed. The patient's willed efforts should be slight because too much effort can evoke a flexor response rather than the desired extensor response. Excessive muscle tension in the limb and entire body has to be avoided, or finger extension will not occur.

Many patients with hemiplegia never achieve good voluntary extension or coordinated fine hand motions. If semivoluntary extension can be well established, voluntary extension usually follows so that the patient can open the hand in all positions.[3] The accomplishment of palmar prehension and fine hand movements requires the achievement of voluntary opening of the hand, opposition of the thumb to the fingers, and ability to release objects in contact with the palm of the hand.

Lower Limb Training

Lower limb training is directed toward restoring safe standing and development of a gait pattern that is as nearly normal as possible. The goal is to modify the gross movement synergies and facilitate movement combinations that are more nearly like those used during normal ambulation. Lower limb training includes trunk balance and activation of specific muscle groups, followed by gait training. Training procedures for the LE are primarily the domain of the physical therapist. When training the patient in functional activities, however, the occupational therapist uses procedures that are in concert with the work of the physical therapist—for example, transfer training, dressing, toileting, and ambulating that involves the lower limb. Therefore it is important for the occupational therapist to know which LE training procedures are in progress, which movement patterns are to be encouraged or inhibited, and which methods facilitate the desired gait pattern when assisting or accompanying the patient during functional tasks.

OCCUPATIONAL THERAPY APPLICATIONS

Controlled movements achieved in upper limb training have more significance if the patient can use them for functional activities. Even with limited control, the affected limb can be used in many ways to assist with function. Encouraging the use of the affected arm in everyday activities decreases the possibility of the patient's functioning strictly as a one-handed person.

During stages three and four, when the patient has voluntary control of the synergies and can begin to use movement combinations that deviate from the synergies, the occupational therapist helps the patient to use the newly learned movement for functional and purposeful activities. Some of the activities that can be adapted to use the synergy patterns or gross combined movement patterns are skateboard or powder board exercises, sanding, leather lacing, braid weaving, finger painting, sponging off tabletops, and using a push broom or carpet sweeper. Activities that demand too much conscious effort tend to increase fatigue and hypertonicity and should be avoided.

Brunnstrom[3] described several possible uses for the flexor and extensor synergies in stage three. The extensor synergy may be used to stabilize an object on a table while the unaffected arm is performing a task; examples are stabilizing stationery while writing letters or stabilizing fabric for sewing. The extensor synergy can also be used to stabilize a jar against the body while unscrewing the lid or to hold a handbag or newspaper under the arm. When pushing the affected arm through the sleeve of a garment, the individual can position the garment so that the arm follows the path of the extensor synergy. The forearm has to be pronated first, however, to facilitate elbow extension.

The flexor synergy or its components can be used for such tasks as carrying a coat or handbag over the forearm or holding a toothbrush while the unaffected hand squeezes the toothpaste. Bilateral pushing and pulling activities that alternate the paths of both synergies can be helpful for some patients. Examples are sweeping, vacuuming, and dusting. Such activities can be performed with the unaffected hand stabilizing the affected one. The affected hand can be more hindrance than help until greater control is gained. Strongly motivated patients try to use available movements under the guidance and encouragement of the occupational therapist.

To promote transition from stage three to stage four, movement combinations are facilitated and practiced in upper limb training. These movements are (1) hand to chin, (2) hand to ear on the same side and opposite side, (3) hand to opposite elbow, (4) hand to opposite shoulder, (5) hand to forehead, (6) hand to top of head, (7) hand to back of head, and (8) stroking movements from top to back of head and from dorsum of the forearm to the shoulder and toward the neck on the normal side. As soon as possible, these movement patterns are translated to functional activities. Success at functional tasks increases motivation and establishes a purpose for the training. Contact with body parts where sensation is intact is instrumental in guiding the hand to its goal.

Examples of these movements in daily activities are eating finger foods, combing hair, washing the face, washing the unaffected arm, and reaching the opposite axilla for washing or application of deodorant.[3] The therapist's role is to analyze activities for movement patterns that are possible for the patient, and to select activities that have meaning and are interesting to the patient.

At this point the occupational therapist stresses the use of any voluntary movement of the affected limb in performance of activities of daily living. Using the arm for dressing and hygiene skills translates the movements to purposeful function. The patient's sensory status, and not only the motor recovery achieved, influences the degree to which purposeful, spontaneous use of the arm is possible. If the patient surpasses stage four, the number of activities that can be performed increases, and more movement combinations are possible. The involvement of the affected limbs in activities of daily living is encouraged. The activities mentioned earlier can be performed in their usual manner, and may be graded to demand finer and more complex movement patterns. Gardening, furniture refinishing, leather tooling, rolling out dough, sweeping, dusting, and washing dishes are a few of the activities that are used to engage the affected arm purposefully if hand recovery is adequate.

SUMMARY

Signe Brunnstrom was a physical therapist who developed a treatment approach for CVA called movement therapy. The approach is based in neurophysiological principles of successive levels of CNS integration. Brunnstrom described stages of motor recovery following CVA and developed treatment methods designed to enhance the progress of the patient from one stage to the next, to higher levels of motor skill. Her approach uses techniques of facilitation such as synergies, reflexes, associated reactions, resistance, tapping, and stretch.

The use of reflexes or synergistic movement in treatment is controversial, and the concept of the hierarchical organization of the nervous system has been modified in neurophysiology in recent years. However, Brunnstrom's observations of motor recovery and motor behavior are valid, and many of the techniques are still useful in treatment. Some similarities can be seen between Brunnstrom's methods and those of other sensorimotor theorists. The assessment of motor recovery and some elements of treatment methodology continue to be used in the treatment of CVA.

REVIEW QUESTIONS

1. List the stages of recovery of arm function after CVA, as described by Brunnstrom.

2. List the motions in the flexor and extensor synergies of the arm.

3. What is the most hypertonic component of the flexor synergy of the arm?

4. What is the least hypertonic component of the extensor synergy of the arm?

5. What is the basis of the Brunnstrom approach to the treatment of hemiplegia?

6. For what purposes does Brunnstrom recommend the use of reflexes and associated reactions in the early recovery stages after onset of hemiplegia?

7. Define or describe the following terms: limb synergy, associated reactions, imitation synkinesis, proximal traction response, grasp reflex, and the Souques' finger phenomenon.

8. Describe or demonstrate the procedure that Brunnstrom recommended to maintain or achieve pain-free ROM at the glenohumeral joint.

9. What is the aim of treatment for functional recovery of the arm during stages one and two? Stages two and three? Stages three and four?

10. List two treatment methods that could be used to achieve each of the aims in the previous question.

11. Describe three activities other than those listed in the text that may be used in occupational therapy to enhance voluntary control of the flexor and extensor synergies.

12. What is the effect of the proximal traction response on muscle function?

13. Describe or demonstrate the procedure that Brunnstrom recommends to establish wrist fixation in association with grasp.

14. Describe the procedure that may be used to relax hypertonic finger flexors and facilitate finger extension.

15. Which muscle group is thought to play a substantial role in maintaining glenohumeral joint stability?

16. Describe proper bed positioning for the patient with a dominant extensor synergy of the leg. What is the rationale for this position?

REFERENCES

1. Bobath B: *Adult hemiplegia: evaluation and treatment*, London, 1978, Heinemann.
2. Brunnstrom S: Motor behavior in adult hemiplegic patients, *Am J Occup Ther* 15(1):6-12, 1961.
3. Brunnstrom S: *Movement therapy in hemiplegia*, New York, 1970, Harper & Row.
4. Cailliet R: *The shoulder in hemiplegia*, Philadelphia, 1980, FA Davis.
5. Fiorentino MR: *Reflex testing methods for evaluating CNS development*, Springfield, Ill, 1973, Charles C Thomas.
6. Ghez C: The control of movement. In Kandel ER, Schwartz JH, Jessel TM: *Principles of neural science*, New York, 1991, Elsevier.
7. Giuliani CA: Theories of motor control: new concepts for physical therapy. *In Contemporary management of motor control problems: proceedings of the II Step Conference*, Alexandria, Va, 1991, Foundation for Physical Therapy.

8. Perry C: Principles and techniques of the Brunnstrom approach to the treatment of hemiplegia, *Am J Phys Med* 46:789, 1967.
9. Sawner K: *Brunnstrom approach to treatment of adult patients with hemiplegia: rationale for facilitation procedures,* Buffalo, State University of New York. Unpublished manuscript, 1969.
10. Schleichkorn J: *Signe Brunnstrom, physical therapy pioneer, master clinician and humanitarian,* Thorofare, NJ, 1990, Slack.
11. Taylor J, editor: Selected writings of Hughlings Jackson, New York, 1958, Basic Books (abstract). Cited in Brunnstrom S: *Movement therapy in hemiplegia,* New York, 1970, Harper & Row.
12. Twitchell TE: The restoration of motor function following hemiplegia in man, *Brain* 74:443-480, 1951 (abstract). Cited in Brunnstrom S: *Movement therapy in hemiplegia,* New York, 1970, Harper & Row.

CHAPTER 35

Proprioceptive Neuromuscular Facilitation Approach

SARA A. POPE-DAVIS

KEY TERMS

Proprioceptive neuromuscular facilitation
Mass movement patterns
Diagonal patterns
Stretch
Verbal commands
Verbal mediation
Manual contacts
Part-task practice
Whole-task practice
Stepwise procedures
Unilateral patterns
Bilateral patterns
Symmetrical patterns
Asymmetrical patterns
Reciprocal patterns
Combined movements
Traction
Approximation
Maximal resistance
Repeated contractions
Rhythmic initiation
Slow reversal
Rhythmic stabilization
Contract-relax
Hold-relax
Slow reversal-hold-relax
Rhythmic rotation

LEARNING OBJECTIVES

After studying this chapter the student or practitioner will be able to do the following:
1. Name the theorists who developed the proprioceptive neuromuscular facilitation (PNF) approach
2. Define PNF
3. List the principles of PNF
4. Describe the influence of sensory input on motor learning
5. List the elements of the PNF evaluation
6. Identify and perform upper and lower extremity (LE) diagonal patterns
7. Describe applications of PNF principles and methods in occupation therapy
8. Define key terms associated with this approach

The purpose of this chapter is to introduce the reader to **proprioceptive neuromuscular facilitation** (PNF) and its application to evaluation and treatment in occupational therapy (OT). This chapter includes the basic principles, diagonal patterns, and a few of the more commonly used facilitation techniques of PNF. A case study is used to apply the concepts discussed. To use PNF effectively, it is necessary to understand normal development, learn the motor skills to use the techniques, and apply the concepts and techniques to OT activities. This chapter should form the basis for further reading and training under the supervision of a therapist experienced in PNF.

PNF is based on normal movement and motor development. In normal motor activity the brain registers total movement and not individual muscle action.[12] Encompassed in the PNF approach are **mass movement patterns** that are spiral and diagonal in nature and that resemble movement seen in functional activities. In this multisensory approach, facilitation techniques are superimposed on movement patterns and postures through the therapist's manual contacts, verbal commands, and visual cues. PNF is effective in the treatment of numerous conditions, including Parkinson's disease, spinal cord injuries, arthritis, stroke, head injuries, and hand injuries.

HISTORY

PNF originated with Dr. Herman Kabat, physician and neurophysiologist, in the 1940s. He applied neurophysiological principles, based on the work of Sherrington, to the treatment of paralysis secondary to poliomyelitis and multiple sclerosis. In 1948 Kabat and Henry Kaiser founded the Kabat-Keiser Institute in Vallejo, California. Here Kabat worked with physical therapist Margaret Knott to develop the PNF method of treatment. By 1951 the **diagonal patterns** and several techniques were established. Essentially no new techniques have been developed since 1951, although new methods have been applied. PNF is now used to treat numerous neurological and orthopedic conditions.

In 1952 Dorothy Voss, a physical therapist, joined the staff at the Kaiser-Kabat Institute. She and Knott undertook the teaching and supervision of staff therapists. In 1954 Knott and Voss presented the first 2-week course in Vallejo. Two years later, the first edition of *Proprioceptive Neuromuscular Facilitation* by Margaret Knott and Dorothy Voss was published by Harper & Row.

During this same period several reports in the *American Journal of Occupational Therapy* described PNF and its application to OT treatment.[3,5,6,13,19,23] It was not until 1974 that the first PNF course for occupational therapists, taught by Dorothy Voss, was offered at Northwestern University. Since then, Beverly Myers, an occupational therapist, and others have offered courses for occupational therapists throughout the United States. In 1984 PNF was first taught concurrently to both physical and occupational therapists at the Rehabilitation Institute in Chicago.[15,22] Today combined courses are offered throughout the United States.

PRINCIPLES OF TREATMENT

Voss presented 11 principles of treatment at the Northwestern University Special Therapeutic Exercise Project in 1966. These principles were developed from concepts in the fields of neurophysiology, motor learning, and motor behavior.[20]

1. *All human beings have potentials that have not been fully developed.* This philosophy is the underlying basis of PNF. Therefore in evaluation and treatment planning, the patient's abilities and potentials are emphasized. For example, the patient who has weakness on one side of the body can use the intact side to assist the weaker part. Likewise, the hemiplegic patient who has a flaccid arm can use the intact head, neck, and trunk musculature to begin reinforcement of the weak arm in weight-bearing activities.

2. *Normal motor development proceeds in a cervicocaudal and proximodistal direction.* The cervicocaudal and proximodistal direction is followed in evaluation and treatment. When severe disability is present, attention is given to the head and neck region, with its visual, auditory, and vestibular receptors, and to the upper trunk and extremities. If the superior region is intact, an effective source of reinforcement for the inferior region is available.[22] The proximodistal direction is followed by developing adequate function in the head, neck, and trunk before developing function in the extremities. This approach is of particular importance in treatment that often facilitates fine motor coordination in the upper extremities. Unless there is adequate control in the head, neck, and trunk region, fine motor skills cannot be developed effectively.

3. *Early motor behavior is dominated by reflex activity. Mature motor behavior is supported or reinforced by postural reflexes.* As the human being matures, primitive reflexes are integrated and available for reinforcement to allow for progressive development such as that of rolling, crawling, and sitting. Reflexes also have been noted to have an effect on tone changes in the extremities. Hellebrandt and associates[10] studied the effect of the tonic neck reflex (TNR) and the asymmetrical tonic neck reflex (ATNR) on changes in tone and movement in the extremities of

I want to thank Beverly Myers and Diane Harsch for their assistance in reviewing and editing this chapter. I also want to thank Barbara Gale for using her technical skills to take photographs for the illustrations and Diane Harsch for her patience in posing for them.

normal adults. They found that head and neck movement significantly affected arm and leg movement. In applying this finding to treatment, weak elbow extensors can be reinforced with the ATNR by having the patient look toward the side of weakness. Likewise, the patient can be assisted in assuming postures with the influence of reflex support. For example, the body-on-body righting reflex supports the patient in assuming a side-sitting position from the side-lying position.

4. *Early motor behavior is characterized by spontaneous movement, which oscillates between extremes of flexion and extension. These movements are rhythmic and reversing in character.* In treatment it is important to attend to both directions of movement. When the OT practitioner is working with the patient on getting up from a chair, attention also must be given to sitting back down. Often with an injury the eccentric contraction (e.g., sitting down) is readily lost and becomes very difficult for the patient to regain. If not properly treated, the patient may be left with inadequate motor control to sit down smoothly and thus may "drop" into a chair. Similarly, in training for activities of daily living (ADL) the patient must learn how to get undressed, as well as how to get dressed.

5. *Developing motor behavior is expressed in an orderly sequence of total patterns of movement and posture.* In the normal infant the sequence of total patterns is demonstrated through the progression of locomotion. The infant learns to roll, to crawl, to creep, and finally to stand and walk. Throughout these stages of locomotion the infant also learns to use the extremities in different patterns and within different postures. Initially the hands are used for reaching and grasping within the most supported postures, such as supine and prone. As postural control develops, the infant begins to use the hands in side-lying, sitting, and standing. To maximize motor performance the patient should be given opportunities to work in a variety of developmental postures.

   The use of extremities in total patterns requires interaction with component patterns of the head, neck, and trunk. For example, in swinging a tennis racquet in a forehand stroke, the arm and the head, neck, and trunk move in the direction of the swing. Without the interaction of the distal and proximal components, movement becomes less powerful and less coordinated.

6. *The growth of motor behavior has cyclic trends, as evidenced by shifts between flexor and extensor dominance.* The shifts between antagonists help to develop muscle balance and control. One of the main goals of the PNF treatment approach is to establish a balance between antagonists. Developmentally the infant establishes this balance before creeping (i.e., when rocking forward [extensor dominant] and

backward [flexor dominant] on hands and knees). Postural control and balance must be achieved before movement can begin in this position. In treatment it is important to establish a balance between antagonistic muscles by first observing where imbalance exists and then facilitating the weaker component. For example, if the stroke patient demonstrates a flexor synergy (flexor dominant), extension should be facilitated.

7. *Normal motor development has an orderly sequence but lacks a step-by-step quality. Overlapping occurs.* The child does not perfect performance of one activity before beginning another, more advanced activity. In trying to ascertain in which total pattern to position the patient, normal motor development should be heeded. If one technique or developmental posture is not effective in obtaining the desired result, it may be necessary to try the activity in another developmental posture. For example, if an ataxic patient is unable to write while sitting, it may be necessary to practice writing in a more supported posture, such as prone on the elbows. Just as the infant reverts to a more secure posture when attempting a complex fine motor task, so must the patient. On the other hand, if the patient has not perfected a motor activity such as walking on level surfaces, he or she may benefit from attempting a higher-level activity such as walking up or down stairs, which in turn can improve ambulation on level surfaces. It is natural for the patient to move up and down the developmental sequence, and this allows multiple and varied opportunities for practicing motor activities. The cognitive demands of the task in relation to the developmental posture also must be considered. When the patient's position is varied, either by changing the base of support or by shifting weight on different extremities, the quality of visual and cognitive processing is influenced.[1]

8. *Locomotion depends on reciprocal contraction of flexors and extensors, and the maintenance of posture requires continual adjustment for nuances of imbalance. Antagonistic pairs of movements, reflexes, and muscles and joint motion interact as necessary with the movement or posture.* This principle restates one of the main objectives of PNF—to achieve a balance between antagonists. An example of imbalance is the head-injured patient who is unable to maintain adequate sitting balance for a tabletop cognitive activity because of a dominance of trunk extensor tone. Another example is the hemiplegic patient with tight finger flexors secondary to flexor-dominant tone in the hand. In treatment, emphasis is placed on correcting the imbalances. In the presence of spasticity, first the spasticity is inhibited and then the antagonistic muscles, reflexes, and postures are facilitated.

9. *Improvement in motor ability is dependent upon motor learning.* Multisensory input from the therapist facilitates the patient's motor learning and is an integral part of the PNF approach. For example, the therapist may work with a patient on a shoulder flexion activity such as reaching into the cabinet for a cup. The therapist may say, "Reach for the cup," to add verbal input. This approach also encourages the patient to look in the direction of the movement to allow vision to enhance the motor response. Thus tactile, auditory, and visual input are used. Motor learning has occurred when these external cues are no longer needed for adequate performance.

10. *Frequency of stimulation and repetitive activity are used to promote and retain motor learning and to develop strength and endurance.* Just as the therapist who is learning PNF needs the opportunity to practice the techniques, the patient needs the opportunity to practice new motor skills. In the process of development the infant constantly repeats a motor skill in many settings and developmental postures until it is mastered, as becomes apparent to anyone who watches a child learning to walk. Numerous attempts fail, but efforts are repeated until the skill is mastered. After the activity is learned, it becomes part of the child. He or she is able to use the activity automatically and deliberately as the occasion demands.[22] The same is true for the person learning to play the piano or to play tennis. Without the opportunity to practice, motor learning cannot successfully occur.

11. *Goal-directed activities coupled with techniques of facilitation are used to hasten learning of total patterns of walking and self-care activities.* When facilitation techniques are applied to self-care, the objective is improved functional ability, but improvement is obtained by more than instruction and practice alone. The correction of deficiencies is accomplished by directly applying manual contacts and techniques to facilitate a desired response.[11] In treatment this approach may mean applying **stretch** to finger extensors to facilitate release of an object or providing joint approximation through the shoulders and pelvis of an ataxic patient to provide stability while the patient is standing to wash dishes.

MOTOR LEARNING

Motor learning requires a multisensory approach. Auditory, visual, and tactile systems are all used to achieve the desired response. The correct combination of sensory input with each patient should be ascertained, implemented, and altered as the patient progresses. The developmental level of the patient and the ability to cooperate also should be taken into consideration.[22] The

approach used with an aphasic patient differs from the approach used with a hand-injured patient. Similarly, the approach used with a child varies greatly from that used with an adult.

Auditory System

Verbal commands should be brief and clear. It is important to time the command so that it does not come too early or too late in relation to the motor act. Tone of voice may influence the quality of the patient's response. Buchwald[4] states that tones of moderate intensity evoke gamma motor neuron activity and that louder tones can alter alpha motor neuron activity. Strong, sharp commands simulate a stress situation and are used when maximal stimulation of motor response is desired. A soft tone of voice is used to offer reassurance and to encourage a smooth movement, as in the presence of pain. When a patient is giving the best effort, a moderate tone can be used.[22]

Another effect of auditory feedback on motor performance was studied by Loomis and Boersma.[14] They used a "verbal mediation strategy to teach wheelchair safety before transferring out of the chair to patients with right cerebrovascular accident (CVA). Loomis and Boersma taught patients to say aloud the steps required to leave the wheelchair safely and independently. They found that only patients who used verbal mediation learned the wheelchair drill sufficiently to perform safe and independent transfers. These patients also had better retention of the sequence of steps, suggesting that verbal mediation is beneficial in reaching independence with better sequencing and fewer errors.

Visual System

Visual stimuli assist in initiation and coordination of movement. Visual input should be monitored to ensure that the patient is tracking in the direction of movement. For example, the therapist's position is important because the patient often uses the therapist's movement or position as a visual cue. If the desired direction of movement is forward, the therapist should be positioned diagonally in front of the patient. In addition to the therapist's position, placement of the OT activity also should be considered. If the treatment goal is to increase head, neck, and trunk rotation to the left, the activity is placed in front and to the left of the patient. Because OT is activity oriented, an abundance of visual stimuli is offered to the patient.

Tactile System

Developmentally the tactile system matures before the auditory and visual systems.[7] Furthermore, the tactile system is more efficient. This is because it has both temporal and spatial discrimination abilities, as opposed to the visual system, which can make only spatial discriminations, and the auditory system, which can make only temporal discriminations.[8] Affolter[2] states that during development, processing of tactile-kinesthetic information can be considered fundamental for building cognitive and emotional experience. Looking at and listening to the world does not result in change; however, the world cannot be touched without some change taking place. A Chinese proverb often cited at PNF courses reinforces this viewpoint: "I listen and I forget, I see and I remember, I do and I understand."

It is important for the patient to feel movement patterns that are coordinated and balanced. With the PNF approach, tactile input is supplied through the therapist's **manual contacts** to guide and reinforce the desired response. This approach may involve gently touching the patient to guide movement, using stretch to initiate movement, and providing resistance to strengthen movement. The type and extent of manual contacts depend on the patient's clinical status, which is determined through evaluation and reevaluation. For example, the use of stretch or resistance in the presence of musculoskeletal instability may be contraindicated. Likewise, stretch or resistance should not be used if they cause increased pain or tone imbalance.

To increase speed and accuracy in motor performance, the patient needs the opportunity to practice. Through repetition, habit patterns that occur automatically without voluntary effort are established. The PNF approach uses the concepts of **part-task practice** and **whole-task practice.** In other words, to learn the whole task, emphasis is placed on the parts of the task that the patient is unable to perform independently. The term **stepwise procedures** is descriptive of the emphasis on a part of the task during performance of the whole.[22] Performance of each part of the task is improved by combining practice with appropriate sensory cues and techniques of facilitation. For example, the patient learning to transfer from a wheelchair to a tub bench may have difficulty lifting the leg over the tub rim. This part of the task should be practiced, with repetition and facilitation techniques to the hip flexors, during performance of the transfer. When the transfer becomes smooth and coordinated, it is no longer necessary to practice each part individually. It is also unnecessary for the therapist to provide continued facilitation.

In summation, several components are necessary for motor learning to occur. In the PNF treatment approach, these components include multisensory input from the therapist's verbal commands, visual cues, and manual contacts. Touch is the most efficient form of stimulation and provides the opportunity for the patient to feel normal movement. Current motor-learning theory argues that for motor learning to occur, the patient cannot be a passive recipient of treatment.

Therefore the patient needs opportunities to practice motor skills in the context of functional life situations. Initially the therapist's manual contacts and sensory input are needed. These should be decreased, however, as the patient demonstrates and learns skilled movement. The amount of feedback from the therapist should also be decreased as the patient learns to rely on his or her own internal feedback system for error detection and correction.

ASSESSMENT

Assessment of the patient requires astute observational skills and knowledge of normal movement. An initial assessment is completed to determine the patient's abilities, deficiencies, and potential. After the treatment plan is established, ongoing assessment of the patient is necessary to ascertain the effectiveness of treatment and to make modifications as the patient changes.

The PNF assessment follows a sequence from proximal to distal. First, vital and related functions are considered, such as breathing, swallowing, voice production, facial and oral musculature, and visual-ocular control. Any impairment or weakness in these functions is noted.

The head and neck region is observed after vital functions. Deficiencies in this area directly affect the upper trunk and extremities. Head and neck positions are observed in varying postures and total patterns during functional activities. It is important to note (1) dominance of tone (flexor or extensor), (2) alignment (midline or shift to one side), and (3) stability and mobility (more or less needed).[15]

After observation of the head and neck region, the assessment proceeds to the following parts of the body: upper trunk, upper extremities, lower trunk, and lower extremities. Each segment is assessed individually in specific movement patterns, as well as in developmental activities in which the body segments interact. For example, shoulder flexion can be observed in an individual upper-extremity movement pattern, as well as during a total developmental pattern such as rolling.

During assessment of developmental activities and postures, the following issues should be addressed:

1. Is there a need for more stability or mobility?
2. Is there a balance between flexors and extensors, or is one more dominant?
3. Is the patient able to move in all directions?
4. What are the major limitations (e.g., weakness, incoordination, spasticity, and contractures)?
5. Is the patient able to assume a posture and to maintain it? If not, which total pattern or postures are inadequate?
6. Are the inadequacies more proximal or distal?
7. Which sensory input does the patient respond to most effectively—auditory, visual, or tactile?

8. Which techniques of facilitation does the patient respond to best?

Finally the patient is observed during self-care and other ADL to determine whether performance of individual and total patterns is adequate within the context of a functional activity. The patient's performance may vary from one setting to another. After the patient leaves the structured setting of the OT or physical therapy clinic for the less structured home or community environment, deterioration of motor performance is not unusual. Thus the treatment plan must accommodate the practice of motor performance in a variety of settings in locations appropriate to the specific activity.

TREATMENT IMPLEMENTATION

After assessment a treatment plan is developed that includes goals the patient hopes to accomplish. The techniques and procedures that have the most favorable influence on movement and posture are used. Similarly, appropriate total patterns and patterns of facilitation are selected to enhance performance.

Diagonal Patterns

The diagonal patterns used in the PNF approach are mass movement patterns observed in most functional activities. Part of the challenge in OT assessment and intervention is recognizing the diagonal patterns in ADL. Knowledge of the diagonals is necessary for identifying areas of deficiency. Two diagonal motions are present for each major part of the body: head and neck, upper and lower trunk, and extremities. Each diagonal pattern has a flexion and extension component, together with rotation and movement away from or toward the midline.

The head, neck, and trunk patterns are referred to as (a) flexion with rotation to the right or left and (b) extension with rotation to the right or left. These proximal patterns combine with the extremity diagonals. The upper and lower extremity diagonals are described according to the three movement components at the shoulder and hip: (1) flexion and extension, (2) abduction and adduction, and (3) external and internal rotation. Voss[20] introduced shorter descriptions for the extremity patterns in 1967 and referred to them as diagonal 1 (D_1) flexion/extension and diagonal 2 (D_2) flexion/extension. The reference points for flexion and extension are the shoulder and hip joints of the upper and lower extremities, respectively.

The movements associated with each diagonal and examples of these patterns seen in self-care and other ADL are presented in the following sections. Note that in functional activities, not all components of the pattern or full range of motion (ROM) are necessarily seen. Furthermore, the diagonals interact during func-

tional movement, changing from one pattern or combination to another, when they cross the transverse and sagittal planes of the body.[17]

Unilateral Patterns

1. *Upper extremity (UE) D_1 flexion (antagonist of D_1 extension):* Scapula elevation, abduction, and rotation; shoulder flexion, adduction, and external rotation; elbow in flexion or extension; forearm supination; wrist flexion to the radial side; finger flexion and adduction; thumb adduction (Fig. 35-1, A). Examples in functional activity: hand-to-mouth motion in feeding, tennis forehand, combing hair on the left side of the head with right hand (Fig. 35-2, A), rolling from supine to prone.

2. *UE D_1 extension (antagonist of D_1 flexion):* Scapula depression, adduction, and rotation; shoulder extension, abduction, and internal rotation; elbow in flexion or extension; forearm pronation; wrist extension to the ulnar side; finger extension and abduction; thumb in palmar abduction (Fig. 35-1, B). Examples in functional activity: pushing a car door open from the inside (Fig. 35-2, B), tennis backhand stroke, rolling from prone to supine.

3. *UE D_2 flexion (antagonist of D_2 extension):* Scapula elevation, adduction, and rotation; shoulder flexion, abduction, and external rotation; elbow in flexion or extension; forearm supination; wrist extension to the radial side; finger extension and abduction; thumb extension (Fig. 35-3, A). Examples in functional activity: combing hair on the right side of the head with the right hand (Fig. 35-4, A), lifting a racquet in tennis serve, back stroke in swimming.

4. *UE D_2 extension (antagonist of D_2 flexion):* Scapula depression, abduction, and rotation; shoulder extension, adduction, and internal rotation; elbow in flexion or extension; forearm pronation; wrist flexion to the ulnar side; finger flexion and adduction; thumb opposition (Fig. 35-3, B). Examples in functional activity: pitching a baseball, hitting a ball in tennis serve, buttoning pants on the left side with the right hand (Fig. 35-4, B). The rotational component in LE D_2 flexion and extension parallel the UE patterns.

5. *LE D_1 flexion (antagonist of D_1 extension):* Hip flexion, adduction, and external rotation; knee in flexion or extension; ankle and foot dorsiflexion with inversion and toe extension. Examples in functional activity: kicking a soccer ball, rolling from supine to prone, putting on a shoe with legs crossed (Fig. 35-5, A).

6. *LE D_1 extension (antagonist of D_1 flexion):* Hip extension, abduction, and internal rotation; knee in flexion or extension; ankle and foot plantar flexion with eversion and toe flexion. Examples in functional activity: putting leg into pants (Fig. 35-5, B), rolling from prone to supine. The rotational

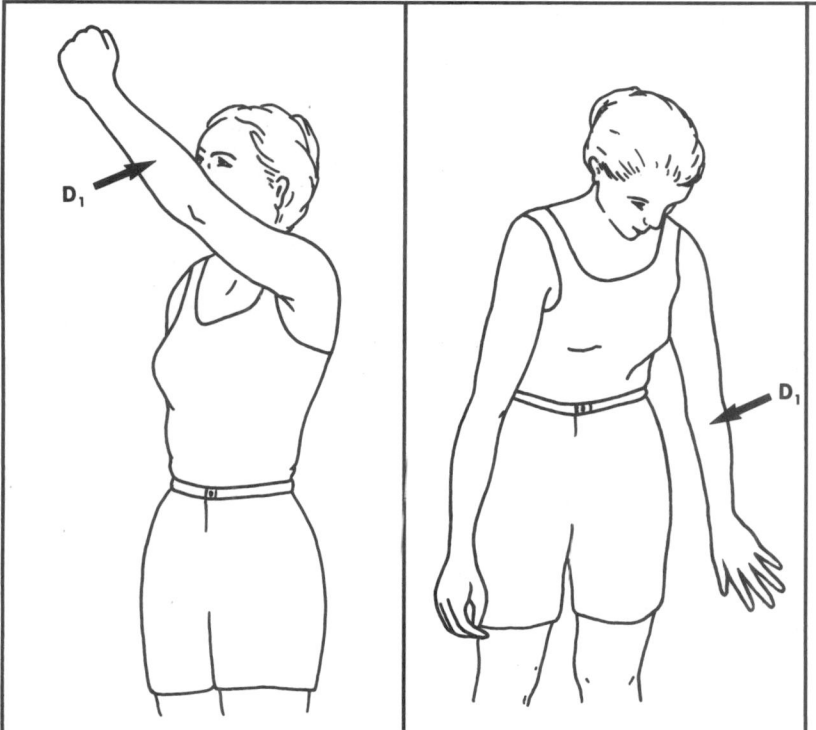

Diagonal One
(D₁)

- D_1 extension begins in the shortened range of D_1 flexion with hand closed toward radial side.
- Diagonal 1 (D_1) extension leads with hand opening toward ulnar side.
- Eyes follow hand of leading arm so that head and hand cross midline.
- Elbows may remain straight, may flex or extend.

FIG. 35-1
A, Upper extremity D_1 flexion pattern. **B,** Upper extremity D_1 extension pattern. (From Myers BJ: *Unit I: PNF diagonal patterns and their application to functional activities,* videotape study guide, Rehabilitation Institute of Chicago, 1982.)

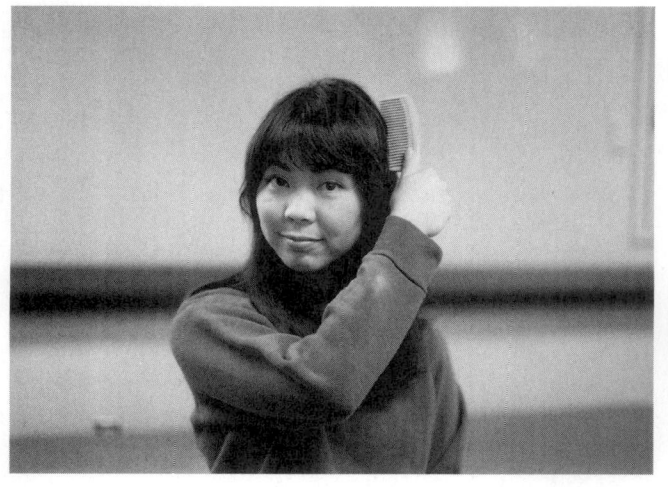

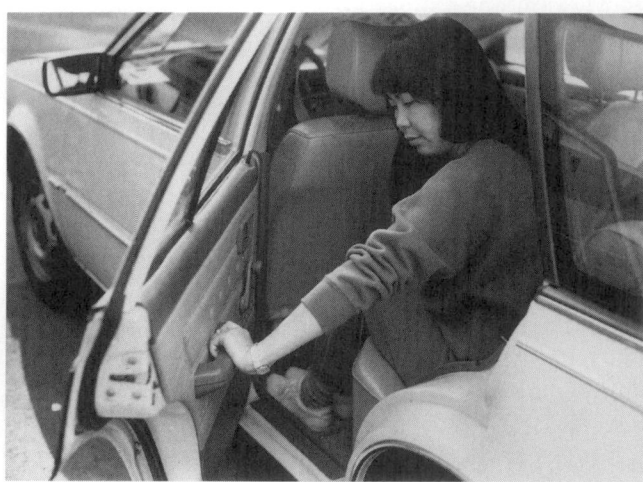

A

B

FIG. 35-2
A, Upper extremity D_1 flexion pattern is used in combing hair, opposite side. **B,** Upper extremity D_1 extension pattern is used in pushing a car door open.

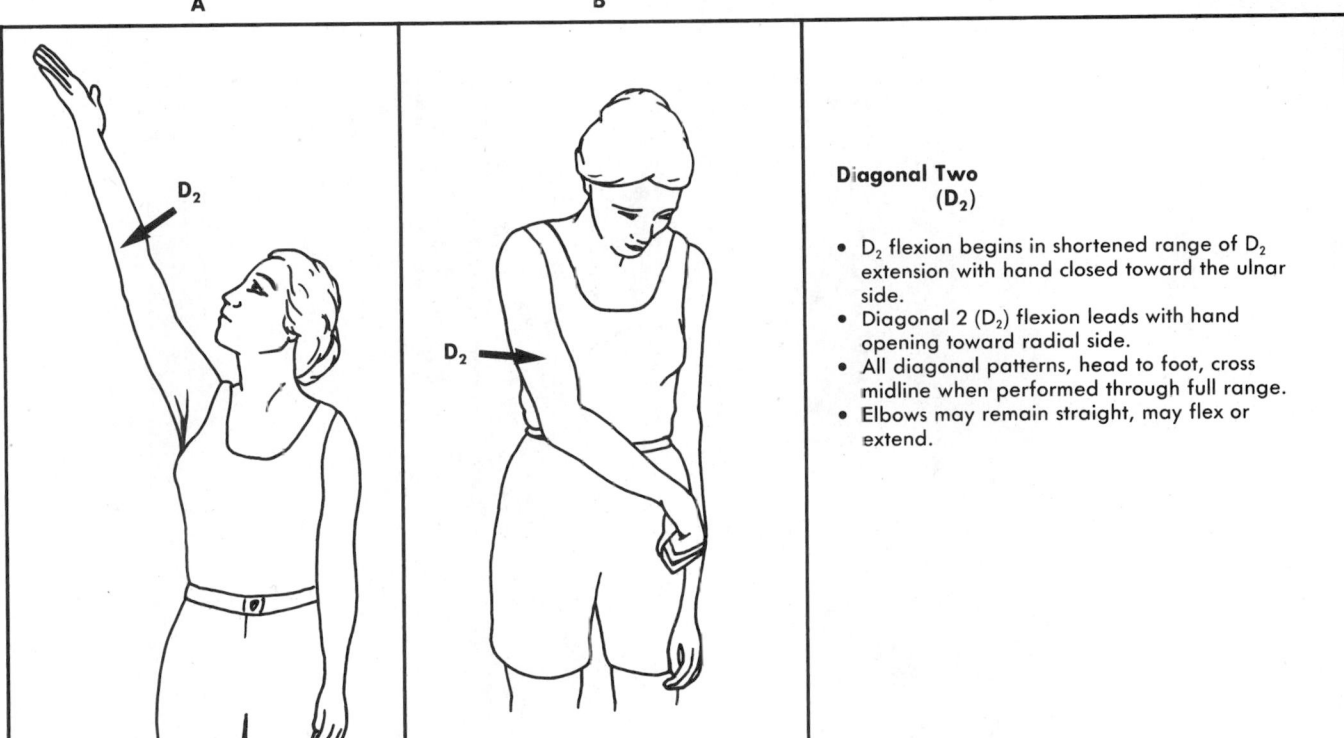

Diagonal Two (D₂)

- D₂ flexion begins in shortened range of D₂ extension with hand closed toward the ulnar side.
- Diagonal 2 (D₂) flexion leads with hand opening toward radial side.
- All diagonal patterns, head to foot, cross midline when performed through full range.
- Elbows may remain straight, may flex or extend.

FIG. 35-3
A, Upper extremity D₂ flexion pattern. **B,** Upper extremity D₂ extension pattern. (From Myers BJ: *Unit I: PNF diagonal patterns and their application to functional activities,* videotape study guide, Rehabilitation Institute of Chicago, 1982.)

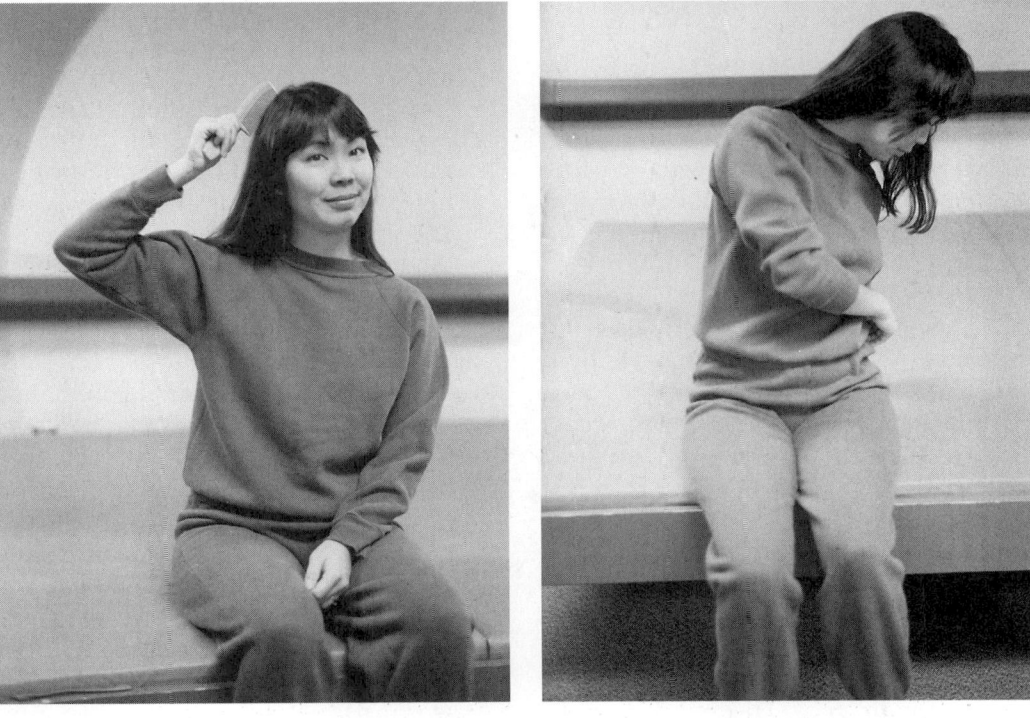

FIG. 35-4
A, Upper extremity D₂ flexion pattern is used in combing hair, same side. **B,** Upper extremity D₂ extension pattern is used in buttoning trousers, opposite side.

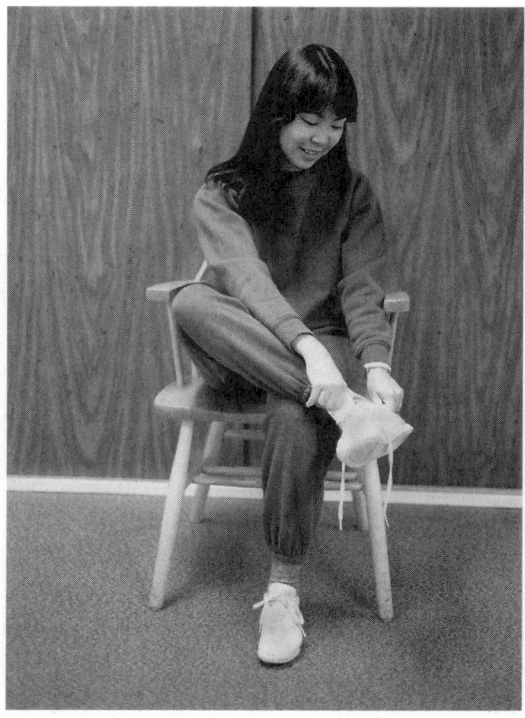
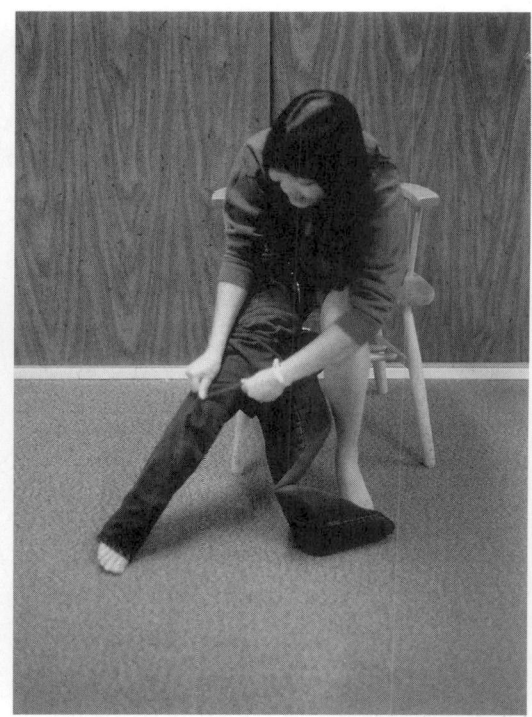

A   B

FIG. 35-5
A, Lower extremity D₁ flexion pattern is demonstrated in crossed leg when putting on shoe.
B, Lower extremity D₁ extension pattern is used when pulling on trousers.

component of LE D_2 flexion and extension is opposite to the UE patterns.

7. *LE D_2 flexion (antagonist of D_2 extension):* Hip flexion, abduction, and internal rotation; knee in flexion or extension; ankle and foot dorsiflexion with eversion and toe extension. Examples in functional activity: karate kick (Fig. 35-6, *A*), drawing the heels up during the breaststroke in swimming.

8. *LE D_2 extension (antagonist of D_2 flexion):* Hip extension, adduction and external rotation: knee in flexion or extension; ankle and foot plantar flexion with inversion and toe flexion. Examples of functional activity: push-off in gait, the kick during the breaststroke in swimming, long sitting with legs crossed (Fig. 35-6, *B*).

Bilateral Patterns
Movements in the extremities may be reinforced by combining diagonals in **bilateral patterns** as follows:

1. Symmetrical patterns: Paired extremities perform similar movements at the same time (Fig. 35-7, *A*). Examples: bilateral symmetrical D_1 extension, such as pushing off a chair to stand (Fig. 35-8, *A*); bilateral symmetrical D_2 extension, such as starting to take off a pullover sweater (Fig. 35-8, *B*); bilateral symmetri-

cal D_2 flexion, such as reaching to lift a large item off a high shelf (Fig. 35-8, *C*). Bilateral symmetrical UE patterns facilitate trunk flexion and extension.

2. *Asymmetrical patterns:* Paired extremities perform movements toward one side of the body at the same time, which facilitates trunk rotation (Fig. 35-7, *B*). The **asymmetrical patterns** can be performed with the arms in contact, such as in the chopping and lifting patterns in which greater trunk rotation is seen (Figs. 35-9 and 35-10). Furthermore, with the arms in contact, self-touching occurs. This is frequently observed in the presence of pain or in reinforcement of a motion when greater control or power is needed.[22] This phenomenon is observed in the baseball player at bat and in the tennis player who uses a two-handed backhand to increase control and power. Examples of asymmetrical patterns are bilateral asymmetrical flexion to the left, with the left arm in D_2 flexion and the right arm in D_1 flexion, such as when putting on a left earring (Fig. 35-11), and bilateral asymmetrical extension to the left, with the right arm in D_2 extension and the left arm in D_1 extension, such as when zipping a left-side zipper.

3. *Reciprocal patterns:* Paired extremities move in opposite directions simultaneously, either in the same di-

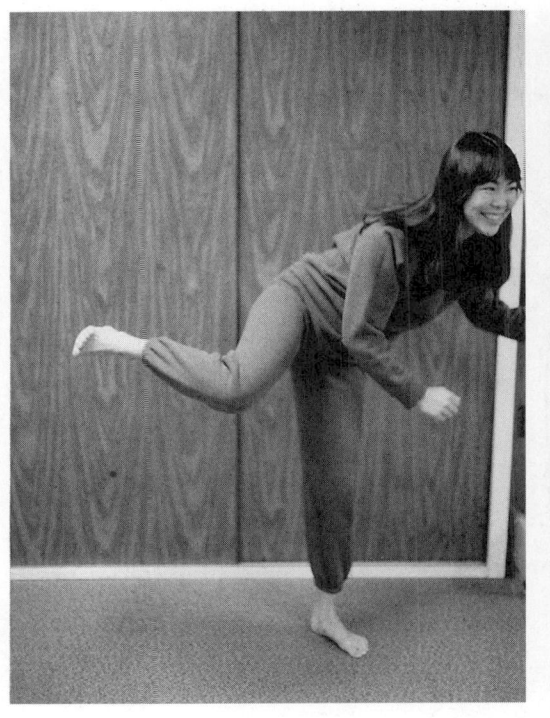 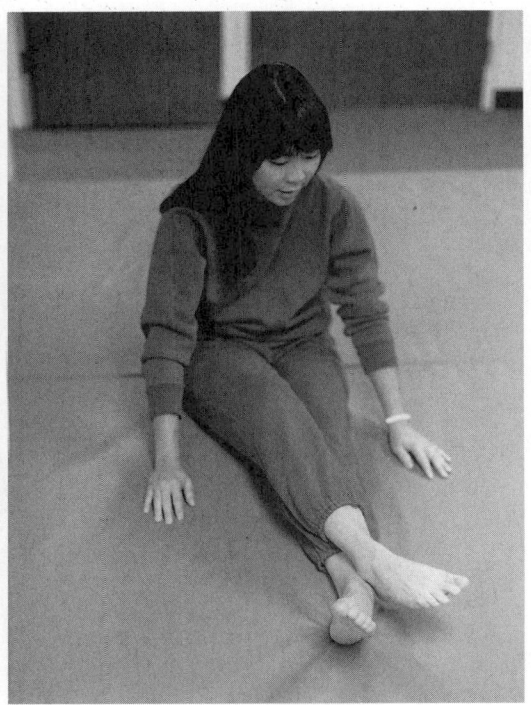

A   B

FIG. 35-6
A, Lower extremity D_2 flexion pattern is shown in karate kick. **B,** Lower extremity D_2 extension pattern is used in long sitting with legs crossed.

agonal or in combined diagonals. If paired extremities perform movements in combined diagonals (Fig. 35-7, *C*), there is a stabilizing effect on the head, neck, and trunk because movement of the extremities is in the opposite direction while head and neck remain in midline. During activities requiring high-level balance, the **reciprocal patterns** with combined diagonals come into play with one extremity in D_1 extension and the other extremity in D_2 flexion. Examples of this are pitching in baseball, sidestroke in swimming, and walking a balance beam with one extremity in a diagonal flexion pattern and the other in a diagonal extension pattern (Fig. 35-12). In contrast, reciprocal patterns in the same diagonal, such as D_1 in arm swing during walking, facilitate trunk rotation.

Combined Movements of Upper and Lower Extremities

Interaction of the upper and lower extremities results in (1) ipsilateral patterns, with extremities of the same side moving in the same direction at the same time, (2) contralateral patterns, with extremities of opposite sides moving in the same direction at the same time, and (3) diagonal reciprocal patterns, with contralateral extremities moving in the same direction at the same time

while opposite contralateral extremities move in the opposite direction (Fig. 35-7, *D, E,* and *F*).

The **combined movements** of the upper and lower extremities are observed in such activities as crawling and walking. Awareness of these patterns is important in the assessment of the patient's motor skills. The ipsilateral patterns are more primitive developmentally and indicate a lack of bilateral integration. Less rotation also is observed in ipsilateral patterns. Therefore the goal in treatment is to progress from ipsilateral to contralateral to diagonal reciprocal patterns.

There are several advantages to using the diagonal patterns in treatment. First, crossing of midline occurs. This movement is of particular importance in the remediation of perceptual motor deficits such as unilateral neglect, in which integration of both sides of the body and awareness of the neglected side are treatment goals. Second, each muscle has an optimal pattern in which it functions. For example, the patient who has weak thumb opposition benefits from active movement in D_2 extension. Similarly, D_1 extension is the optimal pattern for ulnar wrist extension. Third, the diagonal patterns use groups of muscles, which is typical of movement seen in functional activities. For example, in eating, the hand-to-mouth action is accomplished in one mass movement pattern (D_1 flexion) that uses several

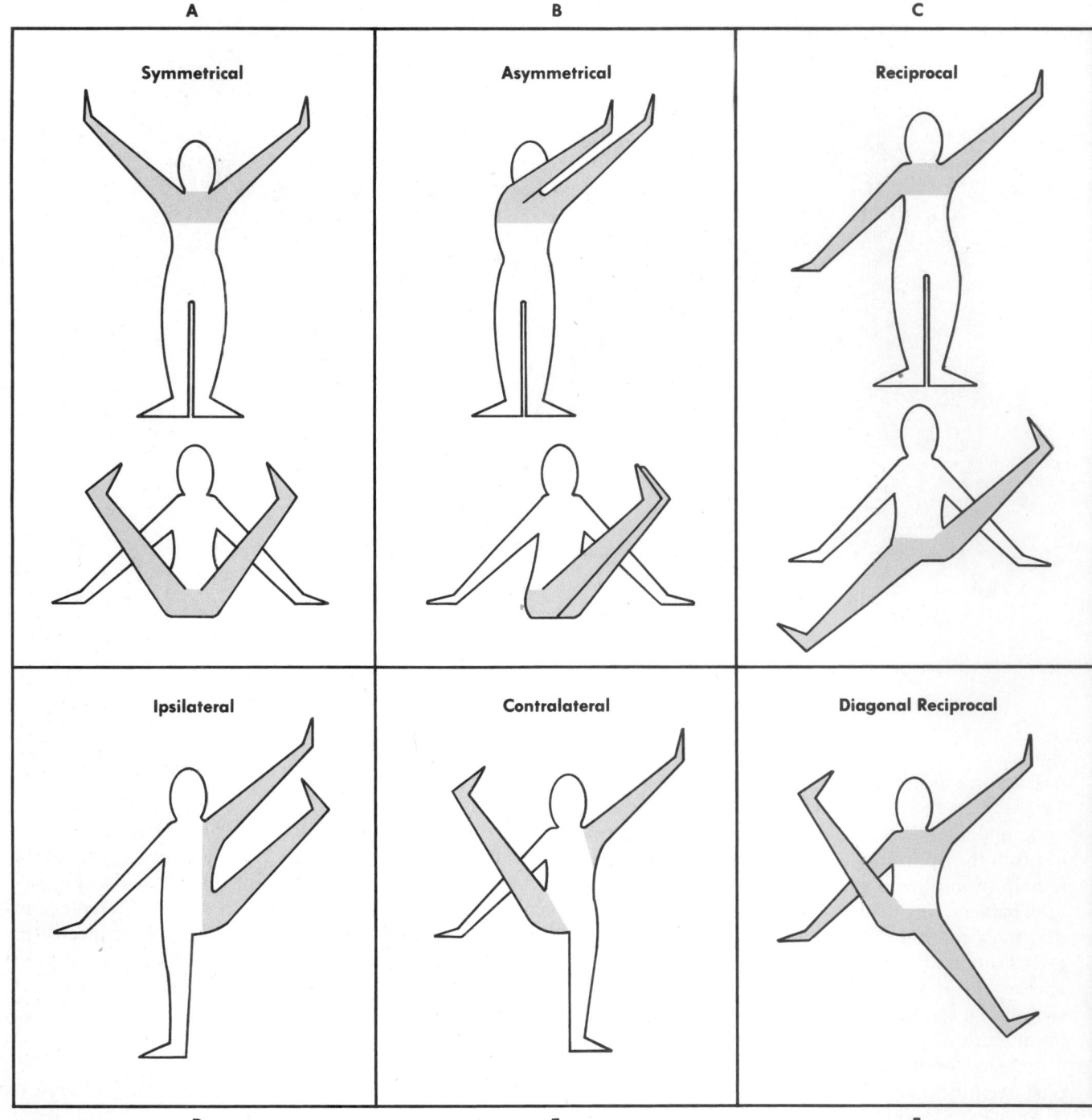

FIG. 35-7

A, Symmetrical patterns. **B,** Asymmetrical patterns. **C,** Reciprocal patterns. **D,** Ipsilateral pattern. **E,** Contralateral pattern. **F,** Diagonal reciprocal pattern. (From Myers BJ: *Unit I: PNF diagonal patterns and their application to functional activities,* videotape study guide, Rehabilitation Institute of Chicago, 1982.)

muscles simultaneously. Therefore movement in the diagonals is more efficient than movement performed at each joint separately. Finally, rotation is always a component in the diagonals (e.g., trunk rotation to the left or right and forearm pronation and supination). With

an injury or the aging process, rotation frequently is impaired and can be facilitated with movement in the diagonals. In treatment, attention should be given to the placement of activities so that movement occurs in the diagonal. For example, if the patient is working on a

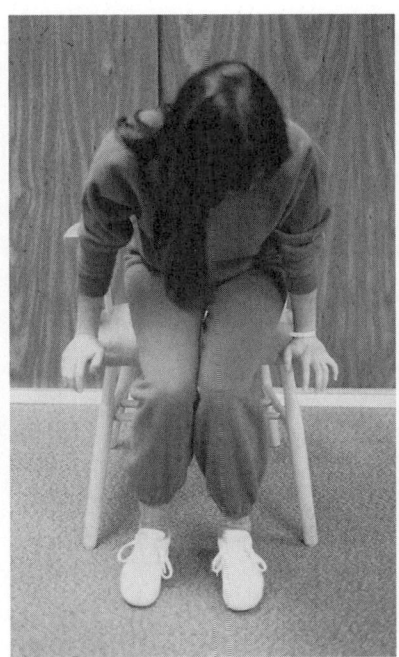 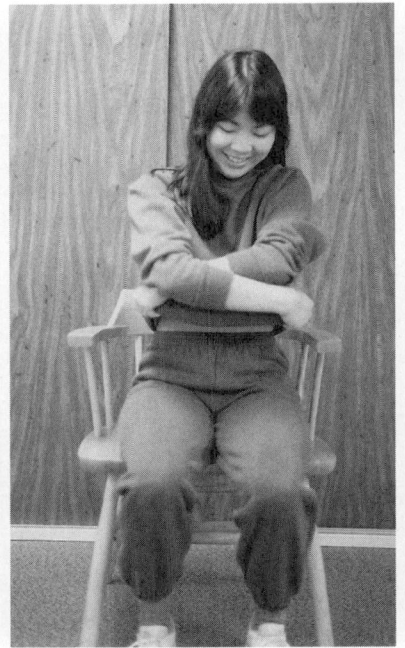 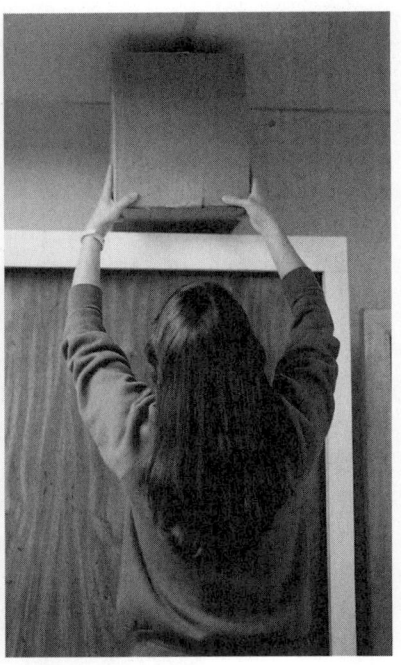

A   B   C

FIG. 35-8
A, Upper extremity bilateral symmetrical D$_1$ extension pattern is shown in pushing off from chair.
B, Upper extremity bilateral symmetrical D$_2$ extension pattern is used when starting to take off pullover shirt. **C,** Upper extremity bilateral symmetrical D$_2$ flexion pattern is used when reaching to lift box off high shelf.

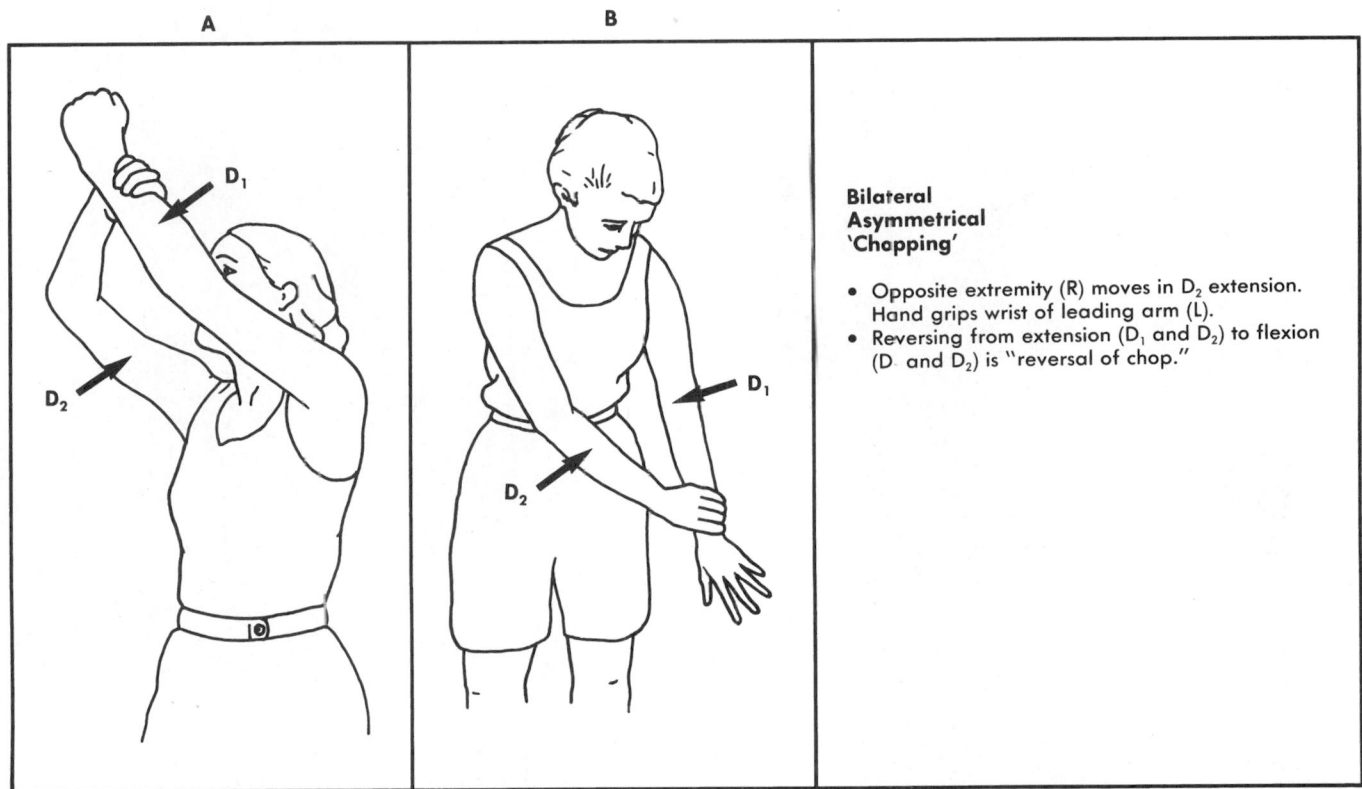

A   B

Bilateral Asymmetrical 'Chopping'

- Opposite extremity (R) moves in D$_2$ extension. Hand grips wrist of leading arm (L).
- Reversing from extension (D$_1$ and D$_2$) to flexion (D$_1$ and D$_2$) is "reversal of chop."

FIG. 35-9
Bilateral asymmetrical chopping. (From Myers BJ: *Unit I: PNF diagonal patterns and their application to functional activities,* videotape study guide, Rehabilitation Institute of Chicago, 1982.)

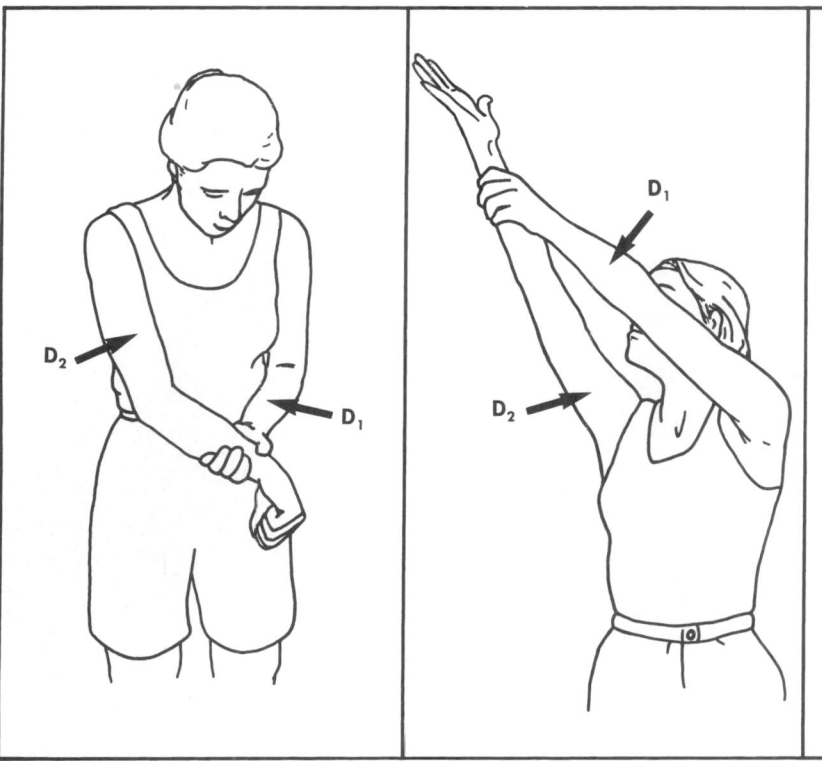

A   B

D₂   D₁

D₁

D₂

**Bilateral
Asymmetrical
'Lifting'**

- In lifting the hand opens with abduction, D_1 flexion, and D_2 flexion, and closes with adduction, D_1 extension and D_2 extension. Reversing from flexion (D_1 and D_2) to extension (D_1 and D_2) is "reversal of the lift."
- Contact with opposite extremity, self-touching, promotes stability and perception.

FIG. 35-10
Bilateral asymmetrical lifting. (From Myers BJ: *Unit I: PNF diagonal patterns and their application to functional activities,* videotape study guide, Rehabilitation Institute of Chicago, 1982.)

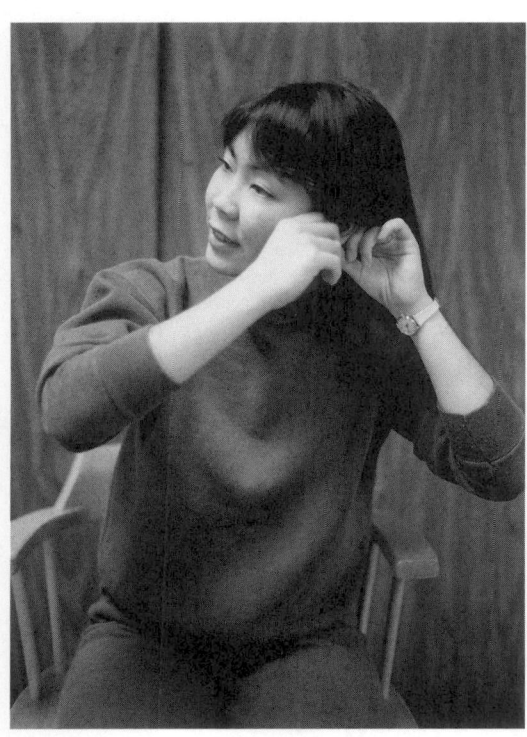

FIG. 35-11
Putting on earring requires use of upper extremity bilateral asymmetrical flexion pattern.

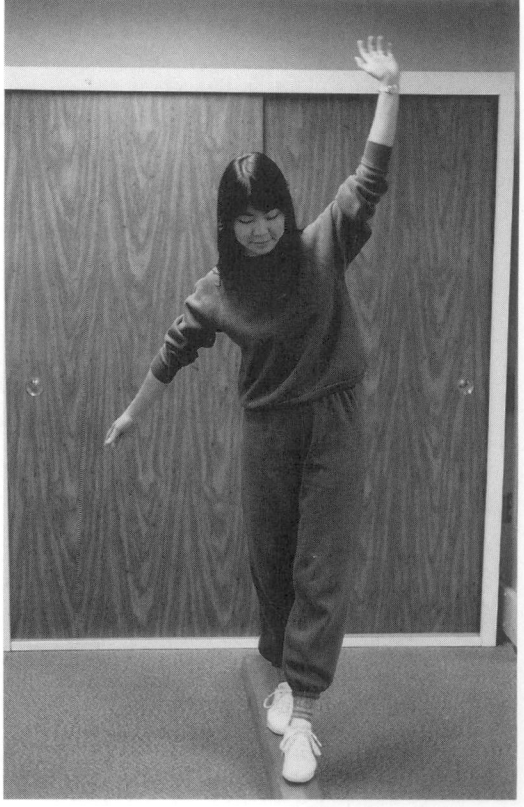

FIG. 32-12
Bilateral reciprocal pattern of upper extremities is used to walk balance beam.

wood-sanding project, trunk rotation with extension can be facilitated by placing the project on an inclined plane in a diagonal.

Total Patterns

In PNF, developmental postures also are called total patterns of movement and posture.[16] Total patterns require interaction between proximal (head, neck, and trunk) and distal (extremity) components. The assumption of postures is important, as is the maintenance of postures. When posture cannot be sustained, emphasis should be placed on the assumption of posture.[21] For example, before the patient can be expected to sustain a sitting posture, he or she must have ability in lower developmental total patterns of movement, such as rolling and moving from side-lying to side-sitting.

The active assumption of postures can be included in OT activities. For example, a reaching and placing activity could be set up so that the patient must reach for the object in the supine posture and place the object in the side-lying posture. The use of total patterns also can reinforce individual extremity movements. For example, in an activity such as wiping a tabletop, wrist extension is reinforced when the patient leans forward over the supporting arm.

Several facts support the use of total patterns in the PNF treatment approach.[16] First, total patterns of movement and posture are experienced as part of the normal developmental process in all human beings. Therefore recapitulation of these postures is meaningful to the patient and acquired with less difficulty. Second, movement in and out of total patterns and the ability to sustain postures enhance components of normal development, such as reflex integration and support, balance between antagonists, and development of motor control in a cephalocaudal, proximodistal direction. Third, the use of total patterns improves the ability to assume and maintain postures, which is important in all functional activities.

The sequence and procedures for assisting patients with the developmental postures were developed by Voss. In 1981 Myers developed a videotape showing use of the sequence and procedures in OT.[16] This video demonstrates more information on the application of the total patterns and postures to OT.

Procedures

PNF techniques are superimposed on movement and posture. Among these techniques are basic procedures considered essential to the PNF approach. Two procedures, verbal commands and visual cues, were discussed previously. Other procedures are described in the following sections.

Manual contacts refers to the placement of the therapist's hands on the patient. These contacts are most ef-

fective when applied directly to the skin. Pressure from the therapist's touch is used as a facilitating mechanism and serves as a sensory cue to help the patient understand the direction of the anticipated movement.[22] The amount of pressure applied depends on the specific technique being used and on the desired response. The location of manual contacts is chosen according to the groups of muscles, tendons, and joints responsible for the desired movement patterns. If the patient is having difficulty reaching to comb the back of the hair because of scapular weakness, the desired movement pattern is D_2 flexion. Manual contacts should be on the posterior surface of the scapula to reinforce the muscles that elevate, adduct, and rotate the scapula.

Stretch is used to initiate voluntary movement and enhance speed of response and strength in weak muscles. This procedure is based on Sherrington's neurophysiological principle of reciprocal innervation.[18] When a muscle is stretched, the Ia and II fibers in the muscle spindle send excitatory messages to the alpha motor neurons, which innervate the stretched muscle. Inhibitory messages are sent to the antagonistic muscle simultaneously.[7]

When stretch is used in the PNF approach, the part to be facilitated is placed in the extreme lengthened range of the desired pattern (or where tension is felt on all muscle components of a given pattern). This range is the completely shortened range of the antagonistic pattern. Special attention is given to the rotatory component of the pattern because it is responsible for elongation of the fibers of the muscles in a given pattern. After the correct position for the stretch stimulus has been achieved, stretch is superimposed on the pattern. The patient should attempt the movement at the exact time that the stretch reflex is elicited. The use of verbal commands also should coincide with the application of stretch, to reinforce the movement. Discrimination should be exercised when using stretch, to prevent an increase in pain or muscle imbalances.

Traction facilitates the joint receptors by creating a separation of the joint surfaces. It is thought that traction promotes movement and is used for pulling motion.[22] In activities such as carrying a heavy suitcase or pulling open a jammed door, traction can be felt on joint surfaces. Although traction may be contraindicated for patients with acute symptoms, such as after surgery or a fracture, it can sometimes provide relief of pain and promote greater ROM in painful joints.

Approximation facilitates joint receptors by creating a compression of joint surfaces. It promotes stability and postural control and is used for pushing motion.[22] Approximation is usually superimposed on a weight-bearing posture. For example, to enhance postural control in the prone on elbows posture, approximation may be given through the shoulders in a downward direction.

Maximal resistance is a procedure that involves Sherrington's principle of irradiation—namely, that stronger muscles and patterns reinforce weaker components.[18] This procedure is frequently misunderstood and applied incorrectly. The procedure is defined as the greatest amount of resistance that can be applied to an active contraction while allowing full ROM to occur, or to an isometric contraction without defeating or breaking the patient's hold.[22] Maximal resistance is *not* the greatest amount of resistance that the therapist can apply. The objective is to obtain maximal effort on the part of the patient because strength is increased by movement against resistance that requires maximal effort.[9]

If the resistance applied by the therapist results in uncoordinated or jerky movement or if it breaks the patient's hold, too much resistance has been given. Movement against maximal resistance should be slow and smooth. To use this technique effectively, the therapist must sense the appropriate amount of resistance. For patients with neurological impairment or pain, the resistance may be very light, and light resistance is probably maximal for the patient's needs. The therapist's manual contacts may offer light resistance that actually assists by providing the patient with a way to track the desired movement. In the presence of spasticity, resistance may increase existing muscle imbalance and thus needs to be monitored. For example, if an increase in finger flexor spasticity is noted with resisted rocking in the hands-knees position, resistance should be decreased or eliminated or an alternate position should be used.

Techniques

Specific techniques are used in conjunction with these basic procedures. A few have been selected for discussion. These techniques are divided into three categories: those directed to the agonists, those that are a reversal of the antagonists, and those that promote relaxation.[22]

Techniques Directed to the Agonist

Repeated contractions is a technique based on the assumption that repetition of an activity is necessary for motor learning and helps develop strength, ROM, and endurance. The patient's voluntary movement is facilitated with stretch and resistance, using isometric and isotonic contractions. Repeated contractions could be used to increase trunk flexion with rotation in the patient who has difficulty reaching to put on a pair of shoes from the sitting position. The patient bends forward as far as possible. At the point where active motion weakens, the patient is asked to "hold" with an isometric contraction. This action is followed by isotonic contractions, facilitated by stretch, as the patient

is asked to "reach toward your feet." This sequence is repeated either until fatigue is evident or until the patient is able to reach the feet. The pattern can be reinforced further by asking the patient to hold with another isometric contraction at the end of the sequence.

Rhythmic initiation is used to improve the ability to initiate movement, which may be a problem with Parkinson's disease or apraxia. This technique involves voluntary relaxation, passive movement, and repeated isotonic contractions of the agonistic pattern. The verbal command is, "Relax and let me move you." As relaxation is felt, the command is, "Now you do it with me." After several repetitions of active movement, resistance may be given to reinforce the movement. Rhythmic initiation allows the patient to feel the pattern before beginning active movement. Thus the proprioceptive and kinesthetic senses are enhanced.

Reversal of Antagonists Techniques

Reversal of antagonists techniques employ a characteristic of normal development—namely, that movement is reversing and changes direction. These techniques are based on Sherrington's principle of successive induction, according to which the stronger antagonist facilitates the weaker agonist.[18] The agonist is facilitated through resistance to the antagonist. The contraction of the antagonist can be isotonic, isometric, or a combination of the two. These techniques may be contraindicated for patients in whom resistance of antagonists increases symptoms such as pain and spasticity. For example, the facilitation of finger extension (agonist) would not be achieved effectively through resistance applied to spastic finger flexors (antagonist). In this situation, finger extension may be better facilitated through the use of repeated contractions, in which the emphasis is only on the extensor surface.

Slow reversal is an isotonic contraction (against resistance) of the antagonist followed by an isotonic contraction (against resistance) of the agonist. Slow reversal-hold is the same sequence, with an isometric contraction at the end of the range. For the patient who has difficulty reaching his mouth for oral hygiene because of weakness in the D_1 flexion pattern, the slow reversal procedure is as follows: an isotonic contraction against resistance in D_1 extension with the verbal command, "Push down and out," followed by an isotonic contraction of D_1 flexion against resistance with the verbal command, "Pull up and across." An increase or buildup of power in the agonist should be felt with each successive isotonic contraction.

Rhythmic stabilization is used to increase stability by eliciting simultaneous isometric contractions of antagonistic muscle groups. Cocontraction results if the patient is not allowed to relax. This technique requires repeated isometric contractions, leading to increased circulation or the tendency for the patient to hold his or her breath, or both. Therefore rhythmic stabilization may be contraindicated for patients with cardiac involvement, and no more than three or four repetitions should be done at a time on any patients.

In rhythmic stabilization manual contacts are applied on both agonist and antagonist muscles, with resistance given simultaneously. The patient is asked to hold the contraction against graded resistance. Without allowing the patient to relax, manual contacts are switched to opposite surfaces. Rhythmic stabilization is useful with patients lacking postural control because of ataxia or proximal weakness. Used intermittently during an activity requiring postural stability, such as meal preparation in standing posture, this technique enhances muscle balance, endurance, and control of movement.

Relaxation Techniques

Relaxation techniques are an effective means of increasing ROM, particularly in the presence of pain or spasticity, which may be increased by passive stretch.

Contract-relax involves passive motion to the point of limitation in movement patterns. This is followed by an isotonic contraction of the antagonist pattern against maximal resistance, with only the rotational component of the diagonal movement allowed. This action is followed by relaxation, then by further passive movement into the agonistic pattern (e.g., contract-relax could involve passive motion to the point of limitation in D_2 flexion, which would be followed by an isotonic contraction of D_2 extension, then by further passive movement into D_2 flexion). This procedure is repeated at each point in the ROM in which limitation is felt to occur.[22] Contract-relax is used when no active range in the agonistic pattern is present. However, the ultimate goal is active movement through the full range. Therefore once relaxation and increased ROM occur, active movement should be facilitated.

Hold-relax is performed in the same sequence as contract-relax but involves an isometric contraction (no movement allowed) of the antagonist, followed by relaxation and then active movement into the agonistic pattern. Because this technique involves an isometric contraction against resistance, it is particularly beneficial in the presence of pain or acute orthopedic conditions. For the patient with reflex sympathetic dystrophy (RSD) who has pain with shoulder flexion, abduction, and external rotation, the therapist asks the patient to hold against resistance in the D_2 extension pattern, then to initiate active movement into the D_2 flexion pattern. This technique is beneficial for the patient with RSD

during self-care activities such as shampooing hair and zipping a shirt in back.

Slow reversal-hold-relax begins with an isotonic contraction, followed by an isometric contraction, relaxation of the antagonistic pattern, and then by active movement of the agonistic pattern. When the patient has the ability to move the agonist actively, the technique is preferred. For example, to increase active elbow extension in the presence of tight elbow flexors, the therapist asks the patient to perform D_1 flexion with elbow flexion as resistance is applied. When the ROM is complete, the patient is asked to hold with an isometric contraction, followed immediately by relaxation. When relaxation is felt, the patient moves actively into D_1 extension with elbow extension. This technique helps increase elbow extension for such activities as reaching to lock the wheelchair brakes or picking up an object off the floor.

Rhythmic rotation is effective in decreasing spasticity and increasing ROM. The therapist passively moves the body part in the desired pattern. When tightness or restriction of movement is felt, the therapist rotates the body part slowly and rhythmically in both directions. After relaxation is felt, the therapist continues to move the body part into the newly available range. This technique is effective in preparing the paraplegic patient with LE spasticity or clonus to put on a pair of pants. The technique is also effective in preparing for splint fabrication on a spastic extremity.

SUMMARY

The PNF approach emphasizes the patient's abilities and potential so that strengths assist weaker components. Strengths and deficiencies are assessed and addressed in treatment within total patterns of movement and posture. A battery of techniques is superimposed on these total patterns to enhance motor response and facilitate motor learning.

PNF uses multisensory input. The coordination and timing of sensory input are important in eliciting the desired response from the patient. The patient's performance should be monitored, and sensory input should be adjusted accordingly.

To use PNF effectively, the therapist must understand the developmental sequence and the components of normal movement. The therapist must learn the diagonal patterns and how they are used in ADL, must know when and how to use the techniques of facilitation and relaxation, and must be able to apply patterns and techniques of facilitation to OT evaluation and treatment. Attaining these skills requires observation and practice under the supervision of a therapist experienced in the PNF approach.

CASE STUDY 35-1

CASE STUDY

A 50-year-old woman was referred for OT services with a right cerebrovascular accident (CVA) resulting in left hemiplegia. Before the CVA she had a history of hypertension but otherwise good health. Referral to OT was made 10 days after onset of CVA for evaluation and treatment in ADL, visual perceptual skills, and left UE function.

Assessment

An initial assessment revealed intact vital and related functions, such as oral and facial musculature and swallowing. Voice production was good. The patient had a tendency to hold her breath during activities, and subsequent decreased endurance was noted. Visual tracking was impaired, with an inability to scan past midline and apparent left-side neglect.

The head and neck were observed to be frequently rotated to the right and slightly flexed because of weak extensors. The trunk was noted to be asymmetric in sitting posture, with most of the weight supported on the right side. The patient's posture was flexed because of weak extensors. Static sitting balance was fair and dynamic sitting balance was poor with the patient listing forward and left.

The patient's right arm was normal in sensation and strength, although motor planning was impaired. The left arm was essentially flaccid, with impaired sensation of light touch, pain, and proprioception. The patient complained of mild glenohumeral pain during passive movement at the end ranges of shoulder abduction and flexion. Scapular instability was noted. No active movement could be elicited in the left arm.

Perceptual testing showed apraxia (especially during activities requiring crossing of midline) and left-side neglect. The patient was alert and oriented, with good attention span and memory. Carryover in tasks was adequate.

The patient needed moderate assistance in ADL and moderate to maximum assistance with transfers. Impaired balance and apraxia were the most limiting factors in performance of ADL.

Treatment implementation

Following the cervicocaudal direction of development, alignment of the head and neck was the appropriate starting point for treatment. Left-side awareness, sitting posture, and trunk balance were directly influenced by the position of the head and neck. Before the start of self-care activities, the patient performed head and neck patterns of flexion and extension with rotation. To reinforce rotation to left, the therapist was positioned to the left of the patient. Clothing and hygiene articles also were placed to the left of the patient.

A lack of trunk control was another problem. During bending activities, the patient reported a fear of falling and was unsure of her ability to return to the upright position. Consequently, the patient had difficulty leaning forward to transfer from wheelchair. Slow reversal-hold technique was used to reinforce trunk patterns during ADL. For example, as the patient prepared to don her left pant leg, the therapist was positioned in front and to the left of the patient. Manual contacts were on the anterior aspect of either scapula. The therapist moved with the patient and applied resistance as the patient leaned forward to don her

pants. At the end of the range, the patient was instructed to hold with isometric contraction. After the pants were donned, manual contacts were switched to the posterior surface of either scapula. Resistance was applied as the patient returned to the upright position. The verbal command was, "Look up and over your right shoulder." When the patient was upright, she was again instructed to hold with isometric contraction. In addition to reinforcing trunk control, this technique alleviated the patient's fear of leaning forward, because the therapist was in continual contact with the patient.

An indirect benefit of the flexion and extension patterns of the head, neck, and trunk was the reinforcement of respiration. The patient was encouraged to inhale during extension and exhale during flexion. This approach eliminated the patient's tendency to hold her breath.

Treatment consisted of total patterns and techniques to facilitate proximal stability in the left UE and to provide proprioceptive input. Weight-bearing activities were selected because no active movement was available in the left arm. The patient used the right UE in diagonal patterns to perform perceptual tasks such as a mosaic tile design, paper and pencil activities, and board games. These activities were performed to include the side-lying posture on the left elbow, the prone posture on elbows, the side-sitting posture with weight on the left arm, and on all fours. To reinforce stability at the shoulder girdle, approximation and rhythmic stabilization were used with manual contacts at both shoulders and then at the shoulder and pelvis. The performance of perceptual tasks in diagonals improved the patient's motor planning, left-side awareness, and trunk rotation.

The patient was instructed in bilateral asymmetrical chopping and lifting patterns to support the scapula and left UE in rolling and other activities. These patterns also enhanced left-side awareness and trunk rotation. To facilitate scapular movement during chop and lift patterns, the therapist applied stretch to initiate movement, followed by slow reversal technique. In preparation for the lift pattern, manual contacts were placed on the posterior surface of the scapula. Stretch was applied in lengthened range. As the patient initiated the lifting pattern, resistance was given and maintained throughout the ROM. This procedure was repeated for antagonistic or reverse of lift pattern, with manual contacts switching to the anterior surface of the scapula.

About 3 to 4 weeks after the injury the patient was able to initiate left UE movement in synergy with predominance of flexor tone. Weight-bearing activities and rhythmic rotation were helpful in normalizing tone, and both techniques were used with ADL such as dressing and bathing. Wrist and finger extensions were facilitated in the D_1 extension and D_2 flexion patterns using repeated contractions.

Outcomes

Reevaluation after 5 weeks of OT revealed increased endurance and ability to coordinate breathing with activity, and consistency in crossing midline during visual scanning activities. The patient was able to turn her head and neck to the left without cues from the therapist. The fear of falling forward with bending had diminished, and the patient automatically turned her head to look up and over her shoulder to reinforce assumption of the upright position. As trunk strength continued to improve, reinforcement with head and neck rotation was no longer necessary. Visual tracking alone, in the direction of movement, was sufficient to reinforce assumption of the upright position. Eventually the patient was able to obtain an upright position without apparent visual or head and neck reinforcement. Sitting balance improved with bilat-

eral weight-bearing through both hips. Shoulder pain decreased and scapular stability improved during weight-bearing activities. The patient initiated left UE movement out of flexor synergy pattern. Right UE motor planning was within functional limits for ADL. Transfers and self-care required only minimal assistance, and cues were no longer needed for left UE awareness.

REVIEW QUESTIONS

1. Give examples of how the TNR and the ATNR reinforce motor performance.
2. Is rolling from prone to supine a flexor- or extensor-dominant activity?
3. In the presence of pain, what tone of voice should be used when giving verbal commands?
4. Discuss the significance of auditory, visual, and tactile input in motor learning.
5. Which UE diagonal pattern is used for the hand-to-mouth phase of eating? For zipping front-opening pants?
6. Discuss the advantages of using the chop and lift patterns.
7. Which trunk pattern is used when donning a left sock?
8. List three advantages of using the diagonal patterns.
9. What is the developmental sequence of total patterns?
10. If a patient needs more stability, which of the following total patterns should be chosen: side-lying or prone posture on elbows?
11. Which PNF technique facilitates postural control and cocontraction?
12. Discuss the neurophysiological principles of Sherrington upon which the PNF techniques of facilitation are based.
13. What is an effective technique to prepare the patient with UE flexor spasticity to don a shirt?
14. Define *maximal resistance*.
15. Name two PNF techniques that facilitate initiation of movement.

REFERENCES

1. Abreu BF, Toglia JP: Cognitive rehabilitation: a model for occupational therapy, *Am J Occup Ther* 41(7):439-448, 1987.
2. Affolter F: Perceptual processes as prerequisites for complex human behavior, *Int Rehabil Med* 3(1):3-10, 1981.
3. Ayres JA: Proprioceptive neuromuscular facilitation elicited through the upper extremities. I. Background, *Am J Occup Ther* 9(1):1. II. Application, *Am J Occup Ther* 9(2):57. III. Specific application to occupational therapy, *Am J Occup Ther* 9(3):121, 1955.
4. Buchwald JS: Exteroceptive reflexes and movement, *Am J Phys Med* 46(1):121-128, 1967.
5. Carroll J: The utilization of reinforcement techniques in the program for the hemiplegic, *Am J Occup Ther* 4(5):211, 1950.
6. Cooke DM: The effects of resistance on multiple sclerosis patients with intention tremor, *Am J Occup Ther* 12(2):89, 1958.
7. Farber SD: *Neurorehabilitation: a multisensory approach*, Philadelphia, 1982, WB Saunders.
8. Hagbarth KE: Excitatory and inhibitory skin areas for flexor and extensor mononeurons, *Acta Physiol Scand* 26(suppl 94):1, 1952.
9. Hellebrandt FA: Physiology. In Delorme TL, Watkins AL: *Progressive resistance exercise*, New York, 1951, Appleton, Century, & Crofts.
10. Hellebrandt FA, Schade M, Carns ML: Methods of evoking the tonic neck reflexes in normal human subjects, *Am J Phys Med* 4(90):139, 1962.
11. Humphrey TL, Huddleston OL: Applying facilitation techniques to self care training, *Phys Ther Rev* 38(9):605, 1958.
12. Jackson JH: *Selected writings*, vol 1, London, 1931, Hodder & Staughton (edited by J Taylor).
13. Kabat H, Rosenberg D: Concepts and techniques of occupational therapy for neuromuscular disorders, *Am J Occup Ther* 4(1):6, 1950.
14. Loomis JE, Boersma FJ: Training right brain damaged patients in a wheelchair task: case studies using verbal mediation, *Physiother Can* 34(4):204, 1982.
15. Myers BJ: Proprioceptive neuromuscular facilitation: concepts and application in occupational therapy as taught by Voss. Notes from course at Rehabilitation Institute of Chicago, September 8-12, 1980.
16. Myers BJ: *Assisting to postures and application in occupational therapy activities*, Chicago, Rehabilitation Institute of Chicago, 1981 (videotape).
17. Myers BJ: *PNF: patterns and application in occupational therapy*, Chicago, Rehabilitation Institute of Chicago, 1981 (videotape).
18. Sherrington C: *The integrative action of the nervous system*, New Haven, Conn, 1961, Yale University Press.
19. Voss DE: Application of patterns and techniques in occupational therapy, *Am J Occup Ther* 8(4):191, 1959.
20. Voss DE: Proprioceptive neuromuscular facilitation, *Am J Phys Med* 46(1):838-899, 1967.
21. Voss DE: Proprioceptive neuromuscular facilitation: the PNF method. In Pearson PH, Williams CE, editors: *Physical therapy services in the developmental disabilities*, Springfield, Ill, 1972, Charles C Thomas.
22. Voss DE, Ionta MK, Myers BJ: *Proprioceptive neuromuscular facilitation*, ed 3, Philadelphia, 1985, Harper & Row.
23. Whitaker EW: A suggested treatment in occupational therapy for patients with multiple sclerosis, *Am J Occup Ther* 4(6):247, 1950.

CHAPTER 36

Neurodevelopmental Treatment: The Bobath Approach

JAN ZARET DAVIS

KEY TERMS

Neurodevelopmental treatment
Symmetry
Mixed tone
Weight bearing
Associated movement
Associated reactions
Inhibition
Facilitation
Key points of control
Trunk rotation
Subluxation

LEARNING OBJECTIVES

After studying this chapter the student or clinician will be able to do the following:

1. State the primary goal of the neurodevelopmental treatment (NDT) approach.
2. List the advantages of the NDT approach.
3. Describe the typical hemiplegic posture.
4. List the key elements of the NDT assessment.
5. List factors that can increase spasticity.
6. Describe the elements of a vicious circle that can contribute to the maintenance of spasticity.
7. List possible causes of asymmetrical shoulder height seen in patients with hemiplegia.
8. Describe treatment methods designed to normalize tone.
9. List the purposes of trunk rotation and bilateral activities.
10. Describe bed positioning for the patient with hemiplegia.
11. Discuss how the affected upper extremity (UE) can be incorporated into activity.
12. Discuss why real life activities, rather than simulated or contrived activities, are advantageous in the treatment program.
13. Perform and teach methods of dressing described in this chapter.
14. Discuss the importance of scapula protraction in positioning and movement of the hemiplegic arm.
15. List possible causes of shoulder subluxation.
16. Discuss the treatment of subluxation recommended in the NDT approach.
17. List the problems with use of the hemiplegic sling.
18. Describe the role of the occupational therapist in preparing the patient to go home.

The ultimate goal of occupational therapy (OT) for the patient with hemiplegia is to regain as much independence as possible, under safe conditions, regardless of the therapy setting or length of treatment. A foundation of treatment should be established that allows the patient to make positive changes beyond the time limitations of therapy. Changes often occur for many months or even years after a cerebrovascular accident (CVA). Working within the confines of the current health care system, most therapists will not have the opportunity to follow a patient throughout the recovery process. The limitations of a therapist's time with the patient should not dictate the theme of the treatment program.

Occupational therapists want to establish a program that facilitates optimal learning and promotes recovery. **Neurodevelopmental treatment (NDT)** provides a sound foundation for such a program. First developed in the 1940s by Berta Bobath, a physical therapist, and her husband, Dr. Karel Bobath,[2] NDT is based on normal development and movement. The term *neurodevelopmental treatment* was coined by the Bobaths from their work with children with cerebral palsy. Also known as the Bobath approach, NDT has been used successfully in the treatment of adult hemiplegia.

During recovery a patient typically overuses the uninvolved side, compensating for the loss of sensory and motor function on the hemiplegic side. Resulting problems in posture, alignment, balance, strength, tone, and coordination often lead to less effective patterns of movement and may eventually cause orthopedic problems, pain, or decreased safety. If patients are trained only in the use of adaptive equipment, compensatory movement is reinforced and the potential for obtaining the highest level of function is hindered.

In NDT the therapist develops a program to help the patient avoid these abnormal patterns of movement. The program provides a foundation that promotes the highest level of functional recovery based on relearning normal movement rather than on compensation. NDT techniques are intended for more than just the movements of an arm or leg. The client is encouraged to use both sides of the body. One of the central principles of NDT is that alignment and **symmetry** of the trunk and pelvis are necessary for good alignment and symmetry of the extremities. Adaptive equipment is used when absolutely necessary for safety, but not as a first resort and not as a replacement for treatment.

With good handling and treatment skills the occupational therapist can facilitate positive changes for the patient with hemiplegia at any stage of recovery. It is important to know what to avoid in treatment, as well as what to promote and facilitate. Therapists must become efficient in problem-solving and prioritizing patient needs to design an effective treatment program

that will best serve the needs of the patient throughout recovery.

TYPICAL PROBLEMS OF HEMIPLEGIA
Motor Problems

The major motor problem in hemiplegia is the lack of postural control affecting voluntary movement. Flaccidity is most common at the onset of a CVA. During this time the patient is often passive, displaying low endurance and low tolerance to activity. This condition may last a few days or as long as several months. Although the patient does not display movement in the affected extremities at this time, a proper treatment program can have a strong impact on the eventual functional outcome.[2]

After the flaccid stage, patients enter a stage of **mixed tone,** displaying a combination of flaccidity and spasticity. For example, the upper extremity (UE) may have an increase in tone proximally (scapular retraction, depression or downward rotation, internal rotation of the humerus) but a decrease in tone distally (at the wrist, hand, or fingers). During the mixed-tone phase, trauma to the shoulder is common. If treatment does not address the problems of high tone at this stage, the patient progresses to the next stage.

Spasticity is the most commonly identified problem and the most difficult motor problem to treat after a CVA. If not treated correctly, spasticity can progress until independent living is nearly impossible. Spasticity interferes with the patient's selective motor function. It produces abnormal sensory feedback and contributes to weakness of the antagonist muscles. It can cause contractures, pain, and an all-consuming fear in many patients. Fear, pain, and spasticity are often so intertwined that they cause a vicious circle. The spasticity causes an increase in pain, which causes an increase in fear, which in turn increases the amount of spasticity.[5]

If measures are taken to reduce pain and fear, the therapist has a much better chance for success with the methods used to reduce spasticity. Other factors that may influence the amount of spasticity are emotional stress, physical effort (on the hemiplegic side or the unaffected side), temperature, and the rate at which an activity is performed.

The typical posture in the adult patient with hemiplegia (Fig. 36-1) can be described as follows:

Head: Lateral flexion toward the involved side with rotation away from the involved side

UE: A combination of the strongest components of the flexion and extension synergies
  1. Scapula—depression, retraction
  2. Shoulder—adduction, internal rotation
  3. Elbow—flexion
  4. Forearm—pronation
  5. Wrist—flexion, ulnar deviation
  6. Fingers—flexion

Trunk: Lateral flexion toward the involved side (trunk shortening)

Lower extremity: Typical posture in adult with hemiplegia is the extension synergy

1. Pelvis—posterior elevation, retraction
2. Hip—internal rotation, adduction, extension
3. Knee—extension
4. Ankle—plantar flexion, supination, inversion
5. Toes—flexion

Additional Problems

In addition to motor problems, patients often have many problems that can be debilitating either alone or in combination. The following are some of the most common problems.

Weight bearing

Most patients avoid **weight bearing** on the affected side of the body. Instead of the weight being equally distributed over both hips (in sitting) or over both feet (in standing), it is usually shifted to the nonhemiplegic

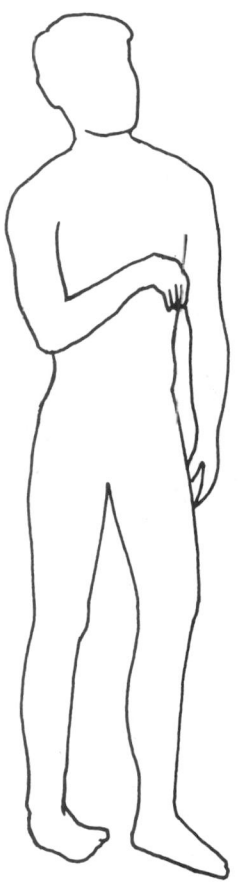

FIG. 36-1
Typical posture of adult with hemiplegia in standing position. (Courtesy of Graphic Arts Department, Harmarville Rehabilitation Center, Pittsburgh, Pa.)

side. Many factors make weight-bearing difficult over the weak side. Loss of sensation, loss of strength, and fear of falling contribute to this problem.

Fear

Fear may be the most debilitating factor for many patients. Fear magnifies other problems that cause the patient to be dependent rather than independent. Fear can be caused by loss of sensation, poor balance reactions, lack of protective extension (i.e., fear of falling), and perceptual or cognitive problems. Fear is a major factor influencing spasticity.[5]

Sensory Loss

Sensory loss may include loss of stereognosis, kinesthetic awareness, light touch, and pressure. A patient's extremity may remain useless because of sensory loss even though there is good motor control.[2,5]

Neglect

Unilateral neglect may be a combination of one or more of the following: sensory loss, perceptual or cognitive dysfunction, or visual field deficit (homonymous hemianopsia). The patient may have good motor recovery but is unable to use it functionally because of the neglect.[1,5]

Many other problems are related to CVA, such as aphasia, apraxia, perceptual motor and cognitive deficits, and psychological dysfunction. These conditions are discussed in Chapters 25 to 28.

ASSESSING THE PATIENT

When the patient is assessed, emphasis is placed on the quality of movement (i.e., the way the patient moves). The therapist observes coordination, changes of tone, and postural reactions rather than looking at specific muscles and joints.[2] The therapist must have knowledge of normal posture and movement, to identify patterns that may be abnormal. Each patient presents a different picture, based upon age, premorbid physical condition, and normal degenerative changes.

Importance of Observation

Good observation skills are the foundation for a good assessment. Therapists must learn to be specific in their observations and in their analysis of these observations. Although certain characteristics are common to most patients with hemiplegia, each patient demonstrates a unique set of problems. Therapists with the most advanced skills see problems that others may miss.

Basic Observation Process

During assessments, patients must be observed from the front, back, and side. Most information about patient symmetry is gained by observing both the hemiplegic and nonhemiplegic sides from head to toe. Observations should be both static and dynamic; the patient should be sitting, standing, or supine in a static position, and the observation should be made while the patient tries to move for dynamic changes in the trunk, head and neck, and both upper extremities.

To assess asymmetry in posture and pelvic and shoulder girdles, the therapist should have the patient in an upright position. If the patient is unable to maintain the sitting posture, the assessment may be performed in a supine position, but observations will be limited. It helps to have the patient's shirt off to detect asymmetries in the trunk, shoulder girdle, and upper extremities. For privacy the therapist may want to perform the assessment in the patient's room. It is also helpful to keep a tank top in the OT department for female patients. Outpatients often wear a bathing suit, halter top, or tank top under their shirts.

A good way to structure observation is to imagine reference lines, as shown in Fig. 36-2, which will help to identify deviations. The first line of reference is vertical at midline (Fig. 36-2, A). The therapist should look for asymmetries by comparing the right and left sides of the patient. Is the head centered in midline? Are the medial borders of both scapulae equidistant from the spine? Is the trunk shifted to one side? Next the therapist visualizes a level, horizontal line at the top of the shoulders (Fig. 36-2, B). Is one shoulder higher than the other? Is one shoulder abnormally high or the other abnormally low? The third reference is a level horizontal line at the height of the hips (Fig. 36-2, C). Is one hip higher or lower? Is the patient bearing weight equally over both hips? The therapist also should look for unilateral creases or folds on the trunk (Fig. 36-2, D), that might indicate additional problem areas.

Observations of asymmetry do not necessarily indicate what the problem is; asymmetry indicates only that there is a problem. To understand the cause of the problem, the therapist continues the assessment. The therapist should never assume the obvious. The detective work begins as the pieces of the puzzle come together. In problem solving, information from observations is combined with information about the medical history and premorbid conditions and, most important, the handling by the therapist.

To identify the underlying cause when asymmetries are noted, the therapist takes the affected limb through passive range of motion (PROM). It is important for the therapist to move the UE within normal patterns of movement and in normal alignment to avoid orthopedic problems (e.g., microtearing of structures or soft-tissue impingement). Any pain or discomfort on movement should be noted, and the limb should not be moved past the point of pain or discomfort. If able, the patient should be asked to describe the pain (e.g., stabbing, aching, dull, or pulling) and show its specific loca-

Observation Guide

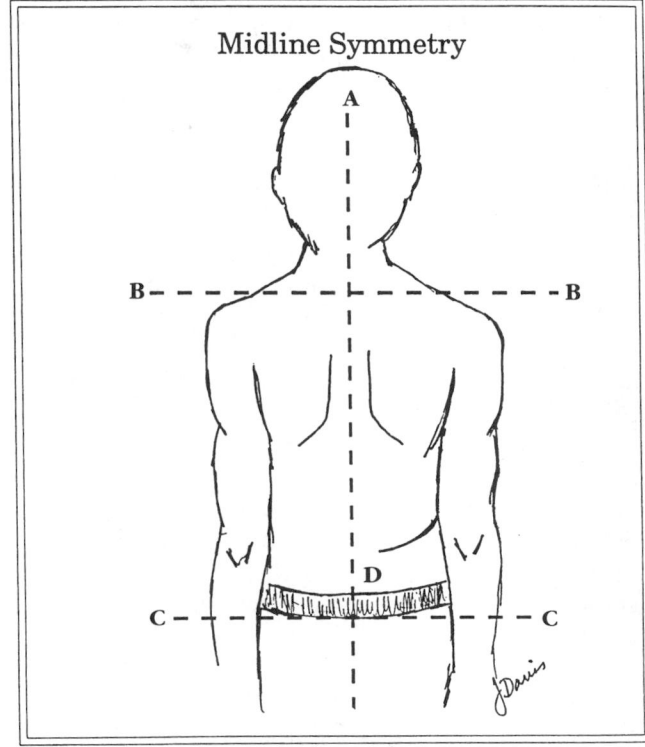

FIG. 36-2
Observation guide. (Courtesy of International Clinical Educators, Inc, 1993.)

tion. This information will help the therapist determine the cause of the pain.

As the patient is passively moved, the therapist feels deviations from normal. If resistance is felt, the patient probably has abnormally high tone. It is important to take the limb slowly through ROM to prevent a quick stretch followed by clonus, which increases the problem of high tone. If no resistance is felt but the arm feels heavy, the patient probably has abnormally low tone.

For the dynamic assessment the therapist observes any movement initiated by the patient on the weak side. As the patient attempts to move the weak side, sometimes the strong side attempts to make the same movements. The effect, called **associated movement**, is normal. Everyone has associated movements at one time or another. These movements are most commonly identified in children; for example, when cutting with scissors, the child's tongue protrudes. The patient may use compensatory movements or movements influenced by abnormal synergy patterns. These abnormal patterns of movement, called **associated reactions**, can be caused by excessive effort on the sound side that "overflows" to the weak side or by excessive effort on the weak side, which causes a synergy pattern. Associated reactions are abnormal and should be discouraged or inhibited.[6]

By comparing the patient's movement pattern with the normal pattern, the therapist can identify problem areas interfering with normal movement. For example, when the patient with a hemiplegic arm reaches for an object, the shoulder elevates and retracts, the elbow maintains a flexed position, and the forearm is in partial pronation with wrist and finger flexion; the trunk flexes forward to position the hand nearer the object (Fig. 36-3). In comparison, in a normal pattern of movement trunk stability with scapular protraction, selective elbow extension with pronation, wrist extension, and finger flexion might be displayed (Fig. 36-4). The therapist must thoroughly understand the components of normal movement to compare it with abnormal movement for assessment. Table 36-1 lists a few common problems observed during static assessment, along with their possible causes.

Integrating Assessment and Treatment

When the therapist observes the patient both statically and dynamically, the information collected is followed by the identification of specific problem areas. Next the therapist determines what to do in treatment. According to Bobath, "Every evaluation is a treatment and every treatment is an evaluation."[2]

The primary goal of NDT is to relearn normal movements. The methods used are intended to treat the person as a whole, encouraging the use of both sides of the body. The patient makes less use of adaptive equipment (e.g., slings, braces, and canes) and is more able to move about freely with more normal muscle tone.[2] This approach creates a better atmosphere for the psychosocial adjustment to family life and everyday living. The more normal a person appears to others, with less deformity from spasticity, the better he or she is accepted.

Fluctuations in Tone

Under stressful conditions anyone's muscle tone might be higher; for example, muscle tension increases when a person is presenting a paper in front of the class for the

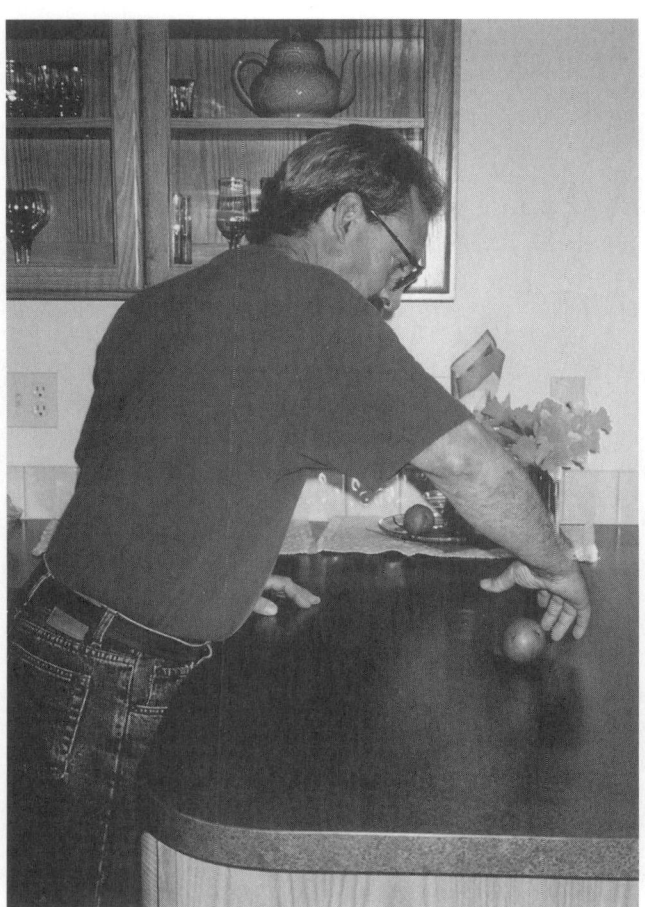

FIG. 36-3
Patient reaching forward using abnormal movement patterns.

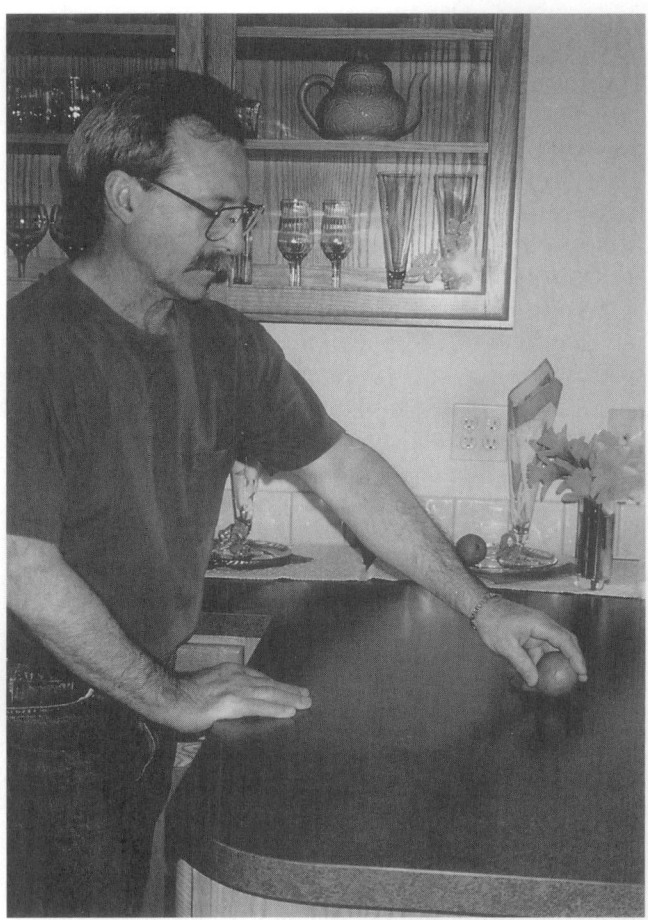

FIG. 36-4
Patient using normal movement patterns while reaching forward with the uninvolved side.

TABLE 36-1
Observations and Possible Causes

STRUCTURED OBSERVATION (STATIC)		
Area Observed	Observation	Possible Causes of Problem*
Head	Lateral flexion to affected side	Shortened upper trapezius Poor head righting Midline orientation deficit
Shoulder	Hemiplegic shoulder lower	Weak trunk with lateral flexion to the hemiplegic side Low tone in shoulder girdle with arm hanging to the side Increased tone in depression and downward rotation of the scapula
	Unaffected shoulder higher	Bracing or holding with strong side caused by poor sitting balance, weak trunk control, or fear
Scapular position	Downward rotation of scapula	Increased tone of muscles acting on scapular downward rotation (rhomboids, levator scapulae, serratus anterior) Decreased tone of stabilizing muscles of the scapula allowing it to fall into downward rotation
	Winging of the scapula	Weakness of serratus anterior Increased tone of the subscapularis pulling the scapula and causing it to wing
Trunk	Unilateral crease on affected side	Lateral flexion of trunk caused by weak abdominals or increased tone in scapular retraction and depression with pelvic retraction and elevation causing shortening on the hemiplegic side

*These are some examples. A problem may have one or more causes.

first time. Conversely, tone may be lower during relaxing experiences such as after a big lunch or when the instructor turns down the lights for a slide presentation. Patients with a neurological insult, on the other hand, demonstrate abnormally high tone and abnormally low tone. It is the therapist's job to determine where the patient displays abnormally high or low tone and then to implement a treatment program designed to normalize tone. Decreasing abnormally high tone is called **inhibition;** increasing abnormally low tone is called **facilitation.**

The points of contact or hand placement of the therapist that are most effective in regulating tone are called **key points of control.** Proximal key points are the shoulder and pelvic girdles, helpful with more gross patterns of movement. Distal key points of control are the hand, thumb, or foot. These can be helpful for more refined movement patterns. Abnormal patterns (synergies) must be suppressed or inhibited before normal, selective isolated movement can take place. It is impossible to superimpose normal movement on abnormal tone.[2] Muscle tone may be normalized by using one or more of the following techniques[2,5,7]:

1. Weight bearing over the affected side
2. Trunk rotation
3. Scapular protraction
4. Positioning of the pelvis forward toward an anterior pelvic tilt

5. Facilitation of slow, controlled movements
6. Proper positioning

These six techniques, discussed in the paragraphs that follow, provide the foundation for treatment of the adult patient with hemiplegia using the Bobath (NDT) approach. The techniques are most effective and provide the best potential in rehabilitation when they are started in the acute phase but can be useful in any phase of the treatment program.

NEURODEVELOPMENTAL TREATMENT
Weight Bearing Over Affected Side

Weight bearing over the hemiplegic side is the most effective way of helping to regulate tone, or bring the muscle tone into a more normal range. With patients displaying low tone it is facilitative, and with patients displaying high tone it can be inhibitory. Weight bearing not only helps to regulate tone, but also provides sensory input to the hemiplegic side through proprioception. Additionally this approach improves the patient's awareness of that side and helps to decrease neglect. As the awareness of the weak side improves, the patient is often less fearful, thus establishing a better foundation for the recovery process.

The positive effects of weight bearing can be observed in nearly every stage of recovery. Correct weight bearing can be as simple as positioning the patient in a side-lying position on the hemiplegic side in bed or as difficult as the facilitation of stance phase in gait training. When weight bearing is introduced early, the benefits can be seen throughout the rehabilitation program. The patient should be taught to bear weight equally through both hips in sitting and through both feet in standing.

Weight bearing through the UE in sitting or standing can help to regulate tone throughout the UE. This is most effective with patients displaying a flexion synergy of the UE. The patient can be brought into a weight-bearing position before or during treatment in functional daily living tasks.

Before the patient begins weight bearing through the UE, the UE and shoulder girdle must be prepared. The therapist must make sure the scapula is gliding in forward protraction, elevation, and upward rotation. After mobilization of the scapula the patient's hand should be placed on the mat or bench several inches from the hip; if the hand is placed next to the hip, extreme hyperextension of the wrist may occur. The humerus is in external rotation with the elbow in extension. As the patient shifts weight over the hemiplegic side, the therapist should be careful not to allow internal rotation of the upper arm and not to allow the elbow to collapse. Weight bearing is not allowed if the patient complains of pain or if the hand is edematous. The patient should not be allowed to hang on the arm in weight bearing, but instead should move the body over the arm to regulate tone without putting undue stress on the joint (Fig. 36-5).

When the therapist facilitates weight bearing during functional activities, he or she normally allows the patient's elbow to bend slightly. The best rule of thumb is to check the position usually assumed by nondisabled persons for the activity and then see if the patient's position is similar.

Trunk Rotation

Trunk rotation, or dissociation of the upper and lower trunk, is another very effective way of regulating tone and facilitating normal movement throughout the upper and lower extremities. Patients with hemiplegia often move in a block-like pattern, with little separation of the shoulder girdle and pelvic girdle. To facilitate normal movement the therapist should set up activities to stimulate or facilitate trunk rotation, which activates trunk musculature and aids in trunk stability. Without stabilization of the trunk the patient will be unable to use the upper extremities effectively.

When facilitating trunk rotation in sitting or standing the therapist should vary the height of the task. This approach not only helps to incorporate the rotational components of movement, but also mobilizes the shoulder girdle and pelvic girdle and improves weight

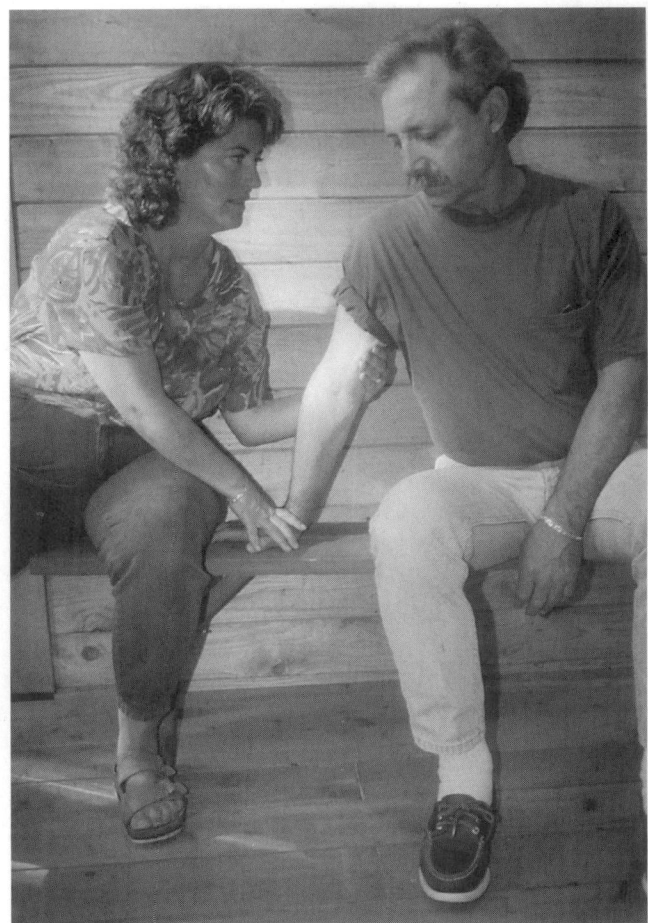

FIG. 36-5
Proper position for weight bearing over hemiplegic side.

shift to the hemiplegic side. Additional benefits from activities facilitating trunk rotation include increased sensory input to the hemiplegic side, improved awareness of the hemiplegic side, and trained compensation for visual field deficit (Figs. 36-6 to 36-8). It is easiest and most effective to facilitate trunk rotation during functional daily activities.

Scapular Protraction

Scapular protraction benefits patients who display a flexion synergy of the UE. High tone involving finger flexion, wrist flexion, or elbow flexion with either supination or pronation of the forearm can be difficult to inhibit. The therapist must remember the basic principle of treatment and work from proximal to distal; before trying to pry open clenched fingers the therapist first brings the scapula forward into protraction and does not pull on the arm. Instead, the arm is gently cradled while the therapist's other hand is placed along the medial border of the scapula and the scapula is brought forward. Once the scapula is forward, the posi-

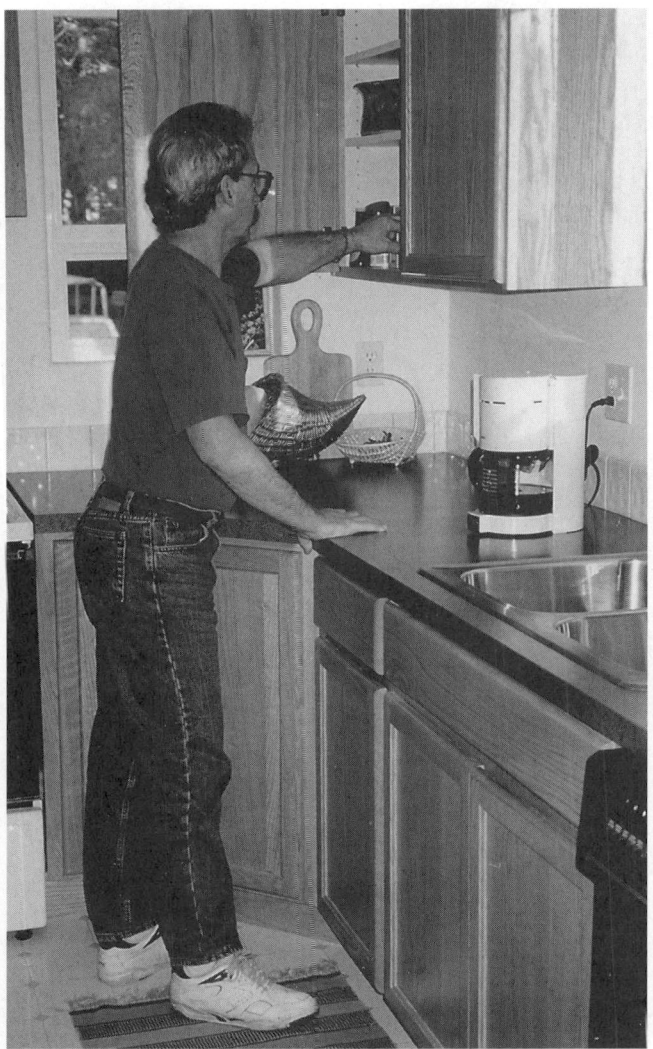

FIG. 36-6
Trunk rotation, side to side, to a high surface.

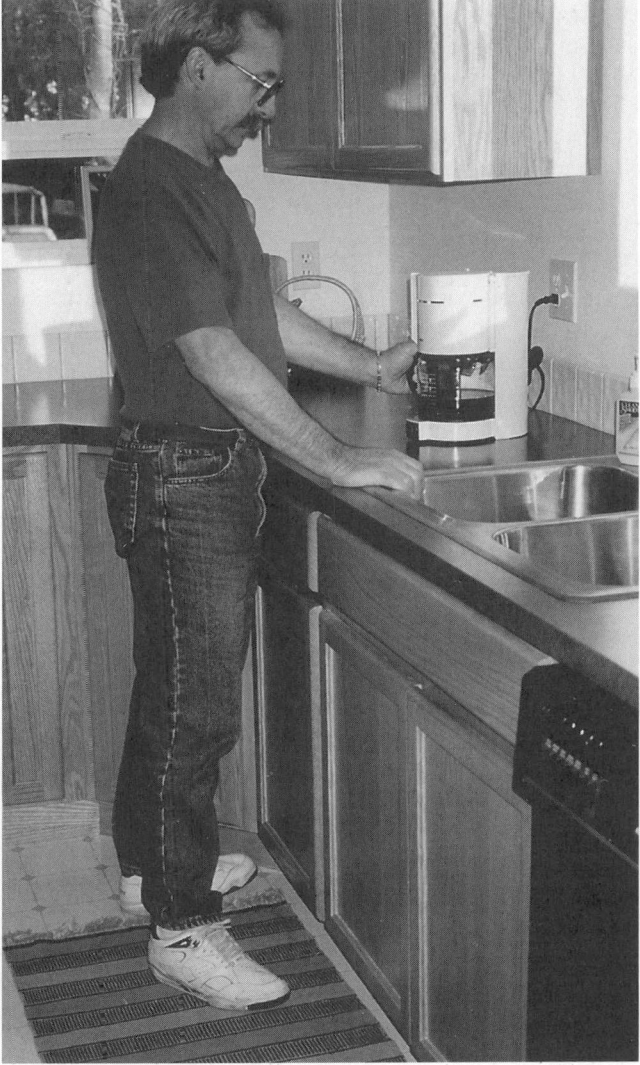

FIG. 36-7
Trunk rotation, side to side, to counter height.

tion should be maintained for a few seconds before the arm is returned to the starting position. The therapist must remember never to force the arm into scapular retraction.

Positioning Pelvis Forward

The neutral position of the pelvis is the preferred sitting position for patients with hemiplegia. Patients are often seen in the posterior pelvic tilt position, and these patients look as if they are sliding out of the wheelchair. Sitting in this position encourages abnormal posture, resulting in increased hip extension (often associated with extension synergy of the lower extremity) and rounding of the upper thoracic region (kyphosis), with resultant head and neck extension. This posture has an adverse affect on swallowing (see Chapter 40), impedes normal and proper alignment of the scapula and

humerus, and encourages flexion synergy of the UE. If the pelvis is brought forward into a more neutral position, proper alignment of the pelvis, shoulder, and head position in sitting can be attained.

In addition to facilitating the pelvis into a more forward position, the therapist can bring the patient forward to help inhibit extensor tone at the hip. The patient should be sitting with both feet flat on the floor. The therapist is on the weak side and helps guide the patient's hands toward the shoes. The benefits of this position are that it (1) inhibits extension synergy of the lower extremity, (2) promotes weight bearing equally through both lower extremities, (3) permits gravity assistance in bringing both scapulae into forward protraction, (4) facilitates thoracic and neck extension for patients who fall forward in a sitting position, and (5) helps to decrease the fear factor for patients fearful of coming forward.

Facilitation of Slow, Controlled Movements

Slow, controlled movements benefit patients with high tone. Patients who move too quickly should be slowed down. Whether they are doing home exercise programs, changing position (e.g., moving from side-lying to sitting or coming from sit to stand), or trying to use the affected UE functionally, quick movements increase tone and tend to set off an associated reaction, resulting in a flexion synergy of the UE. To be most effective in bringing muscle tone within a normal range, the therapist must teach the patient to use slower and more controlled movements. Another basic treatment principle is that the therapist must act as the patient's biofeedback, that is, give feedback appropriate to the patient's response. The patient is told that he or she has done something well if it is so; otherwise, the patient will not learn to distinguish proper movements from compensatory movements.

Proper Positioning

Proper position of the patient in the side-lying, supine, sitting, or standing position facilitates more normal movement throughout the recovery process. Abnormal postures manifested in flexion or extension synergies of the upper or lower extremities promote compensatory movement and should be avoided. Proper positioning in bed is extremely important during the acute stage but is effective at any stage of recovery. In sitting, excessive posterior pelvic tilt, lower extremity external rotation, asymmetry of the trunk and head, and scapular retraction should be avoided. The patient should have the feet flat on the floor, hips near 90° of flexion, knees and ankles at less than 90° of flexion, and trunk extended (thoracic flexion is discouraged). The head should be in midline and the arm fully supported when the patient is working at a table. In standing, the head should be in midline, the trunk symmetrical, and weight equally distributed on both lower extremities.[2]

Incorporating the Upper Extremity Into Activity

The involved UE can be incorporated into functional activities in three ways: weight bearing through the involved UE (Fig. 36-9), bilateral activities, and guiding.

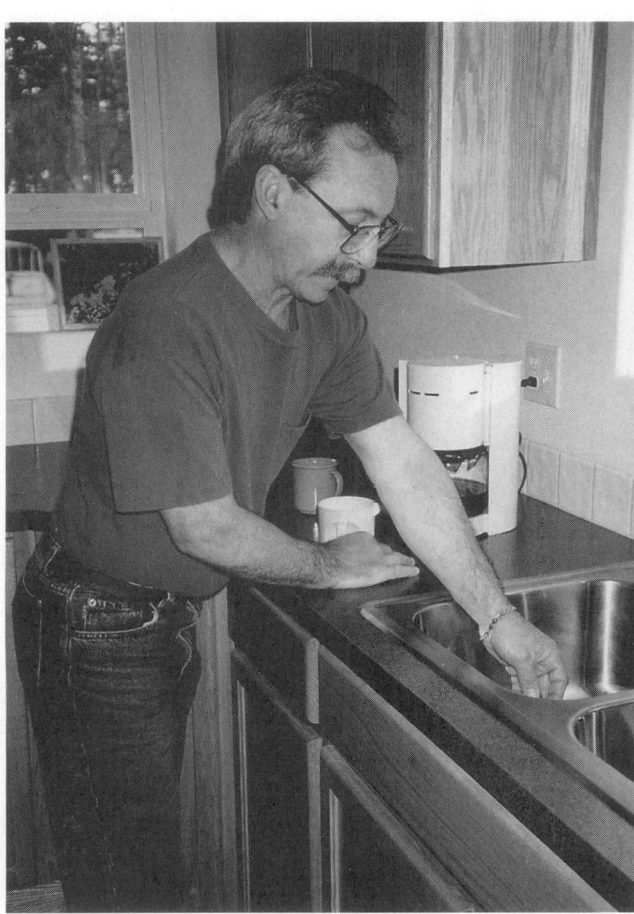

FIG. 36-8
Trunk rotation, side to side, to a lower surface.

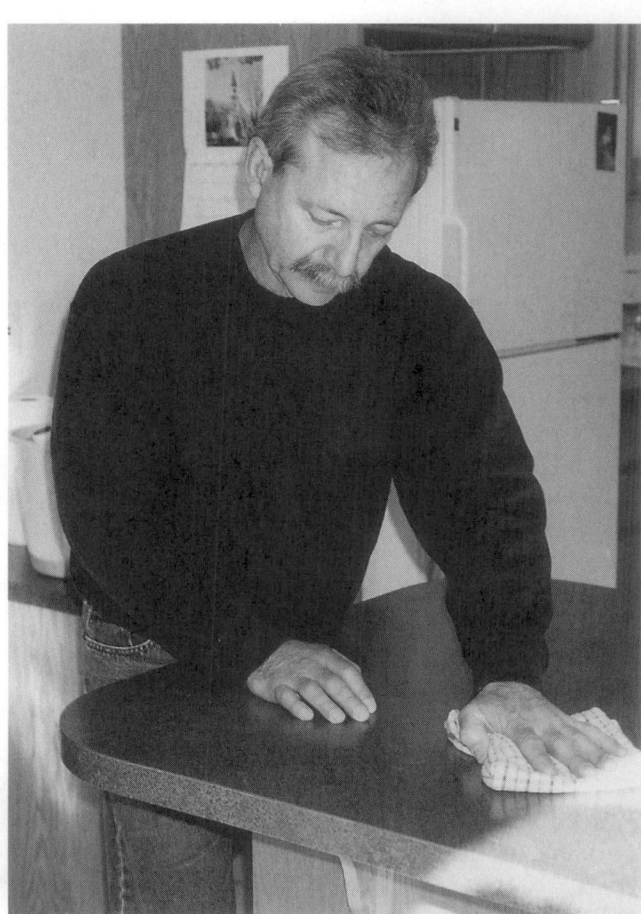

FIG. 36-9
Proper position for weight bearing over hemiplegic side during functional activity.

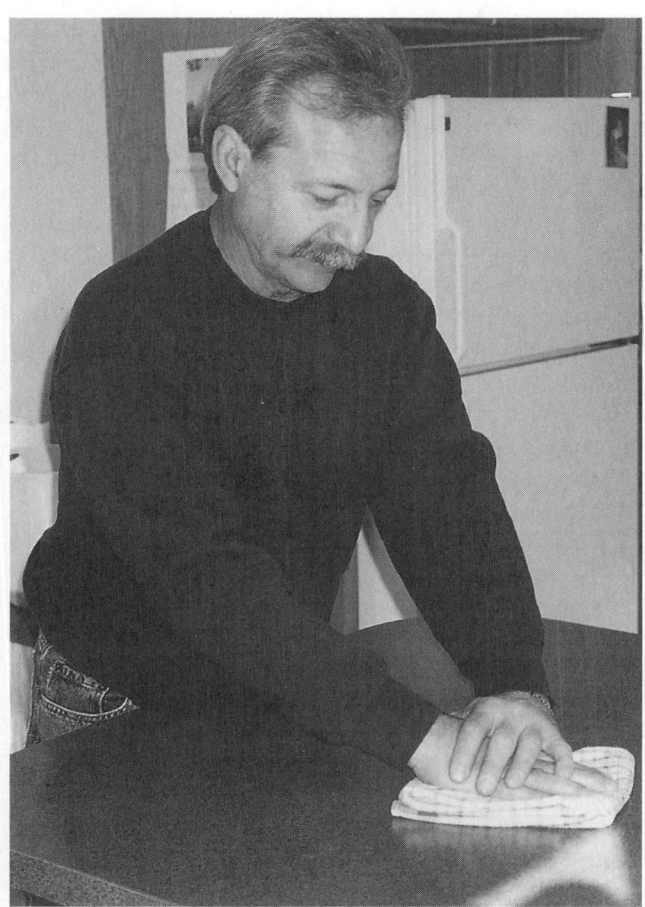

FIG. 36-10
Bilateral use of upper extremity during functional activity.

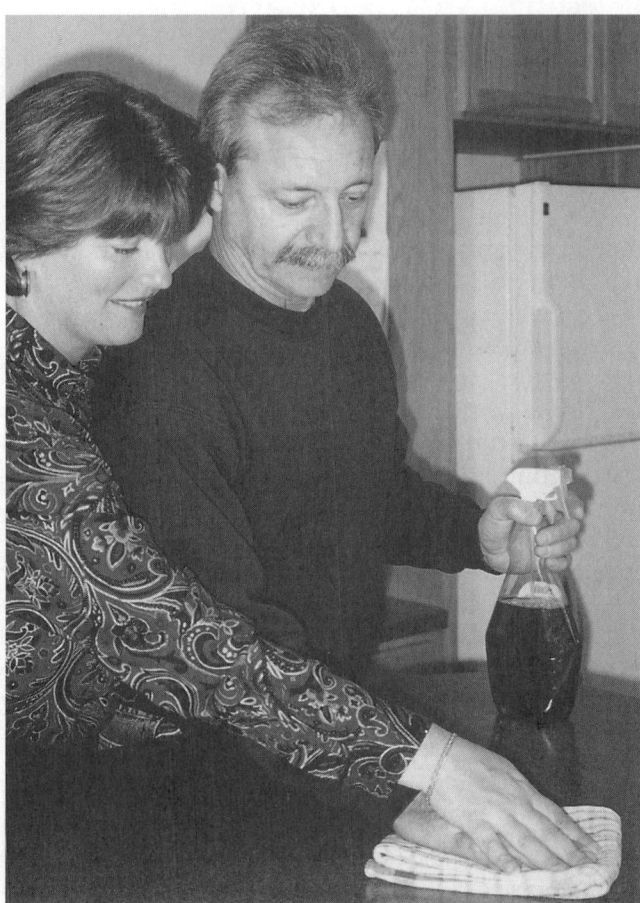

FIG. 36-11
Guiding upper extremity during functional activity.

Weight bearing was discussed previously. Bilateral activities with hands clasped together (Fig. 36-10) are used to do the following:

1. Increase awareness of the hemiplegic side
2. Increase sensory input to the hemiplegic side
3. Bring the affected arm into the visual field
4. Begin purposeful movement of the hemiplegic arm
5. Discourage flexion synergy by protraction of the scapula and extension of the elbow and wrist
6. Develop abduction of fingers and thumb that discourages spasticity of the hand
7. Teach the patient reflex-inhibiting patterns that can be performed without help

To guide the patient's hand (Fig. 36-11) through normal patterns of movement during functional activities, the therapist can place his or her hand over the patient's hand and perform firm but not forceful movements.[6]

Each therapeutic activity can be performed in the sitting or standing position, depending on the patient's level of function. At every possible opportunity the patient should be treated in a straight chair (or standing), rather than the wheelchair, to obtain maximal benefit. During NDT the therapist must advise the patient specifically whether he or she is moving correctly (normally) or incorrectly (abnormally, with compensatory movements). If the patient is unable to move selectively when the therapist asks, the therapist should take the patient through the normal pattern of movement, either during isolated movement or during functional activities and tasks, so that the patient can experience the movement.

NEURODEVELOPMENTAL TREATMENT IN EVERYDAY LIVING

It may be difficult to bridge the gap between facilitation of selective UE control and incorporation of these movements and NDT principles into daily living skills. The patient's inability to function independently is extremely complex, involving much more than just movement and motor control. Problems of perception, cognition, sensation, motor planning, and language can complicate the rehabilitation process, making it especially difficult for the therapist to treat something as specific and refined as motor control.

Selecting a Therapeutic Activity

To incorporate the desired movement into functional activity, the therapist should think of a functional activity that will require or elicit the movement. There are a great number of variations on normal movement. If a patient attempts the task with a movement sequence different from the therapist's, it is important to determine if the sequence is abnormal or just a variation of normal. This task sounds simple, but it is critical to bridging the gap between movement and function.

The best learning experiences come from real life situations that are practical, functional, and familiar.[1] Contrived (simulated) activities are exercises or tasks that have little or no direct relation to real-life situations. Contrived activities weaken the carryover from movement to functional performance. Stacking cones, using parquetry cubes, and tossing beanbags are contrived activities that are often difficult for perceptually disturbed patients to translate into functionally significant tasks. It is much easier for patients to attend to and be motivated by activities that are purposeful and relate to real-life situations. When a patient relates to an activity, more normal movement patterns are displayed, as well as increased attention and endurance.

A primary goal of therapy is independence. A great deal of treatment time is spent practicing skills that do not relate to actual daily tasks or routines. Teaching problem solving allows the patient to transfer and adapt those skills to any situation. In rehabilitation programs therapists must make sure they are teaching problem solving, rather than splinter skills with little if any carryover. Part of the problem-solving process is anticipating problems before they occur. Therapists are often guilty of planning an activity that is contrived or that fixes a problem before the patient has an opportunity to solve it. This approach does not encourage learning and does not promote carryover into functional daily life tasks.

When a functional activity is being selected, the following questions should be asked:
1. Is the activity meaningful to the patient?
2. Does the patient see the purpose of the activity?
3. Does the activity require problem solving?

With the most effective activities the answer is "yes" to all questions.

Initiating Treatment

The therapist introduces the patient to the activity. If possible, the patient should take part in preparing for the activity. For example, the patient can help get the supplies from the cabinet. The additional cues from the environment often help the patient understand what is expected, especially for patients with aphasia. The therapist gets the patient in a good starting position: feet flat on the floor, good base of support, and good pelvic alignment with trunk, shoulder, neck, and head posi-

tion. As the patient moves through the functional activity, the therapist facilitates, inhibits, or guides as needed to elicit normal movement patterns. The therapist does not just modify the patient's movements, but modifies the activity to elicit better movements or modifies the position of the patient to elicit more appropriate movements. The speed of movement is monitored; a good pace is usually slightly slower than normal. Patients need time to process incoming information and motor responses. The therapist increases the difficulty of the activities as the patient improves, to stimulate both problem-solving and motor skills.

A number of factors influence the quality of a patient's movement within a functional context:
1. How the patient is positioned, and on which surface(s)
2. The patient's base of support
3. The patient's response when the base of support changes (e.g., are there any associated reactions?)
4. Where the activity is set up in relation to the patient (to facilitate the desired movement and weight shift)
5. Where weight shifts are initiated
6. Physical properties of the objects to be manipulated.

As the patient moves within the context of function, the therapist gains additional information and insight into the patient's problem areas and observes where the specific difficulties are.

During each treatment session the therapist should constantly be asking the following questions:
1. Was the patient able to do the task?
2. How did the patient do the task?
3. Which components of the task appeared to be normal?
4. Which components were in abnormal movement patterns?

The activity is broken down into its components. What is lacking? Movement? Stability? Weight shift? Sensation? Motor planning? Treatment priorities are redefined as new problem areas are identified.

NEURODEVELOPMENTAL TREATMENT IN ACUTE CARE, REHABILITATION, OR LONG-TERM CARE

NDT is more than muscle reeducation for a specific limb; it is 24-hour management of the patient with hemiplegia. NDT principles should be incorporated into the daily management of the patient, whether in the hospital, in long-term care (skilled nursing facility), or at home. The following tips help the patient to (1) become more aware of the hemiplegic side, (2) better integrate both sides of the body, and (3) increase sensory stimulation to the hemiplegic side. By following these tips, family members and all members of the health care team can help prevent or minimize some problems that are characteristic of hemiplegia.

Room Arrangement

The hemiplegic side of the patient should face the source of stimulation. The patient's hemiplegic side should face the door and be positioned so that the telephone, night stand, and television encourage the patient to turn toward that side, thus increasing integration of both sides of the body (Fig. 36-12). The one exception is the call light for the nurse.[4,6]

Approach

Always approach the patient from the hemiplegic side to encourage eye contact. Sometimes the patient has difficulty turning his or her head and may need assistance. The therapist should simply assist the patient by gently but firmly turning the patient's head until the patient is able to establish eye contact. Family members can be encouraged to give tactile input to the patient by holding the patient's hand or stroking the arm.

Naming

During nursing tasks such as washing, each body part is named to increase the patient's awareness of the part.

Encouraging Independence

The patient should begin to assist in simple ADL. If the patient is unable to complete a task independently, the therapist or caregiver can guide the patient's hands so the patient can feel the movement pattern necessary to complete an activity. This approach encourages the patient to learn to carry out the task sooner.[1]

In each medical setting the roles of OT and physical therapy may differ slightly. Yet the methods described are imperative for proper patient treatment, and all persons in professional services should be aware of the methods and be able to apply them appropriately. The Bobaths strongly emphasized that this approach is not a series of exercises and that the upper and lower extremities must not be treated independently.[2] The occupational therapist must be constantly aware of the tonus, motor patterns, positions, and reflex mechanisms of both the upper and lower extremities.

Bed Positioning

The patient should be properly positioned (Figs. 36-13 to 36-15). The benefits of positioning patients in the proper manner are that (1) weight bearing normalizes tone and inhibits spasticity, (2) weight bearing increases awareness of the hemiplegic side and increases sensory input, (3) weight bearing on the weak side helps the patient to be less fearful, and (4) lengthening of the hemiplegic side inhibits spasticity.

The three basic positions are listed in order of their therapeutic value: lying on the hemiplegic side, lying on the nonhemiplegic side, and lying supine. Patients should be repositioned as often as nursing procedures require (usually every 2 hours) for the prevention of decubiti.

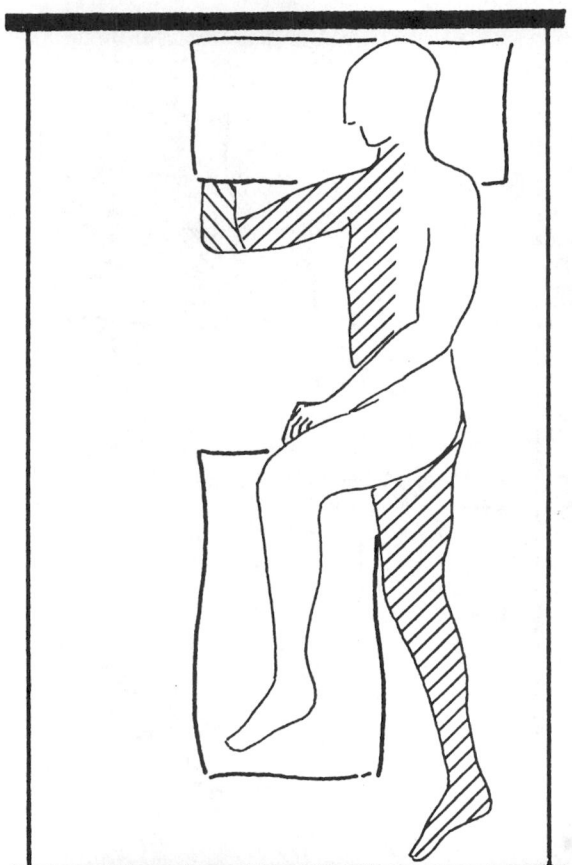

FIG. 36-13
Bed position when lying on affected side.

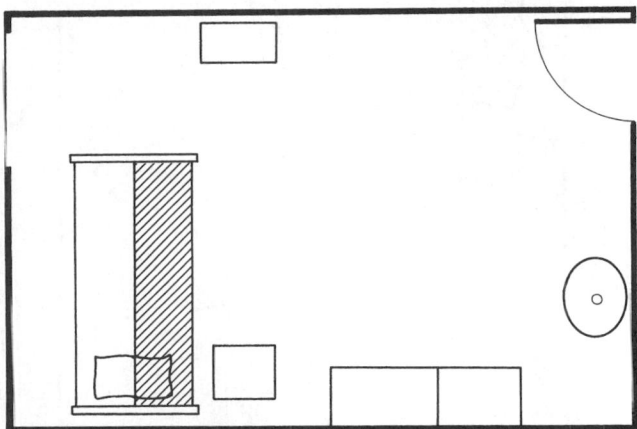

FIG. 36-12
Room arranged so that patient must turn to affected side. Shaded area represents affected side of body.

Lying on the Hemiplegic Side

This position is preferred for the hemiplegic patient (Fig. 36-13). [2,7] The patient's back should be parallel with the edge of the bed. The patient's head is placed on the pillow symmetrically but not in extreme flexion. The shoulder is fully protracted with at least 90° of shoulder flexion (less than 90° encourages a flexion synergy). The forearm is supinated, and the elbow is flexed. The patient's hand is placed under the pillow. An alternative position is with the elbow extended and the wrist either supported on the bed or slightly off the bed, which encourages wrist extension. These positions are familiar to most patients and encourage external rotation at the shoulder. The unaffected leg is placed on a pillow. The affected leg is slightly flexed at the knee with hip extension. A pillow can be placed behind the patient to prevent the patient from rolling onto the back.

Lying on the Nonhemiplegic Side

In this position the back should be parallel with the edge of the bed (Fig. 36-14). [2,5] The head is placed symmetrically on the pillow. The shoulder is in full protraction, with the shoulder in at least 90° of flexion. The arm and hand are fully supported on a pillow. The wrist should not be allowed to drop off the pillow into flexion. The affected lower extremity is in hip flexion and knee flexion and fully supported on a pillow. The foot and ankle must be supported to keep the foot from inverting.

Lying Supine

The head should be symmetrical on the pillow (Fig. 36-15). [2,5] The body and trunk are also symmetrical to prevent the shortening of the hemiplegic side of the trunk. A pillow is placed under the affected shoulder, supporting the shoulder so that it is no more than level with the nonhemiplegic shoulder. If the affected shoulder is higher, an anterior **subluxation** may occur at the glenohumeral joint. The affected arm is fully supported, with the elbow extended and forearm in supination and entirely supported in elevation on a pillow. A small pillow may be placed under the hip to reduce retraction of the pelvis. The therapist should not place a pillow under the knees or a foot board at the end of the bed because the former encourages knee flexion contractures and the latter encourages an extension synergy of the lower extremity.

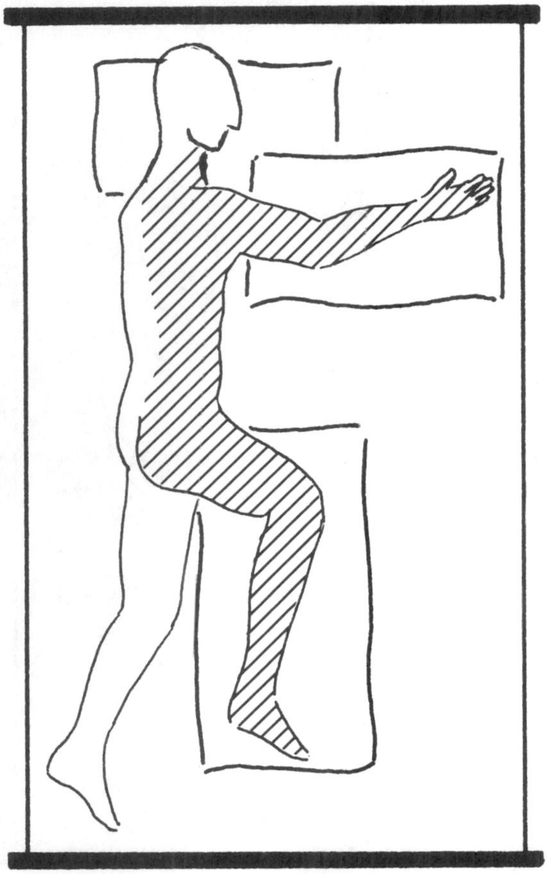

FIG. 36-14
Bed position when lying on unaffected side.

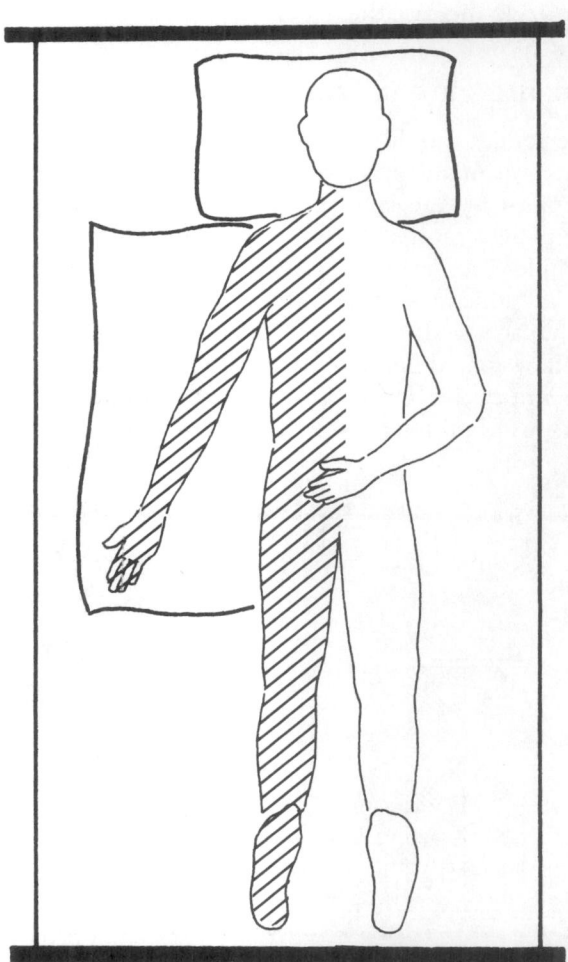

FIG. 36-15
Bed position when lying supine.

Dressing Activities

Dressing and grooming activities are a part of every OT program. These activities are purposeful, functional, familiar to the patient, and necessary for improving the patient's level of independence. Relearning how to dress may be one of the most frustrating activities requested of the patient. Dressing requires not only trunk stability in sitting, but also the ability to perform motor planning, sequencing, and problem solving. Dressing is one of the most difficult tasks required by the occupational therapist, yet it is nearly always the first one introduced.[1]

With the difficulty of dressing in mind, the therapist should grade a dressing-training activity to the sitting balance, endurance, frustration level, and cognitive-perceptual status of the patient. As the patient learns to bear weight over both hips in sitting and to shift weight to either side (or forward) as necessary, he or she moves more normally and with less compensation. The patient learns to inhibit his or her own spasticity. The procedure breaks up typical hemiplegic patterns of LE extension synergy and UE flexion synergy. With the NDT approach, dressing is learned faster than by traditional, one-handed methods, especially for patients with perceptual problems. The patient learns to carry over techniques of inhibition into daily living skills. The following methods are examples of how the principles of NDT can be used in ADL training. The facilitation of each task should be modified to fit each patient's abilities and problem areas.

Tips

The patient should not attempt to get dressed in bed. Instead the patient should be seated on a chair, preferably a straight chair next to the bed. The therapist should always assist from the affected side and should always begin dressing with the hemiplegic side. The same sequence in dressing is maintained to increase learning. Following are specific instructions for the patient to follow when dressing.

DONNING SHIRT

1. Position the shirt across the knees with the armhole visible and the sleeve between the knees (Fig. 36-16).
2. Bend forward at the hips (inhibiting extension synergy of the LE), placing the affected hand in the sleeve (Fig. 36-17).
3. Drop the arm into the sleeve; shoulder protraction and gravity inhibit UE flexion synergy.
4. Bring the collar to the neck.
5. Sit upright; dress the nonhemiplegic side.
6. Button the shirt from bottom to top.

DONNING UNDERCLOTHES AND PANTS (FIG. 36-18)

1. Clasp hands and cross the affected leg over the non-hemiplegic leg (the therapist helps when needed).
2. Release hands. The hemiplegic arm can dangle and should not be trapped in the lap. When able, use the affected hand as needed.
3. Pull the pant leg over the hemiplegic foot.
4. Clasp hands to uncross the leg.
5. Place the nonhemiplegic foot in the pant leg (no need to cross legs). This step is difficult because the patient must bear weight on the hemiplegic side.
6. Pull pants to the knees.
7. While holding onto the waistband, stand with the therapist's help.

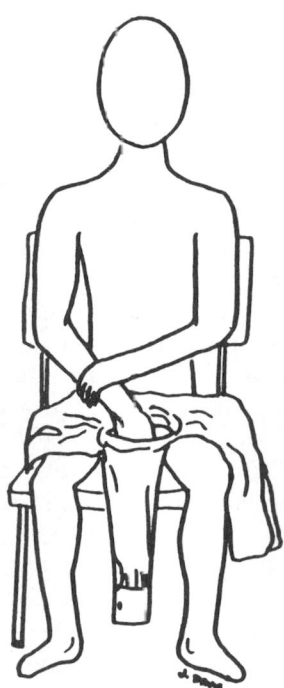

FIG. 36-16
Dressing training. Shirt positioned across patient's knees, armhole visible, and sleeve dropped between knees.

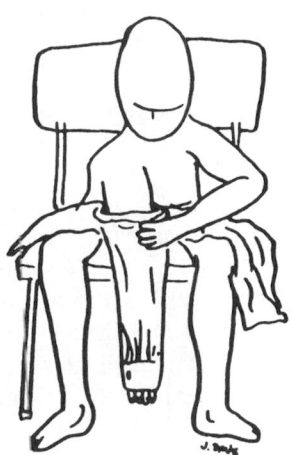

FIG. 36-17
Patient bends forward at hips (inhibiting extension synergy of lower extremity) and places affected hand into sleeve.

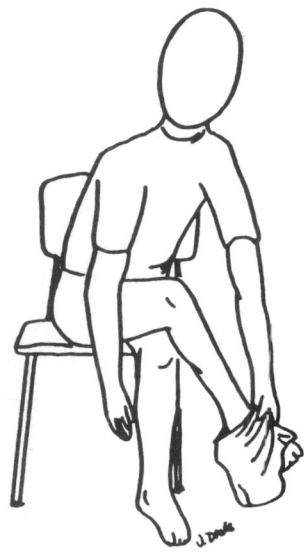

FIG. 36-18
Proper position while putting on pants and underclothes.

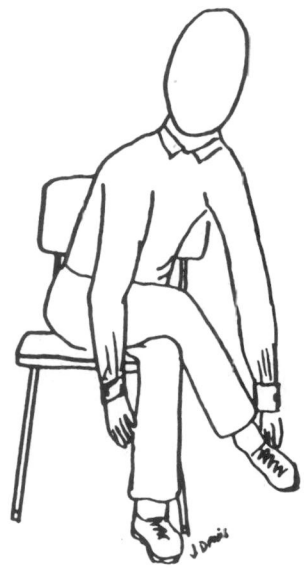

FIG. 36-19
Proper position while putting on shoes and socks.

8. Zip and snap the pants.
9. Return to sitting position with the therapist's help.

DONNING SHOES AND SOCKS (FIG. 36-19)
1. Clasp hands and cross legs (as before).
2. Put sock and shoe on hemiplegic foot.
3. Cross the nonhemiplegic leg and put on sock and shoe.

SHOULDER IN HEMIPLEGIA

Problems of the hemiplegic shoulder are often frustrating and confusing to the occupational therapist. Pain

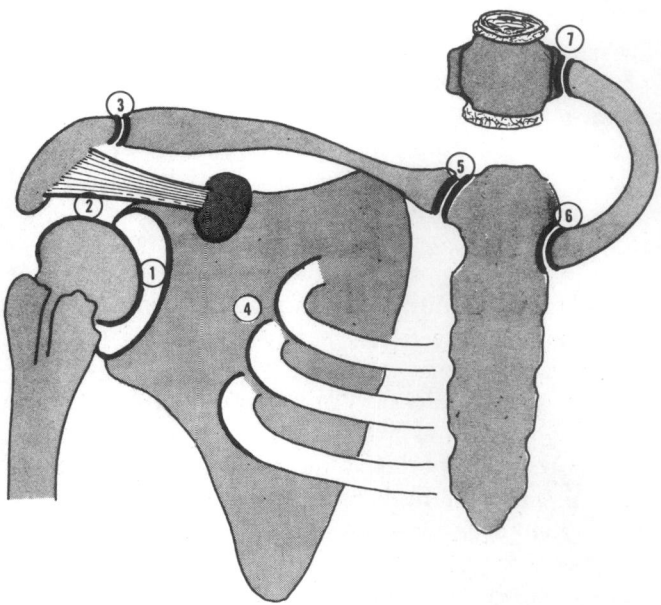

FIG. 36-20
Composite drawing of shoulder girdle. (From Cailliet R: *The shoulder in hemiplegia*, Philadelphia, 1980, FA Davis.)

can hinder the entire rehabilitation program. The responsibility of the therapist is to learn how to evaluate these problems and prepare a treatment program that is effective in dealing with them. An understanding of the basic anatomy and functional mechanism of the shoulder girdle is important. Those interested in expanding their knowledge in this area are directed to the references, particularly *The Shoulder in Hemiplegia* by Rene Cailliet.[3] The shoulder girdle is made up of seven joints (Fig. 36-20): glenohumeral, suprahumeral, acromioclavicular, scapulocostal, sternoclavicular, costosternal, and costovertebral.

For full pain-free range of motion (ROM), all seven joints need to work synchronously. The glenohumeral joint allows considerable mobility but lacks stability. It is dependent on the proper alignment of the scapula and humerus for mechanical support and on the supraspinatus for muscular support.

The therapist must understand the relationship of the scapula to the humerus and the significance of that relationship in pain-free shoulder flexion and abduction. When the arm is raised in forward flexion or abduction, the scapula must glide and rotate upward. The humerus and the scapula work in unison; more specifically, they work in a 2:1 ratio pattern. In other words, if the shoulder moves into 90° of abduction, the humerus moves 60° and the scapula moves 30°. As another example, when there is 180° of shoulder flexion, the humerus moves 120° and the scapula moves 60° (again, a 2:1 ratio).[3]

If for any reason, the arm is raised in shoulder flexion or abduction without the scapula's gliding along, joint trauma and pain can occur. The therapist must be aware of this effect and take it into consideration during ROM, ADL, transfers, and all other activities.

In the hemiplegic shoulder the scapula can fall into downward rotation because of a heavy, flaccid UE or because the muscles that move the scapula in downward rotation (rhomboids, latissimus dorsi, and levator scapulae) are spastic. This condition makes it difficult for the scapula to glide upward, which is necessary for pain-free movement. The scapula must first be mobilized and the spasticity reduced to regain the ROM and allow selective movement. The arm must never be raised over 90° before the scapula has been mobilized and the therapist can feel its gliding movements. Even in a seemingly flaccid arm the scapula can be influenced by spasticity of the rhomboids, trapezius, and latissimus dorsi. The techniques previously described assist the therapist.

Because the hemiplegic shoulder can often be pulled back into retraction by hypertonicity, the emphasis of treatment is placed on forward gliding of the scapula. By protracting the scapula, the patient is able to reduce the hypertonicity of the UE, allowing more isolated movement and selective control. When the spasticity is too strong for the patient to obtain protraction of the shoulder, the therapist must assist. The therapist should use reflex-inhibiting patterns to control and reduce spasticity. As Bobath stated, "The main reflex-inhibiting pattern counteracting spasticity in the trunk and arm is the extension of neck and spine and external rotation of the arm at the shoulder with elbow extended. Further reduction of flexor spasticity can be obtained by adding extension of the wrist with supination and abduction of the thumb."[2]

Subluxation

Many health care professionals are particularly concerned about the subluxed shoulder. Numerous efforts are made to protect the shoulder and prevent subluxation, but subluxation cannot be prevented. If the muscles around the shoulder girdle (which are attached to the humerus and scapula) are weak enough, the shoulder will be subluxed. Slings do not help subluxation. They keep the arm in a poor position and may contribute to pain and swelling. Subluxation itself does not cause pain; the pain is caused by improper handling of a subluxed arm. Forcing the head of the humerus back into place before moving the arm above 90° of shoulder flexion or abduction can cause trauma and pain. Performing standard ROM procedures on an arm without a gliding scapula can also cause pain. Treatment of the subluxed arm should include proper sitting, weight bearing, mobilization of the scapula, and proper positioning in bed (Figs. 36-13 to 36-15).

Slings

The application of a sling to the hemiplegic arm is a source of considerable controversy. It has been demonstrated over the past several years that "the commonly used hemiplegic sling has no appreciable effect on ultimate ROM, subluxation, pain, or peripheral nerve traction injury."[9] It has also been stated that "there is no need to support a pain free shoulder in order to prevent or correct subluxation since the sling does not prevent, improve, cure or reduce such a deformity."[8] The use of a sling on the hemiplegic arm can actually contribute to subluxation and lead to a painful, disabling condition called shoulder-hand syndrome. The therapist should realize that when a patient wears a sling, the arm is supported in a position that is compatible with the typical hemiplegic posture, which discourages the patient from using the arm either bilaterally or unilaterally. Even the sling that was previously described by the Bobaths is no longer being used.[2] This sling was found to hinder the circulation of the arm and to push the head of the humerus into lateral subluxation. If the patient has a painful shoulder or swollen hand, a thorough assessment should be done to determine the cause. Then appropriate treatment can be started.

PREPARING THE PATIENT FOR HOME

The benefits of the treatment program are lost if the patient is not adequately prepared for returning home. This preparation should include (1) prescribing a home exercise program, (2) providing family education, and (3) communicating with the follow-up therapist when applicable. The hospital or clinic is a very secure setting, and both the patient and family must feel comfortable and confident on the return home. The home exercise program is important for maintaining mobility and movement. The therapist should select exercises that can be performed easily and correctly without assistance. If stress or excessive effort is used to complete the exercises, the patient is likely to form bad habits and spasticity will increase.

After selecting exercises the therapist must train the patient in each exercise. To encourage consistency the patient should follow the same sequence of exercises each day. This program should begin long before discharge from OT so that it is a well-established part of the daily routine.

A description of the exercises should be written down in proper sequence. The description should include how often the exercises should be done (e.g., twice a day) and the number of repetitions (e.g., 10 times each). Diagrams should be used if necessary. Some family members have found videotape to be especially helpful in following through with a home program. During a treatment session the therapist can videotape the home program (exercises, bed positioning, or other tasks important to continue at home); the family then has a copy to use at home.

Next, the family should be trained so that they are also well acquainted with each exercise and thus can guide the home program properly. For best results in family teaching, the occupational therapist should demonstrate and explain the importance of tasks, emphasize each major point (e.g., position of arm and placement of hands), have the family work with the patient under the therapist's guidance, and repeat instructions as often as needed until the family and patient are confident enough to do the exercises at home alone.

Family education should include a home exercise program and ADL training in the areas of dressing, eating, grooming, hygiene, bathing, transfers, and cooking. This program should also include instruction in proper position (lying, sitting, and standing) and the proper use of equipment. Before discharge from the treatment center the therapist should give the family his or her name and telephone number at work, set up a date for a reevaluation if necessary, and contact the therapist treating the patient after discharge from the treatment facility to ensure proper carryover.

SUMMARY

Neurodevelopmental treatment, developed by Karel and Berta Bobath, is used successfully in the treatment of adult hemiplegia. This treatment emphasizes relearning normal movement and avoiding abnormal movement patterns. Quality of movement, control, and coordination are emphasized through the use of treatment methods to normalize abnormal muscle tone and the avoidance of abnormal patterns of movement.

REVIEW QUESTIONS

1. What is the primary goal of the NDT approach?
2. List three advantages of the NDT approach stated in the text.
3. Describe and assume the typical posture of the adult patient with hemiplegia.
4. List the key points of control used to normalize tone
5. What is the key element of an NDT assessment?
6. List four factors that can cause or increase spasticity.
7. Describe the observation process using the NDT approach in evaluating a patient.
8. Why is skilled observation critical to treatment effectiveness?
9. Describe the elements of the vicious circle that may contribute to the maintenance of spasticity.
10. What are some of the possible causes of asymmetrical shoulder height observed in the patient with hemiplegia?

11. List and describe at least three treatment methods designed to normalize tone and promote normal movement.
12. What are the purposes of trunk rotation? Bilateral activities?
13. Describe recommended positioning and mobilization procedures to prevent shoulder pain and severe spasticity around the shoulder and shoulder girdle.
14. How can the affected upper extremity be incorporated into activity? What effects will this approach have?
15. Why is it important to use functional activities from real life in the treatment program?
16. List at least four factors that will influence the quality of the patient's movement when performing functional activities.
17. How should the therapist evaluate the effectiveness of the treatment session?
18. Describe and assume the recommended positions for the patient with hemiplegia in the supine, prone, and side-lying positions on the affected and unaffected sides. What is the rationale for these postures?
19. When using the NDT approach, what is the recommended method for donning a shirt? Put on your own shirt using this method, and then teach it to another person.
20. Why is scapula protraction stressed in positioning and movement of the hemiplegic arm?
21. What are some possible causes of shoulder subluxation in hemiplegia?
22. What is the recommended treatment for shoulder subluxation in the NDT approach?
23. Why is the common hemiplegic sling contraindicated?
24. What is the role of the occupational therapist in preparing the patient to go home?

REFERENCES

1. Affolter F: *Perceptual processes as requisites for complex human behavior,* Bern, Switzerland, 1980, Hans Huber.
2. Bobath B: *Adult hemiplegia: evaluation and treatment,* London, 1978, Heinemann.
3. Cailliet R: *The shoulder in hemiplegia,* Philadelphia, 1980, FA Davis.
4. Cash J: *Neurology for physiotherapists,* London, 1977, Faber & Faber.
5. Davies P: *Treatment techniques for adult hemiplegia:* study course, Valens, Switzerland, 1979, Klinik Valens.
6. Davies P: *Steps to follow,* Berlin, 1985, Springer-Verlag.
7. Eggers O: *Occupational therapy in the treatment of adult hemiplegia,* Rockville, Md, 1984, Aspen Systems.
8. Friedland F: Physical therapy. In Licht S, editor: *Stroke and its rehabilitation,* Baltimore, 1975, Williams & Wilkins.
9. Hurd MM, Farrell KH, Waylonis FW: Shoulder sling for hemiplegia: friend or foe? *Arch Phys Med Rehabil* 55:519, 1974.

CHAPTER 37

Cerebrovascular Accident

GLEN GILLEN

KEY TERMS

Ischemia
Transient ischemic attack
Dysarthria
Client-centered assessment
Top-down approach to assessment
Postural control
Balance strategies
Aphasia
Neurobehavioral deficits
Motor control
Weight bearing
Subluxation

LEARNING OBJECTIVES

After studying this chapter the student or practitioner will be able to do the following:

1. List and describe evaluation procedures for survivors of a stroke.
2. Discuss the neuropathology of a stroke.
3. Identify risk factors associated with a stroke.
4. Identify multiple factors that impede task performance after a stroke.
5. Describe evaluation procedures for neurobehavioral deficits.
6. Identify balance strategies that support functional performance.
7. Describe motor control dysfunction associated with stroke.
8. Identify standardized stroke assessments for multiple areas of dysfunction.
9. Apply a client-centered approach to stroke rehabilitation.
10. Develop comprehensive function-based treatment plans to remediate or compensate for underlying deficits.

Cerebrovascular accident (CVA), or stroke, continues to be a national health problem despite recent advances in medical technology. The American Heart Association[4] publishes stroke statistics that demonstrate the severity of this problem. Selected statistics include the following[4]:

1. Stroke ranks as the third leading cause of death behind heart disease and cancer.

2. On average, a United States citizen suffers a stroke every 53 seconds; every 3.3 minutes someone dies of a stroke.
3. Each year, 600,000 people suffer a new or recurrent stroke. Approximately 500,000 strokes are first attacks, and 100,000 are recurrent.
4. About 4,400,000 stroke survivors are alive today.
5. The percentage of strokes that result in death within 1 year is about 29%, less if the stroke occurs before age 65.

The author would like to acknowledge the contribution of Michael Lawrence to this chapter.

6. Twenty-eight percent of people who suffer a stroke are under age 65. For people over 55, the incidence of stroke more than doubles for each successive decade.

7. The incidence of stroke is about 19% higher for males than for females.

In addition, the aftermath of stroke is a substantial public health and economic problem. For example:

1. Stroke is a leading cause of serious, long-term disability in the United States.

2. Stroke accounts for more than half of all patients hospitalized for acute neurological disease.

3. The average cost of a stroke from hospital admission to discharge is $18,244. In a survey year, $3.7 billion was paid to Medicare beneficiaries who survived a stroke.

4. Among long-term stroke survivors, 48% have hemiparesis, 22% cannot walk, 24% to 53% report complete or partial dependence on activities of daily living (ADL) scales, 12% to 18% are aphasic, and 32% are clinically depressed.

Obviously, stroke rehabilitation as a practice area for occupational therapists is a specialization that crosses multiple settings, from the intensive care unit to community-based programs. The Agency for Health Care Policy and Research has critically reviewed the practice area of stroke rehabilitation.[65] The agency has published guidelines to "improve the effectiveness of stroke rehabilitation in helping the person with disabilities from a stroke to achieve the best possible functional outcome and quality of life."[65]

DEFINITION OF CEREBROVASCULAR ACCIDENT

CVA is a complex dysfunction caused by a lesion in the brain. The World Health Organization[88] defines stroke as an "acute neurologic dysfunction of vascular origin . . . with symptoms and signs corresponding to the involvement of focal areas of the brain." CVA results in upper motor neuron dysfunction that produces hemiplegia or paralysis of one side of the body, including limbs and trunk and sometimes the face and oral structures that are contralateral to the brain hemisphere that has the lesion. Thus a lesion in the left cerebral hemisphere (left CVA) produces right hemiplegia. Conversely, a lesion in the right cerebral hemisphere (right CVA) produces a left hemipleia. When reference is made to the patient's disability as right or left hemiplegia, the reference is to the paralyzed body side and not to the locus of the lesion.[75]

Accompanying the motor paralysis may be a variety of dysfunctions other than the motor paralysis. Some of these are sensory disturbances, perceptual dysfunction, visual disturbances, personality and intellectual changes, and a complex range of speech and associated language disorders.[76,85] The neurological deficits persist longer than 24 hours.

CAUSES OF CEREBROVASCULAR ACCIDENT

"Stroke is essentially a disease of the cerebral vasculature in which failure to supply oxygen to the brain cells, which are the most susceptible to ischemic damage, leads to their death. The syndromes that lead to stroke comprise two broad categories: ischemic and hemorrhagic stroke. Ischemic strokes account for approximately 80% of strokes, whereas hemorrhagic strokes account for the remaining 20%."[9]

Ischemia

Ischemic strokes may be the result of embolisms to the brain from cardiac or arterial sources. Cardiac sources include atrial fibrillation (pooling of blood in the dysfunctional atrium leads to emboli production), sinoatrial disorders, acute myocardial infarction, endocarditis, cardiac tumors, and valvular (both native and artificial) disorders. Cerebral **ischemia** caused by perfusion failure occurs with severe stenosis of the carotid and basilar arteries, as well as when there is microstenosis of the small deep arteries.[4,9]

Age, gender, race, ethnicity, and heredity are considered nonmodifiable risk factors for ischemic strokes. In contrast, a major focus of stroke prevention and education programs is on the potentially modifiable risk factors discussed in the following list[4,44]:

1. *Hypertension* is considered the single most important modifiable risk factor for ischemic stroke. Forty percent of strokes have been attributed to systolic blood pressures greater than 140 mm Hg.[69]

2. Management of *cardiac diseases*, particularly atrial fibrillation (a-fib), mitral stenosis, and structural abnormalities (patent foramen ovale and atrial septal aneurysm), can reduce the risk of stroke.

3. Management of *diabetes and glucose metabolism* can also reduce the risk of stroke.

4. *Cigarette smoking* increases the relative risk of ischemic stroke nearly two times.

5. Although *excessive use of alcohol* is a risk factor for many other diseases, *moderate consumption of alcohol* may reduce incidence of cardiovascular disease, including stroke.

6. *Use of illegal drugs*, particularly cocaine, is commonly associated with stroke. Other drugs linked to stroke include heroin, amphetamines, LSD, PCP, and marijuana.

7. *Lifestyle factors* such as obesity, physical inactivity, diet, and emotional stress are associated with stroke risk.

"The realization that the probability of stroke is increased several fold by the presence of multiple risk factors may help the patient . . . fully appreciate the need for serious risk factor management."[4] The responsibility for stroke prevention education (including the prevention of recurrence) falls on each member of the stroke rehabilitation team.

Hemorrhage

Hemorrhagic strokes include subarachnoid and intracerebral hemorrhage, which accounts for only 15% to 25% of total strokes.[4] This type of stroke has numerous causes. The four most common causes are deep hypertensive intracerebral hemorrhages, ruptured saccular aneurysms, bleeding from arteriovenous malformations, and spontaneous lobar hemorrhages.[51]

Related Syndromes

Cerebral anoxia and aneurysm can also result in hemiplegia.[75] Some of the treatment approaches outlined in this chapter may be applicable to hemiplegia that results from causes other than CVA or stroke, such as head injuries, neoplasms, and infectious diseases of the brain.

Transient Ischemic Attacks

Vascular disease of the brain can result in a completed CVA or cause **transient ischemic attacks** (TIAs). A TIA occurs as mild, isolated, or repetitive neurological symptoms that develop suddenly, last from a few minutes to several hours but not longer than 24 hours, and clear completely. The TIA is seen as a sign of impending CVA. Most TIAs occur in people with atherosclerotic disease. Of those who experience TIAs and do not seek treatment, an estimated one third will sustain a completed stroke, another third will continue to have additional TIAs without stroke, and one third will experience no further incidence.[67] If the TIA is caused by extracranial vascular disease, surgical intervention to restore vascular flow (carotid endarterectomy) may be effective in preventing the CVA and the resultant disability.[76]

EFFECTS OF CEREBROVASCULAR ACCIDENT

The outcome of the CVA depends on which artery supplying the brain was involved (Fig. 37-1). Dysfunction of performance components and performance areas depends on various pathological conditions resulting in CVA and the different anatomical structures involved. Stroke diagnostic workups help localize the lesion and find a cause of the stroke. Techniques include such cerebrovascular imaging techniques as computerized tomography (CT scanning), magnetic resonance imaging (MRI), and more recently, positron emission tomography (PET) and single photon emission computerized tomography (SPECT).[9] The information collected using these techniques (e.g., the extent of damage and location of the lesion) may help the occupational therapist iden-

tify neurological deficits that affect function. The information may also help the therapist develop hypotheses regarding recovery and plan appropriate treatment. Initial information may be collected during a medical record review that focuses on the chief complaint of the patient on admission, previous medical and surgical history, results of diagnostics, and current pharmacological management. The following section and Tables 37-1 and 37-2 explain patterns of impairment resulting from CVA in both cortical and noncortical areas.

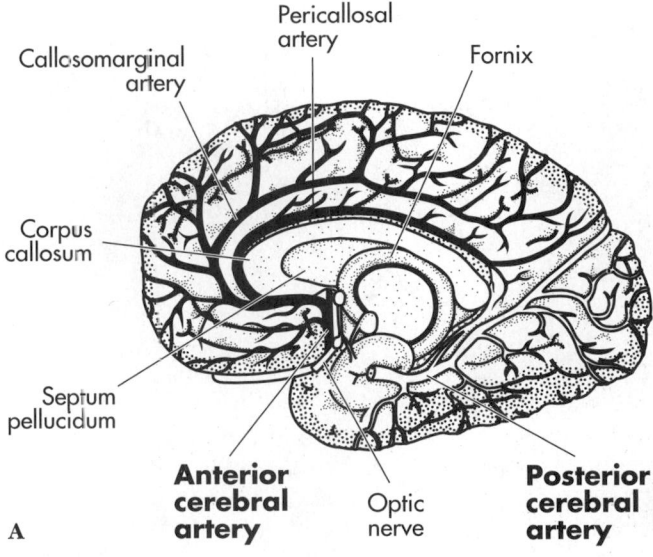

The Cerebral Hemispheres

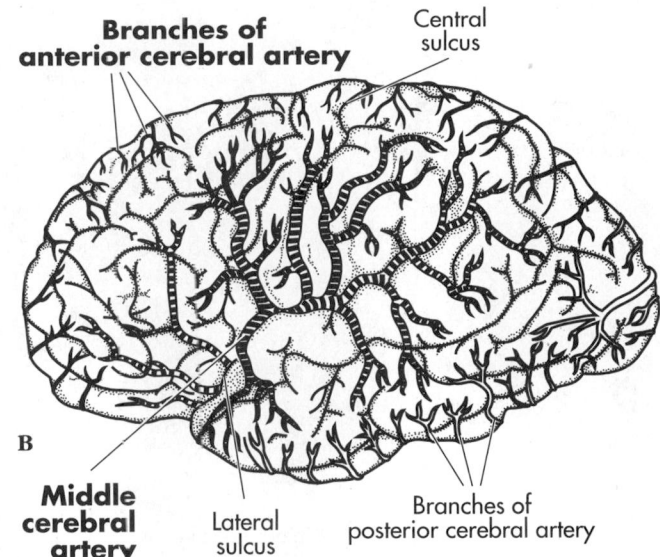

FIG. 37-1

Blood supply to brain. Middle cerebral, anterior cerebral, and posterior cerebral arteries supply blood to cerebral hemispheres. **A,** Medial surface. **B,** Lateral surface. (From Nolte J: *The human brain,* ed 3, St Louis, 1993, Mosby.)

Artery	Location	Possible Impairments
Middle cerebral artery: upper trunk	Lateral aspect of frontal and parietal lobe	**Dysfunction of Either Hemisphere** Contralateral hemiplegia, especially of the face and the upper extremity Contralateral hemisensory loss Visual field impairment Poor contralateral conjugate gaze Ideational apraxia Lack of judgment Perseveration Field dependency Impaired organization of behavior Depression Lability Apathy **Right Hemisphere Dysfunction** Left unilateral body neglect Left unilateral visual neglect Anosognosia Visuospatial impairment Left unilateral motor apraxia **Left Hemisphere Dysfunction** Bilateral motor apraxia Broca's aphasia Frustration
Middle cerebral artery: lower trunk	Lateral aspect of right temporal and occipital lobes	**Dysfunction of Either Hemisphere** Contralateral visual field deficit Behavioral abnormalities **Right Hemisphere Dysfunction** Visuospatial dysfunction **Left Hemisphere Dysfunction** Wernicke's aphasia
Middle cerebral artery: both upper and lower trunks	Lateral aspect of the involved hemisphere	Impairments related to both upper and lower trunk dysfunction as listed in previous two sections
Anterior cerebral artery	Medial and superior aspects of frontal and parietal lobes	Contralateral hemiparesis, greatest in foot Contralateral hemisensory loss, greatest in foot Left unilateral apraxia Inertia of speech or mutism Behavioral disturbances
Internal carotid artery	Combination of middle cerebral artery distribution and anterior cerebral artery	Impairments related to dysfunction of middle and anterior cerebral arteries as listed above
Anterior choroidal artery, a branch of internal carotid artery	Globus pallidus, lateral geniculate body, posterior limb of the internal capsule, medial temporal lobe	Hemiparesis of face, arm, and leg Hemisensory loss Hemianopsia
Posterior cerebral artery	Medial and inferior aspects of right temporal and occipital lobes, posterior corpus callosum and penetrating arteries to midbrain and thalamus	**Dysfunction of Either Side** Homonymous hemianopsia Visual agnosia (visual object agnosia, prosopagnosia, color agnosia) Memory impairment Occasional contralateral numbness

Artery	Location	Possible Impairments
		Right Side Dysfunction Cortical blindness Visuospatial impairment Impaired left-right discrimination **Left Side Dysfunction** Finger agnosia Anomia Agraphia Acalculia Alexia
Basilar artery proximal	Pons	Quadriparesis Bilateral asymmetrical weakness Bulbar or pseudobulbar paralysis (bilateral paralysis of face, palate, pharynx, neck, or tongue) Paralysis of eye abductors Nystagmus Ptosis Cranial nerve abnormalities Diplopia Dizziness Occipital headache Coma
Basilar artery distal	Midbrain, thalamus, and caudate	Papillary abnormalities Abnormal eye movements Altered level of alertness Coma Memory loss Agitation Hallucinations
Vertebral artery	Lateral medulla and cerebellum	Dizziness Vomiting Nystagmus Pain in ipsilateral eye and face Numbness in face Clumsiness of ipsilateral limbs Hypotonia of ipsilateral limbs Tachycardia Gait ataxia
Systemic hypoperfusion	Watershed region on lateral side of hemisphere, hippocampus and surrounding structures in medial temporal lobe	Coma Dizziness Confusion Decreased concentration Agitation Memory impairment Visual abnormalities as a result of disconnection from frontal eye fields Simultanognosia Impaired eye movements Weakness of shoulder and arm Gait ataxia

From Arnadottir G: Impact of neurobehavioral deficits of activities of daily living. In Gillen G, Burkhardt A, editors: *Stroke rehabilitation: a function-based approach*, St Louis, 1998, Mosby.

TABLE 37-2

Cerebrovascular Dysfunction in Noncortical Areas: Patterns of Impairment

Location	Possible Impairments	Location	Possible Impairments
Anterolateral thalamus, either side	Minor contralateral motor abnormalities Long latency period Slowness **Right side** Visual neglect **Left side** Aphasia	Caudate	Dysarthria Apathy Restlessness Agitation Confusion Delirium Lack of initiative Poor memory Contralateral hemiparesis Ipsilateral conjugation deviation of the eyes
Lateral thalamus	Contralateral hemisensory symptoms Contralateral limb ataxia	Putamen	Contralateral hemiparesis Contralateral hemisensory loss Decreased consciousness Ipsilateral conjugate gaze Motor impersistence
Bilateral thalamus	Memory impairment Behavioral abnormalities Hypersomnolence		
Posterior thalamus	Numbness or decreased sensibility of face and arm Choreic movements Impaired eye movements Hypersomnolence Decreased consciousness Decreased alertness **Right Side** Visual neglect Anosognosia Visuospatial abnormalities **Left Side** Aphasia Jargon aphasia Good comprehension of speech Paraphasia Anomia		**Right Side** Visuospatial impairment **Left Side** Aphasia
		Pons	Quadriplegia Coma Impaired eye movement
		Cerebellum	Ipsilateral limb ataxia Gait ataxia Vomiting Impaired eye movements

From Arnadottir G: Impact of neurobehavioral deficits of activities of daily living. In Gillen G, Burkhardt A, editors: *Stroke rehabilitation: a function-based approach*, St Louis, 1998, Mosby.

Internal Carotid Artery

In the absence of adequate collateral circulation, occlusion of the internal carotid artery results in contralateral hemiplegia, hemianesthesia, and homonymous hemianopsia.[8,9] Additionally, involvement of the dominant hemisphere is associated with aphasia, agraphia or dysgraphia, acalculia or dyscalculia, right-left confusion, and finger agnosia. Involvement of the nondominant hemisphere is associated with visual perceptual dysfunction, unilateral neglect, anosognosia, constructional or dressing apraxia, attention deficits, and loss of topographic memory. A tendency to tilt space in a counterclockwise direction is seen in some persons with left

hemiplegia, making ambulation and two-dimensional constructional tasks difficult.[76]

Middle Cerebral Artery

Involvement of the middle cerebral artery (MCA) is the most common cause of CVA.[8,9,20] Ischemia in the area supplied by the MCA results in contralateral hemiplegia with greater involvement of the arm, face, and tongue; sensory deficits; contralateral homonymous hemianopsia; and aphasia if the lesion is in the dominant hemisphere. There is a pronounced deviation of the head and neck toward the side on which the lesion is located.[20,27,75,76] Perceptual deficits such as anosognosia, unilateral neglect, impaired vertical perception, visual spatial deficits, and perseveration are seen if the lesion is in the nondominant hemisphere.[8]

Anterior Cerebral Artery

Occlusion of the anterior cerebral artery (ACA) produces contralateral lower extremity weakness that is more severe than that of the arm. Apraxia, mental changes, primitive reflexes, and bowel and bladder incontinence may be present. Total occlusion of the ACA results in contralateral hemiplegia with severe weakness of the face, tongue, and proximal arm muscles and marked spastic paralysis of the distal lower extremity. Cortical sensory loss is present in the lower extremity. Intellectual changes such as confusion, disorientation, abulia, whispering, slowness, distractibility, limited verbal output, perseveration, and amnesia may be seen.[8,9,76]

Posterior Cerebral Artery

The scope of posterior cerebral artery (PCA) symptoms is potentially broad and varied because this artery supplies the upper brainstem region, as well as the temporal and occipital lobes. Possible results of PCA involvement depend on the arterial branches involved and the extent and area of cerebral compromise. Some possible outcomes are sensory and motor deficits, involuntary movement disorders (e.g., hemiballism, postural tremor, hemichorea, hemiataxia, and intention tremor), memory loss, alexia, astereognosis, dysesthesia, akinesthesia, contralateral homonymous hemianopsia or quadrantanopsia, anomia, topographic disorientation, and visual agnosia.[8,9,27,76]

Cerebellar Artery System

Cerebellar artery occlusion results in ipsilateral ataxia, contralateral loss of pain and temperature sensitivity, ipsilateral facial analgesia, dysphagia and **dysarthria** caused by weakness of the ipsilateral muscles of the palate, nystagmus, and contralateral hemiparesis.[8,9,20,27]

Vertebrobasilar Artery System

A CVA in the vertebrobasilar artery system affects brainstem functions. The outcome of the stroke is some combination of bilateral or crossed sensory and motor abnormalities, such as cerebellar dysfunction, loss of proprioception, hemiplegia, quadriplegia, and sensory disturbances, with unilateral or bilateral cranial nerve involvement of nerves III to XII.[76]

MEDICAL MANAGEMENT

Specific treatment of CVA depends on the type and location of the vascular lesion, the severity of the clinical deficit, concomitant medical and neurological problems, availability of technology and personnel to administer special types of treatment, and the cooperation and reliability of the patient.

Early medical treatment involves maintenance of an open airway, hydration with intravenous fluids, and treatment of hypertension. Appropriate steps should be taken to evaluate and treat coexisting cardiac or other systemic diseases. Measures should be taken to prevent the development of deep venous thrombosis (DVT). DVT is the formation of emboli (blood clots) in the deep veins of the lower extremities, a common risk for patients who have prolonged periods of bed rest and immobility. The incidence of DVT in stroke ranges from 22% to 73%. Emboli that are released from deep veins and subsequently lodge in the lungs are referred to as pulmonary emboli. A pulmonary embolus is the most common cause of death in the first 30 days after the CVA.[9,18]

The physician oversees routine surveillance for thrombosis that includes daily evaluation of leg temperature, color, circumference, tenderness, and appearance. Preventive treatments for DVT may involve medication, the use of elastic stockings, the use of reciprocal compression devices, and early mobilization of the patient.

Respiratory problems and pneumonia may complicate the early poststroke course. The National Survey of Stroke reported that one third of stroke patients studied had respiratory infections.[66]

Symptoms are a low-grade fever and increased lethargy. Medical management involves the administration of fluids and antibiotics, aggressive pulmonary hygiene, and mobilization of the patient. Ventilatory insufficiency is a major factor contributing to the high frequency of pneumonia. The hemiparesis of stroke involves the muscles of respiration. Exercise programs that involve strengthening and endurance training of both inspiratory and expiratory muscles help improve breathing and cough effectiveness and reduce the frequency of pneumonia.[18]

Cardiac disease is another frequently occurring condition that complicates the poststroke course. The stroke itself may cause the cardiac abnormality, or the patient may have had a preexisting cardiac condition. The former is treated like any new cardiac diagnosis. A preexisting cardiac condition is reevaluated and the treatment regime modified as appropriate. Monitoring of heart rate, blood pressure, and an electrocardiogram (ECG) during self-care evaluations is frequently indicated to determine cardiac response to activity.[62,63]

During the acute phase bowel and bladder dysfunction is common. The physician is responsible for ordering a specific bowel program that includes a time schedule, adequate fluid intake, stool softeners, suppositories, oral laxatives, and medications or procedures to treat fecal impaction. A timed or scheduled toilet program is essential in treating urinary incontinence. Catheterization may be necessary in stroke rehabilitation.

EVALUATION PROCEDURES FOR STROKE SURVIVORS

The evaluation of a stroke survivor is a complicated process requiring the assessment of the multiple performance components and performance areas[5] that may be affected by the CVA. Therapists may have two or three stroke survivors assigned to their caseloads, each with completely different patterns or impairment and resulting functional deficits. Therefore the most logical starting point in the evaluation process is the use of a client-centered approach to evaluation.

Client-Centered Assessments

"Client-centered practice is an approach to providing occupational therapy which embraces a philosophy of respect for, and partnership with, people receiving services. Client-centered practice recognizes the autonomy of individuals, the need for client choice in making decisions about occupational needs, the strengths clients bring to a therapy encounter, the benefits of client-therapist partnership, and the need to ensure that services are accessible and fit the context in which a client lives."[53]

Law, Baptiste, and Mills[54] and Pollack[64] suggest that the therapist implementing this approach to evaluation include the following concepts:
1. Recognizing that the recipients of occupational therapy (OT) are uniquely qualified to make decisions about their occupational functioning
2. Offering the patient a more active role in defining goals and desired outcomes
3. Making the patient-therapist relationship an *interdependent* one to enable the solution of performance dysfunction
4. Shifting to a model in which occupational therapists work with patients to enable them to meet their own goals
5. Evaluation (and intervention) focusing on the contexts in which patients live, their roles and interests, and their culture
6. Allowing the patient to be the "problem-definer," so that in turn the patient will become the "problem-solver."
7. Allowing the client to evaluate his or her own performance and set personal goals[54,64]

Through the use of these strategies the evaluation process becomes more focused and defined, patients become immediately empowered, the goals of therapy are understood and agreed on, and a patient-tailored treatment plan may be established. The Canadian Occupational Performance Measure[53] is a standardized tool that uses a client-centered approach to allow the recipient of treatment to identify performance areas of difficulty, rate the importance of each area, and rate his or her satisfaction with current performance.

Top-Down Approach to Assessment

A **top-down approach to assessment** process has been described in the literature[82] and is applicable to the evaluation of the stroke survivor. Principles of this approach include the following:
1. Inquiry into role competency and meaningfulness is the starting point for evaluation.
2. Inquiry is focused on the roles that are important to the stroke survivor, particularly those in which the patient was engaged before the stroke.
3. Any discrepancy of roles in the past, present, or future is identified to help determine a treatment plan.
4. The tasks that define a person are identified, as well as whether those tasks can be performed and the reasons that the task is problematic.
5. A connection is determined between the components of function and occupational performance.

A top-down approach to evaluation is in contrast to a bottom-up approach that first focuses on performance component dysfunction.[82]

Effects of Neurological Deficits on Activity Performance

Using activity analysis and keen observation allows therapists to identify errors during task performance and to analyze the errors and determine the underlying deficits blocking independent functioning. "A systematic evaluation of daily activities can be used as a structure for clinical reasoning that helps therapists detect neurobehavioral dysfunction or impaired neurologic performance components and assess functional independence in self-care activities. This method allows the therapist to analyze the nature or cause of a functional problem that requires occupational therapy intervention, so the analysis is made from the view of occupations" (Fig. 37-2).[8]

Since the performance of a single functional task (e.g., donning a shirt) requires the use of multiple underlying skills that may have been affected by a stroke, multiple performance components may be evaluated in the context of one patient-chosen activity (Fig. 37-3).[7,8]

Standardized Tools

The Clinical Practice Guidelines for Post-Stroke Rehabilitation[65] encourages the use of tools that are reliable, valid, and sensitive to change. In addition, the assessment

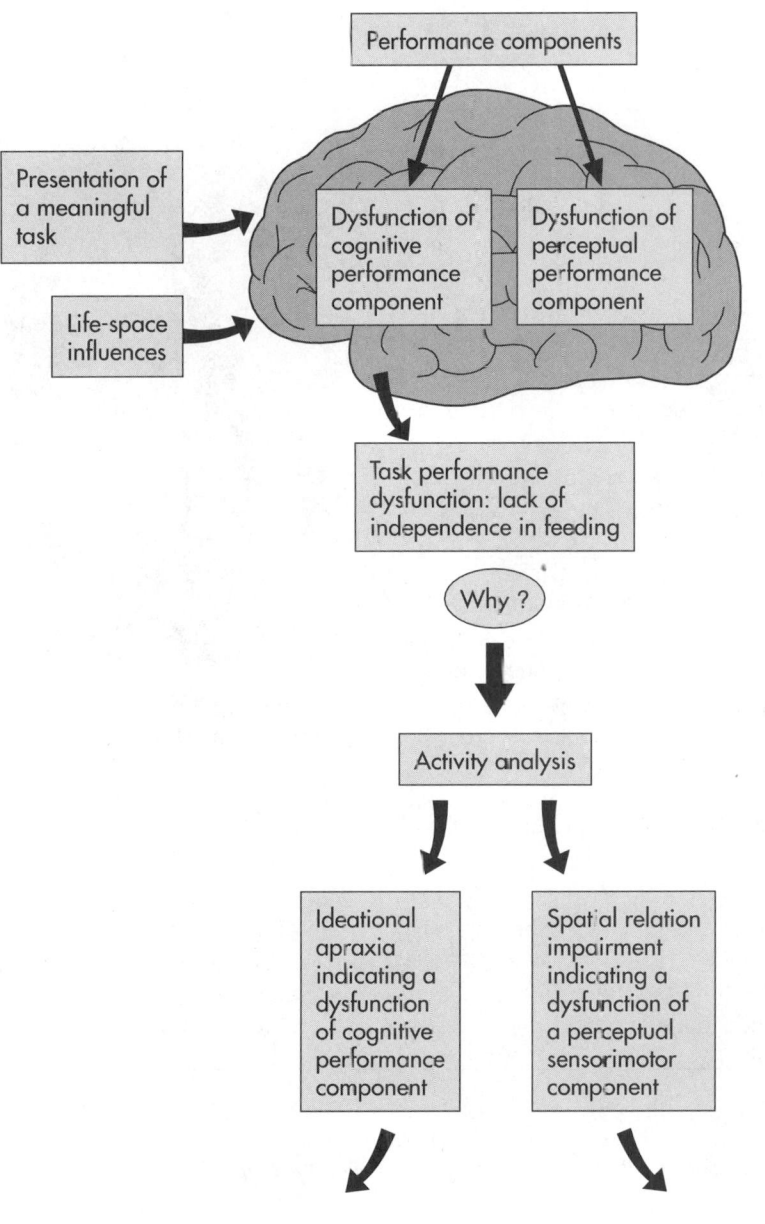

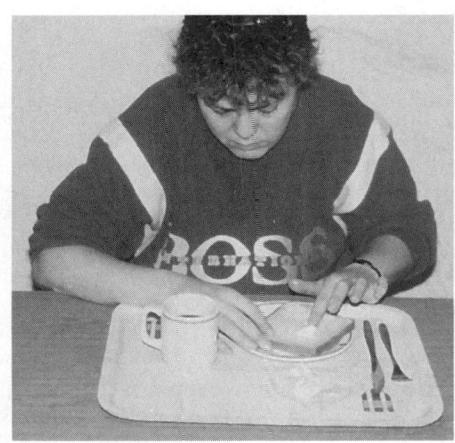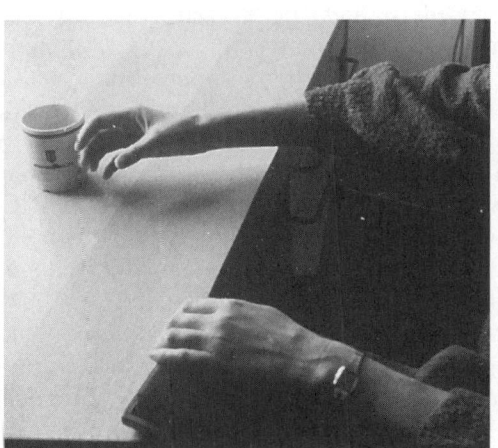

FIG. 37-2

Dysfunction of multiple performance components such as ideational apraxia and spatial relations can be revealed by activity and error analysis during functional tasks such as feeding. (Modified from Arnadottir G: *The brain and behavior: assessing cortical dysfunction through activities of daily living,* St Louis, 1990, Mosby.)

Possible behavioral deficits interfering with function

Premotor perseveration: pulling up sleeve

Spatial-relation difficulties: differentiating front from back on shirt

Spatial-relation difficulties: getting an arm into the right armhole

Unilateral spatial neglect: not seeing shirt located on neglected side (or a part of the shirt)

Unilateral body neglect: not dressing the neglected side or not completing the dressing on that side

Comprehension problem: not understanding verbal information related to performance

Ideational apraxia: not knowing what to do to get shirt on or not knowing what the shirt is for

Ideomotor apraxia: having problems with the planning of finger movements in order to perform

Tactile agnosia (astereognosis): having trouble buttoning shirt without watching the performance

Organization and sequencing: dressing the unaffected arm first and getting into trouble with dressing the affected arm; inability to continue the activity without being reminded

Lack of motivation to perform

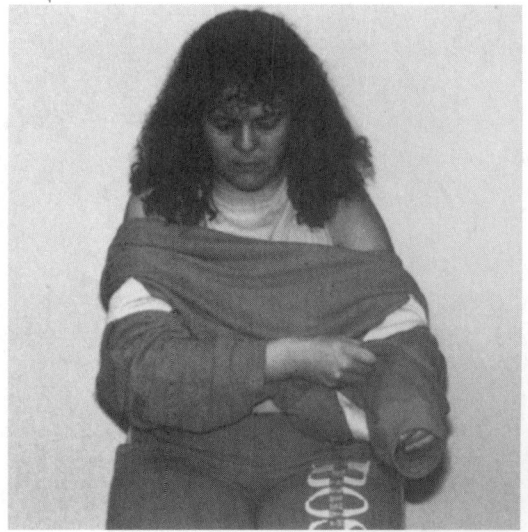

Distraction: becomes interrupted by other things

Attention deficit: difficulty attending to task and quality of performance

Irritated or frustrated when having trouble performing or when not getting the desired assistance

Aggressive when therapist touches patient in order to assist her (tactile defensiveness)

Difficulties recognizing foreground from background or a sleeve of a unicolor shirt from the rest of the shirt

FIG. 37-3
Possible behavioral deficits interfering with function during donning a shirt. (From Arnadottir G: *The brain and behavior: assessing cortical dysfunction through activities of daily living*, St Louis, 1990, Mosby.)

tools focused on task performance should be used. Tools that are focused on performance component evaluation in isolation from task performance, that use novel nonfunctional tasks, and that do not consider the affect of environmental context should be interpreted with caution. Tools are available to the occupational therapist that directly relate performance dysfunction observed during activities of daily living (ADL) with the effect of underlying skills necessary for independent performance of activities.

The *Arnadottir Occupational Therapy Neurobehavioral Evaluation*[7] (A-ONE) correlates the dysfunction of performance components (e.g., left neglect, apraxia, and spatial dysfunction) with self-care and mobility tasks. The *Assessment of Motor and Process Skills*[35] (AMPS) uses instrumental activities of daily living (IADL) to evaluate underlying motor function (e.g., reaching, grasping, and posture) and process skill dysfunction (e.g., using items and searching and locating). See Table 37-3 for a summary of evaluation tools used with stroke survivors.

FUNCTIONAL LIMITATIONS COMMONLY OBSERVED AFTER STROKE

Multiple factors can impede effective and efficient performance of various tasks on which the patient desires to focus in OT. The following section reviews blocks to function that are typically observed during work with stroke survivors.

Inability to Perform Chosen Tasks While Seated

A commonly observed deficit after stroke is the loss of trunk and **postural control.**

Impairment in trunk control may lead to the following problems[40]:
1. Dysfunction of limb control
2. Increased risk for falls
3. Impaired ability to interact with the environment
4. Visual dysfunction secondary to resultant head and neck malalignment

TABLE 37-3

Instrument	Description and Usage
NIH Stroke Scale*[21]	Stroke deficit scale that scores 15 items (e.g., consciousness, vision, extraocular movement, facial control, limb strength, ataxia, sensation, and speech and language)
Canadian Neurological Scale*[26]	Stroke deficit scale that scores 8 items (e.g., consciousness, orientation, speech, motor function, and facial weakness)
Rankin Scale*[17]	Global disability scale with six grades indicating degrees of disability
Canadian Occupational Performance Measure[53] (CCPM)	Client-centered assessment tool based on clients' identification of performance area dysfunction; clients rate importance of self-care, productivity, and leisure skills, as well as their perception of performance and satisfaction with performance Used as outcome measure, as well as patient satisfaction survey
Barthel Index*[57]	Measure of BADL disability that ranges from 0 to 20 or 0 to 100 (by multiplying each item by 5); includes 10 items: bowels, bladder, feeding, grooming, dressing, transfer, toileting, mobility, stairs, and bathing
Kohlman Evaluation of Living Skills (KELS)[79]	Living skills evaluation that includes ratings of 17 tasks (e.g., safety awareness, money management, phone book use, and money and bill management)
Functional Independence Measure* (FIM)[48]	Measure of BADL disability that includes 18 items scored on a seven-point scale; includes subscores for motor and cognitive function; performance areas include self-care, sphincter control, mobility, locomotion, cognition, and socialization
Frenchay Activities Index*[45]	15-item IADL scale that evaluates domestic, leisure, work, and outdoor activities
PCG Instrumental Activities of Daily Living*[55]	IADL evaluation of telephone use, walking, shopping, food preparation, housekeeping, laundry, public transportation, and medication management
Assessment of Motor and Process Skills[35]	16 motor skills (e.g., reach, manipulation, calibration, coordination, posture, and mobility) and 20 process skills (e.g., attends, organizes, searches and locates, initiates, and sequences) evaluated within context of patient-chosen IADL skills; patients choose familiar and culturally relevant tasks from list of 50 standardized activities of various difficulties
Mini-Mental State Examination*[36]	Mental status screening test of orientation to time and place, registration of words, attention, calculation, recall, language, and visual construction
Glasgow Coma Scale*[78]	Level of consciousness scale that includes three sections scoring eye opening, motor, and verbal responses to voice commands or pain
Arnadottir Occupational Therapy Neurobehavioral Evaluation (A-ONE)[7]	Evaluates apraxias, neglect syndromes, body scheme disorders, organization/sequencing dysfunction, agnosias, and spatial dysfunction via BADL and mobility tasks; directly correlates impairment and disability levels of dysfunction
Neurobehavioral Cognitive Status Examination*[50]	Mental status screening test that includes the domains of orientation, attention, comprehension, naming, construction, memory, calculation, similarities, judgment, and repetition
Fugl-Meyer Test*[38]	Motor function evaluation that uses a 3-point scale to score the domains of pain, range of motion, sensation, volitional movement, and balance
Functional Test for the Hemiparetic Upper Extremity[87]	Arm and hand function are assessed via 17 hierarchical functional tasks based on Brunnstrom's view of motor recovery; sample tasks are folding a sheet, screwing in a light bulb, stabilizing a jar, and zipping a zipper
Arm Motor Ability Test (AMAT)[52]	Arm function evaluated by functional ability and quality of movement; test involves performance of 28 tasks (e.g., eating with a spoon, opening jar, tying shoelace, and using telephone)
TEMPA[30,31]	Upper extremity performance test composed of nine standardized tasks (bilateral and unilateral) measured by three criteria: length of execution, functional rating, and task analysis; sample tasks are handle coins, pick up a pitcher and pour water, write and stamp an envelope, and unlock a lock

From references 7, 11-13, 17, 21, 23, 24, 26, 29-31, 33-38, 42, 45, 47-50, 52, 53, 55, 57, 78-80, 86, 87, and 90.
*Recommended in AHCPR's Clinical Practice Guidelines #16, *Post-Stroke Rehabilitation,* 1995.

Continued

TABLE 37-3

Assessments Used with the Stroke Survivor Population—cont'd

Instrument	Description and Usage
Jebsen Test of Hand Function[47]	Hand function evaluation; includes seven test activities: writing a short sentence, turning over index cards, simulated eating, picking up small objects, moving empty and weighted cans, and stacking checkers during timed trials
Motor Assessment Scale*[23]	Motor function evaluation; includes disability and impairment measures; includes arm and hand movements, tone, and mobility (bed, upright, and ambulation)
Motricity Index*[29]	Measures impairments of limb strength with a weighted ordinal scale
Trunk Control Test[37]	Trunk control evaluated on a 0-100 point scale; tasks used: rolling, supine to sit, and balanced sitting
Berg Balance Scale*[12]	Balance assessment of 14 items scored on a 0- to 4-point ordinal scale
Tinetti Test[80]	Evaluates balance and gait in the older adult population
Rivermead Mobility Index*[24]	Measures bed mobility, sitting, standing, transfers, and walking on a pass or fail scale
Functional Reach Test[33]	Balance evaluation; objectively measures length of forward reach in the standing posture
Boston Diagnostic Apnasia Examination*[42]	Assesses sample speech and language behavior, including fluency, naming, word finding, repetition, serial speech, auditory comprehension, reading and writing
Western Aphasia Battery*[49]	Includes an "Aphasia Quotient" and "Cortical Quotient" scored on a 100-point scale: assesses spontaneous speech, repetition, comprehension, naming, reading, and writing
Beck Depression Inventory*[11]	21-item, self-rating scale with attitudinal, somatic, and behavioral components
Geriatric Depression Scale*[90]	Self-rated depression scale of 30 items with a yes-or-no format
Family Assessment Device*[34]	Family assessment of problem solving, communication, roles, affective responsiveness, affective involvement, behavioral control, and general functioning
Medical Outcomes Study/Short Form Health Survey*[86]	Quality of life measure that includes the domains of physical functioning, physical and emotional problems, social function, pain, mental health, vitality, and health perception
Sickness Impact Profile*[13]	Quality of life measure in the format of a 136-item scale with 12 subscales that measure ambulation mobility, body care, emotion, communication, alertness, sleep, eating, home management, recreation, social interactions, and employment

From references 7, 11-13, 17, 21, 23, 24, 26, 29-31, 33-38, 42, 45, 47-50, 52, 53, 55, 57, 78-80, 86, 87, and 90.
*Recommended in AHCPR's Clinical Practice Guidelines #16, *Post-Stroke Rehabilitation,* 1995.

5. Symptoms of dysphagia secondary to proximal malalignment
6. Decreased independence in ADL

The loss of trunk control after a stroke may be observed as an inability to sit in proper alignment, the loss of righting and equilibrium reactions, the inability to reach beyond the arm span because of lack of postural adjustments, and falling during attempts to function.

Stroke survivors who lose trunk control need to use the more functional upper extremity (UE) for postural support to remain upright and prevent falls. In these cases the patient effectively eliminates the ability to engage in ADL and mobility tasks because lifting the more functional arm from the supporting surface can result in a fall. "Trunk control appears to be an obvious prerequisite for the control of more complex limb activities that in turn constitute a prerequisite to complex behavioral skills."[37] Studies have found trunk control to be a predictor of gait recovery,[25] sitting balance,[15] Func-

tional Independence Measure scores,[37] and scores on the Barthel Index[71] after stroke.

Specific effects of a stroke on the trunk include the following:

1. Inability to perceive midline as a result of spatial relations dysfunction and resulting in sitting postures that are misaligned from the vertical
2. Assumption of static postures that do not support engagement in functional activities (e.g., posterior pelvic tilt, kyphosis, and lateral flexion)
3. Multidirectional trunk weakness[16]
4. Spinal contracture secondary to soft-tissue shortening
5. Inability to move the trunk segmentally (i.e., the trunk moves as unit) (Examples of this phenomenon are patients using "log rolling" patterns during bed mobility and an inability to rotate the trunk while reaching for an item across the midline.)
6. Inability to shift weight through the pelvis anteriorly, posteriorly, and laterally.

Specific deficits in trunk control are evaluated during observation of task performance (Box 37-1). Observing tasks allows the therapist to evaluate trunk control in many directions (i.e., isometric, eccentric, and concentric control of the trunk muscle groups [extensors, abdominal muscles, and lateral flexors]) and the patient's limits of stability. *Limits of stability* refers to "boundaries of an area of space in which the body can maintain its position without changing the base of support"[73] or "an area about which the center of mass may be moved over any given base of support without disrupting equilibrium."[32] The therapist must differentiate between the patient's perceived limits of stability and the actual limits of stability. After a stroke it is common to have a disparity between the two because of body scheme disorder, fear of falling, or lack of insight into or awareness of disability. If the patient's perceived limits are greater than his or her actual limits, there is a risk for falls. In other cases the patient's perceived limits are less than actual limits. In such instances the patient will not attempt more dynamic activities or will overrely on adaptive equipment.

Treatment interventions aimed at increasing the patient's ability to perform chosen tasks in seated postures include the following[40]:

1. *Establishing a neutral yet active starting alignment, i.e. a position of readiness to function.* This starting alignment (similar to a typist's posture) is a prerequisite to engaging the limbs in an activity. The desirable posture is as follows:
   - Feet flat on floor and bearing weight
   - Equal weight bearing through both ischial tuberosities
   - A neutral to slight anterior pelvic tilt
   - An erect spine
   - Head over the shoulders and shoulders over the hips

   The reader should attempt reaching activities from the above posture and do the same activities with a posterior pelvic tilt and flexed spine (a typical trunk pattern after stroke). The freedom of movement and the available range for each posture should be compared (Fig. 37-4).

2. *Establishing the ability to maintain the trunk in midline using external cues.* Many patients have difficulty assuming and maintaining the correct posture. The therapist can provide verbal feedback (e.g., "Sit up nice and tall"). Visual feedback (e.g., using a mirror or the therapist assuming the same postural misalignment as the patient) may be helpful. Environmental cues may be used to correct the posture For example, the patient may be instructed to maintain contact between the shoulder and an external target such as a bolster or wall, positioned so that the trunk is in the correct posture.

3. *Maintaining trunk range of motion (ROM) by wheelchair and armchair positioning that maintains the trunk in proper alignment.* The therapist can provide an exercise program focused on trunk range of motion and flexibility. Activities that elicit the desired movement patterns can be chosen, and hands-on mobilization of the trunk can be used if needed. Trunk ranges that should be addressed include flexion, extension, lateral flexion, and rotation.

4. *Prescribing dynamic weight-shifting activities to allow practice of weight shifts through the pelvis.* The most effective way to train weight shifts is to coordinate the trunk and limbs. Positioning of objects during reach beyond the span of either arm requires the patient to adjust the posture to be successful. The reader is encouraged to reach beyond arm span in all directions while seated (preferably while reaching for an object) and to analyze the corresponding postural adjustment of the pelvis and trunk. The position and goal of the task will dictate the required weight shift.

5. *Strengthening the trunk, best achieved by using tasks that require the patient to control the trunk against gravity.* Some examples are bridging of the hips in the supine position to strengthen the back extensors and initiating a roll with the arm and upper trunk to strengthen the abdominal muscles. Strengthening occurs within the context of an activity.

BOX 37-1

Trunk Control Evaluation During Task Performance: Examples of Postural Adjustments That Support Participation in Chosen Activities

Feeding
Anterior weight shift occurs to bring upper body toward table, to prevent spillage of food from utensils, and to support a hand-to-mouth pattern.

Dressing
Lateral weight shift to one side of the pelvis occurs so that pants and underwear can be donned over hips.

Oral Care
Anterior weight shift occurs so that saliva and paste may be expectorated.

Transfer
Trunk extends with concurrent hip flexion to initiate a sit-to-stand transition.

Meal Preparation
Trunk flexes into gravity in a controlled fashion to support a reach pattern to the lower shelf of the refrigerator.

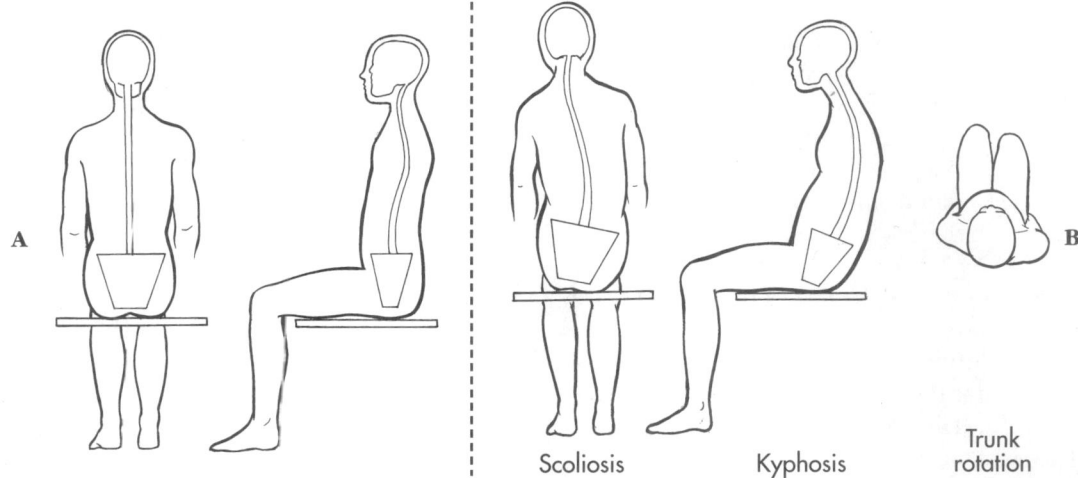

Scoliosis   Kyphosis   Trunk rotation

FIG. 37-4

Normal and poststroke sitting alignment. (From Donato SM, Pulaski KH: Overview of balance impairments: functional implications. In Gillen G, Burkhardt A, editors: *Stroke rehabilitation: a function-based approach,* St Louis, 1998, Mosby.)

6. *Using compensatory strategies and environmental adaptations when trunk control does not improve to a sufficient level and the patient is at risk for injury.* Examples of interventions include wheelchair seating systems (e.g., lateral supports, lumbar rolls, chest straps, and tilt-in-space frames with head supports) and adaptive ADL equipment (e.g., reachers, long-handled equipment) to decrease the amount of required trunk displacements (see Chapter 13).

Inability to Engage in Chosen Activities in Standing

The inability to assume and maintain a standing posture has a significant effect on the type of activities a person may engage in and may play a significant role in the eventual discharge destination for the inpatient recovering from stroke. Impaired upright control has been correlated with an increased risk of falls,[89] as well as with less than optimal functional outcomes[57] on the Barthel Index. Because many basic and instrumental ADL and work and leisure skills require control of standing postures, early training in upright control is a necessary component of stroke rehabilitation programs.

Similar to the deficits seen in sitting, upright standing postures are characterized by asymmetrical weight distribution; unlike deficits in sitting, the weight distribution in standing is seen through the lower extremities[89] in addition to the trunk. Stroke survivors commonly have an inability to bear weight through the affected leg. There may be several reasons for this, including a fear of falling or buckling, patterns of weakness that will not support the weight of the body, spasticity that impedes proper alignment (i.e., plantar flexion spasticity that

effectively blocks weight bearing through the sole of the foot),[41] and perceptual dysfunction.

In addition to asymmetry and an inability to bear weight or shift weight through the affected leg, many stroke patients lose upright postural control and **balance strategies.** Effective upright control depends on the following automatic postural reactions[32,73]:

1. *Ankle strategies* are used to maintain the center of mass over the base of support when movement is centered around the ankles. These strategies control small, slow, swaying motions such as standing in a movie line, engaging in conversations while standing, and stirring a pot on a stovetop. They are most effective when the support surface (floor) is firm and longer than the foot. Ankle weakness, loss of ankle range of motion, and proprioceptive deficits may all contribute to ineffective ankle strategies and balance.

2. *Hip strategies* are used to maintain or restore equilibrium. These strategies are used specifically in response to larger, faster perturbations, when the support surface is compliant, or when the surface is smaller than the feet (e.g., walking on a beam).[46]

3. A *stepping strategy* is used when ankle and hip strategies are, or are perceived to be, ineffective. This strategy results in movement of the base of support toward the center of mass movement. A step is taken to widen the base of support. Tripping over an uneven sidewalk or standing on a bus that unexpectedly stops elicits this strategy.

Both the loss of postural reactions and the inability to bear and shift weight onto the affected leg will result in such functional limitations as gait deviations or dysfunction, an inability to climb stairs, transfer, and perform upright basic ADL (BADL) and IADL, and an increased risk of falls. The assessment process provides the therapist with more specific information regarding the cause of dysfunction. "Specifically, therapists should observe what happens when patients have to move their center of mass over their base of support, move their head, stand on uneven surfaces, function in lower lighting, move from one type of surface to another, or function on a narrower base of support. Therapists should also observe patients' postural alignment, whether a bias in posture exists and in which direction that bias occurs, patients' limits of stability, the width between their feet during functional tasks, and what patients do after losing their balance."[32]

Treatment strategies aimed at improving the patients' ability to perform chosen tasks in standing postures include the following[32,73,89]:

1. *Establishing a symmetrical base of support and proper alignment to prepare to engage in activities.* This starting alignment is assumed to provide ample proximal stability and to support engagement in functional tasks. The therapist may use hands-on support or visual or verbal feedback to establish proper alignment as follows:
   - Feet approximately hip width apart
   - Equal weight bearing through the feet
   - A neutral pelvis
   - Both knees *slightly* flexed
   - Aligned and symmetrical trunk
2. *Establishing the ability to bear weight and shift weight through the more affected lower extremity.*[28] The ability to bear weight may be graded at first. For example, if a patient cannot assume standing because of postural insecurity or imbalance, sitting on a high surface (e.g., stool or raised therapy mat) allows the patient to begin to bear weight but does not require bearing full body weight. As the patient improves, full standing is encouraged, followed by graded weight shifts and progressing to full weight bearing on the affected leg. For example, a modified soccer activity requires the patient to fully shift weight to kick the ball. The environment (e.g., work surface height and placement of objects) is manipulated in conjunction with the patient's positioning to elicit the required weight shift.
3. *Encouraging dynamic reaching activities in multiple environments to develop task-specific weight-shifting abilities.* For example, kitchen activities that require retrieval of cleaning supplies under the sink, in a broom closet, and in overhead cabinets require mastery of multiple postural adjustments and balance strategies.
4. *Using the environment to grade task difficulty and provide external support.* Proper use of the environment can decrease the patient's fear of falling and simultaneously improve confidence and challenge underlying balance skills. Examples include working in front of a high countertop, using one hand for weight bearing as a postural support, and using a walker for support. The patient must not rely too much on external supports because balance strategies may not be fully challenged to reach optimal recovery.
   - *Training upright control within the context of functional tasks that are graded.* Tasks are graded in relation to length of required reach, speed, and progressively more challenging bases of support. Examples include making a bed, changing a pet's food bowl, setting a table, stepping up a curb, cleaning a wall mirror, playing horseshoes or shuffleboard, and doffing slippers in a standing posture. All of these activities require various weight shifts, balance strategies, and the ability to bear weight through both lower extremities. The activity choice is driven by the patient's desires, and the therapist designs positioning and setup of the activity to elicit the desired postural strategies (Fig. 37-5).

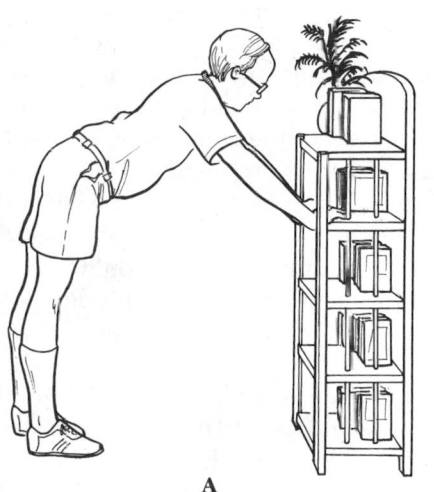
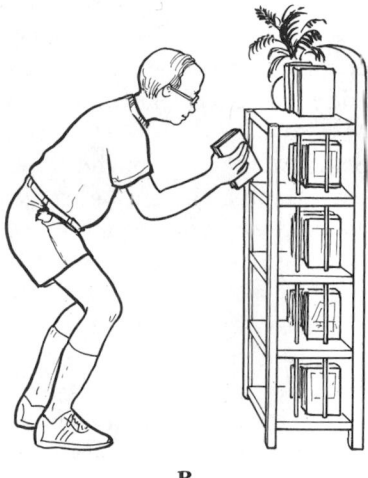

A   B

FIG. 37-5
Activity is positioned to elicit the desired postural strategies. (From Donato SM, Pulaski KH: Overview of balance impairments: functional implications. In Gillen G, Burkhardt A, editors: *Stroke rehabilitation: a function-based approach,* St Louis, 1998, Mosby.)

Inability to Communicate Secondary to Language Dysfunction

CVA may result in a wide variety of speech or language disorders that may vary from mild to severe. These deficits occur most frequently in CVA resulting from damage to the left hemisphere of the brain. They can also occur less frequently with damage to the right hemisphere. All persons with CVA should be evaluated by the speech pathologist for the presence of speech and language disorders. The speech pathologist can provide valuable information to other members of the rehabilitation team and to the family regarding the best techniques for communicating with a particular patient. The occupational therapist should carry over the work of the speech therapist in the treatment sessions, as appropriate. Carryover may occur in reinforcing communication techniques the patient is learning and in presenting instruction in ways the patient is able to understand and integrate.

The specific speech and language dysfunctions described below can exist in mild to severe form and in combination with one another.

Aphasia

Aphasia is a language disorder that results from neurological impairment. It can affect auditory comprehension, reading comprehension (alexia), oral expression, written expression (agraphia), and the ability to interpret gestures. Mathematical deficits (acalculia) can also be present in aphasia. There are several different types of aphasia.

GLOBAL APHASIA. Global aphasia is characterized by a loss of all language skills. Oral expression is lost, except for some persistent or recurrent utterance. Global aphasia is usually the result of involvement of the middle cerebral artery of the dominant cerebral hemisphere. The patient with global aphasia may be sensitive to gestures, vocal inflections, and facial expression. Consequently, the patient may appear to understand more than he or she actually does.[43]

BROCA'S APHASIA. Speech apraxia and agrammatism characterize Broca's aphasia. The apraxia is manifested by slow, labored speech with frequent misarticulations. Syntactical structure is simplified because of the agrammatism, sometimes referred to as telegraphic speech. The patient with this aphasia has good auditory comprehension, except when speech is rapid, grammatically complex, or lengthy. Reading comprehension and writing may be severely affected, and the patient with Broca's aphasia usually has deficits in monetary concepts and the ability to do calculations.[43]

WERNICKE'S APHASIA. Wernicke's aphasia is characterized by impaired auditory comprehension and feedback, with fluent, well-articulated paraphasic speech. Paraphasic speech consists of word substitution errors. Speech may occur at an excessive rate and may be hyperfluent. The patient uses few substantive words and many function words. The patient produces running speech composed of English words in a meaningless sequence. English-speaking patients produce neologisms (non-English nonsense words) interspersed with real words. Reading and writing comprehension is often limited, and mathematical skills may be impaired.[43]

ANOMIC APHASIA. Persons with anomic aphasia have difficulties with word retrieval. Anomia, or word-finding difficulty, occurs in all types of aphasia. However, patients in whom word-finding difficulty is the primary or only symptom may be said to have anomic aphasia. The speech of these patients is fluent, grammatically correct, and well articulated, but there is significant difficulty with word finding. This problem can result in hesitant or slow speech and the substitution of descriptive phrases for actual names of things. Mild to severe deficits in reading comprehension and written expression occur, and mild deficits in mathematical skills may be present.[2,43]

Dysarthria

Patients with dysarthria have an articulation disorder, in the absence of aphasia, because of a dysfunction of the central nervous system (CNS) mechanisms that control speech musculature.[85] This disorder results in paralysis and incoordination of the organs of speech, causing the speech to sound thick, slurred, and sluggish.

Communication with Patients Who Have Aphasia

Although the speech pathologist is responsible for the treatment of speech and language disorders, the occupational therapist can facilitate communication and meaningful interaction with patients who have aphasia.

Patients respond best to intelligent and empathetic understanding from professional staff and family members. Staff and family members communicating with patients should adopt an attitude of patience, relaxation, and acceptance. When talking to the patient, the staff or family member should use simple, short, concrete sentences. Instructions and explanations should be kept simple. The patient should be encouraged, but not pressured, to respond in any way possible. The use of gestures for communication should be encouraged. Having the patient demonstrate through performance is the best way to ensure that instructions are understood.

The occupational therapist can use routine ADL as opportunities to encourage speech. The patient needs to be reassured that the language disorder is part of the disability and is not a manifestation of mental illness. In addition, Rubio[68] has outlined strategies for the occupational therapist to use with patients and their caregivers:

1. Understanding is facilitated when one person talks at a time. Extra noise creates confusion.
2. Give the patient time to respond.
3. Carefully phrase questions to make it easier for the patient to respond; for example, use "yes-no" and "either-or" questions.
4. Use visual cues or gestures with speech to help the patient understand.
5. Never force a response.
6. Use concise sentences.

Do not rush communication because this may increase frustration and decrease the effectiveness of communication.[68]

Inability to Perform Chosen Tasks Secondary to Neurobehavioral Impairments

Neurobehavioral deficit is defined as "a functional impairment of an individual manifested as defective skill performance resulting from a neurologic processing dysfunction that affects performance components such as affect, body scheme, cognition, emotion, gnosis, language, memory, motor movement, perception, personality, sensory awareness, spatial relations, and visuospatial skills."[8] A major responsibility of the occupational therapist treating a stroke survivor is evaluating which neurobehavioral deficits are blocking independent performance of chosen tasks.

Arnadottir[8] has proposed a relationship between the ability to perform daily activities, neurobehavioral impairments, and the CNS origin of the neurobehavioral dysfunction (a CVA, for the purposes of this chapter). She supports this theory with the following relational statements:

1. Behaviors required for task performance are related to neuronal processing at the CNS level. Therefore a relationship also exists between the defective behavioral responses of an individual with CNS damage during performance of ADL and the dysfunction of neuronal processing and performance components resulting from CNS damage.
2. Performance of daily activities requires adequate function of specific parts of the nervous system. Consequently, CNS impairment may result in dysfunction of specific aspects of ADL. For example, a CVA that causes a lesion of the posteroinferior parietal lobe of the left hemisphere commonly results in bilateral motor apraxia. "This neurobehavioral impairment may make manipulation of objects difficult during functional activities such as combing hair, brushing teeth, or holding a spoon while eating."[8]
3. Neurological impairment can be observed through the patient's engagement in daily activities. Thus

---

BOX 37-2

Tooth Brushing Task: Treatment of Neurobehavioral Impairments

Spatial Relations and Spatial Positioning
Positioning of toothbrush and toothpaste while applying paste to brush.
Placement of toothbrush in mouth
Positioning of bristles in mouth
Placement of brush under faucet

Spatial Neglect
Visual search for and use of brush, paste, and cup in affected hemisphere
Visual search and use of faucet handle in affected hemisphere

Body Neglect
Brushing of affected side of mouth

Motor Apraxia
Manipulation of toothbrush during task performance
Manipulation of cap from toothpaste
Squeezing of toothpaste onto brush

Ideational Apraxia
Appropriate use of objects (brush, paste, cup) during task.

Organization and Sequencing
Sequencing of task (removal of cap, application of paste to brush, turning on water, and putting brush in mouth)
Continuation of task to completion

Attention
Attention to task (for greater difficulty, distractions such as conversation, flushing toilet, or running water may be added)
Refocus on task after distraction

Figure-Ground
Distinguishing white toothbrush and toothpaste from sink

Initiation and Perseverance
Initiation of task on command
Cleaning parts of mouth for appropriate period of time, then moving bristles to another part of mouth
Discontinuation of task when complete

Visual Agnosia
Use of touch to identify objects

Problem Solving
Search for alternatives if toothpaste or toothbrush is missing

From Gillen G, Burkhardt A: *Stroke rehabilitation: a function-based approach*, St Louis, 1998, Mosby.

through the analysis of ADL the integrity of the CNS can be evaluated (Box 37-2).

To properly evaluate the effect of neurobehavioral deficits on task performance, the therapist must develop activity analysis skills with the goal of analyzing which performance components are necessary to achieve an outcome that is satisfactory to the patient. Even the "simplest" of BADL tasks challenge multiple underlying skills (Fig. 37-3 and Boxes 37-3 and 37-4).[8,68]

BOX 37-3
Examples of Environmental and Task Manipulation to Challenge Component Skills During Meal Preparation

Spatial Neglect
Place ingredients in both visual fields
Choose a task that requires use of right and left burners

Figure-Ground
Place necessary utensils in a cluttered drawer
Use utensils that match the color of the counter

Spatial Dysfunction
Prepare items that require the patient to pour ingredients from one container to another (e.g., pour pasta into a bowl or fill a pot with water)

Motor Apraxia
Choose recipes that require manipulation of food items
Choose recipes that require control of distal extremity adjustments (e.g., using a ladle, whisking, and stirring)

BOX 37-4
Sample Compensatory Strategies for Neurobehavioral Deficits Affecting Dressing Skills

Spatial Neglect
Place necessary clothing on right side of closet and drawers
Move dresser to right side of room

Motor Apraxia
Utilize loose-fitting clothing without fasteners
Use Velcro closures

Spatial Dysfunction
Use shirts with a front emblem to identify proper orientation
Lay out clothing in the proper orientation

Arnadottir[7,8] proposed a system of observing patients engaged in functional activities, allowing errors (as long as they are safe) to occur, analyzing the errors, and, finally, detecting the impairments that are interfering with task performance so that an appropriate treatment plan can be developed. She cautioned that when the therapist analyzes errors and observed behaviors, knowledge of neurobehavior, cortical function, activity analysis, and clinical reasoning must be considered in the results of the evaluation (Table 37-4).

Treatment aimed at counteracting the effects of neurobehavioral dysfunction may be based upon an adaptive and compensatory approach or a restorative and remedial approach.[59,61,68] A combination of approaches has also been suggested (Table 37-5).[1]

Decisions regarding choosing a treatment approach may be difficult. Neistadt[59,60] suggested evaluating a patient's learning potential in the context of ADL evaluation and training, focusing on such issues as the number of repetitions needed to learn new approaches to tasks and the type of transfer of learning that is demonstrated.

Toglia[81] has suggested that the transfer of learning from one context to another (e.g., transferring skills learned from making a cup of tea in the OT clinic to meal preparation at home) may be facilitated by the therapist through the following methods:
1. Varying treatment environments
2. Varying the nature of the task
3. Helping patients become aware of how they process information
4. Teaching processing strategies
5. Relating new learning to previously learned skills

Toglia[81] has identified degrees of transfer of learning. The degree of transfer is defined by the number of task characteristics that differ from those of the original task. Examples of these characteristics are spatial orientation, mode of presentation (e.g., auditory or visual), movement requirements, and environmental context.

A near transfer of learning involves transfer between two tasks that are different by one to two characteristics. Intermediate transfer involves transfer of learning to a task that varies by three to six characteristics. A far transfer involves a task that is conceptually similar but has one or no characteristics in common. Finally, a very far transfer involves the "spontaneous application of what has been learned in treatment to everyday living."[81]

From her review of the literature, Neistadt[61] reached the following conclusions:
1. Near transfer from remedial tasks to similar tasks is possible for all patients with brain injury.
2. Intermediate, far, and very far transfer from remedial to functional tasks will occur only with localized brain lesions and good cognitive skills and after training with a variety of treatment tasks.

TABLE 37-4
Evaluating the Effect of Neurobehavioral Dysfunction on Task Performance

Performance Area	Observed Behavior	Possible Impairment
Grooming	Difficulty adjusting grasp on razor or toothbrush	Motor apraxia
	Using a comb to brush teeth	Ideational apraxia
	Repetitive brushing of one side of the mouth	Premotor perseveration
Feeding	Not eating food on the left side of the plate	Spatial neglect
	Overestimating or underestimating distance of glass results in knocking over glass	Spatial relations dysfunction
	"Forgetting" that a glass of orange juice is in the hand results in spillage as the patient attends to another aspect of the meal	Body neglect
	Hand is placed in cereal bowl	Body neglect
Dressing	Patient attempts to put socks on after he or she has put on sneakers	Organization and sequencing dysfunction
	Patient cannot locate armholes in an undershirt	Spatial relations dysfunction
	Only the right side of the body is dressed	Body neglect
	Patient attempts to dress the therapist's arms instead of his or her own	Somatoagnosia
Mobility	Patient not able to locate the bathroom in his or her hospital room	Topographic disorientation
	Patient does not lock brakes or remove wheelchair footrests before attempting to transfer	Organization and sequencing dysfunction
	After a transfer, only the intact buttock is on the seat of the chair	Body neglect

From Arnadottir G: *The brain and behavior: assessing cortical dysfunction through activities of daily living*, St Louis, 1990, Mosby; Anadottir G: Impact of neurobehavioral deficits of activities of daily living. In Gillen G, Burkhardt A, editors: *Stroke rehabilitation: a function-based approach*, St Louis, 1998, Mosby.

TABLE 37-5
Treatment Approaches for Neurobehavioral Deficits After Stroke

Compensatory and Adaptive Approach	Restorative and Remedial Approach	Combination Approach
Repetitive practice of tasks	Restoration of component skills	Rejects dichotomy between compensatory and restorative approaches
Top-down approach	Bottom-up approach	
Emphasizes intact skill training	Deficit-specific	Uses optimally relevant occupations and environments as the treatment modality to challenge components
Emphasizes modification	Targets cause of symptoms and emphasizes components	
Uses environmental or task modifications to support optimal performance	Assumes transfer of training will occur	Treatment choice is driven by tasks relevant to patient needs; tasks are presented so that the underlying deficits are challenged via the task
Activity choice driven by performance challenges, not component deficits	Assumes improved component performance will result in increased skill	
Treats symptoms, not the cause	Activity choice driven by component deficits	Rejects usage of contrived activities
Patient-driven compensatory strategies		
Caregiver-therapist environmental adaptations	Research demonstrates short-term results with skills generalizable to very similar tasks	
Task-specific and not generalizable		

3. Far and very far transfer from remedial to functional tasks will not occur for clients with diffuse injury and severe cognitive deficits.

Using a functional and meaningful task as a treatment modality promotes acquisition of a desired skill, and the therapist may use this task to challenge multiple underlying performance components.[1,68] It is up to the therapist to present the task by manipulating the environment in a way that challenges the underlying skills. If a compensatory approach is chosen, adaptive techniques are used to counteract the effects of the underlying neurobehavioral deficits.

Inability to Perform Chosen Tasks Secondary to Upper Extremity Dysfunction

The loss of UE control is common after stroke, with 88% of stroke survivors having some level of UE dysfunction.[65] The stroke survivor's ability to integrate the affected arm into chosen tasks may be limited by such multiple factors as the following:[39]

1. Pain
2. Contracture and deformity
3. Loss of selective **motor control**
4. Weakness[19]
5. Tonal dysfunction[14]
6. Superimposed orthopedic limitations
7. Loss of postural control to support UE control
8. Learned nonuse[77]
9. Loss of biomechanical alignment[22]
10. Inefficient and ineffective movement patterns

Integration into Function

UE evaluation procedures should focus primarily on assessing the patient's ability to integrate the UE into performance of functional tasks. Standardized evaluations such as the TEMPA,[30,31] AMAT,[52] Jebsen,[47] and AMPS[35] (Table 37-3) are available to objectively measure the patient's ability to use the affected extremity during task performance.

The UE may be used during functional performance in different ways, including but not limited to the following[39]:

1. *Weight bearing.* Weight bearing through the hand and forearm with an extended elbow is a pattern used during ADL and mobility tasks. The establishment of weight bearing is a goal of UE rehabilitation.[14] Effective control of weight bearing depends on enough trunk and scapula stability to accept partial body weight, control of *active* elbow extension, and ability of the hand to bear weight without losing the palmar arches. Once weight bearing is established, the patient can effectively use the arm as a postural support (e.g., by supporting the upper body weight with the affected arm while wiping crumbs from the table with the more functional arm), as an assist during transitional movements (e.g., while pushing up from side-lying to sitting), and for fall prevention (increased postural support is provided).

2. *Moving objects across a work surface with a static grasp.* Such activities as ironing, opening or closing a drawer, polishing, and sliding a paper across the table are all examples of UE control of movement that does not occur with the arm in space. The hand is in contact with the objects involved in the task or is supported on the work surface; therefore these types of tasks do not require the same control as, and may require less effort than, activities performed while the patient is reaching in space, such as removing dishes from a cabinet or reaching for food in the refrigerator. This movement pattern can be used in multiple tasks and at the same time strengthens various muscle groups used to eventually support reach in space.

3. *Reach and manipulation.* Reviews of research on UE motor control[2,39] have identified two components of function during reaching activities. The first component is the transportation component, which is defined as the trajectory of the arm between the starting position and the object. The second component is the manipulation component, which is the formation of grip by combined movements of the thumb and the index finger during arm movement. Finger posturing anticipates the real grasp and occurs during transportation of the hand toward the object.[2] The shaping of the hand is independent of the manipulation itself. Trombly's[84] reaching studies of patients with left hemiparesis documented that the ability to reach smoothly and with coordination was significantly less on the affected than on the unaffected side. The continuous movement strategy was lost, movement time was longer, peak velocity occurred earlier, and weakness indicators were present.

Trombly[83] demonstrated that although muscular activity did not improve in the patients in her study, the discontinuity improved over time. She stated that the "level and pattern of muscle activity of these subjects depended on the biomechanical demands of the task rather than any stereotypical neurological linkages between the muscles."

Patients are commonly observed demonstrating the use of stereotypical movement patterns of the UE. These patterns are characterized by scapula elevation and fixation, humeral abduction, elbow flexion, and wrist flexion. Mathiowetz and Bass Haugen[56] suggested that the use of these movement patterns is evidence of attempts to use remaining systems to complete tasks. They gave an example of a patient with weak shoulder flexors trying to lift an arm. The patient flexes the elbow when trying to raise the arm because this movement strategy shortens the lever arm and makes shoulder flexion easier.

The following are examples of using treatment activities to improve the patient's ability to integrate the UE into tasks[2,6,14,22,39,41,70,74]:

1. Using objects of different sizes and shapes to encourage control of the hand during reach and manipulation

2. Choosing activities that are appropriate to the patient's level of available motor control

3. Using constraint-induced movement techniques: a technique in which the *less affected* UE is constrained (e.g., with a sling and splint) to force use of the affected extremity, providing massed practice of graded activities for the affected side to increase functional use[77]

4. Specifically training the arm to be used in **weight bearing**, reach, and manipulation situations within the context of ADL and mobility
5. Presenting the patient with graded tasks related to the number of degrees of freedom, the level of required antigravity control, and the resistance involved in the task (Fig. 37-6)

Upper Extremity Complications After Stroke

SUBLUXATION. Subluxation, or malalignment caused by instability of the glenohumeral joint, is a common occurrence after stroke. The subluxation may be inferior (head of the humerus below the glenoid fossa), anterior (head of the humerus anterior to the fossa), or superior (head of the humerus lodged under

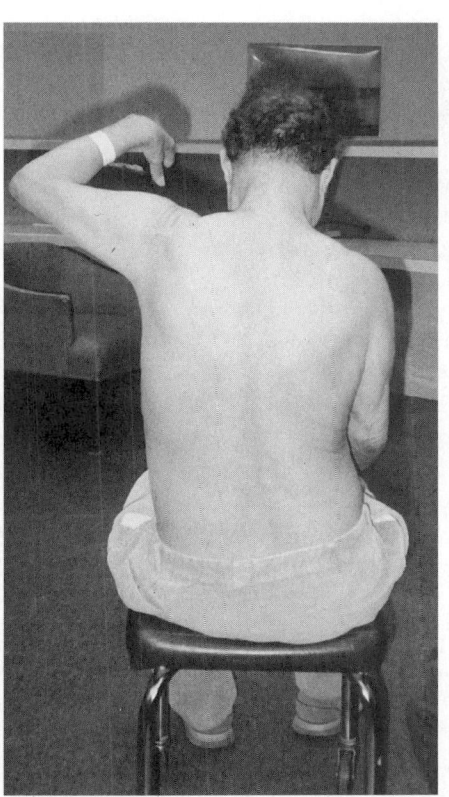

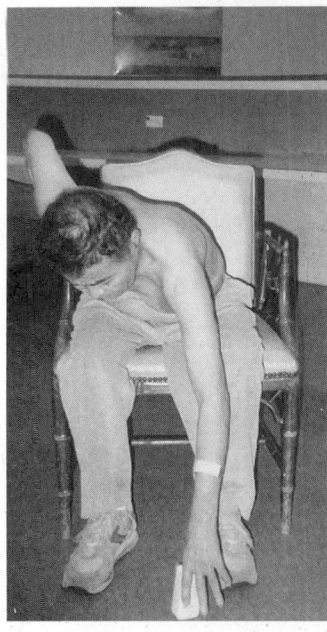
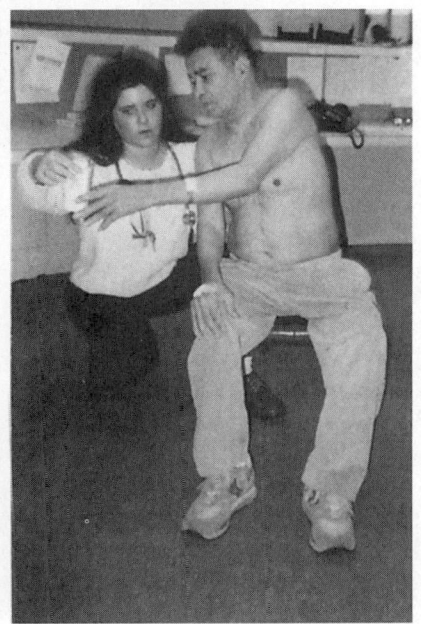

FIG. 37-6
The task is designed to elicit the desired motor pattern; purpose of the activity drives the motor output. (From Gillen G: Upper extremity function and management. In Gillen G, Burkhardt A, editors: *Stroke rehabilitation: a function-based approach,* St Louis, 1998, Mosby.)

the acromion-coracoid).[70] Cailliet[22] and Basmajian[10] have described the mechanism of inferior subluxation, in which the head of the humeral head drifts inferior to the glenoid fossa. This common subluxation occurs as a result of malalignment of the scapula and the trunk. The normal position of the scapula is one of upward rotation, an orientation that "cradles" the head of the humerus and stabilizes it in alignment. After stroke the scapula commonly assumes a position of downward rotation, resulting in subluxation of the glenohumeral joint (Fig. 37-7).

A common misunderstanding about subluxation is that it is associated with pain. The literature does not support this relationship.[91] Because the shoulder is unstable after a stroke, care must be taken to support the flail shoulder in bed (e.g., using pillows to maintain alignment), wheelchair (e.g., with lap boards or pillows), and in upright position (e.g., putting the hands in a pocket or taping the shoulder). Treatment to reduce a subluxation should focus on achieving trunk alignment and scapula stability in a position of upward rotation.[70]

ABNORMAL SKELETAL MUSCLE ACTIVITY. A change in the resting state of the limb and postural muscles is common after stroke.[14] Immediately after a stroke, there is a change in available/resting skeletal

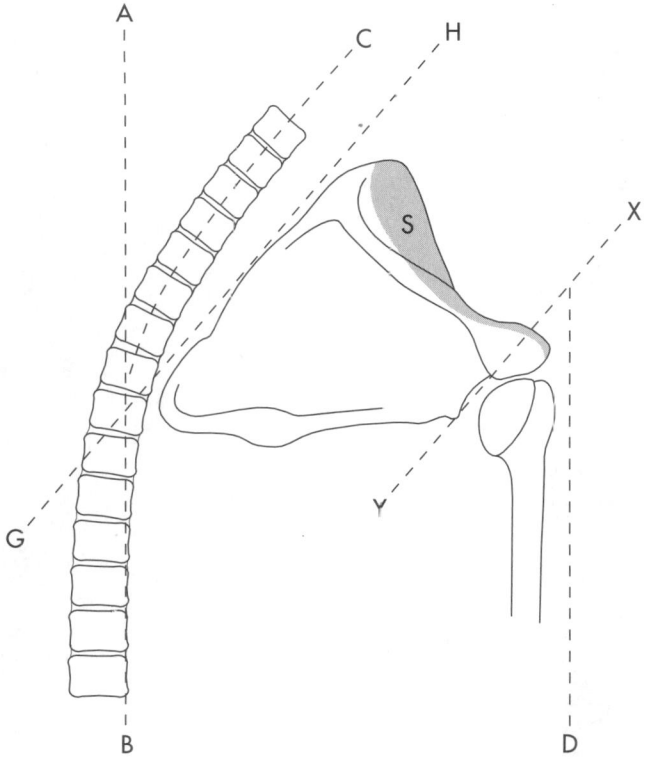

FIG. 37-7
Biomechanics of subluxation. (From Gillen G: Upper extremity function and management. In Gillen G, Burkhardt A, editors: *Stroke rehabilitation: a function-based approach,* 1998, Mosby.)

muscle activity. Most commonly, in the acute state there is low tone ("low-tone stage"). During this low-tone stage the limbs and trunk become increasingly influenced by the pull of gravity. Little or no available muscle activity is available at this stage, resulting in deviations from the normal resting alignment of the musculoskeletal system.

Generally the inability to recruit and maintain muscle activity is the greatest limiting factor at this stage. Because of the generalized lack of muscle activity and the dependent nature of the trunk and limbs, secondary problems can occur.[41] These include the following:
1. Edema of the dorsal surface of the hand that pools under the extensor tendons, effectively blocking active or passive digit flexion
2. Overstretching of the joint capsule of the glenohumeral joint
3. Eventual shortening of muscles that are passively positioned, in an effort to support a weak limb (Commonly, flaccid upper extremities are positioned in the patient's lap, on a pillow, on a lap tray, or in a sling. These static positions, although they support the arm, result in prolonged positioning of certain muscle groups [internal rotators, elbow flexors, and wrist flexors] in a shortened position, placing them at risk for mechanical shortening. Interestingly, these are the muscle groups that tend to become spastic as time progresses.)
4. Overstretching of the antagonists to the previously mentioned muscles
5. Risk of joint and soft-tissue injury during ADL and mobility tasks (Because of the lack of control associated with a low-tone stage, the arm dangles and is not positioned appropriately during dynamic activities. Common examples include an arm being caught in the wheel during wheelchair mobility, pinning of the arm during bed mobility or rest, sitting on the arm after a transfer, or weight bearing through a flexed wrist during engagement in self-care activities.)

The progression to a state of increased or excessive skeletal muscle activity (increased tone) with clonus, stereotypical posturing of the trunk and limbs, hyperactive stretch reflexes, and increased resistance to passive limb movements that are velocity dependent may occur within several days or months of the stroke.[41]

As spasticity increases, the risk for soft-tissue shortening is heightened. This factor may lead to a vicious circle of spasticity to soft-tissue shortening to overrecruitment of shortened muscles to increased stretch reflexes. Secondary problems that may occur if the spasticity is not managed in a therapy program include the following[41]:
1. Deformity of the limbs, specifically the distal upper limb (elbow to digits)
2. Tissue maceration of the palm
3. Possible "masking" of underlying selective motor control

4. Pain syndromes resulting from loss of normal joint kinematics (These syndromes are usually related to soft-tissue contracture that blocks full joint excursion. A typical example is the loss of full passive external rotation of the glenohumeral joint. Attempts at forced abduction in these cases will result in a painful impingement syndrome of the tissues in the subacromial space.)

5. Impaired ability to manage BADL tasks, specifically UE dressing and bathing of the affected hand and axilla when flexor posturing is present

6. Loss of reciprocal arm swing during gait activities

In the past, the sensorimotor approaches were used to treat patients with abnormal skeletal muscle activity (see Chapters 32 through 36). These approaches were developed by Rood, Bobath, Knott and Voss, and Brunnstrom and are based on an understanding of CNS dysfunction at the time these clinicians were doing their research (the mid-1900s). Although these interventions may be used, their effectiveness is being challenged as occupational therapists move toward models of evidence-based practice. When choosing treatment techniques or a treatment approach, therapists must consider that "neither research evidence nor expert consensus adequately supports recommendations concerning the superiority of one type of exercise regimen over another. . . ."[65]

PREVENTION OF PAIN SYNDROMES AND CONTRACTURE

PROTECTION OF UNSTABLE JOINTS. During the low-tone stage, joints tend to become malaligned secondary to loss of muscular stabilization. In these cases patients are at risk for injury to unstable joints (traction injuries and joint trauma) because of the joint instability. The glenohumeral and wrist joints are particularly at risk. The glenohumeral joint (usually already inferiorly subluxated at this stage) is at risk for a superimposed orthopedic injury if another individual unknowingly pulls on the affected arm during self-care and mobility or during unskilled passive range of motion (PROM) of the joint. The unstable glenohumeral joint is in a malaligned state, putting the patient at risk for an impingement syndrome during PROM if normal joint mechanics is not addressed. Key joint motions of concern are upward rotation of the scapula and external (lateral) rotation of the shoulder. If these motions are not present and range of motion is forced, the patient is at risk for the development of an impingement and pain syndrome.[41]

Patients with low tone also have an unstable wrist. Care should be taken to protect the wrist if the patients are not controlling the joint during ADL and mobility tasks. Patients commonly practice a bed mobility or lower extremity dressing sequence, then complete the task while bearing weight through a malaligned flexed wrist. These patients are at risk for orthopedic injury (traumatic synovitis) and may be considered candidates for splinting to protect the wrist.[39]

MAINTAINING SOFT-TISSUE LENGTH. Patients who have both increased and decreased skeletal muscle activity are at risk for soft-tissue contracture secondary to the immobilization that occurs during both low-tone and increased tone stages. The maintenance of tissue length is a 24-hour regimen. This regimen involves frequent variations in resting postures during waking hours, teaching the patient and significant others *appropriate* ROM procedures, daytime and nighttime positioning programs, and staff and family education so that positioning and exercise programs may be carried out in the home environment.[41]

There must be no prolonged static positioning (e.g., prolonged use of a sling). Rather, teaching patients to adjust their resting postures during the day will help prevent soft-tissue tightness.

POSITIONING PROGRAMS. The same wheelchair and bed positioning programs should not be applied to every patient. Instead positioning should be individualized and focus on (1) promoting normal resting alignment of the trunk and limbs in an effort to maintain tissue length on both sides of the joints and (2) providing stretch to muscle groups that have been identified as contracture prone or already shortened.

SOFT-TISSUE ELONGATION. If soft-tissue shortening and length-associated changes have already developed, the treatment of choice is low-load prolonged stretch (LLPS). LLPS involves placing the soft tissues in question on submaximal stretch for prolonged periods. This technique is quite different from the common passive range of motion with terminal stretch (high-load brief stretch) programs commonly used to treat this population.[58]

LLPS programs can be implemented in various ways, including splinting, casting, and positioning programs. For example, during a UE assessment, a patient is noted to have tightness in the internal rotators, overactive internal rotation during attempts to move, and weakened external rotators. An effective LLPS would involve having the patient rest in a supine position with both hands behind his or her head, allowing the elbows to drop toward the bed. This is a normal resting posture during recumbent leisure activities (e.g., watching television) and effectively elongates the muscle group identified as a contracture risk for a prolonged period.[41]

LLPS can also be achieved through splinting programs. A common example is that of a splint designed to elongate the long flexors of the hand during sleeping hours.

SPLINTING. Commonly a controversial subject in the management of stroke, splinting should be considered on a case-by-case basis and may be quite effective for many clients.[58] In the low-tone stage the most common uses for splints are maintaining joint alignment, protecting the tissues from shortening or overstretching, preventing injury to the extremity, and serving as an adjunctive treatment for edema control.[58] Specifically, splinting support may be needed to provide palmar arch support and maintain neutral wrist deviation and the neutral position of the wrist between flexion and extension. For most cases the fingers do not require splinting in this stage of recovery.[58]

Splints may also be effective for patients developing spasticity. In these cases the splints may be used to maintain soft-tissue length, provide LLPS, place muscles at their resting lengths on both sides of the joints, and attempt distal relaxation by promoting proximal alignment.[58]

PATIENT MANAGEMENT. In addition to the interventions already described, it is helpful to train the patient to manage his or her UE. For a patient with low tone the most important information to share with the patient and significant others is the method for protecting the unstable joints and maintaining full range of motion. In the spastic stage the treatment of choice is to teach positioning that will provide prolonged elongation to the overactive muscles and that will prevent contracture. Examples of positions that may be prescribed during leisure or self-care activities include the following[41]:

1. Weight bearing on the extended arm (elongates commonly shortened UE musculature)
2. In supine position, hands behind the head while allowing the elbows to drop toward the bed (provides stretch to the internal rotators)
3. In supine position, a pillow protracting the scapula and under the elbow to promote glenohumeral joint alignment
4. Lying on a protracted scapula to maintain stretch of the retractors and maintain scapulathoracic mobility
5. Supporting the involved wrist with the more functional hand and reaching down toward the floor with both hands (This pattern will elongate muscles that tend to contract during difficult activities, which is particularly helpful after gait activities or difficult self-care activities.)

The keys to prescribing a proper resting posture are to identify muscle groups in the trunk and upper limb that are shortening, overactive, or at risk to develop shortening, and to select a comfortable posture that elongates the muscle group for a prolonged period.

The Nonfunctional Upper Extremity

Although the restoration of UE control is a realistic goal for some patients, many patients will not regain enough control to integrate the affected UE into ADL and mobility tasks. Patients who will not regain enough control require extensive retraining in BADL and IADL[65] (see Chapter 13) using one-handed techniques and prescription of appropriate assistive devices (Box 37-5). Persons

---

BOX 37-5

Examples of Assistive Devices Used After Stroke to Improve Task Performance

Rocker knife
Elastic laces and lace locks
Adapted cutting board
Dycem
Plate guards
Pot stabilizer
Playing card holder
Suction devices to stabilize mixing bowls, cleaning brushes

---

in this population are also candidates for dominance retraining. Deformity control to prevent body image issues is paramount for these patients.

Inability to Perform Chosen Tasks Secondary to Visual Impairment

The processing of visual information is a complex act that requires intact functioning of multiple peripheral and CNS structures to support functional independence. The site of the lesion determines the visual dysfunction and the effect on task performance (Fig. 37-8).[7]

Visual dysfunction and its treatment are detailed in Chapter 24. In general, treatment may focus on remediation such as eye calisthenics, fixations, scanning, visual motor techniques, and bilateral integration. Adaptive techniques are also used, including a change in working distance, the use of prisms, adaptations for driving, adaptations for reading, changes in lighting, and enlarged print.[3,72]

Psychosocial Adjustment

An important role of the occupational therapist is helping in the patient's adjustment to hospitalization and, more important, to disability. Much patience and a supportive approach by the therapist are essential. The therapist must be sensitive to the fact that the patient has experienced a devastating and life-threatening illness that has caused sudden and dramatic changes in the patient's life roles and performance. The therapist must be cognizant of the normal adjustment process and must gear the approach and performance expectations to the patient's level of adjustment. Frequently the patient is not ready to engage in rehabilitation measures with wholehearted effort until several months after onset of the disability.

Family education is extremely important throughout the treatment program. The family can be better equipped to assist their loved one with the adjustment

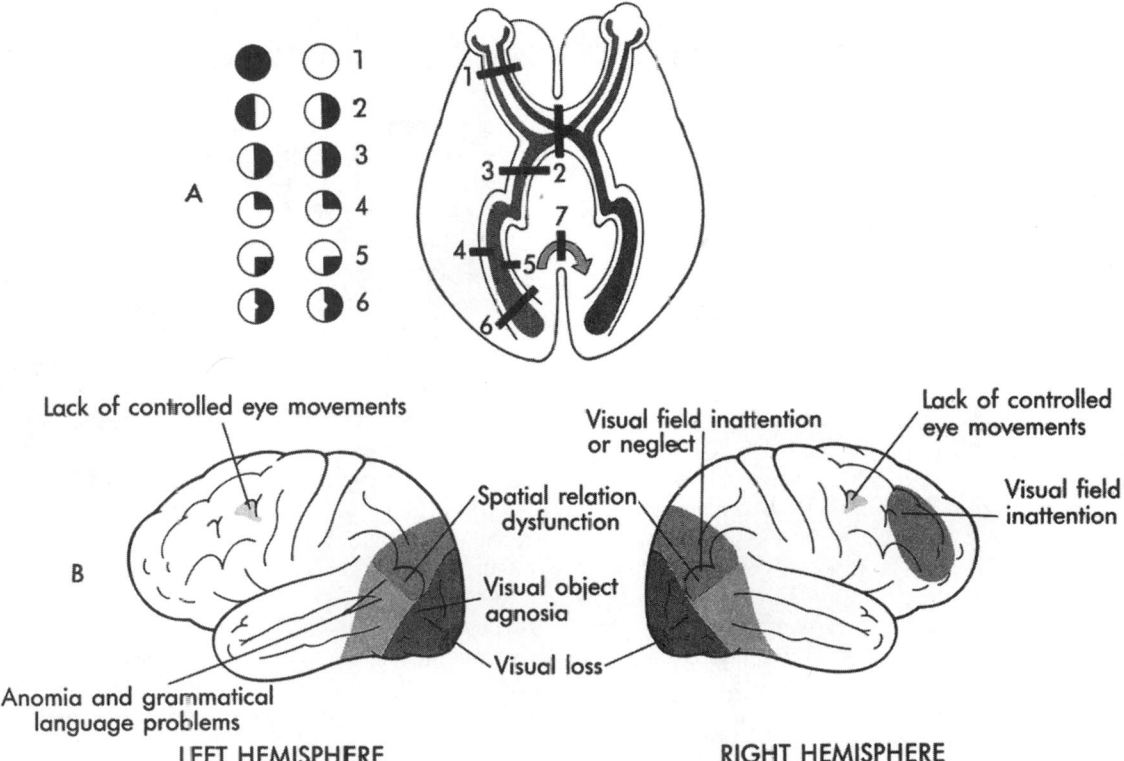

FIG. 37-8
Visual processing deficits. (From Arnadottir G: *The brain and behavior: assessing cortical dysfunction through activities of daily living,* St Louis, 1990, Mosby.)

to disability if they have knowledge and understanding of the disability and its implications.

Many patients dwell on the possibility of full recovery of function and need to be made aware gradually that some residual dysfunction is likely. The therapist may approach this probability by discussing in objective terms what is known about prognosis for functional recovery from CVA. This information may have to be reviewed many times with the patient before the patient begins to apply it to his or her recovery, and it should be done in a way that is honest and yet does not destroy all hope.

The OT program should focus on the skills and abilities of the patient. The patient's attention should be focused, through the performance of activity, on his or her remaining and newly learned skills. The OT program can also involve therapeutic group activities for socialization and sharing of common problems and their solutions. The discovery that there are residual abilities, and perhaps new abilities and success at performing many daily living skills and activities that were initially thought to be impossible, can improve the patient's mental health and outlook.

SUMMARY

CVA is a complex disability that challenges the skills of professional health care workers. Although the number and effectiveness of approaches for the remediation of affected motor, sensory, perceptual, cognitive, and performance dysfunctions have increased considerably, many limitations in treatment remain. The occupational therapist must bear in mind that the degree to which the patient achieves treatment goals depends on the CNS damage and recovery, psychoneurological residuals, psychosocial adjustment, and the skilled application of appropriate treatment by all concerned health professionals.

Some patients remain severely disabled in spite of the noblest efforts of rehabilitation workers, whereas others recover quite spontaneously with minimal help in a short period. Most patients benefit from the professional skills of occupational therapists and other rehabilitation specialists and achieve improvement of performance skills and resumption of meaningful occupational roles.

CASE STUDY 37-1

CASE STUDY—Mr. L.

Mr. L. is a 64-year-old man who lives in an elevator apartment by himself. He works as a manager for a garden center and was looking forward to retiring next year to enjoy his lifelong hobbies of furniture refinishing and antiquing.

Mr. L. has a medical history of atrial fibrillation and one morning woke up with slurred speech and an inability to move his left side. His medical workup revealed a large right cerebrovascular accident of the middle cerebral artery. Mr. L. was medically stabilized and admitted to the local rehabilitation center.

Mr. L. was seen by occupational therapy (OT), as well as by physical therapy, speech-language pathology, and respiratory therapy. His OT evaluation revealed that he was cognitively intact except for mild, short-term memory loss that was attributed to his being overwhelmed with his situation. The evaluation also revealed the appearance of depression (poor eye contact, no initiation of conversation), 0/5 strength in his left upper extremity with an inferior subluxation, loss of trunk control characterized by falling to the left, and an impaired ability to stand secondary to knee buckling. He required moderate assistance for basic ADL (except being independent with oral care and shaving while seated) and maximal assistance for instrumental ADL requiring bilateral upper extremities.

Mr. L. was a private person and identified the desire to toilet, bathe, and dress in at least his undergarments independently as an initial focus of OT intervention. Activities of interest, such as plant care and modified sports activities, were chosen in conjunction with Mr. L. These activities were presented in such a manner as to remediate trunk control and standing balance. The activities were graded to promote increasing amounts of weight shifting and tolerance for sitting and standing postures.

Specific one-handed techniques for dressing and toileting were taught to Mr. L. He was encouraged to practice independently. Durable medical equipment (tub bench and commode) was prescribed to increase Mr. L.'s safety during bathroom activities and to compensate for his balance dysfunction. As he mastered his chosen tasks, Mr. L.'s affect brightened, he was able to continue his participation in treatment, and his outlook related to his future remained optimistic.

Although Mr. L. did not regain use of his upper extremity, adaptive techniques and equipment allowed him to be independent in his chosen activities. He was provided with a home exercise program to maintain upper extremity flexibility and prevent pain. He continued to work on instrumental ADL and leisure task participation during his rehabilitation stay and with his home care occupational therapist.

REVIEW QUESTIONS

1. Define *CVA* and list three of its causes.
2. List the disturbances that can result from occlusion of the ACA, MCA, PCA, and cerebellar arteries.
3. Name three modifiable risk factors associated with stroke.
4. Define *transient ischemic attack*.
5. Name three functional deficits that occur as a result of loss of trunk control.
6. Besides the paralysis of limbs and trunk after CVA, what important motor disturbances can result?
7. Name two components of a "client-centered approach" to evaluation.
8. What are two frames of reference used to treat neurobehavioral impairments after stroke?
9. Name three postural reactions that support standing activities.
10. How does aphasia differ from dysarthria?
11. Describe four ways to aid effective communication with an aphasic patient.
12. What is the importance of comprehensive occupational therapy evaluation of patients with hemiplegia?
13. Describe two methods used to maintain range of motion.
14. List four major elements of the occupational therapy program for hemiplegia. Describe the purposes of each.
15. How can occupational therapy assist with the psychosocial adjustment of the hemiplegic patient?

REFERENCES

1. Abreu B et al: Occupational performance and the functional approach. In Royeen C: *AOTA self-study: cognitive rehabilitation*, Bethesda, Md, 1994, American Occupational Therapy Association.
2. Ada L et al: Task-specific training of reaching and manipulation. In Bennett KMB, Castiello U, editors: *Insights into the reach to grasp movements*, New York, 1994, Elsevier Science.
3. Aloisio L: Visual dysfunction. In Gillen G, Burkhardt A, editors: *Stroke rehabilitation: a function-based approach*, St Louis, 1998, Mosby.
4. American Heart Association: *1999 Heart and stroke statistical update*, Dallas, 1998, The Association.
5. American Occupational Therapy Association: Uniform terminology for occupational therapy, ed 3, *Am J Occup Ther* 48(11):1047-1054, 1994.
6. Andersen LT: Shoulder pain in hemiplegia, *Am J Occup Ther* 39(1):11-19, 1985.
7. Arnadottir G: *The brain and behavior: assessing cortical dysfunction through activities of daily living*, St Louis, 1990, Mosby.
8. Arnadottir G: Impact of neurobehavioral deficits of activities of daily living. In Gillen G, Burkhardt A, editors: *Stroke rehabilitation: a function-based approach*, St Louis, 1998, Mosby.
9. Bartels MN: Pathophysiology and medical management of stroke. In Gillen G, Burkhardt A, editors: *Stroke rehabilitation: a function-based approach*, St Louis, 1998, Mosby.
10. Basmajian JV: The surgical anatomy and function of the arm-trunk mechanism, *Surg Clin North Am* 43:1471-1482, 1963.
11. Beck AT, Steer RA: *Beck Depression Inventory Manual*, rev ed, New York, 1987, Psychological Corp.

12. Berg K et al: Measuring balance in the elderly: preliminary development of an instrument, *Physiother Can* 41:304-311, 1989.

13. Bergner M, Bobbitt RA, Carter WB, et al: The sickness impact profile: development and final revision of a health status measure, *Med Care* 19(8):787-805, 1981.

14. Bobath B: *Adult hemiplegia: evaluation and treatment*, ed 3, Oxford, 1990, Butterworth-Heinemann.

15. Bohannon RW: Recovery and correlates of trunk muscle strength after stroke, *Int J Rehabil Res* 18(4):162-167, 1995.

16. Bohannon RW, Cassidy D, Walsh S: Trunk muscle strength is impaired multidirectionally after stroke, *Clin Rehabil* 9(1):47-51, 1995.

17. Bonita R, Beaglehole R: Recovery of motor function after stroke, *Stroke* 19(12):1497-1500, 1988.

18. Bounds JV, Wiebers DO, Whisnant JP: Mechanisms and timing of deaths from cerebral infarction, *Stroke* 12(4):414-477, 1981.

19. Bourbonnais D, Vanden Noven S: Weakness in patients with hemiparesis, *Am J Occup Ther* 43(5):313-319, 1989.

20. Branch EF: The neuropathology of stroke. In Duncan PW, Badke MB: *Stroke rehabilitation: the recovery of motor control*, Chicago, 1987, Year Book Medical.

21. Brott T et al: Measurements of acute cerebral infarction: a clinical examination scale, *Stroke* 20(7):864-870, 1989.

22. Cailliet R: *The shoulder in hemiplegia*, Philadelphia, 1980, FA Davis.

23. Carr JH, Shepherd RB, Nordholm L, et al: Investigation of a new motor assessment scale for stroke patients, *Phys Ther* 65(2):175-180, 1985.

24. Collen FM et al: The Rivermead mobility index: a further development of the Rivermead motor assessment, *Int Disabil Stud* 13(2): 50-54, 1991.

25. Collins C, Wade D: Assessing motor impairment after stroke: a pilot reliability study, *J Neurol Neurosurg Psychiatry* 57(7):576-579, 1983.

26. Cote R et al: The Canadian Neurological Scale: a preliminary study in acute stroke, *Stroke* 17(4):731-737, 1986.

27. Chusid J: *Correlative neuroanatomy and functional neurology*, ed 19, Los Altos, Calif, 1985, Lange Medical Publications.

28. Daleiden S: Weight shifting as a treatment for balance deficits: a literature review, *Physiother Can* 42(2):81-87, 1990.

29. Demeurisse G, Demol O, Robaye E: Motor evaluation in vascular hemiplegia, *Eur Neurol* 19(6):382-389, 1980.

30. Desrosiers J et al: Development and reliability of an upper extremity function test for the elderly: the TEMPA, *Can J Occup Ther* 60(1):9-16, 1993.

31. Derosiers J et al: Upper extremity performance test for the elderly (TEMPA): normative data and correlates with sensorimotor parameters, *Arch Phys Med Rehabil* 76(12):1125-1129, 1995.

32. Donato SM, Pulaski KH: Overview of balance impairments: functional implications. In Gillen G, Burkhardt A, editors: *Stroke rehabilitation: a function-based approach*, St Louis, 1998, Mosby.

33. Duncan P et al: Functional reach: a new clinical measure of balance, *J Gerontol* 45(6):M192-M197, 1990.

34. Epstein NB et al: The McMaster family assessment device, *J Marital Fam Ther* 9(2):171-180, 1983.

35. Fisher AG: *Assessment of motor and process skills*, Fort Collins, Colo, 1995, Three Star Press.

36. Folstein MF et al: Mini-mental state: a practical method for grading the cognitive state of patients for the clinician, *J Psychiatr Res* 12(3):189-198, 1975.

37. Franchigoni FP et al: Trunk control test as an early predictor of stroke rehabilitation outcome, *Stroke* 28(7):1382-1385, 1997.

38. Fugl-Meyer AR et al: The post-stroke hemiplegic patient: a method for evaluation of physical performance, *Scand J Rehabil Med* 7:13-31, 1975.

39. Gillen G: Upper extremity function and management. In Gillen G, Burkhardt A, editors: *Stroke rehabilitation: a function-based approach*, St Louis, 1998, Mosby.

40. Gillen G: Trunk control: a prerequisite to functional independence. In Gillen G, Burkhardt A, editors: *Stroke rehabilitation: a function-based approach*, St Louis, 1998, Mosby.

41. Gillen G: Managing abnormal tone after brain injury, *OT Pract* 3:8, 1998.

42. Goodglass H, Kaplan E: *Boston Diagnostic Aphasia Examination*, Philadelphia, 1983, Lee & Febiger.

43. Halper AS, Mogil SI: Communication disorders: diagnosis and treatment. In Kaplan PE, Cerullo LJ, editors: *Stroke rehabilitation*, Boston, 1986, Butterworth.

44. Helgason CM, Wolf PA: *American Heart Association prevention conference IV: prevention and rehabilitation of stroke*, Dallas, 1997, American Heart Association.

45. Holbrook M, Skilbeck CE: An activities index for use with stroke patients, *Age Ageing* 12(2):166-170, 1983.

46. Horak FB, Nashner L: Central programming of postural movements: adaptation to altered support surface configurations, *J Neurophysiol* 55(6):1369-1381, 1986.

47. Jebsen RH et al: An objective and standardized test of hand function, *Arch Phys Med Rehabil* 50(6):311-319, 1969.

48. Keith RA, Granger CV, Hamilton BB, et al: The functional independence measure: a new tool for rehabilitation. In Eisenberg MG, Grzesiak RC, editors: *Advances in clinical rehabilitation*, vol 1, New York, 1987, Springer-Verlag.

49. Kertesz A: *Western Aphasia Battery*, New York, 1982, Grune & Stratton.

50. Kiernan RJ: *The Neurobehavioral Cognitive Status Examination*, 1987, Northern California Neuro Group.

51. Kistler JP, Ropper AH, Martin JB: Cerebrovascular disease. In Isselbacher KJ et al, editors: *Harrison's principles of internal medicine*, New York, 1994, McGraw-Hill.

52. Kopp B et al: The arm motor ability test: reliability, validity, and sensitivity to change of an instrument for assessing disabilities in activities of daily living, *Arch Phys Med Rehabil* 78(6):615-620, 1997.

53. Law M et al: *The Canadian Occupational Performance Measure*, ed 2, Ottawa, 1994, CAOT Publications ACE.

54. Law M, Baptiste S, Mills J: Client-centered practice: what does it mean and does it make a difference? *Can J Occup Ther* 62(5):250-257, 1995.

55. Lawton MP: Instrumental activities of daily living scale: self-rated version, *Psychopharmacol Bull* 24(4):785-787, 1988.

56. Mathiowetz V, Bass Haugen J: Motor behavior research: implications for therapeutic approaches to central nervous system dysfunction, *Am J Occup Ther* 48(8):733-745, 1994.

57. Mahoney FI, Barthel DW: Functional evaluation: the Barthel index, *Maryland State Med J* 14:61-65, 1965.

58. Milazzo S, Gillen G: Splinting applications. In Gillen G, Burkhardt A, editors: *Stroke rehabilitation: a function-based approach*, St Louis, 1998, Mosby.

59. Neistadt ME: Perceptual retraining for adults with diffuse brain injury, *Am J Occup Ther* 48(3):225-233, 1994.

60. Neistadt ME: Occupational therapy treatments for constructional deficits, *Am J Occup Ther* 46(2):141-148, 1992.

61. Neistadt ME: A critical analysis of occupational therapy approaches for perceptual deficits in adults with brain injury, *Am J Occup Ther* 44(4):299-304, 1990.

62. Ogden LD: *Procedure guidelines for monitored self-care evaluation and monitored task evaluation*, Downey, Calif, 1981, Cardiac Rehabilitation Resources.

63. O'Leary SS: *Monitored showers during inpatient rehabilitation following cardiac events*, master's thesis, San Jose, Calif, 1986, San Jose State University.

64. Pollock N: Client-centered assessment, *Am J Occup Ther* 47(4): 298-301, 1993.

65. Post-Stroke Rehabilitation Guideline Panel: *Post-stroke rehabilitation: clinical practice guidelines # 16*, Rockville, Md, 1995, U.S.

Department of Health and Human Services, Agency for Health-care Policy and Research.

66. Roth EJ: Medical complications encountered in stroke rehabilitation, *Phys Med Rehabil Clin North Am* 2(3):563-577, 1991.

67. Rubenstein E, Federman D, editors: *Neurocerebrovascular diseases,* New York, 1994, Scientific American.

68. Rubio KB: Treatment of neurobehavioral deficits: a function-based approach. In Gillen G, Burkhardt A, editors: *Stroke rehabilitation: a function-based approach,* St Louis, 1998, Mosby.

69. Rutan GH et al: Mortality associated with diastolic hypertension and isolated systolic hypertension among men screened for the Multiple Risk Factor Intervention Trial, *Circulation* 77(3):504-514, 1988.

70. Ryerson S, Levit K: The shoulder in hemiplegia. In Donatelli RA, editor: *Physical therapy of the shoulder,* ed 2, Edinburgh, 1991, Churchill Livingstone.

71. Sandin KJ, Smith BS: The measure of balance in sitting in stroke rehabilitation prognosis, *Stroke* 21(1):82-86, 1990.

72. Scheiman M: *Understanding and managing vision deficits: a guide for occupational therapists,* Thorofare, NJ, 1997, Slack.

73. Shumway-Cook A, Horak FB: Balance rehabilitation in the neurological patient. NERA, 1992.

74. Shumway-Cook A, Woollacott M: *Motor control: theory and practical applications,* Baltimore, 1995, Williams & Wilkins.

75. Spencer EA: Functional restoration. In Hopkins HL, Smith HD, editors: *Willard & Spackman's occupational therapy,* ed 8, Philadelphia, 1993, JB Lippincott.

76. Sutin JA: Clinical presentation of stroke syndromes. In Kaplan PE, Cerullo LJ, editors: *Stroke rehabilitation,* Boston, 1986, Butterworth.

77. Taub E et al: Technique to improve chronic motor deficit after stroke, *Arch Phys Med Rehabil* 74(4):347-354, 1993.

78. Teasdale G, Jennett B: Assessment of coma and impaired consciousness: a practical scale. *Lancet* 2(7872):81-84, 1974.

79. Thomson-Kohlman L: *The Kohlman Evaluation of Living Skills,* ed 3, Bethesda, Md, 1992, American Occupational Therapy Association.

80. Tinetti ME: Performance-oriented assessment of mobility problems in elderly patients, *J Am Geriatr Soc* 34(2):119-126, 1986.

81. Toglia J: Generalization of treatment: a multicontext approach to cognitive perceptual impairment in adults with brain injury, *Am J Occup Ther* 45(6):505-516, 1991.

82. Trombly CA: Anticipating the future: assessment of occupational function, *Am J Occup Ther* 47(3):253-257, 1993.

83. Trombly CA: Observations of improvements in five subjects with left hemiparesis, *J Neurol Neurosurg Psychiatry* 56(1):40-45, 1993.

84. Trombly CA: Deficits in reaching in subjects with left hemiparesis: a pilot study, *Am J Occup Ther* 46(10):887-897, 1992.

85. Turner A: *The practice of occupational therapy,* ed 2, New York, 1987, Churchill Livingstone.

86. Ware JE, Sherbourne CD: The MOS 36-item short form health survey: conceptual framework and item selection, *Med Care* 30(6):473-483, 1992.

87. Wilson DJ, Baker LL, Craddock JA: Functional test for the hemiparetic upper extremity, *Am J Occup Ther* 38:159-164, 1984.

88. World Health Organization: *International classification of impairments, disabilities, and handicaps,* Geneva, 1980, The Organization.

89. Wu S et al: Effects of a program on symmetrical posture in patients with hemiplegia: a single-subject design, *Am J Occup Ther* 50(1): 17-23, 1996.

90. Yesavage JA, et al: Development and validation of a geriatric depression screening scale: a preliminary report, *J Psychiatr Res* 17(1):37-49, 1982-1983.

91. Zorowitz RD et al: Shoulder pain and subluxation after stroke: correlation or coincidence? *Am J Occup Ther* 50(3):194-201, 1996.

CHAPTER 38

Traumatic Brain Injury

SHARON A. GUTMAN

Closed head injury
Open head injury
Substance use
Neuroplasticity
Posttraumatic amnesia
Decorticate rigidity
Decerebrate rigidity
Spasticity
Unilateral neglect syndrome
Disinhibition
Behavioral management
Sensory stimulation

After studying this chapter the student or practitioner will be able to do the following:

1. Describe the pathology underlying traumatic brain injury (TBI).
2. State current medical, surgical, and pharmaceutical interventions for acute TBI.
3. Identify levels of consciousness in TBI patients using standard scales.
4. Describe the clinical picture of individuals with TBI, including common physical, cognitive, and psychosocial sequelae.
5. Identify occupational therapy (OT) evaluation methods for beginning, intermediate, and advanced patients with TBI.
6. Identify several standard OT assessments for physical, cognitive, and psychosocial impairment after TBI.
7. Describe OT treatment methods for beginning, intermediate, and advanced patients with TBI.
8. Describe the continuum of care services available for a patient with TBI in the acute, subacute, and postacute stages of rehabilitation.

Traumatic brain injury (TBI) is an insult to the brain resulting from an external physical force (as differentiated from a degenerative or congenital condition), often causing impairment of cognitive, perceptual, and physical functioning. There are two basic categories of TBI: **closed head injury** (CHI), in which the skull remains intact, and **open head injury** (OHI), in which the skull is fractured or penetrated. CHI usually results from motor vehicle accidents (MVAs) and falls that cause rapid acceleration and deceleration of the head. The stress of acceleration and deceleration causes the brain to be jolted back and forth and bounce off the bony prominences located on the underside of the skull. Such rapid movement of the brain pulls apart and damages nerve fibers that regulate all sensations traveling to the brain and all motor signals emerging from the brain and leading to all body parts. OHI is a visible injury that often results from gunshot and knife wounds and accidents causing penetration of the skull and exposure of brain substance.[9]

Nontraumatic brain injury may result from organic, degenerative, and congenital conditions. Cardiac arrest, stroke, and drowning accidents all can cause anoxia or loss of oxygen to the brain, leading to brain injury. Tumors, toxic substances (e.g., carbon monoxide poisoning and drug overdose), and infection (e.g., encephalitis) can also cause brain injury.[22] This chapter focuses on brain injury of the traumatic categories (CHI and OHI).

Medical technology to prolong the lives of individuals who sustain TBI emerged in the 1980s with the invention of high-powered imaging tools such as magnetic resonance imaging (MRI), computed tomography (CT), positron emission tomography (PET), and more effective clinical pathways and medical practices.[36] Each year, approximately 373,000 Americans are hospitalized as a result of TBI. Of these, 99,000 individuals sustain moderate to severe brain injuries that result in lifelong disabling conditions. It is estimated that 56,000 Americans die each year as a result of TBI.[9]

The cost of TBI in the United States is estimated to be $48.3 billion annually. Approximately $31.7 billion of this figure is attributed to postacute hospitalization and supportive living arrangements because individuals with moderate to severe TBI often require lifelong rehabilitative assistance.[9]

POPULATION

Eighty percent of individuals who sustain TBI are men between the ages of 18 and 30. TBI occurs more frequently in men than in women by a ratio of 4:1. It is suggested that males are more likely to sustain TBI because of lifestyle and risk exposure activities. Most young men sustain TBI as a result of MVAs, violence, and sports that have a safety-risk element. Alcohol use is a leading contributor to TBI. Two thirds of individuals who have sustained TBI have measurable blood alcohol levels. Although substance abuse is a major concomitant of TBI, very few TBI rehabilitation programs are prepared to address adequately both the physical and cognitive sequelae of TBI and the precipitating alcohol abuse. This is a serious problem because one third of all individuals with TBI who are released from rehabilitation services return to **substance use**.[9]

The risk of TBI is also great among infants, toddlers, and the elderly. According to the National Pediatric Trauma Registry, more than 30,000 children sustain permanent disability as a result of TBI. Mortality, however, is higher in adults than in children because of a child's greater **neuroplasticity**, the ability for the central nervous system (CNS) to reorganize neurological pathways to compensate for damaged brain areas.[32] Appropriate rehabilitation treatment for the cognitive, perceptual, psychosocial, and physical sequelae of TBI is vital because a second head injury occurs in 15% to 20% of those who sustain TBI.[9]

PATHOPHYSIOLOGY

Two commonly described categories of TBI are *diffuse* and *focal*. Both are considered to be primary damage re-

sulting from TBI. Primary damage is the original physical impairment resulting directly from the event that caused the TBI. Secondary damage is produced as a consequence of the original primary tissue damage.

Primary Damage

The first category of primary damage, focal brain injury, is localized, meaning that damage to specific brain areas can be identified on imaging scans (e.g., CT and MRI scans). A focal brain injury is commonly caused by penetrating wounds (e.g, gunshot and knife wounds) and is often a result of an open head injury.

A diffuse brain injury is not localized, but rather involves widespread damage to brain tissue; this damage is more difficult to pinpoint on imaging scans. A diffuse axonal injury (DAI) often results from high-speed auto accidents that cause severe strain and shearing of axons throughout the white matter (neuronal axons) and damage to small capillaries and veins. Shearing occurs as the brain accelerates, decelerates, or rotates against the sharp bony prominences (the sphenoid wings, the petrous bones, and the orbital bones) on the underside of the skull, causing tearing of the gray matter (cell bodies). Shearing of brain structures that are more loosely connected to the underneath of the skull and the gray matter causes axonal stretching and tearing.[34]

Both focal and diffuse brain injury may involve skull fractures. Three basic types of skull fractures occur with TBI: linear, depressed, and basilar. Linear skull fractures occur most frequently. These fractures are considered to be the least serious and extend from the site of impact in a linear fashion. Depressed skull fractures occur when a small object contacts the skull with great force, resulting in a depression or cavitation of the bone at the point of impact. Basilar skull fractures are fracture lines that radiate from the point of contact to the base of the skull. Basilar skull fractures create an abnormal pathway between air contained in the neural sinuses and the subarachnoid space, leading to cerebrospinal fluid (CSF) leakage. Depressed and basilar skull fractures place patients at a higher risk for infection. Such patients are treated prophylactically with antibiotics. Because basilar skull fractures frequently involve the petrous bone, cranial nerve damage often results. The most commonly damaged cranial nerves as a result of TBI are I, II, III, VI, VII, and VIII because of their position within the skull.[6]

Secondary Damage

After the initial primary damage of a TBI occurs, various secondary responses are produced. The most common of these secondary responses is an increase in intracranial pressure (ICP). Because intracranial contents (e.g., brain matter, sinuses, CSF, arteries, and veins) are enclosed within a rigid skull, ICP increases as a result of cerebral edema, hematoma, or obstruction of CSF. As ICP increases, cerebral blood flow is compromised and anoxic brain damage can occur. Uncontrolled increased ICP causes diffuse hypoxia (lack of oxygenated blood to brain areas), eventually leading to cardiovascular and renal failure, brain herniation, and death. Uncontrolled ICP accounts for 50% of TBI-related deaths.[15]

Cerebral edema is a natural body response resulting from hypoxia. Again, because brain contents are encased in a rigid, nonexpandable skull, there is no natural way for the body to accommodate increased volume. Uncontrolled cerebral edema is a major factor that causes increased ICP, leading to morbidity.[17]

Posttraumatic hydrocephalus is an abnormal accumulation of CSF that can also cause increased ICP. A common treatment for obstructive hydrocephalus is ventroperitoneal shunting, in which a tube is placed to circumvent the ventricular blockage and discharge excess CSF to the peritoneal cavity.[6,15] Normal-pressure hydrocephalus occurs when the ventricles enlarge without an increase in CSF pressure. Normal-pressure hydrocephalus is indicated by a slow onset of symptoms, including dementia, incontinence, and an unsteady gait. Such symptoms can progress over weeks to months following TBI.[34]

A hematoma is a collection of blood in a space-occupying lesion. In other words the pooling of blood displaces areas where brain tissue should normally lie. Hematomas may result in distortion of brain tissue, obstruction of CSF, and decreased cerebral circulation. Treatment may involve evacuation of the blood through burr holes.[6,34]

A subarachnoid hemorrhage involves bleeding into the subarachnoid space and ventricles and often results from contusions over orbital surfaces. Hemorrhages—rather than hematomas—form because the pooling blood does not clot as it is diluted by the CSF. Symptoms include blood in the CSF, painful stiff neck, headache, and restlessness. The most common treatment of a subarachnoid hemorrhage is drainage through a ventroperitoneal shunt.[17]

Posttraumatic epilepsy is a sudden abnormal discharge of cerebral neurons that is characterized by brief attacks of altered consciousness, motor activity, or sensory phenomena. Medication is commonly prescribed for this condition.[19]

Further secondary damage includes brain distortion, shift, and herniation. In the presence of expanding fluid and increased ICP, the brain will eventually attempt to compensate by distorting its normal shape. Treatment may involve surgery and control of the increased ICP and edema.[6,34]

MEDICAL MANAGEMENT OF ACUTE TBI

Few emergency trauma units are set up to adequately handle the acute medical management of TBI. Thus the patient should be transported as quickly as possible to a trauma unit that specializes in TBI care. Upon the patient's admission to the emergency room the first concern is to address the ABCs: airway, breathing, and blood circulation. An obstructed airway may require suctioning, intubation, or tracheostomy. The patient may be in shock and need intravenous (IV) fluids, plasma, blood transfusions, or vasopressor agents. Imaging (e.g., MRI or CT) is performed to evaluate the extent of damage and detect focal abnormalities. It is often difficult to evaluate the extent of damage soon after a TBI because CT scans may not identify a diffuse type of brain injury.

Traditional methods of treating acute TBI involved restricting fluids to prevent further swelling. However, research has shown that IV fluids are critical for adding volume to increase pressure to the circulatory system. A strong blood pressure forces oxygenated blood to the brain. Restricting fluids causes blood pressure to drop, resulting in poorer patient outcomes.[11]

Standards of care for acute TBI have changed over the years. Medical professionals now know that the secondary damage from TBI (i.e., increased ICP, cerebral edema, hydrocephalus, hematoma, subarachnoid hemorrhage, and seizures) causes more impairment to brain structures and functioning than does the initial primary damage. It is therefore critical to treat the secondary damage of TBI aggressively in the first week of hospitalization.[17] Two of the newest critical pathways (or guidelines for practice) for acute TBI that have been shown to be effective through scientific research methods are ventriculostomy with continued monitoring of ICP and cooling hypothermia treatment.

Ventriculostomy involves the insertion of a tube into the brain (where the CSF is produced) to drain the increased fluid and relieve swelling. The surgeon drills a hole into the skull and punctures the dura until the CSF sinus is tapped. A catheter is placed 5 to 7 mm into the CSF canal. The catheter is then connected to a monitor that continuously measures fluid pressure for several days. A normal ICP level is 0 to 10. Patients exhibiting an ICP of 20 or higher are at severe risk for further brain damage. When brain swelling cannot be controlled, the brain chokes off the supply of oxygenated blood. In the ventriculostomy procedure, medications are used to raise and maintain the blood pressure at 70 points higher than the ICP. A raised blood pressure will force oxygenated blood through the brain.[48]

If the ICP does not decrease and a hematoma occurs, a hole must be drilled through the skull to drain the fluid and remove the hematoma. Either the patient's removed skull section is replaced, or a metal brain plate is secured over the surgically removed skull section. Signs that the acute crisis is over include the patient's opening the eyes with visual tracking and responding to commands (e.g., "squeeze my hand"). Because research has demonstrated that these guidelines for the acute treatment of TBI are effective, the World Health Organization approved and adopted them as standard care practices in 1997.[48]

One other method that has been shown to be effective in the treatment of acute TBI is the cooling hypothermia treatment. The cooling hypothermia method involves the use of ice water to decrease the patient's metabolism, thereby diminishing the cascade of neurochemical reactions that immediately follows TBI and culminates in further destruction of brain cells. After TBI a flood of a neurotransmitter called glutamate is released throughout the brain at 1000 times its normal level. It is believed that this flood of glutamate initiates a series of biochemical events that further damages and destroys brain cells.[7]

The conventional method for preventing the mass destruction of brain cells resulting from abnormal glutamate levels involves the administration of medications to lower ICP and the placing of the patient on a respirator to increase oxygenated blood levels. High ICP and low oxygen levels are thought to initiate the overproduction of glutamate. In hypothermia treatment the patient is placed in a specialized bed in which the arms and legs are wrapped in cool packs that are attached to pumps providing a constant infusion of ice. For 8 hours the body temperature is gradually lowered to 89° to 90° F—a temperature low enough to slow metabolism but not cause life-threatening complications such as irregular heartbeat. By slowing the metabolism, the cooling decreases ICP and inhibits the release of glutamate. Patients remain in a state of hypothermia for 48 hours, the longest time possible before dangerous reactions ensue. Then the patient's body temperature is gradually warmed to normal, and ICP continues to be monitored until normal. For cooling hypothermia to be most effective, it must begin within the first 6 hours after injury.[7,51]

Drug therapy is among the experimental methods being used to treat acute TBI. One such drug, aptiganel hydrochloride, is designed to prevent the destruction of brain cells by breaking one link in the chain of chemical reactions that follows excessive glutamate production. Research is needed to demonstrate the effectiveness of aptiganel hydrochloride.[51]

Nutrition begins by IV within the first few days after injury. Later, parenteral nutrition (nasogastric [NG] tube) or enteral nutrition (gastric tube) is often needed to ensure that the patient receives adequate nutrition if the level of awareness is decreased or oral-bulbar function is impaired. In these procedures either an NG tube is inserted through the nose or a gastrostomy tube is surgically placed within the stomach cavity.[6] Bowel and bladder function is often impaired, necessitating catheterization. Later in rehabilitation, as bowel and bladder function begins to return, a bowel and bladder program is initiated.

As mentioned, posttraumatic epilepsy is a common occurrence with TBI. Seizures may begin immediately at the time of injury or even several years later. Prophylactic treatment with anticonvulsants in comatose patients should be started in the emergency room because research suggests that the risk of early posttraumatic seizures may be reduced by the administration of such medication.[6] The patient is transferred to a subacute rehabilitation service when he or she is considered medically stable—that is, the cardiovascular, respiratory, and neurological status have stabilized and there are no acute signs and symptoms of serious infection.

COMA AND LEVELS OF CONSCIOUSNESS

A TBI typically results in an altered level of consciousness. The continuum of consciousness includes coma at one end, a stuporous state in the middle, and consciousness at the opposite end. The individual's progression along this continuum of consciousness is unique and depends on age, prior health status, substance abuse history, and, especially, severity of injury.

Coma is a state of sleeplike (eyes closed) unarousability as a result of extensive brain damage. Coma that involves severe damage to the brainstem often indicates a poor prognosis. The brainstem contains the reticular activating system, which is the arousal system for the entire brain. When severe damage occurs to the reticular activating system, all communication between the body and the cerebral hemispheres is disrupted. The brainstem controls vegetative functions such as respiration and primitive stereotyped reflexes such as cough reflex, gag reflex, and swallowing reflex. Because individuals with severe brainstem involvement lose the cough, gag, and swallowing responses, they are likely to have fatal respiratory infections in 6 months to 1 year.[26]

Persistent vegetative state is a form of coma in which the brunt of neurological destruction has occurred to the cerebral hemispheres but the brainstem has remained intact. A persistent vegetative state often results from hypoxia, or a lack of oxygen to the brain for a period of minutes. Because the brainstem is fairly resistant to hypoxia, it is often spared, although cerebral hemisphere tissue is commonly destroyed. Sparing of the brainstem allows the continued functions of respiration and the cough, gag, and swallowing reflexes, which significantly decreases the likelihood of fatal respiratory infections. As a result, individuals can live for years in persistent vegetative states. A persistent vegetative state may be a transient coma that continues for a period of days to months (or longer). When the patient begins to emerge from a vegetative state, he or she will awaken into a condition of eyes-open, unresponsive unconsciousness but demonstrate a reflexive response to painful or vigorous stimulation. This state is particularly difficult for family members because the patient appears

TABLE 38-1
Glasgow Coma Scale

Examiner's Test		Patient's Response	Assigned Score
Eye opening	Spontaneous	Opens eyes on own	4
	Speech	Opens eyes when asked to in a loud voice	3
	Pain	Opens eyes when pinched	2
	Pain	Does not open eyes	1
Best motor response	Commands	Follows simple commands	6
	Pain	Pulls examiner's hand away when pinched	5
	Pain	Pulls a part of body away when examiner pinches patient	4
	Pain	Flexes body inappropriately to pain (decorticate posturing)	3
	Pain	Body becomes rigid in an extended position when examiner pinches victim (decerebrate posturing)	2
	Pain	Has no motor response to pinch	1
Verbal response (talking)	Speech	Carries on a conversation correctly and tells examiner where he is, who he is, and the month and year	5
	Speech	Seems confused or disoriented	4
	Speech	Talks so examiner can understand victim but makes no sense	3
	Speech	Makes sounds that examiner can't understand	2
	Speech	Makes no noise	1

From Rosenthal M and associates: *Rehabilitation of the head-injured adult*, Philadelphia, 1984, FA Davis.

conscious (eyes open) but does not interact with any person or object in the environment.[26]

If the patient emerges from a vegetative state, he or she will have a clouding of consciousness characterized by reduced wakefulness, reduced clarity of thought, confusion, decreased attention span, and memory lapses. Conversely, in complete consciousness the individual possesses awareness of the self and the surrounding environment, is able to perceive and correctly interpret his or her perceptions, and displays appropriate responses. Complete consciousness is a function of an intact cortex.

The Glasgow Coma Scale (GCS) has been the traditional method used by health care professionals to assess levels of consciousness after a TBI (Table 38-1). The GCS has been used to quantify the severity of brain injury and predict outcome. Three behavioral areas assessed in the GCS are motor responses, verbal responses, and eye opening. Although more recent studies have suggested that the GCS is not an effective predictor of long-term TBI outcomes, the GCS *is* an effective indicator of acute TBI status.[25]

Posttraumatic amnesia (PTA) has traditionally been used as another predictor of outcome (Table 38-2). PTA is the length of time from the injury to the moment when the patient regains ongoing memory of daily

TABLE 38-2
Duration of Posttraumatic Amnesia and Severity of Injury

PTA Duration	Severity
Less than 5 min	Very mild
5 to 60 min	Mild
1 to 24 hr	Moderate
1 to 7 days	Severe
1 to 4 weeks	Very severe
More than 4 weeks	Extremely severe

From Rosenthal M and associates: *Rehabilitation of the head-injured adult*, Philadelphia, 1984, FA Davis.
PTA, Posttraumatic amnesia.

events. There is evidence that the duration of PTA is highly correlated with patient outcomes. Longer PTAs are associated with poorer long-term cognitive and motor abilities. A PTA of 4 weeks or greater is correlated with significant long-term disability.[26]

The Ranchos Los Amigos Scale is an assessment that measures levels of awareness and cognitive function.[41]

BOX 38-1
Levels of Cognitive Functioning

I. No response. Patient appears to be in a deep sleep and is completely unresponsive to any stimuli presented to him or her.

II. Generalized response. The patient reacts inconsistently and nonpurposefully to stimuli in a nonspecific manner. Responses are limited in nature and are often the same, regardless of the stimulus presented. Responses may be physiological changes, gross body movements, or vocalization. Often the earliest response is to deep pain. Responses are likely to be delayed.

III. Localized response. The patient reacts specifically but inconsistently to stimuli. Responses are directly related to the type of stimulus presented, as in turning the head toward a sound or focusing on an object presented. The patient may withdraw an extremity or vocalize when presented with a painful stimulus. He or she may follow simple commands in an inconsistent, delayed manner, such as in closing the eyes, squeezing, or extending an extremity. After the external stimulus is removed, the patient may lie quietly. He or she may also show a vague awareness of self and body by responding to discomfort by pulling at a nasogastric (NG) tube or catheter or resisting restraints. The patient may show bias by responding to some persons (especially family, friends) but not to others.

IV. Confused-agitated. The patient is in a heightened state of activity with a severely decreased ability to process information. He or she is detached from the present and responds primarily to his or her own internal confusion. Behavior is frequently bizarre and nonpurposeful relative to the immediate environment. The patient may cry out or scream out of proportion to stimuli even after removal and may show aggressive behavior, attempt to remove restraints or tubes, or crawl out of bed in a purposeful manner. The patient does not, however, discriminate among persons or objects and is unable to cooperate directly with treatment effort. Verbalization is frequently incoherent and inappropriate to the environment. Confabulation may be present; the patient may be euphoric or hostile. Thus gross attention is very short and selective attention is often nonexistent. Being unaware of present events, the patient lacks short-term recall and may be reacting to past events. He or she is unable to perform self-care (e.g., feeding and dressing) without maximum assistance. If not disabled physically, the patient may perform motor activities as in sitting, reaching, and ambulating, but as part of the agitated state and not as a purposeful act or on request.

V. Confused, inappropriate, nonagitated. The patient appears alert and is able to respond to simple commands fairly consistently. However, with increased complexity of commands or lack of any external structure, responses are nonpurposeful, random, or at best fragmented toward any desired goal. The patient may show agitated behavior, not on an internal basis (as in Level IV), but rather as a result of external stimuli, and usually out of proportion to the stimulus. He or she has gross attention to the environment, but is highly distractible and lacks the ability to focus attention to a specific task without frequent redirection back to it. With structure, the patient may be able to converse on a social, automatic level for short periods of time. Verbalization is often inappropriate; confabulation may be triggered by present events. Memory is severely impaired, with confusion of past and present in his or her reaction to ongoing activity. The patient lacks initiation of functional tasks and often shows inappropriate use of objects without external direction. He or she may be able to perform previously learned tasks when they are structured for him or

---

An abridged version of the scale appears below; for a complete description of the assessment, see Box 38-1.

Level I	No response. Unresponsive to any stimulus.
Level II	Generalized response. Nonspecific, inconsistent, and nonpurposeful responses to stimuli (often only to pain).
Level III	Localized response. Response directly related to the type of stimuli presented, yet responses still inconsistent and delayed.
Level IV	Confused-agitated. Heightened state of activity, confusion, disorientation; may exhibit aggressive behaviors; agitation appears related to internal confusion.
Level V	Confused-inappropriate. Appears alert, responds to simple commands, distractible; does not concentrate on task; agitated responses to external stimuli; verbally inappropriate; does not learn new information.

The Ranchos Los Amigos Scale can be used at any time after injury to assess level of awareness and cognitive function. However, it is not meant to be used as a predictive scale.

No accurate predictive measures of long-term outcome have been developed. The GCS predicts outcome more accurately in patients with a GCS score of 7 or more.[52] In addition to severity of injury, age, and prior health status, social factors can significantly determine an individual's long-term prognosis. Individuals who have large and committed supportive networks and can access financial and material resources fare the best, particularly if they receive aggressive and effective acute care. For individuals with histories of alcohol abuse, a return to substance use after injury appears to be a predictor of a possible second brain injury. Patients who receive substance abuse counseling and who do not return to alcohol use have better prognoses.[29] Studies have also suggested that although cognitive, perceptual, psychosocial, and physical gains occur most rapidly in

BOX 38-1

Levels of Cognitive Functioning—cont'd

her, but the patient is unable to learn new information. He or she responds best to self, body, comfort—and often family members. The patient can usually perform self-care activities with assistance and may accomplish feeding with maximum supervision. Management on the ward is often a problem if the patient is physically mobile, as he or she may wander off either randomly or with vague intention of "going home."

VI. **Confused-appropriate.** The patient shows goal-directed behavior but is dependent on external input for direction. The response to discomfort is appropriate and the patient is able to tolerate unpleasant stimuli (e.g., NG tube) when the need is explained. The patient follows simple directions consistently and shows carryover for tasks that have been relearned (such as self-care). He or she is at least supervised with old learning and is unable to maximally assist for new learning with little or no carryover. Responses may be incorrect because of memory problems, but they are appropriate to the situation. Responses may be delayed, and the patient shows a decreased ability to process information with little or no anticipation or prediction of events. Past memories show more depth and detail than recent memory. The patient may show beginning awareness of his or her situation by realizing he or she doesn't know an answer. The patient no longer wanders and is inconsistently oriented to time and place. Selective attention to tasks may be impaired, especially with difficult tasks and in unstructured settings, but the patient is now functional for common daily activities (30 min with structure). He or she shows at least vague recognition of some staff, has increased awareness of self, family, and basic needs (e.g., food), again in an appropriate manner, as in contrast to Level V.

VII. **Automatic-appropriate.** The patient appears appropriate and oriented within hospital and home settings, goes through the daily routine automatically, but is frequently robot-like. The patient has minimal to absent confusion but has shallow recall of what he or she has been doing. He or she shows increased awareness of self, body, family, foods, people, and interaction in the environment. The patient has superficial awareness of, but lacks insight into, his or her condition, demonstrates decreased judgment and problem solving, and lacks realistic planning for the future. He or she shows carryover for new learning, but at a decreased rate. He or she requires at least minimal supervision for learning and for safety purposes and is independent in self-care activities and supervised in home and community skills for safety. With structure the patient is able to initiate tasks in social and recreational activities in which he or she now has interest. Judgment remains impaired, such that the patient is unable to drive a car. Prevocational or avocational evaluation and counseling may be indicated

VIII. **Purposeful and appropriate.** The patient is alert and oriented, is able to recall and integrate past and recent events, and is aware of and responsive to his or her culture. He or she shows carryover for new learning if it is acceptable to him or her and his or her life role. The patient needs no supervision after activities are learned within his or her physical capabilities. He or she is independent in home and community skills, including driving. Vocational rehabilitation, to determine ability to return as a contributor to society (perhaps in a new capacity), is indicated. The patient may continue to show a decreased ability, relative to premorbid abilities, in reasoning, tolerance for stress, judgment in emergencies, or unusual circumstances. His or her social, emotional, and intellectual capacities may continue to be at a decreased level, but are functional for society.

From Rancho Los Amigos Medical Center, Downey, Calif, Adult Brain Injury Service: Original Scale, Levels of Cognitive Functioning, 1980.

the first 2 years after injury, subtle and slow recovery from deficits can continue throughout an individual's life.[6]

CLINICAL PICTURE OF INDIVIDUALS WITH TRAUMATIC BRAIN INJURY

Physical Status

Most individuals with moderate to severe TBI exhibit primitive reflexes, impaired muscle tone, decreased motor control and coordination, decreased muscular strength and endurance, postural deficits, decreased range of motion (ROM) in one or more joints, decreased sensation, and impaired proprioception.

Decorticate and Decerebrate Rigidity

Comatose individuals often display one of two common positions: decorticate rigidity and decerebrate rigidity. In **decorticate rigidity** the upper extremities (UEs) are in a spastic flexed position with internal rotation and adduction. The lower extremities (LEs) are in a spastic extended position, but also internally rotated and adducted. Decorticate rigidity results from damage to the cerebral hemispheres (particularly the internal capsules), causing an interruption in the corticospinal tracts—the spinal cord tracts that emerge from the cortex and send voluntary motor messages to all extremities.

In **decerebrate rigidity** both the UEs and LEs are in a position of spastic extension, adduction, and internal rotation. The wrist and fingers flex, the feet plantar flex and invert, the trunk extends, and the head retracts. Decerebrate rigidity occurs as a result of damage to the brainstem and extrapyramidal tracts—the tracts that send involuntary motor messages from the brainstem to the extremities. Patients with decerebrate rigidity have a poorer prognosis than do those exhibiting decorticate rigidity.[11,17]

Generally, patients emerging from coma have a reduction in **spasticity** as neurological recovery progresses. However, patients with moderate to severe spasticity tend to experience some degree of spasticity or abnormal tone for the remainder of their lives.

Abnormal Muscle Tone and Spasticity

Although decorticate rigidity and decerebrate rigidity are the most severe types of abnormal muscle tone caused by TBI and tend to occur in comatose individuals, spasticity in a patient with TBI may range from minimal to severe in any muscle group. Patients who are functioning at a higher cognitive level than coma generally display a combination of both hypotonicity (decreased tone, or flaccidity) and hypertonicity (increased tone, or spasticity). Depending on the injury site, spasticity and flaccidity can occur on one side of the body in both the UEs and LEs, bilaterally in any of the four extremities, or unilaterally in one limb (either upper or lower extremity). It is important to understand and to teach family members and the patient that tone fluctuates as a result of changes in position, volitional movement, medication, infection and illness, hormonal changes (particularly the monthly hormonal changes that occur in female patients), pain, and changes in emotional state.[5]

Primitive Reflexes

If present beyond their usual time of disappearance, primitive reflexes are indicative of moderate to severe brain injury. The adult patient with a TBI often displays one or more CNS levels of primitive reflexes. The absence of primitive reflexes on reevaluation is a sign of progress in recovery. Primitive reflexes emerge from the five CNS levels: spinal cord, brainstem (medulla and lower pons), midbrain, basal ganglia, and the cerebral hemispheres.[5] The level of primitive reflexes that emerge in the patient with TBI depends on the injury site and interruption of nerve signals to the body (Box 38-2). For example, an individual with brain damage interrupting signals to the spinal cord may experience extensor thrust when the heel is stimulated by contact with the floor. This extensor thrust reflex will interfere with transfers to a seated position. It is common to observe an asymmetrical tonic neck reflex, a positive supporting reaction, and associated reactions if damage has occurred to the brainstem area. The asymmetrical tonic neck reflex prevents rolling from a supine to a prone position to get out of bed. The presence of a positive supporting reaction will inhibit the ability to flex the LEs alternatively in walking. Associated reactions are stereotyped movement patterns, in which one extremity influences the posture of another extremity. Individuals with TBI

BOX 38-2
Primitive Reflex Levels

Spinal Cord Level Reflexes
Flexor withdrawal
Extensor thrust
Crossed extension

Brainstem Level Reflexes
Asymmetrical tonic neck
Symmetrical tonic neck
Tonic labyrinthine reflex
Positive supporting reaction
Associated reactions

Midbrain
Righting reactions

Basal Ganglia
Protective extension
Equilibrium reactions
Cortical reactions
Optical righting

---

who display associated reactions commonly have increased spasticity in their involved extremity when they attempt volitional movement with their opposite extremity.

If damage has occurred to the midbrain, impaired righting reactions are commonly observed. Similarly, damage to the basal ganglia can result in the absence of equilibrium reactions and protective extension. The absence of righting reactions, equilibrium reactions, and protective extension places the patient at a significant risk for further injury from falls during such activities as transfers, getting out of bed, toileting, bathing, and dressing.

Muscle Weakness

A decrease in muscular strength—without spasticity—can occur in the patient with TBI. Often such deconditioning results from a lack of physical activity or extended bed rest caused by secondary factors associated with the TBI (e.g., compromised respiration, fractures, and infection).

Decreased Endurance

Decreased endurance and vital capacity usually accompany reduced muscular strength as a result of medical complications such as pneumonia or infections, and as a result of prolonged bed rest. Increasing the patient's muscular strength and endurance are primary goals in the intensive care unit and in the initial stages of rehabilitation.

Ataxia

Ataxia is a movement abnormality characterized by incoordinated movements and decreased tone. Ataxia results from impairment of the cerebellum or the sensory pathways leading to and from the cerebellum. Thus impaired sensation often accompanies ataxia.[5,47] Ataxia can occur in the entire body, in the trunk, or in the UEs and LEs. The patient with ataxia has lost the ability to perform minute adjustments in the distal and proximal extremities that are necessary for smooth, coordinated movement. The degree of ataxia can range from mild to severe. The patient with truncal ataxia displays decreased postural stability in standing and sitting. He or she has difficulty maintaining the trunk in a stable position to free the UEs for activities. The patient may compensate for this deficit by holding onto a stable surface such as a tabletop. Ataxia in the UEs causes dysfunction in activities in which the patient attempts to perform gross or fine motor movements, such as bringing a glass of water to the mouth. The UE oscillates back and forth, causing spillage of the water. Ataxia in the LEs results in an impaired ability to ambulate while maintaining balance; falls can easily occur with this condition.

Postural Deficits

Postural deficits develop as a result of an imbalance in muscle tone throughout the body. A patient may inadvertently accentuate postural deficits by using ineffective strategies to compensate for impaired motor control, delayed or absent righting reactions or impaired vision, cognition, or perception. The therapist must possess a thorough knowledge of the patient's postural deficits to properly position the patient in a wheelchair with the appropriate seating equipment, which is necessary to obtain an upright posture, maintain good postural alignment, and prevent further postural deformities. Abnormal postures frequently exhibited in adults with moderate to severe TBI include the following:

1. *Head and neck.* Many patients with TBI exhibit forward flexion or hyperextension of the neck. The head may be laterally flexed to the involved side. Lateral flexion of the head often accompanies lateral flexion of the trunk because the muscle groups on the involved side may be spastic and commonly pull the head, neck, and trunk into lateral flexion. Because equilibrium reactions and kinesthesia are often impaired, the patient does not have conscious knowledge of this postural deformity and will not voluntarily attempt to correct it. Primitive reflexes such as the asymmetric tonic neck reflex may be exhibited.

2. *Scapula.* The scapula may be depressed, protracted or retracted, downwardly rotated, or all of these at once. This results from an imbalance in scapular muscle tone; some muscles are hypertonic, whereas others are hypotonic.

3. *Upper extremities.* Depending on the area and severity of brain damage, the UEs may be bilaterally or unilaterally involved. When both UEs are involved, it is common to see asymmetry between the UEs. For example, one extremity may be hypertonic, whereas the other displays hypotonicity. In unilateral involvement it is common to see variations in ROM, tone, and strength in each muscle group and joint of the arm, forearm, wrist, and hand. For example, the biceps may exhibit reduced strength and a moderate degree of hypertonicity, whereas the digits may be nonfunctional because of extreme spastic flexion. Primitive reflexes such as the asymmetrical tonic neck and associated reactions commonly reinforce UE postural deformities.

4. *Lower extremities.* Severe extension patterns are often observed in both LEs in the comatose patient. Patients exhibiting a higher cognitive level may display bilateral or unilateral involvement of the LEs. In bilateral involvement it is common to see muscular weakness in one LE and moderate to severe spastic extension in the other. In unilateral involvement the involved LE may display some degree of spastic extension and primitive reflexes that reinforce postural deformities, such as a positive supporting reaction. Other commonly observed postural deficits include hip adduction and internal rotation, knee flexion, plantar flexion, and inversion of the feet.

5. *Trunk:* Kyphosis, scoliosis, and lordosis may all be present secondary to weak or spastic muscles (e.g., abdominal, spinal, and paraspinal). It is also common to observe lateral flexion and rotation of the involved side as a result of hypertonicity.

6. *Pelvis:* A posterior pelvic tilt is common because of hypertonicity of the intrinsic back muscles (e.g., the iliocostalis and longissimus). A posterior pelvic tilt results in sacral sitting and facilitates kyphosis. Another typical pattern is retraction of one side of the pelvis with a pelvic obliquity, in which one side of the pelvis sits lower than the other side as a result of hypertonicity of the quadratus lumborum on the involved side.

Limitations of Joint Motion

Patients with TBI frequently exhibit loss of ROM in the joints in the involved extremities. It is often difficult to distinguish between several possible causes of decreased ROM, such as the following: increased muscle tone, spastic contractures, heterotopic ossification (in which abnormal bone substance forms in the joint capsule, causing immobility of the joint), fractures or dislocations, and tissue pain. Because the treatment of decreased ROM depends on the cause, it is important for the therapist to determine the cause of the decreased ROM before initiating treatment.

Loss of Sensation

Patients with TBI may display absent or diminished sensation. Lost or diminished light touch, sharp-dull differentiation, proprioception, kinesthesia, and vibration result from brain damage that interrupts the signals from the dorsal columns (or medial lemniscus tracts) leading to the postcentral gyrus. Lost or diminished temperature and pain sensations result from brain damage that interrupts the signals from the lateral spinothalamic tracts leading to the postcentral gyrus. Lost or diminished stereognosis, two-point discrimination, and graphesthesia (the ability to interpret letters written on the hand without visual input) result from damage to the parietal lobe (specifically the sensory association areas). Lost or diminished taste, smell, and sensation of the face result from cranial nerve damage.[5]

Loss of the Integration of Total Body Movements

Total body movements include the integration of head, neck, and trunk control, with dynamic sitting and standing balance while reaching, bending, stooping, and ambulating. To perform total body movements, the patient must coordinate and modulate gross and fine motor movements of the trunk-head-neck and the limbs while performing activities of daily living (ADL). A patient with severe physical involvement often displays poor sitting and standing balance and is unable to maintain an upright position in order to free the UEs for activities. The patient at a more advanced level may exhibit subtle deficits in total body movements, making it difficult to bend down, to reach overhead to retrieve items in a cabinet, or to stoop to retrieve an item fallen to the floor. Integrated total body movements are necessary for the performance of almost all ADL.

Dysphagia and Self-Feeding

Dysphagia is a difficulty in the four stages of chewing and swallowing, caused by cranial nerve damage (see Chapter 40). There is a higher incidence of oral preparatory, oral, and pharyngeal stage dysphagia than esophageal stage dysphagia. Typically, more than one stage of chewing and swallowing is impaired.[4]

With dysphagia the cognitive, visual-perceptual, and neurological problems evident in the patient with TBI further complicate the ability to self-feed. A patient may display oral muscular hypotonicity or hypertonicity as a result of cranial nerve damage. A patient may exhibit instability of the jaw because of cranial nerve damage and secondary fractures. A patient may also possess abnormal oral reflexes, such as rooting, biting, sucking, gagging, or coughing, that prevent the activity of eating. Cognitively, the patient may experience difficulty in sequencing chewing, swallowing, and breathing. The patient may also be unable to sustain attention long enough to self-feed. If impulsivity is apparent, the patient will have difficulty monitoring the amount and rate of food brought to the mouth, thus causing coughing and possible aspiration. Oral apraxia, the inability to perform an intended action or execute an act on command with the mouth or lips, may occur. If the patient possesses an ideational apraxia, he or she will have difficulty understanding the demands required of the self-feeding activity and will be unable to recognize utensils as tools for eating. A patient may also have lost the motor plan for self-feeding (ideomotor apraxia) and be unable to access the neurological motor pattern for bringing food to the mouth. A hemianopsia (visual field cut) may prevent a patient from seeing one half of the plate of food.

Cognitive Status

Cognitive deficits in the patient with TBI are always evident to varying degrees. The most common include decreased attention and concentration, impaired memory, impaired initiation and termination of activities, decreased safety awareness and poor judgment, impulsivity, and difficulty with executive functions and abstract thinking (e.g., problem solving, planning, the integration of new learning, and generalization).

Reduced Attention and Concentration

Reduced attention and concentration impair the ability to maintain an activity without distractibility and to resume an activity when interrupted. The patient with TBI often loses both the ability to concentrate for a length of time and the ability to filter out distractions from the surrounding environment. A patient who is conversing with one individual may detect a peripheral conversation (among others in the environment) and incorporate pieces of that conversation into his or her own sentences. The inability to attend to and concentrate on activities severely impedes the ability to function at work and school and to complete ADL. Although deficits in attention and concentration can diminish as neurological recovery progresses, such deficits can remain in varying degrees throughout an individual's life. Even patients who experience mild TBI can demonstrate subtle deficits in attention and concentration that often linger for years after injury.

Impaired Memory

Impaired memory is the most frequently observed cognitive deficit in the patient with TBI and can remain a problem for the remainder of the individual's life. Memory impairment can range from the inability to recall several words just heard (immediate memory), to forgetting which family members visited the patient last night (short-term memory), to having lost memory of events that occurred years before the injury (long-term memory). Despite neurological recovery, most patients with moderate to severe TBI continue to demonstrate short-term memory deficits. Often, patients recover long-term memory of events that occurred years before the injury. This can be emotionally devastating because the individual with TBI commonly has a clear memory of who he or she was before the injury, as well as his or her accomplishments, goals, and plans for the future—all of which were severely disrupted and perhaps lost as a result of TBI.

Impaired Initiation and Termination of Activities

Impaired initiation and termination of activities affect the ability to start and end activities. The inability to initiate activities without assistance significantly affects the individual's ability to live independently. In general, the patient who exhibits deficits in initiation progresses best in a rehabilitation setting that provides assistance and structure. Patients discharged home rather than to a supportive living arrangement commonly regress if left alone to complete daily activities. Similarly, patients may exhibit difficulty terminating an activity once it is started. Perseveration may develop, in which the patient cannot end the neurological motor pattern started for a specific activity. For example, a client with a TBI in a vocational program may refuse to end his work task to break for lunch because he or she feels compelled to continue. Sometimes perseveration involves a thought process. A patient may be unable to concentrate on one activity because he or she is perseverating on the idea that another activity (e.g., the laundry) must be completed.

Decreased Safety Awareness and Poor Judgment

Frontal lobe damage often results in an impairment of insight regarding a person's limitations, as well as impulsivity, or the inability to consider consequences before acting. These results cause the patient to demonstrate poor safety awareness and judgment. For example, a patient may attempt to rise out of a wheelchair without locking the brakes or moving the foot plates. A higher-level client who has been reintegrated into the community may attempt to cross streets without observing traffic signals or remove pots from the stove or oven without using protective oven mitts or pot holders. It is important for the occupational therapist to structure the patient's environment to reduce accidents and increase the patient's awareness of his or her limitations through repeated opportunities to practice and relearn safe and appropriate behaviors.

Delayed Processing of Information

Most individuals with TBI have some degree of difficulty with the processing of external information from the environment. A delay in response time is often noted and can range from a few seconds to several minutes. It is important for the therapist to recognize the presence of delayed processing and to distinguish the delay from the absence of function. For example, during a sensory evaluation a patient may exhibit a delay in response to a dull stimulus. The therapist may mistakenly interpret the patient's delayed processing time as an absence of sensory awareness. A delay in the processing of external information from the environment can include visual, auditory, sensory, and perceptual processing.

Impaired Executive Functions and Abstract Thinking

Executive function skills include the ability to plan, set goals, understand the consequences of one's actions, and modify behaviors in accordance with environmental responses. Abstract thinking is the ability to hold and manipulate a concept in one's mind using critical reasoning and analytical skills. Many patients with TBI exhibit concrete thinking, in which they are able to interpret information only at the most literal level. For example, a patient with impaired executive and abstract functions may be able to complete a meal preparation activity accurately and safely only if step-by-step directions are provided. If the directions do not specifically state to modify the cooking temperatures, the patient may burn the food because he or she is unable to foresee the consequences of maintaining the stove on a high setting.

Generalization

Generalization of new learning is the ability to learn a specific task and transfer the skills needed for that task to a similar activity. Deficits in executive functions, abstract thinking, and short-term memory significantly impair the generalization of new learning. For example, a patient who has learned in a group home the skills for completing a laundry task may be unable to transfer the skills to an unfamiliar laundromat. Often this occurs as a result of concrete thinking and the inability to make abstractions. Although the cognitive pattern for completing laundry tasks using the laundry machine in the group home is established, the patient cannot transfer that cognitive pattern to a similar but unfamiliar laundry machine in a different environment. Impaired generalization of new learning is one of the most significant problems impeding the individual's ability to resume independent functioning in a community setting.

Visual Status

Visual skills involve the ability to accurately see stimuli from the external environment (see Chapter 24). Visual skills do not involve the identification of objects, which is a function of perception. Among the many deficits in visual skills that may result from TBI are accommodative dysfunction (causing blurred vision), convergence insufficiency (the inability to maintain a single vision while fixating on an object), lateral or medial strabismus, nystagmus, hemianopsia, and impairment of scanning and pursuits. Saccades (fast, jerky movements of the eyes as they change from one position of gaze to another, as are needed to track the puck in a hockey game) may also be compromised by TBI. Reduced blink rate, ptosis of the eyelid (drooping of the eyelid), and lagophthalmos (incomplete eyelid closure) are also common visual deficits resulting from oculomotor nerve damage.[5,47]

A dysfunction in any of these visual elements can profoundly affect daily life function. Individuals rely on vision indirectly in social and interpersonal interactions. Vision is used as a cueing and feedback system in motor skills such as ambulation and in eye-hand coordination activities. Deficits in vision can affect all daily life activities, including the areas of hygiene and grooming, meal preparation and eating, wheelchair mobility, reading and writing, and driving.

Perceptual Skills

Perception is the ability to interpret stimuli from the external environment (see Chapter 26). Perception is a function of the secondary cortical areas of the right hemisphere, including the secondary visual area, the secondary somatosensory area, the secondary auditory area, and the multimodal parietal-occipital-temporal area. Perceptual deficits are more often a result of right hemisphere damage but also sometimes occur in left hemisphere lesions. Perception can be categorized into *visual* perception, *body schema* perception, *motor* perception, and *speech and language* perception. A patient with visual perceptual impairments may exhibit difficulty with right-left discrimination, figure-ground discrimination, form constancy, position in space, and topographical orientation. Visual perceptual deficits also include visual agnosia, in which the patient displays difficulty recognizing familiar objects and people. For example, prosopagnosia is the inability to connect faces with names. Prosopagnosia results from damage to the multimodal association area.[5]

Body schema perception is the awareness of the spatial characteristics of a person's own body. This awareness is derived from a neural synthesis of tactile, proprioceptive, and pressure sensory associations about the body and its individual parts. A common problem in persons with TBI is anosognosia, a failure to recognize defects or limitations. This may lead to the body schema perceptual dysfunction of **unilateral neglect syndrome**, in which the individual has lost the ability to integrate perceptions from one side of the body or environment (usually the left). A unilateral neglect is commonly caused by a lesion to the right parietal lobe but also can occur as a result of frontal and occipital lobe damage. The patient with a left unilateral neglect may disown his or her left extremities as though they belonged to someone else. For example, a patient may shave only the right side of his face or dress only the right side of his body.[5,47]

Perceptual-speech and language dysfunctions, or the aphasias, involve impairment in the expression and comprehension of language. There are two primary types of aphasia: receptive and expressive. The aphasias can result from both left and right occipital, parietal, and temporal lobe damage. Wernicke's aphasia is a type of receptive aphasia that results from left temporal-parietal lesions. In Wernicke's aphasia the individual cannot comprehend what others have said to him or her; however, the person's own speech is fluid and intact. If receptive aphasia results from a right hemisphere lesion, aprosodia occurs. Aprosodia causes impaired comprehension of the tonal inflections or emotional tone of another's speech. For example, a receptive aphasic with a left hemisphere disorder can still accurately interpret the emotional tone of a conversation but cannot understand the literal meaning of the words spoken (Wernicke's aphasia). A receptive aphasic with a right hemisphere disorder can understand the concrete meaning of the words spoken but cannot accurately interpret the emotional tone of the conversation (aprosodia). This latter type of patient may miss the point of a joke or story because he or she could not comprehend the subtle innuendoes and the implicit meanings conveyed through tonal qualities and inflections.[46]

Receptive aphasias also include alexia, or dyslexia (difficulty comprehending the written word), and asymbolia (difficulty comprehending the meaning of gestures and symbols such as shaking the head no). Expressive aphasia includes Broca's aphasia (the inability to express and transfer thoughts to spoken words), anomia (the inability to transfer the word or name for a specific object or person from the mind into spoken words), and agrommation (a difficulty arranging words in a sentence in an accurate sequence).[46] Patients with TBI commonly display one or more aphasias, making communication with others difficult. The inability to communicate needs often causes added frustration and agitation.

Perceptual-motor dysfunction is an impairment in motor planning, or an apraxia. The apraxias are usually a result of impairment to the premotor cortex and the primary motor area of the frontal lobe. It is in these cortical areas that established motor patterns for specific activities are stored and accessed for the execution of common movement patterns. Ideational apraxia is the inability to understand the demands of a task or the use of the wrong motor plan for a specific task. For example, a patient may not understand that a shirt is an item of clothing to be placed on the torso and UEs. Not understanding the demands of the task, he may be unable to activate the motor plan for UE dressing, or he may activate the wrong plan and attempt to place his legs through the sleeve holes. Sometimes this is referred to as a dressing apraxia. Ideomotor apraxia is the loss of the kinetic memory of a movement pattern for a specific activity. The patient may understand that a shirt is an item of clothing to be placed on the torso and UEs but be unable to execute the appropriate movement plan because it is no longer accessible. Constructional apraxia is the inability to accurately put together pieces of an object to form a three-dimensional whole. For example, a patient whose profession was carpentry may now be unable to put together the wooden pieces of a birdhouse kit.[2]

Psychosocial Factors

Researchers have found that the greatest concerns of individuals 1 or more years after injury are the psychosocial deficits that prevent them from rebuilding a satisfactory postinjury quality of life. As time after injury increases, patients and family members view such psychosocial factors as more detrimental than both the physical and cognitive sequelae of TBI.

Self-Concept

One of the most difficult psychosocial sequelae of TBI is the alteration in the individual's self-concept. Self-concept is the internal image a person holds about personal human identity, sexual and gender identity, body image, personal strengths and limitations, and position in the family, peer group, and community systems. An individual's self-concept changes drastically after TBI. One of the most difficult characteristics of TBI is that although short-term memory is often impaired, long-term memory commonly remains intact. The individual has a clear memory of who he or she was before injury and must now resolve the emotional conflict of having to let go of the preinjury self-concept to rebuild a postinjury self-concept that is both meaningful and satisfying. Some patients describe this process as an unwanted death and rebirth. They say that the person who lived before the injury is now gone, replaced by another who is very different from the individual they remember themselves to be.[39]

Social Roles

Self-concept is derived largely from the social roles the person attains in the family, peer group, and larger community systems. Commonly the individual with TBI loses most preinjury roles and the activities that supported those roles. Family and peer group roles change. Family members and friends are often readily visible during the acute and subacute stages of TBI rehabilitation. However, as time after injury increases, family and friends become less and less involved with the individual, leaving him or her feeling isolated and abandoned.

Many individuals with TBI report that the feeling of isolation and the inability to form and maintain social relationships is their most troubling postinjury concern. The loss of the roles of dating or of partner or spouse commonly leave the individual feeling a deep sense of loss and failure if he or she cannot rebuild a postinjury life that includes intimacy with another human being, partnership in a committed relationship, and parenting of children. The loss of the work role and the inability to support oneself are intimately tied to the feelings of dependence and lack of personal control.[28]

Independent Living Status

As a result of the physical, cognitive, and psychosocial sequelae of TBI, many individuals find that they require supportive living arrangements or that they must live with their parents. The loss of the ability to live independently in the community further reinforces feelings of dependence and decreased personal control. As a result of these role losses, adults who sustain a TBI commonly experience role strain and feel that they cannot reenter their communities. The TBI, particularly if it occurred between the ages of 18 and 30, disrupts the developmental transition from adolescence to adulthood, leaving individuals feeling inadequate and unable to attain a postinjury adult status. Depression, withdrawal, and apathy are common psychosocial sequelae of the alterations in self-concept discussed earlier and of the loss of desired social roles.[33]

Dealing With Loss

Individuals with TBI often experience a process that is similar to the stages of death and dying experienced by terminally ill patients.[30] These stages begin with denial, in which the individual denies that he is experiencing physical, cognitive, or psychosocial deficits. Denial can impede therapy because the patient may refuse to participate, believing that therapy is unnecessary. Denial subsides (by degrees) as the patient is continually confronted with his or her limitations in daily life activities. Anger follows denial. The patient grows increasingly aware of his or her deficits and becomes frustrated and angry because recovery is slower than desired. Bargaining is the next stage. The patient strikes a deal with the Creator or the fates, offering to work as diligently as possible in therapy if the creator will restore the individual's preinjury lifestyle. Often this stage is marked by increased motivation and optimism. Depression tends to emerge next. The patient begins to realize the severity of the injury and the meaning that the injury holds for the rest of the individual's life. Acceptance of the injury and resultant limitations is the next stage in the process and is necessary for the individual to become sufficiently motivated to attempt to build a postinjury life that, although drastically different from preinjury goals and expectations, is nevertheless meaningful and personally valuable. These stages may require years of transition. Often denial, anger, and bargaining occur in the first months to a year after the injury. Depression sets in as the individual is able to let go of some of the denial and becomes aware of the effect the injury will have on his or her future life. It may take years before an individual can truly accept the injury and the alterations in personality, skill, and lifestyle and move on to rebuild a new life. The process of denial, anger, depression, and acceptance does not generally proceed in a linear fashion. Patients commonly experience repeated periods of denial, anger, and depression throughout their years of rehabilitation. Renewed denial, anger, and depression may occur in response to a new environmental demand, such as a change in life condition (e.g., a need to move from the parental home to a community group home) or the development of further physical, cognitive, or psychosocial deterioration over time (e.g., the need for increased ambulatory assistance because of a deterioration in visual skills).

Affective Changes

Depression, increased emotional lability, and decreased affect can result from the neurological damage itself. Patients with left hemisphere damage tend to exhibit increased depression and emotional lability. Lesions of the left orbitofrontal lobe often cause severe depression and heightened affect (including excitement, agitation, and tearfulness). Lesions of the left dorsolateral frontal lobe commonly result in a decreased or flat affect. A patient with these lesions may appear depressed to the observer even though he or she may feel fine. Neurological damage to the right hemisphere often causes a strange sense of euphoria or lack of emotional response to the severity of injury.[39]

Behavioral Factors

Behavioral disturbance is common in TBI recovery. Most behavioral disturbances are organically based and result from specific neurological damage. Cognitive levels IV and V of the Ranchos Los Amigos Scale describe the patient who is confused and agitated and behaves in a socially inappropriate manner. Patients may exhibit behavioral problems on a continuum from severely verbally and physically combative to mildly confused and agitated. Patients who are experiencing severe confusion are often impatient, easily irritated, and combative (both physically and verbally). They may shout, scream, and be restless. Such agitation is neither purposeful nor permanent, but rather results from the patient's inability to correctly interpret events in the environment. Displays of anger are often quickly forgotten, allowing the therapist to redirect the patient to another, less confusing activity.

Social inappropriateness and **disinhibition** are also common behavioral problems in some patients with TBI and may involve using obscenities, making indiscriminate sexual advances to staff or strangers in the community, and removing clothing in public settings. Such disinhibition results from damage to the frontal lobe areas that mediate behavioral control according to learned social norms.

A patient's agitation may occur sporadically in isolated contexts. Many patients experience periods of agitation and confusion for weeks or months during the subacute recovery period. These periods tend to be replaced by more appropriate behaviors as neurological recovery progresses. However, some patients experience severe behavioral disturbances that do not change with time. It is important to provide a **behavioral management** program for patients displaying long-term and chronic behavioral problems.

EVALUATION OF THE BEGINNING-LEVEL PATIENT

A beginning-level patient with TBI (Ranchos Los Amigos Scale score of 1 to 3) may be comatose, exhibit minimal arousal, or display severe confusion and attentional deficits. Evaluation of such patients may have to be completed in short segments because of the patients' low level of functioning. A quiet environment with minimal distractions will enhance the patients' concentration and ability to attend to the therapist's requests. Evaluation will include assessment of the following items:

1. *Cognition.* Is the patient oriented and alert? Can the patient respond to simple verbal commands, such as "Squeeze my finger"? Can the patient communicate through verbalizations or eye movements?
2. *Vision.* Is the patient able to scan an object or maintain eye contact with the therapist? Does the patient's eye open in response to the sound of a human voice?
3. *Sensation.* Does the patient respond to external stimulation such as pain or cold?
4. *Joint ROM.* Has the patient lost ROM in certain joints as a result of decorticate or decerebrate rigidity, increased tone and spasticity, contractures, or heterotopic ossification?
5. *Muscular strength.* Does the patient demonstrate weakness in muscle groups without accompanied changes in tone?
6. *Motor control.* Is the patient exhibiting decorticate or decerebrate rigidity? Is the patient experiencing increased tone and spasticity bilaterally, unilaterally, or in one or more limbs? Does the patient have decreased tone and hypotonicity? Are deep tendon responses present, diminished, or absent? Does the patient exhibit the presence of primitive reflexes?
7. *Dysphagia.* If the patient is self-feeding, can he or she eat without aspirating? Is the patient able to exhibit oral motor control without pocketing the food in his or her cheeks or drooling?

8. *Psychosocial and behavioral factors.* Is the patient's affect flat, agitated, or emotionally labile?

Evaluation of the beginning-level patient with TBI is generally accomplished with such tools as a goniometer and with manual muscle testing, a traditional neurological screening, and clinical observation. Many TBI acute facilities use their own initial evaluation forms. The Glasgow Coma Scale and the Ranchos Los Amigos Scales are often used to assess cognitive status in the beginning level patient.

TREATMENT OF THE BEGINNING-LEVEL PATIENT WITH TRAUMATIC BRAIN INJURY

The general aims of treatment for the beginning-level patient are to increase the patient's level of response and awareness of self and the environment. All stimulation must be well structured, broken down into simple steps and commands. Sufficient time must be allowed for a patient's response because cognitive processing is often significantly delayed during this phase of rehabilitation. Treatment at this stage can be grouped into six areas: sensory stimulation, wheelchair positioning, bed positioning, casting or splinting, dysphagia management, behavioral and emotional management, and family and caregiver education.

Sensory Stimulation

Treatment of the beginning-level patient should start as soon as the patient is medically stable. Treatment generally begins in the ICU. At this stage the patient often lacks responsiveness to pain, touch, sound, or sight. The patient also may exhibit a generalized response to pain that appears reflexive (e.g., attempting to push away a painful stimulus). The goal of treatment is to increase the patient's level of awareness by presenting controlled **sensory stimulation.** Sensory stimulation increases neurological signals to the reticular activating system, the structure of the brainstem that alerts the brain to important sensory input from the external environment.[5] Stimulation of the reticular activating system is believed to decrease the threshold necessary for cortical responsiveness in the beginning-level patient with TBI.

Traditional methods of sensory stimulation include introducing isolated visual, auditory, tactile, olfactory, and gustatory stimulants to the patient to heighten arousal of the reticular activating system. For example, a flashlight may be used to elicit eye opening and visual tracking. A therapist may ring a bell or play music and observe the patient's response to auditory stimulation. During olfactory stimulation a variety of scents (e.g., vanilla and banana) may be placed under the patient's nose to stimulate arousal. The therapist waits for the patient to respond in some way, such as opening the

eyes. Gustatory stimulation involves the controlled presentation of tastes to the patient's lips and tongue using a cotton swab. Such stimulants include salty tastes (sodium chloride solution), sweet tastes (sucrose solution), bitter tastes (quinine), and sour tastes (vinegar or lemon juice). Any response from the patient is noted. Treatment progresses from the introduction of isolated sensory stimulants to the presentation of multisensory stimuli to activate the integration of several structures of the brain simultaneously. For example, a therapist may use tactile stimulation on the patient's face while soft music is playing. The most effective types of sensory stimulants are those that have personal meaning to the patient. The therapist could play the patient's favorite songs, present the perfume worn by his girlfriend or mother, or introduce tastes for which the patient has particular preferences. The therapist should learn about the patient's preinjury history, personality, and interests so as to introduce meaningful sensory stimulation. Often patients respond more readily to the verbal commands, touch, and scents of family members than those of unfamiliar health care professionals. For this reason and others, it is helpful to include family members in therapy from the beginning of the patient's treatment.

The functional approach to sensory stimulation may be used for the patient who displays some response to sensory stimulation and verbal commands. The patient is actively assisted by the therapist to perform simple functional activities, such as rolling in bed, cleaning the face with a damp washcloth, combing the hair, and applying lotion to the skin. The theoretical aim of the functional sensory stimulation approach is to reactivate highly processed neural pathways that had been established before the injury. Some therapists use the functional sensory stimulation approach in sequence, following the presentation of isolated and multisensory stimulation. The therapist observes the patient during the activity for any changes, such as the following:

1. Turning of the patient's head toward the direction of sound
2. Visual attention and tracking of objects used in the activity
3. Physical responses (e.g., changes in respiration, muscle tone, voluntary use of the extremities, and posture)
4. Vocalizations (e.g., groans, sighs, or one word)
5. The following of oral commands

Wheelchair Positioning

Seating and positioning are important components. Because wheelchair ambulation provides the first opportunity for the patient to interact with the immediate environment in an upright posture, positioning aims to help the patient keep the head erect and see people and objects in the environment. A proper wheelchair seating position helps prevent skin breakdown and joint contractures, facilitate normal tone, inhibit primitive reflexes, promote safety, and enhance cognitive skills (Fig. 38-1).

Effective seating and positioning require a stable base of support at the pelvis, maintenance of the trunk in midline, and placement of the head in an upright posture. This position frees the UEs for use and allows the patient to visually scan the environment.

Pelvis

Wheelchair positioning should begin at the pelvis, since poor hip placement adversely alters trunk and head alignment and influences tone in the extremities. Because sling-seat wheelchairs contribute to internal rotation and adduction of the hips, it is important to insert a hard, solid seat (padded with foam and covered by vinyl) to facilitate a neutral to slightly anterior pelvic tilt. A lumbar support will also help to maintain the natural curve in the lumbar spine. A wedged seat insert (with the downward slope pointing toward the back of the chair) can be used to facilitate hip flexion and inhibit extensor tone in the hips and LEs. The patient's

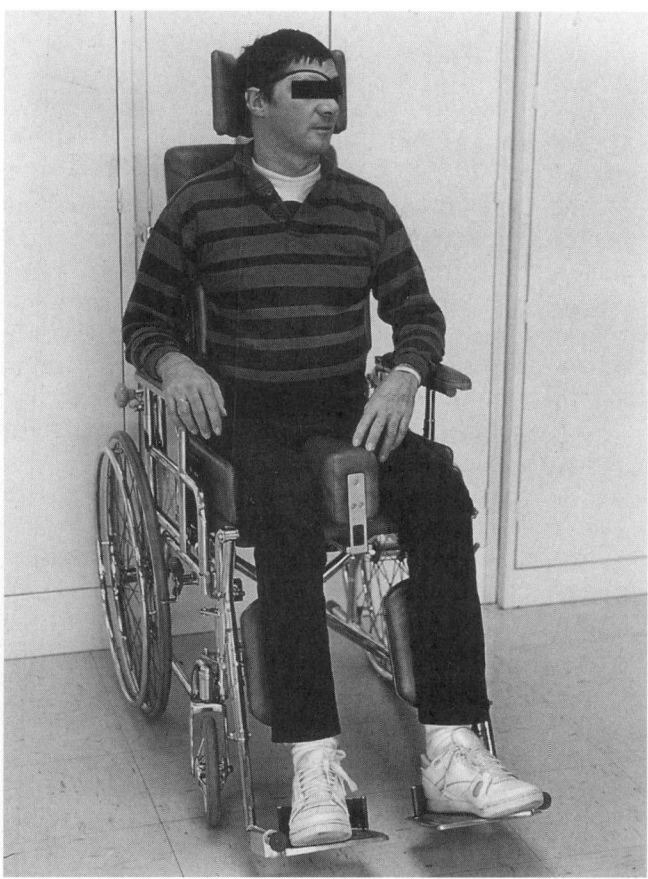

FIG. 38-1
Improved posture and trunk alignment is achieved with positioning devices.

buttocks should bear weight evenly, with both ischial tuberosities firmly resting on the wheelchair seat; sacral sitting is contraindicated. A seat belt angled across the pelvis helps maintain this desired position. The patient must be able to release the seat belt because restraining devices are illegal and could cause agitation in the confused patient.

Trunk

The trunk should be positioned after the pelvis because it is the next most proximal body structure. A solid back insert or solid contoured back should be placed behind the patient's back to maintain the spine in an erect posture. A back insert that is contoured to the curves in the spine will maintain the lumbar and thoracic curves. Lateral trunk supports can be used to reduce scoliosis and lateral trunk flexion caused by imbalanced tone of the intrinsic muscles of the back. A chest strap (with easily opened Velcro fasteners) can be used to decrease kyphosis, facilitate shoulder retraction and abduction, and expand the upper chest for proper diaphragmatic breathing.

Lower Extremities

An abductor wedge placed between the LEs just proximal to the knees may be used to decrease hip adduction and internal rotation. If hip abduction is present, foam pads can be placed along the lateral aspect of the thigh to reduce LE abduction. Ideally the knees should be positioned at 90°, with the heels slightly behind the knees in sitting. However, many patients with TBI exhibit LE extensor spasticity and need adjustable, raised foot plates that can place the knee in a position of extension or a flexed position greater than 90°. It is desirable to maintain both feet securely on the foot plates to provide proprioceptive input and facilitate weight bearing in both heels to normalize tone.

Upper Extremities

The UEs should be positioned with the scapulae in a neutral position (neither elevated nor depressed), the shoulders slightly externally rotated and abducted, the elbows in a neutral position of slight flexion with forearm pronation, and the wrists and digits in a functional position. This position is often difficult to achieve because of severe spasticity and soft-tissue contractures of the UEs. A splint or cast (discussed later) may be applied to decrease spasticity and facilitate a functional position of the UEs. Frequently a lap tray is used to provide support for the UEs and to encourage bilateral UE use.

Head

The beginning-level patient with TBI often has little or no active head control. Attaining a neutral-midline head position, which affords the patient optimal visual contact with the environment, is difficult. A U-shaped device that cradles the head posteriorly and laterally may be used to support the head in a midline position. A forehead strap (fabricated from soft, padded material) may be used to prevent the head from falling forward. Slightly reclining the patient's back (in an adjustable wheelchair) also prevents the head from falling forward and facilitates visual interaction with the environment. The patient should be reclined between 10° to 15°; reclining the patient beyond this point reduces weight bearing through the trunk and pelvis and tends to facilitate a posterior pelvic tilt and sacral sitting.

As the patient progresses in rehabilitation, wheelchair seating and positioning should be reevaluated continually to better meet the needs of the patient. Devices should be modified gradually or removed as the patient begins to control his or her body actively and manipulate more items in the environment. A schedule is necessary to indicate the length of time the patient should be seated in the wheelchair. Keeping the patient in a wheelchair longer than can be tolerated will increase behavioral problems and decrease the patient's cognitive awareness.

Bed Positioning

Proper bed positioning is also difficult to maintain because of spasticity, primitive reflexes, and abnormal posturing. Other complications that prevent proper bed positioning include UE and LE casts or splints, IV tubes, NG tubes, heterotopic ossification, fractures with open reduction, compressive neuropathies, and active movement of the patient by other staff who need to clean the patient, perform neurological examinations, administer medications, and access IV and NG tubes. Prolonged use of any one position may lead to decubitus ulcers, particularly over bony prominences. Thus a bed positioning program must include several appropriate positions that can be alternated during an 8-hour rest period to reduce this risk.

If the patient is exhibiting abnormal posturing, a side-lying or semi-prone position is preferable. A supine position will elicit the tonic labyrinthine reflex, and a supine position with the head in a lateral position will elicit the asymmetrical tonic neck reflex. Because the patient with TBI commonly has bilateral involvement, it is best to create a bed positioning program that involves alternate side-lying on both sides. This may be impossible, however, given the placement of IV tubes. In the side-lying position the patient's head should rest on a small pillow in a neutral, midline position, aligned with the trunk. The bottom UE should be moved into scapular protraction and shoulder external rotation. The top UE also should be moved into scapular protraction with slight shoulder flexion, supported on a pillow to avoid horizontal adduction. The bottom elbow should be flexed; the top elbow extended. Both wrists and all digits should be maintained in extension, often with the aid of splints. The top LE should be moved into slight hip and knee flexion, supported with pillows or bolsters. A foam wedge placed between the knees will decrease hip internal rotation and adduction. The bottom hip and knee should also be slightly flexed. This side-lying position may be maintained with bolsters or pillows behind the back, pelvis, and shoulders. The feet should not extend to the bed footboard because this could elicit extensor thrust.

If the patient must be maintained in a supine bed position, a small pillow under the head with lateral foam wedges will keep the head in midline. The patient's shoulders should be positioned in slight abduction and external rotation. Both elbows are extended, and splints may be used to maintain the wrist and digits in a neutral position. The use of cones or rolled towels between the digits and the palmar surface is contraindicated because these devices will easily move against the muscle bellies of the finger flexors and elicit further flexor spasticity. Both hips should be maintained in slight external rotation and abduction, with the support of lateral bolsters placed between the patient's legs. The patient's knees should be slightly flexed by placing pillows or small bolsters under the distal thigh just above the knee joint.

Splinting and Casting

Splinting or casting is indicated when (a) spasticity has limited functional movement and ADL independence, (b) joint ROM limitations are present, and (c) there is potential for soft-tissue contractures. Splinting of the hands and wrists is often implemented to maintain a functional position at rest and to reduce tone. Serial casting is a more aggressive intervention to increase joint ROM in the elbow when severe spasticity is present. Both splinting and serial casting are used to prevent skin breakdown (particularly when severe finger flexor spasticity has caused the fingers and nails to embed in the palmar surface) and to maintain ROM for self-care (bathing, dressing, and bowel and bladder care).

The stretch splint is a resting splint that is worn when the patient is not involved in functional activities (Fig. 38-2). Once the splint has been fabricated, a splint schedule must be established for nursing staff and caregivers to follow. A typical splint schedule has the patient wearing the splint for repeated, alternating 2-hour periods (2 hours on, followed by 2 hours off). The patient must be monitored frequently for skin breakdown or irritation caused by wearing the splint. If irritation is noted, the splint must be modified. Nursing staff and caregivers should be trained in application and removal of each splint. It is also advisable to post the splint schedule above the patient's bed and on the patient's wheelchair and to mark each splint (in permanent marker) "right" and "left."

Other splints that may be indicated include a wrist cock-up splint, used to stabilize the wrist while enhancing finger prehension, and a thumb opposition splint. used to facilitate palmar pinch or three-point pinch. Splints are modified as needed and may eventually be discontinued if the patient's motor control and tone improve.

A serial casting program is indicated when severe spasticity cannot be managed by splints (i.e., when the spasticity is so great that it breaks the splint). The goal of serial casting is to increase ROM and decrease tone gradually using a progressive succession of separately fabricated casts, each worn continuously for a period of weeks. Successive casts are designed to increase ROM further until a functional joint range is achieved and maintained. The common difficulty that prevents the success of serial casting is skin breakdown. If skin breakdown occurs because of a cast that is worn for several days, the cast must be removed until the skin has healed. While wound healing is occurring, spastic-

ity again increases and any gain in joint ROM is often lost.

The most common UE casts are the elbow cast, used for decreased ROM in the elbow flexors, and the wrist, thumb, and finger cast, used for decreased ROM in the wrist, thumb, and finger flexors. Other variations of casts include elbow and wrist casts and wrist and thumb casts. However, the casting of more than one joint at a time often leads to skin breakdown as a result of multiple pressure points. It is thus recommended that casting be applied to one joint at a time.

Casting is frequently used in conjunction with motor point blocks and baclofen pumps. Blocks involve the injection of a chemical substance (e.g., Lidocaine, Marcaine, phenol, *Botulinum* toxin) into the nerve or motor point to inhibit the innervation of spastic muscles temporarily. A baclofen pump is surgically inserted into a patient's abdomen and time-releases the chemical to inhibit the nerve innervation of spastic muscles. Motor point blocks and baclofen pumps are inserted by physicians before the initiation of serial casting. The combination of blocks and casting is more effective than casting alone[23,40] (see Chapter 23).

Indications for the completion of a casting program include obtaining a functional ROM or plateauing (i.e., the patient has not gained significant improvement in ROM after two consecutive casts). When improvement has been made and the goal has been reached, the final cast is cut in half, the edges are finished, and the cast is used as a bivalved cast with Velcro straps (Fig. 38-3). A wearing schedule is then established. The wearing of a cast is often ended if continual treatments with baclofen are sufficient to maintain ROM.

Dysphagia

The patient emerging from coma is fed through an NG tube or gastrointestinal tube. Once the patient is alert and more oriented, the physician decides when tube feeding can be stopped, and a dysphagia evaluation is then initiated. Dysphagia programs usually begin in the intermediate- to advanced-level stages of rehabilitation (see Chapter 40).

Behavioral and Emotional Management

A patient who has begun to become more alert and aware of his or her environment will often display confusion, emotional lability, or a flat affect. For the beginning-level patient the therapist should provide orientation and a calming presence. The therapist should reintroduce himself or herself to the patient at each session, describe the therapist's role, indicate how he or she will work with the patient, clarify why the patient is in the hospital (if the patient cannot remember), and orient the patient to the place (the hospital), date, time,

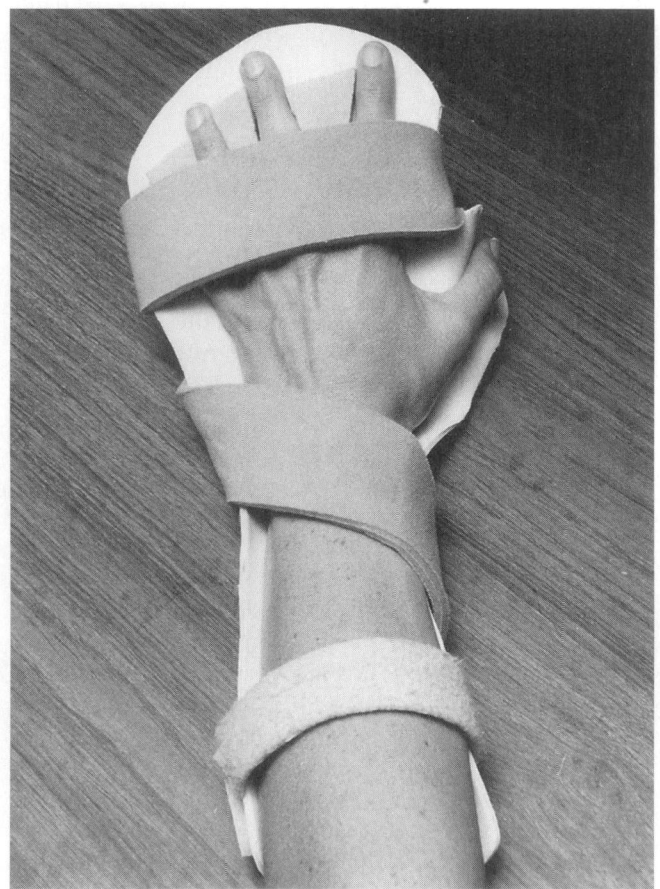

FIG. 38-2
Stretch splint.

and season. If the patient is emotionally labile, care providers should take the time necessary to allow the patient to express his or her emotions, help the patient to feel that he or she has been heard by an empathic listener (the therapist), and reassure the patient that the hospital staff are there to help him or her get better. To reduce confusion and enhance cooperation in the beginning-level patient, therapy should be provided in a quiet setting (e.g., bedside or in a private therapy room), and no more than one family member should be present. Stimuli in the environment (e.g., other people, extraneous noise, and personal items) should be kept to a minimum.

Family and Caregiver Education

The therapist is in a position to provide information and emotional support to family members and caregivers. Family members may display confusion, anger, and grief. At times family members direct their anger and emotional responses toward the therapist, but these actions stem from fear, feelings of lost control, and a lack of knowledge regarding TBI. The therapist should always respect a family member's need to express anger and grief and should address the family member's questions without personalizing any expression of anger. It is important for family members to feel that their concerns have been heard by an understanding therapist. The unfamiliarity of the hospital setting and the serious condition of a loved one often heighten fear in family members. A therapist who can act as a calming presence while providing the family member with information is best able to establish the rapport necessary to elicit family cooperation and assistance in the patient's rehabilitation process.

Involving family members in therapy is a particularly beneficial way of providing information about the loved one's condition while alleviating their confusion and anger. Family members (or one primary family member who is integral to the patient's well-being, such as a parent or spouse) should be involved in therapy from the beginning of the patient's hospital stay. Frequently the patient responds first to the familiar faces of relatives when emerging from a coma. Family members should be involved in therapy to elicit patient responses, assist in the sensory stimulation program, maintain proper bed positioning, and contribute to the ROM program. Later, when the patient is more alert and mobile, family members can be involved in wheelchair positioning, feeding programs, and ADL retraining.

EVALUATION OF THE INTERMEDIATE- TO ADVANCED-LEVEL PATIENT

The intermediate- to advanced-level patient (Rancho Los Amigos Scale score of 4 to 8) is alert but often displays confused, agitated, and inappropriate responses. The patient may be able to follow simple two- to three-step verbal commands but is easily distracted. Often, minimal or moderate cues are necessary to assist the patient in the performance of ADL. Generally, the intermediate- to advanced-level patient with TBI can complete most components of the OT evaluation, but because of distractibility or agitation the patient may need several breaks during the evaluation process. The evaluation for the intermediate to advanced patient with TBI is similar to that for the beginning-level patient, in that physical status, dysphagia, psychosocial and behavioral factors, vision, sensation, and perception are assessed. Additionally, the intermediate- to advanced-level patient requires more extensive evaluation of ADL (including driving), work readiness, and ability to reintegrate into the community.

Physical Status

The physical status evaluation includes an assessment of joint ROM, muscular strength, sensation, proprioception, kinesthesia, fine and gross motor control, and

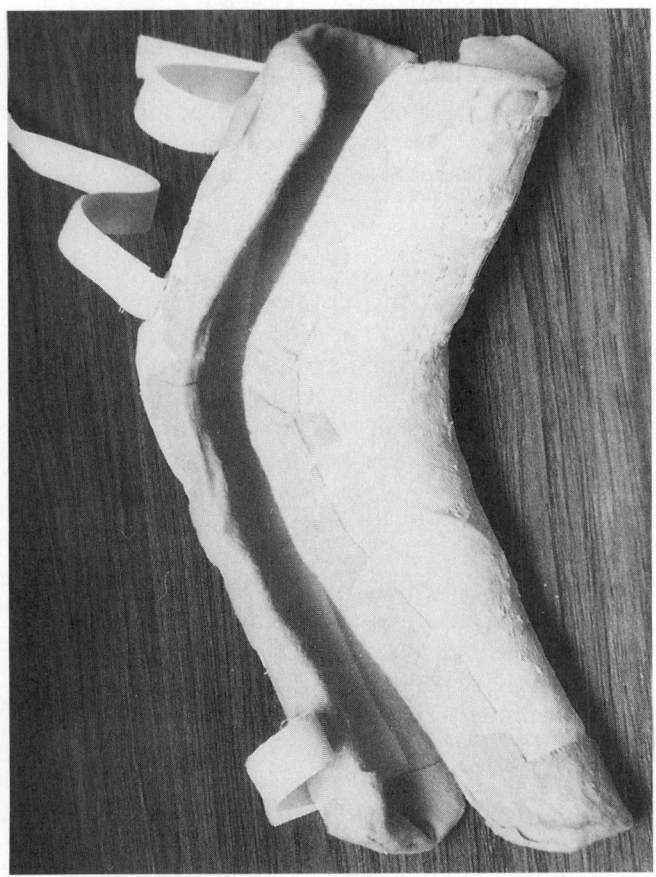

FIG. 38-3
Bivalved cast.

total body control (i.e., the patient is able to integrate movement of separate body parts during the performance of an activity that requires bilateral integration and dynamic sitting or standing balance). Limitations in physical status will probably be the result of abnormal tone, spasticity, muscle weakness without abnormal tone, heterotopic ossification, fractures, soft-tissue contractures, and peripheral nerve compression. Tools to evaluate physical status include goniometers, dynamometers, manual muscle testing, and clinical observation. Standard assessments may include the Jebsen Hand Function Test,[24] the Minnesota Rate of Manipulation Tests,[35] the Minnesota Manual Dexterity test,[35] and the Purdue Pegboard.[45]

Dysphagia

Assessment of the patient with TBI should include both a clinical (bedside) dysphagia assessment and videofluoroscopy. The bedside examination will provide the therapist with information regarding impulsivity (does the patient gulp large portions of food quickly, thus causing aspiration?), and oral motor control (can the patient make a bolus, or does the patient pocket food in cheeks; can the patient manage saliva production while eating, or is drooling apparent; does the patient chew with both sides of his jaw, or is one used to compensate for decreased function on the opposing side?). The bedside dysphagia examination will also provide the therapist with information regarding cognitive status (does the patient appear to understand what to do with the utensils and food items?), perceptual skills (is a neglect present, causing the patient to leave one side of the plate untouched?), and language functioning (does the patient know the names of the utensils and food items, or is aphasia suspected?).

The videofluoroscopy must be performed by a physician and will provide information regarding the anatomy and physiology of the oral, pharyngeal, and esophageal stages of swallowing. Videofluoroscopy is the only dysphagia assessment tool that can provide information regarding the patient's ability to manage liquids and solid foods. This information will be used to design a feeding program that may require a diet of thick liquids and pureed foods. Reevaluation should be made as the patient improves in rehabilitation and can progress to thin liquids and solid foods. (See Chapter 40 for more information on dysphagia.)

Improper positioning, behavioral disorders, and cognitive-perceptual impairment have all been implicated as factors contributing to swallowing disorders. Dysphagia treatment must address seating and positioning, behavioral management while self-feeding, and cognitive-perceptual distortions. Formal assessments to evaluate dysphagia include the Dysphagia Evaluation Protocol[3] and the Evaluation of Oral Function in Feeding.[44]

Cognition

Cognitive skills of the patient with TBI should be assessed within a functional task (e.g., ADL) because paper and pencil tasks do not provide the real-life situations that will reveal cognitive deficits. For example, a therapist may assess a patient's cognitive skills during a cold meal preparation that requires the ability to (1) follow two- to three-step written or spoken directions, (2) correctly sequence the order of steps, (3) attend to the task with minimal distraction, and (4) display good safety and judgment. When the therapist is evaluating the patient's cognitive status during ADL, measurement of cognitive skills can be assessed by (1) counting the number of errors and correct responses, (2) assessing the amount of assistance or cueing needed (minimal, moderate, or maximal), and (3) totaling the percentage of the task completed correctly. Assessment of the complexity of the activity (simple versus multistep) and the conditions of the environment (isolated versus multistimulus) is also important.

When assessing a patient's cognitive skills, it is important to consider other factors that may affect performance. These include language barriers (e.g., the presence of aphasia, a primary language other than English), visual-perceptual deficits, the effects of medication on cognitive level, educational and cultural background, and previous experience with the task. Formal cognitive assessments that may be used with a TBI population include the Allen Cognitive Level Test,[1] the Loewenstein Occupational Therapy Cognitive Assessment,[31] the Rivermead Behavioural Memory Test,[49] and the Cognitive Assessment of Minnesota.[42]

Vision

Adults with TBI should undergo a vision screening. The vision screening should be completed as early as possible in the rehabilitation process, since early detection of vision deficits will allow the treatment team to obtain more reliable information regarding the patient's overall health status. For example, diplopia (double vision) or accommodative dysfunction (inability to adjust focus for changes in distance) will probably influence the results of the neuropsychology or speech-language pathology assessments.

A vision screening is a tool that allows therapists to identify potential vision deficits. Although therapists cannot diagnose conditions of vision dysfunction, they can determine if a patient passes or fails a visual screening based on standard criteria. The screening is a means to determine which patients require a referral to an optometrist or ophthalmologist for a complete evaluation and treatment. A comprehensive vision treatment program is designed by an optometrist and implemented by an occupational therapist or vision therapist. A vision history questionnaire should be completed as well. The vision history questionnaire should contain an ophthalmologic history, questions regarding the use of glasses and contact lenses, and questions regarding the presence of blurred vision, dizziness, headaches, eye strain, diplopia, and visual field loss.

Common areas evaluated in a vision screening include visual attention, near and distant acuities, ocular movement (e.g., pursuits and saccades), convergence, accommodation, ocular alignment, depth perception (stereopsis), and visual field function. Vision dysfunction can also be identified during the clinical observation of the patient's performance in functional activities. Tilting the head as a result of a field deficit, closing or covering one eye to decrease blurred vision, and bumping into walls or objects in the environment because of a field deficit or unilateral neglect are all easily observed behaviors indicative of vision dysfunction.

Perceptual Function

The perceptual evaluation should be administered when the therapist has obtained a clear understanding of the patient's cognitive, sensory, motor, and language status because deficits in these areas may skew the patient's performance on a perceptual evaluation. Evaluation of visual perception should include right-left discrimination, form constancy, position in space, topographical orientation, and the naming of objects. Evaluation of perceptual-speech and language function should assess for aphasia, agrommatism, and anomia. Evaluation of perceptual motor function should include the functions of ideational praxis, ideomotor praxis, three-dimensional constructional praxis, and body schema perception (including the identification of unilateral neglect). Formal perceptual assessments that can be used with a population of adults with TBI include the Hooper Visual Organization Test,[20] Motor-Free Visual Perception Test—Revised,[12] Rivermead Perceptual Assessment Battery,[8] Loewenstein Occupational Therapy Cognitive Assessment,[31] and Behavioural Inattention Test.[50]

Activities of Daily Living

The intermediate-level patient with TBI should be assessed in all basic ADL—grooming, oral hygiene, bathing, toileting, dressing, functional mobility (including transfers), and emergency response. The advanced-level patient with TBI should also be assessed with regard to instrumental activities of daily living (IADL)—hot and cold meal preparation, money management, community shopping, household maintenance, cleaning and clothing care, safety procedures, medication routine, and work readiness. During assessment the therapist will have ample opportunity to observe cognitive skills, perceptual skills, and behavioral appropriateness.

The patient with a history of alcohol abuse requires assessment of leisure patterns. An interest history and interest checklist may reveal healthful leisure interests that can replace alcohol use. The combination of leisure skills development and substance abuse rehabilitation will help the patient manage time more effectively, so as to avoid a return to alcohol use after discharge. Formal assessments that can be used with a population with TBI to assess ADL skills include the Arnadottir OT-ADL Neurobehavioral Evaluation,[2] Assessment of Motor and Process Skills,[13] Functional Independence Measure,[18] and Klein-Bell Activities of Daily Living Scale.[27]

Driving

Many states require physicians to report to the Department of Motor Vehicles any patient who has lapses of consciousness, seizure disorders, and cognitive, visual, and perceptual dysfunction caused by TBI. Regulations regarding such disorders often mandate that the driver's license be revoked until further assessment confirms that the patient can drive without posing a safety risk to self or others.

Advanced-level patients with TBI who do not have seizure disorders or severe cognitive deficits must undergo a comprehensive driving evaluation to assess their ability to resume driving. Two types of driving evaluations are completed for the patient with TBI: a clinical assessment (evaluation of the patient's visual, cognitive, perceptual, and physical status as it relates to driving) and an on-road assessment. Both driving evaluations are necessary because the patient may fail the clinical assessment but pass the on-road assessment using compensatory strategies. Conversely, the patient may perform successfully on the clinical assessment but fail the on-road assessment (see Chapter 14).

Patients with TBI frequently exhibit deficits (e.g., visual processing disorders, figure-ground discrimination dysfunction, and impulsivity) that significantly affect the ability to drive safely. When visual processing is delayed, the patient hesitates during driving maneuvers and stops unsafely (e.g., in the middle of the road or at a corner) to allow adequate time to process visual information. A patient with figure-ground impairments may be unable to identify stop signs and traffic signals at intersections or locate the gearshift near the dashboard. An impulsive patient may respond aggressively rather than defensively when driving, increasing the risk of accidents. The patient may use poor judgment when making driving decisions and may be unable to inhibit inappropriate responses. The Elemental Driving Simulator[16] and Driving Assessment System[16] constitute an off-the-road clinical driving assessment that can be used, with an on-road assessment, to determine a patient's ability to resume driving after brain injury.

Vocational Rehabilitation

An advanced-level patient with TBI may be evaluated for return to work. It has been well documented that the return to work after a moderate to severe brain injury is generally unsuccessful. High unemployment rates have been attributed to the adverse emotional, behavioral, and neuropsychological changes arising from brain injury. Substance abuse in the TBI population is also a major factor inhibiting the ability to return to and maintain employment.[21]

The vocational assessment for the advanced-level patient with TBI must involve assessment in the actual work setting because psychometric tests and job simulations do not accurately determine work potential. The individual with TBI is often able to compensate in the work setting for deficits that may appear as significant impairments on a psychometric test. The therapist's vocational evaluation should summarize the patient's interests, strengths, and areas of deficit. The report should conclude with recommendations that state the patient's realistic job goals and a plan for achieving those goals with professional assistance.

Psychosocial Skills

The advanced-level patient with TBI who will be discharged to home or a community-supported living residence should also receive a psychosocial skill evaluation. Such an evaluation should assess role loss, social conduct, interpersonal skills, self-expression, time management, and self-control. The therapist should also assess the patient's social support system, the patient's ability to form and maintain friendships, and resources to decrease feelings of isolation (such as TBI support groups). The ability to form and maintain intimate and sexual relationships after TBI will be of paramount concern to single individuals who sustained their TBI between the ages of 18 and 30. Child rearing and care of family members will be of concern for patients responsible for children and other family members.

The assessment of psychosocial skills in the patient with a brain injury is critical, since a year or more after injury individuals with TBI report that their psychosocial deficits significantly diminish life satisfaction and are a greater problem than physical and cognitive deficits combined. Often psychosocial impairment is neglected in the rehabilitation setting as the treatment of acute physical, cognitive, and perceptual deficits is prioritized. Psychosocial difficulties appear more readily after discharge, when the individual has left the structured and safe setting of the rehabilitation hospital to reenter the community. It is important to address psychosocial difficulties before the patient is discharged. Psychosocial assessment tools that can be used for a population with TBI include the Assessment of Communication and Interaction Skills,[43] the Occupational Role History,[14] and the Role Checklist.[38]

TREATMENT OF THE INTERMEDIATE-TO ADVANCED-LEVEL PATIENT

Treatment of the intermediate- to advanced-level patient with TBI involves two primary approaches: the *rehabilitative* model and the *compensatory* model. The rehabilitative model is supported by the theory of neuroplasticity, which holds that the brain can repair itself or reorganize its neural pathways to allow the relearning of functions that had been lost as a result of neural damage sustained in the accident. The compensatory model holds that the repair of damaged brain tissue either has occurred to its full extent or cannot occur, leaving the patient unable to perform lost functions without external assistance. Tools used in the compensatory model are adaptive equipment, environmental modification, and compensatory strategies that allow the patient to perform ADL. Treatment using both the rehabilitative and compensatory approaches can address neuromuscular impairment, cognitive deficits, perceptual deficits, vision dysfunction, and behavioral disorders. Generally a rehabilitative approach is used in the acute stages of TBI recovery until the patient has plateaued or has been unable to progress, at which time a compensatory approach is attempted.

Neuromuscular Impairments

As with a beginning-level patient with TBI, numerous types of neuromuscular impairment can be present in the intermediate- to advanced-level patient with TBI. Spasticity, rigidity, soft-tissue contractures, the presence of primitive reflexes, diminished or lost postural reactions, muscular weakness (without accompanying spasticity), and impaired sensation affect the patient's ability to perform activities independently and with normal control. The prerequisites for normal movement include normal postural tone, a balanced integration of flexor control (reciprocal innervation), normal proximal stability, and the ability to implement selective movement patterns.

The common principles of treatment for neuromuscular impairment are to facilitate control of muscle groups, progressing proximally to distally; encourage symmetrical posture; facilitate integration of both sides of the body into activities; encourage bilateral weight bearing; and introduce a normal sensory experience. The variety of effective rehabilitation techniques for the intermediate- to advanced-level patient with TBI include neurodevelopmental treatment (NDT), proprioceptive neuromuscular facilitation (PNF), myofascial release, Rood techniques, and some physical agent modalities (see Chapters 30 and 32 through 36). These clinical treatments require education beyond the entry level and must be either incorporated into or followed by a meaningful functional activity that requires the same movement. The following brief overview of principles is not meant to substitute for training in the specific techniques.

The treatment of impaired neuromuscular control should begin at the pelvis, since positioning of the pelvis affects motor control of all other body parts. A variety of approaches may be used to normalize pelvic positioning. For example, it is common for a patient with TBI to have a posterior pelvic tilt. To move the patient to a more functional erect pelvic position, a therapist trained in NDT might use an anterior pelvic tilt mobilization. A therapist with a different approach might use a bedsheet behind the pelvis to lift and rotate the pelvis forward over the heads of the femurs. In either case the patient would be directed to "sit up tall."

The trunk is positioned after the pelvis. Proper positioning of the trunk frees the UEs for functional activities. Major principles include (1) facilitating trunk alignment, (2) stimulating reciprocal trunk muscle activity (balancing the dorsal and ventral flexor-extensor muscle groups), (3) encouraging the patient to shift weight out of a stable posture into all directions (bending forward, bending backward, reaching to each side while laterally flexing the trunk), and (4) helping the patient move the lower trunk on a stable upper trunk, or to move the upper trunk on a stable lower trunk. Once trunk control improves, treatment should progress to the UEs.

Rehabilitative techniques may be applied in various ways by the service-competent practitioner. The patient with soft-tissue contractures or spasticity in a particular muscle group may benefit from NDT mobilizations and inhibitory techniques of the agonistic muscle group. The patient with low tone or weak muscles (without the presence of spasticity) may benefit from NDT, PNF, Rood, and physical agent modalities. Neuromuscular electrical stimulation can effectively stimulate UE muscle groups, including the triceps, pronators, supinators, and wrist and finger extensors, to enhance muscle strength, increase sensory awareness, and assist in motor learning and coordination.[10]

Many advanced-level patients with TBI have fairly intact motor control. These patients ambulate independently and incorporate both UEs in functional activities. However, close observation reveals subtle trunk and extremity deficits related to coordination and speed of movement. The treatment for trunk control with these patients focuses on developing full isolated movements of the trunk and extremities, good dynamic standing balance for all activities (including reaching and bending to high and low surfaces), and the ability to shift weight naturally from one LE to the other during activities. UE treatment programs are designed to increase scapular stability and improve fine motor control. A goal of treatment is to improve the patient's speed while maintaining good coordination.

Ataxia

Ataxia is a common motor dysfunction that occurs primarily as a result of damage to the cerebellum or to the neural pathways leading to and from the cerebellum. Ataxia develops early in the acute stages of recovery and may remain permanently. Ataxia is a clinical problem for which rehabilitation methods are generally ineffective. More often, therapists use compensatory strategies to control the effects of ataxia. For example, weighting of body parts and the use of resistive activities often improve control during the performance of tasks but show inconsistent carryover of muscular control when the weights or resistance is removed. When applying weights to the patient, the therapist must identify at which joint(s) the tremor originates. Applying weights to a patient's wrists when the tremor emerges from the trunk and shoulders is ineffective.

Weighted eating utensils and cups are also used as compensatory aids to reduce effects of ataxia in the UEs. These assistive devices are limited in their effectiveness. Another alternative used more successfully in the LEs than the UEs is to wrap Theraband in a figure-eight pattern around the extremity during treatment. The Theraband provides increased proprioceptive input to the extremity and decreases the degree of ataxia.

Cognition

Treatment designed to enhance cognitive skills should be implemented through functional ADL and IADL. Because impairment of cognition often results in concrete thinking, the patient with TBI is likely to have difficulty with abstract concepts. Activities that require the generalization of skills from one task to another will also present difficulty for the patient with TBI. It is best to engage the patient in activities needed in his or her everyday life. For example, if the patient will return to a community environment in which she or he needs to use public transportation, interpreting bus schedules is a meaningful and relevant activity that addresses concentration, frustration tolerance, sequencing, and categorization. Planning a trip to the hardware store to purchase supplies to install a hand-held shower addresses organization, problem solving, and money management.

Advanced-level patients with TBI who demonstrate high-level cognitive skills often display subtle cognitive deficits in the areas of organization, planning, sequencing, and short-term memory. Activities such as establishing a monthly budget to live independently in the community and negotiating the community public transportation system to pay a bill at the electric company provide a context for cognitive retraining to address subtle cognitive deficits. Activities should be challenging, age appropriate, and relevant to the patient's real-life needs. The activities mentioned earlier are based on the rehabilitative approach. Compensatory strategies include the use of a schedule or memory book, the use of a monthly budget chart, and the use of simplified maps of the patient's community.

The use of computers in cognitive retraining has been implemented largely by neuropsychologists and cognitive educators. Computer programs have been designed to enhance sequencing, categorization, cognitive processing time, and concentration. Such programs, however, bear no functional relevance and have not been shown to generalize to the cognitive skills needed to improve performance in IADL.[37] Computers should be used in therapy only if the patient needs to use a computer for work, school, word processing, e-mail exchange, and Internet access. Software programs that do not represent functional activities should be avoided. Therapy should address the individual's specific computer needs. For example, therapists may reprogram a patient's home computer to make it less complicated to use, by simplifying tool bars and menus and programming step-by-step written directions that appear on screen.

Vision

Treatment alternatives for the patient with TBI and vision dysfunction include the use of corrective lenses, occlusion (patching one eye), prism lenses, vision exercises, environmental adaptations, and corrective surgery. An optometrist or ophthalmologist can evaluate and prescribe glasses for patients with accommodative dysfunction caused by brain injury. However, the glasses should not be prescribed until the patient has passed the subacute phase of rehabilitation because an accommodative dysfunction that presents in the acute stages of brain injury may improve during the recovery process.

A common technique to eliminate double vision (diplopia) is patching, or occlusion. The patient wears a patch over one eye that blocks the image seen by that eye, eliminating diplopia. Patching is a temporary compensatory strategy. Prism glasses or binasal occluders may be prescribed by an optometrist for patients with consistent diplopia resulting from permanent oculomotor nerve damage. The prisms assist the eyes in fusing images. Prism glasses are not effective for patients with a significant lateral strabismus or for patients with exotropia (outward eye turn). Binasal occluders encourage the malaligned eye to fixate centrally. Prism glasses and binasal occluders are used conjointly with vision exercises. The goal of this treatment is to decrease the diplopia and eventually eliminate the need for prisms or occluders.

Vision exercises consist of a series of activities that (1) maximize residual vision, (2) enhance impaired vision skills (the rehabilitative approach), (3) increase the patient's awareness of his or her vision deficits, and (4) help the patient learn compensatory strategies. Treatment progresses from monocular to binocular vision and follows a developmental progression (supine to sitting to standing). Exercises initially address basic skills such as visual attention, pursuits, and saccades and may progress to more difficult skills such as fusion and stereopsis. These vision exercises are based on the rehabilitative model that holds that impaired vision skills can improve with training.

Environmental adaptations for vision deficits are based on the compensatory model. Compensatory strategies for vision deficits include using a colored border along one side of a page to facilitate reading, using a colored strip of tape along one side of a plate or meal tray to promote self-feeding, using large objects such as a clock with bold numbers or a telephone with enlarged buttons, using contrasting colors to highlight controls and knobs (e.g., marking a TV/VCR remote control buttons with fluorescent paint), increasing lighting in an environment, and using textures as cues (e.g., adhering textured tape to a banister by the bottom step to cue the individual that the bottom step is coming, to reduce falls). This last compensatory strategy is particularly valuable for patients with vertical gaze paralysis who can look neither up nor down. Patients who have lost pupil constriction should wear sunglasses whenever they are in bright light.

Corrective surgery performed by an ophthalmologist may be indicated to align the eyes and eliminate double vision; however, the patient must wait at least a year after the injury to allow for any improvement that may occur naturally in the course of recovery.

Perception

Treatment of perceptual deficits involves both rehabilitative and compensatory approaches. For example, impairment of figure-ground perception might be treated using a rehabilitative approach through repeated practice of locating objects against a similar background (e.g., finding a white shirt on a bed with white sheets or finding a spoon in a drawer of similar stainless-steel utensils). Using a compensatory approach, the therapist would help the patient to arrange the kitchen drawers so that utensils were categorized (perhaps color-coded) and distinctly divided to facilitate identification.

Aphasia (a perceptual-speech disorder) can also be treated using both rehabilitative and compensatory approaches. An expressive aphasia may be treated rehabilitatively through repeated conversation exercises in which the patient is provided with feedback regarding his or her incorrect spoken words and challenged to express the correct words that he or she meant to verbalize. If the patient has not made significant gains in expressive speech through the use of the rehabilitative approach, the compensatory approach should be used to help the patient articulate his or her needs to caregivers. For example, a chart with letters, words, or pictures (or a combination of the three) of important items in the patient's environment can be used to help the patient identify such needs as eating, toileting, and medications. Such a chart may be used concomitantly with rehabilitative approaches.

Through a rehabilitative approach, apraxia can be treated by helping the patient perform specific tasks (such as dressing) hand-over-hand (i.e., the therapist's hands guide the patient's hands during the performance of dressing). The rehabilitative approach holds that through repeated hand-over-hand exercise the patient's brain can repair the neural pathways that mediate specific motor patterns (such as those needed in dressing) or can reorganize pathways so that different areas of the brain (that have not been damaged) can establish new pathways for specific motor patterns. Using a compensatory approach, the patient may perform dressing by following the steps through the visual interpretation of pictures sequentially depicted (pictures) or listed (words) on a poster or note card.

Neglect syndrome (a disorder of body schema) can also be addressed using rehabilitation and compensatory strategies. Severe neglect syndromes tend to decrease as a natural part of the recovery process. However, some neglect syndromes may continue into the postacute rehabilitation stage. In a rehabilitative approach the patient is encouraged to use the neglected extremity in all ADL. The patient's room may be rearranged to encourage interaction with the neglected part of the environment (e.g., placing the television or standing-bed tray in the left side of the room if a patient has a left neglect). A compensatory model is used when the patient has not demonstrated significant improvement in attending to the neglected side of the body or environment. Colored tape may be placed along the side of the meal tray to cue the patient to attend to the food on the neglected side of the tray. Similarly, a colored border may be placed on the left side of book pages to cue the patient to read the entire page. The patient's home environment is set up to maximize safety; for example, all objects that the patient could bump into (e.g., furniture legs) are moved to the nonneglected side.

Behavioral Management

The types of intervention strategies used to decrease and eliminate problem behaviors may be divided into two categories: *environmental* and *interactive*. Environmental interventions alter objects or other environmental features to facilitate appropriate behaviors, inhibit unwanted behaviors, and maintain patient safety. The agitated patient should be placed in a quiet, isolated room without a roommate. All extraneous stimuli (e.g., radios and televisions) should be removed. Similarly, therapy is provided in a private, quiet room away from other patients and extraneous stimuli.

An agitated patient who demonstrates severe behavioral problems may require one-to-one care. The patient is assigned a rehabilitation aide who remains with the patient throughout the day (including during therapy) to monitor and regulate the patient's behavior. Such a patient may also wear an alarm bracelet that signals staff when the patient attempts to wander off the appropriate floor or out of the building. Walkie-talkies and pagers may be used with patients who are at risk of eloping. One walkie-talkie or pager remains in the nursing station; the other is held by the rehabilitation aide who is providing one-to-one care to the patient. If the patient begins to act aggressively or attempts to elope, the rehabilitation aide can alert the staff that assistance is needed.

Interactive interventions are the approaches that the staff and caregivers use to interact with the patient. These interventions should be implemented in a consistent way by the entire team. These include speaking in a calm, soothing, and concise manner to an agitated patient, deliberately avoiding detailed explanations that will only increase the patient's confusion. For safety's sake, therapists should also keep the bedroom door open when working with the patient at bedside and should maintain an awareness of the patient in relation to self.

The patient who is in the postacute stages of rehabilitation and who continues to exhibit behavioral problems should be placed on a behavioral modification program. Such a program should allow the patient to experience the natural consequences of inappropriate behavior (such as losing community recreational privileges) in an effort to help the patient learn more appropriate responses. Drug therapy may be used for a patient who has not made significant improvement in his or her behaviors and presents a safety risk to self and others.

Dysphagia and Self-Feeding

Treatment strategies for dysphagia follow the same guidelines as for other neurological impairments; intervention, however, may be more complex in the population with TBI as a result of bilateral neurological involvement, cognitive and behavioral issues, and severe muscular spasticity. A self-feeding program begins in isolated areas such as the patient's bedroom. Eating is graded to more social situations such as the hospital dining room. Common pieces of adaptive equipment, such as a rocker knife, plate guard, and nonspill mug, may be used if a patient demonstrates diminished strength, coordination, or perceptual deficits. If a patient displays decreased attention, introducing one piece of adaptive equipment at a time may help. A patient who displays heightened impulsivity may benefit from the strategy of placing the fork down after each bite to ensure that the patient chews and swallows completely before initiating the next bite. Depending on the patient's level of dysphagia (preoral, oral, pharyngeal, and esophageal), a diet of thick liquids or pureed foods may be indicated until the patient progresses in recovery.

Functional Mobility

Mobility training can be subdivided into bed mobility, transfer training, wheelchair mobility, functional ambulation in ADL, and community travel. The NDT principles of bilateral extremity use, equal weight bearing, and tone normalization are used in intervention strategies that address functional mobility. The rehabilitation model, based on the principles of NDT and PNF, should be used with the intermediate patient with TBI in the acute and subacute stages of rehabilitation. Allowing the patient with loss of function to use compensatory strategies, such as grabbing a bed rail with one hand and rolling or standing on one leg to transfer, may appear to enable the patient to function more independently earlier. However, the use of such strategies diminishes the patient's ability to perform activities using a bilateral UE pattern at a later point. In time, the unilateral performance of activities results in hemiplegic postures, contractures, and abnormal gait deviations. Compensatory strategies should be used only in the later stages of recovery and when the patient has not been able to demonstrate significant improvement in functional mobility skills and so must learn compensatory strategies to enhance the ability to live independently in the community.

Bed Mobility

An intermediate-level patient with TBI may require training in bed mobility skills. These include (1) scooting up and down in bed, (2) rolling, (3) bridging, and (4) moving from a supine position to and from sitting and standing positions.

Wheelchair Management

Wheelchair management includes the ability to manage wheelchair parts (e.g., removing foot plates and locking brakes) and propel the wheelchair both indoors and outdoors on a variety of surfaces (e.g., low-pile carpeting, sidewalks, and ramps). If a patient needs to use a wheelchair but is cognitively and perceptually intact, he

or she may need to learn how to lift the wheelchair in and out of a car. Such a skill, however, is infrequently required by a population with TBI. Customized wheelchairs may be ordered for the patient who is in the postacute stages of rehabilitation and exhibits neuromuscular impairment that requires use of a wheelchair for long-term ambulatory needs. A custom wheelchair provides a seating and positioning design that contours the individual's body for comfort and decubiti reduction, includes adaptive supports for proper pelvis and trunk alignment, and offers a seating position that enhances the individual's ability to interact with the environment. Electric wheelchairs are ordered for the patient who cannot control the wheelchair manually and needs an electric chair for independent distance ambulation.

Functional Ambulation

Functional ambulation refers to the patient's ability to walk during functional activities. Whereas physical therapists address gait training, occupational therapists facilitate the carryover of ambulation skills into daily life activities. Often ambulation during ADL requires the integrated use of UEs and LEs to carry and manipulate objects (e.g., carrying a plate to a table, holding a book bag or purse, sweeping with a broom or vacuum cleaner, or carrying an infant). Functional ambulation also requires the ability to negotiate an ambulatory device (e.g., straight or quad cane and walker) with one or both UEs during ADL. This is a high-level activity that requires eye-hand coordination and the integration of total body movements. Compensatory aids to improve the individual's ability to negotiate an ambulatory device while performing ADL include walker bags and baskets, wheeled carts (to provide balance and support while transporting items such as plates to a table), canes with built-in reachers, and pouch belts worn abdominally (to hold keys, wallet, and memory books). See also Chapter 14, Section 1.

Community Travel

For the advanced-level patient who will be discharged to home or a community supportive living arrangement, the ability to negotiate uneven sidewalks and curb cuts and to correctly interpret traffic light signals and the direction and speed of oncoming traffic is important for independent community travel. Functional ambulation in the community requires the client to respond quickly, initiate actions (to cross the street when the light turns green quickly enough, before it turns red), perceive depth and spatial relations (to correctly judge the distance and speed of oncoming and turning traffic), and visually identify and avoid environmental hazards that could cause falls (e.g., pot holes and broken sidewalks). Electric mobile scooters are often recommended for individuals who must perform long-distance ambulation in the community but who fatigue easily or are unable to walk independently. The use of an electric mobile scooter requires good static sitting balance and the ability to quickly integrate UE hand control and cognitive decisions regarding the environment.

Transfers

Because patients with TBI commonly have memory deficits and limited carryover of information, transfer training should be consistent (in technique and sequence) among all staff members treating the patient. It is preferable that transfers for the intermediate- and advanced-level patient be practiced moving to both the right and left sides. Without this practice a patient who becomes proficient in a transfer toward the uninvolved side (in the hospital) may be dismayed to find that the home setting or public restroom requires transfers toward the opposite side. Additionally, teaching patients to transfer to both sides provides weight bearing on both LEs, the use of bilateral trunk muscles, and bilateral sensory input.

Family members and caregivers should be trained in proper transferring techniques (including proper body mechanics) and cleared by a therapist before transferring a patient alone. The decision about when to begin caregiver training depends on the patient's functional level and ability to cooperate, the discharge date, and the caregiver's physical and cognitive abilities.

Home Management

As the patient's skills and independence in self-care, dressing, self-feeding, and functional mobility increase, treatment is expanded to include home management skills in preparation for discharge to the community. Home management skills include meal preparation, laundry, cleaning, money management (e.g., balancing a checkbook, paying bills, and budgeting), home repairs (e.g., changing a washer in a leaking faucet), and community shopping (which includes planning a shopping list, locating the correct items in the store, and paying the correct amount of money at the cash register). Examples of high-level activities include planning a monthly budget, organizing a file cabinet, ordering from a catalogue or the Internet, and filing income taxes. These are skills that adults need to live independently in the community and are thus relevant for most patients with TBI.

The degree to which individuals participate in home management activities varies. For example, some individuals prepare only simple meals, using a microwave oven. For patients who must prepare meals to live independently in the community but who do not possess an interest in cooking, the goal is to help the patient to safely prepare simple hot and cold meals at home.

Some patients do not perform household cleaning activities except for making their bed and doing the laundry. Common sense dictates that therapy first address the activities that individuals performed before their injury.

As in all other areas of treatment, home management skills are graded to accommodate the patient's functional level. Beginning meal preparation tasks may involve the completion of a cold sandwich, whereas beginning money management skills may involve learning to read and interpret a utility bill. As the patient progresses in home management skills, the meal preparation task may be graded to the completion of a hot meal using a microwave and preparation of microwave-packaged foods. Money management skills may be graded to writing checks and balancing a checkbook. As the patient continues to gain skills, activities requiring higher-level demands are made until the patient reaches desired goals.

Child care is an often overlooked area of treatment. Family involvement is critical if a mother or father is to return effectively to his or her role as a spouse and parent. Sensory overload and its resultant agitation in the parent with a TBI is a commonly reported problem for patients and their children. OT sessions should gradually reintroduce the parent to the role of caring for his or her children. Some hospitals have a patient and family suite where the family members can practice ADL and interpersonal skills with the patient on weekends, in preparation for the patient's discharge home. This provides the opportunity for family members to gain a greater awareness of their loved one's impairments and need for assistance. It also makes the transition from hospital to home less stressful for both patients and family members.

The occupational therapist can also assist the parent with TBI in the adaptation of strollers, cribs, and child care equipment to make the handling of such items easier for an adult parent with a disability. Safely bathing a baby, preparing a meal while simultaneously caring for children, one-handed diapering and dressing techniques, and carrying a child are examples of the areas that could be addressed by OT services.

Community Reintegration

Patients who will be discharged from the subacute rehabilitation hospital to home or to a postacute, residential supportive-living arrangement should receive training to facilitate the transition from the hospital to the community. A patient who achieves a maximal level of independence in the protected and structured environment of the rehabilitation hospital may find that community reintegration holds even greater challenges. Community trips—in which the advanced-level patient with TBI is accompanied in the community by the occupational therapist (and perhaps one family member) to practice IADL in the natural environment—should be implemented to provide the patient with the opportunity to rebuild daily life skills. Depositing or withdrawing money from the bank or ATM, using the public transportation system, and planning a shopping list and purchasing items at the grocery or hardware store are activities that will facilitate the beginning of the patient's community reentry. Having the patient perform daily life activities within the community setting will also allow the therapist to observe the patient's social interaction skills and social appropriateness. The patient will be provided with a chance to receive feedback from others in the community regarding his or her behaviors.

Some patients are discharged from the subacute rehabilitation center to a transitional living center for individuals with TBI. Transitional living centers are designed to develop daily life skills by providing the patient an opportunity to live temporarily in a community group setting with 24-hour staff supervision and assistance. The goal of transitional living centers is to facilitate the patient's progression from supervised living to greater independence in community living. The patient is usually discharged from the transitional living center to a relative's home or to a residential supportive-living facility that provides various levels of living arrangements (e.g., community apartments and shared community group homes). Because long-term residential community facilities for people with brain injury are expensive for insurance companies, many patients are discharged home and then receive continued treatment in outpatient rehabilitation or in day treatment programs that provide community reentry services.

Psychosocial Skills

As mentioned previously, a year or more after injury individuals with TBI commonly report that psychosocial impairment is the greatest obstacle to rebuilding a meaningful postinjury lifestyle. Individuals report feeling a deep sense of isolation and loneliness. Loss of such roles as date, partner or spouse; worker or student; independent home maintainer; friend; and community member often leaves individuals feeling as though they have lost their identity. The goal of the occupational therapist, particularly in postacute TBI centers (e.g., day treatment programs, outpatient rehabilitation, transitional living sites, and long-term community supportive living arrangements) is to help clients rebuild desired occupational and social roles. This involves a three-step process: (1) identifying the desired roles that the individual lost secondary to TBI; (2) identifying the activities that would support desired roles; and (3) identifying rites of passage that the individual either lost or never

made a transition through as a result of TBI. Rites of passage are socially recognized events that mark the transition from one life stage to another. Common rites of passage in Western society include obtaining a driver's license, graduating from secondary school or obtaining a higher education degree, securing full-time employment, living independently in the community, dating, marrying, and parenting.

Once desired occupational and social roles, activities, and rites of passage have been identified by the individual, the therapist helps the person to approach these using adaptation, compensatory strategies, and the integration of new learning. The therapist will also help the client enhance interpersonal skills, self-expression, social appropriateness, time management, and self-control. Such psychosocial skills will be critical for the individual to reintegrate into the community—to live in a neighborhood setting, hold a job, perform volunteer work in the community, and participate in desired recreational opportunities along with other adult community members.

Group treatment is beneficial, because it enables the individual to meet others experiencing the same life concerns (thus decreasing feelings of isolation), offers exposure to peer reactions to behaviors (particularly helpful if the individual exhibits socially inappropriate behaviors), and facilitates problem solving by providing the opportunity to speak with others who have successfully dealt with the same or similar problems. Individuals who have been in the group for a while can become peer mentors to new group members. The opportunity to help others—to share one's experience of having a brain injury with others who can benefit from that knowledge—has been shown to enhance an individual's life satisfaction, feelings of competency, and sense of usefulness. Many states have support groups for individuals with TBI, run by state associations for brain injury.

Substance Use

If a patient's preinjury history includes substance use, the individual should receive drug and rehabilitation services specifically designed for patients with TBI. Patients with histories of substance use may not display any signs of a desire to return to substance use while in the structured and protective environment of the subacute rehabilitation facility. Substance use may become a problem only after the individual has been discharged to home, a community supported-living arrangement, or any residential situation in which long periods of time may be spent alone and unsupervised. Drug rehabilitation services are critical for the patient with a substance abuse history because a return to substance use after brain injury has been implicated in the occurrence of a second TBI.

Discharge Planning

Planning for the patient's discharge from OT services begins at the initial evaluation and continues until the last day of treatment. Components of discharge planning include a home safety evaluation (if the patient will be discharged home), equipment evaluation and ordering, family and caregiver education, recommendations for a driver's training program (if indicated), and recommendations for vocational retraining and work skills.

Home Safety

If a patient is to be discharged home, the therapist should visit the home (or transitional living setting) to recommend modifications to enhance the patient's safety. For example, a patient with balance difficulties should have grab bars in the shower stall or tub, around the toilet and sink, in hallways, and by all interior and exterior steps. Increased lighting should be added in dark interiors for a patient with vision deficits because low lighting has been linked to falls. Recommendations should also be made regarding the patient's ability to handle sharp items (e.g., knives and glass items that could shatter easily), use of the stove, and the ability to remember to turn off the water, stove, and other appliances. The temperature setting on the hot water system should be set at or below 120° F to prevent scalding. Anything that the patient could trip over (e.g., throw rugs, appliance cords, furniture legs, or objects placed on steps) should be removed. If feasible, nonslip flooring should be added to slippery surfaces (e.g., bathroom and kitchen tiles). If the patient needs a wheelchair, the therapist should recommend modifications to doorways and bathroom spaces and should suggest the replacement of high-pile carpeting with tiles, wood, or other surfaces that can be easily traversed by a wheelchair. Additionally, family members and caregivers should be educated in the appropriate steps to follow during a seizure, should understand how to evacuate the patient in case of emergency, and should practice how to transfer the patient safely. Caregivers should be able to identify unsafe activities in which their loved one should not participate and should know the length of time the patient can safely be left alone (if the patient can be left alone).

Equipment Evaluation and Ordering

A patient who will be discharged from the subacute rehabilitation facility will require an evaluation for equipment needed in the next setting. This may necessitate a reevaluation of the patient's equipment needs because many of the adaptive devices that were valuable in the beginning and intermediate stages of rehabilitation may be discarded as the patient improves. For example, a patient may initially have needed a tub bench to shower because of dynamic standing balance difficulties. This

patient may have progressed sufficiently during the course of rehabilitation to stand in the shower while using only a grab bar.

Family and Caregiver Education

Family members and caregivers should be involved in the patient's rehabilitation and should be considered members of the treatment team. Education of the caregivers in such activities as transfers, wheelchair mobility, ADL, bed positioning, splint schedules, equipment usage, ROM exercises, and self-feeding techniques will facilitate follow-through with the skills that the patient learned in the rehabilitation hospital. As mentioned previously, patient safety is of primary importance for caregiver education. If a home program is to be given to the patient (in either written or videotape form), the caregivers should be trained in the implementation of the home program. Home programs may include the areas listed earlier, as well as specific activities for the improvement of cognition, vision, perception, and motor control.

Recommendations for Driver's Training

If the patient passes the clinical and on-road driver's evaluation, a specific number of hours of driver's training may be recommended by the occupational therapist. Driver's training should be implemented by an occupational therapist or a driving instructor who has experience working with individuals with TBI (see Section 3 of Chapter 14).

Recommendations for Vocational Training and Work Skills

An occupational therapist may make recommendations for vocational training if the individual is discharged to an outpatient rehabilitation center or to a transitional living site. Vocational training of the patient with TBI is an extended process requiring the involvement of an occupational therapist and a vocational counselor. The patient's eventual return to work may require the assistance of a job coach. The occupational therapist in the subacute rehabilitation center may make vocational training recommendations to be implemented by an occupational therapist working in an outpatient site, a transitional living site, a day treatment program, or a community supportive-living residence.

SUMMARY

Treatment of the adult with TBI is challenging and requires flexibility, stamina, and creativity. Behavioral and psychosocial deficits greatly influence recovery. Substance abuse may be a contributing factor and must be assessed and addressed. Most patients have a multitude of problems requiring intervention. Coordination of evaluation and goal setting with the interdisciplinary

CASE STUDY 38-1

CASE STUDY—JOE

Joe is an 18-year-old Caucasian man who sustained a mild brain injury in a motor vehicle accident. He is a high school senior who lives at home and is planning to attend college next fall. As a result of the injury, Joe demonstrates mild cognitive deficits, including short-term memory loss, decreased concentration, and increased distractibility. He also demonstrates word-finding and word-generation difficulties. Joe is presently taking Dilantin for a seizure disorder secondary to the brain injury. He plans to return home with his parents and shortly thereafter move into his own community apartment. Joe also plans to take several community college courses and work part time as a clerk in a hardware store.

Results of the OT evaluation indicate that Joe is independent in all basic self-care skills (e.g., bathing, dressing, grooming, and toileting) but requires minimal assistance in several instrumental ADL (e.g., laundry, use of public transportation, meal preparation, money management and banking, and computer use). Joe demonstrates no insight into his deficits. Occupational therapy was initiated to accomplish the following: (1) minimize the effects of short-term memory deficits; (2) enhance Joe's use of public transportation, since he is no longer able to drive because of his seizure disorder; (3) help Joe use compensatory strategies to in-

crease his concentration for a return to school and work; (4) help Joe learn compensatory strategies to enhance his study skills as a student; (5) teach time management and stress-reduction skills in preparation for a return to school and work; (6) help Joe to adopt an organizational system for budgetary and money management skills; and (7) reprogram Joe's personal computer to simplify tool bars, menus, and commands to accommodate his decreased concentration and increased distractibility.

Joe received 3 months of OT, during which he learned how to use a memory and schedule book to keep appointments and organize his daily occupations. He learned to use three different bus routes from his parents' house (1) to and from a small local community college, (2) to and from the hardware store, where he returned to his part-time job, and (3) to and from the rehabilitation hospital for outpatient services. Joe also learned to use a computer program independently for money management, budgeting, and bill paying. The time management and study skill habits he learned in OT helped him prepare for his enrollment in several part-time community college courses. Upon discharge Joe was referred to outpatient OT to help him make the transition from his parents' home to an independent apartment located in the community near his parents' home.

---

team (including the patient and family) is assumed. Treatment should be individualized and oriented toward functional outcomes that are important to the patient. Effective transition of the patient from acute care to intermediate care and then to the community requires the therapist to plan thoughtfully and to communicate clearly. For the patient, recovery and adjustment may be a lifelong challenge.

REVIEW QUESTIONS
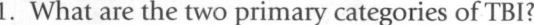

1. What are the two primary categories of TBI?
2. Name five types of neuromuscular impairment that may be present in the patient with TBI.
3. Describe the types of care settings available for patients with TBI in the acute, subacute, and postacute stages of rehabilitation.
4. Describe the psychosocial deficits that may be present in an individual with TBI.
5. List two components of a behavioral management program.
6. Name three standard assessments for a population with TBI and describe what performance components and areas they assess.
7. List four vision skills that are evaluated in a vision screening.
8. Why is it important for the patient with TBI to complete an on-road driving assessment?

9. What are the goals of a proper wheelchair-positioning program?
10. What are the indications for splinting? Casting?
11. Describe three areas that should be addressed during discharge planning.
12. Why is it important to address substance use with a population with TBI?

REFERENCES

1. Allen CK: *Occupational therapy for psychiatric diseases*, Boston, 1984, Little, Brown.
2. Arnadottir G: *The brain and behavior*, Philadelphia, 1990, Mosby.
3. Avery-Smith W, Brod Rosen A, Dellarosa DM: *Dysphagia evaluation protocol*, San Antonio, 1996, Therapy Skill Builders.
4. Avery-Smith W, Dellarosa DM: Approaches to treating dysphagia in patients with brain injury, *Am J Occup Ther* 48(3):235-239, 1994.
5. Bennett SE, Karnes JL: *Neurological disabilities*, Philadelphia, 1998, JB Lippincott.
6. Berker E: Diagnoses, physiology, pathology and rehabilitation of traumatic brain injuries, *Int J Neurosci* 85(3-4):195-220, 1996.
7. Biagas KV, Gaeta ML: Treatment of traumatic brain injury with hypothermia, *Curr Opin Pediatr* 19(3):271-277, 1998.
8. Bhavnani G et al: *Rivermead Perceptual Assessment Battery*, Los Angeles, 1985, Western Psychological Services.
9. Brain Injury Association: *Fact sheets*, Washington, DC, 1997, The Association.
10. Carmick J: Clinical use of neuromuscular electric stimulation for children with cerebral palsy, *Phys Ther* 73(8):514-522, 1993.
11. Chestnut RM: The management of severe traumatic brain injury, *Emerg Med Clin North Am* 15(3):581-604, 1997.

12. Colarusso RP, Hammill DD, Mercier L: *Motor-Free Visual Perception Test—Revised*, Novato, Calif, 1995, Academic Therapy Publications.
13. Fisher AG: *Assessment of motor and process skills*, Fort Collins, Colo, 1994, Colorado State University.
14. Florey L, Michelman SM: The occupational role history, *Am J Occup Ther* 36(5):301-308, 1982.
15. Gale SD et al: Nonspecific white matter degeneration following traumatic brain injury, *J Int Neuropsychol Soc* 1(1):17-28, 1995.
16. Giatnutsos R et al: *Elemental driving simulator and driving assessment system*, Bayport, NY, 1994, Life Sciences Associates.
17. Graham DI et al: The nature, distribution and causes of traumatic brain injury, *Brain Pathol* 5(4):397-406, 1995.
18. Granger CV et al: Functional assessment scales, *Arch Phys Med Rehabil* 74(2):133-138, 1993.
19. Habermann B: Post-traumatic brain injury seizures, *J Neurosci Nurs* 30(4):269, 1998.
20. Hooper HE: *Hooper Visual Organization Test*, Los Angeles, 1983, Western Psychological Services.
21. Hunstiger T, Thompson G: Vocational rehabilitation of people with traumatic brain injury, *Hawaii Med J* 57(9):618-620, 622-623, 1998.
22. Ito H et al: Cerebral perfusion changes in traumatic diffuse brain injury, *Ann Nucl Med* 11(2):167-172, 1997.
23. Jankovic J, Brin MF: Therapeutic uses of botulinum toxin, *N Engl J Med* 324(17):1186-1194, 1991.
24. Jebsen RH et al: An objective and standardized test of hand function, *Arch Phys Med Rehabil* 50(6):311-319, 1969.
25. Jennett B, Teasdale G: *Management of head injuries*, Philadelphia, 1981, FA Davis.
26. Kampfl A: The persistent vegetative state after closed head injury, *J Neurosurg* 88(5):809-816, 1998.
27. Klein RM, Bell BJ: *Klein-Bell Activities of Daily Living Scale*, Seattle, Wash, 1982, Health Science Center for Educational Resources.
28. Kreuter M et al: Partner relationships, functioning, mood and global quality of life in persons with spinal cord injury and traumatic brain injury, *Spinal Cord* 36(4):252-261, 1998.
29. Kreutzer JS et al: A prospective longitudinal multicenter analysis of alcohol use among persons with traumatic brain injury, *J Head Trauma Rehabil* 11(5):58-69, 1996.
30. Kubler-Ross E: *On death and dying*, New York, 1969, Macmillan.
31. Loewenstein Rehabilitation Hospital, Israel: *Loewenstein Occupational Therapy Cognitive Assessment*, Pequannock, NJ, 1990, Maddak.
32. Max JE et al: Traumatic brain injury in children and adolescents, *J Am Acad Child Adolesc Psychiatry* 36(9):1278-1285, 1997.
33. Mazaux JM et al: Long-term neuropsychological outcome and loss of social autonomy after traumatic brain injury, *Arch Phys Med Rehabil* 78(12):1316-1320, 1997.
34. McIntosh TK et al: Neuropathological sequelae of traumatic brain injury, *Lab Invest* 74(2):315-342, 1996.
35. *Minnesota rate of manipulation tests*, Circle Pines, Minn, 1969, American Guidance Service.
36. Newberg AB, Alavi A: Neuroimaging in patients with traumatic brain injury, *J Head Trauma Rehabil* 11(6):65-79, 1996.
37. Novak TA et al: Focused versus unstructured intervention for attentional deficits after traumatic brain injury, *J Head Trauma Rehabil* 11(3):52-60, 1996.
38. Oakley FM: The role checklist, *Occup Ther J Res* 6(3):157-169, 1986.
39. Ownsworth TL: Depression after traumatic brain injury, *Brain Inj* 12(9):735-751, 1998.
40. Penn RD et al: Intrathecal baclofen for motor disorders, *Mov Disord* 10(5):675-677, 1995.
41. Ranchos Los Amigos Medical Center: *Levels of cognitive functioning*, Downey, Calif, 1980, The Center.
42. Rustad RA et al: *Cognitive Assessment of Minnesota*, San Antonio, Therapy Skill Builders.
43. Salamy M et al: *Assessment of communication and interaction skills*, Chicago, 1993, Model of Human Occupational Clearinghouse, University of Illinois at Chicago.
44. Stratton M: Behavioral assessment scale of oral functions in feeding, *Am J Occup Ther* 35(11):719-721, 1981.
45. Tiffan J: *Purdue pegboard*, Lafayatte, Ind, 1960, Lafayette Instruments.
46. Tucker FM, Hanlon RE: Effects of mild traumatic brain injury on narrative discourse production, *Brain Inj* 12(9):783-792, 1998.
47. Weiner WJ, Goetz CG: *Neurology for the non-neurologist*, ed 3, Philadelphia, 1994, JB Lippincott.
48. Nova: *Coma*, Boston, 1997, WGBH-TV, PBS (videotape).
49. Wilson B, Cockburn J, Baddeley A: *The Rivermead Behavioural Memory Test*, Gaylord, Mich, 1991, National Rehabilitation Services.
50. Wilson B, Cockburn J, Halligan P: *Behavioural Inattention Test*, Gaylord, Mich, 1987, National Rehabilitation Services.
51. Vespa P et al: Increase in extracellular glutamate caused by reduced perfusion pressure and seizures after human traumatic brain injury, *J Neurosurg* 89(6):971-982, 1998.
52. Zasler ND: Prognostic indicators in medical rehabilitation of traumatic brain injury, *Arch Phys Med Rehabil* 78(8):12-16, 1997.

CHAPTER 39

Degenerative Diseases of the Central Nervous System

WINIFRED SCHULTZ-KROHN
DIANE FOTI
CAROLYN GLOGOSKI

KEY TERMS

Section 1
Amyotrophic Lateral Sclerosis (ALS)
Upper motor neuron
Lower motor neuron
Bulbar
Fasciculations
Dysphagia

Section 2
Alzheimer's Disease
Executive function
Apraxia
Aphasia
Agnosia

Section 3
Huntington's Disease (HD)
Choreiform movements
Chorea
Rigidity
Dysarthria
Akinesia

Section 4
Multiple Sclerosis (MS)
Exacerbation
Myelin sheath
Remission

Section 5
Parkinson's Disease (PD)
Resting tremor
Bradykinesia
Festinating gait
Micrographia

LEARNING OBJECTIVES

After studying each section, the student or practitioner will be able to do the following:

Section 1
1. Describe the course of ALS.
2. Describe the differences between FALS and SALS.
3. Describe the role of the occupational therapist for a client with ALS.
4. Describe the three subtypes of ALS.

Section 2
1. Identify the symptoms and incidence of Alzheimer's disease.
2. Describe the pathophysiology of Alzheimer's disease.
3. Describe the overall model of medical management used by primary care providers and other health professionals.
4. Describe an approach to evaluation used by occupational therapists.
5. Identify stages of disease progression and general methods of treatment interventions associated with stages of dementia.

Section 3
1. Describe the course and stages of HD.
2. Identify current research regarding the etiology of the disease.
3. Describe the medical management of HD.
4. Describe the purpose of occupational therapy for a client with HD.

Section 4
1. Describe the three typical forms of multiple sclerosis.
2. Describe current research regarding the etiology of the disease.
3. Describe the symptoms of multiple sclerosis.
4. Describe complications that may occur as a result of the disease.
5. Describe the role of the occupational therapist for the person with multiple sclerosis.

Section 5
1. Describe the course and stages of PD.
2. Identify current research regarding the etiology of the disease.
3. Describe the medical management of PD.
4. Describe the role of the occupational therapist for a client with PD.

Introduction

WINIFRED SCHULTZ-KROHN

This chapter addresses the impact of degenerative neurological disorders on a person's occupational performance and outlines the role of occupational therapy (OT) in treating clients with these disorders. The specific disorders are discussed in this chapter are amyotrophic lateral sclerosis (ALS), Alzheimer's disease (AD), Huntington's disease (HD), multiple sclerosis (MS), and Parkinson's disease (PD).

In degenerative neurological disorders the disease progresses and an individual's performance areas and components are increasingly compromised. Occupational therapy aims to help the client compensate and adapt as function declines secondary to the disease process. Environmental adaptations and modifications are often necessary to maintain functional skills for as long as possible.

Degenerative neurological diseases may occur because of structural or neurochemical changes within the central nervous system (CNS).[4] In the disorders discussed in this section, the client's CNS most often functions normally during the childhood and adolescent years. After these years the client then experiences signs and symptoms indicating that CNS functions are deteriorating. The progressive nature of the disorder varies from person to person. Some clients have a rapid decline in function, whereas others maintain functional skills for many years.

The decline in function may compromise the individual's sense of self-efficacy in performing various tasks.[7] No longer is the individual able to perform personal or instrumental activities of daily life at the same level of independence. Dependence on others can alter the client's concept of self-worth and self-control. The OT practitioner serves an important role in reframing the client's sense of self even though functional independence may be deteriorating. A man with PD who is unable to dress independently may now direct a personal care attendant (PCA) or home health aide (HHA) to perform these tasks. A woman with MS who was previously responsible for household finances may need to instruct a member of the family to complete these activities.

The disorders discussed in this chapter are most often diagnosed during adult or later adult life, after habits and patterns of independent behavior are well established. A client may encounter a significant change in social relationships and interactions secondary to a decline in functional abilities. The OT practitioner must consider how progressive loss of function affects the person's social and occupational roles, whether those roles are as husband, wife, parent, adult child, worker, sibling, or friend. Occupational therapy must address the needs of the client within the context of his or her social, physical, and cultural environment.

OT intervention aims to support the client's ability to function within his or her environment. The rate of a client's symptom progression influences the intervention plan. A client who displays a progressive loss of fine motor skills over 20 years has a much different profile from a client who loses all upper extremity function within 2 years. Use of adaptive equipment must be carefully considered against the rate of deteriorating skills.

The OT practitioner needs to be knowledgeable about support services and respite care available to clients with a degenerative neurological disorder. A PD support group may provide the needed social support both for a man with this disorder and for his family. MS support groups may offer clients information regarding new treatments available, along with the opportunity to share experiences of living with this disorder.

An OT intervention plan should address not only the physical limitations associated with various disorders but also the cognitive, social, and emotional implications of the disorder. Many individuals with neurodegenerative disorders have concomitant depression. Depression can be reactive to the loss of function in some disorders or may be the primary symptom of other disorders. Occupational therapists should regularly screen for depressive features. An instrument such as the Beck Depression Inventory can effectively evaluate this component.[1,2] In addition to the evaluation of depression in clients with neurodegenerative disorders, cognitive abilities should be evaluated. Patients may have concomitant cognitive problems because of the destruction of neurological structures, and these deficits can have a dramatic effect on intervention. Brief assessments such as the Mini Mental State Examination (MMS)[3] or the Cognistat[6] can be used to determine cognitive abilities and establish a baseline of performance.

Most often the occupational therapist is a member of a team providing services to the individual with a degenerative neurological disorder.[5] As a team member, the occupational therapist must consider the roles other professionals and family members play in the client's life and incorporate this knowledge into the intervention plan. Occupational therapy practitioners provide a unique and needed service to individuals with degenerative neurological disorders. A client who is able to engage in meaningful occupations despite deteriorating skills reflects the significant contribution of occupational therapy.

SECTION 1
Amyotrophic Lateral Sclerosis

DIANE FOTI

The term *amyotrophic lateral sclerosis* (ALS) is used to identify a group of progressive, degenerative neuromuscular diseases. The underlying neurological process involves destruction of the motor neurons within the spinal cord, brainstem, and motor cortex.[2,4] There is a combination of both **upper motor neuron** (UMN) and **lower motor neuron** (LMN) deficits at some point in the progression of the disease.

The term *motor neuron disease* is used interchangeably with ALS. In the United States ALS is also known as Lou Gehrig's disease, and in France it is referred to as Charcot's disease.[1] As mentioned initially, the term *ALS* refers to a group of diseases. This group of diseases consists of progressive **bulbar** palsy (PBP), progressive spinal muscular atrophy (PSMA), and primary lateral sclerosis (PLS). See Table 39-1 for a description of each of these distinct subtypes of ALS. The classic forms of ALS are presented in this section.

The incidence of ALS is estimated to be between 1.4 and 2.0 per 100,000 people. There are two forms of ALS, familial (FALS) and sporadic (SALS). Between 5% and 10% of individuals with ALS are found to have a family history of the disease. Families with FALS have been found to have an autosomal dominant transmission pattern.[2] There is no difference in symptoms of clients with FALS and those with SALS. Differences between FALS and SALS pertain to age of onset and incidence. Onset for FALS is between 45 and 52 years of age, and onset for SALS is between 55 and 65 years of age. The ratio of male to female incidence for FALS is 1:1, but with SALS the ratio is between 1.5:1 and 2:1.[2]

PATHOPHYSIOLOGY

The etiology of ALS has not been established. There are multiple theories regarding the cause of the motor neuron destruction, including metabolic disorders of glutamate insufficiency, metal toxicity, autoimmune factors, genetic factors, and viral infection.[5]

CLINICAL PICTURE

The symptoms of ALS are variable, depending on the initial area of motor neuron destruction. The individual with ALS typically has a focal weakness beginning in the arm, leg, or bulbar muscles. The individual may trip or drop things and may have slurred speech, abnormal fatigue, and uncontrollable periods of laughing or crying (emotional lability). With progression of the disease there are marked muscle atrophy, weight loss, spasticity, muscle cramping, and **fasciculations** (twitching of the muscle body at rest). The individual may have greater difficulty with walking, dressing, fine motor activities, swallowing, and breathing. In the end stages the individual may need tube feedings and the support of a ventilator for respiration. ALS is fatal, and the mean duration of the disease after onset is between 2 and 4 years.

ALS does not affect eye function, cognition, or bowel and bladder function. There is no loss of sensory function.

Prognosis is difficult to predict. Generally, individuals with early bulbar involvement have a poorer prognosis. A more positive prognosis is usually associated with the following factors: young age of onset; onset involving the spine; deficits of either UMN or LMN, not a combination of both areas; absent or slow changes in respiratory function; fewer fasciculations; and a longer time from onset of symptoms to diagnosis. In some cases the patient's condition has stabilized with little progression of the disease.[4]

MEDICAL MANAGEMENT

Symptoms such as muscle cramping, excessive saliva, and depression are managed with medication. The individual's swallowing status should be reevaluated frequently to prevent aspiration when and if symptoms of **dysphagia** progress.

TABLE 39-1
Clinical Subtypes of ALS

Name	Area of Destruction	Symptoms
Progressive bulbar palsy (PBP) ("Bulbar form")	Corticobulbar tracts and brainstem motor nuclei involved	Dysarthria, dysphagia, facial and tongue weakness and wasting
Progressive spinal muscular atrophy (PMA) or (PSMA) (LMN form)	Lower motor neurons in the spinal cord and sometimes the brainstem	Marked muscle wasting of the limbs, trunk, and sometimes the bulbar muscles
Primary lateral sclerosis (PLS) (UMN form)*	Destruction of the cortical motor neurons, may involve both corticospinal and corticobulbar	Progressive spastic paraparesis

From Belsh JM, Schiffman PL, editors: *ALS diagnosis and management for the clinician*, Armonk, NY, 1996, Futura Publishing; Guberman A: *An introduction to clinical neurology, pathophysiology, diagnosis, and treatment*, Boston, 1994, Little, Brown.
*The World Federation of Neurology Classification of SMAs and other disorders of the motor neurons does not identify PLS as a subtype of ALS.[1] I include PLS in the list because many other articles, texts, and clinicians recognize it as a subtype of ALS.

In 1995 the Federal Drug Administration approved the drug riluzole (Rilutek). This is the first drug used specifically to alter the course of the disease by prolonging survival. Riluzole is an antiglutamate. It inhibits the release of glutamate from nerve endings and blocks the amino acid receptors on the cell bodies.[5] Researchers believe the success of riluzole indicates that an excess of glutamate leads to the death of the motor neuron.

Three other medications, grouped as neurotrophic factors, are undergoing clinical trials for treatment of ALS. These medications are ciliary neurotrophic factor (CNTF), insulin-like growth factor-1 (IGH-1), and brain-derived neurotrophic factor (BDNF). Exactly how these factors act on the motor neuron is unclear.[2]

It is essential to work with the client and family throughout the progression of the disease as needs change. The client and family must often update decisions about care. Decisions range from when or if to use a wheelchair or adaptive eating device to whether to undergo a tracheostomy, choose tube feeding, or use a ventilator.[3] Psychosocial support regarding decisions about the extent of life support and medical intervention should be provided by the entire health care team, with the physician and patient having primary responsibility. The family's and client's cultural and social values must be understood as they struggle to make ongoing decisions about personal care and life support.

Cobb and associates[3] found that physicians frequently tell patients "nothing can be done," and that families often are not informed of services that can be provided by occupational, physical, and speech therapy. Education is needed for nursing staff and physicians to improve understanding of the occupational therapist's role with the client with ALS. Ongoing OT assessment is also essential to provide the client with needed information regarding choices about available therapy services as the disease progresses.

ROLE OF THE OCCUPATIONAL THERAPIST

ALS progresses rapidly. The occupational therapist needs to determine which form of ALS the client has because this suggests the most pertinent areas to evaluate. The intervention plan should focus on occupational performance, since the client's functional status is frequently changing and intervention with physical performance components is limited. As the client's physical status declines, there is a greater need for environmental support through providing durable medical equipment, modifying the home, and providing adaptive equipment. Depending on the client's understanding, life support choices, and acceptance of the disease, the OT intervention may focus on death and dying issues through structuring the client's environment to support

independence. Some clients with ALS may choose to have the maximum environmental and life support provided to extend life. In this case the occupational therapist may provide periodic reevaluations to determine the client's need for adapting self-care, work, and leisure activities. Table 39-2 gives a list of the functional deficits at various stages of the disease and interventions that may be required.

SUMMARY

ALS is a rapidly progressing, fatal condition of unknown etiology. Occupational therapy intervention aims to maximize functional independence by providing stage-specific compensatory strategies.

SECTION 2
Alzheimer's Disease

CAROLYN GLOGOSKI

Alzheimer's disease (AD), the most common form of dementia, is an insidious and progressive neurological disorder. Alzheimer's disease is labeled as a mental disorder by the American Psychiatric Association.[3] The exact etiology of AD is unknown. Because of the disease's damaging effects on the brain, higher mental processes are impaired, behavior is altered, and mood is disturbed. The onset of the disorder is gradual, with multiple cognitive deficits, a significant decline from previous levels of functioning, and noticeable impairment in social and occupational functioning. Effects on the motor and sensory systems are not apparent until later in the disease process. Dementia is a significant health care problem because of the increasing number of individuals who are living longer, the higher incidence of dementia among older persons, the very high cost of supervised care, and the extensive use of medical resources.[34] Early recognition of cognitive decline by physicians, occupational therapists, and all other health care professionals is critical. The AD diagnosis is often overlooked or mistaken for other disorders, especially in the early stages. Occupational therapists have an essential role in helping the individual with AD experience quality of life and remain as self-sufficient as possible and in supporting families and care providers over the course of this difficult disease.

INCIDENCE

Alzheimer's disease accounts for almost two thirds of the cases of dementia, and the incidence increases dramatically as people age.[23,72] Approximately 6% to 8% of adults aged 65 and older have AD. The disease

TABLE 39-2

ALS Interventions

Patient Characteristics	Interventions With Occupation as a Focus	Interventions With Occupational Performance Components as a Focus
Phase I (Independent)		
Stage I		
■ Mild weakness ■ Clumsiness ■ Ambulatory ■ Independent with ADL	■ Continue normal activities or increase activities if sedentary to prevent disuse atrophy and prevent depression ■ Integrate energy conservation into daily activities, work, and leisure ■ Provide opportunity for individual to voice concerns (provide psychological support as needed)	■ Begin program of ROM (stretching, yoga, tai chi) ■ Add strengthening program of gentle resistance exercises to all musculature with caution not to cause overwork fatigue
Stage II		
■ Moderate, selective weakness ■ Slightly decreased independence in ADL: for example, difficulty climbing stairs, difficulty raising arms, or difficulty buttoning clothing	■ Assess self-care, work, and leisure skills impaired by loss of function; if patient continues to work, focus on how to adapt tasks with current deficits; assist with balance between work, home, and leisure activities; include significant others in treatment ■ Use adaptive equipment to facilitate ADL (e.g., button hook, reacher, built-up utensils, shower seat, grab bar) ■ Integrate hand orthotic use into daily activities ■ Baseline dysphagia evaluation; reevaluation throughout each stage of the disease	■ Continue stretching to avoid contractures ■ Continue cautious strengthening of muscles with MMT grades above F+ (3+). Monitor for overwork fatigue. ■ Consider orthotic support (e.g., AFOs, wrist or thumb splints—short opponens splint)
Stage III		
■ Severe, selective weakness in ankles, wrists, and hands ■ Moderately decreased independence in ADL ■ Becomes easily fatigued with long-distance ambulation ■ Ambulatory ■ Slightly increased respiratory effort	■ Prescribe manual or power wheelchair with modifications to allow eventual reclining back with head rest, elevating leg rests, adequate arm and trunk support ■ Help patient prioritize activities and provide work simplification ■ Reassess for adaptive equipment needs (universal cuff to eat) ■ Assess and adapt use of communication devices such as phone to cordless or speaker phone; writing to using computer to type; and adapted typing aid ■ Provide support if there is loss of employment or other activities; explore alternative activities ■ Begin discussing need for home modification, such as installing ramps or moving the bedroom to the lowest floor ■ Instruct in type of bathroom equipment available for energy conservation and safety	■ Keep patient physically independent as long as possible through pleasurable activities and walking ■ Encourage deep breathing exercises, chest stretching, and postural draining if needed

Modified from Yase Y, Tsubaki T, editors: *Amyotrophic lateral sclerosis: recent advances in research and treatment*, Amsterdam, 1988, Elsevier Science. In Umphred DA, editor: *Neurological rehabilitation*, ed 3, St Louis, 1995, Mosby.

TABLE 39-2—cont'd

ALS Interventions

Patient Characteristics	Interventions With Occupation as a Focus	Interventions With Occupational Performance Components as a Focus
Phase II (partially independent) *Stage IV* ■ Hanging-arm syndrome with shoulder pain and sometimes edema in the hand ■ Wheelchair dependent ■ Severe lower extremity weakness (with or without spasticity) ■ Able to perform ADL but fatigues easily	■ Try arm slings, deltoid aids, overhead slings, ball-bearing feeders for eating, typing, page turning ■ If arm supports are not used, provide arm troughs or wheelchair lap tray for wheelchair positioning; wrist cock-up splints or full resting hand splints may be needed for positioning ■ Motorized chair if the patient wants to be independently mobile; adapt controls as needed ■ Evaluate the need for high-tech devices such as environmental control systems, voice-activated computer ■ Help the patient prioritize activities and consider negotiating roles with significant others ■ Reinforce the need for home modifications ■ Reinforce the need for shower seat or transfer tub bench and shower hose ■ Assist with patient's ability to participate in closure activities such as writing letters or making tapes for children, life history, writing a log on household management for the family	■ Heat, massage as indicated to control spasm ■ Preventive antiedema measures ■ Active assisted or passive ROM exercises to the weak joints; caution to support, rotate shoulder during abduction and joint accessory motions ■ Encourage isometric contractions of all musculature to tolerance
Stage V ■ Severe lower extremity weakness ■ Moderate to severe upper extremity weakness ■ Wheelchair dependent ■ Increasingly dependent in ADL ■ Possible skin breakdown secondary to poor mobility	■ Instruct family in methods to assist patient with self-care, especially bathing and dressing; aim to minimize caregiver's burden and stress ■ Family training to learn proper transfer, positioning principles, and turning techniques ■ Instruct in use of mechanical lift if needed for transfers out of bed (sling needs head support) ■ Adapt and select essential control devices for telephone, stereo, television, electric hospital bed controls for independent use ■ Adapt wheelchair for respiratory unit if needed to allow for continued community access ■ Instruct family and patient in skin inspection techniques	■ Instruct in use of electric hospital bed and antipressure device ■ Adapt wheelchair for respiratory unit if needed; reassess adequacy of wheelchair cushion for pressure relief
Phase III (dependent) *Stage VI* ■ Bedridden/dependent with wheelchair positioning ■ Completely dependent in ADL	■ Eating: evaluate dysphagia, recommend appropriate diet; may discuss tube feedings if high-risk for aspiration; recommend suction machine for handling secretions/aspiration precaution ■ Augmentative speech devices may be recommended (speech therapy may be requested if not providing services)	■ Continue with PROM to all joints ■ Provide sensory stimulation with massage, skin care

Modified from Yase Y, Tsubaki T, editors: *Amyotrophic lateral sclerosis: recent advances in research and treatment,* Amsterdam, 1988, Elsevier Science. In Umphred DA, editor: *Neurological rehabilitation,* ed 3, St Louis, 1995, Mosby.

affects approximately 4 million people in the United States. Age is a primary risk factor. The incidence of AD doubles every 5 years after age 65, and AD is expected to occur in 20% to 40% of the population of old-old (85+ years) adults.[72] Family history is another primary risk factor for AD. Early-onset, familial forms of AD are linked to genetic mutations on chromosomes 1, 14, and 21.[31,47,71] Late-onset AD has been linked to the apolipoprotein E-4 (APOE-4) allele on chromosome 19, but it should be noted that this allele has also been found in older persons who do not have AD.[20,72] Previous head trauma, lower educational levels, Down's syndrome, and female sex are other potential risk factors.

Although the incidence of dementia is growing rapidly, it does not occur in all older adults. Many older adults experience a normal slowing of information processing but do not develop clinically significant cognitive deficits. *Senility* is a misleading and nonspecific term that has been used in conjunction with older persons and aging. Early signs of what could really be a dementing illness have been erroneously attributed to the normal aging process[72] and identified as senility. The use of the term *senility* perpetuates stereotypical impressions that progressive cognitive decline occurs in normal aging. Such ideas prevent early recognition and accurate diagnosis of dementia.

PATHOPHYSIOLOGY

Alzheimer's disease is the result of degenerative changes in the CNS. Neuroanatomical (structural) and neurochemical changes occur in genetically or environmentally susceptible brains. The result of these changes is progressive and diffuse neuronal loss in the cerebral cortex and the hippocampus.[54,67] Pathological changes have been found through microscopic examination of brain tissue after death. These changes include increased neuritic plaques and neurofibrillary tangles, with loss of neurons and synapses. Early AD is associated with decreased cholinergic markers in areas of the brain where there is also increased distribution of plaques and tangles. Many of the changes in the brains of persons with AD can be seen only at autopsy, though neuroimaging techniques (e.g., CT, MRI, and PET) provide further diagnostic information.

Degenerative changes in the brain involve several processes that affect neurotransmission and result in neuronal death.[67] An inflammatory process causes the tau proteins in the cortical and limbic neurons to undergo microtubular dysfunction, preventing the neurons from sending nutrients and hormones along the axons. The paired filaments of these intracellular proteins actually become cross-linked in an abnormal metabolic process. These filaments form neurofibrillary tangles that eventually lead to neuron death. Neurofib-

rillary tangles are also seen in the temporal areas and to a lesser degree in the parietal association areas.

Neuritic plaques are large, extraneuronal bodies consisting of accumulated β-amyloid and neuronal debris—small axons and dendrites. This material degenerates, taking up cellular space. Extracellular accumulation of too much insoluble β-amyloid into neuritic plaques contributes to neuron degeneration. Distribution of neuronal plaques predominates in the temporal and parietal areas in early AD. The production of high levels of insoluble β-amyloid, associated with familial AD, has been linked to genetic markers on chromosomes 14,1, and 21.[31,47,71] The accumulation of amyloid deposits may be affected by APOE-4 on chromosome 19 and can also affect the development of neurofibrillary tangles.[69]

The ongoing neurodegenerative process itself may lead to further damage to cell membranes, enzymes, DNA, and proteins through the excess production of oxygen-based free radicals.[67] The metabolic processes triggering excess free radicals may further be associated with activation of the amyloid precursor protein (APP) gene and the formation of insoluble β-amyloid.

Cholinergic dysfunction is the process responsible for the expression of clinical symptoms, such as memory deficits and word-finding problems, in early AD. Specifically, cholinergic deficits, thought to be linked to APOE-E4, include less choline acetyltransferase (ChAT) activity in the frontal cortex and less ChAT activity in the hippocampus and temporal cortex.[59,60,67] These areas of the brain are associated with the symptoms of AD, such as recent memory impairment and problems with **executive functions**.

CLINICAL PICTURE

Symptoms and patterns of behavior in AD are most often described in terms of stages. The simplest description of staging, useful for caregivers and consumers, defines the progression of AD either in terms of a three-point scale using early, middle, and late stages or in terms of a four-point scale (Table 39-3).[29,32,55] More clinically and diagnostically complex scales, such as the seven-point Global Deterioration Scale,[63,64] are used in research or modified for diagnostic purposes and used as part of an assessment battery.

The primary symptom of AD is impairment in recent memory that worsens as time goes on, followed by at least one other cognitive deficit such as **apraxia, aphasia, agnosia,** or impaired executive function, according to the American Psychiatric Association.[3] Memory impairment involves increased difficulty learning new information and recalling information after more than a few minutes.[72] Over time the ability to learn deteriorates further and the ability to recall old memories also declines. Symptoms such as speech and

TABLE 39-3

Progression of Alzheimer's Disease and Intervention Considerations

Patient Characteristics	Intervention Using Occupation	Intervention Using Occupational Performance Components
Stage I: Very mild to mild cognitive decline		
■ Feels loss of control, less spontaneous; may become more anxious and hostile if confronted with losses ■ Mild problems with memory and less initiative; difficulty with word choice, attention, and comprehension; need for repetition at times; conversation more superficial; mild problems with gnosis or praxis may be first noticed ■ Socially and physically seems intact except to intimates, job performance declines	■ Listen to client concerns; collaborate with client on identifying areas that are challenging and identify associated feelings (depression or anxiety) ■ Begin training the caregiver to serve as a case manager[7] ■ Provide educational and other resources for disease information, support and relaxation, groups or activities for both client and caregiver ■ Identify roles, activity frequency and configuration; encourage continuation of or increase in enjoyable activities by keeping a log and planning enjoyable activity daily or weekly[74]; use activity or task as a focus in socialization ■ Explore meaning of occupations and occupational role changes with client and caregiver ■ Identify needs, preferences, and goals of the caregiver ■ Discuss driving skills and plan for future evaluation and restrictions	■ Encourage physical exercise and wellness behavior ■ Help client and caregiver establish a daily routine and post it in a central place ■ Use environmental aids such as calendars, appointment books, adhesive notes, and notebooks to enhance memory and reinforce engagement in occupation ■ Identify appropriate environments or adapt for activities that are currently challenging ■ In learning new tasks use auditory, visual, and kinesthetic input and provide supportive or positive feedback; grade activity for success to decrease anxiety ■ Communication training, rehearse with client how to use "I" statements and assertively express self and needs in response to changed ability and the feelings aroused ■ Educate and train caregiver on how to empower client to keep active and facilitate initiation of tasks
Stage II: Mild to moderate decline (problems from Stage I are exacerbated)		
■ Use of denial, labile moods, anxious or hostile at times; excessive passivity and withdrawal in challenging situations; paranoia may develop ■ Moderate memory loss with some gaps in personal history and for recent or current events; concentration decreases; may lose valued objects; difficulty with complex information and problem solving; difficulty learning new tasks; visuospatial deficits more apparent ■ Need for supervision slowly increases; decreased sociability; moderate impairment in IADL that are complicated and mild impairment in some ADL (finances, marketing, medications, community mobility, cooking complex meals); no longer employed; complicated hobbies dropped	■ Emphasize to caregiver the importance of environment in managing dementia at home[19] ■ Analyze and adapt meaningful leisure, home management, and other productive activities so as to allow the client to safely participate and exert initiation, independence, and control ■ Identify needs and design ways to adapt and grade activity by simplifying complex tasks, train the caregiver to provide cognitive support (verbally) with the client on IADL and some ADL[7] ■ Encourage look at family structure and resources to respond to increasing need for supervision, consider outside resource (e.g., day care, legal planning, friendly visitor volunteer, public transportation for the disabled)	■ Maintain routines and design environmental support (e.g., lists, posters, and pictures) and level of assistance for cues to remember daily routine and important events ■ Avoid tasks involving new learning; help to simplify surroundings and tasks, make objects accessible, establish expectations for object use, simplify instructions and clarify what is "success" ■ Help caregiver interpret behavioral problems by understanding source of frustration because of the effects of memory loss on behavior ■ Maintain socialization and structure opportunities in which others initiate socialization to ensure satisfying relationships in group activity and other social activities

Adapted from Baum C: Addressing the needs of the cognitively impaired elderly from a family policy perspective, *Am J Occup Ther* 45:594-596, 1991; Morscheck P: An overview of Alzheimer's disease and long term care, *Pride J Long-Term Health Care* 3:4-10, 1934; Glickstein J: *Therapeutic interventions in Alzheimer's disease*, Gaithersburg, Md, 1997, Aspen Publishers; Gwyther L, Matteson M: Care for the caregivers, *J Gerontol Nurs* 9, 1983.

Continued

TABLE 39-3—cont'd

Progression of Alzheimer's Disease and Intervention Considerations

Patient Characteristics	Intervention Using Occupation	Intervention Using Occupational Performance Components

Stage II: Mild to moderate decline (problems from Stage I are exacerbated)—cont'd

		■ Use reality orientation activities, photo albums, pictures around the home as a reminder of the past and past competence and for socializing
		■ Encourage stretching, walking, and other balance activities

Stage III: Moderate to moderately severe decline in cognition (problems from Stage II are exacerbated—difficulties involving physical status more prominent)

Patient Characteristics	Intervention Using Occupation	Intervention Using Occupational Performance Components
■ Reduced affect, increased apathy; sleep disturbances; repetitive behaviors; hostile behavior, paranoia, delusions, agitation and violence may surface if overwhelmed	■ Maintain involvement in meaningful activity and reactivate alternative roles; identify and design tasks in home management activity; client can assist caregiver with design of productive activity related to former work role[44,46,75]	■ In managing problem behaviors such as assaultiveness teach caregivers to identify problem, understand and consider possible precipitants for the behavior (e.g., feelings; antecedent events; who, where, when; medical problem or task; environment; or communication problem), and adapt own behavior or change the environment[16,21,80]
■ Progressive memory loss for well-known material; some past history retained; unaware of most recent events; disorientation to time and place and sometimes extended family; progressively impaired concentration; deficits in communication severe; apraxia and agnosia more evident	■ Help caregiver problem solve and recognize degree of need for initiation, verbal cues, and physical assistance and completion with ADL; provide time orientation; simplify environment	■ Essential to maintain consistent daily routines as means of facilitating participation in overlearned tasks, maintain function, and continue to define the self[16]
■ Slowed response, impaired visual and functional spatial orientation	■ Support socialization at home and with family or in structured settings outside of the home	■ Educate and train family that overlearned tasks are possible but require safe environment; overall, tasks take longer, need to be simplified, require setup and grading to comprise two steps or less
■ Unable to perform most IADL; in ADL, assistance eventually needed with toileting, hygiene, eating, and dressing; urinary and fecal incontinence begins; wandering behavior	■ Ensure safety in the home environment and other environments by making adaptations suited to level of client functioning (e.g., alarms, restrict use of heating devices and sharps, cabinet latches, ID bracelet, visual cues for item location, and visual camouflaging)[17,26,35,70]	■ Make further environmental adaptations to compensate for perceptual deficits and ensure safe mobility
		■ Rehearse and review names of family and others with pictures
		■ Encourage standby or assisted ambulation, stretching, and exercise on a regular basis
		■ In new environments cue and assist client in navigation and provide more light and pictorial representations to cue

Adapted from Baum C: Addressing the needs of the cognitively impaired elderly from a family policy perspective, *Am J Occup Ther* 45:594-596, 1991; Morscheck P: An overview of Alzheimer's disease and long term care, *Pride J Long-Term Health Care* 3:4-10, 1984; Glickstein J: *Therapeutic interventions in Alzheimer's disease,* Gaithersburg, Md, 1997, Aspen Publishers; Gwyther L, Matteson M: Care for the caregivers, *J Gerontol Nurs* 9, 1983.

TABLE 39-3—cont'd
Progression of Alzheimer's Disease and Intervention Considerations

Patient Characteristics	Intervention Using Occupation	Intervention Using Occupational Performance Components
Stage IV: Severe cognitive decline and moderate to severe physical decline		
■ Memory impairment severe, may forget family member name but recognizes familiar people; can become confused even in familiar surroundings	■ For ADL (hygiene, feeding), instruct care providers (family or nursing assistants) on need for simple communication, one-step commands, step-by-step verbal cues and physical guidance	■ Encourage and support caregiver to use respite programs and maintain recreation and leisure activity for himself or herself
■ Gait and balance disturbances, difficulty negotiating environmental barriers, generalized motoric slowing	■ Encourage continued socialization by family; socialization dependent on initiation of conversation by others and may not consistently include a response from the client	■ Encourage assisted ambulation until patient/client no longer able
■ Often unable to communicate except for word or grunt, psychomotor skills deteriorate until unable to walk; incontinent of both urine and feces; inability to eat; nursing home placement often occurs at this time	■ Use dysphagia techniques to promote swallowing, prevent choking, and encourage eating	■ Maintain proper positioning in bed and wheelchair; instruct family in skin inspection
	■ Instruct family on transfer techniques	■ Provide controlled sensory stimulation involving sound, touch, vision, and olfaction to maintain contact with reality
		■ Begin program of active and assisted and passive ROM

Adapted from Baum C: Addressing the needs of the cognitively impaired elderly from a family policy perspective, *Am J Occup Ther* 45:594-596, 1991; Morscheck P: An overview of Alzheimer's disease and long term care, *Pride J Long-Term Health Care* 3:4-10, 1984; Glickstein J: *Therapeutic interventions in Alzheimer's disease*, Gaithersburg, Md, 1997, Aspen Publishers; Gwyther L, Matteson M: Care for the caregivers, *J Gerontol Nurs* 9, 1983.

language problems, impaired recognition of previously familiar objects, and impaired ability to perform planned motor movement are more variable and may not be seen in all persons with AD. The expression of symptoms depends on the areas of the brain most affected by the disease. Executive function (the ability to initiate, plan, organize, safely implement, and judge and monitor performance) inevitably deteriorates as AD progresses. Visuospatial dysfunction is common. Mood and behavioral changes are often observed in the early stages of AD, with personality shifts and the development of depression, anxiety, and increased irritability. Later in the course of the disease, troubling behavior problems such as agitation, psychosis (delusions and hallucinations), aggression, and wandering can emerge.[53,66,73] Motor performance areas such as gait and balance may become impaired, and sensory changes usually arise in the mid to later stages in the course of AD (Table 39-3). Frequently delirium and depression complicate the clinical picture. The average duration of AD is from 8 to 10 years but can range from 3 to 20 years with a variable rate of progression.

Deterioration in the individual's functional performance usually occurs in a hierarchical pattern. This pattern of decline consists of a gradual progression from mild impairments in work and leisure performance to more moderate difficulties in performing instrumental activities of daily living (IADL) to a progressive loss of the ability to perform even basic self-care tasks in activities of daily living (ADL). The trend is for cognitive deficits to increase and executive function to become more impaired (Table 39-3).[15,27,28,68] Motivation and perception can influence functional performance but may not be routinely considered in individuals with AD.[28]

MEDICAL MANAGEMENT

According to Larson,[39] medical management of the individual with AD in primary care settings generally includes several areas. Many aspects of what is termed medical management may also be performed by certain other members of an interdisciplinary health care team, including the nurse, social worker, physical therapist, or occupational therapist. First, there is a need for early recognition and diagnosis of AD.[39] Second, there is the issue of how to treat the person with AD who is living in the community, before institutionalization or more restrictive care. The third area concerns treatment issues as the disease progresses. Last is the role of health care providers in recognizing and addressing treatment of other conditions that lead to excess disability in the person with AD.

Although dementia is a relatively common disease in persons over 80 years of age, such individuals often are not diagnosed until approximately 2 to 4 years after the onset of dementia symptoms.[38,39,41,51] A comprehensive physical examination, laboratory evaluation, mental status examination, brief neurological examination, and informant interview are essential in diagnosing AD. It is important to identify and treat medical conditions (e.g., metabolic disturbances, infections, alcohol use, vitamin deficiencies, chronic obstructive pulmonary disease, heart disease, and drug toxicity) that can contribute to comorbidity. MRI, PET, and CT scan results can be useful, but overreliance on these techniques should avoided because their value is in identifying relatively uncommon, treatable causes of cognitive impairment. A comprehensive and skillful interview with a reliable informant is essential to the evaluation and diagnostic process in order to recognize decline by comparing current changes with past performance. Informant questionnaires, interviews, and screening measures may be performed by many health care professionals other than physicians and are important to the diagnostic process.

The goal of health care providers in the successful management of an individual with dementia, whether in the community or in a semiinstitutional or institutional setting, is to "minimize behavior disturbances, maximize function and independence, and foster a safe and secure environment"[72] (p. 1367). Increased mortality is associated with dementia.[12] Regular health maintenance visits in primary care settings are important for all older adults, but especially those with AD, to identify treatable illnesses such as depression, Parkinson's disease, low folate levels, arthritic conditions, urinary tract infections, and other conditions that may exacerbate dementia.[41,72]

Depression and dementia easily may be mistaken for each other, or they may coexist.[72] Careful attention to whether the onset of symptoms has been gradual (dementia) or more recent (depression) is an important diagnostic issue because affective and cognitive symptoms frequently occur together.[62] Cognitive impairments and especially functional performance may improve in individuals with both dementia and depression after they are treated for depression. Delirium (impairment in attention, alertness, and perception) and dementia frequently coexist as well, especially in hospital settings.[72] Both conditions involve global cognitive impairment, but delirium is usually acute in onset, shows fluctuating symptoms, disrupts consciousness and attention, and interferes with sleep. Adverse drug reactions are more common in AD because of the vulnerable, impaired brain.[40] Often a cause of delirium, such as drug toxicity, is treatable.

Hearing, vision, and other sensory impairments are known to make dementia worse and cause greater strain on the caregiver.[76,77] Falls with hip fractures are 5 to 10 times more common in persons with AD than in normal persons of the same age and often result in earlier institutionalization for the individual and the need for higher levels of care.[13] Unsafe mobility quickly

becomes an overwhelming burden for caregivers, especially those who are aged.

According to Small and colleagues,[72] pharmacotherapy for the treatment of individuals with AD should be assessed carefully and justified at regular intervals. Although OT practitioners do not prescribe medications, knowledge of pharmacotherapy is useful. Cholinesterase inhibitors such as tacrine and donepezil may improve cognition and functional performance, at least in the short term. Promising research is under way in this area. Other agents that may improve cognitive function include estrogen, nonsteroidal antiinflammatory agents, gingko biloba, and vitamin E.[56] Evidence about the benefits of these agents is inconclusive. Antidepressant medications, especially selective serotonin reuptake inhibitors (SSRIs), are often prescribed.[72] However, some of the tricyclic antidepressants (amitriptyline, imipramine, and clomipramine) and monoamine oxidase inhibitors (MAOIs) can have troublesome side effects in older adults. Atypical antipsychotics such as clozapine, risperidone, and olanzapine may be used to reduce agitation and psychosis.[72,50] Benzodiazepines are prescribed for treating anxiety and infrequent agitation but have been found to be less effective than antipsychotics when the symptoms are severe.[72]

ROLE OF THE OCCUPATIONAL THERAPIST

In the early stages of Alzheimer's disease most individuals with the disorder live alone or with family and friends, rather than in institutions. A predominant feature of AD is significant and progressive deterioration of function from previous levels of performance because of advancing brain atrophy and pathological tissue changes. These changes cause deficits in occupational performance components, which in turn lead to deterioration in occupational performance areas and major changes in occupational roles. Over time, more structured and supervised living environments are needed. Increased difficulties in everyday functioning create challenges for the individual with the disorder and have an impact on the quality of life for the patient, the family, and caregivers as the disease progresses. Effective OT interventions must be directed at the changing meaning of occupation for the individual. Priority interventions include maintaining capabilities and adapting tasks and environments or otherwise compensating for declining function in individuals with Alzheimer's disease while trying to help them retain as much control as possible over their lives in the least restrictive environment.[4]

Support for the caregiver is a must. Collaboration with and training of the caregiver is essential in the management of persons with dementia. Family members should encounter an open and encouraging environment in which to discuss safety, security, and dependence issues. Legal, financial, and health concerns that require advance directives (medical and legal), trusts, activity restrictions (e.g., driving, financial, and medication management), and contingency and transitional care plans (e.g., day care, residential care, and long-term care) are important in preparation for the inevitable progression of the disease. [39,72] Behavior problems can be expected in the client with AD until the terminal or bed-bound stage. Encouragement to use respite care, in-home support services, and support groups is important. Caregivers also need effective strategies for dealing with behavioral disturbances and disruptions in mood. The use of environmental adaptations, therapeutic interpersonal approaches, referral to other disciplines, and resource sharing helps in collaborating with the patient's family and handling these problems. Health professionals use education, training, counseling, and support to help caregivers deal with their feelings, manage behaviors, and maintain quality of life for themselves and for the client with AD. Awareness of the multidimensional effects of this illness on the individual and on the family and the society at large is important to promote more effective and efficient care. [61]

EVALUATION

An OT screening is often performed before the evaluation. Occupational therapy services are indicated for individuals who have demonstrated a recent decline in function; pose a safety hazard to family, staff, other residents, or self because of their behaviors; or may experience improved quality of life. [11] Much of the therapist's time in community settings and in long-term care is spent helping families and caregivers develop strategies and environmental adaptations to cope with the overwhelming stresses of safely managing a cognitively impaired individual. [7]

The type of assessment and the depth of the evaluation process used depends on the setting, the stage of progression of AD, the reimbursement process, the presence of other medical and mental health disorders, and the cooperation and interest of the caregiver or care staff. The consequences of caregiving and the needs of the caregiver can vary greatly, depending on gender, family relationships, culture, and ethnicity. The caregiver's understanding of dementia, reaction to dementia-related behaviors, use of problem-solving skills, use of the environment, use of formal and informal support systems, and decision-making style greatly affect the caregiver's ability to participate in the care plan and treatment of persons with dementia. [6,18,22,48,78]

Evaluation should be comprehensive despite changing reimbursement. Much information can be gathered before an interview and treatment session by asking caregivers, family members, and staff informants to complete questionnaires and rating scales. These scales are used to assess occupational performance, functional abilities, and skills, using measures such as the Functional Behavior Profile, [9] the Activity Profile, [7] the Caregiver's Strain Questionnaire, [65] the Katz Activities of Daily Living Scale (KADL), [37] and the Instrumental Activities of Daily Living Scale (IADL). [42] Informant rating measures should routinely be followed by an interview either before or during the first visit. The use of a few brief screening instruments for mental status (e.g., the MMS), [25] depression, [10,79] and anxiety [43] provides baseline data and a wealth of information about factors that are likely to influence performance.

The functional evaluation of an individual with AD depends on the stage of cognitive decline. [4] The American Occupational Therapy Association's statement on services for persons with Alzheimer's disease suggests that tasks involving work, home management, driving skills, and safety should be targeted in the early stages of the disease. In the later stages, the focus shifts to self-care, mobility, communication, and leisure skills. The concerns and observations of the caregiver are important, but the therapist's observation of task performance is also necessary. Unfortunately, many of the functional ADL scales developed for use with older adults have targeted physical performance and are not appropriate for persons experiencing cognitive decline. [28] Fortunately, several excellent, standardized measures that determine whether individuals are able to use their cognitive skills to perform tasks in ADL and IADL have been developed over the last 15 years. The Kitchen Task Assessment (KTA) determines the level of cognitive support a person with AD needs to complete a cooking task successfully. [8] The Allen Cognitive Level (ACL) [1] test determines the quality of problem-solving an individual uses while engaged in perceptual motor tasks. Levy [45,46] has written at great length about the use of the ACL for clients with cognitive impairments. Consistent with the Allen theoretical approach, the Cognitive Performance Test (CPT) [2,14] was developed to identify cognitive deficits that are predictive of functional capacity, using several ADL and IADL tasks. Another measure, the Assessment of Motor and Process Skills (AMPS), [89] has been used with individuals who have dementia. [24,56] The AMPS measures motor (posture, mobility, and strength) and process (attentional, organizational, and adaptive) skills by using task performance in IADL. A promising new measure, the Disability Assessment for Dementia (DAD), [28] uses informant ratings to determine the ability of the individual with AD to complete tasks in both ADL and IADL. The DAD also provides information relevant to executive functioning, such as the person's ability to initiate, plan, and execute the activity. Further information regarding the evaluation of cognitive function and ADL performance is given in Chapters 13 and 27. After obtaining through evaluation a good understanding of the disease process and the functional level of the person with AD, the therapist can begin to look at the all-important question of what aspects of the occupational performance context, especially the environment and care provider interactions, must be modified to optimize function of the person with AD.[56]

TREATMENT METHODS

The goals of OT are to provide services to persons with dementia and their families and caregivers so as to emphasize remaining strengths, maintain physical and mental activity for as long as possible, decrease caregiver stress, and keep the person in the least restrictive setting possible.[3,90,96] Treatment planning takes into account the progressive nature of the disorder, the expected decline in function, and the care setting itself. Occupational therapy interventions for persons with dementia are directed toward maintaining, restoring, or improving functional capacity; promoting participation in occupations that are satisfying and that optimize health and well-being; and easing the burdens of caregiving.[7] The methods therapists use in the intervention process include activity analysis, caregiver training, behavior management techniques, environmental modification, use of purposeful activity, and the provision of resources and referrals. Treatment takes place in many different settings, such as home care, adult day care, and semiinstitutional or institutional long-term care. The treatment setting and the stage of the illness help frame the focus of intervention, determine the recipients of service, and prescribe the methods used (Table 39-3).

SUMMARY

Alzheimer's disease (AD) is a neurological condition characterized by the development of multiple cognitive impairments with a gradual onset. The effect of these impairments is a significant and progressive decline from previous levels of functioning. The course of the disorder is variable, but loss of function generally occurs in a hierarchical pattern, beginning with work and progressing to difficulties with home management, driving, and safety until even basic self-care skills such as dressing, functional mobility, toileting, communication, and feeding are affected.

OT interventions should be directed at enhancing the abilities of the person with AD by continually adapting tasks of daily living and modifying the physical and social environment as the individual experiences progressive loss of function. Given many of the current limitations in treatment time imposed by third-party payment, therapists may find it useful to employ some of the self-report and informant report measures identified in this chapter as a means of gathering information more efficiently during the evaluation process. Several standardized measures also have been identified to assist with the assessment of functional per-

formance and the establishment of a baseline of performance. Recommendations for OT treatment for AD have been identified. The focus of treatment must be flexible and depends on an understanding of the particular expression of the disease process in the individual, the specific treatment setting, and the needs of the person giving care. Generally, the goal of OT services for persons with dementia are to maintain or enhance function, promote continued participation in meaningful occupation, and optimize health and quality of life, and work collaboratively with the caregiver to ease the burden of caregiving.

SECTION 3
Huntington's Disease

WINIFRED SCHULTZ-KROHN

INCIDENCE

Huntington's disease (HD) is a fatal, degenerative neurological disorder that affects 5 to 10 of every 100,000 individuals.[12] The disorder is transmitted in an autosomal dominant pattern. Each offspring of an affected parent has a 50% chance of having HD. Genetic studies have identified a mutation on chromosome 4 as the cause of this.[7,12,13,15] Presymptomatic diagnosis of HD is possible with genetic testing when the family history shows this disease.[10,12] Diagnosis is also made through clinical examination when the family history is unavailable or unknown.

PATHOPHYSIOLOGY

The neurological structure associated with HD is the corpus striatum. Deterioration of the caudate nucleus is more severe and occurs earlier than atrophy of the putamen.[2,9] The corpus striatum plays an important role in motor control. The caudate nucleus is also linked to cognitive and emotional function through connections with the cerebral cortex. A progressive loss of tissue occurs in the frontal cortex, globus pallidus, and thalamus as the disease advances.[12] The degeneration of the corpus striatum results in a decrease in the neurotransmitter gamma-aminobutyric acid (GABA). Additional deficiencies in acetylcholine and substance P, both neurotransmitters, are noted in clients with HD. The triggering mechanism for the neuronal degeneration has not been clearly identified, but it is linked to genetic coding on chromosome 4.[15]

CLINICAL PICTURE

Huntington's disease is characterized by progressive disorders of both voluntary and involuntary movement, in addition to a significant deterioration of cognitive and behavioral abilities.[12,17] A client usually experiences an insidious onset of symptoms in the third to fourth decade of life, but cases have been reported in teenage and younger clients.[18] The symptoms progress over a 15- to 20-year period, ultimately necessitating long-term care or hospitalization for the client.[12] Death is often the result of "secondary causes, such as pneumonia"[10] (p. 341).

The initial symptoms vary but are most often reported as alterations in behavior, changes in cognitive function, and **choreiform movements** of the hands.[18] The early symptoms of cognitive disturbances are probably related to the degeneration of the caudate nucleus. The client may appear forgetful or display difficulty in concentrating. During the initial stages of HD a client may have difficulty maintaining adequate work performance. Family members often identify the initial behavioral changes seen in the person with HD as increased irritability or depression. Irritability and depression may be attributed inappropriately to the decline in work performance rather than to the disease process. Emotional and behavioral changes are often the earliest symptoms of HD.[3] **Chorea**, seen in clients with HD, consists of rapid, involuntary, irregular movements.[12] During the early stages of HD, chorea is often limited to the hands. These irregular movements are exacerbated during stressful conditions and decrease during voluntary motor activities. Chorea is absent when the client is sleeping. Onset of HD in teenage years is associated more often with early symptoms of **rigidity** than with chorea.[18]

Cognitive and emotional abilities progressively deteriorate over the course of the disease.[18] Disturbances in memory and in decision-making skills become more apparent during the middle stages of HD. A patient may be able to complete familiar tasks at work or in the home, but if the environment is changed or if additional demands are placed on the individual, task performance is significantly compromised. Further deterioration of cognitive abilities may result in dismissal from employment for the person with HD. The cognitive deficits most frequently associated with HD are problems with mental calculations, the performance of sequential tasks, and memory.[3] Verbal comprehension often is spared until the later stages of the disease and even then appears to be more compromised by **dysarthria** than by difficulty in comprehension.

As HD progresses, depression often worsens and suicide is not uncommon.[18] Clients with HD are often hospitalized because of various psychiatric problems, including depression, emotional lability, and behavioral outbursts. Although the loss of function may contribute to the client's level of depression, depression is clearly identified as a specific characteristic of HD.[3] This affective disorder frequently is treated with various anti-depressants. Periods of mania have also been reported in approximately 10% of patients with HD.

As the disease progresses, the chorea becomes more severe and may be observed throughout the entire body, including the face.[12] Disturbances in gait are often observed during the middle stages of the disease, and balance is frequently compromised.[3] The individual with HD may display a wide-based gait pattern and have difficulties walking on uneven terrain. This staggering gait is at times misinterpreted by others in the client's life as evidence of alcoholism.[11] The client also has progressive difficulty with voluntary movements.[12] The performance of voluntary motor tasks is slowed (bradykinesia), and the initiation of movement is compromised (**akinesia**). Although handwriting ability may be spared initially, the client displays increasing difficulties with this task as the disease progresses. Letter size is enlarged, and letter formation, such as slant and shape, is distorted. Saccadic eye movements and ocular pursuits may be slowed at this stage of HD.[10] Slight dysarthria may be noted, which compromises communication.[3] **Dysphagia** is seen, and the client may choke on various foods. Difficulties may be noted with the coordination of both chewing and breathing while eating.

In the later stages of HD, choreiform movements may be reduced because of the further deterioration of the corpus striatum and globus pallidus.[12] Hypertonicity often replaces the chorea, and the client experiences a severe reduction in voluntary movements. Severe difficulties in eye movement are common during the final stage of the disease.[10] At this stage the client often needs significant support from others or resides in a long-term care facility. The client is usually unable to talk, walk, or perform basic ADL without significant assistance.[7]

MEDICAL MANAGEMENT

Medical management of clients with HD can address symptoms, but no effective course of treatment has been identified to arrest the progression of this disease.[14] Intervention based on replacing the deficient neurotransmitters has not been effective in changing the course or rate of progression of HD. Tricyclic antidepressants are often used to treat the depression seen in clients with HD, but monoamine oxidase inhibitors (MAOIs) are contraindicated because of possible exacerbation of chorea.[18] Haloperidol may be used to decrease the negative effects of chorea on the performance of functional activities.[12] Haloperidol is prescribed cautiously and only when the chorea significantly compromises a person's daily activities.

Systematic evaluation of a client with HD must be performed at regular intervals to identify the rate of symptom progression and modify intervention strategies. Standardized instruments are available for determining the presence and severity of various symptoms.[5,16] One evaluation tool, known as the Unified Huntington's Disease Rating Scale (UHDRS), combines aspects from several instruments into a scale that can be administered within 30 minutes. The UHDRS is often administered by a team. This tool provides an accurate means of determining a change in the areas of "motor function, cognitive function, behavioral abnormalities and functional capacity."[5] The occupational therapist should complete additional assessments before an intervention plan is developed. An evaluation would address functional daily living skills; cognitive abilities such as problem solving, motor performance, and strength; and personal interests and values. The occupational therapist must consider the client's role within the family and community and incorporate these data into the intervention plan. An evaluation at both the home and work site would provide needed information that could be modified if necessary.

ROLE OF OCCUPATIONAL THERAPY

The role of the OT practitioner varies, depending on the stage of the disease.[6] During the early stages of HD an occupational therapist should address the cognitive components of memory and concentration. At this stage a client may still be employed. Strategies such as establishment of a daily routine, the use of checklists, and task analysis to break tasks down into manageable steps can be very helpful. These strategies provide the external structure and support to help the person with HD maintain functional abilities at both the workplace and home. A work-site evaluation can identify changes that would allow the person with HD to continue working. The use of a kitchen timer or a watch with a beeper can serve as a reminder to perform a specific task. Family members should be instructed in the use of these techniques. Environmental modifications such as providing a quiet workplace and reducing extraneous stimuli will decrease the impact of compromised memory and concentration on functional tasks.

Psychological issues during this stage of the disease often include anxiety, depression, and irritability.[3,4] A client may express guilt that any of his or her children have a 50% chance of having HD.[11] The diagnosis of HD often is not confirmed until a person is 30 to 40 years old. The patient may already be married and have children by that time. Decisions on whether to complete predictive genetic testing on children may be a significant stress for the client with HD and for his or her family members.

Maintaining social contacts and engaging in purposeful activities is important in the treatment of patents with HD.[11] Changes in cognitive abilities and emotional responses may result in the loss of a job and decreased income for the family, even during this early stage of the disease.[3] This additional stress should also be considered when developing an intervention plan.

The OT intervention plan must include community support services for the client with HD.

The motor disturbances during the early stages of HD are usually limited to fine motor coordination problems.[3] The characteristic chorea may be noticed only as a twitching of hands when the patient is anxious. OT should provide modifications to diminish the effect of chorea and fine-motor incoordination on performance of functional activities.[6] Home modifications should be instituted at this stage to allow the person with HD to become familiar with the changes. Typical modifications are the use of cooking and eating utensils with built-up handles, unbreakable dishes, a shower bench or seat with tub safety bars, and sturdy chairs with high backs and armrests. Throw or scatter rugs should be eliminated wherever possible in the home, and walkways should be kept free of clutter. The occupational therapist should establish a home exercise program with the client to address the flexibility and endurance of the entire body. These exercises will be incorporated into the client's daily routine. As the movement disorder progresses, the client will have to discontinue driving a car. These further losses of independent function and control must be considered within the OT intervention plan. Alternative community mobility must also be explored.

As HD progresses, the role of OT changes to meet the client's needs.[6] During the middle stages of HD, further deterioration of cognitive abilities is noted, often requiring the person to terminate a job. Engagement in purposeful activities is greatly needed at this stage and should be a focus of the OT intervention plan.[4,11] Decision-making and arithmetic skills show further deterioration, and family members may need to arrange for others to handle the client's financial matters.[3,8] Generally, comprehension of verbal information is better preserved than ability to complete sequential tasks during this stage. The occupational therapist should encourage the family to use simple written cues or words to help the family member with HD complete self-care and simple household activities. For example, selecting clothing items for the person with HD and placing the clothes in a highly visible area can provide the prompt to change from pajamas to clothes in the morning.

During the middle stage of HD the client may display increasing levels of irritability and depression.[18] Patients with HD may attempt suicide. The OT intervention plan should focus on the client's engagement in purposeful activities, particularly leisure activities. Selection of craft activities should always consider the client's interests but should avoid the use of sharp instruments.[4,8] Modification of craft activities allows the client with HD to successfully complete a task with minimal support.

Motor problems become more apparent during the middle stage of HD, necessitating further modifications in daily living tasks.[6,16] The client's compromised balance may require that tasks such as dressing, brushing teeth, shaving, and combing hair be performed while seated. The client may require the use of a walker or wheelchair at this stage. A rollator walker is preferred to a standard walker without wheels. The walker may need to be fitted with forearm supports to provide additional support when the client is ambulating. When a wheelchair becomes necessary, it should have a firm back and seat; however, additional padding is often required on the armrests because of the chorea. Many clients with HD are better able to move the wheelchair with their feet than with their hands. The seat height of the wheelchair should be fitted to allow the client to use his or her feet to move the chair, if possible.

Fatigue is a common issue during the middle stage of HD and can be addressed by taking frequent breaks during the day. Breaks must be scheduled, because the person with HD may not readily recognize fatigue. Clothing should have few or no fasteners, and shoes should be sturdy with low heels.[8] Additional adapted equipment that may prove helpful for the patient with HD includes shower mitts, electric razor or chemical hair removal, covered mugs, and nonskid placemats.[6] The choreic movements may become so severe as to necessitate the use of a bed with railings. Padding should be used on the railings, and additional cushions should be used in the bed.

Because of excessive movements associated with chorea, the client with HD often needs to consume 3000 to 5000 calories per day to maintain weight.[8] Smaller, high-calorie meals should be provided five times a day. This schedule may require additional support from family members or a personal care attendant. Dysphagia, poor postural control, and deficient fine motor coordination compromise the client's ability to eat.[6] Positioning during feeding is crucial, and the trunk should be well supported during mealtime. The person with HD should be able to support his or her arms on the table while the feet are stabilized. Feet may be supported on the floor, or the person may wrap the feet around the legs of the chair for additional support. Problems with dysphagia can be addressed with positioning, oral motor exercises, and changes in diet consistency. Soft foods and thickened fluids are preferable to chewy foods and thin liquids.

During the final stages of HD the client is often dependent upon others for all self-care tasks because of the lack of voluntary motor control.[6,7] The chorea may diminish in some clients, to be replaced by rigidity. The occupational therapist provides important input on positioning and the use of splints to prevent contractures at this stage. Because of the risk of aspiration, oral feedings are provided by trained personnel; alternatively, the client may receive nutrition through a feeding tube.[8] A combination of oral feedings and tube feedings may be used during this stage.

Although cognitive abilities continue to deteriorate, the level of functional decline is difficult to assess because of dysarthria and the loss of motor control.[3]

Dementia is part of the HD profile and must be considered in development of the intervention plan. A patient may still recognize family members and enjoy watching television. The occupational therapist should explore the use of various environmental controls to allow the client control of and access to the immediate environment.[1] Providing a touch pad or switch for selecting television channels may prove successful for the client.

Behavioral outbursts have been reported in approximately one third of patients with HD living in long-term care facilities.[7] Occupational therapy can decrease the frequency of these outbursts by organizing consistent daily schedules and routines for the client with HD.

SUMMARY

Although HD is a progressive, degenerative process, OT has much to offer the client with this disease.[4,6,8,11] The diminishing ability to control the environment has been identified as one of the variables contributing to the deterioration of function in patients with HD. Throughout the course of the disease, OT addresses the ability of the person with HD to exercise a degree of control over the environment and to engage in purposeful activity.

SECTION 4
Multiple Sclerosis

DIANE FOTI

INCIDENCE

Multiple sclerosis (MS) is a progressive neurological disease that damages the **myelin sheath** in the CNS. Onset usually occurs between the ages of 20 and 40 years.[11] The disease affects 60 to 100 people per 100,000.[8] It is more prevalent in women than in men.[5] Five percent of people with MS have a brother or sister with the same diagnosis, and approximately 20% have a close relative with the same diagnosis. The highest prevalence of the disease is in Caucasians of northern European ancestry.

The myelin is typically damaged in discrete regions of the white matter, with the axon remaining preserved. Disruption of the myelin sheath has differing effects on the axonal conduction, depending on the degree of breakdown and the length of the damaged segment.[8] When axons are conducting in a slower manner because of inflammation of the myelin sheath, the individual with MS may have intermittent symptoms of sensory distortions, incoordination, or weakness. This inflammatory process results in the remitting and relapsing form of MS.

In advanced cases of MS acute and chronic plaques develop throughout the white matter, especially in the the spinal cord, optic nerve, and periventricular white matter, including the corpus callosum.[8] Axons may be damaged and severed in advanced cases, resulting in extensive loss of function.

ETIOLOGY

The specific cause of MS is unknown, although it is suspected to be the result of a combination of environmental and genetic factors. The most current theory is that MS is an immune system reaction that acts on the nervous system. Recent studies have shown that 30% to 60% of the new clinical attacks of the disease occur after a cold, flu, or common viral illness. Some researchers theorize that the immune system mistakes a portion of the myelin protein for a virus and destroys it. Other researchers believe that the viral infection damages the myelin and releases small amounts into the body, resulting in an autoimmune reaction.[14]

CLINICAL PICTURE

The symptoms that occur with MS are related to the area of the CNS affected.[2] Early symptoms may be paresthesias, diplopia, or visual loss in one eye; fatigability, emotional lability; and sensory loss in the extremities. Cognitive deficits have also been documented in individuals with a disease duration of less than 2 years and with few neurological signs.[1] Other initial symptoms are trigeminal neuralgia and a worsening of symptoms when the body temperature is elevated. These symptoms may be temporary and may resolve.

In advanced stages the individual may have varying degrees of paralysis, from total lower extremity paralysis to involvement of the upper extremities, dysarthria, dysphagia, severe visual impairment, ataxia, spasticity, nystagmus, neurogenic bladder, and impaired cognition. Cognitive deficits are reported to occur in 30% to 70% of persons with MS but do not necessarily correlate with a physical decline.[1,7] Emotional changes such as depression may also be present; less commonly seen are euphoria and a sense of indifference. Dementia may develop in individuals who exhibit euphoria and indifference. Dementia occurs in less than 5% of the population with MS.[8]

The course of MS is unpredictable. It is marked by episodes of **exacerbation** and **remission.** An exacerbation may be an episode as minor as fatigue and sensory loss or as extensive as total paralysis in all extremities and loss of bladder control. Remissions may involve a total resolution of the symptoms, may result in a short plateau, or may result in some loss of function.

The three typical patterns seen in MS are: (1) relapsing and remitting, (2) secondary-progressive, and (3) primary-progressive.[2] The relapsing and remitting form of MS involves episodes of exacerbation and remission resulting in a slow, stepwise progression as the deficits accumulate. The secondary-progressive course begins with a pattern of relapses and remissions but evolves into the progressive form of the disease. The primary-progressive form of MS is distinguished by a downward course and little recovery after exacerbations. Individuals with this form eventually are nonambulatory and incontinent of urine and may have dysphagia and dysarthria, little lower extremity function, and varying degrees of upper extremity function. For individuals with the primary-progressive form of MS the average time to reach the stage of severe disability is 10 to 25 years. Overall, life expectancy is near normal for those with MS.[14]

The two atypical patterns of MS are the benign course and the progressive-relapsing form. The clinical signs of a benign course are a younger age at onset, female sex, and onset with sensory symptoms. The symptoms usually resolve within 6 weeks, and there may be only a few residual deficits. If the disability is minimal after five years, the course is considered benign.[8] The progressive-relapsing form of MS is rare. It is identified as steadily progressive but has specific relapses.[2]

MEDICAL MANAGEMENT

In recent years new treatments have been introduced to limit inflammation during periods of exacerbation and to slow the immune system response. Medical management centers primarily on treating the symptoms of the disease.

Antiinflammatory medications such as prednisone or methylprednisolone are used during an exacerbation. These medications are usually given in high doses for short periods because of their extensive side effects. In lower doses that can be tolerated for long periods, these medications have not demonstrated the ability to prevent further exacerbations or change the long-term course of the disease but are effective primarily for shortening the duration of an exacerbation.[14]

In the relapsing and remitting form of MS several new medications are being used and are thought to have an effect in preventing the slow, stepwise decline. Three different medications for this group have recently been introduced: interferon β-1 b (Betaseron), interferon β1 a (Avonex), and glatiramer (Copaxone).[9] Individuals treated with these medications, given by subcutaneous self-injection, showed a one-third reduction in frequency of exacerbations. Studies are ongoing regarding the effects of these medications for individuals with the progressive form of the disease.

Symptom management includes treatment of spasticity, bladder management, prevention of bladder infection, management of pain, and management of fatigue. Spasticity is often managed with medication; unfortunately, this may also worsen muscle weakness. Bladder management may involve the use of incontinence pads or catheters, along with the prevention of bladder infections. Fatigue should be managed with good nutrition, the prevention of overfatigue with energy conservation methods, regular exercise, and control of stress.[12] Bowel incontinence is rarely a problem related to a neurological deficit but is usually a functional impairment as a result of immobility.

ROLE OF THE OCCUPATIONAL THERAPIST

The OT practitioner may treat the person with MS in a number of settings. The type and degree of intervention provided will be determined by the setting, the type of reimbursement, and the patient's and caregiver's response to treatment.

The evaluation should include the gathering of information about all performance areas: work and productive activities, self-care, and leisure. All performance components should be evaluated: motor, psychological, sensory-perceptual, and social. Optimally, a home evaluation should be completed. Since not all treatment settings allow a home evaluation, the occupational therapist should interview the client and caregiver regarding the home environment and potential barriers. Because MS has an unpredictable course, the client may need referral for other resources and periodic reevaluation by an occupational therapist.

The evaluation of performance components and performance areas is generally accomplished with a combination of standardized and nonstandardized assessments, through the use of interviews with the family and client, and through observation. If the client has a cognitive deficit, a family member or significant other should be included in the evaluation process to provide accurate information.

Evaluation of the sensorimotor components is discussed thoroughly in previous chapters of this text. Since endurance is such a significant factor, it is important not to rely solely on the results of an evaluation of performance components. Observing a client performing a functional activity over a period of time will provide the clinician with a more accurate evaluation of fatigue.[9] Perceptual processing and cognition should be included in each reassessment to determine specific deficits and the functional impact and to incorporate this information into family training. The client's perceptual and cognitive deficits may determine whether that client can stay home alone or needs close, constant supervision. Various standardized cognitive and perceptual assessments are included in previous chapters of the text. Basso developed a screening tool for cognitive dysfunction for individuals with MS. Basso's tool was found to be both sensitive to functional impairment and cost effective.[4] This tool could be used by an occupational therapist or recommended to another discipline when evaluating the person with MS for cognitive deficits.

ADL may be evaluated with a check-off list, a standardized assessment such as the Assessment of Motor and Process Skills,[6] or other standardized assessments for ADL.[3] The most widely accepted tool to measure clinical impairment for the person with MS is the Expanded Disability Status Scale (EDSS).[13] The scale should be completed by a physician because it includes a detailed neurological examination. The EDSS combines an assessment of neurological function and a scale to measure a client's ambulatory and functional mobility status. There are limitations with this tool; it does not allow for detail in measuring all ADL and has been found to be insensitive to cognitive deficits in MS.[13] The OT practitioner should be familiar with the EDSS because it is mentioned often in much of the literature as a baseline for evaluating disability and has been adopted by the International Federation of MS Societies.[10,15]

Evaluation of the social environment is important to consider with each client. MS is usually identified during the phase of life in which a person is raising a family and developing a career. Because the disease is unpredictable and fluctuating, it leads to disruptions in normal daily activities and in family life. This places stress on the spouse or partner, children, and other family members. The occupational therapist must determine what type of support the client can expect from family members.

Behavioral issues for the person with MS vary depending on the person's premorbid personality, progression of the disease, coping skills, and social environment. Cognitive deficits and denial of the progressive nature of the disease may lead to behavior that places the individual at risk and makes management difficult. If families do not understand or recognize the client's behavioral problems, there may be further complications when the behavior is not restricted or modified by the family. For example, an individual with MS is able to ambulate to the car but has cognitive deficits that are exacerbated with fatigue in the afternoon. Because the client has already had to discontinue work, the family members do not want to take away driving privileges as well. Continuing to drive places the client and others at risk of injury. The occupational therapist may need to educate the family about the deficits by providing examples of how cognition is evaluated and by discussing the client's performance on the assessment and how the deficits relate to driving and other daily activities. Also, in this example the occupational therapist is responsible for reporting the driving risk to the client's physician. Other behavioral examples include the client who is depressed or labile, has poor memory, refuses assistance from outside caregivers, or uses poor judgment regarding safety with medications and transfers. Each client demonstrates a unique set of behavioral issues and requires individual evaluation and a treatment approach that encompasses the family, client, and caregivers.

GOAL SETTING

For the individual with a progressive disease such as MS, goal setting focuses on the need for the client to adapt as the disability progresses. Families often need to negotiate role changes to accommodate the individual with MS, who may not be able to participate consistently in a previously established family role. A client may initially be capable of working outside the home and may be able to complete household management tasks. The individual with the progressive form of MS may have such a significant decline that work is eventually given up, and then household management, so that finally the client is responsible only for basic self-care activities. Eventually the client may become totally dependent for basic self-care. The adaptation of roles requires working not only with the client but also with family members and significant others. The occupational therapist may identify areas of difficulty the family and client are experiencing and provide training in methods to better handle those situations. The therapist may also refer the client and family to a social worker or psychologist for further support.

SUMMARY

MS affects each person in a unique way, necessitating individual evaluation to determine the affected person's deficits and strengths. Working with an individual with MS requires the practitioner to use expertise in the evaluation and treatment of all performance areas and performance components. Because of exacerbations and remissions, developing an intervention plan involves particularly difficult challenges. The client may be expecting the return of function and therefore deny deficits, creating safety problems or refusing to adapt to a change in status as he or she waits for further return of function. The OT practitioner focuses on assessing the current level of functioning and the best methods for the client to adapt to current changes in status. The occupational therapist may also assist the family with making long-range, realistic plans. For example, if the family is planning to remodel the bathroom, the therapist may help the family consider a roll-in shower and not just a standard shower stall with a shower seat.

Working with the individual with MS requires a multidisciplinary approach. The physician, physical therapist, registered nurse, and social worker may be involved as team members. Because the social environment may create complex and difficult problems, good communication among all team members is needed to ensure that the team goals are congruous. The occupational therapist has a unique perspective to offer to the team as cognition, perception, psychosocial, and motor abilities are assessed in a functional context.

SECTION 5
Parkinson's Disease

WINIFRED SCHULTZ-KROHN

INCIDENCE

Parkinson's disease (PD) is one of the most common adult-onset, degenerative neurological disorders.[6] Three classic symptoms are associated with PD: tremor, rigidity, and bradykinesia. The prevalence rate for PD varies greatly, from 10 to over 400 per 100,000.[33] Incidence increases with age, and the disease affects 1.4% of the population over the age of 55.[27] Gender differences have been noted, and the prevalence of PD in men between the ages of 55 and 74 is slightly higher than in women of the same age. After the age of 74, women show a slightly greater prevalence of PD than do men. Diagnosis is most often made after the age of 60.

The etiology for PD has not been definitively established.[1,12] Although a positive family history has been established as a risk factor for PD, a clear genetic marker has not been identified. Twin studies have not conclusively identified a genetic factor as the cause for PD. Current genetic work is looking at a specific gene mutation on chromosome 4 in familial PD, but whether this genetic mutation will also be identified as the causal factor in sporadic occurrences of PD is unknown. A mutation on the gene that encodes a specific protein has also been linked to PD.[1]

Environmental factors have been considered as a possible cause of PD.[12] The possibility of an exogenous agent's producing PD gained considerable recognition when narcotic addicts began using 1-methyl-4-phenyl-1,2,3,6-tetrahydropyridine (MPTP). After use of MPTP many addicts quickly exhibited parkinsonism that "strictly mimics the clinical and anatomical features of Parkinson's disease"[12] (p.143). Other toxins, such as manganese and hydrocarbon solvents, produced more widespread neurological damage and lacked the selective deterioration in the basal ganglia.

Researchers have also considered dietary habits as a potential risk factor for PD. The incidence of PD was higher among persons with a diet high in animal fat. The incidence of PD was inversely related to a diet high in nuts, legumes, and potatoes. Many researchers are now investigating a possible interactional effect between a genetic predisposition and environmental agents as the possible cause of PD. Although many possible etiologies are being considered, the majority of individuals with diagnosed PD are identified as having idiopathic parkinsonism.[7]

PATHOPHYSIOLOGY

The neurological structure associated with PD is the substantia nigra, specifically the pars compacta portion.[20] The pars compacta receives input from other basal ganglia nuclei and appears to serve as a modulator of striatal activity.[22] The substantia nigra nuclei undergo significant deterioration as the disease progresses. The significant reduction in the dopaminergic neurons in the substantia nigra pars compacta produces a decrease in activity within the basal ganglia and an overall "reduction in spontaneous movement"[22] (p. 426). The substantia nigra serves as one of the major output nuclei for the basal ganglia to other structures.[21] In addition to the loss of dopaminergic neurons, intracytoplasmic inclusions are found on postmortem examination within the substantia nigra.[20] These intracytoplasmic inclusions are also known as *Lewy bodies*.[7] Although the greatest amount of neurodegeneration is found in the pars compacta substantia nigra, destruction of other neurological structures has been reported.[20] Deterioration is also seen in the remainder of the substantia nigra, locus ceruleus, nucleus basilis, and hypothalamus.

CLINICAL PICTURE

PD is characterized as a slowly progressive, degenerative movement disorder.[22] The diagnosis of PD is most often made after the age of 55. Although PD is not considered fatal, the degeneration of various neurological structures severely compromises performance of functional tasks. A person with PD may live for 20 to 30 years with progressive loss of motor function, ultimately requiring specialized care.[7] This person then has an increased risk for the development of pneumonia, which may be fatal.

PD is characterized by dysfunction in both voluntary and involuntary movements.[22] A classic triad of symptoms includes a tremor, rigidity, and a voluntary movement disorder. The disturbances in voluntary movement are identified as difficulty initiating movement (**akinesia**) and slowness in maintaining movement (**bradykinesia**). The bradykinesia and akinesia are often the most disabling motor symptoms for the client with PD.[5] The delay in initiating movement patterns and the slowness in executing the motion compromise functional tasks such as driving, dressing, and eating.

In addition to the slowness of movement, rigidity is seen in individuals with PD. Rigidity is the stiffness within a muscle that impedes smooth movement. This stiffness is not isolated to one direction but occurs in both directions for each plane of motion at a specific joint.[25] The characteristic **resting tremor** with a rate between 4 and 5 Hz is a disturbance of involuntary movement.[17] This tremor often diminishes with activity, but in some clients the tremor persists during performance of functional activities.

Additional symptoms of PD are disturbances in gait and postural reactions and masked face with decreased facial expressions and depression.[22] Deterioration in gait is seen throughout the course of the disease.[28] Initially gait may be fairly normal, but as the disease progresses, changes in stride length and speed of gait are noted. The characteristic **festinating gait** is often seen; as the client walks, the stride length decreases in length and the speed slightly increases. This produces a shuffling appearance. A reduced arm swing during ambulation is noted. Another motor disturbance associated with gait is the phenomenon of "freezing."[11] Freezing occurs when the person ceases to move, often after attempting to initiate, maintain, or alter a movement pattern. During gait, freezing may be seen as the client attempts to change directions or approaches a narrow hallway or stairs. Freezing can also be seen during other motor tasks such as writing, brushing teeth, and speaking.

Postural abnormalities associated with PD include a flexed, stooped posture with the head positioned forward.[18] The client tends to stand with flexion at the knees and hips. In addition to the stooped posture, balance reactions are compromised.[24] Righting and equilibrium reactions are markedly reduced in effectiveness, and the person with PD may experience frequent falls.

Approximately 50% of individuals with diagnosed PD exhibit depression,[24] which is not merely reactive to the severity of symptoms or the chronic nature of the disease.[7] The depression seen in individuals with PD appears to be related to a serotonergic deficit, which is similar to that in patients without PD who have depression. Complicating the feature of depression is a decrease in facial expressiveness caused by akinesia.[24] This "masked face" or decrease in spontaneous facial expressions is characteristic of clients with PD. Initially, decreased facial expressions are seen unilaterally, but as the disease progresses, spontaneous expression decreases on both sides of the face.[7] Individuals with PD may also self-limit social interaction because of their embarrassment at decreased facial expressions and movement disorders.

Mental status is fairly normal throughout the early stages of PD, but visual-spatial perception is often compromised.[24] Higher-order cognitive disorders are common in patients with PD. The person with PD often has difficulty shifting attention between various stimuli. Processing simultaneous information is often difficult for the individual with PD, and tasks that require a sequential process are somewhat easier to perform. Although dementia is seldom seen in the younger-onset person with PD, approximately one third of patients over 70 years old display dementia.

Additional symptoms associated with PD include autonomic dysfunction, **dysphagia,** and dysarthria.[24] A patient with PD may have bowel and bladder problems, with reduced intestinal motility producing constipation.

Patients often report an increase in the frequency and urgency of urination. Patients also frequently complain of orthostatic hypotension, but syncope is rare.[7] Individuals with PD occasionally report periods of sweating and abnormal tolerances of heat and cold.[24] Speech volume is often decreased, and the person with PD seems to whisper. Articulation is imprecise and speech is monotone. Dysphagia tends to occur in the later stages of PD, and the individual may be at risk for choking and aspiration pneumonia resulting from the dysphagia.

The course of the disease varies from person to person, but the first clinical symptom identified is typically a unilateral resting tremor in the hand.[17] Hoehn and Yahr[13] established a scale identifying the progression of symptoms in PD. A client at stage I exhibits unilateral involvement, typically a hand tremor, but no impairment of functional abilities is reported. During this stage the client's handwriting may become very small with letters that are cramped together.[7] This change in handwriting is referred to as **micrographia.** The client may also complain of muscle cramping when required to write for extended periods. Slight rigidity may be seen when the client is asked to rapidly open and close the involved hand. Stage II denotes a progression of symptoms, and in this stage the person has bilateral motor disturbances. Although the course of PD is variable, this stage is usually seen 1 to 2 years after initial diagnosis. Even though tremors or rigidity may be noted bilaterally, the client is still independent in ADL skills. Posture becomes slightly stooped, with flexion at the knees and hips. The person with stage II PD is still able to ambulate independently. As PD progresses to stage III, the client experiences delayed righting and equilibrium reactions. Balance is impaired; the client will have difficulty performing daily tasks that require standing, such as showering and meal preparation. A person in Stage IV PD has significant deficits in completing daily living tasks. The client is still able to ambulate at this stage, but motor control is severely compromised and negatively affects dressing, feeding, and hygiene skills. Stage V is the final stage of PD. The client is typically confined to a wheelchair or bed and depends on others for most self-care activities. The rate of progression through these stages varies from person to person, but PD is a slowly progressive disorder.

The extent of PD symptoms in individual clients has been measured using the Unified Parkinson's Disease Rating Scale.[8] This scale evaluates a patient's motor skills, functional status, and extent of disability. Motor skills are evaluated by a trained observer.[26] The functional status and extent of disability are measured through a patient interview that includes items addressing ADL skills and cognitive and emotional factors.[16] This instrument has been used for research and clinical practice to measure the effectiveness of various interventions in reducing PD symptoms.

MEDICAL MANAGEMENT

The most frequently used medical management strategy for PD is the provision of a dopamine agonist to make up for the depletion of dopamine caused by the destruction of the substantia nigra.[6,29] Levodopa is the medication most commonly used in the treatment of PD.[23] This oral medication is actually a precursor to dopamine because dopamine is too large to cross the blood-brain barrier. Levodopa provides substantial relief from tremors and rigidity during the initial stages of PD. After approximately 5 to 10 years of chronic use of levodopa, motor side effects are reported.[24] Those most often reported are dyskinesias and motor fluctuations. This so-called on-off phenomenon is related to the levodopa dosage. A decrease in tremors and rigidity occurs during the "on" period after administration of levodopa, but the patient also has various dyskinesias, such as abnormal movements of the limbs. As the dosage of levodopa wears off, the motor symptoms associated with PD return. Timing of the medication and the periods of "on-off" are important considerations in planning the client's daily activities. Even though abnormal movements are observed during the "on" period, the client has greater freedom of movement to complete functional activities.

As PD progresses, control of various motor symptoms through the use of levodopa becomes less effective.[24] Surgical intervention, known as **stereotactic surgery**, has been used. In this surgery, specific lesions are made in neurological structures to decrease the severity of PD symptoms. Stereotactic surgery of the globus pallidus internus has been used to decrease the severity of motor symptoms associated with PD and thus reduce the needed dosage of levodopa.[14,19] This surgical procedure is known as a *pallidotomy*. Pallidotomies have also been shown to reduce the dyskinesias associated with long-term use of levodopa.[24] Stereotactic surgery has also been used to create lesions in portions of the thalamus to reduce tremor and rigidity associated with PD.[15]

Neural transplantation has been used selectively for patients with PD.[2] This process involves harvesting fetal mesencephalic neural tissue and then transplanting this tissue into the basal ganglia of patients with PD.[3] The results of fetal brain transplants have been varied. The best success for this procedure has been reported when bilateral implants are placed in the putamen from multiple fetuses. The transplanted fetal tissue produces dopamine and thereby reduces the debilitating symptoms of progressive PD. Patients must continue to use levodopa, but at a reduced dosage.

ROLE OF OCCUPATIONAL THERAPY

Occupational therapy services vary, depending on the client's stage of PD. Typically, an OT program would provide compensatory strategies, patient and family education, environmental and task modifications, and community involvement.

During the initial stages of the disease, OT services should establish a daily, routine exercise program addressing full range of motion.[30] It is preferable to have a client with PD perform a short exercise program for 5 to 10 minutes daily rather than a longer program three times a week. Postural flexibility exercises should be included in the program, with specific attention given to trunk extension. The most common postural change noted with the progression of PD is a stooped posture. In addition to the flexibility exercises, occupational therapists should instruct patients in the use of relaxation techniques and controlled breathing. Inhaling slowly through the nose and exhaling through pursed lips two or three times in succession, combined with improved postural alignment, can promote relaxation.

Modification of household items may decrease the impact of tremors during the initial stage of the disease process. The use of built-up handles for eating and for writing utensils should be introduced during the initial stages of PD. Handwriting often becomes small and difficult to read during the initial stage of PD. Time management techniques should be introduced at this stage. Paying bills, signing forms, or other written work should be done soon after taking levodopa, using the built-up handle writing utensil. Even though tremors are not severe during the early stages of PD, clothing fasteners should be modified. The use of slip-on shoes or Velcro closures for clothing should be considered at this time. Although a client may be able to complete the fastening of clothing during this stage of PD, the occupational therapist must consider the amount of energy and time needed to perform such a task. In addition to the modification of specific tasks, household changes should be made at this time. Loose rugs should be removed from floors and furniture placed close to the wall to decrease obstacles. Chairs should have armrests to allow the client to push up to stand from the chair. Although balance is not significantly compromised during the early stages of PD, the family and client should become familiar with the new arrangement of furniture before it is a necessity. Bath and toilet railings and a raised toilet seat should be provided within the home. Fatigue is a common complaint, and clients should develop a habit of taking frequent breaks during the day. Modifying the household setting early in the course of PD allows the client and family members to adjust to changes and incorporate these changes into daily routines before they become a necessity.

During the early stages of the disease the client and family should be informed of community resources and support groups. In one study, clients with PD were found to be far more dependent on others for personal care and household activities than were same-age peers without PD.[32] This dependence can place additional stress on the family. Involvement in a community-based group may provide the support needed to accommodate the changes in family roles and interaction.

As the disease progresses, additional exercises can improve gait.[31] Rhythmic auditory stimulation in the form of music with an accentuated initial beat has been found to significantly improve stride length and speed in clients with PD. Dancing can also enhance gait patterns, in addition to providing a social environment for the client with PD. As akinesia becomes more apparent, the client with PD should be instructed to use a rocking motion to begin movement activities. Rocking forward and backward a few times while seated can produce the momentum needed to rise from a chair.

During the middle stages of PD a person may have decreased oral motor control.[24] Dysphagia and drooling may embarrass a client and further restrict social engagements. The occupational therapist should encourage oral motor exercises and provide education regarding food selection. Food consistencies can be altered to improve the client's ability to eat.

As PD progresses, the client has further deterioration of motor skills, particularly the execution of skilled, sequential movements.[4] These types of movements are needed to complete personal care and household tasks. Curra and associates[4] found that external cues improved the speed and sequential performance of novel motor tasks. The occupational therapist should suggest modifications to activities to include visual cues, verbal prompts, and rehearsal of movements. These strategies increase a client's ability to perform personal care and household activities.

The ability to complete personal care tasks has been identified as a critical variable in a client's perception of quality of life.[9] Although progressive movement problems are characteristic of PD, the occupational therapist can minimize the impact the movement disorder has on functional activities. Tremors have less effect on the completion of personal care tasks than does postural instability.[10] The use of group OT sessions has been demonstrated to be effective in reducing the impact of postural instability in patients with PD. An additional benefit of these group sessions is the reported improvement in the perception of quality of life in clients attending the sessions.

Access to community mobility and support programs should be included in the OT intervention plan during the middle stages of PD. A client with PD is often dependent on others for transportation. The use of community mobility services can decrease the client's dependence on family members for shopping and errands.

During the last stages of PD a client's movement disorder and rigidity may eliminate the ability to perform personal care tasks such as dressing and grooming.[13] Depression caused by the decreased ability to perform these tasks can significantly compromise a person's quality of life.[9] OT services should be provided to further modify the home environment for access and control. The use of environmental control units such as a switch-operated television or radio can be helpful. The switch plate should be activated with only light touch. Voice- or sound-activated environmental control units may not be as useful because of decreased vocal volume and poor articulation control during speech production. The client's ability to control the immediate environment can compensate for the loss experienced during the final stages of PD. The person with PD may no longer be able to dress himself or herself, but through the use of various switches the client can select preferred television or radio programs, access room lighting, and control a computer using minimal motor action.

SUMMARY

Although PD is a progressive, neurodegenerative disorder, OT has much to offer the client with this disease.[9,10] The diminishing ability to perform personal care and engage in self-selected tasks has been identified as one of the variables contributing to depression and the decreased quality of life in patients with PD. Throughout the progressive course of PD, OT addresses the ability of the person to engage in meaningful activities. The client's wishes and the family circumstances are incorporated into the OT intervention plan at every stage of the disease process.

CASE STUDY 39-1

CASE STUDY—DEGENERATIVE DISEASES OF THE CENTRAL NERVOUS SYSTEM: PARKINSON'S DISEASE

Mr. S is a 62-year-old college professor in whom Parkinson's disease was diagnosed at the age of 57. He is married and lives in a small one-story home with his wife. He has two adult children who live in another state. Mr. S reports that he enjoys traveling, reading, painting, and attending concerts.

Mr. S has recently considered early retirement because of the increase in tremors in both hands and difficulties with correcting papers. He also reports some problems with endurance as a result of stiffness. Mr. S indicates that he is no longer able to paint because of the tremors. He also reports that he is unsure if he should continue driving because of the tremors in both hands.

Results of the OT evaluation indicate that Mr. S is cooperative and motivated for therapy. Although he does not indicate that he is depressed, his wife reports features of depression such as a decreased interest in going to concerts or planning summer vacations to see their adult children and grandchildren. His wife also reports that Mr. S seems depressed about his possible early retirement and loss of status as a college professor.

Mr. S is able to complete most personal ADL independently but has difficulties stepping into and out of the tub and shower. His wife reports that she is afraid he will fall and that she often assists him in getting into and out of the shower. Mr. S also has difficulty tying his tie and buttoning his shirt. Tremors are noted bilaterally in his hands, and slight rigidity is present during PROM. Dynamic balance is slightly compromised on uneven surfaces and stairs.

Mr. S has been taking Sinemet (levodopa and carbidopa medication) for the past 3 years to decrease the rigidity and tremors. He does not report any dyskinesias.

When asked about his personal goals, Mr. S replies, "I guess I'll have more time to read now."

OT was initiated to accomplish the following:
1. Improve ADL performance
   a. Instruct in use of a buttonhook
   b. Give suggestions regarding clothing modifications such as clip-on ties and slip-on shoes
   c. Instruct in use of momentum to initiate movement, such as rocking back and forth to rise from a chair
2. Modify home environment
   a. Remove throw rugs and obstacles in walkways
   b. Provide a tub seat and shower extension hose
   c. Provide a raised toilet seat
   d. Provide a cushion on dining room chairs
3. Assess work setting for modifications
   a. Assess for computer access
   b. Instruct in energy conservation to take frequent breaks and schedule activities during "on" phase of medications
4. Investigate leisure pursuits
   a. Provide modifications to his easel using forearm supports to allow him to continue to paint
   b. Provide information regarding community-based Parkinson's disease support groups
5. Instruct in daily AROM exercise program
   a. Trunk extension and rotation exercises
   b. Bilateral upper extremity exercise
   c. Use of music during exercise program

Mr. S responded well to OT intervention. He was able to complete the academic school year but decided to retire after that year. He stopped driving, but his wife began to drive them to concerts and art exhibits. He was able to complete personal ADL safely with the use of adapted equipment and home modifications. He resumed painting during the "on" periods of his medications schedule, using the forearm supports attached to an angled table. He attended a Parkinson's support group two times a week and began to socialize with members from that group. Mr. S reported that the daily exercises seemed to decrease his stiffness, and he and his wife took frequent "strolls" in the park when weather permitted. He and his wife also joined a book club.

REVIEW QUESTIONS

SECTION 1

1. What are the symptoms of ALS at onset?
2. What is the underlying neurological process in ALS?
3. What bodily functions remain intact throughout the disease process?
4. What is the prognosis for ALS? With this in mind, what is the goal of the occupational therapist?
5. What are the symptoms at each stage of the disease?
6. What interventions are appropriate at each stage of the disease?

SECTION 2

1. What are the initial symptoms of AD?
2. What is the underlying degenerative neurological process associated with AD?
3. What changes in symptoms occur over the course of the disease?
4. How do the changes in symptoms affect occupational performance?
5. What is the prognosis for a client with AD?
6. What OT interventions are appropriate for the client at each stage of AD?
7. What environmental modifications should be made to accommodate the client with AD?

SECTION 3

1. What are the symptoms of MS at onset?
2. What is the underlying neurological process in MS?
3. What are the three typical patterns of MS? How do they differ?
4. What symptoms of MS are managed with medication? What are the side effects of the medication management?
5. How is medication management in the relapsing and remitting form of MS different than in the other forms of MS?
6. What does the OT evaluation include for the person with MS?
7. Why is it important to include the family in the evaluation and treatment process for the person with MS?

SECTION 4

1. What are the initial symptoms of HD?
2. What is the underlying degenerative neurological process associated with HD?
3. What changes in symptoms occur over the course of the disease?
4. How do the changes in symptoms affect occupational performance?
5. What is the prognosis for a client with HD?
6. What OT interventions are appropriate for the client with HD at the various stages of the disease?
7. What environmental modifications should be made to accommodate the client with HD?

SECTION 5

1. What are the initial symptoms of PD?
2. What is the underlying degenerative neurological process associated with PD?
3. What changes in symptoms occur over the course of the disease?
4. How do the changes in symptoms affect occupational performance?
5. What is the prognosis for a client with PD?
6. What OT interventions are appropriate for the client with PD?
7. How does the medication schedule of levodopa affect a client's daily routine?
8. What environmental modifications should be made to accommodate the client with PD?

REFERENCES
Introduction

1. Beck AT, Steer RA: *Beck Depression Inventory*, rev ed, San Antonio, 1987, Psychological Corporation.
2. Beck AT, Ward CM, Mendelson M, et al: An inventory for measuring depression, *Arch Gen Psychiatry* 4:561-571, 1961.
3. Folstein MF, Folstein SE, McHugh PR: Mini-Mental State: a practical method for grading the cognitive state of patients for the clinician, *J Psychiatr Res* 12(3):189-198, 1975.
4. Gelb DJ: *Introduction to clinical neurology*, Boston, 1995, Butterworth-Heinemann.
5. Imbriglio S: *Physical and occupational therapy for Huntington's disease*, New York, 1997, Huntington's Disease Society of America.
6. Northern California Neurobehavioral Group: *Cognistat: the neurobehavioral cognitive status examination*, Fairfax, Calif, 1995, The Group.
7. Schwartz CE, Coulthard-Morris L, Zeng Q, et al: Measuring self-efficacy in people with multiple sclerosis: a validation study, *Arch Phys Med Rehabil* 77(4):394-398, 1996.

SECTION 1
Amyotrophic Lateral Sclerosis

1. Belsh JM: Definitions of terms, classifications, and diagnostic criteria of ALS. In Belsh JM, Schiffman PL, editors: *ALS diagnosis and management for the clinician*, Armonk, NY, 1996, Futura Publishing.
2. Belsh JM, Schiffman PL, editors: *ALS diagnosis and management for the clinician*, Armonk, NY, 1996, Futura Publishing.
3. Cobb AK, Hamera E, Festoff BW: The decision-making process in amyotrophic lateral sclerosis. In Charash L, Lovelace RE, Wolf SG, et al, editors: *Coping with progressive neuromuscular diseases*, Philadelphia, 1987, Charles Press.
4. Guberman A: *An introduction to clinical neurology, pathophysiology, diagnosis, and treatment*, Boston, 1994, Little, Brown.
5. Robberecht W. Brown RH: Etiology and pathogenesis of ALS: biochemical, genetic, and other theories. In Belsh JM, Schiffman PL, editors: *ALS diagnosis and management for the clinician*, Armonk, NY, 1996, Futura Publishing.

RECOMMENDED READING
Bello-Haas VD, Kloos AD, Mitsumoto H: Physical therapy for a patient through six stages of amyotrophic lateral sclerosis, *Phys Ther* 78(12):1312-1324, 1998.

WEB SITES
Amyotrophic Lateral Sclerosis Association
http://www.alsa.org

SECTION 2
Alzheimer's Disease

1. Allen C: *Allen Cognitive Level (ACL) test*, Rockville, Md, 1991, American Occupational Therapy Foundation.
2. Allen CK, Earhart CA, Blue T: Occupational therapy treatment goals for the physically and cognitively disabled, Rockville, Md, 1992, American Occupational Therapy Association.
3. American Psychiatric Association: *DSM IV: Diagnostic and statistical manual of mental disorders*, ed 4, Washington, DC, 1994, the Association.
4. American Occupational Therapy Association: Statement: occupational therapy services for persons with Alzheimer's disease and other dementias, *Am J Occup Ther* 48(11):1029-1031, 1994.
5. Atchison P: Helping people with Alzheimer's and their families preserve independence, *OT Week* 8:16-17, 1994.
6. Barusch A, Spaid W: Gender differences in caregiving: why do wives report greater burden? *Gerontologist* 667-676, 1989.
7. Baum C: Addressing the needs of the cognitively impaired elderly from a family policy perspective, *Am J Occup Ther* 45(7):594-606, 1991.
8. Baum C, Edwards D: Cognitive performance in senile dementia of the Alzheimer's type: the kitchen task assessment, *Am J Occup Ther* 47(5):431-436, 1993.
9. Baum C, Edwards D: Identification and measurement of productive behaviors in senile dementia of the Alzheimer's type, *Gerontologist* 33(3):403-408, 1993.
10. Beck AT, Ward CM, Mendelson M, et al: An inventory for measuring depression, *Arch Gen Psychiatry* 4:561-571, 1961.
11. Birnesser L: Treating dementia: practical strategies for long-term care, *OT Practice* 2(6):16-21, June 1997.
12. Bowen J, Malter A, Sheppard L, et al: Predictors of mortality in patients diagnosed with probable Alzheimer's disease, *Neurology* 47(2):433-439, 1996.
13. Buchner D, Larsen E: Falls and fractures in patients with Alzheimer's-type dementia, *JAMA* 257(11):1492-1495, 1987.
14. Burns T, Mortimer JA, Merchak P: Cognitive performance test: a new approach to functional assessment in Alzheimer's disease, *J Geriatr Psychiatry Neurol* 7(1):46-54, 1994.
15. Carswell A, Eastwood R: Activities of daily living, cognitive impairment and social function in community residents with Alzheimer disease, *Can J Occup Ther* 60:130-136, 1993.
16. Cherry D: Teaching others how to manage the challenging behaviors of dementia. In *Summer series on aging*, San Francisco, Calif, 1997, American Society on Aging.
17. Christenson M: Environmental design, modification and adaptation. In Larson O, Stevens-Ratchford L, Pedretti LW, et al, editors: *Role of occupational therapy and the elderly*, Rockville, Md, 1996, American Occupational Therapy Association.
18. Corcoran M, Gitlin L: Dementia management: an occupational therapy home based intervention for caregivers, *Am J Occup Ther* 46(9):801-807, 1992.
19. Corcoran M, Gitlin L: A home environmental intervention to manage dementia-related problems, *Maximizing human potential* 2-7, 1998.
20. Corder E, Saunders A, Strittmatter W, et al: Gene dose of apolipoprotein E type allele and the risk of Alzheimer's disease in late onset families, *Science* 261(5123):921-923, 1993.
21. Dixon C: Preventing striking out behavior by a geriatric resident, *OT Practice* 1(2):39, 1996.
22. Edwards D, Baum C: Caregiver burden across stages of dementia, *OT Practice* 2:17-31, 1990.
23. Evans D: Estimated prevalence of Alzheimer's disease in the U.S., *Milbank Quarterly* 68:267-289, 1990.
24. Fisher A: *The assessment of motor and process skill (AMPS) in assessing adults: functional measures and successful outcomes*, Rockville, Md, 1991, American Occupational Therapy Foundation.
25. Folstein MF, Folstein SE, McHugh PR: Mini-Mental State: a practical method for grading the cognitive state of patients for the clinician, *J Psychiatr Res* 12(3):189-198, 1975.
26. Foti D: Gerontic occupational therapy: specialized intervention for the older adult. In Larson O, Larson R, Stevens-Ratchford L, et al, editors: *Role of occupational therapy and the elderly*, Rockville, Md, 1996, American Occupational Therapy Association.
27. Galasko D, Edland S, Morris J, et al: The consortium to establish a registry for Alzheimer's disease (CERAD). XI. Clinical milestones in your patients with Alzheimer's disease followed over 3 years, *Neurology* 45(8):1451-1455, 1995.
28. Gelinas I, Gauthier L, McIntyre M, et al: Development of a functional measure for persons with Alzheimer's disease: the disability assessment for dementia, *Am J Occup Ther* 53(5):471-481, 1999.
29. Glickstein J: *Therapeutic interventions in Alzheimer's disease*, Gaithersburg, Md, 1997, Aspen Publishers.
30. Glogoski-Williams C, Foti D, Covault M: Dementia. In Cara E, MacRae A, editors: *Psychosocial occupational therapy: a clinical practice*, Albany, NY, 1998, Delmar Publishing.
31. Goate A, Chartier-Harlin MC, Mullan M, Segregation of a missense mutation in the amyloid precursor protein gene with familial Alzheimer's disease, *Nature*, 349(6311):973-977, 1991.
32. Gwyther L, Matteson M: Care for the caregivers, *J Gerontol Nurs* 9(2):93-95, 1983.
33. Hasselkus B: Occupation and well being in dementia: the experience of day-care staff, *Am J Occup Ther* 52(6):423-434, 1998.
34. Hendrie H: Epidemiology of dementia and Alzheimer's disease, *Am J Geriatric Psychiatry* 6(2):S3-S18, 1998.
35. Hussian R: Modification of behaviors in dementia via stimulus manipulation, *Clin Gerontol* 8:37-43, 1988.
36. Joiner C, Hansel M: Empowering the geriatric client, *OT Practice*, 34-39, 1996.
37. Katz S, Ford A, Maskowitz R, et al: Studies of illness in the aged. The index of ADL: a standardized measure of biological and psychological function. *JAMA* 135:75-86, 1963.
38. Kukull W, Larsen E, Teri L, et al: The Mini-Mental Status Examination and the diagnosis of dementia, *J Clin Epidemiol* 47(9):1061-1067, 1994.
39. Larson E: Management of Alzheimer's disease in primary care settings, *Am J Geriatr Psychiatry* 6(2):S34-S40, 1998.
40. Larson E, Kukull W, Buchner D, et al: Adverse drug reactions associated with global cognitive impairment in elderly persons, *Ann Intern Med* 107(2):169-173, 1987.
41. Larson E, Reifler B, Featherstone H, et al: Dementia in elderly outpatients: a prospective study, *Ann Intern Med* 100(3):417-423, 1984.
42. Lawton M, Brody E: Assessment of older people: self-maintaining and IADL, *Gerontologist* 9(3):179-186, 1969.
43. LeBarge E: A preliminary scale to measure degree of worry among mildly demented Alzheimer disease patients, *Phys Occup Ther in Geriatrics* 11:43-57, 1993.
44. Levy L: Activity, social role retention and the multiply disabled aged: strategies for intervention, *Occup Ther in Mental Health* 10:1-30, 1990.
45. Levy LL: Cognitive treatment. In Davis LJ, Kirkland M, editors: *The role of occupational therapy with the elderly*, Rockville, Md, 1988, American Occupational Therapy Association.
46. Levy LL: Cognitive integration and cognitive components. In Larson KO, Stevens-Ratchford RG, Pedretti LW, et al, editors: *The role of occupational therapy with the elderly*, Bethesda, Md, 1996, American Occupational Therapy Association.
47. Levy-Lahad E, Wasco W, Poorkaj P, et al: Candidate gene for chromosome 1 familial Alzheimer's disease locus, *Science* 269(5226):973-977, 1995.
48. Lewis I, Kirchen S, editors: *Dealing with ethnic diversity in nursing homes*, Washington, DC, 1996, Taylor & Francis.

49. Liu L, Gauthier L, Gauthier S: Spatial disorientation in persons with early senile dementia of the Alzheimer's type, *Am J Occup Ther* 45(1):67-74, 1991.
50. Madhusoodanan S, Brenner R, Araujo L, et al: Efficacy of risperidone treatment for psychoses associated with schizophrenia, bipolar disorder or senile dementia in 11 geriatric patients: a case series *J Clin Psychiatry* 56(11):514-518, 1995.
51. McCormick W, Kukull W, van Belle G, et al: Symptom patterns and co-morbidity in the early stages of Alzheimer's disease, *J Am Geriatr Soc* 42:517-521, 1994.
52. McCormick W, Kukull W, van Belle G, et al: The effect of diagnosing Alzheimer's disease on frequency of physician's visits: a case control study, *J Gen Intern Med* 10(4):187-193, 1995.
53. Mega M, Cummings J, Fiorello T, et al: The spectrum of behavioral changes in Alzheimer's disease, *Neurology* 46(1):130-135, 1996.
54. Mirra S, Heyman A, McKeel D, et al: The consortium to establish a registry for Alzheimer's disease (CERAD). II. Standardization of the neuropathologic assessment of Alzheimer's disease, *Neurology* 41(4):479-486, 1991.
55. Morscheck P: An overview of Alzheimer's disease and long term care, *Pride J Long-Term Health Care* 3:4-10, 1984.
56. Nygard L, Bernspang B, Fisher A, et al: Comparing motor and process ability of persons with suspected dementia in home and clinic settings, *Am J Occup Ther* 48(8):689-696, 1994.
57. Nygard L, Borell L: A life-world of altering meaning: expressions of illness experience of dementia in everyday life, *Occup Ther J Res* 18:109-136, 1998.
58. Oakley F, Fisher A, Sunderland T: Assessing motor and process skills in people with Alzheimer's disease. In 73rd Annual Conference of the American Occupational Therapy Association, Seattle, Wash, 1995, American Occupational Therapy Association.
59. Poirier J: Apolipoprotein E in animal models of CNS injury and in Alzheimer's disease, *Trends Neurosci* 17(12):525-530, 1994.
60. Poirier J, Delisle M, Quirion R, et al: Apolipoprotein E4 allele as a predictor of cholinergic deficits and treatment outcome in Alzheimer's disease. In *Proceedings of the National Academy of Science* 92:12260-12264, Washington, DC, the Academy.
61. Rabins P, Cummings J: Introduction, *Am J Geriatr Psychiatry* 6(2):S1, 1998.
62. Reifler B: Detection and treatment of mixed cognitive and affective symptoms in the elderly: is it dementia, depression or both? *Clin Geriatrics* 6:17-33, 1998.
63. Reisberg B, Ferris S, Anand R: Functional staging of dementia of the Alzheimer's type *Ann New York Acad Sci* 435:481-483, 1984.
64. Reisberg B, Ferris S, DeLeon M, et al: The Global Deterioration Scale for assessment of primary degenerative dementia, *Am J Psychiatry* 139(9):1136-1139, 1982.
65. Robinson B: Validation of caregiver strain index, *J Gerontol* 38(3):99-110, 1983.
66. Sano M, Ernesto C, Thomas R, et al: A controlled trial of selegiline, alpha-tocopherol or both as treatment for Alzheimer's disease, *New Engl J Med* 336(17):1216-1222, 1997.
67. Schneider LS: Cholinergic deficiency in Alzheimer's disease: pathogenic model, *Am J Geriatr Psychiatry* 6(2):S49-S55, 1998.
68. Sclan S Reisberg B: (1992). Functional Assessment Staging (FAST) in Alzheimer's disease: reliability, validity, and ordinality, *Int Psychogeriatrics* 4(suppl 1):55-69, 1992.
69. Seshadri S, Drachman D, Lippa C: Apolipoprotein E epsilon 4 allele and lifetime risk of Alzheimer's disease: what physicians know and what they should know, *Arch Neurol* 52(11):1074-1079, 1995.
70. Shamberg S, Shamberg A: Blueprints for independence, *OT Week* June, 24-29, 1996.
71. Sherrington R, Rogaev E, Liang Y, et al: Cloning of a gene bearing missense mutations in early-onset familial Alzheimer's disease, *Nature* 375(6534):754-760, 1995.
72. Small GW, Rabins PV, Barry PP, et al: Diagnosis and treatment of Alzheimer's disease and related disorders. Consensus statement of the American Association of Geriatric Psychiatry, the Alzheimer's Association, and the American Geriatrics Society, *JAMA* 278(16):1363-1371, 1997.
73. Stern Y, Hesdorffer D, Sano M, et al: Measurement and prediction of functional capacity in Alzheimer's disease, *Neurology* 40(1):8-14, 1990.
74. Teri L, Logsdon R: Identifying pleasant activities for Alzheimer's disease patients: the pleasant events schedule, *Gerontologist* 31:124-127, 1990.
75. Trace S, Howell T: Occupational therapy in geriatric mental health, *Am J Occup Ther* 45(9):833-838, 1991.
76. Uhlmann R, Larson E, Koepsell T: Visual impairment and cognitive dysfunction in Alzheimer's disease, *J Gen Intern Med* 6(2):126-132, 1991.
77. Uhlmann R, Larson E, Rees T: Relationship of hearing impairment to dementia and cognitive dysfunction in older adults, *JAMA* 261(13):1916-1919, 1989.
78. Yeo G, editor: *Background*, Washington, DC, 1996, Taylor & Francis.
79. Yesavage JA, Brink TL, Rose TL, et al: Development and validation of a geriatric depression scale: a preliminary report, *J Psychiatr Res* 17(1):37-49, 1982-1983.
80. Zarit S, Orr N, Zarit J: *The hidden victims of Alzheimer's disease*, New York, 1985, NYU Press.
81. Zgola J, editor: *Therapeutic activity*, Baltimore, 1990, Johns Hopkins University Press.

SECTION 3
Huntington's Disease

1. Bain BK: Switches, control interfaces, and access methods. In Bain BK, Leger D, editors: *Assistive technology*, New York, 1997, Churchill Livingstone.
2. Cicchetti F, Parent A: Striatal interneurons in Huntington's disease: selective increase in the density of calretinin-immunoreactive medium-sized neurons, *Mov Disord* 11(6):619-626, 1996.
3. Folstein SE: *Huntington's disease: a disorder of families*, Baltimore, 1989, Johns Hopkins University Press.
4. Hayden MR: *Huntington's chorea*, New York, 1996, Springer-Verlag.
5. Huntington Study Group: Unified Huntington's Disease Rating Scale: reliability and consistency, *Mov Disord* 11(2):136-142, 1996.
6. Imbriglio S: *Physical and occupational therapy for Huntington's disease*, New York, 1997, Huntington's Disease Society of America.
7. Nance MA, Sander G: Characteristics of individuals with Huntington's disease in long-term care, *Mov Disord* 11(5):542-548, 1996.
8. National Institutes of Health: *Huntington's disease: hope through research*, NIH Publication No. 98-19, Bethesda, Md, 1998, the Institutes.
9. Parent A, Cicchetti F: The current model of basal ganglia organization under scrutiny, *Mov Disord* 13(2):199-202, 1998.
10. Penney JB, Young AB: Huntington's disease. In Jankovic J, Tolosa E, editors: *Parkinson's disease and movement disorders*, ed 3, Baltimore, 1998, Williams & Wilkins.
11. Phillips DH: *Living with Huntington's disease*, Madison, Wis, 1982, University of Wisconsin Press.
12. Phillips JG, Stelmach GE: Parkinson's disease and other involuntary movement disorders of the basal ganglia. In Fredericks CM, Saladin LK, editors: *Pathophysiology of the motor systems*, Philadelphia, 1996, FA Davis.
13. Quinn N, Brown R, Craufurd D, et al: Core assessment program for intracerebral transplantation in Huntington's disease, *Mov Disord* 11(2):143-150, 1996.
14. Ranen NG, Peysser CE, Coyle JT, et al: A controlled trial of idebenone in Huntington's disease, *Mov Disord* 11(5):549-554, 1996.

15. Reddy PH, Williams M, Tagle DA: Recent advances in understanding the pathogenesis of Huntington's disease, *Trends Neurosci* 22(6):248-255, 1999.

16. Shoulson I, Fahn S: Huntington's disease: clinical care and evaluation, *Neurology* 29(1):1-3, 1979.

17. Siesling S, Zwinderman AH, van Vugt JP, et al: A shortened version of the motor section of the Unified Huntington's Disease Rating Scale, *Mov Disord* 12(2):229-234, 1997.

18. Wiederholt W: Parkinson's disease and other movement disorders. In *Neurology for non-neurologists*, ed 3, Philadelphia, 1995, WB Saunders.

SECTION 4
Multiple Sclerosis

1. Amato MP, Ponziani G, Pracucci G, et al: Cognitive impairment in early-onset multiple sclerosis, *Arch Neurol* 52(2):168-172, 1995.

2. American Occupational Therapy Association: *Occupational therapy practice guidelines for adults with neurodegenerative diseases: multiple sclerosis, transverse myelitis, and amyotrophic lateral sclerosis*, Bethesda, Md, 1999, the Association.

3. Asher IE: *Occupational therapy assessment tools: an annotated index*, ed 2, Bethesda, Md, 1996, American Occupational Therapy Association.

4. Basso MR, Beason-Hazen S, Lynn J, et al: Screening for cognitive dysfunction in multiple sclerosis, *Arch Neurol* 53(10):980-984, 1996.

5. Comptson A, editor: *McAlpine's multiple sclerosis*, ed 3, New York, 1998, Churchill.

6. Doble SE, Fisk JD, Fisher AG, et al: Functional competence of community-dwelling persons with multiple sclerosis using the Assessment of Motor Process Skills, *Arch Phys Med Rehabil* 75(8):843-851, 1994.

7. Grigsby J, Kravcisin N, Ayarbe S, et al: Prediction of deficits in behavioral self-regulation among persons with multiple sclerosis, *Arch Phys Med Rehabil* 74(12):1350-1353, 1993.

8. Guberman A: *An introduction to clinical neurology, pathophysiology, diagnosis, and treatment*, Boston, 1994, Little, Brown.

9. Hugos C, Copperman L: Workshop: the new multiple sclerosis guidelines, delivering effective comprehensive therapy services, Monterey, Calif, 1999.

10. International Federation of Multiple Sclerosis Societies: *Symposium on a minimal record of disability for multiple sclerosis, Acta Neurol Scand* 70:169-190, 1984.

11. Matthews WB, Acheson ED, Batchelor JR, et al, editors: *McAlpine's multiple sclerosis*, New York, 1985, Churchill.

12. Multiple Sclerosis Council: *Fatigue and multiple sclerosis*, Washington, DC, 1998, Paralyzed Veterans of America.

13. Paty D, Willoughby E, Whitaker J: Assessing the outcome of experimental therapies in multiple sclerosis patients. In Rudick RA, Goodkin DE, editors: *Treatment of multiple sclerosis trial design, results, and future perspectives*, London, 1992, Springer-Verlag.

14. Sibley W: *Therapeutic claims in multiple sclerosis: a guide to treatments*, ed 4, New York, 1996, Demos Medical Publishing.

15. Weinshenker BG, Issa M, Baskerville J: Long-term and short-term outcome of mulitple sclerosis, *Arch Neurol* 53(4):353-358, 1996.

SUGGESTED READINGS

Frankel D: Multiple Sclerosis. In Umphred DA, editor: *Neurological rehabilitation*, ed 3, St Louis, 1995, Mosby.

Kraft GH, Freal JE, Coryell JK: Disability, disease duration, and rehabilitation service needs in multiple sclerosis: patient perspectives, *Arch Phys Med Rehabil* 67(3):353-358, 1986.

LaBan MM, Martin T, Pechur J, et al: Physical and occupational therapy in the treatment of patients with multiple sclerosis, *Phys Med Rehabil Clin North Am* 9(3):603-614, 1998.

Newman EM, Echevarria ME, Digman G: Degenerative diseases. In Trombly CA, editor: *Occupational therapy for physical dysfunction*, ed 4, Boston, 1995, Williams & Wilkins.

Pulaski KH: Adult neurological dysfunction. In Neistadt ME, Crepeau EB, editors: *Willard & Spackman's occupational therapy*, ed 9, Philadelphia, 1998, Lippincott.

Struifbergen AK, Rogers S: Health promotion: an essential component of rehabilitation for persons with chronic disabling conditions, *Adv Nurs Sci* 19(4):1-2, 1997.

WEB SITES

Http://www/nmss.org
National Multiple Sclerosis Society
Http://www.mswatch.com
Sponsored by Shared Solutions, a service designed to help people with multiple sclerosis.
Http://http 1 brunel.ac.uk:8080/~hssrsdn/papers/pap-ms.htm
From the Centre for the Study of Health, Sickness and Disablement, The Department of Human Sciences, Brunel, The University of West London, Uxbridge, Middlesex, UB8 3PH, UK.

SECTION 5
Parkinson's Disease

1. Bandmann O. Marsden CD, Wood NW: Genetic aspects of Parkinson's disease, *Mov Disord* 13(2):203-211, 1998.

2. Borlongan CV, Sanberg PR, Freman TB: Neural transplantation for neurodegenerative disorders, *Lancet* 353(suppl 1):29-30, 1999.

3. Collier TJ, Kordower JH: Neural transplantation for the treatment of Parkinson's disease: present-day optimism and future challenges. In Jankovic J, Tolosa E, editors: *Parkinson's disease and movement disorders*, ed 3, Baltimore, 1998, Williams & Wilkins.

4. Curra A, Berardelli A, Agostino R: Performance of sequential arm movements with and without advanced knowledge of motor pathways in Parkinson's disease, *Mov Disord* 12(5):646-654, 1997.

5. Delwaide PJ, Gonce M: Pathophysiology of Parkinson's signs. In Jankovic J, Tolosa E, editors: *Parkinson's disease and movement disorders*, ed 3, Baltimore, 1998, Williams & Wilkins.

6. Dodel RC, Eggert KM., Singer MS, et al: Cost of drug treatment in Parkinson's disease, *Mov Disord* 13(2):249-254, 1998.

7. Duvoisin RC, Sage JI: The spectrum of parkinsonism. In Chokroverty S, editor: *Movement disorders*, New Brunswick, NJ, 1990, PMA Publishing.

8. Fahn S, Elton RL: The Unified Parkinson's Disease Rating Scale. In Fahn S, Marsden CD, Calne DB, et al, editors: *Recent developments in Parkinson's disease, volume 2*, Florham Park, NJ: Macmillian Healthcare Information.

9. Fitzpatrick R, Peto V, Jenkinson C: Health-related quality of life in Parkinson's disease: a study of outpatient clinic attenders, *Mov Disord* 12(6):916-922, 1997.

10. Gauthier L, Dalziel S, Gauthier S: The benefits of group occupational therapy for patients with Parkinson's disease, *Am J Occup Ther* 41(6):360-365, 1987.

11. Giladi N, Kao R, Fahn S: Freezing phenomenon in patients with parkinsonian syndromes, *Mov Disord* 12(3):302-305, 1997.

12. Goldman SM, Tanner C: Etiology of Parkinson's disease. In Jankovic J, Tolosa E, editors: *Parkinson's disease and movement disorders*, ed 3, Baltimore, 1998, Williams & Wilkins.

13. Hoehn MM, Yahr MD: Parkinsonism: onset, progression and mortality, *Neurology* 17(5):427-442, 1967.

14. Kelly PJ: Pallidotomy in Parkinson's disease, *Neurosurgery* 36(6):1154-1157, 1995.

15. Krauss JK, Grossman RG: Surgery for hyperkinetic movement disorders. In Jankovic J, Tolosa E, editors: *Parkinson's disease and movement disorders*, ed 3, Baltimore, 1998, Williams & Wilkins.

16. Louis ED, Lynch T, Marder K, et al: Reliability of patient completion of the historical section of the Unified Parkinson's Disease Rating Scale, *Mov Disord* 11(2):185-192, 1996.

17. Misulis KE: *Neurologic localization and diagnosis*, Boston, 1996, Butterworth-Heinemann.

18. Muller V, Mohr B, Rosin R, et al: Short-term effects of behavioral treatment on movement initiation and postural control in Parkinson's disease: a controlled clinical study, *Mov Disord* 12(3):306-314, 1997.
19. Olanow CW: Gpi pallidotomy—have we made a dent in Parkinson's disease? *Ann Neurol* 40(3):341-343, 1996.
20. Olanow CW, Jenner P, Tatton NA, et al: Neurodegeneration and Parkinson's disease. In Jankovic J, Tolosa E, editors: *Parkinson's disease and movement disorders*, ed 3, Baltimore, 1998, Williams & Wilkins.
21. Parent A, Cicchetti F: The current model of basal ganglia organization under scrutiny, *Mov Disord* 13(2):199-200, 1998.
22. Phillips JG, Stelmach GE: Parkinson's disease and other involuntary movement disorders of the basal ganglia. In Fredericks CM, Saladin LK, editors: *Pathophysiology of the motor systems*, Philadelphia, 1996, FA Davis.
23. Poewe W, Wenning G: Levodopa in Parkinson's disease: mechanisms of action and pathophysiology of late failure. In Jankovic J, Tolosa E, editors: *Parkinson's disease and movement disorders*, ed 3, Baltimore, 1998, Williams & Wilkins.
24. Pollak P: Parkinson's disease and related movement disorders. In Bogousslasky J, Fisher M, editors: *Textbook of neurology*, Boston, 1998, Butterworth Heinemann.
25. Prochazka A, Bennett D, Stephens M, et al: Measurement of rigidity in Parkinson's disease, *Mov Disord* 12(1):24-32, 1997.
26. Richards M, Marder K, Cote L, et al: Interrater reliability of the Unified Parkinson's Disease Rating Scale Motor Examination, *Mov Disord* 9(1):89-91, 1994.
27. de Rijk MC, Breteler MM, Graveland GA, et al: Prevalence of Parkinson's disease in the elderly: the Rotterdam study, *Neurology* 45(12):2143-2146, 1995.
28. Rosin R, Topka H, Dichgans J: Gait initiation in Parkinson's disease, *Mov Disord* 12(5):682-690, 1997.
29. Sage JI, Duvoisin RC: The modern management of Parkinson's disease. In Chokroverty S, editor: *Movement disorders*, New Brunswick, NJ, 1990, PMA Publishing.
30. Stern G, Lees A: *Parkinson's disease*, Oxford, 1990, Oxford University Press.
31. Thaut MH, McIntosh GC, Rice RR, et al: Rhythmic auditory stimulation in gait training for Parkinson's disease patients, *Mov Disord* 11(2):193-200, 1996.
32. Tison F, Barberger-Gateau P, Dubroca B, et al: Dependency in Parkinson's disease: a population-based survey in nondemented elderly subjects, *Mov Disord* 12(6):1073-1074, 1997.
33. Zhang Z, Roman GC: Worldwide occurrence of Parkinson's disease: an updated review, *Neuroepidemiology* 12(4):195-208, 1993.

CHAPTER 40

Dysphagia

KAREN NELSON JENKS

KEY TERMS

Deglutition
Dysphagia
Sulcus
Bolus
Viscosity
Faucial arches
Velum
Velopharyngeal port
Pyriform sinuses
Aspiration
Nasogastric tube
Gastrostomy tube
Videofluoroscopy
Tracheostomy
Fenestrated
Cannula
Fiberoptic endoscopy
Diet progression

LEARNING OBJECTIVES

After studying this chapter the student or practitioner will be able to do the following:

1. Define key terms.
2. Name and locate oral structures concerned with swallowing.
3. Name and describe the stages of the normal swallow.
4. List the components of the swallowing assessment.
5. Name and describe normal and abnormal oral reflexes.
6. Describe the role of the occupational therapist in the clinical assessment of swallowing.
7. Describe four steps in the swallowing assessment.
8. Describe the appropriate progression of foods and liquids in the assessment and treatment of dysphagia.
9. Name two types of tracheostomy tubes, and list the advantages and disadvantages of each.
10. List symptoms of swallowing dysfunction.
11. List treatment goals for patients with dysphagia.
12. Describe the roles of the dysphagia treatment team members.
13. Describe proper positioning for treatment.
14. Describe and demonstrate two hand-hold techniques for head stabilization during treatment.
15. Describe two methods of nonoral feeding.
16. List principles of oral feeding.
17. List and describe treatment techniques for management of dysphagia.

Eating is the most basic activity of daily living, necessary for survival from birth until death. The components of eating include seeing and reaching for food, placing it in the mouth, chewing the food, and swallowing. **Deglutition** refers to the normal consumption of solids or liquids. **Dysphagia** is difficulty with swallowing or the inability to swallow.

Occupational therapists are trained to assess and treat all components of eating. These components are motor control; muscle tone; positioning of the trunk, head, and upper and lower extremities; inhibition of primitive reflexes; oral and pharyngeal function; and sensory, perceptual, and cognitive dysfunction, which may interfere with the eating process. *Continuing education and special training are required for competence in treatment of dysphagia.*

This chapter provides the occupational therapist with a foundation for the assessment and treatment of the adult patient with an acquired dysphagia. Some of the conditions that can result in an acquired dysphagia are cerebrovascular accident (CVA), head injury, brain tumor, anoxia, Guillain-Barré syndrome, multiple sclerosis, amyotrophic lateral sclerosis, Parkinson's disease, myasthenia gravis, poliomyelitis, and quadriplegia. Anatomic or developmental dysphagia is beyond the scope of this chapter.

ANATOMY AND PHYSIOLOGY OF NORMAL SWALLOW

Deglutition, the normal consumption of solids or liquids, is a complex sensorimotor process involving the brainstem, the cerebral cortex, six cranial nerves, the first three cervical nerve segments, and 48 pairs of muscles.[7,25,34] A normal swallow requires all these structures to be intact (Fig. 40-1). Therefore the occupa-

tional therapist treating the patient with dysphagia must have a thorough understanding of the anatomy, including the muscle origin and insertion and the physiology of swallowing (Table 40-1). The swallowing process can be divided into four stages: oral preparatory phase, oral phase, pharyngeal phase, and esophageal phase (Fig. 40-2).[31]

Oral Preparatory Phase

The oral preparatory phase of swallowing begins with the act of looking at and reaching for food.[13,31] Visual and olfactory information stimulates salivary secretions. Salivation plays an important role as a triggering mechanism for the entire swallowing process.[7,39] As tactile contact is made with the food, the jaw comes forward to open. The lips close around a glass or utensil to remove the food or liquid. The labial musculature forms a seal to prevent any material from leaking out of the oral cavity.

As chewing begins, the mandible and tongue move in a strong, combined rotary and lateral direction. The upper and lower teeth shear and crush the food. The tongue moves laterally to push the food between the teeth. The buccinator muscles of the cheeks contract to act as lateral retainers, to prevent food particles from

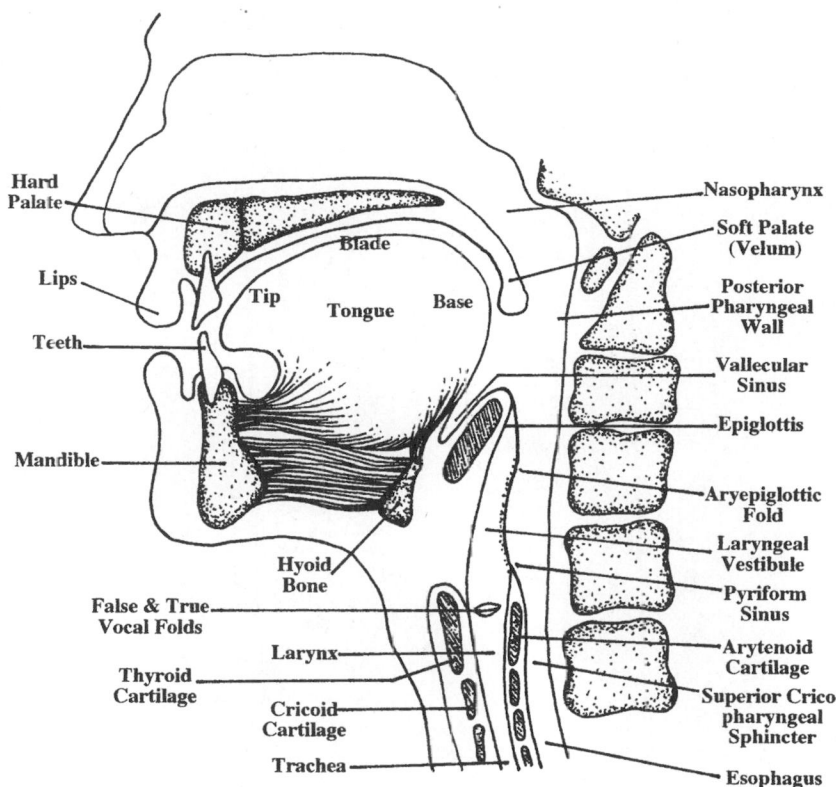

FIG. 40-1
Oral structures, swallowing mechanism at rest. (Courtesy of Rene Padilla, MS, OTR, Occupational Therapy Department, Creighton University, 1994.)

TABLE 40-1
Swallowing Process

Structure	Muscle	Movement	Cranial Nerve	Sensation
Oral Preparatory Stage				
Jaw	Pterygoideus medialis	Opens jaw	←Trigeminal (V)→	Face, temple, mouth, teeth, mucus
	Pterygoideus medialis and lateralis	Protrudes lower jaw; moves jaw laterally		
	Masseter	Closes jaw		
	Digastricus; mylohyoideus; geniohyoideus	Depresses lower jaw		
Mouth	Orbicularis oris	Compresses and protrudes lips	←Facial (VII)	
	Zygomaticus minor	Protrudes upper lip		
	Zygomaticus major	Raises lateral angle of mouth upward and outward (smile)		
	Levator anguli oris	Moves angle of mouth straight upward		
	Risorius	Draws angle of mouth backward (grimace)		
	Depressor labii inferioris	Draws lower lip downward and outward		
	Mentalis	Protrudes lower lip (pouting)		
	Depressor anguli oris	Draws down angles of mouth		
Tongue	Superior longitudinal	Shortens tongue; raises sides and tip of tongue	Facial (VII)→	Taste, anterior two thirds of tongue
	Transverse	Lengthens and narrows tongue	←Glossopharyngeal (IX)→	Taste, posterior third of tongue
	Vertical	Flattens and broadens tongue	←Hypoglossal (XII)	
	Inferior longitudinal	Shortens tongue Turns tip of tongue downward		
ORAL STAGE				
Tongue	Styloglossus	Elevates and pulls tongue posteriorly	←Accessory (XI)	

From Bass N: The neurology of swallowing. In Groher M, editor: *Dysphagia: diagnosis and management,* ed 3, Newton, Mass, 1997, Butterworth-Heinemann Publishers; Davies P: *Steps to follow,* New York, 1985, Springer-Verlag; Hislop H, Montgomery J, Connelly B: *Daniels & Worthington's muscle testing: techniques of manual examination,* ed 6, Philadelphia, 1995, WB Saunders; Liebman M: *Neuroanatomy made easy and understandable,* Rockville, Md, 1986, Aspen Publishers; Netter F, Dalley A: *Atlas of human anatomy,* ed 2, 1998, Ciba-Geigy.
←, Movement function; →, sensory function.

TABLE 40-1—cont'd
Swallowing Process

733

Structure	Muscle	Movement	Cranial Nerve	Sensation
	Palatoglossus	Elevates and pulls tongue posteriorly; narrows fauces		
	Genioglossus	Depresses, protrudes, and retracts tongue; elevates hyoid	←Hypoglossal (XII)	
	Hyoglossus	Depresses and pulls tongue posteriorly		
Soft palate	Tensor veli palatini	Tenses soft palate	←Trigeminal (V)→	Mouth
	Levator veli palatini	Elevates soft palate	←Accessory (XI)	
	Uvulae	Shortens soft palate		

PHARYNGEAL STAGE

Structure	Muscle	Movement	Cranial Nerve	Sensation
Fauces	Palatoglossus	Narrows fauces	←Vagus (X)→	Membranes of pharynx
	Palatopharyngeus	Elevates larynx and pharynx		
Hyoid	Suprahyoidei	Elevates hyoid anteriorly, posteriorly	←Trigeminal (V)	
	Stylohyoideus			
	Sternothyroideus	Depresses thyroid cartilage	←Cervical segments 1, 2, 3	
	Omohyoideus	Depresses hyoid		
Pharynx	Salpingopharyngeus	Pharynx elevation	←Glossopharyngeal (IX)	
	Palatopharyngeus	Pharynx elevation		
	Stylopharyngeus	Pharynx and larynx elevation		
	Constrictor pharyngeus superior	Sequentially constricts the nasopharynx, oropharynx, laryngopharynx	←Vagus (X)→	Membranes of pharynx
	Constrictor pharyngeus medius			
	Constrictor pharyngeus inferior			
	Cricopharyngeus	Relaxes during swallow; prevents air from entering esophagus		
Larynx	Aryepiglotticus Thyroepiglotticus	Closes inlet of larynx	←Vagus (X)→	Membranes of larynx
	Thyroarytenoideus	Closes glottis; shortens vocal cords		

From Bass N: The neurology of swallowing. In Groher M, editor: *Dysphagia: diagnosis and management*, ed 3, Newton, Mass, 1997, Butterworth-Heinemann Publishers; Davies P: *Steps to follow*, New York, 1985, Springer-Verlag; Hislop H, Montgomery J, Connelly B: *Daniels & Worthington's muscle testing: techniques of manual examination*, ed 6, Philadelphia, 1995, WB Saunders; Liebman M: *Neuroanatomy made easy and understandable*, Rockville, Md, 1986, Aspen Publishers; Netter F, Dalley A: *Atlas of human anatomy*, ed 2, 1998, Ciba-Geigy.
←, Movement function; →, sensory function.

Continued

TABLE 40-1—cont'd

Swallowing Process

Structure	Muscle	Movement	Cranial Nerve	Sensation
	Arytenoid-oblique, transverse	Adducts arytenoid cartilages		
	Lateral cricoarytenoid	Adducts and rotates arytenoid cartilage		
	Vocalis	Controls tension of vocal cords		
	Postcricoary-tenoideus	Widens glottis		
	Cricothyroideus-straight, oblique	Elevates cricoid arch		
Esophageal Stage				
Esophagus	Smooth	Peristaltic wave	←Vagus (X)	

From Bass N: The neurology of swallowing. In Groher M, editor: *Dysphagia: diagnosis and management*, ed 3, Newton, Mass, 1997, Butterworth-Heinemann Publishers; Davies P: *Steps to follow*, New York, 1985, Springer-Verlag; Hislop H, Montgomery J, Connelly B: *Daniels & Worthington's muscle testing: techniques of manual examination*, ed 6, Philadelphia, 1995, WB Saunders; Liebman M: *Neuroanatomy made easy and understandable*, Rockville, Md, 1986, Aspen Publishers; Netter F, Dalley A: *Atlas of human anatomy*, ed 2, 1998, Ciba-Geigy.
←, Movement function; →, sensory function.

falling into the **sulcus** between the jaw and cheek.[31] The tongue sweeps through the mouth, gathering food particles and mixing them with saliva.[7] Sensory receptors throughout the oral cavity carry information of taste, texture, and temperature of the food or liquid through the seventh and ninth cranial nerves to the brainstem. The chewing action of the mandible and tongue is repeated rhythmically, repositioning the food until a cohesive **bolus** is formed. The length of time needed to form a swallowable bolus varies. A short time is needed for soft foods, and a longer time is needed for hard foods.[24] Large amounts of thick liquids or thick and hard foods require the tongue to divide the food into smaller parts to be swallowed one at a time.[31] The posterior portion of the tongue forms a tight seal with the velum, preventing slippage of the bolus or liquid into the pharynx.[10,15,31]

In preparation for the next stage, the solid or liquid bolus, having been formed into a cohesive and swallowable mass, may be held between the anterior tongue and palate, with the tongue tip elevated or with the tongue tip dipped toward the floor of the mouth.[31] The tongue cups around the bolus to seal it against the hard palate. The larynx and the pharynx are at rest during this phase of the swallowing process. The airway is open.

Oral Phase

The oral phase of swallowing begins when the tongue moves the bolus toward the back of the mouth.[3] The tongue elevates to squeeze the bolus up against the hard palate. The tongue forms a central groove to funnel the food posteriorly. The amount of food swallowed is inversely related to the **viscosity** of the food. For less viscous foods, such as thin liquids, larger amounts may be swallowed. In contrast, more viscous foods or thick liquids require that a smaller amount be swallowed. This is necessary to make it easier for the bolus to pass through the pharynx.[31]

The oral stage of the swallow is voluntary, requiring the person to be alert.[10,31,34] A normal voluntary swallow is necessary to elicit a strong swallow response during the pharyngeal stage that follows. Overall, the oral phase takes approximately 1 second to complete with thin liquids and slightly longer with thick liquids.

Pharyngeal Phase

The pharyngeal phase of swallowing begins when the bolus passes through the anterior **faucial arches** and the middle of the tongue base into the pharynx, marking the start of the involuntary component of the swallow. After the swallow response has been triggered, it continues with no pause in bolus movement until the total act is completed. The swallow response is controlled by the medulla oblongata of the brainstem.[34] Within the medulla oblongata the medullary reticular formation is responsible for screening out all extraneous sensory patterns and for responding only to those patterns that indicate the need to swallow. The reticular formation also assumes control of all motor neurons and related muscles needed to complete the swallow. Higher brain

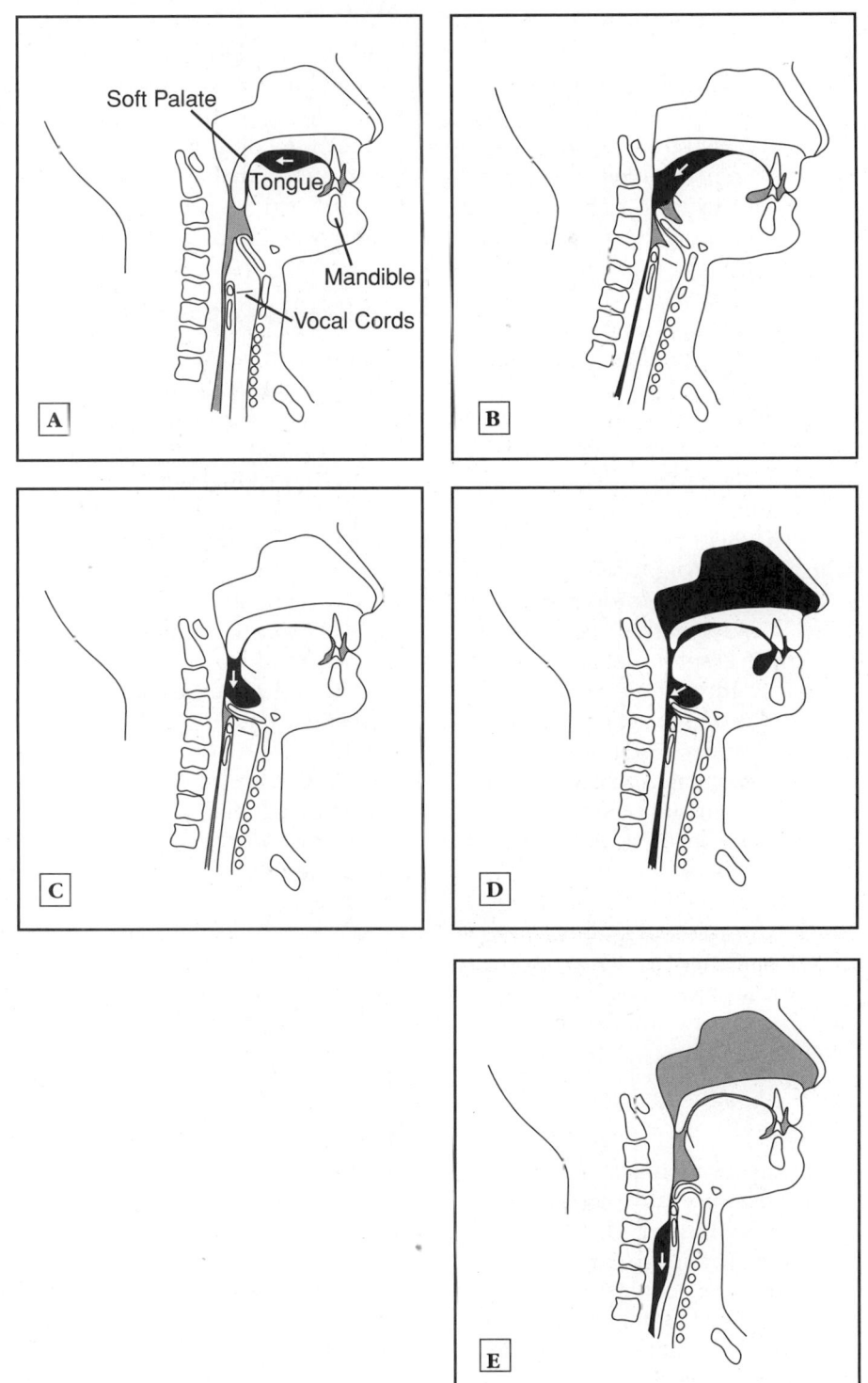

FIG. 40-2
The normal swallow. **A,** Lateral view of bolus propulsion during the swallow, beginning with the voluntary initiation of the swallow by the oral tongue. **B,** Triggering of the pharyngeal swallow. **C,** Arrival of the bolus in the vallecula. **D,** Tongue base retraction to the anteriorly moving pharyngeal wall. **E,** Bolus in the cervical esophagus and the cricopharyngeal region. (From Logemann J: *Evaluation and treatment of swallowing disorders,* Austin, Texas, 1998, ProEd Publishers)

functions such as speech, in addition to the respiratory reflex center, are preempted.[34]

When the swallow response is triggered, several physiological functions occur simultaneously. The **velum** elevates and retracts, closing the **velopharyngeal port** to prevent regurgitation of material into the nasal cavity. The tongue base elevates to direct the bolus into the pharynx. The entire pharyngeal tube elevates and contracts from the top to the bottom in the pharyngeal constrictors, carrying the bolus into and through both sides of the pharynx to the upper esophageal sphincter.[10] This movement must be rapid and efficient so that respiration is interrupted only briefly.

Concurrently, the larynx elevates beneath the back of the tongue base, protecting the airway. Three actions occur to facilitate closure of the larynx. These are: soft palate elevation and retraction and closure of the nasopharynx; laryngeal displacement anteriorly and superiorly with obliteration of the laryngeal vestibule and closure at the epiglottis and true vocal cords, preventing food from entering the airway; and relaxation and opening of the upper esophageal sphincter.[10,23,31] As the sphincter relaxes, food passes through the pharynx, dividing in half at the valleculae and moving down each side through the **pyriform sinuses.** The bolus reforms into a whole at the top of the esophagus and then passes through the esophagus. If the involuntary swallow response does not occur, neither do these physiological functions, thus preventing a safe, normal swallow.[27,31]

The pharyngeal phase of the swallow takes about 1 second to complete for thin liquids. Both voluntary and involuntary components are needed in a normal swallow. Neither mechanism alone is sufficient to produce the immediate, consistent swallow necessary for normal eating.[31]

Esophageal Phase

The esophageal phase of the swallow starts when the bolus enters the esophagus through the cricopharyngeal juncture or upper esophageal sphincter. The esophagus is a straight tube, about 10 inches long, that runs from the pharynx to the stomach. The pharynx is separated from the esophagus by the upper esophageal sphincter. The lower esophageal sphincter separates the esophagus from the stomach.[12,31] The upper third of the esophagus is composed of striated muscle and is innervated by the central nervous system. The middle section is made up of striated and smooth muscle and is innervated by the enteric nervous system that is visceral. The lower third of the tube is composed of smooth muscle.[12,23,34] The bolus is transported through the esophagus by peristaltic wave contractions. The overall transit time needed for the bolus to reach the stomach varies from 8 to 20 seconds.

SWALLOWING ASSESSMENT

When a referral is received from a physician, a thorough swallowing assessment for possible dysphagia must be completed. The occupational therapist reviews the patient's medical history and assesses the patient's visual, perceptual, and cognitive skills; physical control of head, trunk, and extremities; oral structures; and swallowing ability.

Medical Chart Review

A review of the patient's medical chart before the assessment often reveals important information. The therapist should take note of the patient's diagnosis, pertinent medical history, prescribed medications, and current nutritional status.

The medical diagnosis may indicate the cause or type of swallowing problem the patient is experiencing. For example, the presence of a neurological disorder should alert the therapist that dysphagia problems could exist. It is important to learn whether the dysphagia was of sudden or gradual onset. The therapist should seek information regarding the onset and duration of the patient's swallowing difficulties. The therapist also should note any previous surgeries involving the head, neck, and gastrointestinal tract that affect deglutition.

Particular attention should be paid to reported episodes of pneumonia or **aspiration** (entry of material into the airway).[31,35] Aspiration pneumonia is a complication that occurs when food enters or penetrates the lungs. An elevated temperature may indicate that a patient is aspirating.

A description of the patient's current nutritional status may be found in the dietary section of the chart or in the nursing progress notes. Consideration should be given to prescribed medications that may alter the patient's alertness, orientation, and muscle control.[38] How the patient is receiving food is important—for example, whether the patient is taking food orally or through a **nasogastric tube** (NG tube) or **gastrostomy tube,** (G tube) and whether the patient is able to take all nutrients orally or is receiving supplemental tube feedings. The nurses' notes may indicate whether the patient has difficulty managing certain food or liquid consistencies and whether the patient coughs or chokes during eating or when taking medication. The patient's intake and output (I & O) record provides additional information about hydration status.

Cognitive-Perceptual Status

The patient's cognitive and perceptual functions must be assessed to determine the patient's ability to participate actively in a feeding assessment or treatment program. The therapist should establish whether the patient is alert; oriented to name, day, and date; and able to follow simple directions, either verbal or with manual guidance. The therapist should also establish whether the patient is able to see the food clearly and motor plan hand-to-mouth and oral movements. The patient who exhibits confusion, dementia, poor awareness, or poor perception may require close supervision during eating or may not even be a good candidate for eating, since chewing and swallowing require voluntary control.[5,6,10,35]

Physical Status

Control of head and trunk is an important component of a safe swallow. To assess head control, the therapist asks the patient to turn the head from side to side and up and down. Assessment should include the quality of head movement, whether it is smooth and coordinated and whether it is adequate to allow the patient to maintain control with assistance. The therapist also should move the head passively from side to side and up and down to look for stiffness or abnormal muscle tone. Poor head control may indicate decreased strength, decreased or increased muscle tone, or decreased awareness. Head control is important because it develops first, followed by jaw movement and, last, by quality tongue movement. Head control is also necessary to provide adequate jaw and tongue movement for an optimal swallow response.

In assessing the patient's trunk control, the therapist observes whether the patient is sitting in midline with equal weight bearing on both hips. Thus the therapist learns whether the patient can maintain the midline position when provided with postural supports (such as wheelchair trunk supports or a lap board) and whether a return to midline is possible if loss of balance occurs. To participate in an eating and swallowing training program, the patient must maintain an upright position with head and trunk in midline to provide correct alignment of the swallowing structures.[5,9] If the patient has poor head or trunk control, the therapist may assist the patient during assessment and treatment.

Oral Assessment

Outer Oral Status

The face and mouth are sensitive areas to assess. Most adults are cautious about or even threatened by having another person touch their faces. Therefore each step of the assessment process should be carefully explained, using terms that the patient understands. The therapist also should tell the patient how long he or she will be touching the face; for example, "For a count of three." The therapist assesses the outer oral structures, including the facial musculature and mobility of the cheeks,

jaw, and lips. Working within the patient's visual field, the therapist moves his or her hand(s) slowly toward the patient's face. This allows the patient time to process and acknowledge the approach. If the patient is hypersensitive or resistant to the therapist's touch, the therapist can first guide the patient's hand as needed to evaluate that area.

It is important for the patient to feel comfortable with the therapist's touch during the assessment. If a patient is not comfortable with the face or lips being touched, he or she will certainly be less inclined to allow the therapist's hand inside his or her mouth.

SENSATION. Indications of poor oral sensation are drooling, food on the mouth, and food falling out of the mouth of which the patient is unaware. To assess the patient's awareness of touch, the therapist occludes the patient's vision and uses a cotton-tipped swab to touch the patient gently with a quick stroke to different areas of the face. The patient is asked to point to where he or she was touched. If pointing is difficult for the patient, the patient is asked to nod or say yes or no when touched. The patient with intact sensation responds accurately and quickly.

The patient's ability to sense hot and cold should be assessed. The therapist may use two test tubes, one filled with hot water and one with cold water. A laryngeal mirror that is first heated and then cooled with hot and cold water may also be used. The patient is touched on the face or lips in several places and is asked to indicate whether the touch was hot or cold. An aphasic patient may have difficulty answering correctly. In this instance the therapist must make an assessment from clinical observations.

Poor sensory awareness affects the patient's ability to move facial musculature appropriately. The patient's self-esteem also may be affected, especially in social situations, if decreased awareness causes the patient to ignore saliva, food, or liquids remaining on the face or lips.

MUSCULATURE. An assessment of the facial muscles provides the therapist with information about the movement, strength, and tone available to the patient for chewing and swallowing. The therapist first observes the patient's face at rest and notes any visible asymmetry. If a facial droop is obvious, the therapist should observe whether the muscles feel slack or taut. A masked appearance, with little change in facial expression, may also be observed. The therapist should observe whether the patient appears to be frowning or grimacing with jaw clenched and mouth pulled back. These symptoms may indicate increased or decreased muscle tone. Information obtained through clinical observations should be compared with that seen during actual movement.

TABLE 40-2
Outer Oral Motor Assessment

Function	Instruction to Patient	Testing Procedure*
Facial expression	Lift your eyebrows as high as you can	Place one finger above each eyebrow. Apply downward pressure.
	Bring your eyebrows toward your nose in a frown.	Place one finger above each eyebrow. Apply pressure outward.
	Wrinkle your nose upwards.	Place one finger on tip of nose and apply downward pressure.
	Suck in your cheeks.	Apply pressure outward against each inside cheek.
Lip control	Smile.	Observe for symmetrical movement. Palpate over each cheek.
	Press your lips together tightly and puff out your cheeks.	Place one finger above and one finger below lips. Apply pressure, moving fingers away from each other; check for ability to hold air.
	Pucker your lips as in a kiss.	Apply pressure inwardly against lips (toward teeth).
Jaw control	Open your mouth as far as you can.	Help patient maintain head control. Apply pressure from under chin upward and forward.
	Close your mouth tightly. Don't let me open it.	Help patient maintain head control. Apply pressure on chin downward.
	Push your bottom teeth forward.	Place two fingers against chin and apply pressure backward.
	Move your jaw from side to side.	Place one finger on left cheek and apply pressure to right.

From Alta Bates Hospital Rehabilitation Services: *Bedside dysphagia evaluation protocol,* Berkeley, Calif, 1999; Community Hospital of Los Gatos, Rehabilitation Services: *Dysphagia protocol,* Los Gatos, Calif, 1999; Logemann J: *Evaluation and treatment of swallowing disorders,* Austin, Tex, 1998, Pro-Ed Publishers; Miller R: Clinical examination for dysphagia. In Groher M: *Dysphagia diagnosis and management,* ed 3, Newton, Mass, 1997, Butterworth-Heinemann Publishers.
*Apply resistance only in the absence of abnormal muscle tone.

The therapist tests the facial musculature by asking the patient to perform the movements listed in Table 40-2. The therapist should note how much assistance the patient needs to perform these movements. As the patient moves through each task, bilateral symmetry is assessed. Asymmetry could indicate weakness or increased tone. Musculature is palpated for abnormal resistance to the movement. Resistance, which feels as if the patient is fighting the movement, is caused by hypertonicity in the antagonistic muscle group.

If the patient is able to hold the position at the end of the movement, the therapist applies pressure against the muscle to determine the muscle's strength. The patient with normal strength is able to hold the position throughout the applied resistance. The patient who is able to hold the position briefly against pressure may have adequate strength for chewing and swallowing with assistance. The patient who is unable to move into the testing position independently or with assistance will have difficulty with eating and with facial expression.

ORAL REFLEXES. A patient with clearly documented neurological involvement may demonstrate primitive oral reflexes that interfere with a dysphagia retraining program. The rooting, bite, and suck-swallow reflexes, normal from 0 to 5 months of age, may reappear in adults when higher cortical structures are damaged. The gag, palatal, and cough reflexes, which should be present in adults and act to protect the airway, may be impaired. Specific assessment techniques can be found in Table 40-3. Persistence of these primitive oral reflexes interferes with the patient's development of isolated motor control, which is needed for chewing and swallowing.

Inner Oral Status
An assessment of the patient's inner oral status includes an examination of oral structures, tongue musculature, palatal function, and swallowing. By performing the outer oral status assessment first, the therapist has established a rapport and trust with the patient. Each proce-

TABLE 40-3
Oral Reflexes

Reflex	Assessment	Functional Implications
Rooting (0-4 months)	*Stimulus:* touch patient on right or left corner of mouth	Limits isolated motor control of lip muscles
	Response: patient moves lips and head in direction of stimulus	Moves head out of midline altering alignment of swallowing mechanism
Bite (4-7 months)	*Stimulus:* touch crowns of teeth with unbreakable object	Prevents normal forward, lateral, and rotary movements of jaw necessary for chewing
	Response: patient involuntarily clamps teeth shut.	
Suck-swallow (0-4 months)	*Stimulus:* introduction of food and liquid	Prevents development of normal voluntary swallow
	Response: sucking	
Tongue thrust (abnormal)	*Stimulus:* introduction of food and liquid	Interferes with ability to keep lips and mouth closed
	Response: tongue comes forward to front of teeth	Prevents tongue from propelling food to back of mouth in preparation for swallow; prevents formation of bolus, loss of tongue lateralization
Gag (0-adult)	*Stimulus:* pressure on back of tongue	Protects airway (not always present in normal adult); hypersensitive gag reflex can interfere with chewing, swallowing.
	Response: tongue humping, pharyngeal constriction	
Palatal (0-adult)	*Stimulus:* stroke along faucial arches	Protects airway, closes off nasal passages, triggers swallow response
	Response: constriction of faucial arches; elevation of uvula	

From Avery-Smith W: Management of neurologic disorders: the first feeding session. In Groher M, editor: *Dysphagia: diagnosis and management,* ed 3, Newton, Mass, 1997, Butterworth-Heinemann; Farber S: *Neurorehabilitation, a multisensory approach,* Philadelphia, 1982, WB Saunders; Logemann J: *Evaluation and treatment of swallowing disorders,* Austin, Tex, 1998, Pro-Ed Publishers; Schulze-Delrieu K, Miller R: Clinical assessment of dysphagia. In Perlman A, Schulze-Delrieu K, editors: *Deglutition and its disorders: anatomy, physiology, clinical diagnosis and management,* San Diego, Calif, 1997, Singular Publishing; Silverman EH, Elfant IL: *Am J Occup Ther,* 1979.

dure is first explained to the patient. The therapist works within the patient's visual field and gives the patient time to process the instructions found in Table 40-4.

It is important that the therapist place only a wet finger or tongue blade into the patient's mouth, because the mouth is normally a wet environment. A dry finger or tongue blade is uncomfortable.[13] After a count of three, the therapist removes the finger and allows the patient to swallow the saliva. The therapist should wear latex gloves for protection from infections. Appropriate hand washing techniques are also necessary.

DENTITION. Because the adult uses teeth to shear and grind food during bolus formation, the therapist needs to assess the condition and quality of the patient's teeth and gums.[13,38]

For assessment purposes, the mouth is divided into four quadrants: right upper, right lower, left upper, and left lower. Each quadrant is assessed separately, as is each side (e.g., assess right upper side, then right lower side). First the therapist slides a wet fifth finger under the patient's upper lip and moves it back toward the cheek, rubbing the gums three times.[13] The therapist notes whether the patient's gums are bleeding, tender, or inflamed and whether the gums feel spongy or firm. Loose teeth and sensitive or missing teeth are also noted. *The therapist should take caution to avoid placing his or her finger between the patient's teeth until it has been determined that the patient does not have a bite reflex.*

After assessing the gums, the therapist turns over his or her finger, sliding the pad of the finger against the inside of the patient's cheek and gently pushing the

TABLE 40-4
Inner Oral Motor Assessment

Function	Instruction to Patient	Testing Procedure*
Tongue		
Protrusion	Stick out your tongue.	Apply slight resistance toward the back of the throat with tongue blade after patient exhibits full range of motion.
Lateralization	Move your tongue from side to side.	Apply slight resistance in opposite direction of motion with tongue blade.
	Touch your tongue to your inside cheek—right, then left; move your tongue up and down.	Using finger on outside of cheek, push against tongue inwardly.
Tipping	Touch your tongue to your upper lip.	With tongue blade between tongue tip and lip, apply downward pressure.
	Open your mouth. Touch your tongue behind your front teeth.	With tongue blade between tongue and teeth, apply downward pressure on tongue.
Dipping	Touch your tongue behind your bottom teeth.	With tongue blade between tongue and bottom teeth, apply upward pressure.
Humping	Say, "ng"; say, "ga."	Observe for humping of tongue against hard palate. Tongue should flow from front to back.
	Run your tongue along roof of your mouth, front or back.	Observe for symmetry and ease of movement.
Swallow		
Hard palate	Open your mouth and hold it open.	Using flashlight, gently examine for sensitivity by walking finger from front to back.
Soft palate	Say, "ah" for as long as you can (5 seconds). Change pitch up an octave.	Observe for tightening of faucial arches, elevation of uvula. Using laryngeal mirror, stroke juncture of hard and soft palate to elicit palatal reflex. Observe for upward and backward movement of soft palate.
Hyoid Elevation (base of tongue)	Can you swallow for me?	Place finger at base of patient's tongue underneath the chin, and feel for elevation just before movement of the larynx.
Laryngeal		
Range of motion	I am going to move your Adam's apple side to side.	Grasp larynx by placing fingers and thumb along sides. Move larynx gently side to side; evaluate for ease and symmetry of movement.
Elevation	Can you swallow for me?	Place fingers along the larynx: first finger at hyoid, second finger at top of larynx, and so on. Feel for quick and smooth elevation of larynx as the patient swallows.
Cough		
Voluntary	Can you cough?	Observe for ease and strength of movement, loudness of cough, swallow after cough.
Reflexive	Take a deep breath.	As patient holds breath, using palm of hand, push downward (toward stomach) on the sternum. Evaluate strength of reaction.

From Community Hospital of Los Gatos, Rehabilitation Services: *Dysphagia protocol,* Los Gatos, Calif, 1999; Coombes K: *Swallowing dysfunction in hemiplegia and head injury,* course presented by International Clinical Educators, Aug 24-27, 1986, and Aug 24-28, 1987, Los Gatos, Calif; Hislop H, Montgomery J, Connelly B: *Daniels & Worthington's muscle testing: techniques of manual examination,* ed 6, Philadelphia, 1995, WB Saunders; Miller R: Clinical examination for dysphagia. In Groher M: *Dysphagia diagnosis and management,* ed 3, Newton, Mass, 1997, Butterworth-Heinemann Publishers; Schulze-Delrieu K, Miller R: Clinical assessment of dysphagia. In Perlman A, Schulze-Delrieu K, editors: *Deglutition and its disorders: anatomy, physiology, clinical diagnosis and management,* San Diego, Calif, 1997, Singular Publishing.

*Apply resistance in absence of abnormal muscle tone.

cheek outward to feel the tone of the buccal musculature. The therapist notes whether the cheek is firm with an elastic quality, too easy to stretch, or tight without any stretch. The therapist observes the condition of the inside of the patient's mouth, checking for bite marks on the tongue, cheeks, and lips. Next, the therapist should remove the finger from the patient's mouth, allow or assist the patient to swallow saliva, and assist the patient to move the lip and cheek musculature into the normal resting position. This procedure is repeated for each quadrant. The therapist should avoid moving the finger across midline from the right to the left side of the patient's gums because this practice can be annoying.

If the patient has dentures, the therapist must discern whether the fit is adequate for chewing. Because dentures are held in place and controlled by normal musculature and sensation, changes in these areas, or marked weight loss, affect the patient's ability to use dentures effectively.[16] The dentures should fit over the gums without slipping or sliding during eating or talking. Because the patient needs to wear dentures throughout the dysphagia training period, necessary corrections or repairs should be completed quickly.[35,39] A dental consultation may be needed to ensure appropriate fit if dentures cannot be held firmly with commercial adhesive creams or powders. Patients who have gum or dental problems require appropriate follow-up and good oral hygiene to participate in a feeding program. Loose dentures or teeth may necessitate changes in food consistencies that the patient might have otherwise managed.

TONGUE MOVEMENT. The tongue is an intricate part of the normal chewing and swallowing process. Controlled tongue movement is necessary for moving and shaping food in the mouth. The tongue propels the food back in preparation for swallowing; therefore a thorough assessment of the tongue's strength, range of motion, control, and tone is needed.[10,13,38,41]

The patient is asked to open the mouth, and the therapist can assess the appearance of the tongue with a flashlight and note whether the tongue is pink and moist, very red, or a heavily coated white. A heavily coated tongue may decrease the patient's sensations of taste, temperature, and texture and may indicate poor tongue movement or be a sign of infection.

When examining the shape of the tongue, the therapist notes whether it is flattened out, bunched up, or rounded. Normally the tongue is slightly concave with a groove running down the middle. The therapist observes the position of the tongue. The therapist should determine whether it is at midline, resting just behind the front teeth in the normal position, retracted or pulled back away from the front teeth, or deviated to the right or left side. A retracted tongue may indicate an increase of abnormal muscle tone or a loss of range of motion as a result of soft-tissue shortening. The patient

exhibiting tongue deviation with protrusion may have muscle weakness on the affected side, causing the tongue to deviate toward the unaffected side because the stronger muscles dominate. The patient also may have abnormal tone, which results in the tongue deviating toward the affected side.

Grasping the tongue gently between the forefinger and thumb, the therapist can pull the tongue slowly forward. A wet gauze square wrapped around the tip of the tongue may help the therapist to grip it.[13] Next, the therapist walks a wet finger along the tongue from front to back, to determine whether the tongue feels hard, firm, or mushy. The right side of the tongue is compared with the left side. An abnormally hard tongue may be the result of increased muscle tone.

While continuing to grip the tongue between forefinger and thumb, the therapist can assess the patient's range of motion by moving the tongue forward, side to side, and up and down. The tongue with normal range will move freely in all directions without resistance.[13,38] Moving the tongue through its range, the therapist can simultaneously evaluate tone. As the therapist pulls the tongue forward, he or she determines whether it comes easily or whether resistance feels as if the tongue were pulling back against the movement, indicating increased tone. A tongue that seems to stretch too far beyond the front teeth is indicative of decreased tone. When moving the tongue side to side, the therapist notes whether it is easier to move in one direction or the other. Increased abnormal tone makes it difficult for the therapist to move the tongue in any direction without feeling resistance against the movement. The amount of assistance needed to decrease or increase tone to within normal limits should be noted. Patients who are confused or apraxic may resist this passive motion but not have an actual increase in tone.

To assess the tongue's motor control (strength and coordination), the therapist asks the patient to elevate, stick out, and move the tongue laterally (Table 40-4). If the patient has difficulty following verbal directions, the therapist can use a wet tongue blade to guide the patient through the desired movements. The patient is asked to place the tongue against the tongue blade and to keep it there. The therapist then moves the tongue blade slowly, guiding the patient's tongue in the testing direction.[13] Ease of movement, strength of movement, and coordination of movement are assessed for each direction.

Poor muscle strength or abnormal tone decreases the ability of the tongue to sweep the mouth and gather particles to form a cohesive bolus. If the tongue loses even partial control of the bolus, food may fall into the valleculae, the pyriform sinuses, or the airway, possibly leading to aspiration before the actual swallow.[31] The back of the tongue must also elevate quickly and strongly to propel the bolus past the faucial arch into the pharynx to trigger the swallow response.[13,38] The therapist must carefully assess the tongue's function. The patient with poor tongue control may not be a candidate for eating. The therapist must first normalize tone and improve tongue movement before attempting to feed the patient. The correct selection of appropriate foods also facilitates motor control when the patient is ready for eating. Close supervision by an experienced therapist is required for this type of patient to participate in eating.

Clinical Assessment of Swallowing

Because aspiration is a primary concern in swallowing, the occupational therapist must carefully assess the patient's ability to swallow safely. Before the therapist presents the patient with material to swallow, he or she should assess the ability of the patient to protect the airway. The patient must have an intact palatal reflex, elevation of the larynx, and a productive cough. Directions for assessing all the components of the swallow are described in Table 40-4. The therapist should note the speed and strength of each component. The patient with intact cognitive skills may accurately report to the therapist where and when there is difficulty with the swallow.[31]

The occupational therapist must assimilate all the information from the assessment process. Clinical judgment plays an important role in the accurate assessment of dysphagia.[3,5,13] The following are questions that must be asked:

1. Is the patient alert enough to follow through with bolus formation and an immediate swallow when presented with food?
2. With assistance, does the patient maintain adequate trunk and head control, normalizing tone and facilitating quality movement?
3. Does the patient display adequate tongue control to form a partially cohesive bolus and to regulate the speed with which the bolus enters the pharynx?
4. Is the larynx mobile enough to elevate quickly and strongly?
5. Can the patient handle the saliva with minimal drooling?
6. Does the patient have a productive cough, strong enough to expel any material that may enter the airway?

If the answer is yes to all of the above questions, the therapist may assess the patient's oral and swallow control with a variety of food consistencies.

The therapist should request an assessment tray from dietary services. The tray should contain a sample of pureed food such as pudding or applesauce, soft food such as a banana or macaroni and cheese, and ground tuna with mayonnaise or chopped meat with gravy. The tray also should include a thick drink such as nectar blended with one half banana for a seven-ounce drink,

a semithick drink such as fruit nectar or a yogurt drink, and a thin liquid such as water.[1,11]

To minimize the risk of aspiration, pureed foods are chosen for patients with decreased motor control and chewing difficulties or apraxia. Soft foods are easily formed into a bolus and require less chewing than ground meat for patients who have poor oral motor control. Soft foods also stay together in a cohesive bolus. Ground foods allow the therapist to assess a patient's ability to chew, form a cohesive bolus, and move it in the mouth. Thick liquids move more slowly from front to back, giving the patient with a delayed swallow more time to control the liquid until the swallow response is triggered. Thin liquids are the most difficult to control because they require an intact swallow to prevent aspiration.

For the patient who appears to have some ability to chew, the therapist should start with pureed and soft foods and introduce solid materials if the patient is doing well.[11,13,37,39] The following procedures should be completed after each swallow of food or liquid:

1. Using a fork, the therapist places a small amount (⅓ teaspoon) on the middle of the patient's tongue. A fork allows the therapist greater control of food placement in the mouth.[11,13,31] This procedure is repeated for each substance for two or three bites to check for fatigue.
2. The therapist palpates for the swallow by placing the index finger at the hyoid notch, the second finger at the top of the larynx, and the third finger along the midlarynx. The therapist can feel the strength and smoothness of the swallow and also notes whether the patient needs subsequent or additional swallows to clear the bolus.[13,31] The therapist can also evaluate the oral transit time by noting when food entered the mouth, when tongue movement was initiated, and when the elevation of the hyoid notch was felt, indicating the beginning of the swallow process. The therapist can time the swallow from the time that hyoid movement begins to when laryngeal elevation occurs, indicating triggering of the swallow response.[31] A normal swallow takes only 1 second to complete for thin liquids.
3. The therapist asks the patient to open the mouth to check for remaining food. Food is commonly seen in the lateral sulci, under the tongue, on the base of the tongue, and against the hard palate.[10,31] Food remaining in the mouth indicates decreased or poor oral transit skills. The patient who exhibits oral motor deficits has increasing difficulty with chewing, shaping a bolus, and channeling food backward as harder consistencies of food are introduced.[13]
4. The therapist asks the patient to say, "ah." By listening carefully, the therapist can assess the patient's voice quality and classify the sound production as strong, clear, or gurgly or gargling.[13,31]

A gurgly voice may result from a delayed swallow response, which allows material to collect in the larynx. The therapist asks the patient to take a second "dry" swallow to clear any pooling of material. Asking the patient to say, "ah" again enables the therapist to assess whether the voice quality remains gurgly or gargling for any length of time after the dry swallow. In addition, the therapist asks the patient to pant for a few seconds. This will shake loose any material that may remain in the pyriform sinuses or valleculae.[11] If the voice is still gurgly, the therapist should be concerned with the possibility that material has come into contact with or is sitting on the vocal cords.[31]

If the patient has significant coughing episodes, particularly before the therapist feels the initiation of the swallow (elevation of hyoid notch) with any consistency, the procedure should not be continued. If there is coughing from food with a pureed consistency, the therapist may try a soft food such as a banana, if the patient has good anterior to posterior tongue movement.[13] If problems persist, a videofluoroscopy may be indicated.

A neurologically impaired patient with poor sensation may have difficulty with a food of pureed consistency because it does not stay together as a bolus. The weight of soft foods may adequately trigger the swallow response. If the patient continues to cough even with soft foods, the swallow assessment should be discontinued. In this instance videofluoroscopy is indicated. If a patient is having difficulty at this level, only a prefeeding treatment program can be considered appropriate.

A patient who has difficulty managing solid consistencies may or may not have difficulty with liquids. To assess the patient's swallow with liquids, the therapist starts with a thickened (thick) nectar, then a pure nectar (semithick), and finally a thin liquid such as water or juice (see Table 40-8). Small amounts of the liquid are placed on the middle of the patient's tongue with a spoon. The therapist proceeds by following the four-step sequence described earlier for solid foods. The therapist assesses the patient's skill at moving material from front to back, the time of oral transit and swallow, and the voice quality after each swallow. Each liquid consistency is assessed for two or three swallows to check for fatigability. If the patient tolerates and swallows liquids by spoon without difficulty, the therapist assesses the ability to tolerate liquids from a cup or with a straw.[11] Again, the patient's voice quality is checked.

A patient with a poor swallow may aspirate directly or pool liquids in the pyriform sinuses and valleculae, which, when full, overflow into the laryngeal vestibule and down into the trachea. If a patient continues to have a gurgling or gargling voice after a second dry swallow or substantial coughing with any of the liquid consistencies, the assessment should be discontinued (Fig. 40-3).

The therapist must also assess the patient's ability to alternate between liquids and solids, which occurs naturally during meals. The therapist presents the patient with an easily managed food bolus, followed by the safest type of liquid tolerated, and then assesses the patient for coughing when the consistency of the food is changed.

A patient with a tracheostomy tube in place can be assessed as previously described. The same criteria must be met before the therapist assesses the patient's eating and swallowing of food or liquids. The therapist must have a thorough understanding of the types of tracheostomy tubes and varied functions.

There are two main types of tracheostomy tubes: fenestrated and nonfenestrated (Figs. 40-4 and 40-5).[18,31,42] A fenestrated tube is designed with an opening in the middle to allow increased air flow. This type of tube is frequently used for patients being weaned from a tube because it allows a patient to breathe nasally as he or she relearns a normal breathing pattern. Placement of an inner cannula piece into the tracheostomy tube allows the fenestrated opening to be closed off. With the inner cannula removed, a trachea button may be used to allow the patient to talk. A nonfenestrated tube has no opening. A fenestrated tube is preferred for treating a patient with dysphagia.

A tracheostomy tube may be cuffed or uncuffed. A cuffed tube has a balloonlike cuff surrounding the bottom of the tube.[18,31] When inflated, the cuff comes into contact with the trachea wall, preventing the aspiration of secretions into the airway. A cuffed tube is used in cases in which aspiration has occurred. The therapist should consult with the patient's attending physician to see whether the patient is still at risk of aspirating, or if it is safe to deflate the cuff for an eating and swallowing assessment.

Before the therapist presents any food matter to the patient with a tracheostomy who has a fenestrated tube, the inner cannula should be in place. If the patient has a cuffed tube, the therapist should thoroughly suction orally and around the cuff, present food, and slowly deflate the cuff while suctioning to prevent substances from penetrating the airway. The airway again needs to be suctioned orally and through the tracheostomy to ensure that all secretions have been cleared.[10,19,31] The nursing staff or a therapist who has been trained and is considered competent can perform the suctioning procedure.

After presenting food or liquids the therapist should check for oral transit skills and swallow as previously described. Blue food coloring added to food or liquids can help the therapist identify material in the trachea. The patient can use a gloved finger to cover the trachea opening, to achieve a more normal tracheal pressure during the swallow.[31]

If the tracheostomy tube is cuffed, the cuff is slowly deflated. The airway is suctioned through the tracheostomy tube to determine whether any material entered the airway. The swallow assessment should not

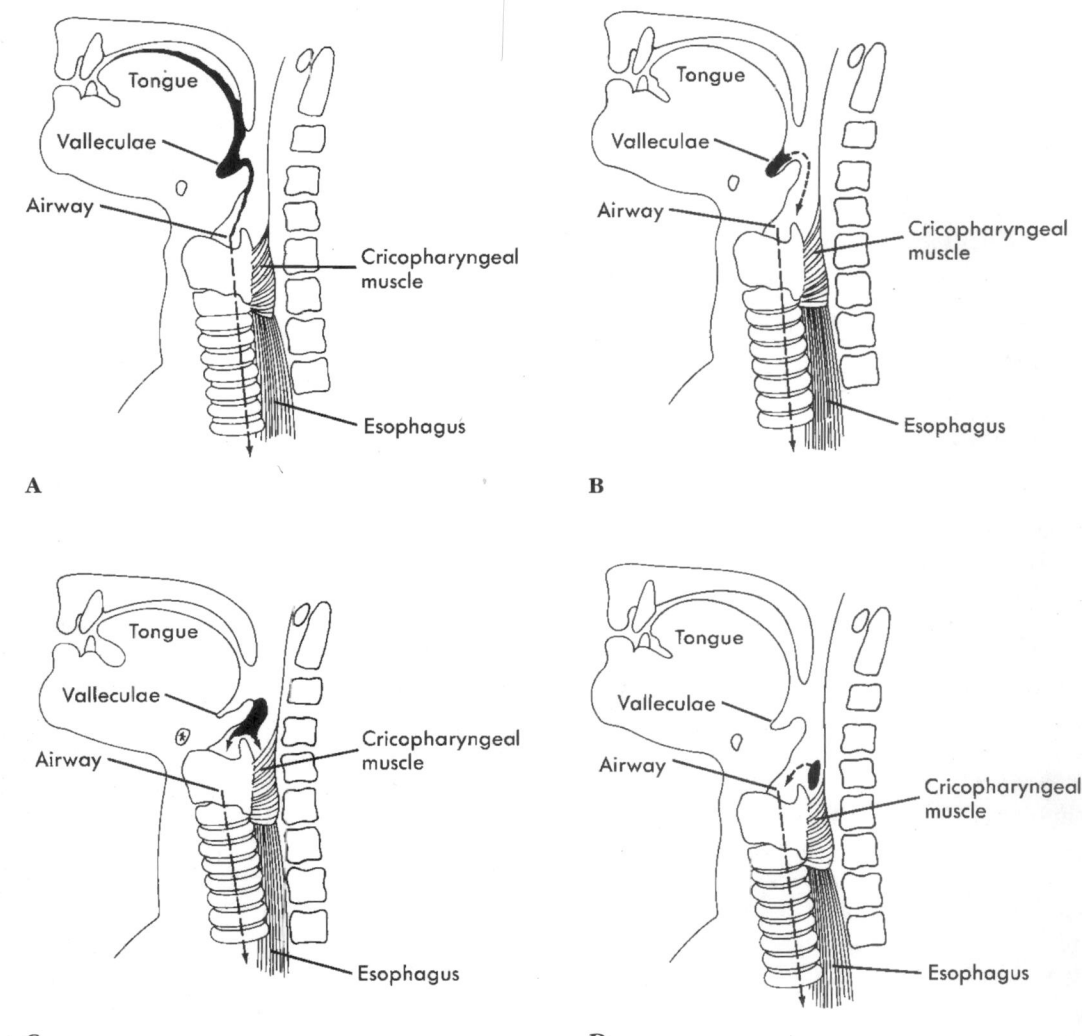

FIG. 40-3

Types of aspiration. **A,** Aspiration before swallow caused by reduced tongue control. **B,** Aspiration before swallow caused by absent swallow response. **C,** Aspiration during swallow caused by reduced laryngeal closure. **D,** Aspiration after swallow caused by pooled material in pyriform sinuses overflowing into airway. (From Logemann J: *Evaluation and treatment of swallowing disorders,* San Diego, 1983, College-Hill Press).

be continued if material is found in the trachea.[10,19,31] The presence of a tracheostomy tube may affect a patient's swallow as secretions are increased and laryngeal mobility is decreased. When assessment is complete, the airway is thoroughly suctioned. The inner cannula is removed from the fenestrated tube, or the cuff inflated to the level prescribed by the physician.[18,19]

The patient's performance on the swallowing assessment determines whether the patient is able to participate in a feeding program and at which food and liquid consistencies he or she is able to function efficiently. The therapist must decide which consistency is the safest for the patient. The safest consistency is that which the patient is able to chew, move through the oral cavity, and swallow with the least risk of aspiration.

Indicators of Eating and Swallowing Dysfunction

The indicators of swallowing dysfunction include the following[10,13,31,38,40]:

1. Difficulty with bringing food to the mouth
2. The inability to shape food into a bolus
3. Coughing or throat clearing before, during, or after the swallow
4. Gurgling voice quality
5. Changes in breathing pattern
6. Delayed or absent swallow response
7. Poor cough
8. Reflux of food after meals

The presence of any swallowing dysfunction can lead to aspiration pneumonia. The following are acute

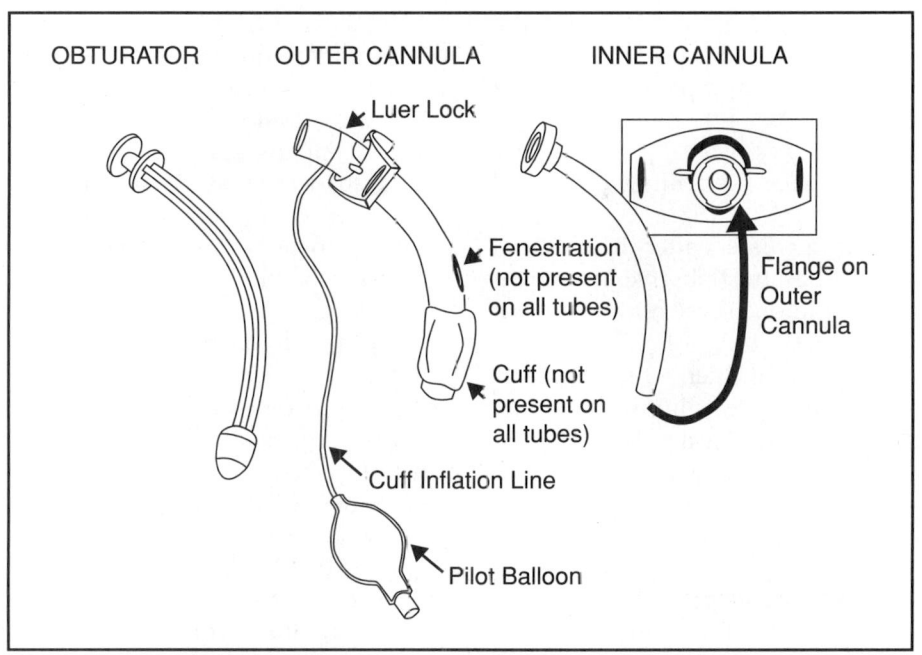

FIG. 40-4
Tracheostomy tube components. (From Logemann J: *Evaluation and treatment of swallowing disorders,* Austin, Tex, 1998, ProEd Publications.)

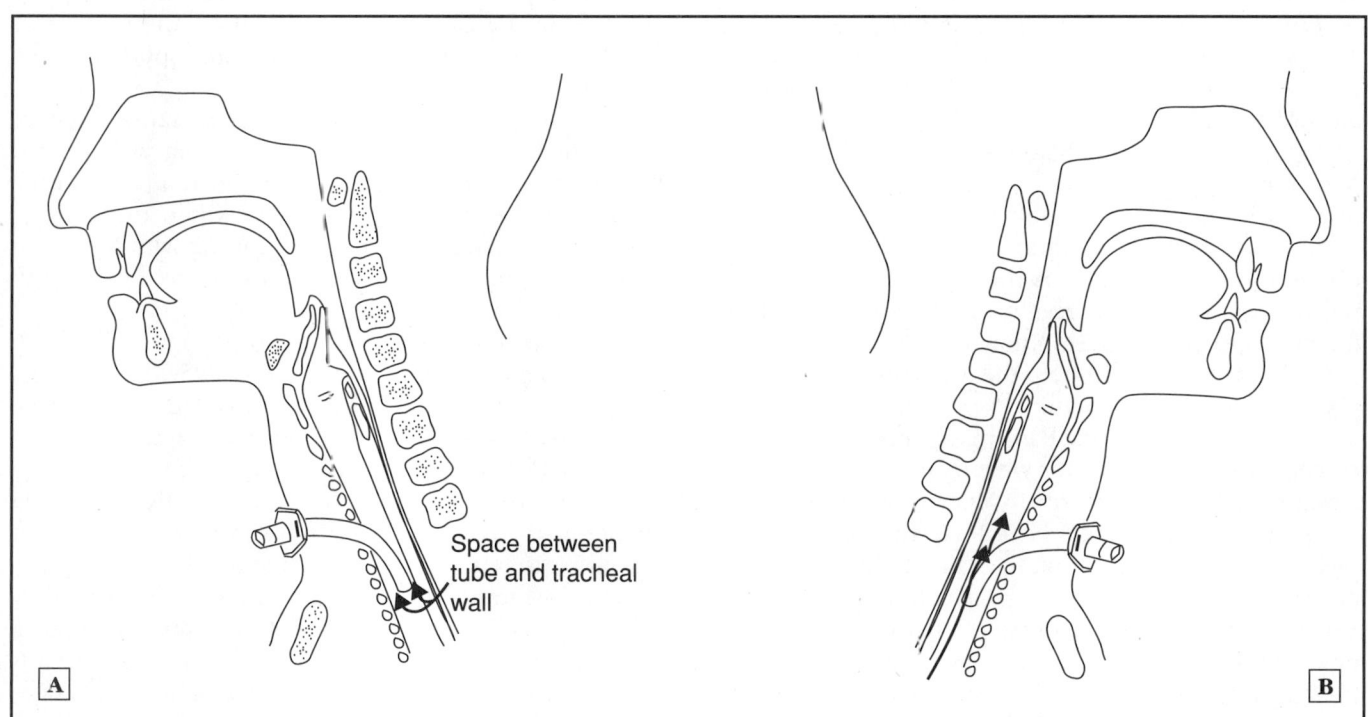

FIG. 40-5
A, Midsagittal section of the head and neck showing the position of an uncuffed tracheostomy tube. **B,** Midsagittal section of the head and neck showing the passage of air between the tracheostomy tube and the tracheal wall. (From Logemann J: *Evaluation and treatment of swallowing disorders,* Austin, Tex, 1998, ProEd Publications.)

symptoms of aspiration occurring immediately after the swallow[13,18,19,40]:

1. Any change in the patient's color, particularly if the airway is obstructed
2. Prolonged coughing
3. Gurgling voice, and extreme breathiness or loss of voice

During the 24 hours immediately after the swallow, the therapist and medical staff must observe the patient for additional signs of aspiration. These may be a nasal drip, an increase to profuse drooling of a clear liquid, and temperatures of 100° F or greater, which may not have been evident during the clinical examination.[13,22,31] If aspiration pneumonia develops, the patient must be reevaluated for a change in diet levels or taken off the feeding program, if necessary. An alternative feeding method is required.

Assessment With Videofluoroscopy

Videoflouroscopy is an important technique for assessing a patient's swallow. Videofluoroscopy is a radiographic procedure using a modified barium swallow recorded on videotape.[31] This technique allows the therapist to see the patient's jaw and tongue movement, to measure the transit times of the oral and pharyngeal stages, see the swallow, see any residue in the valleculae and the pyriform sinuses, and observe any aspiration. With videofluoroscopy the therapist can determine the cause of aspiration. Videofluoroscopy may also be used to determine which treatment techniques to use and the safest diet level to help the patient achieve a safe swallow.

Aspiration can occur before the swallow because of poor tongue control, pooled material in the valleculae, or a delayed or absent swallow response. Poor laryngeal closure can result in aspiration during the swallow. Aspiration after the swallow is the result of pooled material in the pyriform sinuses or of the valleculae overflowing into the trachea. Knowing the reason why a patient is aspirating can help the occupational therapist plan appropriate treatment.[31,32]

A fluoroscopy machine has three components: a fluoroscopy tube, a monitor for viewing the picture, and an elevation table or platform. A television videocassette recorder is set up to record the image. Other necessary pieces of equipment normally available in a radiology department are lead-lined aprons, lead-lined gloves, and foam positioning wedges.[31,32] Because it may not be possible to lower the fluoroscopy machine enough to view a patient seated in a wheelchair, a special plywood seat system or wheelchair platform with a ramp may be needed. Commercially made seating systems are also available.

Videofluoroscopy is necessary for ruling out silent aspiration. Forty to sixty percent of patients with neurological impairment who have dysphagia are found to be silent aspirators during the clinical assessment.[31,40] It is important to rule out the occurrence of aspiration.

Other indicators for videofluoroscopy are difficulties with liquid consistencies and a need to identify specific pharyngeal problems. Some clinicians, however, advocate that all patients be evaluated by videofluoroscopy, regardless of these indicators. Contraindications to performing videofluoroscopy include rapid progress of the patient, a poor level of awareness or poor cognitive status, oral stage problems only, and the physical inability of the patient to undergo the test.

Three people are involved in performing videofluoroscopy: the radiologist, the occupational therapist, and the video technician. The patient should be positioned to allow a lateral view, with the fluoroscopy tube focused on the lips, hard palate, and posterior pharyngeal wall. The lateral view is most frequently used because it allows the therapist to evaluate all four stages of the swallow. This view clearly shows the presence of aspiration. A posterior-anterior view also may be needed to evaluate asymmetry in the vocal cords and pooling of the valleculae or pyriform sinuses.

During a videofluoroscopy assessment the therapist presents the patient with food or liquid to which barium paste or powder has been added.[11,31,32] The therapist mixes or spreads small amounts of paste or powder onto or into each food or liquid consistency. Premixing the consistencies with the barium paste or powder prevents time-consuming interruptions during the actual assessment procedure.

Food and liquids are presented in the same sequence used for the clinical assessment. Starting with pureed foods, the patient is given ½ teaspoon at a time of each consistency and asked to swallow when instructed.[11] Liquids are tested separately, beginning with the thickened substance. Material is given in small amounts to reduce the risks of aspiration, if it occurs. An experienced dysphagia therapist may choose to use only foods or liquids that the patient had difficulty with during the clinical examination, rather than to proceed through the entire sequence. The therapist continues to assess with each consistency until aspiration occurs.

If the patient aspirates during the swallow, allowing material to fall directly into the airway, the therapist should discontinue the assessment with that consistency. If aspiration occurs before the swallow, secondary to poor tongue control or a delayed swallow reflex, a thicker or denser substance should be tried because it is easier for the patient to control. If the patient aspirates after the swallow because of pooling in the valleculae or pyriform sinuses, the assessment with that consistency is discontinued.

The videofluoroscopy procedure can also be used to observe for fatigue. The patient is asked to take repeated, or *serial*, swallows of solids and liquids. The therapist should assess the patient's ability to control mixed consistencies of solids and liquids such as soups and to alternate between solids and liquids. Various compensatory techniques may also be assessed to determine if the airway can be protected, which may allow the therapist to initiate a feeding program.[31,32]

The solid and liquid consistency that the patient manages without aspiration is selected as the starting point for feeding training. A patient aspirating on pureed or soft foods is not suited for an oral program. The patient who is aspirating thick liquids is not a candidate for liquid intake.

Videofluoroscopy is a valuable tool to be used in conjunction with the clinical examination. It can provide the therapist with additional information regarding the patient's difficulties. By identifying silent aspirators, the therapist can feel comfortable with the decisions made in determining a course of treatment. Because videofluoroscopy exposes the patient to radiation, the therapist should exercise good clinical judgment when deciding whether videofluoroscopy is needed. The therapist must keep in mind that videofluoroscopy records the patient's performance in an isolated instance and is not a conclusive indicator of the patient's potential ability in a feeding program. If a patient continues to progress without difficulty, a second videofluoroscopy is not necessary. A second videofluoroscopy may be needed, however, to reevaluate a patient who shows signs of readiness to participate in a feeding program or to determine whether a patient can progress to thin liquids.[13,31]

When the results of a videofluoroscopy test are documented, foods that were presented, problems that occurred at each stage, and the number of swallows taken to clear the food or liquid are recorded. The therapist also should document any facilitation techniques that worked effectively.[11,31,32] *This assessment procedure requires advanced training and should be done only by appropriately trained therapists.*

Assessment With Fiberoptic Endoscopy

Fiberoptic endoscopy (FEES) is an alternative technique used to assess swallowing. This technique is valuable when it is not possible for the patient to participate in videofluoroscopy or when it is used as a follow-up assessment for the patient making rapid progress. It can be repeated as often as necessary without exposure to radiation.[28,29,37]

The equipment needed for a FEES includes a flexible fiberoptic nasopharyngolaryngoscope, a portable light source, a video camera, a video recorder, and a television monitor. Placed on a rolling cart, this system can be brought directly to the patient. The therapist first topically anesthetizes one nasal fossa. After a brief amount of time the therapist passes a flexible fiberoptic tube through the nasal fossa, positioning the tip just above the palate.[28] The therapist initially examines the oral

cavity and swallowing structures. Food and liquids are then introduced as described previously. The therapist notes bolus formation, tongue movement, swallow, and aspiration, if it occurs. The FEES allows the therapist to see the pharynx and the larynx before and after the swallow, assessing for the possibility of aspiration.[29] *The evaluation procedure requires advanced training and should be performed only by appropriately trained therapists.*

The results of a thorough assessment determine the course of treatment to increase a patient's ability to eat. Upon completion of the entire dysphagia assessment, the therapist should clearly document the patient's major problems, treatment goals and objectives, and treatment plan. The objectives should be concise and measurable. The treatment plan should include the type of diet needed, the training and facilitation that the patient requires, positioning techniques to be used during feeding, and the type of supervision that must be provided. Treatment recommendations should be communicated to the appropriate nursing and medical staff.

TREATMENT

Because a patient may display more than one problem at each stage of deglutition, the intervention program for dysphagia is multifaceted. Treatment of the patient with dysphagia involves trunk and head positioning and control, hand-to-mouth skills, oral motor skills, and swallowing. Perceptual and cognitive deficits that interfere with eating are also addressed. To treat the patient the occupational therapist needs to devote 35% to 45% of the patient's total daily treatment time to oral motor and swallowing retraining.[22] A patient with severe problems can require up to 6 months of intense intervention before he or she reaches optimal recovery. In preparing a treatment plan for the patient with acquired dysphagia, the therapist must identify the symptoms and causes of the patient's deficits.[4,6,13,16,31,33]

Goals

The overall goals of OT in the treatment of dysphagia are as follows[2,3-5,13,17,31]:

1. Facilitation of appropriate positioning during eating
2. Improvement of motor control at each stage of swallow, through normalization of tone and the facilitation of quality movement
3. Maintenance of an adequate nutritional intake
4. Prevention of aspiration
5. Reestablishment of oral eating to the safest, optimum level

Team Management

Because of the complex nature of dysphagia treatment, the patient's optimal progress is facilitated by development of a team approach. The dysphagia team should consist of the patient's attending physician, the occupational therapist, the dietitian, the nurse, the physical therapist, the speech-language pathologist, the radiologist, and the patient's family. Each professional contributes expertise toward patient improvement. All members of the dysphagia team should have a thorough working knowledge of treating patients with dysphagia. Interdepartmental inservice education is frequently required so that team members have a similar frame of reference.

The occupational therapist's role is to assess the patient and implement the appropriate course of treatment. The occupational therapist is also responsible for coordinating the team effort, which includes obtaining physician's orders as needed, communicating with all other team members and staff, providing family education to ensure proper follow-through, and selecting the appropriate diet. The occupational therapist initiates changes in the patient's program whenever necessary.[4,6,13,39]

The attending physician's role involves the medical management of the patient's health and safety. The physician oversees all decisions regarding treatment for diet level selection, oral and nonoral feeding procedures, and the progression of treatment as recommended by the team. The physician should reinforce the course of treatment with the patient and the family.[19,22,31,39]

The dietitian is responsible for monitoring the patient's caloric intake. He or she makes recommendations to ensure that the patient receives a balanced, nutritional diet in accordance with the medical condition. The dietitian is involved in suggesting types of feeding formulas for the nonoral patient. Diet supplements to augment oral intake may be recommended. In conjunction with the occupational therapist, the dietitian ensures that the proper food and liquid consistencies are served to the patient. Additional training may be necessary for the dietary staff because dysphagia diets vary from traditional medical diets.

The patient's physical therapist is involved in muscle reeducation and tone normalization techniques of the trunk, neck, and face. The patient receives treatment in balance, strength, and control. The physical therapist is involved in increasing the patient's pulmonary status for breath support, chest expansion, and cough.[1]

The role of the speech-language pathologist involves the reeducation of the oral and laryngeal musculature used in speaking and voice production. Because these muscles are also used in swallowing, a therapist with dysphagia experience may participate in oral motor and swallowing training during prefeeding and feeding sessions.[22]

The nurse is another key member of the dysphagia team. The nursing staff is responsible for monitoring the patient's medical and nutritional status. The nurse usually is the first to notice changes in the patient's condition, such as an elevated temperature, an increase in pulmonary congestion, and an increase in secretions indicating swallowing dysfunction.[19] The nurse informs the physician and occupational therapist of these changes. The patient's oral and fluid intake is recorded in the nursing notes, and the nurse notifies the dysphagia team when the patient's nutritional status is adequate or inadequate. Supplemental tube feedings that have been ordered by the physician are administered by the nursing staff, which also provides oral hygiene, tracheostomy care, and supervision for appropriate patients during meals.[1,11,19,31]

The patient's family is included on the team to act as program supporters. The family frequently underestimates the danger of aspiration. Therefore it is important to educate the family and the patient from the first day of assessment. The family and patient should understand which food consistencies are safe to eat and which foods must be avoided.[2,37]

The roles of the various team members may vary from one treatment facility to another. Designated roles must be clearly defined to ensure a coordinated team approach. Therapists who are responsible for direct treatment should have advanced knowledge and training in the treatment procedures.

Positioning

Proper positioning is essential for treating the patient with dysphagia. The patient should be positioned symmetrically with normal alignment between the head, neck, trunk, and pelvis. The ideal position is as follows[3,5,6,8,16]:

1. The patient is seated on a firm surface, such as a chair.
2. The patient's feet are flat on the floor.
3. The patient's knees are at 90° flexion.
4. There is equal weight bearing on both ischial tuberosities of the hips.
5. The patient's trunk is flexed slightly forward (100° hip flexion) with the back straight.
6. Both of the patient's arms are placed forward on the table.
7. The head is erect, in midline, and the chin is slightly tucked.

For the patient who may be bed bound, the same principles apply: equal weight bearing on both ischial tuberosities for the hips, the trunk flexed slightly forward (100° hip flexion) with the back straight, knees slightly flexed, and both arms placed forward on a bedside table.

Fig. 40-6 shows two hand-hold techniques that allow the therapist to help the patient maintain head control. Correct positioning normalizes tone, thereby facilitating quality motor control and function of the facial musculature, jaw and tongue movement, and the swal-

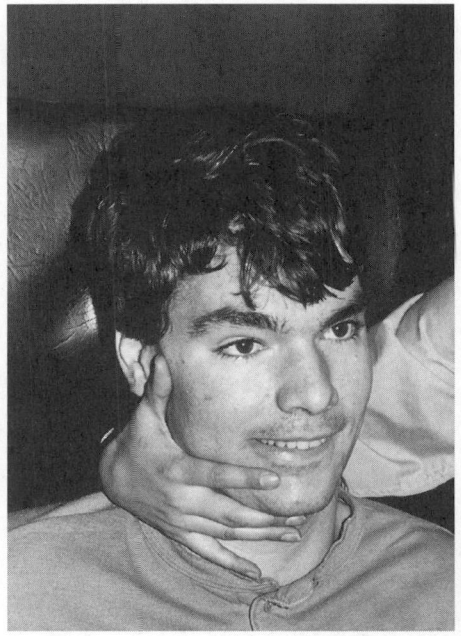
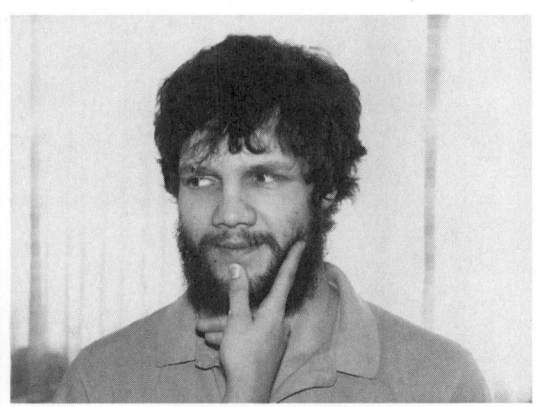

A   **B**

FIG. 40-6
Head control. **A,** Side hold position for patients requiring maximum to moderate assistance. **B,** Front hold position for patients requiring minimal assistance. (From Meadowbrook Neurological Care Center, San Jose, Calif, 1988.)

lowing process, all of which minimize the potential for aspiration.

A patient who has difficulty moving into the correct position or maintaining the position presents a challenge to the occupational therapist. A more careful analysis of the patient is needed to determine the major problem preventing good positioning. Poor positioning may be a result of decreased control or balance secondary to hypertonicity or hypotonicity or poor body awareness in space secondary to perceptual dysfunction (Fig. 40-7).[3,8,13,16] After the cause is identified, the therapist can treat it accordingly. Specific treatment suggestions are described later in this chapter. To assist in maintaining trunk position, the therapist may consider the use of an adaptive lateral trunk support. Seating the patient at a table provides forward trunk support.

Oral Hygiene

Oral care by nursing and therapy team members prevents gum disease, the accumulation of secretions, the development of plaque, and the aspiration of food particles that remain after eating. The appropriate therapy team member begins the oral hygiene process by positioning the patient upright and symmetrically. The patient who is apprehensive or who displays a hypersensitive oral cavity may first require preparation by the therapist. Preparation steps may include firmly stroking outside the patient's mouth or lips with the patient's or therapist's finger. Sensitive gums can also be firmly rubbed, preparing the patient for the toothbrush.

For cleaning purposes, the mouth can be divided into four quadrants. A toothbrush with a small head and soft bristles is used to clean each quadrant, starting with the top teeth and moving from front to back. When brushing the bottom teeth, the therapist brushes from back to front. Next, holding the toothbrush at a vertical angle, the therapist brushes the inside teeth downward from gums to teeth. Finally, the cutting surfaces of the teeth are brushed. An electric toothbrush can be more effective, if the patient can tolerate it.

After each procedure the patient is allowed to dispose of secretions. After brushing, the patient is carefully assisted in rinsing the mouth. If the patient can tolerate thin liquids, small amounts of water can be given. Having the patient flex the chin slightly toward the chest helps prevent the water from being swallowed. The therapist can help the patient expel the water, by placing one hand on each cheek and, simultaneously, pushing inward on the cheeks while the chin remains slightly tucked. If the patient has no ability to manipulate liquids, a dampened sponge toothette can be used. The therapist and nursing staff also can consider using small amounts of baking soda instead of toothpaste because it is easier to rinse out.[13,16]

Oral hygiene for the nonoral or oral patient can be used as effective sensory stimulation of touch, texture, temperature, and taste. It can be used to facilitate

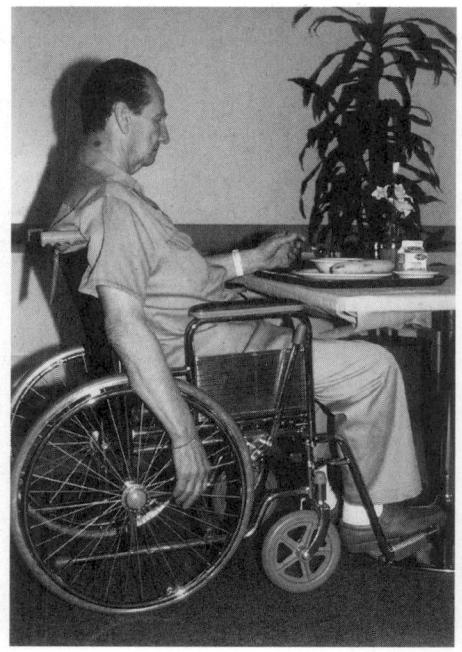
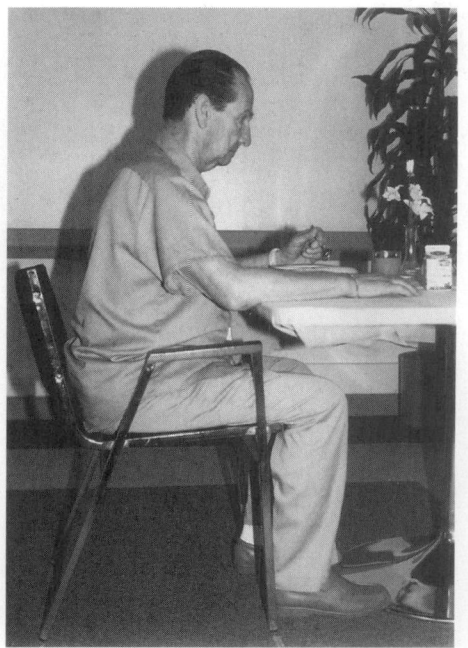

A   B

FIG. 40-7
Positioning of the patient with dysphagia. **A,** Incorrect positioning. **B,** Correct positioning. (From Meadowbrook Neurological Care Center, San Jose, Calif, 1988.)

beginning jaw and tongue movements and to encourage an automatic swallow.[14] Lack of oral stimulation over a prolonged time leads to hypersensitivity within the oral cavity. Patients who display poor tongue movement and who are eating, frequently have food remaining on their teeth or dentures or between the cheek and gum. A patient with decreased sensation is not aware of the remaining food. A thorough cleaning should follow each time the patient eats.

Nonoral Feedings

A patient who is aspirating more than 10% of food or liquid consistencies or whose combined oral and pharyngeal transit time is more than 10 seconds, regardless of positioning or facilitation techniques, is an inappropriate candidate for oral eating.[14,31] Such a patient needs a nonoral nutritional method until eating and drinking capability is regained. Patients who lack the endurance to take in sufficient calories also may require nonoral feedings or supplements.

The two most common procedures for nonoral feedings involve the NG tube and the G tube.[18,19] The NG tube is passed through the nostril, through the nasopharynx, and down through the pharynx and esophagus to rest in the stomach.[19] The NG tube is a temporary measure that should not be used for longer than 1 month.[31] There are several advantages to using the NG tube:

1. The NG tube can be inserted and removed nonsurgically, if necessary.
2. The NG tube allows the physician to choose between continuous or bolus feedings (a feeding that runs no more than 40 minutes).
3. The NG tube allows the therapist to begin prefeeding and feeding training while the tube is in place.

There are also some disadvantages of the NG tube[19,21,31]:

1. It can desensitize the swallow response.
2. It can interfere with a positioning program (the patient needs to be elevated to 30° during feeding).
3. It can increase aspiration risk, pharyngeal secretions, and nasal reflux.
4. It can decrease the patient's self-esteem.

Placement of a G tube is a minor surgical procedure. The patient receives a local anesthetic, and a small skin incision is made to create an external opening in the abdominal wall for a percutaneous endoscopic gastrostomy (PEG) procedure. A tube is passed through the opening into the stomach. There are several advantages of using a G tube:

1. Using a G tube allows the physician to choose between continuous or bolus feedings.
2. It allows the therapist to begin a prefeeding or feeding program while the tube is in place.
3. It carries less risk of reflux and aspiration.
4. It does not irritate or desensitize the swallowing mechanisms.

5. It does not interfere with a positioning program.
6. It can be removed when the patient no longer requires supplemental feedings or liquids.

There are some disadvantages of using a G tube[19,21,42]:
1. The stoma site can become irritated or inflamed.
2. The family can perceive the tube as being permanent.

A G tube is the ideal choice for the patient who may require tube feeding or supplemental feedings for longer than 1 month.[14,31]

A commercially prepared liquid formula that provides complete nutrition usually is used for tube feedings. Many types and brands are available. The physician and dietitian determine which formula is best suited to the patient. The feedings are administered by either a bolus or a continuous method. A bolus feeding takes 20 to 40 minutes to run through either the NG tube or the G tube. It can be gravity assisted or run through a feeding pump. Bolus feedings can be scheduled at numerous times throughout a 24-hour period.

Continuous feedings, which may be better tolerated by the patient, are smaller amounts that are administered continuously by a feeding pump. The feeding pump can be set to regulate the rate at which the formula is dripped into the tube. A disadvantage of continuous feedings is that the patient is less mobile because the pump always accompanies the patient.

While the patient is on a nonoral program, the occupational therapist concentrates efforts on retraining the patient in oral motor control and swallowing. The prefeeding retraining can occur whether the patient is on bolus or on continuous feedings. As a patient begins to eat enough to require an adjustment in the intake amount of formula, however, bolus feedings become the preferred method. A bolus feeding allows the therapist to work with the physician to wean the patient from formula feeding. A bolus feeding can be held back before a feeding session, and the number of bolus feedings per day can be decreased as the patient improves. If satisfied by the tube feedings, the patient will not have an appetite and will have decreased motivation to eat.

As the patient improves, oral intake can be increased, and the formula feeding can be used to supplement the patient's caloric intake. An accurate calorie count, determined by recording the percentage of oral intake, assists the physician in decreasing the calories received through the tube feedings as the patient begins to meet nutritional needs orally. If the patient has progressed only enough to handle solids, the NG or G tube can be used to meet the patient's total or partial fluid requirements. Either tube can be removed when the patient is safely able to eat and drink enough to meet caloric and fluid needs.[1,11,31]

Oral Feedings

For a patient to be an appropriate candidate for oral feeding, several criteria must be met. The therapist can use the criteria for evaluating a patient's swallow with foods or liquids. To participate in an oral feeding program, a patient must (1) be alert, (2) be able to maintain adequate trunk and head positioning with assistance, (3) have beginning tongue control, (4) manage secretions with minimal drooling, and (5) have a reflexive cough. The therapist needs to identify the food or liquid consistency that is most appropriate for the patient. The safest consistency with which to initiate the oral program is one that enables the patient to complete the oral and pharyngeal stages combined in less than 10 seconds and to swallow with minimal aspiration (10% or less).[31] The ultimate goal of an oral feeding program is for the patient to achieve swallowing without any aspiration.

Diet Selection

A dysphagia diet must be carefully selected to reflect the needs of the patient. In general, foods chosen for dysphagia diets should (1) be uniform in consistency and texture, (2) provide sufficient density and volume, (3) remain cohesive, (4) provide pleasant taste and temperature, and (5) be easily removed or suctioned when necessary.[13,14,19] The following foods are contraindicated for dysphagia diets: foods with multiple textures, such as vegetable soup and salads; fibrous and stringy vegetables, meats, and fruits; crumbly and flaky foods; foods that liquefy, such as gelatin and ice cream; and foods with skins and seeds.[11] Garnishes such as lettuce, parsley, and orange wedges should also be avoided because they may be unsafe for the confused patient.

The occupational therapist should work closely with the dietitian to develop dysphagia diet levels. Using specific dysphagia diets facilitates ordering appropriate foods consistently. Once the diets are developed, the medical, nursing, and therapy staff should be educated about which foods are in each level, to ensure the patient's safety. Liquid diet levels should also be established. When requesting a dysphagia diet, the therapist should specify both levels desired, liquid and solid, because a patient may handle each differently.

Diet Progression

Tables 40-5 through 40-7 list foods in three progressive dysphagia stages.[1,11,14,37] After mastering stage III, or ground food items, the patient may progress to a regular diet. Stage I foods are pureed. This food group is best for patients with little or no jaw or tongue control, a moderately delayed swallow, and a decreased pharyngeal transit, resulting in pooling in the valleculae and pyriform sinuses.[13,31] Pureed foods move more slowly past

TABLE 40-5

Dysphagia, Stage I Food Level (Pureed)

Food Groups	Foods Allowed	Foods to Avoid
Cereals and breads	Cooked refined cereals; creamed wheat or rice; Malt-o-Meal	All others
Eggs	Custard; pureed egg salad (without onions or celery)	All others
Fruits	Pureed fruit; applesauce	Whole fruits; juicy fruits; all others
Potatoes or substitutes	Mashed (white or sweet) potatoes mixed with thick gravy	All others
Vegetables	Pureed asparagus; beets; carrots; green beans; peas; spinach; squash	All others
Soups	Thickened, strained cream soups, with consistency of a pureed vegetable	All others
Meat, fish, poultry, cheese	Pureed meat; pureed poultry with gravy	All others
Fats	Butter; margarine; cream mixed with pureed foods	All others
Desserts	Plain puddings; smooth yogurt without fruit; custard	Any with nuts, coconut, seeds; all others
Sugars and sweets	Honey; sugar; syrup; jelly mixed in with pureed food	All others

From American Occupational Therapy Association: *AOTA resource guide: feeding and dysphagia,* Rockville, Md, 1997; Avery-Smith W: An occupational therapist co-ordinated dysphagia program, *Occup Ther Pract* 3:10, 1998; Community Hospital of Los Gatos, Rehabilitation Services: *Dysphagia protocol,* Los Gatos, Calif, 1999; Curran J: Nutritional consideration. In Groher M, editor: *Dysphagia: diagnosis and management,* ed 3, Newton, Mass, 1997, Butterworth-Heinemann; Rader T, Rende B: *Swallowing disorders: what families should know,* Tucson, Ariz, 1993, Communication Skill Builders.

the faucial arches and into the pharynx, allowing time for the swallow response to trigger. Because pureed foods cannot be formed into an adequate bolus, they offer little opportunity for increasing oral motor control.[13] Stage I foods are best used only to increase the patient's oral intake. The patient should be advanced to the next level as soon as possible.

Stage II items are soft foods that stay together as a cohesive bolus; thus the possibility of particles spilling into the airway is decreased. Stage II foods are best for patients with a beginning rotary chew, enough tongue control with assistance to propel food back toward the pharynx, and a minimally delayed swallow.[13,14] Mechanical soft foods reduce the risk of aspiration in patients who have both a motor and a sensory loss affecting the start of the swallow response.[5,20,40] Mechanical soft foods with a density provide increased proprioceptive input throughout the mouth. These foods also stay together as a cohesive bolus rather than crumbling and falling uncontrolled into the airway. Because patients who are at this diet stage display improved tongue control, the swallow response may be triggered faster as the back of the tongue elevates toward the hard palate. For the patient who is just beginning to chew, mashing the food with a fork enhances the patient's ability to keep the food together as a bolus.[13]

Stage III, chopped ground food items, requires chewing, controlled bolus formation, and a fair or delayed swallow. This food group offers a wider variety of consistencies. Meats should be finely cut to facilitate a controlled swallow. Smaller particles are less likely to obstruct the airway and are less of a health risk than large pieces, if minimal aspiration occurs. These foods are safer than items found on a regular diet, yet require work on the part of the patient. Stage III foods work well for the patient who has minimal problems with jaw or tongue control and a mildly delayed but intact swallow response. The patient who has reached a stage III level needs to be concerned with a delayed swallow only when fatigued.

When a patient is ready to progress to the next diet level, the therapist can adjust the meals by requesting one or two items from the higher group, enabling assessment at the new level. This technique is also appropriate for patients who become fatigued. The patient is thus able to work with the therapist on the harder food item first and continue the meal with foods that are easier. The therapist also may consider arranging several small meals throughout the day for the patient who fatigues, rather than three traditional meals.

A patient should progress to a regular diet when oral motor control is within functional limits, allowing the patient to chew and form any consistency into a bolus and propel it back toward the faucial arches. The patient at this level should be able to swallow any food or liquid consistency with only occasional coughing. Continuing dietary precautions for a patient with a history

TABLE 40-6
Dysphagia, Stage II Food Level (Mechanical Soft)

Food Groups	Foods Allowed	Foods to Avoid
Cereals and breads	Cooked refined cereals; creamed wheat or rice; Malt-o-Meal; oatmeal; white, wheat, or rye bread (without crust or seeds); graham crackers; soft French toast without crust	Hard rolls; bread with nuts, seeds, coconut, and fruit; bread with cracked wheat particles; sweet rolls; waffles; Melba toast; English muffins; popcorn; cereals such as Rice Krispies, corn flakes, puffed rice
Eggs	Custard; boiled, poached, and scrambled eggs; minced egg salad (without onions or celery)	All others
Fruits	Pureed fruit; applesauce; ripe banana and avocado; soft, canned and cooked fruits such as peaches, pears, apricots, pitted plums, stewed prunes, grapefruit, and orange sections (no membrane),* baked apple (no skin), cranberry sauce	Fruits with seeds, coarse skins, and fibers; fruits with pits; all raw fruit except those listed as allowed; raisins; grapes; fruit cocktail
Potatoes or substitute	Mashed potatoes (white or sweet); baked potatoes (no skin); soft noodles, spaghetti, and macaroni, finely chopped	Fried potatoes; potato or corn chips; rice
Vegetables	Cooked or canned artichoke hearts, asparagus tips, beets, carrots, mushrooms, squash, pumpkin, green beans, tomato puree and paste (no skins or seeds)	All other raw, stringy, fried, and dried vegetables; pickles
Soups	Thickened, strained, cream soups made with pureed allowed vegetables	All others
Meat, fish, poultry, cheese	Finely ground meat; poultry; tuna (without celery or onions); soft casseroles; soft sandwiches (without crust); cream or cottage cheese; American cheese	Fish (because of bones); meat, any consistency other than finely ground; bacon; all other cheeses
Fats	Butter; margarine; cream; mayonnaise mixed with food; thick gravy; thick cream sauce	Nuts; olives; all other
Desserts	Plain puddings; custard; tapioca; fruit whip; smooth yogurt; soft cake; cream pie with graham cracker crust	Cookies; cake with nuts, seeds, raisins, dates, coconuts, and fruits not on allowed list; all others
Sugars and sweets	Honey; sugar; syrup; jelly; plain, soft milk chocolate bars	Marmalade; coconut; all others

From American Occupational Therapy Association: *AOTA resource guide: feeding and dysphagia,* Rockville, Md, 1997, The Association; Avery-Smith W: *Occup Ther Pract* 3:10, 1998; Community Hospital of Los Gatos, Rehabilitation Services, *Dysphagia protocol,* Los Gatos, Calif, 1999; Rader T, Rende B: *Swallowing disorders: what families should know,* Tucson, Ariz, 1993, Communication Skill Builders Publishers.
*Allowed only if thin liquids are appropriate.

of dysphagia include avoiding raw vegetables, stringy foods, and foods containing nuts or seeds.[1,11,14]

Because a patient may exhibit a difference in ability to manage different liquids, a progression of liquid levels, separate from the solid levels, should be developed. The liquid progression is divided into three groups: thick, semithick, and thin liquids.[1,11,14] Examples of liquids in these levels are given in Table 40-8.

Thick liquids are made by adding such thickening agents as banana, pureed fruit, yogurt, dissolved gelatin, baby cereal, cornstarch, or a commercial thickener to achieve an added "honeylike" viscosity. A dietitian can provide the occupational therapist with specific recipes. These substances are usually added to the liquids and power-blended for smoothness. The thick drink or soup should stay blended and not be allowed to separate or liquefy. Thick liquids are the appropriate choice for patients with markedly delayed swallow. A thick liquid moves more slowly through the faucial arches, giving some time for the swallow response to be triggered. Semithick liquids such as fruit nectars, buttermilk, tomato juice, and yogurt drinks, which have a natural

TABLE 40-7
Dysphagia, Stage III Food Level (Chopped or Ground)

Food Groups	Foods Allowed	Foods to Avoid
Cereals and breads	Cooked cereals, ready-to-eat cereals* such as Rice Krispies, corn flakes, puffed rice; pancakes, French toast, white, wheat, and rye bread (with crust), salt crackers, soda and graham crackers; sweet rolls, English muffins, Melba toast, donuts	Hard rolls, bread with nuts, seeds, coconut, and fruit, coarse cereals such as granola, Grapenuts; popcorn
Eggs	Soft- and hard-boiled, poached, fried, scrambled eggs; egg salad (without onions and celery)	All others
Fruits	Banana, avocado; soft, canned, and cooked fruit, ripe fruit	Fruits with seeds, coarse skins and fibers, pits; fruit cocktail
Potatoes or substitute	Mashed potatoes (white or sweet), creamed potatoes, baked potatoes (without skin), noodles, spaghetti, and macaroni	Fried potatoes, potato and corn chips, rice without gravy
Vegetables	Cooked and canned vegetables (without skins, seeds, and stringy fibers), drained	All raw, stringy, fried, and dried vegetables
Soups	Thickened, creamed soups made with pureed or whole allowed vegetables only*	All others
Meat, fish, poultry, cheese	Finely diced or minced meat, poultry, tuna (without onions or celery), flaked fish, fish sticks; soft casseroles, sandwiches, and cheeses	Bacon; fish with bones; poultry with skin
Fats	Butter, margarine, cream, mayonnaise, gravy, cream sauces	Nuts; all others
Desserts	Soft cookies, cakes, pies, puddings, custard, yogurt	Cookies, cake with nuts, seeds, coconuts, and fruits not on allowed list; hard pies, crusts, and pastries; all others
Sugars and sweets	Honey, sugar, syrup, jelly; plain soft milk chocolate bars	Marmalade, coconut; all others

From American Occupational Therapy Association: *AOTA resource guide: feeding and dysphagia,* Rockville, Md, 1997; Avery-Smith W: An occupational therapist co-ordinated dysphagia program, *Occup Ther Pract* 3:10, 1998; Community Hospital of Los Gatos, Rehabilitation Services: *Dysphagia protocol,* Los Gatos, Calif, 1999; Curran J: Nutritional considerations. In Groher M, editor: *Dysphagia: diagnosis and management,* ed 3, Newton, Mass, 1997, Butterworth-Heinemann Publishers; Rader T, Rende B: *Swallowing disorders: what families should know,* Tucson, Ariz, 1993, Communication Skill Builders Publishers.
*Allowed only if thin liquids are appropriate.

TABLE 40-8
Liquids

Thin Liquids	Semithick Liquids	Thick Liquids
Water	Extrathick milkshake	Nectar thickened with banana
Coffee, tea	Extrathick eggnog	Nectar with pureed fruit
Decaffeinated coffee	Strained creamed soup	Regular applesauce with juice
Milk	Tomato juice, V-8 juice	Eggnog with baby cereal
Hot chocolate	Plain nectars	Creamed soup thickened with mashed potatoes
All fruit juices	Yogurt and milk blended	Commercial thickener
Broth or consomme		
Gelatin dessert		
Ice cream		
Sherbert		

From American Occupational Therapy Association: *AOTA resource guide: feeding and dysphagia,* Rockville, Md, 1997; Avery-Smith W: An occupational therapist co-ordinated dysphagia program, *Occup Ther Pract* 3:10, 1998; Community Hospital of Los Gatos, Rehabilitation Services: *Dysphagia protocol,* Los Gatos, Calif, 1999; Curran J: Nutritional considerations. In Groher M, editor: *Dysphagia: diagnosis and management,* ed 3, Newton, Mass, 1997, Butterworth-Heinemann Publishers; Rader T, Rende B: *Swallowing disorders: what families should know,* Tucson, Ariz, 1993, Communication Skill Builders Publishers.

medium viscosity, are used with patients who have a moderate swallow delay of 3 to 5 seconds.[13,24,31] Thin or low-viscosity liquids, the highest liquid level, require intact swallowing ability.

Principles of Oral Feeding

The therapist should incorporate certain principles into the oral feeding program. First, an important aspect of the oral preparation stage is looking at and reaching for food. The patient must actively participate in the eating process. Food should be presented within the patient's visual field. If the patient has a severe visual field deficit or unilateral neglect, the therapist needs to assist the patient to scan the plate or tray visually.

When physically possible the patient should be allowed self-feeding. If the patient does not have a normal hand-to-mouth movement pattern, the therapist must help the patient achieve one by guiding the extremity in the correct pattern. Abnormal movement of the upper extremity facilitates abnormal movement in the trunk, head, face, tongue, and pharynx and decreases the patient's functioning.

If the patient is not capable of self-feeding, the therapist can keep the patient actively involved by allowing the patient to choose which food or liquid is preferred for each bite. Food is presented by moving the utensil slowly from the front, toward the mouth, so that the patient can see the food the entire time. The utensil should not be brought in from the side because the patient will have less preparation time. The patient should be allowed as much control of the situation as possible.

The patient should eat in a normal setting, if possible. For adults, eating is a social activity shared with friends and family. The patient can be redirected if distracted and can use environmental cueing when eating in a dining room with others. Adjustments, such as eating in the dining room but at a separate table, can be made to facilitate patient concentration. The therapist must be conscious of how the patient appears to others, and help the patient to eat in a normal manner.

The occupational therapist must continually assess the patient's positioning, upper extremity movement, muscle tone, oral control, and swallow. The therapist helps the patient perform the task correctly and does not allow eating while the patient exhibits an abnormal pattern. If the patient displays poor oral motor skills, the therapist looks for food pocketing after every few bites. The rate of the patient's intake is monitored. The therapist should determine when too much food is in the mouth and when the patient puts food into the mouth before the previous bite has been cleared. The therapist feels for the swallow with a finger at the hyoid notch if the patient displays abnormal laryngeal tone or a delayed swallow.[13,31] The therapist also as-sesses the patient's voice quality upon completion of the swallow.

The frequency with which the therapist must check each component depends on the skill level and performance of the patient. The more difficulty the patient exhibits, the more frequent the assessment. The therapist may find it necessary to assess after each bite or sip, after a few bites or sips, or after each food item. Use of good observational skills allows the therapist to make the appropriate clinical decision. Specific techniques for assessment during feeding trials can be found in the swallowing assessment section of this chapter. After completing the feeding process, the patient should remain in an upright position for 15 to 30 minutes to reduce the risk of refluxing food and of aspirating small food particles that may remain in the throat.[1,5,11]

The therapist also must continue to monitor the patient for signs of aspiration while eating and for the development of aspiration pneumonia over time. Although a conservative estimate of aspiration is 10% of material swallowed, measurement is difficult while a patient eats. Patients vary in the amount of aspiration they can tolerate before developing aspiration pneumonia, according to age, health, and pulmonary status. The signs of acute and chronic aspiration were outlined previously.

When a patient is participating in oral feedings, careful monitoring of the nutritional status is necessary. The patient's caloric needs are determined by the dietitian and the physician and depend on the patient's height, weight, activity level, and medical condition.[14,31] Fluid intake is monitored by having the physician order a calorie count and a liquid intake and output hydration count (I and O).[11] Each person who supervises or works with the patient should record, in percentages, the caloric amount of each item the patient eats or drinks. The dietitian converts the percentages into a daily calorie total. The patient also should be monitored for physical signs of nutritional deficiency and dehydration. These symptoms are weakness, irritability, decreased alertness, changes in eating habits, hunger, thirst, decreased turgor, and changes in amounts or color of urine.[14,21,39] If a patient is not able to take in the necessary calories (50% of the determined total), supplemental feedings are necessary to make up the difference.[11] The physician and dietician decide on the number of supplemental feedings.

Techniques for the Management of Dysphagia

Tables 40-9 through 40-12 provide treatment techniques for the management of dysphagia. These techniques are not intended to be used in all situations. Each patient

TABLE 40-9
Dysphagic Treatment: Oral Preparatory Stage

Structure	Symptoms	Problem	Prefeeding Technique	Feeding Technique
Trunk	Leaning to one side	Decreased trunk tone Ataxia Increased trunk tone Poor body awareness in space	Facilitate trunk strength Exercises at midline Have patient clasp hands, lean down, and touch foot, middle, other foot; rotate trunk with hands clasped and shoulders flexed to decrease or normalize tone	Assist patient to hold correct position; assist with head control Assist patient to hold correct feeding position; provide with perceptual boundary; consider lateral trunk support
	Hips sliding forward out of chair	Increased tone in hip extensors Poor body awareness in space	See previous entry above Provide firm seating service	Adjust positioning so that patient leans slightly forward at hips, arms forward on table
Head	Inability to hold head in midline	Decreased tone Weakness	Facilitate strength through neck and head exercises in flexion, extension, and lateral flexion	Assist with head control
	Inability to move head	Increased tone Poor range of motion	Tone reduction of head, shoulders, and trunk Facilitate normal movement Myofascial release techniques Soft tissue mobilization	Assist with head control
Upper extremity	Spillage of food from utensils	Decreased tone Apraxia Decreased coordination	Facilitate increased tone through weight bearing, sweeping, or tapping muscle belly of desired muscle	Guide patient through correct movement pattern Provide adaptive equipment or utensils as needed
	Inability to self-feed	Increased tone Abnormal movement patterns Weakness or decreased motor control	Reduce proximal tone with scapula mobilization, weight bearing through arm Strengthening exercises Facilitation of normal movement	Guide patient through correct movement pattern Provide adaptive equipment or utensils as needed
Face	Drooling, food spillage from mouth	Decreased lip control Poor lip closure secondary to decreased tone, poor sensation Apraxia	Place a wet tongue blade between patient's lips; ask patient to hold tongue blade while therapist tries to pull it out Vibrate lips with back of electric toothbrush down cheek and across lips Lip exercises: movements described in outer oral motor evaluation; patient performs repetitions 2-3 times daily Blow bubbles into glass of liquid with straw	Using side handgrip for head control, the therapist approximates lip closure by guiding and assisting with jaw closure Have patient use a straw when drinking liquids until control improves Place food to unimpaired side Use cold food or liquids

From American Occupational Therapy Association: *Am J Occup Ther,* 1996; Avery-Smith W: Management of neurologic disorders: the first feeding session. In Groher M, editor: *Dysphagia: diagnosis and management,* ed 3, Newton, Mass, 1997, Butterworth-Heinemann Publishers; Bobath B: *Adult hemiplegia: evaluation and treatment,* ed 2, London, 1978, William Heinemann Medical Books; Community Hospital of Los Gatos, Rehabilitation Services: *Dysphagia protocol,* Los Gatos, Calif, 1999; Coombes K: *Swallowing dysfunction in hemiplegia and head injury.* Course presented by International Clinical Educators, Aug 24-27, 1986, and Aug 24-28, 1987, Los Gatos, Calif; Davies P: *Steps to follow,* New York, 1985, Springer-Verlag; Farber S: *Neurorehabilitation: a multisensory approach,* Philadelphia, 1982, WB Saunders; Logemann J: *Manual for the videofluorographic study of swallowing,* ed 2, Austin, Tex, 1993, Pro-Ed Publishers.

TABLE 40-9—cont'd
Dysphagic Treatment: Oral Preparatory Stage

Structure	Symptoms	Problem	Prefeeding Technique	Feeding Technique
		Decreased sensation	Fan lips so that patient feels drool or wetness on lips or chin to increase awareness	Teach patient to pat mouth (versus wiping mouth) and chin every few bites or sips
Tongue	Pocketing of food in cheeks or sulci Poor bolus formation	Poor tongue control for lateralization or tipping Decreased tone Poor sensation	Tongue exercises: use movements described in inner oral motor evaluation	Avoid crumbly foods Stroke patient's outside cheek where pocketing occurs with index finger back and up toward patient's ear; instruct patient to check cheek for pocketing
	Retracted tongue	Increased tone Retracted jaw	Tongue range of motion: wrap tip of tongue in wet gauze; gently pull tongue forward, side to side and up and down; move slowly Pull tongue wrapped in wet gauze forward past front teeth, using index and middle finger to vibrate tongue back and forth sideways to decrease tone and facilitate protrusion	Avoid crumbly foods Reduce tone as needed during meal Double swallow Resist head flexion to facilitate jaw closure Resist head extension to facilitate jaw opening

From American Occupational Therapy Association: *Am J Occup Ther,* 1996; Avery-Smith W: Management of neurologic disorders: the first feeding session. In Groher M, editor: *Dysphagia: diagnosis and management,* ed 3, Newton, Mass, 1997, Butterworth-Heinemann Publishers; Bobath B: *Adult hemiplegia: evaluation and treatment,* ed 2, London, 1978, William Heinemann Medical Books; Community Hospital of Los Gatos, Rehabilitation Services: *Dysphagia protocol,* Los Gatos, Calif, 1999; Coombes K: *Swallowing dysfunction in hemiplegia and head injury.* Course presented by International Clinical Educators, Aug 24-27, 1986, and Aug 24-28, 1987, Los Gatos, Calif; Davies P: *Steps to follow,* New York, 1985, Springer-Verlag; Farber S: *Neurorehabilitation. a multisensory approach,* Philadelphia, 1982, WB Saunders; Logemann J: *Manual for the videofluorographic study of swallowing,* ed 2, Austin, Tex, 1993, Pro-Ed Publishers.

presents a different clinical picture and may display one deficit or a combination of deficits. After careful assessment the therapist must determine the primary cause of the patient's deficits, and treat accordingly. The patient must be assessed and treated as a whole person, rather than treated as a person with a single deficit.

Treating a patient with dysphagia requires a logical and consistent approach.[3,13] Abnormal tone, for example, should be normalized before the therapist can expect good motor control. Motor control must be improved before a patient can shape food into a cohesive bolus and achieve an effective swallow. Individualized prefeeding techniques can prepare the patient for eating. The therapist should strive toward facilitating the return of normal eating patterns in each patient.

Ongoing assessment of treatment by the therapist is essential. The therapist must continually assess the patient's response, which should reflect desired change. Therefore the therapist must develop good clinical observation skills.[4,13,31] The clinician needs to adapt treatment to performance and progress. For difficult patients the clinician should seek a consultation with an experienced dysphagia therapist. To develop expertise in dysphagia management, it is recommended that the therapist continue education in this area.

Text continued on p. 762

TABLE 40-10
Dysphagic Treatment: Oral Stage

Structure	Symptoms	Problem	Prefeeding Techniques	Feeding Technique
Tongue	Slow oral transit Tongue retraction	Poor anterior to posterior movement; decreased tone, poor sensation Increased tone	Practice "ng-ga" sounds Grasping tongue wrapped in gauze, pull it forward past front teeth; use finger or tongue blade to vibrate base of tongue back and forth sideways Improve tongue range of motion	Tuck chin toward chest Position food in center, midtongue Avoid crumbly foods Use cold or hot foods instead of warm Correct positioning Place index finger at base of tongue under chin; stroke up and forward
	Slow oral transit time Inability to channel food back toward pharynx	Inability to form central groove in tongue Apraxia	Grasping tongue wrapped in gauze, pull forward to front teeth; stroke firmly down middle of tongue with edge of tongue blade	Tuck chin toward chest Position food in center, midtongue Avoid crumbly foods Use cold or hot foods instead of warm Correct positioning Place index finger at base of tongue under chin; stroke up and forward
	Repetitive movement of tongue; food is pushed out front of mouth	Tongue thrust	Facilitate tongue retraction to bring tongue back into normal resting position; vibrate on either side of the frenulum found inside the mouth, under the tongue with finger Increase jaw control; teach isolated tongue movements	Correct positioning Place food away from midline of tongue toward back of mouth Provide downward and forward pressure to back of tongue with spoon after food placement
	Food falls off tongue into sulci or food remains on tongue without patient awareness	Poor sensation	Ice tongue with ice chips placed in gauze to prevent ice chips from slipping into pharynx Brush tongue with toothbrush to stimulate receptors	Use foods with high viscosity or density Alternate presentation of cold and hot foods during meal

From Community Hospital of Los Gatos, Rehabilitation Services: *Dysphagia protocol,* Los Gatos, Calif, 1999; Coombes K: *Swallowing dysfunction in hemiplegia and head injury.* Course presented by International Clinical Educators, Aug 24-27, 1986, and Aug 24-28, 1987, Los Gatos, Calif; Davies P: *Steps to follow,* New York, 1985, Springer-Verlag; Farber S: *Neurorehabilitation: a multisensory approach,* Philadelphia, 1982, WB Saunders; Logemann J: *Evaluation and Treatment of Swallowing Disorders,* ed 2, Austin, Tex, 1998, Pro-Ed Publishers; Martin BJW: Treatment of dysphagia in adults. In Cherney L, editor: *Clinical management of dysphagia in adults and children,* Gaithersburg, Md, 1994, Aspen Publishers; Silverman EH, Elfant IL: *Am J Occup Ther,* 1979.

TABLE 40-10—cont'd
Dysphagic Treatment: Oral Stage

Structure	Symptoms	Problem	Prefeeding Techniques	Feeding Technique
	Slow oral transit time; food remains on hard palate; coughing before swallow	Poor tongue elevation; decreased tone	Ask patient to practice "k," "g," "n," "d," and "t" sounds. Lightly touch tongue blade or soft toothbrush to roof of mouth at back of tongue, instruct patient to press spot with tongue; resist movement with blade or brush to increase strength. Vibrate tongue at base below chin; provide quick stretch by pushing down on base of tongue	Correct positioning. With finger under chin at base of tongue, move finger upward and forward to facilitate elevation. Avoid crumbly foods. Double swallow
	Slow oral transit time. Food remains on back of tongue as patient is unable to elevate tongue to push food to hard palate. Coughing before the swallow. Retracted tongue	Decreased sensation. Increased tone. Decreased range of motion. Soft tissue shortening	Tone reduction; grasping tongue with gauze wrapped around tip, pull tongue forward with finger or tongue blade. Apply pressure to base of tongue right to left. Grasping base of tongue under chin between two fingers, move it back and forth to decrease tone. Tone reduction. Range of motion exercises. Place a variety of tastes on lips to facilitate tongue-licking lips	Adjust correct positioning by increasing forward flexion at hips, arms forward to decrease tone. Reduce tone as needed; give patient breaks because tone increases with effort. With finger under chin at base of tongue, move finger upward and forward to facilitate tongue elevation

From Community Hospital of Los Gatos, Rehabilitation Services: *Dysphagia protocol,* Los Gatos, Calif, 1999; Coombes K: *Swallowing dysfunction in hemiplegia and head injury.* Course presented by International Clinical Educators, Aug 24-27, 1986, and Aug 24-28, 1987 Los Gatos, Calif; Davies P: *Steps to follow,* New York, 1985, Springer-Verlag; Farber S: *Neurorehabilitation: a multisensory approach,* Philadelphia, 1982, WB Saunders; Logemann J: *Evaluation and Treatment of Swallowing Disorders,* ed 2, Austin, Tex, 1998, Pro-Ed Publishers; Martin BJW: Treatment of dysphagia in adults. In Cherney L, editor: *Clinical management of dysphagia in adults and children,* Gaithersburg, Md, 1994, Aspen Publishers; Silverman EH, Elfant IL: *Am J Occup Ther,* 1979.

TABLE 40-11

Dysphagia Treatment: Pharyngeal Stage

Structure	Symptoms	Problem	Prefeeding Technique	Feeding Technique
Soft palate	Tight voice; nasal regurgitation Air felt through nose or mist seen on mirror when patient says "ah" Decreased tone Nasal speech	Increased tone Decreased tone Rigidity	Facilitate normal head/neck positioning Have patient tuck chin into therapist's cupped hand, then push into hand as therapist applies resistance; patient says, "ah" afterward; speed and height of uvula elevation should increase; follow by thermal application	Facilitate normal head and neck positioning With head and neck in midline, have patient tuck chin slightly to decrease rate of food entering into pharynx
	Delayed swallow	Decreased triggering of swallow response	Thermal application: using a laryngeal mirror #00 after being placed in ice water or chips for 10 seconds, touch base of faucial arch; repeat up to 10 times; process can be repeated several times a day	Alternate presentation of food; start very cold substance, then warm; cold substance can increase sensitivity of faucial arches; tuck chin slightly forward to prevent bolus entering airway
Hyoid	Delayed elevation of hyoid bone Poor tongue elevation	Delayed swallow Incomplete swallow	Increase tongue humping as elevation of tongue and hyoid stimulates triggering of response	Place index finger under chin at base of tongue and push up forward to facilitate tongue elevation
	Tongue retraction	Abnormal tongue tone; poor range of motion	Tone reduction	
Pharynx	Coughing after swallow	Decreased pharyngeal movement Penetration into laryngeal vestibule	None	If appropriate, alternate presentation of liquid with stage II or stage III solids; liquid material moves solids through pharynx
	Coating of pharynx seen on videofluoroscopy Gurgling voice	Pharyngeal weakness	Isometric or resistive head and neck exercises	Have patient take second dry swallow to clear valleculae and pyriform sinuses Tilt head to stronger side Supraglottic swallow

From Community Hospital of Los Gatos, Rehabilitation Services, *Dysphagia protocol,* Los Gatos, Calif, 1999; Coombes K: *Swallowing dysfunction in hemiplegia and head injury.* Course presented by International Clinical Educators, Aug 24-27, 1986, and Aug 24-28, 1987, Los Gatos, Calif; Davies P: *Steps to follow,* New York, 1985, Springer-Verlag; Kaatzke-McDonald M, Post E, Davis P: *Dysphagia,* 1996; Logemann J: *Evaluation and treatment of swallowing disorders,* Austin, Tex, 1998, Pro-Ed Publishers; Martin BJW: Treatment of dysphagia in adults. In Cherney L, editor: *Clinical management of dysphagia in adults and children,* Gaithersburg, Md, 1994, Aspen Publishers; Schulze-Delrieu K, Miller R: Clinical assessment of dysphagia. In Perlman A, Schulze-Delrieu, editors: *Deglutition and its disorders: anatomy, physiology, clinical diagnosis and management,* San Diego, Calif, 1997, Singular Publishing; Smith C, Logemann J, Colangelo L, et al: *Dysphagia* 14(1):1-7, 1999.

TABLE 40-11—cont'd

Dysphagia Treatment: Pharyngeal Stage

Structure	Symptoms	Problem	Prefeeding Technique	Feeding Technique
	Seen on videofluoroscopy, anteroposterior view; material residue seen on one side; weak or hoarse voice	Unilateral pharyngeal movement	None	Compensatory technique for patients with low tone: have patient turn head toward affected side during swallow to prevent pooling in affected pyriform sinuses; evaluate technique against its effect on patient positioning and tone in trunk, upper extremities
Larynx	Coughing, choking after swallow	Decreased laryngeal elevation Decreased tone Weakness	Quickly ice up sides of larynx; ask patient to swallow; assist movement by guiding larynx upward Vibrate laryngeal musculature from under chin, downward on each side to sternal notch	Teach patient to clear throat immediately after swallow to move residual Use supraglottic swallow, Mendelsohn maneuver, effortful swallow
	Noisy or audible swallow	Increased tone Rigidity Uncoordinated swallow	Range of motion—place fingers and thumb along both sides of larynx and gently move it back and forth until movement is smooth and easy, tone decreased Using chipped ice, form pack in washcloth and place around larynx for 5 min	Placing fingers and thumb along both sides of larynx, assist patient with upward elevation before swallow Double swallow
Trachea	Continuous coughing before, during, after swallow	Aspiration—before: poor tongue control; during: delayed swallow response; after: decreased pharyngeal movement	Teach patient how to produce a voluntary cough; ask patient to take a deep breath and cough while breathing out; therapist uses palm of hand to push downward (toward stomach) on the sternum	Encourage patient to keep coughing; facilitate reflexive cough; push downward on sternum as patient breathes out; suction patient if problem increases Push into patient's sternal notch to assist with cough
	Patient grabs or reaches for throat Reddening in the face No voice or cough	Blocked airway	None	Perform Heimlich maneuver Seek medical assistance

From Community Hospital of Los Gatos, Rehabilitation Services, *Dysphagia protocol,* Los Gatos, Calif, 1999; Coombes K: *Swallowing dysfunction in hemiplegia and head injury.* Course presented by International Clinical Educators, Aug 24-27, 1986, and Aug 24-28, 1987, Los Gatos, Calif; Davies P: *Steps to follow,* New York, 1985, Springer-Verlag; Kaatzke-McDonald M, Post E, Davis P: *Dysphagia,* 1996; Logemann J: *Evaluation and treatment of swallowing disorders,* Austin, Tex, 1998, Pro-Ed Publishers; Martin BJW: Treatment of dysphagia in adults. In Cherney L, editor: *Clinical management of dysphagia in adults and children,* Gaithersburg, Md, 1994, Aspen Publishers; Schulze-Delrieu K, Miller R: Clinical assessment of dysphagia. In Perlman A, Schulze-Delrieu, editors: *Deglutition and its disorders: anatomy, physiology, clinical diagnosis and management,* San Diego, Calif, 1997, Singular Publishing; Smith C, Logemann J, Colangelo L, et al: *Dysphagia* 14(1):1-7, 1999.

TABLE 40-12

Dysphagia Treatment: Esophageal Stage

Structure	Symptoms	Problem	Prefeeding Technique	Feeding Technique
Esophagus	Frequent regurgitation of food or liquid and coughing or choking after the swallow: material collecting in a side pocket in esophagus	Esophageal diverticulum	Requires a medical diagnosis; problem can be seen through traditional barium x-ray examination Surgical correction is needed	Report symptoms to medical staff (therapist cannot treat)
	Regurgitation of food, coughing, or choking on food after the swallow: inability of food to pass through the pharynx, esophagus, or stomach	Partial or total obstruction of the pharynx or esophagus Impaired esophageal peristalsis	Requires a medical diagnosis; problem can be seen through traditional barium x-ray examination Surgical correction is needed	Report symptoms to medical staff (therapist cannot treat)

From Coombes K: *Swallowing dysfunction in hemiplegia and head injury.* Course presented by International Clinical Educators, Aug 24-27, 1986, and Aug 24-28, 1987, Los Gatos, Calif; Davies P: *Steps to follow,* New York, 1985, Springer-Verlag; Logemann J: *Evaluation and treatment of swallowing disorders,* Austin, Tex, 1998, Pro-Ed Publishers; Smith C, Logemann J, Colangelo L, et al: *Dysphagia,* 1999; Martin B: Treatment of dysphagia in adults. In Cherney L, editor: *Clinical management of dysphagia in adults and children,* Gaithersburg, Md, 1994, Aspen. Workman J, Pillsbury H, Hulka G: Surgical interventions in dysphagia. In Groher M: *Dysphagia: diagnosis and management,* ed 3, Newton, Mass, 1977, Butterworth-Heinemann.

SUMMARY

Eating is the most basic activity of daily living. Several performance components are required for the patient to eat and swallow effectively. *Dysphagia* refers to difficulty with swallowing or an inability to swallow. The occupational therapist is trained to treat many of the problems that interfere with normal eating. An understanding of the normal anatomy of swallowing and special training are required to treat dysphagia.

Assessment of the patient with dysphagia includes testing of head and trunk control, sensation, perception, cognition, inner and outer oral structures, oral reflexes, and swallowing. Assessment may also include videofluoroscopy or fiberoptic endoscopy.

Several members of the rehabilitation team are involved in the treatment of the patient with dysphagia. Positioning, selection of appropriate feeding procedures, diet selection, diet progression, and special techniques to facilitate normal patterns of swallowing are part of the treatment program. The social and psychological aspects of eating are important considerations in the treatment program.

as vice president of a local marketing company. Mr. B. lives with his wife. He and his wife have two grown children living in the area. Before the onset of the CVA, Mr. B. was independent in all activities of daily living and instrumental activities of daily living. He was an active member of the community.

Results of the occupational therapy evaluation indicate that Mr. B. needs moderate to maximum assistance in dressing, toileting, bathing, eating and swallowing, and transfers.

The clinical assessment of eating indicates that the patient has a mild to moderate increase in jaw and facial tone with poor rotary chew, poor isolated tongue control, and mild increase in laryngeal tone with delayed swallow.

The videofluoroscopy confirmed that the patient had a mildly delayed swallow with minimal pooling in the valleculae and pyriform sinuses. Aspiration was less than 10% on pureed foods. The patient was seen three times a day for 6 weeks by occupational therapy. A summary of evaluation results and treatment plan are shown in Fig. 40-8.

The patient responded well to treatment. The G tube was removed after 5 weeks. The patient achieved all treatment goals by the time of discharge. He went home with family supervision for correct diet, positioning, and swallowing techniques during meals. The patient was referred to home health occupational therapy for 2 to 3 weeks for activities of daily living and home modification so that independence at home could be achieved. The patient returned for follow-up outpatient visits.

CASE STUDY 40-1

CASE STUDY: MR. B.

Mr. B. is a 65-year-old man who suffered a right cerebrovascular accident (CVA) with left hemiplegia 2 weeks ago. He has a G tube in place for nutrition. He recently retired from his position

Dysphagia Evaluation and Treatment Plan

Pt: _65 y. male_

Dx: _Ⓡ CVA_

Onset: _2 weeks ago_

Medical hx: _Elevated BP — 5 years. Elevated blood lipids. Otherwise unremarkable. Independent in ADL & IADL prior to onset._

Current nutritional status: _gastrostomy tube, NPO_

	WNL	Adequate— without assistance	Unable	Comments
Mental status:				
Alert/oriented		c̄ assist		oriented to name, max assist for date
Direction following		c̄ assist		appropriate c̄ guiding
Physical status (symmetry, control, tone):				
Head control		c̄ assist		slight ↑'d tone c̄ head turning
Trunk control		c̄ assist		ataxic, TLR present
Endurance		c̄ assist		fatigues after 30 min.
Respiratory				
Suctioning required	N/A			
Tracheostomy	N/A			
Outer oral status:				
Facial expressions		c̄ assist		flat affect 2° ↑'d tone to moderate degree
Jaw movement			✓	poor rotary chew, poor jaw glide, pt. uses up & down movt.
Lip movement		c̄ assist		unable to purse & retract, poor lip compression
Sensation		c̄ assist		delayed 2° ↓'d attention
Abnormal reflexes		c̄ assist		suck-swallow present, others absent
Inner oral status (symmetry, control, tone):				
Dentition	✓			good, slightly inflammed gums
Tongue				
Appearance		c̄ assist		slight white coating & mid Ⓡ tongue laceration
Tone		c̄ assist		↑'d c̄ retraction
Movement: Protrusion		c̄ assist		deviated to Ⓡ
Lateralization		c̄ assist		mild weakness
"ng" → "ga"			✓	poor anterior to posterior
Soft palate/gag reflex:	✓			uvula rises symmetrically
Cough (reflexive/voluntary):	✓			
Swallow:				
Spontaneous	✓			intact
Voluntary		c̄ assist		delayed 2° to tone
Laryngeal movement				
Tongue		c̄ assist		requires tone reduction
Elevation		c̄ assist		delayed fatigue factor after serial swallows
Food management:				
Puree		c̄ assist		Overall pt. shows ↓'d cognitive aware-ness of food in mouth & requires cueing pt. uses suck-swallow
Mechanical soft		c̄ assist		pocketing assist
Chopped/ground		c̄ assist		needed c̄ rotary chew
Regular diet			N/A	
Liquids: Thick		c̄ assist		c̄ straw, 5 sec. delay, ∅ cough
Semithick		c̄ assist		c̄ straw, 5 sec. delay, coughing
Thin			N/A	

FIG. 40-8

Case study: dysphagia evaluation and treatment plan.

Dysphagia Evaluation and Treatment Plan

Major problems:

① ↓'d cognition for attention and awareness of food in mouth s̄ cueing.

② ↑'d jaw & facial tone resulting in poor rotary chew.

③ Poor isolated tongue movements for lateralization, humping.

④ ↑'d laryngeal tone resulting in delayed swallow.

⑤ Poor sitting balance.

Recommendations / treatment plan:
(positioning, diet level, environment, techniques)

① Positioning - upright on solid seating surface, slight forward lean.

② Tone reduction techniques for jaw, tongue, & larynx before & during meal.

③ Diet level - pureed & mechanical soft foods, thickened liquids 2x daily c̄ therapist only.

④ Therapeutic feeding in quiet setting.

⑤ No food or liquid in pts. room.

⑥ Monitor patient for signs of aspiration.

⑦ Videofluoroscopy for confirmation.

Long-term goals:

① Independent trunk and head control for self feeding.

② ↑ attention and awareness of food in mouth to WFL.

③ ↑ isolated motor control of facial expression to WNL.

④ ↑ isolated motor control of jaw, tongue, & larynx to WFL.

⑤ ↑ oral intake for solids from pureed to regular diet for all meals with family supervision.

⑥ ↑ oral intake for liquids from thick to thin.

⑦ Calorie and hydration count, wean from gastrostomy.

⑧ Family ① in swallowing & diet follow through.

FIG. 40-8—cont'd
Case study: dysphagia evaluation and treatment plan.

REVIEW QUESTIONS

1. List the components of dysphagia.
2. List the four stages of swallowing and the characteristics of each.
3. List the physiological functions that occur when the swallow response triggers, and explain why these functions are necessary.
4. Why is it necessary to assess a patient's mental status during a dysphagia evaluation?
5. Describe what the therapist should look for when evaluating the trunk and head during the dysphagia evaluation.
6. What information can the therapist gain when assessing the patient's facial motor control?
7. How does poor tongue control contribute to aspiration?
8. Name the components required to protect the airway.

9. What is the safest food sequence to follow for a swallowing evaluation?
10. Describe the finger placement that a therapist can use to feel the strength and smoothness of the swallow.
11. Why should the therapist assess voice quality after a swallow?
12. Will a patient who has difficulty handling solids also have difficulty with liquids?
13. What options does the occupational therapist have when a patient coughs?
14. List the indicators of swallowing dysfunction.
15. List the acute symptoms of aspiration.
16. When is videofluoroscopy necessary?
17. List the elements in treatment of the patient with dysphagia.
18. Describe the position in which a patient should be treated, and give the rationale for this position.
19. What are the indications for placing a patient on a nonoral treatment program?
20. Name five important criteria a patient must meet to participate in an oral feeding program.
21. List the properties of food preferred for diets for patients with dysphagia.
22. Describe the effect that poor hand-to-mouth movements have on the patient's swallow.
23. Why is it important to involve the patient in the eating process?
24. What are the symptoms of nutritional deficiency?
25. Describe two possible treatment techniques used for a patient who displays a masked appearance.
26. Name three treatment techniques the occupational therapist can use for poor rotary jaw movement and increased tone.
27. Describe two ways a therapist can decrease abnormally high tone in the tongue.
28. Describe thermal application as a treatment technique. For which problem is it used?
29. When is use of the dry swallow technique appropriate?
30. How can the therapist facilitate a cough?

REFERENCES

1. Alta Bates Hospital Rehabilitation Services: *Bedside dysphagia evaluation protocol*, Berkeley, Calif, 1999, the Hospital.
2. American Occupational Therapy Association: *AOTA resource guide: feeding and dysphagia*, Rockville, Md, 1997, The Association.
3. American Occupational Therapy Association: Eating dysfunction: position paper, *Am J Occup Ther* 50(10):846-847, 1996.
4. Avery-Smith W: An occupational therapist coordinated dysphagia program, *Occup Ther Pract* 3(10):20-23, 1998.
5. Avery-Smith W: Management of neurologic disorders: the first feeding session. In Groher M, editor: *Dysphagia: diagnosis and management*, ed 3, Newton, Mass, 1997, Butterworth-Heinemann.
6. Avery-Smith W, Dellarosa D: Approaches to treating dysphagia in patients with brain injury, *Am J Occup Ther* 48(3):235-239, 1994.
7. Bass N: The neurology of swallowing. In Groher M, editor: *Dysphagia: diagnosis and management*, ed 3, Newton, Mass, 1997, Butterworth-Heinemann.
8. Bobath B: *Adult hemiplegia: evaluation and treatment*, ed 2, London, 1978, William Heinemann Medical Books.
9. Buchholz D, Bosma J, Donner M: Adaption, compensation, and decompensation of the pharyngeal swallow, *Gastrointest Radiol* 10(3):235-239, 1985.
10. Cherney L, Pannell J, Cantieri C: Clinical evaluation of dysphagia. In Cherney L, editor: *Clinical management of dysphagia in adults and children*, Gaithersburg, Md, 1994, Aspen Publishers.
11. Community Hospital of Los Gatos, Rehabilitation Services: *Dysphagia protocol*, Los Gatos, Calif, 1999.
12. Conklin JL: Control of esophageal motor function, *Dysphagia* 8(4):311-317, 1993.
13. Coombes K: *Swallowing dysfunction in hemiplegia and head injury*. Course presented by International Clinical Educators, Aug 24-27, 1986, and Aug 24-28, 1987, Los Gatos, Calif.
14. Curran J: Nutritional considerations. In Groher M, editor: *Dysphagia: diagnosis and management*, ed 3, Newton, Mass, 1997, Butterworth-Heinemann.
15. Curtis D, Cruess D, Wilgress E: Normal solid bolus swallowing: erect position, *Dysphagia* 1:63, 1986.
16. Davies P: *Steps to follow*, New York, 1985, Springer-Verlag.
17. Farber S: *Neurorehabilitation: a multisensory approach*, Philadelphia, 1982, WB Saunders.
18. Fleming S.: Treatment of mechanical swallowing disorders. In Groher M, editor: *Dysphagia: diagnosis and management*, ed 3, Newton, Mass, 1997, Butterworth-Heinemann Publishers.
19. Griggs B: Nursing management of swallowing disorders. In Groher M, editor: *Dysphagia: diagnosis and management*, ed 3, Newton, Mass, 1997, Butterworth-Heinemann Publishers.
20. Groher M: Bolus management and aspiration pneumonia with pseudobulbar dysphagia, *Dysphagia* 1:215, 1987.
21. Groher M: Ethical dilemmas in providing nutrition, *Dysphagia* 5(2):102-109, 1990.
22. Groher M: Establishing a swallowing program. In Groher M, editor: *Dysphagia: diagnosis and management*, ed 3, Newton, Mass, 1997, Butterworth-Heinemann Publishers.
23. Hendrix TR: Coordination of peristalsis in pharynx and esophagus, *Dysphagia* 8(2):74-78, 1993.
24. Hiiemae K, Palmer JB: Food transport and bolus formation during complete feeding sequences on foods of different initial consistency, *Dysphagia* 14(1):31-42, 1999.
25. Hislop H, Montgomery J, Connelly B: *Daniels & Worthington's muscle testing: techniques of manual examination*, ed 6, Philadelphia, 1995, WB Saunders.
26. Kaatzke-McDonald M, Post E, Davis P: The effects of cold, touch and chemical stimulation of the anterior faucial pillar on human swallowing, *Dysphagia* 11(3):198-206, 1996.
27. Kahrilas PJ: Pharyngeal structure and function, *Dysphagia* 8(4):303-307, 1993.
28. Langmore S, McCulloch T: Examination of the pharynx and larynx and endoscopic examination of pharyngeal swallowing. In Perlman A, Schulze-Delrieu K, editors: *Deglutition and its disorders: anatomy, physiology, clinical diagnosis, and management*, San Diego, Calif, 1997, Singular Publishing.
29. Leder S, Sasaki C, Burrell M: Fiberoptic endoscopic evaluation of dysphagia to identify silent aspiration, *Dysphagia* 13(1):19-21, 1998.
30. Liebman M: *Neuroanatomy made easy and understandable*, Rockville, Md, 1986, Aspen Publishers.
31. Logemann J: *Evaluation and treatment of swallowing disorders*, Austin, Tex, 1998, Pro-Ed Publishers.
32. Logemann J: *Manual for the videofluorographic study of swallowing*, ed 2, Austin, Tex, 1993, Pro-Ed Publishers.

33. Martin BJW: Treatment of dysphagia in adults. In Cherney L, editor: *Clinical management of dysphagia in adults and children*, Gaithersburg, Md, 1994, Aspen Publishers.

34. Miller A, Bieger D, Conklin JL: Functional controls of deglutition. In Perlman A, Schulze-Delrieu K, editors: *Deglutition and its disorders: anatomy, physiology, clinical diagnosis, and management*, San Diego, Calif, 1997, Singular Publishing.

35. Miller R: Clinical examination for dysphagia. In Groher M: *Dysphagia diagnosis and management*, ed 3, Newton, Mass, 1997, Butterworth-Heinemann Publishers.

36. Netter F, Dalley A: *Atlas of human anatomy*, ed 2, 1998, Ciba-Geigy Corp.

37. Rader T, Rende B: *Swallowing disorders: what families should know*, Tucson, Ariz, 1993, Communication Skill Builders Publishers.

38. Schulze-Delrieu K, Miller R: Clinical assessment of dysphagia. In Perlman A, Schulze-Delrieu K, editors: *Deglutition and its disorders: anatomy, physiology, clinical diagnosis and management*, San Diego, Calif, 1997, Singular Publishing.

39. Silverman EH, Elfant IL: Dysphagia: an evaluation and treatment program for the adult, *Am J Occup Ther* 33(6):382-392, 1979.

40. Smith C, Logemann J, Colangelo L, et al: Incidence and patient characteristics associated with silent aspiration in the acute care setting, *Dysphagia* 14(1):1-7, 1999.

41. Stone M, Shawker T: An ultrasound examination of tongue movement during swallowing, *Dysphagia* 1(2):78-83, 1986.

42. Workman J, Pillsbury H, Hulka G: Surgical interventions in dysphagia. In Groher M: *Dysphagia: diagnosis and management*, ed 3, Newton, Mass, 1977, Butterworth-Heinemann Publishers.

CHAPTER 41

Spinal Cord Injury

CAROLE ADLER

KEY TERMS

Quadriplegia
Tetraplegia
Paraplegia
ASIA impairment scale
Neurological classification
Decubitus ulcer
Vital capacity
Hypotension
Autonomic dysreflexia
Spasticity
Heterotopic ossification
Tenodesis
Durable medical equipment
Rehabilitation technology supplier

LEARNING OBJECTIVES

After studying this chapter the student or practitioner will be able to do the following:

1. Understand the difference between complete and incomplete spinal cord injury and the classification system used to describe such levels of injury.
2. Recognize and identify the various spinal cord injury syndromes.
3. Briefly describe the medical and surgical management of the individual who has experienced a traumatic spinal cord injury.
4. Identify some of the complications that can limit optimal functional potential.
5. Describe the changes in sexual functioning in males and females after spinal cord injury.
6. Identify the specific assessment tools that must be considered before developing treatment objectives.
7. Analyze the critical issues in what to consider when developing treatment objectives during the acute, active, and discharge phases of the rehabilitation process.
8. Identify in detail the functional outcomes, including equipment considerations and attendant care needs, that can be reached at each level of complete injury under optimal circumstances.
9. Analyze how the normal aging process is accelerated by the effects of spinal cord injury and explain how functional status may change.

Rehabilitation of the individual with a spinal cord injury (SCI) is a lifelong process that requires readjustment to nearly every aspect of life. Occupational therapists play a significant role in physical and psychosocial restoration and help the individual achieve maximum independence. Through accurate assessment, retraining, and adaptive techniques and equipment, occupational

therapists provide their patients with the tools and resources needed to achieve their maximal physical and functional potential.

Spinal cord injuries have many causes. Trauma is the most common cause. Trauma can result from motor vehicle accidents, violent injuries such as gunshot and stab wounds, falls, sports accidents, and diving accidents.[5,13] Normal spinal cord function may also be disturbed by diseases such as tumors, myelomeningocele, syringomyelia, multiple sclerosis, and amyotrophic lateral sclerosis. Some of the treatment principles outlined in this chapter may have application to these conditions; however, the emphasis is on rehabilitation of the individual with a traumatic spinal cord injury.

RESULTS OF SPINAL CORD INJURY

Spinal cord injury results in **quadriplegia** (more recently labeled **tetraplegia** by the American Spinal Cord Injury Association) or **paraplegia**. Tetraplegia is any degree of paralysis of the four limbs and trunk musculature. There may be partial upper extremity (UE) function, depending on the level of the cervical lesion. Paraplegia is paralysis of the lower extremities (LEs) with some involvement of the trunk, depending on the level of the lesion.[5,13]

Spinal cord injuries are referred to in terms of the regions (cervical, thoracic, and lumbar) of the spinal cord in which they occur and the numerical order of the neurological segments. The level of spinal cord injury designates the last fully functioning neurological segment of the cord. For example, C6 refers to the sixth neurological segment of the cervical region of the spinal cord as the last fully intact neurological segment.[5,12] Complete lesions result in the absence of motor or sensory function of the spinal cord below the level of the injury. Incomplete lesions may involve several neurological segments, and some spinal cord function may be partially or completely intact.[3,12] For example, C5-6 refers to C5 as being the last intact neurological level and C6 as having incomplete innervation of musculature and absence of neurological function below C6.

Complete Versus Incomplete Neurological Classifications

The extent of neurological damage depends on the location and severity of the injury (Fig. 41-1). In a complete injury, total paralysis and loss of sensation result from a complete interruption of the ascending and descending nerve tracts below the level of the lesion. In an incomplete injury there is some degree of preservation of the sensory or motor nerves below the lesion.

The Frankel classification scale[3,4] has been replaced by the **American Spinal Injury Association (ASIA) Impairment Scale**[1]:

ASIA impairment scale classification A indicates a complete lesion; there is no motor or sensory function preserved in the sacral segments S4-5.

ASIA classification B indicates an incomplete lesion in which only sensation is present below the neurological level, including the sacral segments S4-5.

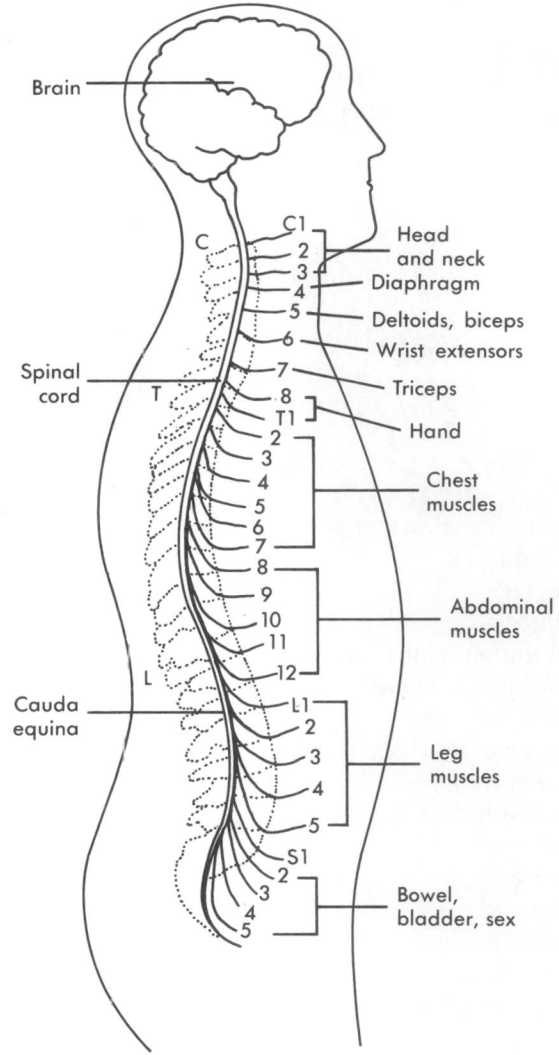

FIG. 41-1
Spinal nerves and major areas of body they supply. (From Paulson S, editor: *Santa Clara Valley Medical Center spinal cord injury home care manual,* ed 2, San Jose, Calif, 1994, Santa Clara Valley Medical Center.)

ASIA classification C indicates an incomplete lesion with motor function below the neurological level and the majority of key muscles below the level having a grade less than 3.

ASIA classification D indicates an incomplete lesion with motor function preserved below the neurological level and the majority of key muscles below the level having a muscle grade of 3 or greater.

ASIA classification E indicates that motor and sensory functions are normal.[1]

Incomplete injuries are categorized according to the area of damage: central, lateral, anterior, or peripheral.

Central Cord Syndrome

Central cord syndrome occurs when there is more cellular destruction in the center of the cord than in the periphery. Paralysis and sensory loss are greater in the UEs because these nerve tracts are more centrally located than nerve tracts for the LEs. This syndrome is often seen in older people in whom arthritic changes have caused a narrowing of the spinal canal; in such cases cervical hyperextension without vertebral fracture may precipitate central cord damage.

Brown-Sequard Syndrome (Lateral Damage)

Brown-Sequard syndrome results when only one side of the cord is damaged, as in a stabbing or gunshot injury. Below the level of injury there is motor paralysis and loss of proprioception on the ipsilateral side and loss of pain, temperature, and touch sensation on the contralateral side.

Anterior Spinal Cord Syndrome

Anterior spinal cord syndrome results from injury that damages the anterior spinal artery or the anterior aspect of the cord. This syndrome involves paralysis and loss of pain, temperature, and touch sensation. Proprioception is preserved.

Cauda Equina (Peripheral)

Cauda equina injuries involve peripheral nerves rather than directly involving the spinal cord. Because peripheral nerves possess a regenerating capacity that the cord does not, there is better prognosis for recovery with this injury. Patterns of sensory and motor deficits are highly variable and asymmetrical.

After spinal cord injury the victim enters a stage of spinal shock that may last from 24 hours to 6 weeks. This period is one of areflexia, in which reflex activity ceases below the level of the injury.[12] The bladder and bowel are atonic or flaccid. Deep tendon reflexes are decreased, and sympathetic functions are disturbed. This disturbance results in decreased constriction of blood vessels, low blood pressure, a slower heart rate, and no perspiration below the level of injury.[10,16]

The spinal cord is usually not damaged below the level of the lesion. Therefore muscles that are innervated by the neurological segments below the level of injury usually develop spasticity, because the monosynaptic reflex arc is intact but separated from higher inhibitory influences. Deep tendon reflexes become hyperactive, and spasticity may be evident. Sensory loss continues, and the bladder and bowel usually become spastic ("upper motor neuron" bladder) in patients whose injuries are above T12. The bladder and bowel usually remain flaccid ("lower motor neuron" bladder) in patients whose lesions are at L1 and below. Sympathetic functions become hyperactive. Spinal reflex activity (mass muscle spasms) usually becomes evident in the areas below the level of the lesion.[3,13,15]

PROGNOSIS FOR RECOVERY

The prognosis for substantial recovery of neuromuscular function after spinal cord injury depends on whether the lesion is complete or incomplete. If there is no sensation or return of motor function below the level of lesion 24 to 48 hours after the injury in carefully assessed complete lesions, motor function is less likely to return. However, partial to full return of function to one spinal nerve root level below the fracture can be gained and may occur in the first 6 months after injury. In incomplete lesions progressive return of motor function is possible, yet it is difficult to determine exactly how much and how quickly return will occur.[15] Frequently, the longer it takes for recovery to begin, the less likely it is that it will occur.

MEDICAL AND SURGICAL MANAGEMENT OF THE PERSON WITH SPINAL CORD INJURY

After a traumatic event in which spinal cord injury is likely, the conscious victim should be carefully questioned about cutaneous numbness and skeletal muscle paralysis before being moved. Emergency medical technicians, paramedics, and air transport personnel are trained in spinal cord injury precautions and extrication techniques for moving a possible SCI victim from an accident site. Movement of the spine must be prevented during the transfer procedures. A firm stretcher or board to which the victim's head and back can be strapped should be procured before moving the victim. After the victim is transferred to the stretcher or board, he or she should be strapped to the board or stretcher and carefully transferred via air or ground transport to the nearest hospital emergency room. Axial traction on the neck should be maintained and any movement of the spine and neck prevented during this process. Careful examination, stabilization, and transportation of the patient may prevent a temporary or slight spinal cord injury from becoming more severe or permanent. Initial care is directed toward preventing further damage to the spinal cord and reversing neurological damage, if possible, by stabilization or decompression of the injured neurological structures.[5,10,13] Antiinflamatory and steroidal drugs are now being administered immediately after injury in an effort to minimize the neurological damage, although the significance of their effect on neurological recovery is still unclear.

A careful neurological examination is carried out by the examining physician to aid in determining the site and type of injury. The patient is in a supine position for this procedure, with the neck and spine immobilized. A catheter is usually placed in the patient's bladder for drainage of urine. Anteroposterior and lateral x-ray films may be taken, with the patient's head, neck, or spine immobilized, to help determine the type of injury. A computed tomography (CT) scan or magnetic resonance imaging (MRI) may be needed for further evaluation. In early medical treatment the goals are to restore normal alignment of the spine, maintain stabilization of the injured area, and decompress neurological structures that are under pressure.

Bony realignment and stabilization are usually achieved by placing the patient on a rotating kinetic bed (Fig. 41-2) that allows skeletal traction and immobilization. The bed's constant rotation allows continuous pressure relief, mobilization of respiratory secretions, and easy access to the patient's entire body for bowel, bladder, and hygiene care. Open surgical reduction with wiring and spinal fusion may be indicated.

The goals of surgery are to decompress the spinal cord and to achieve spinal stability and normal bony alignment.[5,13] Surgery is not always necessary, and adequate immobilization may allow the patient to heal. As soon as possible, a means of portable immobilization is provided, usually a halo vest for cervical injuries (Fig. 41-3, *A*) and a thoracic brace or body jacket for thoracic injuries (Fig. 41-3, *B*). This approach enables the patient to be transferred to a standard hospital bed and, subsequently, to be up in a wheelchair and involved in an active therapy program in as little as 1 to 2 weeks after injury. Initiating an upright sitting tolerance program shortly after injury can substantially reduce the incidence and severity of further medical complications such as deep vein thrombosis, joint contractures, and the general deconditioning that can result from prolonged bed rest.

The benefits of early transport to a spinal cord injury center have been documented.[7] Patients treated initially in a spinal cord acute-care unit rather than a general hospital had shorter acute-care lengths of stay. Patients treated in general hospitals tended to have a higher incidence of skin problems and spinal instability. It has been found that patients sent to rehabilitation centers specializing in the treatment of SCI made functional gains with greater efficiency.[16] Spinal cord centers are able to offer a complete, multidisciplinary program executed by an experienced team of professionals who specialize in this unique and demanding disability.

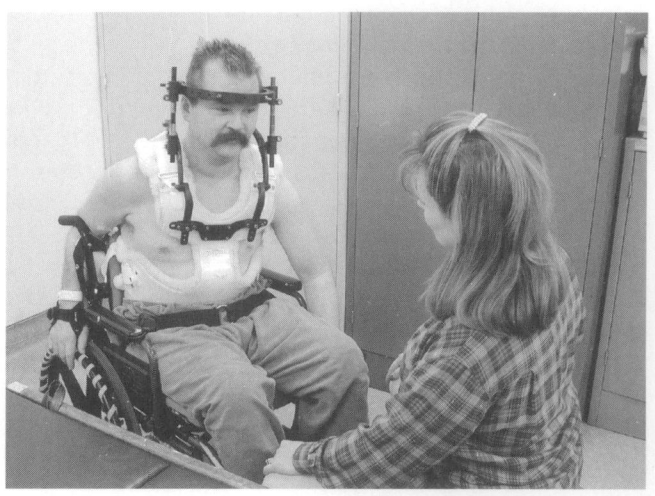

A

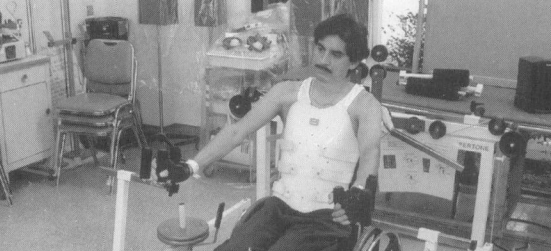

B

FIG. 41-3
A, Halo vest, neck immobilization device for patients with quadriplegia and high level paraplegia (T1 to T4). **B,** Body jacket, one type of immobilization device for paraplegia. (Courtesy of Luis Gonzalez, Media Resource Department, Santa Clara Valley Medical Center.)

FIG. 41-2
Kinetic bed with custom arm positioner. Designed and fabricated by the Occupational Therapy Department, Santa Clara Valley Medical Center, San Jose, Calif. (Courtesy of Luis Gonzalez, Media Resource Department, Santa Clara Valley Medical Center.)

COMPLICATIONS OF SPINAL CORD INJURY

Skin Breakdown, Pressure Sores, or Decubitus Ulcers

Sensory loss increases the risk of skin breakdown. The patient with sensory loss cannot feel the pressure and shearing of prolonged sitting or lying in one position or the presence of pain or heat against the body. Pressure causes the loss of blood supply to the area, which can ultimately result in necrosis. Heat can quickly burn and destroy tissues. Shearing can destroy underlying tissue. Any combination of the above will hasten skin breakdown. The areas most likely to develop skin breakdown are bony prominences over the sacrum, ischium, trochanters, elbows, and heels; however, other bony prominences such as the iliac crest, scapula, knees, toes, and rib cage are also at risk.

It is important for all rehabilitation personnel to be aware of the signs of developing skin problems. At first the area reddens, yet blanches when pressed. Later, the reddened or abraded area does not blanch, which indicates that necrosis has begun. Finally, a blister or ulceration appears in the area. Often the problem is more severe below the level of the skin surface. The visible sore may only be the tip of the iceberg. If allowed to progress, a sore can become severe, destroying underlying tissues even as deep as the bone.

Skin breakdown can be prevented by relieving and eliminating pressure points and protecting vulnerable areas from excessive shearing, moisture, and heat. Turning in bed on a routine basis, specialized mattresses and wheelchair seat cushions, protection of bony prominences with various types of padding, and performing weight shifts are some of the methods used to prevent pressure sores.

The use of hand splints, body jackets, and other orthoses can also cause skin breakdowns. The therapist must inspect the skin, and the patient must be taught to examine his or her skin on a consistent, daily basis, using a mirror or caregiver assistance to watch for signs of developing problems. Skin damage can develop within 30 minutes, so frequent weight shifting, repositioning, and vigilance are essential if skin breakdown is to be prevented.[13,15]

Decreased Vital Capacity

Decreased **vital capacity** is a problem in people who have sustained cervical and high thoracic lesions. Such individuals have markedly limited chest expansion and decreased ability to cough because of weakness or paralysis of the diaphragm and the intercostal and latissimus dorsi muscles. This can result in a tendency toward respiratory tract infections. Reduced vital capacity affects the overall endurance level for activity. Endurance can be improved by assisted breathing and by vigorous respiratory and physical therapy. Strengthening of the sternocleidomastoids and the diaphragm, manually assisted cough, and deep breathing exercises are essential to maintain optimal vital capacity.[13,15]

Osteoporosis of Disuse

Osteoporosis is likely to develop in patients with spinal cord injuries because of disuse of long bones, particularly of the lower extremities. Osteoporosis may be sufficiently advanced for pathological fractures to occur a year after the injury. Pathological fractures are most common in the supracondylar area of the femur, proximal tibia, and distal tibia, the intertrochanteric area of the femur, and the neck of the femur. Pathological fractures are usually not seen in UEs. Daily standing with a standing frame may slow the onset of osteoporosis[13,15]; however, this is a controversial method and not embraced in all rehabilitation programs. A standing program must fit into the patient's activities of daily living (ADL) routine after discharge to be effective on an ongoing basis. Not all reimbursement sources will cover the cost of standing equipment.

Orthostatic Hypotension

A lack of muscle tone in the abdomen and LEs leads to pooling of blood in these areas, with a resultant decrease in blood pressure (**hypotension**). This problem occurs when the patient moves from a supine to upright position or changes body position too quickly. Symptoms are dizziness, nausea, and loss of consciousness.[4] The patient must be reclined quickly and, if sitting in a wheelchair, should be tipped back with legs elevated until symptoms subside. With time this problem can diminish as sitting tolerance and level of activity increase; however, some people continue to have hypotensive episodes. Abdominal binders, leg wraps, antiembolism stockings, and medications can aid in reducing symptoms.

Autonomic Dysreflexia

Autonomic dysreflexia is a phenomenon seen in persons whose injuries are above the T4 to T6 level. It is caused by reflex action of the autonomic nervous system in response to some stimulus, such as a distended bladder, fecal mass, bladder irritation, rectal manipulation, thermal or pain stimuli, or visceral distention. The symptoms are immediate pounding headache, anxiety, perspiration, flushing, chills, nasal congestion, paroxysmal hypertension, and bradycardia.

Autonomic dysreflexia is a medical emergency and life threatening. The patient should not be left alone.[5,13,15] The condition is treated by placing the patient in an upright position and removing anything restrictive, such as abdominal binders or elastic stockings, to reduce blood pressure. The bladder should be drained or legbag tubing checked for obstruction. Blood pressure and other symptoms should be monitored until they return to normal. The occupational therapist must be aware of symptoms and treatment because dysreflexia can occur at any time after the injury.

Spasticity

Spasticity is a nearly universal complication of spinal cord injury.[15] It is an involuntary muscle contraction below the level of injury that results from lack of inhibition from higher centers. Patterns of spasticity change over the first year, gradually increasing in the first 6 months and reaching a plateau about 1 year after the injury. A moderate amount of spasticity can be helpful in the overall rehabilitation of the patient with a spinal cord injury. It helps to maintain muscle bulk, assists in joint range of motion (ROM), and can be used to assist during wheelchair and bed transfers and mobility. A sudden increase in spasticity can alert the patient to other medical problems, such as bladder infections, skin breakdown, or fever.

Severe spasticity can be very frustrating to both the patient and the therapist, in that it can interfere with function. It may be treated more aggressively with a variety of medications. In select instances local injections and surgical procedures that involve cutting or lengthening involved muscles may benefit some patients. In severe cases neurosurgical procedures such as nerve blocks or rhizotomies (the lesioning of spinal roots) have been performed.[5,13,15]

Heterotopic Ossification

Heterotopic ossification (HO), also called *ectopic bone*, is bone that develops in abnormal anatomical locations.[16] It most often occurs in the muscles around the hip and knee, but occasionally it can be noted also at the elbow and shoulder. The first symptoms are swelling, warmth, and decreased joint ROM. The onset of HO is usually 1 to 4 months after injury. Early diagnosis and initiation of treatment can minimize complications. Treatment consists of medication and the maintenance of joint ROM during the early stage of active bone formation, to preserve the functional ROM necessary for good wheelchair positioning, symmetrical position of the pelvis, and maximal functional mobility. If HO progresses to the phase of substantially limiting hip flexion, pelvic obliquity while in the sitting position is likely to occur. This problem contributes to trunk deformities such as scoliosis and kyphosis, with subsequent skin breakdown at the ischial tuberosities, trochanters, and sacrum.[5,13]

SEXUAL FUNCTION

The sexual drive and the need for physical and emotional intimacy are not altered by SCI. However, problems of mobility, functional dependency, and altered body image, as well as complicating medical problems and the attitudes of partners and society, affect social and sexual roles, access, and interest and satisfaction. Education is essential for the spinal cord-injured individual and is a critical part of the rehabilitation process.

Lack of sensation over one part of the body is accompanied by increased or altered sensation over other parts of the body. The sexual response of the body after SCI needs to be explored in the same way a person learns what muscles are working and where he or she can feel.

In males, erections and ejaculations are often affected by SCI. However, this problem is variable and needs to be evaluated individually. Frequently the viability of sperm in men with SCI is decreased, even when other function is near normal.[1] Research is under way to investigate the possible sources of infertility caused by SCI and to reverse the problem.

In women menstruation usually ceases for an interval of weeks to months after injury. It will usually start again and return to normal in time. There may also be changes in lubrication of the vagina during sexual activity. In contrast to males, however, there is no change in female fertility. Females with SCI can conceive and give birth. Special attention must be given to the interaction of pregnancy and childbirth with SCI, especially in regard to blood clots, respiratory function, bladder infections, dysreflexia, and the use of medications during pregnancy and breast feeding.

To avoid pregnancy, women with SCI must take precautions, and the type of birth control used must be considered carefully. Birth control pills are associated with blood clots, especially when combined with smoking, and probably should not be used. The intrauterine device (IUD) is not recommended, even for able-bodied females. Diaphragms may be difficult to position properly when there is loss of sensation in the vagina or decreased hand function. Foams and suppositories are not very effective. The use of condoms by the male partner is probably the safest method.

Individuals with disability quickly sense the attitudes of professionals and caregivers toward their sexuality. Awareness and acceptance by professionals is increasing, and sexual counseling and education are a regular part of many rehabilitation programs for all types of physical disabilities. Some patients lack basic sex education. Others feel asexual because of their disability and altered self-esteem and are isolated from peers; thus they may feel uncomfortable with any type of sexual interaction. For these reasons sexual education and counseling must be geared to the needs of the individual patient and his or her significant other. In some instances, social interaction skills need improvement before sexual activity can be considered, and occupational therapists play an important role in providing information and a forum to deal with these issues. (See Chapter 15 for more information on sexuality with physical dysfunction.)

OCCUPATIONAL THERAPY INTERVENTION
Evaluation

Assessment of the patient is an ongoing process that begins on the day of admission and continues long after discharge on an outpatient follow-up basis. Depending on whether the patient is in an acute inpatient rehabilitation, outpatient, or home setting, the occupational therapist should continually assess the patient's functional progress and the appropriateness of treatment and equipment. An accurate and comprehensive formal initial evaluation is essential to determine baseline neurological, clinical, and functional status from which to formulate a treatment program and substantiate progress. Initial data gathered from the medical chart will provide personal information, a medical diagnosis, and a history of other pertinent medical information. Input from the multidisciplinary team will enhance the occupational therapist's ability to predict realistic optimal outcomes accurately.

Discharge planning begins during the initial evaluation. Therefore the patient's social and vocational history, as well as past and expected living situations, are necessary for planning a treatment program that meets the patient's ongoing needs. Treatment should begin as soon as possible. It is possible to gather enough information quickly to begin addressing high-priority areas such as splinting, positioning, and family training without having to wait for the evaluation to be completed.

Physical Status

Before evaluation of the patient's physical status, very specific medical precautions should be obtained from the primary and consulting physicians. Skeletal instability and related injuries or medical complications will affect the way in which the patient is moved and the active or resistive movements allowed.

Passive range of motion (PROM) should be measured before specific manual muscle testing to determine available pain-free movement. This evaluation also identifies the presence of or potential for joint contractures, which could suggest the need for preventive or corrective splinting and positioning.

Shoulder pain, which ultimately causes decreased shoulder and scapular ROM, is extremely common in C4-7 tetraplegics. Among the possible causes are scapular immobilization resulting from prolonged bed rest and nerve root compression subsequent to the injury. Shoulder pain should be thoroughly assessed and diagnosed so that proper treatment can be provided before the onset of chronic discomfort and functional loss.

Accurate assessment of the patient's muscle strength is critical in determining a precise diagnosis of neurological level and establishing a baseline for physical recovery and functional progress. Because the occupational therapist's skills with activity analysis greatly enhance his or her effectiveness in treating the individual with SCI, a precise working knowledge of musculoskeletal anatomy and specific manual muscle testing techniques is essential. Using accepted muscle testing protocols ensures accurate technique while performing this complex evaluation. The muscle test should be repeated as often as is necessary to provide an ongoing picture of the patient's strength and progress.

Sensation is evaluated for light touch, superficial pain (pinprick), and kinesthesia, which determines areas of absent, impaired, and intact sensation. These findings are useful in establishing the level of injury and determining functional limitations (Fig. 41-4).[1]

If the patient is evaluated in the acute stage, spasticity is rarely noted, because the patient is still in spinal shock. When spinal shock subsides, increased muscle tone may be present in response to stimuli. The therapist should then determine whether the spasticity interferes with or enhances function.

An evaluation of wrist and hand function determines the degree to which a patient can manipulate objects. This information is used to suggest the need for equipment such as positioning splints or universal cuffs or, later, consideration of a **tenodesis** orthosis (wrist-driven flexor hinge splint). Gross grasp and pinch measurements indicate functional abilities and may be used as an adjunct to manual muscle testing to provide objective measurements of baseline status and progress for patients who have active hand musculature.[8]

Clinical observation is used to assess endurance, oral motor control, head and trunk control, LE functional muscle strength, and total body function. More specific assessment in any of these areas may be required, depending on the individual.

An increased number of combined spinal cord injury–head injury diagnoses suggests that a specific cognitive and perceptual evaluation may be necessary.[9] Assessing a patient's ability to initiate tasks, follow directions, carry over learning day to day, and do problem solving contributes to the information base needed for appropriate and realistic goal setting. Understanding the patient's learning style, coping skills, and communication style is also essential.

Functional Status

Observing the patient performing ADL is an important part of the OT evaluation. The purpose of this

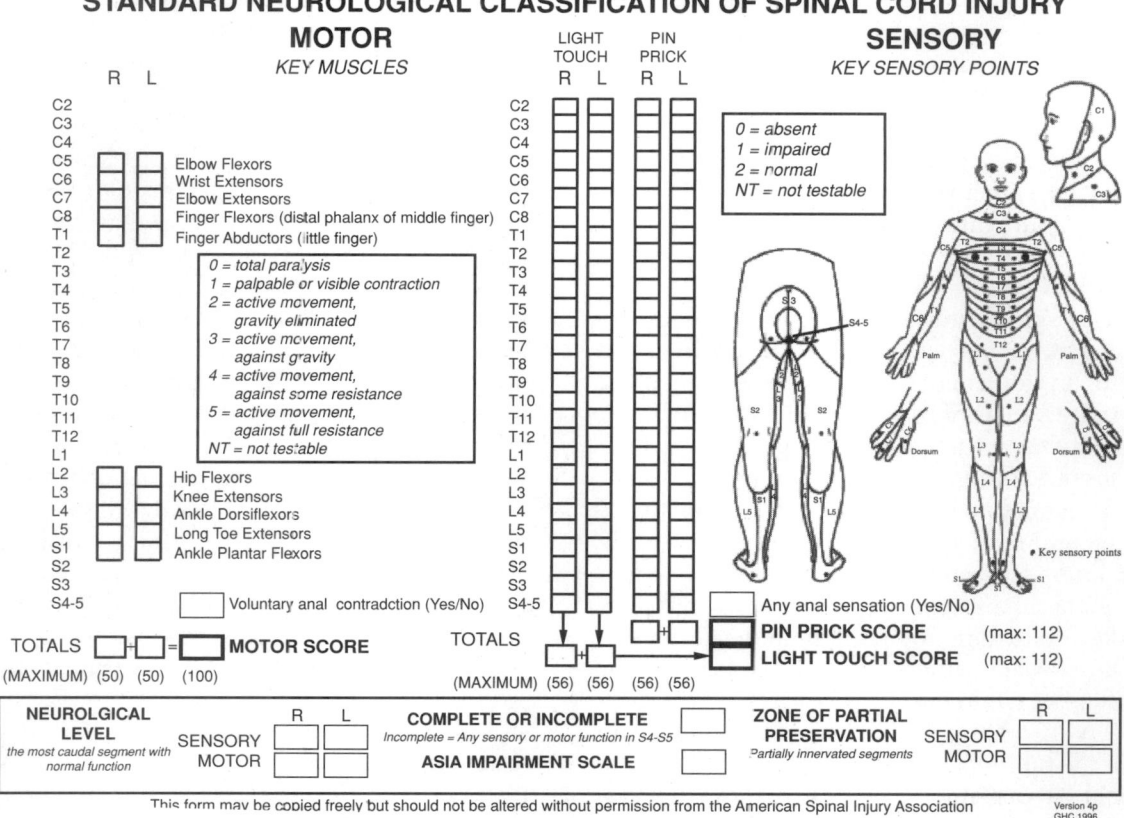

FIG. 41-4

Standard neurological classification of spinal cord injury. (Courtesy of American Spinal Injury Association, 1992.)

observation is to determine present and potential levels of functional ability. If the patient is cleared of bed rest precautions, evaluation and simultaneous treatment should begin as soon as possible after injury. Light activities such as feeding, light hygiene at the sink, and object manipulation may be appropriate, depending on the level of injury.

Direct interaction with the patient's family and friends provides valuable information regarding the patient's support systems while in the hospital and, more important, after discharge. This information is relevant to later caregiver training in areas in which the patient may require the assistance of others to accomplish self-care and mobility tasks.

In addition to physical and functional assessments, the occupational therapist has the opportunity to observe the patient's psychosocial adjustment to the disability and life in general through the nature of activities in which the patient participates.[13] The evaluation phase is important for establishing rapport and mutual trust, which will facilitate participation and progress in later and more difficult phases of rehabilitation. An individual's motivation, determination, socioeconomic background, education, family support, acceptance of disability, problem-solving abilities, and financial resources can prove to be invaluable assets or limiting factors in determining the outcome of rehabilitation. A therapist must carefully observe the patient's status in each of these areas before recommending the course of treatment.[8]

ESTABLISHING TREATMENT OBJECTIVES

Establishing treatment objectives in concert with the patient and with the rehabilitation team is important. The primary objectives of the rehabilitation team may not be those of the patient. Psychosocial factors, cultural factors, cognitive deficits, environmental limitations, and individual financial considerations must be identified and integrated into a treatment program that will meet the unique needs of each individual. Every patient is different; therefore a variety of treatment approaches and alternatives may be necessary to address each factor that may affect goal achievement.[7] More participation can be expected if the patient's priorities are respected to the extent that they are achievable and realistic.

The therapist's general objectives for treatment of the person with SCI are as follows:

1. To maintain or increase joint ROM and prevent deformity via active and passive ROM, splinting, and positioning

2. To increase the strength of all innervated and partially innervated muscles through the use of enabling and purposeful activities
3. To increase physical endurance via functional activities
4. To maximize independence in all aspects of self-care, mobility, and homemaking and parenting skills
5. To explore leisure interests and vocational potential
6. To aid in the psychosocial adjustment to disability
7. To evaluate, recommend, and train the patient in the use and care of necessary **durable medical and adaptive equipment**
8. To ensure safe and independent home accessibility through home modification recommendations
9. To instruct the patient in the communication skills necessary for training caregivers to provide safe assistance

The patient's length of stay in the inpatient rehabilitation program and the ability to participate in outpatient therapy determine the appropriateness and priority of the just-named activities.

TREATMENT METHODS
Acute Phase

During the acute, or immobilized, phase of the rehabilitation program the patient may be in traction or wearing a stabilization device such as a halo brace or body jacket. Medical precautions must be in force during this period. Flexion, extension, and rotary movements of the spine and neck are contraindicated.

Evaluation of total body positioning and hand splinting needs should be initiated at this time. In patients with tetraplegia, scapular elevation and elbow flexion (as well as limited shoulder flexion and abduction while on bed rest) cause potentially painful shoulders and ROM limitations. Upper extremities should be intermittently positioned in 80° of shoulder abduction, external rotation with scapular depression, and full elbow extension to assist in alleviating this common problem. The forearm should be positioned in forearm pronation, since the patient is at risk for supination contractures such as at the C5 level. At Santa Clara Valley Medical Center a device has been designed and fabricated by the Occupational Therapy Department to maintain the arm in an appropriate position while the patient is immobilized on a kinetic bed (Fig. 41-2).

Selection of appropriate splint style and accurate fabrication and fit of the splint by the occupational therapist enhance patient acceptance and optimal functional gain. If musculature is not adequate to support the wrist and hands properly for function or cosmesis, splints should be fabricated to support the wrist properly in extension and the thumb in opposition and to maintain the thumb web space while allowing the fingers to flex naturally at the metacarpophalangeal

(MP) and proximal interphalangeal (PIP) joints. Splints should be dorsal rather than ventral in design to allow maximal sensory feedback while the patient's hand is resting on any surface. If at least F+ (3+) strength of wrist extension is present, a short opponens splint should be considered to maintain the web space and support the thumb in opposition. This splint can be used functionally while the patient is trained to use a tenodesis grasp.

Active and active-assisted ROM of all joints should be performed within strength, ability, and tolerance levels. Muscle reeducation techniques for wrists and elbows should be employed when indicated. Progressive resistive exercises for wrists may be carried out. The patient should be encouraged to engage in self-care activities such as feeding, writing, and hygiene if possible, using simple devices such as a universal cuff or a custom writing splint. Even though the patient may be immobilized in bed, discussion of anticipated durable medical equipment (DME), home modifications, and caregiver training should be initiated to allow sufficient time to prepare for discharge.

Active Phase

During the active, or mobilization, phase of the rehabilitation program, the patient can sit in a wheelchair and should begin developing upright tolerance. A high priority at this time is determining a method of relieving sitting pressure for the purpose of preventing **decubitus ulcers** on the ischial, trochanteric, and sacral bony prominences. If the patient has quadriplegia yet has at least F+ (3+) shoulder and elbow strength bilaterally, pressure can be relieved on the buttocks by leaning forward over the feet. Simple cotton webbing loops are secured to the back frame of the wheelchair (Fig. 41-5).

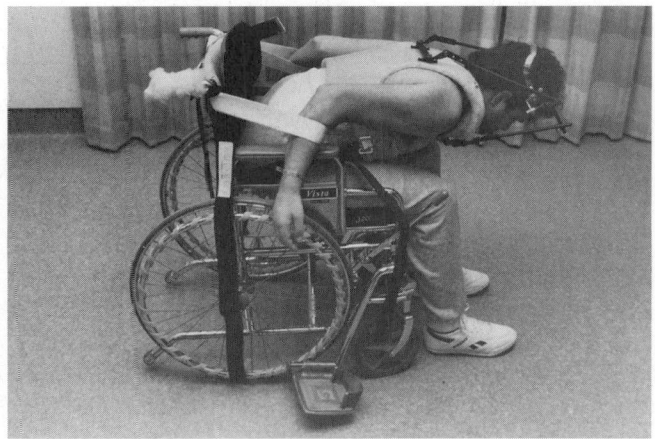

FIG. 41-5
Forward weight shift using loops attached to wheelchair frame. A patient with C6 quadriplegia with symmetrical grade 4 deltoids and biceps and wrist extensors.

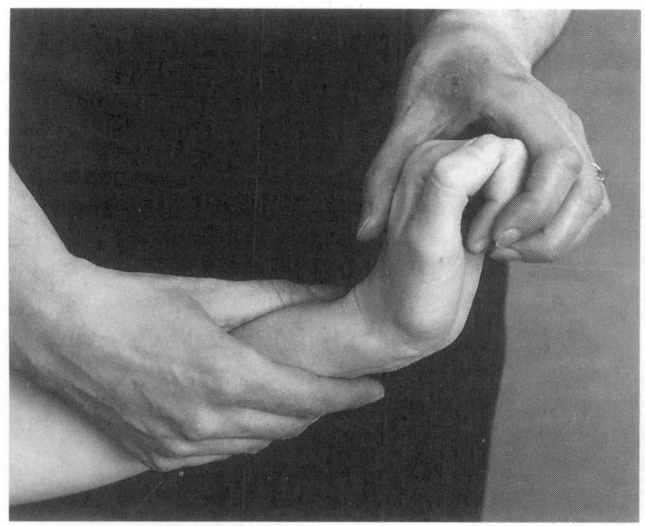

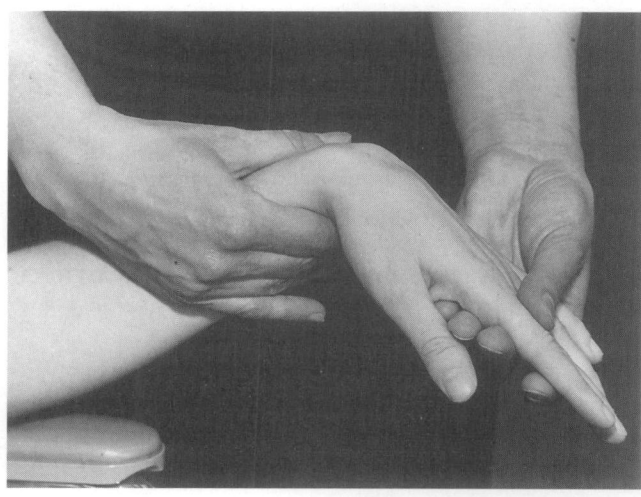

A   B

FIG. 41-6

Tenodesis action. **A,** Wrist is extended when fingers are passively flexed. **B,** Wrist is flexed when fingers are passively extended.

A person with low quadriplegia (C7) or a person with paraplegia with intact UE musculature can perform a full depression weight shift off the arms or wheels of the wheelchair. Weight shifts should be performed every 60 minutes until skin tolerance is determined.

Active and passive ROM exercises should be continued regularly to prevent undesirable contractures. Splinting or casting of the elbows may be indicated to correct contractures that are developing. Some patients will have wrist extension, which will be used to substitute for absent grasp through tenodesis action of the long finger flexors. With these patients it is desirable to develop some tightness in these tendons to give some additional tension to the tenodesis grasp. The desirable contracture is developed by ranging finger flexion with the wrist fully extended and finger extension with the wrist flexed, thus never allowing the flexors or extensors to be in full stretch over all of the joints that they cross (Fig. 41-6).[15]

Elbow contractures should never be allowed to develop. Full elbow extension is essential for allowing propping to maintain balance during static sitting and for assisting in transfers. With zero triceps strength a person with C6 quadriplegia can maintain forward sitting balance by shoulder depression and protraction, external rotation, full elbow extension, and full wrist extension (Fig. 41-7).

Progressive resistive exercise and resistive activities can be applied to innervated and partially innervated muscles. Shoulder musculature should be exercised so as to promote proximal stability, with emphasis on the latissimus dorsi (shoulder depressors), deltoids (shoulder flexors, abductors, and extensors), and the remainder of the shoulder girdle and scapular muscles. The

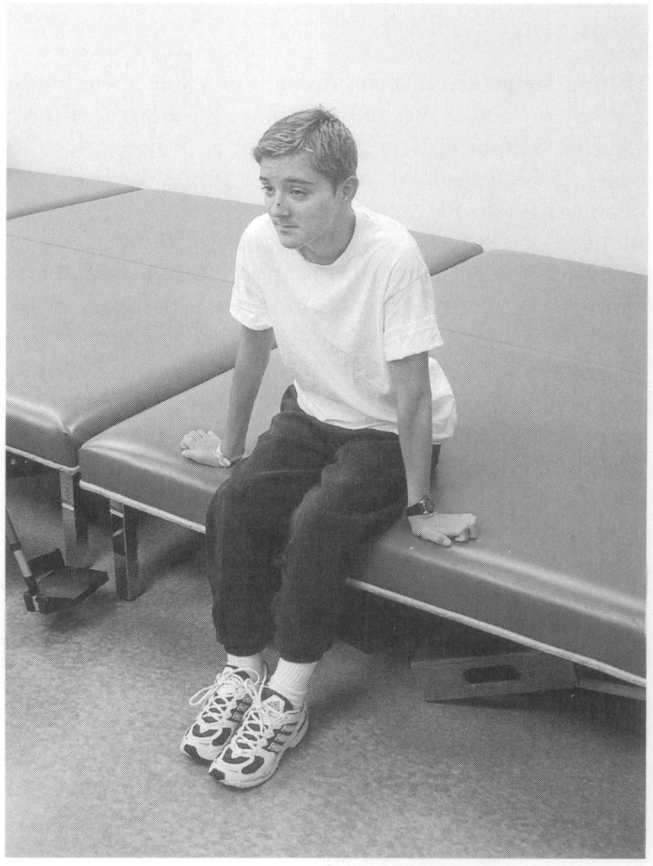

FIG. 41-7

A patient with C6 quadriplegia; forward sitting balance is maintained (without triceps) by locking elbows. This is a valuable skill for maintaining sitting balance, bed mobility, and transfers. (Courtesy of Luis Gonzalez, Media Resource Department, Santa Clara Valley Medical Center.)

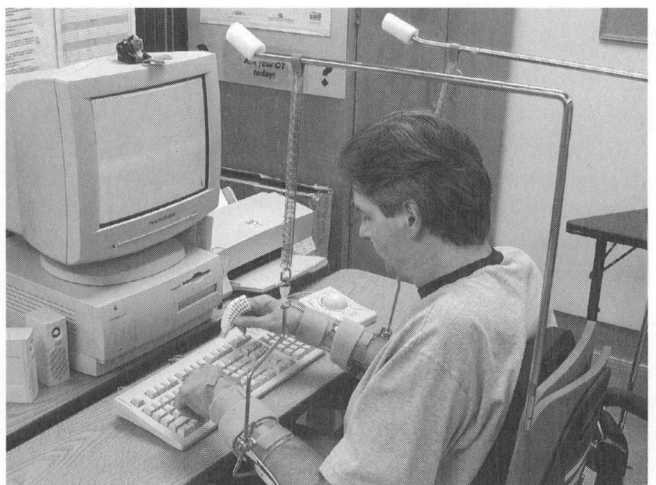 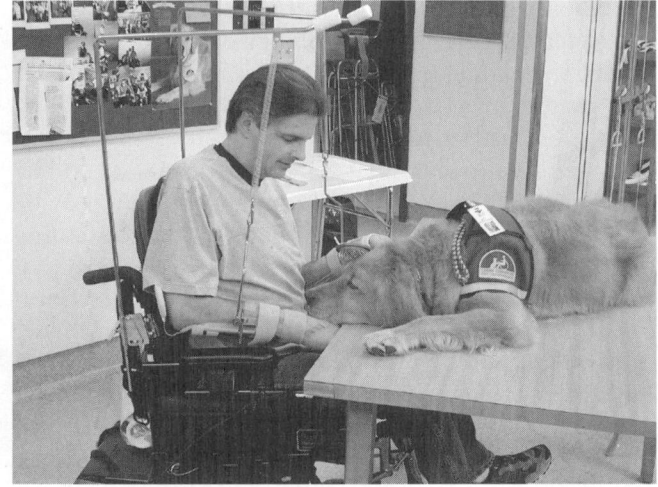

FIG. 41-8

A, Patient with injury at C4-5 typing at keyboard with bilateral overhead slings, bilateral wrist splints, and typing splints. **B,** Use of a service dog as a treatment option to facilitate bilateral upper extremity use. (Courtesy of Luis Gonzalez, Media Resource Department, Santa Clara Valley Medical Center.)

triceps, pectoralis, and latissimus dorsi muscles are needed for transfers and for shifting weight when in the wheelchair. Wrist extensors should be strengthened to maximize natural tenodesis function, thereby maximizing the necessary prehension pattern in the hand for functional grasp and release.

The treatment program should be graded to increase the amount of resistance that can be tolerated during activity. As muscle power improves, increasing the amount of time in wheelchair activities will help the patient gain upright tolerance and endurance.

Many assistive devices and equipment items can be useful to the person with SCI. However, every attempt should be made to have the patient perform the task with no equipment or with as little as possible. Modified techniques are available that enable an individual to perform efficiently without the need for expensive or bulky equipment.

When appropriate, the universal cuff for holding eating utensils, toothbrushes, pencils, and paintbrushes is a simple and versatile device that offers increased independence. A wrist cock-up splint to stabilize the wrist with attachment of the universal cuff may be useful for persons with little or no wrist extension. A plate guard, cup holder, extended straw with straw clip, and nonskid table mat can facilitate independent feeding. A wash mitt, soap holder, or soap-on-a-rope appears to make bathing easier; however, the added difficulty of donning and doffing such equipment must be considered. Many people with quadriplegia can use a button hook to fasten clothing. A transfer board is a valuable option for safe transfers. Through treatment, optimal muscle strength and coordination can occur, enabling the patient to outgrow the use of initially necessary equipment.

The ADL program may be expanded to include independent feeding with devices, oral hygiene and upper-body bathing, bowel and bladder care, such as digital stimulation and application of the urinary collection device, UE dressing, and transfers using the sliding board. Communication skills in writing and using the telephone, tape recorder, stereo equipment, computer, and calculator keyboard should be an important part of the treatment program (Fig. 41-8). Training in the use of the mobile arm support and overhead slings (see Chapter 31), wrist-hand orthosis (flexor hinge or tenodesis splint), and assistive devices is also part of the OT program.

The occupational therapist should continue to provide psychological support by allowing and encouraging the patient to express frustration, anger, fears, and concerns.[13] The OT clinic in a spinal cord center can provide an atmosphere where patients can establish support groups with other inpatients and outpatients who can offer their experiences and problem-solving advice to those in earlier phases of their rehabilitation.

The assessment, ordering, and fitting of DME such as wheelchairs, seating and positioning equipment, mechanical lifts, beds, and bathing equipment are extremely important parts of the rehabilitation program. Such equipment should be specifically evaluated, however, and ordered only when definite goals and expectations are known. Inappropriate equipment can impair function and cause further medical problems, such as skin breakdown or trunk deformity; the therapist must take into account all functional, positioning, environmental, psychological, and financial considerations in evaluating the patient's equipment needs. The desired equipment, especially wheelchairs, seat cushions, back supports, positioning devices and bathing equipment, should be available for demonstration and trial by the patient before final ordering. It is imperative that the therapist involved in the evaluation and ordering of this costly and highly individualized equipment be familiar with what is currently on the market and be knowledgeable in ordering equipment that will provide the patient with optimal function and body positioning on a short- and long-term basis. A good working relationship with an experienced **rehabilitation technology supplier** (RTS), an equipment supplier specializing in custom rehabilitation equipment, is imperative. Advancements in technology and design have provided a wide variety of equipment from which to choose, and working with another professional specializing in such equipment will help ensure correct selection and fit. See Chapter 14 for a more detailed discussion of wheelchairs, seating, and positioning equipment.

In addition to enhancing respiratory function by supporting the patient in an erect, well-aligned position that maximizes sitting tolerance and optimizes upper-extremity function, wheelchair seating must assist in the prevention of deformity and pressure sores. An appropriate and adequate wheelchair cushion helps distribute sitting pressure, assists in the prevention of pressure sores, stabilizes the pelvis as necessary for proper trunk alignment, and provides comfort. Whether it is the occupational therapist's or the physical therapist's role to evaluate and order the wheelchair and cushion, both should work closely together to ensure consistent training and use for the individual needs of each patient.

An increasing number of individuals with high-level SCI, C4 and above, are surviving and participating in active rehabilitation programs. The treatment and equipment needs of these individuals are unique and extremely specialized, ranging from mouthsticks and environmental control systems to ventilators and sophisticated electric wheelchairs and drive systems (see Table 41-1, levels C1-3 and C3-4, at the end of this chapter). The use of experienced resources in determining appropriate short- and long-term goals and equipment needs enhances the quality and functional ability of an individual who otherwise would be quite dependent. Rehabilitation centers specializing in the care of ventilator-dependent patients should be sought for their expertise in addressing all aspects of care for this unique patient population.

When place of discharge is determined and the patient can tolerate leaving the hospital for a few hours, a home evaluation should be performed. The therapist, patient, and family members can then view and attempt activities in the home in anticipation of return to a safe and accessible environment. The therapist must be knowledgeable about safety and accessibility options for a variety of environments and often must advise architects or contractors to ensure that appropriate modifications are made. The therapist must be aware of accessibility requirements in the home, as well as those required in the workplace by the Americans with Disabilities Act of 1990 (ADA) (see Chapter 17).

Decreases in the time of inpatient rehabilitation have moved the extended phase of treatment to an outpatient basis or home therapy. Adaptive driving, home management, leisure activities, or workshop skill assessments using hand- or power-based tools are feasible and appropriate treatment modalities for evaluating and increasing UE strength, coordination, and trunk balance; however, they may not be a priority during inpatient hospitalization. Such activities can improve socialization skills and can also assess problem-solving skills and potential work habits.

OT services can offer valuable evaluation and exploration of the vocational potential of persons with SCI. By the sheer magnitude of the physical disability, vocational possibilities for individuals with high levels of SCI are limited. Many patients must change their vocation or alter former vocational goals. Low aptitude, poor motivation, loss of health benefits, and lack of perseverance on the part of many patients make vocational rehabilitation challenging.

The occupational therapist can assess the patient's level of motivation, functional intelligence, aptitudes, attitudes, interests, and personal vocational aspirations during the process of the treatment program and through the use of ADL, mobility, and work simulation activities. The therapist can observe the patient's attention span, concentration, manual ability with splints and devices, accuracy, speed, perseverance, work habits, and work tolerance level. The therapist can serve as a liaison between the client and the vocational rehabilitation counselor by offering valuable information from observations during activities. When suitable vocational objectives have been selected, they may be pursued in an educational setting or in a work setting, usually out of the realm of OT.

AGING WITH SPINAL CORD INJURY

Following survival of acute SCI, the primary goal of rehabilitation is independence. Independence as the measure of quality of life for people with disabilities is an idea accepted and often perpetuated by professionals and survivors alike.[14]

Occupational therapists treating patients with SCI have considerable responsibility in influencing the level of independence, whether in the acute setting, during active rehabilitation, or in follow-up care throughout the life of a spinal cord–injured individual. Understanding the aging process in both able-bodied and disabled individuals is necessary for providing appropriate options and fostering attitudes that enhance the quality of the patient's life at any age.

Physical aging is a natural, nonpreventable process encountered by all humans. The signs of the process can occur at varying rates for each individual, and aging affects most systems of the body. In spinal cord–injured individuals, aging is usually accelerated by the secondary effects of the disability, such as the presence of muscle imbalance, infections (urinary and respiratory), deconditioning, pain, and joint degeneration secondary to overuse.[13]

Twenty years after injury appears to be a point at which some of the aging problems begin to increase. Since at least one of four SCI survivors is over 20 years postinjury,[14] a significant portion of SCI survivors are prematurely experiencing the problems of aging. Individuals with SCI onset in their later years have very different patterns of functional outcomes, program needs, and financial resources than do those with onset in their earlier years. For someone who acquired quadriplegia in his or her 20s, when the majority of spinal cord injuries occur, the degenerating conditions of normal aging become evident prematurely, usually before the 40s.[4] Thus someone who was independent in transfers at home and loading a wheelchair in and out of the car may now require assistance getting in and out of bed; this person may have to trade the car for a van requiring costly modifications because his or her shoulders have given out. Likewise, someone at a level at which one would assume functional independence (e.g., T10 paraplegia) may, in fact, need personal care assistance because of aging. The occupational therapist should make good trunk alignment and seating a priority from the outset to prevent fixed trunk and pelvic deformities such as kyphosis and scoliosis, which can lead to considerable skin problems and uncorrectable cosmetic deformities years later. In addition, it is necessary to be aware of how manual wheelchair propulsion can affect a weak shoulder complex, as well as the advantage of the cardiopulmonary conditioning that such an activity can provide.

When SCI is compounded by the increased fatigue and weakness often associated with normal aging, the functional status of the individual affected with SCI may decline. Occupational therapists may cite this change to justify additional services or equipment. Many considerations must be weighed to make appropriate short- and long-term decisions. Contacting experienced resources who have a perspective of both acute and long-term injuries and issues can offer valuable insight into treatment decisions.

RESEARCH

Research is being conducted in clinical settings and scientific laboratories around the world, focusing on understanding the nature of SCI and defining the nervous system's response to this injury. There is now a sense of

CASE STUDY 41-1

Mr. S. is a 44-year-old Caucasian man who sustained a C7-8 complete (ASIA A) spinal cord injury as a result of a fall. He also sustained facial lacerations and bilateral radial wrist fractures, which necessitated casting without internal fixation. Mr. S is divorced with no biological children. He is a firefighter and has a background in auto mechanics. Mr. S is very athletic, a triathlete and marathon runner. Just before his accident, Mr. S had moved into a second-story apartment.

Mr. S was referred to OT on the day of his injury and was initially evaluated in the ICU within 24 hours of injury. He was immobilized in cervical traction and bilateral wrist casts on a kinetic bed. His specific manual muscle test revealed 3+ to 4 strength in deltoids, biceps, and triceps. Wrists could not be tested secondary to bilateral wrist casts, and finger and thumb flexion and extension was noted to be at least 2–bilaterally. Sensory examination was intact to the C7 dermatome. Vital capacity was low secondary to the absence of innervation of intercostal and abdominal musculature, and Mr. S required respiratory treatments 4 times per day to mobilize lung secretions. Because of his immobilization, he required assistance for all aspects of his self-care and mobility.

OT treatment objectives included (1) maintaining optimal range of motion (ROM) in all joints for optimal upper extremity function and seated positioning, (2) achieving optimal strength and endurance in available musculature, (3) achieving optimal independence in all self-care skills, including bathing, toileting, and skin care, (4) achieving independent wheelchair mobility on all indoor and outdoor surfaces, (5) receiving appropriate durable medical equipment (DME) to meet both short- and long-term needs (e.g., manual and power wheelchair, cushion, and bathing and toileting equipment), (6) returning to safe and accessible housing, and (7) being educated in all aspects of care and independently instructing caregivers in assistance needed.

Mr. S has had a very difficult time accepting the fact that he has a complete spinal cord injury. He could not imagine how he could function at work and in his community as a quadriplegic. His college and church community offered a tremendous amount of support, yet he continued to be depressed and angry over his loss of mobility and independence. He received regular psychological counseling and attended a weekly peer support group.

On discharge from acute rehabilitation, Mr. S returned to a newly rented single-story home that required ramps at the front and back entrances and bathroom modifications. Mr. S initially received 4 hours of attendant care daily. He required assistance only for completion of his daily bath and bowel program, as well as for some homemaking tasks. After Mr. S received in-home OT for home setup and community transition issues, his need for personal care diminished and he now requires only homemaking assistance. He regularly visits a neighborhood gym to maintain upper extremity strength and endurance, and he will soon be driving a modified van. His vocational plans are on hold until his van and driving training are completed.

optimism in the scientific community that it will be possible someday to restore function after SCI. This optimism is based on the combined research efforts of scientists in many different disciplines. It is important for occupational therapists treating spinal cord injury to be aware of the scientific and technological advances so as to better educate patients, while at the same time providing them with the most realistic and comprehensive rehabilitation interventions for their immediate and long-term needs.

SUMMARY

SCI can result in substantial paralysis of the limbs and trunk. The degree of residual motor and sensory dysfunction depends on the level of the lesion, whether the lesion was complete or incomplete, and the area of the spinal cord that was damaged.

Following a spinal cord injury, bony realignment and stabilization are established surgically, via an external immobilization device, or through a combination of both methods. The many possible complications of SCI include skin breakdown, rapid loss of bone density, and spasticity.

OT is concerned with facilitating the patient's achievement of optimal independence and functioning. Areas of focus are physical restoration of available musculature, self-care, independent living skills, short- and long-term equipment needs, and educational, work, and leisure activities. The psychosocial adjustment of the patient is important, and the occupational therapist offers emotional support toward this end in every phase of the rehabilitation program.

Table 41-1 presents expectations of functional performance of SCI at 1 year after injury and at each of eight levels of injury (C1-3, C4, C5, C6, C7-8, T1-9, T10-L1, L2-S5). The outcomes reflect a level of independence that can be expected of a person with motor complete SCI, given optimal circumstances.

The categories presented reflect expected functional outcomes in the areas of mobility, activities of daily living, instrumental activities of daily living, and communication skills. The guidelines are based on consensus of clinical experts, available literature on functional outcomes, and data compiled from Uniform Data Systems (UDS) and the National Spinal Cord Injury Statistical Center (NSCISC).

Within the functional outcomes for people with SCI listed in Table 41-1, a series of essential daily functions and activities, as well as the attendant care likely to be needed to support the predicted level of independence at 1 year after injury, have been identified. These outcome areas include the following:

- *Respiratory, bowel, and bladder function*. The neurological effects of spinal cord injury may result in deficits in the ability of the individual to perform basic body functions. Respiratory function includes the ability to breathe with or without mechanical assistance and to adequately clear secretions. Bowel and bladder function includes the ability to manage elimination, maintain perineal hygiene, and adjust clothing before and after elimination. Adapted or facilitated methods of managing these bodily functions may be required to attain expected functional outcomes.
- *Bed mobility, bed/wheelchair transfers, wheelchair propulsion, and positioning/pressure relief*. The neurological effects of spinal cord injury may result in deficits in the ability of the individual to perform the activities required for mobility, locomotion, and safety. Adapted or facilitated methods of managing these activities may be required to attain expected functional outcomes in standing and ambulation.
- *Standing and ambulation*. Spinal cord injury may result in deficits in the ability to stand for exercise or psychological benefit or to ambulate for functional activities. Adapted or facilitated methods of management may be outcomes in standing and ambulation.
- *Eating, grooming, dressing, and bathing*. The neurological effects of spinal cord injury may result in deficits in the ability of the individual to perform these ADL. Adapted or facilitated methods of managing ADL may be necessary to attain expected functional outcomes.
- *Communication (keyboard use, handwriting, and telephone use)*. The neurological effects of spinal cord injury may result in deficits in the ability of the individual to communicate. Adapted or facilitated methods of communication may be required to attain expected functional outcomes.
- *Transportation (driving, attendant-operated vehicle, and public transportation)*. Transportation activities are critical for individuals with SCI to become maximally independent in their community. Adaptations may be required to help the individual meet the expected functional outcomes.
- *Homemaking (meal planning and preparations and home management)*. Adapted or facilitated methods of managing homemaking skills may be required to attain expected functional outcomes. Individuals with complete SCI at any level will require some level of assistance with some homemaking activities. The hours of assistance with homemaking activities are presented in Table 41-1.
- *Assistance required*. Table 41-1 lists the number of hours that may be required from a caregiver to assist with personal care and homemaking activities in the home. Personal care includes hands-on delivery of all aspects of self-care and mobility, as well as safety interventions. Homemaking assistance is also included in the recommendation for hours of assistance and includes activities previously presented. The number of hours presented in both the

panel recommendations and the self-reported CHART data is representative of skilled and unskilled and paid and unpaid hours of assistance. The 24-hour-a-day requirement noted for the C1-3 and C4 levels includes the expected need for unpaid attendant care to provide safety monitoring.

Adequate assistance is required to ensure that the individual with SCI can achieve the outcomes set forth in Table 41-1. The hours of assistance recommended by the panel do not reflect changes in assistance required over time as reported by long-term survivors of SCI[6] nor do they take into account the wide range of individual variables mentioned throughout this document that may affect the number of hours of assistance required. The Functional Independence Measure (FIM) estimates are widely variable in several of the categories. Whether the representative individuals with SCI in the individual categories attained the expected functional outcomes for their specific level of injury is unclear, as is whether there were mitigating circumstances, such as age, obesity, or concomitant injuries, that would account for variability in assistance reported. An individualized assessment of needs is required in all cases.

■ *Equipment requirements.* Minimum recommendations for durable medical equipment and adaptive devices are identified in each of the functional categories. The most commonly used equipment is listed, with the understanding that variations exist among SCI rehabilitation programs and that use of such equipment may be necessary to achieve the identified functional outcomes. Additional equipment and devices that are not critical for the majority of individuals at a specific level of injury may be required for some individuals. The equipment descriptions are generic to allow for variances in program philosophy and financial resources. Rapid changes and advances in equipment and technology will be made and therefore must be considered.

Healthcare professionals should keep in mind that the recommendations set forth in Table 41-1 are not intended to be prescriptive, but rather to serve as a guideline. The importance of individual functional assessment of people with SCI before making equipment recommendations cannot be overemphasized. All durable medical equipment and adaptive devices must be thoroughly assessed and tested to determine medical necessity, to prevent medical complications (e.g., postural deviations, skin breakdown, or pain), and to foster optimal functional performance. Environmental control units and telephone modifications may be needed for safety and maximal independence, and each person must be individually evaluated for the need for this equipment. Recommendations for

disposable medical products are not included in this document.

■ *FIM.* Evidence for the specific levels of independence provided in Table 41-1 relies both on expert consensus and on data from FIM in large-scale, prospective, and longitudinal research conducted by NSCISC. FIM is the most widely used disability measure in rehabilitation medicine, and although it may not incorporate all of the characteristics of disability in individuals recovering from SCI, it captures many basic disability areas.

FIM consists of 13 motor and 5 cognitive items that are individually scored from 1 to 7. A score of 1 indicates complete dependence and a score of 7 indicates complete independence (Table 41-1). The sum of the 13 FIM motor score items can range from 13, indicating complete dependence for all items, to 91, indicating complete independence for all items. FIM is a measure usually completed by healthcare professionals; different observers, including the patient, family members, and caregivers, can contribute information to the ratings. Each of these reporters may represent a different type of potential bias.

Although the sample sizes of FIM data for certain neurological level groups are quite small, the consistency of the data adds confidence to the interpretation. Other pertinent data regarding functional independence must be factored into outcome analyses, including medical information, patient factors, social role participation, quality of life, and environmental factors and supports.

In Table 41-1, FIM data, when available, are reported in three areas. First, the expected FIM outcomes are documented based on expert clinical consensus. The second number reported is the median FIM score, as compiled by NSCISC. The interquartile range for NSCISC FIM data is the third set of numbers. In total, the FIM data represent 1-year postinjury FIM assessments of 405 survivors with complete SCI and a median age of 27 years. The NSCISC sample size for FIM and Assistance Data is provided for each level of injury. Different outcome expectations should clearly apply to different patient subgroups and populations. Some populations are likely to be significantly older than the referenced one. Functional abilities may be limited by advancing age.[15,19]

■ *Home modifications.* To provide the best opportunity for individuals with SCI to achieve the identified functional outcomes, a safe and architecturally accessible environment is necessary. An accessible environment must take into consideration, but not be limited to, entrance and egress, mobility in the home, and adequate setup to perform personal care and homemaking tasks.

Text continued on p. 790

TABLE 41-1

Expected Functional Outcomes

	Expected Functional Outcomes	Equipment	FIM/Assistance Data		
			Exp	Med	IR

Level C1-3

Functionally relevant muscles innervated: sternocleidomastoid: cervical paraspinal; neck accessories
Movement possible: neck flexion, extension, rotation
Patterns of weakness: total paralysis of trunk, upper extremities, lower extremities; dependent on ventilator
NSCISC sample size: FIM = 15\assist = 12

	Expected Functional Outcomes	Equipment	Exp	Med	IR
Respiratory	Ventilator dependent Inability to clear secretions	Two ventilators (bedside, portable) Suction equipment or other suction management device Generator/battery backup			
Bowel	Total assist	Padded reclining shower/commode chair (if roll-in shower available)	1	1	1
Bladder	Total assist		1	1	1
Bed Mobility	Total assist	Full electric hospital bed with Trendelenburg feature and side rails	1	1	1
Bed/wheelchair transfers	Total assist	Transfer board Power or mechanical lift with sling	1	1	1
Pressure relief/positioning	Total assist; may be independent with equipment	Power recline and/or tilt wheelchair Wheelchair pressure-relief cushion Postural support and head control devices as indicated Hand splints may be indicated Specialty bed or pressure-relief mattress may be indicated			
Eating	Total assist		1	1	1
Dressing	Total assist		1	1	1
Grooming	Total assist		1	1	1
Bathing	Total assist	Handheld shower Shampoo tray Padded reclining shower/commode chair (if roll-in shower available)	1	1	1
Wheelchair propulsion	Manual: total assist Power: independent with equipment	Power recline and/or tilt wheelchair with head, chin, or breath control and manual recliner Vent tray	6	1	1-6
Standing/ambulation	Standing: total assist Ambulation: not indicated				
Communication	Total assist to independent, depending on work station setup and equipment availability	Mouth stick, high-tech computer access, environmental control unit Adaptive devices everywhere as indicated			
Transportation	Total assist	Attendant-operated van (e.g., lift, tie downs) or accessible public transportation			
Homemaking	Total assist				
Assist required	24-hour attendant care to include homemaking Able to instruct in all aspects of care		24*	24*	12-24*

From Consortium for Spinal Cord Medicine, Paralyzed Veterans of America: *Outcomes following traumatic spinal cord injury: clinical practice guidelines for health-care professionals,* Washington, D.C., 1999, The Consortium. (Carole Adler was a member of the guideline development panel.)

FIM/assistance data: *Exp,* expected FIM score; *Med,* NSCISC median; *IR,* NSCISC Interquartile Range.

*Hours per day

TABLE 41-1—cont'd
Expected Functional Outcomes

	Expected Functional Outcomes	Equipment	FIM/Assistance Data		
			Exp	Med	IR
Level C4					

Functionally relevant muscles innervated: upper trapezius; diaphragm; cervical paraspinal muscles
Movement possible: neck flexion, extension, rotation; scapular elevation; inspiration
Patterns of weakness: paralysis of trunk, upper extremities, lower extremities; inability to cough, endurance and respiratory reserve low secondary to paralysis of intercostals
NSCISC sample size: FIM = 28/assist = 12

	Expected Functional Outcomes	Equipment	Exp	Med	IR
Respiratory	May be able to breathe without a ventilator	If not ventilator free, see C1-3 for equipment requirements			
Bowel	Total assist	Reclining shower/commode chair (if roll-in shower available)	1	1	1
Bladder	Total assist		1	1	1
Bed mobility	Total assist	Full electric hospital bed with Trendelenburg feature and side rails			
Bed/wheelchair transfers	Total assist	Transfer board Power or mechanical lift with sling	1	1	1
Pressure relief/positioning	Total assist; may be independent with equipment	Power recline and/or tilt wheelchair Wheelchair pressure-relief cushion Postural support and head control devices as indicated Hand splints may be indicated Specialty bed or pressure-relief mattress may be indicated			
Eating	Total assist		1	1	1
Dressing	Total assist		1	1	1
Grooming	Total assist		1	1	1
Bathing	Total assist	Shampoo tray Handheld shower Padded reclining shower/commode chair (if roll-in shower available)	1	1	1
Wheelchair propulsion	Power: independent Manual: total assist	Power recline and/or tilt wheelchair with head, chin, or breath control and manual recliner Vent tray	6	1	1-6
Standing/ambulation	Standing: total assist Ambulation: not usually indicated	Tilt table Hydraulic standing table			
Communication	Total assist to independent, depending on work station setup and equipment availability	Mouth stick, high-tech computer access, environmental control unit			
Transportation	Total assist	Attendant-operated van (e.g., lift, tie-downs) or accessible public transportation			
Homemaking	Total assist				

From Consortium for Spinal Cord Medicine, Paralyzed Veterans of America: *Outcomes following traumatic spinal cord injury: clinical practice guidelines for health-care professionals,* Washington, D.C., 1999, The Consortium. (Carole Adler was a member of the guideline development panel.)
FIM/assistance data: *Exp,* expected FIM score; *Med,* NSCISC median; *IR,* NSCISC Interquartile Range.
*Hours per day

Continued

TABLE 41-1—cont'd
Expected Functional Outcomes

	Expected Functional Outcomes	Equipment	FIM/Assistance Data		
			Exp	Med	IR
Assist required	24-hour attendant care to include homemaking Able to instruct in all aspects of care		24*	24*	16-24*

Level C5

Functionally relevant muscles innervated: deltoid, biceps, brachialis, brachioradialis, rhomboids, serratus anterior (partially innervated)
Movement possible: shoulder flexion, abduction, and extension; elbow flexion and supination; scapular adduction and abduction
Patterns of weakness: absence of elbow extension, pronation, all wrist and hand movement; total paralysis of trunk and lower extremities
NSCISC Sample size: FIM = 41/assist = 35

	Expected Functional Outcomes	Equipment	Exp	Med	IR
Respiratory	Low endurance and vital capacity caused by paralysis of intercostals; may require assist to clear secretions				
Bowel	Total assist	Padded shower/commode chair or padded transfer tub bench with commode cutout	I	I	I
Bladder	Total assist	Adaptive devices may be indicated (electric leg bag emptier)	I	I	I
Bed mobility	Some assist	Full electric hospital bed with Trendelenburg feature with patient control Side rails			
Bed/wheelchair transfers	Total assist	Transfer board Power or mechanical lift	I	I	I
Pressure relief/positioning	Independent with equipment	Power recline and/or tilt wheelchair Wheelchair pressure-relief cushion Hand splints Specialty bed or pressure-relief mattress may be indicated Postural support devices			
Eating	Total assist for setup, then independent eating with equipment	Long opponens splint Adaptive devices as indicated	5	5	2.5-5.5
Dressing	Lower extremity: total assist Upper extremity: some assist	Long opponens splint Adaptive devices as indicated	I	I	I-4
Grooming	Some to total assist	Long opponens splint Adaptive devices as indicated	I-3	I	I-5
Bathing	Total assist	Padded tub transfer bench or shower/commode chair Handheld shower	I	I	I-3
Wheelchair propulsion	Power: independent Manual: independent to some assist indoors on noncarpeted, level surface; some to total assist outdoors	Power recline and/or tilt with arm drive control Manual: lightweight rigid or folding frame with handrim modifications	6	6	5-6
Standing/ambulation	Total assist	Hydraulic standing table			

From Consortium for Spinal Cord Medicine, Paralyzed Veterans of America: *Outcomes following traumatic spinal cord injury: clinical practice guidelines for health-care professionals,* Washington, D.C., 1999, The Consortium. (Carole Adler was a member of the guideline development panel.)
FIM/assistance data: *Exp,* expected FIM score; *Med,* NSCISC median; *IR,* NSCISC Interquartile Range.
*Hours per day

TABLE 41-1—cont'd
Expected Functional Outcomes

	Expected Functional Outcomes	Equipment	FIM/Assistance Data		
			Exp	Med	IR
Communication	Independent to some assist after setup with equipment	Long opponens splint Adaptive devices as needed for page turning, writing, button pushing			
Transportation	Independent with highly specialized equipment; some assist with accessible public transportation; total assist for attendant-operated vehicle	Highly specialized modified van with lift			
Homemaking	Total assist				
Assist Required	Personal care: 10 hours/day Homecare: 6 hours/day Able to instruct in all aspects of care		16*	23*	10-24*

Level C6

Functionally relevant muscles innervated: clavicular pectoralis; supinator; extensor carpi radialis longus and brevis; serratus anterior; latissimus dorsi
Movement possible: scapular protractor; some horizontal adduction, forearm supination, radial wrist extension
Patterns of weakness: absence of wrist flexion, elbow extension, hand movement; total paralysis of trunk and lower extremities
NSCISC sample size: FIM = 43/assist = 35

	Expected Functional Outcomes	Equipment	Exp	Med	IR
Respiratory	Low endurance and vital capacity secondary to paralysis of intercostals; may require assist to clear secretions				
Bowel	Some total assist	Padded tub bench with commode cutout or padded shower/commode chair Other adaptive devices as indicated	1-2	1	1
Bladder	Some total assist with equipment; may be independent with leg bag emptying	Adaptive devices as indicated	1-2	1	1
Bed mobility	Some assist	Full electric hospital bed Side rails Full to king standard bed may be indicated			
Bed/wheelchair transfers	Level: some assist to independent Uneven: some to total assist	Transfer board Mechanical lift	3	1	1-3
Pressure relief/positioning	Independent with equipment and/or adapted techniques	Power recline wheelchair Wheelchair pressure-relief cushion Postural support devices Pressure-relief mattress or overlay may be indicated			
Eating	Independent with or without equipment; except cutting, which is total assist	Adaptive devices as indicated (e.g., U-cuff, tendenosis splint, adapted utensils, plate guard)	5-6	5	4-6
Dressing	Independent upper extremity; some assist to total assist for lower extremities	Adaptive devices as indicated (e.g., button-hook; loops on zippers, pants; socks, velcro on shoes)	1-3	2	1-5

From Consortium for Spinal Cord Medicine, Paralyzed Veterans of America: *Outcomes following traumatic spinal-cord injury: clinical practice guidelines for health-care professionals*, Washington, D.C., 1999, The Consortium. (Carole Adler was a member of the guideline development panel.)
FIM/assistance data: *Exp*, expected FIM score; *Med*, NSCISC median; *IR*, NSCISC Interquartile Range.
*Hours per day

Continued

TABLE 41-1—cont'd
Expected Functional Outcomes

	Expected Functional Outcomes	Equipment	FIM/Assistance Data		
			Exp	**Med**	**IR**
Grooming	Some assist to independent with equipment	Adaptive devices as indicated (e.g., U-cuff, adapted handles)	3-6	4	2-6
Bathing	Upper body: independent Lower body: some to total assist	Padded tub transfer bench or shower/commode chair Adaptive devices as needed Handheld shower	1-3	1	1-3
Wheelchair propulsion	Power: independent with standard arm drive on all surfaces Manual: independent indoors; some total assist outdoors	Manual: lightweight rigid or folding frame with modified rims Power: may require power recline or standard upright power wheelchair	6	6	4-6
Standing/ambulation	Standing: total assist Ambulation: not indicated	Hydraulic standing frame			
Communication	Independent with or without equipment	Adaptive devices as indicated (e.g., tendenosis splint; writing splint for keyboard use, button pushing, page turning, object manipulation)			
Transportation	Independent driving from wheelchair	Modified van with lift Sensitized hand controls Tie-downs			
Homemaking	Some assist with light meal preparation; total assist for all other homemaking	Adaptive devices as indicated			
Assist Required	Personal care: 6 hours/day Homecare: 4 hours/day		10*	17*	8-24*

Level C7-8

Functionally relevant muscles innervated: latissimus dorsi; sternal pectoralis; triceps; pronator quadratus; extensor carpi ulnaris; flexor carpi radialis; flexor digitorum profundus and superficialis; extensor communis; pronator/flexor/extensor/abductor pollicis; lumbricals (partially innervated)

Movement possible: elbow extension; ulnar/wrist extension; wrist flexion; finger flexions and extensions; thumb flexion/extension/abduction

Patterns of weakness: paralysis of trunk and lower extremities; limited grasp and dexterity secondary to partial intrinsic muscles of the hand

NSCISC sample size: FIM = 43/assist = 35

Respiratory	Low endurance and vital capacity secondary to paralysis of intercostals; may require assist to clear secretions				
Bowel	Some to total assist	Padded tub bench with commode cutout or shower/commode chair Adaptive devices as indicated	1-4	1	1-4
Bladder	Independent to some assist	Adaptive devices as indicated	2-6	3	1-6
Bed mobility	Independent to some assist	Full electric hospital bed or full to king standard bed			

From Consortium for Spinal Cord Medicine, Paralyzed Veterans of America: *Outcomes following traumatic spinal cord injury: clinical practice guidelines for health-care professionals,* Washington, D.C., 1999, The Consortium. (Carole Adler was a member of the guideline development panel.)
FIM/assistance data: *Exp,* expected FIM score; *Med,* NSCISC median; *IR,* NSCISC Interquartile Range.
*Hours per day

TABLE 41-1—cont'd
Expected Functional Outcomes

	Expected Functional Outcomes	Equipment	FIM/Assistance Data		
			Exp	Med	IR
Bed/wheelchair transfers	Level: independent Uneven: independent to some assist	With or without transfer board	3-7	4	2-6
Pressure relief/positioning	Independent	Wheelchair pressure-relief cushion Postural support devices as indicated Pressure-relief mattress or overlay may be indicated			
Eating	Independent	Adaptive devices as indicated	6-7	6	5-7
Dressing	Independent in upper extremities; independent to some assist in lower extremities	Adaptive devices as indicated	4-7	6	4-7
Grooming	Independent	Adaptive devices as indicated	6-7	6	4-7
Bathing	Upper body: independent Lower body: some assist to independent	Padded tub transfer tub bench or shower/commode chair Handheld shower Adaptive devices as needed	3-6	4	2-6
Wheelchair propulsion	Manual: independent on all indoor surfaces and level outdoor terrain; some assist with uneven terrain	Manual: rigid or folding lightweight or folding wheelchair with modified rims	6	6	6
Standing/ambulation	Standing: independent to some assist Ambulation: not indicated	Hydraulic or standard standing frame			
Communication	Independent	Adaptive devices as indicated			
Transportation	Independent in car if independent with transfer and wheelchair loading/unloading; independent in driving modified van from captain's seat	Modified vehicle Transfer board			
Homemaking	Independent light meal preparation and homemaking; some to total assist for complex meal preparation and heavy housecleaning	Adaptive devices as indicated			
Assist required	Personal care: 6 hours/day Homecare: 2 hours/day		8*	12*	2-24*

Level T1-9

Functionally relevant muscles innervated: intrinsics of the hand including thumbs; internal and external intercostals; erector spinae; lumbricals; flexor/extensor/abductor pollicis

Movement possible: upper extremities fully intact; limited upper trunk stability; endurance increased secondary to innervation of intercostals

Patterns of weakness: lower trunk paralysis; total paralysis of lower extremities

NSCISC sample size: FIM = 144/assist = 122

Respiratory	Compromised vital capacity and endurance				
Bowel	Independent	Elevated padded toilet seat or padded tub bench with commode cutout	6-7	6	4-6

From Consortium for Spinal Cord Medicine, Paralyzed Veterans of America: *Outcomes following traumatic spinal cord injury: clinical practice guidelines for health-care professionals*, Washington, D.C., 1999, The Consortium. (Carole Adler was a member of the guideline development panel.)
FIM/assistance data: *Exp,* expected FIM score; *Med,* NSCISC median; *IR,* NSCISC Interquartile Range.
*Hours per day

Continued

TABLE 41-1—cont'd
Expected Functional Outcomes

	Expected Functional Outcomes	Equipment	FIM/Assistance Data		
			Exp	**Med**	**IR**
Bladder	Independent		6	6	5-6
Bed mobility	Independent	Full to king standard bed			
Bed/wheelchair transfers	Independent	May or may not require transfer board	6-7	6	6-7
Pressure relief/positioning	Independent	Wheelchair pressure-relief cushion Postural support devices as indicated Pressure-relief mattress or overlay may be indicated			
Eating	Independent		7	7	7
Dressing	Independent		7	7	7
Grooming	Independent		7	7	7
Bathing	Independent	Padded tub transfer bench or shower/commode chair Handheld shower	6-7	6	5-7
Wheelchair propulsion	Independent	Manual rigid or folding lightweight wheelchair	6	6	6
Standing/ambulation	Standing: independent Ambulation: typically not functional	Standing frame			
Communication	Independent				
Transportation	Independent in car, including loading and unloading wheelchair	Hand controls			
Homemaking	Independent with complex meal preparation and light housecleaning; total to some assist with heavy housecleaning				
Assist Required	Homemaking: 3 hours/day		2*	3*	0-15*

Level T10-L1

Functionally relevant muscles innervated: fully intact intercostals; external obliques; rectus abdominis
Movement Possible: food trunk stability
Patterns of weakness: paralysis of lower extremities
NSCISC Sample Size: FIM = 71/assist = 57

Respiratory	Intact respiratory function				
Bowel	Independent	Padded standard or raised padded toilet seat	6-7	6	6
Bladder	Independent		6	6	6
Bed mobility	Independent	Full to king standard bed			
Bed/wheelchair transfers	Independent		7	7	6-7

From Consortium for Spinal Cord Medicine, Paralyzed Veterans of America: *Outcomes following traumatic spinal cord injury: clinical practice guidelines for health-care professionals*, Washington, D.C., 1999, The Consortium. (Carole Adler was a member of the guideline development panel.)
FIM/assistance data: *Exp*, expected FIM score; *Med*, NSCISC median; *IR*, NSCISC Interquartile Range.
*Hours per day

TABLE 41-1—cont'd
Expected Functional Outcomes

	Expected Functional Outcomes	Equipment	FIM/Assistance Data		
			Exp	Med	IR
Pressure relief/positioning	Independent	Wheelchair pressure-relief cushion Postural support devices as indicated Pressure-relief mattress or overlay may be indicated			
Eating	Independent		7	7	7
Dressing	Independent		7	7	7
Grooming	Independent		7	7	7
Bathing	Independent	Padded transfer tub bench Handheld shower	6-7	6	6-7
Wheelchair propulsion	Independent all indoor and outdoor surfaces	Manual rigid or folding lightweight wheelchair	6	6	6
Standing/ambulation	Standing: independent Ambulation: functional, some assist to independent	Standing frame Forearm crutches or walker Knee, ankle, foot orthosis (KAFO)			
Communication	Independent				
Transportation	Independent in car, including loading and unloading wheelchair	Hand controls			
Homemaking	Independent with complex meal prep and light housecleaning; some assist with heavy housecleaning				
Assist required	Homemaking: 2 hours/day		2*	2*	0-8*

Level L2-S5

Functionally relevant muscles innervated: fully intact abdominals and all other trunk muscles; depending on level, some degree of hip flexors, extensor, abductors; knee flexors, extensors; ankle dorsiflexors, plantar flexors.
Movement possible: good trunk stability; partial to full control of lower extremities.
Patterns of weakness: partial paralysis of lower extremities, hips, knees, ankle, foot
NSCISC sample size: FIM = 20/assist = 16

Respiratory	Intact function				
Bowel	Independent	Padded toilet seat	6-7	6	6-7
Bladder	Independent		6	6	6-7
Bed mobility	Independent				
Bed/wheelchair transfers	Independent	Full to king standard bed	7	7	7
Pressure relief/positioning	Independent	Wheelchair pressure-relief cushion Postural support devices as indicated			
Eating	Independent		7	7	7
Dressing	Independent		7	7	7
Grooming	Independent		7	7	7

From Consortium for Spinal Cord Medicine, Paralyzed Veterans of America: *Outcomes following traumatic spinal cord injury: clinical practice guidelines for health-care professionals,* Washington, D.C., 1999, The Consortium. (Carole Adler was a member of the guideline development panel.)
FIM/assistance data: *Exp,* expected FIM score; *Med,* NSCISC median; *IR,* NSCISC Interquartile Range.
*Hours per day

Continued

TABLE 41-1—cont'd
Expected Functional Outcomes

	Expected Functional Outcomes	Equipment	FIM/Assistance Data		
			Exp	Med	IR
Bathing	Independent	Padded tub bench Handheld shower	7	7	6-7
Wheelchair propulsion	Independent all indoor and outdoor surfaces	Manual rigid or folding lightweight wheelchair	6	6	6
Standing/ambulation	Standing: independent Ambulation: functional, independent to some assist	Standing frame Knee-ankle-foot orthosis (KAFO) or ankle-foot orthosis (AFO) Forearm crutches or cane as indicated			
Communication	Independent				
Transportation	Independent in car, including loading and unloading wheelchair	Hand controls			
Homemaking	Independent with complex meal preparation and light housecleaning; some assist with heavy housecleaning				
Assist required	Homemaking: 0-1 hour/day		0-1*	0*	0*

From Consortium for Spinal Cord Medicine, Paralyzed Veterans of America: *Outcomes following traumatic spinal cord injury: clinical practice guidelines for health-care professionals*, Washington, D.C., 1999, The Consortium. (Carole Adler was a member of the guideline development panel.)
FIM/assistance data: *Exp*, expected FIM score; *Med*, NSCISC median; *IR*, NSCISC Interquartile Range.
*Hours per day

TABLE 41-2
Functional Independence Measure Levels

(7) Complete independence (timely, safely)	No helper
(6) Modified independence (device)	
Modified Dependence	Helper
(5) Supervision	
(4) Minimal assist (subject = 75% or more)	
(3) Moderate assist (subject = 50% to 74%)	
Complete Dependence	
(2) Maximal assist (subject = 25%-49%)	
(1) Total assist (subject = 0%-24%)	

From *Guide for the uniform data set for medical rehabilitation (including the FIM instrument)*, Version 5.0, Buffalo, NY, State University of New York at Buffalo

REVIEW QUESTIONS

1. List three causes of spinal cord injury. Which is most common?
2. Describe the patterns of weakness in quadriplegia and paraplegia.
3. Describe the functional and prognostic differences between complete and incomplete lesions.
4. When reference is made to C5 in quadriplegia, what is meant in terms of level of injury and functioning muscle groups?
5. What are the characteristics of spinal shock?
6. What physical changes occur following the spinal shock phase?
7. What is the prognosis for recovery of motor function in complete lesions and incomplete lesions?
8. What are the purposes of surgery in management of spinal injury?
9. What are some medical complications, common to patients with spinal cord injuries, that can limit achievement of functional potential?
10. How should postural hypotension be treated?
11. How should autonomic dysreflexia be treated?
12. What is the role of the occupational therapist in the prevention of pressure sores?
13. Why is vital capacity affected in patients with spinal cord injuries?
14. What effect does reduced vital capacity have on the rehabilitation program?
15. Which level of injury has full innervation of the rotator cuff musculature, biceps, and extensor carpi radialis and partial innervation of the serratus anterior, latissimus dorsi, and pectoralis major?

16. What additional muscle power does the patient with C6 quadriplegia have over the patient with C5 quadriplegia? What is the major functional advantage of this additional muscle power?

17. What are the additional critical muscles that the patient with C7 quadriplegia has, as compared with the patient with C6 quadriplegia?

18. What additional functional independence can be achieved because of this additional muscle power?

19. What is the first spinal cord lesion level that has full innervation of the UE musculature?

20. Which assessments does the occupational therapist use to evaluate the patient with a spinal cord injury? What is the purpose of each?

21. List five goals of occupational therapy for the patient with a spinal cord injury.

22. How is wrist extension used to effect grasp by the patient with quadriplegia?

23. How does the patient with C6 quadriplegia substitute for the absence of elbow extensors?

24. What is the contracture that is encouraged in patients with spinal cord injuries? Why? How is it developed?

25. What is the splint that allows the C6 quadriplegic to achieve functional prehension?

26. What are some of the first self-care activities that the patient with a C6 spinal cord injury should be expected to accomplish?

27. List four assistive devices commonly used by persons with quadriplegia, and tell the purpose of each.

28. How can ordering an ill-fitting wheelchair affect the UE function and skin care of a C6 quadriplegic?

29. Describe the role of occupational therapy in the vocational evaluation of a patient with a spinal cord injury.

30. What are two considerations when predicting the future functional outcomes for a 25-year-old individual with T4 paraplegia?

31. Why would a person with paraplegia require homemaking assistance if he is independent in all self-care and mobility?

REFERENCES

1. Amador J: Contemporarary information regarding male infertility following spinal cord injury, SCI Nursing 15(3):61-65, 1998.
2. American Spinal Injury Association (ASIA): Standards for neurological and functional classification of spinal cord injury, Chicago, 1992, The Association.
3. Bromley I: Tetraplegia and paraplegia: a guide for physiotherapists, ed 3, New York, 1985, Churchill Livingstone.
4. Frankel H and associates: The value of postural reduction in the initial management of closed injuries to the spine with paraplegia and tetraplegia, Paraplegia 7:179, 1969.
5. Freed MM: Traumatic and congenital lesions of the spinal cord. In Kottke FJ, Lehmann JF, editors: Krusen's handbook of physical medicine and rehabilitation, Philadelphia, 1990, WB Saunders.
6. Gerhart KA, Koziol-McClain J, Lowenstein SR, et al: Quality of life following spinal cord injury: knowledge and attitudes of emergency care providers, Ann Emerg Med 23(4):807-812, 1994.
7. Hanak M, Scott A: An illustrated guide for health care professionals, New York, 1983, Springer-Verlag.
8. Heinemann AW et al: Mobility for persons with spinal cord injury: an evaluation of two systems, Arch Phys Med Rehabil 68(2):90-93, 1987.
9. Hill JP, editor: Spinal cord injury, a guide to functional outcomes in occupational therapy, Rockville, Md, 1986, Aspen.
10. Institute for Medical Research, Santa Clara Valley Medical Center: Severe head trauma, a comprehensive medical approach, Project 13-9-59156/9, report to National Institute for Handicapped Research, Nov 1982.
11. Malick MH, Meyer CMH: Manual on the management of the quadriplegic upper extremity, Pittsburgh, 1978, Harmarville Rehabilitation Center.
12. Consortium for Spinal Cord Medicine, Paralyzed Veterans of America: Outcomes following traumatic spinal cord injury: clinical practice guidelines for health-care professionals, Washington, D.C., 1999, The Consortium.
13. Paulson S, editor: Santa Clara Valley Medical Center spinal cord injury home care manual, ed 3, San Jose, Calif, 1994, Santa Clara Valley Medical Center.
14. Pierce DS, Nickel VH: The total care of spinal cord injuries, Boston, 1977, Little, Brown.
15. Penrod LE, Hegde SK, Ditunno JF Jr: Age effect on prognosis for functional recovery in acute traumatic central cord syndrome (CCS), Arch Phys Med Rehabil 71(12):963-968, 1990.
16. Spencer EA: Functional restoration. In Hopkins HL, Smith HD, editors: Willard and Spackman's occupational therapy, ed 8, Philadelphia, 1993, JB Lippincott.
17. Whiteneck G et al, editors: Aging with spinal cord injury, New York, 1993, Demos.
18. Wilson DJ, McKenzie MW, Barber LM: Spinal cord injury: a treatment guide for occupational therapists, rev ed, Thorofare, NJ, 1984, Slack.
19. Yarkony GM, Roth EJ, Heinemann AW, et al: Spinal cord injury rehabilitation outcomes: the impact of age, J Clin Epidemiol 41(2):173-177, 1988.
20. Yarkony GM: Spinal cord injury: medical management and rehabilitation, Gaithersburg, Md, 1994, Aspen.

CHAPTER 42

Neurogenic and Myopathic Dysfunction

REGINA M. LEHMAN
GUY L. McCORMACK

KEY TERMS

Neurogenic
Myopathic
Motor unit
Lower motor neuron dysfunction
Poliomyelitis
Contracture
Postpolio syndrome
Guillian-Barré syndrome
Peripheral nerve injury
Neuropraxia
Neurotmesis
Axonotmesis
Atrophy
Regeneration
Paresthesias
Wrinkle test
Causalgia
Peripheral nerve pain syndrome
Nociceptors
Myasthenia gravis
Muscular dystrophy

LEARNING OBJECTIVES

After studying this chapter the student or practitioner will be able to do the following:
1. Describe the characteristics of neurogenic and myopathic dysfunctions.
2. Discuss the clinical manifestations of neurogenic and myopathic dysfunctions.
3. Discuss the impact of neurogenic and myopathic dysfunctions on physical and psychosocial function.
4. Identify the goals and treatment techniques for an occupational therapy program for the various neurogenic and myopathic dysfunctions

The symptoms, course, medical treatment, and occupational therapy (OT) intervention for the **neurogenic** and **myopathic** disorders most commonly seen in OT practice are presented in this chapter. Neurogenic and myopathic disorders are diseases of the motor unit. The **motor unit** is the elementary functional unit in the motor system. It consists of four elements: the cell body of the motor neuron in the anterior horn of the spinal cord, the axon of the motor neuron which travels via spinal nerves and peripheral nerves to muscle, the neuro-muscular junction, and the muscle fibers innervated by the neuron.

Diseases of the motor unit generally cause muscle weakness and atrophy of skeletal muscle that may be of neurogenic or myopathic origin. Those with a neurogenic basis are the lower motor neuron disorders, affecting the cell bodies, and peripheral neuropathies, affecting peripheral nerves. Those with a myopathic basis affect the neuromuscular junction or the muscle itself.[34]

NEUROGENIC DISORDERS

The motor neurons in the anterior horn cells of the spinal cord mediate all voluntary movement and reflexes that promote motor behavior. Variations in range of motion, muscle strength, and the characteristics of movement are determined by the pattern and firing frequency of specific motor units. Therefore muscle contraction is the output of the motor system.

The lower motor neuron system includes the cell bodies in the anterior horn of the spinal cord and their axons (which pass by way of the spinal nerves and peripheral nerves to the neuromuscular junction) and the nuclei of cranial nerves III through X (located in the brainstem) and their axons.[8,10] The motor fibers of the lower motor neurons are divided into the somatic and autonomic components. The somatic motor components include the alpha motor neurons, which innervate skeletal muscles (extrafusal fibers), and gamma motor neurons, which innervate muscle spindles (intrafusal fibers). The autonomic component innervates the glands, smooth muscles, and heart musculature.[9,35] A lesion to any of these neurological structures results in neurogenic motor unit disease or a **lower motor neuron dysfunction**.[9,34]

Lesions of lower motor neuron systems may be located in the anterior horn cells of the spinal cord, spinal nerves, peripheral nerves, and cranial nerves or their nuclei in the brainstem. Such lesions can result from nerve root compression; trauma (e.g., bone fractures and dislocations, lacerations, traction, or penetrating wounds and friction); toxins (e.g., lead, phosphorus, alcohol, benzene, or sulfonamides); infections (e.g., poliomyelitis or Guillain-Barré syndrome); neoplasms (e.g., neuromas and multiple neurofibromatosis); vascular disorders (e.g., arteriosclerosis, diabetes mellitus, peripheral vascular anomalies, and polyarteritis nodosa); degenerative diseases of the central nervous systems (e.g., amyotrophic lateral sclerosis); and congenital malformations.[10,18,45,50]

Poliomyelitis

The active immunization program (Salk and Sabin vaccines) in the United States since the mid-1950s has essentially eradicated poliomyelitis in the Western Hemisphere, and new cases of the disease are rare.[45,53] However, some new cases have been identified among persons who have not been immunized.

Poliomyelitis is a contagious viral disease that affects the anterior horn cells of the gray matter of the spinal cord and the motor nuclei of the brainstem. The cervical and lumbar enlargements of the cord are primarily affected. Poliomyelitis results in a flaccid paralysis that may be local or widespread. The lower extremities, accessory muscles of respiration, and muscles that promote swallowing are primarily affected, but there

may also be upper extremity involvement. Marked atrophy may be seen in the involved extremities, and deep tendon reflexes may be absent. Because poliomyelitis destroys the anterior horn cells, sensory roots are spared and sensation is intact. **Contractures** can occur early in the course of the disease. In cases of local paralysis the asymmetry of muscles pulling on various joints may promote deformities, such as subluxation, scoliosis, and contractures. In severe cases osteoporosis (bone atrophy) may weaken the long weight-bearing bones and pathological fractures can occur.[26]

The medical treatment for poliomyelitis during the acute phase involves bed rest, positioning, and applications of warm packs to reduce pain and promote relaxation. Because there is no known cure for poliomyelitis, the disease must run its course. It has an incubation period of 1 to 3 weeks, and recovery depends on the number of nerve cells destroyed. Paralysis may begin in 1 to 7 days after the initial symptoms appear. The medical aspects of rehabilitation include reconstructive surgery, such as tendon transfer, arthrodesis, and surgical release of fascia, muscles, and tendons. Other medical procedures include therapeutic stretching, casts, muscle reeducation, orthoses, and bracing for standing or stability.[20]

Postpolio Syndrome

Occupational therapists are seeing more patients with **postpolio syndrome** in rehabilitation centers. Persons who had polio earlier in life may have the onset of additional weakness and other disabling symptoms years after the initial disease.[45,53] The number of such persons has increased, in part, because of the influx of immigrants from Southeast Asia and Latin America who contracted the original infection in their native lands.[15]

The cause of postpolio syndrome is not fully understood. Motor unit dysfunction, musculoskeletal overuse, and musculoskeletal disuse are three factors, thought to contribute, singly or in combination, to the onset of postpolio syndrome.[15] Several theories have been postulated about the cause of postpolio syndrome; however, none has proved to be the explanation for the syndrome. Postpolio syndrome causes health and functional problems, and patients who are affected are likely to be referred for OT services.[53]

The primary symptom of postpolio syndrome is progressive weakness.[15] Muscles that were thought to be spared in the original illness may exhibit slowly progressive weakness, as well as previously affected muscles. Pain, fatigue, cold intolerance, and new breathing difficulties may accompany the muscle weakness. Such musculoskeletal problems as joint, limb, or trunk deformities can cause pain, decreased endurance, nerve entrapment, degenerative arthritis, falls, and unsteady gait.[53]

Fatigue is the most debilitating symptom because it limits activity, yet is not apparent to others. The fatigue may be severe and out of proportion to the apparent physical demands of the activity and can be overwhelming.[15,53] An increase in difficulties with activities of daily living (ADL) accompanies the symptoms. Problems with ambulation, transfers, using stairs, home management, driving, dressing, eating and swallowing, and bladder and bowel control may occur.[53]

Unless there is severe pulmonary or swallowing involvement in postpolio syndrome, the symptoms are not life threatening. The symptoms can range from very mild weakness that is only slightly annoying to profound weakness that is severely incapacitating, with risks of additional disabling problems such as fractures, osteoporosis, contractures, and depression. In general, however, patients who adjust their lifestyles by incorporating the recommendations that prevent muscle fatigue, improve body mechanics, and conserve energy will have an improvement of symptoms and stabilization of function.[15] OT has an important role to play in achieving these goals.[53]

Guillain-Barré Syndrome

Guillain-Barré syndrome (also known as acute idiopathic neuropathy, infectious polyneuritis, and Landry's syndrome) is an acute inflammatory condition involving the spinal nerve roots, peripheral nerves, and in some cases selected cranial nerves. Guillain-Barré syndrome often follows a viral illness, immunization, or surgery. It produces a hypersensitive response resulting in patchy demyelination of lower motor neuron pathways. The axons are generally spared, so recovery often follows a predictable course. In severe cases, however, wallerian degeneration of the axon results in a slow recovery process. Guillain-Barré syndrome affects both sexes at any age.[6,8,18,36,41,42,45,50]

Guillain-Barré syndrome is characterized by a rapid onset. Initially there is no fever, but pain and tenderness of muscles, generalized weakness, and decrease in deep tendon reflexes occur. As the disease progresses, it produces motor weakness or paralysis of the limbs, sensory loss, and muscle atrophy. The prognosis is varied. In severe cases cranial nerves VII, IX, and X may be involved and the patient may have difficulty speaking, swallowing, and breathing. If vital centers in the medulla are affected, the patient may have respiratory failure and require tracheostomy or assisted ventilation. In most cases the patient recovers completely within a few weeks to a few months with relatively few residual effects.[18,45]

Occupational Therapy Intervention: Common Factors

Although specific strategies may be required for OT intervention for each of the neurogenic disorders, there are some similarities in both the evaluation process and the selection of therapeutic modalities. The occupational therapist assesses occupational performance, ADL, psychosocial and cognitive status, range of motion (ROM), muscle strength, and endurance. Functional activities are used in combination with passive and active ROM exercises, muscle reeducation, rest, proper positioning for function, and training in the use of assistive and adaptive devices and mobility aids. In all cases, fatigue is carefully monitored and avoided. Treatment goals should be coordinated with the nurse, physical therapist, and other members of the interdisciplinary team for a comprehensive rehabilitation program. Prognosis depends on the progression of the disorder.

Poliomyelitis

During the acute phase the poliomyelitis virus is infectious. Therefore all personnel involved in the care of the patient must carefully follow isolation procedures. During this phase the patient is confined to bed and receives symptomatic treatment. Hot packs and positioning are used to relieve muscle spasm and to prevent contracture and deformity. The therapist can assist the nurse in providing good bed positioning to prevent contractures and protect weakened muscles. The therapist should provide gentle passive ROM at the patient's physical tolerance level. Care should be taken not to grasp the involved muscle bellies because they will be extremely tender and painful. The muscles may also be prone to spasm when stimulated to the point of pain.[42]

Muscle fatigue, which can result in further weakness, should be avoided throughout the treatment program. If the patient has bulbar poliomyelitis, which affects the muscles of respiration, a respirator may be used or a tracheostomy performed to provide an airway. If the muscles necessary for swallowing are impaired, tube feeding may also be prescribed. The therapist should collaborate with the nursing staff when carrying out treatment to ensure proper functioning of the equipment necessary for life support.[8,20,23,42]

Psychological support for the patient and family is part of the treatment program. The patient's fears and anxieties about the disabling effects of the disease should not be underestimated. The patient may need encouragement and positive experiences to promote an optimistic outlook during the rehabilitation process. The family may also need assistance in adjusting to the patient's disability. Psychosocial issues may be addressed by the occupational therapist during treatment, with additional support from the psychologist sought as needed.

Assistive devices, splints, and mobile arm supports may be used to gain independence in daily activities. The long-range rehabilitation program should follow a functional course of action. After the acute medical problems have subsided, the recovery stage may last as long as 2 years.[8] Because the damage to the anterior horn cells is permanent, the therapist should help the patient make the best possible use of whatever muscular function remains. Manual muscle tests should be repeated monthly for the first 4 months and bimonthly for the next 4 months. After 8 months of therapeutic exercises the average patient has probably responded maximally.[6,18]

For the patient recovering from acute poliomyelitis, movement proceeds from passive to active ROM depending on the patient's level of voluntary control. Muscle reeducation should be preceded by gentle stretching exercises. All active motions should be performed under careful supervision of the therapist. Compensatory movement should be avoided. A limited but correct movement is preferred to an ampler but incorrect movement. Active movements should be performed in front of a mirror to enable the patient to monitor and correct motions accordingly.[20,23,41]

Muscle reeducation is accomplished in a graded fashion. At first the patient should learn "muscle-setting" exercises—that is, alternating contraction and relaxation of muscles without moving the joints. Isometric exercises and electromyographic (EMG) biofeedback may be beneficial. As the patient progresses, light resistance can be applied manually by the therapist before the use of resistance equipment. This approach allows the therapist to accurately assess the patient's physical strengths and weaknesses.

Weakened muscles must be protected at all times. Muscles that cannot resist the forces of gravity are supported during exercise and rest periods. As a rule, resistive exercises are not attempted until the muscle is able to carry out a complete ROM against gravity. Weakened or flaccid muscles can be splinted at night to counteract the forces of gravity or the pull of the stronger antagonist muscles. During resistive exercises the therapist should stress correct body positioning, joint alignment, and energy conservation. Periods of rest should be included in the exercise program. Functional activities that incorporate the same movements and musculature are encouraged.[14]

The goals for resistive exercises in the rehabilitation of the patient who has poliomyelitis are to strengthen undamaged muscles and give usefulness to the slightest contraction by integrating it into the global movement that permits the performance of a given activity. If the muscle is unable to contract completely against gravity after the 8-month period, it is doubtful that additional muscle strength will return. At this point the emphasis should be placed on maintenance of existing muscles and functional ADL. A self-care assessment should be administered to determine a baseline of functioning. Assistive devices should be tailored to meet the needs of the patient.[32]

Postpolio Syndrome

As part of the initial evaluation process, the therapist performs an interview with the patient to ascertain valued occupational roles and obtain an activity profile of daily life. Activities that cause pain or fatigue, those that have been curtailed or eliminated because of symptoms, the time and circumstances in which symptoms are most likely to occur, and the kinds of aids, equipment, and human assistance currently used are identified. This information is used to prioritize and select valued, relevant activities for the patient with postpolio syndrome.

Postpolio muscles may actually function at levels of strength lower than estimated from scores on the manual muscle test, and upper extremity strength varies markedly throughout the ROM.[53] Joint ROM measurements are important if the patient has contractures and muscle imbalances.

The psychosocial assessment will help the therapist select a treatment approach that will facilitate rehabilitation efforts and the patient's adjustment to new limitations. Changes in physical capacities and curtailment of valued life skills confront the individual with psychological issues of coping, adjustment, and adaptation. These changes may be as traumatic as they were at the time of the original illness. Feelings of denial, anger, frustration, and hopelessness must be identified and worked through as a part of the OT intervention program.[15]

As a group, persons who originally had polio assumed that the disease was over, that disability was in the past, and that any residual weakness was static. They worked hard to overcome the effects of the initial paralysis and often performed well, achieved high levels of personal fulfillment, became well integrated into society, and so "disappeared" as a disabled group. The onset of new symptoms disrupts the performance and lifestyle achieved by years of hard work. Such individuals must deal with the onset of new limitations, and old remedies do not work to ameliorate the effects of these limitations. It is often difficult for the patient to confront the reality of these circumstances. Thus, to facilitate changes in activity patterns and introduce needed equipment, the therapist should introduce these changes gradually. Small changes may be more acceptable than major ones, even if the latter are obviously necessary.[15]

The patient is confronted for a second time, years after the disability was thought to be stabilized, with the notion of being "disabled" and with a limitation of function and valued life activities. A supportive and realistic approach and patient education are the keys to lifestyle modification.[53]

The benefits of exercise are controversial. Exercise may aggravate pain. Overwork of muscles that have a decreased number of motor units may be damaging. Muscles weakened by disuse, however, may benefit from a nonfatiguing trial of gentle exercises for strengthening purposes. Strength may be maintained by performance of ADL. Muscles being used for ADL should not be stressed further.[53] Patients should be encouraged to be active within limits of comfort and safety. A regular routine of activity or nonfatiguing exercise is important and affords the patient the feeling of doing something positive. Exercise programs must be carefully supervised, and long-term strengthening or maintenance exercise is recommended only in muscles that show no EMG evidence of prior polio involvement. Further weakness, discomfort, pain, muscle spasm, and chronic fatigue resulting from exercise are signs of excessive activity.[15,53]

Pain can be managed or alleviated by improving body mechanics, supporting weakened muscles, and promoting lifestyle modification. The occupational therapist can teach correct body mechanics in such daily living tasks as work and home management, ambulation, and transfers. Orthoses are indicated for the support of weakened muscles, and lifestyle modification reduces fatigue, stress, and activity that can cause overuse of muscles. Weight reduction is necessary for some patients.[15]

Perhaps the most important contribution of the occupational therapist is the guiding and facilitating of lifestyle modifications. Patients must avoid overuse of muscles. Assessment and retraining in all aspects of ADL are important. Assistive devices for self-care and home management may be indicated. Home and workplace modifications can be important for preventing muscle overuse and decreasing fatigue and potential deformity. Energy conservation and work simplification techniques should be taught. The patient and therapist should set priorities on occupational role performance. Energy conservation for the most valued activities may mean allowing less valued ones to be performed by others or with the assistance of equipment such as orthoses, assistive devices, or ambulation aids.[53]

Guillian-Barré Syndrome

Rehabilitation is initiated once the patient is medically stabilized. The patient may be referred to OT while still totally paralyzed. During this initial phase of treatment, passive ROM, positioning, and splinting to prevent contracture and deformity and protect weak muscles are indicated. Passive activities such as watching television and light social activities such as visits from friends are encouraged. As improvement occurs and more active motion is possible, gentle, nonresistive activities and light ADL can be introduced to alleviate joint stiffness and muscle atrophy and prevent contractures. The activity program is graded according to the patient's physical tolerance level. Fatigue is avoided, and psychological support is provided.[42]

Since the assessment process itself may be fatiguing, it is best to spread it over the course of a few days. The manual muscle test or functional motion test should not be performed in one session. It is best to test a few muscles or motions at a time and allow the patient periods of rest.

Particular attention should be paid to determining residual weakness in the intrinsic muscles of the hands. If swallowing or speech is impaired, an assessment of cranial nerve functions is indicated (Chapter 40). Sensory testing, including light touch, pressure, two-point discrimination, pain and temperature, proprioception, and stereognosis, should be conducted because the sensory pathways are often affected.

Passive ROM should begin with gentle movement of the proximal joints and should proceed only to the point of pain. As the patient's tolerance level increases, active ROM and light exercises may be introduced. The exercise program should stress joint protection, and the therapist should look for muscle imbalance and substitution patterns. Progressive resistive exercises should be used conservatively. Throughout the course of recovery the therapist should guard against fatigue and irritation of the inflamed nerves. As the patient's strength and tolerance level increase, resistance can be gradually and moderately increased.

The therapist may also introduce sedentary or table-top activities during the early stages of recovery. As the patient's strength increases, activities promoting more resistance can be incorporated into the treatment regimen. Grooming, self-care, and other ADL should be included as soon as the patient is capable of some independence and should be graded to include more activities as strength and endurance improve. Slings and mobile arm supports may be used to alleviate muscle fatigue and promote independence. Activities should be varied between gross and fine and resistive and nonresistive to prevent undue fatigue.

Psychological support is important throughout the treatment program. The therapist should try to facilitate the feeling of self-worth, a positive attitude, and encouragement throughout the therapeutic process. Because the prognosis for recovery is good, the activities should be mentally stimulating and purposeful to the patient. The therapist should also respect the patient's level of pain tolerance during stretching and ROM exercises.[48]

Peripheral Nerve Injuries

General Characteristics

Trauma to the shoulder complex, upper extremity, or hand may result in **peripheral nerve injury.** Regardless of the origin of the injury, peripheral nerve lesions produce similar clinical manifestations. Specific clinical findings will vary with the underlying cause of the lesion. Peripheral nerve injuries may be placed in three categories: neuropraxia, neurotmesis, and axonotmesis.[37]

Neuropraxia is a nerve lesion that is usually caused by orthopedic injuries (e.g., compression, concussion, and traction injuries). It results in a block of neuronal transmission, usually in the larger myelinated nerve fibers. Although it produces muscle paralysis, there is usually some sparing of sensory modalities and an absence of peripheral nerve degeneration. In general, neuropraxia has a good prognosis for recovery if causal factors are removed.[5]

Neurotmesis is a complete severance of the nerve root or division of all the essential neuronal structures. This injury usually results from such traumatic mechanisms as severe traction forces or open lacerations.

Axonotmesis represents disruption of nerve fibers (axons) causing peripheral (wallerian) degeneration. Because the epineurium and surrounding connective tissues are preserved, spontaneous regeneration is likely to occur. Axonotmesis usually follows traction injuries or closed fractures or dislocations or results from ischemia.[28,37]

The most obvious manifestation of peripheral nerve injury is muscle weakness or flaccid paralysis, depending on the extent of the nerve damage. Because of the loss of muscle innervation, **atrophy** follows, and deep tendon reflexes are absent or depressed. Sensation along the cutaneous distribution of the nerve is also lost. Trophic changes, such as dry skin, hair loss, cyanosis, brittle fingernails, painless skin ulcerations, and slow wound healing in the area of involvement, may be present.

Occasionally, minute muscle contractions called *fasciculations* may be seen on the surface of the skin overlying the denervated muscle belly. As a result of disturbances of sympathetic fibers of the autonomic nervous system, ability to sweat above the denervated skin surfaces is lost. The patient may experience paresthesias— that is, such sensations as tingling, numbness, and burning or pain (causalgia)—particularly at night. In addition, if the nerve damage was caused by trauma, edema is a prominent clinical manifestation. EMG examinations may reveal extremely small muscle contractions called *fibrillations*.[3,4,8,9,13,21]

Extensive peripheral nerve damage may produce deformity if contractures, joint stiffness, and poor positioning are allowed to occur. Disfigurement of the hands is particularly noticeable and may produce some psychological complications. Other complications may include osteoporosis of bone and epidermal fibrosis of the joints.

The medical and surgical management of peripheral nerve lesions depends on the type of injury that has occurred. Management may include microsurgery to suture the severed nerve, nerve grafts or transplants for severe traumatic injuries, and injections of alcohol, vitamin B_{12}, and phenol to alleviate the pain that might accompany peripheral neuropathy.[6,8,14]

Peripheral nerve **regeneration** begins about 1 month after the injury has occurred. The rate of regeneration depends on the nature of the nerve lesion. If the nerve root has been cleanly severed and surgically repaired, the rate of regeneration ranges from ½ inch (1.3 cm) to 1 inch (2.5 cm) per month. Peripheral nerve injuries caused by burns, sepsis, or crushing will present other complications to the healing process. Age is another factor: children usually have a faster rate of regeneration than adults.[29]

Proximal lesions regenerate faster than distal lesions, and injuries to mixed nerves are slower to recover than single nerves.[5,27] Early medical treatment may involve suturing the nerve and immobilizing the affected extremity to ensure good apposition of the severed nerves. In the past, full recovery of muscles was not probable because regenerated fibers lose about 20% of their original diameter and conduct impulses at a slower rate.[9,28] Advancements in microsurgery in recent years have improved the regenerative process.

Because peripheral nerves have the capacity to regenerate, the course of recovery is somewhat predictable. The clinical signs of regeneration do not always follow a specific sequence. The following clinical signs of nerve regeneration can be expected:

- *Skin appearance.* As the edema subsides and collateral blood vessels develop, the circulatory system should become more normalized. Skin color and texture should improve.
- *Primitive protective sensations.* The first sign of cutaneous sensation is usually the gross recognition of crude pain, temperature, pressure, and touch.
- *Paresthesias (Tinel's sign).* Tapping or percussing from distal to proximal along the course of the damaged nerve route can be used to detect recovery. If the patient feels **paresthesias** (pins and needles) distal to the presumed site of lesion, regeneration is occurring, whereas a painful Tinel's sign at the lesion may indicate neuroma formation.[5,18]
- *Scattered points of sweating.* As the parasympathetic fibers of the autonomic nervous system regenerate, the sweat glands recover their functions.
- *Discriminative sensations.* The more refined sensations, such as the ability to identify and localize touch, joint position (proprioception), recognition of objects in the three-dimensional form (stereognosis), movement (kinesthesia), and two-point discrimination, should be returning at this point.
- *Muscle tone.* Flaccidity decreases and muscle tone increases. An important principle is that paralyzed muscles must first sense pressure before tone and movement can be realized.
- *Voluntary muscle function.* The patient is able to move the extremity, first in the gravity-lessened plane. As strength increases, active movement of the extremity through full ROM may be possible, although full recovery of muscle power is unlikely. At this point graded exercises can begin.

For complete laceration of peripheral nerves, the two-point discrimination test and the **wrinkle test** are good methods of monitoring sensory return.[29] The two-point discrimination test provides a quantitative measure of sensation. The normal distance to discriminate one point from two points on the distal fingertip is 2 to 4 mm. A two-point discrimination of greater than 15 mm denotes tactile agnosia (absent sensation). This test can be performed with a commercially available two-point discrimination instrument or a high-quality caliper with tips blunted so that the pain sensation is not elicited. Light application of the instrument to the patient's skin in a random pattern can help the therapist map the cutaneous, topographical areas that are innervated and denervated.

Another test that can be clinically significant is the wrinkle test. This test is performed by immersing the patient's hand in plain water at 108° F. The hand remains submerged for about 20 to 30 minutes, until wrinkling occurs. At this point the patient's hand is dried, graded on a scale of 0 to 3, and photographed. The "0" on the scale represents an absence of wrinkling, whereas "3" represents normal wrinkling. The wrinkle test appears to provide an objective method of testing innervation of the hand with recent complete and partial peripheral nerve injuries. The actual physiological mechanism that causes the wrinkling is not fully understood, and the test is not appropriate for patients with traumatic peripheral nerve compression injuries.[29] Nevertheless, the test can help determine the rate of sensory regeneration and can provide a graphic record of denervated areas.

Brachial Plexus Injury

The nerve roots that innervate the upper extremity originate in the anterior rami between the C4 and T1 spinal segments. This network of lower anterior cervical and upper dorsal spinal nerves is collectively called the *brachial plexus*. This important nerve complex can be palpated just behind the posterior border of the sternocleidomastoid as the head and neck are tilted to the opposite side.[6,8,20,40]

Lesions to the brachial plexus usually result from a variety of traumatic injuries. Most brachial plexus injuries in children are caused by birth trauma. Such injuries are called *Erb's palsy* and *Klumpke's paralysis*. Erb's palsy is indicative of lesions to the fifth and sixth brachial plexus roots. Paralysis and atrophy occur in the deltoid, brachialis, biceps, and brachioradialis muscles. Clinically the arm hangs limp, the hand rotates inward, and functional movement is extremely limited.

Klumpke's paralysis affects the more distal aspect of the upper extremity. The disorder results from injury to the eighth cervical and first thoracic brachial plexus roots. Consequently there is paralysis to the distal musculature of the wrist flexors and the intrinsic muscles of the hand.[6,8]

Long Thoracic Nerve Injury

The long thoracic nerve (C5-7) innervates the serratus anterior muscle, which anchors the apex of the scapula to the posterior of the rib cage. Although injury to this nerve is not common, the nerve can be injured by carrying heavy weights on the shoulder, neck blows, and axillary wounds. The resulting clinical picture involves winging of the scapula, difficulty flexing the outstretched arm above shoulder level, and difficulty protracting the shoulder or performing scapula abduction and adduction.

Injuries involving the long thoracic nerve are usually treated by stabilizing the shoulder girdle to limit scapula motion. The therapist must avoid using activities that promote shoulder movements. If nerve regeneration is not complete, surgery may be indicated to relieve the excessive mobility of the scapula. After medical treatment the occupational therapist encourages maximal functional independence during activities and teaches the patient to use long-handled devices to compensate for shoulder limitations.

Axillary Nerve Injury

The axillary nerve is composed of the C5-6 spinal nerves and derived from the posterior region of the brachial plexus. The motor branches of the axillary nerve innervate the superior aspect of the deltoid muscle and the teres minor muscle. Although the axillary nerve is rarely damaged by itself, it is often damaged along with traumatic lesions to the brachial plexus. As a result the patient has weakness or paralysis of the deltoid muscle, which causes limitations in horizontal abduction and hyperesthesia on the lateral aspect of the shoulder. In addition to the loss of muscle power, atrophy of the deltoid muscle produces asymmetry of the shoulders. If the nerve damage is permanent, muscle transplantation may be necessary to provide some abduction of the arm.[6,8,36]

The occupational therapist should maintain ROM to prevent deformity and improve circulation. Passive abduction of the shoulder should be performed daily. The teres minor and deltoid muscles should be protected from stretch during the passive ROM activities. The patient may be taught to use long-handled assistive devices to compensate for the abduction deficit. If a surgical transplant is performed, the therapist should be familiar with the surgical procedure and assist in muscle reeducation. An EMG biofeedback machine can be beneficial in providing the patient with visual and auditory incentives during muscle reeducation sessions.

The occupational therapist may also assist the patient in dressing activities. If the asymmetry of the shoulders presents a cosmetic problem when wearing shirts or jackets, a foam rubber or thermoplastic pad can be fabricated to fill in the space that was once occupied by the deltoid muscle. The patient should be encouraged to learn self-ranging techniques and to implement an exercise program, to maintain the integrity of the unimpaired muscles of the involved extremity.

Lesions of the radial, median, and ulnar nerves and cumulative trauma disorders affecting the hand are discussed in Chapter 44.

Volkmann's Contracture
A fracture of the lower end of the humerus (supracondylar region) may result in a diminished supply of well-oxygenated blood to the muscles of the forearm. This phenomenon can occur when the fracture has been tightly cast and bandaged. Edema occurs near the site of the injury and shuts down the blood supply to the muscle bellies because the site of injury cannot swell outward. Ischemia deprives tissues of oxygen and nourishment. The muscle can become necrotic, causing atrophy and contractures of the wrist, fingers, and forearm. The flexor digitorum profundus and flexor pollicis longus muscles are severely affected. The median nerve is often more impaired than the ulnar nerve.[8,20]

Shortly after a fracture of the humerus has been immobilized, the patient may have a cold, distal extremity with a smooth, glossy, or dusky appearance of the skin. If the therapist observes these symptoms and cannot detect a radial pulse, the physician should be informed immediately and the cast should be removed. Early detection and prevention of this problem can eliminate a severe deformity. If, for example, the ischemia lasts 6 hours, some contracture will follow. Ischemia lasting 48 hours or more results in a permanent deformity of the forearm. If mild ischemia has occurred, the physician may prescribe vigorous, active exercises to increase circulation, activate the musculature, and prevent joint stiffness.[6]

Peripheral Nerve Pain Syndromes
Pain is a common complication in peripheral nerve injuries.[7,52] For some patients the pain itself becomes an overwhelming disability. The pain syndromes that have been associated with peripheral nerve injuries are **causalgia** and neuroma pain.[37,43,52] Causalgia is pain of great intensity originating from peripheral lesions affecting the fibers of the autonomic nervous system.[13] Causalgia most commonly results from injury to the brachial plexus or the sciatic, tibial, median, or ulnar nerve.[5] Because the sympathetic and parasympathetic fibers travel in the walls of blood vessels until they reach their respective organs, the pain can radiate to quadrants of the body served by these major blood vessels.[12,27]

In the upper extremity, causalgia is described as an intense burning sensation so excruciating that the patient holds the affected limb immobile for fear of stimulating the pain. The affected limb becomes extremely sensitive to temperature change, wind, and even noise.[12,27] Causalgia is also exacerbated by emotional stress. Because of the origin of the pain in the sympathetic division of the autonomic nervous system, even mood changes alter the pain sensitivity levels.[12]

Neuromas are incompletely regenerated nerve endings and fibers at the site where the peripheral nerve was damaged. Neuromas are a particular problem in nerve endings serving the fingers and in amputated limbs. Phantom limb pain is often the result of neuroma formation. Neuromas are exquisitely painful and tender when they develop in the extremities that bear weight or are easily traumatized. In some cases, surgical resection is necessary to remove neurons that adhere to fascia and subcutaneous tissue.

Occupational Therapy Intervention
Peripheral Nerve Injuries
The aim of the treatment of peripheral nerve injuries is to help the patient regain the maximal level of motor function and independence in all occupational performance areas. Treatment is directed to the stage of recovery and to remediation and compensation for sensory, motor, and performance deficits. The rate of return and the residual impairments depend largely on the severity of the lesion and the quality of care during the rehabilitation process. For treatment to be effective, the therapist must know the anatomy and innervation of the affected part and be able to assess the pattern of paralysis and its effects on function. Table 42-1 is a useful summary of the major nerve roots and the clinical manifestations of their lesions.

The occupational therapist may be involved during the acute and rehabilitation phases of treatment. During the acute postoperative phase, treatment is aimed at preventing deformity. Static splints are used initially to immobilize the extremity and protect the site of injury. (Chapter 44 provides more information on postoperative management of peripheral nerve repair.[41,46]) During this phase the reduction of edema is important, and this is achieved by elevating the extremity above the level of the heart. This decreases the hydrostatic pressure in the blood vessels and promotes venous and lymphatic drainage.

Manual massage while the extremity is elevated may also reduce edema. The massage should entail centripetal strokes to gently force the excess fluids toward the proximal aspects of the body. Care must be taken not to disturb the healing process of the site of injury. External elastic support can also be used to alleviate the edema, and passive ROM will help prevent edema by promoting venous return.[49]

As the patient's muscle function returns, an appropriate exercise program can be established. Functional activities that involve resistance are used in conjunction with isometric and isotonic exercises when muscle

TABLE 42-1

Clinical Manifestations of Peripheral Nerve Lesions

Spinal Nerves	Nerve Roots	Motor Distribution	Clinical Manifestations
Brachial plexus			
C5-7	Long thoracic	Shoulder girdle, serratus anterior	Winged scapula
C5-6	Dorsal scapular	Rhomboid major and minor, levator, scapulae	Loss of scapular adduction and elevation
C7-8	Thoracodorsal	Latissimus dorsi	Loss of arm adduction and extension
C5-6	Suprascapular	Supraspinatus, infraspinatus	Weakened lateral rotation of humerus
C5-6	Subscapular	Subscapularis, teres major	Weakened medial rotation of humerus
C6-8, T1	Radial	All extensors of forearm, triceps	Wrist drop, extensor paralysis
C5-6	Axillary	Deltoid, teres minor	Loss of arm abduction, weakened lateral rotation of humerus
C5-6	Musculocutaneous	Biceps brachii, brachialis, coracobrachialis	Loss of forearm flexion and supination
C6-8, T1	Median	Flexors of hand and digits, opponens pollicis	Ape hand deformity, weakened grip, thenar atrophy, unopposed thumb
C8, T1	Ulnar	Flexor of hand and digits, opponens pollicis	Claw hand deformity, interosseus atrophy, loss of thumb adduction
Lumbosacral Plexus			
L2-4	Femoral	Iliopsoas, quadriceps femoris	Loss of thigh flexion, leg extension
L2-4	Obturator	Adductors of thigh	Weakened or loss of thigh adduction
L4-5, S1-3	Sciatic	Hamstrings, all musculature below the knee	Loss of leg flexion, paralysis of all muscles of leg and foot
L4-5, S1-2	Common peroneal	Dorsiflexors of foot	Foot drop, steppage gait, loss of eversion
L4-5, S1-3	Tibial	Gastrocnemius, soleus, deep plantar flexors of foot	Loss of plantar flexion and inversion of foot

Data from references 3, 4, 6, 8, 9, 13, 21, 28, 36, 41, 45, 50.

function is adequate. The therapist should not overtax the returning musculature and should protect the weaker muscle groups from stretch and fatigue. The therapist may fabricate splints or slings to protect weakened musculature, prevent overstretching, and maintain functional position.

ADL assessment is necessary to identify difficulties with essential performance tasks. One-handed methods of dressing, eating, and hygiene activities may be necessary on a temporary or permanent basis. Assistive devices, such as long-handled reaching aids and one-handed kitchen tools, can be provided to increase independence in self-care ADL and IADL skills.

Sensory reeducation is used to help the patient establish appropriate responses to sensory stimuli. Sensory reeducation for peripheral nerve injuries is discussed in Chapters 25 and 44.

Peripheral Nerve Pain Syndromes

Pain is perceived by the conscious mind when painful stimuli travel from pain receptors (**nociceptors**) along ascending pathways to the thalamus and to the cerebral cortex. Research on pain management has revealed that certain activities and noninvasive techniques can modulate pain perception.[22,43,44] A better understanding of pain control mechanisms and the discovery of endogenous opiate-like substances (e.g., endorphins, enkephalins, and substance P) in the body have provided therapists with new techniques for patients with peripheral nerve pain.[1,7,22,30,39]

Since pain resulting from peripheral nerve injury can interfere with compliance with therapeutic intervention, it is important for the occupational therapist to be able to participate in and assist the patient with pain management strategies.

The therapist must first assess the intensity, quality, and location of pain. This can be done by having the patient mark the point of pain on an anatomical drawing and then estimate pain intensity on a numerical scale. The patient is asked to describe the personal perception of pain using terms such as sharp, dull, aching, throbbing, sore, or burning. Factors that seem to contribute to pain should also be explored during the interview. These factors might include specific foods and drinks, positions, and activities.[22]

Several intervention techniques can alter pain messages or neuronal transmission within these pathways. Peripheral pain emitting from neuromas can be alleviated by increased input to mechanoreceptors in the skin. The therapist can increase mechanoreceptor input using one or more of the following techniques:

1. Graded light, local percussion, and therapeutic vibration over neuromas.[1,24,25]
2. Transcutaneous electrical nerve stimulation (TENS) to provide relief from pain related to neuromas, peripheral nerve injuries, residual limb pain, and phantom limb syndromes[19,38] The occupational therapist who has been appropriately trained can use TENS when it is prescribed by a physician. With appropriate training, localized stimulation to acupoints and trigger points can also be used to modify neuroma pain.[39,43]
3. Protection of the painful regions of the body. The therapist can fabricate protective devices from splinting materials.
4. Some patients find relief when the extremity is wrapped with a cloth material that has been soaked in water.[5]

These approaches work because when the sensory neurons transmitting pain messages synapse in the dorsal horn of the spinal cord to secondary neurons in the dorsal gray matter, substance P, one of the opiate-like neurotransmitters, is released. Increased input to the mechanoreceptors in the skin inhibits the release of substance P.[30,43]

Pain management for causalgia uses a different rationale and different neurophysiological systems. Causalgia arises from the autonomic nervous system. Increased activity in the sympathetic division of the autonomic nervous system exacerbates causalgia. In addition, the neuronal connections to the limbic system suggest that emotions play an important role in causalgia.[5,12,27,30]

The neurophysiological rationale for alleviating causalgia is complex because it involves at least two distinct systems. Both systems originate in areas of the cortex. One system is more direct, in that it projects to neurons in the reticular formation and to motor pathways terminating on excitatory and inhibitory neurons in the dorsal gray matter of the spinal cord. The other system includes neurons in the cortex projecting to cell bodies in the limbic system, which go on to transmit to the midbrain.[1,7,39,43]

The first cortical modulating system is very responsive to physical and emotional stress. Consequently, stress increases blood concentrations of catecholamines (dopamine, epinephrine, and norepinephrine) via the autonomic nervous system, which triggers the release of enkephalins that inhibit transmission of afferent interneurons in the dorsal gray matter. The second cortical modulating system, involving the limbic system and midbrain, responds by releasing endorphins to inhibit pain transmission.[1,7,39,43] The release of these endogenous opiates (enkephalin and endorphins) demonstrates the effectiveness of purposeful activities to modulate the perception of pain.

By involving the patient in successful and purposeful activities, the occupational therapist provides cognitive diversion from the pain experience. Engagement in purposeful activities can influence moods and emotions, an effect that in turn alters the perception of pain intensity and ultimately modifies the pain threshold.[16,22,27,43] The therapist can also use background music or music delivered via headphones as a therapeutic modality. While the patient is engaged in activities, the volume of the music can be increased or decreased to accommodate pain intensity. This provides a control factor over the pain stimulus because concentration on music affects the cortical modulating system through connections with the limbic system.[22]

Causalgia is related to tension and stress. To decrease feelings of stress and anxiety, the therapist can instruct the patient in such relaxation techniques as deep breathing, progressive relaxation, and visualization.[7,12]

When the relaxation response is elicited, the patient's muscles relax, the heart rate and respiration rate decrease, and the patient experiences a sense of well-being. By learning relaxation techniques, the patient can control emotional tension and depression, both contributors to causalgia and the perception of pain.[22]

DISEASE OF THE NEUROMUSCULAR JUNCTION
Myasthenia Gravis

Myasthenia gravis is a disease of chemical transmission at the nerve-muscle synapse or neuromuscular junction. It is caused by an autoimmune response in which antibodies are produced against nicotinic acetylcholine (ACh) receptors and interfere with synaptic transmission at the nerve-muscle junction. Because neurotransmission is defective, there is weakness of skeletal muscle.[33] Myasthenia gravis occurs at all ages but primarily affects younger women and older men.[18,45]

A majority of patients with myasthenia gravis have enlarged thymus glands, and some have tumors of the thymus gland. Removal of the thymus gland (thymectomy) reduces symptoms or causes remission in about 50% of patients, and this procedure has become standard therapy. Patients are also treated with anticholinesterase drugs, glucocorticoids, and other immunosuppressive pharmacological agents.[33,51] Plasmapheresis, a procedure that entails filtering the blood to remove the IgG autoantibodies, is sometimes used for patients with severe disease who have failed to respond to other therapeutic measures and in seriously ill patients before thymectomy.[2,17,18,45]

Myasthenia gravis is characterized by abnormal fatigue of voluntary muscle.[14] The disease can affect any of the striated skeletal muscles of the body, but it has an affinity for the muscles of the eyelids and eyes and oropharyngeal muscles. Therefore the muscles most often affected are those that move the eyes, eyelids, tongue, jaw, and throat. The limb muscles may also be affected. The muscles that are used most often fatigue sooner.[14,33,51] Therefore the patient may have double vision, drooping of the eyelids, and difficulty with speech or swallowing as muscles fatigue. Patients with myasthenia gravis may experience life-threatening respiratory crises, which require hospitalization and use of a ventilator. The incidence of these crises has declined significantly in recent years, probably because of increased use of thymectomy.[33,51] The intensity of the disease fluctuates, and its course is unpredictable.[51]

Spontaneous remissions occur frequently, but relapse is usual.[8] Remissions or a decrease in symptoms and an improvement in strength and function can last for years. However, exertion, infection, or childbirth may induce exacerbations of unpredictable severity.[42] The prognosis for myasthenia gravis varies with each individual. For most people it is a progressively disabling disease, and the patient may ultimately become confined to bed with severe permanent paralysis. Death usually occurs as a result of respiratory complications.[8,42,45]

Occupational Therapy Intervention

The primary role of the occupational therapist is to help the patient regain muscle power and build endurance. The therapeutic program should not cause fatigue; therefore the therapist must be aware of the patient's medication regimen and ability to tolerate activity and the time of day that the patient has the most energy. The patient's muscle strength must be monitored on a regular basis; however, the therapist need not assess all of the muscles during one session because the evaluation contributes to fatigue. Instead, the therapist can test the strength of a few muscles during each visit and keep a running record to note any important changes.

If the patient is taking oral cholinergic drugs, optimal strength is expected about 1 or 2 hours after the medication has been ingested.[2] Therefore the therapist should coordinate muscle testing with the drug treatment regimen so the test results are not confounded by the medication. The therapist should also report to the physician any changes in the patient's physical appearance, such as ptosis of the eyelids, drooping facial muscles, or alterations of breathing or swallowing.

The therapist should provide gentle, nonresistive activities that are intellectually and psychologically stimulating. The activities should be graded so they do not fatigue the patient. Overexertion must be avoided and respiratory problems prevented. The treatment plan should include energy conservation, work simplification, and adaptive and assistive devices necessary to reduce effort during daily activities. If appropriate, electronic communication devices can be installed in the patient's home so that contact with community agencies can be maintained. In addition, the therapist may assist with home planning to determine architectural barriers, bathroom adaptations, and furniture rearrangements. Mobile arm supports and splints may be used to protect weakened musculature from overstretching and aid in positioning for function.[42]

The therapist should assist in educating the patient about the disease. The patient should avoid emotional stress, overexertion, fatigue, and excessive heat or cold because they may exacerbate the symptoms of the disease. The therapist should also follow infection control procedures because minor infections can also exacerbate the symptoms.

MYOPATHIC DISORDERS
Muscular Dystrophies

The muscular dystrophies are a group of uncommon inherited conditions. There are four major types of muscular dystrophy (MD).[34,51] They have in common the progressive degeneration of muscle fibers while the neuronal innervation to muscle and sensation remain intact. As the number of muscle fibers declines, each axon innervates fewer and fewer of them, resulting in progressive weakness.[31]

Duchenne's Muscular Dystrophy

Duchenne's MD is inherited as an X-linked recessive trait and affects males only. The disease begins at birth and is usually diagnosed between the ages of 18 and 36 months. It begins in the muscles of the pelvic girdle and legs, then spreads to the shoulder girdle. Calf muscles appear hypertrophic because of the infiltration of fat cells that accompanies degeneration of muscle fibers. The child has difficulty walking, has a waddling gait, and usually must use a wheelchair by age 12. Ultimately the child becomes confined to bed; death usually occurs by the age of 30.[34,42,51]

Facioscapulohumeral Muscular Dystrophy

Facioscapulohumeral MD has its onset in adolescence and affects primarily the muscles of the face and shoulder girdle—hence its descriptive name. It progresses slowly, and there is a normal life expectancy for those affected.[51] The disease is inherited through an autosomal dominant gene and affects males and females equally.[34]

Myotonic Muscular Dystrophy

Myotonic MD not only causes weakness but has another component, myotonia (tonic spasm of muscles), that makes relaxation of muscle contraction difficult. It is inherited through an autosomal dominant gene and affects males and females. Its unique features, besides the myotonia, are that it involves the cranial muscles and that the limb weakness tends to be distal rather than proximal. Associated symptoms are cataracts, found in almost all patients, and testicular atrophy and baldness in men. The disease may be mild or severe and can occur at any age.[34,51]

Limb-Girdle Dystrophy

Limb-girdle MD is a group of disorders that do not fit readily in the other types described. Affected persons differ in age at onset, extent of weakness, and familial inheritance patterns. The disease is inherited as an autosomal recessive gene.[34,51]

OCCUPATIONAL THERAPY INTERVENTION. Because this group of diseases is degenerative, the decline of muscle function cannot be prevented. Medical management is largely supportive, and rehabilitation measures are vital in delaying deformity and achieving maximal function within the limits of the disease and its debilitating effects. The primary goal of OT is to help the patient attain maximal independence in ADL for as long as possible. Self-care activities and assistive devices for independence and leisure activities are a vital part of the treatment program.[42]

Wheelchair prescription and mobility training in either a manual or power wheelchair are included in the OT program. The wheelchair may require a special seating system or supports to minimize the development of scoliosis, hip and knee flexion contractures, and ankle plantar flexion deformity. A wheelchair lap board, suspension slings, or mobile arms supports are indicated to facilitate self-feeding, writing, reading, use of a computer, and tabletop leisure activities when there is substantial shoulder girdle and upper limb weakness. Built-up utensils may be helpful when grip strength declines.[42] Home and workplace modification may be necessary for some patients.[11]

Active exercise may be helpful, but overexertion and fatigue must be avoided. For patients with respiratory involvement, exercise for breathing control may be administered by the physical therapist.[47]

The occupational therapist also addresses psychosocial problems and educational and vocational requirements. Deficits in cognitive function and verbal intelligence have been reported in some types of MD. Depression and other personality abnormalities may be concomitant problems.[11] Patient and family education is an important part of the OT program. A supportive approach to the patient and family is helpful as function changes and new mobility aids, assistive devices, and community resources become necessary.[42]

SUMMARY

The motor unit consists of the lower motor neuron, neuromuscular junction, and muscle. Some motor unit dysfunctions are reversible, and others are degenerative. The role of the occupational therapist is to assess functional capabilities in all occupational performance areas. ADL and IADL skills (including self-care, home management, mobility, and work-related tasks), energy conservation, work simplification, and joint protection techniques are used to restore function. Proper positioning, exercise programs, and pain management techniques are used as indicated to facilitate recovery and increase functional capacity. Orthoses, assistive devices, communication aids, and mobility equipment and training in their use may be necessary. Psychosocial considerations and patient and family education are important aspects of the OT program.

CASE STUDY 42-1

CASE STUDY—MS. J.

Ms. J. is a 23-year-old, African-American woman who received a diagnosis of Guillian-Barré syndrome 6 weeks before her admission to rehabilitation. She was admitted to the acute care hospital with progressive weakness of both the upper and lower extremities. She reported the presence of flu-like symptoms for 1 week prior to the onset of weakness in her hands and feet.

Ms. J. is unmarried and has two children; one is 7 years old and the other is 4 months old. She lives in a two-bedroom apartment that is in a wheelchair accessible building. She and her children are presently living with her parents. Ms. J. worked as a waitress in a coffee shop near her home. Her leisure interests include reading to her children, watching television, shopping, and sewing. She has 11 years of formal education and was pursuing a general education development certificate (GED). Ms. J. was referred to occupational therapy for evaluation and treatment. During the initial interview it became apparent that she was having some difficulty accepting the loss of physical ability and function. She did not understand the nature of her disease or its prognosis. Her goals for the rehabilitation program included returning to her own apartment, caring for her children, returning to work, and continuing to pursue a GED. She stated that her family is involved and would be willing to provide assistance should she require it.

Results of the occupational therapy (OT) evaluation indicated that Ms. J. is alert, oriented, cooperative, and motivated. Cognition is intact. Before her illness she was independent in all areas of ADL and IADL. Active and passive range of motion are within

Continued

CASE STUDY 42-1—cont'd

normal limits (WNL) and muscle strength is fair (F or 3) for both upper extremities (BUE). Lower extremity strength is fair (3). Sensation is intact. However, she complains of numbness, tingling and burning in BUE. Fine motor coordination is impaired, as evidenced by inability to do clothing fasteners. Dynamic sitting balance is minimally impaired because of trunk weakness and deconditioning. Standing balance is severely impaired because of lower extremity (LE) weakness. Ms. J. is able to roll in bed and move from supine to sitting using the bed rails. Transfers to all surfaces require moderate assistance because of generalized weakness and LE pain. Ms. J. is independent in feeding. She requires set up for grooming, minimal assistance with UE dressing, and moderate assistance with LE dressing, bathing, and toileting. She complains of pain and generalized weakness that interfere with performance of activities. Ms. J. is not ambulatory at this time because of weakness and deconditioning.

OT was initiated to improve mobility and transfers; improve functional performance of ADL and IADL activities; improve patient's awareness of the disease process and prognosis for recovery of function; increase muscle strength and coordination in both UEs; decrease pain in LEs.

OT intervention included transfer training, ADL and IADL training, patient education related to Guillian-Barré Syndrome, energy conservation and work simplification techniques, a therapeutic exercise program, and participation in a pain management regimen.

Ms. J. responded well to treatment. Her strength, mobility, and endurance improved so that she is now independent in ADL and IADL, including caring for her infant son, with the use of equipment and energy conservation techniques. She requires a tub bench for safety in the shower. She gained sufficient endurance and UE strength for modified work activities (cashier rather than waitress duties) up to 4 hours per day. She is ambulatory with a narrow base quad cane in her home and outdoors for up to 500 feet, and transfers to all surfaces independently. Pain issues have been resolved. She no longer complains of LE pain interfering with performance of functional activity. She and her children continue to live with her parents, but Ms. J. plans to return to her apartment when there are further gains in strength and independence. She returned to modified work on a part-time basis and was referred back into the GED program in the community.

REVIEW QUESTIONS

1. Name the components of the motor unit and three causes of lesions that may result in motor unit dysfunction.
2. Describe the major clinical findings and the characteristics of the occupational therapy program for patients with poliomyelitis.
3. Describe the symptoms of postpolio syndrome.
4. What are the elements of the occupational therapy program for the patient with postpolio syndrome?

5. Describe Guillain-Barré syndrome and the occupational therapy interventions used for patients with this disorder.
6. List at least six clinical manifestations of peripheral nerve injury.
7. Describe the sequential signs of recovery following peripheral nerve injury.
8. Describe the occupational therapy treatment strategies, including any contraindications, for peripheral nerve injuries.
9. Differentiate between causalgia and neuroma.
10. Describe four noninvasive methods of modulating pain perception that may be used by the occupational therapist.
11. Discuss the clinical signs of myasthenia gravis.
12. Describe the role of occupational therapy for patients who have myasthenia gravis.
13. What is the primary treatment precaution in myasthenia gravis?
14. Name and differentiate four types of muscular dystrophy. Which one primarily affects children?
15. What are the treatment goals for muscular dystrophy?

REFERENCES

1. Adler M: Endorphins, enkephalins and neurotransmitters, *Med Times* 110:32, 1982.
2. Barone D: Steroid treatment for experimental autoimmune myasthenia gravis, *Arch Neurol* 37(10):663-666, 1980.
3. Barr ML: *The human nervous system*, ed 2, New York, 1974, Harper & Row.
4. Bateman J: *Trauma to nerves in limbs*, Philadelphia, 1962, WB Saunders.
5. Birch R, Grant C: Peripheral nerve injuries: clinical. In Downie P, editor: *Cash's textbook of neurology for physiotherapists*, ed 4, Philadelphia, 1986, JB Lippincott.
6. Brashear RH, Raney RB: *Shands' handbook of orthopaedic surgery*, ed 9, St Louis, 1978, Mosby.
7. Brena SF, editor: *Chronic pain: America's hidden epidemic*, New York, 1978, Atheneum.
8. Chusid JG: *Correlative neuroanatomy and functional neurology*, ed 19, Los Altos, Calif, 1985, Lange Medical Publications.
9. Clark RG: *Clinical neuroanatomy and neurophysiology*, ed 5, Philadelphia, 1975, FA Davis.
10. deGroot J: *Correlative neuroanatomy*, ed 21, Norwalk, Conn, 1991, Appleton & Lange.
11. Fowler WF, Goodgold J: Rehabilitation management of neuromuscular diseases. In Goodgold J, editor: *Rehabilitation medicine*, St Louis, 1988, Mosby.
12. Gandhavadi B: Autonomic pain: features and methods of assessments, *Postgrad Med* 71(1):85-90, 1982.
13. Gardner E: *Fundamentals of neurology*, ed 6, Philadelphia, 1975, WB Saunders.
14. Gilroy J, Meyer J: *Medical neurology*, ed 3, New York, 1979, Macmillan.
15. Halstead LS: Late complications of poliomyelitis. In Goodgold J, editor: *Rehabilitation medicine*, St Louis, 1988, Mosby.
16. Heck SA: The effect of purposeful activity on pain tolerance, *Am J Occup Ther* 42(9):577-581, 1988.
17. Kornfeld P: Plasmapheresis in refractory generalized myasthenia gravis, *Arch Neurol* 38(8):478-481, 1981.

18. Krupp MA, Chatton MJ: *Current medical diagnosis and treatment,* 1984, Los Altos, Calif, 1984, Lange Medical Publications.

19. Lampe G: Introduction to the use of transcutaneous electrical nerve stimulation devices, *Phys Ther* 58(12):1450-1454, 1975.

20. Larson CB, Gould M: *Orthopedic nursing,* ed 9, St Louis, 1978, Mosby.

21. Laurence TN, Pugel AV: Peripheral nerve involvement in spinal cord injury: an electromyographic study, *Arch Phys Med Rehabil* 59(7):309-313, 1978.

22. McCormack GL: Pain management by occupational therapists, *Am J Occup Ther* 42(9):582-590, 1988.

23. Melville ID: Clinical problems in motor neurone disease. In Obeham P, Rose FC, editors: *Progress in neurological research,* London, 1979, Pitman Publishing.

24. Melzack R: Prolonged relief from pain by brief, intense transcutaneous somatic stimulation, *Pain* 1(4):357-373, 1975.

25. Melzack R, Wall PD: Psychophysiology of pain, *Int Anesthesiol Clin* 8(1):3-34, 1970.

26. Morrison D, Pathier P, Horr K: *Sensory motor dysfunction and therapy in infancy and early childhood,* Springfield, Ill, 1955, Charles C Thomas.

27. Newburger P, Sallan S: Chronic pain: principles of management, *J Pediatr* 98(2):180-189, 1981.

28. Noback CR, Demares RJ: *The nervous system: introduction and review,* ed 2, New York, 1977, McGraw-Hill.

29. Phelps PE, Walker C: Comparison of the finger wrinkling test results to establish sensory tests in peripheral nerve injury, *Am J Occup Ther* 31(9):565-572, 1977.

30. Piercey MF, Folkers K: Sensory and motor functions of spinal cord substance P, *Science* 214(4527):1361-1363, 1981.

31. Portney L: Electromyography and nerve conduction velocity tests. In O'Sullivan SB, Shmitz TJ: *Physical rehabilitation: assessment and treatment,* ed 2, Philadelphia, 1988, FA Davis.

32. Robinault I: *Functional aids for the multiply handicapped,* New York, 1973, Harper & Row.

33. Rowland LP: Diseases of chemical transmission at the nerve-muscle synapse: myasthenia gravis. In Kandel ER, Schwartz JH, Jessell TM: *Principles of neural science,* New York, 1991, Elsevier.

34. Rowland LP: Diseases of the motor unit. In Kandel ER, Schwartz JH, Jessell TM: *Principles of neural science,* New York, 1991, Elsevier.

35. Schmidt RF: *Fundamentals of neurophysiology,* ed 2, New York, 1978, Springer-Verlag.

36. Schumacher B, Allen HA: *Medical aspects of disabilities,* Chicago, 1976, Rehabilitation Institute.

37. Seddon HJ: *Surgical disorders of the peripheral nerves,* ed 2, Edinburgh, 1975, Churchill Livingstone.

38. Shealy C: Transcutaneous electrical nerve stimulation for control of pain, *Surg Neurol* 2(1):45-47, 1974.

39. Sjolund B, Erikson M: Electroacupuncture and endogenous morphines, *Lancet* 2(7994):1085, 1976.

40. Smith B: *Differential diagnosis in neurology,* New York, 1979, Arco.

41. Spencer EA: Functional restoration, specific diagnoses. In Hopkins HL, Smith HD, editors: *Willard & Spackman's occupational therapy,* ed 6, Philadelphia, 1983, JB Lippincott.

42. Spencer EA: Functional restoration, section 2. In Hopkins HL, Smith HD, editors: *Willard & Spackman's occupational therapy,* ed 8, Philadelphia, 1993, JB Lippincott.

43. Swerdlow M: *The therapy of pain,* Philadelphia, 1981, JB Lippincott.

44. Tappan FM: *Healing massage techniques: a study of eastern and western methods,* Reston, Va, 1978, Reston.

45. Tierney LM, McPhee SJ, Papadakis MA: *Current medical diagnosis and treatment,* ed 33, Norwalk, Conn, 1994, Appleton & Lange.

46. Trombly CA, Scott AD: *Occupational therapy for physical dysfunction,* Baltimore, 1977, Williams & Wilkins.

47. Turner A: *The practice of occupational therapy,* ed 2, New York, 1987, Churchill Livingstone.

48. Van Dam A: Guillain-Barré syndrome: a unique perspective, *Occup Ther Forum* 2:6, 1987.

49. Vasudevan S, Melvin JL: Upper extremity edema control: rationale of the techniques, *Am J Occup Ther* 33(8):520-523, 1979.

50. Walter JB: *An introduction to the principles of disease,* Philadelphia, 1977, WB Saunders.

51. Walter JB: *An introduction to the principles of disease,* ed 3, Philadelphia, 1992, WB Saunders.

52. Wynn-Parry CB, Withrington R: Painful disorders of peripheral nerves, *Postgrad Med J* 60(710):869-875, 1984.

53. Young G: Occupational therapy and the postpolio syndrome, *Am J Occup Ther* 43(2):97-103, 1989.

CHAPTER 43

Arthritis

WENDY STORM BUCKNER

KEY TERMS

Connective tissue
Inflammation
Chronic
Autoimmune
Systemic
Synovitis
Osteophytes
Crepitation
Joint laxity

LEARNING OBJECTIVES

After studying this chapter the student or practitioner will be able to do the following:

1. Identify common symptoms and differences between arthritis, osteoarthritis, and fibromyalgia.
2. Identify common joint and hand deformities seen in osteoarthritis and rheumatoid arthritis.
3. Recognize medications commonly used in the treatment of arthritis and the side effects of the medications.
4. Recognize surgical interventions commonly performed on persons with rheumatoid arthritis.
5. Identify the psychological effects of arthritis.
6. Identify important areas to evaluate in patients with arthritis.
7. Identify treatment objectives of occupational therapy intervention for persons with arthritis.
8. Identify appropriate preventive, compensatory, and restorative treatment methods for persons with arthritis, based on diagnosis, stage of disease, functional limitations, type of deformity(ies), and lifestyle.
9. Identify resources helpful to persons with arthritis.
10. Identify treatment precautions.

Although arthritis literally means *joint inflammation*, the term is used to describe many different conditions that cause aching and pain in joints and **connective tissues** throughout the body. Many of these diseases, such as osteoarthritis, do not involve **inflammation**. Three of the most prevalent forms of arthritis are rheumatoid arthritis, osteoarthritis, and fibromyalgia.[1,4,18]

DESCRIPTION OF MAJOR ARTHRITIC DISEASES

Rheumatoid Arthritis

Rheumatoid arthritis (RA) is a **chronic**, systemic **autoimmune** disorder. In response to the body's immune system activity, the joint lining becomes inflamed. The chronic inflammation causes pain, deterioration of the joint, and limited movement.[1] The course of the disease is different for each person. Some people have a single episode of joint inflammation and a long-lasting remission. The majority of persons with RA have inflammation of the joints over long periods of time. The disease process may progress continuously and slowly or may consist of series of "flare-ups," or exacerbations, and complete or incomplete remissions. Remissions provide a period of pain relief, but this does not mean the condition has been cured; it may flare up again. In addition, any damage done during an active stage remains. The patient's functional skills may vary, depending on the course of the disease and the severity of the symptoms.[3,6,18]

The **systemic** symptoms characteristic of RA include fatigue, loss of appetite, fever, overall aching or stiffness, and weight loss. Morning stiffness, an overall stiffness that occurs on awakening, is another indicator of systemic involvement. The severity of the systemic symptoms usually matches the severity of joint involvement. As in many chronic diseases, there may also be a resulting depression or lack of motivation. In a small percentage of persons the blood vessels, heart, lungs, or eyes are involved.[3,6,18]

The cause of RA is unknown. It occurs most frequently between the ages of 30 and 40, and women are three times more commonly affected than men.[3,6] Its outstanding clinical feature is **synovitis,** or inflammation of the synovial tissue surrounding the joints. The function of the synovial tissue is to produce fluid to lubricate the joint. Joint swelling results from an abundance of synovial fluid, enlargement of the synovium, and thickening of the joint capsule. This weakens the joint capsule, tendons, and ligaments. Inflamed joints will be warm, swollen, tender, often red, and difficult or painful to move. The affected person usually has a loss of range of motion (ROM), strength, and endurance. As the inflammation continues, it invades the cartilage, bone, and tendons and secretes enzymes that damage them. If the inflammation is not stopped, the cartilage, bone, tendons, and ligaments surrounding the involved joint(s) can be destroyed. Scar tissue can form between the bone ends, and the joint can become fused, permanently rigid, and immovable.[3,5,6,18]

Joint involvement is frequently bilateral.[5] If one hand is involved, the other one is also. However, the disease progression is often different on the two sides. One side may be more involved and have different deformities than the other. The joints most affected by RA are the wrist, thumb, and hand. RA is frequently seen in the proximal interphalangeal (PIP) and metacarpophalangeal (MP) joints, while the distal interphalangeal (DIP) joints are usually spared severe damage. The elbows, shoulders, neck, jaw, hips, knees, ankles, and feet also may be involved. The spine is usually not directly affected.[3,5,18]

Osteoarthritis (Degenerative Joint Disease)

Osteoarthritis (OA) is a disease that causes the breakdown of cartilage in joints, leading to joint pain and stiffness. Unlike RA, OA is not inflammatory or systemic, but limits its attack to individual joints. It is often referred to as the "wear and tear" disease, because the involved joints wear down with age or overuse. Up to the age of 45, OA is more common in men; beyond age 54, it is more common in women.[3] It is also interesting to note that because rheumatoid arthritis may cause malalignment or instability of the weight-bearing joints, it often results in premature osteoarthritis.[7]

In osteoarthritis the breakdown of joint tissue occurs in several stages. First, the smooth cartilage softens and loses its elasticity. This allows it to be more easily damaged. Eventually, large sections of the cartilage wear away completely and permit the bones to rub together, causing pain. The joint may lose its normal shape. As the ends of the bone thicken, spurs (bony growths) are formed where the ligaments and capsule attach to the bone (Fig. 43-1). These are also referred to as **osteophytes.** Fluid-filled cysts may form in the bone, near the joint. Bits of bone or cartilage may float loose in the joint space. The joint becomes stiff or unstable, and joint motion becomes restricted and painful. Occasionally the process of osteoarthritis causes irritation of the joint, and local inflammation may occur.[2,18]

Osteoarthritis can affect any joint and is most frequently seen in the weight-bearing joints of the hips, knees, and spine and the metatarsophalangeal joint of the big toe, producing bunions.[2,5] In the hand, the DIP joints, PIP joints, and the carpometacarpal (CMC) joint at the base of the thumb are most likely to be affected. Hip and knee involvement causes the most severe disability and may necessitate surgery for joint replacement.

The symptoms of OA usually begin slowly and may appear as a minor ache or soreness with movement. Pain is most frequently felt in the affected joint(s) after overuse or long periods of inactivity. The joint becomes stiff, although movement is possible. If the joint is not moved, surrounding musculature becomes weak. Coordination and posture may also be impaired.[2,5]

Degenerative joint disease occurs to some degree among many people over the age of 60. Although it is most common in the elderly, other factors such as obesity, heredity, injury, and overuse of joints can aggravate the disease process.[2,5,18]

Fibromyalgia

The use of the term *fibromyalgia* and its definition are relatively recent events, although its symptoms have been discussed since the early 1900s.[28] In fibromyalgia,

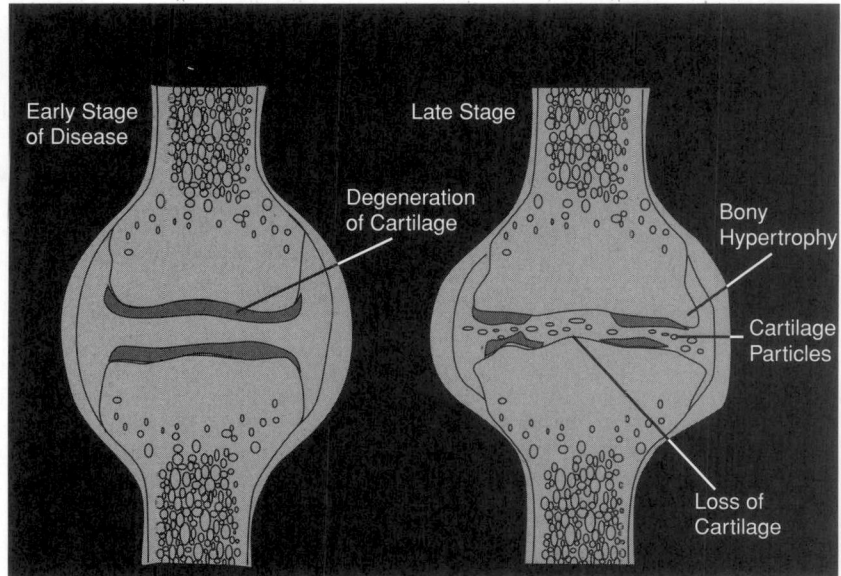

FIG. 43-1
Joint involvement in osteoarthritis. (From ARHP Arthritis Teaching Slide Collection, American College of Rheumatology.)

widespread pain affects the muscles and attachments to the bones. In addition to pain, symptoms may include fatigue, sleep disturbance, depression and anxiety, headaches, morning stiffness, irritable bowel syndrome, bladder irritability, numbness and tingling in extremities, circulatory problems, and cold intolerance.[28]

Some 3.7 million Americans have fibromyalgia, and the condition affects men, women, and children. It occurs most often in people between the ages of 20 and 55 and affects women 10 times more frequently than men.[28] The presence of other rheumatic diseases puts one at greater risk of having fibromyalgia. For example, in 20% of those with RA, fibromyalgia develops.[28]

The cause of fibromyalgia is not known. Theories to explain the underlying cause include (1) previous trauma affecting the central nervous system's response to pain, (2) infections, (3) lack of or overuse of exercise, and (4) hormonal influences.[28]

Diagnosis

Physicians diagnose arthritic diseases based on the overall pattern of symptoms, a medical history, and the results of a physical examination, x-ray examinations, and laboratory tests. Definitive diagnosis may not be possible at onset because of the large number of connective tissue disorders with similar symptoms. In most cases, it takes weeks or even months for the constellation of symptoms to develop and eventually be diagnosed.[18,16]

Rheumatoid Arthritis

The American College of Rheumatology criteria for classification of RA require that the patient show four of

seven criteria or clinical manifestations of the disease for the diagnosis of RA to be made (Table 43-1).[1] One criterion is the presence of rheumatoid factors in the blood. Rheumatoid factors are autoantibodies that appear in 75% to 90% of patients with RA. These patients are said to have seropositive RA. The presence of rheumatoid factors in the blood correlates with increased severity of symptoms and increased involvement of systemic symptoms.[16]

Osteoarthritis

A thorough physical examination confirms typical symptoms, and lack of systemic symptoms rules out an inflammatory joint disorder. X-ray examination of the affected joint can confirm joint damage. However, the degree of radiological evidence of joint involvement does not necessarily correlate with the amount of pain and discomfort experienced by the patient.[18] The classification criteria for osteoarthritis of the hand may be seen in Box 43-1.[16]

Fibromyalgia

Classic symptoms of fibromyalgia include a history of widespread pain that is present for at least 3 months on both sides of the body, above and below the waist. Another classic symptom is pain in at least 11 of 18 "tender point" sites (Box 43-2).[28] Tender points are areas of the body that are painful when pressed. The most distinctive characteristic of fibromyalgia is the presence of tender points at the base of the skull, above and between the shoulder blades, below the elbows, in the lower back, on the hips, and behind the knees.

TABLE 43-1

Criteria for the Classification of Rheumatoid Arthritis

Criterion	Definition
Morning stiffness	Morning stiffness in and around the joints, lasting at least 1 hour before maximal improvement
Arthritis of three or more joint areas	At least 3 joint areas simultaneously have had soft-tissue swelling or fluid (not bony overgrowth alone) observed by a physician. The 14 possible areas are right or left PIP, MP, wrist, elbow, knee, ankle, and MTP joints.
Arthritis of hand joints	At least 1 area swollen (as defined above) in a wrist, MP, or PIP joint.
Symmetrical arthritis	Simultaneous involvement of the same joint areas (as defined in 2) on both sides of the body (bilateral involvement of PIPs, MP, or MTPs is acceptable without absolute symmetry)
Rheumatoid nodules	Subcutaneous nodules over bony prominences or extensor surfaces or in juxtaarticular regions, observed by a physician
Serum rheumatoid factor	Demonstration of abnormal amounts of serum rheumatoid factor by any method for which the result has been positive in more than 5% of normal control subjects
Radiographic changes	Radiographic changes typical of rheumatoid arthritis on posteroanterior hand and wrist radiographs that must include erosions or unequivocal bony decalcification localized in or most marked adjacent to the involved joints (osteoarthritis changes alone do not qualify)

From Arnett FC, Edworthy SM, Bloch DA, et al: The American Rheumatism Association 1987 revised criteria for the classification of rheumatoid arthritis, *Arthritis Rheum* 31:315-324, 1988.
MP, Metacarpophalangeal; *MTP*, metatarsophalangeal; *PIP*, proximal interphalangeal.

BOX 43-1

American College of Rheumatology Classification Criteria for Osteoarthritis of the Hand

Hand pain, aching, or stiffness and three or four of the following features:
- Hard-tissue enlargement of two or more of 10 selected joints.
- Hard-tissue enlargement of two or more DIP joints.
- Fewer than three swollen MP joints.
- Deformity of at least 1 of 10 selected joints.

From http://www.rheumatology.org/classifi/oshand.html.
The 10 selected joints are the second and third distal interphalangeal (DIP), the second and third proximal interphalangeal, and the first carpometacarpal joints of both hands. This classification method yields a sensitivity of 94% and a specificity of 87%.
MP, Metacarpophalangeal.

Description of Common Upper Extremity Joint and Hand Deformities

The destructive processes seen in arthritis can result in tendon, muscle, and nerve dysfunction and many joint deformities. A brief explanation of some of the most common deformities and the associated disease follows.

Crepitation is seen in both RA and OA and occurs as the joints degenerate. It is characterized by a grating, crunching, or popping sensation (or sound) that occurs during joint or tendon motion. When the presence of crepitus is documented, the location and motion that caused the sensation should be noted.[2,18]

OSTEOARTHRITIS

In osteoarthritis, osteophytes may form in the fingers or at the base of the thumb.[2,5,18] This indicates that cartilage damage has occurred. Osteophytes are hard to the touch and generally not painful. They are most commonly seen at the DIP joint and are called *Heberden's nodes* (Fig. 43-2). If seen at the PIP joint, they are called *Bouchard's nodes* (Fig. 43-2).

Osteoarthritis may also involve the CMC joint at the base of the thumb. This joint is highly mobile and is subject to significant stress during pinch activities. The most common symptom is pain with motion. Patients may be limited in many activities, since the thumb accounts for 45% of hand function.[18] As the disease process progresses, osteophytes may form; the joint can subluxate, giving a squared appearance to the joint (Fig. 43-3).[2]

RHEUMATOID ARTHRITIS

The hands are the most severely affected sites of RA.[3,5,18] A typical sign of RA is the *fusiform* (spindle-shaped) *swelling* in the PIP joints (Fig. 43-4). Swan neck and boutonniere deformities may also result from muscle and tendon contractures.

BOX 43-2
American College of Rheumatology 1990 Criteria for the Classification of Fibromyalgia

1. History of widespread pain.
   Definition: Pain is considered widespread when all of the following are present: pain in the left side of the body, pain in the right side of the body, pain above the waist, and pain below the waist. In addition, axial skeletal pain (cervical spine or anterior chest or thoracic spine or low back) must be present. In this definition, shoulder and buttock pain is considered as pain for each involved side. "Low back" pain is considered lower segment pain.
2. Pain in 11 of 18 tender point sites on digital palpation.
   Definition: Pain, on digital palpation, must be present in at least 11 of the following 18 sites:
   Occiput: Bilateral, at the suboccipital muscle insertions.
   Low cervical: Bilateral, at the anterior aspects of the intertransverse spaces at C5-C7.
   Trapezius: Bilateral, at the midpoint of the upper border.
   Supraspinatus: Bilateral, at origins, above the scapula spine near the medial border.
   Second rib: Bilateral, at the second costochondral junctions, just lateral to the junctions on upper surfaces.
   Lateral epicondyle: Bilateral, 2 cm distal to the epicondyles.
   Gluteal: Bilateral, in upper outer quadrants of buttocks in anterior fold of muscle.
   Greater trochanter: Bilateral, posterior to the trochanteric prominence.
   Knee: Bilateral, at the medial fat pad proximal to the joint line.
   Digital palpation should be performed with an approximate force of 4 kg.
   For a tender point to be considered "positive," the subject must state that the palpation was painful.
   "Tender" is not to be considered as "painful."

From http://www.rheumatology.org/classifi/fibro.html.
For classification purposes, patients will be said to have fibromyalgia if both criteria are satisfied. Widespread pain must have been present for at least 3 months. The presence of a second clinical disorder does not exclude the diagnosis of fibromyalgia.

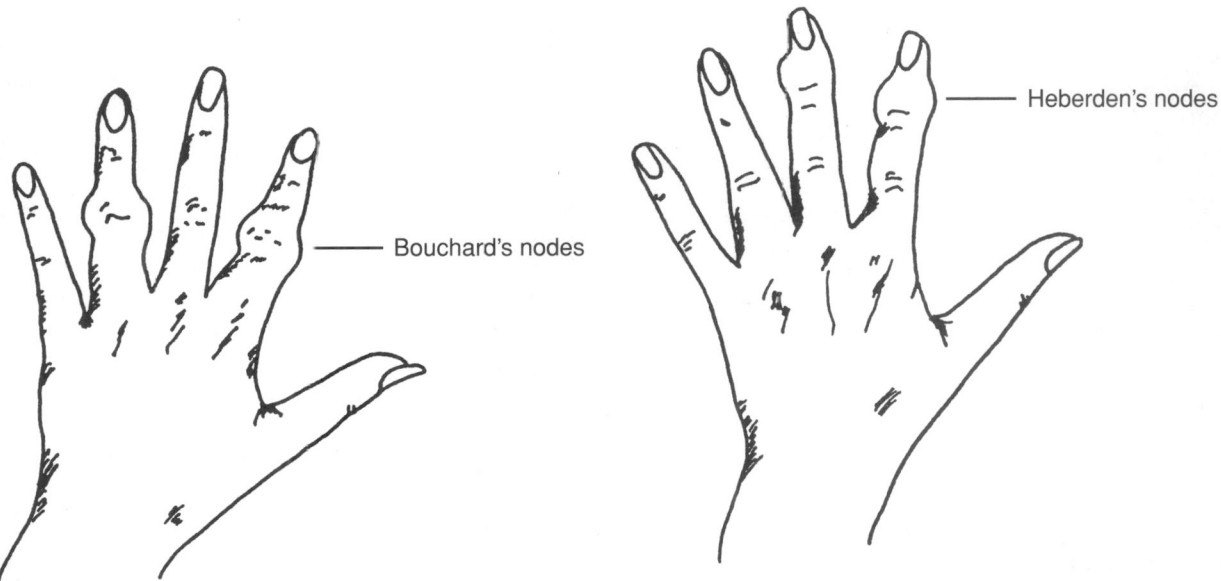

FIG. 43-2
Osteophyte formation in the proximal interphalangeal joints (Bouchard's nodes) and distal interphalangeal joints (Heberden's nodes) is characteristic of osteoarthritis.

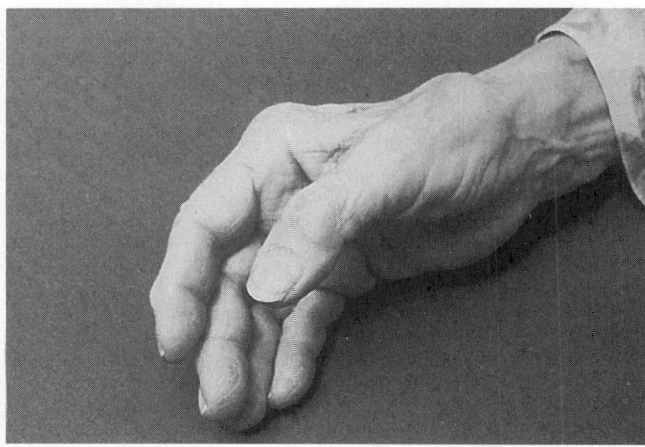

FIG. 43-3
Arthritic changes in the carpometacarpal joint of thumb result in a squared appearance. (From ARHP Arthritis Teaching Slide Collection, American College of Rheumatology.)

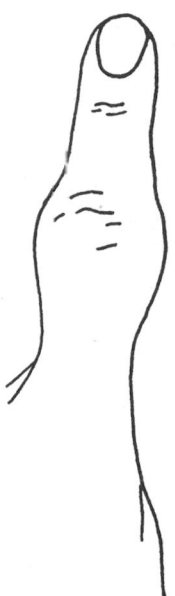

FIG. 43-4
Fusiform swelling.

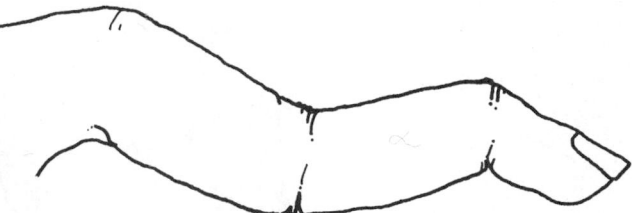

FIG. 43-5
Swan-neck deformity results in proximal interphalangeal hyperextension and distal interphlangeal flexion.

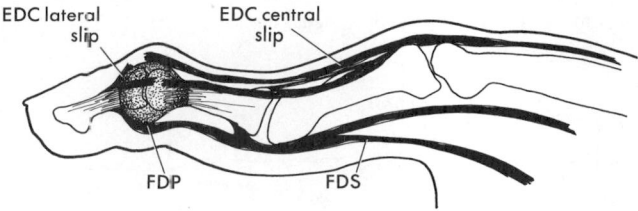

FIG. 43-6
Swan-neck deformity resulting from rupture of lateral slips of extensor digitorum communis tendon.

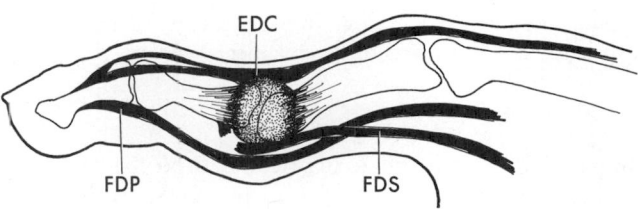

FIG. 43-7
Swan-neck deformity as a result of rupture of flexor digitorum superficialis tendon.

The *swan-neck deformity* involves a flexion contracture of the MP joint, hyperextension of the PIP joint, and flexion of the DIP joint (Fig. 43-5). There are several types of swan-neck deformity, three of which are discussed here. One type of swan-neck deformity is caused by initial involvement at the MP joint and results in intrinsic muscle tightness.[18] Another type of swan-neck deformity is a result of initial involvement at the DIP joints and rupture of the lateral slips of the extensor tendons (Fig. 43-6).[18] A swan-neck deformity with initial involvement at the PIP joint is caused by chronic synovitis, which leads to stretching of supporting structures or rupture of the flexor digitorum superficialis

(FDS) tendon (Fig. 43-7).[18] Bony spurs producing tendon erosion may also cause the tendon to rupture.[18] With progression of a swan-neck deformity, the patient may lose active flexion and will be unable to make a fist or flex the PIP joint to hold small objects.

The *boutonniere deformity* may look worse than a swan-neck deformity, but it generally does not impair function as much. The deformity is a combination of PIP flexion and DIP hyperextension (Fig. 43-8). A boutonniere deformity can occur when synovitis at the wrist, MP, or PIP joints weakens or destroys the central slip of the extensor tendon, which inserts into the base of the middle phalanx. There is often associated PIP joint arthritis. The result is incomplete and weak-to-absent extension at the PIP joint when the lateral slips of the extensor tendon, which insert into the base of the distal phalanx, slip below the axis of the PIP joint, becoming flexors of that joint and hyperextending the DIP joint where they insert (Fig. 43-9).[3,5,18] The central slip of the extensor tendon is the major extensor of the

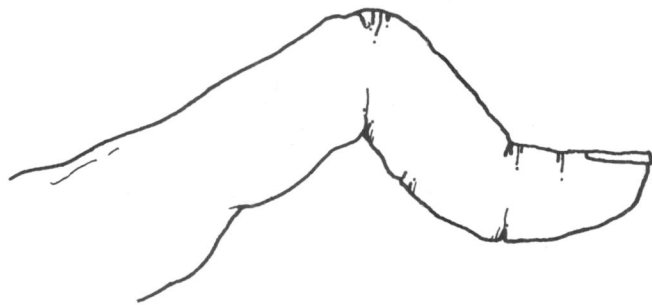

FIG. 43-8
Boutonniere deformity results in distal interphalangeal hyperextension and proximal interphalangeal flexion.

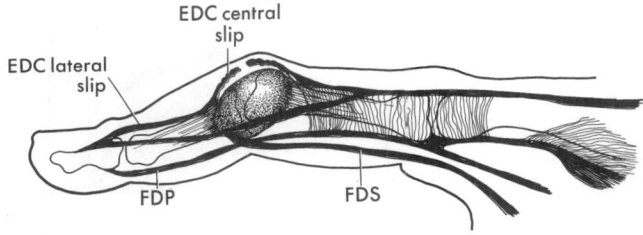

EDC central slip

EDC lateral slip

FDP   FDS

FIG. 43-9
Boutonniere deformity caused by rupture or lengthening of central slip of extensor digitorum communis tendon.

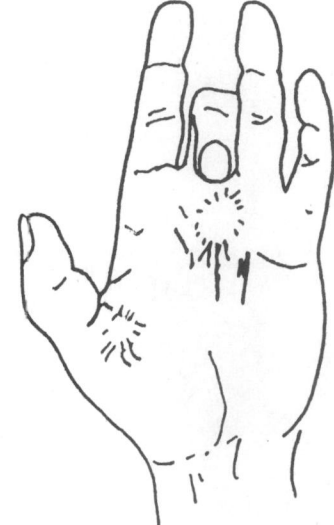

FIG. 43-10
Trigger finger.

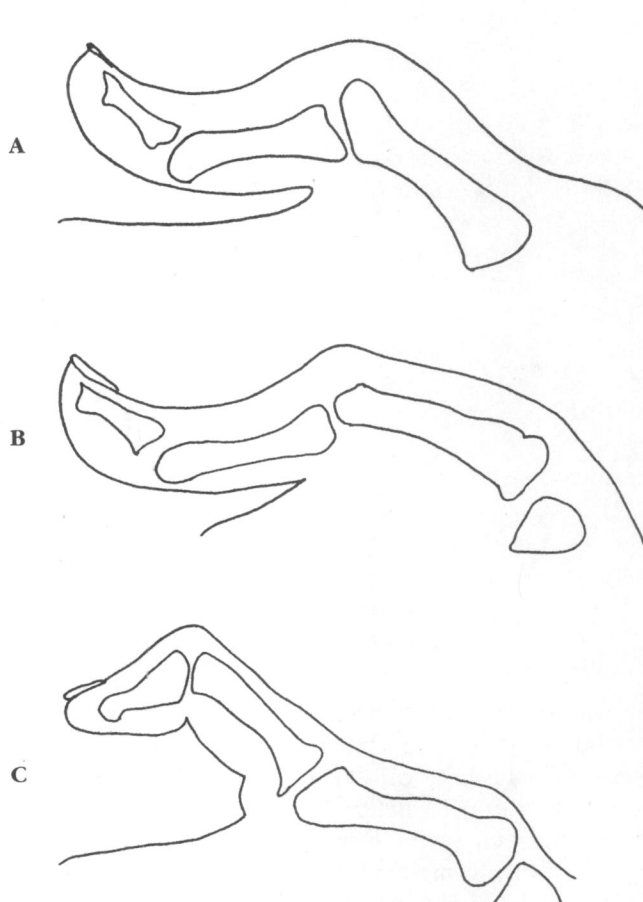

FIG. 43-11
Common rheumatoid thumb deformities. **A,** Type I is the most common deformity seen in rheumatoid arthritis, followed by **C,** type III. **B,** Although type II is seen infrequently in rheumatoid arthritis, it is a common sequela of osteoarthritis of the carpometacarpal joint.

finger. If the occurrence of these symptoms is recent (days) and if the physician does not know of it, he or she should be informed immediately. Invariably a flexion contracture of the PIP joint and hyperextension of the DIP joint with loss of flexion range will ensue. Function of the finger will be seriously compromised because of an inability to straighten the finger and loss of flexion at the tip for pinch or making a fist.

Trigger finger is caused by a nodule or thickening of the flexor tendons of the fingers or thumb as they pass through the digital pulleys. The nodule on the FDS tendon or thickening of the synovium blocks or hinders the tendon's gliding motion through its sheath. This results in a snapping or catching of the finger during active flexion or extension (Fig. 43-10). If persistent triggering occurs, it may result in lost ROM or tendon rupture.[5,18]

As with the fingers, the MP and CMC joints are the most common sites of inflammation in the thumb.[3,5,18] *Thumb deformities* are referred to by several names. Many clinicians use the same terms that are used when describing the fingers. The revised Nalebuff classification uses five categories (Fig. 43-11). *Type I* (Fig. 43-11, *A*) is the most commonly seen deformity in RA. It begins with chronic synovitis of the MP joint, which leads to stretching of the joint capsule and flexion of the MP joint with hyperextension of the interphalangeal (IP) joint. The *type II* deformity (Fig. 43-11, *B*) is rarely seen. It involves subluxation of the CMC joint and leads to a

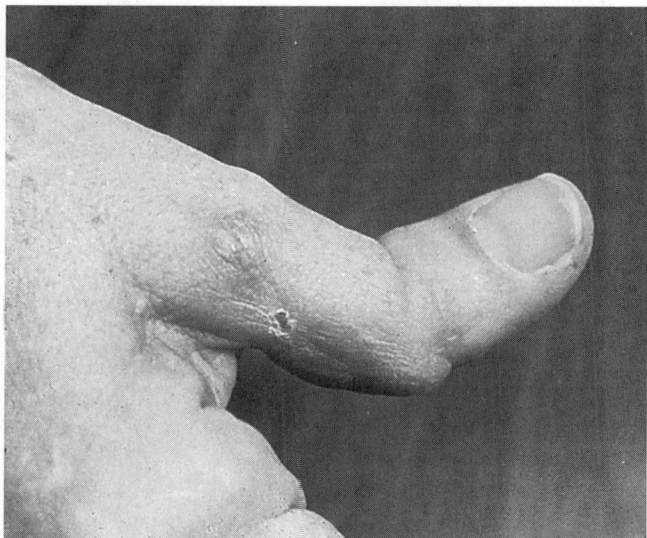

FIG. 43-12
Joint laxity, or instability. (From ARHP Arthritis Teaching Slide Collection, American College of Rheumatology.)

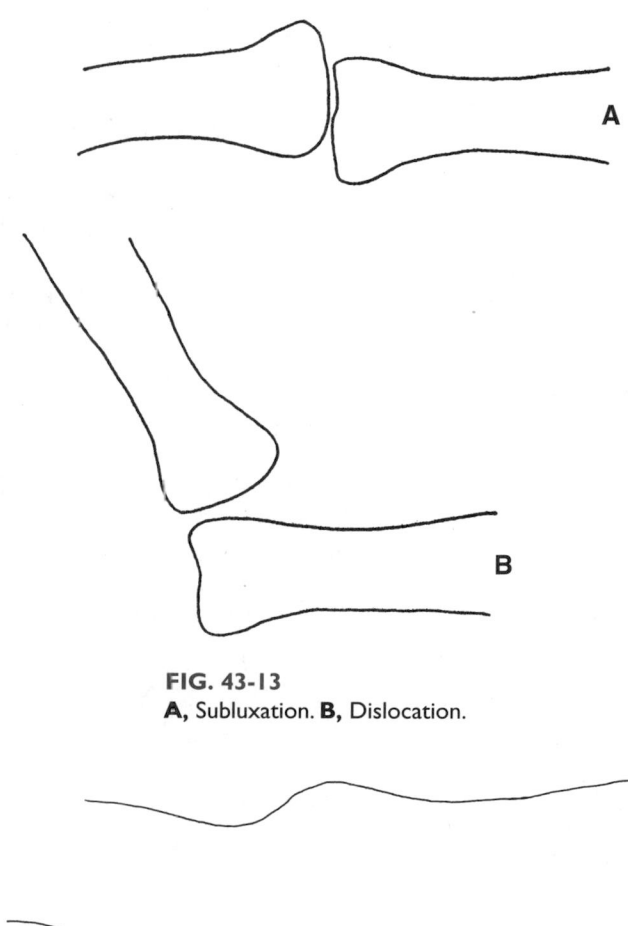

FIG. 43-13
A, Subluxation. **B,** Dislocation.

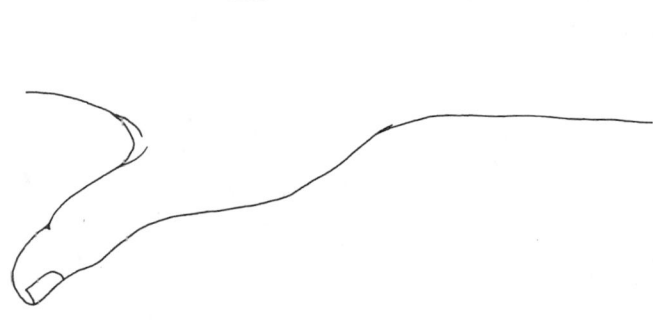

FIG. 43-14
Flexion subluxation of wrist.

fixed adduction contracture with hyperextension of the distal phalanx.[18] The *type III* deformity (Fig. 43-11, C) is seen in both RA and OA. It is characterized by MP hyperextension and flexion of the DIP joint.[18,21] The *type IV* looks similar to the *type II* deformity but does not involve the CMC joint. The *type V* deformity is a collapse and shortening of the phalanges with total instability.[20]

Joint laxity is a term that describes ligamentous instability. Joint laxity is a major cause of loss of hand function. In the fingers and thumb the collateral ligaments support the joint capsule on either side. Chronic synovitis can result in stretching or lengthening of the ligaments and abnormal lateral movement. When the thumb IP joint becomes unstable, the thumb tip can easily be wiggled by the therapist, but the patient loses the ability to oppose the thumb and manipulate small objects (Fig. 43-12).

Joints may also become *subluxated* or *dislocated* (Fig. 43-13) because of weakened ligaments. The most common sites of subluxation are the wrist and MP joints.[5,18] Subluxation of the wrist is a volar slippage of the carpal bones on the radius. It is caused by the chronic synovitis that weakens the supporting ligaments.

Carpal tunnel syndrome is caused by pressure on the median nerve where it passes through the carpal tunnel of the wrist. The carpal tunnel under the transverse flexor carpal ligament is a tightly closed space, and inflammation can lead to increased pressure and subsequent pain and sensory disturbances over the median nerve distribution in the hand. Initial symptoms may be numbness and tingling in the thumb, index, and middle fingers. Median nerve motor weakness and atrophy of the opponens pollicis and abductor pollicis brevis may result in thenar atrophy. *If its presence is not already known by the*

physician, this condition should be promptly brought to his or her attention for treatment. Untreated median nerve compression can progress to permanent loss of feeling in the hand and weak to lost thumb opposition, which are serious impairments to hand use.

Synovial invasion of the wrist may also involve the extensor tendons, carpal bones, and radioulnar joint. If the *extensor tendons* are involved, there will be dorsal swelling that can lead to tendon weakness or rupture, resulting in weak to lost extension of the fingers at the MP, PIP, and DIP joints, flexor contractures, and serious loss of hand function. Synovial invasion of the *carpal bone* results in erosion and destruction of the intercarpal ligaments and joints. It can cause progressive loss of wrist motion, contracture of the wrist in a nonfunctional position, or, in flexion, subluxation-dislocation of the wrist (Fig. 43-14). *Radioulnar joint* involvement usually results in progressive loss of pronation and supination, particularly if there is associated elbow disease. This can lead to severe functional impairment.

A characteristic sign of RA is *ulnar drift* or *deviation* of the MP joint (Fig. 43-15). In the normal hand the MP ligaments, particularly when the MP joints are flexed at 45°, give medial and lateral stability. Both the extensor and flexor tendons of the fingers are bowed to produce an ulnar drift tendency of the tendons at the MP joints during normal contraction. Forced contractions and especially forceful hand grips accentuate this tendency. With MP ligaments weakened, normal forces result in ulnar drift. The fifth MP joint buttresses the remainder of fingers from static, postural ulnar drift. However, when the fifth MP ligament loses stability, ulnar drift can occur with gravity and posture, even at rest.

If the MP ligament damage is mild or if the stability of the fifth joint is preserved, the ulnar drift may be less evident and may occur only dynamically with finger extension-flexion. This condition gives weak pinch, which may result in thumb adduction and lateral pinch being substituted for true opposition. If the MP ligament damage is severe or if the stability of the fifth MP joint is lost, there will be ulnar drift even at rest (posturally), and impairment of opposition will be severe.

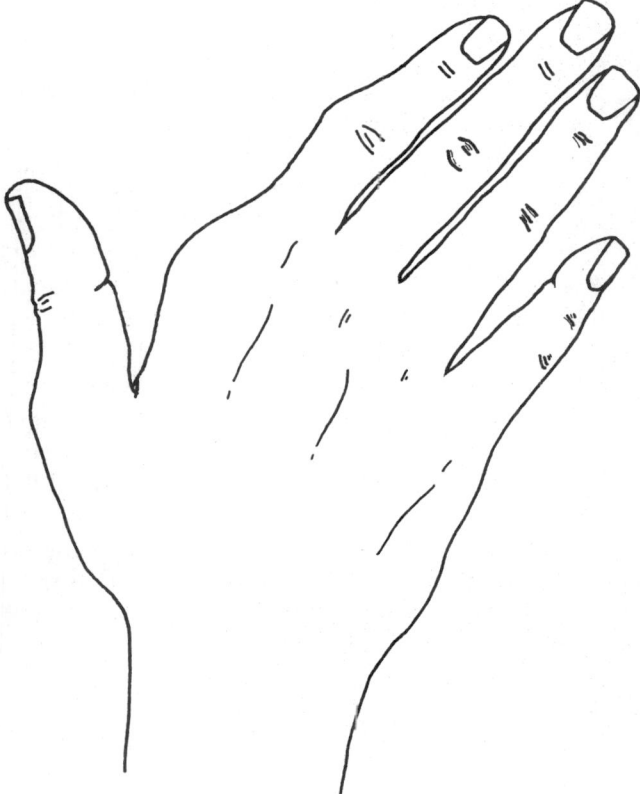

FIG. 43-15
Metacarpophalangeal joint ulnar drift.

The dynamic and static ulnar drift, combined with lifting of the extensor hood by MP synovitis, results in dislocation of the extensor tendons from the extensor hood over the metacarpal heads into the space between the heads. This may lead to tendon injury and loss of ability to completely extend the MP joints. The lateral pinching of the thumb results in radial subluxation and deformity of the IP joint of the thumb.[5,18]

The loss of elbow and shoulder motion as a result of weakness, pain, and contractures is also a common occurrence in RA. Secondary conditions such as tendinitis and bursitis are frequent causes of pain. *Elbow synovitis* may result in the loss of pronation, supination, flexion, and extension, which may severely limit self-care activities. Frozen shoulder is a complication of shoulder synovitis characterized by very restricted ROM.[18] Other commonly seen shoulder problems include bursitis and rotator cuff dysfunction.[7] Additionally, most patients with RA have muscle weakness as a result of disuse, bed rest, and drug effects.[13]

MEDICAL MANAGEMENT

There is no known cure for arthritis. Treatment is aimed toward reducing inflammation, pain, and joint damage. Treatment methods include medication, exercise, the use of heat and cold, joint protection techniques, weight control, surgery (when necessary), and coping strategies.[18,26] When making treatment decisions, one must consider both the benefits and risks (or costs) of one form of treatment over another.

Drug Therapy

Traditionally, the approach to medical management of RA has followed the pyramid model, with well established and less toxic treatment methods forming the foundation of treatment, or the base of the pyramid (Fig. 43-16).[23] With this approach, all patients with RA receive treatment described at the base of the pyramid. These treatment methods include rest, education, and what are referred to as *first-line medications*. If these methods are not effective in preventing disease progression, treatment progresses up the pyramid to agents that can be more toxic to the patient. At the apex of the pyramid are the more experimental and cytotoxic medications, which are generally reserved for patients who have severe disease not responding to other medication. Supportive measures such as therapy and cortisone injections form the sides of the pyramid and can be used throughout treatment.[1] More recently, an "inverted pyramid" approach has been suggested.[27] This approach calls for more aggressive treatment for patients with early, active inflammatory disease in an effort to prevent severe deformity.[16,27]

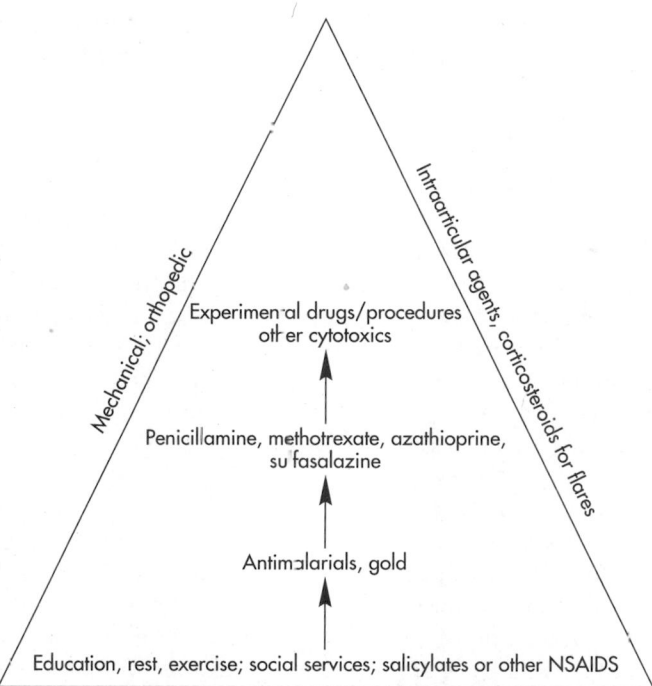

Experimental drugs/procedures other cytotoxics

Penicillamine, methotrexate, azathioprine, sulfasalazine

Antimalarials, gold

Education, rest, exercise; social services; salicylates or other NSAIDS

Intraarticular agents, corticosteroids for flares

Mechanical, orthopedic

FIG. 43-16

Treatment pyramid for arthritis. (From *Primer on the rheumatic diseases,* ed 10, Atlanta, 1993, Arthritis Foundation.)

Drug therapy is constantly changing, and no single method is recommended over all other methods.[18] Patients' needs and reactions change, and each physician develops his or her own philosophy and regimen. Allied health professionals need to be aware of the medical protocols used in their facilities and of the specific medications (and the side effects) taken by their patients.

The medications used in the treatment of RA are divided into two groups. The first group, or first-line drugs, are fast-acting drugs such as nonsteroidal antiinflammatory drugs (NSAIDs), intraarticular corticosteroid injections, and aspirin, which can suppress inflammation but cannot alter the progression of the disease. These drugs cannot prevent joint destruction.[16] Because they are less toxic, they are often prescribed at the initial diagnosis of RA.

In large doses, aspirin is one of the most frequently prescribed medications because it reduces pain and inflammation with tolerable side effects. Inflammation can also be reduced with NSAIDs that are used either individually or in conjunction with others. Some side effects to be aware of are stomach pain, diarrhea, dizziness, headache, nausea, ringing in the ears, and dark stools caused by bleeding.[3,18]

The second group of drugs include disease-modifying antirheumatic drugs (DMARDs). These drugs may actually have an effect on the course of the disease, although this possibility is still in question. The drugs in this group include gold salts, penicillamine, hydroxy-

chloroquine, and methotrexate, among others. All of these medications require careful medical monitoring because of potentially serious side effects.[18] Frequent blood and urine tests may be needed to rule out adverse effects. DMARDs and cytotoxic agents are slow acting, with 2 to 3 months of drug therapy needed before their full benefit is realized. During this time first-line drugs to control synovitis and the addition of steroids may improve the patient's functional status. It is also important that supportive measures such as joint protection, energy conservation, and splinting be employed until synovitis is controlled. Side effects include diarrhea, skin rashes, mouth ulcers, bone marrow suppression, and possible blindness. Any of these symptoms should be promptly reported to the physician.

Steroids are effective as antiinflammatory and pain-reducing agents but have serious side effects, such as bone erosion, diabetes, weight gain, emotional problems, and hypertension. Steroids are used most frequently on a temporary basis if the disease is not adequately controlled by other medications alone.[3,18]

For OA and fibromyalgia, medication for pain is generally limited to aspirin, NSAIDS, or acetaminophen. Additionally, patients with fibromyalgia may benefit from antidepressants used to promote sleep.[28]

Surgical Intervention

Treatment of the patient with long-term RA will often include operative procedures to repair soft tissue or replace joints destroyed by the rheumatoid process.[4,18] Surgeries are often delayed and are used only when more conservative methods fail to control the inflammation and subsequent soft-tissue damage. Several different surgical procedures may be of benefit to patients with RA. *Synovectomy* (removal of the diseased synovium) and *tenosynovectomy* (removal of diseased tendon sheath) are performed to prevent further complications. The removal of the excessive tissue does not prevent the progression of the disease. The surgeries are performed to relieve symptoms and slow the process of joint destruction or tendon rupture and to help preserve vascular supply to the joint. A synovectomy may be performed on the ankle, knee, hip, MP, wrist, elbow, or shoulder.[4,18]

Tendon surgery, including tendon relocation, tendon repair, tendon transfer, and tendon release, is considered a corrective strategy for specific hand impairments. Tendon surgery is most frequently performed on the extensor tendons of the hand and wrist.[4,18]

Arthroplasty (joint reconstruction) and *arthrodesis* (joint fusion) may be done when joint restoration is not possible. Both types of surgery may be performed to relieve pain, provide stability, correct deformity, and improve function. Common sites for these types of surgery are the ankle, knee, hip, first MP, PIP, and wrist.[4,18] Patients with OA are often seen by the occupational therapist after total hip or total knee replacement surgeries. These surgeries are described in Chapter 45.

PSYCHOLOGICAL FACTORS

Anyone who has a chronic illness must develop coping strategies to deal with the disability. This is especially true of the person with any type of arthritis. The person may have suffered a serious change in physical function and life roles, and even appearance is altered by deformity and drug side effects. These changes evoke an adjustment process similar to the grief process after a death. Because the disease is both unpredictable and characterized by pain, it is normal to respond to the disability with depression, denial, a need to control the environment, and dependence.[1,18,28] Psychological stressors may also result in an exacerbation of the disease.[22]

Some aspects of the illness that may contribute to the psychological state are constant pain and fear of pain; changed body image and perception of self as a sick person; continuous uncertainty about the course and prognosis of the disease because of remissions and flares; sexual dysfunction because of the pain or deformity or associated depression; and altered social, vocational, and leisure roles.

Rehabilitation workers need to be aware of the patient's response to disability and the adjustment that is in progress. All the factors and the behaviors just cited will have an influence on rehabilitation. The interaction of personnel with the patient may facilitate the development of healthy coping mechanisms and acceptance of disability (see also Chapter 28).

Family relationships and culture will also influence the patient's response to the disability. OT practitioners should work with both the patients and their families to help them learn all they can about the disease and to give them opportunities to share their concerns.[5,18] The support groups available through the Arthritis Foundation will be helpful for many. (See address at end of chapter.)

OCCUPATIONAL THERAPY INTERVENTION

Rehabilitation of the patient with arthritis is somewhat different from that of a patient with an acute or traumatic condition.[18] Because of the chronic and progressive nature of the disease, rehabilitation intervention may be needed periodically for months or even years, depending on the course of the disease and the individual patient.

Because many of the treatment principles are similar for patients with RA, OA, and fibromyalgia, this section identifies general treatment strategies and discusses specific suggestions for each disease when applicable.

Evaluation

Medical History
An initial intake should include a review of medical charts or records if they are available. If these are not available, a brief medical history should be taken, because the therapist must be aware of all health problems. Current medications should also be noted. The patient's report of which joints are currently involved or have been involved in the past, as well as any other systems affected, should be recorded.

Functional Abilities
The functional abilities of the patient with arthritis must be the first consideration in evaluation. Impaired ROM measurements and the presence of joint deformities do not necessarily mean that the patient cannot function independently. The patient may use substitute motions to complete tasks. On the other hand, the patient may display no apparent deformities but be severely disabled for routine tasks because of pain, fatigue, edema, or joint laxity.[5,18] It is also important to consider the effect of medication on performance.[18]

Interview
The initial interview should involve such factors as the medical history, joints involved, presence of pain, medication, functional abilities, and current symptoms.[18] It is also important to find out how much the patient already knows about the disease and if any treatment regimen is being followed. If the patient reports pain, the practitioner should ask, "Where is it?," "When does it occur?," and "How does it limit your abilities?" The patient may also be asked to complete a pain rating on a scale of "0" (no pain) to "10" (greatest pain) at different times of the day or with different activities (see Chapter 29). The patient should be asked if he or she has morning stiffness. Morning stiffness that lasts less than an hour would be more characteristic of OA. With RA, the stiffness would last for longer than an hour. The stiffness associated with fibromyalgia is generally worse in the morning and, although diminished, usually remains throughout the day.[18]

The OT practitioner should also ask the patient about present abilities and attempt to estimate the potential for independence in self-care. The patient's tolerance for activity should be included. An example of an Arthritis Evaluation Checklist for RA may be seen in Figure 43-17.

Observation
The occupational therapist should observe the appearance of joints for heat, redness, edema, deformity,

ARTHRITIS EVALUATION CHECKLIST

Name: _____   Diagnosis: _____

Referral: _____

Initial Interview:

Which joints bother you the most? _____

Pain at rest ___ on movement ___ constant ___ Description _____

Do you experience morning stiffness? _____ Duration? _____

What medications are you presently taking? _____

Since taking the medication have you noticed any of the following? (circle)

headaches   nausea   itching   rash   ringing in ears   other _____

Surgeries? _____

Exercise Program? _____

Splints? _____

What do you know about arthritis? _____

What are your goals? _____

UPPER EXTREMITY JOINT INVOLVEMENT:

	RIGHT	LEFT
NECK		
SHOULDER		
ELBOW		
FOREARM		
WRIST		
DIGITS 1 2 3 4 5		

HAND PLACEMENT EVALUATION

KEY: 0 - EASILY   2 - WITH MODERATE DIFFICULTY
       1 - WITH MINIMAL DIFFICULTY   3 - UNABLE

	RIGHT	LEFT	COMMENTS
REACH OVERHEAD			
TOUCH TOP OF HEAD			
TOUCH MOUTH			
TOUCH BACK OF NECK			
TOUCH BEHIND BACK			

FIG. 43-17

Arthritis evaluation checklist.

Continued

ARTHRITIS EVALUATION CHECKLIST

HAND	RIGHT	LEFT	COMMENTS
9 Hole Peg (seconds)			
Grip Strength			
Pinch lateral, 3-jaw			
Opposition			

SENSATION: _____

SOFT TISSUE & HAND DEFORMITIES NOTED: (Include Flexion Contractures, Swan Neck, Boutonniere, Ulnar
Deviation, Subluxation, Edema, Redness, Warmth)

_____

_____

FUNCTIONAL ABILITIES: KEY: 0 - EASILY   2 - WITH MODERATE DIFFICULTY
                              1 - WITH MINIMAL DIFFICULTY   3 - UNABLE

	COMMENTS
Grasp Spoon or Fork	
Carry to Mouth	
Cut Meat	
Drink from Glass/Cup	
BILATERAL ACTIVITIES	
Button	
Manipulate Coins	
Turn Key in Lock	
Write Name	
Turn Pages	
Use Telephone	
Open doors	
Open jars	

Endurance: _____

Marital Status: _____ Family Members/Supportive Persons at Home: _____

Household Responsibilities: _____

Do you have difficulty in ADL? _____

Architecture: _____

Vocational Responsibilities: _____

RECOMMENDATIONS:Adaptive Equipment (circle): Key Extension Feeding Device Writing Device Telephone Device
                Car Door Opener Dressing Stick Buttonhook   Other_____

Splints:_____

Joint Protection: _____

Home Program: _____

Evaluation Completed By: _____   Date: _____

FIG. 43-17 cont'd
Arthritis evaluation checklist.

deforming tendencies on motion, skin quality, and joint enlargement. In the early stages of RA, joints may appear puffy and soft. If the disease is active, joints may be red and hot. Patients with fibromyalgia may also display swelling of the hands. This is considered "subjective swelling" and may be a type of paresthesia.[18] The therapist should record the location of such observations so that later comparisons may be made. Actual photographs of the hands and wrist may be useful. Evaluation procedures for the previously described deformities of the hand and wrist seen in RA and OA are shown in Table 43-2.

Sensorimotor Components

The OT evaluation of sensorimotor components may take considerable time. If there is discomfort or pain in

---

TABLE 43-2

Tests for Specific Deformities of the Hand and Wrist

Deformity	Test
Synovial thickening or nodules (seen in trigger finger)	Ask the patient if the fingers ever catch or stay closed when attempting to open the hand. Determine whether this happens rarely, occasionally, or consistently and whether there is any pain or loss of function because of it. Observe the patient actively move the finger. Note any snapping or catching of the finger during motion. Look for discrepancy between AROM and PROM. If these clinical signs are observed or reported, palpate along the tendon surface and feel for the presence of a nodule. Flexor nodules are often felt near the distal palmar crease.
Tendon rupture	Observed as a detached tendon, and the patient is unable to actively move the joint.
Extrinsic tightness	Position the patient's wrist at neutral. Passively flex the MP joint to different positions while simultaneously flexing the PIP and DIP joints. If the position of the MP joint influences the degree of flexion possible at the distal joints, the extrinsics are tight..*
Intrinsic tightness	First perform a test for extrinsic tightness to rule out adhesions of extensor tendons. Passively extend the MP joint and flex the PIP joint. Repeat the action with the MP joint in flexion. Intrinsic tightness is noted if there is more resistance when the MP joint is extended.*
MCP ulnar drift	Measure the angle between the PIP and the MP joints during active extension and compare it with the normal ROM. The index finger normally has 10° to 20° of ulnar deviation during active extension. Ulnar drift is described as follows:

SEVERITY	INDEX FINGER	FINGERS 3-5
Mild	20° to 30°	0° to 10°
Moderate	30° to 50°	10° to 30°
Severe	50° or more	30° or more

Deformity	Test

MP palmar subluxation-dislocation	Palpate over the dorsum of the joint when it is at the 0° neutral position. Subluxation is felt if there is a step between the metacarpal and the first phalanx. Subluxation is described as follows:
	   Mild: step is felt, full extension is possible
	   Moderate: the step is both felt and visible, extension is limited
	   Severe: gross malalignment and definite limitation of ROM[20]

Swan-neck deformity	May be observed with intrinsic muscle tightness. To test if the deformity is caused by initial involvement at the DIP joints and rupture of the lateral slips of the extensor tendons, first test for extrinsic tightness. Then move the MP joint into extension and flex the PIP joint to prove that there is no intrinsic tightness. Then the patient should extend the finger actively. If there is a rupture of the lateral slips of the extensor tendon, the DIP joint will drop into flexion because ruptured lateral slips of the EDC cannot function to extend the joint. The middle slip of the EDC, acting on the PIP joint, pulls too hard and hyperextends the joint when active extension is attempted, resulting in the swan-neck appearance. To test if the deformity is caused by stretching of supporting structures or rupture of the FDS tendon, first test for extrinsic tightness. Move the MP joint into hyperextension, and flex the PIP joint to rule out intrinsic tightness. The patient is then asked to flex the finger into the palm actively while the examiner holds the adjacent fingers in extension. If the FDS tendon is ruptured, it will not be possible to flex the PIP joint.
Boutonniere and thumb deformities	Observation.

*Perform all movements gently to avoid causing further damage, including tendon rupture.

AROM Active range of motion; *DIP,* distal interphalangeal; *EDC,* extensor digitorum communis; *FDS,* flexor digitorum superficialis; *MP,* metacarpophalangeal; *PIP,* proximal interphalangeal; *PROM,* passive range of motion; *ROM,* range of motion.

the joints, the assessments may have to be performed gradually over two or three treatment sessions.

Sensory evaluation is indicated if there is potential nerve damage or compression caused by swelling. Modalities that should be tested are senses of touch, pain, temperature, and proprioception. Paresthesias should be noted.

When performing ROM measurements, the therapist should note whether the joints feel stiff, unstable, or crepitant. A major discrepancy between active and passive ROM may be caused by pain secondary to inflammation in the joint or soft tissue, as well as by weakness or tendon involvement.

For patients with RA, manual muscle testing may not be possible because of joint instability and alterations in the line of muscle pull. If muscle testing is indicated, the usual procedures will need to be adapted. Resistance should be applied within the patient's pain-free ROM rather than at the end of the ROM, as is usual in manual muscle testing. It is not unusual for patients with arthritis to have pain in the last 30° to 40° of joint motion. Therefore if resistance is applied within the pain-free range, the inhibition of muscle strength by pain will be avoided.[18]

The use of the manual muscle test is controversial because some physicians prohibit any resistance that can cause harm to diseased tissue and joints or place deforming forces on the joint.[7] Functional muscle or motion testing may be used if resistance is prohibited.

In both the ROM assessment and the muscle strength test the therapist should make note of the time of day and the amount of antiinflammatory or analgesic medication taken. These medications may influence results of the evaluation.[18] In addition, future reevaluations should be performed under the same conditions as the initial evaluation.

Hand function testing is important, but the therapist should be careful not to stress the joints during the assessment. For this reason, grip and pinch strength may be tested with an adapted blood pressure cuff and measured in millimeters of mercury.[5,18] Specific devices for measuring grip strength for the arthritic hand are also commercially available. A test of hand function that evaluates grasp and prehension patterns, such as the Jebsen Test of Hand Function,[15] or observation of hand use with common functional tasks should be done. Hands that have severe involvement and obvious deformity may, in fact, have very good function.

The patient's physical *endurance* should be evaluated by observation and an assessment of the daily or weekly schedule. Lack of sleep, chronic pain, weakness, deconditioning, and emotional stress are factors that may lead to decreased endurance in patients with arthritis. Fatigue may be one of the most disruptive factors in lifestyle for patients with fibromyalgia.[18,28]

Screening for lower extremity (LE) involvement may be carried out by the occupational or physical therapist. Specific LE joint problems or problems with the feet may benefit from physical therapy or orthotic assessment.[2] The footwear should be noted so that shoes that will provide good support to arthritic feet can be recommended.

Strength of the LEs can be observed in the patient's gait pattern and when the patient rises from a chair. If the patient must use arms and hands to push off, this is indicative of LE weakness. The patient's need for assistive devices and safety in ambulation should also be assessed. The therapist should observe for any obvious joint limitations and weakness in the LEs and should have data from specific evaluation of ROM, strength, and deforming tendencies in the legs. These factors are important considerations when planning treatment, presenting joint protection and energy conservation techniques, and positioning to prevent loss of ROM in the LEs.

Cognitive and Psychosocial Components

Patients with arthritis should be screened for problems in cognitive and psychosocial components. The associated pain, lack of sleep, and depression may cause deficits in attention span, short-term memory, and problem-solving skills.[18] It is also important to understand how patients manage stress in their lives.

Occupational Performance

The evaluation of activities of daily living (ADL) for patients with arthritis is similar to ADL evaluations for other physical disabilities. However, the evaluation should consider such factors as morning stiffness, medication schedule, activity tolerance, and proper positioning.[18] Patients with arthritis may report both "good days" and "bad days." It is important to find out the relative percentage of each and how the patient's functional abilities differ on good and bad days. Such information may help the patient learn how to prevent pain and stress to the joints and to increase functional independence.[18]

Evaluations for ADL and work and leisure activities should consider both psychological and social factors. What is the patient's attitude toward the disability? What specific goals does the patient have? What strategies are used to deal with pain and fear? The patient's abilities may be determined, in part, by interview. The actual performance should be observed at the normal time each activity is performed because the patient's abilities may change at different times of the day. Ideally, a home evaluation should be done in the patient's home. On-site or simulated experiences may be used to assess job performance. The job tasks can be analyzed, and joint protection principles can be applied, if possible. Pacing of work responsibilities may help the patient incorporate required rest periods into the working day. In all areas of ADL it is essential to determine whether the patient is using energy conservation and joint protection techniques.[5,18]

Treatment Objectives

Treatment of the patient with arthritis must take into account the chronic and progressive nature of the disease.[7] An overall goal of treatment for patients with RA is to decrease pain and inflammation. Patients with OA may be seen by the occupational therapist because of hand, hip, or knee involvement or as a part of a postoperative rehabilitation program after total hip or total knee replacement surgery (see Chapter 45). Patients with fibromyalgia will benefit from a holistic approach that focuses on the psychological conflicts that create stress, as well as on the physical factors.[18,28]

The general objectives of treatment in occupational therapy are to (1) maintain or increase joint mobility and strength; (2) increase physical endurance; (3) prevent, correct, or minimize the effect of deformities; (4) maintain or increase the ability to perform ADL; (5) increase knowledge about the disease and the best methods of dealing with the physical, psychological, and functional effects; and (6) assist with stress management and adjustment to physical disability.

The treatment plan should be designed for the individual patient and be based on the severity of the symptoms and the general health status, lifestyle, and personal goals of the patient. The patient should be an active participant in the treatment process. Both the patient and significant others need to understand the disease process and treatment methods. Rehabilitation intervention will most likely be intermittent, so the patient's ability to follow through with the treatment methods will greatly influence the success of the treatment.[5,18]

Treatment Methods

Many treatment strategies are used in OT for the management of arthritis. Traditional methods include rest, positioning, physical agent modalities, exercise, therapeutic activity, splinting, and ADL training. The choice of methods will depend upon the patient's condition and reaction to the various procedures. When indicated, methods for the specific type of arthritis will be provided.

Rest

Rest is an important part of treatment and should be considered an active way of reducing inflammation and pain. Frequently, patients with RA and OA will develop fibromyalgia, which is believed to be related to sleep disturbances.[16] Rest and relaxation effectively break the vicious circle of pain, stress, and depression by allowing the body time to heal itself. Rest can take several forms. The amount of systemic rest needed varies with individuals, from complete bed rest to a short nap during the day. Localized rest to individual joints may include wearing a splint to support the involved joint during activity or lying in non–weight-bearing positions to prevent joint stress. Psychological rest is experienced when a person takes a short diversion from routine activities or focuses attention on enjoyable, instead of stressful, events.[7,13]

Positioning

Positioning against the patterns of deformity is recommended to reduce pain and prevent contractures. To prevent flexion contractures, persons with RA should not sleep with a pillow under the knees and should use only a small pillow under the neck. Prone lying is recommended for both the hip and knee joints. Maintaining good postural alignment when standing and sitting will discourage the development of deformities and prevent undue stress on the muscles and joints. Patients with both RA and OA may benefit from using chairs with high seats and armrests, which will make it easier to stand up.[18]

Physical Agent Modalities

Physical agent modalities (PAMs) such as heat, transcutaneous electrical nerve stimulation (TENS), and biofeedback are helpful in relieving pain.[17,28] Local applications of heat, including paraffin wax treatments and moist or dry heat packs, help to reduce stiffness and increase mobility. At home, patients may enjoy the benefits of heat by taking a warm bath or shower. The application of heat should be limited to 20 minutes because longer periods of warmth can cause an increase in inflammation and edema.[17,19] Ice packs are used both for pain relief and to decrease edema. Practitioners must be aware of their state licensure requirements and be trained in the use of PAMs if they plan to use these modalities with their patients.

Massage

Massage is helpful in relieving muscle spasm and in increasing blood flow to the area. Patients may purchase electrical massage devices to assist with self-massage.[28]

Therapeutic Activity and Exercise

Therapeutic activity and exercise are used to promote joint function, muscle strength, and endurance. Exercise, in particular, may reduce the morning stiffness associated with RA and fibromyalgia, and exercise also reduces the risk of cardiovascular disease and osteoporosis.[28]

For patients with fibromyalgia, exercise is also helpful in diminishing pain and improving sleep.[28] Any functional program should be coordinated with the physical therapy program to avoid overworking the same muscles.

The Arthritis Foundation (see the address at end of chapter), in cooperation with the YMCA, sponsors aquatic programs designed to meet the needs of people with arthritis throughout the United States. These programs are run by certified instructors, and pools are maintained at the recommended 83° F water temperature. Studies suggest that these programs improve function and reduce pain. Exercises performed under water are less stressful to the joints and rarely exacerbate arthritis-related symptoms.[16] For this reason patients may also be instructed to perform their exercises while bathing.

RHEUMATOID ARTHRITIS. The specific types of activity that might be prescribed for patients with RA will depend primarily on the stage of disease the patient is experiencing. The stages of the inflammatory process have been described as *acute, subacute, chronic active,* and *chronic inactive.*[18]

Clinical symptoms seen in the *acute* stage include limited movement, pain and tenderness at rest that increases with movement, overall stiffness, weakness, tingling or numbness, and hot, red joints. In the *subacute* stage, limited movement and tingling remain. A decrease in pain and tenderness indicates that inflammation is subsiding. Stiffness is limited to morning stiffness, and the joints appear pink and warm. The *chronic-active* stage is characterized by less tingling, pain, and tenderness and increased activity tolerance, although endurance remains low. No signs of inflammation are present in the *chronic-inactive* stage. The patient's low endurance and pain and stiffness at this stage result from disuse. Overall functioning may be decreased as a result of fear of pain and limited ROM, muscle atrophy, and contractures.[18,22]

Any treatment program should begin slowly and gradually increase in intensity, duration, and frequency of the various activities.[5] Splints, braces, and positioning devices may be used throughout the stages to provide joint rest and stability. The patients may perform self-care activities as tolerated.

Preservation of function of the hips, knees, elbows, and MP joints is essential in the treatment program. Therefore exercise to other joints must not interfere with functions of these joints or be done at their expense.

During the acute stage, active assistive exercises and exercises with gravity eliminated may be performed within the limits of pain tolerance. As the patient's abilities improve, the activities will progress to include active and resistive exercises. The exercises should be done at the best time of the day for the patient (i.e., when the patient feels most limber and has the least pain). This might be after a warm shower or a short time after receiving pain medication.[5,18]

In the acute stage gentle passive and active ROM exercises to the point of pain (without stretch) should be done twice a day. As little as one to two repetitions of complete joint range are needed to prevent loss of ROM.[18] However, several attempts at movement may be needed before full range is achieved. The patient may perform ROM exercises of the neck, elbows, and hands, but the therapist should passively exercise the shoulder to promote muscle relaxation.[18] Isometric exercises without resistance may be attempted to preserve strength. The patient should be instructed to tighten each muscle without moving the joint and maintain tension for 6 seconds once or twice per day.[7] Resistive exercise and stretching at the end range should be avoided.[18]

Active and passive ROM exercises that include a gentle passive stretch may be started in the subacute stage. Isotonic exercises may be done, provided there is minimal stress to the joints.[18] The number of repetitions performed may range from three to five and should be done once or twice per day. The number of repetitions should be decreased if pain or swelling increases.[7] Graded isometric exercises may be performed once a day. Patients should exert about three quarters of their maximum strength (or less if pain occurs) and perform one to three repetitions.[7]

In the chronic-active and chronic-inactive stages, stretch at the end of the range may be included during ROM. Resistive isotonic and isometric exercises may be done as long as they do not overstress the joints.[5,18] Endurance exercises are most important in this stage to improve overall cardiovascular fitness.[7]

There is some controversy over the use of isotonic resistive exercise for patients with RA.[18] The occupational therapist must determine if that patient has stable, inactive joints that would benefit from a strengthening program without jeopardizing other joints. If pain resulting from exercise lasts longer than 1 hour, the vigor of the exercise should be reduced.[18]

OSTEOARTHRITIS. Exercise will not increase ROM limited by osteophytes, but it may help decrease generalized stiffness. Exercise helps lessen the symptoms of OA by increasing the strength of the muscles that stabilize the joints.[2] Low-impact activities such as flexibility and strengthening exercises, brisk walking, biking, and swimming or water aerobics may help to ease the pain and prevent disability. Patients should avoid exercising tender, injured, or inflamed joints.[2]

FIBROMYALGIA. A program of flexibility and endurance exercise is the best defense for combating the pain associated with fibromyalgia.[28] Some of the benefits include decreased stiffness, increased strength and energy, improved sleep patterns, and decreased depression. Going without exercise can lead to deconditioning and result in increased pain. Low-impact or nonimpact aerobic exercises such as brisk walking, biking, swimming, and water aerobics are a few ways to start exercising without jarring painful joints.[28] Aerobic exercise appears to be more beneficial than simple stretching.[16] It is very important to watch the pace at which patients advance their exercise, because if performed incorrectly, exercise may exacerbate patients' conditions. Exercise should begin at low intensity, include stretching, and then progress to more strenuous aerobic exercise.[16]

Whether choosing therapeutic activities or exercise, the therapist should apply the same principles.[18] Activities should not overstress the joints but should offer enough repetition of movement to help improve ROM and strength. The activities should be nonresistive and avoid patterns of deformity. For patients with RA, resistive squeezing of the hand should be avoided because it can promote ulnar deviation, MP subluxation, and extensor tendon displacement.[12,18] When choosing an activity, the therapist should consider how it will affect all joints. Although sanding a piece of wood on an inclined board may be helpful in increasing shoulder and elbow range, it could be harmful for the hand to grip a piece of sandpaper. This could be remedied by using a sanding block.

Patients with RA should avoid activities that require the use of the hand in prolonged static contractions. However, sometimes the psychological benefits of doing activities one enjoys may outweigh the risks involved, especially if the risks can be minimized. According to Melvin, activities such as knitting and crocheting are contraindicated only if there is active MP synovitis, developing swan-neck deformity, or thumb CMC joint involvement.[18] Problems may be prevented by having the patient wear a hand or thumb splint while performing the activity. Additionally, frequent rest breaks and stretching exercises for the intrinsic muscles will help to limit complications.[6,18]

Other leisure activities may be introduced to patients as a means of helping them cope with their disabilities. An interest survey completed by the patient can be analyzed to determine appropriate activities. The patient may need help modifying tools or tasks or substituting similar activities.

Splinting

The goals of splinting are to support the joint in an optimal position for function and to reduce inflammation by providing rest or support to the joint.[18] Dynamic splints are also used to correct deformity. Splints can be useful for the wrist, fingers, neck, elbows, knees, and ankles. The therapist should determine the need for splinting based on a thorough evaluation and consultation with the patient's physician. The inappropriate use of splints can be harmful.[10,24] The splinting of one joint may put added stress on the surrounding joints. An example of this is the increased stress to the MP joints when the wrist is splinted.[18]

Some of the more commonly used splints in the treatment of the arthritic hand include the resting hand splint, wrist immobilization splint, wrist cock-up splint with MP support, and ulnar drift positioning splint. Specific directions for these and other splints may be found in several sources.[18,24,29] Additionally, several splints designed for the arthritic hand are available commercially.

The *resting hand splint* (see Chapter 31) is useful for the treatment of acute synovitis of the wrist, fingers, and thumb because it helps to prevent ulnar drift and maintains the thumb web space. The primary use of this splint is to provide rest to the involved joints, but it may also help prevent multiple joint contractures from developing. Because it prevents movement, it is usually worn during sleep. If the patient needs resting splints for each hand, each splint should be worn on alternate nights so the patient has one free hand.[18,29]

A *wrist immobilization splint* (Fig. 43-18) is used to immobilize a painful wrist while allowing the hand to remain functional. This splint supports the wrist in extension, which relieves compression of the carpal tunnel.[18,29] If the MPs are also involved, a *wrist cock-up splint with MP support* may be necessary (Fig. 43-19). This splint places the MP joints in normal alignment, allowing them 0° to 25° of MP flexion.

During pinch and grasp activities, an *ulnar drift positioning splint* (Fig. 43-20) may be used to prevent ulnar drift. A *CMC splint* may be used to provide support and reduce stress to the CMC joint. This may help to decrease pain during activities involving the thumb.

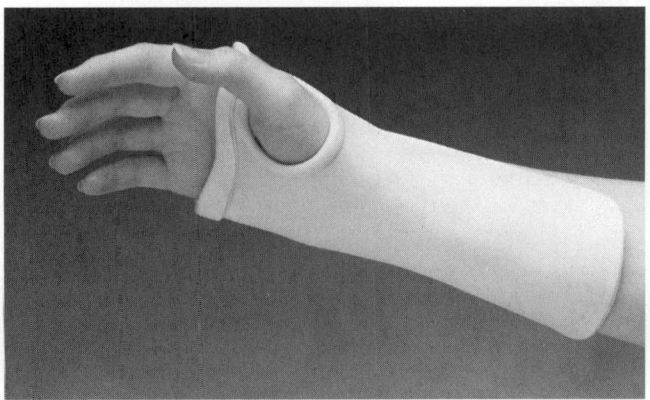

FIG. 43-18

Wrist immobilization splint. (Courtesy of North Coast Medical, Inc, Morgan Hill, Calif.)

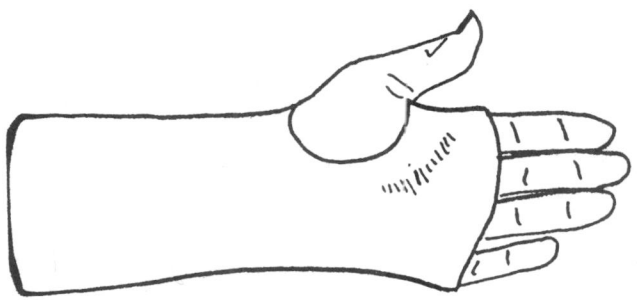

FIG. 43-19
Wrist cock-up splint with metacarpophalangeal support.

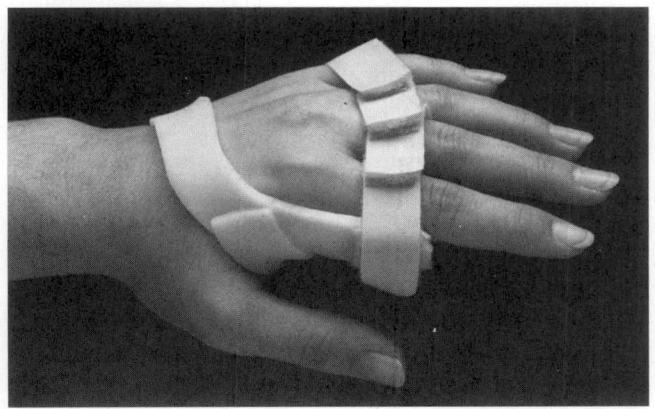

FIG. 43-20
Ulnar drift positioning splint. (Courtesy of North Coast Medical, Inc, Morgan Hill, Calif.)

To prevent stiffness from occurring, it is important to remove splints and other orthoses on a regular basis to complete ROM exercises to the involved joints.[18,29] Table 43-3 describes specific splinting and treatment strategies for upper extremity deformities previously described.[14]

Occupational Performance

An effective method of minimizing the effects of disuse and bed rest is to have patients perform ADL throughout their hospitalization.[5,6,18] When the patient's condition is acute, activities may be limited to feeding and facial hygiene. As the patient's condition improves, ADL should be resumed because this will help to maintain muscular tone and improve endurance. Adaptive equipment and methods may be used with bathing, dressing, feeding, work and home management, and leisure activities to promote independence and to prevent pain and further injury to the joints. Therapists working with this population should be familiar with adaptive equipment and joint protection and work simplification techniques described in this chapter. Additional resources are provided at end of the chapter.

An important but often neglected aspect of self-care training is sexual counseling. Patients may approach any member of the health care team with questions related to sexual concerns. In addition to open discussion of sexual problems, patients and their partners are often helped by illustrations of more comfortable positions for intercourse. Several excellent treatments of this subject are available.[8,25] Additional information may be found in Chapter 15.

ENERGY CONSERVATION. Because patients with arthritis have a decreased energy supply and may need more energy to do things, they can benefit from using *energy conservation techniques* (Box 43-3).[13,18] OT practitioners can teach the techniques to their patients and help the patients apply the principles to daily activities. Patients may have difficulty fitting the principles into their lifestyle, which often necessitates a change in life-long habits. Practice in using the techniques during hospitalization will help with carryover after discharge.

ASSISTIVE DEVICES. *Assistive devices* should be used only when necessary and must be selected with the patient's needs in mind.[5,17,18] Patients are less likely to use equipment that is expensive or difficult to use. Patients will need to be taught to use some of the assistive devices (such as those that compensate for loss of ROM) when they have a flare-up. When the inflammation has subsided, patients should be encouraged to stop using the devices and to begin using their own ROM and muscle power to maintain their strength and mobility. Table 43-4 describes the principles used in selecting devices, and examples for each.[5,18]

JOINT PROTECTION. Joints affected by arthritis are at risk for further damage. *Joint protection* (or joint saver) techniques are taught to patients in order to minimize their risk of injury during daily activities. These techniques are especially helpful for patients with RA or with OA involving the hands.[7,9,26]

1. *Respect pain.* Pain is one way the body signals there is something wrong. Many patients with arthritis may feel that they can "tough it out," but ignoring pain will often lead to more pain. As a rule of thumb, pain that lasts for more than 1 or 2 hours after completion of a task indicates that the activity was too stressful and the activity should be changed. This change might include breaking the task into steps or using less effort to complete the task. Activities that put strain on an already painful joint should be avoided.[6,7,14,26]

2. *Maintain muscle strength and joint ROM.* This may be accomplished by using each joint to its maximal available ROM and strength during daily activities. When ironing, sweeping, or mopping, the patient should use long, flowing strokes, straightening and

TABLE 43-3

Treatment for Specific Deformities

Deformity	Possible Medical Care	Treatment Methods	Splinting	Methods to Avoid
Swan neck	Synovectomy in early stages	Daily PROM and gentle stretching for the DIPs Daily AROM to each finger joint Active muscle contraction with stretch for flexion contractures	Small, short dynamic splint for the PIPs during daily activity to prevent hyperextension Three-point finger splint[18] to maintain range of PIP flexion	Isotonic, isometric and resistive exercise Passive or device stretch to flexion contractures
Boutonniere	Synovectomy for the second and third fingers	Daily PROM to all joints of the involved finger(s)	Dynamic extension splints[18] for second and third fingers may improve function and opposition	Isotonic, isometric, and resistive exercise
Trigger finger	Steroid injections Surgery	Tendon protection techniques Heat and ice for mobility and inflammation	Trigger finger splint[18]	
MP ulnar drift	Synovectomy Tendon replacement Joint replacement	Daily PROM to MP joints if AROM lacks full flexion and extension Joint protection	Dynamic ulnar deviation splints during the day Static splints with the MPs in neutral deviation and 45° of flexion at night	Isotonic, isometric, and resistive exercise Positions of deformity
MP palmar subluxation-dislocation	Joint replacement or repair	PROM and AROM of the MPs Joint protection		
Wrist subluxation	Arthroplasty		Flexible splint during the day and rigid splint at night	
Elbow synovitis	Steroid injections Synovectomy and resection of the radial head Arthroplasty	Rest for acute synovitis Use of cold Daily AROM and PROM exercises Isotonic or isometric exercise	Splint to provide joint rest or for instability	Overuse
Shoulder synovitis	Steroid injections Applicable surgery	AROM and isotonic exercises preceded by hot packs Joint protection		Slings

AROM, Active range of motion; *MP,* metacarpophalangeal; *PIP,* proximal interphalangeal; *PROM,* passive range of motion.

bending the arms as much as possible (Fig. 43-21). Light items, such as cereal or noodles, can be stored in high cabinets so that full shoulder ROM will be used when reaching.[6,7,14,26]

3. *Avoid positions that put stress on involved joints.* The "normal" way of doing things may need to be changed so that joints are used in their most stable position. Activities involving a tight grip can be avoided by using items with enlarged handles.[6,7,14,26]

Holding a knife in the traditional manner puts too much direct pressure on the fingers. Instead, the patient should use the knife as if it were a dagger or use a pizza cutter. A vegetable peeler should be held parallel to MP joints and not diagonally across the palm. A butter knife can be used to open milk cartons. The palm of the hand (not just the fingers) should be used when pushing from a chair to stand up (Fig. 43-22).[6,7,14,26]

BOX 43-3
Principles of Energy Conservation

Attitudes and Emotions
Remove yourself from stressful situations.
Avoid concentrating on things that make you tense.
Close your eyes and visualize pleasant places and thoughts.

Body Mechanics
When lifting something that is low, bend your knees and lift by straightening your legs. Try to keep your back straight.
Avoid reaching (use reachers). Avoid stretching, bending, carrying, and climbing. If you have to bend, keep your back straight.
Incorporate good posture into your activities.
Sit to work whenever possible.
To get up from a chair, slide forward to the edge of the chair. With your feet flat on the floor, lean forward and push with your *palms* on the arms or seat of the chair. Stand by straightening your legs.
Before you get tired, stop and rest.

Work Pace
Plan on getting 10 to 12 hours of rest daily (naps and nights).
Work at your own pace.
Spread tedious tasks throughout the week.
Do the tasks that require the most energy at the times you have the most energy.
Alternate easy and difficult activities and take a 10- to 15-minute rest break each hour.

Leisure Time
Devote a portion of your day to an activity that you enjoy and find relaxing.
Check out what's available in the community.

Work Methods
Keep items within easy reach.
Use good light and proper ventilation and room temperature.
Use joint protection techniques.
Work surfaces should be at a correct height.

Organization
Plan ahead; don't rush or push yourself.
Decide which jobs are absolutely necessary.
Share the workload with family and friends.

How to Begin
Plan ahead by charting your daily routine.
Make a list of tasks and spread them out in your schedule.
Include daily rest periods and rest breaks during energy-consuming times.

Other hand positions to avoid are those that involve tight pinching, squeezing, or twisting motions. A dusting mitt will help keep the fingers extended while dusting. Sponges or rags may be wrung out by spreading the hand flat over them or by squeezing them between the palms. Several methods may be used to open a screw-top jar, such as leaning on the jar with the palm of the hand and turning the lid with shoulder motion (Fig. 43-23), or holding the jar in a drawer as the cap is twisted.[7,18,26]

To discourage the development of ulnar drift deformities, patients are taught to turn the hand toward the thumb when turning doorknobs. Patients should use the right hand to open a jar and the left hand to close it. When stirring, the patient should move the spoon counter-clockwise if using the right hand or clockwise if using the left hand (Fig. 43-24). Patients should be discouraged from leaning their chins on the hands or fingers and from using their fingers to pick up a mug because pressure

BOX 43-3
Principles of Energy Conservation—cont'd

Weekly Schedule

TIME:	SUN.	MON.	TUES.	WED.	THUR.	FRI.	SAT.
7:00							
8:00							
9:00							
10:00							
11:00							
12:00							
1:00							
2:00							
3:00							
4:00							
5:00							
6:00							
7:00							
8:00							
9:00							
10:00							

Check your schedule for the following factors:
Is there one day longer than another?
Are heavier tasks distributed through the week?
Is there a long task that could be done in several steps?
Will your plan allow for flexibility?
Have you devoted part of your day to a relaxing activity?
Does your plan use the principles of energy conservation?

on the thumb side of the fingers may promote ulnar deviation.[7,26]

4. *Avoid staying in one position for a long time.* Staying in the same position for a long time can cause excess fatigue and stiffness. Instead, the patient should use a book stand to hold a book. When stirring, the patient should place the bowl in a partially opened drawer or on a rubber mat to eliminate holding. The patient should never begin an activity that cannot be stopped immediately if pain or fatigue sets in.[7,26]

5. *Use the strongest joints and muscles available.* Using the larger joints reduces the stress on the smaller joints. One example of this is carrying a purse on the shoulder instead of in the hands (backpacks and fanny packs are also helpful). The weight should be either balanced between both shoulders or frequently

TABLE 43-4

Assistive Devices

Problem	Principle	Examples
Decreased range of motion	Lengthen the handle on objects Organize objects within easy reach	Reachers, long-handled shoe horn, extended mop handle Revolving space saver, pegboards
Impaired grasp	Enlarge the circumference of handles	Built-up soft handles, large pens, universal cuffs, stocking aids
Instability	Stabilize objects and provide support for safety	Nonskid mats, suction brushes, handrails, grab bars
Decreased energy	Facilitate ease of performance	Lightweight tools, electrical tools Zim jar opener
Potential for joint deformities	Increase leverage	Extended faucet handles, adapted key holder, vegetable peeler held at metacarpophalangeal joints
	Prevent static or prolonged holding	Book stand, bowl holder
Decreased strength	Modify work heights Raise the height of beds and chairs to make it easier to stand.	Raised toilet seats

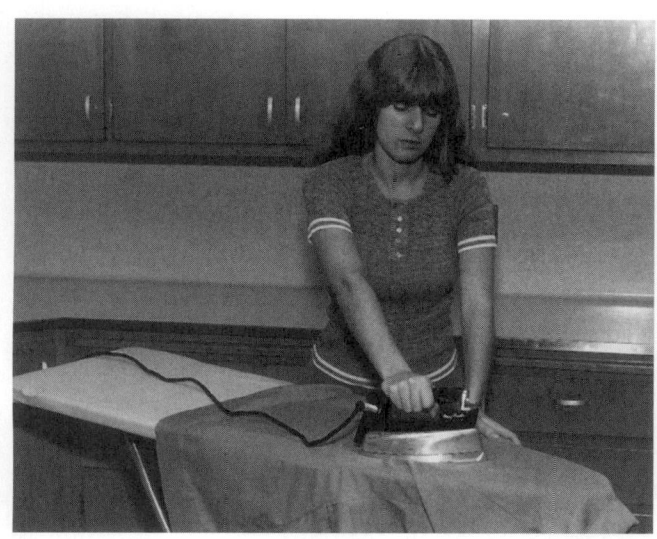

FIG. 43-21
During ironing, full extension at elbow can be practiced.

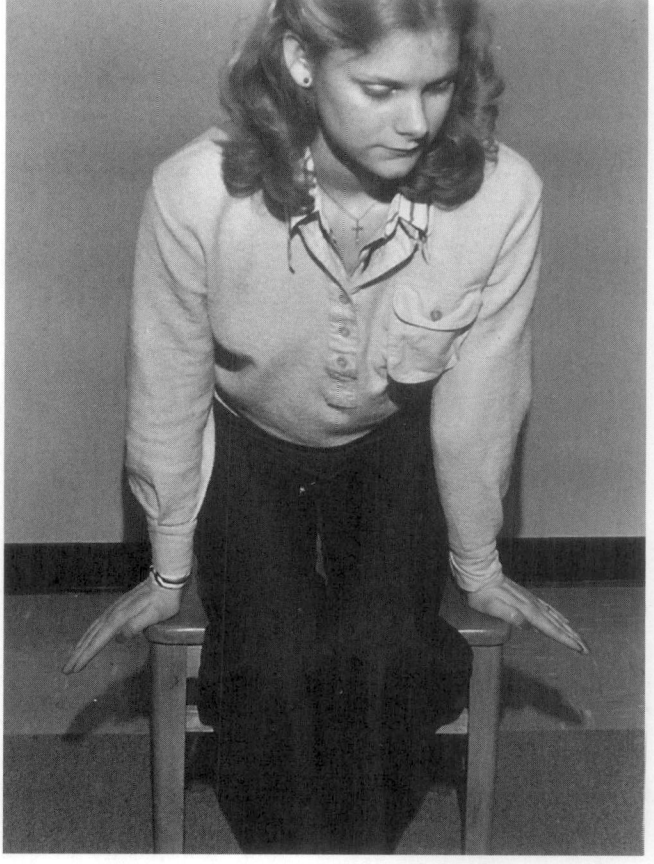

FIG. 43-22
Use of palms to push off chair helps to prevent dislocation of finger joints.

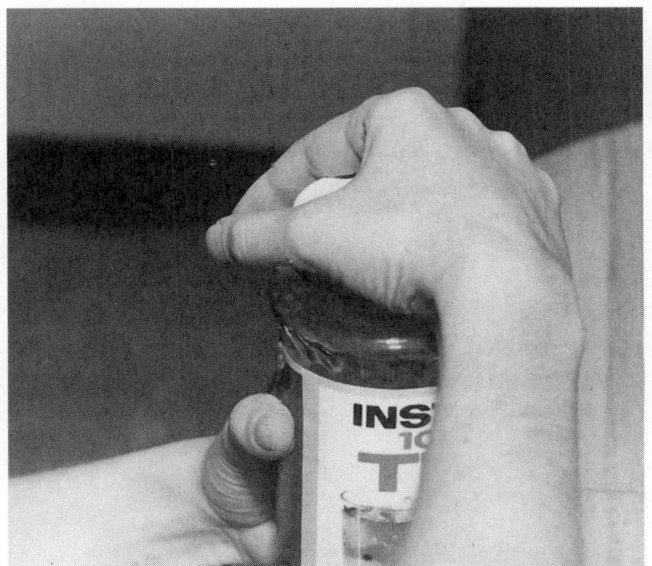

FIG. 43-23
Jar cap is twisted off, using palm of hand, and opened with right hand to prevent ulnar drift.

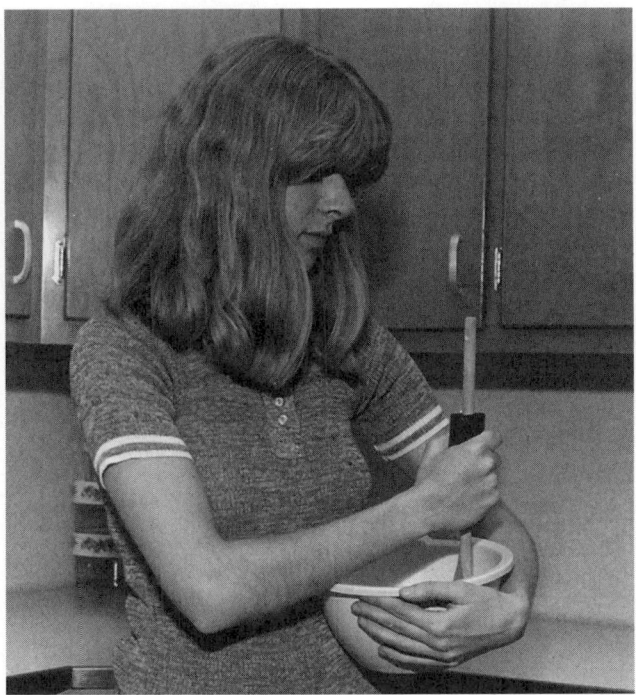

FIG. 43-24
Mixing bowl is stabilized with forearm. Spoon with soft, built-up handle is held so that pressure is toward radial side of the hand.

alternated between the two sides. Other examples include pushing doors open with the side of the arm instead of the hand; adding cloth loops to drawer pulls so they can be opened with the forearm; using palms, instead of fingers, to pick up a coffee mug; and using the stronger leg to go first up the stairs and last down the stairs. It is also important to keep weight under control to prevent stress on the weight-bearing joints.[7,18,26]

6. *Distribute the workload over several joints.* The patient should distribute the workload over several joints. For example, the patient should use the palms of both hands to lift and hold cups, plates, pots, and pans instead of grasping them with the fingers. The patient should also use oven mitts to carry hot dishes and carry heavy loads close to the body, in the arms, instead of holding them with the hands. He or she should slide objects along the counter instead of carrying them. If necessary, the patient should lift objects by scooping them up with both palms turned upward. Stress may also be reduced by wearing a wrist splint.[7,18,26]

Discharge Planning

Discharge planning begins as soon as the patient is referred to OT. Patients must be active participants throughout their treatment program so that they will follow through with the treatment once discharged.[16,18] Patient education helps patients use the many appropriate resources available to them.

Education of the patient and family should include information about the disease process, including signs of inflammation, the range of potential disability, and realistic treatment options.[6] It is important for families to understand the patient's abilities and when they should help (or not help) the patient do things.[16] They must be cautioned against medical quackery, which promotes worthless arthritis remedies. Over 30 million Americans have arthritis, helping to make health fraud a very lucrative business.[2]

When providing patient education, the occupational therapist should pay particular attention to questions the patient may ask. Information should be reviewed even if the patient may have heard it before.[5] Repetition and reinforcement are the keys to education. Topics should be approached in a variety of ways, and using examples that relate directly to the patient's interest and experiences.[5]

Group treatment, such as movement or exercise classes, home management classes, or arthritis education classes, can provide mutual support and promote problem solving. Seeing others with similar problems may serve as a powerful motivational tool.[5,11,18] OT practitioners may lead or participate with other members of the rehabilitation team in such activity groups.

One group program, designed by an occupational therapist, is the ROM Dance Program.[12] Based on the principles of T'ai-chi ch'uan, this program promotes involvement in daily exercise and rest. Components include the ROM dance itself, relaxation techniques, group sharing, and health education. Information on

ARTHRITIS RANGE OF MOTION EXERCISES

The following exercises will help you to maintain your mobility. Do only those checked by the therapist.

INSTRUCTIONS:

1.   Start doing five of each exercise two times per day.
2.   Progress to ten of each, two times per day.
3.   Do all exercises **slowly** and while sitting.
4.   If in an active flare up, cut down or eliminate exercises. After the flare, start at the beginning to build up tolerance.

SHOULDER

_____   Hold your hands on your shoulders and make small to large circles with your elbows. Go clockwise and then counterclockwise.

_____   With your hands on your shoulders, bring your elbows together in front of you and then spread elbows apart to the side and as far back as you can reach.

_____   Roll up a newspaper and hold onto the ends of it with each hand facing down. Rest the paper on your knees. Bend your elbows to bring the paper to your right shoulder and back to your knees. Bend your elbows to your left shoulder and back to your knees.

ELBOW

_____   Hold your hands on your shoulders. Bring them out straight in front of you with your palms up.

_____   With your elbows bent at your side, turn your palms up and down.

WRIST

_____   Hold your hands facing down. Make a fist as you bend your wrist up. Open your fingers as you bend your wrist down.

_____   Hold your hands together like you're praying. Keeping your hands together, and moving only your wrist, point your fingertips away from and toward you.

HANDS

_____   Touch your thumb to each finger.

_____   Make a fist and stretch your fingers open and out.

Please call if you have any questions.

Instructed by: _____   Phone: _____

FIG. 43-25
Arthritis range of motion exercises.

the ROM Dance Program can be obtained from the address given at the end of the chapter.

Treatment should include the development of a home program and training of the patient in its use. A variety of topics, including energy conservation, joint protection, and appropriate activities and exercises, may be included. An example of a home exercise program for RA can be found in Fig. 43-25. Verbal and written directions should be geared to the patient's level of understanding. The patient should be made aware of the resources available from the local or national chapter of the Arthritis Foundation. The Foundation supports research and offers a variety of publications and classes designed to improve the quality of life for patients with arthritis. (See the address at the end of the chapter.)

Treatment Precautions

The following is a list of treatment precautions to be used when working with patients with arthritis.[14] More specific information on each can be found in the appropriate sections in this chapter.

1. Avoid fatigue.
2. Respect pain.
3. Avoid static, stressful, or resistive activities.
4. Limit the application of heat to 20 minutes.
5. Use resistive exercises with caution and never with unstable joints.[7]
6. Be aware of sensory impairments.

SUMMARY

Three of the more common forms of arthritis are rheumatoid arthritis, osteoarthritis, and fibromyalgia. Although their causes and symptoms differ, methods for treating the joint involvement are similar. The potential for further injury can be reduced by proper medication, a balance between rest and activity, exercise, and surgery. In occupational therapy, patients learn how to protect their joints while performing day-to-day tasks at work and at home. Successful treatment depends on early intervention and ongoing care and reassessment.

CASE STUDY 43-1

CASE STUDY—MRS. J.

Mrs. J. is a 36-year-old woman with a diagnosis of rheumatoid arthritis, with onset 3 years ago. She is a wife and the mother of an 8-year-old girl. She lives with her husband and daughter in a three-bedroom, single-level tract home. Mrs J.'s primary role is that of homemaker. She also holds a part-time job at a florist shop doing wreath design and construction and flower arranging. She both enjoys this work and sees her salary as a necessary adjunct to the family income.

Mrs. J. was referred to OT during the acute phase of her most recent episode for prevention of deformity and loss of ROM and maintenance of maximal function. Medical precautions are: no strenuous activity, no resistive exercise or activity, and avoidance of fatigue.

In the OT evaluation , the therapist found Mrs. J. to be pleasant, cooperative, and motivated for therapy. During periods of remission, she is independent in light housekeeping, self-care, and work. She fatigues after 2 hours of light to moderate activity and requires a 20-minute rest period. During flare-ups she is severely limited in ADL, tends to withdraw from social situations, leaves home management tasks to her family, and is unable to work. She also displays limited patience when fatigued and in pain. She manages to do only light self-care activities independently.

Analysis of her job tasks revealed that some aspects of her job may contribute to the development of deformity. Cutting and twisting floral wire, forcing stems and stem supports into Styrofoam, and binding wreaths are contraindicated, while wreath design and layout and fresh flower arrangement are possible alternatives. Mrs. J.'s employer is willing to retain her on a part-time basis to perform these duties.

The evaluation revealed weakness in wrist and finger extensors (F +) and to a lesser degree in flexor groups (G). Mild ROM limitations are present in elbows, wrists, and fingers, with some MP instability noted (10° ulnar drift). No subluxation or other deformities are noted. Difficulty with fingertip prehension is noted, and pinch and grip are good but not normal in strength. Forceful use of the thumb in opposition enhances ulnar drift and produces MP discomfort. Mrs. J.'s sensation is intact. She is intelligent and motivated.

OT was initiated to (1) maintain ROM and strength of affected joints during the acute stage, (2) increase muscle strength by ½ grade, (3) prevent potential deformity, and (4) teach the patient to independently perform ADL, home management, and work tasks without causing fatigue and stress to involved joints. The OT program provided instruction and practice in using joint protection techniques and adaptive equipment, graded therapeutic exercises and activities for the involved joints, education about rheumatoid arthritis and methods of dealing with its effects, and job simulation tasks.

Mrs. J. responded well to treatment. Upper extremity ROM was maintained and strength was increased by ½ grade. Mrs. J. was happy to modify the way she had always done things if it meant having less pain and deformity. She was given a home exercise program and the phone number for the local chapter of the Arthritis Foundation. She plans to join a PACE (People with Arthritis Can Exercise) class within the month.

REVIEW QUESTIONS

1. What is the outstanding clinical feature that causes joint damage in rheumatoid arthritis?
2. What are the major differences between osteoarthritis and rheumatoid arthritis?
3. When is occupational therapy indicated for the treatment of patients with fibromyalgia?
4. What are three systemic signs of rheumatoid arthritis?
5. What are the clinical signs of joint inflammation?
6. When is resistive exercise appropriate for persons with rheumatoid arthritis?
7. Why are activities such as crocheting and knitting controversial for patients with rheumatoid arthritis?
8. What adaptive equipment would be useful for patients with arthritis?
9. Why is it important to know the type and schedule of medication the patient is taking?
10. Why should patients with rheumatoid arthritis avoid opening doors in the usual method?
11. What are important areas to evaluate in patients with arthritis?

12. Why is grip strength measured with an adapted blood pressure cuff for patients with rheumatoid arthritis?
13. Why is rest an important part of treatment for patients with arthritis?
14. Identify five principles of joint protection.
15. Describe how energy conservation techniques can be applied to daily activities.
16. Identify five assistive devices and describe why they are useful for patients with arthritis.

REFERENCES

1. Arthritis Foundation: *Arthritis fact sheet,* Atlanta, 1998, The Foundation.
2. Arthritis Foundation: *Arthritis information: osteoarthritis,* Atlanta, 1994, The Foundation.
3. Arthritis Foundation: *Arthritis information: rheumatoid arthritis,* Atlanta, 1993, The Foundation.
4. Arthritis Foundation: *Arthritis surgery information: information to consider,* Atlanta, 1981, The Foundation.
5. Arthritis Health Professions Section Task Force: *Arthritis teaching slide collection for teachers of allied health professionals,* New York, 1980, Arthritis Foundation.
6. Batts C: Rheumatoid arthritis. In Hansen RA, Atchison B, editors: *Conditions in occupational therapy: effect on occupational performance,* Baltimore, 1993, Williams & Wilkins.
7. Chang RW: *Rehabilitation of persons with rheumatoid arthritis,* Gaithersburg, Md, 1996, Aspen Publishers.
8. Comfort A: *Sexual consequences of disability,* Philadelphia, 1978, George F Stickley.
9. Cordery JC: Joint protection: a responsibility of the occupational therapist, *Am J Occup Ther* 19(5):285-294, 1965.
10. Hanten DW: The splinting controversy in rheumatoid arthritis, *Physical Disabilities Special Interest Newsletter* 5:4, 1982.
11. Harkcom TM et al: Therapeutic value of graded aerobic exercise training in rheumatoid arthritis, *Arthritis Rheum* 28(1):32-39, 1985.
12. Harlowe D: The ROM dance program, *Physical Disabilities Special Interest Newsletter* 5:4, 1982.
13. Harris E: Rheumatic arthritis: the clinical spectrum. In Kelly WH, editor: *Textbook of rheumatology,* Philadelphia, 1981, WB Saunders.
14. Hittle JM, Pedretti LW, Kasch MC: Rheumatoid arthritis. In Pedretti LW: *Occupational therapy practice skills for physical dysfunction,* ed 4, St Louis, 1995, Mosby.
15. Jebsen RH et al: An objective and standardized test of hand function, *Arch Phys Med Rehabil* 50:311, 1969.
16. Klippel JH, editor: *Primer on the rheumatic diseases,* ed 11, Atlanta, 1997, Arthritis Foundation.
17. Mann WC, Hurren D, Tomita M: Assistive devices used by home-based elderly persons with arthritis, *Am J Occup Ther* 49(8):810-820, 1995.
18. Melvin JL: *Rheumatic disease in the adult and child: occupational therapy and rehabilitation,* ed 3, Philadelphia, 1989, FA Davis.
19. Michlovitz SL: *Thermal agents in rehabilitation,* ed 3, Philadelphia, 1996, FA Davis.
20. Nalebuff EA: Diagnosis, classification and management of rheumatoid thumb deformities, *Bull Hosp Joint Dis* 24:119, 1968.
21. Nalebuff EA: The rheumatoid thumb, *Clin Rheum Dis* 10(3):589-607, 1984.
22. Rudolph M: The psychosocial affects of rheumatoid arthritis, *OT Forum* 2:24, 1987.
23. Schumacher HR, editor: *Primer on the rheumatic diseases,* ed 10, Atlanta, 1993, Arthritis Foundation.
24. Seeger M: Splints, braces and casts. In Riggs G, Gall E, editors: *Rheumatic diseases: rehabilitation and management,* Boston, 1984, Butterworth Publishers.
25. Sidman JM: Sexual functioning and the physically disabled adult, *Am J Occup Ther* 31(2):81-85, 1977.
26. Slonaker D: *Arthritis information: using your joints wisely,* Atlanta, 1992, Arthritis Foundation.
27. Wilske KR, Healey LA: Remodeling the pyramid: a concept whose time has come, *J Rheumatol* 16(5):565-567, 1989.
28. Arthritis Foundation: *Your personal guide to living with fibromyalgia,* Atlanta, 1997, The Foundation.
29. Ziegler EM: *Current concepts in orthotics: a diagnosis-related approach to splinting,* Chicago, 1984, Rolyan Medical Products.

RECOMMENDED READING

Lorig K, Fries J: *The arthritis help book,* Reading, Mass, 1990, Addison-Wesley.
Marx H, producer: *Arthritis: best use of the hands,* Phoenix, 1988, Video Education Specialist (Video).
Melvin JL: *Rheumatic disease in the adult and child: occupational therapy and rehabilitation,* ed 3, Philadelphia, 1989, FA Davis.
Arthritis Foundation: *Your personal guide to living well with fibromyalgia,* Atlanta, 1997, Longstreet Press.

RESOURCES

American College of Rheumatology
 (www.rheumatology.org)
Arthritis Foundation
 (www.arthritis.org)
 PO Box 7669
 Atlanta, GA 30357-0669
 (1-800-283-7800)
The National Council on Independent Living
 (provides information on assistive devices)
 (703) 525-3406
The ROM Dance Program
 ROM Institute
 New Ventures of Wisconsin, Inc.
 3601 Memorial Drive
 Madison, WI 53704
 (608) 249-6670
A Workbook for Persons with Arthritis
 Superintendent of Documents
 US Government Printing Office
 Washington, DC 20402
AOTA Consumer Pamphlets
 American Occupational Therapy Association, Inc.
 4720 Montgomery Lane, PO Box 31220
 Bethesda, MD 20824-1220
 Consumer line 1-800-668-8255
 http:/www.aota.org/nonmembers.html
Mayo Foundation for Medical Education and Research
 http:/www.mayohealth.org

CHAPTER 44

Hand and Upper Extremity Injuries

MARY C. KASCH
ED NICKERSON

MARY C. KASCH
ED NICKERSON

KEY TERMS

Upper quadrant
Edema
Provocative tests
Splinting
Peripheral nerve injuries
Tendon injuries
Complex regional pain syndrome
Cumulative trauma disorders
Functional capacity evaluation
Ergonomics

LEARNING OBJECTIVES

After studying this chapter the student or practitioner will be able to do the following:

1. Discuss the incidence and effect of upper extremity (UE) injuries in the United States.
2. Identify three upper quarter screening tests, and explain their significance in developing a treatment plan.
3. Discuss the importance of joint mobility in regaining hand function.
4. Describe the four categories of tests used to evaluate peripheral nerve function, and explain how the results would be used in treatment planning.
5. Compare the standardized tests used to assess hand function.
6. Describe the sensory and motor innervation patterns of the three major nerves, and differentiate between the effects of proximal and distal lesions in each of the nerves.
7. Discuss complex regional pain syndrome and treatment techniques that should be included in the occupational therapy (OT) program for that disorder.
8. Compare techniques used in the rehabilitation of tendon injuries.
9. Describe the significance of edema on wound healing and joint mobility.
10. Discuss the role of the occupational therapist in evaluation and rehabilitation of injured workers.

Treatment of the upper extremity (UE) is important to all occupational therapists who work with physically disabled persons. The incidence of UE injuries is significant and accounts for about one third of all acute injuries. About 63% of the 90,000 work-related repetitive motion injuries per year in the United States involve the wrist, hand, and shoulder. Combined, these injuries account for 98 million days of restricted activity. The UEs are involved in about one third of work-related farm injuries and one quarter of all disabling injuries. In addition, disease and congenital anomalies contribute to UE dysfunction, and it is estimated that only about 15% of those suffering from severe cerebrovascular accident recover hand function. The total cost of UE disorders in the United States in 1995 was estimated to be almost $19 billion.[53]

The hand is vital to human function and appearance. It flexes, extends, opposes, and grasps thousands of times daily, allowing the performance of necessary daily activities. The hand's sensibility allows feeling without looking and provides protection from injury. The hand touches, gives comfort, and expresses emotions. Loss of hand function through injury or disease thus affects much more than the mechanical tasks that the hand performs. Hand injury may jeopardize a family's livelihood, and at the least affects every daily activity. The occupational therapist with training in physical and psychological assessment, prosthetic evaluation, fabrication of orthoses, assessment and training in the activities of daily living (ADL), and functional restoration is uniquely qualified to treat UE disorders.

Hand rehabilitation, or hand therapy, has grown as a specialty area of both physical therapy and occupational therapy (OT). Many of the treatment techniques used with hand-injured patients have evolved from the application of therapy and knowledge of both specialties to be used by the hand therapist. It is not the purpose of this chapter to instruct the OT student in physical agent modalities. Rather, treatment techniques that have been found to be beneficial to hand injury patients are presented. It is assumed that therapists best trained to provide them will provide these techniques.

As used in this chapter, hand therapy is a term that includes treatment of the entire **upper quadrant**, which includes the scapula, shoulder and arm. Upper quadrant and upper extremity are used interchangeably. UE rehabilitation requires advanced and specialized training by both physical and occupational therapists. A practice analysis study of the theory and knowledge that serves as the underpinning for hand therapy has been reported.[21,87] Treatment techniques, whether thermal modalities or specifically designed exercises, are used as a bridge to reach a further goal of restoring functional performance. Thus some modalities may be used as adjunctive or enabling modalities in preparation for functional use. It is within this context that treatment techniques will be presented in this chapter.

Treatment of the injured UE is a matter of timing and judgment. Following trauma or surgery, a healing phase must occur in which the body performs its physiological function of wound healing. Following the initial healing phase when cellular restoration has been accomplished, the wound enters its restorative phase. It is in this phase that hand therapy is most beneficial. Early treatment that occurs in this restorative phase is ideal, and in some cases essential for optimal results.

Although sample timetables may be presented, the therapist should always coordinate the application of any treatment with the referring physician. Surgical techniques may vary, and inappropriate treatment of the patient with hand injury can result in failure of a surgical procedure.

Communication between the surgeon, therapist, and patient is especially vital in this setting. A comfortable environment in which group interaction is possible may increase patient motivation and cooperation. The presence of the therapist as an instructor and evaluator is essential, but without the patient's cooperation limited gains will be achieved. Treating the psychological loss suffered by the patient with a hand injury is also an integral part of the rehabilitative therapy.

Hand therapy is provided in a number of treatment settings, ranging from private therapy offices to outpatient rehabilitation clinics and hospitals. Reimbursement for services may come directly from the patient, or through private medical insurance, workers' compensation insurance, or a variety of managed care programs. Changes in reimbursement have driven changes in the market place and employment patterns. In the future, OT will be provided in a variety of new settings and OT intervention will continue to evolve.

In UE rehabilitation, these changes have been manifested as changes in delivery of services. In some cases therapists are not members of the approved provider panel and are no longer able to treat patients who are members of a health maintenance organization. Reimbursement patterns have altered the provision of services by limiting the number of visits authorized. Therapists are also being asked to provide outcome data that support the need for services. It is likely that outcome-based treatment plans with functional goals and analysis of goal achievement will become the standard for the reimbursement of OT services. In addition, patient satisfaction and perception of health status have become crucial in the delivery of medical care in a consumer-based economy. Continuous quality improvement documentation is often required for participation in managed care programs. With fewer authorized visits the therapist must be more adept at instructing the patient in self-management of the condition being treated. Occupational therapists should anticipate a greater need to justify treatment in the future as part of the national challenge to control medical costs. Aides, certified assistants, and other support personnel will be used increasingly, but the quality of service provided must continue to meet all professional and ethical standards. This climate of change will present unique opportunities for the occupational therapist. Clinical specialists may find new roles as consultants and trainers. Just as OT teaches an individual to adapt to changes in health status, the profession of OT will need to adapt to social and economic changes to remain a leader in health management.

EXAMINATION AND EVALUATION

When approaching a patient who has a hand injury, the therapist must be able to evaluate the nature of the injury and the limitations it has produced. First the injured structures must be identified by consulting with the hand surgeon, reviewing operative reports and x-ray films, and discussing the injury with the patient. Assessment of bone, tendon, and nerve function must be ascertained, using standardized assessment techniques whenever possible.

The patient's age, occupation, and hand dominance should be taken into account in the initial evaluation. The type and extent of medical and surgical treatment that has been received and the length of time since such treatment are important in determining a treatment plan. Any further surgery or conservative treatment that is planned should also be noted. A written treatment plan should have the approval of the referring physician. Most physicians welcome observations and evaluation-based recommendations from the therapist regarding the patient's care.

The purposes of hand evaluation are to identify[1] physical limitations, such as loss of range of motion (ROM); functional limitations, such as an inability to perform daily tasks,[3] substitution patterns to compensate for loss of sensibility or motor function,[4] and established deformities, such as joint contracture.

The movement of the arm and hand must be coordinated for maximum function. Shoulder motion is essential for positioning the hand and elbow for daily activities.[20] The wrist is the key joint in the position of function.[13] Skilled hand performance depends on wrist stability. Although a mobile wrist is preferable, function is possible as long as the wrist is positioned to maximize movement of the fingers. Function also depends on arm and shoulder stability and mobility for fixing or positioning the hand for activity. The thumb is of greater importance than any other digit. Effective pinch is almost impossible without a thumb, and attempts will be made to salvage or reconstruct an injured thumb whenever possible. Within the hand the proximal inter-

phalangeal (PIP) joint is critical for grasp and is considered to be the most important small joint.[13] Limitations in flexion or extension will result in significant functional impairment.

Observation and Topographical Assessment

The occupational therapist should observe the appearance of the entire UE. The position of the hand and arm at rest and the carrying posture can yield valuable information about the dysfunction. How the patient treats the disease or injury should be observed. The therapist should note if the hand and arm is overprotected and carefully guarded or ignored, and if the patient carries the arm close to the body, in an awkward posture, or even covered.

The cervical and shoulder area posture should be observed for evidence of abnormalities in cervical and thoracic curvature that may reduce the potential for shoulder movement. Muscle atrophy may be observable in the scapular area if there has been significant long-term weakness or if the rotator cuff is torn. The scapula may appear asymmetrical or altered if muscle imbalances of length or strength are present.

The skin condition of the hand and arm should be noted. In particular, the therapist should note any lacerations, sutures, or evidence of recent surgery; whether the skin is dry or moist; if scales or crusts are present; and if the hand appears swollen or has an odor. Palmar skin is less mobile than dorsal skin normally. The therapist should determine the degree of mobility and elasticity and the adherence of scars. The therapist should also observe trophic changes in the skin. The vascular system is assessed by observing the skin color and temperature of the hand and evaluating for presence of **edema**. Any contractures of the web spaces should be noted. The therapist should observe the relationship between hand and arm function as the patient moves about and performs test items or tasks.

The therapist should ask the patient to perform some simple bilateral ADL, such as buttoning a button, putting on a shirt, opening a jar, and threading a needle, and observe the amount of spontaneous movement and use of the affected hand and arm. Similar screening tests can be used to determine shoulder mobility, such as reaching overhead, as well as placing the hand behind the back and behind the head.

Physical Assessment

A number of standardized tests can be used to determine physical limitations in the UE. ROM and manual muscle testing are crucial and are described in other chapters of this text. Special tests used by the hand therapist are described in a general sense, but the student should consult other textbooks for detailed instructions in such areas as assessment of adverse neural tension.[16]

Screening the Cervical Neck and Shoulder

Screening examination of the cervical neck and shoulder regions should be included in evaluation of hand conditions to determine if these areas are contributing to the patient's symptoms or limitations in function.

Active movements of the neck should be conducted, with attention paid to complaints of UE symptoms during cervical extension or lateral flexion to the same side. Complaints during these movements may be suggestive of nerve root irritation. Hand symptoms with opposite side bending may be a sign of adverse neural tension. Few occupational therapists are knowledgeable in the treatment of cervical conditions, and care must be taken not to aggravate an existing condition. The therapist should return the patient to the referring physician with recommendations for referral to an appropriate practitioner if the results of this testing are positive.

Assessment of Movement

The effect of trauma or dysfunction on anatomical structures is the first consideration in evaluating hand function. The joints must be assessed for active and passive mobility, fixed deformities, and any tendency to assume a position of deformity. The ligaments must be assessed for laxity or contracture and their ability to maintain joint stability. Tendons must be examined for integrity, contracture, or overstretching; muscles are tested for strength and function.

Limited Movement in the Shoulder

Examples of conditions in the shoulder region leading to reduced strength, reduced ROM, or pain in the shoulder are outlined in Table 44-1. Comparing initial responses with the results of follow-up evaluation will help document a positive response to treatment. Patterns of impairments in UE ROM and strength, as well as a positive response to provocative testing, should be reported to the referring physician if they would affect the patient's planned treatment or outcome. Therapists must not attempt to treat conditions that are beyond their scope of knowledge. Referral to an appropriate practitioner should be discussed with the physician if indicated.

IMPINGEMENT TESTS. The examiner passively overpressures the patient's arm into end-range elevation. This movement causes a jamming of the greater tuberosity against the anterior inferior acromial surface.[78] The test is positive if the patient's facial expression shows pain. An alternative test is described by Hawkins and Kennedy.[44] The examiner forward flexes the arm to 90°, then forcibly internally rotates the arm. Pain indicates a positive test result.

DROP ARM TEST. The patient's arm is passively abducted by the examiner to 90° with the patient's palm down. The patient is then asked to lower the arm actively. Pain or inability to lower the arm smoothly with good motor control is considered a positive test result.[65,84]

Soft-Tissue Tightness

Joints may develop dysfunction after trauma, immobilization, or disuse. Mennell emphasizes the importance of the small, involuntary motions of the joint, which he refers to as "joint play."[73] Others[66] describe these as "accessory motions." Joint play or accessory motions are

---

TABLE 44-1

Clinical Tests for Specific Dysfunction in the Shoulder

Condition	Pattern of Impairment	Characteristic Findings/Special Tests
Adhesive capsulitis	Loss of active and passive shoulder motion with the most pronounced loss in external rotation, and to a lesser degree abduction and internal rotation	Capsular end feel to passive motions in restricted planes of movement.
Subacromial impingement	Painful arc of motion between approximately 80° to 100° elevation and/or at end range of active elevation.	In early stages, muscle tests may be strong and painless despite positive impingement test.
Rotator cuff tendinitis	Painful active or resistive rotator cuff muscle use	Painful manual muscle test of scapular plane abduction and/or external rotation Nonpainful passive motion end ranges Tenderness at tendons of supraspinatus or infraspinatus.
Rotator cuff tear	Significant substitution of scapula with attempted arm elevation	Positive drop arm test Very weak, less than $\frac{3}{5}$ abduction and/or external rotation

those movements that are involuntary and physiological and can be performed only by someone else.[54] Examples of accessory motions are joint rotation and joint distraction. If accessory motions are limited and painful, the active motions of that joint cannot be normal. Therefore it is necessary to restore joint play through the use of joint mobilization techniques before attempting passive or active ROM.[74]

Joint mobilization may date back to the fourth century BC, when Hypocrites first described the use of spinal traction.[54] In the 1930s an English physician, James Mennell, encouraged physicians to perform manipulation without anesthesia, a practice that is advocated today by James Cyriax,[27] who explored the use of manipulation of the intervertebral disks. Current theorists include Cyriax, Robert Maigne, F.M. Kaltenborn, G.D. Maitland, Stanley Paris, and John Mennell, son of the late James Mennell. Although physicians originally practiced manipulation, therapists have adapted the techniques, which are now called *joint mobilization.*

The techniques used to assess joint play are also used in the treatment of joint dysfunction. During assessment the evaluator determines the range of accessory motion and the presence of pain by taking up the slack only in the joint. Some practitioners advocate use of a high-velocity, low-amplitude thrust or graded oscillation to regain motion and relieve pain.[66]

Guidelines must be followed in applying joint mobilization techniques, and the untrained or inexperienced practitioner should not attempt to use the techniques. Postgraduate courses are offered in joint mobilization of the extremities, and the therapist must be familiar with the orthokinematics of each joint, as well as with the techniques used.

Joint mobilization is generally indicated with restriction of accessory motions or the presence of pain caused by tightness of the joint capsule, meniscus displacement, muscle guarding, ligamentous tightness, or adherence. It is contraindicated in the presence of infection, recent fracture, neoplasm, joint inflammation, rheumatoid arthritis, osteoporosis, degenerative joint disease, and many chronic diseases.[54]

Limitations in joint motion may also be caused by tightness of the extrinsic or intrinsic muscles and tendons. If the joint capsule is not tight and accessory motions are normal, the therapist should test for extrinsic and intrinsic tightness.

To test for extrinsic extensor tightness the metacarpophalangeal (MP) joint is passively held in extension and the PIP joint is moved passively into flexion. Then the MP joint is flexed, and the PIP joint is again passively flexed. If the PIP joint can be flexed easily when the MP joint is extended but not when the MP joint is flexed, the extrinsic extensors are adherent.[4]

If there is extrinsic flexor tightness, the PIP and distal interphalangeal (DIP) joints will be positioned in flexion, with the MP joints held in extension. It will not be possible to pull the fingers into complete extension. If the wrist is then held in flexion, the IP joints will extend more easily because slack is placed on the flexor tendons.

Tightness of the intrinsic musculature is tested by passively holding the MP joint in extension and applying pressure just distal to the PIP joint. This action is repeated with the MP joint in flexion. If there is more resistance when the MP joint is extended, intrinsic tightness is indicated.[4]

If passive motion of the PIP joint remains the same whether the MP joint is held in extension or flexion and there is limitation of PIP joint flexion in any position, tightness of the joint capsule is indicated. The therapist should assess the joint for capsular tightness if this has not already been done.

Provocative tests that are used to assess ligament, capsule, and joint instability are summarized in Table 44-2. The reader is referred to more comprehensive textbooks for details on the administration of these tests.[65,84]

Assessment of Peripheral Nerve Status

Nerve dysfunction can occur at any point from the nerve roots through the digital nerves in the fingers. A good understanding of the peripheral nervous system is essential for appropriate treatment of the UE. Determining the approximate location of nerve dysfunction can assist in treatment planning.

CATEGORIES OF TESTS. A variety of tests may be required to assess nerve function adequately. These tests can be divided into four categories[1]: modality tests for pain, heat, cold, and touch pressure[2]; functional tests to assess the quality of sensibility, or what Moberg[76] described as "tactile gnosis"[3]; objective tests that do not require active participation by the patient[4]; and provocative tests that reproduce symptoms.

Examples of functional tests are stationary and moving two-point discrimination and the Moberg pickup test; objective tests include the wrinkle test, the Ninhydrin sweat test, and nerve-conduction studies.[18] Electrodiagnostic testing is the most conclusive and widely accepted method of determining nerve dysfunction.

Provocative tests are highly suggestive of a nerve lesion if results are positive but not do rule out a problem if results are negative. Tests of nerve dysfunction are summarized in Table 44-3. Instructions for administration of the most common tests are described in the following paragraphs.

ADSON MANEUVER. The examiner palpates the radial pulse on the arm to be tested. The patient then rotates the head toward the arm being tested. The patient then extends the head and holds a deep breath while the arm is being laterally rotated and extended. Disappearance or slowing of pulse rate is considered a positive test result.[1,65]

TABLE 44-2
Clinical Tests for Specific Dysfunction in the Wrist

Condition	Pattern of Impairment	Special Tests
Thumb ulnar collateral ligament instability (gamekeeper's or skier's thumb)	Pain and instability of the thumb MP joint	Movement greater than 35° when valgus stress is applied to the thumb MP joint
Instability of the scaphoid	Pain in the area of the scaphoid bone (anatomical snuffbox) or "clunking" with movement of the wrist	Watson Test Pain or sound associated with subluxation of the dorsal pole of the scaphoid while performing test
Instability of the distal radioulnar joint	Pain and tenderness in the wrist	"Piano Keys" Test Hypermobility and pain associated with pressure on the distal ulna
Lunate dislocation	Pain or instability in the central wrist	Murphy's sign The head of the third metacarpal is level with the second and fourth metacarpals while making a fist
Lunotriquetral instability	Pain or instability in the central or ulnar wrist	Lunotriquetral Ballottement Test Crepitus, laxity or pain with isolated movement of the lunate
TFCC tear	Pain and instability in the ulnar wrist	Wrist arthrogram or MRI

TABLE 44-3
Clinical Tests for Specific Nerve Dysfunction in the Upper Extremity

Condition	Pattern of Impairment	Characteristic Findings/Special Tests
Thoracic outlet syndrome	Nonspecific paresthesias or heaviness with sustained positioning or activity above shoulder level or behind the plane of the body	Adson test Roos test
Adverse neural tension	Nonspecific pain or paresthesias with reaching in positions that places tension on brachial plexus nerves	Positive upper limb screening test
Carpal tunnel syndrome	Pain and numbness, primarily in the thumb, index, and middle fingers Usually worse at night and may be associated with activity	Tinel's sign at the wrist Phalen's test Reverse Phalen's test Carpal compression test
Cubital tunnel syndrome	Compression of ulnar nerve at elbow	Elbow flexion test
Ulnar nerve paralysis	Paralysis of the adductor pollicis muscle	Froment's sign Jeanne's sign Wartenberg's sign

Roos Test. In this test the patient maintains a position of bilateral arm abduction to 90°, shoulder external rotation, and elbow flexion to 90° for 3 minutes while slowly alternating between an open hand and a clenched fist. Inability to maintain this position for the full 3 minutes or onset of symptoms is considered a positive test result.[65,86]

Upper Limb Tension Test (Brachial Plexus Tension Test). This test is designed to screen for symptoms that are produced when tension stress is placed on the brachial plexus. The maneuver described primarily stresses the median nerve and C5-C7 nerve roots. Adverse neural tension in the ulnar or radial nerves may also be tested. However, we have found that using the median nerve test as a screening device establishes a marker against which to gauge the success of treatment. Although some authors recommend using the neural tension tests for treatment as well as assessment, this has not been the practice of the authors. This screening process should be used by the occupational therapist to rule out or confirm the involvement of more proximal structures.

The patient is positioned supine, and the examiner takes the patient's arm into abduction and external rotation behind the coronal plane at the shoulder. The shoulder girdle is fixed in depression. The elbow is then passively extended with the wrist in extension and the forearm in supination. Symptoms of stretch or ache in the cubital fossa or tingling in the thumb and first three fingers indicates tension on the median nerve. Lateral flexion of the neck to the opposite side will amplify symptoms by increasing tension on the dura mater. Elbow extension ROM should be compared with the uninvolved side to indicate the degree of restriction.[65]

TINEL'S SIGN. The test is performed by tapping gently along the course of the nerve, starting distally and moving proximally to elicit a tingling sensation in the fingertip. The point at which tapping begins to elicit a tingling sensation is noted and indicates the approximate location of nerve compression. This test is also used after nerve repair, to determine the extent of sensory axon growth.

PHALEN'S TEST AND REVERSE PHALEN'S TEST. Phalen's Test is performed by fully flexing the wrists with the dorsum of the hands pressing against each other. Reverse Phalen's is performed by holding the hands in the "prayer" position for 1 minute. The test results are positive if the patient reports tingling in the median nerve distribution (thumb, index, middle and radial aspect of ring finger) within 1 minute.

CARPAL COMPRESSION TEST. The examiner places pressure over the median nerve in the carpal tunnel for up to 30 seconds. The test result is positive if tingling occurs in the median nerve distribution. The combination of wrist flexion and compression of the median nerve for 20 seconds has been found to be more sensitive than other provocative tests used alone.[95]

ELBOW FLEXION TEST. The elbow flexion test is used to screen for cubital tunnel syndrome (compression of the ulnar nerve in the cubital tunnel). The patient is asked to fully flex the elbows with the wrists fully extended for a period of 3 to 5 minutes. The test result is positive if tingling is reported in the ulnar nerve distribution of the forearm and hand (ulnar ring finger and small finger).[65]

QUICK TESTS FOR MOTOR FUNCTION IN THE PERIPHERAL NERVES. The ulnar nerve may be tested by asking the patient to pinch with the thumb and index finger and palpating the first dorsal interosseous muscle. Another test for ulnar nerve paralysis involves asking a patient to grasp a piece of paper between the thumb and index finger. When the examiner pulls away the paper, the tip of the thumb flexes because of absence of the adductor pollicis muscle (Froment's sign). If the MP joint of the thumb also extends at the same time, it is known as

Jeanne's sign. Wartenberg's sign is positive if the patient is unable to adduct the small finger when the hand is placed palm down on the table with the fingers passively abducted.

The radial nerve may be tested by asking the patient to extend the wrist and fingers. Median nerve function is tested by asking the patient to oppose the thumb to the fingers and flex the fingers.[25]

SENSORY MAPPING. Detailed sensibility testing can begin with sensory mapping of the entire volar surface of the hand.[18] The hand must be supported by the examiner's hand or be resting in a medium such as therapy putty. Either the examiner or the patient can draw a probe, usually the eraser end of a pencil, lightly over the skin from the area of normal sensibility to the area of abnormal sensibility. The patient must immediately report the exact location where the sensation changes. This is done from proximal to distal and radial and ulnar to medial directions. The areas are carefully marked and transferred to a permanent record. Mapping should be repeated at monthly intervals during nerve regeneration.

SYMPATHETIC FUNCTION. Recovery of sympathetic response such as sudomotor (sweating), vasomotor (temperature discrimination), pilomotor (gooseflesh), and trophic (skin texture, nail, and hair growth) may occur early but does not correlate with functional recovery.[29] O'Rain[81] observed that denervated skin does not wrinkle. Therefore nerve function may be tested by immersing the hand in water for 5 minutes and noting the presence or absence of skin wrinkling. This test may be especially helpful in diagnosing a nerve lesion in young children. The ability to sweat is also lost with a nerve lesion. A Ninhydrin test[76] evaluates sweating of the finger.

The wrinkle test and the Ninhydrin test are objective tests of sympathetic function. Recovery of sweating has not been shown to correlate with the recovery of sensation, but the absence of sweating correlates with the lack of discriminatory sensation. Other signs of sympathetic dysfunction are smooth, shiny skin; nail changes; and "pencil-pointing" or tapering of the fingers.[102]

NERVE COMPRESSION AND NERVE REGENERATION. Sensibility testing is performed to assess the recovery of a nerve following laceration and repair, as well as to determine the presence of a nerve compression syndrome and the return of nerve function after surgical decompression, or the efficacy of conservative treatment to reduce compression. Therefore tests such as vibratory tests may be interpreted differently, depending on the mechanism of nerve dysfunction. In the following section, tests will be described and differences drawn as appropriate to assist the therapist in selecting the correct assessment technique, as well as in planning treatment based on the evaluative measures.

During the first 2 to 4 months after nerve suture, axons regenerate and travel through the hand at a rate of about 1 mm per day, or 1 inch (2.54 cm) per month. Tinel's sign may be used to follow this regeneration.[59] As regeneration occurs, hypesthesias develop. Although this hypersensitivity may be uncomfortable to the patient, it is a positive sign of nerve growth. A treatment program for desensitization of hypersensitive areas can be initiated as soon as the skin is healed and can tolerate gentle rubbing and immersion in textures. Desensitization is discussed further in the treatment section.

VIBRATION. Dellon was an early advocate of the use of 30-cycles-per-second (30-cps) and 256-cps tuning forks for assessing the return of vibratory sensation after nerve repair, as regeneration occurs and as a guideline for initiating a sensory reeducation program.[30,31] However, many clinicians found that use of a tuning fork was not discrete enough to detect sensory abnormalities.

Lundborg[62] has described the use of commercial vibrometers to detect abnormal sensation. This method was less subjective and thought to be more reliable. In a study of induced median nerve compression, Gelberman[41] found that vibration and touch perception as measured by the Semmes-Weinstein monofilaments are altered before two-point discrimination because they measure a single nerve fiber innervating a group of receptor cells. Two-point discrimination is a test of innervation density that requires overlapping sensory units and cortical integration. Thus two-point discrimination is altered after nerve laceration and repair but remains normal if the nerve is compressed, as long as there are links to the cortex. Bell[10] has also found normal two-point values in the presence of decreased sensory function.

Vibration and the Semmes-Weinstein Test are more sensitive in picking up a gradual decrease in nerve function in the presence of nerve compression where the nerve circuitry is intact. They also correlate with decreases in the potential amplitude of sensory nerve action as measured by nerve conduction studies.[94] Therefore vibration, Semmes-Weinstein, and electrical testing are reliable and sensitive tests for early detection of carpal tunnel syndrome and other nerve compression syndromes. Vibration and Semmes-Weinstein can be performed in the clinic with no discomfort to the patient and are excellent screening tools when nerve compression is suspected.

TOUCH PRESSURE. Moving touch is tested using the eraser end of a pencil. The eraser is placed in an area of normal sensibility and, pressing lightly, is moved to the distal fingertip. The patient notes when the perception of the stimulus changes. Light and heavy stimuli may be applied and noted.[29]

Constant touch is tested by pressing with the eraser end of a pencil, first in an area with normal sensibility and then moving distally. The patient responds when the stimulus is altered; again, light and heavy stimuli may be applied.[29]

The Semmes-Weinstein monofilaments are the most accurate instruments for assessing cutaneous pressure thresholds.[10] The testing equipment consists of 20 nylon monofilaments housed in plastic handheld rods. The diameter of the monofilaments increases, and when applied correctly exert a force ranging from 4.5 mg to 447 g. Markings on the probes range from 1.65 to 6.65 but do not correspond to the grams of force of each rod. Normal fingertip sensibility has been found to correspond to the 2.44 and 2.83 probes.

The monofilaments must be applied perpendicularly to the skin and are applied just until the monofilament bends. The skin should not blanch when the monofilament is applied. Probes 1.65 through 2.83 are bounced three times. Probes marked 3.22 to 4.08 are applied three times with a bend in the filament, and probes marked 4.17 to 6.65 are applied once. The larger monofilaments do not bend, and therefore skin color must be observed to determine how firmly to apply the probe.

The examiner should begin with a probe in the normal range and progress through the rods in increasing diameters to find the patient's threshold for touch throughout the volar surface.[10] A grid should be used to record the responses so that varying areas of touch perception can be demonstrated. Two correct responses out of three applications are necessary for an area to be considered as having intact sensibility. It is preferable to place the monofilaments randomly rather than to concentrate on an area, to allow the nerves recovery time. When a filament is placed three times, it should be held for a second, rested for a second, and reapplied. Results can be graded from normal light touch (probes 2.83 and above) to loss of protective sensation (probes 4.56 and below). Diminished light touch and diminished protective sensation are in the range reflected by the central probes.[10]

TWO-POINT AND MOVING TWO-POINT DISCRIMINATION. Discrimination, the second level of sensibility assessment, requires the subject to distinguish between two direct stimuli. Static or stationary two-point discrimination measures the slowly adapting fibers. The two-point discrimination test, first described by Weber in 1853, was modified and popularized by Moberg,[76] who was interested in a tool that would assess the functional level of sensation. A variety of devices have been proposed to use in measuring two-point discrimination. The bent paper clip is inexpensive but often has burrs on the metal tip. Other devices include industrial calipers* and the Disk-Criminator.†[63] A device with parallel prongs of variable distance and blunted ends should produce replicable results.

---

*Central Tool Company of Germany (available from Anthony Products, Indianapolis, Ind).
†Disk-Criminator (available from Smith & Nephew, Germantown, Wis).

The test is performed as follows[59]:

1. The patient's vision is occluded.
2. An area of normal sensation is tested as a reference, using blunt calipers or a bent paper clip.
3. The calipers are set 10 mm apart and are randomly applied, starting at the fingertip and moving proximally and longitudinally in line with the digital nerves, with one or two points touching. The skin should not be blanched by the caliper.
4. The distance is decreased until the patient no longer feels two distinct points, and that distance is measured.

Three to four seconds should be allowed between applications, and the patient should have four correct responses out of five administrations. Because this test indicates sensory function, it is usually administered at the tips of the fingers. It may be used proximally to test nerve regeneration. Normal two-point discrimination at the fingertip is 6 mm or less.

Moving two-point discrimination measures the innervation density of the quickly adapting nerve fibers for touch. It is slightly more sensitive than stationary two-point discrimination. The test is performed as follows[29]:

1. The patient's vision is occluded.
2. An area of normal sensation is tested as a reference, using blunt calipers or a bent paper clip.
3. The fingertip is supported by the examining table or the examiner's hand.
4. The caliper, separated 5 mm to 8 mm, is moved longitudinally from proximal to distal in a linear fashion along the surface of the fingertip. One and two points are randomly alternated. The patient must correctly identify the stimulus in seven out of eight responses before proceeding to a smaller value. The test is repeated down to a separation of 2 mm.

Two-point values increase with age in both sexes, with the smallest values occurring between the ages of 10 and 30. Women tend to have smaller values than men, and there is no significant difference between dominant and nondominant hands.[60]

MODIFIED MOBERG PICK-UP TEST. Recognition of common objects is the final level of sensory function. Moberg used the phrase tactile gnosis to describe the ability of the hand to perform complex functions by feel. Moberg described the Pick-Up Test in 1958,[76] and it was later modified by Dellon.[29] This test is used with either a median nerve injury or injury to a combination of median and ulnar nerves. It takes twice as long to perform the tests with vision occluded as with vision unimpaired. The test is performed as follows:

1. Nine or ten small objects (e.g, coins or paper clips) are placed on a table, and the patient is asked to place them, one at a time, in a small container as quickly as possible, while looking at them. The patient is timed.
2. The test is repeated for the opposite hand with vision.
3. The test is repeated for each hand with vision occluded.
4. The patient is asked to identify each object one at a time, with and then without vision.

It is important to observe any substitution patterns that may be used when the patient cannot see the objects.

Edema Assessment

Hand volume is measured to assess the presence of extracellular or intracellular edema. Volume measurement is generally used to determine the effect of treatment and activities. By measuring volume at different times of the day, the therapist can measure effects of rest versus activity, as well as the effects of **splinting** or treatment designed to reduce edema.

A commercial volumeter[25] may be used to assess hand edema. The volumeter has been shown to be accurate to 10 ml[103] when used in the prescribed manner. Variables that have been shown to decrease the accuracy of the volumeter include the use of a faucet or hose that introduces air into the tank during filling, movement of the arm within the tank, inconsistent pressure on the stop rod, and the use of a volumeter in a variety of places. The same level surface should always be used.[103] The evaluation is performed as follows (Fig. 44-1):

1. A plastic volumeter is filled and allowed to empty into a large beaker until the water reaches spout level. The beaker is then emptied and dried thoroughly.
2. The patient is instructed to immerse the hand in the plastic volumeter, being careful to keep the hand in the midposition.
3. The hand is lowered until it rests gently between the middle and ring fingers on the dowel rod. It is important that the hand not press onto the rod.
4. The hand remains still until no more water drips into the beaker.
5. The water is poured into a graduated cylinder. The cylinder is placed on a level surface, and a reading is made.

A method of assessing edema of an individual finger or joint is circumferential measurement using either a circumference tape* or jeweler's ring-size standards. Measurements should be made before and after treatment and especially after the application of thermal modalities or splinting. Although patients often have subjective complaints relating to swelling, objective data of circumference or volume will help the therapist to assess the response of the tissues to treatment and

---

*DeRoyal/LMB, DeRoyal Industries, Powell, TN.

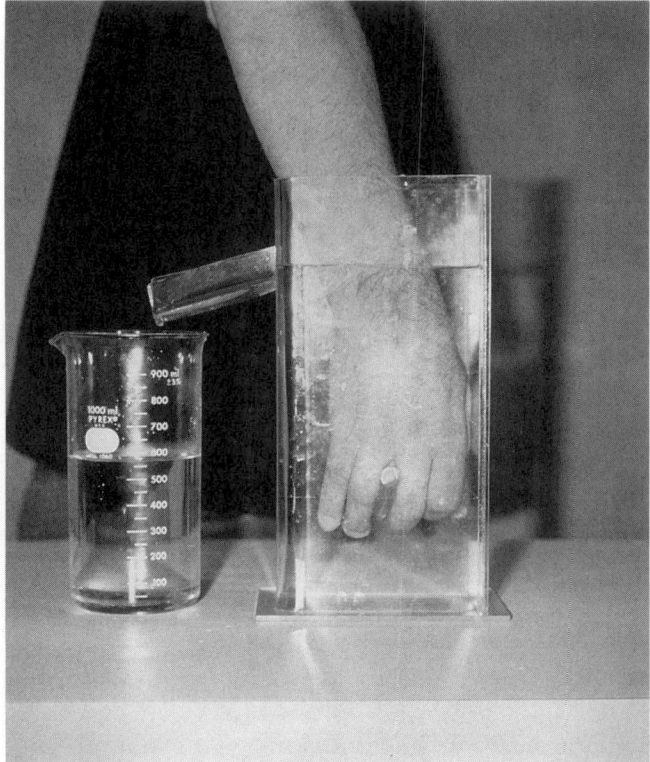

FIG. 44-1
Volumeter is used to measure volume of both hands for comparison. Increased volume indicates presence of edema.

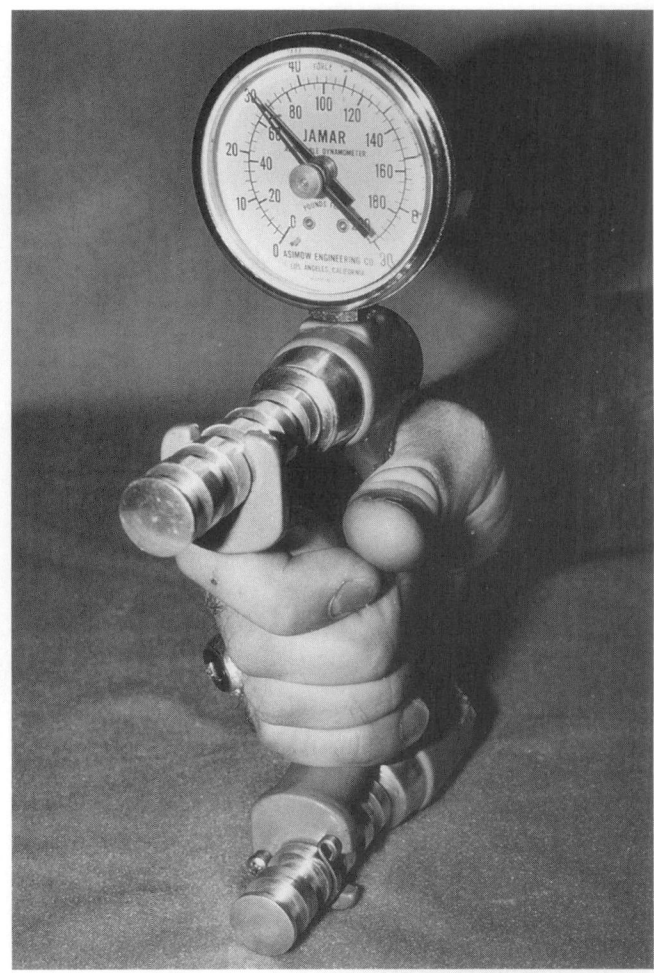

FIG. 44-2
Jamar dynamometer is used to evaluate grip strength in both hands.

activity. Edema control techniques are discussed later in this chapter.

Circulation

The Allen Test is used to assess patency in the radial and ulnar arteries to the hand, which form the superficial and deep palmar arches. The test is performed by having the patient open and close the hand quickly, then make a tight fist. The examiner applies pressure over both arteries, then releases the pressure on one artery to see if hand color returns. The test is repeated for the other artery.[65]

Grip and Pinch Strength

UE strength is usually assessed after the healing phase of trauma. Strength testing is not indicated after recent trauma or surgery. Testing should not be performed until the patient has been cleared for full-resistive activities, usually 8 to 12 weeks after injury.

A standard adjustable-handle dynamometer is recommended for assessing grip strength (Fig. 44-2). The subject should be seated with the shoulder adducted and neutrally rotated, the elbow flexed at 90°,[68] forearm in the neutral position, and wrist between 0° and 30° extension and between 0° and 15° of ulnar de-

viation. Three trials are taken of each hand, with the dynamometer handle set at the second position.[71] The dynamometer should be lightly held by the examiner to prevent accidental dropping of the instrument. A mean of the three trials should be reported. The noninjured hand is used for comparison. Normative data may be used to compare strength scores.[52,70] Variables such as age will affect the strength measurements.

Pinch strength should also be tested, using a pinch gauge. The pinch gauge made by B & L Engineering has been found to be the most accurate.[71] Two-point pinch (thumb tip to index fingertip), lateral or key pinch (thumb pulp to lateral aspect of the middle phalanx of the index finger), and three-point pinch (thumb tip to tips of index and middle fingers) should be evaluated. As with the grip dynamometer, three successive trials should be obtained and compared bilaterally (Fig. 44-3).[39]

Manual muscle testing is also used to test UE strength. Accurate assessment is especially important

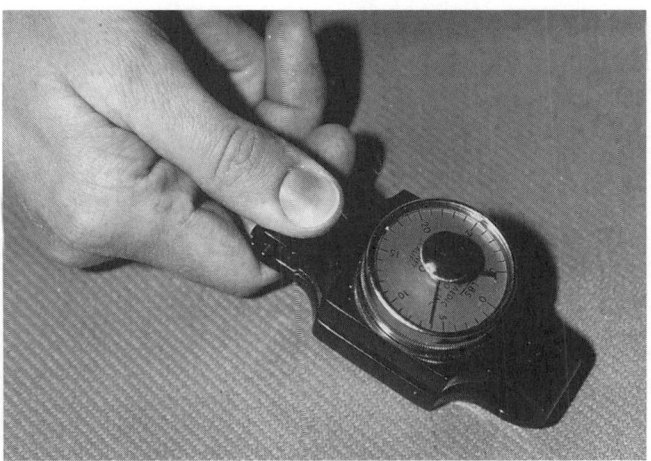

FIG. 44-3
Pinch gauge is used to evaluate pinch strength to variety of prehension patterns of pinch.

when the patient is being prepared for tendon transfers or other reconstructive surgery. The student who wishes to study kinesiology of the UE is referred especially to Brand's work.[15]

Maximum voluntary effort during grip, pinch, or muscle testing will be affected by pain in the hand or extremity, and the therapist should note if the patient's ability to exert full force is limited by subjective complaints. Localization of the pain symptoms and consistency in noting pain will help the therapist to evaluate the role that pain is playing in the recovery from injury. Pain problems are discussed in more detail later in this chapter.

Functional Assessment

Assessment of hand function or performance is important because the physical assessment does not measure the patient's ingenuity and ability to compensate for loss of strength, ROM, or sensation or the presence of deformities.[20]

The physical assessment should precede the functional assessment because awareness of physical dysfunction can result in a critical analysis of functional impairment and an understanding of why the patient functions as he or she does.[72]

The occupational therapist should observe the effect of the hand dysfunction on the use of the hand in ADL. In addition, some type of a standardized performance test, such as the Jebsen Test of Hand Function[46] or the Carroll Quantitative Test of Upper Extremity Function,[20] should be administered.

The Jebsen Test of Hand Function[46] was developed to provide objective measurements of standardized tasks with norms for patient comparison. It is a short test that is assembled by the administrator. It is easy to administer and inexpensive. The test consists of seven subtests, which test writing a short sentence, turning over 3- × 5-inch cards, picking up small objects and placing them in a container, stacking checkers, simulated eating, moving empty large cans, and moving weighted large cans. Norms are provided for dominant and nondominant hands for each subtest and also are divided by sex and age. Instructions for assembling the test, as well as specific instructions for administering it, are provided by the authors.[46] This has been found to be a good test for overall hand function.

The Quantitative Test of Upper Extremity Function described by Carroll[20] was designed to measure ability to perform general arm and hand activities used in daily living. It is based on the assumption that complex UE movements used to perform ordinary ADL can be reduced to specific patterns of grasp and prehension of the hand, supination and pronation of the forearm, flexion and extension of the elbow, and elevation of the arm.

The test consists of six parts: grasping and lifting four blocks of graduated sizes to assess grasp; grasping and lifting two pipes of graduated sizes to test cylindrical grip; grasping and placing a ball to test spherical grasp; picking up and placing four marbles of graduated sizes to test fingertip prehension or pinch; putting a small washer over a nail and putting an iron on a shelf to test placing; and pouring water from pitcher to glass and glass to glass. In addition, to assess pronation, supination, and elevation of the arm, the therapist instructs the subject to place his or her hand on top of the head, behind the head, and to the mouth, and write his or her name. The test uses simple, inexpensive, and easily acquired materials. Details of materials and their arrangement, test procedures, and scoring can be found in the original source.[20]

Other tests that are useful in the assessment of hand dexterity are the Crawford Small Parts Dexterity Test,[24] the Bennett Hand Tool Dexterity Test,[11] the Purdue Pegboard Test,[97] and the Minnesota Manual Dexterity Test.[75] The VALPAR Corporation* has developed a number of standardized tests that measure an individual's ability to perform work-related tasks. They provide information about the test taker's results, compared with industry performance standards. All of these tests include comparison with normal subjects working in a variety of industrial settings. This information can be used in predicting the likelihood of successful return to a specific job. The tests are especially useful when administering a work capacity evaluation. Tests may be purchased and come with instructions for administration of the test and the standardized norms. Melvin[72] lists a variety of additional hand function tests.

---

*VALPAR Assessment Systems (available from VALPAR International, Tuscon, Ariz).

TREATMENT
Fractures

In treating a hand or wrist fracture the surgeon attempts to achieve good anatomical position through either a closed (nonoperative) or open (operative) reduction. Internal fixation with Kirschner wires, metallic plates, or screws may be used to maintain the desired position. External fixation may also be used with internal fixation. The hand is usually immobilized in wrist extension and MP joint flexion, with extension of the distal joints whenever the injury allows this position. Trauma to bone may also involve trauma to tendons and nerves in the adjacent area. Treatment must be geared toward the recovery of all injured structures, and this fact may influence treatment of the fracture.

OT may be initiated during the period of immobilization, which is usually 3 to 5 weeks. Uninvolved fingers of the hand must be kept mobile through the use of active motion. Edema should be carefully monitored, and elevation is required whenever edema is present.

As soon as there is sufficient bone stability, the surgeon allows mobilization of the injured part. The surgeon should provide guidelines for the amount of resistance or force that may be applied to the fracture site. Activities that correct poor motor patterns and encourage use of the injured hand should be started as soon as the hand is pain free. Early motion will prevent the adherence of tendons and reduce edema through stimulation of the lymphatic and blood vessels.

As soon as the brace or cast is removed, the patient's hand must be evaluated. If edema remains present, edema control techniques can be initiated using techniques described later in this chapter. A baseline ROM should be established, and the application of appropriate splints may begin. A splint may be used to correct a deformity that has resulted from immobilization, or it may be used to protect the finger from additional trauma to the fracture site. An example of this type of splinting would be the application of a Velcro "buddy" splint (Fig. 44-4). A dorsal block splint that limits full extension of the finger may be used following a fracture or dislocation of the PIP joint. A dynamic splint may be used to achieve full ROM or to prevent the development of further deformity at 6 to 8 weeks after fracture.

Intraarticular fractures may result in injury to the cartilage of the joint, causing additional pain and stiffness. An x-ray examination will indicate whether the joint surface has been damaged, which might limit the treatment of the joint. Joint pain and stiffness after fracture without the presence of joint damage should be alleviated by a combination of thermal modalities, restoration of joint play, or joint mobilization and corrective and dynamic splinting followed by active use. Resistive exercise can be started when bony healing has been achieved.

Wrist fractures are common and may present special problems for the surgeon and therapist. Colles fractures

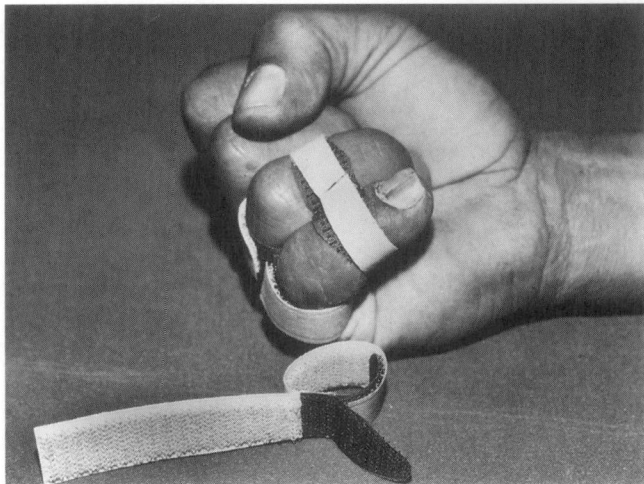

FIG. 44-4
Velcro "buddy" splint may be used to protect finger following fracture or to encourage movement of stiff finger. (Splint available from Smalley and Bates, Inc.)

of the distal radius are the most common injury to the wrist[13] and may result in limitations in wrist flexion and extension, as well as pronation and supination resulting from the involvement of the distal radioulnar joint. External fixators, which may be used with or without internal fixation, are now common in the reduction of distal radius fractures. The external fixator maintains the anatomical relationship between the radius and ulna by maintaining the length of the radius, often with excellent results. The therapist must carefully instruct the patient in active ROM of the fingers and proper care of the pin sites while the fixator is in place. Use of splints, active motion that emphasizes wrist movement, and joint mobilization may be beneficial after removal of the fixator or cast. The weight well may be used to provide resistance to wrist motions (Fig. 44-5).

The scaphoid is the second most commonly injured bone in the wrist[13] and is often fractured when the hand is dorsiflexed at the time of injury. Fractures to the proximal pole of the scaphoid may result in nonunion because of poor blood supply to this area. Scaphoid fractures require a prolonged period of immobilization, sometimes up to several months in a cast, with resulting stiffness and pain. Care should be taken to mobilize uninvolved joints early.

Trauma to the lunate may result in avascular necrosis of the lunate or Kienböck's disease,[13] which may result from a one-time accident or may be caused by repetitive trauma. Lunate fractures are usually immobilized for 6 weeks. Kienböck's disease may be treated with a bone graft, removal of the proximal carpal row, or partial wrist fusion.

Stiffness and pain are common complications of fractures. The control of edema coupled with early

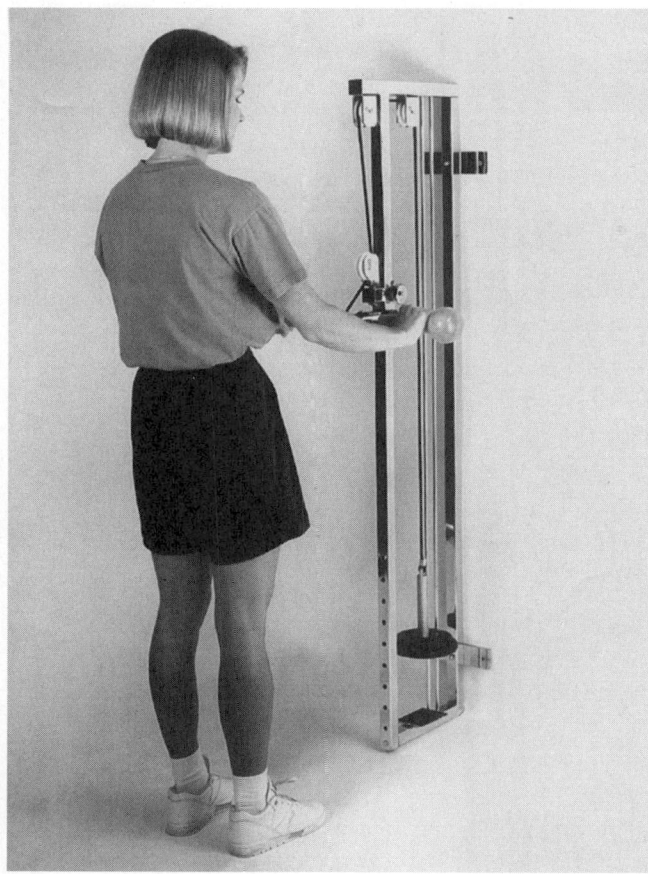

FIG. 44-5
Weight well is used for strengthening upper extremity with progressive resistance applied to weakened musculature and is also useful in retraining prehension of pinch and grip. (Photo courtesy of Karen Schultz Johnson)

motion and good patient instruction and support will minimize these complications, however.

Nerve Injuries

Nerve injury may be classified into the following three categories:

1. Neurapraxia is contusion of the nerve without wallerian degeneration. The nerve recovers function without treatment within a few days or weeks.
2. Axonotmesis is an injury in which nerve fibers distal to the site of injury degenerate, but the internal organization of the nerve remains intact. No surgical treatment is necessary, and recovery usually occurs within 6 months. The length of time may vary, depending on the level of injury.
3. Neurotmesis is a complete laceration of both nerve and fibrous tissues. Surgical treatment is required. Microsurgical repair of the fascicles is common. Nerve grafting may be necessary in situations in which there is a gap between nerve endings.[90]

Peripheral nerve injuries may occur as a result of disruption of the nerve by a fractured bone, laceration, or crush injury. Symptoms of nerve injuries include weakness or paralysis of muscles that are innervated by motor branches of the injured nerve and sensory loss to areas that are innervated by sensory branches of the injured nerve. Before evaluating the patient for nerve loss, the therapist must be familiar with the muscles and areas that are innervated by the three major forearm nerves. A summary of UE peripheral neuropathic conditions can be found in Table 44-4.

Radial Nerve

The radial nerve innervates the extensor-supinator group of muscles of the forearm, including the brachioradialis, extensor carpi radialis longus, extensor carpi radialis brevis, extensor digitorum communis, extensor digiti minimi, extensor indicis, extensor carpi ulnaris, supinator, abductor pollicis longus, extensor pollicis brevis, and extensor pollicis longus. The sensory distribution of the radial nerve is a strip of the posterior upper arm and the forearm; dorsum of the thumb; and index and middle fingers and radial half of the ring finger to the PIP joints. Sensory loss of the radial nerve does not usually result in dysfunction.

Clinical signs of a high-level radial nerve injury (above the supinator) are pronation of the forearm, wrist flexion, and the thumb held in palmar abduction resulting from the unopposed action of the flexor pollicis brevis and the abductor pollicis brevis.[82] Injury to the posterior interosseous nerve spares the extensor carpi radialis longus and brevis. Posterior interosseous nerve syndrome includes normal sensation and wrist extension with loss of finger and thumb extension. Clinical signs of low-level radial nerve injury include incomplete extension of the MP joints of the fingers and thumb. The interossei extend the interphalangeal (IP) joints of the fingers, but the MP joints rest in about 30° of flexion.

A dorsal splint that provides wrist extension, MP extension, and thumb extension should be provided to protect the extensor tendons from overstretching during the healing phase and to position the hand for functional use (Fig. 44-6). A dynamic splint is commonly provided.

Median Nerve

The median nerve innervates the flexors of the forearm and hand and is often called the "eyes" of the hands because of its importance in sensory innervation of the volar surface of the thumb, index, and middle fingers. Median nerve loss may result from lacerations, as well as from compression syndromes of the wrist, such as carpal tunnel syndrome.

Motor distribution of the median nerve is to the pronator teres, palmaris longus, flexor carpi radialis,

TABLE 44-4

Nerve Injuries of the Upper Extremity

Nerve	Location	Affected	Test
Radial nerve (posterior cord, fibers from C5, C6, C7, C8)	Upper arm	Triceps and all distal motors Sensory to SRN	MMT Sensory test
Radial nerve	Above elbow	Brachioradialis and all distal motors Sensory to SRN	MMT Sensory
Radial nerve	At elbow	Supinator, ECRL, ECRB, and all distal motors Sensory to SRN	MMT Sensory
Posterior interosseous nerve	Forearm	ECU, ED, EDM, APL, EPL, EPB, EIP No sensory	Wrist extension—if present, indicates PIN rather than high radial nerve
Radial nerve at ECRB, radial artery, arcade of Frohse, origin of supinator	Radial tunnel syndrome	Weakness of muscles innervated by PIN No sensory loss	Palpate for pain over extensor mass Pain with wrist flexion and pronation, Pain with wrist extension and supination Pain with resisted middle finger extension
Median nerve (lateral from C5, C6, C7, medial cord from C8, T1)	High lesions (elbow and above)	Paralysis/weakness of FCR, PL, all FDS, FDP I and II FPL, pronator teres and quad., opponens pollicis, APB, FPB (radial head), lumbricals I and II Sensory cutaneous branch of median nerve	MMT Sensory
Median nerve	Low (at wrist)	Weakness of thenars only	Inability to flex thumb tip and index fingertip to palm Inability to oppose thumb Poor dexterity
Median nerve under fibrous band in PT, beneath heads of pronator, arch of FDS, origin of FCR	Pronator syndrome	Weakness in thenars, but not muscles innervated by AIN Sensory in median nerve distribution in hand	Provocative tests to isolate compression site
Median nerve under origin of PT, FDS to middle	Anterior interosseous nerve syndrome	Pure motor, no sensory Forearm pain precedes paralysis Weakness of FPL, FDP I and II, PQ	Inability to flex IP joint of thumb and DIP of index Increased pain with resisted pronation Pain with forearm pressure
Median nerve at wrist	Carpal tunnel syndrome	Weakness of medial intrinsics Sensory	Provocative tests Tinel's Sensory
Ulnar nerve at elbow (branch of medial cord from C7, C8, T1)	Cubital tunnel syndrome	Weakness/paralysis of FCU, FDP III and IV, ulnar intrinsics Numbness in palmar cutaneous and dorsal cutaneous distribution Loss of grip and & pinch strength	Pain with elbow flexion and extension
Ulnar nerve at wrist	Compression at canal of Guyon	Weakness and pain in ulnar intrinsics	Reproduced by pressure at site

AIN, Anterior interosseus nerve; *APB,* abductor pollicis brevis; *APL,* abductor pollicis longus; *ECRB,* extensor carpi radialis brevis; *ECRL,* extensor carpi radialis longus; *ECU,* extensor carpi ulnaris; *ED,* extensor digitorum; *EDM,* extensor digitorum minimus; *EIP,* extensor indicis proprius; *FDS,* flexor digitorum superficialis; *EPB,* extensor pollicis brevis; *EPL,* extensor pollicis longus; *FCR,* flexor carpi radialis; *FDP,* flexor digitorum profundus; *FPB,* flexor pollicis brevis; *FPL,* flexor pollicis longus; *MMT,* manual muscle test; *PIN,* posterior interosseus nerve; *PQ,* pronator quadratus; *PT,* pronator teres; *SRN,* superficial radial nerve.

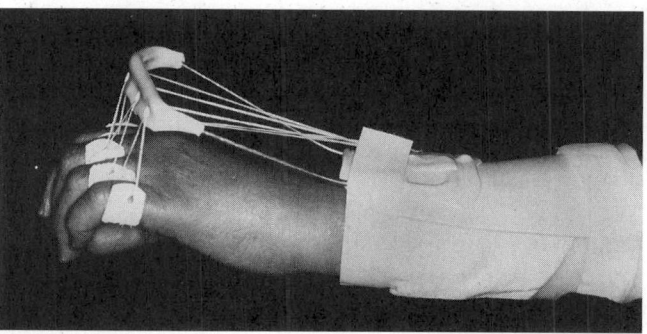

FIG. 44-6

Low-profile radial nerve splint is carefully balanced to pull metacarpophalangeal (MP) joints into extension when wrist is flexed and allows the MP joints to fall into slight flexion when wrist is extended, thus preserving normal balance between two joints and preserving joint contracture. (Splint courtesy of Judy C Colditz, Raleigh Hand Rehabilitation Center.)

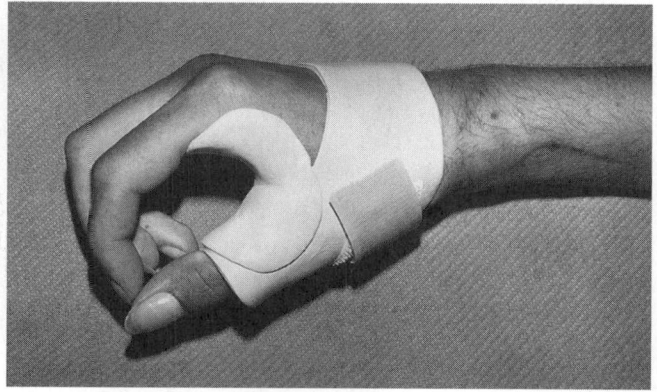

FIG. 44-7

Thumb stabilization splint may be used with median nerve injury to protect thumb and to improve functioning by placing thumb in position of pinch. Normal pinch cannot be achieved with median nerve injury because of paralysis of thumb musculature.

flexor digitorum profundus of the index and middle fingers, flexor digitorum superficialis, flexor pollicis longus, pronator quadratus, abductor pollicis brevis, opponens pollicis, superficial head of the flexor pollicis brevis, and first and second lumbricals.

Sensory distribution of the median nerve is to the volar surface of the thumb, index, and middle fingers; radial half of the ring finger and dorsal surface of the index and middle fingers; and radial half of the ring finger distal to the PIP joints.

Clinical signs of a high-level median nerve injury are ulnar flexion of the wrist caused by loss of the flexor carpi radialis, loss of palmar abduction, and opposition of the thumb. Active pronation is absent, but the patient may appear to pronate with the assistance of gravity. In a wrist-level median nerve injury the thenar eminence appears flat and there is a loss of thumb flexion, palmar abduction, and opposition.[82]

The sensory loss associated with median nerve injury is particularly disabling because there is no sensation to the volar aspects of the thumb and index and middle fingers and the radial side of the ring finger. The patient when blindfolded substitutes pinch to the ring and small fingers to compensate for this loss. An injury in the forearm that involves the anterior interosseous nerve does not result in sensory loss. Motor loss includes paralysis of the flexor pollicis longus, the flexor digitorum profundus of the index and middle fingers, and the pronator quadratus. The pronator teres is not affected. Pinch is affected.

Splints that position the thumb in palmar abduction and slight opposition increase functional use of the hand (Fig. 44-7). If clawing of the index and middle fingers is present, a splint should be fabricated to prevent hyperextension of the MP joints. Patients report that they avoid use of the hand with a median nerve injury because of lack of sensation rather than because

of muscle paralysis. Nevertheless, the weakened or paralyzed muscles should be protected.

Ulnar Nerve

The ulnar nerve in the forearm innervates only the flexor carpi ulnaris and the median half of the flexor digitorum profundus. It travels down the volar forearm through the canal of Guyon, innervating the intrinsic muscles of the hand, including the palmaris brevis, abductor digiti minimi, opponens digiti minimi, flexor digiti minimi, dorsal and volar interossei, third and fourth lumbricals, and medial head of the flexor pollicis brevis. The sensory distribution of the ulnar nerve is the dorsal and volar surfaces of the small finger ray and the ulnar half of the dorsal and volar surface of the ring finger ray.

A high-level ulnar nerve injury results in hyperextension of the MP joints of the ring and small fingers (also called clawing) resulting from overaction of the extensor digitorum communis that is not held in check by the third and fourth lumbricals.[82] The IP joints of the ring and small fingers do not demonstrate a great flexion deformity because of the paralysis of the flexor digitorum profundus. The hypothenar muscles and interossei are absent. The wrist assumes a position of radial extension caused by the loss of the flexor carpi ulnaris. In a low-level ulnar nerve injury the ring and small fingers claw at the MP joints, and the IP joints exhibit a greater tendency toward flexion because the flexor digitorum profundus is present. Wrist extension is normal.

Clinical signs of a high-level ulnar nerve injury may include clawhand with a loss of the hypothenar and the interosseus muscles. In a low-level ulnar nerve injury the flexor digitorum profundus and flexor carpi ulnaris are present and unopposed by the intrinsic muscles. There is a positive Froment's sign. Long-standing compression of the ulnar nerve in the canal of Guyon results in a flattening of the hypothenar area and conspicuous atrophy of the first dorsal interosseus muscle.[13]

With a low-level ulnar nerve injury a small splint may be provided to prevent hyperextension of the small and ring fingers without limiting full flexion at the MP joints. Stabilization of the MP joints will allow the extensor digitorum communis to extend the IP joints fully (Fig. 44-8).

Sensory loss of the ulnar nerve results in frequent injury to the ulnar side of the hand, especially burns. Patients must be instructed in visual protection of the anesthetic area.

Postoperative Management After Nerve Repair

After nerve repair the hand is placed in a position that minimizes tension on the nerve. For example, after repair of the median nerve, the wrist is immobilized in a flexed position. Immobilization usually lasts for 2 to 3 weeks, after which protective stretching of the joints may begin. The therapist must exercise great care not to put excessive traction on the newly repaired nerve. A repaired digital nerve will also be protected with flexion of the PIP joint.

Correction of a contracture may take 4 to 6 weeks. Active exercise is the preferred method of gaining full extension, although a light dynamic splint may be applied with the surgeon's supervision. Splinting to assist or substitute for weakened musculature may be necessary for an extended period during nerve regeneration. Splints should be removed as soon as possible to allow active exercise of the weakened muscles. It is important to instruct the patient in correct patterns of motion, however, so that substitution is minimized.

Initially treatment is directed toward the prevention of deformity and correction of poor positioning during the acute and regenerative stages. Patients must be instructed

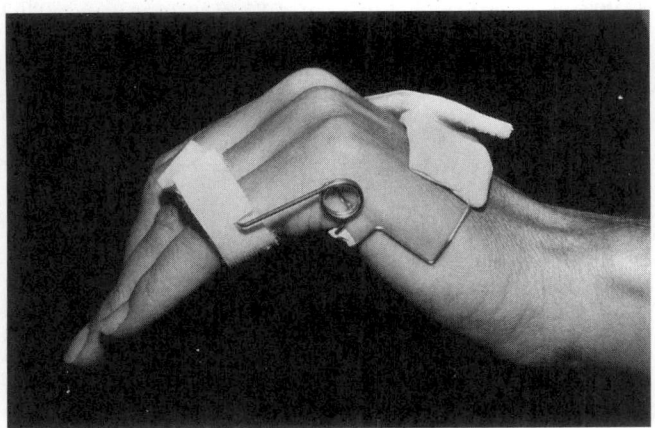

FIG. 44-8
Dynamic ulnar nerve splint blocks hyperextension of metacarpophalangeal (MP) joints that occurs with paralysis of ulnar intrinsic muscles and allows MP flexion, which maintains normal range of motion of MP joints. (Splint courtesy of Mary Dimick, University of California-San Diego Hand Rehabilitation Center.)

in visual protection of the anesthetic area. ADL should be assessed, and new methods or devices may be needed for independence. Use of the hand in the patient's work should be assessed, and the patient should be returned to employment, with any necessary job modifications or adaptations of equipment, as soon as possible.

Careful muscle, sensory, and functional testing should be done frequently. As the nerve regenerates, splints may be changed or eliminated. Exercises and activities should be revised to reflect the patient's new gains, and adapted equipment should be discarded as soon as possible.

As motor function begins to return to the paralyzed muscles, a careful program of specific exercises should be devised to facilitate the return. Proprioceptive neuromuscular facilitation techniques, such as hold-relax, contract-relax, quick stretch, and icing, may assist a fair-strength muscle and increase ROM. Neuromuscular electrical stimulation (NMES) can also provide an external stimulus to help strengthen the newly innervated muscle. When the muscle has reached a good rating, functional activities should be used to complete the return to normal strength.

SENSORY REEDUCATION. Assessment of sensibility is described in some detail earlier in this chapter. This information should be used to prepare a program of sensory reeducation following nerve repair.

When a nerve is repaired, regeneration is not perfect and results in fewer and smaller nerve fibers and receptors distal to the repair. The goal of sensory reeducation is to maximize the functional level of sensation or tactile gnosis.

Parry first described sensory reeducation in 1966,[82] and Dellon reported a highly structured sensory reeducation program in 1974.[31] Dellon divided his program into early- and late-phase training, based on vibratory sensation for early phase and perception of moving and constant touch sensation for late-phase reeducation. Localization of stimuli and recognition of objects were used by both Parry and Dellon. Higher cortical integration was achieved by focusing attention on the stimuli through visual clues and by employing memory when vision was occluded. The patients were taught to compensate for sensory deficits by improving specific skills and generalizing them to other sensory stimuli. Daily repetition appears to be a necessary component of reeducation.

Callahan[18] has outlined a program of protective sensory reeducation and discriminative sensory reeducation if protective sensation is present and touch sensation has returned to the fingertips. Waylett-Rendall[102] has also described a sensory reeducation program using crafts and functional activities, as well as desensitization techniques. All programs emphasize a variety of stimuli used in a repetitive manner to bombard the sensory receptors. A sequence of eyes-closed, eyes-open, eyes-closed is used to provide feedback during the training process. Sessions are limited in length to avoid fatigue and frustration. Objects must not be potentially harmful to the insensate areas, to avoid further trauma. A home program should be provided to reinforce learning that occurs in the clinical setting.

Researchers[18,28,102] have found that sensory reeducation can result in improved functional sensibility in motivated patients. Objective measurement of sensation following reeducation must be performed and then accurately compared with initial testing to assess the success of the program.

TENDON TRANSFERS. If after a minimum period of 1 year after nerve repair, a motor nerve has not reinnervated its muscle, the surgeon may consider tendon transfers to restore a needed motion. The rules of tendon transfer are to evaluate what is absent, what is needed for function, and what is available to transfer.[88]

Some muscles, such as the extensor carpi radialis longus and the sublimis to the ring finger, are commonly used for transfers because their motions are easily substituted by the extensor carpi radialis brevis and flexor digitorum profundus, respectively, to the ring finger. The pronator teres is often used to restore wrist extension for radial nerve paralysis. The surgeon may request assistance from the therapist in evaluating motor status to determine the best motor transfer. Therapy before tendon transfer is essential if the motor being used is not of normal strength. A muscle loses a grade of strength when transferred, and a strengthening program of progressive resistive exercises, NMES, and isolated motion will help ensure success of the transfer. There must be full passive ROM of all joints before tendon transfer can be attempted.

Following transfer, many patients require instruction to perceive the correct muscle during active use of the transfer. Use of surface EMG-biofeedback, careful instruction, and supervised activity to note any substitution patterns during active use usually help the patient to use the transfer correctly. Therapy must be initiated before the patient has time to develop incorrect use patterns. NMES may be used to isolate the muscle and to strengthen it postoperatively.

Tendon Injuries

Flexor Tendons

Tendon injuries may be isolated or may occur in conjunction with other injuries, especially fractures or crushes. Flexor tendons injured in the area between the distal palmar crease and the insertion of the flexor digitorum superficialis are considered the most difficult to treat because the tendons lie in their sheaths in this area beneath the fibrous pulley system and any scarring causes adhesions. This area is often referred to as zone two or "no-man's-land."

Primary repair of the flexor tendons within zone 2 is most frequently attempted after a clean laceration. Several methods of postoperative management have been proposed with the common goals of promoting gliding of the tendons and minimizing the formation of scar adhesions.

CONTROLLED MOBILIZATION OF ACUTE FLEXOR TENDON INJURIES: LOUISVILLE TECHNIQUE. Dr. Harold Kleinert of the University of Louisville School of Medicine was an early advocate of rubberband traction after repair of flexor tendons in zone two. This technique is often referred to as the Kleinert technique. The doctor and therapist do not actively participate in moving the tendon or finger when this protocol is followed as outlined by Kutz.[56]

After surgical repair, rubberbands are attached to the nails of the involved fingers, using a suture through the nail or a hook held in place with cyanoacrylate glue. A dorsal blocking splint is fabricated of low-temperature thermoplastic material, with the MP joints held in about 60° of flexion. The splint is constructed so that the IP joints are able to extend fully to the splint. The rubberbands are passed through a safety pin in the palm and are attached to the distal strap of the splint. The rubberbands should be placed in sufficient tension to hold the PIP joints in 40° to 60° of flexion without tension on the rubberbands. The patient must be able to fully extend the IP joints actively within the splint, or joint contractures will develop (Fig. 44-9).

The patient wears the splint 24 hours a day for 3 weeks and is instructed to actively extend the fingers several times a day in the splint, allowing the rubberbands to pull the fingers into flexion. This movement of the tendon through the tendon sheath and pulley

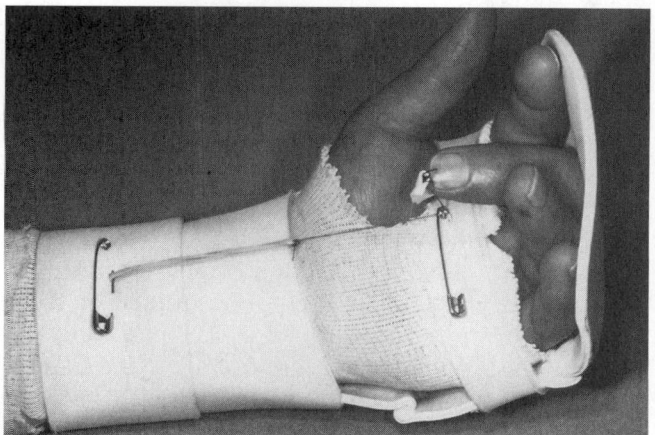

FIG. 44-9

Following flexor tendon repair, wrist is placed in 30° flexion with traction applied from the nail through a safety pin pulley in the palm and attached to proximal strap of splint. Metacarpophalangeal joints should be maintained in about 70° flexion, allowing full passive interphalangeal joint flexion and active extension.

system minimizes scar adhesions, while enhancing tendon nutrition and blood flow.

The dorsal blocking splint is removed at 3 weeks, and the rubberband is attached to a wristband, which is worn for 1 to 5 additional weeks, depending on the judgment of the surgeon. The primary disadvantage of this technique is that contractures of the PIP joints frequently occur as a result of too much tension on the rubberband or incomplete IP extension within the splint.

Dynamic extension splinting of the PIP joint can be started at 5 to 6 weeks if a flexion contracture is present. To be successful, this technique requires a motivated patient who thoroughly understands the program.

CONTROLLED PASSIVE MOTION: DURAN AND HOUSER TECHNIQUE.

Duran and Houser[33] suggested the use of controlled passive motion to achieve optimal results after primary repair, allowing 3 to 5 mm of tendon excursion. They found this amount sufficient to prevent adherence of the repaired tendons. On the third postoperative day the patient begins a twice-daily exercise regimen of passive flexion and extension of six to eight motions for each tendon. Care is taken to keep the wrist flexed and the MPs in 70° of flexion during passive exercise. Between exercise periods the hand is wrapped in stockinette. At 4½ weeks the protective dorsal splint is removed and the rubberband traction is attached to a wristband. Active extension and passive flexion are performed for an additional week and gradually increased over the next several weeks.

IMMOBILIZATION TECHNIQUE.

A third postoperative program involves complete immobilization for 3½ weeks after tendon repair. Good results have not been consistently achieved with immobilization, and this technique may lead to a great incidence of tendon rupture after repair because a tendon gains tensile strength when submitted to gentle tension at the repair site. It is still the preferred method when treating young children or with a noncompliant patient.[93]

As methods of tendon suturing and the suture materials themselves have evolved, some clinicians have begun to prescribe active movement of the repaired tendon within days of surgery. This technique is usually performed only with the most experienced surgeons and therapists working closely together. The condition of the tendon and the technique of repair must be communicated to the therapist, and the patient must be closely monitored. As the rate of rupture decreases with more sophisticated repairs, the results after tendon injury have improved.[92] Many practitioners have modified the tendon protocols, using a combination of passive flexion and active extension techniques, based on their clinical experience. Protocols are suggested as guidelines but vary in actual practice.

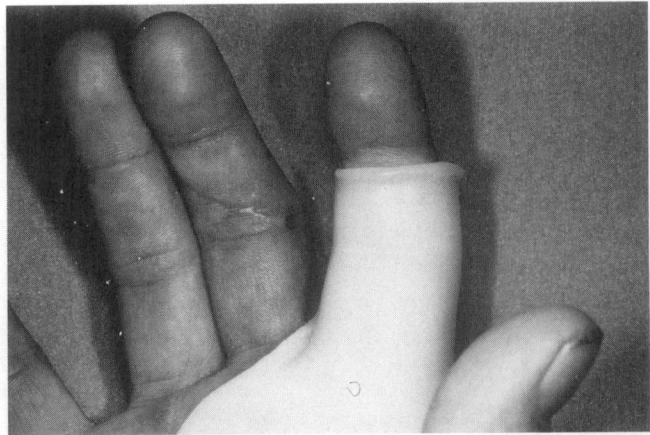

FIG. 44-10
Blocking splint can be used to isolate tendon pull-through and joint range of motion by blocking out proximal joints. This splint is being used to facilitate motion at distal interphalangeal joint following repair of flexor digitorum profundus tendon.

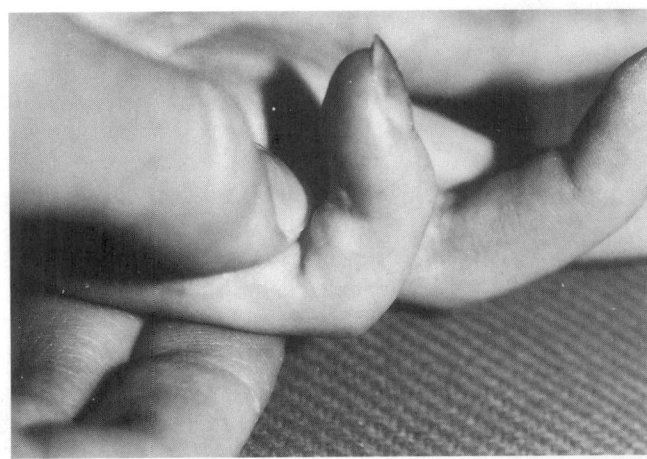

FIG. 44-11
Manual blocking of metacarpophalangeal joint during flexion of proximal interphalangeal joint.

POSTACUTE FLEXOR TENDON REHABILITATION.

When active flexion is begun out of the splint after any of the postoperative management techniques described previously, the patient should be instructed in exercises to facilitate differential tendon gliding.[104] Wehbe[105] recommends three positions—hook, straight fist, and fist—to maximize isolated gliding of the flexor digitorum superficialis and the flexor digitorum profundus tendons, as well as stretching of the intrinsic musculature and gliding of the extensor mechanism. Tendon gliding exercises should be done for 10 repetitions of each position, two or three times a day.

Isolated exercises to assist tendon gliding may also be performed using a blocking splint (Fig. 44-10)[35] or the opposite hand (Fig. 44-11). The MP joints should be held in extension during blocking so that the intrinsic

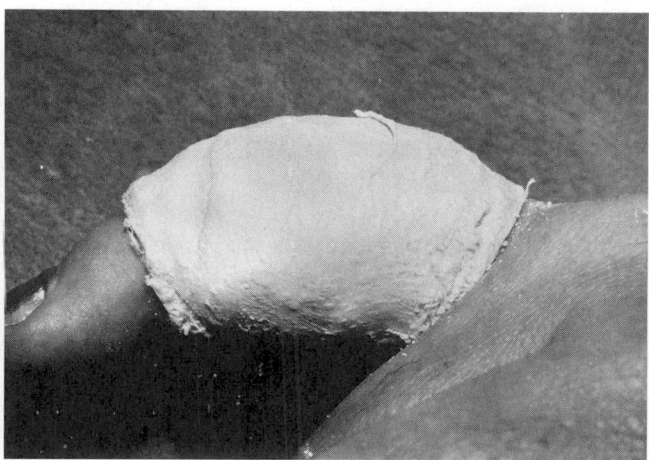

FIG. 44-12
Plaster cylindrical splint is used to apply static stretch of proximal interphalangeal joint contracture. It is not removed by patient and must be replaced frequently by therapist with careful monitoring of skin condition.

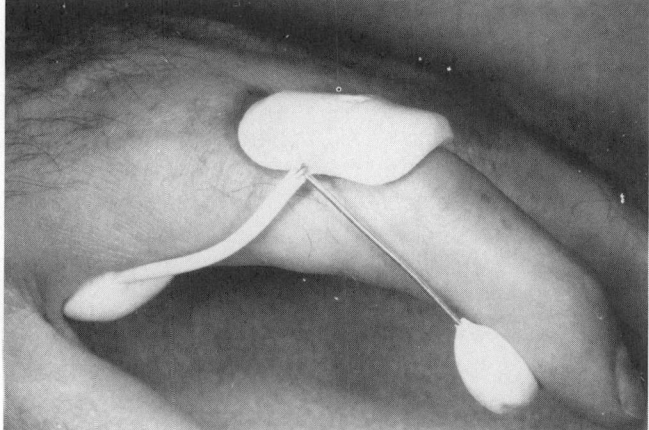

FIG. 44-13
This finger splint is used to increase extension of proximal interphalangeal joint. Splint available from DeRoyal/LMB, DeRoyal Industries, Inc, Powell, TN.

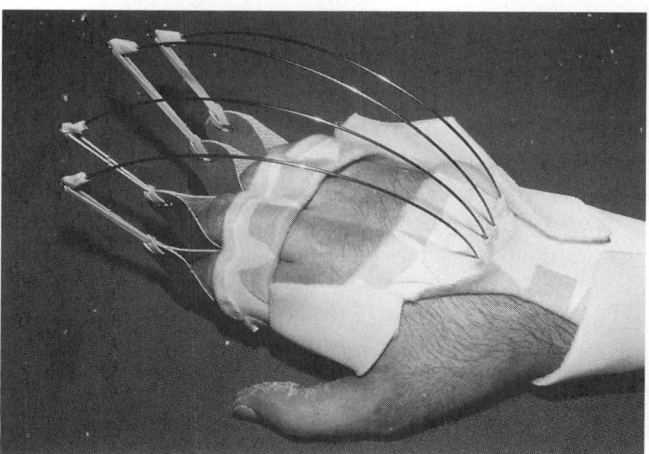

FIG. 44-14
Dynamic outrigger splint using spring-steel outriggers with a lumbrical block can be used to assist proximal interphalangeal (PIP) joint extension, stretch against scar adhesions of extrinsic flexors, or reduce PIP joint contractures. Proper fit and tension of rubber bands must be assessed frequently by therapist.

muscles that act on it cannot overcome the power of the repaired flexor tendons. Care should be taken not to hyperextend the PIP joints and overstretch the repaired tendons.

After 6 to 8 weeks passive extension may be started and splinting may be necessary to correct a flexion contracture at the PIP joint. A cylindrical plaster splint may be fabricated to apply constant static pressure on the contracture, as described by Bell (Fig. 44-12).[9] Static splinting may be especially effective with a flexion contracture greater than 25°. A finger gutter splint may be made using $\frac{1}{16}$-inch (0.16-cm) thermoplastic material for static extension at night, which will help maintain extension gains made during the day. Gentle dynamic traction may be applied using a commercial splint such as a spring finger extension assist (Fig. 44-13) or one that is fabricated by the therapist (Fig. 44-14). Dynamic flexion splinting may be necessary if the patient has difficulty regaining passive flexion.

At about 8 weeks the patient may begin light resistive exercises and activities. The hand can now be used for light ADL, but the patient should continue to avoid heavy lifting with the affected hand or excessive resistance. Sports activities should be discouraged. Such activities as clay work, woodworking, and macramé are excellent, however. Full resistance and normal work activities can be started at 3 months following surgery.

After a hand that has sustained a tendon injury, passive versus active limitations of joint motion must be evaluated. Limitations in active motion may indicate joint stiffness, muscle weakness, or scar adhesions.[83] If passive motion is greater than active motion, the therapist should consider that tendons may be caught in the scar tissue. The therapist should be able to determine if a tendon is adhering and causing a flexion contracture or if the tendon is free but the joint itself is stiff. Treatment should be based on this type of evaluation.

ROM, strength, function, and sensibility testing (if digital nerves were also injured) should be performed frequently, with splints and activities geared to progress. Although performance of ADL is generally not a problem, the therapist should ask the patient about any problems he or she may have or anticipate. Disuse and neglect of a finger, especially the index finger, are common and should be prevented.

Gains in flexion and extension may continue to be recorded for 6 months postoperatively. A finger with limber joints and minimal scarring preoperatively will function better after repair than one that is stiff and scarred and has trophic skin changes.[14] Therefore it is important that all joints, skin, and scars be supple and movable before reconstructive surgery is attempted. A functional to excellent result is obtained if the combined loss of extension is less than 40° in the PIP and DIP joints of the index and middle fingers and less than 60° in the ring and small fingers[76] and if the finger can flex to the palm.[14]

FLEXOR TENDON RECONSTRUCTION. If the tendon is damaged as a result of a crush injury or the laceration cannot be cleaned up enough to allow for a primary repair, staged flexor tendon reconstruction may be performed. At the first operation a Silastic rod is inserted beneath the pulley system and attached to the distal phalanx. Other reconstructive procedures, such as pulley reconstruction, are performed at the same time. A mesothelial cell–lined pseudosheath is formed about the rod, and a fluid similar to synovial fluid is formed in the postoperative recovery phase.[58] The second stage is performed about 4 months later when the digit can be moved passively to the palm. A tendon graft is inserted and the Silastic rod removed. The postoperative program is carried out in the same manner as for a primary tendon repair.[45]

Following a two-stage tendon reconstruction or primary repair, a tenolysis may be performed if there is a substantial difference between the active and passive motion. Tenolysis is usually not performed for 6 months to 1 year after tendon repair. At the time of tenolysis surgery, scar adhesions are removed from the tendon and gliding of the tendons is assessed. Patients are often asked to move their fingers in the operating room at the time of lysis to determine the extent of scar removal. Active motion is begun within the first 24 hours using bupivacaine (Marcaine) blocks[89] or transcutaneous electrical nerve stimulation (TENS)[19] to control pain.

LaSalle and Strickland[58] have recommended a system for evaluating the results of tenolysis surgery by comparing the preoperative passive IP joint motion with the postoperative IP joint motion. Based on this comparison LaSalle and Strickland found that in one group of patients undergoing tenolysis, 40% had an improvement in motion of 50% or better, compared with their preoperative status.

Extensor Tendons

Dorsal scar adherence is the most difficult problem after injury to the extensor tendons because of the tendency of the dorsal extensor hood to become adherent to the underlying structures and thus limit its normal excursion during flexion and extension.

Extensor tendons in zones V, VI, and VII (proximal to the MP joints) become adherent because they are encased in paratenon and synovial sheaths and respond to injury in a way similar to flexor tendons, resulting in either incomplete extension, also known as extensor lag, or incomplete flexion caused by loss of gliding of the extensor tendon.

Evans[36,37] studied the normal excursion of the extensor digitorum communis in zones V, VI, and VII to suggest guidelines for early passive motion of extensor tendons. She concluded that 5 mm of tendon glide after repair was safe and effective in limiting tendon adhesions and designed a postoperative splint that allows slight active flexion while providing passive extension.[37] The splint is worn for 3 weeks, with the initiation of active motion between the third and fourth weeks. A removable volar splint is used between exercise periods to protect the tendon for 2 additional weeks. Dynamic flexion splinting may be started at 6 weeks after surgery to regain flexion if needed.

Injuries to extensor tendons proximal to the MP joint may be immobilized for 3 weeks. After this period the finger may be placed in a removable volar splint that is worn between exercise periods for an additional 2 weeks. Progressive ROM is begun at 3 weeks, and if full flexion is not regained rapidly, dynamic flexion may be started at 6 weeks.

Extensor tendon injuries that occur distal to the MP joint require a longer period of immobilization, usually 6 weeks. A progressive exercise program is then initiated with dynamic splinting during the day and a static night splint to maintain extension.

Dynamic splints may include a PIP-DIP splint, first described by Hollis and now available commercially (Fig. 44-15),* a web strap made of lamp wick or elastic, a fingernail hook with rubber band traction, a traction glove, or another splint.

If a lysis of scar tissue is required because of persistent scar adhesion, the surgeon may place a thin sheet of Silastic between the tendon and bone at the time of surgery to reduce further scar adherence. The patient begins exercising within the first 24 hours, and splints are applied as needed. Active exercise is essential, and the patient must be carefully instructed in a home program. The patient is encouraged to use the hand for all activities except those requiring heavy resistance. After 4 to 6 weeks the Silastic sheet is removed and ROM should be maintained.

Total Active Motion and Total Passive Motion

Total active motion (TAM) and total passive motion (TPM) are mthods of recording joint ROM that are used

---

*DeRoyal/LMB, DeRoyal Industries, Powell, Tenn.

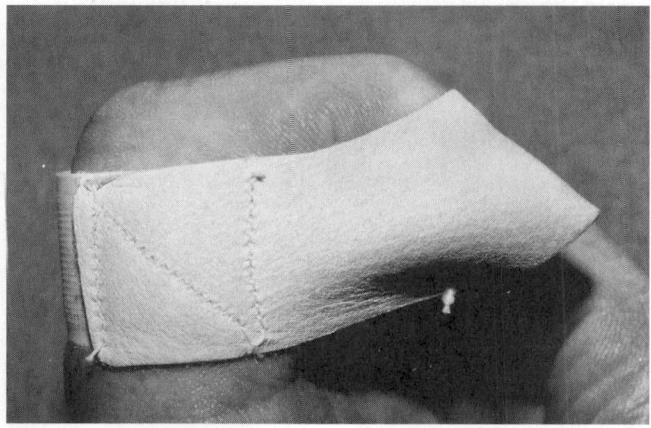

FIG. 44-15
Proximal interphalangeal (PIP)-distal interphalangeal (DIP) splint may be used to increase flexion of both PIP and DIP joints. Tension can be adjusted with Velcro closure. Wearing time should be determined by therapist.

to compare tendon excursion (active) and joint mobility (passive). It is the measure of flexion minus extensor lag of three joints. TAM and TPM have been recommended for use in reporting joint motion by the American Society for Surgery of the Hand.[4]

TAM is computed by adding the sum of the angles formed by the MP, PIP, and DIP joints in flexion, minus incomplete active extension at each of the three joints. For example, MP joint flexion is 85° with full extension, PIP is 100° and lacks 15° extension, and DIP is 65° with full extension; therefore

$$TAM = 85 + 100 + 65 - 15 = 235°.$$

TAM should be measured while making a fist. It is used for a single digit and should be compared with the same digit of the opposite hand or subsequent measurements of the same digit. It should not be used to compute a percentage of loss of impairment. TPM is calculated in the same manner but measures only passive motion.

Edema

Edema is a normal consequence of trauma but must be quickly and aggressively treated to prevent permanent stiffness and disability. Within hours of trauma, vasodilatation and local edema occur, with an increase in white blood cells to the damaged area.[64] The inflammatory response to the injury results in a decrease in bacteria to control infection.

Early control of edema should be achieved through elevation, massage, compression, and active ROM. The patient is instructed at the time of injury to keep the hand elevated, and a compressive dressing is used to reduce early swelling. Pitting edema is present early and can be recognized as a bloated swelling that "pits" when

pressed. Pitting may be more pronounced on the dorsal surface where the venous and lymphatic systems provide return of fluid to the heart. Active motion is especially important to produce retrograde venous and lymphatic flow.

If the swelling continues, a serofibrinous exudate invades the area. Fibrin is deposited in the spaces surrounding the joints, tendons, and ligaments, resulting in reduced mobility, flattening of the arches of the hand, tissue atrophy, and further disuse.[64] Normal gliding of the tissues is eliminated, and a stiff, often painful hand is the result. Scar adhesions form and further limit tissue mobility. If untreated, these losses may become permanent.

Early recognition of persistent edema through observation and volume and circumference measurement is important. It may be necessary to use several of the suggested edema control techniques.

Elevation
Early elevation with the hand above the heart is essential. Slings tend to reduce blood flow and should be avoided. Resting the hand on pillows while seated or lying down is effective. Resting the hand on top of the head or using devices that elevate the hand with the elbow in extension has been suggested. Suspension slings may be purchased or fabricated.

The patient should use the hand for ADL, within the limitations of resistance prescribed by the physician. Light ADL that can be accomplished while the hand is in the dressing are permitted.

Contrast Baths
Alternating soaks of cold and warm water that is 66° and 96° F (18.9° and 35.6° C) have been recommended as a method preferred over warm water soaks or whirlpool baths. The contrast baths can be done for 20 minutes, alternating the hand between cool water for 1 minute and warm water for 1 minute, starting and ending with cool water. A sponge can be placed in each tub so that the hand is moved during the soaking period. The tubs should be placed as high as possible to provide elevation of the extremity. The alternating warm and cool water cause vasodilatation and vasoconstriction, resulting in a pumping action on the edema. Combined with elevation and active motion, edema may be reduced and pain is often alleviated by this technique.

Manual Edema Mobilization*
"Manual edema mobilization (MEM) is a method of edema reduction based on the role of the lymphatics for moving tissue fluid, protein molecules, and other large molecule substances not permeable to the venous

---

*Material used courtesy of Sandra Artzberger, Hartford, Wis.

system out of an edematous area. MEM specifically addresses how to activate lymph uptake and the uniqueness of the lymphatic system.

"Recent European and Australian studies have given new insights into lymphatic pathways (routes); pressures which collapse or damage lymphatics preventing protein absorption; functional anatomical characteristics differentiating lymphatics from the venous system; the role of stagnant high protein fluid in the interstitium and chronic edema; formation of lymphatics in scar tissue, etc. These studies plus Manual Lymphatic Treatment principles associated with post cancer lymphedema form the foundation for Manual Edema Mobilization. MEM is a technique used on the patient with sub acute edema to either prevent edema from moving into a chronic state or to reduce an existing chronic edema."[6]

PRINCIPLES AND CONCEPTS OF MANUAL EDEMA MOBILIZATION

- Provide light massage, less than 40 mm Hg pressure to prevent collapse of the lymphatic pathways.
- Incorporate exercise before and after massage in a specific sequence when possible.
- Massage, done in segments, is proximal to distal, then distal to proximal, always following movement of the therapist's hand in proximal direction.
- Massage follows the flow of lymphatic pathways.
- Massage reroutes around the incision area.
- Method does not cause additional inflammation.
- Include a patient home self-massage program.
- Guide treatment to avoid increased edema from other treatment techniques.
- Incorporate low stretch compression bandaging and warmth to soften hardened tissues, especially at night.

Active Range Of Motion

Normal blood flow is dependent on muscle activity. Active motion does not mean wiggling the fingers, but rather maximum available ROM, performed firmly. Casts and splints must allow mobility of uninjured parts while protecting newly injured structures. The shoulder and elbow should be moved several times a day. The importance of active ROM for edema control, tendon gliding, and tissue nutrition cannot be overemphasized.

Compression

Light compression using Coban wraps* of the affected area (Fig. 44-16) or light compressive garments such as those made by Aris† or Jobst[47] (Fig. 44-17) will help to control swelling, especially at night.

---

*Coban (available from Smith & Nephew, Inc, Germantown, Wis).
†Aris Isotoner gloves (available from North Coast Medical, Morgan Hill, Calif).

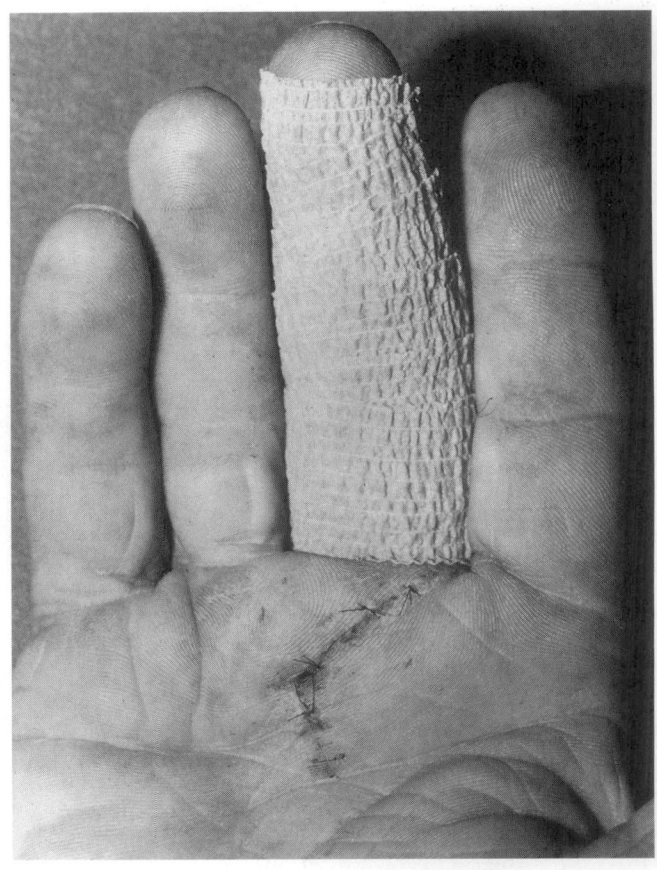

FIG. 44-16
One-inch Coban is wrapped with minimal pressure from distal end to proximal crease of digit. Patient is instructed to be aware of vascular compression or tingling. Coban may be worn several hours a day to reduce edema. Product available from Medical Products Division/3M, St. Paul, Minn.

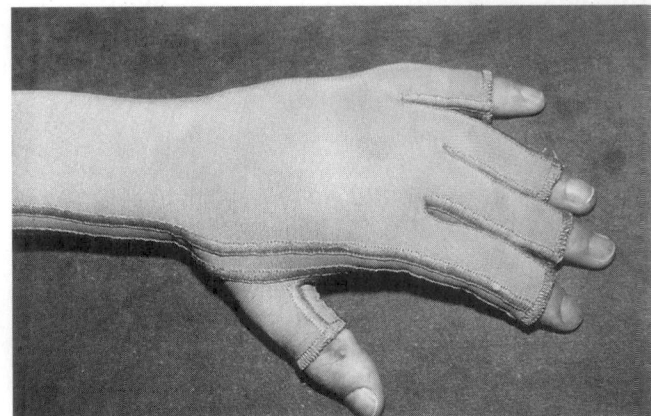

FIG. 44-17
Custom-fit Jobst garment may be used to reduce edema and to reduce and prevent hypertrophic scar formation after burns or trauma. Inserts may be used with garment to increase pressure over natural curves, such as dorsum of wrist.

Wound Healing and Scar Remodeling

The basis of hand therapy is the histology of wound healing. Acute treatment must be planned using the foundation of tissue healing as a guide. Bones, tendons, nerves, and skin follow a progression of healing phases. Treatment must respect healing tissue to promote recovery and prevent further damage. The therapist must take care to do no harm, and that can be accomplished only with a thorough understanding of the physiology of healing.

The first phase of wound healing, the acute inflammatory phase, is initiated within hours, when the tissues are disrupted through injury or surgery, causing vasodilatation, local edema, and migration of white blood cells and phagocytic cells to the area. The phagocytes remove tissue fragments and foreign bodies and are critical to healing. The inflammatory process can subside or persist indefinitely, depending on the degree of bacterial contamination.[64]

Fibroblasts in combination with associated capillaries begin to invade the wound within the first 72 hours and gradually replace the phagocytes, leading to the second phase: the collagen or granulation phase, between the fifth and fourteenth days. Collagen fiber formation follows the invasion by fibroblasts, so that by the end of the second week the wound is rich with fibroblasts, a capillary network, and early collagen fibers. This increased vascularization results in the erythema of the new scar.

During the third to sixth weeks fibroblasts are slowly replaced with scar collagen fibers, and the wound becomes stronger and more able to withstand progressive stresses, leading to the last phase of scar maturation. Tissue strength continues to increase for 3 months or longer. The collagen metabolizes and synthesizes during this period, so that new collagen replaces old while the wound remains relatively stable. Covalent bonding between collagen molecules leads to dense scar adhesions and the formation of whorl-like patterns of collagen deposits, which may be altered as the scar architecture and collagen fiber organization within the wound change over time.[32]

Myofibroblasts, which are fibroblasts with properties similar to smooth muscle cells, are contractile and cause a shortening of the wound.

Tissues that have restored gliding have different scar architecture from those that do not develop the ability to glide. With gliding, the scar resembles the state of the tissues before injury, whereas the nongliding scar remains fixed on surrounding structures. Controlled tension on the scar has been shown to facilitate remodeling. Scar formation is also influenced by age and the quantity of scar deposited.[64]

Wound Care and Dressings

Wounds may be described using a "three-color concept" of red, yellow, or black wounds.[38] This system simplifies wound description and treatment. Guidelines for treating the three wound types help the therapist choose the proper method of cleansing and dressing wounds. The reader is encouraged to review this material before treating open wounds.

Topical treatment such as antimicrobials, may be used to control bacteria. There are a variety of dressings that can be placed on a wound, including gauze that has been impregnated with petroleum, such as Xeroform gauze or Adaptic. Ointments such as Polysporin are also commonly applied. N-Terface* is a dry mesh fabric that looks and feels like the interfacing used in sewing. Because it is nonadherent, it can be used directly over wounds and will not stick to them. Sterile dressings can be applied directly over the N-Terface without ointments or gels. The selection of materials depends on the amount of exudate and the goal of the dressing (which may include removing debris, absorbing exudate, or protecting new cells).

Spenco Second Skin* is an inert gel sheeting made from 96% water and 4% polyethylene oxide. It removes friction between two moving surfaces and is said to clean wounds by absorbing secretions. It comes in sterile and nonsterile packs and is encased in a light plastic covering. It is especially effective with abrasions or areas of skin loss because it is cool and reduces itching. It can be used after burns.

Spenco Dermal Pads* are artificial fat pads that can be used to prevent pressure sores or can be cut to size to use around an existing pressure sore or wound to allow it to heal. Dermal pads are ⅛ inch thick (0.32 cm) and will adhere to the skin when the protective film is removed. The pad can be held in place with a dressing or with a pressure garment. It also can be washed without reducing its adherence. Dermal pads can be cut and placed around a healing wound to protect it under a splint or dressing. They are generally not needed after the wound is healed.

The wound can be cleaned with a solution of hydrogen peroxide and sterile saline, with dead tissue then being gently removed with sterile swabs. Sterile saline solution can be used to soak off adherent bandages rather than pulling them off the patient. The therapist should pour a very small amount of saline on the area that is sticking, wait a few moments, and gently pry the dressing off. Dead skin can be debrided using iris scissors and pickups. Betadine-impregnated scrub sponges may be used for cleaning and desensitization of the wound once it is healed and the stitches have been removed. The patient also can do this procedure at home. Sterile whirlpool may be used for debridement, especially if the wound is infected.

---

*N-Terface, made by Winfield Laboratories (available from North Coast Medical, Morgan Hill, Calif).
*Spenco Medical Corp, Waco, Tex.

Pressure

A hypertrophic scar or a scar that is randomly laid down and thickened is reduced by the application of pressure, often by means of pressure garments.*[47] Use of an insert of neoprene† fabric or molds made from Silastic elastomer‡[67] under the pressure garment increases the conformity of the garment. Pressure should be applied for most of the 24-hour period, and with a hypertrophic burn scar this treatment should continue for 6 months to 1 year after the injury. Silicone Gel Sheets§ have been found to reduce hypertrophic scarring when worn on a regular basis for up 12 to 24 hours a day.

Massage

Gentle to firm massage of the scarred area using a thick ointment rapidly softens scar tissue and should be followed immediately with active hand use so that tendons glide against the softened scar.[27] Vibration to the area with a small, low-intensity vibrator will have a similar effect.[48] Active exercise, using facilitation techniques and against resistance, or functional activity, should follow vibration. Massage and vibration may be started 4 weeks after injury.

Thermal heat in the form of paraffin dips, hot packs, or fluidotherapy, immediately followed by stretching while the tissue cools, provides stretch to the scar tissue. Wrapping the scarred or stiff digit into flexion with Coban during the application of heat often increases mobility in the area. Heat should not be used with insensate areas or if swelling persists.[49]

Active Range of Motion and Electrical Stimulation

Active ROM provides an internal stretch against resistant scar, and its use cannot be overemphasized. If the patient is unable to achieve active motion because of scar adhesions or weakness, use of a battery-operated NMES may augment the motion.[107] Stimulation may be performed by the patient for several hours at home and has been shown to increase ROM and tendon excursion.[77]

Many hand therapists use high-voltage direct current as a treatment to increase motor activity, and it may be used for scar remodeling.[2] Ultrasound treatments are often prescribed but may be more effective if done within the first few months after trauma. A continuous passive motion (CPM) device may be used at home to maintain passive ROM and promote tendon gliding. It should be used for several hours a day for maximum benefit.

*Bio-Concepts, Phoenix, Ariz.
†Neoprene (available from Benik Corp, Silverdale, Wash).
‡Silicone elastomers (available from Smith & Nephew, Germantown, Wis).
§Cica-Care Silicone Gel Sheets (available from Smith & Nephew, Germantown, Wis).

Pain Syndromes

Pain is the subjective manifestation of trauma transmitted by the sympathetic nervous system, which may interfere with normal functioning. Because pain leads to overprotection of the affected part and disuse of the extremity, it should be treated early.

Desensitization

Stimulation of the large afferent A nerve fibers leads to a reduction of pain by decreasing summation in the slowly adapting, small, unmyelineated C fibers, which carry pain sensation. The A-axons can be stimulated mechanically with pressure, rubbing, vibration, TENS, percussion, and active motion. Desensitization techniques are based on the amplification of inhibitory mechanisms.

Yerxa[109] has described a desensitization program that "employs short periods of contact with three sensory modalities: dowel textures, immersion or contact particles, and vibration." This program allows the patient to rank 10 dowel textures and 10 immersion textures on the degree of irritation produced by the stimulus. Treatment begins with a stimulus that is irritating but tolerable. The stimulus is applied for 10 minutes, three or four times a day. The vibration hierarchy is predetermined and is based on cycles per second of vibration, the placement of the vibrator, and the duration of the treatment. Complete instructions for assembling the Downey Hand Center desensitization kit can be found in the literature in the references. The Downey Hand Center Hand Sensitivity Test can be used to establish a desensitization treatment program and to measure progress in decreasing hypersensitivity.[7,109]

Neuromas

Neuromas are a complication of nerve suture or amputation. A traumatic neuroma is an unorganized mass of nerve fibers that results from accidental or surgical cutting of the nerve. A neuroma in continuity occurs on a nerve that is intact.[96] Neuromas may be clinically identified by a specific, sharp pain. Stimulation of a neuroma usually causes the patient to pull the hand away quickly; many patients report a burning pain that radiates up the forearm. Neuromas are disabling because any stimulation causes intense pain and the patient avoids the sensitive area.

A generalized desensitization program may not work because the patient never develops a tolerance for stimulation of the neuroma. Injection of cortisone acetate may help break up the neuroma, making desensitization techniques more effective. Surgically excising the neuroma or burying the nerve endings deeper may be necessary.

Complex Regional Pain Syndrome

Complex regional pain syndrome (CRPS) is the new term that replaces "reflex sympathetic dystrophy (RSD)" to describe a group of disorders that "involve pain and dysfunction of severity or duration out of proportion to those expected from the initiating event."[108]

"Complex" denotes the complex nature of the pain response, which may include inflammation, autonomic, cutaneous, motor and dystrophic changes. "Regional" refers to the wide distribution of symptoms beyond the area of the original lesion. "Pain" is the primary characteristic of this syndrome. It includes spontaneous pain, thermal changes, and at times burning pain. CRPS, type I, corresponds to RSD. Type II corresponds to causalgia, a severe, burning pain first described during the Civil War.

Diagnostic criteria for CRPS must include spontaneous pain beyond the territory of a single peripheral nerve and disproportionate to the inciting event. There is generally edema, skin blood-flow abnormality, or abnormal sudomotor activity in the area of the pain. The diagnosis is excluded by existence of conditions that would otherwise account for the pain. The hallmarks of CRPS are pain; edema; blotchy-looking, shiny skin; and coolness of the extremity. Sensory changes may occur. There may be excessive sweating or dryness if there is associated sympathetic dysfunction. The degree of trauma does not correlate with the severity of the pain and may occur after any injury. CRPS, Type I may be triggered by a cycle of vasospasm and vasodilatation after an injury. Abnormal edema and constrictive dressings or casts may be a factor in initiating the vasospasm. A vasospasm "causes tissue anoxia and edema and therefore more pain, which continues the abnormal cycle."[79] Circulation is decreased, which causes the extremity to become cool and pale.

Fibrosis after tissue anoxia and the presence of protein-rich exudates result in joint stiffness. The patient may cradle the hand and prefers to keep it wrapped. There may be an exaggerated reaction to touch, especially light touch. Osteoporosis may be apparent on x-ray films by 8 weeks after trauma after active use of the hand. Burning pain associated with causalgia (CRPS, type II) is a symptom that may be alleviated by interruption of the sympathetic nerve pathways.

There are three stages of CRPS. Stage I (traumatic stage) may last up to 3 months; it is characterized by pain, pitting edema, and discoloration. Stage II (dystrophic stage) may last an additional 6 to 9 months. Pain, brawny edema, stiffness, redness, heat, and bony demineralization are usually found in this stage. The hand usually has a glossy appearance. Stage III (atrophic stage) may last up to several years or indefinitely. Pain usually peaks in Stage II and decreases in stage III. Thickening around the joints occurs, and fixed contractures may be present. If there is swelling, it is hard and not responsive to techniques such as elevation. The hand may be pale, dry, and cool. There may be substantial dysfunction of the limb.

CRPS is treated by decreasing sympathetic stimulation. It is most responsive in stage I. The first goal of treatment is reduction of the pain and hypersensitivity to light touch. This goal may be accomplished with application of warm (not hot), moist heat, fluidotherapy, gentle handling of the hand, acupressure, desensitization, and TENS before active ROM. Treatment that increases pain (such as passive ROM) should be avoided. Many patients respond well to gentle manual edema mobilization,[6] which reduces the edema and reintroduces touching of the hand. Stellate ganglion blocks to eliminate the pain are effective early. They should be coordinated with therapy so that the patient can perform active ROM and functional activities during the pain-free period after the blocks. Active ROM is crucial. Gravity-eliminated exercise either in water or on a tabletop may be easier for the patient to tolerate.

A variety of drugs may be used, including sympatholytic drugs[57] that reduce the vasoconstrictive action of the peripheral vessels. Neurontin is often effective in reducing pain and increasing temperature in the extremity. Calcium channel blockers are also effective. Carefully monitored use of narcotics may interrupt the pain cycle and allow active use of the hand. A stress-loading program that has been used effectively to reduce symptoms of RSD (CRPS, type I) has been described.[101] It can easily be adapted for home use.

Edema control techniques should be started immediately. Elevation, manual edema mobilization, contrast baths, and high-voltage direct current in water have been found to be effective. Surface EMG-biofeedback training for relaxation may help muscle spasms and increase blood flow, in addition to reducing anxiety.

CRPS frequently triggers shoulder pain and stiffness, resulting in shoulder-hand syndrome or adhesive capsulitis of the shoulder ("frozen shoulder"). Therefore active ROM and functional activities should include the entire upper quadrant. Use of skateboard exercises is helpful in the early stages for active-assisted exercise of the shoulder. Splints that reduce joint stiffness should be used as tolerated. Splints must not be painful or increase swelling. Reliance on immobilization splinting should be avoided because patients with CRPS prefer not to move the affected part, which ultimately makes their symptoms worse.

A tendency to develop CRPS should be suspected in any patient who seems to complain excessively about pain, appears anxious, and complains of profuse sweating and temperature changes in the hand. Some patients report nausea associated with touching the hand. Patients tend to overprotect the hand. Early intervention with a structured therapy program of functional activities, group interaction, and exercises that include the hand and shoulder may prevent the occurrence of a fully developed CRPS. This problem is best recognized early and treated with tempered aggressiveness and empathy.

Transcutaneous Electrical Nerve Stimulation

TENS is a treatment technique that is thought to stimulate the afferent A nerve fibers in the high-frequency mode and stimulate the release of morphinelike neural hormones, the enkephalins, in the low-frequency mode. Its efficacy as a treatment for pain control is well documented in medical literature. As with other electrical modalities that may be used by hand therapists, TENS should be correlated with functional use of the hand.

TENS should be used for treatment periods not to exceed 60 minutes at a time to achieve pain control.[51] A TENS diary should be used to record the level of pain on a scale of 1 to 10 before and after treatment, as well as activities that exacerbate the pain. To prevent overuse, TENS may be tapered as the pain-free periods increase. Treatment can be continued as long as necessary to provide pain control.

Joint Stiffness

Joint stiffness has been discussed in other sections of this chapter because it is seen after almost any hand trauma or disease. In the acute phase it may also result from "internal splinting" done unconsciously by the patient to avoid pain. It may be prevented by early mobilization, pain control, reduction of edema, active and passive ROM, use of a continuous passive motion device, and appropriate splinting techniques. Grade I and II joint mobilization are especially helpful in preparing for passive and active motion and for pain relief.

Treatment of established joint stiffness is more difficult. Thermal modalities, joint mobilization, ultrasound and electrical stimulation, dynamic splinting, serial casting, and active and passive motion in preparation for functional use should all be included in the treatment regimen.

Cumulative Trauma Disorders

A number of terms are used throughout the world to describe injuries to the musculoskeletal system, including overuse syndromes, repetitive strain injuries, cervicalbrachial disorders, repetitive motion injuries, and in the United States, **cumulative trauma disorders** (CTDs). The incidence of CTDs in the United States is on the rise, with 281,800 cases reported in private industry in 1992.[53] Between 1981 and 1992, CTDs increased from 18% to 62% of all worker's compensation claims filed.[91] Women account for about two thirds of work-related repetitive motion injuries.

The term "cumulative trauma disorder" should be viewed as a description of the mechanism of injury and not a diagnosis. Even when the presenting symptoms are confusing, attempts to define a specific diagnosis are necessary because "each disorder has a different cause, treatment, and prognosis."[85] Diagnoses associated with cumulative trauma usually fall into one of three categories: tendinitis (such as lateral epicondylitis or de Quervain's tenosynovitis), nerve compression syndromes (such as carpal tunnel syndrome or cubital tunnel syndrome), or myofascial pain.

Cumulative trauma occurs when force is applied to the same muscle or muscle group, causing an inflammatory response in the tendon or muscle.[85] Muscle fatigue is an important aspect of cumulative trauma. Excessive use of the muscle or body system (overuse or overexertion) is experienced as a muscle cramp. Acute overuse is relieved by rest, but chronic fatigue is not relieved by rest. The amount of fatigue is related to the amount of force and the duration of force application.

Fatigue occurs more quickly with high force. If force is maintained, repetitions must be reduced to allow recovery. Therefore if the force is decreased while repetitions are maintained and recovery time is adequate, harm is less likely to occur. The combination of repetitions without adequate recovery time and high force establishes an environment that is likely to lead to injury. Byl[17] has found that repetitive hand opening and closing may lead to motor control problems and the development of focal hand dystonias through a degradation of the cortical representation. Applying this research may help therapists develop more effective treatment programs for cumulative trauma and chronic pain.

Treatment may be divided into phases. Acute-phase treatment is geared toward decreasing the inflammation through dynamic rest. Splints are used for immobilization. Splinting alone may relieve symptoms; splinting is often combined with cortisone injections to reduce inflammation. Icing, contrast baths, ultrasound phonophoresis, iontophoresis, and interferential and high-voltage electrical stimulation have all been found to be effective in reducing pain and decreasing inflammation. Nonsteroidal antiinflammatory drugs are also frequently used. Newer medications such as Celebrex and Vioxx seem to be more effective clinically in reducing symptoms than previous antiinflammatory drugs.

When splints are used, they should be removed three times a day for stretching of the affected musculature (e.g., the extensor group with lateral epicondylitis) to maintain or increase muscle length and to prevent joint stiffness. Painful activities should be avoided during the dynamic rest phase. Vibration is contraindicated because vibration may contribute to inflammatory problems.

As the acute symptoms decrease, the patient begins the exercise phase of treatment. After warmup of the muscles by slow stretching, the patient begins controlled progressive exercise. Resistance should be given at the end of range when progressive resistive exercise is performed. A tennis-elbow armband can be worn over the extensor muscle bellies to limit full excursion of the muscle during active use of the arm. Resistance should be increased slowly and should not cause an increase in pain.

Patients are instructed to continue stretching three times a day, especially before activity, for an indefinite time. Proper body mechanics are critical in the long-term control of inflammatory problems, so patients must become aware of what triggers their symptoms and learn early intervention if symptoms reappear. Icing, splints, stretching, and modified activities combined with correct body mechanics are usually effective. The key is that the patients learn self-management techniques and take an active role in their treatment.

Work-related risk factors for CTDs include the following[5]:
- Repetition
- High force
- Awkward joint posture
- Direct pressure
- Vibration
- Prolonged static positioning

An assessment of the job site, tools used, and hand position during work activities may be indicated with the patient whose symptoms are related to job demands. Modification of the equipment used and strengthening of the dominant muscle groups and their antagonist muscles may permit continued employment and control the inflammatory problem.

Tendinitis and tenosynovitis are frequently seen in cumulative trauma. The cycle of overuse leading to microtrauma, swelling, pain, and limitations in movement is followed by rest, disuse, and weakness. Normal activity is resumed, and the cycle begins again.

Patients usually have a combination of localized pain, swelling, pain with resisted motion of the affected musculotendinis unit, limitations in motion, weakness, and crepitation of the tendons. Symptoms are reproduced with activity or work simulation. Using functional grades to describe the associated symptoms assists in evaluation, as well as monitoring of improvement (Table 44-5).[50] Although isometric grip strength may be normal, wrist and forearm strength are often decreased and out of balance. Dynamic grip strength may be more limited because tendon gliding is more likely to increase inflammation and pain. Muscle imbalance leads to positioning and substitution patterns that may result in worsening or spreading of symptoms.

Nerve compression syndromes, especially carpal tunnel syndrome, are frequently seen.[61] Carpal tunnel syndrome is caused by pressure on the median nerve as it travels beneath the transverse carpal ligament at the volar surface of the wrist.[40] The syndrome is associated with increased pressure in the carpal canal because of trauma, edema, retention of fluids as a result of pregnancy, flexor tenosynovitis, repetitive wrist motions, or static loading of the wrist.

Symptoms are night pain that is severe enough to waken the patient; tingling in the thumb and index and middle fingers; and, if advanced, wasting of the thenar

TABLE 44-5
Functional Grading of Cumulative Trauma Disorders

Grade I	Pain after activity; resolves quickly with rest No decrease in amount or speed of work Objective findings usually absent.
Grade II	Pain in one site while working Pain is consistent while working, but resolves when activity stops Productivity may be mildly affected May have objective findings
Grade III	Pain in one or more sites while working Pain persists after activity is stopped Productivity affected and multiple breaks may be necessary to continue working May affect other activities away from work May have weakness, loss of control and dexterity, tingling, numbness, and other objective findings May have latent or active trigger points
Grade IV	All common uses of hand/upper extremity cause pain, which is present 50% to 75% of the time May be unable to work or works in limited capacity May have weakness, loss of control and dexterity, tingling, numbness, trigger points, and other objective findings
Grade V	Loss of capacity to use upper extremities because of chronic, unrelenting pain Usually unable to work Symptoms may persist indefinitely.

From Kasch MC: Therapist's evaluation and treatment of upper extremity trauma disorders. In Hunter JM et al, editors: *Rehabilitation of the hand*, ed 4, St Louis, 1995, Mosby.

musculature caused by pressure on the motor branch of the nerve. Early carpal tunnel syndrome may be recognized during a thorough nerve evaluation.

Conservative treatment is usually attempted first and includes splinting of the wrist in no more than 20° extension, contrast baths to reduce edema, wearing of Isotoner gloves, and activity analysis. A semiflexible or neoprene splint rather than a completely rigid splint may be used to provide support while allowing a small amount of flexion and extension for greater functional use in carpal tunnel syndrome.

Ultrasound phonophoresis and iontophoresis may be used to reduce inflammation, and icing techniques are beneficial. Specific strengthening exercises of the wrist, fingers, and thumb should be given when the pain and inflammation have been controlled.

In 1988, 35,000 carpal tunnel releases were performed in the United States. In 1993, this number climbed to over 250,000 releases.[53] Most patients report a relief of numbness, but many have persistent pain. Therapy is often provided after surgical release and may include a combination of ultrasound to the scar, massage, manual edema mobilization, desensitization, dexterity activities, and strengthening.

Myofascial pain and fibrositis are also conditions of pain elicited by activation of trigger points within the muscles and resulting in pain referred to a distal area; these are frequently encountered conditions. Travell[98] has studied myofascial pain and mapped out the traditional trigger points and their referral patterns. Poor posture and positioning of the body out of normal alignment are often the mechanisms of injury in myofascial pain, so careful examination of the patient and his or her normal daily activities is indicated. The therapist should observe the patient performing the activity rather than rely on a verbal description.

Myofascial pain should be considered if direct treatment of the painful area does not relieve the pain. Evaluation for trigger points must be done meticulously, and mapping of the trigger points and the referral areas must be documented. Because the pain is referred, the trigger point must be treated, not the referral area. The treatments used for other inflammatory problems, such as ice and ultrasound phonophoresis, can be used. In addition, there are specific treatments for the trigger points, such as friction massage and TENS, that may relieve the pain. Activity analysis is an essential part of treatment to relieve the stresses on the affected tissues.

Strengthening Activities

Acute care is followed by a gradual return of motion, sensibility, and preparation to return to normal ADL.

The patient usually cannot strengthen the injured and neglected extremity at home because of the fear of further injury and pain. Because every hand clinic has its own armamentarium of strengthening exercises and media, only a few suggestions are provided here.

Computerized Evaluation and Exercise Equipment

Baltimore Therapeutic Equipment (BTE) has made available the BTE Work Simulator (Fig. 44-18),[26] an electromechanical device that has more than 20 interchangeable tool handles and can be used for both work evaluation and UE strengthening. Resistance can vary from no resistance to complete static resistance, with tool height and angle also adjustable. When the device is used for strengthening, the resistance is usually set low and gradually increased. Length of exercise is increased when a base level of strength has been achieved. The BTE Work Simulator allows for close simulation of real-world tasks that are easily translatable into physical demands common to manual work.

Other computerized evaluation equipment allows the therapist to record the results of assessment and print a report. Percentage of impairment can also be determined electronically. Portable systems are being developed that allow the therapist to record daily treatment and download the information into a computer-

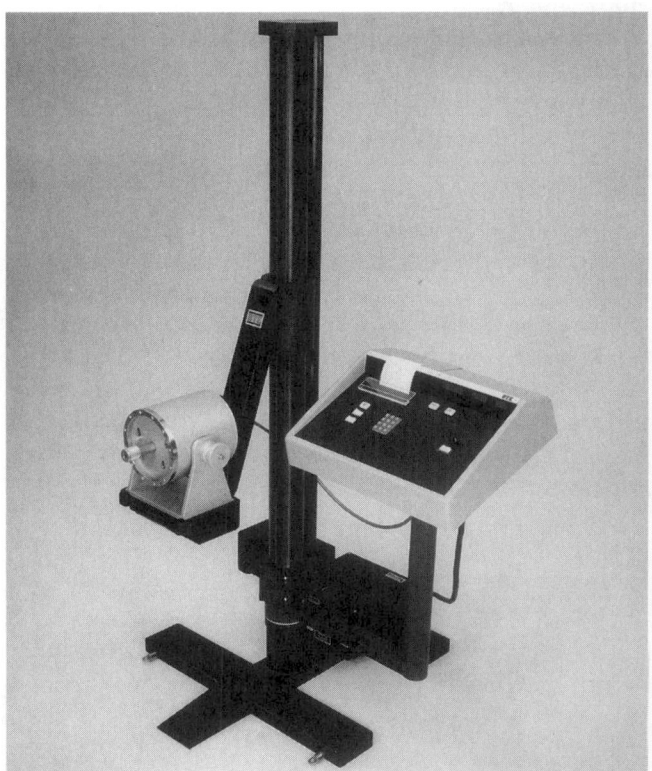

FIG. 44-18

BTE Work Simulator is electromechanical device used to simulate real-life tasks for upper extremity evaluation and strengthening. Patient's progress is monitored through computerized print-out, and program can be modified to increase resistance and endurance.

ized network. Outcome data from many sources can then be compared. The advancement of technology in rehabilitation will allow the therapist to be more efficient and also capture important information that is not available through traditional means.

Weight Well
The Weight Well[7] was developed at the Downey Community Hospital Hand Center in Downey, California, and is available commercially.* Rods with a variety of handle shapes are placed through holes in the box and have weights suspended. The rods are turned against resistance throughout the ROM to encourage full grasp and release of the injured hand, wrist flexion and extension, pinch, and pronation and supination patterns. The Weight Well can be graded for resistance and repetitions and is an excellent tool for progressive resistive exercise.

Theraband
Theraband† is a 6-inch (15.2-cm) wide rubber sheet that is available by the yard and is color coded by degrees of resistance. It can be cut into any length required and used for resistive exercise for the UE. Use of Theraband is limited only by the therapist's imagination, and it can be adapted to diagonal patterns of motion, wrist exercises, follow-up treatment of tennis elbow, and other uses. The Theraband can be combined with dowel rods and other equipment to provide resistance throughout the ROM. It is inexpensive and easy to incorporate into a home treatment program.

Hand-Strengthening Equipment
Hand grips of graded resistance are available from rehabilitation supply companies and sporting goods stores. They can be purchased with various resistance levels and can be used for progressive resistive hand exercises.

The therapist is cautioned against using overly resistive spring-loaded grippers often sold in sporting goods stores. These devices may be beneficial to the seasoned athlete but are usually too resistive for the recently injured.

Therapy putty can be purchased in bulk, and the amount given to the patient is geared to hand size and strength. Putty is also available in grades of resistance, and some provide chips that can be added to progressively increase resistance. It can be adapted to most finger motions and is easily incorporated into a home program.

Household items such as spring-type clothespins have been used to increase strength of grasp and pinch.

*Upper Extremity Technology Weight Well (available from Upper Extremity Technology, Glenwood Springs, Colo).
†Theraband (available from Smith & Nephew, Germantown, Wis).

Imaginative use of common objects should present a challenge to the hand therapist.

Functional Activities
Functional activities are an integral part of rehabilitation of the hand. Functional activities may include crafts, games, dexterity activities, ADL, and work samples. Many of the treatment techniques described previously are used to condition the hand for normal use.

Activities should be started as soon as possible at whatever level the patient can perform them with adaptations to compensate for limited ROM and strength. They should be used in conjunction with other treatments. The occupational therapist must continually assess the patient's functional capacities and initiate changes in the treatment program to incorporate activities as soon as possible in the restorative phase.

Vocational and leisure goals should be established at the time of initial evaluation and taken into account when planning treatment. The needs of a brick mason may be quite different from those of a mother with small children, and the environmental needs of the patient must not be neglected.

Crafts should be graded from light resistance to heavy resistance and from gross dexterity to fine dexterity. Crafts that have been found to work extremely well with hand injuries include macramé, Turkish knot weaving, clay, leather, and woodworking. All of these crafts can be adapted and graded to the patient's capabilities and have been found to have a high level of patient acceptance. When integrated into a program of total hand rehabilitation, they are viewed as another milestone of achievement and not as a diversion to fill up empty hours. For example, the pride of accomplishment for a patient who sustained a Volkmann's contracture caused by ischemia and who completed her first project in nearly 4 years is evidence that crafts belong in hand rehabilitation.

Activities that do not have an end product but provide practice in dexterity and ADL skills also fit into the category of functional activities. Developmental games and activities that require pinch or grasp and release may be graded and timed to increase difficulty. ADL boards that have a variety of opening and closing devices provide practice for use of the hand at home and increase self-confidence. String and finger games are challenging coordination activities that can be done in pairs and are fun to do.

Many times a hobby can be adapted for use in the clinic. Fly-tying is a difficult dexterity activity but one that will be enjoyed by an avid fisherman. Golf clubs and fishing poles can be adapted in the clinic to allow early return to a favorite form of relaxation.

Humor and interaction with the therapists and the other patients are vital but intangible benefits of treatment. Treatment should be planned to promote both.

FUNCTIONAL CAPACITY EVALUATION

The ultimate goal of therapy for an injured worker is to return to full employment. Many weeks or months may have elapsed between the time of the injury and the point at which the physician feels a return to work is appropriate from a medical standpoint. Despite the fact that x-ray examinations may show full healing and restored ROM, many patients do not feel they have the strength, dexterity, or endurance to return to their former jobs. Pain may continue to be a limiting factor, especially with heavy activities. Light duty or part-time positions may not be available, and the physician, therapist, industrial insurance carrier, and most of all the patient are frustrated by the lack of an objective method of evaluating an individual's physical capacity for work. Occupational therapists with training in evaluation, kinesiology, and adaptation of environmental factors coupled with a functional approach to the patient may play a key role in **functional capacity evaluation**.

A renewed interest in evaluation of prevocational factors has brought the profession of OT full circle (see Chapter 16). Although one of the cornerstones of the profession in its early years, prevocational evaluation has been neglected in many centers during the last two decades. Since the early 1980s, however, occupational therapists have rediscovered a need that the profession is in a unique position to provide. The term "prevocational evaluation" ambiguously implied that occupational therapists were involved in assessing the vocational needs of patients they treated. The terms functional capacity evaluation (FCE) and work tolerance screening (WTS), however, more clearly describe the process of measuring an individual's ability to perform the physical demands of work.

The results of the functional capacity evaluation allow the therapist, worker, physician, and vocational counselor to establish a specific, attainable employment goal using reliable data. This approach relieves the physician of the responsibility of returning the patient to work without objective information about the patient's ability to do a job. It also allows the patient to test his or her own abilities and may result in increased self-confidence about returning to work.

Many techniques for performing a functional capacity evaluation have been proposed.[8,43,68,69,90] Some basic steps may be followed regardless of the specific technique adopted. The patient should be evaluated for grip and pinch strength, sensation, and ROM. Edema and pain must also be assessed and reassessed during the course of the evaluation.

The GULHEMP (general physique, UE, lower extremity, hearing, eyesight, mentality, and personality) Work Capacity Evaluation Worksheet[68] may be used as a general method of determining functional abilities. The GULHEMP Physical Development Analysis Worksheet[68] may be used to evaluate the job.

Job analysis may also be provided by a rehabilitation counselor, and through information provided by the patient. The therapist should consult the *Dictionary of Occupational Titles* (DOT)[99] to obtain information about the worker traits required for the expected job. This dictionary contains 12,900 job descriptions and 20,000 job titles. If sufficient information about the job is not available through these methods, an on-site job analysis by the therapist may be necessary. Once the physical demand characteristics of work have been documented, it is possible to evaluate the patient's ability to perform them.

Schultz-Johnson[90] described a functional capacity evaluation adapted for UE injuries based on the physical demands established by the U.S. Department of Labor. After evaluation, the therapist may recommend a work therapy program.[90] Work therapy can include simulated job tasks to increase job performance.

Matheson[63,69] has written several manuals and articles that describe work capacity evaluation (WCE). This 8- to 10-day work assessment includes evaluation of the patient's feasibility for employment (worker characteristics, such as safety and dependability), employability, work tolerances (such as strength, endurance, and the effect of pain on work performance), the physical demand characteristics of the job, and the worker's ability to "dependably sustain performance in response to broadly defined work demands."[69]

Tests with well-accepted reliability, such as the Purdue Pegboard Test,[97] the Crawford Small Parts Dexterity Test,[24] the Minnesota Manual Dexterity Test,[75] and the Jebsen Hand Dexterity Test,[46] may be administered as a screening process. These tests will give the therapist valuable information through observation, whether the normal tables are used or the test is adapted to an individual worker.

Many assessments and job simulation devices are available and should be reviewed before a physical capacity evaluation program is established. To choose appropriate work samples the therapist should determine the job market in a specific area. This can be done by consulting with vocational schools, rehabilitation counselors, and employment agencies in the area.

Work samples, available through Jewish Employment and Vocational Service,[100] Singer,* VALPAR,† and Work Evaluation Systems Technology (WEST),‡ may be used to test specific skills. The therapist may also develop job samples by using information on jobs in the local area. Discarded electronic assembly boards, a lawn mower motor, an automobile engine, or other items from the local hardware store may provide valuable information about the worker's ability.

---

*Singer Education Division, Career Systems, Rochester, NY.
†VALPAR Assessment Systems (available from VALPAR International, Tuscon, Ariz).
‡Work Evaluation Systems Technology, Fort Bragg, Calif.

Work simulation using job samples or the BTE Work Simulator assesses the worker's specific physical capacities, as well as endurance and symptoms that become cumulative with prolonged use of the injured part (called symptom response to activity, or SRA). Monitoring the client's SRA may prevent loss of time and money expended in training for an inappropriate vocational goal. King[55] has written about the analysis of test results to determine the consistency of effort and veracity of evaluation findings, which assists in identifying patients who may be magnifying their symptoms.

A combination of "normed" tests, job samples, job simulation, and work capacity evaluation devices may provide the therapist with the best information about a worker's physical capacity. For more information about vocational evaluation and rehabilitation, the therapist should write to the Materials Development Center at the University of Wisconsin-Stout in Menomonie, Wisconsin.*

Work Hardening

Work hardening is the progressive use of simulated work samples to increase endurance, strength, productivity, and often feasibility. Work hardening may be performed for a period of weeks, and the progressive ongoing nature of the work usually results in improvements in physical capacity. It is an important contribution to return to work.

Because FCE is also performed over time, it may be difficult to identify the difference between FCE and work hardening. An FCE is generally done when the patient has stopped improving with traditional therapy methods and may have been released from acute medical care. The patient may be unable to return to his or her former employment, or it may be questionable if the patient would be able to do the former work. An FCE may be initiated by a physician, rehabilitation counselor, insurance adjustor, or attorney.

Work hardening or work conditioning may be initiated earlier in the rehabilitation process, perhaps by the treating physician or therapist who recognizes that an individual may have difficulty returning to the former employment. It is performed before the end of medical care and may serve as a final checkout before discontinuing treatment.

Standards for work hardening services have been developed by the Commission on Accreditation of Rehabilitation Facilities (CARF)[23] to ensure that injured workers are offered high-quality programs that are maximally effective in returning them to gainful employment. The Employment and Rehabilitation Institute of California (ERIC)[34] has many publications and re-

sources available to therapists interested in establishing work capacity evaluation, work tolerance screening, or work hardening services. A publications and equipment list is available on request.

FCE and work hardening are adjuncts to the vocational rehabilitation process. Occupational therapists are trained to observe behavior and have the skills necessary to translate that observation into useful data. FCE and work hardening should not be a process that is in competition with the work of rehabilitation or vocational counselors, but rather one that provides critical information about a worker's physical functioning and may serve as a program to foster reentry into the job market.

CONSULTATION WITH INDUSTRY

Occupational therapists may be asked to visit the job site to make recommendations for ergonomic adaptations, including tool modification, ergonomic furniture and accessories, and training of workers in proper positioning to reduce the incidence of CTDs. Prevention substantially reduces the costs to industry, which presents occupational therapists with a unique opportunity to apply their training in activity analysis and adaptation of the environment in a new setting. The Americans with Disabilities Act (ADA) mandates reasonable accommodations for workers with disabilities (see Chapter 17). Many occupational therapists have become active in helping companies comply with the requirements of the ADA. The American Occupational Therapy Association is an excellent resource for information about how therapists can be involved in these efforts in their communities.[3]

This chapter provides an overview of treatment of the UE. Evaluation procedures are discussed, as well as the basic treatment techniques. Management of both acute injuries and cumulative trauma is included, as well as information on strengthening and programs for industrial injuries. References for additional study are provided.

Most occupational therapists should be familiar with the basic treatment approaches because they work with patients who have some limitation in the UEs. Specialization in hand therapy requires both academic study and clinical experience. Therapists who have specialized in this area of practice and who meet minimum requirements may choose to take the Hand Therapy Certification Examination and become a Certified Hand Therapist (CHT). Both levels of expertise are needed in the profession. For more information on becoming a CHT, contact the Hand Therapy Certification Commission.[42]

*Materials Development Center, Stout Vocational Rehabilitation Institute, University of Wisconsin-Stout, Menomonie, Wis.

CASE STUDY 44-1

CASE STUDY—MS. L.

Ms. L. is a 42-year-old, right-handed administrative manager for an insurance company. She has had numbness and pain in both hands for about 2 years. She first consulted a physician about a year ago. Nerve conduction studies were positive for carpal tunnel syndrome in both hands, right greater than left. She had a right carpal tunnel release, open technique, 2 months ago and a left carpal tunnel release 10 days ago. She had therapy following the first surgery until the second hand was operated on. She has been referred for postoperative management of the left hand.

Ms. L. is divorced and lives alone. Her interests are gardening, needlework, and reading. She has had difficulty using the right hand since surgery, since she still had residual weakness from the first surgery. She has been sitting at home watching television since the most recent surgery and has not moved her arm. She expressed fear that she will not be able to return to work because she uses a computer for about six hours a day. She is having difficulty cooking for herself, and she has not been able to garden for two months. She stated that she cries frequently.

It was observed that Ms. L. was holding the left arm close to her body and not initiating movement with the arm. There were limitations in active range of motion of the left shoulder and wrist. Ms. L. was able to make a full fist, but she stated that her fingers felt stiff and sore. Volume measurements revealed that the left hand was 15% larger than before surgery, indicating significant swelling. She reported that her numbness was nearly gone, although she had occasional shooting pain to the tip of the middle finger. The scar was sensitive to touch, and she had difficulty wearing long-sleeved blouses.

OT was initiated to increase wrist and shoulder range of motion, reduce edema, decrease pain and hypersensitivity, soften the scar, and improve her tolerance for use of the hand. The OT program included active range of motion of the shoulder and wrist, tendon gliding exercises, edema reduction techniques, desensitization techniques, scar massage, and kinetic activities to improve strength and endurance.

Ms. L. responded well to treatment. As the swelling decreased, her hand and wrist felt less stiff. After doing pendulum and pulley exercises for two weeks she was able to reach to the cereal shelf in her kitchen without difficulty. She worked on simulated activities on the BTE Work Simulator, and once she was able to "open a jar" on the BTE, she was able to do it at home. As her strength reached a functional level, she was able to build endurance. She began to spend 30 minutes of each therapy session working on a computer. Her employer asked the therapist to perform an ergonomic assessment of her workstation before she returned to work. It was decided to provide her with an ergonomic keyboard and wrist rest with an adjustable keyboard tray. She was given a trackball to use instead of a mouse. The employer was investigating use of voice activation software for some of her work tasks so she would not have to type the entire day. She returned to work four hours a day six weeks after surgery. She continued in therapy for conditioning. Within a month she had resumed full-time work, and therapy was discontinued.

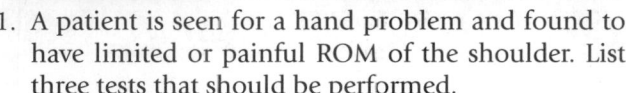

REVIEW QUESTIONS

1. A patient is seen for a hand problem and found to have limited or painful ROM of the shoulder. List three tests that should be performed.
2. Discuss three approaches to postoperative care of flexor tendon injuries, and compare how the differences between the methods would influence the initiation of OT.
3. To what does *joint dysfunction* refer? What are its causes?
4. Discuss the three classifications of nerve injury.
5. Define the area referred to as "no-man's land." What distinguishes injury to this area?
6. What techniques are used to evaluate the physical demand characteristics of work?
7. List three methods of applying pressure to a hypertrophic scar.
8. Which functional activities could be used for restoration of hand function following laceration and repair of the extrinsic finger flexors?
9. Which assessments should be included in a functional capacity evaluation?
10. List five tests used to assess joint integrity in the hand.
11. List three objectives of splinting as they relate to injury of the radial, median, and ulnar nerves.
12. What are the characteristics of complex regional pain syndrome, type I? What are the treatment goals?
13. Define "work hardening." How can work hardening be incorporated into OT?
14. How is the presence of edema evaluated? List three methods used to reduce edema.
15. What are the primary work-related risk factors associated with cumulative trauma? How can the occupational therapist intervene to prevent the development of cumulative trauma?

REFERENCES

1. Adson A, Coffey J: Cervical rib—a method of anterior approach for relief of symptoms by division of scalenus anticus, *Ann Surg* 85:834, 1927.
2. Alon G: *High voltage stimulation*, Chattanooga, Tenn, 1984, Chattanooga.

3. American Occupational Therapy Association, ADA Network, Practice Division, Bethesda, Md.

4. American Society for Surgery of the Hand: *The hand examination and diagnosis*, ed 3, New York, 1990, Churchill Livingstone.

5. Armstrong TJ: Cumulative trauma disorders of the upper limb and identification of work-related factors. In Millender LH, Louis DS, Simmons BP, editors: *Occupational disorders of the upper extremity*, New York, 1992, Churchill Livingstone.

6. Atrzberger S: *Manual edema mobilization.* Presented at the annual meeting of the American Society of Hand Therapists, Orlando, Fla, 1991.

7. Barber LM: Occupational therapy for the treatment of reflex sympathetic dystrophy and post-traumatic hypersensitivity of the injured hand. In Fredericks S, Brody G, editors: *Symposium on the neurologic aspects of plastic surgery*, St Louis, 1978, Mosby.

8. Baxter-Petralia P, Bruening L, Blackmore S: The work tolerance program of the Hand Rehabilitation Center in Philadelphia. In Hunter JM et al, editors: *Rehabilitation of the hand*, ed 3, St Louis, 1990, Mosby.

9. Bell-Krotoski J: Plaster cylinder casting for contractures of the interphalangeal joints. In Hunter JM et al, editors: *Rehabilitation of the hand*, ed 4, St Louis, 1995, Mosby.

10. Bell-Krotoski J: Sensibility testing: current concepts. In Hunter JM et al, editors: *Rehabilitation of the hand*, ed 4, St Louis, 1995, Mosby.

11. Bennett G: *Hand-tool dexterity test*, New York, 1981, Harcourt, Brace, Jovanovich.

12. Benton LA et al: *Functional electrical stimulation: a practical clinical guide*, ed 2, Downey, Calif, 1981, Rancho Los Amigos Hospital.

13. Boyes JH: *Bunnell's surgery of the hand*, ed 5, Philadelphia, 1970, JB Lippincott.

14. Boyes JH, Stark HH: Flexor-tendon grafts in the fingers and thumb, *J Bone Joint Surg Am* 53(7):1332-1342, 1971.

15. Brand PW, Hollister A: *Clinical mechanics of the hand*, ed 3, St Louis, 1999, Mosby.

16. Butler D: *Mobilisation of the nervous system*, New York, 1991, Churchill Livingstone.

17. Byl N, Melnick M: The neural consequences of repetition: clinical implications of a learning hypothesis, *J Hand Ther* 10(2):160-174, 1997.

18. Callahan A: Sensory assessment: prerequisites and techniques for nerve lesions in continuity and nerve lacerations. In Hunter JM et al, editors: *Rehabilitation of the hand*, ed 4, St Louis, 1995, Mosby.

19. Cannon N et al: Control of immediate postoperative pain following tenolysis and capsulectomies of the hand with TENS, *J Hand Surg Am* 8:625, 1983.

20. Carroll D: A quantitative test of upper extremity function, *J Chronic Dis* 18:479, 1965.

21. Chai S et al: A role delineation study of hand therapy, *J Hand Ther* 1:7, 1987.

22. Chusid J: *Correlative neuroanatomy and functional neurology*, ed 19, Los Altos, Calif, 1985, Lange Medical Publications.

23. Commission on Accreditation of Rehabilitation Facilities (CARF), Tuscon, Ariz.

24. Crawford J, Crawford D: *Crawford small parts dexterity test manual*, New York, 1981, Harcourt, Brace, Jovanovich.

25. Creelman G: Volumeters Unlimited, Idyllwild, Calif.

26. Curtis RM, Engalitcheff J: A work simulator for rehabilitating the upper extremity: preliminary report, *J Hand Surg* 6(5):499-501, 1981.

27. Cyriax J: Clinical applications of massage. In Basmajian JV, editor: *Manipulation, traction and massage*, ed 3, Balimore, 1985, Williams & Wilkins.

28. Dellon AL: Clinical use of vibratory stimuli to evaluate peripheral nerve injury and compression neuropathy, *Plast Reconstr Surg* 65(4):466-476, 1980.

29. Dellon AL: *Evaluation of sensibility and reeducation of sensation in the hand*, Baltimore, 1981, Williams & Wilkins.

30. Dellon AL: The vibrometer, *Plast Reconstr Surg* 71(3):427-431, 1983.

31. Dellon AL, Curtis RM, Edgerton MT: Reeducation of sensation in the hand after nerve injury and repair, *Plast Reconstr Surg* 53(3):297-305, 1974.

32. Donatelli R, Owens-Burkhart H: Effects of immobilization on the extensibility of periarticular connective tissue, *J Orthop Sports Phys Ther* 3:67, 1981.

33. Duran R et al: Management of flexor tendon lacerations in zone 2 using controlled passive motion postoperatively. In Hunter JM et al, editors: *Rehabilitation of the hand*, ed 3, St Louis, 1990, Mosby.

34. Employment and Rehabilitation Institute of California (ERIC), Anaheim, Calif.

35. English CB, Rehm RA, Petzoldt RL: Blocking splints to assist finger exercise, *Am J Occup Ther* 36(4):259-264, 1982.

36. Evans RB: Therapeutic management of extensor tendon injuries, *Hand Clinics* 2(1):157-169, 1986.

37. Evans RB, Burkhalter WE: A study of the dynamic anatomy of extensor tendons and implications for treatment, *J Hand Surg* 11(5):774-779.

38. Evans RB, McAuliffe J: Wound classification and management. In Hunter JM et al, editors: *Rehabilitation of the hand*, ed 4, St Louis, 1995, Mosby.

39. Fess E, Moran C: *Clinical assessment recommendations*, Indianapolis, 1981, American Society of Hand Therapists.

40. Gelberman RH et al: The carpal tunnel syndrome, *J Bone Joint Surg* 63(3):380-383, 1981.

41. Gelberman RH et al: Sensibility testing in peripheral-nerve compression syndromes, *J Bone Joint Surg* 65(5):632-638, 1983.

42. Hand Therapy Certification Commission, Kansas City, Mo.

43. Harrand G: *The Harrand guide for developing physical capacity evaluations*, Menomonie, Wis, 1982, Stout Vocational Rehabilitation Institute.

44. Hawkins R, Kennedy J: Impingement syndrome in athletes, *Am J Sports Med* 8(3):151-158, 1980.

45. Hunter JM et al: Staged flexor tendon reconstruction using passive and active tendon implants. In Hunter JM et al, editors: *Rehabilitation of the hand*, ed 4, St Louis, 1995, Mosby.

46. Jebsen RH et al: An objective and standardized test of hand function, *Arch Phys Med Rehabil* 50(6):311-319, 1969.

47. Jobst Institute, Toledo, Ohio.

48. Kamenetz H: Mechanical devices of massage. In Basmajian JV, editor: *Manipulation, traction and massage*, ed 3, Baltimore, 1985, Williams & Wilkins.

49. Kasch MC: Clinical management of scar tissue, *OT in Health Care* 4:37, 1987.

50. Kasch MC: Therapist's evaluation and treatment of upper extremity cumulative trauma disorders. In Hunter JM et al, editors, *Rehabilitation of the hand*, ed 4, St Louis, 1995, Mosby.

51. Kasch MC, Hester L: Low-frequency TENS and the release of endorphins, *J Hand Surg* 8:626, 1983.

52. Kellor M et al: *Technical manual of hand strength and dexterity test*, Minneapolis, 1971, Sister Kenney Rehabilitation Institute.

53. Kelsey JL et al: *Upper extremity disorders: frequency, impact and cost*, New York, 1997, Churchill Livingstone.

54. Kessler RM, Hertling D: Joint mobilization techniques. In Kessler RM, Hertling D, editors: *Management of common musculoskeletal disorders*, New York, 1983, Harper & Row.

55. King JW, Berryhill BH: A comparison of two static grip testing methods and its clinical applications: a preliminary study, *J Hand Ther* 1:204, 1988.

56. Kutz JE: Controlled mobilization of acute flexor tendon injuries: Louisville technique. In Hunter JM, Schneider LH, Mackin EJ, editors: *Tendon surgery in the hand*, St Louis, 1987, Mosby.

57. Lankford LL: Reflex sympathetic dystrophy. In Hunter JM et al, editors: *Rehabilitation of the hand*, ed 3, St Louis, 1990, Mosby.

58. LaSalle WB, Strickland JW: An evaluation of the two-stage flexor tendon reconstruction technique, *J Hand Surg* 8:263, 1983.

59. Lister GL: *The hand: diagnosis and indications*, ed 3, New York, 1993, Churchill Livingstone.

60. Louis DS et al: Evaluation of normal values for stationary and moving two-point discrimination in the hand, *J Hand Surg* 9(4):552-555.

61. Lublin JS: Unions and firms focus on hand disorder that can be caused by repetitive tasks, *The Wall Street Journal*, January 14, 1983.

62. Lundborg G et al: Digital vibrogram: a new diagnostic tool for sensory testing in compression neuropathy, *J Hand Surg* 11(5):693-699, 1986.

63. Mackinnon SE, Dellon AL: Two-point discrimination tester, *J Hand Surg* 19(6 pt 1):906-907, 1985.

64. Madden JW: Wound healing: the biological basis of hand surgery. In Hunter JM et al, editors: *Rehabilitation of the hand*, ed 3, St Louis, 1990, Mosby.

65. Magee DJ: *Orthopedic physical assessment*, ed 3, Philadelphia, 1997, WB Saunders.

66. Maitland G: *Peripheral manipulation*, Boston, 1977, Butterworth.

67. Malick MH, Carr JA: Flexible elastomer molds in burn scar control, *Am J Occup Ther* 34(9):603-608, 1980.

68. Matheson LN: *Work capacity evaluation: a training manual for occupational therapists*, Trabuco Canyon, Calif, 1982, Rehabilitation Institute of Southern California.

69. Matheson LN, Ogden LD: *Work tolerance screening*, Trabuco Canyon, Calif, 1983, Rehabilitation Institute of Southern California.

70. Mathiowetz V et al: Grip and pinch strength: normative data for adults, *Arch Phys Med Rehabil* 66(2):69-74, 1985.

71. Mathiowetz V et al: Reliability and validity of grip and pinch strength evaluations, *J Hand Surg* 9(2):222-226, 1984.

72. Melvin J: *Rheumatic disease occupational therapy and rehabilitation*, ed 3, Philadelphia, 1989, FA Davis.

73. Mennell JM: *Joint pain*, Boston, 1964, Little, Brown.

74. Mennell JM, Zohn DA: *Musculoskeletal pain: diagnosis and physical treatment*, Boston, 1976, Little, Brown.

75. Lafayette Instrument: *Minnesota manual dexterity test*, Lafayette, Ind.

76. Moberg E: Objective methods of determining functional value of sensibility in the hand, *J Bone Joint Surg* 40A:454, 1958.

77. Mullins P: Use of therapeutic modalities in upper extremity rehabilitation. In Hunter JM et al, editors: *Rehabilitation of the hand*, ed 4, St Louis, 1995, Mosby.

78. Neer C, Welch R: The shoulder in sports, *Orthop Clin North Am* 8(3):583-591, 1977.

79. Omer G: Management of pain syndromes in the upper extremity. In Hunter JM et al, editors: *Rehabilitation of the hand*, ed 3, St Louis, 1990, Mosby.

80. Nerve response to injury and repair. In Hunter JM et al, editors: *Rehabilitation of the hand*, ed 3, St Louis, 1990, Mosby.

81. O'Riain S: New and simple test of nerve function in the hand, *Br Med J* 3(881):615-616, 1973.

82. Parry C: *Rehabilitation of the hand*, ed 4, London, 1984, Butterworth.

83. Peacock EE, Madden JW, Trier WC: Postoperative recovery of flexor tendon function, *Am J Surg* 122(5):686-692, 1971.

84. Post M: *Physical examination of the musculoskeletal system*, Chicago, 1987, Book Medical Publisher.

85. Rempel DM: Work-related cumulative trauma disorders of the upper extremity, *JAMA* 267(6):838-842, 1992.

86. Roos D: Congenital anomalies associated with thoracic outlet syndrome, *Am J Surg* 132(6):771-778, 1976.

87. Roth L et al: Practice analysis of hand therapy, *J Hand Ther* 9:202, 1996.

88. Schneider LH: Tendon transfers in the upper extremity. In Hunter JM et al, editors: *Rehabilitation of the hand*, ed 3, St Louis, 1990, Mosby.

89. Schneider L, Hunter J: Flexor tenolysis. In Hunter JM et al, editors: *AAOS: symposium on tendon surgery in the hand*, St Louis, 1975, Mosby.

90. Schultz-Johnson K: Upper extremity functional capacity evaluation. In Hunter JM et al, editors: *Rehabilitation of the hand*, ed 4, St Louis, 1995, Mosby.

91. Silverstein S: Preventive medicine standards on cumulative trauma would cover every employee in the state, *LA Times* January 13, 1994.

92. Strickland JW: biologic rationale, clinical application, and results of early motion following flexor tendon repair, *J Hand Ther* 2:71, 1989.

93. Strickland JW, Glogovac SV: Digital function following flexor tendon repair in zone II: a comparison of immobilization and controlled passive motion techniques, *J Hand Surg* 5(6):537-543, 1980.

94. Szabo R et al: Vibratory sensory testing in acute peripheral nerve compression, *J Hand Surg* 9A(1):104-109, 1984.

95. Tetro A et al: A new provocative test for carpal tunnel syndrome: assessment of wrist flexion and nerve compression, *J Bone Joint Surg Br* 80(3):493-498, 1998.

96. Thomas CL, editor: *Taber's cyclopedic medical dictionary*, ed 14, Philadelphia, 1981, FA Davis.

97. Tiffin J: *Purdue pegboard examiner manual*, Chicago, 1968, Science Research Associates.

98. Travell JG, Simons DG: *Myofascial pain and dysfunction: the trigger point manual*, Baltimore, 1983, Williams & Wilkins.

99. US Department of Labor Employment and Training Administration: *Dictionary of occupational titles*, ed 4, Washington, DC, 1991, US Government Printing Office.

100. Vocational Research Institute, Jewish Employment and Vocational Service, Philadelphia.

101. Watson HK, Carlson L: Treatment of reflex sympathetic dystrophy of the hand with an active "stress loading" program, *J Hand Surg* 12(5 pt 1):779-785, 1987.

102. Waylett-Rendall J: Sensibility evaluation and rehabilitation, *Orthop Clin North Am* 19(1):43-56, 1988.

103. Waylett-Rendall J, Seibly D: A study of the accuracy of a commercially available volumeter, *J Hand Ther* 4:10, 1991.

104. Wehbe MA: Tendon gliding exercises, *Am J Occup Ther* 41(3):164-167, 1987.

105. Wehbe MA, Hunter JM: Flexor tendon gliding in the hand. II. Differential gliding, *J Hand Surg* 10(4):575-579, 1985.

106. Wilson RE, Carter MS: Management of joint injuries and intraarticular fractures of the hand. In Hunter JM et al, editors: *Rehabilitation of the hand*, ed 4, St Louis, 1995, Mosby.

107. Wolf SL: *Electrotherapy*, New York, 1981, Churchill Livingstone.

108. Wong G et al: Classification of complex regional pain syndromes, *Hand Clin* 13, 1997.

109. Yerxa EJ et al: Development of a hand sensitivity test for the hypersensitive hand, *Am J Occup Ther* 37(3):176-181, 1983.

CHAPTER 45

Hip Fractures and Lower Extremity Joint Replacement

SONIA COLEMAN

KEY TERMS

Spica cast
Osteoporosis
Open reduction and internal fixation
Weight-bearing restrictions
Arthroplasty
Anterolateral approach
Posterolateral approach
Hip precautions
Knee immobilizer
Critical pathway
Leg lifter
Abduction wedge

LEARNING OBJECTIVES

After studying this chapter the student or practitioner will be able to do the following:
1. Describe the etiology of hip fractures and joint replacements.
2. Describe the medical management for these conditions.
3. Identify occupational therapy treatment goals.
4. Identify the medical precautions associated with hip fractures and joint replacements.
5. Identify and discuss areas of intervention for occupational therapy.
6. Discuss appropriate treatment techniques to address daily occupations and functional mobility.
7. Discuss the impact of hip fractures and joint replacement on occupational performance.

Hip fractures and lower extremity (LE) joint replacements are two orthopedic conditions occurring with more frequency now than in years past. This is in part a result of extended life spans. Older individuals are more likely to have orthopedic problems such as osteoporosis and degenerative joint changes. Medical advances have also made the treatment of hip fractures and LE joint problems safer and easier to manage. LE joint problems can lead to temporary or more long-lasting disability. In both hip and knee conditions a large weight-bearing joint is unstable for a period of time, which limits an individual's mobility and ability to complete meaningful daily occupations.

The elderly population is most at risk for hip fractures. Reduced mobility and the presence of osteoporosis are two specific risk factors. Elderly women, in partic-

ular, develop osteoporosis to a greater degree than men and thus tend to have more hip fractures when they fall.

Mobility is compromised in the elderly population because of decreased flexibility, diminished strength, reduced vision, slowed reaction time, and the use of assistive ambulatory aids such as canes and walkers. Many elderly people become more cautious when moving about and are fearful of falling. In some cases individuals trip over a cane or walker, which causes a fall. Not seeing a step or threshold is also a common cause for falling.

Individuals with a history of arthritis or other joint disease are the primary candidates for LE joint replacement. Individuals who elect to have this surgical procedure performed usually have been living with increasing pain in their joints for many months or years and are already limited in their ability to perform daily tasks. They hope, by having the painful joint replaced, to return to a more active lifestyle that is more satisfying to them.

Occupational therapy (OT) plays a key role in identifying and remediating the many functional problems imposed by these acute and chronic orthopedic conditions, thus sharing in the goal of returning the orthopedic patient to optimal performance of safe, independent, and meaningful occupations.

This chapter discusses hip fractures and LE joint replacements, their medical and surgical management, the psychological implications of hospitalization and disability, and the health care team approach in acute hospital and rehabilitation settings.

GENERAL MEDICAL MANAGEMENT OF FRACTURES

It is important for the occupational therapist working with orthopedic patients to have a good understanding of the site, type, and cause of the fracture before starting treatment. A basic understanding of fracture healing and medical management is also necessary to appreciate risks, precautions, and complications involved. The occupational therapist is advised to consult an orthopedic manual for specific information regarding the fracture healing process.

In general, a fracture occurs when the bone's ability to absorb tension, compression, or shearing forces is exceeded.[8] The healing process begins after the fracture. Osteoblasts, which are cells that form bone, multiply to mend the fractured area. A good blood supply is necessary to supply the cells with oxygen for proper healing. The fracture site is protected during the healing process by pins, plates, and wires. In some cases in which extra protection is needed, a **spica cast** may be used for the hip. A spica cast extends around the pelvis and down the thigh of the fractured hip. Other types of casts may be used for fractures at other parts of the LE. Several months may be needed for a bone fracture to heal completely. The time needed varies with the age and health of the patient, site and configuration of the fracture, initial displacement of the bone, and the blood supply to the fragments.

Etiology of Fractures

Trauma is the major cause of fractures. In most cases the trauma occurs from falling. Poor lighting, throw rugs, and unmarked steps are particular hazards that can lead to a fall. **Osteoporosis** is a common bone disease affecting people over 65 years of age. It results in decreased bone density, most commonly in the vertebral bodies, the neck of the femur, humerus, and distal end of the radius. Because the bone becomes porous and thereby fragile, the affected bones are prone to fracture during a fall or other traumatic event. A pathological fracture can occur in a bone weakened by disease or tumor, as in the cases of osteomyelitis and cancers that have metastasized to the bone.[8]

Medical Management

The goals of fracture treatment are to relieve pain, maintain good position of the bone, allow fracture healing, and restore optimal function to the patient.[19]

Reduction of a fracture refers to restoring the bone fragments to normal alignment.[8] This can be done by a closed procedure (manipulation) or by an open procedure (surgery). The physician performs a closed reduction by applying force to the displaced bone, opposite to the force that produced the fracture. Depending on the nature of the fracture, the reduction is maintained in a cast, brace, traction, or skeletal fixation.[11]

With open reduction the fracture site is exposed surgically so that the bone fragments can be aligned. The fragments are held in place with internal fixation by pins, screws, a plate, nails, or a rod. Further immobilization by a cast or a brace may be necessary. Usually an **open reduction and internal fixation** (ORIF) must be protected from excessive forces, so **weight-bearing restrictions** are indicated.[11]

There are several levels of weight-bearing restrictions. The physician indicates at which level the patient should be placed and changes the restrictions as the fracture site heals and becomes stronger. The levels of weight-bearing restrictions are listed in Box 45-1.[11]

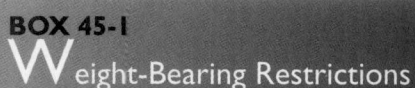

BOX 45-1
Weight-Bearing Restrictions

NWB (nor–weight bearing) indicates that no weight at all can be placed on the extremity involved.

TTWB (tce-touch weight bearing) indicates that only the toe can be placed on the ground to provide some balance while standing–90% of the weight is still on the unaffected leg. In toe-touch weight bearing, patients are instructed to imagine that an egg is under their foot.

PWB (partial weight bearing) indicates that only 50% of the person's body weight can be placed on the affected leg.

WBAT (weight bearing at tolerance) indicates that patients are allowed to judge how much weight they are able to put on the affected leg without causing too much pain.

FWB (full weight bearing) indicates that patients should be able to put 100% of their weight on the affected leg without causing damage to the fracture site.

From Early MB: *Physical dysfunction: practical skills for the OT assistant,* St Louis, 1998, Mosby.

HIP FRACTURES
Types of Hip Fractures and Medical Management

Knowledge of hip anatomy is necessary for understanding medical management of hip fractures. An anatomy and physiology reference should be consulted for details. See Fig. 45-1 for an illustration of the normal hip joint.

The typical levels of fracture lines are shown in Fig. 45-2. The names of the fractures generally reflect the site and severity of injury and may signal which medical treatment will be used. For example, a femoral neck fracture will be treated with femoral neck stabilization.[11]

Femoral Neck Fractures

Femoral neck fractures, which include subcapital, transcervical, and basilar fractures, are common in adults over 60 years old and occur more frequently in women. If the bone is osteoporotic, fracture may result from even a slight trauma or rotational force.[3] Treatment of a displaced fracture in this area is complicated by poor blood supply, osteoporotic bone that is not suited to hold metallic fixation, and a thin periosteum. The type of surgical treatment used is based on the amount of displacement and the circulation in the femoral head.

The age and health of the patient are considered in deciding on the surgical procedure. Generally, hip pinning (application of a compression screw and plate) is used when displacement is minimal to moderate and blood supply is intact. With a physician's approval, a patient is usually able to begin limited out-of-bed activities 1 to 3 days after surgery. Per physician's orders, weight-bearing restrictions may need to be observed

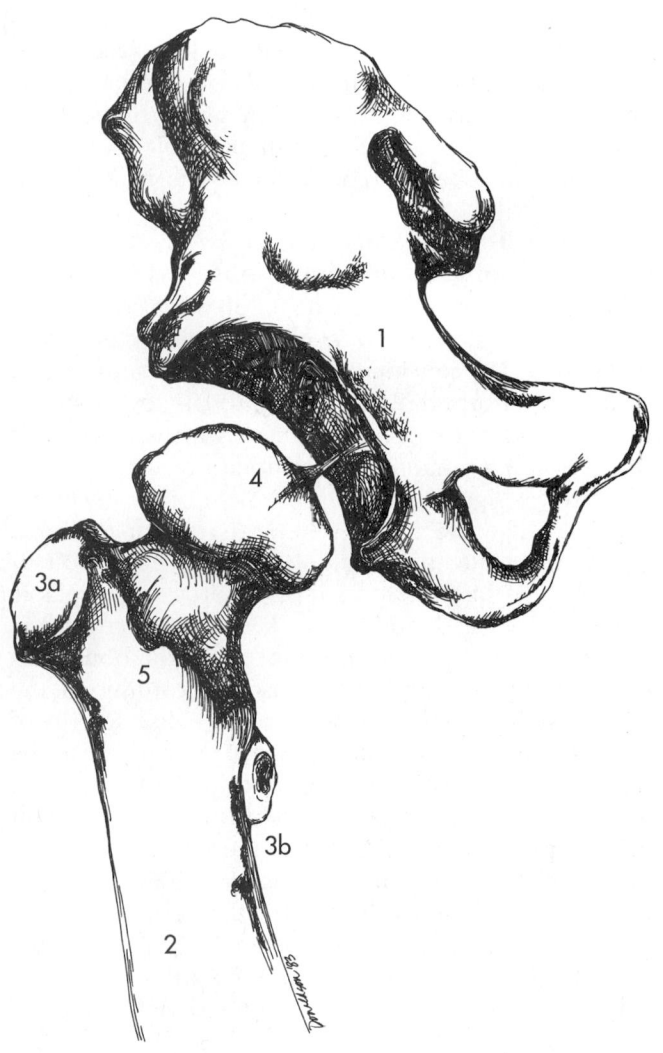

FIG. 45-1
Normal hip anatomy. *1,* Acetabulum. *2,* Femur. *3a,* Greater trochanter. *3b,* Lesser trochanter. *4,* Ligamentum teres. *5,* Intertrochanteric crest. (Modified from Croch JE: *Functional human anatomy,* ed 3, Philadelphia, 1978, Lea & Febiger; Grant LC: *Grant's atlas of anatomy,* ed 6, Baltimore, 1972, Williams & Wilkins.)

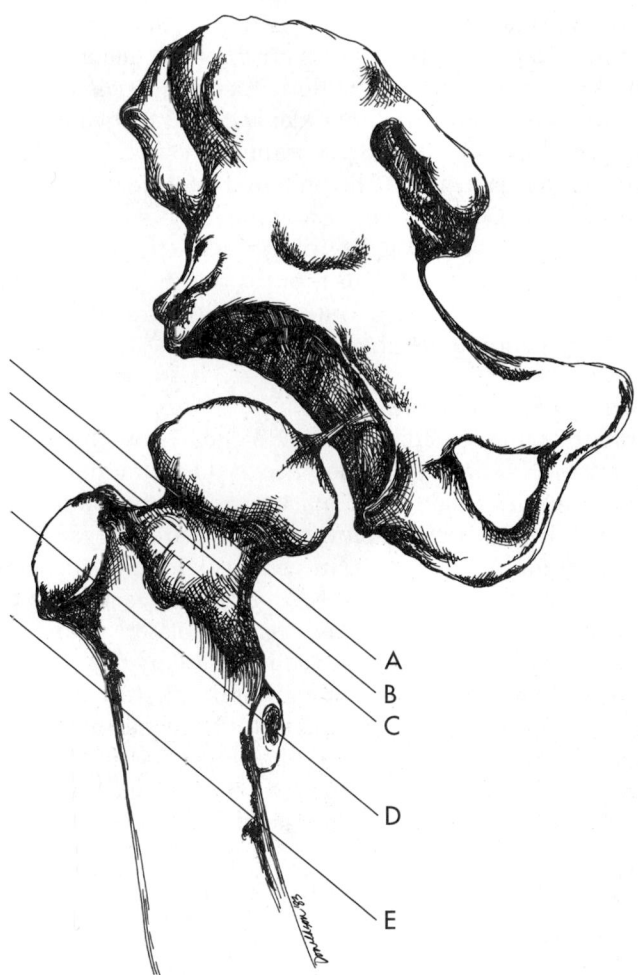

FIG. 45-2
Levels of femoral fracture. **A,** Subcapital. **B,** Transcervical. **C,** Basilar. **D,** Intertrochanteric. **E,** Subtrochanteric. (Modified from Crow I: Fracture of the hip: a self study, *ONA J* 5:12, 1978.)

with the aid of crutches or a walker for at least 6 to 8 weeks while the fracture is healing. Weight bearing may be limited beyond this time if precautions are not observed or if delayed union occurs.[11]

With severe displacement or in the case of a femoral head with poor blood supply (avascular) or nonunion (a poorly healing fracture site where new bone does not form) and degenerative joint disease, the femoral head is surgically removed and replaced by an endoprosthesis. This joint replacement is referred to as a hemipolar or bipolar arthroplasty.[16] Several types of metal prostheses can be used; each has its own shape and advantages. Weight-bearing restrictions are sometimes indicated. Because of the surgical procedure used, precautions for positioning the hip must be observed to prevent dislocation. Patients who have had a prosthesis implanted can usually begin limited out-of-bed activity, with a physician's approval, about 1 to 3 days after surgery.[11]

Intertrochanteric Fractures
Fractures between the greater and lesser trochanter are extracapsular, or outside the articular capsule of the hip joint, and the blood supply is not affected. Like femoral neck fractures, intertrochanteric fractures occur mostly in women but in a slightly older age group. The fracture is usually caused by direct trauma or force over the trochanter, as in a fall. The preferred treatment for these fractures is ORIF. A nail or compression screw with a sideplate is used. Weight-bearing restrictions must be observed for up to 4 to 6 months during ambulation. The patient is allowed out of bed 1 to 3 days after surgery, pending the physician's approval.[11]

Subtrochanteric Fractures
Subtrochanteric fractures 1 to 2 inches below the lesser trochanter usually occur because of direct trauma, as in falls, motor vehicle accidents, or any other situation in which there is a direct blow to the hip area. These fractures are most often seen in persons less than 60 years old. Skeletal traction followed by ORIF is the usual treatment. A nail with a long sideplate or an intramedullary rod is used. An intramedullary rod is a rod inserted through the central part of the shaft of bone to help maintain proper alignment for bone healing.[11]

In all types of hip fractures the practitioner should be aware of the soft-tissue trauma, edema, and bruising that occur around the fracture site.[16]

HIP JOINT REPLACEMENT
Etiology

Restoration of joint motion and treatment of pain by total hip replacement, or **arthroplasty,** is sometimes indicated, primarily in osteoarthritis and rheumatoid arthritis and occasionally in other disease processes. Osteoarthritis or degenerative joint disease may develop spontaneously in middle age and progress as the normal aging process of joints is accelerated. Degenerative changes may also develop as the result of trauma, congenital deformity, or a disease that damages articular cartilage. Weight-bearing joints such as the hip, knee, and lumbar spine are usually affected. In the hip there is a loss of cartilage centrally on the joint surface and formation of osteophytes on the periphery of the acetabulum, producing joint incongruity. Pain originates from the bone, synovial membrane, or fibrous capsule and from muscle spasm. When movement of the hip causes pain and limited mobility, the muscles shorten, which can result in a hip position of flexion, adduction, and internal rotation that causes a painful limp.[12]

Rheumatoid arthritis (see Chapter 43) may involve the hip joint. Surgery is often performed early in the disease process to limit fibrotic damage to joint and tendon structures.[19] Other disease processes (such as lupus and cancer) and some medications (e.g., prednisone) can compromise the blood flow to the hip joint and lead to avascular necrosis (AVN, a condition in which bone cells die because of poor blood supply) or osteoporosis; either condition results in a painful hip.[17]

Medical Management
When other forms of treatment for the pain and decreased mobility have not been successful, a total joint replacement is considered to restore an individual's ability to perform daily occupations. The total joint replacement is not considered for persons who will not comply with a rehabilitation program or who will not experience significant improvement in functional ability.[6] There are two mechanical components to a "total hip." A high-density polyethylene socket is fitted into the acetabulum, and a metallic prosthesis replaces the femoral head and neck. Methylmethacrylate or acrylic cement fixes the components to the bone. Various surgical approaches are used, according to the surgical skill or technique of the orthopedist, severity of the joint involvement, and history of past surgery to the hip. With an **anterolateral approach** the patient will be unstable in external rotation, adduction, and extension of the operated hip and usually must observe precautions to prevent these movements for 6 to 12 weeks. If a **posterolateral approach** is used, the patient must be cautioned not to move the operated hip past specific ranges of flexion (usually 60° to 90°) and not to internally rotate or adduct the leg. Failure to maintain these **hip precautions** during muscle and soft-tissue healing may result in hip dislocation (Box 45-2).

Most surgeons do not restrict weight bearing postoperatively when cement fixation is used. However, one of the major problems with total hip replacement is the loss of fixation at the prothesis interface. The most recent development is the use of biological fixation. Bony

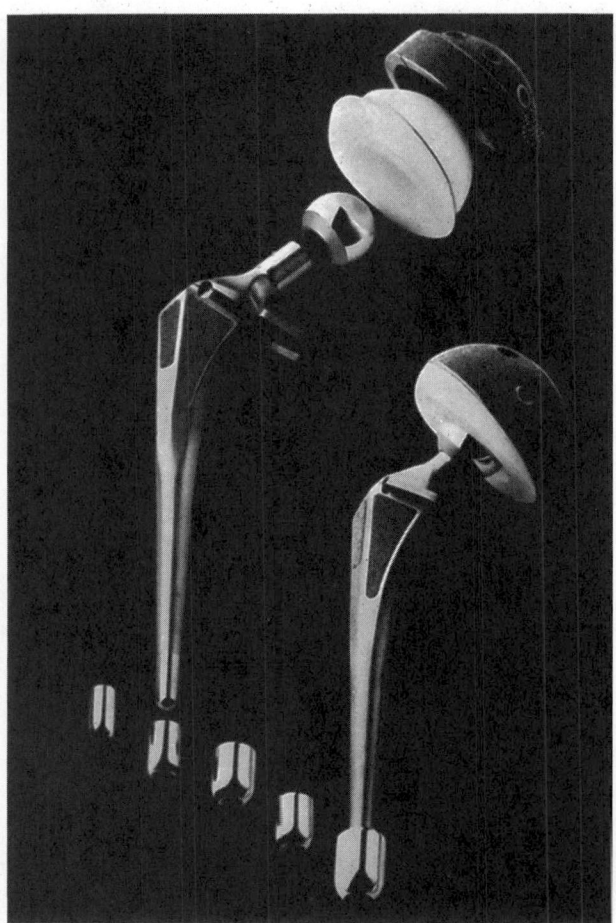

FIG. 45-3
Modular total hip prosthesis designed for bony ingrowth. (From Kottke FJ: *Krusen's handbook of physical medicine and rehabilitation,* ed 4, Philadelphia, 1990, WB Saunders.

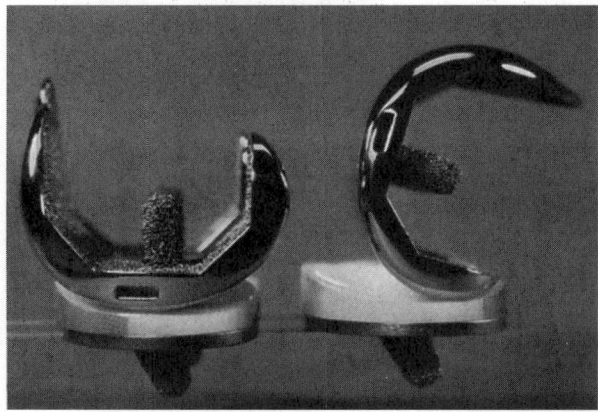

FIG. 45-4
Porous-coated total knee prosthesis. Note resurfacing features of components and beaded surfaces for biological fixation. (From Kottke FJ: *Krusen's handbook of physical medicine and rehabilitation,* ed 4, Philadelphia, 1990, WB Saunders.)

ingrowth, instead of cement, secures the prosthesis. In other words, new bone grows into openings in the prosthesis, and this secures the prosthesis to the bone (Fig. 45-3). The precautions following the surgery are those of the anterior or posterior hip replacements with an additional restriction on weight bearing for 6 to 8 weeks. The restrictions on weight bearing will vary in terms of amount of pressure and length of time. A walking aid, usually a walker or crutches, is necessary for at least the first month while the hip is healing and muscles are becoming stronger. Patients with total joint replacements usually begin out-of-bed activity 1 to 3 days after surgery.[12]

Total joint surface replacements, which are rarely used, are a variation of the total hip replacement.[9] The surface of the femur is capped by a metallic shell, and the acetabular cavity receives a plastic cup. Both are held in place by methylmethacrylate. This technique preserves the femoral head and neck. With this technique no weight-bearing restrictions apply.[12]

KNEE JOINT REPLACEMENT
Etiology and Medical Management

The reason for a total knee replacement is similar to that for the total hip replacement, except that the degenerative changes occur in the knee joint. Total knee replacement, or total knee arthroplasty (TKA), is designed to alleviate pain, increase motion, and maintain alignment and stability of the knee joint. The process involves cutting away the damaged bone (as little bone as possible) and attaching a prosthesis for the new joint. There are various types of prostheses. The type used depends on the severity of joint damage (Figs. 45-4 and 45-5). The prosthesis can be cemented to the bone or not cemented. With a cemented prosthesis, patients are usually able to bear weight at tolerance on the operated leg. With a noncemented prosthesis,

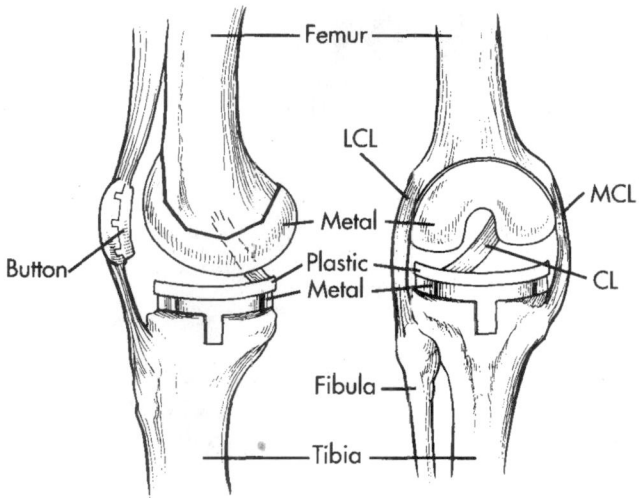

FIG. 45-5
Total knee replacement. The metal aspects of the prosthesis cover the distal portion of the femur and the end of the tibia. There is a polyethylene plastic-bearing surface (*plastic*) between the metallic aspects of the two surfaces. The patella is replaced by a polyethylene button. The medial collateral ligament (*MCL*), lateral collateral ligament (*LCL*), and cruciate ligaments (*CL*) are retained. (From Early MB: *Physical dysfunction: practical skills for the OT assistant*, St Louis, 1998, Mosby; modified from Calliet R: *Knee pain and instability*, ed 3, Philadelphia, 1992, FA Davis.)

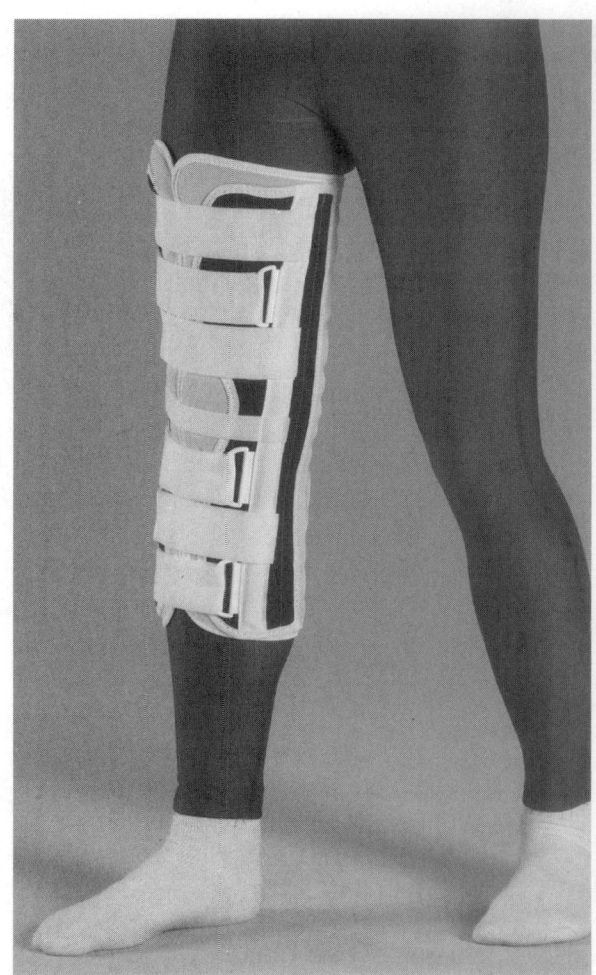

FIG. 45-6
A knee immobilizer is used to support and stabilize the knee joint during mobility. (Courtesy DeRoyal, Powell, Tenn.)

weight bearing is usually avoided initially. Patients may start out-of-bed activities 1 to 3 days after surgery, pending the physician's orders. Patients may use a **knee immobilizer** (Fig. 45-6) when moving in and out of the bed and ambulating to provide support to the knee. The patient should avoid any rotation at the knee up to 12 weeks after surgery. There is usually no restriction on bending the knee. In fact, it is important to maintain the mobility of the knee to ensure good mobility as it heals.[4,18]

GENERAL CONSIDERATIONS FOR LOWER EXTREMITY JOINT REPLACEMENTS

Individuals with joint changes that result in increasing pain may have multiple joint involvement (i.e., both knees or hips). Some patients opt to have both joints replaced during the same hospitalization, with procedures usually 1 week apart. This can complicate the rehabilitation process, since the patient will not have a stronger leg to rely on for walking and performing daily occupations.

It is important to be aware of complications or special procedures that occurred during surgery and to inquire about additional precautions and risks. Common complications include dislocation, wearing out of parts, fracture of bone next to implanted parts, and loosening of parts. A special procedure involves using a spica cast to immobilize the hip joint for individuals at high risk for a dislocation.[12]

Emphasis in rehabilitation is on maintaining or increasing joint motion, slowly increasing the strength of surrounding musculature, decreasing swelling, and increasing independence in activities of daily living (ADL). The occupational therapist's role in this process is primarily in educating the patient who has undergone joint replacement about adaptive techniques for ADL with limited mobility.

PSYCHOLOGICAL FACTORS

Psychological issues are critical in the overall treatment of the orthopedic patient. A large number of patients in this population are faced with a chronic disability (such as rheumatoid arthritis), a life-threatening disease (such as cancer), or the aging process. The loss or potential loss of mobility and physical ability is a major concern for most of these patients. Adjusting to loss is stressful, requiring an enormous amount of physical and emotional energy.[14] An awareness of and a sensitivity toward the orthopedic patient are critical for the delivery of optimal patient care.

Patients with a chronic orthopedic disability often experience one or all of the following: disease of a body part, fear, anxiety, change in body image, decreased functional ability, deformity, and pain. Treatment of a patient with a chronic orthopedic disability must address these issues and provide the support needed for the grieving process to take place. Without an opportunity to confront these issues, the patient is likely to become depressed, filled with guilt and anxiety, and paralyzed with fear. These emotions inhibit the patient's progress and further damage the self-image. Clinicians can help patients acknowledge and experience some of these feelings, ultimately enhancing the treatment process. One way to ease anxiety and fear is to make sure the patient understands the treatment and procedures he or she is receiving. Taking time to answer questions and provide additional information can be crucial for successful adjustment.

The elderly patient experiencing disability deals with additional issues specific to the aging process: fear of dependence and relocation trauma.[2] With the onset of a disability late in life the patient may be forced to let go of independence and self-sufficiency.[14] For some this can be a devastating experience, requiring prolonged grieving before adjustment. Others may use dependence for secondary gain, remaining in the hospital for extra attention or manipulating their support systems to avoid taking responsibility for themselves and others. Relocation may result in confusion, disorientation, and emotional lability when individuals are removed from their familiar environment. Decorating the person's room with familiar items and using a calendar can be helpful in reducing this traumatic event.

Learning to cope and adjust to the changes resulting from chronic disability or the aging process is a critical aspect of recovery. Practitioners must realize that a great deal of a patient's functional independence has been relinquished as a result of disease or disability. The psychosocial issues resulting from this loss must be addressed while focusing on increasing a patient's functional level of independence.[14]

An important area of ADL that is often overlooked is sexual activity. Persons with a hip fracture or LE joint replacement will have difficulty performing sexual activities in their usual manner (See Chapter 15 for a further discussion of sexuality.) It is recommended that persons not engage in sexual activity for 6 weeks so that they maintain the movement precautions applicable to their condition.[6] Patients of all ages and both genders may have questions regarding the level of sexual activity that is allowed. The occupational therapist will need to create an environment in which the patient feels permitted to ask personal questions. The therapist can do this by being open minded and realizing that sexual activity is an important and meaningful occupation. The therapist may need to suggest ways for the patient to position the operated leg during sexual activity to maintain precautions. Side-lying on the nonoperated side is one option. Abduction precautions can be maintained via pillows between the knees. To prevent excessive external rotation at the hips while in the supine position, the patient can place pillows under the knees. Patients with weight-bearing precautions should avoid kneeling.[6] Written information with diagrams can be helpful when addressing such a personal issue. The patient can read it privately or with his or her partner at another time.

REHABILITATION

Good communication and clear role delineation among members of the health care team are essential for an efficient and smooth therapy program. The health care team usually consists of a primary physician, nursing staff, a physical therapist, an occupational therapist or assistant, a nutritionist, a pharmacist, and a case coordinator. Many facilities have a protocol or **critical pathway** that outlines each team member's responsibilities and a time frame for accomplishing assigned tasks related to the patient's rehabilitation. Regular team meetings to discuss each patient's ongoing treatment, progress, and discharge plans are necessary for coordinating individual treatment programs. Members from each service usually attend each meeting to provide information and consultation.

The role of the physician is to inform the team of the patient's medical status. This includes information regarding previous medical history, diagnosis of the present problem, and a complete account of the surgical procedure performed. Information provided may include the type of appliance inserted, the anatomical approach, and any movement or weight-bearing precautions that could endanger the patient. The physician is also responsible for ordering specific medications and therapies. Any change or progression in therapy or change in the patient's medication regimen should be approved by the physician.

The nursing staff is responsible for the physical care of the patient during hospitalization. The orthopedic nurse must have a thorough understanding of the surgical procedures and movement precautions for each patient. Proper positioning using pillows and wedges is carried out by the nurse, especially in the first few days after surgery. As the patient's therapy program progresses, the patient starts to take more responsibility for proper positioning and physical care. The nurse works closely with the physical and occupational therapists to carry through self-care skills that the patient has already learned in therapy.[12]

The physical therapist is responsible for evaluation and treatment in the areas of musculoskeletal status, sensation, pain, skin integrity, and mobility (especially gait). In many cases involving total joint replacement and surgical repair of hip fracture, physical therapy is initiated on the first day after surgery. The physical therapist obtains baseline information, including range of motion (ROM), strength of all extremities, muscle tone, mental status, and mobility, adhering to the prescribed precautions of protocol. A treatment program that includes therapeutic exercises, ROM activities, transfer training, and progressive gait activities is established. The physical therapist is responsible for recommending the appropriate assistive device to be used during ambulation. As the patient's ambulation status advances, instruction in stair climbing, managing curbs, and outside ambulation is given.[12,16]

The nutritionist consults with each patient to ensure that adequate and appropriate nutrition is received to aid the healing process. The pharmacist monitors the patient's drug therapy and provides information and assistance with pain management.[12]

The role of the case coordinator is to ensure that each patient is being discharged to the appropriate living situation or facility. Usually the case coordinator is a registered nurse or social worker with a thorough knowledge of available community resources and nursing care facilities. With input from the health care team the case coordinator makes the arrangements for ongoing therapy after hospitalization, for admission to a rehabilitation facility for further intensive therapy, or for nursing home care if necessary. The case coordinator works closely with the health care team and is instrumental in coordinating the program after the patient's discharge from the hospital.[12,16]

ROLE OF OCCUPATIONAL THERAPY

After a total joint replacement or surgical repair of a fractured hip, OT typically begins when the patient is ready to start getting out of bed, usually 1 to 3 days after surgery. The actual time varies, depending on the age and general health of the patient and on surgical events or medical complications involved. Before any physical assessment it is important for the therapy practitioner to introduce and explain the role of OT and gather any pertinent information regarding the patient's occupational history, including prior functional status, home environment, and living situation. The goal of OT is for the patient to maximize independence in daily occupations, with all movement precautions observed during activities. The role of the occupational therapist and assistant is to teach the patient ways and means of performing daily occupations safely.[12,16]

Evaluation and Treatment Planning

The role of the occupational therapist and occupational therapy assistant can be clearly defined with cases of total joint replacement and hip fractures. The occupational therapist is responsible for performing any evaluations that are needed. In addition to an occupational history, a baseline physical evaluation is necessary for determining whether any physical limitations not related to surgery might prevent functional independence. Upper extremity (UE) ROM, muscle strength, sensation, coordination, and mental status are assessed before a functional evaluation is made. The certified occupational therapy assistant can participate in the ADL evaluation. During evaluation it is also important to observe any signs of pain and fear at rest or during movement.[12,16]

OT involves a progression of functional activities that simulate a normal, daily regimen of occupation that is in accordance with all the movement precautions.[12,16] This is also referred to as ADL training. The therapist introduces and trains patients in the use of assistive devices, proper transfer techniques, and ADL techniques, while maintaining hip precautions. Specific training techniques are discussed later in the chapter. An OT assistant may play a large role in this training. Both the occupational therapist and the OT assistant are involved in treatment planning, documentation, and discharge planning (including recommending equipment and home exercise programs).

Patient Education

Although hip fractures are never a planned occurrence, total joint replacements are usually preplanned and scheduled to be performed on a specific date. Occupational therapists provide education classes for individuals at risk for fractures and those planning joint replacement. For the person who may be at risk for falling, attending a class on fall prevention may be a wise recommendation. Topics may include home modifications (such as removing throw rugs, telephone cords, and clutter), safe transfer techniques, use of public transportation, and community mobility tips. The person who is having an elective total joint replacement may benefit from a class offered before surgery that explains the procedures, introduces assistive devices, and describes therapy procedures.

Specific Training Techniques

Some common assistive devices are useful for many people with hip fractures or joint replacements (Fig. 45-7). Helpful assistive devices or adaptive aides include a dressing stick, sock aid, long-handled sponge, long-handled shoe horn, reacher, elastic shoe laces,

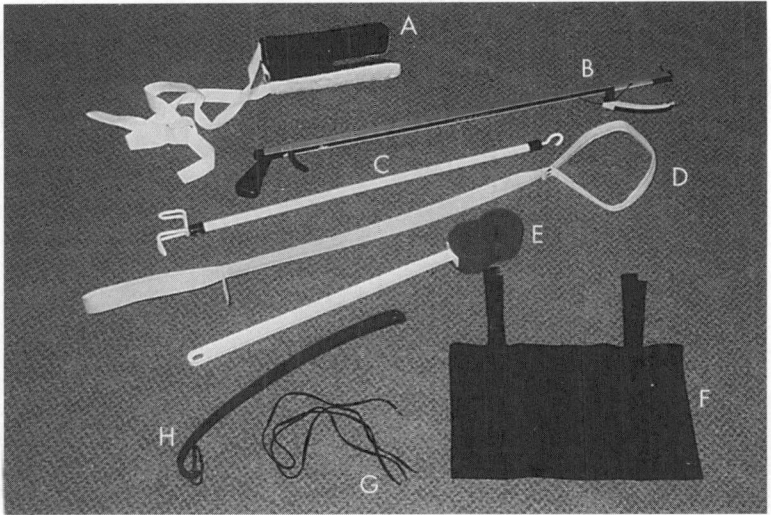

FIG. 45-7
Assistive devices for ADL. **A,** Sock aid. **B,** Reacher. **C,** Dressing stick. **D,** Leg lifter. **E,** Long-handled sponge. **F,** Walker bag. **G,** Elastic shoe laces. **H,** Long-handled shoe horn. (From Early MB: *Physical dysfunction: practical skills for the OT assistant,* St Louis, 1998, Mosby.)

elevated toilet seat or commode seat, leg lifter, and shower chair or bench. Walker bags are helpful for people using walkers who need to carry small items from one place to another. The OT clinic should have samples of these devices and should be able to issue them to patients for use during the training process.

Hip

The training procedures outlined below apply to both types of hip joint replacement (posterolateral and anterolateral) unless otherwise noted. The positions of hip instability for both types of surgical procedures are important to remember. For the posterolateral approach, positions of instability include adduction, internal rotation, and flexion greater than precautions. For the anterolateral approach, positions of instability include adduction, external rotation, and excessive hyperextension.

Bed Mobility

The supine position with the appropriate wedge or pillow in place is recommended. If a patient sleeps in the side-lying position, sleeping on the operated side is recommended if tolerable. When sleeping on the nonoperated side, the patient must keep the legs abducted with the wedge or larger pillows and the operated leg supported to prevent rotation. The patient is instructed in getting out of bed on both sides, although initially it may be easier to observe precautions by moving toward the nonoperated leg. Careful instruction is given to avoid adduction past midline. It is important to determine the type and height of the patient's bed at home. When getting in and out of bed initially, the patient may use a **leg lifter** to help the operated leg move from one surface to another. Some patients have an overhead trapeze placed on the bed to assist with bed mobility. It is important to wean the patient away from using this device because he or she will most likely not have one at home.

Transfers

It is always helpful for the patient to observe the proper technique for transfers first, before attempting the movement.

CHAIR. A firmly based chair with armrests is recommended. The patient is instructed to extend the operated leg forward, reach back for the armrests, and sit slowly. For the person with a posterolateral approach, care should be taken not to lean forward when sitting down (Fig. 45-8). To stand, the patient extends the operated leg and pushes off from the armrests. Because of the hip flexion precaution for the posterolateral approach, the patient should sit on the front part of the chair and lean back (Fig. 45-8, *C*). Firm cushions or blankets may be used to increase the height of chairs and especially may be needed if the patient is tall. Low chairs, soft chairs, reclining chairs, and rocking chairs should be avoided.

COMMODE CHAIR. Three-in-one commode chairs with armrests can be used in the hospital and at home. For the person with a posterolateral approach, the

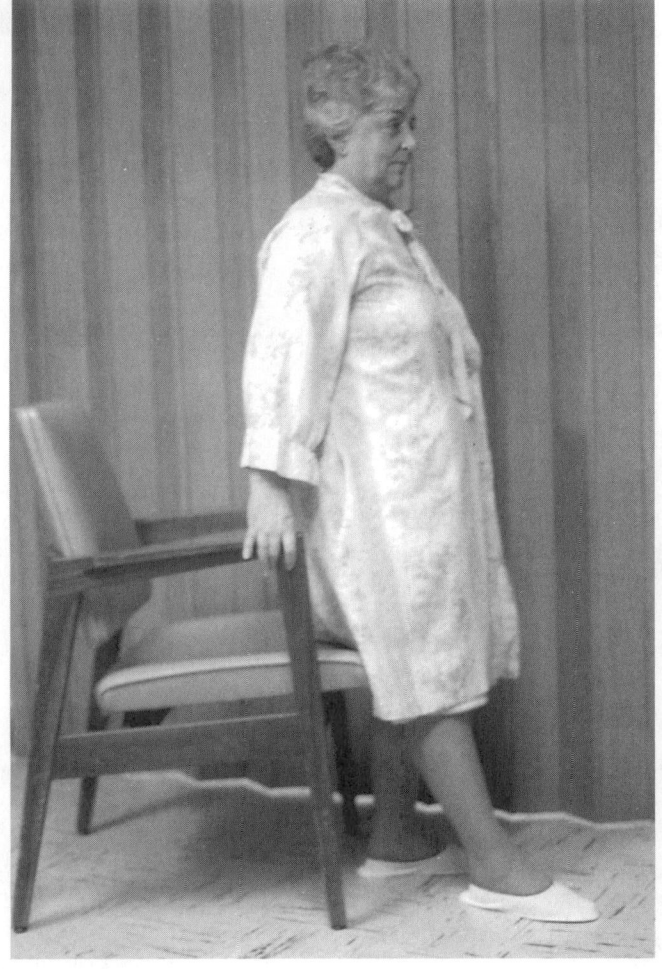

A

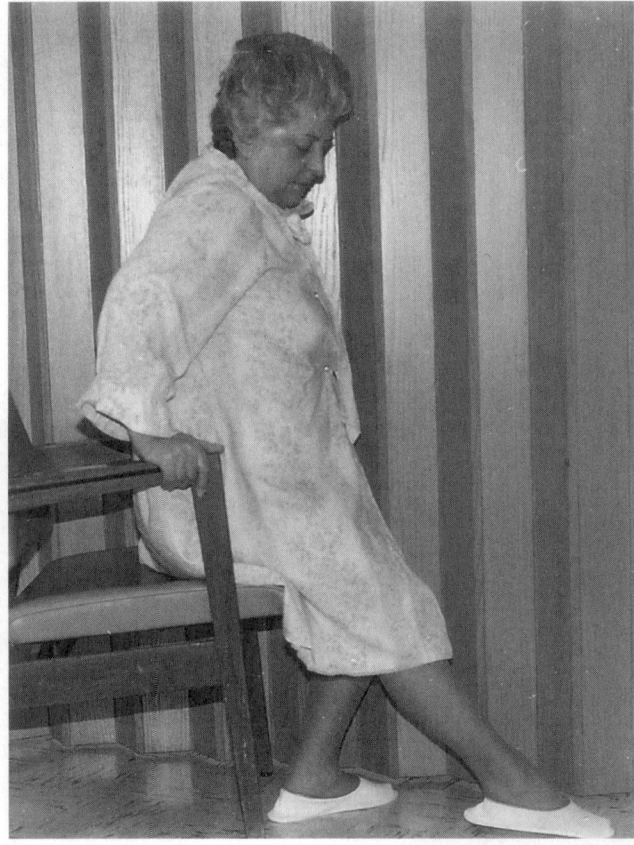

B

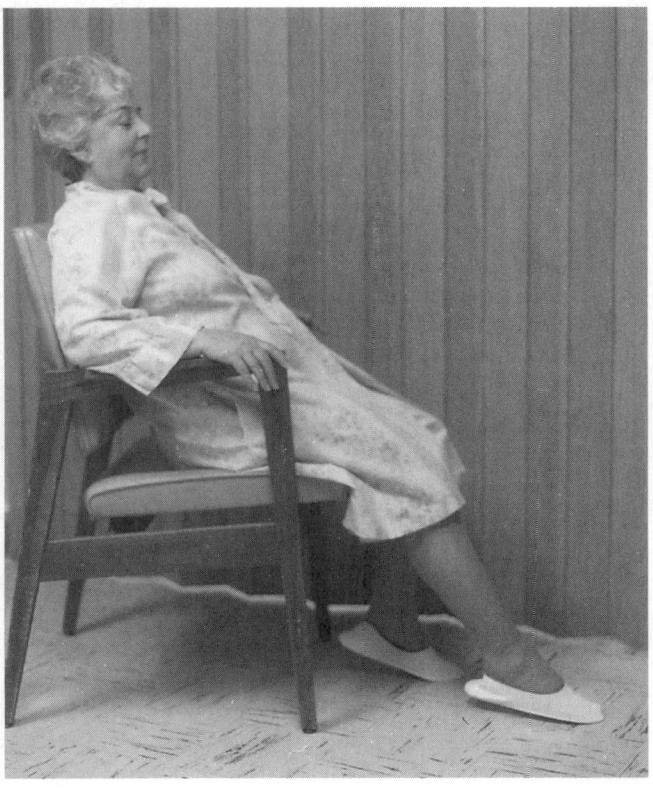

C

FIG. 45-8

Chair transfer technique. **A,** Patient extends operated leg and reaches for armrests. **B** and **C,** Bearing some weight on arms, the patient sits down slowly, maintaining some extension of the operated leg.

height and angle can be adjusted so that the front legs are one notch lower than the back legs; thus with the patient seated, the precautionary hip angle of flexion is not exceeded. A person with an anterolateral approach may have enough hip mobility to use a standard toilet seat safely at the time of discharge. All patients should wipe between the legs in a sitting position or from behind in a standing position and use caution to avoid rotation of the hip. The patient is to stand up and step to turn to face the toilet to flush.

SHOWER STALL. Nonskid strips or stickers are recommended in all shower stalls and tubs. When the patient is entering, the walker or crutches go first, then the operated leg, followed by the nonoperated leg. A shower chair with adjustable legs or a stool and grab bars should be installed if balance is a problem or if weight-bearing precautions are present.

SHOWER-OVER-TUB (WITHOUT SHOWER DOORS). The patient is instructed to stand parallel to the tub facing the shower fixtures. Using the walker or crutches, the patient is to transfer in sideways by bending at the knees, not at the hips. For patients with weight-bearing precautions or poor balance, purchase of a tub bench may be considered, allowing the patient to sit on the edge of the bench and then swing the legs over the tub while observing flexion precautions. Sponge bathing at the sink is an alternative activity.

CAR. Bucket seats in small cars should be avoided. Bench-type seats are recommended. The patient is instructed to back up to the front passenger seat, hold onto a stable part of the car, extend the operated leg, and slowly sit in the car. Remembering to lean back, the patient then slides the buttocks toward the driver's seat. The upper body and LEs move as one unit to turn to face the forward direction. It is helpful to have the seat moved back and reclined to accommodate the hip flexion precaution. Pillows in the seat may be necessary to increase the height of the seat. Prolonged sitting in the car should be avoided. If transferring to the front passenger seat is a problem, transferring to the back seat of a four-door car is an alternative. The patient backs to the seat, extends the operated leg, and slowly sits in the car. Then he or she slides back so that the operated leg is resting on the seat fully supported.

Lower Body Dressing

The patient is instructed to sit in a chair with arms or on the edge of the bed for dressing activities. The patient is instructed to avoid adduction and rotation or crossing the legs to dress. The patient must avoid crossing the operated extremity over the nonoperated extremity at either the ankles or knees. Assistive devices may be necessary for observing precautions (Fig. 45-7). To maintain hip precautions, the patient uses a reacher or dressing stick to don and remove pants and shoes. For pants, the operated leg is dressed first by using the reacher or dressing stick to bring the pants over the foot and up to the knee. A sock aid is used to don socks or knee-high nylons, and a reacher or dressing stick is used to doff them. A reacher, elastic laces, and a long-handled shoehorn can also be provided.

Lower Body Bathing

The section on transfers describes the proper method of getting in and out of the shower or tub. Sponge bathing at the sink is indicated until the patient is approved by the physician to shower. A long-handled bath sponge or back brush is used to reach the lower legs and feet safely. Soap-on-a-rope is used to prevent the soap from dropping, and a towel is wrapped on a reacher to dry the lower legs.

Hair Shampoo

Until able to shower, the patient is instructed to obtain assistance for shampooing hair. If unable to obtain any assistance, the patient may shampoo the hair while standing or sitting on a stool at the kitchen or bathroom sink, observing hip precautions at all times.

Homemaking

Heavy housework, such as vacuuming, lifting, and bed making, should be avoided initially. Kitchen activities are practiced, with suggestions made to keep commonly used items at countertop level. The patient can carry items by using an apron with large pockets, sliding items along the counter top, using a utility cart, attaching a small basket or bag to a walker, or wearing a fanny pack around the waist. Reachers are provided to grasp items in low cupboards or to pick up items from the floor.

Family Orientation

A family member or friend should be present for at least one OT treatment session so that any questions may be answered. Appropriate supervision recommendations and instruction regarding activity precautions are given at this time. Instructional booklets on hip fractures and total hip and knee surgery may be purchased from the American Occupational Therapy Association to supplement training.[12,16]

Total Knee Replacement

Procedures for ADL training for persons with total knee replacement are provided in the following paragraphs. Many of the techniques used with a hip replacement can be used for someone with a knee replacement. Positions of knee instability include internal and external rotation and flexion greater than ROM permits.

Bed Mobility

The supine position is recommended, with the entire leg slightly elevated via balanced suspension or pillows, with or without a knee immobilizer. This will help to reduce edema and prevent knee flexion contractures. It is recommended that a person not sleep on the operated side. As in hip replacement, a pillow or wedge can be placed between the legs if this is necessary for side-lying and the person lies on the nonoperated side.

Transfers

In general, the patient can bend at the hip as much as he or she is able. Because of decreased knee flexion, the patient may need to use the same techniques for commode and car transfers as have been described for hip replacements. Grab bars or a shower chair or bench is recommended, especially for transferring to the shower over the tub, as well as for the individual with decreased standing endurance or inability to bend the knee enough to sit on the bottom of the tub.

Lower Extremity Dressing

This presents a problem only if the patient is unable to reach his or her toes. In such a case, techniques described for the hip replacement can be used. The patient should practice donning and doffing the knee immobilizer.

Homemaking and family training are as for hip replacement.

Special Equipment

The OT practitioner should be familiar with the following equipment that is commonly used in the treatment of hip fracture and total hip replacement.

Hemovac: During surgery a plastic drainage tube is inserted at the surgical site to assist with drainage of blood postoperatively. It has an area for collection of drainage and may be connected to a portable suction machine. The unit should *not* be disconnected for any activity, since this may create a blockage in the system. The Hemovac is usually left in place for 2 days after surgery.

Abduction wedge: Large and small triangular wedges are used when the patient is supine to maintain the LEs in the abducted position.

Balanced suspension: This is fabricated and set up by an orthopedic technician and can be used for about 3 days after surgery. Its purpose is to support the affected LE in the first few postoperative days. The patient's leg can be taken out of the device for exercise only.[18]

Reclining wheelchair: A wheelchair with an adjustable backrest that allows a reclining position is used for patients who have hip flexion precautions while sitting.

Commode chairs: The use of a commode chair instead of the regular toilet aids in safe transfers and allows the patient to observe necessary hip flexion precautions.

Sequential compression devices (SCDs): SCDs are used postoperatively to reduce the risk of deep vein thrombosis. They are inflatable, external leggings that provide intermittent pneumatic compression of the legs.[12]

Antiembolus hose: These are thigh-high hosiery that are worn 24 hours a day and removed only during bathing. Their purpose is to assist circulation, prevent edema, and thus reduce the risk of deep-vein thrombosis.[12]

Patient-controlled administration (PCA) IV: The amount of medication is predetermined and programmed by the physician and nursing staff to allow the patient to self-administer pain medication by pushing a button.

Incentive spirometer: This portable breathing apparatus is used to encourage deep breathing and prevent the development of postoperative pneumonia.

SUMMARY

Hip fractures and LE joint replacement are orthopedic conditions in which OT intervention may speed the patient's return to functional independence safely and comfortably. The protocol for OT is determined by the surgical procedure performed and by the precautions prescribed by the physician. Patients who have weight-bearing precautions must be trained to observe these during all ADL. A simulation of the home environment or a home assessment is helpful in preparing the patient for potential problems that may arise after discharge. Areas to assess include the entry, stairs, bathroom, bedroom, sitting surfaces, and kitchen. Recommendations to remove throw rugs and slippery floor coverings and obstacles are made, since the patient will most likely be going home using an assistive device for ambulation. A kitchen stool or utility cart may be indicated. It is important to assess and instruct the patient and caregiver in ADL with adaptive equipment, as well as in observing any movement precautions.[15] Home therapy may be indicated after a hospital stay to ensure safety and independence in daily occupations if these goals were not met during hospitalization.

Preoperative teaching programs are invaluable in aiding patient adjustment. The class orients and familiarizes the patient with the hospital, nursing, physical therapy, OT, respiratory therapy, and discharge planning. Procedures and equipment, concerns regarding the hospitalization and discharge, and therapy are addressed. Participation in this type of class has been shown to relieve anxiety and fear, empower the patient during the hospitalization, and decrease the hospital length of stay.

CASE STUDY 45-1

CASE STUDY—MRS. T.

Mrs. T. is a 75-year-old woman who sustained a left hip fracture as a result of a fall on ice in front of her home. A hemiarthroplasty was performed to repair the fracture. Currently, she is PWB on the LLE and has ROM precautions for the left hip. She was admitted to the subacute rehabilitation unit 3 days after surgery.

Before the accident, Mrs. T. was independent in ADL and very light housekeeping. She lives in an assisted-living apartment building on the third floor. The building has an elevator and ramp access to the front door. Heavy house cleaning and one meal per day are provided by the center. Mrs. T.'s daily occupations included performing morning ADL, preparing breakfast, watching television, knitting, or getting together with friends or other residents for shopping (van service provided), a movie, or just to socialize in the recreation room. Mrs. T. has a daughter and two grandchildren in the area whom she sees every weekend. Mrs. T. was able to maintain her independence in ADL and light IADL with the use of a straight cane for ambulation and a shower seat in the bathtub.

Results of the OT evaluation reveal that Mrs. T. is anxious about her ability to return home at the same level of independence. She is cooperative in general but has difficulty following weight-bearing precautions. Her UE function is WFL, although she reports joint pain and stiffness in her hands at times. Her endurance is poor, and she is experiencing a great deal of pain in her left hip because of the surgery. She is independent with setup for UE grooming, hygiene, dressing, and eating. She requires MOD assistance for LE dressing and continues to need supervision for transfers and ambulation while using the walker, secondary to her inability to follow weight-bearing precautions.

OT intervention areas include the following: (1) increase level of independence in ADL, particularly in LE dressing, bathing, and toileting; (2) education on hip and weight-bearing precautions; (3) train in use of adaptive equipment; (4) make recommendations to increase safety in her home; and (5) increase UE strength and endurance.

At discharge, Mrs. T. achieved independence in ADL with adaptive equipment. She responded well to treatment after having many opportunities to practice ADL skills and build her confidence. She was trained in the use of a reacher, sock aid, and long-handled sponge. The occupational therapist assisted the patient's daughter in obtaining an elevated toilet seat. Suggestions were given to the patient and her daughter to improve accessibility and safety in her home. Home therapy was recommended for a few visits to do more ADL training in the patient's own home environment.

REVIEW QUESTIONS

1. Explain the difference in precautions for the anterolateral and posterolateral approaches for a hip replacement.
2. When transferring from one surface to another, what is the general procedure to follow to ensure safety and protection of the involved side?
3. List the most common items of adaptive equipment used during rehabilitation of hip fractures and LE joint replacements, and describe their purpose.
4. Describe how the case coordinator and occupational therapist can work together on similar issues.
5. List two specific suggestions for performing sexual activities for someone with a hip replacement.
6. When reviewing the patient's medical and occupational history, what information should be obtained?
7. Identify two factors that affect fracture healing.
8. What is the difference between closed and open reduction procedures?
9. Why are weight-bearing precautions observed with an ORIF?
10. In which diagnoses, other than fractures, is there frequent indication for a total joint replacement? What are the goals of this surgical approach?
11. Compare rehabilitation techniques between patients with a hip replacement and patients with a knee replacement.
12. What are the benefits of conducting patient education preoperative classes for persons who are at risk for falls or who are planning a joint replacement?
13. How might a person's rehabilitation program be affected by bilateral joint replacements?

REFERENCES

1. American Occupational Therapy Association: *Daily activities after your hip surgery*, rev ed, Rockville, Md, 1990, the Association.
2. Butler RN: The life review: an interpretation of reminiscence in the aged. In Kastenbaum R, editor: *New thoughts on old age*, New York, 1964, Springer.
3. Butler RN: *Aging and mental health*, ed 3, St Louis, 1982, Mosby.
4. Calliet R: *Knee pain and disability*, ed 3, Philadelphia, 1992, FA Davis.
5. Crow I: Fractures of the hip: a self study, *ONA J* 5:12, 1978.
6. Delisa J, Gans B: *Rehabilitation medicine: principles and practice*, ed 2, Philadelphia, 1993, JB Lippincott.
7. Ehrlich G: *Rehabilitation of rheumatic conditions*, ed 2, Baltimore, 1986, William & Wilkins.
8. Garland JI: *Fundamentals of orthopedics*, Philadelphia, 1979, WB Saunders.
9. Goodgold J: *Rehabilitation medicine*, St Louis, 1988, Mosby.
10. Gray H: *Gray's anatomy*, Philadelphia, 1974, Running Press

11. Hogshead HP: *Orthopaedics for the therapist,* Gainesville, Fla, 1973, University of Florida (Unpublished).

12. Jones M, Lieberman S, Sitko S, et al: *The total hip replacement protocol,* Stanford, Calif, 1986 and 1982, Stanford University Hospital, Department of Physical and Occupational Therapy (Unpublished).

13. *After total hip replacement and after hip fracture,* Daly City, Calif, 1989, Krames Communications.

14. Lewis SC: *The mature years: a geriatric occupational therapy text,* Thorofare, NJ, 1979, Charles B Slack.

15. Melvin J: *Rheumatic disease: OT and rehabilitation,* ed 2, Philadelphia, 1982, FA Davis.

16. Morawski D: *The total hip replacement protocol and hip fracture protocol,* Los Gatos, Calif, 1990, Community Hospital & Rehabilitation Center of Los Gatos Saratoga, Department of Occupational Therapy (Unpublished).

17. Opitz J: Reconstructive surgery of the extremities. In Kottle F, Lehmann J, editors: *Krusen's handbook of physical medicine and rehabilitation,* ed 4, Philadelphia, 1990, WB Saunders.

18. Richardson JK, Iglarsh ZA: *Clinical orthopaedic physical therapy,* Philadelphia, 1994, WB Saunders.

19. Salter RB: *Textbook of disorders and injuries of the musculoskeletal system,* Baltimore, 1970, Williams & Wilkins.

CHAPTER 46

LOW BACK PAIN

JOAN SMITHLINE
LAURA E. DUNLOP

KEY TERMS

Role blurring
Structural weakness
Cognitive distraction
Self-report
Energy conservation
Pacing
Diagnostic tests
Depression
Social isolation
"Flare-up" plan

LEARNING OBJECTIVES

After studying this chapter, the student or practitioner will be able to do the following:

1. Discuss how low back pain (LBP) disrupts role function.
2. Identify similarities and differences in acute and chronic LBP.
3. Identify appropriate body mechanics for home maintenance and dressing activities.
4. Recognize the inherent structural weakness of the intervertebral disks and ligaments of the lumbar spine.
5. Anticipate **role blurring** between occupational therapy (OT) and physical therapy (PT) in the rehabilitation of LBP.
6. Demonstrate an understanding of diagnostic tests used for determining diagnosis of LBP.
7. Recognize the psychosocial effects of LBP.

Low back pain (LBP) is a complex, multifaceted medical problem that represents an exciting challenge to the occupational therapist. The frequently sudden onset with severe symptoms can be overwhelming to the patient. It is often seen as a narcissistic injury and inherently subjective. LBP affects the physical, psychological, emotional, financial, and social aspects of a person's life.[1,11] The occupational therapist well trained in the psychosocial and physical aspects of rehabilitation is an important member of the health care team.

In the United States approximately 79 billion dollars is spent each year on the direct and indirect costs of LBP.[5] "Back pain is the second-leading reason that Americans visit their doctors."[10] "LBP primarily affects 25- to 55-year-old adults, which places a significant burden on the work force."[4]

Many authors discuss the neuropsychological aspect of the pain experience and how it is compounded by emotional response.[5,12,16] Engel uses the definition of the International Association of the Study of Pain and includes a discussion of acute pain and of numerous differentiations of chronic pain.[5] A practitioner specializing in orthopedics or pain management should explore these and other references, in addition to the basic information presented here.

Diagnosis of LBP is difficult and presents an obstacle to successful treatment.[11] Other obstacles include frequent recurrence, wide variation in patient responses to specific pathological findings, and multiple possible causes of LBP in a patient.[14] LBP is often not the result of one single injury or event, but instead results from (1) participation in activities that are stressful to the joints of the spine, and (2) habitual use of physical positions over several hours, months, or even years that involve inappropriate use of body mechanics. These activities and positions include prolonged static postures such as slouched sitting and forward bending, as well as repetitive tasks like pushing, pulling, lifting, and carrying. The goals in managing LBP are the prevention of prolonged disability and a speedy return to previous function.

The occupational therapist's role in the rehabilitation of the LBP patient may vary, depending on the division of responsibility at the particular health care facility. Patient education and training in maintaining normal spinal alignment while performing functional activities are critical parts of the rehabilitation program. Whether pain is acute or chronic, patients with LBP will respond best to medical professionals who are knowledgeable, positive, and willing to work with them and with each other toward a successful outcome.

SPINAL ANATOMY

To help the therapist understand the medical and rehabilitation management of LBP, a brief review of lumbar anatomy is presented. A more in-depth study of spinal anatomy is recommended for those who will treat this population.

Vertebrae

The spine is composed of 33 stacked spinal vertebrae, 24 of which are movable (7 cervical, 12 thoracic, and 5 lumbar). Below those are five that are fused together to form the sacrum, and four rudimentary fused vertebrae that form the coccyx. The vertebrae are arranged in an S-curve balanced around the line of gravity. The lumbar vertebrae are the largest, reflecting the increasing load from head to pelvis. Each vertebra is made up of two parts: the vertebral body anteriorly and the vertebral arch posteriorly. The vertebral bodies are kidney shaped and separated by intervertebral disks.[9] The vertebral arch is made up of the pedicles, laminae, and seven bony transverse and articular processes.

The vertebral body and arch (Fig. 46-1) form an irregular ring called the *vertebral foramen*. The vertebral foramina of adjacent vertebrae form the spinal canal that encloses the spinal cord and its blood vessels. Facet joints made from the four articular processes above and below the transverse process guide and restrict the movements of the spine: flexion, extension, lateral flexion, and some rotation. The orientation of these facet joints allows considerable movement in trunk flexion and extension but limits lateral flexion and rotation. The transverse processes serve as the attachments for muscles and ligaments. At the junction of the vertebral body and arch, the vertebral notches of adjacent

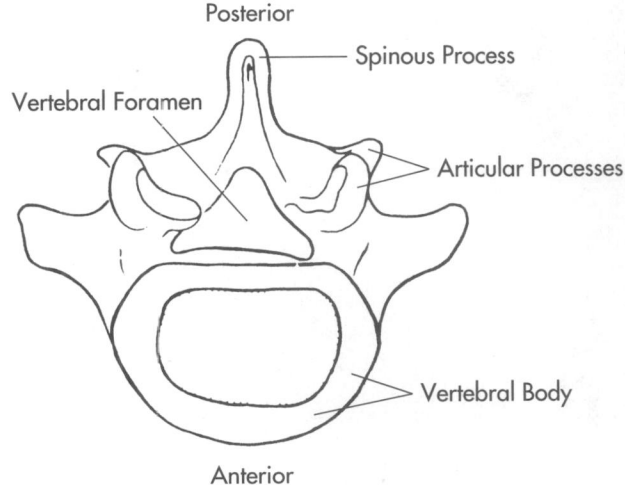

FIG. 46-1

Vertebral body and arch. (From Callahan P et al: *Stanford back school manual*, Stanford, Calif, 1984, Dept. of OT-PT, Stanford University Hospital.)

vertebrae form the intervertebral foramen, where the spinal nerves exit.

Ligaments

Spinal ligaments function to restrain or align the vertebrae. The anterior longitudinal ligament (ALL), a thick, strong band of fibers, runs along the anterior surface of the vertebral bodies, firmly attaching to the bodies and the intervertebral disks. The ALL limits extension of the vertebral column. The posterior longitudinal ligament (PLL) runs along the posterior aspect of the vertebral bodies anterior to the spinal cord. In the lumbar region it narrows considerably, contributing to the inherent **structural weakness** at the lower lumbar levels, where there is the greatest amount of spinal movement. The PLL functions to limit spinal flexion.

The ligamenta flava connect the laminae of adjacent vertebrae and lie posterior to the spinal cord. These ligaments limit flexion of the spinal column, and their elastic quality helps the spine return to upright from a flexed posture.[8]

INTERVERTEBRAL DISKS

Disorders of the intervertebral disks are common causes of LBP. The disks, interposed between adjacent surfaces of the vertebral bodies, are composed of two parts. The central portion, or nucleus pulposus, is a gelatinous substance and is surrounded by the annulus fibrosus, made up of concentric and oblique fibers that encase the nucleus. The nucleus is held under pressure in this casing. During vertebral column movements the nucleus moves posteriorly with flexion, anteriorly with extension, and to the opposite side with lateral flexion. Rotation substantially increases disk pressure and stretches the annular fibers. Static or repetitive flexion forces the nucleus posteriorly, and it can more easily rupture through the annulus. The combination movement of flexion and rotation is even more stressful to the disk.[9]

The lumbar disks are the widest but suffer a substantial loss of height in the aging process; hence the loss of spinal flexibility and height with advancing age. The nucleus pulposus sits more posteriorly in the lumbar spine. The annulus is therefore narrower and offers less support. These anatomical factors make the lumbar disks more vulnerable to injury, which contributes to the high incidence of LBP. Once a load on the disk is removed, it regains its normal height. This process requires a finite amount of time and depends on the health and age of the disk. If the disk is loaded again without time to regain its height, premature aging and potential derangement can result.[9]

When the disk is young and healthy and there is violence to the spine, the bones give way first. After age 25, degenerative changes occur in the annulus fibrosus, and the structure is weakened. Under these conditions, a minor strain can cause internal derangement of the disk, which causes severe pain and muscle spasm. A study by Nachemson[15] demonstrated stress to the L3 disk in various positions and postures (Fig. 46-2), which correlates well with the common histories of patients with LBP and the anatomical considerations described previously.

Nerves

The lumbar nerves exit at the intervertebral foramen at the levels of their respective vertebrae, conveying sensa-

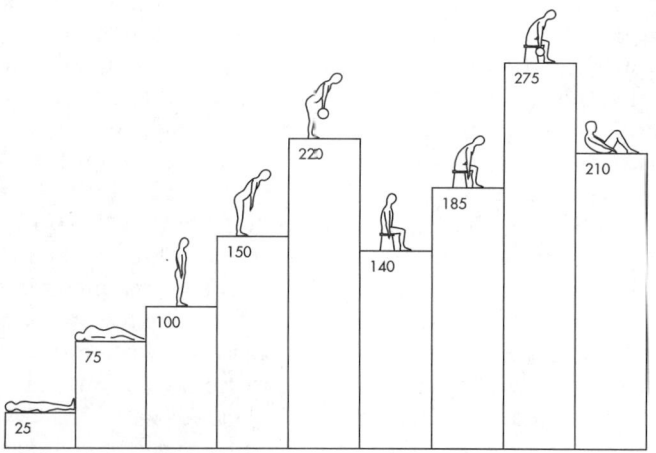

FIG. 46-2
Relative change in pressure in third lumbar disk with various postures and movements. (Adapted from Nachemson A: The lumbar spine: an orthopedic challenge, *Spine* 1[1]:59, 1976.)

tion and motor control to and from the lower extremities (LEs). The three major nerves innervating LE musculature are the femoral, obturator, and sciatic nerves. The close relationship of the disks, ligaments, and facet joints to the nerves complicates the diagnosis of LBP. Patients with LBP who develop LE symptoms should seek medical attention. When pain and symptoms move distally, the spinal nerve root may be compromised, as in sciatica.

Muscles

The muscles of the spine function to move the vertebral column but do little to keep it erect. Erect spinal posture is achieved by the hip and thigh muscles, primarily through the strong ligamentous support of the spine.[8] The muscles of the lower back are divided into three groups: the postvertebral, prevertebral, and lateral trunk muscles. The postvertebral muscles act to extend the spinal column and limit flexion of the trunk, and they accentuate the lumbar lordosis. The postvertebral muscles are categorized as deep, intermediate, and superficial muscles. The deeper they lie, the shorter is their course. The deep muscles include the transversospinalis, interspinalis, spinalis, longissimus, and iliocostalis. At the intermediate level is only one muscle, the serratus posterior inferior. The superficial muscle is the latissimus dorsi. The paravertebral muscles are known as the abdominal muscles and include the rectus abdominis, internal and external obliques, and the transversus abdominis. These muscles flex the spine, flatten the lumbar lordosis, and assist in rotating the spine. The lateral muscles of the trunk are the quadratus lumborum and the psoas. They flex the spine ipsilaterally and rotate it contralaterally, as well as accentuate the lumbar lordosis and flex the vertebral column when the pelvis is fixed.[9]

In summary, the spine is composed of a network of structures: the vertebrae, disks, ligaments, nerves, and muscles. The lumbar spine is subjected to the greatest kinetic strain and, because of the inherent structural weakness of the intervertebral disks and ligaments, is most vulnerable to injury.

REHABILITATION OF THE PATIENT WITH LOW BACK PAIN
Conservative Approach

The past 10 years have brought dramatic changes in health care delivery systems in the United States. In health maintenance organizations and managed care systems the primary care physician (PCP) must screen all patients first. Insurance companies require prior authorization for medical care, including occupational therapy (OT) and physical therapy (PT). Visits are limited, and therapists must evaluate, plan treatment regimens, and establish functional outcomes in a limited time. Patients must demonstrate consistent compliance and motivation and take full responsibility for their medical care. They must understand that with either acute LBP or chronic LBP, the therapist cannot "fix" them or their pain.

The PCP (e.g., an internist or general practitioner) sees patients first. The initial evaluation will vary. The examination should include a thorough medical history, both past and present; a review of the symptoms and functional limitations; observation of posture, gait, trunk mobility, strength, reflexes, and sensation; and palpation of the spine and surrounding soft tissues. A diagnosis is made, and medication (usually a nonsteroidal antiinflammatory drug, or NSAID) is prescribed, along with rest and restrictions on activities.

Unfortunately, pamphlets with instructions for exercise are sometimes given without additional direction. If substantial relief is not achieved in about a week, the physician who is knowledgeable about rehabilitation will prescribe a course of PT and OT.

Role functions for rehabilitation specialists in pain management vary according to the rehabilitation setting. Many factors influence how roles are defined. Therapists may acquire additional skills as a result of interest and studies; the distribution of these skills among practitioners may influence whether an occupational therapist or a physical therapist teaches the skill. A physical therapist who has movement training may be more skilled in teaching moving from sit to stand and from floor to stand. Similarly, an occupational therapist with stress management training will be qualified to teach diaphragmatic breathing, visualization, and other techniques of **cognitive distraction** to help the patient modulate the experience of pain. Open communication and flexibility among practitioners promote effective role function. In rural settings there may be only one therapist for hundreds of miles. By necessity the isolated therapist may perform most of the functions that follow in this chapter.

Evaluation

Physical Therapy

Often the patient is referred first to PT to address pain, muscle spasm, limited joint mobility, and postural defects. The PT evaluation may include a subjective history, including the following information:

1. Mechanism of the injury
2. Progression of symptoms
3. Recent treatment and results
4. The patient's medical history
5. Sleep disturbances, including sleep surface, positions, and use of pillows
6. Work postures
7. Activities of daily living (ADL) postures and the behavior of the symptoms during these postures and activities (Fig. 46-3)

8. Prior level of function in self-care, work, and leisure activities

An objective examination includes analysis of the following items:

1. Static and dynamic posture
2. Gait
3. Active range of motion (ROM) of the spine
4. Active ROM of all extremities
5. Pelvic asymmetry
6. Tension signs
7. Strength, reflexes, and sensation
8. LE muscle flexibility and symmetry
9. Passive movement testing of the spinal segments
10. Palpation of soft tissue restrictions along the spine and surrounding areas

Special tests are performed to help with the differential diagnosis, especially to identify sacroiliac dysfunction and hip pathology.

An analysis of the data will yield a treatment plan, which may include the following components: (1) positioning for relief of muscle spasm and pain; (2) mobilization techniques to improve mobility of specific joints and soft tissues and relieve muscle spasm and pain; (3) muscle stretching to gain symmetry to all musculature, especially the LEs; and (4) training in posture, body mechanics, strengthening, conditioning, and returning to recreational sports and activities. Training in a home program includes first-aid tips for pain and muscle spasm relief, flexibility, mobility, symptom control, posture correction, strengthening, and general conditioning for optimal health and return to the preinjury level of function. The overall goals of PT are to provide symptom relief, to normalize joint and soft-tissue mobility, and to establish an effective exercise regimen to achieve the highest functional level for the patient.

Occupational Therapy

The Stanford Health Services Rehabilitation Services questionnaire (Fig. 46-3) generates information the physical therapist might share with the occupational therapist (this is generally a more efficient use of practitioner time than having both disciplines collect similar information). However, the occupational therapist may prefer to ask the patient some of these questions (1 to 13) directly. These questions could form a "**self-report**" questionnaire, with the patient asked to fill out the information in the presence of the occupational therapist. Patient performance of this task affords the therapist an opportunity to assess comprehension of written material (important if the patient is to follow a home exercise program). This could be graded with answers that best reflect present ability. Concurrently, the therapist can observe the patient's sitting tolerance and pain behaviors.

A functional assessment of the patient's ADL is important. Actual observation of each task enables the

STANFORD HEALTH SERVICES
REHABILITATION SERVICES QUESTIONNAIRE

Name: _____ Age: _____ Date: _____

1. Pain Began: _____ How? _____
   Month   Year
   _____

2. Please draw a picture of your pain <u>today</u>.

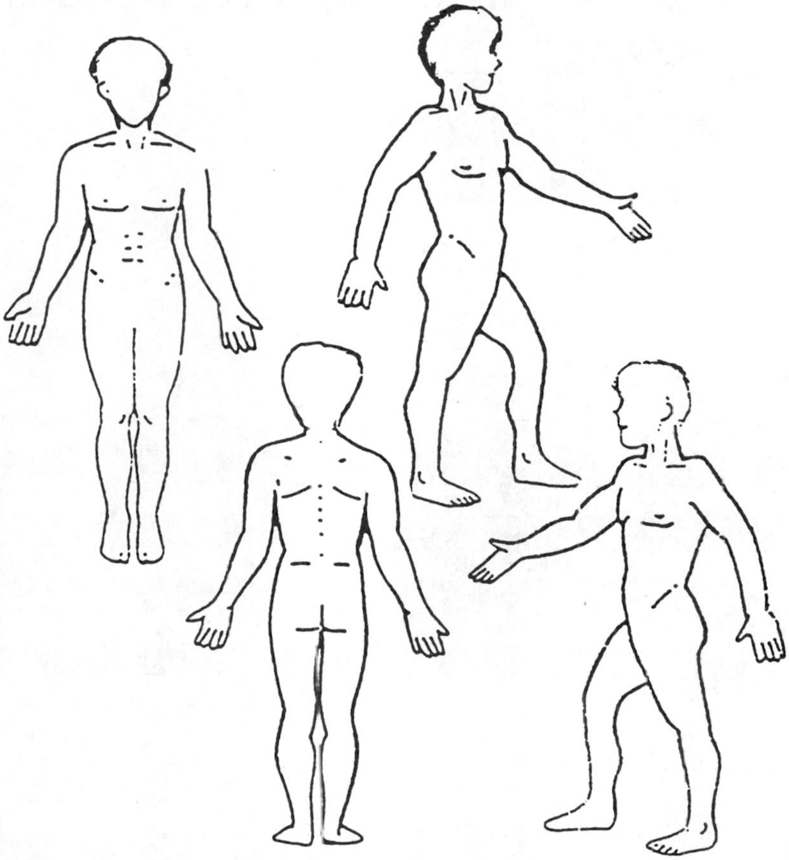

3. Rate your pain:
   0 = Painfree   10 = Severe/Disabling

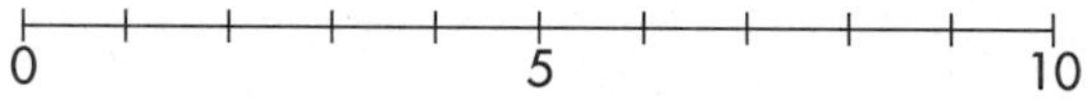

   |————|————|————|————|————|————|————|————|————|————|
   0   5   10

4. Medications: _____
   _____

5. Does rest help decrease your pain?
   yes_____   no_____

6. Please check if you have (or have had):
   ____ High blood pressure   ____ Bowel/Bladder
   ____ Respiratory   ____ Pregnancy
   ____ Heart disease   ____ Allergies
   ____ Diabetes   ____ Skin Disorders
   ____ Arthritis
   ____ Fractures (where?_____)
   ____ Cancer (where?_____)
   ____ Neurological disease

7. Please check if you have had:

√	Test	Results
	CT Scan	
	MRI	
	Myelogram	
	X-Rays	
	EMG/NCV	

8. Please list surgeries/dates: _____
   _____
   _____

9. Doctor's restrictions on activity – please list:
   _____
   _____
   _____

10. A. What is your occupation? _____
    B. Are you currently working? _____Yes _____No Last day worked: _____
    C. What percentage of your day do you sit? _____ Stand? _____

11. Please check if you have difficulty performing the following activities:
    ____ Dressing   ____ Childcare   ____ Gardening   ____ Housekeeping
    ____ Toileting   ____ Cooking   ____ Home or car repair ____ Public transportation
    ____ Bathing   ____ Laundry   ____ Shopping   ____ Keyboard/typing
    ____ Eating   ____ Walking   ____ Telephone   ____ Driving car
    ____ Writing   ____ Other: _____

Continued

FIG. 46-3
Rehabilitation services questionnaire. (Courtesy of J Smithline, Stanford Health Services, Department of Rehabilitation Services, Stanford, Calif.)

12. My pain is	BETTER	WORSE	NO CHANGE	MAX. TIME (MINUTES)
Sitting (soft chair)				
Sitting (hard chair)				
Lying on my stomach				
Lying on my back				
Lying on my side				
Walking				
Standing				
Climbing stairs				
Coughing or sneezing				
Putting on my shoes				
Bending over				
Lifting				
First thing in the morning				
Middle of the day				
Before bedtime				

13. I wake up at night because of pain _____ 0, _____ 1-2, _____ 3 or more times a night.

14. Please check all treatments for pain that you have received and <u>circle</u> those that have helped the most.

√	TREATMENT	√	TREATMENT
	Medication		Chiropractic
	Bed rest		Acupressure
	Hospitalization, but no surgery		Acupuncture
	Injections		Other. Describe:
	Back manipulations		
	Corset or brace		
	Physical therapy, Where?		When?
	Name of P.T. or clinic:		Phone #

15. If you have had physical therapy, what did your treatment include? Please check all that apply:

√	TREATMENT	√	TREATMENT
	Hot packs		Ultrasound
	Ice packs		Massage
	Range of motion exercises		TENS (transcutaneous nerve stimulator)
	Strengthening exercises		Training in posture, body mechanics
	Spinal mobilization		Conditioning program
	Electrical stimulation		Home exercise program. Since:
	Traction (Sitting)		Other. Describe:
	Traction (Lying)		

16. Are you performing a home exercise program? _____ Yes _____ No   How often? _____ × week.

17. What are your leisure activities now? _____

_____

18. What activities (vocational, functional, recreational) do you want to return to? _____

_____

_____

19. If we could do <u>one</u> thing for you, what would it be? _____

FIG. 46-3—cont'd
Rehabilitation services questionnaire. (Courtesy of J Smithline, Stanford Health Services, Department of Rehabilitation Services, Stanford, Calif.)

occupational therapist to evaluate faulty postures and body mechanics. Often patients can verbalize the general principles for minimizing stress to the spine but are not aware that they do not observe these principles in ADL. A kitchen, bedroom, and work simulation area greatly expand the occupational therapist's contexts for evaluation. Activities including dressing, toileting, hygiene and self-care, bed mobility, transfers (from the bed, sofa, chair, bath, and shower), loading and unloading the dishwasher, meal preparation, oven use, refrigerator use, carrying and lifting from various heights, reaching, and simulated work activities can be observed and problems identified. The organization of the kitchen, home, work environment, and frequently used objects can be discussed and modified to minimize spinal stress.

During the evaluation the occupational therapist observes spontaneous movements, such as scratching the foot, posture when sitting, and sequence of movements in rising from a chair. These can be compared to movements performed when the patient knows he or she is being observed. Pain behaviors such as facial grimacing and grunts are noted. Specific lifting and carrying evaluations may be conducted, using work evaluation systems (see Chapter 16) or simulations created by the therapist to mimic a patient's individual occupational demands. Throughout the evaluation the therapist notes the patient's spinal posture, keeping in mind the anatomical constraints of the spinal structures.

Depending on the extent or availability of information from the physical therapist, a physical evaluation including strength, extremity and trunk mobility, general posture, and ambulation may be performed. Finally, the occupational therapist quantifies the information collected, establishing a baseline from which progress can be measured. Probably the greatest advantage of this format for evaluation is that a natural dialogue will ensue, which will provide an opportunity to begin establishing rapport. At the completion of the above the therapist can discuss the difficulties the patient has defined as goals for treatment in OT.

Treatment

Physical Therapy

Finding pain-free positions for rest is the first concern of the physical therapist. Each person is different, but positions of comfort can be found in prone, supine, and side-lying positions by using pillows and towel rolls to support the natural contours of the body. This will allow muscles to relax (Fig. 46-4). Resting should be performed as an exercise. Initially lying down for 10 to 20 minutes three or more times a day can decrease the stress to the spine from sitting, standing, and walking and provide considerable pain relief. Bed rest is rarely prescribed because of the threat of decreased muscle tone. Nonetheless, if an individual is unable to tolerate

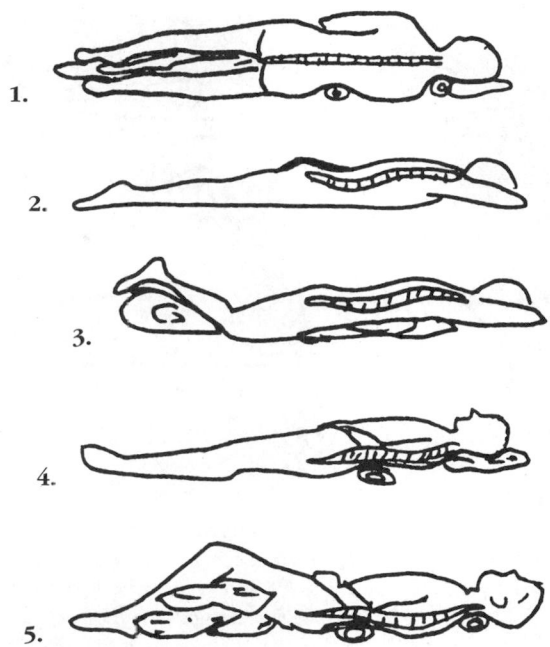

FIG. 46-4

Positions for rest using pillows and towel rolls to support body contours, allowing muscles to relax. (From Smithline J: *First aid tips for back pain*, Stanford, Calif, 1993, Stanford Health Services, Department of Rehabilitation Services.)

the upright position, lying down most of the day is indicated. Pain relief should occur in 1 to 3 days.

Bed mobility techniques and skills could be taught by either the occupational or physical therapist, but collaboration is critical to ensure that sequential learning is taking place. Incorrect performance in bed mobility can contribute to LBP; the patient must learn to eliminate torsion and flexion of the lumbar spine (Fig. 46-5). Lying down on the bed using a prone approach is also helpful. To do this, the patient touches the bed with his or her hands while the leg closest to the bed is elevated to mattress level. The trunk is slowly lowered to the bed surface and the supporting leg is then lifted onto the bed. Spinal alignment must be maintained during this maneuver. Ice (or heat) can be used at home to relieve pain and decrease abnormal muscle tone while resting. Home remedies for ice or heat pack are detailed in Box 46-1. The side-lying and prone positions are most favored and allow ease in using ice or heat pack applications. Supine lying is least favored because of the direct pressure on the lumbar spine and the stress placed on the anatomical structures when the spine flattens to meet the supporting surface. Sitting, especially if prolonged, often aggravates LBP. In addition to using correct posture, patients must learn to use lumbar supports. These can be created by rolling up a towel to fit the lumbar curve (Fig. 46-6). Patients are cautioned against sitting in hot tubs or saunas.

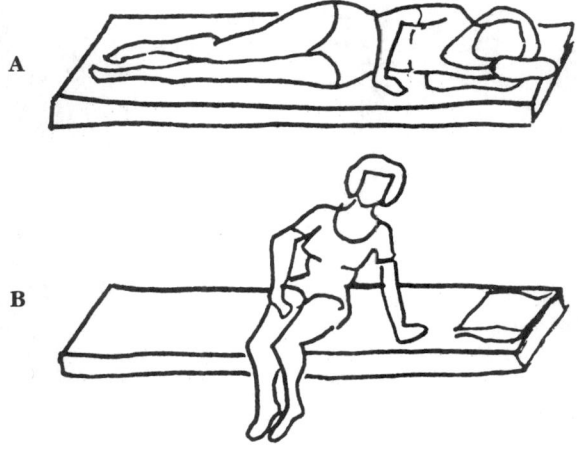

FIG. 46-5
Method for getting up from bed or couch to reduce stress on low back. **A,** Roll to side. **B,** Bend knees forward to bring feet off bed and push up to sitting, using arms and keeping back straight with normal curve. (From Smithline J: *First aid tips for back pain,* Stanford, Calif, 1993, Stanford Health Services, Department of Rehabilitation Services.)

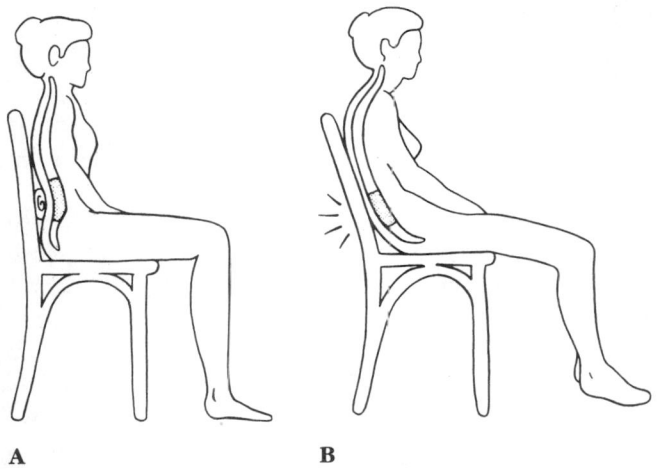

A **B**

FIG. 46-6
Sitting postures. Most important is keeping normal curves in back, preferably by ensuring proper support, especially for low back. (From Callahan P et al: *Stanford Back School Manual,* Stanford, Calif, 1984, Stanford Health Services, Department of Rehabilitation Services.)

Patients with LBP should not exercise because this activity can aggravate the symptoms and prolong the disability. Once pain is controlled, exercise can be initiated. Exercise must be designed for the specific individual and should be performed slowly, gently, and progressively, as the symptoms allow. Exercise must be performed free of pain. If the pain and muscle spasm continue, the therapist may use modalities such as ultrasound or electrical stimulation to normalize muscle tone and decrease pain. Pelvic traction can be helpful in relieving LE radicular symptoms, pain, and paresthesias radiating into one or both LEs.

BOX 46-1
Use of Ice or Heat to Reduce Muscle Spasm

Use ice or heat
Ice or heat, or both, can be helpful in reducing pain and muscle spasm. Ice is usually more effective than heat. Sometimes using heat for 10 minutes, then ice for 10 minutes works well. Below are some preparation techniques.

Remember
1. Use ice or heat when resting, not when sleeping or sitting.
2. Use no longer than 20 minutes.
3. Repeat three to five times per day as pain indicates.

Ice pack preparation

Method 1
Place an unopened bag of frozen peas wrapped in a damp towel on the back. Use as directed above. Return peas to the freezer. Use again and again. DO NOT EAT PEAS.

Method 2
Place cracked ice cubes in a zipper-locking bag. Place on a damp towel on the back. Use as directed above. Return to the freezer. Recrack ice before next application.

Heat pack preparation

Method 1
Place damp towel in microwave to heat. Test temperature, then place on back. Use as directed above.

Method 2
Use heating pad set on LOW. Do *not* sleep on the heating pad. Do not sit in chair with heating pad. Use as directed above.

The physical therapist will perform a variety of manual therapy techniques, including (1) joint mobilization to provide pain relief and reestablish normal physiological and accessory ROM to the lumbar spinal segments; (2) soft-tissue mobilization, including myofascial and massage techniques to alter soft-tissue restrictions that contribute to pain and mobility limitations; and (3) muscle stretching to achieve symmetry and normal length to LE muscles that directly affect spinal function. These muscles include the hamstrings, psoas, tensor fasciae latae, piriformis, rectus femoris, gastrocnemius, and soleus.

Once pain relief is achieved and symptoms are under control, aerobic and strength training can begin, but the training must be very conservative and graded very gently. Recurrence of LBP is frequent and often the result of advancing too rapidly with exercise or activity. Pool exercise is an excellent treatment alternative for patients in the acute stage. The buoyancy of the water and elimination of gravity on the weight-bearing joints allows ease of movement and enables pain-free exercise. Walking and specific exercise are more easily tolerated in water, and patient compliance is very good. Pool temperatures for ambulation and exercise should be 88° to 92° F. Swimming laps, if tolerated, can also be beneficial. Using aqua vests or flotation devices may allow the patient to perform vigorous aerobic activity without loading the spine vertically.

Teaching and modifying a home program will be ongoing during the course of treatment. With health insurance limitations, PT visits may be extended over time to allow musculoskeletal changes to take place, allowing for changes in the program with each visit. An average of three to six visits is commonly authorized by health maintenance organizations and managed care programs. Some insurance benefits limit the duration of treatment to 60 days. These time constraints often make completion of a PT program and the return to work with previous activity expectations difficult for the patient.

Occupational Therapy
The occupational therapist designs a specific treatment plan that could include the following:
1. Education in **energy conservation** and **pacing** skills to be used for symptom control with all self-maintenance, work, and play and leisure tasks

2. Progressive, repetitive tasks to build strength and endurance for specific activities, minimizing spinal stress
3. Discussion of faulty body mechanics and poor postures, with specific education and practice in correct techniques during functional activities
4. Training in the use of assistive devices to increase independence in ADL despite pain and limitation and to minimize recurrence of symptoms
5. Training in simulated work tasks to minimize spinal stress and grade tolerance of these tasks
6. Simulation of body mechanics for play and leisure activities to determine if the activities are appropriate during the rehabilitation phase. The overall goal of OT in treatment of patients with LBP is to achieve the highest level of functional independence in all tasks of role function, including self-care, play and leisure, and work activities.

OT can begin as soon as the patient can tolerate activity in the upright position. Communication with the physical therapist is critical for ensuring that (1) both therapists teach posture and body mechanics with similar principles and (2) suggestions for spinal alignment are coordinated. The occupational therapist also addresses self-care, including hygiene, dressing, and meal preparation. Assistive devices are considered.

Functional training and practice with techniques will be more successful than just discussing them with the patient. Examples include sitting, lifting (Fig. 46-7), carrying, and standing. These activities are monitored to quantify progress. Work simplification and energy

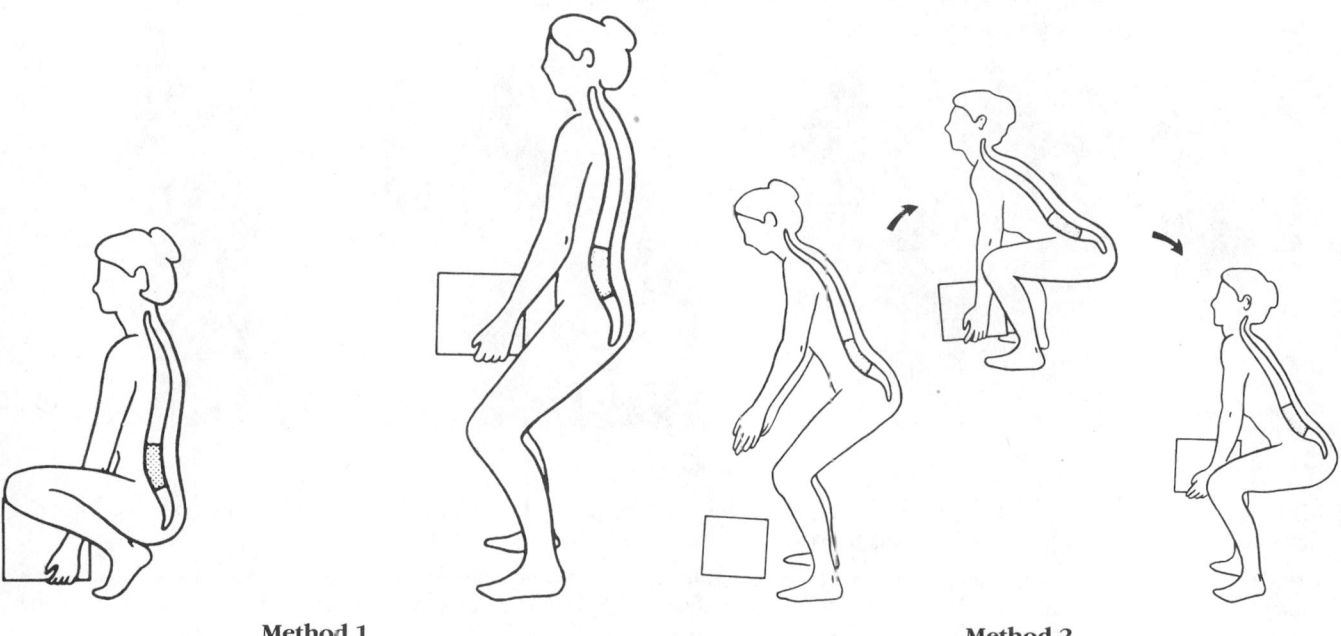

Method 1   Method 2

FIG. 46-7
Lifting methods that protect lumbar spine from injury. (From Callahan P et al: *Stanford back school manual*, Stanford, Calif, 1984, Stanford Health Services, Department of Rehabilitation Services.)

conservation skills are taught and applied to all functional activities. The occupational therapist can perform functional capacity or work tolerance assessment using work assessment systems or simulations created in the OT setting. This information is vital to the physician, patient, and employer and is the foundation for the development of reasonable, achievable goals. Returning to work may mean part-time employment or activity-restricted work. The appropriate activity level can be determined by the occupational therapist through assessment and observation of simulated work tasks.

Helping patients define potential difficulties they may encounter at work is necessary before they attempt to return. This problem identification and problem-solving approach helps prevent exacerbation of symptoms and reinjury. This approach is reinforced as a technique the patients must use after rehabilitation to "problem solve" each "flare-up" in the future. A work hardening program can be initiated and job simulation tasks can be practiced and timed (see Chapter 16).

Body Mechanics Training

Activities of daily living (ADL) must be scrutinized to observe stresses on the lumbar spine. Keeping in mind the anatomical weakness in the lumbar disk and PLL, the occupational therapist must observe patients in all

Forward bending places increased stress on the structures in the back and neck.

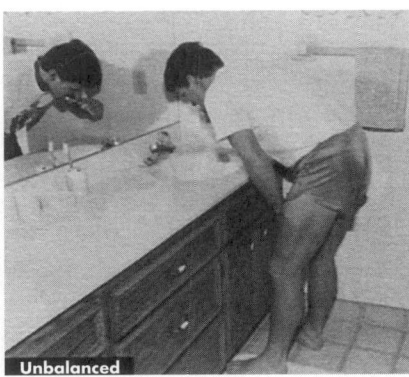 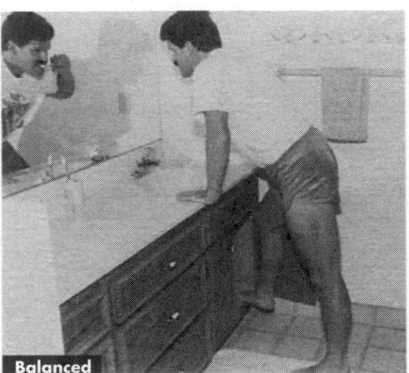 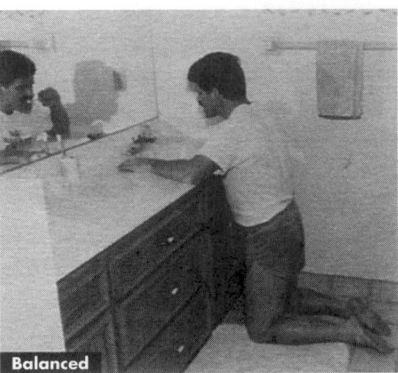

If you are going to work over the bathroom sink, place one hand on the counter to support your weight and bend at the hips, not the back. Elevate one foot and keep your head up and your back in a balanced position.

You can also try performing some of your sink activities in the kneeling position to reduce the temptation to bend forward. Use the counter for support when you come to standing.

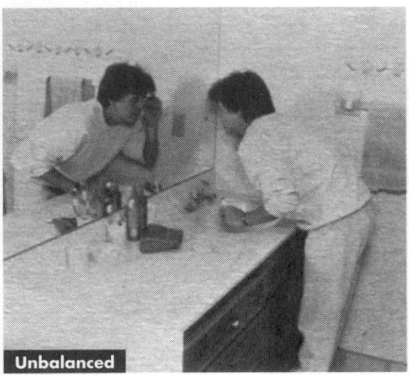 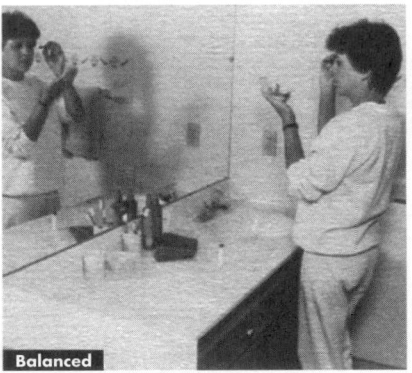 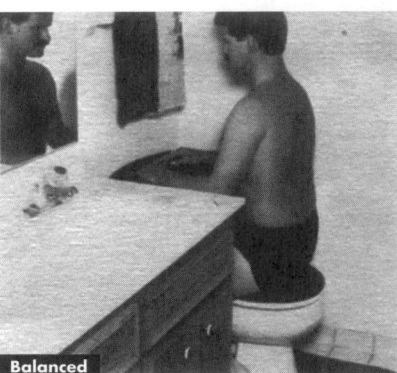

Using a hand-held mirror eliminates the need to bend over the sink.

During an acute episode of back pain you can minimize stress when using the toilet by facing the back of the toilet. This will prevent you from bending forward and will provide you with support when you come to standing.

Additional suggestions: Purchasing an accordion-mounted mirror for shaving and applying make-up allows you to avoid the temptation to lean over the sink. Purchase a good shower caddy and place razor, toothbrush, toothpaste, and face cloth in the shower. Use a tub mirror (not glass) to avoid activities over a low sink.

FIG. 46-8
Bathroom activities. (From Melnick M, Saunders R, Saunders HD: *Managing back pain: daily activities guide for back pain patients*, Minneapolis, Minn, Educational Opportunities.)

daily tasks, especially those that were reported to aggravate symptoms in the subjective assessment.

The following information is adapted from *Managing Back Pain*.[13] Numerous everyday activities are evaluated, and faulty body mechanics are described as "unbalanced." Stressful positions include prolonged static postures with a flexed lumbar spine, repetitive bending with a flexed spine, and lifting and carrying when the normal lumbar curve is not maintained. It is very important to avoid tasks or positions that do not allow a balanced posture. The patient is taught to visualize making the movement necessary to perform the activity before attempting to initiate the activity.

Bathroom Activities

Forward bending places increased stress on structures in the back and neck. To work over the bathroom sink, the patient should place one hand on the counter to support weight and bend at the hips, not the back. The patient should elevate one foot and keep the head up and the back in a balanced position. The patient can also try performing some of the sink activities in the kneeling position to reduce the temptation to bend forward. The counter can be used for support when coming to standing. Using a handheld mirror eliminates the need to bend over the sink. During an acute episode of back pain the patient minimizes stress when using the toilet by facing the back of the toilet to prevent bending forward and to provide support when coming to standing (Fig. 46-8).

Additional suggestions include the following: (1) an accordion-mounted mirror for shaving and applying make-up reduces the temptation to lean over the sink;

(2) a good shower caddy can hold razor, toothbrush, toothpaste, and face cloth in the shower; (3) a tub mirror (not glass) can help the patient avoid activities over a low sink; and (4) a tub bar will promote safety if balance is poor or if patient is elderly.

Bed Making

When making the bed, the patient should not stand on one side and reach across the bed. The temptation to bend forward may be reduced by kneeling or climbing onto the bed, which encourages keeping the back in a balanced position. To complete the task the patient should walk around the bed to finish the far side. Using a lightweight comforter instead of a heavy bedspread decreases spinal stress (Fig. 46-9).

Kitchen Activities

Commonly used items can be arranged between waist and shoulder height to reduce the need to bend over. To reach something from a lower level, the patient can drop down onto one knee, take the object, put the object on the counter, and then use the support of a table, chair, or counter to assist in coming to standing. This support helps maintain the normal curves in the spine (Fig. 46-10). If support is not available, the patient can place the hands on the thighs and push off with the arms.

To load the dishwasher, the patient should place the rinsed dishes on the counter near the dishwasher, go to one knee, and load the dishwasher from this position. This method helps avoid prolonged or repetitive forward bending and twisting movements. The process is reversed to unload the dishwasher. The patient should

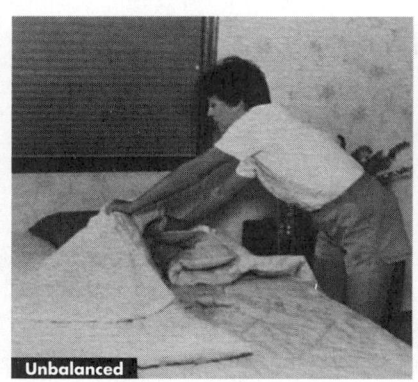 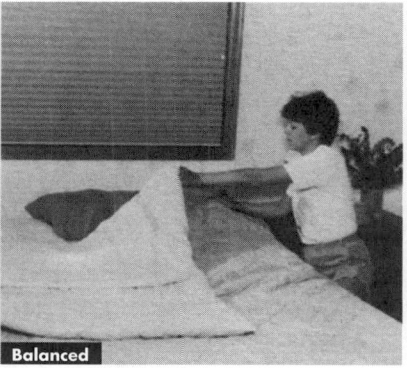 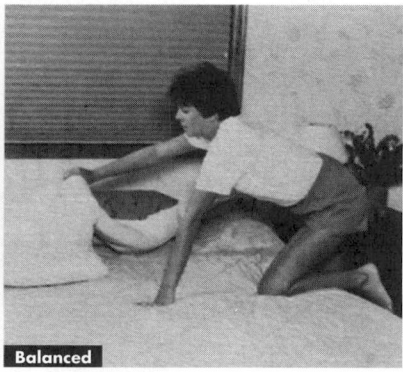

When making the bed, do not stand on one side and reach. The temptation to bend forward can be reduced by kneeling or climbing onto the bed. This will encourage you to keep your back in a balanced position. If you are going to perform the task while standing, walk around the bed to complete the far side.

Additional suggestions: Use a lightweight comforter instead of a heavy bedspread to decrease spinal stress.

FIG. 46-9
Making a bed. (From Melnick M, Saunders R, Saunders HD: *Managing back pain: daily activities guide for back pain patients*, Minneapolis, Minn, Educational Opportunities.)

It is very important to avoid tasks or positions which do not allow a balanced posture. Take a few seconds to approach each task in a way which will minimize the stress to your back.

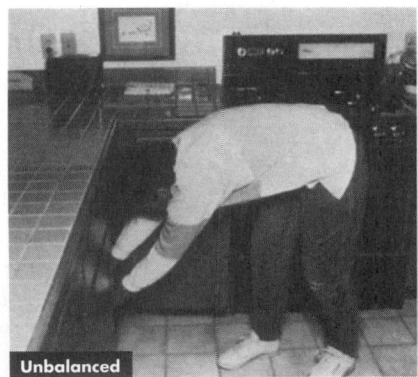 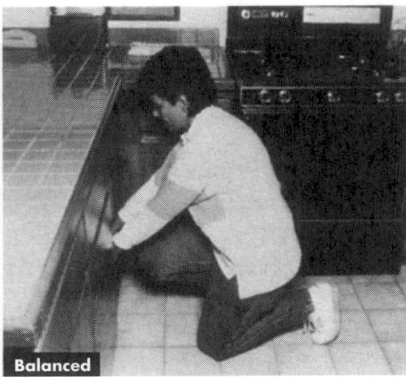 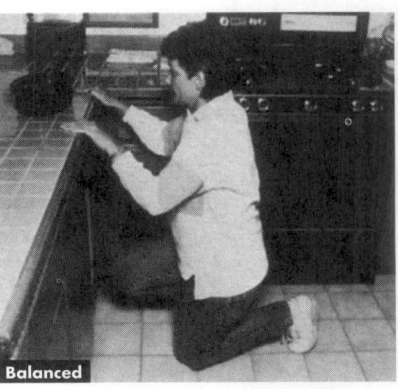

Arrange commonly used items between waist and shoulder height to reduce the need to bend over. If you need to reach something from a lower level, drop down onto one knee, grab the object, put the object on the counter and then use the support of a table, chair or counter to assist you while you come to standing. This support will help you maintain the normal curves in your spine. If you do not have support available, place your hands on your thighs and push off with your arms.

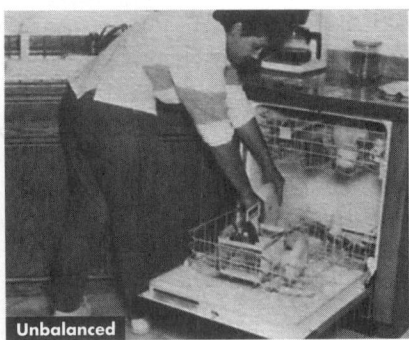 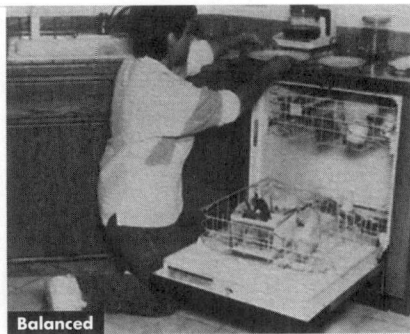 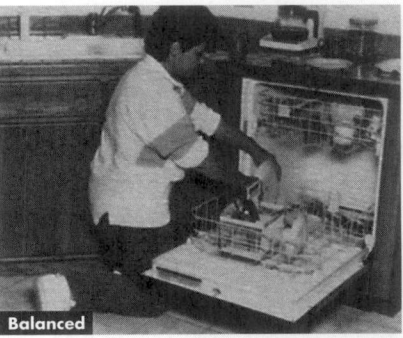

To load the dishwasher, place the rinsed dishes on the counter near the dishwasher. Go to one knee and load the dishwasher from this position. This helps you avoid prolonged or repetitive forward bending and twisting movements. Reverse the process to unload the dishwasher. Use support when you come to standing.

Additional suggestions: Remove silverware basket before loading and place it on the counter. Fill with silverware while standing, then return the basket to the dishwasher. Use top tray only to decrease bending.

FIG. 46-10
Kitchen activities. (From Melnick M, Saunders R, Saunders HD: *Managing back pain: daily activities guide for back pain patients*, Minneapolis, Minn, Educational Opportunities.)

use support when coming to standing. Additional suggestions are to (1) remove the silverware basket before loading and place it on the counter, fill it with silverware while standing, then return the basket to the dishwasher and (2) use only the top tray to decrease the need for bending (Fig. 46-10).

Laundry

When the patient does laundry, loads should be kept small and manageable. Several small loads place less stress on the back than one or two large ones. The patient should avoid bending forward into the machines and should not try to handle large bundles of clothes, particularly if they are wet. When loading or un-

loading a front-loading washer or dryer, the patient should drop to one knee to avoid any forward bending and twisting and should use support when coming to standing (Fig. 46-11).

Home Maintenance

Participation in vacuuming, car maintenance, mowing, and shoveling is not *recommended during the early stages of recovery.* Once the condition has stabilized, the patient may be taught methods for preventing a recurrence of symptoms. Sweeping and vacuuming can be performed as if the vacuum or broom were attached to the body. The patient should move the feet and legs rather than reaching or bending forward and

Keep loads small and manageable. Several small loads will place less stress on your back than one or two large ones.

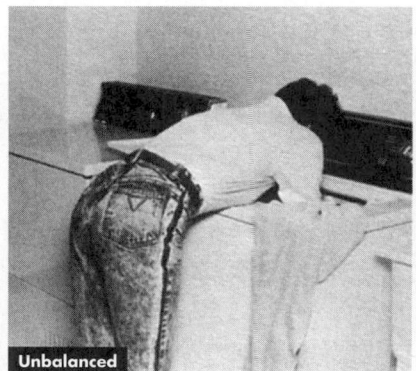 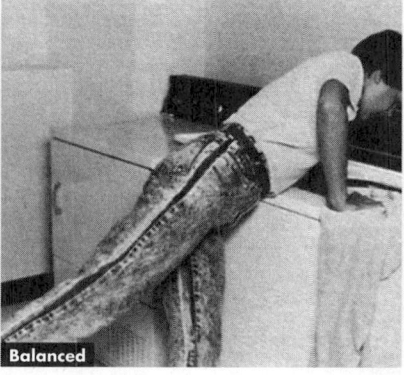 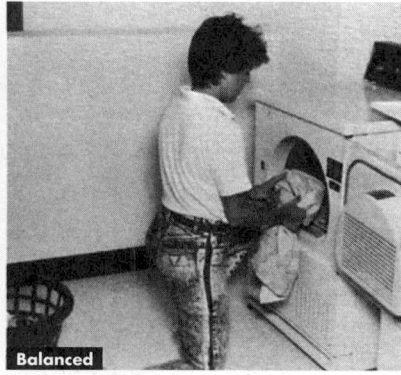

Avoid bending forward into the machines. Do not try to handle large bundles of clothes, particularly if they are wet. When loading or unloading a front-loading washer or dryer, drop to one knee to avoid any forward bending and twisting. Use support when coming to standing

FIG. 46-11
Doing laundry. (From Melnick M, Saunders R, Saunders HD: *Managing back pain: daily activities guide for back pain patients,* Minneapolis, Minn, Educational Opportunities.)

NOTE: Participation in the following activities (vacuuming, car maintenance, mowing and shoveling) is not recommended during the early stages of recovery. These activities are presented to offer methods for preventing a recurrence of your symptoms once your condition has stabilized.

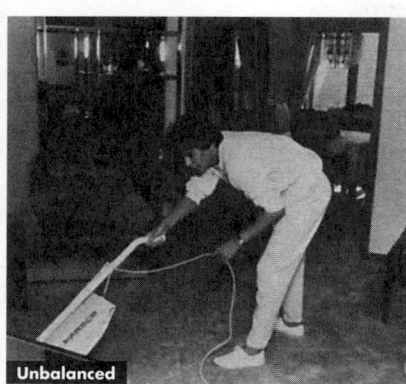 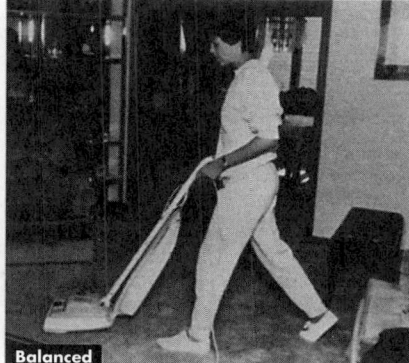 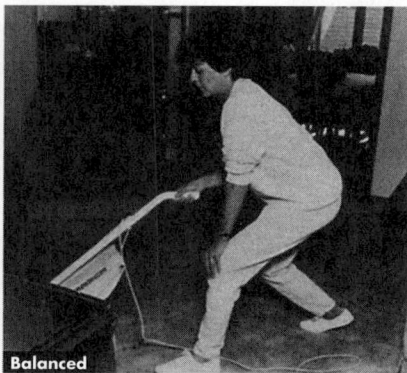

Perform the tasks as if the vacuum or broom were attached to your body. Move your feet and legs rather than reaching or bending forward. Avoid twisting. If you must vacuum or sweep under a table or chair, bend at your hips and knees and keep your back in a balanced position.

Additional suggestions: Lightweight electric brooms make the job much easier. Beware of self-powered vacuum cleaners. They are very heavy!

FIG. 46-12
Sweeping and vacuuming. (From Melnick M, Saunders R, Saunders HD: *Managing back pain: daily activities guide for back pain patients,* Minneapolis, Minn, Educational Opportunities.)

should avoid twisting. If it is necessary to vacuum or sweep under a table or chair, the patient should bend at the hips and knees and keep the back in a balanced position (Fig. 46-12). Lightweight electric brooms make the job much easier.

Gardening may evoke LBP because many people attempt it on the first warm day, after months of sedentary activity indoors. Patients with LBP must learn to prepare by using stretching and conditioning exercises before undertaking extensive gardening. Most gardening catalogues have functional tools such as long-handled rakes, kneeling pads, and knee pads. Some shovels come with hand-controlled jaws to capture and hold the soil. Lightweight gardening stools allow patients to sit while bending forward at the hips to remove dead flowers and perform other similar tasks. Sitting rather than standing helps to conserve energy.

The home can be arranged to meet the needs of the patient with LBP. The following are some suggestions for this arrangement:

1. Place all frequently used items on shelves at waist to chest level.
2. Store refrigerator or freezer items most frequently used on the top shelves of the compartment.
3. Keep a kneeling pad in the kitchen and use it when using the oven, dishwasher, lower shelves of the refrigerator or freezer, and floor-level cupboards.
4. Have a wheeled cart available to conserve energy and avoid unnecessary lifting and carrying.
5. Ask packing clerks in the stores to pack bags lightly and ask for carry-out assistance or delivery service.
6. Line the bottom of the car trunk with boxes, crates, or other means to raise the level of the floor, which will reduce the necessity to lean far into the trunk to place or remove packages. Alternately, use the back seat to hold groceries. (Transporting grocery bags is an awkward activity and should be practiced with supervision.)
7. Shop in stores that offer waist-high, shallow grocery carts.
8. If pain suddenly increases because of a stressful physical position, stand upright and realign the spine to its normal curves and perform stretching exercises (as instructed by therapist) before resuming the same activity.

MEDICAL MANAGEMENT OF LOW BACK PAIN
Diagnostic Tests

If management of acute LBP is not successful with medication, rest, and rehabilitation, further diagnostic testing may be indicated. The PCP then refers the patient to a specialist, usually an orthopedist or neurosurgeon. **Diagnostic tests** are often ordered. These may include the following.

X-Ray Examination
Radiographic evaluation (an x-ray examination) is used to rule out fractures, degenerative disease, possible metastatic disease, and structural abnormalities.

Magnetic Resonance Imaging
Magnetic resonance imaging (MRI) visualizes bones and tissues using a magnetic field and radio waves. The technique is used to localize a problem area and confirm clinical impressions such as herniated disks or spinal stenosis. A study using MRI showed that 66% of people without complaints of LBP had abnormal findings at one or more vertebral levels.[10]

Computed Tomography
Computed tomography (CT) uses cross-sectional x-ray films to define bony and soft-tissue abnormalities. This procedure is used less often for spinal problems now because the MRI is superior at visualizing soft-tissue abnormalities.

Diskogram
In a diskogram, contrast material is injected into the intervertebral disk to see whether symptoms are reproduced and clinical impressions are confirmed.

Myelogram
In a myelogram, iodinated contrast material is injected into the dural sac in order to outline spinal structures on x-ray film. Use of this procedure has declined with the advent of the MRI and CT.

Bone Scan
In a bone scan, radioactive material is injected intravenously and the body is scanned after several hours, making it possible to identify infections or tumors in the skeletal system.

Nerve Conduction Velocity and Electromyography
Nerve conduction velocity and electromyography use electric current to provide physiological data about nerve root dysfunction and peripheral neuropathic conditions, often caused by disk herniation.[17]

INVASIVE, NONSURGICAL PROCEDURES

Epidural corticosteroid injection is an option before surgery. This outpatient procedure can be performed in the hospital with local anesthesia. Relief can occur up to 1 week later, and the corticosteroid medication lasts up to 3 months. By then the patient has resumed activities and often continues to be functional. If partial relief is obtained, another injection may be performed from 1 to 4 weeks later.[6] The patient who feels much better must be cautioned to continue self-pacing and performing exercises recommended by the physical therapist.

Another outpatient procedure performed with local anesthesia is the *percutaneous diskectomy*. Specialized instrumentation is introduced that suctions out the damaged disk material. Very specific criteria are used to determine candidates for this procedure.[3]

SURGICAL PROCEDURES

Indications for surgery include bowel, bladder, and sexual dysfunction, saddle anesthesia, muscle weakness with progressive neurological deficits, and significant pain with the presence of structural deformities. Common procedures include *laminotomy and diskectomy*, in which part of the lamina is excised to expose the nerve root and disk. The extruded material is removed along with the fragmented part of the nucleus.[6]

In a *foraminotomy* small pieces of bone around the intervertebral foramen are excised to allow more room for the spinal nerve. This procedure is usually done in conjunction with a laminotomy. A *decompressive laminectomy* is the removal of the entire lamina and therefore the spinous process, to decompress the spinal canal. It is usually performed in patients with spinal stenosis. A *posterolateral fusion* is performed when there is evidence of spinal instability. Autogenous iliac crest bone graft is used to stabilize the lumbar segments.[6]

Surgery for herniated disk(s) is controversial. Long-term outcome relative to pain and function is similar to that achieved with conservative care.[7] Surgery forms scar tissue, which can be equally painful and inhibiting.

REHABILITATION MANAGEMENT OF THE POSTSURGICAL PATIENT

The OT-PT team initiates treatment on the first postoperative day. Pain is often well controlled through the use of a patient-controlled analgesic device(PCA). This allows the patient to self-administer pain medication in premeasured doses, thus avoiding overdose. Postoperative bandages and surgical tape cover the sutures and help prevent soft-tissue stretching and unwanted pulling on the surgical site.

The goal of inpatient care is to achieve a safe discharge to home with or without supervision from a family member or health care attendant. OT focuses on functional training in bed mobility, self-care, transfers, standing tolerance, dressing, and other daily tasks. With little time for rehabilitation, adaptive equipment such as a commode and shower seat need to be rented in time for discharge to home. Education and training in posture and body mechanics are reviewed and practiced. The emphasis is on maintaining normal spinal alignment during self-care (sitting and standing) to minimize stress on the spine.

The length of stay in the hospital continues to be shortened. Patients with single-level laminotomies are often discharged in 3 days. Patients with multilevel procedures and fusions may stay 5 or 6 days because external stabilization devices sometimes need to be ordered and fitted before discharge.

PT focuses on strengthening, mobility, and ambulation activities, as well as evaluation for ambulation aids such as a walker, cane, or other equipment for neurological deficits that are not resolved after surgery. Functional training is also practiced, and written exercise programs are reviewed and practiced. Home exercise programs usually include standing and bed exercises to improve extremity ROM and strength.

Both the occupational therapist and physical therapist must determine the need for further rehabilitation after discharge. Recommendations for home care and outpatient follow-up are made.

CHRONIC LOW BACK PAIN

The literature reflects that the treatment of chronic pain must be separated from that of acute pain and is most effectively approached by a team of medical and behavioral specialists. The optimum treatment setting is inpatient hospitalization, where all services are coordinated.[16] Although chronic is defined as more than 3 to 6 months' duration, it is functionally determined by disruption of all the patient's chosen life roles. In a center that treats chronic pain, a history of LBP from 3 months to 50 years with multiple surgeries and fusions is not uncommon.

As the intrusiveness and corrosiveness of chronic pain lead to inactivity and a general decline in physical fitness, **depression** and **social isolation** become prominent. Frequently, patients dealing with these problems abuse narcotic analgesics, alcohol, and street drugs. To counteract this decline in function, patients in a pain management program are expected to be out of bed, dressed, and actively involved in their daily rehabilitation program.[16] Many phases of acute LBP rehabilitation can be prescribed to all patients (as in exercises and education in the use of proper body mechanics), but the occupational therapist's evaluation is, by necessity, in greater depth. Of continuing concern is the individual's physical function, time management, ability to pace activities, and cognitive functioning. Additional emphasis is placed on behavioral, cultural, familial, and spiritual aspects of the patent's life.[5]

An interview will yield needed information about the patient's functioning. Even with an interview, a self-report form should be given to the patient, for reasons discussed previously. It may be difficult for the patient to complete such a form because issues such as the abuse of narcotic analgesics, alcoholism, depression, anxiety, and head trauma can depress cognitive function. The practitioner must be aware that in some cases there may be many associated problems that may or may not have been previously diagnosed. (See Chapter 27 on cognitive components and Chapter 28 on the psychological and psychosocial experience of disability.)

Engel discusses the need for accurate, multidimensional evaluations, using instruments that have been validated and are reliable, to establish the effect of treatment.[5] Several methods for pain evaluation have been used to measure clinical pain. Engel discusses overt and covert behavioral approaches, as well as physiological pain responses used in the behavioral evaluations of pain.[5] (See Chapter 29 on pain management.)

All of the evaluation findings are relayed to the pain team. The findings may be indicators for further examination, such as neuropsychological testing. All of this information helps the occupational therapist to structure the patient's experience and thus help maximize acceptance of information and integration of educational experience.

Occupational therapists have many modalities available for individuals with chronic LBP. Engel[5] lists physical activity, communication of pain, relaxation training, biofeedback, cognitive restructuring, distraction, social support, and cutaneous stimulation modalities. Many practitioners see the empowerment of assertive behaviors as a skill critical to management of pain and depression.[16]

One of the major functions of both OT and PT is evaluation of the musculoskeletal system and of the functional capacities of the individual. In addition, the occupational therapist and physical therapist evaluate previous rehabilitation experiences, treatment, and outcomes in order to advise the pain management team about present limitations and the prognosis for positive change with further rehabilitation.

The physical therapist evaluates asymmetries in muscle length, tone, and strength, as well as joint mobility, asymmetry, or changes in soft tissue. Overall function, especially gait and general fitness, are also evaluated. From these findings the physical therapist designs a treatment program that emphasizes muscle stretching and joint mobility to correct or reduce the severe joint restrictions seen in individuals with chronic pain. Often a patient is seen in a "back school" setting for additional education. If movement therapy is available, this is used as an adjunct. The goal of PT is to help the patient return to the highest level of physical function possible.

SUMMARY

The patient with acute or chronic LBP is a challenge to the rehabilitation team of the occupational therapist, physical therapist, physician, psychiatrist, psychologist, nurse, social worker, and vocational rehabilitation counselor. All members of the team must communicate often and realistically with each other, as well as with the patient and family, to facilitate positive change in all aspects of the patient's life.

Understanding the anatomical weaknesses of the lumbar spine, especially with respect to disks and ligaments, enables the occupational therapist to educate patients in ways of moving that minimize spinal stress. This knowledge must become a way of life and must be incorporated into the individual's daily activities now and in the future.

Exacerbation of chronic LBP is common. Patients often disregard safe techniques, only to find that emo-

tional stress and the accumulation of physical stress to the lumbar spine lead to another episode of pain. This is often referred to as a "flare-up." Patients are told that because of human nature, this will probably happen. Patients design a "flare-up plan" for themselves in OT and PT before discharge. Developing this plan reinforces their ability, after education, for self-treatment. Maintaining a positive attitude, planning realistic goals, and taking increasing responsibility for themselves and their own rehabilitation are key ingredients of the ability of LBP patients to decrease pain and pain complaints.

CASE STUDY 46-1

CASE STUDY—MR. C.

Mr. C. is 29 years old. He lives in a two-bedroom, single-story house with his wife and 6-year-old daughter. He worked as a picture framer but was injured at work 3 months ago while lifting a 50-pound box. He complains of pain in his right low back and of an inability to function in normal activities. He appears depressed and admits to becoming more isolated socially since the injury. He states that he would like to return to work but is currently unable to work. He is unable to help his wife with housework, as he once did. He enjoys fishing, skiing, and basketball and would like to do these activities again. His condition is diagnosed as low back strain. He was referred to OT for restoration to maximal functional independence and for instruction in proper body mechanics for self-care, work, and leisure.

The initial evaluation included functional activities such as lifting and carrying, work with LE weights, UE weights, treadmill, and stationary bicycle, and functional analysis of performance of tasks. Tasks evaluated included dressing, housework, and mobility, such as from lying down to standing and sitting to standing. The patient's chief complaint of burning pain in the right lower back interfered with the performance of dressing, particularly the donning of socks and shoes. The patient demonstrated poor body mechanics when sweeping, vacuuming, and lifting and reaching, as well as in sitting to standing and lying to standing. Decreased ROM and poor flexibility were noted in all trunk motions and in hip flexion. The patient's habitual posture showed a flattened lumbar curve with forward head. The patient admitted to watching television all day; he had lost contact with friends and spent much time alone.

The treatment plan focused on the goals of management of pain and stress, increased ROM, flexibility, strength, and endurance, and the consistent use of appropriate body mechanics. Principles of body mechanics were explained and demonstrated; the occupational therapist observed Mr. C. and corrected his posture and body mechanics in the context of activities such as dressing, home maintenance, play and leisure, and work. Simulated tasks of lifting and other functions related to Mr. C.'s job as a picture framer were practiced on the Baltimore Therapeutic Equipment simulator. Tasks were graded for resistance, and time was increased as tolerated. Deep breathing and stress management techniques were taught in a group, and Mr. C. developed friendships with two of the group members.

After 4 weeks of treatment, Mr. C. was able to return to work. He occasionally experiences flare-ups but manages his response by reflecting on what activities or positions might have contributed to the flare-up, by reducing activity level and pacing himself, and by practicing visualization and deep breathing. His employer has accommodated the intermittent LBP by hiring a high-school student to help with lifting heavy frames and by allowing Mr. C. to store frequently used materials so that they are accessible without awkward reaching or lifting. Mr. C. once again helps his wife with the housework, and the family is planning a fishing and camping trip for the coming summer. Mr. C. says he is worried about getting into a tent and a sleeping bag, and he is considering renting a cabin instead.

REVIEW QUESTIONS

1. List three causes of LBP.
2. Name the major components of the spine.
3. Explain the movements of an intervertebral disk with spine flexion, extension, and lateral flexion.
4. List the five areas of physical assessment the therapist evaluates in an individual with LBP.
5. What potential psychosocial stressors may become evident during the evaluation?
6. What emotional responses may a patient demonstrate as a result of LBP?
7. What are some of the physical problems a person with chronic LBP encounters?
8. List the major goals of postsurgical rehabilitation of the patient with LBP.
9. Describe the progression of treatment for the patient with LBP.
10. What is the foundation for good body mechanics?
11. List the general principles of proper body mechanics for ADL.
12. In a team environment, what other disciplines might see or treat the person with LBP?

REFERENCES

1. Bowman JM: The meaning of chronic low back pain, *AAOHN J* 39(8):381-384, 1991.
2. Callahan P et al: *Stanford back school manual*, Stanford, Calif, 1984, Stanford Health Services Department of Rehabilitation Services.
3. Davis G, Onik G, Helms C: Automated percutaneous diskectomy, *Spine* 16(3):359-363, 1991.
4. DeGirolamo G: Epidemiology and social costs of low back pain and fibromyalgia, *Clin J Pain* (suppl 1):S1-S7, 1991 (abstract).
5. Engel JM: Treatment for psychosocial components: pain management. In Willard, Spackman, editors: *Occupational therapy*, ed 9, New York 1998, JB Lippincott.
6. Franklin TD: Personal communication, Dec 10, 1994.
7. Frymoyer JW: Back pain and sciatica, *N Engl J Med* 318(5):291-300, 1988.
8. Gardener W, Osborn W: *Structure of the human body*, Philadelphia, 1967, WB Saunders.
9. Kapandji IA: *The physiology of the joints*. Vol 3. *The trunk and vertebral column*, New York, 1979, Churchill Livingstone.
10. Kolata G: Diagnosis of backache might need more spine, *San Jose Mercury News*, July 14, 1994.
11. Long DM: Failed back surgery syndrome, *Neurosurg Clin North Am* 2(4):899-919, 1991.
12. McCormack GL, Pedretti LW: Motor unit dysfunction. In Pedretti LW, editor: *Practice skills for physical dysfunction*, ed 4, St Louis, 1996, Mosby.
13. Melnick MS, Saunders R, Saunders DH: *Managing back pain: daily activities guide for back pain patients*, Minneapolis, 1989, Educational Opportunities.
14. Moore S, Garg A: Ergonomics: low back pain and carpal tunnel and upper extremity disorder in the workplace, *Occupational Medicine, State of the Art Reviews* 7(4):593-594, 1992.
15. Nachemsom AL: The lumbar spine: an orthopedic challenge, *Spine* 1(1):59, 1976.
16. Snow BR, Lefkowitz M, Lebovits AH, editors: Hospitalization of chronic pain patient. In *A practical approach to pain management*, New York, 1997, Little, Brown.
17. Tollison C, Kriegel M: *Interdisciplinary rehabilitation of low back pain*, Baltimore, 1989, Williams & Wilkins.
18. Warwick P, Williams R: *Gray's anatomy*, ed 35 (British), Philadelphia, 1973, WB Saunders.

CHAPTER 47

Burns and Burn Rehabilitation

SANDRA UTLEY REEVES

KEY TERMS

Epidermis
Dermis
Superficial partial-thickness burn
Deep partial-thickness burn
Full-thickness burn
Hypertrophic scar
Donor site
Ischemia
Escharotomy
Autograft
Split-thickness skin graft
Erythema
Keloid scar
Scar maturation
Boutonniere deformity
Boutonniere precautions
Total active motion
Heterotopic ossification
Ectropion

LEARNING OBJECTIVES

After studying this chapter the student or practitioner will be able to do the following:
1. Recognize and understand the characteristics of the different depths of burn injury.
2. Describe the phases of recovery and focus of occupational therapy (OT) intervention for each phase.
3. Identify factors that increase potential for scar hypertrophy and contractures.
4. Comprehend the impact of ongoing patient and caregiver education on long-term compliance with treatment.
5. Understand the rationale for early involvement of burn patients in their own self-care as a step toward role resumption.
6. Acknowledge and anticipate complications characteristic of a severe burn.
7. Appreciate the impact that a severe burn has on the life roles, self-image, and values of the patient.

It has been estimated that each year 2 million people in the United States sustain a burn injury, approximately 300,000 are burned seriously, and more than 6000 die from burn injuries.[24,67] Since the early 1970s, advances in the medical, surgical, and rehabilitative management of burn victims have expanded the focus of burn care professionals from patient survival to include regaining the quality of life after a burn injury. Although functional recovery may be a long and arduous process, most burn survivors can expect to resume roles and function comparatively close to their preinjury level of independence. However, from the date of injury through the outpatient phase of care, a multidisciplinary team approach is necessary to effectively manage the medical, func-

tional, and psychosocial problems that are encountered during recovery.

SKIN'S FUNCTION

The skin is the largest organ of the body and serves primarily as an environmental barrier. Included in its functions are sensation, temperature regulation, protection from chemical or bacterial invasion and ultraviolet rays, and prevention of loss of body fluids. Anatomically the skin consists primarily of two layers. The **epidermis** is the nonvascular surface layer made up of epidermal cells. The **dermis,** or corium, contains a network of capillaries, sweat glands, sebaceous glands, nerve endings,

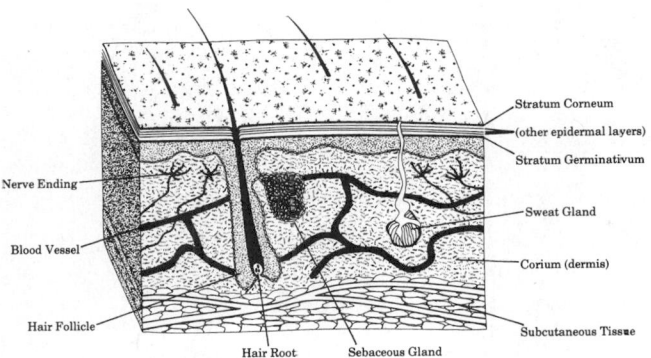

FIG. 47-1
Cross section of skin. (From Iles RL: *Wound care: the skin*, 1988, Marion Laboratories.)

and hair follicles (Fig. 47-1).[17] When the skin is damaged, various systemic, physiological, and functional problems can occur. A burn injury causes a destruction of the environmental barrier. Because of this, a large burn injury is one of the most painful forms of trauma and is life threatening in severe cases.

After a burn injury many factors must be taken into consideration in determining the severity of injury, functional recovery potential, and treatment needs. Primary considerations are the mechanism of injury, the depth and extent of the burn, specific body areas burned, the individual's age, medical history, and preinjury health, and other associated or concurrent injuries such as an inhalation injury or fractures.

MECHANISM OF INJURY

Burns can be thermal, chemical, or electrical in nature and can be caused by flame, steam, hot liquids, hot metals, radiation, or extreme cold.[17] The severity of the injury depends on the area of the body exposed and the duration and intensity of thermal exposure. **Superficial partial-thickness burns** can be caused by prolonged sun exposure or a brief contact with hot liquids or flames. **Deep partial-thickness burns** are caused by longer exposure to intense heat, such as with hot water immersion scalds or contact of the skin with flaming materials. **Full-thickness burns** usually result from prolonged immersion scalds, contact with flaming or high-temperature materials such as hot tar, extended exposure to chemical agents, and contact with electrical current.

BURN DEPTH

The depth of a burn is estimated from clinical observation of the appearance, sensitivity, and pliability of the wound.[62] A burn injury was traditionally classified as first, second, and third degree but now is described as

superficial partial-thickness, deep partial-thickness, or full-thickness injury (Table 47-1). Superficial and deep partial-thickness burns usually heal without surgical intervention. However, once healed they tend to be excessively dry, itchy, and subsequently susceptible to excoriation by shear forces produced during rubbing or scratching. These shear forces can cause blisters and compromised long-term skin integrity caused by repeated reopening of the wound. Partial-thickness and full-thickness burns usually lead to uneven pigmentation of the healed scar. Deep partial- and full-thickness burns have a greater potential for thick, **hypertrophic scar** and contracture formation because of the prolonged period for healing. This is especially true if a burn converts from partial-thickness to full-thickness because of infection or repeated trauma. Most full-thickness wounds necessitate surgical intervention or skin grafting for wound closure. Skin graft **donor sites** usually heal in the same manner that superficial partial-thickness burns heal, with less scarring but uneven pigmentation.

PERCENT TOTAL BODY SURFACE AREA INVOLVED

The extent of a burn is classified as a percentage of the total body surface area (%TBSA) burned. The two most common methods for estimating %TBSA are the "rule of nines" and the Lund and Browder chart.[56] The rule of nines is simple and quick, but relatively inaccurate (Fig. 47-2). It divides the body surface into areas comprising 9%, or multiples of 9%, with the perineum making up the final 1%. The head and neck area is 9%, each upper extremity (UE) is 9%, each leg is 18%, and the front and back of the trunk are each 18%. However, the rule of nines applies only to adults. Body proportions vary with children, depending on their age, especially in the head and legs.[11] The Lund and Browder chart[40] provides a more accurate estimate of the total body surface area and is used in most burn centers. This chart assigns a percent of surface area to body segments (Fig. 47-3), with adjusted calculations for different age groups. For smaller %TBSA injuries the therapist can get a quick, rough estimate using the size of the patient's palm (hand excluding the fingers) to equal approximately 1% of the individual's total body surface area.

SEVERITY OF INJURY

The %TBSA and depth of burn are primary indicators of the severity of injury. A 20% or greater burned surface area is often the determining criterion for admission to a burn intensive care unit. However, depending on the patient's age and preinjury health, partial- or full-thickness burn wounds less than 20% TBSA can still be considered serious enough to warrant admission. A person with deep partial- and full-thickness burns of greater than

TABLE 47-1

Burn Wound Characteristics

Burn Depth	Common Causes	Tissue Depth	Clinical Findings	Healing Time	Scar Potential
Superficial (first degree)	Sunburn, brief flash burns, brief exposure to hot liquids or chemicals	Superficial epidermis	Erythema, dry, no blisters; moderate pain	3-7 days	No potential for hypertrophic scar or contractures
Superficial partial thickness (superficial second degree) and donor sites	Severe sunburn or radiation burns, prolonged exposure to hot liquids, brief contact with hot metal objects	Epidermis, upper dermis	Erythema, wet, blisters; significant pain	Less than 2 weeks	Minimal potential for hypertrophy or contractures if no secondary infection or if trauma does not delay healing
Deep partial thickness (deep second degree)	Flames; firm or prolonged contact with hot metal objects; prolonged contact with hot, viscous liquids	Epidermis and much of dermis nonviable, but skin appendages survive from which skin may regenerate	Erythema; larger, usually broken blisters; on palms and soles of feet, large, possibly intact blisters over beefy red dermis; severe pain to even light touch	Greater than 2 weeks, may convert to full thickness with onset of infection	High potential for hypertrophic scarring and contractures across joints, web spaces, and facial contours; high risk for boutonniere deformities if dorsal fingers involved
Full thickness (third degree)	Extreme heat or prolonged exposure to heat, hot objects or chemicals for extended periods	Epidermis and dermis: skin appendages and nerve endings are nonviable	Pale, nonblanching, dry, coagulated capillaries may be seen; no sensation to light touch except at deep partial-thickness borders	Larger areas require surgical intervention for wound closure; smaller areas may heal in from borders over extended period of time	Extremely high potential for hypertrophic scarring or contractures depending on the method used for wound closure
Subdermal	Electrical burns and severe long-duration burns (e.g., house fires, motor vehicle accidents with a passenger trapped in a burning vehicle or under hot exhaust systems, and smoking in bed or alcohol-related burns)	Full-thickness burn with damage to underlying tissues	Nonviable surface, may be charred or with exposed fat, tendons, muscles; electrical injuries may have small external wounds but significant secondary sub-dermal tissue loss and peripheral nerve damage	Requires surgical intervention for wound closure; may require amputation or significant reconstruction	Similar to full-thickness except where amputation removes the burn site

30% TBSA has a severe burn that usually requires a prolonged period to achieve wound closure and intensive rehabilitation for functional recovery. Burn involvement of certain body areas is also used to classify injury severity, although the %TBSA burn may be limited. For example, deep partial- or full-thickness burns involving the hands, face, or perineum are considered severe burns.[62]

INITIAL MEDICAL MANAGEMENT

Immediately after a burn injury the permeability of blood vessels increases, causing rapid leakage of protein-rich intravascular fluid into surrounding extravascular tissues.[45] In larger burns, hypovolemia or burn shock can occur because of decreased plasma and blood volumes with reduced cardiac output, all results

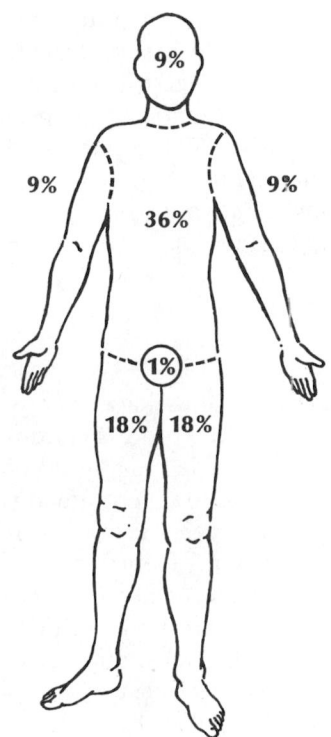

FIG. 47-2
Rule of nines.

AREA	ADULT	2°	3°	DONOR SITE	TOTAL
HEAD	7				
NECK	2				
ANTERIOR TRUNK	13				
POSTERIOR TRUNK	13				
RIGHT BUTTOCK	2.5				
LEFT BUTTOCK	2.5				
GENITALIA	1				
RIGHT UPPER ARM	4				
LEFT UPPER ARM	4				
RIGHT FOREARM	3				
LEFT FOREARM	3				
RIGHT HAND	2.5				
LEFT HAND	2.5				
RIGHT THIGH	9.5				
LEFT THIGH	9.5				
RIGHT LEG	7				
LEFT LEG	7				
RIGHT FOOT	3.5				
LEFT FOOT	3.5				
TOTAL					

FIG. 47-3
Chart for calculating %TBSA. (Adaptation of Lund and Browder chart, from Burn Center at Washington Hospital Center.)

of extensive intravascular fluid loss.[21] Fluid resuscitation with an intravenous fluid such as lactated Ringer's solution is essential for promptly replacing venous fluid and electrolytes. The fluid volume required is determined by various formulas, such as the Parkland and modified Brook formulas,[3] and is based on the extent of the burn and the weight of the patient. The rate of fluid infusion is determined by monitoring pulse rate, central venous pressure, hematocrit, and urinary output.

The lymphatic system, which normally carries away excess tissue fluid, often becomes overloaded, causing subcutaneous edema. With circumferential full-thickness burns, loss of burned skin elasticity combined with increased edema can cause interstitial pressure severe enough to compress vessels. This impairs circulation to the distal extremity and causes limb **ischemia**.[17] **Escharotomy**, or incision through the necrotic burned tissue, is performed to release the binding effect of the tight eschar, relieve the interstitial pressure, and restore distal circulation (Fig. 47-4). In deeper wounds an incision down to and through the fascia, or fasciotomy, may be needed for adequate pressure relief.

A smoke inhalation injury is a common secondary diagnosis with thermal injury and can significantly increase mortality in burn patients. When the face is burned, if the burn occurred in a closed space, or when there is other objective evidence of a possible inhalation injury, bronchoscopy, arterial blood gas, and chest x-ray

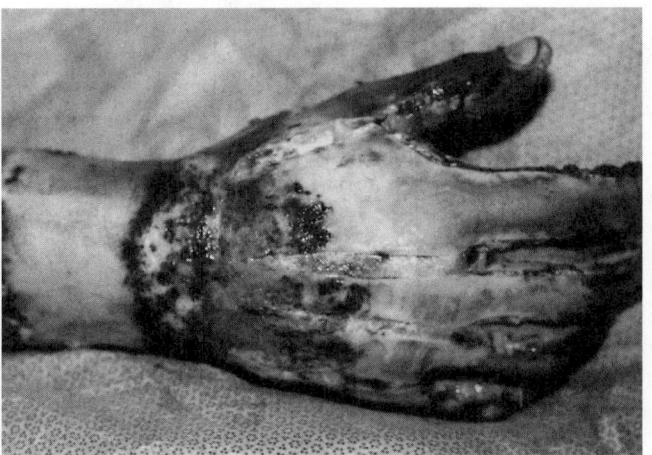

FIG. 47-4
Escharotomies on the dorsum of the hand with full-thickness burn injury.

examinations are used to confirm the diagnosis. Intubation and ventilatory support may be required along with vigorous respiratory therapy. A tracheostomy is performed if the airway is difficult to maintain or ventilatory support is prolonged.[63]

WOUND CARE

After a patent airway and fluid resuscitation have been established, attention is directed to wound care. Hydrotherapy is performed at least once a day via tanking or showering to provide a thorough cleansing of both the wound and uninvolved areas. Various topical agents are applied to delay colonization of organisms and reduce bacterial counts in the burn wounds.[21]

Burn wound colonization begins at the moment of injury, with gram-negative organisms replacing normal bacterial flora. Wound cultures and biopsies are performed to monitor this growth when there are signs of possible serious infection. A severe infection could cause septic shock, which is a state of circulatory collapse and a cardiovascular response to bacterial by-products or endotoxins. Septic shock can be characterized by ischemia, diminished urine output, tachycardia, hypotension, tachypnea, hypothermia, disorientation, or coma.

Although all burn wounds are treated with some type of topical antibacterial agent, when the depth and extent of the wound require 3 or more weeks for healing, surgical intervention is indicated to decrease burn morbidity and mortality. Surgical treatment for burns usually consists of excision of the nonviable burned tissue, or eschar, and placement of biological or synthetic skin grafts.

There are essentially three types of biological grafts. A xenograft, or heterograft, is processed pigskin. A homograft, or allograft, is processed cadaver skin. These are used as biological dressings to provide temporary wound coverage and pain relief. An **autograft** is a permanent surgical transplantation of the upper layers or **split-thickness skin graft** of the person's own skin from an unburned donor site. The graft is applied to the clean, excised tissues of the burn wound graft site. Now that the size of a survivable burn has increased, the amount of available donor sites for autografting has conversely decreased. For this reason, alternatives to autografts are being developed. Examples of such alternatives are epidermal cultured skin substitutes[20] and cultured epidermal autograft (CEA).[5,12] A wound may be limited in size, but the defect may be so deep that bone or tendon survival is at risk. In these instances split-thickness skin graft adherence is difficult to obtain, and a full-thickness skin graft or microvascular skin flap may be indicated.

Adequate nutrition is essential during wound healing because the metabolic rate of the burn patient greatly increases with corresponding increases in protein, vitamin, mineral, and calorie needs.[21,42] Protein is especially important for wound healing and must be provided in substantial amounts. Nutritional requirements are calculated based on the %TBSA and patient's admission weight. Calorie counts and the patient's weight are closely monitored to ensure adequate nutrition. If the patient is unable to meet individual requirements through the diet, high-protein and calorie supplements are given either orally or through a nasogastric or gastric tube. Intravenous hyperalimentation is frequently necessary with severe burns of extensive %TBSA. As wound closure is achieved, nutritional demands decrease and the individual's normal eating habits must be normalized to prevent excessive weight gains.

ASSOCIATED PROBLEMS
Scar Formation

After initial healing, most burn wounds have an **erythemic,** flat appearance. As the healing process continues, the wound's appearance may worsen as a result of scar hypertrophy or contraction. The long-term quality of a mature burn scar can be affected by numerous factors, some of which occur during the early phases of burn care.[25,37] The amount of time needed to achieve wound closure is a strong determinant. Bacterial infections in the wound increase the inflammatory response that can delay wound healing and contribute to scar formation.[31] However, any factor that delays healing will increase the potential for scarring.

Hypertrophic scars are thick, rigid, red scars that become apparent 6 to 8 weeks after wound closure.[1] Histologically, these immature scars have increased vascularity, fibroblasts, myofibroblasts, mast cells, and collagen fibers arranged in whorls or nodules.[6,46] Biochemical investigations of hypertrophic scars have disclosed increased synthesis of collagen fibers and connective tissue. As hypertrophic scars mature, capillaries, fibroblasts, and myofibroblasts decrease significantly, with the collagen relaxing into parallel bands and the scar becoming flatter and more pliable. The time needed for scars to mature differs markedly among individuals. The race and age of the patient, as well as the location and depth of the burn wound, have been reported anecdotally to influence hypertrophic scarring.[16,57] Superficial burns that heal in less than 2 weeks generally will not form hypertrophic scar. Deeper burns that take greater than 2 weeks to heal have a greater potential to form hypertrophic scars. Hypertrophic scars may take from 12 to 24 months to mature.[37] Excessive scar formation, such as a **keloid scar,** may take up to 3 years to mature.

All scars initially have an increased vascularity and red appearance. Scars that remain erythemic for more than 2 months are more likely to develop into hypertrophic scars. They become progressively firmer and thicker, rising above the original surface level of the skin. There is a marked increase in production of fibroblasts, myofibroblasts, collagen, and interstitial material, all with contractile properties that help to draw together the borders of a wound but can also cause scar tightness. Pain and skin tightness cause most patients to become less active. These patients prefer to rest in a flexed, adducted position for comfort. This allows the new collagen fibers in the wound to link and fuse together. The fibers become progressively more compact, coiling up in whorls and nodules and giving the scar surface a textured appearance that can lead to disfigurement. If the scar extends over one or more joints, the progressive tightness leads to a scar contracture and loss of active motion. Fortunately, collagen linkage is less stable in new scars, and an immature hypertrophic scar contracture can be influenced by such sustained mechanical forces as proper positioning, exercise, and splinting.

Psychosocial Factors

During hospitalization the patient is often subject to isolation, dependency, and pain. Because burn injuries and treatment procedures are usually painful, narcotic analgesia is often liberally used.[34] Relaxation and imagery techniques can also be employed to reduce stress and anxiety, which in turn increases the effectiveness of the pain medications. The amount of narcotic analgesia given is gradually decreased as the wound heals, and patients usually require minimal pain medication on discharge.

After a burn injury there is a potential for psychological reactions, including depression, withdrawal reactions because of disfigurement, behavioral regression, and anxiety over the ability to resume work, family, community, and leisure roles.[18] Providing emotional support and education and helping the patient to develop coping mechanisms and self-direction can help with the psychological adjustment of the burn patient. However, a severe burn injury may also result in such positive changes as reassessment of personal values and relationships and a renewed appreciation of life. To help determine how people will adjust psychologically to a severe burn injury, the complex interaction between premorbid personality style, extent of injury, and social and environmental contexts should be considered.[44]

BURN REHABILITATION
The Team

Successful care and rehabilitation of burn victims require a multidisciplinary team approach that begins immediately on the patient's admission to the hospital and continues through and beyond hospitalization.[3,51] Ideally, the burn care team includes physicians, nurses, physical and occupational therapists, dietitians, social workers, respiratory therapists, recreational therapists, clergy, and vocational counselors.[37,54]

Goals of Rehabilitation

The entire burn team is involved in some aspect of burn rehabilitation, whether for verbal support, setting up the patient for self-feeding, or just reinforcing the importance of active motion. The long-term goals of occupational therapy (OT) are quite similar to the long-term goals of the burn team. Although specific goals may be the responsibility of various team members, everyone is focused on the same outcome. Treatment goals should be presented to the patient and family as goals of the entire rehabilitation team. Inherent in this concept are the close communication and cooperation of all burn team members. Role delineation between occupational and physical therapy differs by burn care facility and may be determined by insurance reimbursement rather than by traditional roles or the specialized skills of either individual therapist. Therefore it is especially important that these two disciplines work closely together with ongoing communication, so that patients benefit from the skills and viewpoints of both disciplines. Many occupational and physical therapists who specialize in burn rehabilitation increasingly use cotreatments that promote independence with both mobility and activities of daily living (ADL).

Phases of Recovery

Rehabilitation management of burn victims can be divided into three overlapping phases to aid in categorizing and determining effective treatment goals. These phases of recovery are acute care, surgical and postoperative, and inpatient and outpatient rehabilitation.[37]

The acute care phase is usually the first 72 hours after a major burn injury. However, if the burn is superficial partial thickness and heals spontaneously in less than 2 weeks without surgical intervention, the time from injury until epithelial healing is also considered as an acute care phase.[50]

The surgical and postoperative phase follows the acute phase and continues for varying lengths of time, depending on the size of the burn injury and presence of associated medical complications. During this period, vulnerability to wound infection, sepsis, and septic shock is especially great, and medical treatment is focused on promoting healing and minimizing infection.

The rehabilitation phase covers both inpatient and outpatient care and can extend for an indeterminate length of time. This phase is the postgrafting period, when the patient is medically stable and is affected by the quality of wound healing, scar formation, and need for rehabilitation. It is the most challenging phase for burn patients, their families, and their therapists.

Acute Care Phase
During the acute care phase, medical management is of utmost importance for survival of the patient, and the goal of OT is primarily preventive. As the patient recovers and wound closure progresses, the nature of the activities with the patient also changes, with treatment

being directed at restoring function. Initially, however, when the wounds are partial or full thickness, the acute care rehabilitation goals are as follows:
1. Reduce edema.
2. Prevent loss of joint and skin mobility.
3. Prevent loss of strength and endurance.
4. Promote independence and self-care skills.
5. Provide orientation and begin patient and caregiver education regarding the rehabilitation process.

Surgical and Postoperative Phase
Rehabilitation goals during the surgical and postoperative phase are aimed at preserving or assisting function while supporting surgical objectives. Excision and grafting procedures usually require periods of immobilization of the areas treated. The preferred position and length of immobilization will vary by physician prerogative and burn center protocol, with the average period of immobilization being between 2 and 7 days.[9,22,27,40,55]

During this phase the goals of therapy are as follows:
1. Protect and preserve graft and donor sites by fabricating splints and establishing positioning techniques that support the surgeon's postoperative care orders.
2. Increase self-care by providing or fabricating adaptive equipment as needed.
3. Promote cognitive awareness by providing orientation activities when necessary.
4. Prevent muscular atrophy and loss of endurance and reduce thrombophlebitis risk by providing exercise for areas not immobilized.
5. Educate and reassure the patient and family regarding this phase of recovery.

Rehabilitation Phase
The third phase of recovery is the rehabilitation phase, which begins as wound closure occurs. Individuals with large %TBSA burns frequently enter this phase needing further surgery; however, the majority of their wounds are closed and wound maturation is commencing. The focus of care during this phase is on maximizing self-care, promoting physical and emotional independence, and controlling **scar maturation** to prevent deformity and contracture formation. Patient and family education is especially important for developing competence with wound care and therapy programs in preparation for discharge.

The rehabilitation phase extends past hospital discharge and continues until maturation of both burn wounds and surgical sites is complete. Before discharge from the hospital, emphasis is on independence and education. Once the individual is home, emotional support and intervention are often needed to help restore the self-confidence and motivation needed to cope with the physical, social, and emotional consequences of a severe burn injury.

Wound maturation usually takes from 12 to 18 months following injury; however, it is important to remember that each patient heals differently. Some wounds mature in less than a year, whereas others may take over 2 years.[51] The therapist's goals for this phase are exhaustive, but understandably so, considering the potentially disabling effects of burn scar.[37]

Goals for the rehabilitation phase are as follows:
1. Teach independent self-care skills.
2. Provide education and practice of home care activities, including appropriate exercise, positioning, and skin care.
3. Restore muscle strength, activity tolerance, and endurance.
4. Improve joint mobility and coordination.
5. Fit splints, compression and vascular support garments, and pressure adapters for edema and management of scar maturation.[37]
6. Support reacquisition of social and vocational skills.
7. Provide instruction regarding scar and skin care techniques, including potential changes in sensation and appearance.
8. Control edema and minimize scar hypertrophy, contractures, and disfigurement.
9. Teach compensation techniques for limiting exposure to ultraviolet light, chemical irritants, friction, and extremes of weather and temperature.
10. Guide the implementation of a postdischarge plan that supports resumption of school, work, and leisure roles.

OCCUPATIONAL THERAPY EVALUATION

Although medical issues are a primary concern during acute care, whenever possible the occupational therapist should complete an initial evaluation within the first 24 to 48 hours after hospital admission. Burn cause, medical history, and any secondary diagnoses are obtained from the medical record. The wounds are visually assessed to determine the extent and depth of injury, and any critical areas involved are noted. Patient and family interviews are used to establish rapport and to obtain specific information such as hand dominance, previous functional performance and limitations, preinjury daily routine and activities including job, school, and home responsibilities, and pretrauma psychological status. In the case of a severe burn requiring patient intubation, this information must be obtained from family members to verify and supplement what the patient may relay nonverbally.

Preserving function of the body areas involved is of primary concern; however, a baseline of overall physical function should be established before treatment planning.[37] Involved and uninvolved areas should be evaluated for joint mobility, strength, sensation, and functional use. Before starting, the therapist should explain the purpose of OT and what to expect during the assessment, including the potential for discomfort.

Ideally, the initial OT assessment should take place during a dressing change, when the depth and exact location of the burns can be viewed directly and carefully documented. Distinctions should be made between superficial and deep partial-thickness burns, as well as full-thickness burns, by appearance and presence of sensation. The therapist must view the wounds as soon as possible postinjury, before the development of burn eschar. Eschar causes deep partial-thickness burns to resemble full-thickness burns closely, and makes accurate evaluation of depth difficult. Attention should also be directed to burned joint surface areas and the presence of any circumferential burns. An active or active assistive range of motion (ROM) assessment should be performed without dressings, to evaluate joint mobility and general strength before significant edema develops or restrictive dressings are applied. The dorsum of the hands should be checked for deep burns over the proximal interphalangeal joints that could indicate the need to initiate **boutonniere deformity** precautions or hand splints.

When possible, a goniometer should be used for assessing ROM to accurately document baseline deficits and future changes in recorded measurements. Ongoing instruction and continuous encouragement help reassure patients and decrease anxiety, allowing patients to perform at their best. Instructing the patient regarding the types of movements and the number of repetitions expected while gently guiding the individual through the specific motion can help ensure achievement of full range. If pain, edema, tight eschar, or bulky dressings limit full ROM, this fact should also be documented. Preexisting conditions that may alter expected active ROM should be investigated during the patient and family interview. Although active ROM is preferred, passive ROM should be measured if a patient is unresponsive or unable to move the extremity. When using passive ROM, care must be taken not to apply excessive force, especially with older patients with degenerative joint disease or small children with hypermobile joints. With deeper partial or full-thickness dorsal hand burns, **boutonniere precautions** should be initiated until the integrity of the hand's extensor hood mechanisms can be verified. Composite active or passive flexion of the fingers should be avoided; instead, isolated metacarpophalangeal (MP) flexion is combined with interphalangeal (IP) joint extension to avoid stress and possible damage to a compromised extensor tendon mechanism. All passive proximal interphalangeal (PIP) flexion is avoided, and protective splinting is promptly initiated.

If the individual had normal functional muscle strength before injury, an initial test of gross muscle strength may not be needed if the ROM assessment revealed adequate strength to work against gravity.

Manual muscle testing of major muscle groups is indicated if the burn was an electrical contact injury, severe edema is present causing a possible compartment syndrome, or other musculoskeletal or neurological injuries are suspected.[65] If the hand is not burned or the burn is superficial partial thickness, a dynamometer and pinch gauge are used to measure grip and pinch strength.

A gross sensory screening including all sensory distribution areas should be performed. This is especially important in the case of electrical injury or long-standing diabetes in which peripheral neuropathies may be present.

Assessment of activities of daily living (ADL) is initiated by interviewing the patient or the family to establish preinjury level of functional independence. When the burn injury is severe, an ADL assessment may be inappropriate and should be postponed until the patient is medically stable and able to participate with therapy. Individuals with less severe burns and who are not intubated should be assessed for basic ADL skills, such as the ability to feed self, basic grooming skills, and donning and doffing of hospital gowns. Any compensatory actions or awkward movements used to complete the activity should be noted. Any abnormal patterns should be investigated and discussed to determine if they were present before the burn injury.

After completion of an initial evaluation (Table 47-2), short- and long-term goals should be established with the patient's collaboration. The patient's personal goals, priorities, and previous lifestyle should be taken into account when establishing these goals. After this is done, the treatment plan can be formulated. The OT treatment plan should be practical and should complement and support the goals of the other team members.

Two fundamental principles should be kept in mind when working in burn rehabilitation. First, the main factor that can hinder postburn functional recovery is the formation of scar contractures and hypertrophic scarring. Second, severe scars and contractures are often preventable with prompt therapeutic intervention.[48] Therefore most burn rehabilitation treatment techniques and objectives are directed at prevention, as well as restoration.

OCCUPATIONAL THERAPY INTERVENTION
Acute Care Phase

The purpose of proper positioning is to reduce edema and to maintain involved extremities in an antideformity position. Proper positioning is critical because the position of greatest comfort for the patient is usually the position of contracture.[35,37] The typical position of comfort consists of adduction and flexion of the upper extremities, flexion of the hips and knees, and plantar flexion of the ankles. Hands are held in a dysfunctional position

TABLE 47-2
Burn Rehabilitation Evaluation Components

Initial	Inpatient Rehabilitation	Outpatient Rehabilitation
Burn cause	Graft adherence	
%TBSA, depth of burn	Skin or scar condition	Skin or scar condition
Area(s) involved	Contracture concerns	Compression garment fit
Age, hand dominance	Edema (if present)	Volumetrics if needed
Functional status	ADL performance level	ADL performance level
Occupation	Work skills	Work skills
ROM and strength	Active and passive ROM, TAM	Active and passive ROM, TAM
Mobility and endurance	Strength and endurance	Strength and endurance
Developmental level (child)	Developmental level (child)	Developmental level (child)
Psychological status	Psychological status	Psychological status
Social support	Social support	Social support
Leisure activities	Leisure activities	Leisure activities
	Compression garment needs	Compression garment needs
	Home management	Home management
		Home care understanding
		Return to work capacity
		Return to school potential and need for reentry program

ADL, Activities of daily living; *ROM*, range of motion; *TAM*, total active motion; *TBSA*, total body surface area.

consisting of wrist flexion, metacarpophalangeal extension, interphalangeal flexion, and thumb adduction. This position is often called the "claw hand" position.

During the initial wound assessment, positioning needs are determined by evaluating the surface areas burned and the presence of edema, considering the posture the individual tends to assume, and determining if that posture would limit function if allowed. For example, if the burn injury involves the shoulder, chest, and axillae, the patient's upper extremities should be elevated and positioned in approximately 90° of shoulder abduction, 45° of external rotation, and 60° of horizontal adduction, using pillow inclines, arm boards, or overhead traction (Fig. 47-5). Achieving full shoulder abduction with frequent exercise and activity is critical to preventing axilla web contractures and subsequent loss of abduction as wound healing progresses. Once positioning needs are determined, illustrated guidelines should be posted at bedside and the nursing department should be advised to ensure ongoing correct positioning (Fig. 47-6).

During acute care, positioning is instituted primarily to limit edema formation.[47] Elevation of the entire ex-

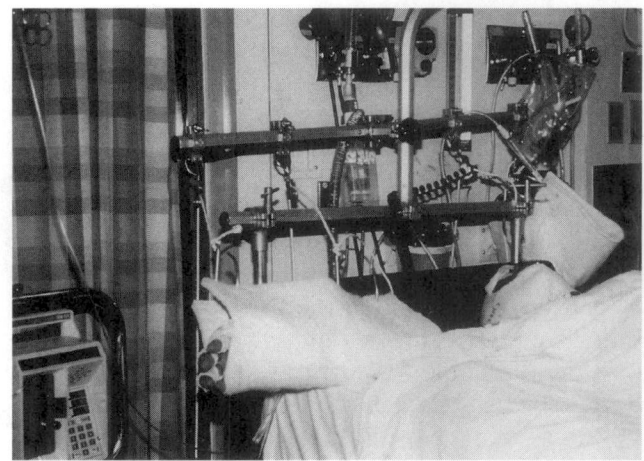

FIG. 47-5
Shoulder positioning using overhead traction and felt slings.

tremity slightly above heart level can reduce the severity of distal edema formation, especially when paired with active ROM exercises. As wound closure progresses, attention should be directed to more proximal body positioning concerns (Table 47-3).[37]

Splinting is initiated to provide positioning assistance and protect compromised tissues. It is not necessary for splints to be worn at all times to prevent contractures. When a splint is used during the acute phase, it is generally static in design and applied when at rest, with activity and exercise emphasized during the day. Volar hand splints are indicated if a burned hand has significant edema, active motion is limited, or unsupervised movement is contraindicated because of deep dorsal burns or other traumatic injury. The typical volar burn hand splint provides approximately 30° wrist extension, 50° to 70° MP joint flexion, full IP joint extension, and the thumb abducted and extended (Fig. 47-7).[37] Elbows or knees should be splinted at 0° to 5° of flexion to avoid joint hyperextension.

When splints are fitted any possible pressure points should be considered and correct positioning ensured. Splints fabricated shortly after injury require daily assessment and possible alterations to accommodate any significant changes in edema. Hand splints are secured in place with a figure-eight wrap of gauze bandage and disposable elastic wraps. Folded 4-by-4 inch gauze sponges are used over the proximal phalanges and under the wrap to keep the fingers extended and secured in the splint. Detachable straps, although convenient for later use, may be inappropriate for use on acute burn splints because of infection control concerns and the potential for constriction during fluctuations in distal edema.

When there is a partial- or full-thickness burn to the external ear, protection is required to prevent further damage caused by pressure from pillows, dressings, or endotracheal tube straps. An ear protection splint

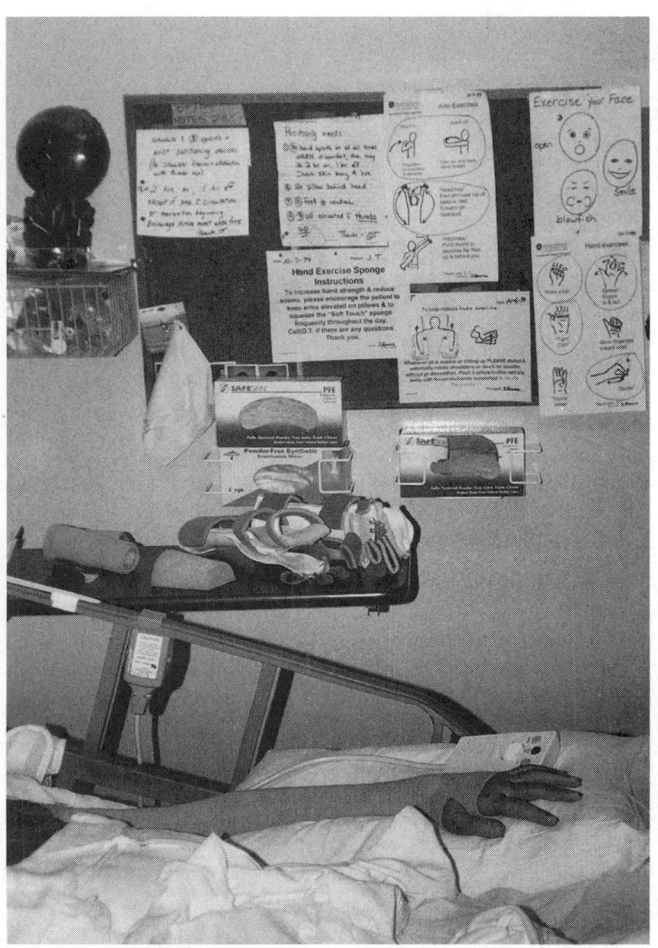

FIG. 47-6
Highly visible posters are beneficial as reminders to patient and staff regarding positioning, exercises, and splinting schedules.

TABLE 44-3

Antideformity Positioning for Specific Body Areas Following Burn Injury

Body Area	Antideformity Position	Equipment and Technique
Neck	Neutral to slight extension	No pillow; soft collar, neck conformer, or triple-component neck splint
Chest and abdomen	Trunk extension, shoulder retraction	Lower top of bed, towel roll beneath thoracic spine, clavicle straps
Axilla	Shoulder abduction 90° to 100°	Armboards, airplane splint, clavicle straps, overhead traction
Elbow and forearm	Elbow extension, forearm neutral	Pillows, armboards, conformer splints, dynamic splints
Wrist and hand	Wrist extension 30°, thumb abducted and extended, MP flexion 50° to 70°, IP extension	Elevate with pillows, volar burn hand splint
Hip and thigh	Neutral extension, hips 10° to 15° abduction	Trochanter rolls, pillow between knees, wedges
Knee and lower leg	Knee extension; anterior burn: slight flexion	Knee conformer, casts, elevate when sitting, dynamic splints
Ankle and foot	Neutral to 0° to 5° dorsiflexion	Custom splint, cast, ankle-foot orthosis (AFO)
Ears and face	Prevent pressure	No pillows; headgear[32]

IP, interphalangeal; *MP*, metacarpophalangeal.

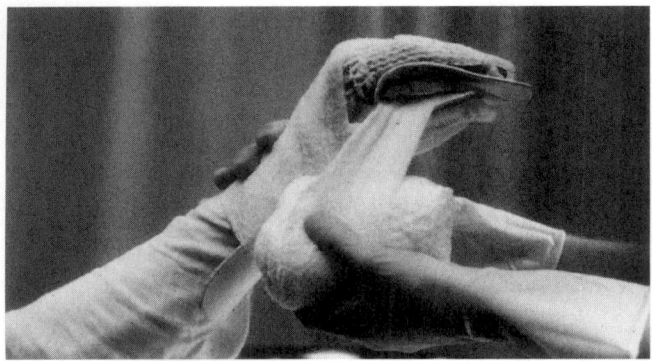

FIG. 47-7
Postburn hand splint. Note wrapping approach for thumb.

should be fitted at the earliest opportunity and worn until the external ear burns have healed. The splint can be fabricated of two thermoplastic ear cups or semirigid oxygen masks secured in place by a three-point stabilizing elastic strapping technique.[15,33]

A patient's ability to perform self-care is often limited during the acute care phase because of individual medical needs. The need for artificial ventilation, multiple lines, catheters, and other supportive equipment interferes with independence with ADL, and patients are dependent on nursing for their self-care. When the patient is extubated and medically cleared to take fluid or food by mouth, the occupational therapist, working in concert with the speech pathologist, should assess self-feeding abilities. Dressings and edema may interfere with self-feeding motions. Temporary use of adaptive equipment may be needed and may include built-up and extended handles on utensils and a plate guard or a travel mug with a lid and a straw. Grooming is another self-care activity that can be encouraged. Temporary adaptations to environment setup, equipment, or the patient's usual technique may be indicated to support independence. Withdrawing adaptations as soon as possible should be a goal of therapy and presented to the patient as a sign of progress. The therapist must convey to the patient that the goal is to be independent with all ADL, using normal movement patterns performed within a normal length of time.

Sitting tolerance and ambulation are initiated as soon as the patient is medically cleared to get out of bed and bear weight on his or her lower extremities. If the patient has lower extremity burns, elastic wraps should be applied before the patient sits up and the feet become dependent. A figure-eight pattern should be used, from the base of the toes, over and including the heel, to at least the knees, and up to the groin as needed. When the patient is sitting in a chair, the lower extremities should be kept elevated. Time spent dangling the feet or static standing should be limited to discourage lower extremity swelling and prevent unnecessary discomfort.

In addition to functional activities, active exercise is a primary component in every burn treatment plan. Exercise techniques used during acute care are not unique to the injury.[37] Active, active-assisted, or passive exercises are used, depending on the patient's condition. The focus of exercise in acute care is to preserve ROM and functional strength, build endurance, and decrease edema.

Strength and endurance activities are introduced into the acute care treatment program as the patient's condition allows. These activities range from simple active movement to resistive activities, as tolerated. The purpose of resistive exercise is to counteract the deconditioning effects of hospitalization.[39] Exercise after a severe burn injury was once thought to overstress an already hypermetabolic patient. However, research and experience have shown that graded, progressive exercise is not deleterious in acute burn recovery.[28]

Although patient education is the responsibility of all burn team members, OT program success depends on patients' understanding of their long-term needs and responsibilities. Initial educational objectives should focus on developing an understanding of stages of burn recovery, the need for and importance of independent activity and motion, and pain and stress management techniques. Meeting these goals promotes the motivation and compliance so essential for successful treatment outcomes.[19]

Surgical and Postoperative Phase

Excision and grafting procedures usually require a period of postoperative immobilization to allow adherence and vascularization of the grafts.[15] It is advantageous for the occupational therapist to discuss postoperative positioning needs with the surgeon before surgery so that splints and positioning devices can be applied in the operating room immediately after the surgical procedure. A wide variety of materials and protocols are available. All have the common purposes of immobilizing the grafted area, preventing edema, and assisting wound healing needs.[50]

Postoperative positioning may use standard positioning techniques or may be unique, designed only for the specific surgical procedure. Although standard burn splints position the extremity in the antideformity position, preoperative or postoperative splints should hold the extremity in the position that promotes the greatest surface area for graft placement. For dorsal hand grafts, the wrist is positioned in neutral, the MP joints in flexion, and the thumb in abduction to maximize the dorsal grafted surface area. Another example is that in which an axillary advancement flap is performed; the shoulder is abducted only 45°. Gaining prior knowledge of the surgical procedure and determining potential postoperative complications enable the therapist to establish effective positioning procedures.

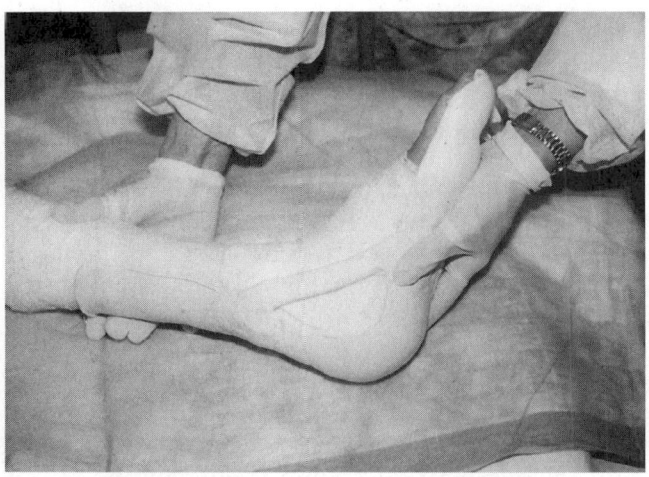

FIG. 47-8
Thermoplastic total-contact ankle dorsiflexion splint.

Although postoperative immobilization is frequently achieved through the use of bulky restrictive dressings and standard positioning equipment, splints are often needed to secure the position. Most splints are regularly made using plaster bandages or thermoplastics (Fig. 47-8). If a wet dressing will cover the graft site, a perforated or open-weave splinting material may be preferred to permit continuous drainage and prevent graft maceration.[15] In some instances movement of adjacent joints may disrupt graft adherence even though the graft does not cover the joint surface. In these cases the splint design should incorporate immobilization of those joints in a functional position. A postoperative thermoplastic splint generally can be made by using a drape and trim technique.[15] Most postoperative splints are for temporary use and are discontinued once graft adherence is ensured. If made of thermoplastics, they can later be remolded into the antideformity position.

Throughout the postoperative phase of care, active and resistive exercise to the uninvolved extremities should be continued when possible, to maintain ROM and strength. Immediately after excision and grafting procedures, exercises for adjacent body areas are usually discontinued for a short time. Although the time varies among burn centers, the average is 3 to 5 days, with 7 to 10 days for cultured epithelium grafts.[9,19,27] Exercises can be resumed as soon as graft adherence is confirmed. Before resuming exercises, the occupational therapist should view the grafts and adjacent areas to determine graft integrity and whether there are any exposed tendons or compromised subcutaneous tissues.

Gentle active ROM is the treatment choice to avoid shearing of the new grafts. If the patient exhibited normal ROM before surgery and was immobilized for only 3 to 5 days, baseline ROM should be expected within 3 days following resumption of activity. Active exercise of a body area with a donor site is generally permitted after 2 to 3 days if there is no excessive bleeding. Lower extremity donor sites are treated similarly to lower extremity burns; therefore elevation and wrapping with elastic bandage are standard treatment.

Ambulation following lower extremity excision and grafting is usually not resumed until 5 to 7 days after surgery. With the physician's consent the patient is then encouraged and assisted to ambulate for short distances and then slowly increase the distance. Before ambulation, double elastic bandage wraps are applied over a fluff gauze dressing to prevent graft shearing or vascular pooling. Wrapping with an elastic bandage, elevation, and avoidance of static stance are particularly important for protecting lower extremity grafts. When the individual is able to walk, exercise on a stationary cycle ergometer is beneficial for increasing endurance.

Environmental stimulation, self-care, and leisure activities should be continued and increased commensurate with the patient's physical abilities and tolerance level. Self-care is often difficult during this phase because of the immobilization positions necessary to ensure graft adherence. Creative ADL adaptations are frequently needed to allow patients some involvement in their care and control over their environment during this time. Although only temporary, simple techniques such as prism glasses for those supine in bed, universal cuffs over splints, or extended handle utensils help preserve current level of independence and foster continued feelings of self-actualization and confidence. Continued emotional support and burn care education are also essential.

Rehabilitation Phase

During the inpatient rehabilitation phase, OT evaluation should emphasize a thorough assessment of performance skills and performance components. Active and passive goniometric measurements should be taken to document any limitations caused by joint restrictions or scar tightness. Individual measurements can be used to document individual joint restriction, but **total active motion** (TAM) measurements should be used if skin tightness affects several joints in the same extremity. Muscle strength can be measured with the manual muscle test (MMT). However, when the MMT is used, caution is needed when the therapist applies resistance, so as not to shear newly healed skin. Other components of the evaluation should include: muscular and cardiorespiratory endurance, performance of self-care and home management activities, skin and scar condition, presence of edema, and the need for compression garments (Table 47-2).

Treatment goals during inpatient rehabilitation are to increase ROM, strength, and endurance, to achieve independence with self-care, to familiarize the patient with the care necessary for discharge from the hospital, to aid psychological adjustment, to begin skin conditioning, and to provide patient and caregiver education. Although these goals are continued and progressively increased during the outpatient rehabilitation phase, many other goals are added as the individual prepares for reintegration into the home and community.

The rehabilitation phase generally begins when a severely burned patient no longer needs the intensive care provided on the burn unit. Most of the wounds are now closed, and the patient may move to a step-down unit or transfer to a rehabilitation setting. Here patients are expected to assume a more active role in establishing treatment goals, demonstrate more independence in their care, and fully participate in their therapy. Specific discussions regarding work, recreation, and self-care skills are necessary to help focus patients on resuming previous roles, returning to normal daily activity routines, and anticipating potential roadblocks to community reentry. An upgraded exercise program, a variety of self-help and rehabilitation equipment, and new techniques are introduced to help increase ROM, strength, endurance, and independence with ADL.

Scar formation begins as wound closure occurs, and consequently patients frequently report increased tightness in joint movements or an inability to perform certain functional activities. Numerous treatment techniques are advocated to counteract the effects of scar maturation. Examples are skin conditioning, scar massage, compression therapy, and therapeutic exercise preceded by slow, sustained stretching.

Skin-conditioning techniques are used to improve scar integrity and durability against minor trauma caused by pressure or shearing forces of garments, to decrease hypersensitivity, and to moisturize dry, newly healed skin. These activities are recommended for any individual whose burns or surgical sites took longer than 2 weeks to heal. Lubrication and massage with a water-based cream or lotion should be performed three to four times a day or whenever the skin feels exceptionally dry, tight, or itchy. This action provides needed lubrication for skin that is dry because of damaged sweat and sebaceous glands. Massage is essential for desensitizing hypersensitive grafted or healed scars and softening tight scar bands during sustained stretching exercises. When massaging a scar band, the therapist should be sure the scar is in full stretch and premoisturized to prevent splitting of immature and often unstable, problematic scar tissue. Massage should be performed using a circular motion, with more pressure applied gradually, as tolerated over time.

Intermediate pressure garments are beneficial for desensitization, general skin conditioning, edema control, and early scar compression. The type of interim garment or compression bandage applied depends on how much pressure and shear force the individual's skin can initially tolerate. The garment or bandage is changed as tolerance gradually increases. The type of interim compression bandage or garments chosen should be based on the amount and consistency of pressure it applies, the ease of application, and the potential for shear forces exerted during application.[8] Elastic bandage wraps, self-adherent elastic wraps, tubular elastic support bandages, presized elastic pressure garments, and spandex garments custom made by the therapist are all commonly employed (Fig. 47-9).[2,43] Tubular elastic bandages, presized elastic garments, and custom-made spandex gloves can be worn over minimal dressings and are routinely applied 5 to 7 days after removal of the postoperative dressing. When patients have small open areas requiring minimal dressings, a woman's nylon stocking can be used over the dressing before the donning of tubular bandages, to reduce shearing forces and preserve correct dressing placement. Intermediate garments are worn consistently day and night, taken off only for bathing and skin care. Independent donning and doffing of interim garments are incorporated into the patient's ADL training.

Newly healed skin tends to blister with shearing forces or splint with overstretching, especially when the skin is dry. Every therapy session should therefore begin with massage to the scars using a moisturizing lotion to prepare the dry or tight skin for increased motion. Patients should learn to perform their own skin care independently before their scheduled therapy. Once the scars are lubricated, stretching is performed to increase flexibility and fluidity of movement.[38] Stretch should be slow and sustained, and forceful dynamic stretch should be avoided, with attention given to the position of adjacent joints during the stretching motion. Massage with additional moisturizers during stretch exercises helps relieve itching and discomfort. Stretching in front of a mirror provides positive feedback for the patient and is helpful for correcting abnormal posturing.

Active ROM, strengthening, and endurance activities should follow stretching exercises. During the rehabilitation phase more complex motions must be emphasized. Flexibility exercises are complex motions that require movement of several joints simultaneously. Most ADL that require complex motions and exercise programs should emphasize not just individual joint ROM but combined joint mobility in functional patterns of movement (Fig. 47-10). An activity that requires hand manipulation skills while reaching overhead is an example of a complex motion for a burn injury that involves the shoulder, elbow, and hand.

For individuals recovering from severe hand burns, treatment activities may involve use of exercise putty, hand manipulation boards, the BTE Work Simulator,[4] Valpar Work Samples,[60] crafts, and other fine motor activities. Strengthening activities may involve the use of

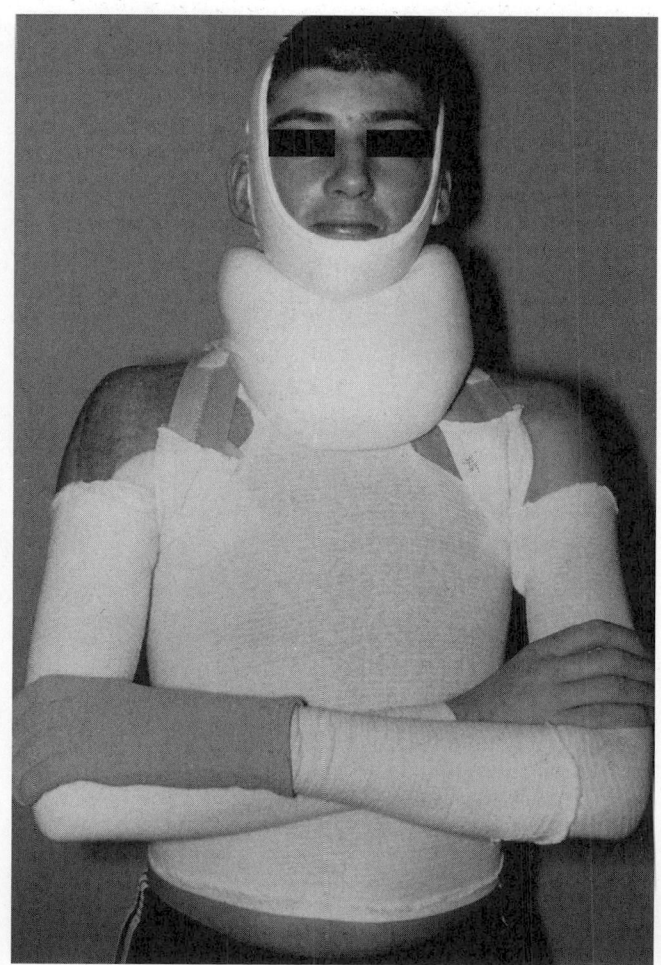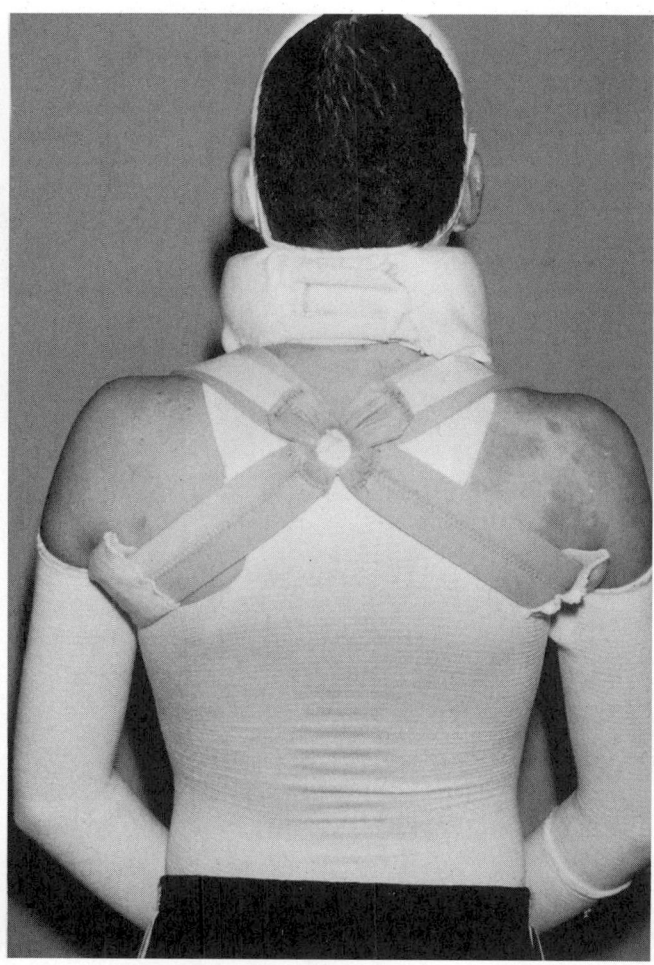

FIG. 47-9
Early compression techniques: tubular elastic dressings, ready-made gloves and chin strap, custom fabricated foam collar, and padded clavicular strap to preserve neck and axillae contours.

cuff weights or dumbbells, the WEST II,[64] or the BTE Work Simulator.[4] The Valpar Full Body ROM Sample provides full body range, as well as finger manipulation.[60]

Following severe hand burns, edema may occur because of decreased function, dependent positioning without adequate external compression, or circumferential scarring to the upper extremity with associated poor lymphatic damage. Dependent edema is also frequently observed in the lower extremities following healing of full-thickness burns. When edema is present, motion is limited and painful, and if allowed to remain, it may lead to fibrosis.[39] Self-adherent elastic bandage material (Coban or Cowrap) is often used as compression dressing to the digits and hand. When self-adherent wrap is applied, before-and-after circumferential or volumetric measurements are recommended to monitor treatment effect (Fig. 47-11).

To treat hand edema, elevation, progressive compression, and activity are recommended. A compression wrap, using a self-adherent bandage (Coban), is applied in a spiral fashion, overlapping the previous turn by one half-turn on each digit and continuing in this manner across the hand and onto the wrist. Strips are also applied to each web space (Fig. 47-12). The wrapped hand should then be used for ADL and other functional motions and elevated just above heart level when the patient is resting. For lower extremity edema, wearing a double layer of elastic wraps when ambulating, elevation when resting, active ankle exercises (e.g., pumping), and avoidance of static standing are recommended. Coban can also be used for treatment of toe edema. Intermittent compression pump therapy is often used to treat chronic edema of the distal extremities.

As patients near discharge from the hospital, stressing independent self-care is extremely important. Eating, dressing, grooming, and bathing skills should be emphasized as part of the normal daily routine. When problems occur, the therapist must determine if the dysfunction originates from a physical limitation, scar contracture, pain, edema, or an assumed abnormal postural reaction. Early identification of abnormal movements helps patients understand their needs and allows an

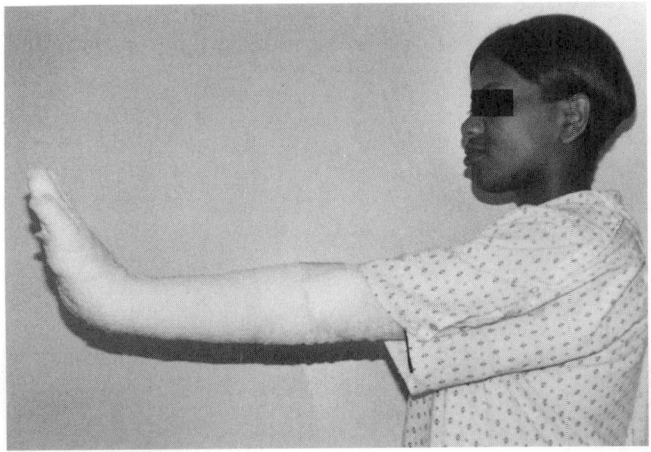
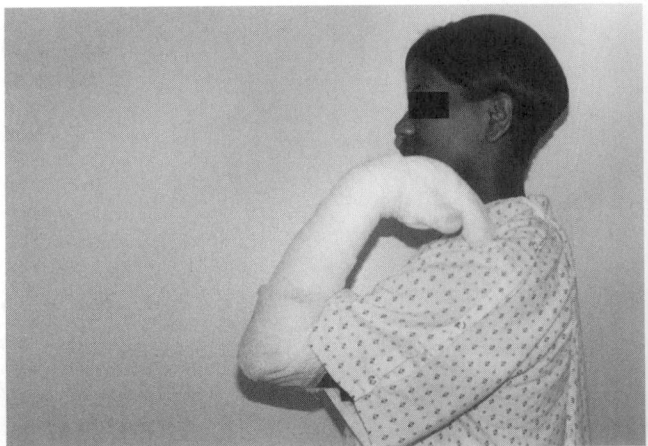
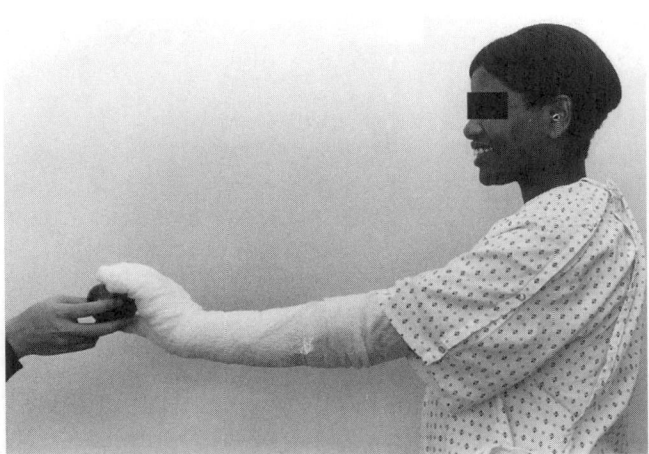
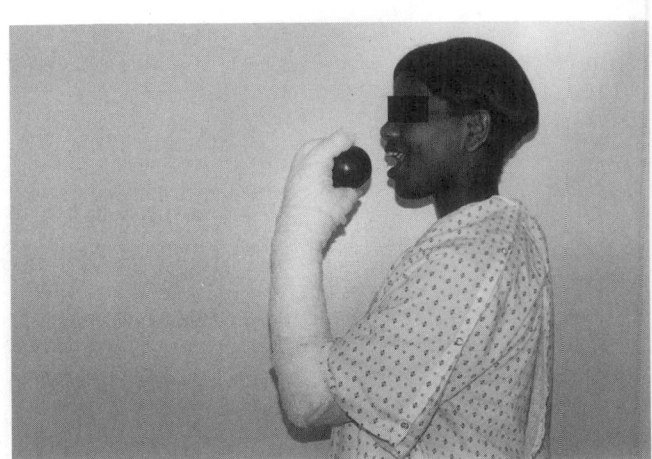

FIG. 47-10
Combined motions in functional patterns of movement help obtain the greatest total active motion.

opportunity for relearning normal movement patterns. Practicing ADL with personal care items and supplies from home can foster a positive attitude toward hospital discharge and feelings about personal abilities. Major burn injuries may require adaptations to support independence initially. Assessing the need for adaptive self-care should differentiate between a scar limitation that can be rehabilitated and a more permanent disabling result.

In addition to self-care, instrumental ADL (IADL), such as home management tasks, should be practiced before discharge. Experience has proven that fears of hot water, the stove, or an iron can hinder functional recovery. For individuals injured during a home activity, counseling, support, and practice of the skills or activity in the clinic should be organized. Prevention techniques taught as part of the inpatient treatment program, should also be part of the home program.[66]

Splinting at this stage is used to limit or reverse potentially disabling or disfiguring contracture formations, to increase ROM, to distribute pressure over problem areas, or to assist function (Fig. 47-13). Static splints, dynamic splints, and casting[7,32,49] may be used, depending on the need. Regardless of the purpose of the splint, every effort should be made to ensure that its purpose is easily understood and that it is simple to apply. Nighttime splinting is preferred because it allows functional use of the extremity during the day and provides treatment of contractures while at rest.

Patient and caregiver education becomes increasingly important during this phase to aid the transition from hospital to home. Increased understanding is needed in the areas of wound healing, the effect of scar contracture, the importance of preserving independence in ADL and IADL, the need for continued activity and exercise, and scar management techniques and principles. Before discharge from the hospital the patient and family should receive comprehensive home care education (Table 47-4).[30,34] To reinforce learning, information should be presented in a variety of ways, such as orally, in writing, as a demonstration, and by video. However, opportunities should be provided for the

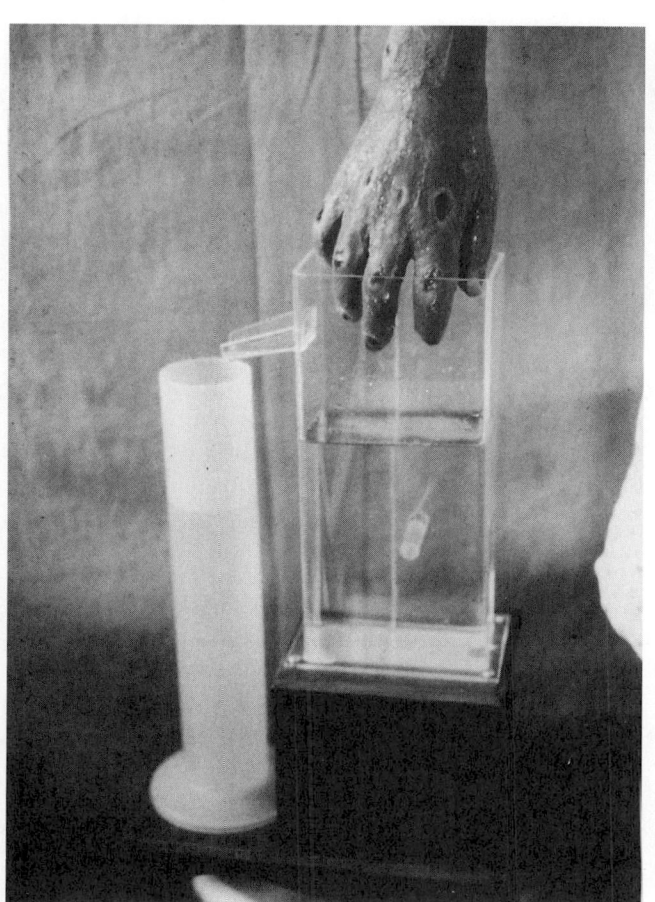

FIG. 47-11
Comparison of sequential volumetric measurements of hand edema substantiates treatment effect.

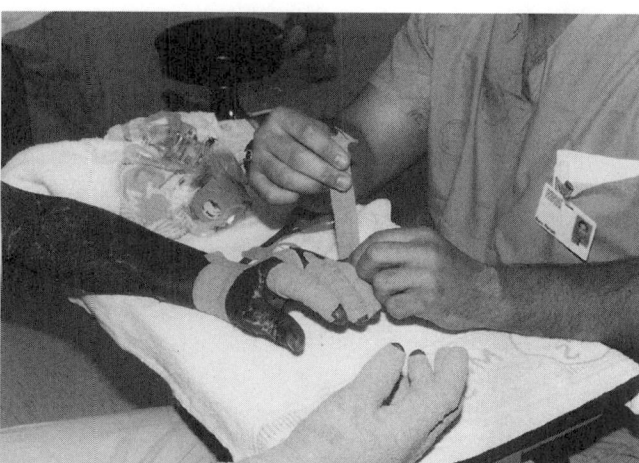

FIG. 47-12
Self-adherent elastic wrap (Coban) applied to hand to provide external compression for treatment of edema.

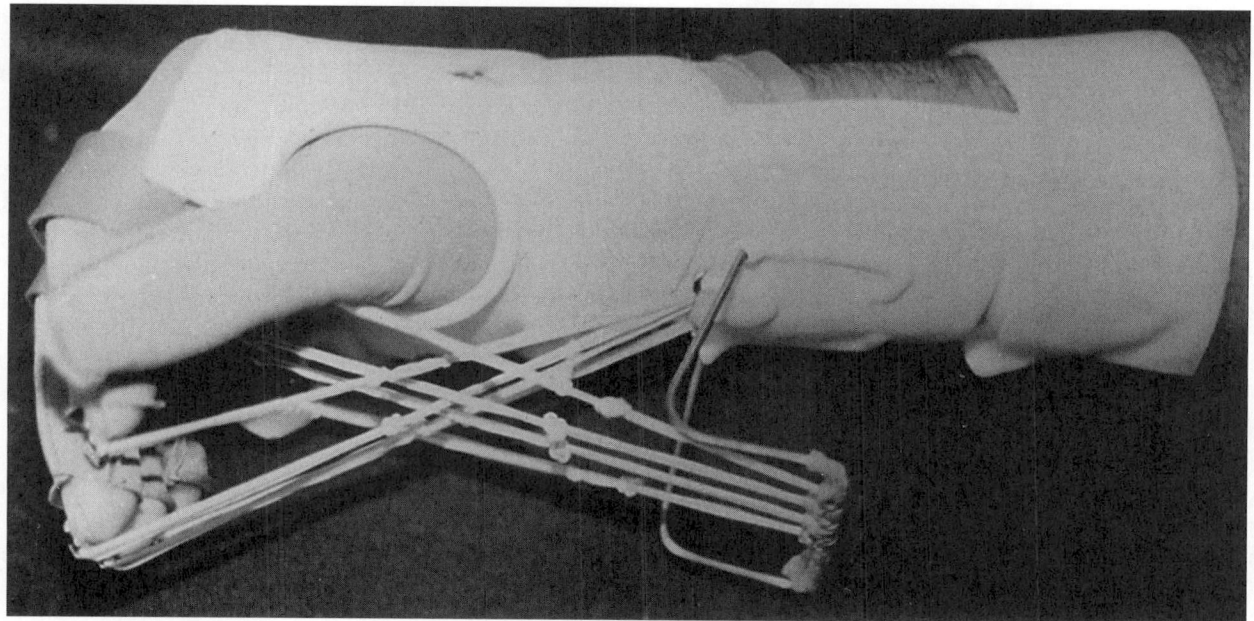

FIG. 47-13
Bivalved dynamic metacarpophalangeal flexion splint. Presized intermediate glove is worn for skin conditioning and edema control.

TABLE 47-4
Home Program Outline

Item	Information Needed
Wound care, positioning	Dressing change technique, precautions, elevation
Skin and scar care	Lubricant frequency, sun protection and trauma precautions
Self-care (ADL)	Techniques and equipment needed
Splints and orthotics	Donning techniques, schedule, precautions
Pressure garments	Purpose, washing, reordering, donning techniques
Exercises	Frequency, techniques for specific areas

patient and caregivers to actually practice wound care, garment and splint application, and all exercises under staff supervision. Only with a detailed understanding of home care techniques and potential outcomes can patients be expected to assume responsibility for their own care and recovery.[66]

Outpatient Rehabilitation

The list of assessment procedures expands during burn recovery. ROM, strength, endurance, ADL, and skin and scar status must be assessed frequently to ensure early identification of specific problem areas. In addition to these physical components, the effectiveness of compression garments, the fit and need for certain splints, home care activities, emotional responses, and coping skills should be constantly monitored.

Physical tolerance and work skills assessment are indicated when patients are ready for return to school, work, or vocational rehabilitation. Driving evaluation and prevocational assessment, using simulated work activities or work sample testing, may also be needed for the more severely injured burn survivor. Vocational counseling and exploration should be undertaken in the later stages of recovery if residual dysfunction necessitates a change in vocational role.

An underlying objective of most burn rehabilitation techniques is the prevention or treatment of hypertrophic scars and scar contractures. For effective treatment of scar problems, scar characteristics must be monitored to recognize when maturation occurs. Active scars have been described as erythemic, raised, and rigid.[30] As they mature, their color, contour, and texture improve, and the scar becomes less vascular in color,

more pliable, and smoother. The time since injury is one evaluation measurement. A rating scale has been designed that allows serial assessment of scar pigment, vascularity, pliability, and height.[58] Although the ratings are somewhat subjective, the scale is a useful clinical tool. Use of high-quality Polaroid photography expedites objective reassessment.

During outpatient rehabilitation, patients may undergo numerous physical and emotional changes. Once discharged from the hospital, they are faced with the overwhelming task of becoming responsible and self-reliant while dealing with the aggravation of developing scars. They may not participate fully with therapy or adequately follow through with home care activities because of the physical and emotional effects of the injury.[31] Noncompliance, apathy, avoidance of pain, scar tightness, and hyperssensitivity all contribute to dysfunction after injury.

In addition to standard treatments such as counseling, support, and relaxation techniques, attending a burn support group can help with adjustment. Experience has shown that burn patients at different stages of recovery tend to provide positive support to each other. Group discussions can facilitate understanding of what they have been through and what they have to do.[31]

Wearing intermediate pressure garments prepares the skin for the fitting of custom-made compression garments. Compression garment use is indicated for all donor sites, graft sites, and burn wounds that take more than 2 to 3 weeks to heal spontaneously.[10,13,40] The occupational therapist is often responsible for the measurement, ordering, fitting, and sometimes adjustments of the custom-made garments. All custom-made garments need to be measured and ordered following the special instructions of each company.*

Ideally, patients should be fitted with custom-made compression garments no later than 3 weeks after wound healing; otherwise, the wearing of interim garments is continued until custom garments can be applied. Garments may need to be ordered "piecemeal" since different areas of the patient may be ready for treating with compression at different points in time. Custom-made compression garments are constructed to provide gradient pressure, starting with 35 mm Hg pressure distally. They must be worn 23 hours a day, being removed only for bathing, massage, or changing into a clean garment (Fig. 47-14). Face masks and gloves also need to be removed for meals. Most patients employed inside are able to return to work and previous activities without interference from the garments. Patients who work outside may find compression garments too hot in

---

* Custom-made garments are available from Jobst Institute, Charlotte, NC (800) 221-7573; Barton Carey, Perrysburg, OH (800) 421-0444; Bio-Concepts, Phoenix, AZ (800) 421-5647; Medical-Z, Seattle, WA (800) 368-7478.

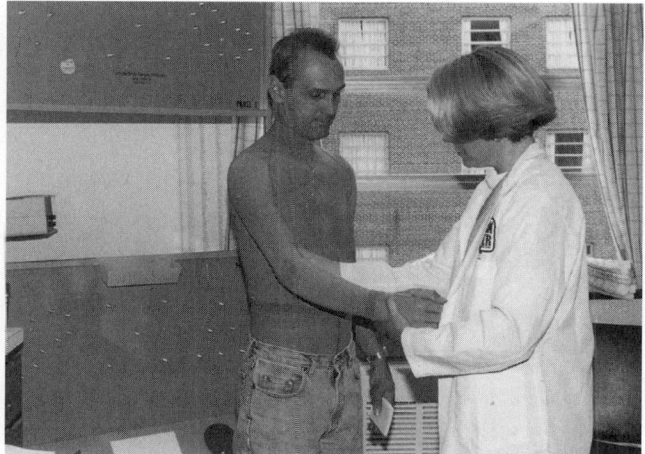

FIG. 47-14

Fit of custom-made compression garments must be frequently assessed to ensure adequate compression for scar management.

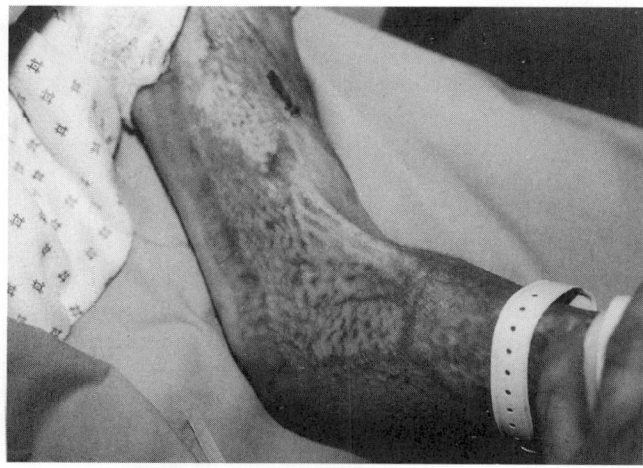

FIG. 47-15

Example of scar contracture of antecubital skin of elbow. Note taut, shortened skin when elbow is extended.

summer months and may need to change their work setting. Because of damaged or lost skin pigment, burn patients are at a greater risk for sun burning and must use sunblock and avoid prolonged sun exposure.

Compression therapy should be applied to the burned area for approximately 12 to 18 months or until scar maturation is complete. Donor sites may also need compression garments, depending on the thickness of the donor skin and whether healing occurred in less than 2 weeks. Once proper fit is established, it is recommended that the patient possess a minimum of two sets of garments at any one time, to allow for both around-the-clock compression therapy and laundering. Because of the resilient construction of the fabric, patients should be instructed to hand wash the garments with mild soap and allow them to air-dry. Washing machines, dryers, direct heat, strong detergents, or bleach should not be used, to prolong the life of the garments. If they are properly cared for, the garments will last approximately 2 months before a new set is needed. Some individuals who have returned to work may need more than two sets of garments at a time; children may need replacements more frequently as a result of their growth and active lifestyle. Toddlers undergoing toilet training and incontinent adults will need extra garments and design options that allow independent toileting.

To be effective, compression garments must exert equal pressure over the entire area. Because of body contours, bony prominences, and postural adjustments, flexible inserts or pressure-adapting conformers are usually needed under the garment to distribute the pressure more evenly. Areas commonly requiring pressure adapters are the supraclavicular region of the chest, between and under the breasts on women, the nasolabial folds, upper and lower lip areas, and the web spaces of the hands and feet.

Pressure inserts were originally made from thermoplastics, but inflexibility and skin reactions limited their use. Inserts and conformers are now made from a variety of materials; the choice is based on the area to be treated and need for flexibility when applied. When one is applied, its fit should be monitored at regular intervals. During the early phases of healing when scar remodeling is possible, conformers need to be replaced frequently to maintain exact contouring. Silicone gel, Silastic elastomer, Otoform-K, Plastazote, and Velfoam are used for hand scars. One-sixteenth-inch Aquaplast and Silastic elastomer are used on face scars; closed cell foams, prosthetic foam elastomer, Elastogel pads, Plastazote, and Velfoam are used for other body areas.*

In addition to skin care and scar management, the outpatient treatment plan should be directed at increasing independence with home care while also emphasizing resumption of past life roles. This includes returning to previous work, school, and leisure activities. Because scar contracture is often the primary cause of dysfunction (Fig. 47-15), activities performed in therapy should emphasize strength, endurance, and functional ROM to counteract the effects of scarring and preserve independence.

Inpatient rehabilitation techniques, equipment, and therapeutic activities are also appropriate for outpatient therapy. However, progressive grading of exercise and activity frequency, intensity, and duration is necessary to successfully regain or improve an individual's strength, endurance, and functional skills. Sequencing the order of treatment activities is necessary to prevent injury and to minimize patient discomfort. Skin lubrication, massage,

---

*Vendors of materials for pressure inserts include the following: Alimed, Dedham, MA (800) 225-2610; North Coast Medical, Inc., Morgan Hill, CA (800) 235-7054; Smith & Nephew, Menomonee Falls, WI (800) 558-8633.

and stretching should precede progressive strengthening exercises and activities.[38] As soon as possible, outpatients should learn how to prepare for exercise and activity by doing their own skin lubrication, massage, and stretching. This approach will maximize actual therapy time and may develop habits that will improve compliance with home activities.

Return to school or work becomes a primary objective during outpatient rehabilitation. Many recovering burn survivors are capable of resuming normal daily routines before their wound maturation is complete. Most burn patients will still be wearing compression garments and inserts, having to avoid prolonged sun exposure and needing to perform skin care while they are in school or at work.

Return to school and association with friends can be an especially difficult process for children who have cosmetic disfigurement or functional loss or restrictions. Many burn centers have developed school reentry programs to educate teachers and students about burn injuries and what the child has been through, and to explain the purpose of compression garments, splints, exercise, and skin care precautions. The goal of a reentry program is to reduce restrictions to the child's activities and ease the transition of returning to school.[53] Summer camps for burned children can help the children adjust by placing them in social settings where all of their peers are also burned. Many such camps are sponsored by local firefighter organizations.

Preparing a burn patient for return to work does not have to be a long-term process. Burn rehabilitation and work skills training have many similarities; therefore it is possible to design treatment activities that simulate not only functional activities but also various work skills. Strength, endurance, and flexibility, often identified as work tolerances, are obvious goals of burn rehabilitation.[36] Physical demands of jobs, as described in the *Dictionary of Occupational Titles*,[59] are also components of functional skills; lifting, stooping, pushing, pulling, handling, and manipulating are a few examples. A job analysis interview, as part of the activity needs analysis, will provide the type of information needed to integrate activities into the treatment plan that should not only improve functional ability but also provide beginning work conditioning.

Preparing an individual for return to work after burn injury also requires attention to two other types of tolerance, skin and temperature. Skin-conditioning activities and exercises performed while wearing garments will improve skin tolerance for friction and shear force demands (Fig. 47-16). Education about the body's response to temperature variations and precautions for dealing with extremes of temperature is the only way to address temperature tolerance abnormalities.

The outpatient therapy program should be reevaluated periodically to determine if the frequency of treat-

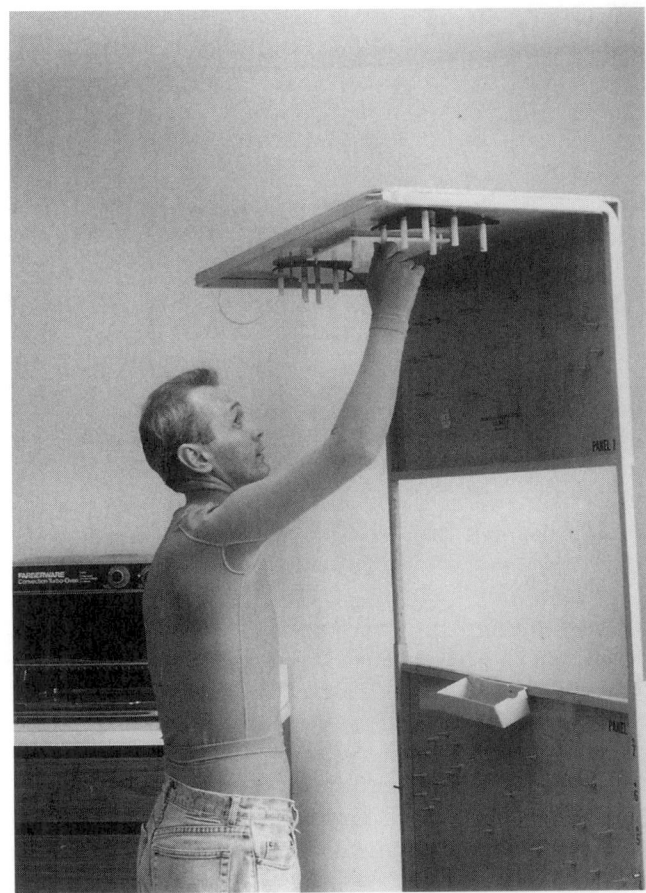

FIG. 47-16
Combined range of motion (ROM) and skin conditioning activity. Use of Valpar Whole Body ROM for upper extremity exercise while wearing compression garments.

ment, program progression, or return to work or school status should be changed.[38] When patients have resumed their preinjury activities, outpatient therapy may be discontinued. Because burn scar maturation may take up to 18 months after injury, some schedule of follow-up care, every 2 to 3 months, is needed until the wearing of compression garments is discontinued.

BURN-RELATED COMPLICATIONS
Heterotopic Ossification

Heterotopic ossification (HO) is new bone formation in tissues that normally do not ossify.[61] Although HO is frequently found in the posterior aspect of the elbow, it may occur in other joint areas, such as the shoulder, wrist, hand, hip, knee, and ankle. It may occur in either extremity or bilaterally, even if both extremities were not burned. It develops either in the soft tissue around the joint or in the joint capsule and ligaments, and often forms a bony bridge across the joint.[26] Signs that HO may be present usually appear during the latter stages of hospitalization, with the patient experiencing increased pain at a certain point in the joint's ROM. The pain is fairly localized and severe and ROM losses are usually rapid. Inflammatory signs, such as redness or swelling, are not easily discernible within healing burn wounds. Once HO has been detected, frequent *active* ROM exercise to the joint should be carried out within the *pain-free range* to maintain joint motion.[14] Use of dynamic splints or forceful passive stretching to the involved joint should be discontinued. The condition may resolve itself with time, or eventual surgical intervention may be required to release fused joints.

Neuromuscular Complications

Peripheral neuropathic conditions are the most common neurological disorder observed in burn patients. They usually occur in high-voltage electrical burns or burns of greater than 20% TBSA.[23] Peripheral nerve damage may be caused by infections, metabolic abnormalities, or neurotoxicities. A peripheral neuropathic condition is generally demonstrated with symmetrical distal weakness, with or without sensory symptoms. Most conditions improve with time; however, patients often complain of fatigue and decreased endurance that may last for months.[23]

In addition to peripheral neuropathic conditions, localized compression or stretch injuries to nerves are encountered during burn recovery. Causes of localized nerve injury include improper or prolonged positioning in bed or on the operating room table, tourniquet injury, and extreme edema. Common injury sites are the brachial plexus and ulnar and peroneal nerves. Prolonged frog-leg positioning can cause a stretch injury, whereas prolonged side lying can cause a compression injury to the peroneal nerve.[23] The ulnar nerve is subject to a compression injury if resting on a firm surface with the elbows flexed and forearms pronated. The brachial plexus is subject to stretch or compression injury if inappropriate shoulder positioning techniques are used. Therapists should be aware of the causes for various nerve injuries, to implement more effective prevention and intervention techniques.

Facial Disfigurement

Facial scars can be devastating, both functionally and psychologically. Hypertrophic scarring not only distorts the smooth contours of the cheeks and forehead, but also can flatten the nasal contours, evert eyelids and lips, and constrict optic and oral commissures. This disfigurement is damaging to an individual's self-image and inhibits social interactions. A considerable amount of communication depends on nonverbal facial expressions and eye contact. Severe facial burn scars not only distort the face and restrict expression, but also inhibit eye contact because of social rejection and loss of self-esteem.

Two main compression therapy methods are used to prevent or manage hypertrophic facial scars. An elastic face mask can be worn with underlying flexible conformers. The other option is a rigid, total-contact transparent facial orthosis.[52] Each has advantages and disadvantages.

Because face masks of elastic fabric usually enclose the entire head and use flexible conformers, they provide more uniform compression during movement or changes in position. However, because they occlude the face, they are cosmetically and socially less acceptable and must be removed before entering facilities such as banks or convenience stores where the patient is not known. Effectiveness of the compression is based on subjective feedback from the patient and observations made by the fabricator between therapy visits. Most types of underlying conformers are easy to modify or replace as needed to provide effective pressure distribution over facial concavities and contours.

Fabrication of the transparent, rigid orthosis is an involved and often expensive process. Fabrication involves taking a negative impression of the patient's face and making a positive plaster mold of the impression. Thermoplastic is heated and stretched over the mold. The edges are finished, elastic straps are applied, and the orthosis is fitted to the patient.[31] The therapist can objectively evaluate the amount of pressure exerted on the scars by noting the presence of scar blanching under the clear mask and make precise adjustments as needed.

With either method, frequent alterations are necessary to achieve and maintain adequate compression of all facial scars (Fig. 47-17). The choice of which method to use is based on patient and physician preference. However, a combination of both is most advantageous with a clear rigid facemask for social settings and the fabric mask with conformers at nighttime or when at home.

Appropriate skin care education is also important. Massage with lotion twice a day will aid scar desensitization and provide necessary lubrication. Facial massage and exercises are performed at least twice a day to stretch tight facial skin, maintain eyelid and mouth flexibility, and maintain nostril openings. Just as with any compression therapy technique, patient compliance is essential to the effectiveness of the treatment. The patient is instructed to wear the face mask(s) at all times, except while eating or bathing. Individuals wearing either type of mask often report feelings of self-consciousness, acute awareness of being stared at, and a fear of going out in public. To successfully manage these social and personal issues, supportive intervention is needed from the family, therapist, and social worker. Compliance is especially critical in controlling facial scar and disfigurement. The therapist must provide

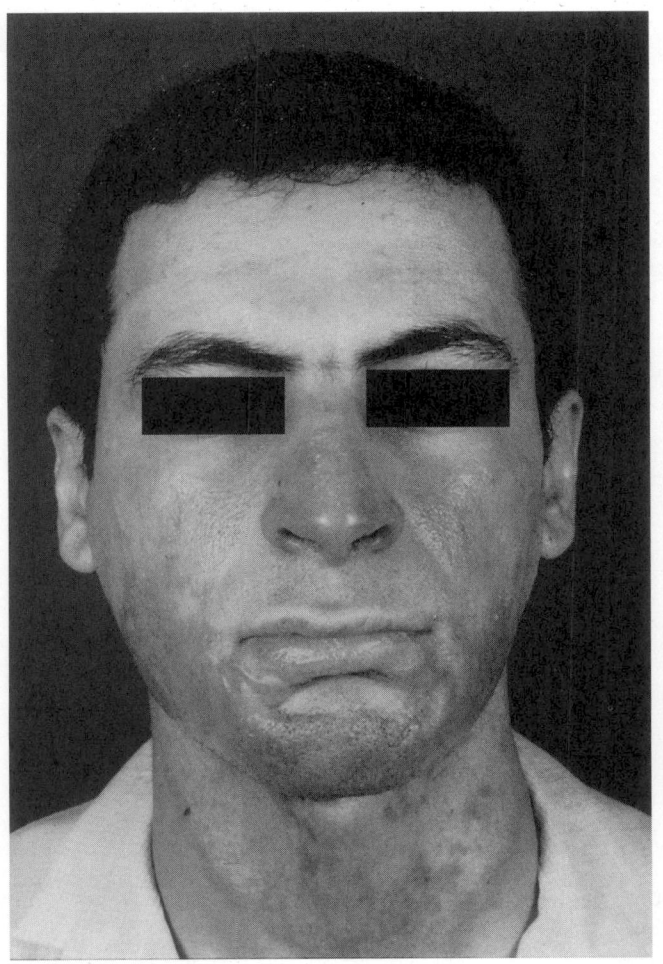

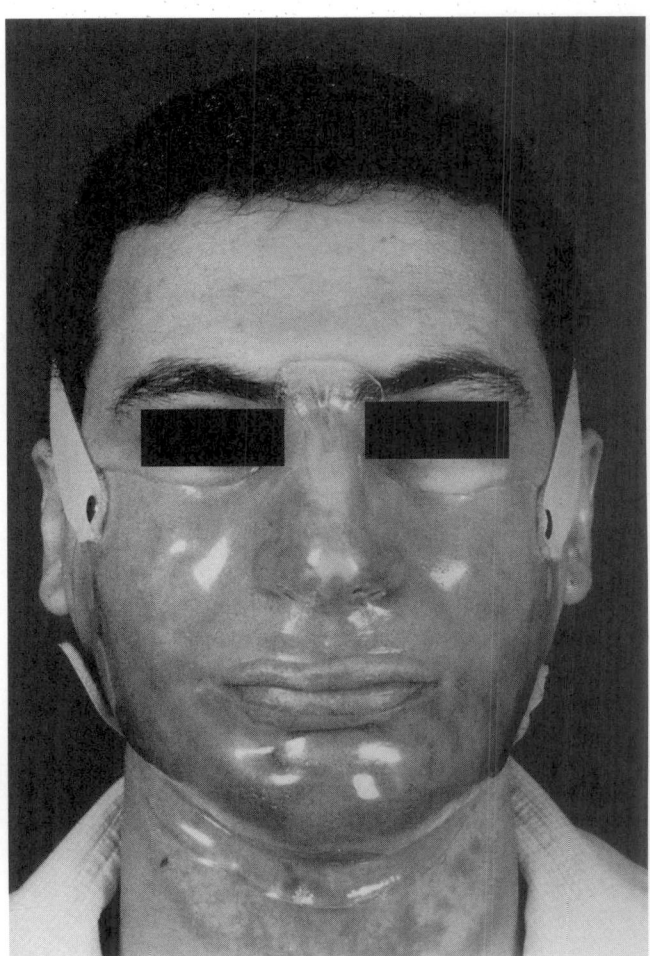

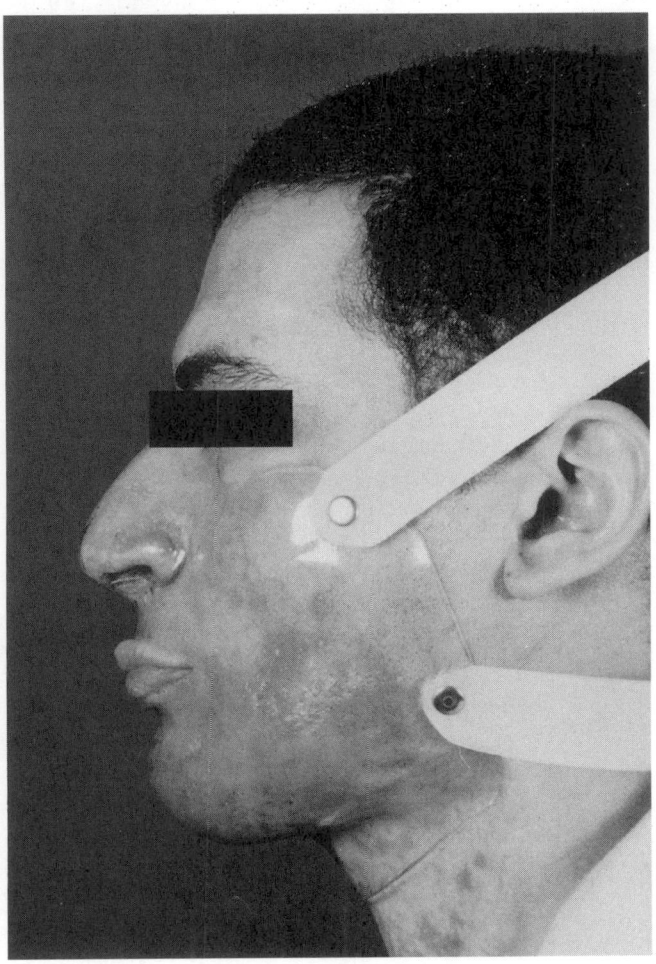

FIG. 47-17
Close-up view of transparent rigid facial orthosis. Mask contours and straps are adjusted to increase pressure over scarred areas (note blanching of lower lip and lateral chin).

encouragement and continual support to ensure perseverance with wearing a facial orthosis, despite the social barrier it can cause. Once the scars are mature and compression therapy is no longer needed, the patient should be instructed in the use of special camouflaging cosmetics such as Covermark that will cover minor texture flaws and correct uneven pigmentation.*

---

*Covermark Cosmetics, Veterans Dr., Suite D, Northvale, NJ 07647, (800)524-1120157, http://www.covermark.com/.

SUMMARY

A thermal injury can be one of the most devastating physical and psychological injuries a person can suffer, especially if appropriate treatment is not received in a timely and comprehensive manner. Successful burn care requires a coordinated, multidisciplinary team approach from the date of the patient's admission to the hospital until wound maturation is complete. The occupational therapist is an integral member of the burn team, providing treatment that promotes recovery of functional skills. Treatment activities include positioning, exercise, ADL, splints, skin conditioning, external compression techniques, patient and family education, and emotional support.

Advancements in medical and surgical burn care have made it possible to expect not only self-care independence, but also early return to school, work, and leisure and social activities. Even when functional recovery is possible, pain, disfigurement, and adverse psychological reactions (noncompliance, apathy, and depression) can contribute to postinjury dysfunction. In addition to progressive physical rehabilitation, ongoing patient education is crucial. A comprehensive patient education program should be initiated early and incorporate information about the physical, psychological, and social components of burn injury to facilitate the patient's cooperation and adjustment to the injury. Frequent reassessment of the patient's physical abilities, emotional status, and social needs is also needed to ensure effective treatment programming.

A basic OT concept that should be observed in all burn care is treatment of the "whole" person. Although this concept is apparent with large, severe burn injuries, it is also important to remember when treating small (less than 20% TBSA) burn injuries. A saying in the burn care field that makes this point is, "There is no such thing as a small burn, unless it is on someone else."

CASE STUDY 47-1

CASE STUDY—S.T.

History

S.T. is a 38-year-old man who received 25% TBSA battery acid burns in a rollover automobile accident in which he was pinned under his vehicle. He had superficial-, deep-, and full-thickness burns to his upper chest, midback, dorsal right hand and forearm, right circumferential upper arm, and right anterior axillary fold, as well as deep partial- and full-thickness burns to his neck, face and dorsal right index finger. Other trauma-related injuries included skin lacerations to his forehead, fracture to his coccyx, right elbow sprain, chest trauma resulting in a lacerated spleen, and a collapsed upper lobe of his right lung. Medical history includes sleep apnea and psoriasis to both lower legs. His right hand is dominant.

S.T. lives alone in a mobile home but shares custody of his 3-year-old son, who stays with him on alternate weekends. He completed high school and had been employed for 18 years as a truck driver for a transportation company until the time of his accident. Leisure interests included fishing, working out at the gym, and competitive power lifting. His previous level of functioning was independent in all ADL and IADL.

S.T. was admitted to the regional burn intensive care unit on 8/1/97. He had not received a significant smoke inhalation injury, but was intubated because of facial swelling, pharyngeal edema, and subsequent airway compromise. Initial nursing care included twice-a-day dressing changes using silver sulfadiazine cream to the torso and arms, antibiotic ointment to the face, and Sulfamylon to the ears. On 8/4 he underwent a tracheostomy to ensure a patent airway. On 8/8 he underwent tangential excision and STSG to the right upper extremity and face with donor sites from his anterior thighs and lower chest. On 8/15 he received tangential excision and grafting again to his face and scalp. His respiratory status improved and he was extubated on 8/20. Initially the patient was incoherent, but by 8/21 his mental status had cleared and he was allowed liquid diet by mouth on 8/21. His tracheostomy was removed on 8/27. He was discharged on 8/29/97 to home, 28 days after injury. At discharge the patient was eating a regular diet but still had unhealed areas on his face and lips.

Evaluation and Goals

An OT evaluation was performed on 8/2. Current status, medical history, and preevaluation background information was obtained from the medical record, family, and nonverbal communication from the patient. Areas of assessment included location and depth of burned surface areas; communication abilities; cognitive and emotional status; active ROM, general strength, and coordination; presence and degree of edema; and screening for changes in neurological function or sensation. The patient's

Continued

CASE STUDY—S.T.—cont'd

functional performance was initially impaired by acute edema of the face and bilateral upper extremities and an acute decline in mental status. Several weeks later, as S.T. became more alert and able to participate in treatment, it was noted that he also had peripheral nerve damage to his right median nerve with subsequent decrease in his right hand strength and sensation. Goals were initially reviewed and discussed with the family and again later with the patient after he became alert and fully cognizant.

Acute phase treatment goals were to:

1. Reduce facial and extremity edema
2. Improve cognitive awareness
3. Preserve functional mobility, strength and coordination of the neck, and both upper extremities
4. Regain independence with basic activities of daily living

A goal was added during the postoperative phase:

1. Protect and immobilize surgical graft sites to maximize graft take

Goals of increased focus in the rehabilitation phase were:

1. Minimize hypertrophic scarring and disfigurement. Preserve facial function.
2. Regain independence with activities of daily living and increase activity tolerance.
3. Develop coping strategies for dealing with pain and facial disfigurement (added later after irreversible facial scarring occurred).

The long-term goal of treatment was to return S.T. to his preinjury level of independence by four months after injury.

Treatment Approaches

Treatment interventions initiated in the acute care phase

1. Positioning guidelines were established with the head of the patient's bed elevated 20° or more; bilateral upper extremities elevated on pillow inclines with right upper extremity abducted to 90°. Illustrated positioning recommendations were posted bedside. As wounds healed, retrograde massage was provided to assist with edema reduction in the hands.
2. Orientation activities were incorporated into the patient's exercise and activity treatment sessions.
3. Passive ROM was provided when the patient was not alert enough to participate. Later, as the patient became more cognizant, an active assistive exercise program was provided to promote edema reduction and return of functional use of the extremities and face. The patient's exercise program was posted bedside. Therapeutic activities of interest were encouraged to increase motivation, activity tolerance, endurance, and fine motor coordination. The patient particularly enjoyed working out on the stationary bicycle.
4. After the patient was fully cognizant, extubated, and allowed food by mouth, the patient began to practice basic oral and facial ADL, sitting supported in bed or in a bedside chair. Sponge handles were initially applied to his eating utensils and toothbrush and removed after his right grip strength improved.

Treatment interventions begun in the postoperative phase

1. A right postoperative elbow extension splint was fabricated and applied, to be worn over dressings full time postoperatively for 5 days and then part time at night until full active ROM (AROM) was regained.

Treatment interventions initiated during the rehabilitation phase

1. After the patient was orally extubated, he was measured and fitted with a Microstomia Prevention Appliance (MPA) mouth splint that he wore initially when sleeping, but later MPA use was increased to include daytime periods because of increased oral tightness. The patient was measured for a manufactured elastic face mask, chin strap, and sleeve. A temporary right compressive sleeve was fabricated and applied. Fabrication of a clear acrylic face mask was initiated before discharge and applied on an outpatient basis. After discharge, the patient continued to receive OT for right upper extremity exercise program, scar management, and monitoring the fit of compression garments. As his scars continued to contract, the tight anterior axilla was treated with moist heat and slow sustained stretch. Facial exercises were intensified with emphasis on patient participation. Horizontal stretch exercises to the healed eyelids and midface were performed by the patient using skin traction. Oral stretch exercises that were initiated by the therapist in the acute phase using plastic thermometer covers, in this phase were performed more aggressively using acrylic straws (horizontal) and tongue depressor stacks (vertical).[28]
2. Practice of ADL was continued, progressing with performing self-care tasks, sitting on the edge of the bed and later standing at the sink in order to increase general strength and activity tolerance while becoming more independent with self-care tasks.
3. Relaxation techniques were taught to help S.T. cope with discomfort during therapy, emotional support was provided, and S.T. was referred for professional counseling while still an inpatient.

Outcomes

In spite of compression therapy, mouth splinting, and facial exercises, S.T.'s facial scars, which were caused by acid burns, continued to contract, causing eye, nasal, and oral constriction, lip eversion, eye **ectropion**, and flattening of his facial features. About 2 months after discharge, S.T. abandoned the use of the acrylic face mask because the frequent long-distance trips for adjustments to the mask could not keep pace with the rapidly changing facial contours. Instead, S.T. preferred using the elastic fabric facemasks and flexible conformers. S.T. continued nighttime use of his MPA for approximately 1 year after discharge to prevent further constriction of his mouth, but continued to have webbing at each oral commissure. S.T.'s right arm graft sites and burn scars responded well to exercise and the consistent use of elastic compression sleeves, with resulting full active ROM, a supple, flattened texture, and acceptable appearance. The scars on his upper shoulders did not receive compression therapy because of his preference to use a sleeve rather a full vest, but these scars, while having a slightly raised texture, were also acceptable to him.

CASE STUDY 47-1—cont'd

CASE STUDY—S.T.—cont'd

Two years later, S.T. has had 10 surgical revisions for treatment of recurrent facial contractures caused by the severe acid burn scarring and an extended period to obtain facial scar maturation. He has regained right hand strength but still lacks sensation in his thumb and forefinger and continues to experience chronic low back pain. He is currently scheduled for a series of surgical reconstruction procedures to establish patent nasal passages and relieve facial tightness. Although improving with multiple surgical procedures and the use of facial compression therapy, the patient's facial appearance is still unacceptable by social standards. Because of limited field of vision caused by distorted eyelids and right eye blurring, S.T. has not been employed as a truck driver since his accident. He is currently self-employed part-time, providing lawn care services for local businesses. His attempts to reenter previous social circles have resulted in mixed responses from individuals, and in some instances led to physical altercations. S.T. and his small son had maintained contact by telephone throughout his hospitalization. Before discharge, the child had been gradually introduced to S.T.'s changed facial features, first with photos, then with the face mask in place, and later without either mask. He was and continues to remain fully accepting of his father, regardless of his altered appearance.

Patient's Personal Long-Term Goals

"Because of my eyes I'll never be able to work as a truck driver again, and because of my back I can't power lift anymore, but I'd like to build up my lawn service into a business with a small crew. Emotionally, I'm doing okay, I have my ups and downs. I won't go out to eat at a restaurant anymore. Sometimes my appearance startles people. What I'd really like is to look halfway normal so that I don't always stand out."

REVIEW QUESTIONS

1. Name the two layers of the skin. In which layer are the nerves and sebaceous glands?
2. Which factors are considered in determining burn severity?
3. What is an escharotomy, and why is it performed?
4. Describe two factors that affect the quality of burn wound healing and promote excessive scar formation.
5. During the acute care phase, which factors may limit full ROM?
6. What is a boutonniere deformity, and what are boutonniere precautions?
7. What are the two basic principles underlying most burn rehabilitation treatment techniques?
8. What is the primary objective for positioning during acute care?
9. What are the indications for initiating splints during the acute care phase?
10. When a splint is indicated, what is the preferred wearing schedule and why?
11. When should patient education about burn injury and rehabilitation begin?
12. Why may a patient need temporary adaptations for self-care during the acute care phase?
13. Why are patients immobilized postoperatively? On the average, how soon after grafting can gentle, active ROM be resumed?
14. How soon postoperatively should an intermediate compression dressing or garment be applied?
15. What are the two main compression therapy options for facial scar treatment?
16. Why are skin conditioning activities used in burn rehabilitation? What are examples of skin conditioning techniques?
17. What is the average length of time required for scar maturation?
18. What are possible causes of limitations in ADL during the rehabilitation phase?
19. Which points should be covered in a home program?
20. What is the primary cause of dysfunction following a burn injury?

REFERENCES

1. Abston S: Scar reaction after thermal injury and prevention of scars and contractures. In Boswick JA, editor: The art and science of burn care, Rockville, Md, 1987, Aspen.
2. Apfel LM et al: Computer-drafted pressure support gloves, J Burn Care Rehabil 9(2):165-168, 1988.
3. Artz CP, Moncrief JA, Pruitt BA: Burns: a team approach, Philadelphia, 1979, WB Saunders.
4. Baltimore Therapeutic Equipment Co, 1201 Bernard Dr., Baltimore, MD, 21223.
5. Bariollo DJ, Nangle ME, Farrell K: Preliminary experience with cultured epidermal autograft in a community hospital burn unit, J Burn Care Rehabil 13(1):158-165, 1992.
6. Baur PS et al: Wound contractions, scar contractures and myofibroblasts: a classical case study, J Trauma 18(1):8-21, 1978.
7. Bennett GB et al: Serial casting: a method for treating burn contracture, J Burn Care Rehabil 10(6):543-545, 1989.
8. Bruster J, Pullium G: Gradient pressure, Am J Occup Ther 37(7):485-488, 1983.
9. Burnsworth B, Krob MJ, Langer-Schnepp M: Immediate ambulation of patients with lower extremity grafts, J Burn Care Rehabil 13(1):89-92. 1992.

10. Carr-Collins JA: Pressure techniques for the prevention of hypertrophic scar. In Salisbury RE, editor: *Clinics in plastic surgery: burn rehabilitation and reconstruction*, Philadelphia, 1992, WB Saunders.

11. Carvajal HF: Resuscitation of the burned child. In Carvajal HF, Parks DH, editors: *Burns in children: pediatric burn management*, Chicago, 1988, Year Book Medical Publishers.

12. Clark JA, Burt AM, Eldad A: Culture epithelium as a skin substitute, *Burns Incl Therm Inj* 13(3):173-180, 1987.

13. Covey MH: Occupational therapy. In Boswick JA, editor: *The art and science of burn care*, Rockville, Md, 1987, Aspen.

14. Crawford CM et al: Heterotopic ossification: are range of motion exercises contraindicated? *J Burn Care Rehabil* 7(4):323-327, 1986.

15. Daugherty MB, Carr-Collins JA: Splinting techniques for the burn patient. In Richard RL, Staley MJ, editors: *Burn care and rehabilitation: principles and practice*, Philadelphia, 1994, FA Davis.

16. Dietch EA and associates: Hypertrophic burn scars: analysis of variables, *J Trauma* 23(10):895-898, 1983.

17. Dyer C: Burn care in the emergent period, *J Emerg Nurs* 6(1):9-16, 1980.

18. Fleet J: The psychological effects of burn injuries: a literature review, *Brit J Occup Ther* 55(5):198-201, 1992.

19. Giuliani CA, Perry GA: Factors to consider in the rehabilitation aspect of burn care, *Phys Ther* 65(5):619-623, 1985.

20. Hansbrough JF: Current status of skin replacements for coverage of extensive burn wounds, *J Trauma* 30(suppl 12):s155-162, 1990.

21. Hartford C: Surgical management. In Fisher S, Helm P: *Comprehensive rehabilitation of burns*, Baltimore, 1984, Williams & Wilkins.

22. Heimbach DM, Engrav LH: *Surgical management of the burn wound*, New York, 1984, Raven Press.

23. Helm PA: Neuromuscular considerations. In Fisher SV, Helm PA, editors: *Comprehensive rehabilitation of burns*, Baltimore, 1984, Williams & Wilkins.

24. Helm PA: Burn rehabilitation: dimensions of the problem. In Salisbury RE: *Clinics in plastic surgery*, Philadelphia, 1992, WB Saunders.

25. Helm PA, Fisher SV: Rehabilitation of the patient with burns. In Delisa J, Currie D, Gans B, editors: *Rehabilitation medicine: principles and practice*, Philadelphia, 1988, JB Lippincott.

26. Hoffer MM, Brody G, Ferlic F: Excision of heterotopic ossification about elbows in patients with thermal injury, *J Trauma* 18(9):667-670, 1978.

27. Howell JW: Management of the acutely burned hand for the nonspecialized clinician, *Phys Ther* 69(12):1077-1089, 1989.

28. Humphrey C, Richard RL, Staley MJ: Soft tissue management and exercise. In Richard RL, Staley MJ, editors: *Burn care and rehabilitation: principles and practice*, Philadelphia, 1994, FA Davis.

29. Hunter JM, Mackin EJ: Management of edema. In Hunter JM, Schneider LH, Mackin EJ, et al, editors: *Rehabilitation of the hand*, St Louis, 1990, Mosby.

30. Johnson CL: Physical therapists as scar modifiers, *Phys Ther* 64(9):1381-1387, 1984.

31. Jordan CL, Allely RA, Gallagher J: Self-care strategies following severe burns. In Christiansen C, editor: *Ways of living: self-care strategies for special needs*, Rockville, Md, 1994, American Occupational Therapy Association.

32. Jordan MH et al: Dynamic plaster casting for burn scar contracture, *Proc Am Burn Assoc* 16:17, 1984.

33. Jordan MH et al: A pressure prevention device for burned ears, *J Burn Care Rehabil* 13(1):673-677, 1992.

34. Kaplan SH: Patient education techniques used at burn centers, *Am J Occup Ther* 39(1):655-658, 1985.

35. Larson DL et al: Techniques for decreasing scar formation and contracture in the burned patient, *J Trauma* 11(10):807-822, 1971.

36. Leman CH: An approach to work hardening in burn rehabilitation, *Top Acute Care Trauma Rehabil* 1(4):62-73, 1987.

37. Leman CJ: Burn rehabilitation. In Hopkins HL, Smith HD, editors: *Willard & Spackman's occupational therapy*, ed 8, Philadelphia, 1993, JB Lippincott.

38. Leman CJ, Ricks N: Discharge planning and follow-up burn care. In Richard RL, Staley MJ, editors: *Burn care and rehabilitation: principles and practice*, Philadelphia, 1994, FA Davis.

39. Leman CJ and associates: Exercise physiology in the acute burn patient: do we really know what we're doing? *Proc Am Burn Assoc* 24:91, 1992.

40. Linares HA: Hypertrophic healing: controversies and etiopathogenic review. In Carvajal HF, Parks DH, editors: *Burns in children: pediatric burn management*, Chicago, 1988, Year Book Medical Publishers.

41. Lund C, Browder N: The estimation of area of burns, *Surg Gynecol Obstet* 79:352-355, 1944.

42. Mahon LM, Neufeld N: The effect of informational feedback on food intake of adult burn patients, *Appl Behav Annal* 17(3):391-396, 1984.

43. Miles WK, Grigsby L: Remodeling of scar tissue in the burned hand. In Hunter JM, Schneider LH, Mackin EJ, et al, editors: *Rehabilitation of the hand*, St Louis, 1990, Mosby.

44. Moss BF, Everett JJ, Patterson DR: Psychologic support and pain management of the burn patient. In Richard RL, Staley MJ, editors: *Burn care and rehabilitation: principles and practice*, Philadelphia, 1994, FA Davis.

45. Nolan WB: Acute management of thermal injury, *Ann Plast Surg* 7(3):243-251, 1981.

46. Peacock EE Jr: *Wound repair*, ed 3, Philadelphia, 1984, WB Saunders.

47. Pullium G: Splinting and positioning. In Fisher SV, Helm PA, editors: *Comprehensive rehabilitation of burns*, Baltimore, 1984, Williams & Wilkins.

48. Richard RL, Staley MJ: Burn patient evaluation and treatment planning. In Richard RL, Staley MJ, editors: *Burn care and rehabilitation: principles and practice*, Philadelphia, 1994, FA Davis.

49. Ricks N, Meagher D: The benefits of plaster casting for lower extremity burns after grafting in children, *J Burn Care Rehabil* 13(4):465-468, 1992.

50. Rivers EA: Rehabilitation management of the burn patient, *Advances in Clin Rehabil* 1:177-214, 1978.

51. Rivers EA, Fisher SV: Rehabilitation for burn patients. In Kottke FJ, Lehmann JF, editors: *Krusen's handbook of physical medicine and rehabilitation*, ed 4, Philadelphia, 1990, WB Saunders.

52. Rivers EA, Strate R, Solem L: The transparent face mask, *Am J Occup Ther* 33(2):108-113, 1979.

53. Rosenstein DL: A school reentry program for burned children. I. Development and implementation of a school reentry program, *J Burn Care Rehabil* 8(4):319-322, 1987.

54. Salisbury RE, Petro JA: Rehabilitation of burn patients. In Boswick JA, editor: *The art and science of burn care*, Rockville, Md, 1987, Aspen.

55. Schmitt MA, French L, Kalil ET: How soon is safe? Ambulation of the patient with burns after lower-extremity skin grafting, *J Burn Care Rehabil* 12(1):33-37, 1991.

56. Solem L: Classification. In Fisher S, Helm P, editors: *Comprehensive rehabilitation of burns*, Baltimore, 1984, Williams & Wilkins.

57. Staley MJ, Richard RL: Scar management. In Richard RL, Staley MJ, editors: *Burn care and rehabilitation: principles and practice*, Philadelphia, 1994, FA Davis.

58. Sullivan T and associates: Rating the burn scar, *J Burn Care Rehabil* 11(3):256-260, 1990.

59. United States Department of Labor: *Dictionary of occupational titles*, ed 4, Washington, DC, 1977, US Government Printing Office.

60. Valpar Component Work Samples, Valpar International Corporation, PO Box 5767, Tucson, Ariz.

61. Varghese G: Musculoskeletal conditions. In Fisher SV, Helm PA, editors: *Comprehensive rehabilitation of burns*, Baltimore, 1984, Williams & Wilkins.

62. Wachtel T: Epidemiology, classification, initial care, and administrative considerations for critically burned patients. In Wachtel T: *Critical care clinics*, Philadelphia, 1985, WB Saunders.

63. Weil R et al: Smoke inhalation injury, *Ann Plast Surg* 4(2):121-127, 1980.
64. Work Evaluation Systems Technology (WEST), PO Box 2477, Fort Bragg, CA 95437.
65. Wright PC: Fundamentals of acute burn care and physical therapy management, *Phys Ther* 64(8):1217-1231, 1984.
66. Yurko L, Fratianne R: Evaluation of burn discharge teaching, *J Burn Care Rehabil* 9(6):643-644, 1988.
67. Burn Survivors Online, http://www.alpha-tek.com/burn/.

ADDITIONAL INFORMATION

American Burn Association
 http://ameriburn.org/home.htm

British Columbia Burn Network Society Homepage
 http://vanserve org/vanservehome.htm
British Columbia Burn Network Society—Burn Related Links on the Internet
 http://vanserve.org/links.html
Burn Survivors Online
 http://www.alpha-tek.com/burn/
Cool the Burn
 http://www.cooltheburn.com/home.html

CHAPTER 48

Amputations and Prosthetics

DENISE D. KEENAN
PATRICIA ANN MORRIS

KEY TERMS

SECTION 1
General Considerations
Preprosthetic
Residual limb
Postprosthetic
Socket
Neuroma
Phantom limb
Phantom pain

SECTION 2
Upper Extremity Amputations
Body-powered prosthesis
Passive prosthesis
Terminal device
Hook
Prepositioning
Wrist flexion unit
Forequarter amputation
Myoelectric prosthesis
Muscle site
Greifer
Pull sock
Control training
Pressure control

SECTION 3
Lower Extremity Amputations
Hemipelvectomy
Above-knee amputation
Below-knee amputation
Symes amputation
Pylon
Ischial weight-bearing prosthesis
SACH foot
Rigid removal dressing

LEARNING OBJECTIVES

After studying each section, the student or practitioner will be able to do the following:

Section 1
1. List the common causes of amputation.
2. Discuss the occupational therapist's role in rehabilitation after amputation.
3. List the goals of amputation surgery.
4. Name two types of surgical procedures.
5. Name four factors that can interfere with prosthetic training.
6. Define neuroma, phantom limb, and phantom pain.
7. Describe typical psychological consequences of amputation surgery.
8. Describe how the occupational therapist facilitates adjustment to amputation.

Section 2
1. Describe the role of the occupational therapist in the rehabilitation of the individual with an upper extremity (UE) amputation.
2. Discuss the impact of the residual limb status on the success of fitting and operating a UE prosthesis.
3. Name the five components common to all body-powered prostheses.
4. List the motions used to operate the body-powered prosthesis.
5. Describe at least two techniques for donning the body-powered prosthesis.
6. Describe the importance of prepositioning the terminal device.
7. List the two phases of training a person to use an UE prosthesis.
8. Appreciate the need to introduce postprosthetic training into three levels.
9. Understand basic operation of an electric prosthesis.
10. Recognize the primary function of any prosthesis in different daily tasks.

Section 3
1. List two major causes of LE amputation.
2. List postsurgical problems that affect prosthetic fitting and rehabilitation.
3. Discuss problems that can occur in postprosthetic rehabilitation.
4. Identify levels of LE amputation and functional losses associated with each.
5. Name and describe at least three types of LE prostheses.
6. List the goals of occupational therapy for the person with LE amputation.
7. Name the members of the rehabilitation team and their respective roles.
8. Describe some treatment strategies used by the occupational therapist.
9. Discuss activities of daily living addressed in the rehabilitation program.
10. Identify typical psychosocial factors affecting the adjustment and rehabilitation program after amputation.

SECTION 1
General Considerations of Upper and Lower Extremity Amputations

DENISE D. KEENAN
PATRICIA ANN MORRIS

Limb loss can result from disease, injury, or congenital causes. Individuals born with congenital limb deficiencies or whose amputations occur early in life usually grow and develop sensorimotor skills and self-images without the limb. The individual who has an amputation in adolescence or adulthood is confronted with the task of adjusting to the loss of a well-integrated part of the body scheme and self-image. These two types of patient populations present different problems for the rehabilitation worker.[32,33]

The occupational therapist's primary responsibility in the rehabilitation program is the formulation and execution of the **preprosthetic** program and prosthetic training. During the preprosthetic phase the treatment plan involves preparing the limb for a prosthesis; during the prosthetic phase, treatment involves increasing prosthesis wearing tolerance and functional use. The rehabilitation program involves an individualized treatment plan that helps the person with the physical and psychological adjustments. This program is designed so that the individual may learn to accept the new body image and function as independently as possible.[1,32,33]

CAUSES AND INCIDENCE OF AMPUTATION

The majority of amputations result from trauma, peripheral vascular disease (PVD), peripheral vasospastic diseases, chronic infections, chemical, thermal, or electrical injuries, and malignant tumors. Elective upper extremity (UE) amputations may occur as a result of a severe or complete brachial plexus injury.[4]

Each year an estimated 40,000 Americans lose a limb. Approximately 4000 to 5500 lose a hand or arm. The incidence of amputation remains fairly constant between the ages of 1 and 15. From 15 to 54 years of age, however, there is a gradual increase in incidence because of work-related injuries and highway accidents. Approximately 75% of UE amputations in adults are caused by trauma.[17,23]

The major cause of lower extremity (LE) amputation is PVD, often associated with smoking and diabetes.[18,21,29] Despite major improvements in noninvasive diagnosis, revascularization, and wound-healing techniques, 2% to 5% of individuals without diabetes but with PVD, and 6% to 25% of those with PVD and diabetes, undergo amputation.[13,14,22,25,35] Perioperative mortality of persons with LE amputation has been variously reported as between 7% and 13% and is usually associated with other medical problems such as cardiac disease and strokes.[9,13,14]

The second leading cause of LE amputation is trauma, usually from motor vehicle accidents or gunshots. Individuals with traumatic amputations are usually young adults and more frequently men.[8,12] Improved imaging techniques, more effective chemotherapy, and better limb salvage procedures have reduced the incidence of amputation from osteogenic sarcoma. Tumor resection followed by limb reconstruction frequently provides as functional an extremity as a prosthesis and does not appear to affect the 5-year survival rate.[15,20,30,34,39]

SURGICAL MANAGEMENT

The surgeon is an important team member. Before surgery the surgeon should consult with the health care team to maximize the functional outcome. The surgeon attempts to preserve as much length as possible and provide a **residual limb** that has good skin coverage and vascularization. Conservation of residual limb length and uncomplicated wound healing are important. During and after surgery the primary goal is to form a residual limb that maintains maximal function of the remaining tissue and allows maximal use of the prosthesis.[1,17,32]

Blood vessels and nerves are severed and allowed to retract so that residual limb pain is minimized during prosthetic use. Bone beveling is a surgical procedure that smoothes the rough edges and prevents spur development of the remaining bone. Muscles are sutured to the bones distally by a surgical process called *myodesis*. The muscles involved in the function of the amputated limb are correspondingly affected by the loss.[27]

Surgical techniques vary with the level and cause of amputation.[31,32] A closed or open surgical procedure may be performed. The open method allows drainage and minimizes the possibility of infection. The closed method reduces the period of hospitalization but also reduces free drainage and increases the risk of infection.[32] The specific type of amputation performed is at the discretion of the surgeon and is often determined by the status of the extremity at the time of amputation. In either case the surgeon must remove the part of the limb that has to be eliminated, allow for primary or secondary wound healing, and construct a residual limb (also called a stump) for optimum prosthetic fitting and function. The residual limb that results should be strong and resilient.[32]

POSTSURGICAL FACTORS AND PROBLEMS

Several factors and potential problems can affect the outcome of rehabilitation. Length of the residual limb, skin integrity, edema, sensation, the time for healing, infections, and allergic reactions to the prosthesis are among the physical factors that affect rehabilitation potential.[19]

Skin

Skin complications account for most postsurgical problems. These complications occur in either the preprosthetic or **postprosthetic** phase. Delayed healing and extensive skin grafting are complications in the preprosthetic phase. Skin breakdown, ulcers, infected sebaceous cysts, and allergic reactions can occur in the postprosthetic phase. Residual limb edema can occur in either phase. Delayed healing of the incision site is one of the earliest preprosthetic complications resulting in postponed prosthetic fitting. Necrotic areas may develop, requiring surgical intervention.[2]

To achieve a residual limb length suitable for prosthetic use, the surgeon may perform extensive skin grafting. If the skin graft adheres to bone, the area may ulcerate and require medical attention.[2] Daily gentle massages by the person or therapist decreases the likelihood of skin graft adherence to bone and the attendant complications.

Immediately after surgery the residual limb is normally edematous as a result of fluid that collects within the soft tissues, especially in its distal portion. Compression wrapping or a rigid dressing helps decrease the edema.[3,10,17]

During the postprosthetic phase an ill-fitting **socket** or wrinkles in the prosthetic sock may cause skin breakdown or scar adhesions.[11] Residual limb ulceration is associated with ischemia and pressure exerted by the prosthesis on the limb. The physician should see the patient in this case, and the prosthesis should not be worn until the area heals. The prosthetist should also examine the prosthesis to determine if the socket should be adjusted. If these problems persist, surgical revision of the limb may be needed before rehabilitation can continue.[27]

The torque forces between the socket and the residual limb cause a predisposition to the development of sebaceous cysts. Treatment involves the application of moist heat. When the cyst becomes infected, drainage ensues and enucleation of the cyst wall may be required.[2]

The development of residual limb edema during the postprosthetic phase is usually indicative of an ill-fitting socket. Proximal tightness of the socket may result in distal edema, which may require a new, well-fitted socket.[2]

Sensory Problems

The loss of sensory feedback from the amputated limb is a major problem that confronts the person. This is especially significant for the person with UE amputation, since sensory feedback from the hand, so essential for function, is lost. Residual limb hyperesthesia, neuromas, and phantom sensation or pain are problems that may interfere with the functional use of the limb either with or without the prosthesis.

Residual limb hyperesthesia, or an overly sensitive limb, limits functional use and causes discomfort. Desensitization consists of tapping and massage, which helps decrease the discomfort.[1,11] Sympathetic nerve blocks may be used to manage residual limb hypersensitivity medically.[28]

The residual limb may have areas of absent or impaired sensation that require special attention and education when the prosthesis is worn. The person must rely on visual and proprioceptive feedback because sensation is functionally lost when the prosthesis is on the residual limb. The person must adjust to new sensations, such as the pressure of the residual limb inside the socket and the feel of the harness system, if used.[32]

Neuromas

Severed peripheral nerves form **neuromas** in the residual limb.[21,24] A neuroma is a small ball of nerve tissue that develops when growing axons attempt to reach the distal end of the residual limb. As the axons grow, they turn back on themselves, producing a ball of nerve tissue. If the neuroma adheres to scar tissue or skin subject to repetitive pressure, it can be painful when pressed. Diagnosis is made by palpating the neuroma.[3] Most neuromas occur 1 to 2 inches (2.5 to 5 cm) proximal to the end of the residual limb and are not troublesome.[2]

So that pain will not interfere with prosthetic wear, the neuroma must be well surrounded by soft tissue. During surgery the surgeon identifies the major nerves, pulls them down under some tension, cuts them clearly and sharply, and allows them to retract into soft tissue of the residual limb. Neuromas that form close to scar tissue or bone generally cause pain.[21,24]

Treatment involves local anesthetic injections or ultrasound. Both treatments should be followed by massage and stretching. Surgical intervention may be necessary. In addition, the residual limb socket may be fabricated or modified to accommodate the neuroma.[1,37,38]

Phantom Limb

The majority of patients who have had an amputation experience **phantom limb.** In its simplest form the phantom is the sensation of the limb that is no longer there. The phantom, which usually occurs initially immediately after surgery, is often described as a tingling, pressure sensation, or sometimes as numbness. The distal part of the extremity is most frequently felt, although sometimes the person feels the whole extremity. The sensation is influenced by external stimuli such as bandaging or rigid dressing. It may dissipate over time, or the person may have the phantom sensation throughout life.

Phantom sensation is painless and usually does not interfere with prosthetic rehabilitation. The patient should be assured that the feeling is quite normal.[31,38]

Desensitization, supportive counseling, and early use of the residual limb with a temporary or permanent prosthesis are effective measures for dealing with phantom sensations.[32] In many cases it is best not to dwell on the discussion of phantom sensation but rather to focus on prosthetic training and the return to a former lifestyle.

Phantom Pain

Phantom pain is different from phantom limb sensation in that it is usually characterized as either a cramping or squeezing sensation, a shooting pain, or a burning pain. Some patients report all three. The pain can be localized or diffuse. It may be continuous or intermittent and can be triggered by external stimuli. It may diminish over time or may become a permanent and often disabling condition. In the first 6 months following surgery, phantom pain is related to preoperative limb pain in location and intensity.[21]

No strict treatment protocol has been established for phantom pain. Isometric exercises begun 5 to 7 days following the amputation and performed several times throughout the day may help control phantom pain. Biofeedback, transcutaneous electrical nerve stimulation (TENS), ultrasound, progressive relaxation exercises, and controlled breathing exercises may reduce phantom pain. Activities such as rubbing, tapping, and applying pressure and heat may be beneficial. The physician may treat the pain by prescribing amitriptyline (Elavil) at bedtime by injecting anesthetics into the tender area or by performing sympathetic nerve blocks. Surgical revision of the residual limb is sometimes necessary to alleviate the pain.[1,37] The appearance of phantom pain or excessive concern with phantom sensation requires the intervention of the team. The therapist can allay the patient's fears about these phenomena by offering support, information, reassurance, and contact with other prosthesis wearers.

Bone Problems

The formation of bone spurs is another complication that may occur during the preprosthetic phase. Because most bone spurs are not palpable, an x-ray examination is needed to confirm their presence or absence. Bone spurs that cause pain or result in persistent drainage require surgical excision.

Delayed Wound Healing and Infection

For the person with LE amputation, delayed wound healing and excessive skin grafting are potential complications during the preprosthetic phase.

Many factors may affect normal wound healing. Postoperative infection from external or internal sources is a major concern. Patients with wounds contaminated from injury, infected foot ulcers, or other causes are at greater risk for infection. Research indicates that smoking is a major deterrent to wound healing. One study reported that cigarette smokers had a 2.5% higher rate of infection and reamputation than nonsmokers.[19] There is some indication that failure of limb revascularization may negatively influence healing at below-knee levels. Other factors that influence wound healing are the severity of the vascular problems, diabetes, renal disease, and other medical conditions such as cardiac disease.[5,21,35,36]

PSYCHOLOGICAL REACTIONS TO AMPUTATION

Profound psychological shock and disbelief are likely to accompany amputation, particularly for those who experience a sudden trauma that causes or necessitates amputation.[6,16,17] Seeing the residual limb for the first time can cause shock, panic, despair, self-pity, suicidal impulses, and even rage.[26] Subsequently there can be feelings of hopelessness, despondency, bitterness, and anger. Some individuals may mourn the possible loss of a job or ability to participate in favorite sports or activities, as well as the lost limb.

The person may feel lonely, isolated, and an object of pity. Concerns about the future, body image and function, the responses of family and friends, and employment all affect the person's emotional status.[26] Reactions to amputation may be less severe in individuals who have had a chance to adjust before the surgery.[6,16,17] Older persons may demonstrate postoperative confusion, whereas younger persons may have a sense of mutilation, emasculation, or castration.[6,16]

The person's personality, age, cultural background, and psychological, social, economic, and vocational resources influence the reaction to amputation. Ultimately, the individual must come to terms with the consequences of limb loss and perceived diminished attractiveness. The person confronts discomfort, inconvenience, economic expense and loss of function, increased energy expenditure, and possible curtailment of favorite activities. He or she may need to change occupations, deal with social discrimination, and cope with resultant medical problems.[6]

Cultural factors are important in the reaction to amputation. In some social, cultural, or religious groups the amputation may be considered a means of punishment or atonement. Such beliefs and society's aversion to amputation can cause the person to adopt the same viewpoint. Such attitudes can result in self-hatred and self-deprecation, which may affect the person's reactions and adjustment to the disability.[6]

Depression and a sense of futility are considered a normal part of the adjustment process.[6] If depression is severe and prolonged, psychological or psychiatric referral is indicated. Medication may be necessary to reduce depression.[6] The preexisting personality of the patient determines the severity and duration of the reactions and ultimately the adjustment to the amputation and to prosthetic use.[6,7]

Psychosocial Adjustment to Amputation

An individual's psychosocial adjustment depends on various factors: the individual's character and inner strength, the quality of the social support systems available, and sociocultural reactions to amputation and the team's management of the rehabilitation.[6]

The process of adjustment to amputations is analogous to the grieving process. The patient experiences identifiable stages of denial, anger, depression, coping, and acceptance.[6] Some patients progress through these stages and ultimately adapt to the loss. The cause of the amputation may contribute significantly to the patient's response.

In any phase the person may have hostile reactions directed toward self and the medical team. Often, overt solicitousness and friendliness may mask such hostility. Caregivers should not react with hostility but should make allowances for such behavior. Positive reinforcement through involvement in the rehabilitation process and contact with people having similar amputations aids in solving the problems of returning to former life roles.[6]

The person may have fear about returning to family, social, vocational, and sexual roles. Frequent discussions of fears and solutions to real or imagined problems, if possible with a similar, successfully rehabilitated person, are important for facilitating adjustment.[6]

After a mourning period, the person may minimize the significance of the amputation and actually joke about it. When this phase of adjustment has subsided, the person begins seriously to consider the future. At this point the therapist can discuss social, vocational, and educational plans with the individual.[6]

Loss of a body part necessitates a revision and acceptance of the body image. Problems with the acceptance of the change in body image may cause difficulties in prosthetic training.[32,33] Fostering acceptance of the prosthesis is a primary way to promote the person's adjustment. Establishing a training program that presents the prosthesis in a manner that meets the person's needs and goals has a beneficial effect in integrating the prosthesis into the body scheme. The prosthesis must become part of the self before it can be used most effectively. The prosthesis contributes to a normal appearance, helping the person identify with able-bodied individuals.[6,32,33]

Long-term adjustment depends on the person's basic personality structure, sense of accomplishment, and place in the family, community, and world. Generally, individuals who have had an amputation may dream of themselves as not being amputated. This image may be so vivid that persons with LE amputation fall as they get up at night and attempt to walk to the bathroom without a prosthesis.[26]

The rehabilitation team members can help the patient understand the importance of the prosthetic training program. The use of new prosthetic technology that addresses different lifestyles and enhances normal

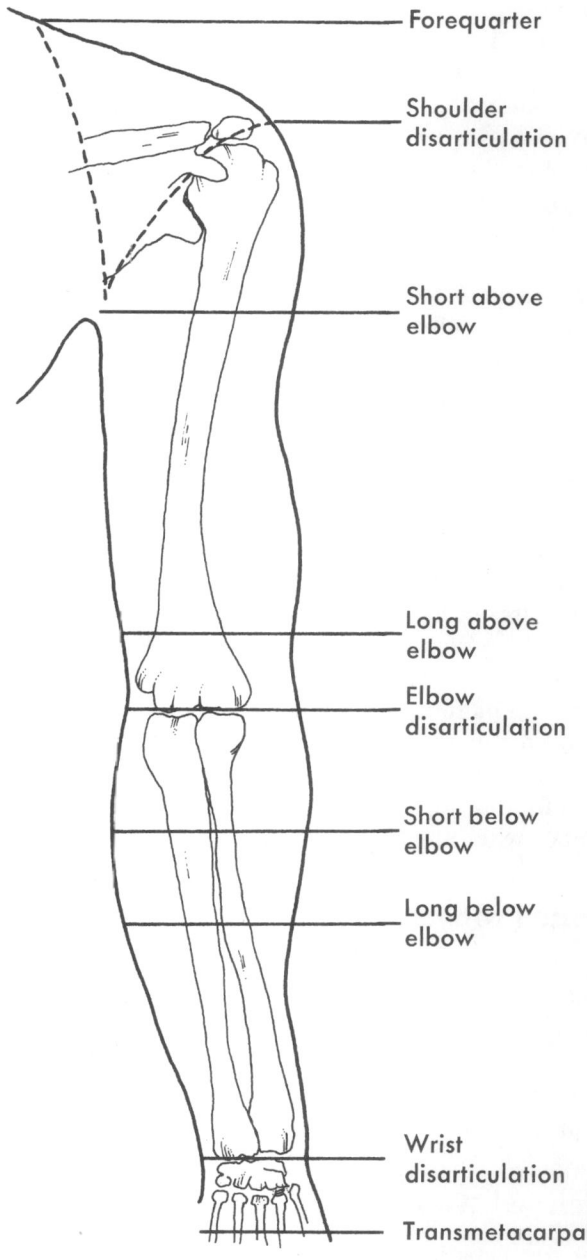

FIG. 48-1
Levels of upper extremity amputation.

appearance should be stressed. The patient needs to receive reassurance and understanding from the entire rehabilitation team.[26]

SECTION 2
Upper Extremity Amputations

I. Body-Powered Prostheses
DENISE D. KEENAN
LYNDA M. ROCK

CANDIDATES FOR PROSTHESES

Information regarding prostheses and the rehabilitation program should be provided before the amputation, if possible, because afterward pain medication and anxiety may interfere with the person's ability to process new information. Team discussion that includes the patient is vital for determining whether to generate a prosthetic prescription and, if so, which components to include, or, alternatively, whether a prosthesis is inappropriate. The person's age, medical status, amputation level, skin coverage, skin condition, cognitive status, and desire for a prosthesis are important factors in making the decision.[8]

LEVELS OF AMPUTATION AND FUNCTIONAL LOSSES IN THE UPPER EXTREMITY

The higher the level of amputation, the greater the functional loss of the arm. Greater functional loss necessitates a more complex prosthesis and more extensive training in operation and use of the prosthesis (Fig. 48-1).[12] Table 48-1 provides an outline of progressively higher UE amputations, associated loss of function, and appropriate components required for a functional **body-powered prosthesis**.[9,12]

COMPONENT PARTS OF THE UPPER EXTREMITY BODY-POWERED PROSTHESIS

Various prosthetic components are available for each level of amputation (Fig. 48-2). Each prosthesis is prescribed according to the patient's needs and lifestyle and is custom made and individually fitted. The prosthesis

TABLE 48-1
Amputation Levels, Functional Losses, and Suggested Prosthetic Components

Level of Amputation	Loss of Function	Suggested Functional Prosthetic Components
Partial hand	Some or all grip functions	Dependent on cosmesis and functional loss
Wrist disarticulation	Hand and wrist function; about 50% of pronation and supination	Harness, control cable, socket, flexible elbow hinges
Long below elbow	Hand and wrist function; most pronation and supination	Same as for wrist disarticulation but circular wrist unit
Short below elbow	Hand and wrist function; all pronation and supination; impaired elbow flexion and extension	Harness, control cable, socket, rigid elbow hinges, and biceps half cuff, wrist unit, and terminal device
Elbow disarticulation	Hand and wrist function; all pronation and supination; elbow flexion and extension	Harness, dual-control cables, socket, externally locking elbow, forearm shell, wrist unit, and terminal device
Long above elbow	Hand and wrist function; all pronation and supination; elbow flexion and extension	Harness, dual-control cables, socket, internally locking elbow, lift assist, turntable, forearm shell, wrist unit, and terminal device
Short above elbow	All of the above; shoulder internal and external rotation	Same as for long above elbow, but socket may partially cover shoulder, restricting its function
Shoulder disarticulation	Loss of all arm and hand functions	Same as for long above elbow, but socket covers shoulder; chest strap; shoulder unit; upper arm shell; chin-operated nudge control for elbow unit
Forequarter	Loss of all arm and hand functions; partial or complete loss of clavicle and scapula	May be same as above but with lightweight materials; when minimal function is attainable, endoskeletal cosmetic prosthesis may be preferred
Bilateral amputation	Dependent on levels of amputation	Appropriate to level of amputation, plus wrist flexion unit and cable-operated wrist rotator

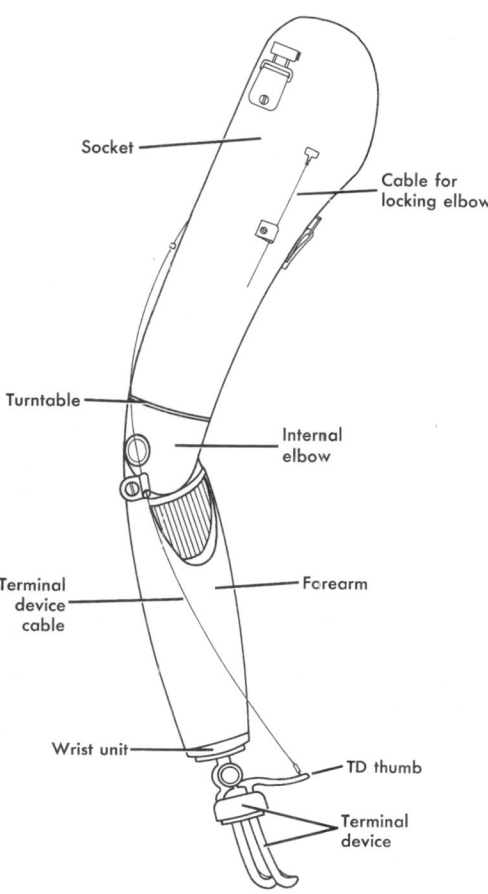

FIG. 48-2
Component parts of standard above-elbow prosthesis. (Adapted from Santschi W, editor: *Manual of upper extremity prosthetics*, ed 2, Los Angeles, 1958, University of California Press.)

can be either a functional prosthesis or a **passive prosthesis.** Passive does not mean nonfunctional; the prosthesis provides postural balance and can act as an assist to secure items for the functional limb.

The first five prosthetic components described below are common to all body-powered prostheses prescribed for wrist disarticulation and higher levels. They are the socket, harness, cable, **terminal device** (TD), and wrist unit. Many people with UE amputations wear a prosthetic sock between the residual limb and the prosthesis.[12]

Prosthetic Sock

A prosthetic sock of knit wool, cotton, or Orlon-Lycra is worn between the prosthesis and the limb (Fig. 48-3). Silipos makes a Silo-Line that assists in minimizing hypertrophic scarring and may be worn as the prosthetic sock or covered with a sock. The function of the prosthetic sock is to absorb perspiration and protect against irritation that could result from direct contact of the skin with the socket. The sock compensates for volume change in the residual limb and contributes to fit and comfort in the socket.[12,14]

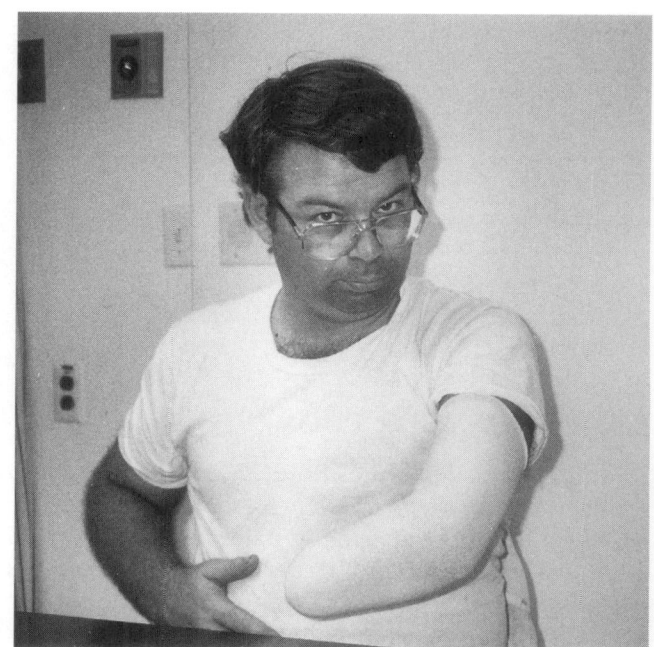

FIG. 48-3
Prosthetic sock worn under the prosthesis.

Socket

The socket is the fundamental component to which the remaining components are attached. A cast molding of the residual limb is used to construct the socket to optimize fit, comfort, and function. It fits snugly over the limb and extends as far as the wrist unit on a below-elbow (BE) prosthesis, or to the elbow unit on an above-elbow (AE) prosthesis. It should cover enough of the residual limb to be stable, but not so much that it unnecessarily restricts movement. Uneven pressure distribution may lead to skin problems.[12,13]

The length of the residual limb determines whether a socket is of single- or double-wall construction. Most sockets have a double wall. The outer wall provides a structurally cosmetic surface. The inner wall maintains total contact with the residual limb's skin surface to distribute the socket pressure evenly. Recently, flexible frame-type sockets have been favored. The inner socket is flexible and is covered with a rigid outer frame that carries the hardware. This type of socket allows for volume and contour changes that occur when muscles contract and relax. Wearers report that this type of socket is cooler than more conventional alternatives.[22] The Utah Dynamic Socket is a unique socket design that provides mediolateral and rotational stability through shaping of the shoulder region.[2]

Harness and Control System

The prosthetic control system functions through the interaction of a Dacron harness and stainless steel cable. The figure-eight harness is commonly used, although others are available. The harness is worn across the back and shoulders or around the chest and fastens to the socket to secure the prosthesis. The higher the level of amputation, the more complex the harnessing system.

Loss of muscle power and range of motion (ROM) may necessitate variations in the harness design. A properly fitted harness is important for both comfort and function.[11-13]

A flexible stainless-steel cable, contained in a Teflon housing, attaches to the harness on one end via a T-bar or hanger fitting and attaches to a functional component of the prosthesis on the other end. Spectra fiber, an ultra strong material, has been used recently instead of the stainless steel cable because it glides through the housing with less friction. A BE prosthesis uses one cable to operate the TD, connected by a ball swivel. An AE prosthesis uses a second cable to lock and unlock the elbow unit. Specific upper body movements create tension on the cables, thereby operating the prosthesis. A properly fitted control system maximizes prosthetic control while minimizing body movements and exertion.[1,11,13]

Terminal Device

The TD, the most distal component, functions to grasp and hold an object. When choosing the most appropriate TD for a prosthesis, team members consider the person's age and life roles.

Two styles of TDs are commonly prescribed: the **hook** and the **hand**. Many TDs and prosthetic hands have the same shaft size at their base, which allows them to be interchangeable. Hooks are of two basic designs: canted or lyre shaped.[6] They may be either voluntary opening (VO) or voluntary closing (VC).[9]

The VO TD opens when the wearer exerts tension on the control cable that connects to the "thumb" of the TD. When tension is released, rubber bands or springs close the fingers of the TD. The number of rubber bands or springs determines the holding force of the TD.

VC TDs close by tension applied to the control cable. The tension may also lock the TD and maintain the grasp on the object. The VC TD automatically opens by spring operation when the cable is relaxed. The VO TD was most commonly prescribed in the past. Since World War II, more modern alternatives have become available (Fig. 48-4).[1,2,5]

VO TDs have several options to better suit the wearer's lifestyle. The option chosen depends on the desired durability, weight, or grip of the TD.

Stainless-steel TDs are prescribed for activities requiring a durable TD, such as yard work or construction. Aluminum TDs are recommended for lighter work and to reduce the total weight of the prosthesis for a person with a higher-level amputation. Most TDs have either a neoprene lining or a serrated grid between their fingers. The

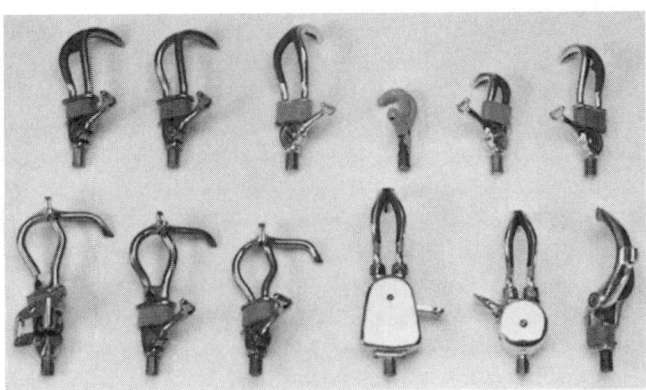

FIG. 48-4
The Hosmer-Dorrance hook terminal devices are available in a variety of materials, shapes, and sizes that can be matched to the particular functional needs of a child or adult. (Courtesy of Hosmer-Dorrance Corp. From Hunter JM, Mackin EJ, Callahan AD: *Rehabilitation of the hand: surgery and therapy*, St Louis, 1995, Mosby.)

neoprene lining increases the holding friction and minimizes damage when holding objects. Neoprene is a high-density rubber that wears out faster than the stainless steel-grid and disintegrates if it comes in excessive contact with some chemical solutions. The TD must be sent back to the manufacturer for neoprene replacement.

A variation of the standard VO TD is the heavy-duty model. This model is made of stainless steel and has a serrated grid between its fingers. The heavy-duty model is designed to hold tools, nails, and such long-handled instruments as a broom or shovel.

A prosthetic hand is also available as a TD. It attaches to the wrist unit and is either passive or cable operated. The passive hand has cosmetic and lightweight appeal, but it is also functional because it is used to push, pull, and stabilize objects. The same control cable that operates the hook activates the functional prosthetic hand. It comes in VO and VC styles. Like the hook style TD, the VO hand is preferred and prescribed more often than the VC hand. A flesh-colored rubber glove fits over the prosthetic hand for protection and a cosmetic appearance.[12]

The person's lifestyle and activities determine the most appropriate TDs. It is important to provide the wearer with certain information regarding the differences between hook- and hand-style TDs. The hook TD is lighter and provides better visibility when grasping objects. It is more durable and functional than prosthetic hands. The hook VO TDs are mechanically simpler than both the VC TDs and functional prosthetic hands. Prosthetic hands provide a more cosmetic appearance than the prosthetic hook TDs. However, the cosmetic glove that covers the hand is easily stained, wears out quickly, and disintegrates if it comes in contact with certain cleaning solutions and chemicals. Many persons with amputations choose an interchangeable hand for social occasions in addition to a hook TD for manual work.[6]

Wrist Unit

The wrist unit connects the TD to the forearm socket and serves as the unit to interchange and to pronate and supinate the TD for **prepositioning** purposes. An individual rotates the TD by turning it with the sound hand, by pushing the TD against an object or a surface, or by stabilizing the TD between the knees and using the arm to rotate it. With bilateral amputations, TD rotation in the wrist unit may be accomplished by cable operation. There are five basic types of wrist units selected according to their ability to meet the person's needs in daily living and vocational activities: the friction-held unit, the locking unit, the **wrist flexion unit,** the oval unit, and the ball-and-socket unit.

The friction-held wrist units hold the TD in place by friction provided by a rubber washer or set-screws. Tightening the washer or screws increases the friction. There is sufficient friction to hold the TD against moderate loads. The friction-held units are mechanically simple but not as strong as the locking unit.

The locking wrist unit allows the TD to be manually positioned and locked into place. The quick-disconnect locking wrist unit is most common. An adapter is permanently attached to the base of the TD. The unit has a button on its side that locks, unlocks, and ejects the TD. Inserting the TD into the wrist unit locks it into place. Another style of TD with the same adapter type on its base may be locked into place. The friction and locking wrist units allow the TD to be rotated up and down, but not deviated in toward the body.

The wrist flexion unit allows the TD to be manually flexed and locked into position. It is generally used on the dominant side of a person with bilateral amputations for facilitating midline activities close to the body, such as dressing and toileting.[1,9,12-14]

The oval unit, which conforms to the shape of the wrist, is used on the wrist disarticulation prosthesis. It is thinner than the other wrist units, so the prosthesis may more closely match the length of the sound arm.

A ball-and-socket wrist unit is also available (Fig. 48-5). The unique aspect of this unit is that it allows prepositioning in multiple wrist positions. It has constant friction, and the magnitude of the loading is adjustable.[6]

The socket, harness, control system, terminal device, and wrist unit are components common to all body-powered prostheses. The remaining body-powered prosthetic components maximize function at specific levels of amputation. These components are the elbow hinges for BE prostheses, elbow units for AE prostheses, and shoulder units designed for shoulder prostheses.

Below-Elbow Hinges

A BE prosthesis employs two hinges, one on each side of the elbow, that attach to the socket below the elbow and to a pad or cuff above the elbow. The hinges stabilize

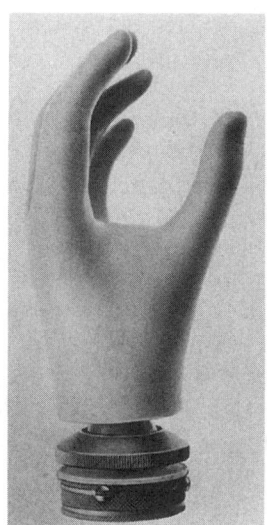

FIG. 48-5
Ball-and-socket wrist unit. (Courtesy of Otto Bock Orthopedic Industry, Inc, Minneapolis. From Bowker JH, Michael JW: *Atlas of limb prosthetics: surgical, prosthetic, and rehabilitation principles,* St Louis, 1992, Mosby.)

and align the BE prosthesis on the residual limb. When properly aligned, the hinges help distribute the stress of the prosthesis on the limb.

Two hinge styles, flexible and rigid, are available for a BE prosthesis. Flexible hinges are used on wrist amputation and long BE prostheses. They are usually made of Dacron and connect the socket to a triceps pad positioned over the triceps muscle. The flexibility permits some forearm rotation, decreasing the need to rotate the TD manually in the wrist.

Medium to short BE prostheses have a socket that covers most of the residual limb below the elbow and rigid hinges to provide stability. Rigid hinges are usually steel and attach to a laminated Dacron biceps half-cuff positioned behind the arm, which is sturdier and provides more support than the triceps pad. Team members consider the amount of residual function and the limb's length when choosing the appropriate style hinge for the BE prosthesis.[9]

Elbow Units for Above-Elbow Prostheses

A prosthetic elbow unit is prescribed for the person who has had an amputation through the level of the elbow or higher. The elbow unit allows 5° to 135° of elbow flexion and locks in various positions. The two main types of elbow units are the internally and externally locking units. The more durable internally locking unit is prescribed for a person who has had an amputation 2 inches or more above the elbow. The unit connects the AE socket to the prosthetic forearm. The locking mechanism is contained within the unit and attaches to a control cable. A lift assist, which consists of a tightly coiled spring attached to the elbow unit and forearm shell, helps

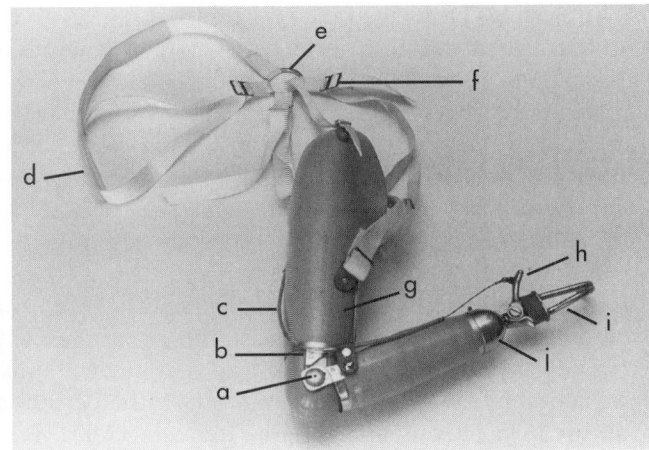

A

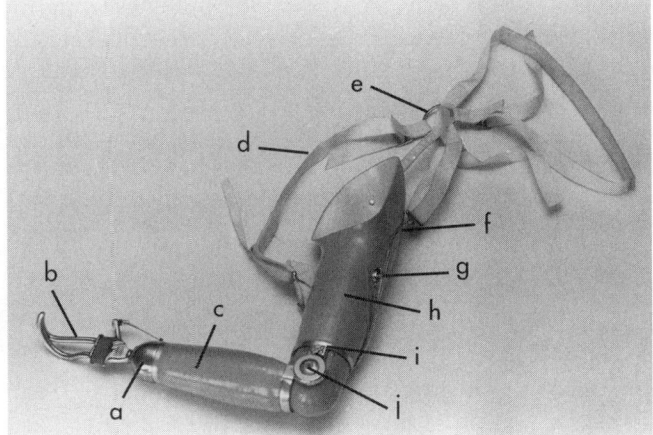

B

FIG. 48-6

A, Lateral side of above-elbow prosthesis: *a,* elbow unit; *b,* turntable; *c,* control cable; *d,* adjustable axilla loop; *e,* harness ring; *f,* figure-of-eight harness; *g,* elbow lock cable; *h,* terminal device (TD) thumb; *i,* hook TD; *j,* wrist flexion unit. **B,** Medial side of AE prosthesis: *a,* wrist unit; *b,* hook TD; *c,* forearm; *d,* harness; *e,* harness ring; *f,* control cable; *g,* baseplate and retainer; *h,* socket; *i,* turntable; *j,* spring-loading device.

reduce the amount of energy required to lift the forearm shell. The lift assist also allows a slight bounce in the forearm when walking with the elbow unlocked, which increases the appearance of a natural arm swing.

A friction-held turntable positioned on top of the elbow unit allows the prosthetic forearm to be rotated manually toward or away from the body. The lateral and medial aspects of an AE prosthesis are shown in Fig. 48-6. The internally locking unit is 2 inches long, and therefore does not fit on a person who has had an amputation close to the elbow.

Correspondingly, the externally locking elbow unit is prescribed for a person who has an elbow disarticulation or an amputation within 2 inches above the elbow. This unit, which consists of a pair of hinges positioned on either side of the prosthesis, attaches the socket to the forearm. The cable attaches to one of the hinges, which locks and unlocks the unit.

Shoulder Units

A person with an amputation at the shoulder requires a prosthesis with a shoulder unit in addition to the TD, wrist unit, forearm shell, elbow unit, socket, harness, and cables. Because of the high level of amputation, however, shoulder and back movements are not sufficient to use a cable-operated shoulder unit. Thus most shoulder units are manually operated and friction held. The TD and elbow units may still be cable operated.

Two shoulder unit styles that are often prescribed are the flexion-abduction unit and the locking shoulder joint. The flexion-abduction (or double-axis) unit provides manual prosthetic positioning in flexion and abduction and is friction held (Fig. 48-7).[6] The locking

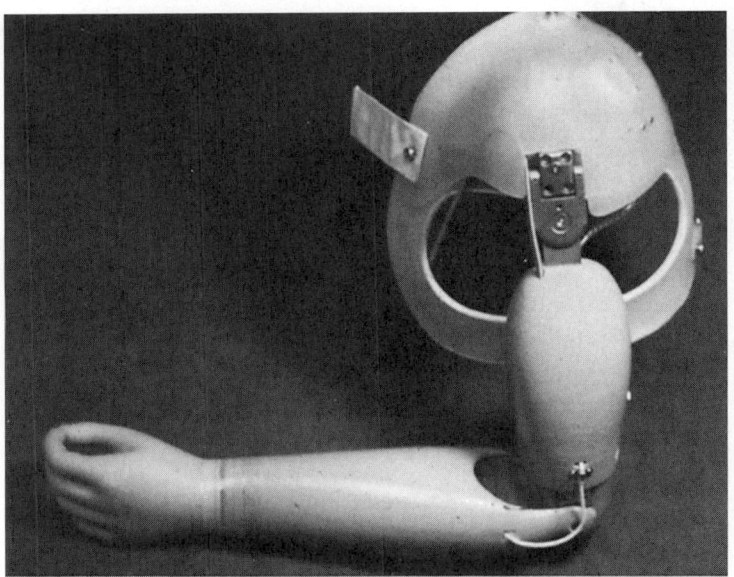

FIG. 48-7

Hosmer-Dorrance "Flexion/Abduction Shoulder Joint," shown attached to a shoulder disarticulation-type prosthesis, provides passive mechanical range of motion in flexion to 90° and abduction to 135°. An extension stop is provided to restrict extension. (From Hunter JM, Mackin EJ, Callahan AD: *Rehabilitation of the hand: surgery and therapy,* St Louis, 1995, Mosby.)

unit allows the prosthesis to be locked in various degrees of shoulder flexion. This feature is helpful because the prosthesis is heavy and the friction style may not be strong enough.

In a **forequarter amputation,** all or a portion of the scapula and clavicle is removed with the arm. If standard prosthetic components were used, the prosthesis might be too heavy for practical use. Therefore an endoskeletal prosthesis made from lightweight materials such as aluminum and dense foam is often prescribed to decrease its weight. The system provides its own style of prosthetic joints, which will not withstand heavy-duty usage. Many of the TDs discussed earlier may be used on the endoskeletal system.

UPPER-EXTREMITY PREPROSTHETIC PROGRAM

The preprosthetic program begins when the decision to perform an amputation is made or when a person is evaluated after a traumatic amputation.[8] Education regarding prostheses, relaxation techniques, and general strengthening may in some cases begin before the surgical amputation. During the period between the amputation and the fitting of the prosthesis, the individual participates in a program designed to prepare the residual limb for a prosthesis, facilitate adjustment to the loss, and achieve maximal independence in self-care.[10,13] It is important for the team to assist the person in securing the financial resources necessary to complete rehabilitation and obtain a prosthesis if desired.

Preprosthetic Evaluation

To establish an individualized treatment plan, the therapist must complete a thorough evaluation. The evaluation includes assessment of the patient's medical history, assessment of family, work, and leisure activities history, and assessment of independent living skills (ILS) status.

A statement of the person's goals is important for orienting the treatment toward meeting the goals and for determining the person's understanding of the program and the prosthesis.[4]

A tape measure is used to record residual limb length and circumference. Care must be taken to measure the limb's circumference at the same place each time. A drawing of the residual limb, with the different levels that were measured marked off in inches or centimeters, will help the therapist chart progress.

Preprosthetic Treatment

The treatment plan is based on evaluation results. Most plans include the following:
- Wound care
- Desensitization techniques
- Wrapping the residual limb to shrink and shape it, and document circumference changes
- Education regarding proper skin hygiene
- Education regarding care of insensate skin
- Maintaining passive and active ROM
- Increasing upper body strength and endurance
- Improving ILS status
- Education regarding prosthetic components and prosthetic prescription

Depending on the level of amputation, medical condition, and ILS status, the decision is made whether to complete the preprosthetic program on an inpatient or outpatient basis. In most cases in which the person has had a unilateral amputation, therapy may be completed on an outpatient basis. A person with bilateral amputations may need to be admitted to the facility because of the amount of therapy and assistance he or she will require. The team closely monitors the residual limb and reports problems to the physician. If the person is followed on an outpatient basis, frequent clinic visits are necessary to monitor progress.

Wound Healing

When the surgical dressing is removed, the residual limb is massaged to discourage scar adhesions, increase circulation, aid in desensitization, and reduce swelling. Massage of the limb also helps the person overcome fear of handling the residual limb. Massage over the incision site begins after the incision has healed.[4] Initially, deep massage over healed areas is performed, followed by lighter pressures as tolerated by the person. If skin grafts have been used, the therapist must communicate with the surgeon to determine the status before performing scar massage.

Desensitization

The residual limb may be hypersensitive after surgery and require a technique known as *desensitization*. Massage is one method of desensitization. Other methods are tapping, vibration, constant pressure, and the application of various textures to the limb, such as terry cloth and cotton. When the therapist performs the techniques, he or she teaches them to the person and family members or caregivers to perform on a home program basis.[4,7]

Wrapping

Shrinking and shaping the residual limb are necessary to form a tapered limb that will tolerate a prosthesis. Compression using an elastic Ace bandage, a tubular bandage, or a shrinker sock applied to the residual limb aids in the shrinking and shaping process. When an elastic bandage is applied to the limb, a figure-eight method (Fig. 48-8) is used, not a circumferential method in which the bandage is wrapped around the limb spirally. Care must be taken to apply the bandage smoothly, evenly, and not too tightly from the distal to the proximal end of the residual limb. Care must also be taken to avoid wrapping skin-grafted areas too tightly or without an inner nonadherent dressing applied, so that the graft is not compromised. A limb that is wrapped incorrectly may not be able to be fitted with a prosthesis or may take longer to shrink and shape. A BE limb

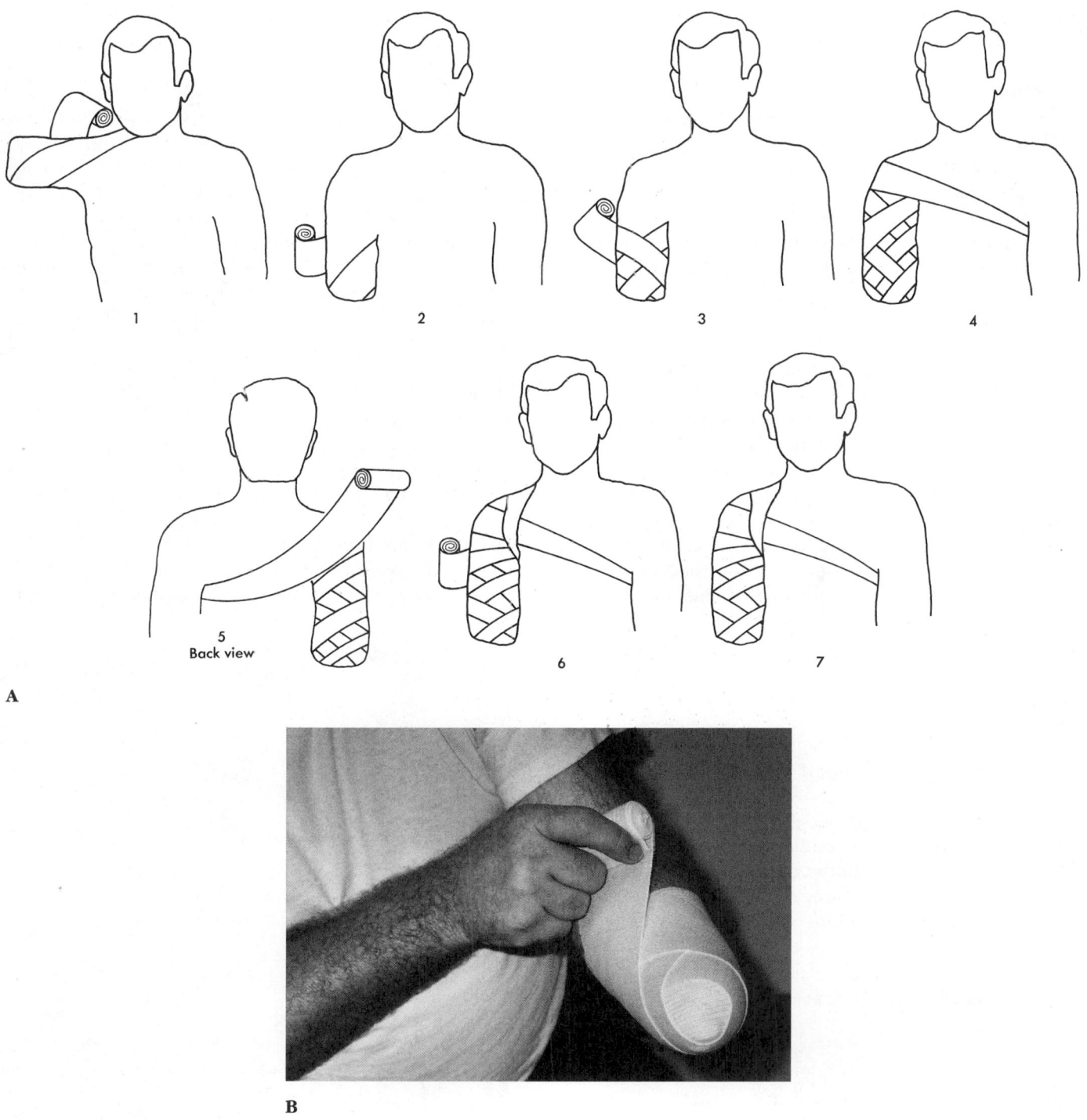

FIG. 48-8
Residual limb bandaging. **A,** Step-by-step procedure. **B,** Bandaging in progress.

should be wrapped up to or above the elbow. An AE limb should be wrapped up to or above the shoulder. Short AE amputations must usually be wrapped around the chest to help stabilize the wrap.[12,13] The elastic bandage should be changed several times a day and the skin checked between wrappings. Several bandages are required so that the limb can be wrapped in a clean bandage at all times, except when bathing. The wraps

should be washed often with a mild soap, rinsed well, and allowed to dry thoroughly lying flat. For longer life, the bandages should not be wrung out after washing.[4]

Shrinker socks have become more favorable than Ace bandage wrapping because the individual with the amputation can more independently don the sock and because changing the sock is much quicker than changing the wrap. Compressogrip tubing with a knot tied in one end is commonly used. The tubing may be attached to a chest strap if necessary.

Circumference Measurements

The residual limb's circumference measurements are taken often and in the same area to determine when the person is ready to be casted for a prosthesis. The therapist uses a tape measure to establish baseline and subsequent measurements (Fig. 48-9). When the edema is gone and the circumference measurements have stabilized, the limb is ready to be casted.

Skin Hygiene

Instruction in proper residual limb hygiene is an important aspect of the preprosthetic program. The limb should be washed daily using a mild soap, rinsed thoroughly, and patted dry. The limb should dry completely before the wrap or sock is reapplied.[3]

Insensate Skin

The person with a UE amputation requires instruction regarding the care and safety of a residual limb that lacks all or partial sensation. The person should learn to inspect the limb when removing the wrap and washing the limb. Problems should be reported to the therapist or physician. The person should also learn to track a sensory-impaired limb when completing activities, and not to use the limb for sensory input, such as by testing water temperature.

Upper Extremity Range of Motion, Strength, and Endurance

Following medical approval, the person begins exercises designed to encourage residual limb usage, maintain ROM, and strengthen upper body muscles. Depending on the level of amputation, the therapist instructs the person to complete specific exercises that mimic and strengthen the movements required to operate the prosthesis. The therapist manually positions and holds the residual limb in the desired posture and asks the person to resist the hold. In the case of a BE amputation, it is important to strengthen the muscles of the shoulder, elbow, and scapula. Pronation and supination movements are also important for long BE amputations. AE amputation strengthening includes a movement combining shoulder depression, extension, and abduction. Isometric exercises are important and enable the individual to engage in a strengthening program without equipment. Exercises may be completed with rubber tubing, elastic band, or strap-on weights. Chest expansion is important for higher-level amputations and when the harness wraps around the chest. A tape measure positioned around the chest helps document increased chest expansion.

A home program should be provided that contains exercises for general strengthening, as well as the specific movements taught during therapy (Fig. 48-10).

Independent Living Skills Status

During the preprosthetic period the person with a unilateral amputation should be encouraged to use the

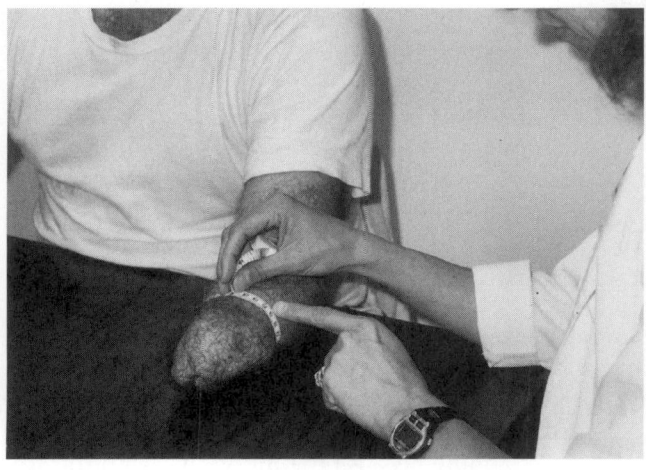

FIG. 48-9
Measuring residual limb circumference.

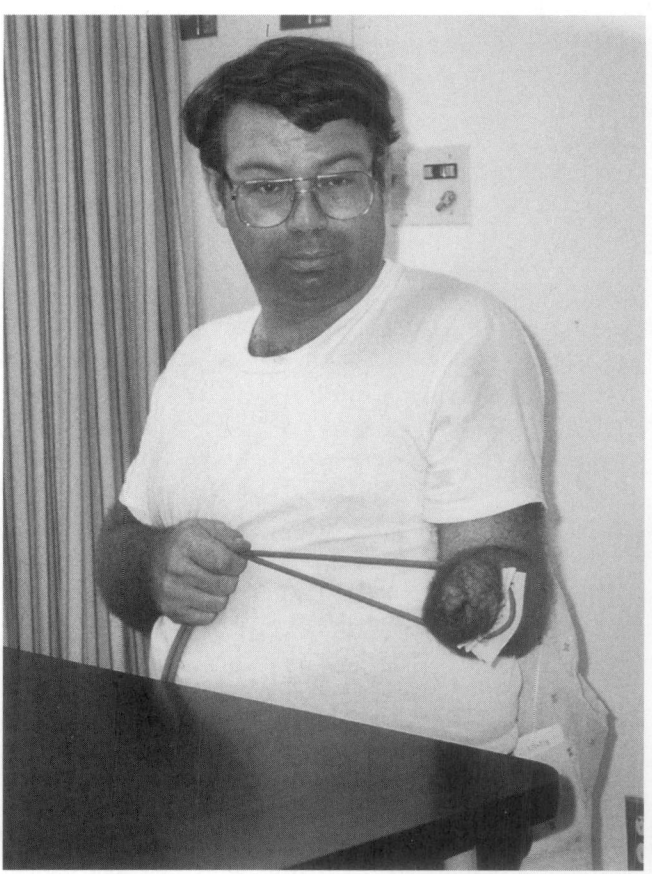

FIG. 48-10
Home program of upper extremity strengthening to prepare arm for prosthesis. Thera-tubing is being used for resistive exercise.

sound arm to perform ILS. If the dominant arm was amputated, training may be required for the nondominant limb to assume the dominant role. Practice in writing and activities requiring dexterity and coordination may be helpful in the retraining process.[10,12,13] Most individuals change dominance to the sound extremity automatically.

In the case of a bilateral amputation, adaptive equipment should be introduced as soon as possible to increase the person's level of independence. The equipment may include a utensil cuff secured by elastic or Velcro to the residual limb to aid in eating, writing, and hygiene; a dressing tree to improve dressing skills; and loops added to items such as socks and towels. The person with a bilateral amputation can also learn to complete activities using foot skills.

PROSTHETIC INFORMATION AND PRESCRIPTION

During the preprosthetic period the person should receive information about the prosthesis and its benefits and limitations. The therapist must be aware of what the amputation and the prosthesis may mean to the person. In selecting prosthetic components and presenting the prosthesis, the therapist must consider whether the person's primary need is function or cosmesis. There are several ways to introduce prosthetic components to the person: an introduction to a person with a similar amputation, slides, video, showing a prosthesis, and scheduling a trip together to the prosthetist.

PROSTHETIC PROGRAM

The amount of training each person needs depends on how fast he or she is able to understand the body mechanics required to operate the prosthesis, the person's problem-solving skills and motivation, the carryover between activities, and the cueing needed to include the prosthesis in an activity. When a long period has elapsed between the amputation and receiving the prosthesis, the person may require more cueing because he or she has become adept at one-handed activities. Some individuals arrive at therapy already able to operate the prosthesis, whereas others require extensive training.

The prosthetist and therapist should coordinate the final fitting of the prosthesis and the initial training session. The therapist may arrange to be present for the final fitting. Communication between the wearer, therapist, and prosthetist is essential to ensure that the prosthesis fits and functions optimally. The therapist should be aware of a possible need for prosthesis adjustment and consult with the prosthetist if this need becomes evident.

The prosthesis will not be as functional as a normal arm, and training should stress that the prosthesis is more like an assist or helper than an arm. If the prosthesis is presented in this manner, the wearer may have an easier time accepting it.

The prosthesis training program begins after the final fitting of the prosthesis. Although a treatment plan focuses on the wearer's prosthetic goals, some information and initial training points are common to all prosthesis training programs. These include the following:

- Residual limb and prosthetic sock hygiene
- Prosthesis terminology and function
- Care of the prosthesis
- Prosthesis wearing schedule
- Prosthesis checkout
- Controls training
- Use training
- Functional training
- Driving
- Home program
- Follow-up appointments

The prosthesis checkout, controls training, and functional training are individualized according to the level of amputation.

Residual Limb and Prosthetic Sock Hygiene

The person is instructed in residual limb hygiene and care of the prosthetic sock in the early phase of prosthesis training. The residual limb and armpit should be inspected, washed, and patted dry, and deodorant should be applied daily. If the person chooses to wear a prosthetic sock, he or she should own several, so that a clean one may be worn daily to decrease chances of skin problems. The socks should be washed, gently squeezed, and placed on a flat surface to dry in their original dimensions. Wearing an undergarment under the harness is often recommended because it will absorb perspiration and protect the axillae and back from irritation. Prosthetic socks and undergarments may need to be changed twice a day in hot weather.[13-14]

Prosthesis Terminology and Function

The wearer should learn the terminology and function of each prosthetic component. This task is important so that the person can communicate with the rehabilitation team, using terminology understood by all, regarding difficulties with or repairs needed to the prosthesis.[3,13,14]

Care of the Prosthesis

Instructions regarding care of the prosthesis are provided and reviewed. The socket should be cleaned daily with a soft cloth and mild soap and rinsed thoroughly with warm water. Cleaning at night is recommended to allow the prosthesis to dry completely. Wearing the prosthesis when the socket is wet may lead to skin problems. Components should be cleaned and maintained according to the manufacturer's or prosthetist's specifications. Daily inspection of the prosthesis will help prevent unnecessary problems.[3]

Prosthesis Wearing Schedule

A prosthesis wearing schedule is provided and reviewed during the first training session. Initially the person wears the prosthesis 15 to 30 minutes, three times a day. The skin must be closely monitored, and wearing time is advanced only if the skin remains in good condition. If there are no skin problems, the three scheduled wearing periods may be increased by 30 minutes each day. By the end of the first week the person should be wearing the prosthesis all day. If skin problems occur, the therapist, prosthetist, or physician must be notified. The prosthesis should not be worn until the skin problem has cleared. Restarting the initial wearing schedule may be necessary to decrease the chance of more skin problems.[3]

As the person's wearing tolerance increases, the number of rubber bands on the TD can be increased. Each rubber band added to the TD increases the pinch force by approximately 1 pound. It is best to wait several days after adding one rubber band before adding another, to allow the residual limb's skin and strength to acclimate. If adding a rubber band substantially increases limb pain or skin irritation, it should be removed until the pain diminishes and skin tolerance increases.

Checkout of the Prosthesis

When the prosthesis is received, team members check it to ensure that it meets prescription requirements, is functioning efficiently, and is mechanically sound. The prosthesis is checked for fit and function against specific mechanical standards developed from actual tests on prostheses worn by individuals. Tests performed are comparative ROM with the prosthesis on and off; control system function and efficiency; TD opening in various positions; amount of socket slippage on the residual limb under various degrees of load or tension; compression fit and comfort; and force required to flex the forearm.[1,11,13] Communication between the wearer, therapist, and prosthetist is essential to ensure an efficiently operating and comfortable prosthesis. The following methods and standards for the prosthesis checkout were adapted primarily from Wellerson.[13] Step-by-step instructions for the prosthetic checkout are available in Wellerson[13] and Santschi.[11]

Checkout of Below-Elbow Prosthesis
The therapist measures elbow flexion with the prosthesis on and off the wearer. The ROM should not differ by more than 10°, except if there are joint or muscle limitations. Pronation and supination of a wrist disarticulation or long BE residual limb with the prosthesis on should not be less than 50% of the rotation possible without the prosthesis.

With the elbow flexed at 90° the person should be able to open the TD fully. The TD is also opened near the mouth (elbow fully flexed), and again near the fly of the trousers (elbow extended). From 70% to 100% of TD opening should be achieved in these two positions.

Checkout of Above-Elbow and Shoulder Prosthesis
With the AE prosthesis on and the elbow locked, the person is instructed to move the residual limb (humerus) into shoulder flexion, extension, abduction, and internal and external rotation. The ROM of each of these is measured. Minimal standards for shoulder ROM with the prosthesis on are as follows: 90° flexion, 30° extension, 90° abduction, and 45° rotation. The previous part of the checkout is not applicable for the shoulder prosthesis.

With the elbow unlocked, the individual is instructed to flex the shoulder slowly, which flexes the mechanical elbow. The elbow ROM should be about 10° to 135°. The therapist measures the amount of shoulder flexion, which should not exceed 45°, required to fully flex the mechanical elbow. The individual should also be able to abduct the prosthesis to 60° without locking of the elbow.

The individual flexes the elbow to 90°, locks the elbow, and then activates the TD. Full TD opening should be attained in this position. The TD is then opened in full elbow flexion with elbow locked (TD at mouth, Fig. 48-11) and extension with elbow locked (TD at fly of trousers). At least 50% of full TD opening should be obtained.

With the elbow unlocked, the individual is asked to walk and practice swinging the prosthesis without locking the elbow. This action mimics a normal arm swing during gait.

The individual flexes the elbow to 90°, locks the elbow, abducts the residual limb to 60°, and then rotates the humerus. The person should be able to control the prosthesis during this motion. The socket should not slip around the residual limb, and the individual should not feel pain or discomfort during these maneuvers. When the prosthesis is removed, the residual limb should not appear discolored or irritated.

The prosthesis checkout also includes a technical inspection of the prosthesis to determine correct length, fit, and mechanical function of all parts. Various forms have been devised to record all information for the complete checkout of the prosthesis. The initial checkout is performed before prosthetic training begins, and the final checkout is done after prosthetic revisions and adjustments and either during or after training.[3,11]

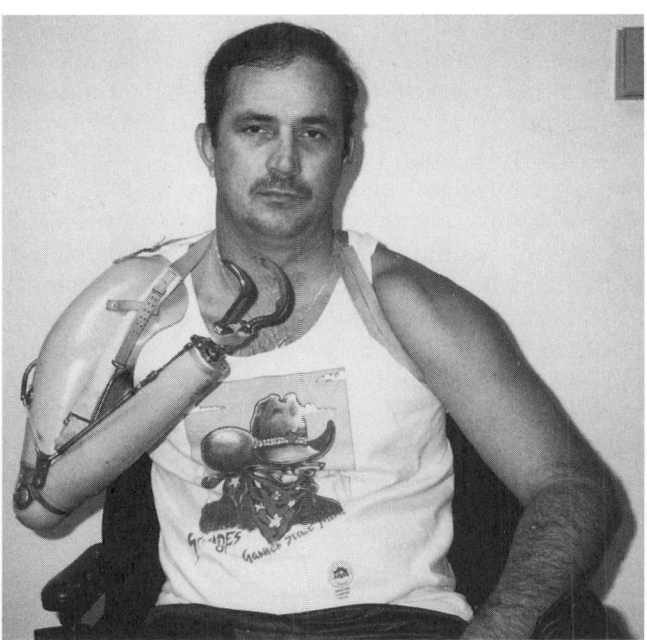

FIG. 48-11
Above-elbow prosthesis checkout: opening terminal device at mouth with elbow locked in full flexion.

Controls Training

Controls training is best accomplished in front of a mirror to help the person learn the minimal motions necessary to operate the prosthesis while maintaining proper body mechanics (Fig. 48-12).

Acquiring skill in the operation of the prosthesis is emphasized in controls training. The therapist educates the wearer in the importance of the practice drills that will ensure more successful function with the prosthesis in daily activities. Joint protection, energy conservation, and work simplification principles and techniques should be stressed during this phase of training. Each prosthetic component should be reviewed separately and understood before the components are combined into functional activities. Such movements as elbow flexion and TD opening are cable operated. Other movements, such as TD or elbow rotation, are passively positioned using the sound hand or an item in the environment, such as a table. Emphasizing external assists from the environment is an important part of this training process.

Donning and Doffing the Prosthesis

The two common methods of donning and doffing the prosthesis are the coat method and the sweater method. Either method can be used with unilateral or bilateral amputations. The method used depends on which is easier for the wearer. Whichever the method, the harness and cables must not be kinked or twisted around the prosthesis before starting. When the pros-

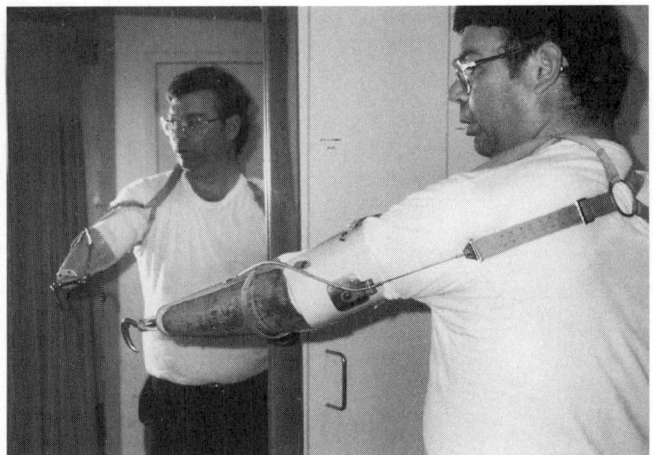

FIG. 48-12
Controls training in front of mirror.

thesis is removed, it should be placed on a surface ready for the person to don again.

Coat Method

The coat method is similar to placing one arm in the coat sleeve and manipulating the coat to a position where the other arm can reach the sleeve. The coat method has two variants. In the first method the person places the prosthesis on a table or bed and pushes the residual limb between the control cable and the Y-strap from the medial side into the socket. By raising the residual limb or leaning sideways, the individual places the harness across the shoulder on the amputated side and dangles the harness down the back. The sound hand reaches around the back and slips into the axilla loop. The person then slips into the harness as if putting on a coat. The shoulders are shrugged to shift the harness forward and into the correct position.

The second method works by placing the axilla loop of the harness on the sound arm first. For example, if the person has an AE amputation, it may be easier to lock the elbow at 90°, position the axilla loop on the sound arm above the elbow, grasp the prosthetic forearm, and raise the prosthesis over the head, allowing the harness to position itself across the back. By raising the residual limb, the individual positions it in the socket (Fig. 48-13).

To remove the prosthesis, the individual uses the TD to slip the axilla loop off the sound side and then slips the shoulder strap off the amputated side. The harness is then slipped off like a coat.[1,11,13]

The person with bilateral amputations can use the coat method by placing the prostheses face up on a surface, placing the longer residual limb into the socket, and elevating the prosthesis, allowing the other prosthesis to hang across the back. The person then leans to the side and places the shorter limb in the prosthesis.[11,14] To remove the prosthesis, the individual shrugs the harness off the shoulders and removes the prosthesis from the shorter side first. Before removing the prosthesis on the longer side, the person should position the prostheses somewhere convenient for the next donning.

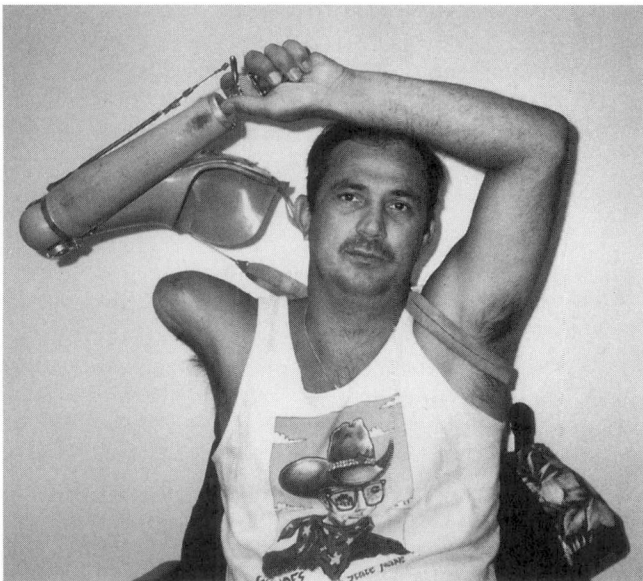

FIG. 48-13
Coat method of donning prosthesis.

Sweater Method

The sweater method (Fig. 48-14) is equivalent to entering both sleeves at the same time and then raising both arms up and out to don the sweater. To apply a unilateral prosthesis using the sweater method, the person places the prosthesis on a surface face up, positions the residual limb in the socket under the Y-strap, and places the opposite arm in the harness. The person then raises both arms above the head, allowing the axilla loop to slide down to the axilla and the harness to be properly positioned across the back and on the shoulders. To remove the prosthesis, the person raises both arms above the head and grasps and removes the prosthesis with the sound arm, while allowing the axilla loop to slide off the arm.[11]

A person with a bilateral amputation dons the prostheses using the sweater method by placing the prostheses on a surface, face up. With the longer limb stabilizing the socket, the shorter residual limb is then positioned under the harness and in the socket. The longer limb is then positioned similarly under the harness in the socket, and the arms are raised, allowing the harness to flip over the head and across the back and shoulders. The individual removes the prostheses by shrugging the shoulders to bring the harness up, grasping it with the TD, and pulling it over the head while allowing the residual limbs to come out of their sockets.

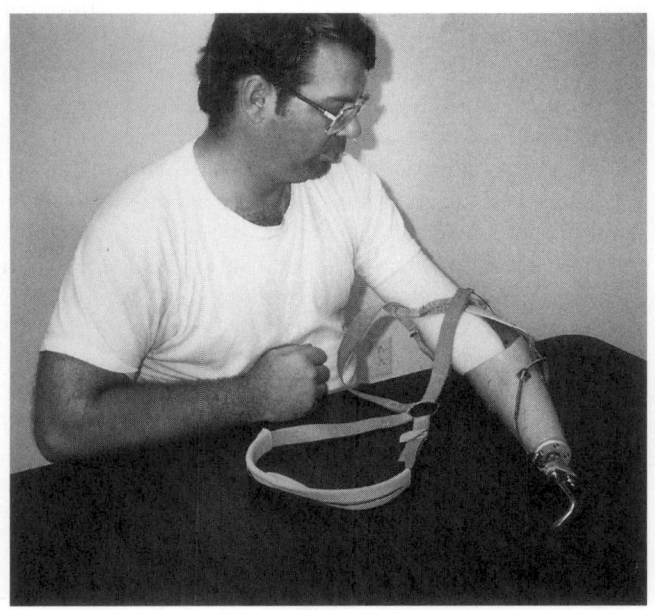

A

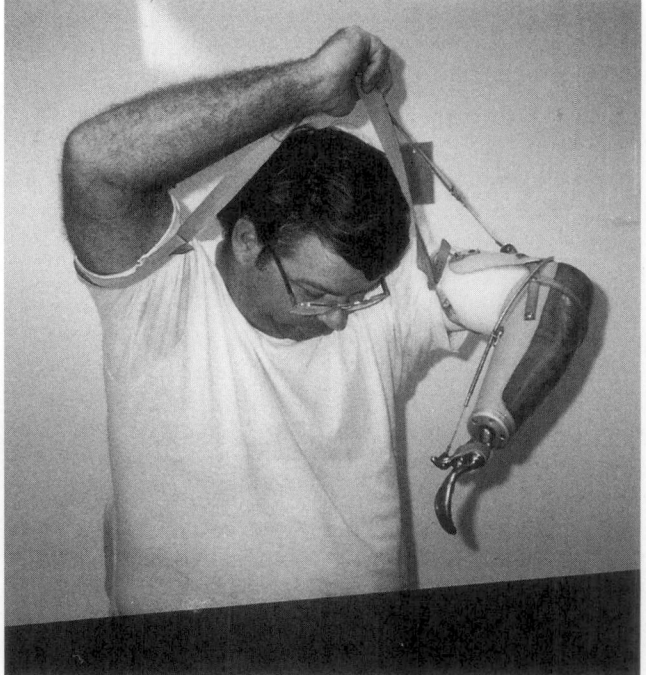

B

FIG. 48-14
Sweater method of donning prosthesis.

Controls Training for the Unilateral Below-Elbow Prosthesis

TERMINAL DEVICE CONTROL. Scapula abduction and glenohumeral flexion are the motions necessary to open and close the TD. The person is instructed to operate the TD first, by flexing the humerus on the amputated side, then by scapula abduction while the humerus remains at the body's side. The therapist instructs the person to operate the TD with the arm in various positions in space, such as overhead and leaning over toward the floor.[14]

PRONATION AND SUPINATION. If the residual limb is long enough for flexible hinges to be prescribed on the prosthesis, pronation and supination should be practiced. The therapist asks the person to stabilize the elbow at 90° and to pronate and supinate the forearm. If rigid hinges were prescribed, the TD is manually rotated in the wrist unit to achieve pronation and supination. Using the opposite hand or stabilizing the TD between the knees and turning the forearm or shoulder accomplishes manual TD rotation.

EXCHANGING TERMINAL DEVICES. The person learns to exchange the TD in the wrist unit if more than one TD is prescribed. Cable slack is needed to release the cable from the TD. To obtain enough slack in the cable, it may be necessary to place an item between the fingers of the hook or hand. The TD is then removed according to the wrist unit prescribed. When the TD has been removed, another TD style may then be positioned in the wrist unit and the cable attached to it.

To complete BE controls training, the therapist instructs the person to repeat the motions required to position and operate the TD, until they are performed in one continuous smooth and natural sequence in both sitting and standing positions.[13] Once controls training is completed, functional training may begin to improve the person's bilateral and ILS activities.

Controls Training for the Unilateral Above-Elbow Prosthesis

Most AE prostheses operate through the use of a dual-control cable system. When tension is applied on the cable attached to the elbow unit, it locks and unlocks. When the elbow unit is unlocked, tension on the second cable attached to the TD raises the prosthetic forearm (flexes the elbow). A spring assist helps reduce the amount of effort required to raise the forearm, and gravity assists in lowering it. When the elbow unit is locked, tension on the second cable is used to operate the TD. The person learns to operate each component separately.

INTERNAL AND EXTERNAL ROTATION. Many internally locking elbow units have a manually operated turntable located between the elbow unit and the socket that allows internal and external forearm rotation. The person operates the turntable, first with the elbow at 90° by manually rotating the forearm medially (toward the body) or laterally (away from the body).

ELBOW FLEXION AND EXTENSION. Flexion and extension of the mechanical elbow are the next steps in the training process. The therapist should protect the person's face when teaching elbow flexion control. This precaution is important because initially the person may have poor control over elbow flexion, which could cause the TD to hit the face.[1]

The therapist makes sure that the elbow unit is unlocked. Then the therapist asks the person to flex the humerus slowly and abduct the scapula to accomplish elbow flexion and slowly extend the shoulder to achieve elbow extension. This movement is repeated until the person gains sufficient control to accomplish elbow flexion and extension smoothly and easily.[1,14]

ELBOW LOCKING. The elbow unit operation has an audible two-click cycle. Both clicks must be heard each time the unit is locked or unlocked. The same body movement both locks and unlocks the unit. The person is instructed to operate the elbow unit by moving the shoulder into a combination of hyperextension, abduction, and scapula depression. This movement places tension on the cable that attaches the harness to the elbow unit and may be difficult to master. The reminder, "Down, out, and away" may be repeated until the person develops a proprioceptive memory. The person is then asked to practice locking and unlocking the elbow in various ranges of elbow flexion and extension (Fig. 48-15).[1,3,14]

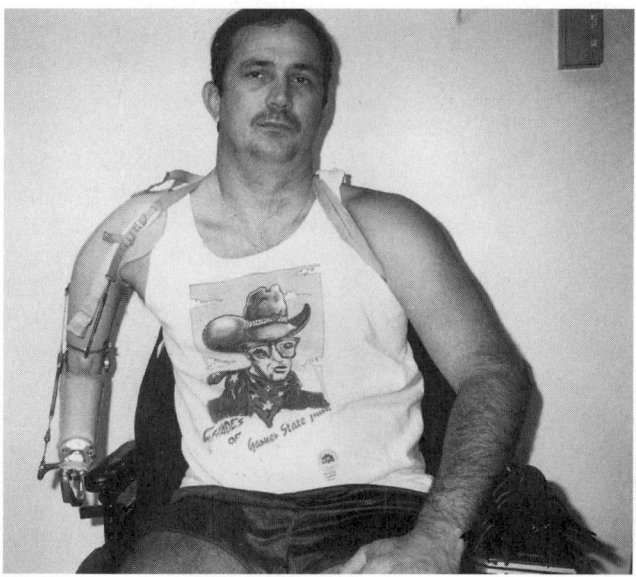

FIG. 48-15
"Down, out, and away" movement used to unlock the elbow unit.

TERMINAL DEVICE CONTROL. The same motions of shoulder flexion and scapula abduction that flex the forearm with the elbow unlocked also control the TD when the elbow is locked. The person is instructed to lock the elbow, first at 90°, and perform the motions to operate the TD. Care must be taken not to unlock the elbow by placing tension on the cable that operates the elbow unit. The sequence of elbow positioning, elbow locking, TD operation, elbow unlocking, elbow repositioning, and locking is repeated at various points in the elbow ROM from full extension to full flexion.[1,14]

The person then learns how to rotate the TD manually in the wrist unit and to exchange TDs in the same manner as described previously for the BE prosthesis. Once the AE prosthesis controls are performed in a smooth manner, functional training begins.

Controls Training for the Shoulder Disarticulation Prosthesis

A prosthesis prescribed for a person with a shoulder disarticulation may have different components and methods of operation than the AE prosthesis. The prosthesis may have a manually operated, friction-held shoulder unit that the person prepositions using the sound arm or a table's edge. A chin-operated nudge control may be used to operate the elbow unit because the person does not have the shoulder movements needed to lock and unlock the elbow (Fig. 48-16). A cable connects the nudge control to the elbow unit. The person still learns the two-click cycle and dual-cable system of operation described previously for the AE prosthesis. The elbow turntable is also available for a shoulder prosthesis.

A chest harness may be needed to secure the prosthesis on the person. It can also assist TD operation by using chest expansion to increase tension on the TD

cable. Shoulder flexion and scapula abduction on the opposite side also assist in TD operation. Wrist operation is the same as explained for the BE prosthesis.

Controls Training for Bilateral Prostheses

A person with bilateral amputations usually receives two prostheses that are attached to one harness (Fig. 48-17). Operating one of the prostheses may transmit tension through the harness to the other prosthesis, causing it to operate also. The person must learn to operate each prosthetic component without affecting the components on either side. This skill is called *separation of controls*, and the individual may need extensive practice to master it. Each prosthesis operates according to the level of amputation as described in the previous sections, with special attention given to relaxing the opposite side (Fig. 48-18).

Two components not generally used on unilateral prostheses may be prescribed on bilateral prostheses to improve the person's independence. These components are the wrist flexion unit and a cable-operated wrist rotation unit. The wrist flexion unit assists completion of midline activities and is prescribed either for both prostheses or for the dominant side. The ability to achieve midline is important for completing many activities such as dressing, grooming, and eating. Depressing the unit's control button and creating tension on the TD cable operate the flexion unit. The opposite TD, a surface edge, the knee, or other surface can depress the button. The TD cable must be medial to the flexion axis of the unit to pull the TD into flexion. A spring in the flexion unit repositions the TD in extension when the button is depressed and slack is provided in the TD cable.

There are several ways to achieve wrist rotation. One is by using the wrist units mentioned earlier and rotat-

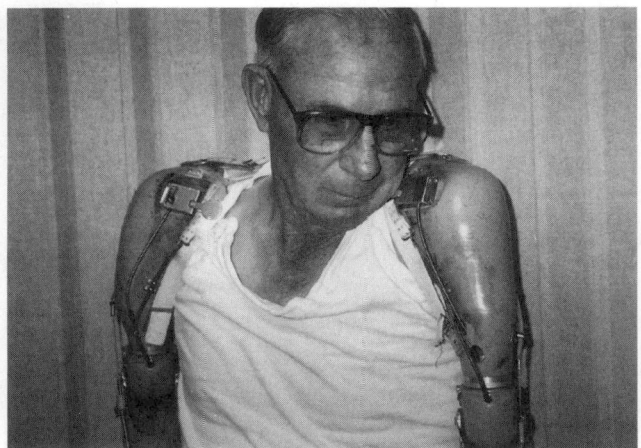

FIG. 48-16
Nudge control used to operate the elbow unit for shoulder disarticulation prosthesis.

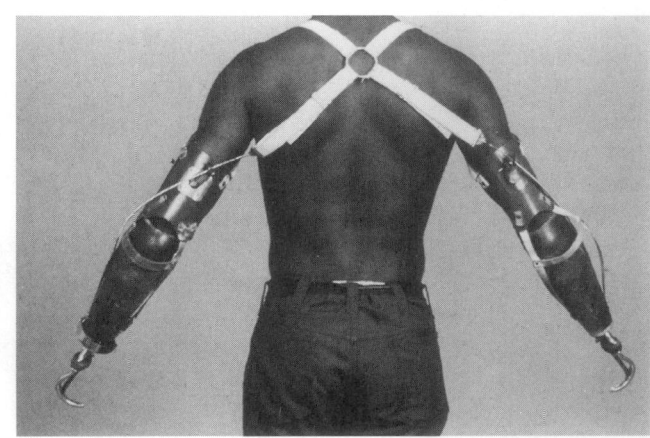

FIG. 48-17
Single harness for bilateral prostheses.

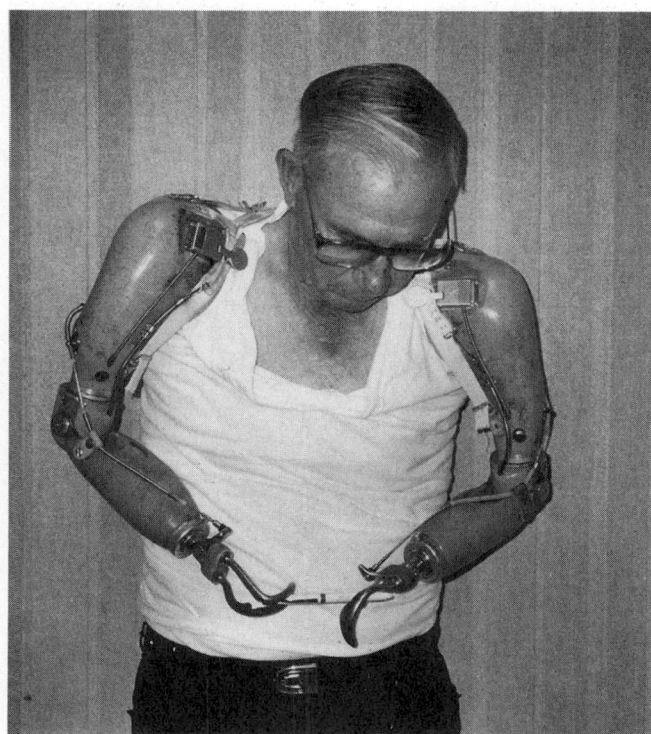

FIG. 48-18
Passing a pen from one prosthesis to the other to practice separation of controls.

ing the TD by placing it between the knees or by pulling on the thumb of one hook with the other. Another method is use of a button on the medial side of the forearm, which controls a cable attached inside the forearm to a wrist-locking device. The wrist is locked and unlocked by pressing the button against the side of the body. When the wrist is unlocked, tension on the TD cable rotates the TD to the desired position.

USE TRAINING

Use training begins after the person understands how to operate and control the prosthetic components. This training applies the mechanics of operation to repetitive activities. Repetition is important for the wearer to gain an understanding of how to preposition the prosthesis and the objects and how to use the environment to help preposition them. Along with prepositioning, prehension training begins.

Prepositioning

Prepositioning involves moving the prosthetic units in their optimum position to grasp an object or perform a given activity. All prosthetic components must be prepositioned in a proximal-to-distal order. Thus the person with the BE prosthesis rotates the TD into the desired degree of pronation or supination to accom-

plish an activity. With an AE prosthesis, the person flexes and locks the elbow and rotates the turntable before prepositioning the TD. The person with a shoulder disarticulation prepositions the shoulder unit before the elbow and wrist components. The person with bilateral prostheses must still preposition all components in the same fashion. The goal of prepositioning is to allow the person to approach the object or activity as one would with a normal hand and thereby avoid awkward body movements used to compensate for poor prepositioning.[11]

Prehension Training

The prosthesis should be regarded as an assistive device and not as the dominant arm.[13] Training objects are used to allow the wearer to practice TD control. The person should first use large, hard objects such as blocks, cans, and jars, and progress to soft, then to crushable objects, such as rubber balls, sponges, paper boxes, cones, and paper cups. These objects should be placed in positions that require elbow and TD prepositioning and TD operation at various heights. The hook TD has a nonmovable and a movable finger. If a hook is used to pick up objects, the person is taught to stabilize the item with the non-movable finger and then release the tension on the movable finger to secure the object. Prehension training should be completed using all prescribed TDs.[13,14]

Use Training for Bilateral Prostheses

After the person understands how the components operate, he or she gains control of the prostheses by practicing passing such items as a ruler or a piece of paper back and forth between the TDs without dropping them (Fig. 48-18). Another activity that helps the person learn separation of controls is holding an object in one prosthesis without dropping it while completing an activity with the other prosthesis.

FUNCTIONAL TRAINING

Functional training applies concepts of control and use training to functional activities. The prosthesis wearer is now introduced to completion of specific tasks important to him or her. Prehension training and methods to complete ILS, including prevocational, leisure, and driving skills, are addressed in this phase. The key to successful functional training is teaching the wearer a problem-solving approach with respect to the activity being performed.

Prehension Training

Prehension training trains the person to use all TDs prescribed in a meaningful manner, such as using the heavy-duty TD with tools and the hand to eat. Such items as a pencil sharpener, lock and key, jar and lid, and bottle opener should be used to challenge the person.[1,13] However, initially there are only two or three rubber bands on the TD, which limit its grip strength. In bilateral activities the person should be encouraged to determine the best position and appropriate use for the prosthesis and the sound arm. For details the therapist is referred to Santschi's work on prosthetic training.[11] Movements become less cognitive and more automatic during this phase, and prepositioning occurs naturally.

Independent Living Skills

Functional training should progress to the performance of necessary ILS. Activities should be introduced in a simple-to-complex order. The therapist should also ask the person what areas are important for him or her to be able to accomplish. The person is encouraged to analyze and perform the activities of personal hygiene and grooming, dressing, feeding, home management, communication, and leisure and vocational activities as independently as possible. The therapist may help the person analyze and accomplish a task or help achieve it by means of adaptive equipment or by encouraging repetitious practice to reach maximum speed and skill. The sound arm or longer prosthesis should complete most of the work while the opposite side acts as a stabilizer.[13] Home management skills and child care should be included as part of the person's assessment when appropriate.[12]

Work-Related Activities

Prevocational evaluation may be included in the rehabilitation program. The therapist assesses the person's potential for returning to a former occupation or a possible change of vocation. A visit to the work site may be necessary to make recommendations that will enable the person to return to work in a safe and efficient environment. It may also be necessary to restrict work activities, such as restricting the amount of weight the person may lift and carry or restricting work on ladders. Initially the person may be able to work only part time, improving work endurance gradually. Training and education for new jobs may be necessary (see Chapter 16).

Driver Training

The ability to drive increases independence and may enhance vocational opportunities. The person should be referred to an adaptive driving program where he or she can be evaluated and trained in using assistive devices such as a driving ring or a steering knob (Fig. 48-19). The controls of the car, such as the ignition switch and turn signals, can be modified to improve safety and comfort. The amount of training and extent

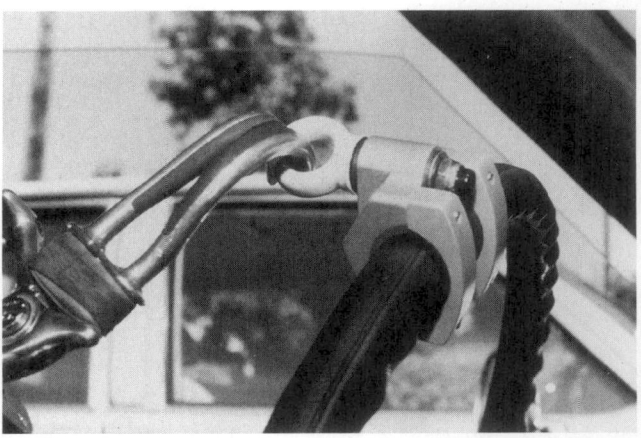

FIG. 48-19
Steering ring used for driving with a prosthesis.

of modifications will vary, depending on the level of amputation.

The occupational therapist is responsible for assessing predriving skills. A predriving evaluation may consist of an assessment of visual acuity, traffic signal recognition, color vision, glare recovery, night vision, peripheral vision, depth perception, reaction time, and UE function. When necessary, additional cognitive, visual, and perceptual skills are evaluated. See Chapter 14, Section 3, for more information on driving.

Upon completion of the predriving evaluation, the therapist is responsible for making driving recommendations. These may include treatment for deficits, referral to a driver education center for training, and installation of assistive devices. The therapist's evaluation should include a statement regarding the person's potential for safe driving. If the person is unable to drive, alternative methods of transportation should be explored.

In some states people are required to report any change in physical health status to the motor vehicle department and to their insurance company. Failure to do so may result in a loss of automobile insurance.

Leisure Activities

The rehabilitation program should include information and training regarding leisure interests. With the person's and the rehabilitation team's joint effort and motivation, the person should be able to return to a meaningful and productive life. A wide variety of specialized prosthetic devices are available for all kinds of sports and recreational hobbies. Therapeutic Recreational Systems (TRS)* provides a catalog of prosthetic devices designed to improve the person's ability to par-

---

* 2450 Central Ave., Unit D, Boulder, CO 80301-2844 // (800) 279-1865.

ticipate in such activities as photography, ball games, and skiing.[3]

Duration of Training

The average adult with a unilateral BE amputation who is otherwise healthy and well adjusted will require approximately 5 hours of training (five to eight treatment sessions) to master control and use of the prosthesis for daily living. The person with a unilateral AE amputation under the same conditions will require approximately 10 hours of training. About 12 hours will be required for bilateral BE prosthetic training, whereas about 20 hours is required for bilateral AE prosthetic training. The initial training session should be about 1 hour long, and subsequent sessions may be more brief, increasing in duration commensurate with the wearer's increased prosthesis tolerance and physical endurance.[3,8,13]

SUMMARY

Acquired UE amputations can occur as a result of trauma, infections, neoplasms, and vascular diseases. Occupational therapists play an essential role in the rehabilitation process by addressing residual limb conditioning and care, preprosthesis exercise, and prosthesis training. The desired outcomes of OT intervention are the independent management of ILS and resumption of work and leisure roles.

Working with an individual who has an amputation can be a real challenge. Careful assessment of the person's needs, a creative approach to therapeutic intervention, and close communication with the team can make the challenge rewarding and successful.

II. Electric-Powered Prostheses
DENISE D. KEENAN
DIANE J. ATKINS

Externally powered electric upper extremity (UE) prostheses have opened a new world of freedom and function for persons with UE amputations. The advent of electronic microminiaturization has allowed the development of prosthetic devices with totally self-contained services of power, motor units, and electrodes.[6] Powered prostheses have existed for decades, but it was not until the 1960s that myoelectrically controlled prostheses were clinically introduced. The activities of the Otto Bock Company in Duderstadt, Germany, began this process, by aiming for the development of an electromechanically driven prosthetic hand that would match both the technical and cosmetic demands of a human hand.[8]

The clinical use of the electric devices began in Europe because of government-supported health care systems and a large patient population of persons with congenital (postthalidomide) amputations. By the late 1970s and early 1980s North America had an increasing but limited experience with myoelectric prostheses.[5] When funding permits, hundreds of myoelectric prostheses are prescribed for children and adults throughout the United States.

The term **myoelectric prosthesis** is often used interchangeably with *electric prosthesis*. A myoelectric prosthesis uses muscle surface electricity to control the prosthetic hand function. The muscle membrane generates an electric potential at the time of contraction. The myoelectric signal is sensed, amplified, and processed by a control unit that generates a motor, which in turn drives a terminal device.[5] This terminal device is often an electromechanical hand (Fig. 48-20).[4] The myoelectric

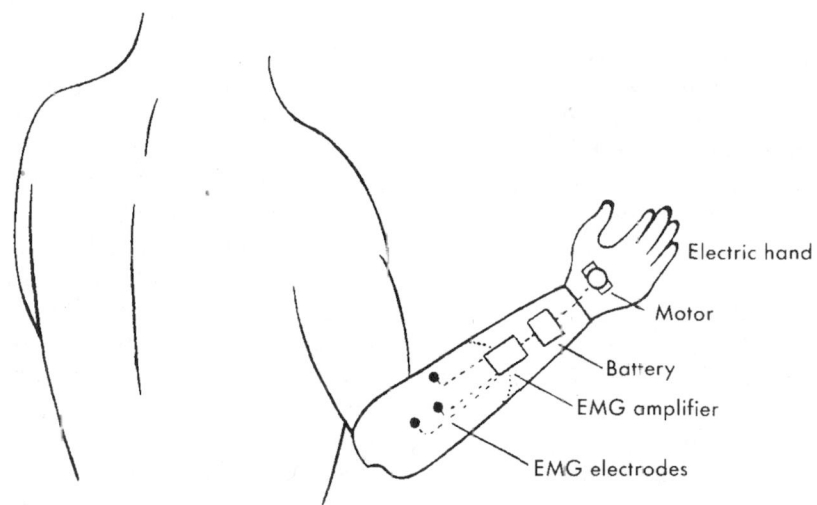

FIG. 48-20

A typical electric-powered myoelectrically controlled, below-elbow prosthesis with an electromechanical hand terminal device activated by electromyographic potentials. (From Billock JN: Upper limb prosthetic terminal devices: hands versus hooks, *Clin Prosthet Orthot* 10[2]:59, 1986.)

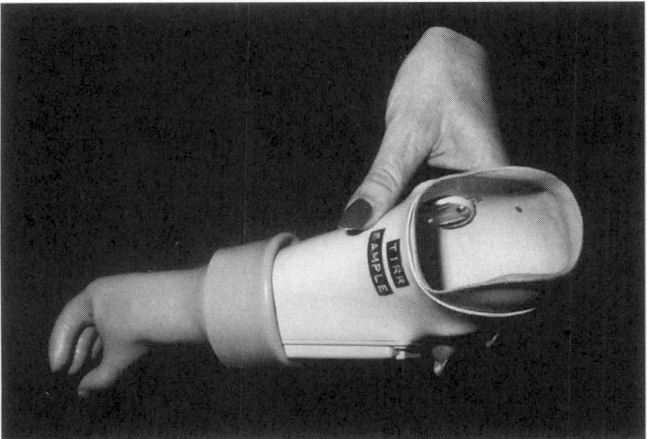

FIG. 48-21
Surface electrodes, recessed within wall of myoelectric socket, detect muscle contractions.

control can be a digital control or a proportional control. Digital systems are operated at only one speed, allowing them to either turn on or turn off. Proportional control means that the myoelectric signal (power) to the hand is proportional to the level of muscle signal the wearer generates, so the wearer's effort directly conrols the speed of the hand.[1]

Myoelectric controls require minimal physical effort for operation and rarely require adjustment. The muscle groups in the below-elbow (BE) area are used according to their physiological function; that is, the wrist extensor muscles are used for hand opening and the wrist flexor muscles for hand closing. Surface electrodes recessed within the wall of the prosthetic socket (Fig. 48-21) detect muscular contractions.

CANDIDATES FOR ELECTRIC-POWERED PROSTHESES

An electric prosthesis might be chosen because of the combination of a natural appearance and the functions of high pinch force without a high level of effort. Also, a myoelectric prosthesis requires no cables for control, so the harnessing can be much more comfortable. The patient's work, home, and recreational needs and activities must all be considered. Previous experience with other prostheses may also be relevant.

In the past, the BE amputation has been the most common condition for which these prostheses were prescribed. For amputation levels above the elbow, the complexity of function and the power level required to accomplish functional movement increases considerably. At the same time, the capability of the patient to operate a prosthesis by harnessing body movement via straps and cables, in the traditional body-powered manner, decreases considerably.[10] More recently, with the advances in technology, there are a greater number

of prescriptions for myoelectric prostheses for higher-level amputees because there functional possibilities are greater.[1]

The task of training a patient with an above-elbow (AE) amputation or shoulder disarticulation to operate and function with a body-powered prosthesis is substantially more challenging than training with an electric-powered prosthesis.

Before a myoelectric prosthesis is prescribed, the patient should have adequate strength and an ability to contract muscles independently. A minimum signal of 5 microvolts will operate the most sensitive system. The candidate with this minimum signal should be capable of developing stronger signals for longer-term prosthesis use. Independent contraction of each muscle is important to produce a smooth and controllable prosthetic function. As a general guideline, the prosthesis can be operated with a 10-microvolt difference, but the wearer will use the prosthesis more easily if a 20- to 30-microvolt difference can be controlled. The surface electric signals are amplified by a miniature electrode and led to the relay system. The relay is responsible for the energy supply to the battery-operated motor in the electric hand. When the alternating contractions of extensor and flexor muscles take place, the direction of the current changes in the electric motor and the hand opens and closes accordingly.[8]

Some rehabilitation professionals who work with patients who have UE amputation believe that electric components may be the only appropriate alternative for high-level unilateral or high-level bilateral amputations.

Conversely, some rehabilitation professionals believe that body-powered prostheses are the most functional and appropriate type of prosthesis for the majority of patients, despite the level of amputation. There are many schools of thought regarding the advantages and disadvantages of myoelectric prostheses. The list in Box 48-1 describes some of the points that differentiate the myoelectric prosthesis from a body-powered, cable-controlled, hook-type terminal device.

HYBRID PROSTHESES

A hybrid prosthesis is one that combines body power with electrical power. These designs have been created and used more and more in the past several years. Hybrid prostheses, using various components and control methods from various systems, can in many cases result in a prosthesis that is more functional and more acceptable to the individual.[4] The improved technology of electric hands has increased the cost of myoelectric prostheses. The hybrid design decreases overall cost of the prosthesis. Some hybrid designs eliminate the cable and harness, therefore eliminating pressure on the sound side when the prosthesis is operated. One hybrid design involves the use of a body-powered elbow flexion device with a myoelectric hand (Fig. 48-22).[4] Another configuration might be the use of a cable elbow

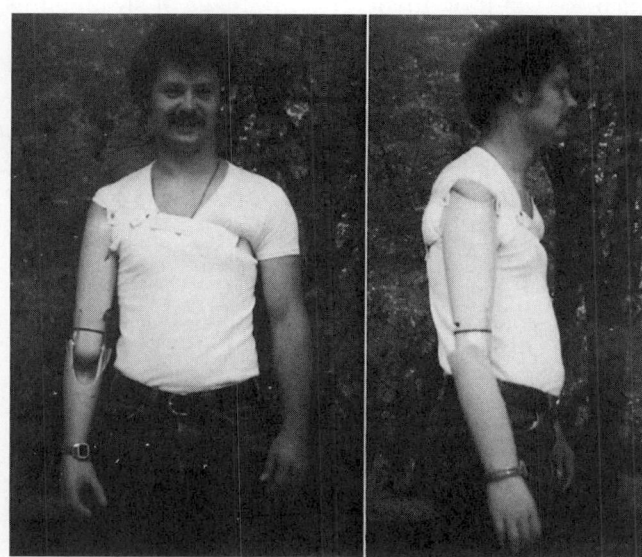

FIG. 48-22
This "hybrid" above-elbow prosthesis uses a thoracic suspension and control harness for total suspension of the prosthesis and actuation of the Bowden cable-controlled mechanical elbow and locking mechanism. The batteries and electronic components for myoelectric control of the hand are self-contained within the upper arm of the prosthesis. (From Hunter JM, Mackin EJ, Callahan AD: *Rehabilitation of the hand: surgery and therapy*, St Louis, 1995, Mosby.)

and hook TD with an electric wrist rotator. For bilateral amputees a powered elbow combined with a cable-hook TD offers a very quick elbow and less overall bulk of the prosthesis and dedicates all excursion of the cable to the TD. A hybrid prosthesis can decrease the overall weight of a prosthesis. It can be less expensive and complex. All excursion of the existing cable is dedicated to one component, as opposed to multiple components. This feature requires less overall force on the part of the amputee for operating the prosthesis.

Training an individual with bilateral limb loss requires extensive rehabilitation experience, and it is not recommended for the therapist with little or no previous exposure to the rehabilitation of patients with amputations. "Centers of excellence," where rehabilitation of persons with amputations is a specialty area of treatment, may be the best rehabilitation choice for the individual with high-level bilateral limb loss.

PREPROSTHETIC THERAPY

Awareness of postoperative and subsequent preprosthetic principles of care is crucial for the successful management of the individual who has sustained traumatic limb loss. The patient has little control over what is happening and must depend on the health care team to provide the best treatment possible.[3]

The rehabilitation team, which should include the physician, nurse, occupational or physical therapist, social worker, and patient, addresses the following goals:
- Promote wound healing
- Control incision pain
- Control residual limb shrinkage and shaping
- Maximize joint ROM
- Increase strength
- Increase ILS independence
- Explore patient's and family's feelings about change in body
- Orient to prosthetic options
- Identify or test potential **muscle sites** for prosthesis control
- Improve muscle site control and strength (once identified)
- Explore the patient's goals regarding the future
- Obtain adequate financial sponsorship for the prosthesis and training[7]

When the sutures are removed, the preprosthetic program can begin. Most of this program has been extensively discussed in Section 1 of this chapter. For the patient receiving a myoelectric prosthesis, the following paragraphs will clarify the last five goals.

Identify Potential Muscle Sites

A myoelectric prosthesis functions by detecting electromyographic (EMG) signals produced by muscles.

Locating appropriate muscle sites superficially is the most important aspect of the successful operation of a myoelectric prosthesis. Physical examination of the forearm can often detect sufficient strength in natural agonist-antagonist pairs, such as the wrist extensor and wrist flexor contractions in the person with a BE amputation and biceps and triceps contractions in the person with an AE amputation. Shoulder amputees often have a pectoralis or deltoid site anteriorly and an infraspinatus or trapezius site posteriorly. It is difficult to identify proximal muscle sites that both are adequate in signal and allow the prosthetist to position the electrodes within the socket and hold them securely against the skin. On occasion, trauma or nerve injuries do not allow the choice of a natural pair. If a particular site could cause tissue breakdown under the pressure for an electrode, avoid it. Often, healed skin or muscle grafts can tolerate such pressure very well. Consult the physician when dealing with repaired tissue. If the best muscle site signals are weak, the therapist and prosthetist require a biofeedback system or myotester (Fig. 48-23). When surface potentials are being measured with the electrodes and a myotester, it is important that all electrodes have good contact with the skin and be aligned along the general direction of the muscle fibers. Moistening the skin slightly with water may improve the EMG signal by lowering skin resistance. EMG testing is begun with the most distal portion of the remnant muscles.

The goal of this testing is to identify two adequate muscle sites with the strongest difference between them, not necessarily the two strongest muscle site signals. The selection can be considered complete when the patient can tolerate a 1-hour training session and is consistently generating sufficient signals to operate the prosthesis in such basic functions as opening and closing of the TD. The therapist should check with the prosthetist for the minimum signal required for operating the myoelectric system chosen for the patient.[9]

Muscle Site Control Training

The more proximal the level of amputation is, the more difficult it becomes for the prosthetist to fit the individual and for the therapist to train that individual. For the patient to understand the desired muscle contraction, the therapist instructs the patient to imitate the desired contraction or movement with both arms. The therapist should ask the patient to raise the sound hand at the wrist (wrist extension) and imagine this motion with the phantom hand on the amputated side (Fig. 48-24). Often a therapist can palpate the wrist flexors and extensors on the residual limb during this exercise. The patient is instructed to contract and relax each muscle group separately and on command. For this step a myoelectric tester is particularly useful because it indicates the magnitude of the EMG signal as the patient contracts the muscle.

The myoelectric tester can be used to train the muscles with both visual and auditory feedback. Various models are available to therapists. The goals of training at this point are to increase muscle strength and to isolate muscle contractions. As confidence and accuracy improve, the visual or auditory feedback should be removed. Practicing muscle contractions without feedback teaches the patient to internalize the feeling of each control movement. The advantage of creating this internalized awareness of proper muscle control is that control and strengthening practice can be continued between treatment sessions without the feedback equipment.[11] The therapist needs to recognize muscle fatigue, which is frequently a side effect in this process, and time must be given to allow that muscle to relax during the treatment session.

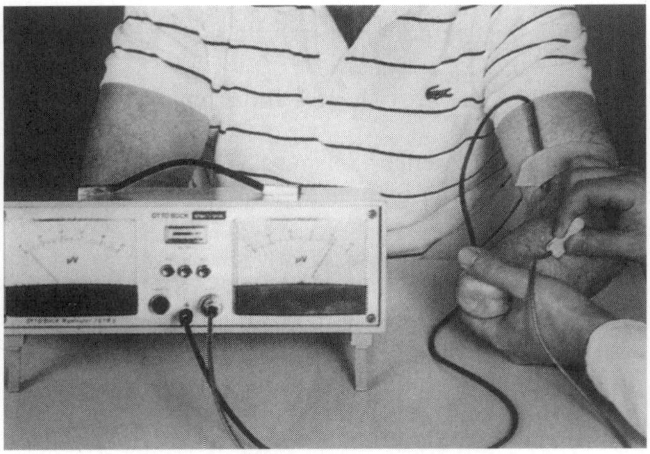

FIG. 48-23
Otto Bock myotester determines magnitude of muscle contraction.

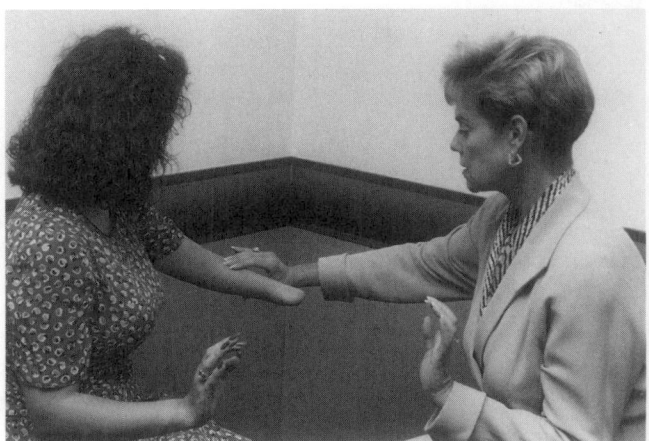

FIG. 48-24
Therapist instructs patient to imitate desired muscle contraction on both sides.

Ideally the individual with an amputation receives adequate training and practice in initiating these muscle contractions before receiving the completed myoelectric prosthesis from the prosthetist. Prosthetists commonly engage a patient in muscle site training with the preparatory socket and prosthesis. This occurs as they strive for optimum electrode placement and socket fit. This training is not adequate for the majority of patients. Anxiety and frustration often accompany training to use a myoelectric prosthesis, and the development of a team approach to training by the therapist and prosthetist can minimize these responses. The patient's success and effectiveness in using the prosthesis are closely related to the quality of the preprosthetic training.

PROSTHETIC PROGRAM

Orientation of the patient to what the prosthesis realistically can and cannot do is an important aspect of a prosthetic training program. If the individual has an unrealistic expectation about the usefulness of the prosthesis as a replacement arm, he or she may be dissatisfied with the ultimate functioning of the prosthesis and may reject it altogether. It is imperative that the therapist be honest and positive about the function of the prosthesis. If he or she believes in and understands the functional potential and limitations of the prosthesis, success can be more realistically achieved.[2]

Orientation and Education

Training with a prosthesis should begin as soon as the prosthesis is received, preferably the same day. An excellent resource in the training process of a patient with a myoelectric hand is in the text *Comprehensive Management of the Upper Limb Amputee.*[3]

Important areas to review during the initial visits are orientation to prosthesis terminology and operation, independence in donning and doffing the prosthesis, orientation to a prosthesis wearing schedule, and care of the residual limb and prosthesis.

Orientation to Prosthesis Terminology

Considering that the prosthesis is a natural extension of the individual's body, it is particularly important to know the function and names of the major parts such as the electrodes, battery, glove, and electric hand. The initial visit is an appropriate time to review the battery-charging procedure with the patient.

The batteries are energy-storing devices, and most are rechargeable. Some prosthesis control systems use a 9-volt disposable battery. The prosthetist supplying the prosthesis will instruct the patient in proper installation and recharging. Rechargers are plugged into a standard electrical outlet. Most manufacturers' rechargers have some indicator to alert the patient when the battery is

fully charged. Some rechargers require 12 hours of charging time, whereas others may take as long as 24 hours (Fig. 48-25). A fast charger, requiring only 1 or 2 hours of charging time, may be available. For best results, the batteries should be just about completely drained before recharging. The prosthesis will begin to operate more slowly when the battery is low, and some unexpected control problems could occur. This is why the first troubleshooting step is always, "Make certain you have installed a fresh battery."[9]

Although the myoelectric hand is the most commonly prescribed electric terminal device, a specially designed gripping device, or **Greifer,** is also recommended at times. The Greifer, designed by the Otto Bock Company, is a universal working tool designed to handle various specialized tasks. It can be used for heavy work in industry or farming and provides quick handling and precise manipulation of small objects. Features of the Greifer include a 38-lb grasp, as well as parallel gripping surfaces and a flexion joint for dorsal and volar flexion (Fig. 48-26).[8]

Instruction manuals from the manufacturer for the battery charger and the prosthesis are often provided for the individual's reference, and they are excellent tools to use for review and education.

Independence in Donning and Doffing the Prosthesis

The individual should be able to put on and remove the prosthesis independently. With proper instruction and the help of the prosthetist in suspension design, the patient should be able to do this. Donning the prosthesis should be performed with the electronics in the off position to prevent any uncontrolled movements. A person with a BE amputation usually has the great advantage of not needing a harness and control cables because a

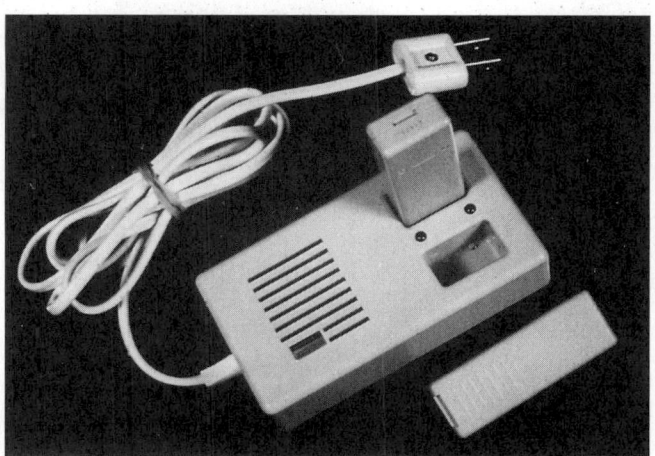

FIG. 48-25
Battery of myoelectric arm is inserted in battery charger and charged overnight.

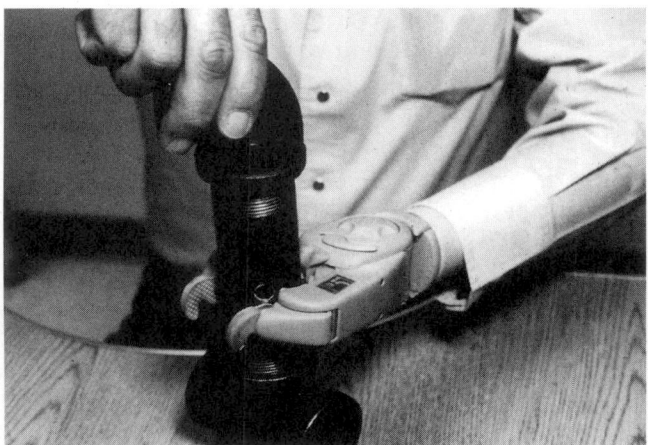

FIG. 48-26
Myoelectric Greifer is designed as universal working tool with parallel gripping force of up to 38 pounds.

supercondylar suspension at the elbow is often used. The wearer can slip the arm directly into the socket.

Suspension designs for the person with an AE amputation frequently require a **pull sock** for donning the prosthesis. This provides close contact with the limb, particularly for very short residual limbs. The wearer must be sure not to start with the stocking too high on the residual limb because this will increase friction during pull and make it harder to pull the sock out of the bottom of the socket. It may be necessary to experiment with different sock materials, powder on the skin, and donning techniques until the most successful materials and techniques are identified.

Good electrical contact is achieved after approximately 1 minute of donning. A wearer can also moisten the skin at the electrode sites to eliminate the waiting period for perspiration to occur. The prosthetic arm should be stored in the off position with the batteries removed. The hand should be fully opened when stored, to keep the thumb web space stretched.

Orientation to a Prosthesis Wearing Schedule
Initial wearing periods should be no longer that 15 to 30 minutes. This limit is particularly important if scarring or insensate areas are present on the residual limb. If redness persists for more than 20 minutes in a particular area after prosthesis removal, the patient should return to the prosthetist for adjustments. If no skin problems exist, the wearing periods can be increased in 30-minute increments two to three times a day. By the end of a week, full-time wearing should be achieved.

Care of the Residual Limb and Prosthesis
Appropriate care of the skin is vitally important. The residual limb should be washed daily with mild soap and lukewarm water. It should be rinsed thoroughly and dried using patting motions with a towel, so as not to irritate sensitive or scar tissue.

The prosthesis may be cleaned with soap and water by using a damp cloth. Rubbing alcohol may be used to clean the inside of the socket if an odor develops. The cosmetic glove stains easily; special attention should be paid to avoiding ink, newsprint, mustard, grease, and dirt. Wiping with soap and water or a glove cleansing cream obtained from the prosthetist will remove general soil but not stains. The average life of a glove is approximately 6 months. Polyvinylchloride (PVC) plastic gloves are the least expensive, most flexible, and toughest. Silicone gloves are being used more frequently because the new silicone formulas are tougher and minimize the yellowing and brittleness that frequently sets in with age, and allow the greatest cosmesis.[4] The prosthesis itself should never be immersed in water because this will seriously damage the internal electronic components. Additionally, it is important to advise myoelectric wearers against excess vibration, sand, dirt, and the extremes of heat and cold. These, too, can seriously impair the electronic components.

The prosthesis should be checked occasionally for loose screws and harness attachments, and these should be brought to the attention of the prosthetist. The covers of the prosthesis should not be opened unless the prosthetist instructs the wearer or therapist to do so.

Control Training

The first function to master is opening and closing the hand. The individual now understands the muscle contractions required to perform these actions. Simple opening and closing of the hand are practiced. The muscles should contract as independently as possible. Next, the patient practices opening the hand halfway, then stopping and relaxing so the hand does not move. If a proportional control system is used, the patient can also practice opening and closing quickly and slowly.

Use Training

Repetitive grasp and release of objects are introduced after **control training.** Simple approach, grasp, and release activities are practiced with objects of various shapes, sizes, and densities. It is important for the individual first to visualize how the object should be approached and grasped, and then to preposition the myoelectric hand. Prepositioning involves placing the terminal device in the optimum position for a specific activity. In approaching a glass, the hand should face in toward the midline to grasp the glass as a normal hand would (Fig. 48-27). The fingers of the hand should not be positioned downward because a normal hand does not approach a glass in this position.

Working on approach, grasp, and release in multiple positions follows practice with more simple activities. The patient with an AE amputation who uses a body-powered or electric elbow should make certain the angle of elbow flexion is appropriate to complete the grasp in a natural manner. Often the patient adjusts the body using compensatory body motions rather than adjusting the elbow position or prepositioning the hand first. It is important to avoid this because it looks unnatural, becomes habitual, and may lead to secondary musculoskeletal problems in the neck, shoulder, or trunk. A mirror can help the patient see the way the body is positioned and visualize how the sound arm would approach a particular object or activity. It is often necessary to remind the patient to maintain an upright posture and avoid extraneous body movements.

Another important goal of training an individual to grasp an object is mastering **pressure control** or the gripping force of the terminal device. This skill involves close visual attention to grade the muscle contraction for a specific result in the myoelectric hand. Foam packaging bubbles, paper cups, and ping-pong balls work well for developing this skill. The individual must learn how to pick up the object without crushing it. Too strong a grasp crushes the object being held (Fig. 48-28). Good grasp control through training with foam, cotton balls, or wet sponges will help develop the control needed to handle paper cups, eggs, potato chips, and sandwiches or even to hold someone's hand.[11]

Release is accomplished by visualizing a wrist extension contraction, or a quick "hand up" or "hand open"

in the patient with a BE amputation. This response should become automatic if there has been good preprosthetic training of the muscles.

Eventually the ability to perform specific movements will take less cognitive effort and the movements become automatic. The wearer now has muscle endurance and prosthesis tolerance for 1-hour therapy sessions. Next, functional use activities are introduced into the therapy program.

Functional Training

The prosthesis is used as a functional assist in the majority of bilateral activities. Therefore most activities of daily living (ADL) will be accomplished with the uninvolved arm and hand. Other than perhaps for practice, it is not appropriate to train a person with a unilateral amputation to eat holding a spoon, write, or brush his teeth using the myoelectric hand. In almost all cases the sound hand becomes the dominant extremity and performs these tasks. Occasionally, if the right arm was dominant and is amputated and the individual is fitted with a myoelectric hand in a timely manner, he or she may prefer to use the myoelectric hand for some of these activities. The critically important component of sensory feedback is often the determining factor in deciding which hand to use. A person with an amputation almost always chooses to

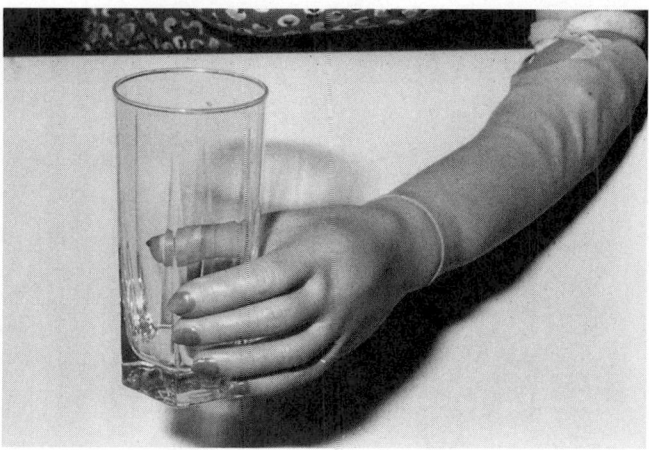

FIG. 48-27
When approaching glass, hand is prepositioned in midline to grasp glass as normal hand.

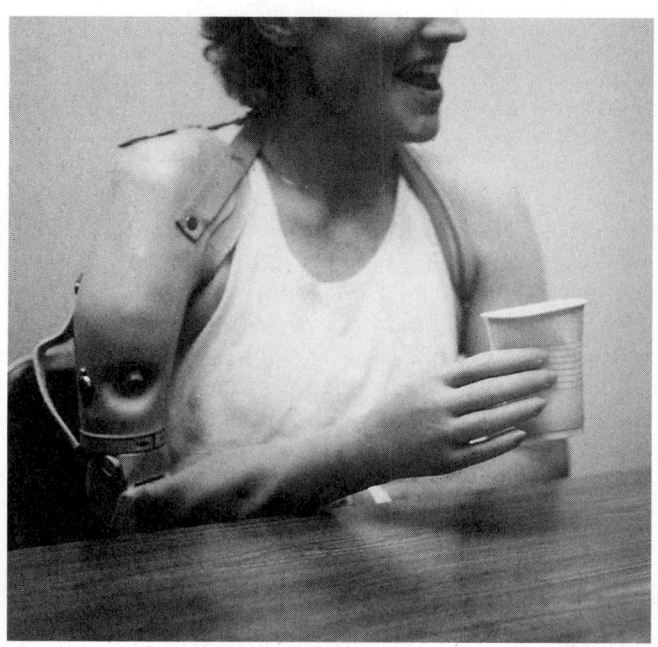

FIG. 48-28
Above-elbow amputee demonstrates how excessive grasp crushes object (plastic cup) being held.

TABLE 48-2

Roles of Myoelectric Hand and Sound Hand in Bilateral Activities of Daily Living

Activity	Myoelectric Hand	Sound Hand
Cutting meat	Hold fork with prongs facing downward; hold knife as grip strength increases	Hold knife Hold fork
Opening a jar (Fig. 48-29)	Hold the jar	Turn the lid
Opening a tube of toothpaste	Hold the tube	Turn the cap
Stirring something in a bowl	Hold the bowl with a strong grip	Hold the mixing spoon or fork
Cutting fruit or vegetables (Fig. 48-30)	Hold the fruit or vegetable firmly	Hold the knife to cut
Using scissors to cut paper	Hold the paper to be cut	Use scissors in normal fashion
Buckling a belt	Hold the buckle end of belt to keep stable	Manipulate long end of belt into buckle
Zipping a jacket from bottom up	Hold anchor tab	Manipulate pull tab at base and pull upward
Applying socks	Hold one side of socks	Hold other side of socks and pull upward
Opening an umbrella (Fig. 48-31)	Hold base knob of umbrella	Open as normal

perform activities with a hand that has feeling. A myoelectric hand lacks this sensory feedback. Feedback is provided more proximally with the action of muscle contraction, yet responding to this is difficult for the wearer.

The therapist should review a list of bilateral ADL tasks with the patient to determine which tasks are most important to accomplish. These are the activities to focus on in training, stressing throughout that the myoelectric hand is used as an assist and stabilizer. If unilateral tasks are presented to the patient, his or her need to operate the prosthesis is minimized or absent. These tasks should be avoided. The bilateral activities listed on Table 48-2 are good examples to review and practice.

With practice, these activities and many others will be easier and automatic to perform. It is important to reinforce and emphasize the fact that bathing, grooming, and hygiene skills involving water must be done without a myoelectric hand because of the damaging effects of water on the electric motor and battery.

Vocational and Leisure Activities

As training proceeds and a sense of self-acceptance and comfort with the amputation is achieved, a therapist should broach the subject of return to work. Ideally the therapist makes an on-site visit. If possible, the various job requirements can be discussed and then practiced in a simulated, step-by-step process. If changes and adjustments to the work environment are necessary, the therapist could advise in these modifications.

Recreational activities are also critically important to discuss at this time because these activities contribute not

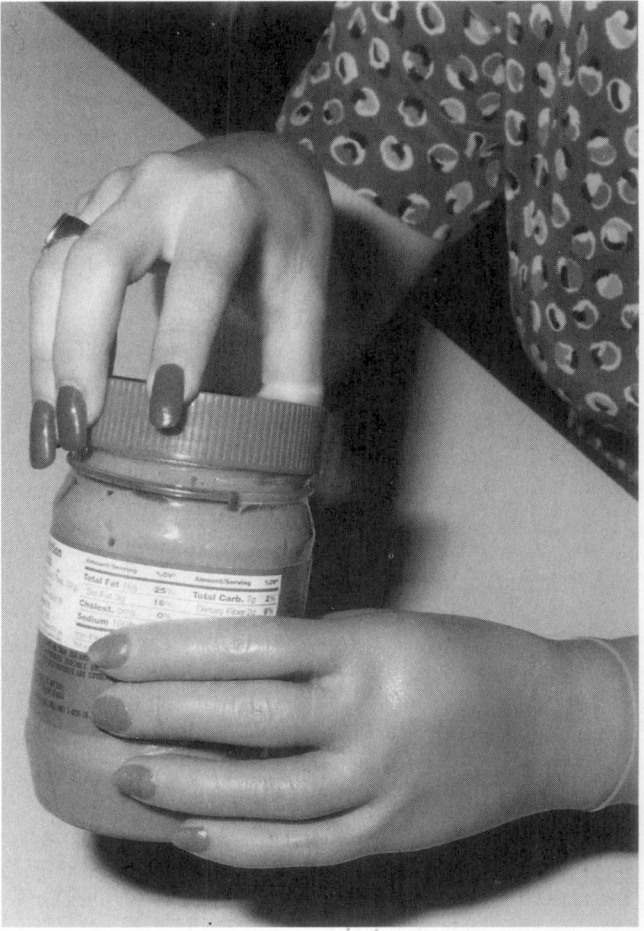

FIG. 48-29

Opening jar is accomplished with myoelectric hand holding jar and sound hand turning lid.

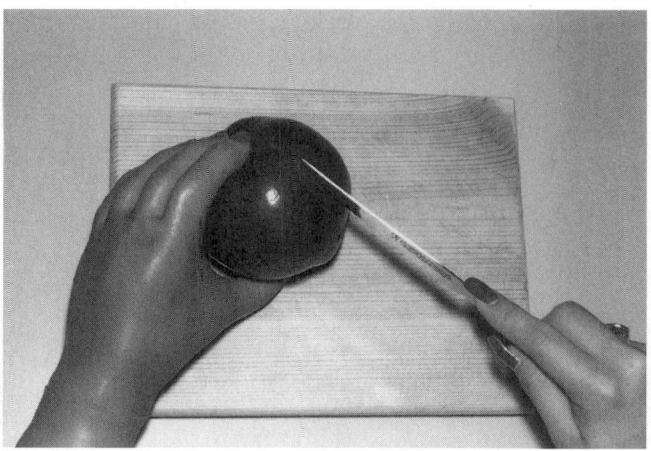

FIG. 48-30
Cutting apple is accomplished with myoelectric hand holding apple while sound hand holds knife to cut.

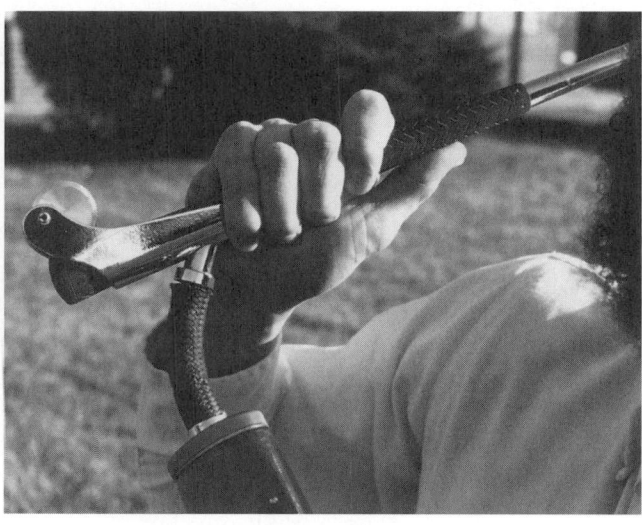

FIG. 48-32
Amputee Golf Grip is high-performance prosthetic golf accessory that allows smooth swings and complete follow-through.

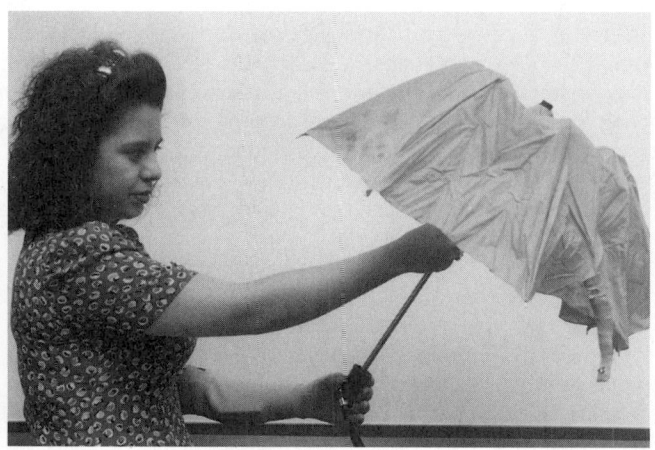

FIG. 48-31
Opening umbrella is accomplished by holding base knob of umbrella with myoelectric hand and using sound hand to open as normal.

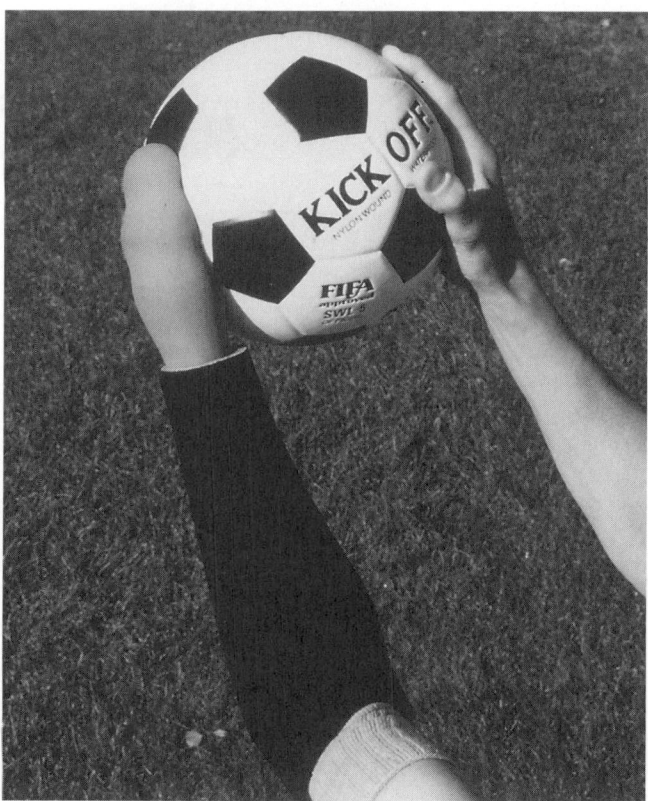

FIG. 48-33
Super Sports terminal device is highly flexible, strong, prosthetic sports accessory for volleyball, soccer, football, floor exercise gymnastics, or any activity in which shock absorption, safety, and bilateral control are important.

only to physical well-being but also to psychological well-being. The terminal devices for recreational activities are not myoelectric. As discussed in Section I, Therapeutic Recreation Systems (TRS) has some excellent TD adaptation components, including an Amputee Golf Grip (Fig. 48-32) and a Super Sports terminal device (Fig. 48-33).

Home Instructions

At the conclusion of training, home instructions that include a wearing schedule, care instructions, and additional tasks to practice should be shared with the patient and his family. A follow-up appointment should be made at this time, as well as a list of the rehabilitation team members and their telephone numbers, to enable the patient to contact the appropriate person when problems arise.

SUMMARY

The rehabilitation process of a person with upper limb loss can be challenging and rewarding. In the instances of AE, shoulder disarticulation, and bilateral limb loss, significant training and expertise on the part of the therapist are essential.

The potential of individuals with amputation is limitless, and often they are able to accomplish activities one never would have predicted. The success of rehabilitation does not rest solely on the quality of training in the use of the prosthesis. Rather, success depends on such complex factors as the quality of medical management, the type and fit of the prosthesis, the patient's interest in learning the use of the prosthesis, and the conscientious follow-up of the individual once the rehabilitation phase is complete. Follow-up is critically important and often overlooked. Perhaps the most important aspect of a successful rehabilitation program is the motivation and the desire of the person with amputation to become more independent. As a team member, this aspect is a pivotal ingredient to cultivate and reinforce. The effect a therapist has during this important process will remain with the patient for life.

CASE STUDY 48-1

CASE STUDY—MR. K.

Mr. K. is 41 years old. He has lived in poverty all his life. He is intellectually limited. Mr. K. recently sustained an above-elbow (AE) amputation of the nondominant left upper extremity (UE) as the result of a traumatic injury. The residual limb is well healed with good shrinkage. There is no pain in the residual limb. There are no medical complications. Mr. K. is performing most self-care activities independently, using the sound right arm, except for bilateral activities such as cutting meat, buttoning the shirt, applying deodorant, carrying large objects, and tying shoes. He needs some assistance in analyzing methods for one-handed performance.

Mr. K. is receiving state aid, and a prosthesis and vocational training have been authorized for him. He has worked as a janitor and as a field hand picking vegetables in the past. He reads the basic vocabulary necessary for everyday life at home and in the street (e.g., signs and newspaper headlines). When employed, Mr. K. is a steady and hard worker. He is married and has four children, all living at home. His interests are watching television, playing cards, and gardening.

Mr. K. is accepting the prosthesis and is no longer depressed about the loss of his arm. He appears to be well motivated for the prosthesis and for return to employment. He was referred to occupational therapy for prosthetic training and vocational evaluation.

Progressive resistive exercises to increase the strength of the shoulder rotators and adductors and manual resistive exercises to strengthen the control movements were initiated. The names and functions of all parts of the prosthesis were reviewed, and Mr. K. practiced putting on and removing the prosthesis smoothly and efficiently. Control training included practice in elbow flexion, elbow locking, elbow and wrist rotation, and terminal device opening and closing in sequence. Training in grasp and release of objects of various weights, textures, sizes, and shapes in a variety of positions (cans, wood cylinders, pencils, cabinet handles, doorknobs) was completed. ADL bilateral activities addressed included fastening trousers, handling a wallet, tying shoes, cleaning fingernails, applying deodorant, tying a necktie, buttoning a shirt, using the phone, cutting food, planting seeds in a pot, and playing cards. Work simulation activities included cleaning the floor, emptying trash, assembling electronic parts, and using hand tools.

Mr. K. tolerates the prosthesis throughout full daytime hours. He has worn it for 100% of his community and social outings. He is incorporating it automatically into 75% of his bilateral ADL tasks. The shoulder muscles have increased in strength to grade 4+/5, but he does fatigue with constant use longer than 2 hours, requiring a brief respite from use. Mr. K. is pleased with the simple household maintenance activities he has been able to perform with the help of the prosthesis. He is anxious to return to gainful employment and has met with the vocational counselor two times, with a third visit for prevocational testing scheduled.

SECTION 3
Lower Extremity Amputations

PATRICIA ANN MORRIS

LEVELS OF AMPUTATION AND FUNCTIONAL LOSSES IN THE LOWER EXTREMITY

The higher levels of lower extremity (LE) amputation result in more functional loss and a greater need for a prostheses for function and cosmesis. They require more complex and extensive prostheses. Levels of amputation are shown in Fig. 48-34.

Hemipelvectomy and hip disarticulation amputations result in loss of the entire LE; hip, knee, ankle, and foot functions are lost.[2] **Above-knee amputation** (AKA) and knee disarticulation amputations result in loss of knee, ankle, and foot motion. The residual limb length of the AKA varies from 10 to 12 inches (5.4 to 30.5 cm) below the greater trochanter.[2,26]

Below-knee amputations (BKA) result in a residual limb that is approximately 4 to 6 inches (10.1 to 15.2 cm) in length from the tibial plateau.[20,26] Other systems classify the levels of amputation into thirds: upper, middle, and lower third indicate the distance below the ischium for AKAs and the distance below the tibial plateau for BKAs.[20] The **Symes amputation** is equivalent to an ankle disarticulation with loss of ankle and foot function. In a transmetatarsal amputation the foot is severed through the metatarsal bones and ankle function remains intact. Loss of the small toes does not result in any significant functional impairment. Loss of the great toe, however, prevents toe-off during ambulation.[27]

TYPES OF PROSTHESES

The **pylon,** a temporary prosthesis, serves as a working prosthesis. It allows the patient to use the proximal musculature of the residual limb and maintains joint ROM, and it provides the sense of pressure, motion, and weight that is similar to that of the actual prosthesis (Fig. 48-35).[28] The immediate postoperative **ischial weight-bearing prosthesis** (IWBP) (Fig. 48-36), designed by Dr. Madan Telikicherla, is an early fitting prosthesis that is fabricated and adjustable to an individual's

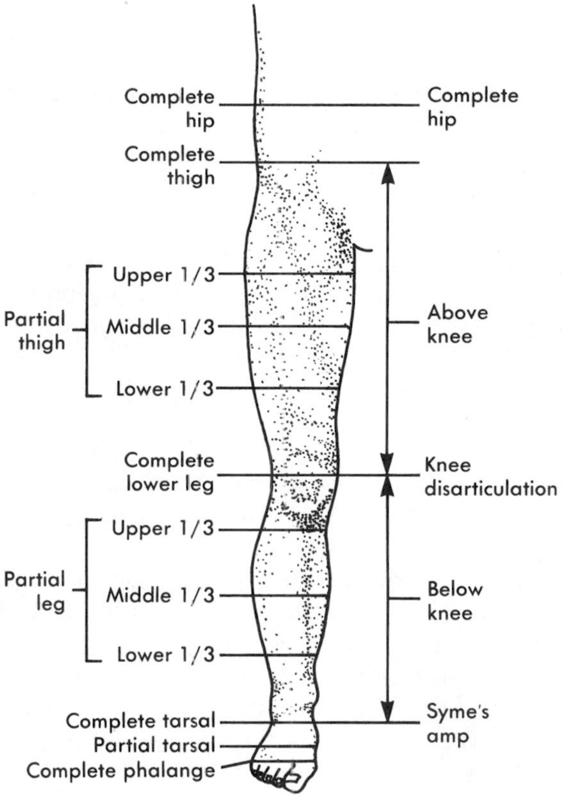

FIG. 48-34
Levels of amputation and functional losses in the lower extremity.

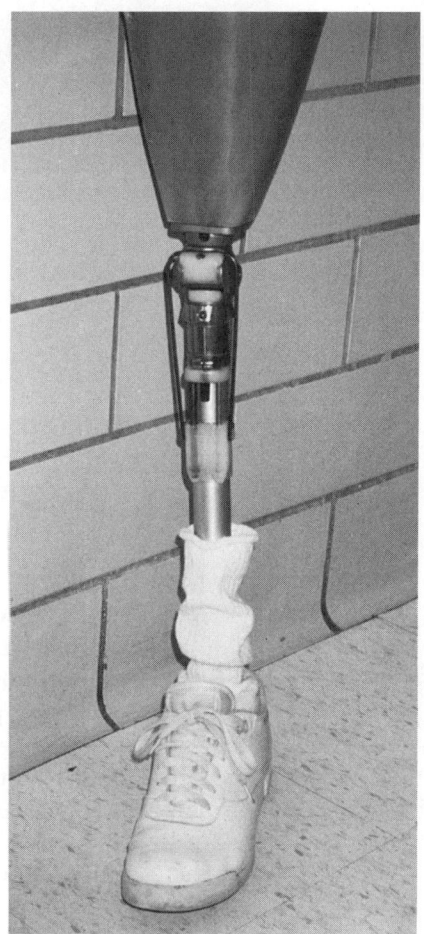

FIG. 48-35
A typical pylon.

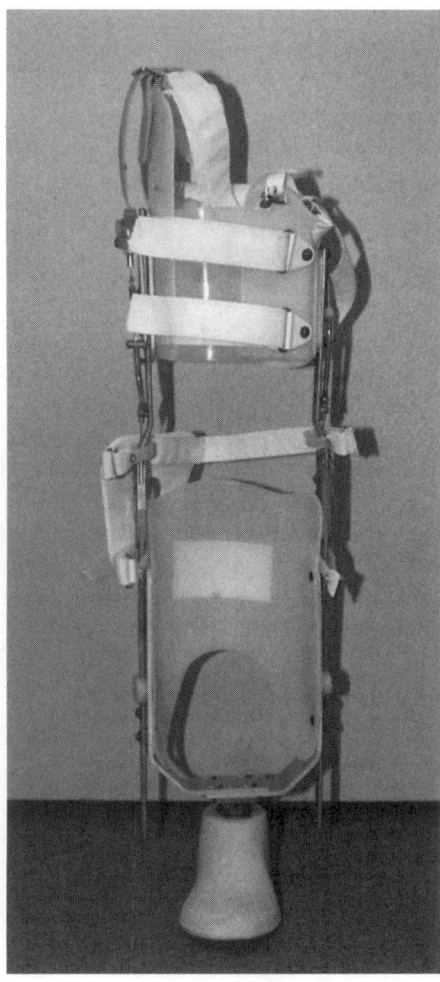

FIG. 48-36
Immediate postoperative ischial weight-bearing prosthesis.

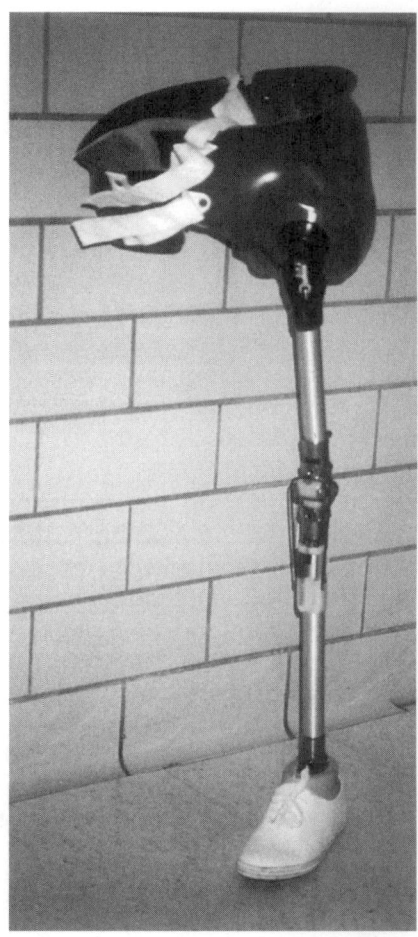

FIG. 48-37
Canadian prosthesis used for the hemipelvectomy and hip disarticulation amputations.

height and weight.[28] It can be fitted to persons with BKA, AKA, and knee disarticulation amputation as early as the first postoperative day. Previous methods of early weight bearing and ambulation have been associated with such complications as separation of the layers of surgical wound (wound dehiscence). The unique design of the IWBP bypasses weight bearing through the residual limb, thus protecting the surgical wound and preventing the pain usually associated with early weight bearing. Use of the IWBP under the supervision of a physician, an occupational therapist, a physical therapist, and a prosthetist enables the patient to achieve functional ambulation and independent mobility. Within a week of surgery, and almost a full month before the patient can be fitted for a regular prosthesis, stairs and uneven terrain can be negotiated. This early independence results in increased self-esteem and dignity and enhances the patient's quality of life. Furthermore, early mobility can potentially reduce the rehabilitation stay and the risk of medical complications associated with immobility.[28]

The Canadian-type hip disarticulation prosthesis meets the needs of patients who have had a hemipelvectomy or hip disarticulation (Fig. 48-37). This prosthesis is suspended from the pelvis by straps and equipped with hip and knee joints and a solid ankle, cushioned heel–type foot (**SACH foot**). Pelvic movements activate the prosthesis.[27]

The patient with an AKA benefits from either a suction socket or a conventional above-knee prosthesis. The conventional socket prosthesis is held in place by a silesian bandage or pelvic belt.[11,21,22] As its name implies, the suction socket is held in place by negative air pressure or suction. Both these prostheses have a quadrilateral socket, a knee joint that permits flexion and extension, a shank, and a SACH foot.

Patients with BKA use either the patella tendon-bearing (PTB) prosthesis or the standard BK prosthesis. The PTB prosthesis has a soft socket for the BK residual limb. It is composed of a strap around the thigh, just above the patella,[11,21] for suspension, a shank, and the ankle-foot assembly.[14] The standard BK prosthesis con-

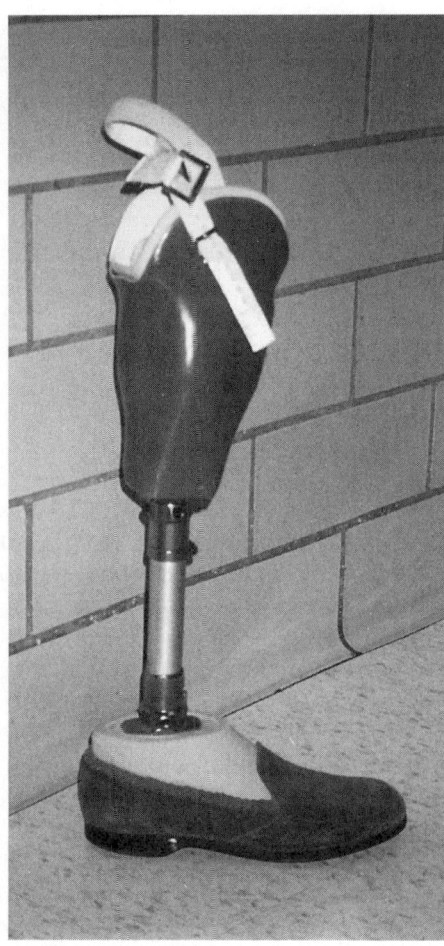

FIG. 48-38
Plastic Syme prosthesis.

sists of a thigh corset, lateral hinges for a knee joint, a shin piece, and the ankle-foot assembly.

The person who has had a Syme's amputation uses the Canadian-type Syme prosthesis or a *plastic* Syme (Fig. 48-38). This prosthesis consists of a total contact plastic socket and SACH foot; there is no ankle joint.[27]

Transmetatarsal and toe or multiple toe amputations do not require prostheses. A shoe-toe-filler is all that is needed.[2,27]

REHABILITATION TEAM

Rehabilitation of the patient with LE amputation is best accomplished with a team approach.[7,8,16] The rehabilitation team consists of a physician, occupational therapist, physical therapist, prosthetist, social worker, vocational counselor, and of course, the patient. Other health professionals who often contribute to the team are the nurse, dietitian, psychologist, and possibly an administrative coordinator.

The physician is responsible for coordinating the team's efforts, making decisions on the patient's general medical condition, and ordering appliances.[22]

The occupational therapist assesses occupational performance areas and performance components. Based on the evaluation, the therapist designs a treatment program, in concert with the patient and the family, to facilitate achievement of maximum independence. Included are recommendations for adaptive devices and durable medical equipment designed to enhance the person's independence and safety for reentry into the community.

The physical therapist evaluates and treats the physical problems (e.g., strength, ROM, coordination, balance, and gait) of patients from the preprosthetic through prosthetic phases of the treatment program. The physical therapist recommends whether to fit the patient with a prosthesis. If a prosthesis is recommended, the physical therapist recommends the prosthetic components. The physical therapist may also act as clinical coordinator of the treatment team.

The prosthetist fabricates and modifies the prosthesis, recommends prosthetic components, and shares data on new prosthetic developments.

The social worker is the financial counselor and coordinator. The social worker acts as liaison with third-party payers and community agencies and helps the family cope with social and financial problems.

The dietitian consults with any patients needing dietary guidance, especially those with diabetes.

The vocational counselor assesses the patient's employment potential and helps with education, training, and job placement.

The nursing staff is responsible for administering medications, monitoring vital signs, and caring for the wound. The nursing staff is also responsible for daily dressing changes, inspection of the surgical site, and helping with prevention of contractures and decubiti.[18] As the patient continues to progress, the nurse encourages performance of activities that have been learned in physical and occupational therapy.

OCCUPATIONAL THERAPY INTERVENTION

The occupational therapist begins the assessment to determine the patient's functional status in the occupational performance areas, performance components, and performance contexts.[1,23] Before the initial assessment the occupational therapist reviews the patient's medical record. The chart contains important medical history such as date and level of amputation, surgical procedure performed, etiology, disease processes that may be associated with the amputation, presence of amputation-associated symptoms, medications, and medical history.[2]

The goals of OT for the patient with lower extremity amputation are as follows:

1. Decrease edema
2. Prevent contractures
3. Maintain or increase ROM
4. Increase strength and endurance
5. Improve posture
6. Decrease pain
7. Increase mobility
8. Educate the patient and family about limb care and prosthesis care and wear
9. Provide adaptive devices and durable medical equipment
10. Assess the home for accessibility

The occupational therapist must be mindful of the importance of eliciting the cooperation and acceptance of the family in order to achieve treatment goals.

Proper positioning, edema reduction techniques, therapeutic exercise and activity, pain desensitization techniques, mobility and transfer training, and support groups with similar patients are some of the methods used to achieve these goals.

Treatment of Occupational Performance Components

Soft Tissue Integrity

The prevention of soft tissue contractures is an immediate postoperative concern.[5] Positioning techniques are used to prevent abduction, flexion, and external rotation of the hip and flexion of the knee.[11,20,27] To prevent hip flexion contractures, patients are instructed in lying prone and are encouraged to sleep and rest in the prone position. A positioning schedule is established in collaboration with the patient and is communicated to the rest of the rehabilitation team. Positions encouraging knee and hip flexion, such as prolonged sitting in a bed or chair, are avoided. In supine or sitting positions, pillows should not be placed under the knee in a BKA, under the residual limb in an AKA, or between the legs, because these positions encourage knee flexion, hip flexion, and hip external rotation, respectively.[8]

The patient with BKA benefits from the use of a support for the residual limb in the wheelchair. The wheelchair padded extension (also called a stump board) allows the patient to be up and reduces the chances of increased edema by not allowing the dependent posture of the residual limb (Fig. 48-39).

To prevent decubiti, the patient is instructed to perform pressure relief and daily skin inspection techniques. The wheelchair-bound patient should relieve pressure every 15 minutes. Pressure relief can be accomplished by weight-shift relief techniques or wheelchair push-ups. When the patient is in bed, prone-lying, side-lying, and supine positions are alternated every 2 hours. Skin inspection techniques, using a long-handled mirror, are conducted once or twice a day.

Edema Reduction

Some edema is a normal postsurgical occurrence. An early rehabilitation goal is to reduce edema. If edema persists, it can cause such secondary complications as pain, contractures, and soft-tissue adhesions. After surgery, elevation is commonly used to reduce edema.[4,9]

Another method used to control edema is a **rigid removal dressing,** developed in the early 1960s by orthopedic surgeons in Europe. The residual limb is fitted with a plaster of Paris socket in the configuration of the final prosthesis (Fig. 48-40). It greatly limits the development of postoperative edema in the residual limb,

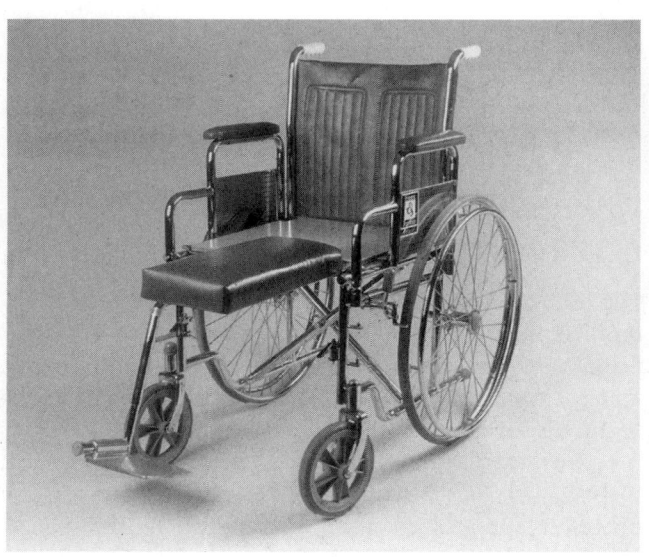

FIG. 48-39
Wheelchair with support for residual limb.

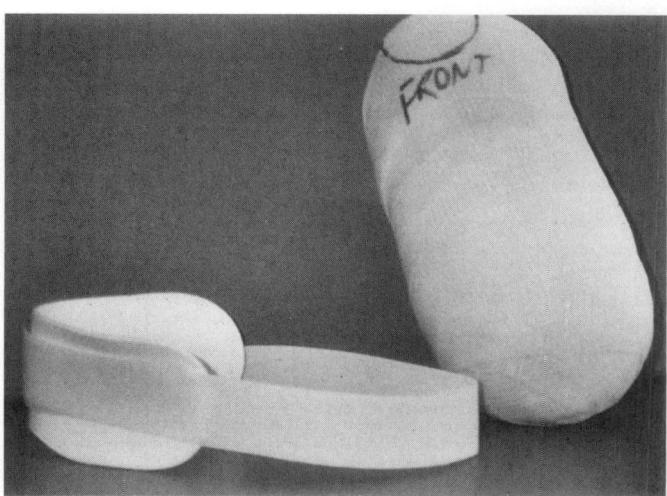

FIG. 48-40
Rigid removal dressing.

thereby reducing postoperative pain and enhancing wound healing.[4] The cast is changed approximately every 10 days, or more often if the cast becomes loose, until the residual limb is healed and ready for a permanent prosthesis.

The cast is held in position with a canvas band and secured with a Velcro strap.[4] The occupational therapist can also incorporate Ace bandage wrapping techniques or the use of a shrinker sock into the patient program. There are several methods of wrapping the limb. Most methods are based on similar principles. These include diagonal bandaging and application of firm, even pressure distally. The pressure decreases as the bandage is applied proximally. The bandage is reapplied as ordered. The advantages of wrapping are that it allows for the patient's contouring and frequent checking of the wound. The disadvantages are that improper wrapping may result in a poorly shaped residual limb and impairment of blood supply to its distal portion.[25]

Because of the disadvantages of wrapping, the clinician may recommend a shrinker sock.[25] The primary advantage of the shrinker sock is that it is easily applied and removed. The shrinker sock is donned as follows:

1. The sock is turned so that the bulky seam at the end is on the outside.
2. The top is turned so that it is folded back on itself about two thirds of the way.
3. The end of the sock is stretched so that it fits smoothly on the end of the residual limb.
4. The sock is gently pulled up over the limb.[3]

The therapist instructs the patient to don and doff the sock and periodically to check its fit. There are two reasons to check the sock: to prevent sock wrinkles and to prevent the top rim of the sock from rolling over onto an elastic band. The latter impairs circulation and causes distal edema; the former may irritate the skin and cause skin breakdown. The major disadvantage of the shrinker sock is that it is available in only a limited number of sizes.

In addition to controlling edema, both wrapping and shrinker socks prevent hemorrhage, promote limb shaping, provide a sense of security, assist in desensitization, and aid in venous return. Ace bandages and shrinker socks should be washed frequently, rinsed thoroughly, and dried on a flat surface. Over time, both Ace bandages and socks lose their elasticity and must be replaced.[21]

Physical Endurance and Strength

At initial evaluation the patient's overall strength usually ranges from good to normal. As the result of a long hospitalization, the patient may lose some muscle strength and a therapeutic exercise program may be indicated.

The goals of the exercise program are to maintain or regain strength in the remaining extremities, condition the cardiovascular system, and increase endurance for performing functional activities. The scapula depressors, elbow extensors, and wrist extensors are required for transfers and ambulation. Trunk exercises are incorporated into the program to facilitate mobility and transfers when performing self-care activities such as hygiene and LE dressing at bed or wheelchair levels. All patients, especially older patients, require close monitoring for signs of fatigue and shortness of breath when exercising.

Some methods to improve the patient's endurance include increasing the number of repetitions of an exercise or activity within the same time allotment, increasing the total time the patient performs the activity, or increasing the distance the patient propels a wheelchair. Wheelchair mobility can be graded from level surfaces to uneven surfaces to ramps. It provides UE exercise and endurance, as well as wheelchair mobility training.

Postural Control

The center of gravity changes in patients with either AKA or BKA. The seating system should be considered when the wheelchair is used for mobility before the final prosthetic fitting. The standard wheelchair has a hammock-type seat, which causes poor postural alignment, unequal distribution of weight, decreased balance, and instability for the patient who sits in the wheelchair for long periods. A solid seating system is recommended to maintain good postural alignment, weight distribution, balance, and stability.

Patients with total hip disarticulation and hemipelvectomy benefit from a hemipelvectomy cushion in the wheelchair. The cushion is made of molded, viscoelastic foam with a polyurethane foam bottom layer and has a contoured seating surface. It provides light pressure relief. These features provide superior weight distribution and pressure relief and improve overall positioning and support.[6,19] For the patient with a BK amputation, proper positioning of the residual limb will require a support system to prevent knee flexion contractures and help control edema.

For patients with bilateral AK amputation, the center of gravity is affected because of the significant change in body weight distribution. The wheelchair must be designed to accommodate the poor posterior alignment and uneven weight distribution. These factors can lead to posterior pelvic tilt and balance problems that can cause the wheelchair to tip over more easily during weight shifts. Antitipping devices address the weight distribution problems of bilateral AKA. These are placed on the rear of the wheelchair to accommodate the change in the center of gravity. The wheelchair's large wheels are placed further back than those on a standard wheelchair to accommodate the change in the patient's center of gravity. It is important for the occupational therapist to have a good working relationship with the wheelchair specialist. It is essential for the patient to achieve good dynamic sitting and standing balance for the safe performance of activities of daily living.[12]

Pain Management

Pain management is a team approach. The physical evaluation will include inspection of the amputated site for poor healing, neuromas, bone fragments, edema, abscesses, and infection. The occupational therapist addresses the physical and psychosocial aspects of pain in the initial evaluation.

Psychosocial issues regarding patient and family customs, emotional support, education, legal issues, and concerns of health care delivery can affect pain status. Phantom pain is an ongoing concern that differs with each person.[2] The physician can consider such various treatment approaches as injection of anesthetics into tender areas, sympathetic nerve blocks, pain medications, positioning, edema reduction techniques, and desensitization techniques. Many patients have found that desensitization techniques such as tapping, rubbing, applying pressure, and heat and cold decrease pain. Biofeedback has been effective in decreasing pain. The effectiveness of a technique varies from patient to patient. The rehabilitation team is concerned with determining the best approaches to pain management.[13]

Occupational Performance Areas

Activities of Daily Living

BED MOBILITY. The patient is taught bed mobility, without using bed rails or an overhead trapeze bar, to promote independence. The movements that are practiced during bed mobility training are rolling from side to side, bridging with knee and hip flexion, using the remaining sound limb for pushing up and down in bed (supine to short sitting and short sitting to supine), and static and dynamic balance training at the bed edge (Fig. 48-41).

WHEELCHAIR MOBILITY AND PARTS MANAGEMENT. After surgery the wheelchair will be the patient's main source of mobility. Wheelchair training consists of propulsion on various surfaces (e.g., even, uneven, smooth, and carpeted) and training in wheelchair navigation (e.g., moving in and around tight spaces, through doorways, and up ramps and curbs). The patient with unilateral LE amputation uses the arms and sound leg to propel the wheelchair. Patients who have bilateral amputations use only the upper extremities.

TRANSFER TRAINING. The patient with a unilateral lower extremity amputation generally uses a standing pivot transfer (90° pivot), transferring toward the sound side when possible. Having the patient practice transfers toward the amputated side or 180° pivots in-

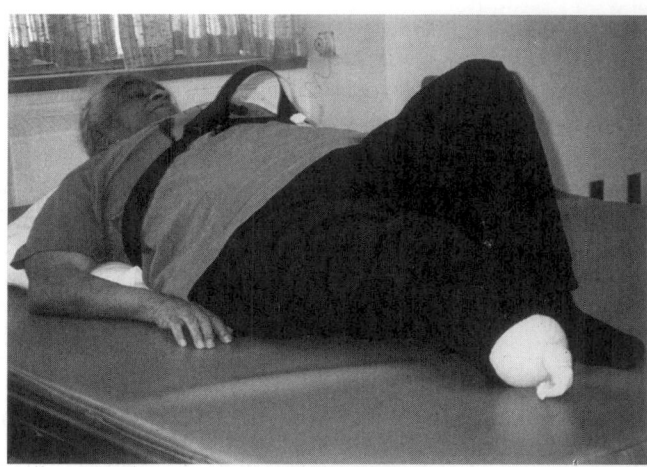

FIG. 48-41
Bridging to perform pushing up in bed and to don lower extremity.

creases independence when transferring in more restrictive environments—for example, in a bedroom or bathroom.

Sliding board transfers may be taught to the patient whose remaining limb is very weak or to the patient with bilateral amputations. Such patients may benefit from a wheelchair with a zippered or removable back. This allows posterior and anterior transfers by sliding backward to a surface, such as the toilet, and by sliding forward to return to the wheelchair.

As the patient progresses, and in collaboration with the physical therapist, ambulation training is incorporated with transfer training. The patient is trained to place hands on the armrests of the chair, scoot forward, place the existing foot backward to avoid several adjustments, and then to stand. Standing pivot and lateral transfers are practiced to and from bed, toilet, and tub. A tub bench and grab bar are used for the tub transfer.

RESIDUAL LIMB HYGEINE. Once the wound is healed and sutures are removed, the residual limb should be washed daily with warm water and dried with a towel. The patient should be instructed in daily skin inspection, using a long-handled inspection mirror to see all surfaces of the limb. The use of lotions or alcohol should be avoided to prevent softening of the residual limb before prosthetic use.[17]

BATHING. Bathing is a self-care activity that requires dressing and undressing, transferring to and from shower chair or tub transfer bench, balancing, and managing body parts while operating the water controls (faucets). Adaptive devices such as the long-handled bath brush, flexible shower hose, and tub transfer bench are helpful for independence and safety.

DRESSING. Most patients with LE amputation are independent in UE dressing but require assistance for LE dressing. LE dressing is graded from performing in bed, to sitting, and then to standing. Socks and shoes should be donned while sitting. A sock aid and elastic shoelaces may ease donning for the person with loss of flexibility, poor dynamic sitting balance, or impaired vision. A footstool may also be used. Using the prosthesis effectively also involves being able to don it correctly and developing good balance and coordination for walking.

Patients with AKA can don the prosthesis in a standing position. The residual limb is pushed into the socket while the prosthesis is steadied against a firm object. The adductor longus tendon fits into the adductor longus tendon groove, and the ischial tuberosity rests on the ischial shelf. The patient must exert weight into the prosthesis while fastening the suspension apparatus to prevent hip internal rotation and a concomitant gait deviation.[2] If the patient has difficulty with sock wrinkling, the sock may be placed in the socket before the prosthesis is donned.

The patient with a BKA dons the prosthesis while sitting. Initially the leg is flexed at the knee. After the limb enters the socket, the knee is extended. To align the limb and socket properly, the patient stands and exerts weight on the prosthesis.

TRANSPORTATION. The ability to resume driving increases mobility and independence. State laws vary regarding driving after LE amputation. The occupational therapist should know the law before recommending that the individual resume driving. When appropriate, the patient should be referred to a driver safety specialist for a driving evaluation. However, the occupational therapist can perform a predriving assessment that includes visual acuity, reaction time, recognition of common traffic signs, color vision, glare recovery, night vision, peripheral vision, depth perception, and transferring to and from the car and wheelchair. Chapter 14, Section 3, provides a further discussion of this issue.

SEXUAL EXPRESSION. There is a lack of literature on sexuality of patients after LE amputation. In a brief interview with a middle-aged woman who lost the left LE as the result of poor circulation, the woman spoke of having to "cope" with her new body image and felt that her spouse would be unwilling to resume a sexual relationship because of her limb loss.

One study found a statistically significant decrease in frequency of sexual intercourse following amputation. The decrease was greater for males than for females. Men cited less interest as the reason for decreased frequency, and women reported fear of injury. None of the respondents cited uncomfortable position as a reason for the decline in frequency. Of the 60 respondents, only 15 discussed sexuality with a health care professional. The authors of the study concluded that there is a risk of sexual dysfunction after amputation and that sexual counseling should be included in the rehabilitation process.[24] The patient needs the reassurance and understanding of the entire rehabilitation team.

Work and Productive Activities

HOME MANAGEMENT. The person with a new amputation usually expresses no interest in performing instrumental activities of daily living (IADL). The occupational therapist can make it possible for the patient to observe other patients who are successfully performing IADL. Performance of such light household tasks as cleaning the tabletop and countertops, stripping the bed, preparing light meals, folding laundry, putting personal things in the closet, and reading recipes while sitting in the wheelchair or kitchen chair is good preparation for doing more complex and physically demanding daily activities later.

ENERGY CONSERVATION AND WORK SIMPLIFICATION. ADL can be performed while sitting or standing. The therapist should provide rest periods and teach graded energy-conserving techniques to increase the patient's productivity and safety. More energy is expended by persons with amputation during ADL than by other individuals of the same sex, age, and stature.[2] Energy expenditure increases with age and obesity.[14] Studies suggest a statistically significant correlation between residual limb length and energy demands.[2] Therefore patients with LE amputation benefit from instruction in work simplification and energy conservation techniques.

PREVOCATIONAL AND VOCATIONAL ACTIVITIES. The vocational evaluator should determine whether the client is able to return to the previous job. The vocational evaluation includes psychological testing, interests, achievement, and work history. The vocational evaluator establishes an initial vocational plan and may provide counseling. Assessing architectural barriers in the work environment, providing driver education and vehicle modification as needed, communicating with state vocational rehabilitation agencies, insurance companies, and other sponsors, and implementing job analysis and modifications are also roles of the vocational evaluator. Follow-up care is an important aspect of the vocational rehabilitation program.

Recreation and Leisure Activities

Recreation and the constructive use of leisure time enhance the quality of life. Many individuals may view mobility limitations as obstacles to returning to previous leisure activities. Thus the rehabilitation program should include using community recreational resources, learning new leisure skills, making adaptations for performance of previous leisure skills and interests, and refining functional abilities related to specific leisure activities. Community groups feature both discussion and reentry trips to develop the skills necessary to take an active role in community recreational opportunities. Special LE prostheses are available for golf, swimming, running, driving a car, and engaging in sports.[15]

Community Reintegration

Ultimately, the person with an LE amputation must gain independence in and accessibility to the community. Management of mobility for curbs, ramps, and inclines, stair climbing, walking on uneven surfaces, and getting on and off public transportation and elevators is essential. The individual should be encouraged to solve problems encountered with specific architectural and community barriers.

Discharge Planning

Discharge planning includes educating the family, providing home exercise programs, and securing necessary durable medical equipment (DME). A home visit may be completed as discharge is anticipated.

Family Education

During family education the occupational therapist demonstrates transfers and encourages the family to practice using recommended DME with the client. The therapist observes how the family and patient perform the activities and corrects any unsafe practices. Exercise programs are reviewed with the family in clear and understandable language, and written instructions are provided. DME and resources for equipment in the community are discussed. To ensure accessibility in and out of the home and tight spaces, a home visit is an essential part of the rehabilitation program before discharge.

PATIENTS WITH MULTIPLE DIAGNOSES AND AGING

In the geriatric population the LE amputation is often complicated by other medical problems such as hypertension, diabetes, congestive heart failure, coronary artery disease, osteoarthritis, cerebrovascular accident (stroke), cognitive deficits (e.g., dementia), and peripheral vascular disease.[10] All or even one of these additional medical problems can cause the geriatric patient additional problems in adjustment to the amputation, and reduce the potential for prosthetic wear and use.

SUMMARY

The rehabilitation of an individual who has had an LE amputation requires the skills of many health care specialists. OT evaluation and training in early rehabilita-

tion are focused on proper positioning to prevent contractures, on basic ADL training, and on improving ROM, strength, and endurance in the residual limb. UE strength and endurance training is also important for the performance of essential occupational performance tasks. In later stages of rehabilitation the occupational therapist can aid in the evaluation of the feasibility of future employment and explore appropriate leisure activities with the client.

Facilitating psychological adjustment is another important goal of all the clinical specialists who work with the client and the family. To help the client achieve the maximum possible independence and function, ongoing collaboration of the rehabilitation team is essential.

CASE STUDY 48-2

CASE STUDY—MR. B.

Mr. B. is a 49-year-old African-American man who sustained a left above-knee amputation as the result of a traumatic injury. He is married and has two small children living in the home. He works as a telephone line man, a job that requires climbing telephone poles. His leisure interests are fishing, camping, traveling with the family to visit parents in Georgia, watching television, gardening, and occasionally reading. Mr. B. lives in a single-family home with four steps up to the front entrance, but there is no railing. The interior of the home is wheelchair accessible.

Mr. B. seems to be accepting the loss of his left leg and is looking forward to returning to the community. He was referred to occupational therapy (OT) for evaluation and treatment. During the initial interview Mr. B. talked freely about the auto accident that caused his amputation. He also expressed doubts about returning to work with a prosthesis and concerns about the need to find new employment.

Results of the OT evaluation indicate that Mr. B. is pleasant, cooperative, and motivated for therapy. Before admission he was independent in activities of daily living. He has normal muscle strength in the upper extremities and the sound right leg. The patient is independent in grooming, hygiene, and dressing. He requires minimal assistance for transfers and can use hopping, with a standard walk-aid in tight spaces such as the bathroom. He is motivated to return to independent living and employment.

OT was initiated to increase activity tolerance and physical endurance, decrease pain and edema in the left residual limb, and improve mobility and transfers. The initial OT program included edema reduction techniques, desensitization techniques, therapeutic exercise for the upper extremities and residual limb, and wheelchair mobility training.

Mr. B. responded well to treatment. Pain was decreased and the edema was eliminated in the residual limb. He became independent in wheelchair mobility and chair-to-bed and chair-to-toilet transfers. He managed tub transfers using a tub bench and stand-by assistance. Upper extremity strength was maintained at normal and strength of the residual limb was increased from F+ to G. The patient was fitted for a prosthesis and referred to physical therapy for ambulation training.

CASE STUDY 48-2—cont'd

CASE STUDY—MR. B.—cont'd

Additional surgery because of venous insufficiency in the left lower extremity interrupted the ambulation training. The vascular problem was corrected, and prosthetic training was resumed with an ischial weight-bearing prosthesis. After healing of the left residual limb there was a final fitting of the prosthesis and plans were made for Mr. B. to return to physical therapy as an outpatient for more intense prosthesis training.

In OT, Mr. B. practiced activities of daily living and functional ambulation within his pain tolerance. He was also referred to vocational rehabilitation for retraining, since he will not be able to return to his former job.

REVIEW QUESTIONS

Section 1: General Considerations for Upper and Lower Extremity Amputations

1. List six causes of amputation.
2. What is the most common cause of LE amputation?
3. What is the second most common cause of LE amputation?
4. What are the primary goals of amputation surgery?
5. Name the two types of surgical procedures that can be performed, and list the advantages of each.
6. Name at least four postsurgical factors that can interfere with prosthetic training and rehabilitation. How is each solved?
7. Define neuroma. How does it affect the wearing of a prosthesis?
8. What is the difference between phantom limb and phantom pain?
9. What are some of the typical and expected psychosocial consequences of limb loss?
10. How can members of the rehabilitation team facilitate adjustment to amputation and prosthesis wear?

Section 2: Upper Extremity Amputations

1. Define the following abbreviations: AE, TD, and BE.
2. Which arm function is lost and which functions are maintained in a long BE amputation?
3. What is the purpose of the preprosthetic program?
4. Describe activities and exercises suitable for the preprosthetic period.
5. Before the TD on an AE prosthesis can be operated, what must the wearer do?
6. How does the prosthesis wearer preposition the TD?
7. Name two types of electric TDs.
8. How is functional training graded?
9. What is the source of power that activates the electric-powered prosthesis?
10. What are some advantages of the electric-powered prosthesis?

11. What is a hybrid prosthesis?
12. What does muscle site control training mean?
13. Describe the relative roles of a prosthesis and a sound arm and hand in the following activities: cutting meat; opening a jar; using scissors; buckling a belt; using an eggbeater; hammering a nail.

Section 3: Lower Extremity Amputations

1. Define AKA, BKA, PVD, and IWBP.
2. Which leg functions are lost after AKA?
3. Which leg functions are lost after a Symes amputation?
4. What are the function and purpose of the rigid dressing?
5. Name three types of prostheses.
6. Which prosthesis allows the AKA and BKA to be trained for transfers?
7. What is included in the initial OT evaluation?
8. Name three additional areas the occupational therapist addresses in the rehabilitation program of the patient with LE amputation.
9. How is residual limb supported in the wheelchair?
10. Identify all members of the rehabilitation team and their roles.
11. Describe a method to decrease edema.
12. What type of wheelchair is needed when there are bilateral LE amputations?
13. Which adaptive devices are helpful for ADL?
14. Which pieces of durable medical equipment are often recommended by the occupational therapist at the time of discharge?
15. Why is family education an important part of the rehabilitation program?
16. List the immediate postoperative concerns. How does OT address these concerns?
17. Which areas are assessed in bed mobility?
18. Which prosthesis is used as a training prosthesis?

REFERENCES

SECTION 1

1. Atkins DJ: Postoperative and preprosthetic therapy programs. In Atkins DJ, Meier RH, editors: *Comprehensive management of the upper-limb amputee*, New York, 1989, Springer-Verlag.
2. Banerjee SJ: *Rehabilitation management of amputees*, Baltimore, 1982, Williams & Wilkins.
3. Bennett JB, Alexander CB: Amputation levels and surgical techniques. In Atkins DJ, Meier RH, editors: *Comprehensive management of the upper-limb amputee*, New York, 1989, Springer-Verlag.
4. Bennett JB, Gartsman GM: Surgical options for brachial plexus and stroke patients. In Atkins DJ, Meier RH, editors: *Comprehensive management of the upper-limb amputee*, New York, 1989, Springer-Verlag.
5. Evans WE, Hayes JP, Vermillion BO: Effect of a failed distal reconstruction on the level of amputation, *Am J Surg* 160(2):217-220, 1990.
6. Friedman LW: *The psychological rehabilitation of the amputee*, Springfield, Ill, 1978, Charles C Thomas.

7. Friedman LW: Rehabilitation of the amputee. In Goodgold J, editor: *Rehabilitation medicine*, St Louis, 1988, Mosby.

8. Glattly HW: A statistical study of 12,000 new amputees, *South Med J* 57:1373-1378, 1964.

9. Harris KA, Van Schie L, Carroll SE, et al: Rehabilitation potential of elderly patients with major amputations, *J Cardiovasc Surg (Torino)* 32(5):648-651, 1991.

10. Hill SL: Interventions for the elderly amputee, *Rehabil Nurs* 10(3):23-25, 1985.

11. Hirschberg G, Lewis L, Thomas D: *Rehabilitation*, Philadelphia, 1964, JB Lippincott.

12. Kay HW, Newman JD: Relative incidence of new amputations: statistical comparisons of 6,000 new amputees, *Orthot Prosthet* 59:109, 1978.

13. Knighton DR, Fylling CP, Fiegel VD, et al: Amputation prevention in an independently reviewed at risk diabetic population using a comprehensive wound care protocol, *Am J Surg* 160(5):466-471, 1990.

14. Krajewski LP, Olin JW: Atherosclerosis of the aorta and lower extremities arteries. In Young JR, Graor RA, Olin JW, et al, editors: *Peripheral vascular diseases*, St Louis, 1991, Mosby.

15. Lane JM, Kroll MA, Rossbach P: New advances and concepts in amputee management after treatment for bone and soft tissue sarcomas, *Clin Orthop* Jul(256):280-285, 1990.

16. Larson CB, Gould M: *Orthopedic nursing*, ed 8, St Louis, 1974, Mosby.

17. Leonard JA, Meier RH: Prosthetics. In DeLisa JA, editor: *Rehabilitation medicine principles and practice*, Philadelphia, 1988, JB Lippincott.

18. Levy LA: Smoking and peripheral vascular disease, *Clin Podiatr Med Surg* 9(1):165-171, 1992.

19. Lind J, Kramhhaft M, Badtker S: The influence of smoking on complications after primary amputations of the lower extremity, *Clin Orthop* 267:211, 1992.

20. Link MP, Goorin AM, Horowitz M, et al: Adjuvant chemotherapy of high grade osteosarcoma of the extremity, *Clin Orthop* 270:8, 1991.

21. Malone JM, Goldstone J: Lower extremity amputation. In Moore WS, editor: *Vascular surgery: a comprehensive review*, New York, 1984, Grune & Stratton.

22. McIntyre KE Jr: The diabetic foot and management of infectious gangrene. In Moore WS, Malone JHM, editors: *Lower extremity amputation*, Philadelphia, 1989, WB Saunders.

23. Meier RH, Atkins DJ: Preface. In Atkins DJ, Meier RH, editors: *Comprehensive management of the upper-limb amputee*, New York, 1989, Springer-Verlag.

24. Michaels JA: The selection of amputation level: an approach using decision analysis, *Eur J Vasc Surg* 5(4):451-457, 1991.

25. Moss SE, Klein R, Klein BE: The prevalence and incidence of lower extremity amputation in a diabetic population, *Arch Intern Med* 152(3):610-616, 1992.

26. Novotny MP: Psychosocial issues, affecting rehabilitation, *Phys Med Rehabil Clin North Am* 2:273, 1991.

27. O'Sullivan S, Cullen K, Schmitz T: *Physical rehabilitation: evaluation and treatment procedures*, Philadelphia, 1981, FA Davis.

28. Raney R, Brashear H: *Shands' handbook of orthopaedic surgery*, ed 8, St Louis, 1971, Mosby.

29. Ritz G, Friedman S, Osbourne A: Diabetes and peripheral vascular disease, *Clin Podiatr Med Surg* 9(1):125-137, 1992.

30. Simon M: Limb salvage for osteosarcoma in the 1980s, *Clin Orthop* 270:264, 1990.

31. Spencer EA: Amputations. In Hopkins HL, Smith HD, editors: *Willard & Spackman's occupational therapy*, ed 5, Philadelphia, 1978, JB Lippincott.

32. Spencer EA: Functional restoration. 3 Amputation and prosthetic replacement. In Hopkins HL, Smith HD, editors: *Willard & Spackman's occupational therapy*, ed 8, Philadelphia, 1993, JB Lippincott.

33. Spencer EA: Musculoskeletal dysfunction in adults. In Neistadt ME, Crepeau EB, editors: *Willard & Spackman's occupational therapy*, ed 9, Philadelphia, 1998, JB Lippincott.

34. Springfield DS: Introduction to limb-salvage surgery for sarcoma, *Orthop Clin North Am* 22(1):1-5, 1991.

35. Taylor LM, Jamre D, Dalman RL, et al: Limb salvage versus amputation for critical ischemia, *Arch Surg* 126(10):1251-1257, 1991.

36. Tsang GM, Crowson MC, Hickey NC, et al: Failed femorocrural reconstruction does not prejudice amputation level, *Br J Surg* 78(12):1479-1481, 1991.

37. Walsh NE, Dumitru D, Ramamurthy S, et al: Treatment of the patient with chronic pain. In DeLisa JA, editor: *Rehabilitation medicine principles and practice*, Philadelphia, 1988, JB Lippincott.

38. Wellerson TL: *A manual for occupational therapists on the rehabilitation of upper extremity amputees*, Dubuque, Iowa, 1958, William C Brown.

39. Yaw KM, Wurtz LD: Resection and reconstruction for bone tumor in proximal tibia, *Orthop Clin North Am* 22(1):133-148, 1991.

SECTION 2 (I)

1. Anderson MH, Bechtol CO, Sollars RE: *Clinical prosthetics for physicians and therapists*, Springfield, Ill, 1959, Charles C Thomas.

2. Andrew JT: Prosthetic principles. In Bowker JH, Michael JW, editors: *Atlas of limb prosthetics: surgical, prosthetic, and rehabilitation principles*, ed 2, St Louis, 1992, Mosby.

3. Atkins DJ: Adult upper limb prosthetic training. In Atkins DJ, Meier RH, editors: *Comprehensive management of the upper-limb amputee*, New York, 1989, Springer-Verlag.

4. Atkins DJ: Postoperative and preprosthetic therapy programs. In Atkins DJ, Meier RH, editors: *Comprehensive management of the upper-limb amputee*, New York, 1989, Springer-Verlag.

5. Billock JN: Prosthetic management of complete hand and arm deficiencies. In Hunter JM, Mackin EJ, Callahan AD, editors: *Rehabilitation of the hand: surgery and therapy*, ed 4, St Louis, 1995, Mosby.

6. Fryer CM, Michael JW: Body-powered components. In Bowker JH, Michael JW, editors: *Atlas of limb prosthetics: surgical, prosthetic, and rehabilitation principles*, ed 2, St Louis, 1992, Mosby.

7. Hirschberg G, Lewis L, Thomas D: *Rehabilitation*, Philadelphia, 1964, JB Lippincott.

8. Leonard JA, Meier RH: Prosthetics. In DeLisa JA, editor: *Rehabilitation medicine principles and practice*, Philadelphia, 1988, JB Lippincott.

9. Muilenburg AL, LeBlanc MA: Body-powered upper-limb components. In Atkins DJ, Meier RH, editors: *Comprehensive management of the upper-limb amputee*, New York, 1989, Springer-Verlag.

10. Olivett BL: Management and prosthetic training of the adult amputee. In Hunter JM et al, editors: *Rehabilitation of the hand*, St Louis, 1984, Mosby.

11. Santschi WR, editor: *Manual of upper extremity prosthetics*, ed 2, Los Angeles, 1958, University of California Press.

12. Spencer EA: Amputation and prosthetic replacement. In Hopkins HL, Smith HD, editors: *Willard & Spackman's occupational therapy*, ed 8, Philadelphia, 1993, JB Lippincott.

13. Wellerson TL: *A manual for occupational therapists on the rehabilitation of upper extremity amputees*, Dubuque, Iowa, 1958, William C Brown.

14. Wright G: *Controls training for the upper extremity amputee* (film), San Jose, Calif, Instructional Resources Center, San Jose State University.

SECTION 2 (II)

1. Andrew JT: Prosthetic principles. In Bowker JH, Michael JW, editors: *Atlas of limb prosthetics: surgical, prosthetic and rehabilitation principles*, ed 2, St Louis, 1992, Mosby.

2. Atkins DJ: Adult myoelectric upper-limb prosthetic training. In Atkins DJ, Meier RH, editors: *Comprehensive management of the upper limb amputee*, New York, 1989, Springer-Verlag.

3. Atkins DJ: Postoperative and preprosthetic therapy programs. In Atkins DJ, Meier RH, editors: *Comprehensive management of the upper limb amputee*, New York, 1989, Springer-Verlag.

4. Billock JN: Prosthetic management of complete hand and arm deficiencies. In Hunter JM, Mackin EJ, Callahan AD, editors: *Rehabilitation of the hand: surgery and therapy*, ed 4, St Louis, 1995, Mosby.

5. Dalsey R et al: Myoelectric prosthetic replacement in the upper extremity amputee, *Orthop Rev* 18(6):697-702, 1989.

6. Jacobsen SC et al: Development of the Utah Artificial Arm, *IEEE Trans Biomed Eng* 29(4):249-269, 1982.

7. Meier RH: Amputations and prosthetic fitting. In Fisher S, editor: *Comprehensive rehabilitation of burns*, Baltimore, 1984, Williams & Wilkins.

8. Nader M, Ing EH: The artificial substitution of missing hands with myoelectric prostheses, *Clin Orthop* 258:9-17, 1990.

9. NovaCare: *Motion control: training the client with an electric arm prosthesis*, King of Prussia, Pa, 1997, NovaCare (videotape).

10. Scott RN, Parker PA: Myoelectric prostheses: state of the art, *J Med Eng Technol* 12(4):143-151, 1988.

11. Spiegal SR: Adult myoelectric upper-limb prosthetic training. In Atkins DJ, Meier RH, editors: *Comprehensive management of the upper-limb amputee*, New York, 1989, Springer-Verlag.

SECTION 3

1. American Occupational Therapy Association: Uniform terminology for occupational therapy, ed 3, *Am J Occup Ther* 48(11):1047-1054, 1994.

2. Banerjee SJ: *Rehabilitation management of amputees*, Baltimore, 1982, Williams & Wilkins.

3. Borcich D, Beukma L, Olives T: *Amputee care: a handout for patients with below knee amputations*, Stanford, Calif, 1986, Department of Physical and Occupational Therapy, Stanford University Hospital (Unpublished).

4. Burgess EM: Amputation of the lower extremities. In Nickel VL, editor: *Orthopedic rehabilitation*, New York, 1982, Churchill-Livingstone.

5. Engstrand JL: Rehabilitation of the patient with a lower extremity amputation, *Nurs Clin North Am* 11(4):659-669, 1976.

6. Everest and Jennings: *Wheelchair catalog*, Camarillo, Calif, 1980.

7. Friedman LW: *The psychological rehabilitation of the amputee*, Springfield, Ill, 1978, Charles C Thomas.

8. Friedman LW: Rehabilitation of the amputee. In Goodgold J, editor: *Rehabilitation medicine*, St Louis, 1988, Mosby.

9. Harrington IJ, Lexier R, Woods J, et al: A plastic pylon technique for below knee amputation, *J Bone Joint Surg Br* 73(1):7676-78, 1991.

10. Harris KA, Van Schie L, Carroll SE, et al: Rehabilitation potential of elderly patients with major amputations, *J Cardiovasc Surg (Torino)* 32(4):463-467, 1991.

11. Hirschberg G, Lewis L, Thomas D: *Rehabilitation*, Philadelphia, 1964, JB Lippincott.

12. Invacare: *Wheelchair catalog*, Elyria, Ohio, 1993.

13. Jensen TS, Krebs B, Nielsen J, et al: Immediate and long-term phantom limb pain in amputees: incidence, clinical characteristics and relationship to pre-amputation limb pain, *Pain* 21(3):267-278, 1985.

14. Kathrins RJ: Lower extremity amputations. In Logigian MK, editor: *Adult rehabilitation: a team approach for therapists*, Boston, 1982, Little Brown.

15. Kegel B, Webster J, Burgess EM: Recreational activities of lower extremity amputees: a survey, *Arch Phys Med Rehabil* 61(6):258-264, 1980.

16. Knighton DR, Fylling CP, Fiegel VD, et al: Amputation prevention in an independently reviewed at risk diabetic population using a comprehensive wound care protocol, *Am J Surg* 160(5):466-471, 1990.

17. Larson CB, Gould M: *Orthopedic nursing*, ed 8, St Louis, 1974, Mosby.

18. May BJ: A statewide amputee rehabilitation programme, *Prosthet Orthot Int* 2(1):24-26, 1978.

19. Metro Medical Seating Systems: *Wheelchair catalog*, Livonia, Mich, 1993.

20. O'Sullivan S, Cullen K, Schmitz T: *Physical rehabilitation: evaluation and treatment procedures*, Philadelphia, 1981, FA Davis.

21. Palmer MI, Toms JE: *Manual for functional training*, ed 3, Philadelphia, 1992, FA Davis.

22. Raney RR, Brashear H: *Shands' handbook of orthopaedic surgery*, ed 8, St Louis, 1971, Mosby.

23. Reed KL, Sanderson SN: *Concepts of occupational therapy*, ed 3, Baltimore, 1972, Williams & Wilkins.

24. Reinstein L, Ashley J, Miller KH: Sexual adjustment after lower extremity amputation, *Arch Phys Med Rehabil* 59(11):501-504, November, 1978.

25. Rusk H, Taylor E: *Rehabilitation medicine: a textbook of physical medicine and rehabilitation*, ed 2, St Louis, 1964, Mosby.

26. Spencer EA: Amputations. In Hopkins HL, Smith HD, editors: *Willard & Spackman's occupational therapy*, ed 5, Philadelphia, 1978, JB Lippincott.

27. Stoner EK: Management of the lower extremity amputee. In Kottke FJ, Stillwell GK, Lehmann JF, editors: *Krusen's handbook of physical medicine and rehabilitation*, ed 3, Philadelphia, 1982, WB Saunders.

28. Telikicherla M: *Immediate postoperative prosthesis for lower extremity amputation*. Detroit, 1993, Rehabilitation Institute of Michigan.

CHAPTER 49

Cardiac and Pulmonary Diseases

MAUREEN MICHELE MATTHEWS

KEY TERMS

Heart rate
Blood pressure
Ischemic heart disease
Myocardial infarction
Cardiac risk factors
Cardiac rehabilitation
Signs and symptoms of cardiopulmonary distress
Rate of perceived exertion
Rate pressure product
Chronic obstructive pulmonary disease
Package year history
Signs and symptoms of respiratory distress
Pulmonary rehabilitation
Dyspnea control postures
Pursed-lip breathing
Diaphragmatic breathing
Cardiovascular response to activity
Basal metabolic equivalent
Energy conservation

LEARNING OBJECTIVES

Study of this chapter will allow the student or practitioner to do the following:
1. Briefly describe the cardiovascular system and its function.
2. Identify the significance of ischemic heart disease and valvular diseases of the heart.
3. Differentiate between modifiable and nonmodifiable risk factors.
4. Identify signs and symptoms of cardiac distress.
5. Describe the course of action one should take if signs and symptoms of cardiac distress are present.
6. List the psychosocial considerations for persons with cardiovascular or pulmonary disease.
7. Describe methods for taking heart rate and blood pressure.
8. Determine rate pressure product, given heart rate and blood pressure.
9. Give a brief overview of the respiratory system and identify its primary function.
10. Define chronic obstructive pulmonary disease (COPD).
11. Identify pulmonary risk factors and psychosocial considerations.
12. Describe dyspnea control postures, pursed-lip breathing, and diaphragmatic breathing.
13. Describe a relaxation technique and explain its purpose.
14. List interview questions that will help the clinician know what the patient understands about treatment.
15. List the principles of energy conservation.
16. Explain the significance of an MET chart in the progression of activity, and describe how to use it.

Individuals with disorders of the cardiovascular or pulmonary system may be severely limited in endurance and performance of activities of daily living (ADL). Occupational therapy (OT) services may benefit such individuals and are available throughout the continuum of health care. An understanding of the normal function of the cardiopulmonary system, the pathology of cardiopulmonary disease, common risk factors, clinical terminology, medical interventions, precautions, and standard treatment techniques will guide the occupational therapist in providing effective care and promoting recovery of function in persons with compromised cardiovascular or pulmonary systems.

Every living cell of the body has three major requirements for life: (1) a constant supply of nutrients and oxygen, (2) continual removal of carbon dioxide and other waste products, and (3) a relatively constant temperature. The cardiovascular and pulmonary systems play key roles in meeting these requirements.

CARDIOVASCULAR SYSTEM[3,13,19]
Anatomy and Circulation

The heart and blood vessels work together to maintain a constant flow of blood throughout the body. The heart, located between the lungs, is pear shaped and about the size of a fist. It functions as a two-sided pump. The right side pumps blood from the body to the lungs; simultaneously the left side pumps blood from the lungs to the body. Each side of the heart has two chambers, an upper atrium and a lower ventricle.

Blood flows to the heart from the venous system. The blood enters the right atrium, which contracts and squeezes the blood into the right ventricle. Next, the right ventricle contracts and ejects the blood into the lungs, where carbon dioxide is exchanged for oxygen. Oxygen-rich blood flows from the lungs to the left atrium. As the left atrium contracts, it forces blood into the left ventricle, which then contracts and ejects its contents into the aorta for systemic circulation (Fig. 49-1). Blood travels from the aorta to the arteries and through progressively smaller blood vessels to networks of very tiny capillaries. In the capillaries, blood cells exchange their oxygen for carbon dioxide.

Each of the ventricles has two valves, an input valve and an output valve. The valves open and close as the heart muscle (myocardium) contracts and relaxes. These valves control the direction and flow of blood. The input valves are the mitral and tricuspid, and the output valves are the aortic and pulmonary.

The heart is living tissue and requires a blood supply (through an arterial and venous system of its own), or it will die. Coronary arteries cross over the myocardium to supply it with oxygen-rich blood. The coronary arteries

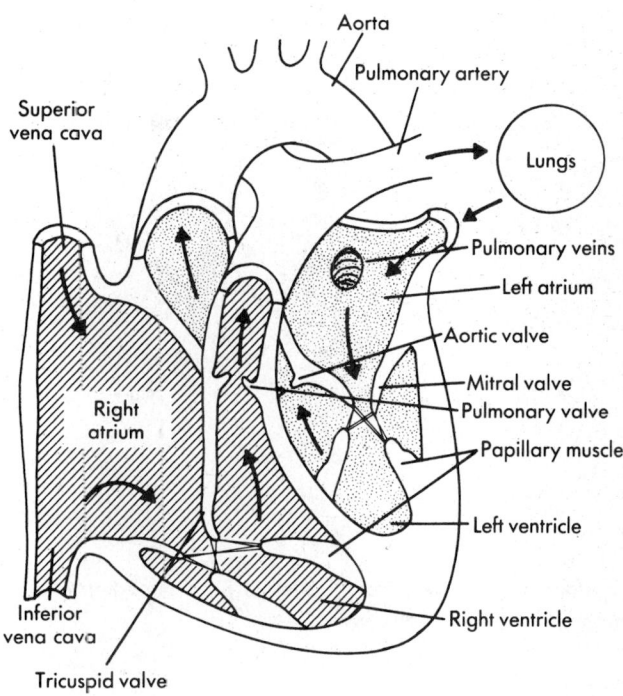

FIG. 49-1
Anatomy of the heart. (Modified from Guyton AC: *Textbook of medical physiology*, ed 8, 1991, WB Saunders.)

are named for their location on the myocardium (Fig. 49-2). Cardiologists generally refer to these arteries by abbreviations, such as "LAD" for "left anterior descending" and "RCA" for "right coronary artery." The LAD is on the left, anterior portion of the heart and runs in a downward direction, supplying part of the left ventricle. A blockage of this coronary artery will interrupt the blood supply to the left ventricle. Because the left ventricle supplies the body and brain with blood, a heart attack caused by LAD blockage can have serious consequences.

What Causes the Heart to Contract?

In addition to the ordinary muscle tissue of the heart, the myocardium is composed of two other types of tissue, *nodal* and *Purkinje*. These tissues are part of a specialized electrical conduction system that causes the heart to contract and relax (Fig. 49-2). An electrical impulse usually originates in the right atrium at a site called the *sinoatrial* (SA) *node*. The impulse travels along internodal pathways to the atrioventricular (AV) node, through the bundle of His, to the left and right bundle branches, and then to the Purkinje fibers. Nerve impulses normally travel this pathway 60 to 100 times every minute, first causing both atria to contract, pushing blood into the ventricles, and then provoking the ventricles to contract. The electrical impulse created by the heart's conduction system can easily be studied.

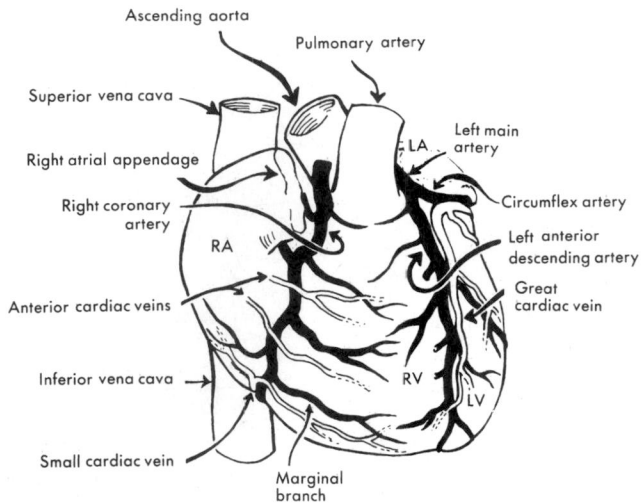

FIG. 49-2
Coronary circulation. (From Underhill SL et al, editors: *Cardiac nursing*, Philadelphia, 1982, JB Lippincott.)

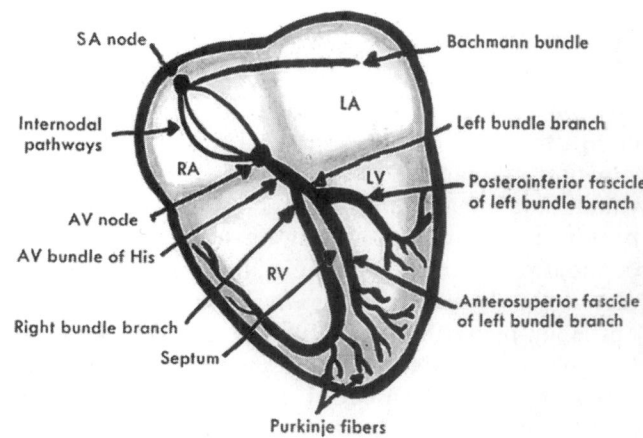

FIG. 49-3
Cardiac conduction. (Modified from Andreoli KG et al: *Comprehensive cardiac care: a text for nurses, physicians, and other health practitioners*, St Louis, 1983, Mosby.)

Electrodes placed on a person's limbs and chest can pick up the heart's electrical impulse, which can be translated to paper via an electrocardiogram (EKG). The resulting EKG tracing is frequently used to help diagnose cardiac disease.

The SA node responds to vagal and sympathetic nervous system input.[3] This is why **heart rate** (HR) increases in response to exercise and anxiety and decreases in response to relaxation techniques, such as deep breathing and meditation. Each cell within the electrical conduction system of the heart can respond to, conduct, resist for a brief period, and generate an electrical impulse. Because of this, electrical impulses causing the heart muscle to contract can be generated from anywhere along the electrical conduction system. This is desirable when part of the conduction system has been damaged and is unable do its job, but it is undesirable when life-threatening conduction irregularities develop.

Cardiac Cycle

The amount of blood ejected by the heart each minute (cardiac output) is controlled by both HR and the **blood pressure** (BP). The cardiac cycle occurs in two phases, input (diastole) and output (systole).

During the input phase, blood flows through the atria and into the ventricles. The atria contract, pushing more blood into the ventricles. Once the pressure inside the ventricles is equal to the pressure in the atria, the input valves (tricuspid in the right ventricle and mitral in the left ventricle) close. The ventricles then contract, resulting in rapidly increasing ventricular pressure. When the pressure inside the ventricles exceeds the pressure in the blood vessels beyond, the output valves (pul-

monary in the right and aortic in the left) open and the diastolic BP is attained.

The ventricles continue to contract, squeezing blood under greater and greater pressure into the pulmonary and body circulation. Systolic BP is attained when pressures in the emptying ventricles fall below pressure in the blood vessels beyond, causing the output valves to close.

PATHOLOGY OF CARDIAC DISEASE
Ischemic Heart Disease

Ischemic heart disease (ischemia) occurs when a part of the body is temporarily deprived of sufficient oxygen to meet its demand. The most common cause of cardiac ischemia is coronary artery disease (CAD). CAD usually develops over a period of many years without causing symptoms. The internal wall of an artery can become injured by years of cigarette smoking or high BP. Once the wall is damaged, it becomes irregular in shape and more prone to collect plaque (fatty deposits like cholesterol). Platelets also gather along the arterial wall and clog the artery, creating a lesion in the same manner in which rust can clog a pipe. The artery gradually narrows, allowing a smaller volume of blood to pass through it. This disease process is called *atherosclerosis*.

If a coronary artery is partially or completely blocked, the part of the heart supplied by that artery may not receive sufficient oxygen to meet its needs. Persons with partial blockage of a coronary artery may be free of symptoms at rest but have angina, a type of chest pain, with eating, exercise, exertion, or exposure to cold. Angina varies from individual to individual and has been described as squeezing, tightness, fullness, pressure, or a sharp pain in the chest. The pain may also radiate to other parts of the body, usually the arm, back, neck, or jaw. Angina has also been confused with indigestion. Rest, medication, or both will frequently relieve angina. Usually no permanent heart damage will result. Angina is a warning sign that should not be ignored. Coronary artery disease is present; the individual may be a candidate for a heart attack. Chest pain that is not relieved by rest or nitroglycerin is indicative of a **myocardial infarction** (MI), or heart attack. The patient who has this type of pain should be evaluated promptly by a physician.

A myocardial infarction is significant because part of the heart muscle dies as a result of lack of oxygen. If a substantial section of the heart is damaged, it will stop pumping (cardiac arrest). Activity restrictions are prescribed for the first 6 weeks after a heart attack, because newly damaged heart muscle, like any injured body tissue, is easily reinjured. During the heart attack, metabolic waste products accumulate in the damaged myocardium, making it irritable and prone to electrical irregularities such as premature ventricular contractions (PVCs). A delicate balance of rest and activity must be maintained to allow the damaged area of myocardium to heal while also maintaining the strength of the healthy part of the heart. To guide the patient toward a safe level of activity during this acute period of recovery, OT may be recommended.

At about 6 weeks after an MI, scar tissue forms and the risk of extending the MI decreases. The scarred part of the heart muscle is not elastic and does not contract with each heartbeat. Therefore the heart does not pump as well. A graded exercise program will help strengthen the healthy part of the myocardium and improve cardiac output, the amount of blood ejected by the heart in 1 minute.

Congestive heart failure (CHF) occurs when the heart is unable to pump effectively, causing fluid to back up into the lungs or the body. Fluid overload is serious because it puts a greater workload on the heart as the heart strains while attempting to clear the excess fluid. This may result in further congestion. Heart size is often enlarged in persons with CHF because the heart muscle thickens (hypertrophy) from working so hard. Diuretics can be prescribed for persons with CHF to promote fluid loss through the urinary system. Low-sodium diets and fluid restrictions reduce the overall amount of fluid in the body. Usually CHF can be controlled with diet, medications, and rest.

Once an acute exacerbation of CHF is controlled, a gradual resumption of activity will promote improved function. If activity is resumed too quickly, another acute episode may follow. Patients who have difficulty resuming their former level of activity may self-limit their recovery. OT can guide persons with acute CHF toward an optimal level of function through graded self-care tasks. Some individuals ultimately eliminate their tendency to develop CHF altogether, whereas others develop severe heart failure.

TABLE 49-1 Functional Classification of Cardiac Disease	
Class 1	Patients have cardiac disease but no limitation of physical activity.
Class 2	Patients have cardiac disease resulting in slight limitation of physical activity. Patients are comfortable at rest. Ordinary physical activity results in fatigue, palpitation, dyspnea, or anginal pain.
Class 3	Patients have cardiac disease resulting in marked limitation of physical activity. Patients are comfortable at rest. Less than ordinary physical activity causes fatigue, palpitation, dyspnea, or anginal pain.
Class 4	Patients have cardiac disease resulting in inability to carry on any physical activity without discomfort. Symptoms of cardiac insufficiency or of the anginal syndrome may be present even at rest. If any physical activity is undertaken, discomfort is increased.

From New York Heart Association: *Nomenclature and criteria for diagnosis of diseases of the heart and great vessels,* ed 8, Boston, 1979, The Association.

Table 49-1 delineates the four functional classifications of heart disease. OT can be of great benefit to persons with stage 3 and 4 disease.

Valvular Disease

The heart valves, which are responsible for controlling the direction and flow of the blood through the heart, may become damaged through disease or infection. Two complications result from valvular disease: volume overload and pressure overload. A fibrous mitral valve will fail to close properly. Blood will be regurgitated back to the atria when the left ventricle contracts. Volume overload results when fluid accumulates in the lungs, causing shortness of breath. Volume overload increases the potential for atrial fibrillation, which causes irregular and ineffective contractions in both atria. Blood flow through the heart slows, and blood clots (emboli) may develop in the ventricles. Many cerebrovascular accidents are caused when emboli ejected from the left ventricle enter the circulatory system of the brain.

If the aortic valve fails to close properly (aortic insufficiency), CHF or ischemia may result. Another disorder of the aortic valve is aortic stenosis (narrowing), which results in pressure overload. The left ventricle, which must work harder to open the sticky valve, becomes enlarged, and cardiac output decreases. Ventricular arrhythmia, cerebral insufficiency, confusion, syncope (fainting), and even sudden death may result from aortic stenosis. Surgery to repair or replace the damaged valves is frequently recommended.

Cardiac Risk Factors

There have been many scientific studies to determine the causes of heart disease. The most famous of these studies, the Framingham study,[8] helped identify many factors that put an individual at risk for atherosclerosis. Risk factors are divided into three major categories: those that cannot be changed (heredity, male gender, and age); those that can be changed (high blood pressure, cigarette smoking, cholesterol levels, and an inactive lifestyle); and contributing factors (diabetes, stress, and obesity). The more risk factors an individual has, the greater is the individual's risk of CAD. All team members should support the patient's attempts to reduce risk factors.

Medical Management

Persons who have a heart attack are initially managed in a coronary care unit, where they are closely observed for complications. Ninety percent of persons who have had an MI will have arrhythmia.[5] Heart failure, the development of blood clots (thrombosis and emboli), aneurysms, ruptures of part of the heart muscle, inflammation of the sac around the heart (pericarditis), and even death are potential outcomes of an MI. Close medical management is imperative.

Generally patients are managed for 2 to 3 days after MI in an intensive care unit. Once their condition is stabilized, they graduate to a monitored hospital bed. Patients stay 4 to 6 days in the hospital after an acute MI. Vital signs are closely monitored while activity is gradually increased. OT personnel may be called on to monitor the patient's response to activity and educate the patient about the disease process, risk factors, and lifestyle modification.

Should the patient not respond well to increased activity, surgical intervention may be necessary. Various surgical procedures can correct circulatory problems associated with CAD. Balloon angioplasty, also called percutaneous transluminal coronary angioplasty (PTCA), and coronary artery bypass graft (CABG) are most common.

In a PTCA a catheter is inserted into the femoral artery and guided through the circulatory system into the coronary arteries. Radioactive dye is ejected into the arteries, and the site of the lesion is pinpointed. A balloon is then inflated at the site of the lesion to push plaque against the arterial wall. When the balloon is deflated and the catheter removed, improved circulation to the myocardium usually results. Eight hours of bed rest after the PTCA helps prevent hemorrhaging from the femoral artery.

If a lesion is too diffuse or an artery reoccludes after a PTCA, a CABG may be performed. The diseased section of the coronary arteries is bypassed with healthy blood vessels (taken from other parts of the body), thus im-

proving coronary circulation. Strict compliance with postsurgical precautions is necessary to avert serious consequences.

When the heart's pumping ability has become too compromised by CHF or cardiomyopathy, a heart transplant or heart-lung transplant may be considered. Healthy tissue of a recently deceased person is harvested; the diseased organ(s) of the patient are removed, and the harvested tissue is transplanted into the patient's body. Transplant patients are typically maintained on special medication to decrease the risk of organ rejection. If the surgery is successful, the patient can generally be rehabilitated to a level of function significantly higher than in the months before surgery.

Cardiac Medications

Knowledge of the purpose and side effects of cardiac medication promotes understanding of the patient's response to activity. Table 49-2 lists common cardiac medications.

Psychosocial Considerations

Persons who have had an MI pass through a number of phases of adjustment to disability. Fear and anxiety develop initially as patients confront their mortality. Sedatives may be prescribed to reduce stress and allow rest so that the cardiovascular system can begin to heal. Once stabilized, patients must confront the reality of their physical limitations. Education and supportive communication will do much to reduce anxiety.[12]

As patients begin to resume more normal activities, such as self-care and walking around the ward, feelings of helplessness may begin to subside. Patients feel more secure when familiar coping mechanisms allow them to respond to the stress, but some former coping mechanisms (e.g., smoking, drinking, or consuming fatty foods) are harmful and should be discouraged.

Denial is common among patients with cardiac disease. Patients in denial must be closely monitored during the acute phase of recovery. Persons in denial may ignore all precautions and could stress and further damage their cardiovascular systems.

Depression is common in the third to sixth day after an MI and may last many months.[4] Forced inactivity during the recovery phase can compromise coping for a person who has previously dealt with stress by exercising until exhaustion. The patient's family must be included in the education so that their misconceptions and anxieties do not compound the patient's fears.

Cardiac Rehabilitation

During the first 1 to 3 days after an MI, stabilization of the cardiac patient's medical condition is usually attained. This acute phase is followed by a period of early mobilization. Phase one of treatment, inpatient cardiac rehabilitation, includes monitored low-level physical

TABLE 49-2
Common Cardiac Medications

Category	Common Names	Purpose and Uses	Side Effects
Diuretics	Lasix (Furosemide) Dyazide HCTZ	Lowers BP Decreases edema	Orthostatic HTN Dehydration Muscle spasms
Vasodilators	Hydralazine Captopril	Lowers BP Controls CHF	Palpitations Tachycardia Orthostatic HTN
Cardiac glycosides	Digoxin Lanoxin	Lowers heart rate Controls ventricular heart rate	Anorexia Nausea Arrhythmia Heart block
Anticoagulants	Coumadin (Warfarin) Heparin Aspirin Persantine	Prevents blood clots	Hemorrhage Nausea and vomiting Abdominal cramps
Antiarrhythmic	Procainamide Quinidine Inderal Lidocaine	Controls heart rhythm	Can aggravate ventricular arrhythmias Bradycardia
Beta blockers	Atenolol (Tenormin) Propranolol (Inderal) Other drugs ending in "olol"	To manage angina, hypertension, and arrhythmia	CHF Worsening of peripheral vascular disease Increased dyspnea
Calcium channel blockers	Verapamil Diltiazem Nifedipine	To manage angina, coronary artery spasms, and arrhythmia	Orthostatic HTN Bradycardia
Nitrates	NTG sublingual Nitropaste Isordil	To manage angina and CHF	Orthostatic HTN Headache

BP, Blood pressure; *CHF,* congestive heart failure; *HCTZ,* hydrochlorothiazide; *NTG,* nitroglycerin; *HTN,* hypotension.

activity, including self-care; reinforcement of cardiac and postsurgical precautions; instruction in energy conservation and graded activity; and establishment of guidelines for appropriate activity levels at discharge. Via monitored activity, the ill effects of prolonged inactivity can be averted, while medical problems, poor responses to medications, and atypical chest pain can be addressed.

Phase two of treatment, outpatient cardiac rehabilitation, usually begins at discharge. During this phase exercise can be advanced while the patient is closely monitored on an outpatient basis. Community-based exercise programs follow in phase three. Some individuals require treatment in their place of residence because they are not strong enough to tolerate outpatient therapy.

Health care costs can be significantly reduced and positive health effects can result from comprehensive cardiac rehabilitation.[17] Additional research indicates reduced mortality among selected patients who have

had cardiac rehabilitation after an acute MI.[22] Cardiac rehabilitation has also been found to benefit patients with left ventricular dysfunction by improving physical work capacity.[14]

Early and accurate identification of the **signs and symptoms of cardiac distress** and modification of treatment to remedy distress are imperative to the well-being of the patient. If the clinician observes any of the signs of cardiac distress (Table 49-3) during treatment, the proper response is to stop the activity, allow the patient to rest, seek emergency medical help if the symptoms do not resolve, report the symptoms to the team, and modify future activity to decrease the workload on the heart.

Table 49-4, the Borg Rate of Perceived Exertion Scale, is a tool used to measure the perceived exertion. The patient is shown the scale before an activity and instructed that a rating of "6" means no exertion at all and a "19" indicates extremely strenuous activity, equal to the most strenuous activity the patient has ever

TABLE 49-3
Signs and Symptoms of Cardiac Distress

Sign/Symptom	What to Look For
Angina	Look for chest pain that may be squeezing, tightness, aching, burning, or choking in nature. Pain is generally substernal and may radiate to the arms, jaw, neck, or back. More intense or longer-lasting pain forewarns of greater ischemia.
Dyspnea	Look for shortness of breath with activity or at rest. Note the activity that brought on the dyspnea and the amount of time that it takes to resolve. Dyspnea at rest, and with resting respiratory rate over 30 breaths per minute, is a sign of acute CHF. The patient may need emergency medical help.
Orthopnea	Look for dyspnea brought on by lying supine. Count the number of pillows the patient sleeps on to breathe comfortably (1, 2, 3, or 4 pillows of orthopnea).
Nausea/emesis	Look for vomiting or signs that the patient feels sick to the stomach.
Diaphoresis	Look for a cold, clammy sweat.
Fatigue	Look for a generalized feeling of exhaustion. The Borg rate of perceived exertion (RPE) scale is a tool used to grade fatigue (Table 49-4).
Cerebral signs	Ataxia, dizziness, confusion, and fainting (syncope) are all signs that the brain is not getting enough oxygen.
Orthostatic hypotension	Look for a drop in systolic blood pressure of greater than 10 mm Hg with change of position from supine to sitting or sitting to standing.

TABLE 49-4
Rate of Perceived Exertion

6		14	
7	Very, very light	15	Hard
8		16	
9	Very light	17	Very hard
10		18	
11	Fairly light	19	Very, very hard
12		20	
13	Somewhat hard		

From Borg et al: *Med Sci Sports Exerc* 14:376, 1982.

performed. After the activity has been completed the patient is asked to appraise his or her feelings of exertion as accurately as possible and give a rating to the activity.

Monitoring Response to Activity

When the patient's response to an activity is being assessed, symptoms provide one indication that the patient is or is not tolerating the activity. HR, BP, **rate pressure product** (RPP), and EKG readings are other measures that may be used to evaluate the cardiovascular system's response to work.

HEART RATE (HR). Heart rate (HR), the number of beats per minute, can be monitored by feeling the patient's pulse at the radial, brachial, or carotid sites. The radial pulse is located on the volar surface of the wrist, just lateral to the head of the radius. The brachial pulse is found in the antecubital fossa, slightly medial to the midline of the forearm. The carotid pulse, located on the neck lateral to the Adam's apple, should be palpated gently; if overstimulated, it can cause the HR to drop below 60 beats per minute (bradycardia). To determine the HR, the clinician applies the second and third fingers (flat, not with the tips) to the pulse site. If the pulse is even (regular), the clinician counts the number of beats in 10 seconds and multiplies the finding by six. The thumb should never be used to take a pulse because it has its own pulse.

All clinicians who take the HR, as well as patients, should be able to note the evenness (regularity) of the heartbeat. HRs can be regular or irregular. Although an irregular heart rate is not normal, many persons function quite well with an irregular rate. Clinicians should note the normal rate pattern for the individual, as well as any variations. A sudden change in HR from regular to irregular should be reported to the physician. An EKG or other diagnostic test may be ordered based on such findings. When the HR is irregular, the number of beats should be counted for a full minute. Patients can be taught to take their own pulse and monitor the response of their HR to activity. As a general rule of thumb, HR should rise in response to activity.

BLOOD PRESSURE. BP is the pressure that the blood exerts against the walls of any vessel as the heart beats. It is highest in the left ventricle during systole and decreases in the arterial system with distance from the heart.[26] A stethoscope and BP cuff (sphygmomanometer) are used to indirectly determine the BP. The BP cuff is placed snugly (but not tightly) around the patient's upper arm just above the elbow, with the bladder of the cuff centered above the brachial artery. The examiner inflates the cuff while palpating the brachial artery to 20 mm Hg above the point at which the brachial pulse is last felt. With the earpieces of the stethoscope angled forward in the examiner's ears, the dome of the stethoscope is placed over the patient's brachial artery. Supporting the patient's arm in extension with the pulse point of the brachial artery and the gauge of the stethoscope at the patient's heart level, the examiner deflates the cuff at a rate of approximately 2 mm Hg per second. Listening is imperative when taking BP. The first two sounds heard correspond to the systolic BP. The examiner continues to listen until the last pulse is heard and the diastolic BP is attained.

Physicians usually indicate treatment parameters for the HR and BP of patients in medical facilities. Parameters are frequently written in abbreviations, such as, "Call HO (house office, or physician on call) if SBP > 150 < 90; DBP > 90 < 60; HR > 120 < 60" (systolic BP greater than 150 or less than 90; diastolic BP greater than 90 or less than 60; HR greater than 120 or less than 60).

HR and BP will fluctuate in response to activity; cardiac output is affected by both HR and BP. **Rate pressure product** (RPP) measurement can give a more accurate indication of how well the heart is pumping. RPP is the product of HR and systolic BP (RPP = HR × SBP). It is usually a five-digit number but is reported in three digits by dropping the last two digits (for example, HR 100 × SBP 120 = 12000 = RPP 120). During any activity RPP should rise at peak and return to baseline in recovery.

EKG reading and interpretation is a skill that requires hours of learning and practice for proficiency. Electrocardiography is not available in most nonacute settings. The reader is referred to Dubin's *Rapid Interpretation of EKG*,[9] which is an excellent resource for persons unfamiliar with the subject.

There are many similarities in the evaluation and treatment of persons with cardiac disease and those with pulmonary dysfunction. A review of the pulmonary system and its disease processes follows.

PULMONARY SYSTEM

Anatomy and Physiology of Respiration[5,19]

While the heart provides oxygen-rich blood to the body and transports carbon dioxide and other waste products to the lungs, the respiratory system exchanges oxygen for carbon dioxide. The cardiac and pulmonary systems are interdependent. If no oxygen were delivered to the bloodstream, the heart would soon stop functioning for lack of oxygen; conversely, if the heart were to stop pumping, the lungs would cease functioning for lack of a blood supply. All body tissues depend on the cardiopulmonary system for their nutrients.

The respiratory system supplies oxygen to the blood and removes waste products, primarily carbon dioxide, from the blood. Air enters the body via the nose and mouth and travels through the larynx to the pharynx or voice box. From there the air continues downward into the lungs by way of the trachea or windpipe. The trachea consists of a ribbed cartilage approximately 10 cm long. The cartilage is lined with a mucous layer and cilia to help to filter out dust. When the trachea or pharynx becomes blocked, a small incision may be made into the trachea to allow air to pass freely into the lungs. This procedure is called a tracheotomy.

Two main bronchi branch off from the trachea, carrying air into the left and right lungs. The bronchi continue to branch off into smaller tubes, called *bronchioles*. Bronchioles are segmented into smaller passages called the *alveolar ducts*. Each alveolar duct is divided and leads into three or more alveolar sacs. The entire respiratory passageway from bronchi to alveolar ducts is often referred to as the *pulmonary tree* because its structure is much like an upside-down tree with the alveolar sacs as its leaves.

Each alveolar sac contains more than 10 alveoli. A very fine, semipermeable membrane separates the alveolus from the capillary network. Across this membrane, oxygen is transported and exchanged for carbon dioxide. Carbon dioxide is exhaled into the air after traveling upward through the "pulmonary tree" (Fig. 49-4).

The musculature of the thorax is responsible for inspiration and expiration. Inspiration, the muscle power for breathing air into the lungs, is provided primarily by the diaphragm. Originating from the sternum, ribs, lumbar vertebrae, and the lumbocostal arches, the diaphragm forms the inferior border of the thorax. The muscle fibers of the diaphragm insert into a central tendon. Innervated by the left and right phrenic nerves, the diaphragm contracts and domes downward when it is stimulated. This downward doming of the diaphragm enlarges the volume of the thorax and causes a drop in pressure in the lungs relative to the air in the environment. Air then enters the lungs to equalize inside and outside pressures. Accessory muscles, the intercostals and scalenes, are also active during inspiration. The intercostals maintain the alignment of the ribs, and the scalene helps elevate the rib cage.

At rest, expiration is primarily a passive relaxation of the inspiratory musculature. The lungs help to draw the thorax inward as the inspiratory muscles relax. Forced expiration requires active contraction of the abdominal muscles to compress the viscera and squeeze the diaphragm upward in the thorax. Expiration can be further forced by flexing the torso forward and pressing with the arms on the chest or abdomen. As the volume of the thorax decreases, air is forced out of the lungs.

Innervation of the Respiratory System

Breathing is mostly involuntary. A person does not have to think to take a breath. The autonomic nervous system

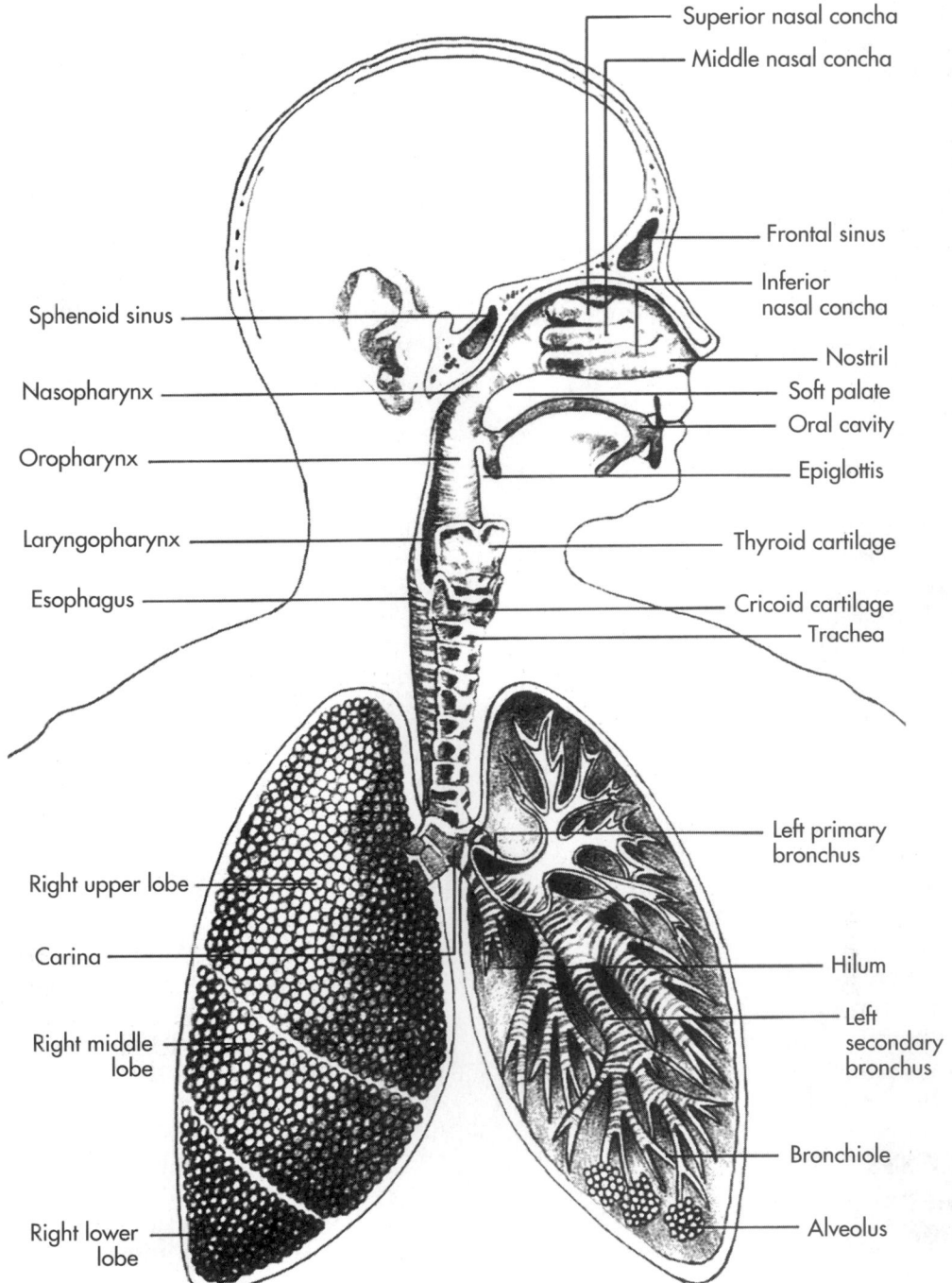

FIG. 49-4

Major structures of the respiratory system. (From *Respiratory support,* Springhouse, Pa, 1991, Springhouse.)

has control over breathing. With anxiety and increased activity the sympathetic nervous system will automatically increase the depth and rate of inspiration.

Inspiration and expiration have a volitional component. This volitional control allows us to control our breathing as we swim and to play the harmonica. Addi-

tionally, receptors within and outside the lungs when stimulated can cause changes in the depth and rate of breathing. Although the pons, medulla, and other parts of the brain provide the central control for breathing, they adjust their response to input from receptors in the lungs, the aorta, and the carotid artery.

Chronic Lung Disease[5,2]

Common chronic disorders of the lungs for which pulmonary rehabilitation is ordered include **chronic obstructive pulmonary disease** (COPD) and asthma.[5] COPD is characterized by "damage to the alveolar wall and inflammation of the conducting airways"[2] and includes emphysema, peripheral airway disease, and chronic bronchitis. COPD has been diagnosed in more than 15 million Americans.

Emphysema is a condition in which the alveoli become enlarged or ruptured, usually because of a restriction during expiration or a decrease in the elasticity of the lungs.[26] Chronic emphysema is most prevalent in men between the ages of 45 and 65 who have a history of chronic bronchitis, smoking, working in areas with high levels of air pollution, or exposure to cold, damp environments. Persons with chronic bronchitis have shortness of breath (dyspnea) on exertion, and as the disease progresses, dyspnea occurs at rest.

Inflammation, fibrosis, and narrowing of the terminal airways of the lungs are the physiological changes that occur with peripheral airway disease. Smoking and other environmental pollutants irritate the airways, leading to the development of abnormal terminal airways. Coughing and spitting up mucus from the lungs are common clinical manifestations of this disorder. The disease process may never progresses beyond this initial phase, or it may evolve into emphysema and full-fledged COPD.

Chronic bronchitis is diagnosed after a 2-year period of repeated episodes, greater than 3 months in length, of mucous-producing cough of unknown origin. A direct relationship exists between the development of chronic bronchitis and a history of cigarette smoking. Clinical manifestations of the disease increase as the **package year history** increases. Package year history is calculated by multiplying the number of packs of cigarettes consumed per day by the numbers of years of smoking. As with other forms of COPD the onset of physical disability is typically gradual, with dyspnea on exertion representing the initial phases of disability, and evolving to shortness of breath at rest.

Asthma is characterized by irritability of the bronchotracheal tree and is typically episodic in its onset. Individuals have wheezing and shortness of breath that may resolve spontaneously or may necessitate the use of medication for calming the airway. Individuals with asthma may be free of symptoms for periods of time between the episodes of wheezing and dyspnea. Some individuals appear to have a genetic predisposition to asthma. Allergenic causes of asthma may include pollens and respiratory irritants such as perfume, dust, pollen, and cleaning agents. Bronchospasms occurring with exposure to cold air or induced by exercise are sometimes the first clinical manifestations of asthma. Irritation of the airway leads to a narrowing of air passages and interferes with ventilation of the alveolar sacs. If the obstruction of the airway is significant enough, a reduction in the oxygen levels in the bloodstream will result in hypoxemia.[11] If left untreated, a severe asthmatic episode may result in death.

Pulmonary Risk Factors

Cigarette smoking is the number one cause of COPD, and smoking cessation will slow the progression of disability in persons with COPD.[20] Since cigarette smoke is a pulmonary irritant, it may also be a causative agent in asthmatic episodes. Other environmental irritants such as air pollution and chemical exposure are contributory risk factors in the development of COPD and asthma.

Medical Management

COPD is a progressive, chronic disease. The onset of the disease is insidious. When patients initially seek medical attention, they are frequently seen in a physician's clinic rather than at a medical center. Besides evaluating the patient's medical history and symptoms and performing a physical examination, the physician will assess the patient's history of smoking and occupational exposure to respiratory irritants. Blood work and an x-ray examination will be performed to further assess the patient's clinical status.

Medications prescribed for persons with pulmonary disease include antiinflammatory agents (e.g., steroids and cromolyn sodium), bronchodilators (e.g., albuterol and theophylline) that help to open the airway, and expectorants (e.g., iodides and guaifenesin) to help loosen and clear mucus. Oxygen therapy may also be prescribed at a specific flow rate. Occasionally persons receiving oxygen therapy may be tempted to increase the liter-per-minute flow, erroneously thinking that more is better. This can result in carbon dioxide retention and lead to failure of the right side of the heart.

Persons with acute respiratory distress may initially be managed with a ventilator before being weaned to oxygen. Ventilators provide a mechanical assist to the process of inspiration and do not increase the number of healthy alveolar sacs. Ventilators will not slow down the end-stage disease process of COPD. Mechanical ventilation is frequently prescribed for persons with an acute exacerbation of the disease process caused by pneumonia, influenza, or CHF.

When a patient's endurance decreases sufficiently enough to impair ADL performance, the physician may refer the patient to OT.

Signs and Symptoms of Respiratory Distress
Dyspnea is probably the most obvious sign that an individual is experiencing some difficulty breathing. In the most severe form of dyspnea the patient is short of

breath even at rest. Persons with this level of dyspnea are unable to utter a short phrase without gasping for air. When reporting that a patient has dyspnea, the practitioner should note the precipitating factors and associated circumstances; for example, "Mr. Smith becomes short of breath when washing his face while seated in front of the sink."

Other signs that the body is not getting enough oxygen include extreme fatigue, a nonproductive cough, confusion, impaired judgment, and cyanosis.

Psychosocial Considerations

Since COPD is a progressive and debilitating physical illness, it is not surprising that the psychosocial effects of the disease are considerable. Depression and anxiety are common; 96% of patients with COPD have reported having disabling anxiety.[1] Other patients with COPD complain of faintness or difficulty concentrating.[10] Training in progressive muscle relaxation can be a successful tool for controlling dyspnea and anxiety and for lowering heart rate.[23]

Most persons with end-stage COPD realize that they will die of their disease. Fear of death from suffocation is misplaced. Persons with such concerns should be referred to their physician, who can reassure them that individuals with CO_2 retention die peacefully in their sleep.[15]

Pulmonary Rehabilitation

The goal of **pulmonary rehabilitation** is to stabilize or reverse the disease process and return the patient's function to its highest capacity. A multidisciplinary rehabilitation team working with the patient can design an individualized treatment program to meet this end. Accurate diagnosis, medical management, therapy, education, and emotional support are components of a pulmonary rehabilitation program. OT personnel are frequently part of the team, which also includes the physician, nurse, and patient. Respiratory therapists, dietitians, physical therapists, social workers, and psychologists may also be team members. Roles of team members vary slightly from facility to facility. Knowledge of specialized pulmonary treatment techniques is imperative when treating persons with pulmonary disease.

TREATMENT TECHNIQUES

DYSPNEA CONTROL POSTURES. Adopting certain postures can reduce breathlessness. In a seated position the patient bends forward slightly at the waist while supporting the upper body by leaning the forearms on the table or thighs. In a standing position relief may be obtained by leaning forward and propping oneself on a counter or shopping cart.

PURSED-LIP BREATHING. Pursed-lip breathing (PLB) is thought to prevent tightness in the airway by providing resistance to expiration. This technique has been shown to increase use of the diaphragm and decrease accessory muscle recruitment.[6] Persons with COPD sometimes instinctively adapt this technique, whereas others may need to be taught it. Instructions for PLB are as follows: (1) Purse the lips as if to whistle. (2) Slowly exhale through pursed lips. Some resistance should be felt. (3) Inhale deeply through the nose. (4) It should take twice as long to exhale as it does to inhale.

DIAPHRAGMATIC BREATHING. Another breathing pattern, which calls for increased use of the diaphragm to improve chest volume, is **diaphragmatic breathing.** Many persons learn this technique by placing a small paperback novel on the abdomen just below the ziphoid process. The novel provides a visual cue for diaphragmatic movement. The patient lies supine and is instructed to inhale slowly and make the book rise. Exhalation through pursed lips should cause the book to fall.

RELAXATION. Progressive muscle relaxation in conjunction with breathing exercises can be effective in decreasing anxiety and controlling shortness of breath. One technique involves tensing muscle groups while slowly inhaling, then relaxing the muscle groups when exhaling twice as slowly through pursed lips. It is helpful to teach the patient a sequence of muscle groups to tense and relax. One common sequence involves tensing and relaxing first the face, followed by the face and the neck, then the face, neck, and shoulders, and so on down the body to the toes. A calm, quiet and comfortable environment is important for the novice in learning any relaxation technique.

OTHER TREATMENTS AND CONSIDERATIONS. Physical therapists are generally called upon to instruct the patient in chest expansion exercises, a series of exercises intended to increase the flexibility of the chest. Percussion and postural drainage use gravity and gentle drumming on the patient's back to loosen secretions and help drain the secretions from the lungs. By isometrically contracting his or her arms and hands while they are placed on the patient's thorax, the therapist may transmit vibration to the patient. Vibration is performed during the expiratory phase of breathing and helps to loosen secretions. Percussion and postural drainage may be contraindicated in acutely ill patients and those who are medically unstable.

Humidity, pollution, extremes of temperature, and stagnant air have deleterious effects on persons with respiratory ailments. The therapist and patient should take these factors into consideration when planning activity.

OCCUPATIONAL THERAPY EVALUATION AND TREATMENT: CARDIOPULMONARY DYSFUNCTION

Individuals with chronic respiratory or cardiovascular limitations are frequently limited in their ability to perform ADL. OT intervention can promote improvements in life management skills and enhance quality of life.

Evaluation

Review of the Medical Record

A review of the medical record will identify the patient's medical history (diagnosis, severity, associated conditions, and secondary diagnoses), social history, test results, medications, and precautions.

Patient Interview

It is common courtesy and good medical practice to begin every encounter with a patient by introducing oneself and explaining the purpose of the evaluation or treatment. Good interviewing skills including asking the right questions, listening to the patient's response, and observing the patient as he or she responds. Thoughtful, probing questions will help the patient and therapist identify areas of concern and lay the groundwork for establishing mutually agreeable goals. The therapist should observe the patient for signs of anxiety, shortness of breath, confusion, difficulty comprehending, fatigue, abnormal posture, reduced endurance, reduced ability to move, and stressful family dynamics. Interview questions should not only seek clarification of information that was unclear in the medical record, but also clarify the patient's understanding of his or her condition and treatment.

A patient with a history of angina should be asked to describe what the angina feels like. If the patient has also had an MI, the patient should be asked if he or she can differentiate between the angina and the MI chest pain. Clarification of symptoms before treatment can prove invaluable should symptoms arise.

Asking patients to describe a typical day, to identify activities that bring on shortness of breath or angina, and to tell how their physical limitations interfere with the things they need to do or enjoy doing most in life will reveal problems that are meaningful and relevant to the patient.

Clinical Assessment

The purpose of the clinical assessment is to establish the patient's present functional ability and limitations. The content of an occupational therapist's clinical assessment will vary from patient to patient and setting to setting. Persons with impairments of the cardiovascular system will require monitoring of their HR, BP, signs and symptoms of cardiac distress, and possibly EKG during an evaluation of tolerance to postural changes and during a functional task. Table 49-5 provides a summary of appropriate versus inappropriate responses to activity. Individuals with disorders of the respiratory system should be closely monitored for signs and symptoms of respiratory distress. The patient's range of motion, strength, and sensation may be grossly assessed within the context of the ADL evaluation. The patient's cognitive and psychosocial status will become apparent to the skilled clinician via interview and observation.

TABLE 49-5

Cardiovascular Response to Activity

	Appropriate	Inappropriate
Heart rate	Increases with activity, to no more than 20 beats/min above resting heart rate	Heart rate more than 20 beats/min above resting heart rate with activity; resting heart rate ≥120 beats/min; pulse drops or fails to rise with activity
Blood pressure	Systolic blood pressure rises with activity	Systolic pressure ≥220 mm Hg; diastolic pressure ≥110 mm Hg; postural hypotension (≥10-20 mm Hg drop in systolic pressure); decrease in systolic pressure with activity
Signs and symptoms	Absence of adverse symptoms	Excessive shortness of breath; angina; nausea and vomiting; excessive sweating; extreme fatigue (RPE ≥15); cerebral symptoms

RPE, Rate of perceived exertion.

Upon completion of the evaluation the clinician has sufficient information to formulate a treatment plan. In establishing the treatment goals and objectives, the clinician verifies that the patient agrees with the treatment plans and projected outcome.

Treatment

Present clinical status, recent functional history, response to current activity, and prognosis guide progression of treatment for persons with cardiovascular or respiratory impairment. Persons with significant cardiac or pulmonary impairment, limited recent functional ability, inappropriate responses to activity or orthostatic change, and a poor prognosis will progress very slowly. Individuals with little impairment of the heart or lungs, a recent history of normal functional ability, appropriate responses to orthostatic change and activity, and a good prognosis will progress rapidly by comparison.

Progression and Energy Costs

The energy costs of an activity and the factors that influence energy costs can further guide the clinician in the safe progression of activity. Oxygen consumption suggests how hard the heart and lungs are working, providing an indication of the amount of energy needed to complete a task. Resting quietly in bed requires the lowest amount of oxygen per kilogram of body weight, roughly 3.5 ml O_2 per kg of body weight. This is also known as 1 **basal metabolic equivalent** (MET). As activity increases, more oxygen is needed to meet the demands of the task. For instance, dressing requires 2.5 METs, or roughly twice the amount of energy that lying in bed requires (Table 49-6). Guided by an MET table, the patient's response to activity, the prognosis, and the patient's goals, the occupational therapist will be able to determine a logical treatment progression. As a general rule of thumb, once a patient tolerates an activity (e.g., seated sponge bathing) with appropriate responses, the patient may progress to the next higher MET-level activity (e.g., standing sponge bath).

The duration of sustained physical activity must be taken into account when activity guidelines are being determined. Obviously, persons who have difficulty performing a 2-MET activity must still use a commode (3.6 METs) or bedpan (4.7 METs) for their bowel management. This is possible because a person can perform at a higher-than-usual MET level for brief periods without adverse effects.

At 5 METs, sexual activity is frequently a grave concern to persons with impaired cardiovascular function and to their partners. Sexual intercourse is intermittent in its peak demands for energy. Patients are frequently able to return to sexual intercourse once they can climb up and down two flights of steps in 1 minute with appropriate cardiovascular responses.[25] Providing the patient with information about when it is safe to resume sexual activity can reduce anxiety surrounding the resumption of sexual intercourse. Anxiety may be further decreased through discussion of sexual activity guidelines with the patient and partner. Besides instructing the patient to monitor heart rate and symptoms of cardiac distress before and after intercourse, the therapist should inform the patient and partner that cardiac medications might affect the patient's libido. The patient should be encouraged to inform the physician of problems related to sexual activity. Frequently the physician can adjust the patient's medications to control symptoms.

Energy Conservation

When patients are taught how to conserve their energy resources, they will be able to perform at a higher functional level without expending more energy. The principles of **energy conservation** and work simplification are based on knowledge of how specific factors cause various cardiovascular responses. Ogden[21] has identified six variables that will increase oxygen demand: increased rate, increased resistance, increased use of large muscles, increased involvement of trunk musculature, raising one's arms, and isometric work (straining). Upper extremity activity has also been shown to require a greater cardiovascular output than lower extremity activity, and standing activity requires more energy than seated activity. Extremes of temperature, high humidity, and pollution make the heart work harder. By applying this information, a skilled clinician can make suggestions for modifying activity that will decrease the amount of energy needed for the task.

TABLE 49-6
Basal Metabolic Equivalent Table of Self-Care and Homemaking Tasks

MET Level	Self-Care	Ambulation and Household Tasks
1.2	Eating, seated[18]	Hand sewing[7]
1.5		Machine sewing or sweeping floors[7]
1.65	Transfers, bed to chair	
2	Washing face and hands, brushing hair[18]	
2.5	Seated sponge bath[24] Standing sponge bath[24] Dressing and undressing[16]	Dusting[18] Kneading dough[7] Hand washing small items[7]
2.6		Vacuuming, electric[18]
3.0	Seated warm shower[24]	Preparing a meal[16]
3.5	Standing shower, warm[16]	Climbing stairs at 24 feet/min[24]
3.6	Bowel movement on toilet[7]	
3.9		Making a bed[16]
4.2	Hot shower[16]	
4.4		Changing bed linens[18]
4.7	Bowel movement on bedpan[16]	
5.0	Sexual intercourse[24]	Walking up stairs at 30 feet/min[24]

MET, Basal metabolic equivalent.

Energy conservation should be individualized for each patient. Time management is an invaluable tool for energy conservation. Time management involves preplanning one's activity so that tasks requiring high energy expenditure are interspersed with lighter tasks and so that rest breaks are scheduled throughout the day, especially after meals. The patient should be actively involved in planning the day. Patient involvement increases the likelihood of realistic goal attainment.

Written material may augment energy conservation instruction. However, until the patient has successfully applied energy conservation principles to activity, the therapist should expect little follow-through with energy conservation recommendations. Practice and practical application of skills are critical to changing behavior.

The specific pulmonary rehabilitation treatment techniques of pursed-lip breathing, diaphragmatic breathing, dyspnea control postures, and relaxation techniques are discussed earlier in this chapter. Exhaling with exertion is another breathing principle for persons with cardiac or pulmonary compromise. This technique is more energy efficient and helps control systolic BP responses to activity. It is important for the patient to practice these skills during treatment. Therapeutic support is often critical in learning.

Patient and Family Education

As members of the health care team, occupational therapists share the responsibility for patient and family education. The team must instruct the patient and family members in cardiac or pulmonary anatomy, the disease process, symptom management, risk factors, diet, exercise, and energy conservation and must reinforce the teaching. Including family members in an education program provides support indirectly to the patient, through the family unit. Such support is critical when the patient is dependent on the assistance of a family member to accomplish everyday tasks.

SUMMARY

Healthy individuals are able to meet the varying demands of their bodies for oxygen because their heart and respiratory rates adjust to meet oxygen demand. When the cardiovascular or pulmonary system is compromised, the ability to perform normal activity declines. This chapter is intended to guide the occupational therapist in the treatment of persons with impairment of the heart or lungs and in designing programs to maximize their independent performance of functional activities.

Sample case studies for both cardiac and pulmonary disability follow.

CASE STUDY 49-1

CASE STUDY—MR. F. (CARDIOVASCULAR DISEASE)

Mr. F. is a 48-year-old auto mechanic who experienced 10/10 substernal chest pain, nausea, and shortness of breath while working under an automobile 2 days ago. He was given a diagnosis of an acute anterolateral MI complicated by subsequent CHF. He is married and the father of three children, ages 9, 5, and 4. His wife works full time and was unable to manage his care at home, so he was placed temporarily in a skilled nursing facility.

Mr. F. is anxious and expresses concern that he will die in the facility, just like his father did. He reports that his wife "is a very desirable woman and a hardworking mother." He wants to return to his home and return to work. He is able to safely walk to the bathroom, according to physical therapy findings.

Results of the OT evaluation indicate that Mr. F., although anxious, was cooperative and motivated to participate in therapy. Although not formally tested, strength, range of motion, and perceptual and cognitive ability were grossly functional during a routine ADL assessment of 2.5-MET seated sponge bathing and dressing. Vital signs were appropriate during the evaluation, except that BP fell 20 mm Hg in recovery (3 minutes after completion of bathing) and Mr. F. became symptomatic (nausea and shortness of breath). Symptoms and vital signs stabilized after 5 minutes of rest. Mr. F. needed frequent cues to pace the activity and demonstrated little knowledge about signs and symptoms of cardiac distress. His risk factors include male gender, family history, and a sedentary lifestyle.

OT was initiated to increase his functional capacity and endurance for self-care and to promote paced activity and management of signs and symptoms. OT treatment included graded ADL, instruction in early identification of fatigue, training in monitoring HR, risk factor education, and the provision of guidelines for resumption of sexual activity. Mr. F. responded well to his therapy program, progressively spending more time each day out of bed and gradually increasing his functional capacity so that he could perform a 3.5-MET standing shower and dress without cues to pace activity and without adverse cardiovascular responses. He learned to monitor his own heart rate and to take rest breaks when fatigued. Both he and his wife met with the occupational therapist to discuss modification of dietary risk factors and resumption of marital relations. He was able to return to his home and continued his cardiac rehabilitation program at a community center.

CASE STUDY 49-2

CASE STUDY—MRS. P. (PULMONARY DYSFUNCTION)

Mrs. P. is a 64-year-old woman with a 3-year history of COPD. She was released from the acute care hospital 3 days ago, her condition having been stabilized after an acute exacerbation of COPD. Mrs. P. has been smoking cigarettes since the age of 20 and currently smokes one pack per day. She is widowed and lives alone in a small one-bedroom apartment. There is a first-floor laundry room in her building. Mrs. P.'s daughter lives three blocks away and checks on Mrs. P. daily. She empties Mrs. P.'s bedside commode and provides groceries and dinner to Mrs. P.

OT results indicated that Mrs. P. became short of breath when combing her hair. She was unable to pace activity, to coordinate pursed-lip breathing with activity, or to assume dyspnea control postures when needed. She was receiving 2 liters of oxygen by nasal cannula at all times. Her primary goals were to be able to empty her bedside commode independently and to prepare most dinners for herself.

OT was initiated to (1) improve endurance and tolerance for activity, (2) promote coordination of pursed-lip breathing and dyspnea control postures with ADL, and (3) improve ADL independence. The OT program included instruction in paced activity, symptom identification and remediation, and graded self-care tasks and provision of smoking cessation information.

Continued

CASE STUDY 49-2—cont'd

At discharge from OT, Mrs. P. was able to empty her bedside commode independently, perform 3-MET seated showering and dressing, and warm up prepared dinners from her refrigerator independently. Her daughter continued to visit daily but was able to decrease visits to twice a week if she desired. Mrs. P. continued to require assistance for laundry and grocery shopping. This was her baseline level of function before the exacerbation. Unfortunately, Mrs. P. continues to smoke.

REVIEW QUESTIONS

1. Describe the heart, including its size, anatomy, and functional parts.
2. Name the heart valves, and give their locations and functions.
3. Discuss the relationship between the coronary arteries and the health of the heart.
4. List and describe the symptoms of cardiac distress.
5. What are the typical psychosocial responses to a diagnosis of heart disease?
6. How is cardiac response to activity monitored? How does the therapist know that a change in activity level is warranted?
7. Describe the functional parts of the pulmonary system.
8. What is COPD, and what is its significance for occupational performance?
9. What can the OT practitioner do to help prevent or reduce the incidence of COPD?
10. Demonstrate the recommended dyspnea control postures.
11. Compare pursed-lip breathing with diaphragmatic breathing. When should one be used rather than the other?
12. Describe appropriate evaluation content and approach for patients with cardiac and pulmonary problems.
13. What is an MET, and what is the clinical value of an MET table for occupational therapists?
14. How would you teach energy conservation techniques to the following individuals who have received diagnoses of cardiac or pulmonary disease?
    - A 40-year-old female marathon runner
    - A 50-year-old homemaker and adoptive mother of eight (including three children under the age of 6)
    - A 60-year-old air conditioner repairman
    - A 72-year-old man who says his main pleasures are riding thoroughbreds, drinking good Kentucky bourbon, smoking cigars, and enjoying the company of lovely women

REFERENCES

1. Agle DP, Baum GL: Psychological aspects of chronic obstructive pulmonary disease, *Med Clin North Am* 61(4):749-758, 1977.
2. American Thoracic Society: Definitions and classifications of chronic bronchitis, asthma, and pulmonary emphysema, *Am Rev Respir Dis* 85:762-768, 1962.
3. Andreoli KG et al: *Comprehensive cardiac care: a text for nurses, physicians and other health practitioners*, St Louis, 1983, Mosby.
4. Bragg TL: Psychological response to myocardial infarction, *Nurs Forum* 14(4):383-395, 1975.
5. Brannon FJ et al: *Cardiopulmonary rehabilitation: basic theory and application*, ed 2, Philadelphia, 1992, FA Davis.
6. Breslin EH: The pattern of respiratory muscle recruitment during pursed-lip breathing, *Chest* 101(1):75-78, 1992.
7. Colorado Heart Association: *Exercise equivalent* (pamphlet), Boston, Mass, 1970, Cardiac Reconditioning & Work Evaluation Unit, Spaulding Rehabilitation Center.
8. Dawber TR: *The Framingham study, the epidemiology of atherosclerotic disease*, Cambridge, Mass, 1980, Harvard University Press.
9. Dubin D: *Rapid Interpretation of EKGs*, ed 5, Tampa, Fla, 1998, COVER Publishing.
10. Dudley DL et al: Psychosocial concomitants to rehabilitation in chronic obstructive pulmonary disease. 2. Psychosocial treatment, *Chest* 77(5):677-684, 1980.
11. Farzan S: *A concise handbook of respiratory diseases*, ed 4, Reston, Va, 1985, Reston Publishing.
12. Gentry WD, Haney T: Emotional and behavioral reaction to acute myocardial infarction, *Heart Lung* 4(5):738-745, 1975.
13. Goldberger E: *Essentials of clinical cardiology*, Philadelphia, 1990, JB Lippincott.
14. Greenland P: Efficacy of supervised cardiac rehabilitation programs for coronary patients: update 1986-1990, *Cardiopulmonary Rehab* 11:190-203, 1991.
15. Hodgkin JE et al: *Pulmonary rehabilitation guidelines to success*, ed 2, Philadelphia, 1993, JB Lippincott.
16. Kottke FJ: Common cardiovascular problems in rehabilitation. In Krusen FH, Kottke FJ, Elwood PM, editors: *Handbook of physical medicine & rehabilitation*, Philadelphia, 1971, WB Saunders.
17. Levin LA, Perk J, Hedback B: Cardiac rehabilitation—a cost analysis, *J Intern Med* 230(5):427-434, 1991.
18. Maloney FP, Moss K: *Energy requirements for selected activities*, Denver, 1974, Department of Physical Medicine, National Jewish Hospital, (Unpublished).
19. Mythos for SoftKey: *BodyWorks 4.0: human anatomy leaps to life*, Cambridge, Mass, 1993-1995, SoftKey International.
20. Nemeny B et al: Changes in lung function after smoking cessation: an assessment from a cross-sectional survey, *Am Rev Respir Dis* 125(2):122-124, 1982.
21. Ogden LD: *Guidelines for analysis and testing of activities of daily living with cardiac patients*, Downey, Calif, 1981, Cardiac Rehabilitation Resources.
22. Oldridge NB, Guyatt GH, Fischer ME, et al: Cardiac rehabilitation after myocardial infarction, *JAMA* 260(7):945-950, 1988.
23. Renfroe KL: Effect of progressive relaxation on dyspnea and state anxiety in patients with chronic obstructive pulmonary disease, *Heart Lung* 17(4):408-413, 1988.
24. Santa Clara Valley Medical Center: *Graded activity sheets*, San Jose, Calif, 1994, The Center.
25. Scalzi C, Burke L: Myocardial infarction: behavioral responses of patient and spouses. In Underhill SL et al, editors: *Cardiac nursing*, Philadelphia, 1982, JB Lippincott.
26. Taber CW: *Taber's cyclopedic medical dictionary*, ed 16, Philadelphia, 1993, FA Davis.

ANN BURKHARDT

KEY TERMS

Cancer
Metastases
Surgery
Chemotherapy
Radiation
Oncology
Hospice
Palliative
Lymphedema
Neoplasm

LEARNING OBJECTIVES

After studying this chapter the student or practitioner will be able to do the following:
1. Describe cancer and its diagnosis and medical and surgical treatments.
2. Identify common psychological conditions associated with life-threatening illness and loss.
3. Identify strategies for helping patients cope with the side effects of the treatments for cancer.
4. Identify common physical dysfunction issues resulting primarily from the cancer and secondarily from the treatment.
5. Identify techniques used in addressing a variety of occupational therapy goals with cancer patients, according to practice setting.
6. Identify problems that may arise as a result of the disease process or the sequelae of disease that could affect a person's occupational roles, activities of importance to those roles, and task performance; identify possible solutions to the problems.

Cancer is a broad grouping of diseases, all of which are linked by the presence of malignant tumor cells in the body. Cancers are described by the type of tissue in which they arise: carcinoma (within an organ), sarcoma (connective tissue), chondroma (cartilage), lymphoma (lymphatic tissue), or leukemia (blood-forming tissue). Malignancies can be low grade (slowly developing) or high grade (rapidly developing) and can adapt within and spread throughout the body (metastasizing). **Metastases** are pieces of tumor that have broken off from the main tumor, traveled in the circulatory system, and reseeded themselves in new organs or tissues in the body. When biopsy of a metastatic lesion is performed (the lesion is sampled to observe its histology or tissue type), the lesion cells appear similar to the cells in the tumor of origin. For example, breast cancer that metastasizes to the lung is breast cancer, not lung cancer, at the cellular level. Tumors occupy space within an organ system and interrupt the function of that organ. For example, liver tumors or lesions can cause the affected person to have abnormal liver function, observed on a blood test or through a clinical sign such as jaundice.

Sometimes tumor cells secrete hormonelike substances. These pseudohormones disrupt the function of organs. The clinical picture may appear as something unrelated to cancer; often there is no tumor mass, just freely circulating tumor cells, resulting in a paraneoplastic syndrome. For example, lung cancer can cause a paraneoplastic syndrome that looks like quadriparesis.

TABLE 50-1
Staging of Cancers

Stage	Tumor	Lymph Nodes	Metastases
I Mean 5-year survival rate: 70%-90%	Tumor present and limited to the organ of its involvement Lesion is operable and prognosis good	No spread of the cancer to the lymph nodes	No metastatic lesions
II Mean 5-year survival rate 50% ± 5%	Tumor has evidence of spread into the localized tissues Tumor is operable and can be fully removed	Lymph nodes have evidence of cancer in the region/body quadrant surrounding the tumor	Local evidence of metastases to the lymphatics; metastases are limited and have not spread to other body organs
III Mean 5-year survival rate 20% ± 5%	Extensive evidence of a primary tumor that has spread elsewhere in the body Tumor can be debulked, but some of the cells remain behind	Lymph node involvement close to the primary tumor and extending to deeper lymphatics	Evidence that the cancer has spread and left other lesions in other organs
IV Mean 5-year survival rate <5%	Inoperable primary lesion Survival depends on depth and extent of the tumor spread	Lymph node involvement that extends to multiple organs and regions of the body	Multiple sites of metastases to organs beyond the one in which the tumor originated

Paraneoplastic syndrome is often considered in a differential diagnosis when polyneuropathy or dermatomyositis is seen. The presence of acute onset quadriparesis without evident physical trauma suggests that lung cancer may be an underlying cause. Blood tests will detect tumor markers, and the cancer can be diagnosed. Once the cancer diagnosis is known, chemotherapy or procedures that can filter the neoplastic cells from the blood (e.g., photophoresis) can rapidly change and possibly improve the functional clinical picture. Cancers are "staged," or classified, in an effort to predict prognosis and identify appropriate intervention (Table 50-1).

PREVENTION

At a number of levels of cancer care it is appropriate for an occupational therapist to work with the person with cancer. Probably the most valuable, yet often overlooked, time for an occupational therapist to intervene is at the level of cancer prevention. For example, influencing a person's choice of and ability to change habits and behaviors that negatively influence health is a starting point. Occupational therapists can give positive health messages to all the people they contact. Children and adolescents may not start smoking if they hear a positive smoking prevention message or if they are involved as role models in an education project focused on communication with their peers or siblings.

Occupational therapists can also intervene by helping smokers quit smoking. In 1998 the Representative Assembly (RA) of the American Occupational Therapy Association (AOTA) voted to support the *Clinical Prac-* *tice Guideline* of the Agency for Healthcare Policy Research.[1] This action supports the role occupational therapists may play in helping their patients set health improvement goals to prevent chronic disease and disability. Smoking cessation initiatives are one example of a cancer prevention intervention. Smoking cessation interventions may be individual, group, or population based and geared to reach any age group across the life span. Other prevention efforts may focus on self-examination and follow-up in scheduling and going for cancer detection tests (e.g., breast self-examinations, mammograms, Pap smears, and colonoscopies). Since the focus in occupational therapy (OT) is on helping people achieve a balanced lifestyle that supports a balance between self-care, work, play and leisure, and rest, occupational therapists are a natural group of professionals to be involved in cancer prevention initiatives.

EARLY POSTDIAGNOSIS PHASE

An occupational therapist also plays an important role in working with persons with cancer who are recovering from such invasive procedures as surgery, chemotherapy, and radiation therapy. This level of OT intervention may occur in a hospital, home health, or community health setting. People who experience a change in their functional status and have difficulty participating in daily activities such as self-care, work, play and leisure activities, or with the ability to rest, may benefit from OT. The prevention of long-term disability, the restoration of normal function, and the support of function through rehabilitative means or through provision of palliative (comfort) care are all appropriate reasons for an OT referral.

The initial treatment for cancer may involve a series of treatments including surgery, chemotherapy, radiation therapy, or immunotherapy. Each of these treatments has side effects. **Surgery** may include removal of a mass, more resection of tissue in addition to the mass (for staging of the disease or for complete removal of tumor-invaded tissue), reconstructive surgery to correct cosmetic or functional defects or the surgical resection, or amputation. Before surgery the therapist can be involved in patient education and training—preparing the patient for what to expect after the surgery. There is some belief that training the patient preoperatively may improve functional outcomes and reduce the rehabilitation needed in the postoperative recovery phase.

POSTOPERATIVE PHASE

In the early postoperative stage the occupational therapist may work with patients to encourage them and enable them to participate safely in daily occupations and goal-directed activities. People may be frightened to move and may need guidance concerning how much is safe to attempt and which movements they need to avoid until healing occurs. Pulling of the incision commonly occurs when patients' bodies are used dynamically in activities. This pulling sensation may be threatening to people who are uncertain about how much movement is too much or too little. The therapist often receives special movement precautions from the surgeon in the early postoperative phase of OT referral and intervention. Postoperative precautions and protocols vary from surgeon to surgeon and facility to facility and must be verified at the time of the referral.

Several types of surgery are used to treat tumors. An en bloc resection is removal of the tumor and surrounding or involved tissues in one block or piece. An en bloc resection can be done when the nerves and vascular structures are patent, unobstructed by tumor growth. Radical surgery, including amputation, is a wide surgical resection. The diseased tissue is removed along with surrounding lymphatic tissue and other soft tissue (skin, nerve, muscle, or bone). If the neurovascular bundle to the limb is involved, the limb has to be amputated.

Amputation is a life-altering event resulting in the loss of a limb or part of a limb (e.g., arm or leg) or of a body part (e.g., breast). The loss always causes a visible change in physical appearance. One difference between amputation as a result of cancer diagnosis and a traumatic amputation in an accident or necessitated by complications of a disease (e.g., diabetes) is that cancer requires further medical management beyond traditional wound care and preprosthetic or prosthetic training. Life span and survival rates and the person's percep-

tion of the relative value of such an investment to them vary and may affect the person's decision about whether to purchase an artificial limb. For example, someone who has a postamputation life expectancy of 2 years or less may decline a prosthesis because of the expense and the time that must be invested in a training regimen. He or she may have other plans for the money or time that are more meaningful to quality of life.

When adapted equipment or techniques are indicated, the therapist may also provide them and train the patient to use them to compensate for motion that is lost or compromised after surgery. If the surgery causes a temporary functional change, the use of adaptation may be only for the immediate, subacute phase of healing. If surgery has caused muscle or bone loss, the functional changes and adaptations may be strategies that will be used for the remainder of life.

CHEMOTHERAPY

Chemotherapy is the use of a variety of toxic chemical substances to kill cancer cells within the body. Each form of chemotherapy has its own pattern of possible side effects. Some of the most common side effects that occupational therapists encounter are alopecia (hair loss), peripheral neuropathy, thrombocytopenia (diminished platelet levels and slow clotting time of the blood), fatigue (associated with such factors as impaired liver function), changes in the red blood cell composition of the blood (e.g., anemia), and function-limiting anxiety and fear.

Chemotherapy-induced neuropathy usually causes wrist-drop and foot-drop, which are transient. Neuropathy can also cause burning, tingling pain. Neuropathic pain can severely limit function, since people are reluctant to hold on to objects or to stand on their feet when pain is serious.

Many people who are receiving chemotherapy contract opportunistic infections because chemotherapy causes immunosuppression. One infection, cytomegalovirus (CMV), can cause blindness, as well as hepatitis. People who have low vision or blindness and chemoneuropathy have a severe handicapping situation, since they cannot use one sensory system (tactile) to substitute for another (vision) functionally. Another infection, a yeast (Candida albicans) infection, can cause dysphagia, an inability to swallow safely. The affected person may have to stop eating by mouth or eat a restricted consistency diet until the infection resolves.

In the acute phase of hospitalization patients receiving chemotherapy may be referred to OT because they have been on prolonged bed rest and may have stopped initiating or participating in their self-care. Also, fatigue may limit their level of participation, since a person who is fatigued may not be able or sufficiently motivated to participate in daily occupations.

Peripheral neuropathy causes weakness and sensory changes in the hands and feet. Often people cannot hold on to objects adequately to use them as intended. Hyperesthesia (tingling, numbness, or burning) and loss of grasp and fine motor hand function can interfere with the ability to do daily tasks and activities, since the person may drop objects or experience pain when trying to use common objects such as a comb or a brush.

The patient who has decreased platelet levels may bleed easily and may have to forgo some normal daily activities for a few days until blood levels improve. When someone's platelet level is below $45,000/mm^3$, for example, the individual may have excessive bleeding of the gums when brushing teeth. While the platelet level is low, using a sponge toothette or a glycerine swab may be all the individual can tolerate until blood levels normalize. Blood levels generally improve as the person's body metabolizes the chemotherapy, in the first few days after a treatment.

Hormone therapy and immunotherapy are also used as forms of chemotherapy. For example, some tumors thrive on estrogens. Hormones such as Lupron or tamoxifen can be used to block estrogen receptors or to prevent the body from producing estrogens. These hormones often have the side effect of inducing menopause. Women may complain about mood swings and hot flashes. Immunotherapy is the use of substances that block the response of the immune system or that heighten the response. For instance, white blood cells phagocytose (ingest) cancer cells and carry them through the lymphatic system to other areas of the body. This response can spread cancer in the local region or carry the cancer cells to other places in the body. Interferon is an immunotherapeutic agent that can be used to fight this spread. People who receive interferon treatment may have a tendency toward hyperactive skin responses, such as forms of eczema. If these individuals are scratched, welts may easily develop. These are normal responses to the drug and should not generate fear or anxiety in the patients who use these substances.

RADIATION THERAPY

Another method of treatment that people may undergo in the acute phase of cancer intervention is **radiation** therapy. Radiation is the use of radioactive materials directly in tumors or the surrounding tissue to kill cancer cells. Radiation is effective when the cancer cells are sensitive to its effects. Radioactive seeds (small pieces or pellets of material) can be directly implanted for a short time in the body (radioactive seed implantation). Sometimes seeds are placed in flexible tubing that is run through the tumor bed (brachytherapy). Another approach involves directing a beam of radioactivity to a generalized area of the body via a linear accelerator

machine. The beam can cover a broad area of a quadrant of the body (wide-beam) or be directed to a more focused area (cone down). An occupational therapist may work collaboratively in some settings with the radiation **oncology** staff to mold body positioners from thermoplastic (splinting) materials. These devices are used to help the patient remain in the position needed for the duration of the radiation treatment. Radiation may also be used in late disease as a form of palliative treatment, particularly to reduce pain.

Burns are a possible side effect of radiation treatment. The topical ointments used to treat a burn caused by radiation are different from those used for burns of other causes. The skin absorbs moisturizing agents. These agents can change the surface composition of the skin and result in an enhancement of the burn at the next radiation treatment. Many interventional radiologists recommend water-based ointments (e.g., Aquaphor) for their patients. Others allow their patients to use silicone gel pads to cover the burn and manage the burn-related pain and discomfort. When people have burns resulting from radiation, they should avoid movement that stretches or pulls the burned area. People may need assistance with range of motion to prevent such complications as frozen shoulder.

REHABILITATIVE PHASE

Therapists who work with cancer patients in the acute care phase of treatment are generally working toward the goal of getting the patient ready to go home or be transferred to an inpatient rehabilitation setting, a subacute center, long-term care, or a hospice setting (at home or in a facility).

Patients who have completed their initial cancer treatment may be well enough to participate in aggressive rehabilitation programs. Sometimes patients are admitted to a rehabilitation unit on a trial therapy basis to test their ability to tolerate 3 hours of therapy per day. After initial healing of a surgery and after or during chemotherapy regimens, cancer patients may be able to tolerate this intensive type of rehabilitation program. On a rehabilitation unit, goals for cancer patients generally involve restoration and support of function within a rehabilitative model of care—learning to live with an acquired handicap. The goal of therapy in a function-based treatment setting is to restore the ability of cancer patients to participate in goal-directed activities that give their lives meaning. Some of the pertinent areas for OT assessment and intervention are analyzed in Table 50-2.

Cancer and cancer treatment can cause a number of functional problems that result in physical disability and handicapping situations. One of the most important issues associated with cancer is impaired mobility. Community mobility—leaving home, crossing the street, getting around the neighborhood, and getting to

Cancer Involvement	Impairment	Activity Restriction	Participation Issues
Brain	Motor	Mobility	Access Architectural barriers Adaptation
	Sensory	Safety Pain	Safety: need for supervision or a helper Pain: intolerance of participation in activities that exacerbate pain to level of intolerance Pain medicine: blurring of senses, inability to drive or operate heavy machinery
	Cognitive	Planning Sequencing Memory Insight Safety	Inability to lead Lack of ability to plan or implement change Social inappropriateness and stigma Loss of occupational roles: work roles, family roles, ability to participate in leisure or sport activities
	Neurobehavioral Visual impairment: hemianopsia, neglect, low vision, cortical blindness, loss of spatial relations perception Motor planning	Interference with ADL/self-care and instrumental activities	Inability to be independently involved in daily occupations
	Communication	Speaking Reading Writing	Loss of or major change in socialization and sharing ideas Severity of participation restriction depends on individual interests and roles
Bone	Loss of motion Pain Impaired mobility Risk of reinjury of affected part	ADL (basic and instrumental)	Diminished ability to dress, bathe, toilet in context Needs adaptation of environment or requires presence of a caregiver Decreased ability to get around—leave home, get around community Possible effect on employment Severity of participation restriction depends on individual interests and roles
Breast	Loss of motion Pain Impaired mobility Risk of reinjury of affected part	ADL (basic and instrumental) Shoulder mobility restrictions (e.g., sports)	Temporary or long-term disruption in ability to do housework, job, leisure activities Risk of injury because of lymphatic compromise Effect on sexuality
Lung	Shoulder mobility impairment (Pancoast tumor; postthoracotomy) Impaired respiratory status Fatigue	ADL (basic and instrumental) Shoulder mobility restrictions (e.g., sports) Respiratory tolerance	Mobility issues related to respiratory tolerance and distance navigated Temporary or long-term disruption in ability to do housework, job, leisure activities Risk of injury because of respiratory compromise Need for oxygen or nebulizing equipment
Colon	Change in how bowels are managed (toileting-colostomy) Change in how body is washed (stomal issues) Cheomoneuropathy impairment potential Fatigue	ADL (basic and instrumental) Fatigue Social stigma of stoma (e.g., odor, bag ruptures) Fine motor impairment related to chemotherapy	Socially stigmatizing in community relationships

Continued

TABLE 50-2—cont'd

Classification of Cancer-Related Sequelae in ICIDH-2 Terminology

Cancer Involvement	Impairment	Activity Restriction	Participation Issues
Prostate	Urinary incontinence Inability to perform sexually	ADL (basic and instrumental)	Loss of sense of self as a sexual being Stigma associated with incontinence
Head and neck	Inability to swallow or eat Loss of voice Neck and shoulder decrease in range of motion, loss of scapular stability	ADL (feeding and eating; swallowing) Respiratory: management of oral secretions Bimanual overhead mobility activities Intimacy issues	Socially stigmatizing in community relationships Need to change contributory habits (e.g., smoking)

and from business or medical appointments—is basic to daily life. A number of factors can contribute to mobility impairments.

Weakness is probably the most common impairment causing disability and restricted activity participation in people with cancer. Weakness leads to a lack of endurance needed for navigating distances and decreased tolerance for sitting or being upright for prolonged periods. Weakness may also limit customary movement within homes or public buildings if there are architectural barriers such as flights of stairs. The inability to get around presents a person with a handicapping situation, since he or she cannot access the venues needed to fulfill occupational roles.

Impaired sensation predisposes people to injury from heat sources or sharp tools. If the sensory impairment is hyperesthetic (intensifying sensation), burning pain can decrease the ability to hold objects, to modulate grasp or pinch to manipulate objects enough to use them, or to tolerate wearing of socks or shoes. The physically disabling condition creates an inability to carry out all of the self-care and other daily activities that involve hand function or foot function.[2]

Impaired cognition is disabling, since a person may not be able to initiate or follow through on tasks. If memory is impaired, a patient may forget what he or she is doing or why he or she is doing it. Impaired judgment, if sufficiently grave, means that a person cannot be left alone. The potential risk of injury or elopement from familiar surroundings may be too great a risk to allow any independence. Impaired cognition may be permanent or transient. If the impairment is associated with a central nervous system structural abnormality, the person may recover only rudimentary cognitive skill and may benefit most from the development of cueing systems to complete daily activities. If the person has a cognitive impairment associated with metabolism of an anesthetic or the introduction of a new pain medication (opiates such as morphine have this property), cognitive abilities may return to normal baseline when the drug is metabolized by the body. The liver's ability to metabolize drugs and anesthesia slows with age, and so many older persons who undergo major surgery experience this phenomenon. Although the acquired cognitive impairments from anesthesia resolve within weeks of surgery, many people need constant supervision during this recovery phase.

Impaired vision is sometimes associated with brain tumors or a CMV infection. Impaired vision of recent onset in a sighted person can be very disorienting. Most sighted people cannot easily orient themselves to daily activities if visual impairment or blindness develops suddenly. The degree of functional impairment will be associated with the daily activities a person enjoys or needs to complete. For example, a person may not be able to resume driving a vehicle. This limits community mobility. A person may not be able to sign or write checks. Other basic and instrumental ADL participation skills and abilities may be lost as a result of vision loss.

Diminished hearing may result from use of metal-based chemotherapy drugs (e.g., cisplatin). These chemotherapy drugs are toxic to auditory nerves. Severe hearing loss or deafness may develop following treatment. Children who receive these drugs may not develop language skills. Adults may have difficulty with social interactions and the use of standard communication devices (e.g., telephones). People who are caregivers for others may have to relinquish their responsibilities or may require training and adapted devices to modify the way they perform essential tasks. People who rely on hearing to work, such as musicians, may need assistance from a therapist to find a new role that is less dependent on hearing.

Chronic fatigue results from a variety of factors after cancer treatment. Chronic fatigue may eventually resolve as factors causing the condition resolve and as the body heals after cancer diagnosis and treatment. However, management of chronic fatigue is necessary for coping during the disease and treatment process. Participation in living can instill hope and the perception that some things can change or be positively managed to give the patient a sense of being able to control his or her own life. Both emotionally and psychologically, hope is crucial to recovery.

Strategies that occupational therapists can use to assist patients who have chronic fatigue include energy conservation and work simplification, as well as scheduling intervals of rest between periods of work or activity. When fatigue is severely disabling, an occupational therapist can help the patient and caregivers prioritize the tasks and activities the patient wants to do, balancing these with the tasks or activities that must be done. Sometimes recognizing the need for help allows people the opportunity to choose the truly important and meaningful occupations that define who they are as people and contributing members of society.

PALLIATIVE CARE

When people have received diagnoses of advanced cancer and are not expected to recover, their physician can declare or certify them as terminally ill. This certification entitles people to have access to **hospice** services. Hospice is a form of **palliative** care. Palliative care is directed toward achieving comfort and ease of participation in activity. Occupational therapists involved in hospice care may adapt the environment, train caregivers to assist with daily life tasks, counsel for psychological or emotional issues related to the disease process, and provide assistance with issues concerning death and dying. Occupational therapists may work with the patient on activities that help the patient plan for death. Reminiscence activities, such as creating memory scrap books, making video "cards," writing letters, making phone calls, and arranging visits are examples of creative tasks that can help the dying person revisit relationships and review life.

In palliative care the occupational therapist may assist with promoting positioning for comfort, treatment to prevent or relieve pain, promoting engagement in activity that is physically tolerable, and creating an opportunity to plan for death. For the patient involved in the active process of dying, having an opportunity to resolve life issues is critical. Creativity still plays a role. When people create and give back something to others, they live in hope. Hope is essential in all phases of life, even in the process of dying, since it motivates us to live each day to the fullest, despite illness and disease.

GENERAL PRINCIPLES OF CANCER CARE
Psychological and Emotional Aspects of Living with Cancer

People with cancer may have social, psychological, and emotional issues that affect their ability to function. Acquaintances may avoid the cancer patient, not knowing how to respond to the news of a life-threatening illness. Some people mistakenly assume that they can catch cancer from the person. Many people, regardless of the stage of their disease, automatically assume they are dying. In reality, more and more people are surviving with diagnoses of cancer for longer and longer periods.

Coping mechanisms are essential for dealing with the stress of having a cancer diagnosis, as well as for facing the inevitability of treatments necessary for seeking control or cure of the cancer. The emotional side effects of the progression of cancer include fear and anticipation of pain, which produces anxiety and stress. Surgery is usually painful. Chemotherapy can cause painful neuropathies. Burns from radiation are painful. Metastatic lesions on bone, muscle, or nerve are painful. Some positive coping mechanisms for dealing with a rational fear of pain are self-hypnosis, meditation, and other relaxation techniques (see Chapter 29).

People who are anxious by temperament often have heightened anxiety when they are trying to cope with cancer diagnoses and treatment. People with anxiety disorders can become too focused on signs or symptoms they experience. They may not be able to sleep. They may be unable to take part in their normal activities, losing perspective on their situation. They may find it difficult to concentrate on normal life tasks. Treatment for an anxiety disorder includes supportive counseling and pharmacological intervention. Once the anxiety is controlled and the fears that underlie the anxiety are addressed, coping behaviors can be developed and improve the person's ability to engage in the rehabilitative process.

Many people living with a diagnosis of cancer experience depression. Depression may be reactive or organic in origin. Depression may also have an organic cause, such as medications, the disease process, or a hereditary predisposition. Depression is characterized by feelings of helplessness and hopelessness. People adjusting to disease or disability go through a normal grieving process. During this time they may experience a number of feelings or stages. The stages of adjustment generally encountered are anger, denial, bargaining, and acceptance. These stages tend to be experienced in combination. Depressed people generally have to be able to see something hopeful concerning their personal circumstances for change to occur and for the effects of the depression to lessen.

Participation in support groups may be helpful for some people. Even people with advanced cancer have been found to benefit from support groups. Women with stage-four breast cancer who participated in support groups lived better and longer than those who did not participate in a support group.[3] Although the exact mechanism is not clear, the experience of knowing that others share what you are feeling and that others care about you can have a positive impact on the immune system. Recent studies have shown that even avoidance of pessimism supports health and well-being.

LONG-TERM AND SPECIAL CHRONIC DISEASE ISSUES

Lymphedema is edema (enlargement of one or more limbs) that results from impaired lymphatic circulation. Lymphatic circulation can be impaired by lymph node dissection, radiation of the lymphatics, or a tumor that has spread into the lymphatic vessels or nodes. Lymphedema is protein-rich edema and is inflammatory in nature. Lymphedema can occur throughout the body but is commonly seen by therapists when it impairs function in a limb by changing the mobility of the extremity or by producing pain in the involved limb. Lymphedema in the arm, in particular, produces a social impairment. A normal approach to social interaction in our society includes extending a hand to shake hands. When a person has lymphedema in an arm and hand, people may react negatively to the appearance of the limb. As discussed previously, publicly sharing knowledge of a diagnosis of cancer can be socially stigmatizing and lead to social rejection.

Treatment for lymphedema usually involves education in skin care and wound precautions. The limb is fitted with a compressive garment or wrap. Light compression can be provided by a tubular support bandage or toning gloves or garments. Moderate (20 to 30 mm Hg) to firm (30 to 40, or 40 to 60 mm Hg) compression can be achieved by using a high-gradient garment (e.g., Jobst, Juzo, Medi, or Sigvarus). Manual lymphatic therapy (massage) can be performed to correct the lymphedema. This is generally followed by bandaging with cotton-based support bandages. A person can be taught self-massage to improve carryover of the treatment program. Also, pneumatic compression pumps may help reduce edema in the limbs.

Lymphedema generally requires treatment that continues over a period of time. When the limb is in an inflammatory state, treatment must be ongoing and aggressive to maximally reduce the size of the limb. In time, and if the person avoids repeat injury, the frequency of treatment may lessen. People with lymphedema must be consistent in their management of the condition. Cellulitis (infection in the subcutaneous tissues of the lymphatically impaired limb) may occur; the person should be taught to recognize the urgent need for antibiotic treatment and reassessment with the therapist. Untreated cellulitis can lead rapidly to a systemic infection. Once infection becomes systemic, the person will require hospitalization and intravenous antibiotic treatment. As a prophylactic measure, physicians who treat people with cancer routinely give their patients antibiotic prescriptions for rapid self-treatment when a crisis occurs.

DISEASE PROGRESSION

One long-term condition that can develop as a result of spread of disease or as an after effect of radiation treatment is brachial plexopathy. The most common complaint associated with the development of brachial plexopathy is progressive loss of function in the arm. Patients complain of clumsiness, inability to hold on to objects, and lack of coordination. Brachial plexopathy associated with cancer treatment or disease progression is irreversible. A person with the condition will lose function and mobility of the arm. The extremity can become flail. When mobility and strength remain, adapted techniques can preserve function for as long as possible. Some patients benefit from functional splinting to preserve function; for example, tenodesis splinting (see Chapter 41 for this concept) may be helpful when a patient is motivated to use a splint to support function. When the limb is flail, positioning for protection is crucial. Sensory loss may develop in addition to the motor loss, including loss of protective sensation. Reinforcing safety issues during activity participation can support safe participation in daily tasks and activities.

SUMMARY

OT is beneficial for many people who have cancer. Occupational therapists may encounter cancer patients in inpatient settings, home care, outpatient settings, community-based settings, work settings, and school or early intervention. This area of OT practice is closely aligned with the medical model, since many people who have cancer-related rehabilitation diagnoses have medical qualifiers that affect their participation in OT treatment. Other OT models are also important in addressing quality of life issues.

The most important tools that we have as OT practitioners are (1) our ability to work with our patients beyond the impairment level of disability and (2) our skills as holistic practitioners that allow us to be effective in intervening with people at the activity and participation levels of their occupational abilities. Given the potential side effects of participation in activities, our knowledge of the medical model will enable us in the future to further develop creative and needed interventions for this population—a population for which we need to document and produce intervention outcome data.

CASE STUDY 50-1

CASE STUDY—MARY

Mary is a 35-year-old married woman and mother of three small children. She has recently received a diagnosis of Hodgkin's lymphoma. Her doctor noticed a lump on palpation of her neck during a routine physical examination. Mary has had chemotherapy and is receiving radiation to the mantle region of the right side of her chest. After the second week of 4 weeks of planned radiation treatment, Mary has been experiencing edema and a glovelike distribution of numbness in her right hand (irradiated side). She has received a diagnosis of lymphedema and radiation-induced brachial plexopathy. Mary is a teacher and uses her right hand to write on the board. In her role as a wife and mother, she does all of the shopping, cooking, and cleaning for her family. Mary is also a "soccer mom" and prides herself on the fact that she hasn't missed one of her children's soccer games in 3 years.

On administration of the COPM, Mary voiced concern about being able to drive, to interact with families (since she can no longer shake hands), and to write on the blackboard. Mary is also concerned about being able to do her basic and instrumental (higher-level) activities of daily living. She states that she expects her husband will assist with grocery shopping, but she wants to be able to do the laundry, dress her children, drive, cook, and do light housekeeping.

The Assessment of Motor and Process Skills (AMPS) suggested that Mary needs some assistance to problem solve and implement strategies to compensate for the functional loss in her arm and hand. She is at risk for injuring her arm and hand because of the sensory loss. She could also benefit from training in energy conservation and work simplification. Since Mary is driving primarily with one hand, she could benefit from adapta-

tions to her car that would increase her safety while driving. Table 50-3 provides an analysis of Mary's situation.

At the end of treatment Mary has returned to work. She uses a high stool to teach the class, so that she conserves her energy for activities she will need to do later in the day with her family. Mary has further adapted her workstation (i.e., classroom) by asking her employer to obtain a specialized overhead projector. She now writes on overheads instead of the blackboard. The students like Mary's class—she always uses colors to write and teaches with fun overheads with comics. Mary has explained to the students that she had an injury that prevents her from using her arm and hand, but that she is trying to do all that she did before, using the new adaptations. Mary has received lots of support from the students and the community.

At home, Mary's husband Tom has been doing the shopping and vacuuming. Mary is able to prepare meals, load the dishwasher, and lift her children into her lap from a seated position. She dresses herself independently and needs only occasional help to put on a necklace or a bracelet when she goes out. Mary has learned to take rest breaks and "power naps." She has joined a SHARE support group and reports that she is so grateful for having found new friends and inspiration from the group.

Mary's doctor has informed her that her cancer is now in remission. She will need to see the doctor every 3 months for the next year. She will need to be watched closely for recurrence for the next 5 years, but the doctor is very positive about her response to treatment.

Mary's lymphedema has been contained at a minimal level. She performs self-massage and wears a gradient compression bandage daily. Although she has permanent nerve damage,

TABLE 50-3
Analysis of Case Study of Mary

Occupation	Impairment	Disability	Handicap
Housewife	Loss of bimanual function Fatigue	Inability to use arm in tasks, goal-directed activities, occupations	Mobility and sensory impairment Energy impairment Needs assistance to do tasks that cannot be adapted to single-hand use
Teacher	Loss of bimanual function Fatigue	Inability to stand to write on the blackboard and lecture for more than 10 minutes at a time	Mobility and sensory impairment Energy impairment Needs assistance to do tasks that cannot be adapted to single-hand use
Mother	Loss of bimanual function Fatigue	Inability to lift and hold children unsupported Difficulty zipping winter coats Difficulty fastening (e.g., car seatbelts)	Mobility and sensory impairment Energy impairment Needs assistance to do tasks that cannot be adapted to single-hand use
Wife	Loss of bimanual function Fatigue	Inability to hug husband using two hands Inability to tie her husband's tie for him (a tradition for this couple)	Mobility and sensory impairment Energy impairment Needs assistance to do tasks that cannot be adapted to single-hand use

Continued

CASE STUDY 50-1—cont'd

preventing return of functional use of her hand, Mary states that people are very supportive and comment less and less on her condition. She says that her lymphedema has become "the least of my problems." Mary recognizes the signs of infection and monitors the measurements of her arm weekly, increasing her self-awareness of any changes in the condition. She seems pleased that the edema has become a background issue in her daily life.

Mary states that she continues to be a "soccer Mom." Her second child is now playing in a junior league. She says her participation in occupational therapy has given her a new lease on life. She is grateful to feel in charge of the things that give her life meaning. Although she is sad about the function she has lost, she looks forward to seeing her children grow and spending years to come with her best friend, her husband.

REVIEW QUESTIONS

1. Contrast the role of the OT practitioner in cancer care during the early postdiagnosis phase versus that in the postoperative phase.
2. List and describe side effects of chemotherapy and radiation therapy.
3. Describe how chemotherapy and radiation therapy may affect occupational performance.
4. What are the causes and effects of impaired sensation and cognition during cancer treatment?
5. What are the psychological and social consequences of a diagnosis of cancer? To what extent do you think these can be affected by the patient's attitude and by social support? How can the occupational therapist assist the patient in facing and managing psychological and social challenges?
6. Describe the protocol for managing lymphedema.

REFERENCES

1. Agency for Health Care Policy and Research: Smoking cessation clinical practice guideline, *JAMA* 275(16):1270-1280, 1996.
2. Burkhardt A, Joachim J: Cancers of the bone. In *A therapist's guide to oncology: medical issues affecting management*, San Antonio, Tex, 1996, Therapy Skill Builders.
3. Spiegel D: Effect of psychosocial treatment on survival of patients with metastatic breast cancer, *Lancet* 2(8668):888-891, 1989.

RECOMMENDED READING

Bates SE, Longo DL: Use of serum tumor markers in cancer diagnosis and management, *Semin Oncol* 14:102-138, 1997.

Calibrisi P, Schein PS: *Medical oncology*, New York, 1993, McGraw-Hill.

Dewys WD, Hall TC: Paraneoplastic syndromes. In Rubin P, editor: *Clinical oncology: a multidisciplinary approach for physicians and students*, Philadelphia, 1993, WB Saunders.

Dimeo F, Steiglitz RD, Novelli Fischer U, et al: Correlation between physical performance and fatigue in cancer patients, *Ann Oncol* 8(12):1251-1255, 1997.

RESOURCES FOR CANCER INFORMATION

National Cancer Institute (NCI)
  1-800-4 CANCER
  www.nci.nih.gov
American Cancer Society
  1-800-ACS-2345
  www.cancer.org
American Lung Association
  1-800-LUNG-USA
  www.lungusa.org
Cancer Care, Inc.
  1-800-813-HOPE
  www.cancercare.org
Cancer Hope Network
  1-877-HOPENET
  email: info@cancerhopenetwork.org
  (on-line cancer support groups)
Coping with Cancer Magazine
  615-790-2400
  email: Copingmag@aol.com
Leukemia Society of America
  1-800-955-4LSA
  www.leukemia.org
National Brain Tumor Foundation
  1-800-934-CURE
  www.braintumor.org
National Breast Cancer Coalition (NABCO)
  202-296-7477
  www.natlbcc.org
Support for People with Oral and Head and Neck Cancer, Inc (SPOHNC)
  516-759-5333
  www.spohnc.org
Y-Me
  1-800-221-3141 (24-hour)
  1-800-986-9505 (en Espanol)
  www.y-me.org

CHAPTER 51

Special Needs of the Older Adult

CAROLYN GLOGOSKI

DIANE FOTI

KEY TERMS

Gerontic therapist
Age-related changes
Memory
Top-down approach
Bottom-up approach
Cognitive screening

LEARNING OBJECTIVES

After studying this chapter the student or practitioner will be able to do the following:

1. Describe the aging population of the future in demographic terms.
2. Identify typical patterns of age-related physical changes.
3. Identify typical patterns of age-related cognitive changes.
4. Describe a style of problem solving that may be common to older adults.
5. Identify typical cognitive impairments of an older adult with dementia.
6. Identify common psychiatric conditions of later life.
7. Analyze personal biases in working with the aging person.
8. Identify performance areas and components that require evaluation for the aging adult with a physical disability.
9. Describe how context affects decisions regarding the focus of treatment.
10. Identify how the focus of a novice clinician during evaluation and treatment might differ from that of an expert clinician.
11. Describe how the learning needs and styles of older adults may differ from those of younger persons.

T he reader may wonder why a separate chapter on the treatment of older adults (OAs) is included in a physical dysfunction book. OAs may receive multiple diagnoses, and they often have deficits in several occupational performance areas, performance components, and performance contexts; for these reasons they present complex clinical issues. Occupational therapy (OT) can help OAs continue or resume participation in everyday activities, thus preserving quality of life and a greater sense of well-being for OAs through competency and control over themselves and their environment.[5] Providing quality care to an OA population is one of the most challenging OT practice areas.

Therapists who work with OAs (**gerontic therapists**) select relevant frames of reference and conceptual models of practice.[54] A developmental frame of reference should be the foundation. Gerontic occupational therapists focus on disruptions in the normal maturational processes of OAs in the physical, psychological, and social realms. The aim is to restore order and help OAs adapt whenever pathology has interfered with occupational performance. An understanding of normal human development and the developmental tasks that relate to age-appropriate life roles, living situations, and occupations is a prerequisite for therapists working in this area. Remember that development across the life span does not occur in distinct, hierarchical stages; rather, it is a dynamic and cyclical process accounting for the great variation found in the OA population.

Clinical reasoning for gerontic OT practice is the focus of this chapter. The first section provides information concerning the OA, aging demographics, age-related health changes, pathological conditions, and psychological adaptation; this review aims to prepare the reader for diagnostic[77] and procedural reasoning.[35] Therapists are encouraged to elicit the OA's personal story in developing therapeutic relationships and to use narrative reasoning.[67] Pragmatic reasoning[88] is highlighted so that the reader can better understand the practical realities of service delivery with OAs. The second section of the chapter illustrates the clinical reasoning process as an interactive process[87] through a case study, "Mrs. N."

The goal of this chapter is to help all practitioners, both novice and expert, better appreciate the complexities involved in working with OAs. It is hoped that readers will broaden their perspectives and employ better clinical reasoning and a multidimensional treatment approach to address the OA's physical, psychological, and occupational performance needs.

OLDER ADULT—DEMOGRAPHICS AND CLINICAL REALITIES

The OA population in the next few decades is expected to have an unprecedented effect on our society as a whole—on politics, economics, family life, and the health and human services industry. Increased numbers of OAs will change the practice of OT in the 21st century.

Who Is the Older Adult?

The OA population consists of individuals 65 years of age or older. The population is further divided into "young-old" individuals aged 65 to 74 years, "old-old"

individuals aged 75+ years, and "very old" individuals older than 85 years. Concerns about the aged population that directly and indirectly affect OT practice include the following:

- Greater life expectancy and increased numbers of OAs
- Differences related to gender and living status
- Increasing diversity within the aging population
- Higher prevalence of chronic conditions
- Greater numbers of functional limitations in daily activity
- Higher incidence of cognitive impairment
- Psychosocial issues
- Complex clinical presentations
- Greater demands for health care services
- More demands for alternative supported living and care facilities
- Need for more social supports
- Higher health care cost
- Increased demands for public funding
- Increased out-of-pocket health expenses

Demographics and Implications for Occupational Therapy

The number of OAs will increase in the next three decades. Currently the older population accounts for close to 13% of the total U.S. population but is expected to reach 20% in the year 2030.[4] In 2000 about half of all OAs were 75 years of age or older. The fastest-growing segment of the older population now and in the future is the very old (85+). Currently OAs use over a third of the nation's health care dollars, account for over a third of all hospital stays, and spend three times more of their total personal expenditures on health than do consumers under age 65.

There are more old-old women than men. Old-old women typically are widowed, live alone, and have lower income, especially after age 85.[100] Many OAs, especially women who are childless or whose children are not available, need formal or agency support services. On average, OAs, especially from non-Caucasian households, have a lower yearly income than all other adult groups. Older men, however, are twice as likely to be married. Being married or living with family in later life is associated with higher household income, assistance with activities of daily living (ADL), social support, and reduced risk of institutionalization.

The demographics and needs of the OA population are expected to change in the second and third decades of the 21st century. Parents of current baby boomers are likely to live with or near family and get support from children when they are very old.[34,43] However, as baby boomers reach old-old age, they may want or need more individualized care services and are likely to wield more political power and expect more social services.

They are likely to seek more supported housing alternatives or environmental adaptations to help them live independently.[19]

The OA population is becoming more racially and ethnically diverse, requiring culturally competent therapists, health care professionals, and service agencies. According to 1998 data from the U.S. Census Bureau,[101] minorities make up 15.7% of the 65+ population. The smallest group is Native Alaskans or American Indians, followed by Asian Americans and Hispanics; African Americans comprise the largest segment of this group. The number of OAs of minority race and ethnicity is expected to double by the year 2030. Future consumers of OT services are much more likely to be ethnically different from the OT practitioner providing treatment. Elders from minority racial and ethnic groups have higher rates of poverty, compared with their Caucasian counterparts.[102] Poverty is often a barrier to obtaining quality health care, including OT.

The following factors are relevant in appreciating the diversity of the OA population:

- Each OA's life experience is unique.
- There are different degrees to which a particular OA may identify with an ethnic group and the cultural traditions of that group (acculturation).
- Particular historical events that occurred during specific age periods in the OA's lifetime can be very influential.[109]

Elders of a particular ethnic group may share similar experiences with other same-age elders of that ethnic group (cohort of interest) but differ greatly from elders who have the same ethnicity but are 10 years younger or 10 years older. Sensitivity to these factors can help the therapist better understand the types of discrimination the OA may have experienced and how history, race, and ethnicity can affect health beliefs, values, illness behaviors, self-image, and the degree of trust in and expectations of health care providers.[107] The OA must at all times be seen as a unique and worthy individual, a person who has a special "story of life" and configuration of occupations to share.

Health in Later Life

Improvements in sanitation, standards of living, access to health care, and medical care and technology have contributed to a longer life span. The price of this longevity has been a higher incidence of chronic medical conditions and limitations in daily activities, primarily for the old-old individual.[99] Functional limitations caused by chronic conditions increase with age. Over one third of persons age 65+ identify a chronic condition that imposes some limitation in everyday living, but only 10% report that the limitation affects a major activity. The four most frequently reported medical conditions in later life are arthritis, heart disease, hearing impairments, and orthopedic impairments. Three fourths of the very old identify one disability; more than half identify two or more disabling conditions. Very old adults have twice as many problems with ADL as do young-old adults. Of the very old, 40% also have problems with instrumental activities of daily living (IADL).[99] Despite chronic medical conditions, OAs in general are able to adapt and maintain function until very late in life.

Age-Related Changes

The process of aging is complex and inescapable, with an increased prevalence of degenerative diseases and the physiological decline in several body systems. Researchers question to what extent decline is a "normal" part of aging. Most biological theories can be grouped according to two major suppositions.[34] Some researchers believe that aging is the result of preprogrammed genes containing a master plan that triggers various mechanisms to cause cells to die.[93] Other theorists believe that aging is the result of accumulated cell damage. A number of accidental events occur, involving free-radical damage to genetic material and damage to cell components.[27,34,70,71] Immune system malfunction may cause cell damage and death.[104] Most experts agree that aging involves both programmed genetic changes and accidental events.[80]

Physical Changes

Age-related change, especially in organ systems, varies. A genetic component is partially responsible; other factors include progressive disease processes, environmental factors (e.g., environmental toxins and poverty), and lifestyle behaviors (e.g., smoking, lack of exercise, and poor nutrition) that can be changed or modified. The ability to adapt to changes in the body system and the effect of those changes on everyday activity are highly dependent on the OA's cognitive state, emotional state, social support systems, and basic physiology. Some of the changes identified in the following paragraphs have functional implications, but it is important to remember that the degree of change and effect on function vary greatly.[61,34]

Sensory losses are common. Vision disturbances include less visual acuity under low light conditions, decreased speed in focusing, presbyopia (farsightedness), poorer color discrimination, and cataract formation (with sensitivity to glare and blurring). These changes can affect driving, leisure performance, mobility, and many IADL and ADL.

Hearing discrimination is reduced, especially for high-frequency sounds and for distinguishing words when there is competing background noise. Hearing impairment affects the ability to interact with the environment and communicate effectively with others, leading to increased social isolation, depression, help-lessness, paranoid thoughts, and cognitive decline.

Decreased efficiency of the kidneys in filtering wastes leads to lower thresholds for drug toxicity.[34] Lungs become less elastic and efficient in the exchange of gases; decreased cardiovascular capacity on exertion affects endurance for demanding activity.[34,61] Many elders have decreased bone strength and mass, decreased muscular strength, and less joint flexibility that can impede movement and mobility. Skin becomes less elastic, more wrinkled, and thinner, increasing the risk of skin breakdown, tearing, and infection.

Changes in the central nervous system (CNS) include fewer neurons in select areas of the brain, a decreased number of dendrites, an increased number of amyloid deposits, more plaques, more neurofibrillary tangles, and reduced levels of certain neurotransmitters. These CNS changes in healthy persons are puzzling, since many are seen to a greater degree in dementia. Overall slowing in response time is common. Mild somatosensory changes occur in somatic receptors, in smell, in taste, and in the vestibular system; these can affect sensitivity thresholds and increase the risk of food poisoning, thermal and mechanical injuries, and falls. Minimal age-associated changes also occur in the gastrointestinal system and the immune system.

Cognitive Changes

Changes in cognition in later life may affect ability to function because information processing and problem solving are so vital to safety and independence in ADL. Therapists find that cognitive capacity greatly affects a person's ability to benefit from rehabilitation. A comprehensive discussion of cognitive aging can be found in other references.[62,63,92] Cognition is also discussed in Chapter 27.

Age differences exist in almost all aspects of cognition in healthy OAs, but this difference is not large enough to have serious implications.[46,47,62] Researchers have found that cognitive processing efficiency, especially for information processing and reaction time, is 1.5 times slower in OAs than in middle-aged or young adults.[47]

Loss of **memory** is a concern of many OAs. Memory involves the retention, storage, and retrieval of information. Memory requires adequate attention to sensory-perceptual cues at the initial stages of reception and encoding.[62,92] Age differences have been found in working memory—one component of short-term memory. OAs exhibit poorer efficiency in complex deliberate processing (simultaneously performing a cognitive task while trying to remember the information for a later task) than they do in automatic processing (remembering how to do a performed activity).[48,84,92] OAs also exhibit a decreased ability to inhibit thoughts not relevant to the task.[41] Age-related deficits have been found in the

recall of information, when information is retrieved from secondary (storage) memory levels, and this deficit worsens with advancing age.[26,28,62] However, the overall effects of age differences in memory on daily function are minimal. Most healthy OAs are able to compensate for reduced processing resources by using the context of situations, environmental cues, environmental supports, and rehearsal.

When impaired cognition (especially memory) interferes with relationships, diminishes daily function, or affects quality of life, the causes should be explored. *The Diagnostic and Statistical Manual of Mental Disorders IV*[6] includes the diagnostic category "Age-Related Cognitive Decline." Among the criteria for this diagnosis is a decline in memory that is sufficient to cause distress but that is not a result of dementia. The decline must be within normal limits when the individual is compared to others who are the same age. It has been suggested that dementia may be the endpoint in a continuum of age-related cognitive decline.[15,62] Therapists will encounter varying degrees of cognitive decline in their elderly clients and will need to screen for cognitive impairments and consider cognition a major factor when planning the treatment approach and making interventions. Occupational therapists can make an important contribution in the early detection and monitoring of cognitive decline by regularly assessing mental status on an informal basis during treatment and formally on the initial evaluation.

PATHOLOGICAL CONDITIONS. Pathological conditions may occur in the aged but are not part of normal aging. Dementia is a progressive, degenerative disease process involving short-term memory deficits that occur with increasing frequency in OAs as they age (see the discussion of Alzheimer's disease in Chapter 39). With an increased number of very old, occupational therapists will see greater numbers of OA clients with dementia and severe cognitive processing impairments. Therapists need to recognize cognitive decline and manage the client's performance context so as to compensate for information-processing deficits; this will allow clients to remain in less restrictive settings longer and to have a better quality of life. Allen's Cognitive Disability Model[2] is useful with this population.

Many chronic medical conditions (e.g., hearing loss, cardiovascular disease, severe high blood pressure, diabetes, and painful orthopedic conditions) and some mental disorders (e.g., depression) predict cognitive decline in later life.[31,32,65,75,85,86] These conditions may also be predictive of functional decline.[29] Cognitive decline becomes more substantial with each new medical condition that develops.

Psychological Adaptation

Most people are able to adapt successfully and manage the many transitions occurring in later life. Researchers and clinicians view OAs as proactive individuals who are able to cope with restrictions and prevail over challenging circumstances by continuously developing and recreating themselves.[81] According to research reviewed by Ruth and Coleman,[81] most OAs rate life events encountered in later years as no more stressful than events experienced earlier. The stresses of previous life events do not seem to have a cumulatively negative effect. The majority of OAs seem able to draw on personal and social resources to cope. Interestingly, their coping strategies (e.g., sublimation, suppression, and humor) are often more successful than the strategies (e.g., hostility, denial, and escapist fantasies) used by younger adults.[25,103]

OAs use such coping strategies as considering themselves to be "better off" than OAs who may be doing less well, changing their priorities from goals that seem less attainable to those that are more attainable, and attributing failure to sources outside of themselves.[9,30,42] OAs also generally cope with threats of illness by using more active strategies.[49,78]

The occupational therapist assessing the relative coping abilities of OAs should consider whether the individual's problem-solving skills match demands and resources. Problem-solving skill may be affected by four elements. The first element is the presence of antecedents such as the following:

- Health (both objective and subjective)
- Basic cognitive ability
- Personality characteristics, such as flexibility versus rigidity

The second element is the approach to the problem and the nature of the problem to be solved. Do clients use an active or a passive individual approach? Can clients clearly identify problems and solutions? Is the problem itself well structured or ill structured?

The third element is the presence of contextual demands. Is the sociocultural and physical environment rich and supportive?

The fourth element concerns whether the individual is likely to experience satisfaction and a sense of well-being when the problem is resolved.[106]

When antecedents are not optimal (diminished cognition or avoidance and high anxiety), when the problem is ill structured, or when the environment is deprived, problem solving with an OA can present many challenges.

Many times the problem-solving approaches used by OAs involve quick decision making and the use of solutions that are low in energy demand. This type of problem solving typically involves a very limited information search, uses fewer pieces of information, emphasizes personalized, episodic knowledge about medical problems, and uses a **top-down approach** for processing information.[106] A top-down approach relies almost exclusively on the extensive knowledge and experience of the individual, with limited or no search for

new information.[91] This may mean that little attention is paid to gathering new data or more objective information. To reduce the distress and anxiety caused by the threat of illness, OAs generally are more vigilant about health problems, respond more quickly to health concerns, and make decisions more quickly than middle-aged adults.[58] OT practitioners can show respect for clients by carefully soliciting their opinions during the clinical encounter and by determining the way in which they look at health and solve problems.[108] OT practitioners should devote attention to eliciting an explanation from OAs and care providers on how they view health, health behaviors, their illness experience, its causes, potential consequences, and possible treatment (see Box 51-1). The practitioner can follow up on information from the client by using the LEARN[13] mnemonic strategies (Box 51-2).

BOX 51-1
Key Questions for Patient-Practitioner Dialogue

1. How would you describe the problem that has brought you to me?
2. What do you think is wrong, or what is causing your problem?
3. Why do you think this problem happened to you?
4. Why do you think this problem started off when it did?
5. What do you think your sickness does to you? How does it work?
6. How bad (severe) do you think your illness is? Do you think it will last a long time, or do you think it get better soon?
7. Why did you decide to come to me for treatment?
8. Apart from me, who else do you think can help you get better?
9. What do you think will help clear up your problem?
10. What are the most important results you hope to get from treatment?
11. Are there things that make you feel better or give you relief that the doctors don't know about?
12. Has anyone else helped you with this problem?
    A. What did that person say was wrong with you?
    B. What did that person say you should do for this problem?
    C. Do you agree?
    D. Did you try?
13. What are the chief problems your illness has caused you?
14. Does it cause problems for your family?
15. What worries you most about your sickness?
16. Is there anyone else that you would like me to talk to about your problem?
17. Is there anything else that you would like to discuss?

Data from: Harwood, 1981; Kleinman, Eisenberg, & Good, 1978; Pfifferling, 1981.

BOX 51-2
LEARN Mnemonic

L *Listen* with sympathy and understanding to the patients perceptions.
E *Explain* your perception of the problem.
A *Acknowledge* and discuss the differences and similarities.
R *Recommend* treatment.
N *Negotiate* agreement.

From Berlin EA for Stanford University Division of Family Medicine and the South Bay Area Health Education Center, DHHS Grant Number 5-UO1-PE-00053-04 (date unknown).

Not enough is known about the coping of the institutionalized or frail elder. As people age, they may become more vulnerable to loss of perceived control and may acquire "learned helplessness."[89] This in turn may make them more susceptible to illness.[79] The use of direct coping strategies has been linked to better physical and psychological health, greater responsibility for managing personal health, and cushioning of the ill effects of stress.[22,59,76,105] The use of direct control strategies works well for many OAs in adapting to changes in later life. Gerontic occupational therapists are encouraged to work collaboratively, empowering their OA clients to be active problem solvers. Clark and colleagues[21] have identified several domains of interest and adaptive strategies used by OAs.[59]

Sometimes, OAs find themselves in uncontrollable situations (e.g., eviction from their homes, chronic illness, or loss of driving privileges). In these circumstances OAs might benefit from using coping mechanisms that render such situations more palatable and reduce internal dissonance.[95] The old-old adult may actually adapt best by accepting change, accommodating to negative events, and framing events in a more positive way.[45,53,82] Occupational therapists are in a unique position to help OA clients take some measure of personal control over their everyday lives by collaboratively constructing meaningful routines that can reduce the health risks of older adulthood.[20] OT offers opportunities to take risks, confront obstacles, achieve personal control, and improve self-efficacy. Through therapeutic use of self and other psychosocial interventions, therapists can facilitate clients' management of dissonant or disturbing thoughts and feelings.

PSYCHIATRIC DISORDERS. Approximately 22% of individuals age 65 or older meet the diagnostic criteria for a mental disorder.[38,39] Mental disorders in OAs may be one of the following:
- A continuation or recurrence of a condition that first emerged earlier in the person's life
- A first appearance of a disorder that was already present in a latent form (e.g., a mental health liability from the past that has been exacerbated in old adulthood, as when developmental issues remain unresolved)
- A new mental disorder occurring in later life

Pathological mental conditions often occur in older adulthood because of physiological brain disorders or because of an inability to adapt to changes, losses, and transitions. OAs who have adjusted poorly to stressors in the past, who are overwhelmed by multiple simultaneous stressors, or who have little social support are particularly vulnerable. After cognitive disorders, depression and anxiety are the two most common mental disorders in later life. Alcohol abuse and personality disorders are less common but are still of concern because they further complicate the clinical picture.

Alcohol abuse may be considered a "hidden" disease in later life, since many OAs who drink alcohol, particularly men, do so at home.[60] OAs are more susceptible to the effects of alcohol because of age-related changes such as decreased liver and kidney function and reduced water content and body mass. Many OAs are taking medications, and the concurrent use of alcohol and use or abuse of medications can lead to greater risk of intoxication or toxicity. Substance abuse leads to increased accidents, a greater risk of falls, poorer nutrition, poor hygiene, increased mental health problems (e.g., depression, delirium, dementia, and psychosis), a higher suicide rate, higher risk of disease (e.g., liver disease, cancer, cardiovascular problems, and diabetes), and increased mortality. Physicians do not regularly assess their OA clients about drinking habits and, if drinking is disclosed, may minimize the severity and consequences.[34] The CAGE[33] questionnaire is useful for screening for alcohol abuse. Effective interventions include Alcoholics Anonymous (AA), counseling, psychotherapy, and medications.

Depression is probably the most frequently reported mental disorder in OAs.[38] Although the rate of major depression is relatively low, subclinical depression and symptoms of dysphoria seem to increase with age.[52] The symptoms most frequently reported by OAs are fatigue, difficulty waking in the early morning and trouble returning to sleep, memory complaints, hopelessness, and thoughts about death; reports of sadness or depressed mood are rare.[37,74] Suicide is a risk. Caucasian men aged 60 to 85 years have an increased risk of suicide, especially if they have a medical illness or live alone.[23] Physical illness is a major risk factor.[74]

The incidence of depression in OAs may be higher than reported because of underreporting or lack of recognition.[57] Many health care providers focus on somatic symptoms, linking patient complaints to a succession of physical problems without screening for depression.

Depression may increase the degree of disability associated with several medical conditions and negatively affect rehabilitation outcomes.[68] Depression can also complicate the clinical picture of dementia or may cause complaints and symptoms that are confused with dementia.[75] Depression can have a major influence on the function of OAs in ADL and IADL, especially in social relationships. OAs are not likely to seek treatment for depressive symptoms, perhaps because of myths about aging, lack of access to care, or the need to be strong and minimize their pain. Therapists in all geriatric settings should screen for depressive symptoms in OAs if this is not done by other disciplines. Screening measures include the Geriatric Depression Scale (GDS)[110] and the Beck Depression Inventory (BDI).[9]

Theories abound as to the causes of depression. One theory proposes that depression is biologically caused and may result from medications (toxicity) and certain somatic illnesses. A second theory suggests that depression is really a reaction to the stress of illness or disability. Depression can be treated successfully with medications in most cases. Clients can return to previous energy levels and again take pleasure in life. OT can help clients regain lost occupations, develop pleasurable and health-promoting routines, learn how to reframe events, change nonproductive thinking, develop social contacts, and experience success.

Anxiety disorders are also common in older adults, but this has received much less attention. Anxiety usually begins earlier in life and is rarely seen for the first time in the later years.[14] Anxiety disorders can take various forms:

- Recurring, sudden episodes of intense apprehension with shortness of breath and chest pain (panic disorders)
- Fear and the disproportionate avoidance of a perceived danger (phobic disorder)
- Chronic, persistent, and excessive anxiety (generalized anxiety disorder)[38]

Biologically based explanations for age-related anxiety suggest that it may be associated with changes in neurotransmitters, decreased noradrenergic function, side effects of some medications, and anxiety-like symptoms of medical conditions (e.g., myocardial infarct or pulmonary embolism).[22,94] OAs may in fact have a realistic basis for their anxiety from a psychological perspective as well.[38] It is not uncommon for anxiety to coexist with depression.[50] Anxiety may be related to concerns about pain, safety, memory loss, fear of the unknown, finances, or caregivers. Anxiety may interfere with attention, memory, enjoyment of pleasurable events, social skills, and the ability to begin or follow through with the therapy program. Therapists should routinely assess the client's level of anxiety and determine to what degree anxiety may affect function. Le Barge[56] provides

a scale to evaluate anxiety in clients with mild cognitive impairments.

Personality disorders (PDs) are lifelong, enduring, inflexible and pervasive tendencies that interfere with the individual's functioning and may cause distress. They are characterized by distorted perception, obliviousness to the effects on others, inappropriate emotional outbursts, and difficulty controlling impulsive behaviors.[6] Although PDs do not develop in later life, they may not be noticed until later life, when an initially vulnerable individual becomes increasingly less adaptive.[83] Older adults with PDs may be at greater risk for depression and other disorders in late life.[1] OAs with PDs can be found in all areas of adult practice and provide an interesting challenge. Individuals with certain PDs make some of the greatest demands on the therapist's time and patience and can disrupt the therapist's emotional equilibrium. Therapists who find themselves feeling frustrated, confused, and guilty (or avoiding particular clients) should consult with a knowledgeable colleague and explore what is going on in the client-therapist relationship. Butin[16] provides a useful description of several characterological types and offers some useful suggestions to OT practitioners.

STEREOTYPES OF OLDER ADULTS

Many of the attitudes and values associated with practice in geriatrics are based on stereotypes and personal experiences. Some stereotypes are negative and others positive (Table 51-1). Taken to extremes, stereotypes can influence clinical reasoning. Because the therapeutic relationship is such a powerful change agent, OT practitioners need to assess their varied motives for working in geriatrics and then assess how these motives, attitudes, and values can affect the client, the therapeutic relationship, and the OT process.

The preceding information should frame the following discussion of the occupational therapy process in gerontic practice.

OCCUPATIONAL THERAPY PROCESS

The remainder of this chapter considers the evaluation and treatment process for the OA with a physical disability. Evaluation and treatment are discussed from the perspective of the novice and of the expert clinician. We believe that effective interventions with OAs require the therapist to consider multiple perspectives and a range of variables simultaneously. Hence the clinician must possess abundant common sense and a fair amount of experience and must (in other words) be an expert. A case study of Mrs. Nelson is presented (see Box 51-3 on p. 999) in segments to illustrate key points and to generate questions for the reader to consider.

TABLE 51-1
Stereotypical Thinking Regarding Older Adults

Myth	Reactions of Care Providers	Facts About Aging
Old people are all alike.	Providers may come to the initial evaluation with a preset idea of an older adult that can influence observations and data collected and lower expectations for treatment results.	Elders demonstrate greater heterogeneity than in any other age group; their collection of experiences and different lifestyles make them a very diverse group.
Old people are lonely and ignored by their family.	Providers might not collaborate with the family in the therapy process. They may not explore the older adult's role in the family. They may ignore the elder's desire for more limited socialization and may make plans for the older adult out of pity or a sense that the therapist knows best.	Elders are generally more satisfied than other groups. The majority are in close contact with their families. Most elders are cared for by their family when possible, rather than institutionalized; if they live alone, it is usually by choice.
Old people are senile. Old people can't learn new things.	Providers may use overly simple words and talk down to the older adult. Providers may talk to the caregiver or adult children instead of allowing older adults to make decisions for themselves. Providers may expect the older adults to "prove" their competence and may act as if the older adults cannot give an accurate history. Providers may not make efforts to use educational or teaching methods.	Older adults show slower cognitive response time than younger adults. Confusion and significant memory loss are not a normal part of aging and should be investigated for such causes as dementia, depression, medication toxicity, or other medical problem.
Most older adults are sickly and end up in nursing homes.	Providers may place an emphasis on illness without considering strengths as well. Providers may have lowered expectations for recovery, may not make the therapy situation challenging enough, and may not educate about wellness, prevention, and maintenance.	Only 5% of older adults are institutionalized at any one time. The risk for institutionalization increases with age. Most older adults do not suffer from activity restrictions despite having at least one chronic medical problem when young-old. Most elders report their health to be good when compared with others their age.
Older people are rigid, don't like change, and live in the past.	Providers may negate the usefulness of reminiscing and stop listening. They may stop planning for new activities and stop active planning for the future, may stop providing older adults with information and talk to their children or others instead, and may negate the experiences of older adults as old fashioned and not scientific.	Most likely, rigid older adults were also rigid when they were younger. Personality characteristics remain very stable over time. Elders have a tendency to conserve cognitive energy when making decisions and may give greater credence to experience at the expense of new information for decisions.
Older people are not attractive or sexy.	Providers may view sexual interest as abnormal. They may expect that desire for sex will stop in late life. They may minimize the importance of grooming and dressing attractively. Providers may make no provisions for privacy for sexual activity and may joke about sexual activity or flirtations from older adults.	Desire and ability for sexual functioning alter but with good health sex can remain satisfying and people can remain active into the 10th decade of life.

Adapted from Ferrini AF, Ferrini RL: *Health in the later years*, ed 3, Boston, 2000, McGraw-Hill.

Top-Down or Bottom-Up Approach

Top-down and **bottom-up approaches** are types of information processing and problem solving, ways of thinking and knowing. Overreliance on either has its drawbacks. Novice therapists lack clinical experience and are more likely to acquire knowledge using a bottom-up approach, working with specific and detailed pieces of information. Novices possess fewer technical skills and are usually less able to shift flexibly from theoretical to practical knowledge because so much energy is focused on the acquisition of information.[87] The novice therapist will use recently learned theory and rule-based procedural learning. With this processing style the novice OT practitioner engages in intense data and information collection. The approach to evaluation and treatment is noncontextual, and the novice practitioner has less skill adapting to fit new situations.

The expert clinician is more likely to use a modified top-down approach, blending highly integrated knowledge and extensive experience (top-down) with identification of need to seek further information (bottom-up) when engaging in the OT process. Chapters 3 and 7 provide a further discussion of clinical reasoning.

Evaluation Process

Experts debate the relative merits of a top-down versus a bottom-up approach to evaluation.[55,98] A top-down evaluation gathers information from the OA regarding current and previous function in performance areas. The methods include interviewing and gathering a life history. In contrast, a bottom-up evaluation approach focuses on performance components and then relates deficits and strengths to function in occupational performance. A novice occupational therapist may choose one approach over the other, taking an "either-or" approach. The expert clinician determines which approach will elicit the needed information most expeditiously. The clinician may blend both approaches and will always aim to develop rapport and trust with the client. Consider the referral information for the case study of Mrs. Nelson (Box 51-3).

A therapist using a top-down approach would begin by interviewing Mrs. Nelson to determine her perception of her illness, areas of interest and activities in which she has been involved (performance areas), her prior level of functioning, and her current level of functioning. An evaluation or standardized assessment of

current functioning might follow. The therapist would interview the family about their perceptions of her illness and needs and would encourage them to express their concerns.

A therapist using a bottom-up approach to evaluation would focus on performance components—for example, evaluating joint limitations. The novice may begin an evaluation at this point, since it is clear that Mrs. Nelson has joint limitations. The disadvantage of this approach is that it does not necessarily reveal to what extent and in what ways joint limitations affect function and, ultimately, the client's occupational roles.

Blending of the two approaches (top-down and bottom-up) requires clinical judgment about how best to develop rapport with the client. Starting the evaluation with performance components while explaining how the results relate to function may be most acceptable to a client who is guarded regarding his personal life and who is very task oriented. On the other hand, beginning with a open question such as, "Tell me what a typical day is like for you," or, "Please tell me how this sickness has affected you and your family," may be more effective for other clients. For example, a client who is uncomfortable being touched, who dislikes the feeling of being "tested," or who has a different cultural perspective might be more comfortable with a top-down approach than with an initial evaluation of performance components. The skillful OT practitioner considers all performance components but uses seasoned observation skills to determine which key performance components should be evaluated.

Prior Level of Function

When working with a younger population with newly acquired physical disability, the occupational therapist may assume the client was independent, active, and healthy before the injury or illness. The typical OA will have a more complex clinical picture, sometimes with multiple chronic conditions (multichronicity) in addition to the main diagnosis. The novice clinician may focus on the newly acquired disability and not consider how other age-related changes, pathological conditions, or the performance context affect function. The expert clinician evaluates for age-related changes, gathers pertinent history of prior pathological conditions, and considers the potential effect. An objective evaluation in conjunction with a medical history and interview with the client and significant others will provide the clinician with the most accurate information about the OA's prior functional level.

Therapists must guard against stereotypical thinking that may lead to erroneous beliefs. For example, a lengthy medical history with multiple diagnoses may conjure up visions of a very limited OA, when in fact the person is quite active. Conversely, the OA client with a newly acquired physical disability, no prior

BOX 51-3
Case of Mrs. Nelson—Referral Information

Mrs. Nelson is a 73-year-old woman admitted to a skilled nursing facility because of a decline in functional status and multiple falls. Mrs. Nelson has rheumatoid arthritis in the upper and lower extremities. She lives with her 40-year-old daughter, her son-in law, and her 10-year-old granddaughter. Her family would like her to return home, but she needs to be safe and independent during the day, when she is alone from 8 AM to 3:30 PM. Her family has expressed concern about her safety in mobility and in meal preparation that involves the use of heated appliances. She was referred to occupational therapy for ADL retraining and safety concerns.

medical history, and minor age-related changes may provide a history that is more limited in activities than the therapist might anticipate.

Performance Context

During the evaluation process the occupational therapist must take into consideration the performance context, including the temporal aspects and the physical, social, and cultural environment. The OA's social, cultural, and physical context affects the degree and type of involvement in performance areas and so is discussed first in the evaluation process.

SOCIAL AND CULTURAL ENVIRONMENT. A person's perception of the aging process, disease, and disability is filtered through the lenses of social and cultural expectations and beliefs. During the interview the occupational therapist asks questions to elicit the OA's views of disability (Box 51-3). Asking open-ended questions demonstrates respect and allows the client to express concerns, ideas, and beliefs; in turn, this gives the therapist a clearer sense of the client's knowledge, values, stereotypes, and motivations.

For example, the therapist observed that Mrs. Nelson (Box 51-3) was sitting and having family members wait on her, when she could help herself. By talking with Mrs. Nelson, the therapist learned that she had cared for her own mother after her mother had experienced several episodes of falling. Mrs. Nelson's mother had progressively declined and was dependent on family members. Mrs. Nelson, unlike her mother, is recovering and improving with treatment and has the potential to be independent from a wheelchair. However, Mrs. Nelson's perception that aging means that an individual does not "recover" and will always need assistance prevents her from imagining the possibility of her own independence. The occupational therapist will need to work carefully with Mrs. Nelson to help her see the progress she is making and identify with other OAs she has known who have recovered from an illness. Additional aspects to consider are the secondary gains Mrs. Nelson realizes from her daughter's attention. The therapist may explore how this attention could be given in other ways.

The OT practitioner must cautiously examine the notion of independence, which is not equally valued by all cultures. The practitioner must consider how to frame the treatment approach so as to best collaborate with the client and family and incorporate their cultural beliefs into the treatment plan. This initially involves listening closely to the family's beliefs and concerns and may involve educating the family about the client's condition and teaching family members how to assist the older client more effectively.

Cultural and social expectations are particularly evident in ADL. Some examples of respectful considera-

tion are being aware of the client's needs for privacy, since culture may dictate issues (gender or age restrictions) regarding private functions, and respecting the decision of which family members are allowed to assist an individual with dressing or bathing. It is important to show sensitivity regarding the type of socially or culturally appropriate clothing that is selected by the OA. The therapist should also be aware of the client's religious or cultural dietary restrictions and traditions for food preparation and consumption, such as vegetarianism or keeping kosher.

Religious or spiritual needs may affect the OA's treatment goals and motivation. Mrs. Rajiv, a client with severe rheumatoid arthritis, had the habit of praying on her knees at the altar in her home every morning for 1 hour. As her arthritis progressed, this became more difficult, but she insisted that it was important to her. The occupational therapist worked with the physical therapist and the family to modify the area where she kneeled so that she had adequate handholds to pull herself up into a chair after her prayer. Kneeling was a meaningful part of her religious occupation, but it occurred at great cost because it prevented Mrs. Rajiv from being able to do other activities at the end of the day. However, she felt it was one of her most important activities.

A fine balance must be maintained in evaluating and considering cultural and social values with people of diverse backgrounds. The therapist must avoid ethnocentric thinking and stereotyping of individuals. The OT practitioner must be sensitive to the degree of acculturation of each person. Even with awareness of cultural diversity, the practitioner must also be sensitive to the uniqueness and the particular value system of each client.

PHYSICAL ENVIRONMENT. The appropriate physical environment may significantly improve the OA's functioning. The evaluation should elicit information about the environment to which the OA will be discharged. If possible, a predischarge home evaluation may be completed by the occupational therapist. In many cases this is not a reimbursable service, so the occupational therapist must work closely with family members to explore potential obstacles in the home environment and determine needed equipment or modifications by interview rather than direct observation. Home evaluations entail consideration not only of the newly acquired physical disability, but also of existing and predicted age-related changes. The evaluation should consider safety and home modifications to promote independent functioning, considering not only the OA's physical deficits but also any sensory or cognitive deficits. Before continuing further, consider the evaluation results for Mrs. Nelson, as reported in Box 51-4.

BOX 51-4
Case of Mrs. Nelson—Occupational Therapy Evaluation Summary

Mrs. Nelson needs minimal verbal cues and moderate physical assistance to initiate bathing and dressing. She needs maximum assistance with brushing and washing her hair. She ambulates with moderate assistance while using a walker. She is unable to lift either leg more than 2 inches off the ground when standing. She is independent in propelling her manual wheelchair on smooth surfaces, with effort. She neglects to lock her brakes 30% of the time. The interview with Mrs. Nelson revealed that she is motivated to return home and receptive to new methods of performing her previous activities. She reported that she has not learned to do meal preparation from the wheelchair but needs to be able to do so in order to prepare her lunch. The occupations she identified as important to her include reading, paying her personal bills, and socializing with her daughter's family and other extended family.

The following deficits were noted during the evaluation: limited bilateral shoulder AROM to 60° of flexion; PROM of bilateral shoulders was full, with generalized weakness in bilateral hand grasp and pinch with arthritic deformities. A gross evaluation of AROM of trunk and lower extremity function showed she is unable to reach down beyond her knees or cross a foot over the opposite knee. A mild visual impairment is present and is corrected with glasses, and a mild hearing loss was reported.

A predischarge home evaluation was completed by the occupational therapist with a family member present. There are four steps to enter the house, measuring a total of 27 inches. The bathroom has a tub-shower combination with glass shower doors. The toilet sits in the corner of the bathroom, separate from the sink or any other surfaces that could be used for support to stand. There is only one bathroom in the house.

Mrs. Nelson complains of feeling "blue" much of the time. She notes forgetfulness and problems with concentration at times. During the beginning of the session, she provides an update of current aches and pains. Conversation is focused on the recent deaths of friends and upcoming birthdays of family members. She is consistently prepared for occupational therapy treatment and rarely forgets the time of a scheduled session. She wheels herself to all physical therapy treatments and is generally prompt.

The therapist must analyze the fit or interaction between person and environment. In the case of Mrs. Nelson, her mild hearing loss may affect her ability to hear the doorbell or a timer set to remind her to take her medication. Visual losses may limit her ability to read without her glasses the keys on the phone pad, emergency phone numbers, or the temperature settings on the oven. The occupational therapist will keep in mind Mrs. Nelson's forgetfulness and consider how the home environment may either exacerbate or compensate for memory deficits.

Much about the home and its effects on Mrs. Nelson's ability to function has not been reported. For example, a neat and structured home environment will provide external structure and improve her ability to function. A specific area for Mrs. Nelson to organize her personal items, such as eyeglasses, cordless phone, bills, memory notebook, and reading material, may reduce or eliminate her need to search for these items. Conversely, a cluttered and disorganized home may contribute to her confusion, increase her anxiety, and limit her ability to compensate for sensory and cognitive deficits.

Mrs. Nelson has preexisting arthritic deformities in her hands; therefore the occupational therapist needs to be sure that she can manipulate doorknobs and has access to various rooms in the house. Because Mrs. Nelson shares the home with three other people, the recommendations for bathroom modifications must also meet the needs of the other family members. Such modifications should allow the easy removal and replacement of any equipment so that all family members may use the facilities. Table 51-2 includes an example of a problem list, suggests recommendations for adaptations, and highlights additional areas to be evaluated during a home evaluation specific to the case study of Mrs. Nelson.

Novice clinicians have the tendency to focus primarily on current problems and may not used a blended approach (i.e., both top-down and bottom-up) that considers the interaction of age-related problems, preexisting deficits, and current problems in thinking about how the OA will function in the discharge environment. A more sophisticated approach is to help the family prioritize the list of recommendations for home modifications. The expert clinician consistently attempts to consider all of the relevant factors in the client's performance context and the effect recommendations may have on both the client and the family.

Evaluation of Performance Areas
The therapist will want to determine the importance the individual places on the three different performance areas: ADL, work and productive activities (home management), and leisure activities. Methods of evaluation may include interviews and performance-based observations and assessments. Both the OA and any significant others should, at some point, participate in the interview. The roles of each person in interrelationships in ADL, home management, or leisure must be considered.

Performance-based evaluations may involve both a standardized assessment and loosely structured observation. A standardized assessment will permit comparing the individual's results with some objective standard. The validity of each assessment should be considered. Among the many resources for assessment

TABLE 51-2

Home Modifications Specific to Case Study for Mrs. Nelson

Problem	Recommendation	Alternative Recommendations
Four stairs into home	Ramp or electric lift	Emergency call system in place
Tub-shower combination	Transfer tub bench	Sponge bath
Glass doors on shower	Remove and replace with shower curtain	Sponge bath
No grab bars in shower	Grab bar installed for easy reach and circumference small enough to fit client's hand	Sponge bath
No grab bars beside toilet	Place commode over toilet	Install grab bars and raised toilet seat to be easily removed by family members Use commode in bedroom and caregiver will empty

Other areas to consider for home evaluation while considering age-related changes, preexisting deficits, and current deficits:
- Location of medications and lighting available to read medications
- Personal space to organize bills, medications, mail, and reading material; evaluate ability to work from wheelchair and evaluate lighting for reading
- Pathway clearance for wheelchair (clear of rugs, furniture, and clutter)
- Nonskid rug outside of shower
- Shower mat and shower hose
- Accessibility of appliances in kitchen from a wheelchair
- Accessible counter to work from a wheelchair
- Functioning smoke or fire alarms
- Telephone access from all rooms
- Calendar within reach and view
- Type of door knobs
- Height of light switches (Mrs. Nelson has difficulty reaching)
- Location of clothing

---

are Asher's[7] *An Annotated Index of Occupational Therapy Evaluation Tools*, Lewis's[64] *Elder Care in OT*, and Beech and Harding's[10] *Assessment of the Elderly*.

Optimally, the evaluation is completed in the same context (time of day and physical environment) in which the OA will be functioning. A matched context allows the OA to use environmental cues to facilitate performance. This is particularly important for OAs with cognitive, perceptual, or sensory deficits. Such individuals typically develop compensatory strategies within their living environment that allow them to function independently. When removed from their living environment, they become more dependent.

Returning to the example of Mrs. Nelson, we recall that she is residing temporarily at a skilled nursing facility. The occupational therapist may choose to evaluate her in her room rather than in the clinic. Mrs. Nelson will then be able to demonstrate how she is managing within the environment where she bathes and dresses daily. Generalization of skills should be more effective if practiced in the environment where she will typically perform these activities.

ACTIVITIES OF DAILY LIVING. The initial evaluation of ADL must consider the mental and physical fatigue of the client, as well as time constraints placed on the therapist, and therefore may not include all aspects of self-care. It is not unusual for a novice therapist to attempt to evaluate all aspects of ADL, perhaps following an ADL checklist from top to bottom without regard for the client's needs. The expert clinician is able to select a few key ADL from the checklist, or alternately to select a key standardized assessment that covers an array of tasks in an efficient manner. The information gathered from a performance evaluation produces data concerning functional activities and abilities and limitations of some performance components. Consider the information gathered from the initial evaluation for Mrs. Nelson, summarized in the following section from the data in Box 51-4.

ACTIVITIES OF DAILY LIVING (DRESSING AND GROOMING)
Results of Performance Evaluation
- Minimal verbal cues needed to initiate dressing
- Moderate physical assistance needed with dressing
- Maximum assistance needed with brushing hair

Discussion of Evaluation Methods, and Interpretation, With Implications. The occupational therapist asked Mrs. Nelson to perform selected dressing tasks—specifically, to don a sweater and comb her hair. This allows assessment of upper extremity function, visuospatial ability, and cognitive abilities. Mrs. Nelson was also asked to don her shoes, for assessment of application of trunk mobility, balance, lower extremity range of motion, and fine and gross upper extremity dexterity. Mrs. Nelson needed minimal verbal cues to initiate dressing, which may indicate the need for a more comprehensive cognitive assessment and evaluation of safety with IADL to determine whether Mrs. Nelson's difficulty with initiation may affect other more complex activities.

ACTIVITIES OF DAILY LIVING (FUNCTIONAL MOBILITY)
Results of Performance Evaluation
- Use of walker with moderate assistance
- Independent with propelling manual wheelchair
- Neglected to lock wheelchair brakes 30% of the time

Discussion and Interpretation of Evaluation Methods, With Implications. Mrs. Nelson was instructed to transfer to the bed and to retrieve a sweater from the closet, using her wheelchair. She was also asked to ambulate with a walker to the bathroom (to assess application of balance, memory for setup of wheelchair and location of clothing, endurance for ambulation with walker and wheelchair, and ability to problem solve how to retrieve a hanging sweater from a seated position). Behaviors related to wheelchair safety were observed in all of these activities. Inconsistent locking of the wheelchair brakes is another indication of the need for further cognitive assessment.

Since Mrs. Nelson had a history of falls, an evaluation of the fall history is appropriate. A falls interview schedule[12] is one way to look for patterns. The cause of Mrs. Nelson's falls could be intrinsic (e.g., dizziness) or extrinsic (e.g., a cluttered hallway).[24] A falls interview will help identify the problem(s) and facilitate a safe discharge home.

ACTIVITIES OF DAILY LIVING (WASHING AND BATHING)
Results of Performance Evaluation
- Assistance needed with bathing
- Maximum assistance needed to wash hair

Discussion and Interpretation of Evaluation Methods, With Implications. The therapist was unable to complete bathing evaluation during the initial session, but from observation of dressing and functional mobility and from the interview, the therapist can make a reasonable judgment regarding Mrs. Nelson's level of functioning with bathing. The occupational therapist uses activity analysis skills to compare the task of hair washing (which was not actually performed by Mrs. Nelson) with the skills required for hair brushing, which was evaluated and found to require maximum assistance.

OCCUPATIONAL PERFORMANCE IN GENERAL
Information Gathered Strictly From Interview
- Client wants to return home.
- Client is motivated to learn new techniques.
- Client identifies valued and necessary occupations, including reading, paying bills, socializing, and preparing meals.

The expert therapist will make indirect observations from the client's behavior and ability to converse. These observations suggest her motivation and concerns, aspects of performance that are not readily apparent during a structured evaluation. Consider the following observations from Box 51-4.

Information Gathered From Observation
- Patient complains of feeling "blue."
- Patient reports being forgetful and having difficulty concentrating.
- Patient focuses on recent deaths and birthdays of family members.
- Patient is punctual in arriving for OT and PT treatments.

Discussion and Interpretation of Evaluation Methods, With Implications. As discussed earlier, depressive symptoms and cognitive deficits are often seen in the OA and affect the treatment process. The observations listed in the preceding sections give an indication that Mrs. Nelson may be experiencing a cognitive deficit or an episode of depression, but these observations do not provide adequate information to support a diagnosis or to distinguish between the two.

Mrs. Nelson's memory complaints, somatic complaints, complaints of feeling blue, and thoughts about dead friends should be queried further. Such measures as the Geriatric Depression Scale[110] are useful in assessing the likelihood of depression, but they should be accompanied by a question about suicidal thoughts. The Beck Depression Inventory (BDI)[9] is useful in assessing depression, suicidal thought, and hopelessness but is sometimes challenging for cognitively impaired OAs. An assessment that screens for memory and concentration can be useful in determining if problems in these cognitive skills are symptoms of depression or evidence of brain impairment such as dementia. Determining baseline mood and talking to the family are important. The fact that Mrs. Nelson attends all therapy sessions promptly indicates that given the appropriate motivation, she is able to remember desirable activities, or that she has developed compensatory strategies to ensure her prompt arrival to therapy. The novice therapist may listen to Mrs. Nelson's concerns but readily dismiss them as situational, a normal part of aging, or not unusual, since Mrs. Nelson is in a skilled nursing facility when she would rather be home. The novice therapist may not recognize the inconsistency between apparent impaired memory and concentration (either of which may be a sign of a cognitive deficit or a symptom of depression) and a behavior that indicates adequate prospective memory (e.g., arriving on time for therapy). The expert therapist will consider performing a screening for depression and a brief screening for cognitive deficits. The expert therapist may also explore environmental cues and attempt to identify Mrs. Nelson's time management strategy. For example, it is possible that Mrs. Nelson uses one or more of the following strategies:

■ Asking the physical therapist to stop by each morning to remind her of her appointment time

■ Asking the nursing aide to write the appointment time on her calendar

■ Using rehearsal to retain appointment information from the previous day by repeating the time over and over, to ensure storage in long-term memory

■ Waiting at the nurses' station and asking the nurse frequently, "Is it time for therapy?"

Determining Mrs. Nelson's strategy will provide insight into how she compensates for what appears to be a memory deficit. If effective, this strategy may be used with other activities.

In summary, ADL are evaluated selectively through observation, standardized assessment, and interview. The occupational therapist is selective regarding activities evaluated, so as to avoid fatiguing the OA mentally or physically.

WORK AND PRODUCTIVE ACTIVITIES. Work and productive activities include home management, care of others, educational activities, and vocational and volunteer activities. Depending on an OA's social and cultural background, roles may be well established in each of these areas or may be very limited. Interviews with the OA, partner, or family member will provide needed information regarding the client's previous involvement with work and productive activities. With a newly acquired disability, compounded by age-related changes, some OAs may be unable to resume their previous roles fully but able to assume a modified role. The occupational therapist may provide instruction to the caregiver and OA regarding how to modify an activity and may educate them about the importance of maintaining involvement and a role in the family. Consider referring information (Box 51-3) from the case study of Mrs. Nelson again.

The goals Mrs. Nelson and her family have identified involve independence with meal preparation so that she can prepare lunch and be safe when home alone. The occupational therapist may also want to explore Mrs. Nelson's role with her 10-year-old granddaughter. De-

pending on interest, Mrs. Nelson may be able to assist with and supervise her granddaughter's homework, given an appropriate setup that allows her to compensate for decreased vision and hearing loss. The granddaughter and Mrs. Nelson could sit down at a well-lit kitchen table with background noise eliminated (the television and stereo turned off) so as to minimize distraction. Alternatively, Mrs. Nelson's involvement with her granddaughter could be less structured, with both of them sharing reading time and with each reading a portion of the book each day.

PLAY OR LEISURE ACTIVITIES. An activity checklist helps determine which of the client's interests are a priority for treatment. Baum's[8] Activity Profile or the Interest Checklist[66] may be useful for this purpose. For a list of leisure activity evaluations, refer to Chapter 18.

In addition to identifying the OA's leisure interests, the evaluation should determine any factors that have restricted the OA from participating in these activities. Many obstacles (e.g., sensory impairments, incontinence, community barriers, lack of transportation, and poor endurance) may limit an individual's participation in leisure activities. Low vision may limit reading or needlework, hearing loss may limit socialization, and incontinence or difficulty with transfers may limit outings in the community. The inability to lift a wheelchair into the car or low endurance for ambulating long distances may limit return to leisure activities. Once the problem is identified, removal of barriers to leisure participation may become a treatment goal.

Evaluation of Performance Components

The therapist evaluating the OA must consider how the performance components interact and how age-related physical and mental changes affect the testing situation and the assessment results. Assessments must have normative data on OAs; if they do not, the results should be viewed cautiously. It is also important to consider each person's motivation, degree of effort expended (Was best effort given that day?), and understanding and valuing of the test.

SENSORIMOTOR COMPONENTS. When assessing sensorimotor components, the therapist must consider what changes have occurred as a result of the normal aging process, concurrent disease processes, or newly acquired disability. Sensory impairments in vision or auditory function will shape the mode of teaching. For the client with visual deficits, the practitioner may need to consider lighting, text size of written instructions, and other aspects of the environmental setup to promote a return to previous activities.[55] Visual acuity, depth perception, visual tracking, and visual fields should all be assessed. Vision impairment is experienced by 15% of the population over age 65, and the incidence increases with age.[72] Because many eye diseases have an insidious onset, the OA may be unaware of losses in visual fields, depth perception, or visual acuity. Therefore the evaluation should consider what deficits the OA has, as well as their potential impact on function (see also Chapter 24). Hearing should be briefly assessed, since the OA may not notify the therapist of problems. If auditory deficits are not identified, a client's inability to follow directions may be mislabeled as a cognitive deficit.

The OA should be screened for tactile and proprioceptive deficits. Preexisting conditions may result in an impairment of which the client is unaware. For example, a client who has recently had a total hip replacement may report frequently dropping items. After further discussion the client might remember having previously received a diagnosis of carpal tunnel syndrome. The expert clinician will do a quick initial screening to determine the status of sensation in the hands and lower extremities because a sensory deficit may affect the client's ability to handle adaptive equipment adequately or may require justification for extra treatment time to compensate for sensory deficits.

Perceptual and cognitive deficits create or contribute to safety issues and frequently determine whether the OA is able to remain at home alone. Perceptual processing may be evaluated with a combination of functional activities and standardized assessments. When evaluating perception the practitioner needs to explain to the client and the family what is being evaluated and connect the evaluation to everyday activities. Family members frequently observe peculiar behaviors (e.g., misjudging where to sit, how to don a shirt, or where to find the toothpaste) but are unable to identify the exact problem or cause. Once family members and the OA understand that some of the difficulties observed are the result of specific perceptual deficits, the family members are more likely to comply with compensatory strategies and safety recommendations.

Neuromusculoskeletal evaluation methods are discussed in depth in previous chapters. In relation to the OA the occupational therapist once again needs to consider preexisting conditions and age-related problems when considering remediation for any deficits in this area. The following information about Mrs. Nelson is given in Box 51-4.

Deficits Noted

- Limited strength in shoulders bilaterally as noted with discrepancy of PROM and AROM
- Generalized weakness in grasp and pinch strength
- Arthritic deformities in the hands
- Limited ROM in trunk and lower extremity flexion and hip external rotation

Discussion and Interpretation of Evaluation Methods, With Implications. The novice may measure all joints

with a goniometer and perform a complete formal muscle test to determine deficits. The expert clinician will do a functional range of motion test (reach above head, behind back, to knees, to toes, make fist, open hand, touch thumb to each finger) and a gross muscle test. The expert clinician will determine how long the deficits have been present and will estimate the effect on function (as noted in the evaluation of performance areas). The expert will try to understand how the disease process of rheumatoid arthritis has affected Mrs. Nelson and what the pattern of the disease has been like.

Postural control may be assessed on a functional basis during activities of daily living and as described earlier with a falls questionnaire.

Soft-tissue integrity is often compromised in the frail OA. The normal aging process, medications (e.g., steroids), incontinence, and immobility all compromise the integrity of the skin. The occupational therapist can use activity analysis to determine sources of skin breakdown. Seating surfaces, bed mattresses, pressure relief techniques and habits, and transfer methods may contribute to skin breakdown.

Screening of oral-motor control is appropriate for the OA. Neurological impairments, changes in dentition, and changes in muscle strength may impair swallowing,[11] placing the OA at risk for inadequate nutrition and aspiration. The OA may also have a preexisting compromised respiratory status, with increased risk for respiratory infection, justifying the time it may take to screen for oral-motor and swallow deficits. Chapter 40 gives specific evaluation methods.

COGNITIVE COMPONENTS. Intact cognition is essential for maintaining independence and autonomy in later life. The clinician's approach to the evaluation of cognitive components in OAs is influenced by several factors:

1. What is the therapist's frame of reference for understanding cognition as it influences occupation? Does the therapist come from a dynamic interaction approach,[95] a cognitive disability model,[2] or a perceptual-motor or deficit-specific approach?[90]

2. What are the client's individual characteristics? When the therapist evaluates older adults, a framework should be maintained that considers the possibility of age-related physical and mental changes (e.g., slowed response, lack of a hearing aid, or forgotten glasses) that may influence the assessment responses, as well as the availability of normative data for OAs on the particular assessment. The clinician may also want to consider the possible influences of culture and ethnicity, as well as motivation and the degree of effort the OA expended in doing the assessment. (Was it important to the OA, and did the OA see it as worthwhile?)

3. What are the questions the therapist wants to answer? Does the therapist need to gather baseline data, identify specific cognitive impairments, understand how impairments affect functional performance, or measure change in the client?

Toglia's[96] Dynamic Interaction Approach proposes that cognition is a dynamic interaction between the internal and external. The therapist should analyze and assess the interaction between the environment (physical aspects, multiple contexts, culture, and familiarity), individual processing strategies and personal characteristics (type of approach to processing information and the skills of self-assessment, self-awareness, problem recognition, problem solving, and self-monitoring), and task demands (complexity, number of decisions, spatial arrangement, and familiarity). Toglia's approach is not designed to assess a particular cognitive component or functional performance area. Rather, this approach is dynamic and offers information on interactions between individual characteristics, cognitive strategies used to perform tasks, and differing conditions that influence task performance.

Allen's[2] Cognitive Disability Model is an information-processing model that estimates the quality of the information-processing abilities of clients. Assessments identify the level and range of sensory cues that are needed to capture attention (input), the quality and type of sensorimotor associations that are intact (throughput), and the type of verbal and motor behavioral responses produced (output). This information is then related to the capacity of the person to perform functional activity safely and effectively. Six hierarchical cognitive levels are defined, and the client is assessed as functioning at a particular level of cognitive ability. This helps the clinician identify the environmental modification needed within the structure of level-specific activity. The goal is to make use of capacities and compensate for limits by providing activity at the appropriate level of the client's performance capacity. Assessments used with this model are standardized and include the Allen Cognitive Level (ACL)[3] test (leather lacing assessment) and the Large Allen Cognitive Level (LACL), an enlarged version for older adults.[97] Much has been written, and research has been done, on the usefulness of this model and assessment with older adults, especially those with dementia.[62,63]

The deficit-specific approach[90] identifies cognitive impairments by testing specific cognitive skills on a variety of cognitive tests. The cognitive skills include attention, orientation, registration of information, short-term memory, concentration, calculation, language (repetition, naming, and written and oral communication), ability to follow multistep directions, and praxis. These tests can measure some of the cognitive components and can be helpful in activity analysis and selection of activities for a client. Other cognitive components (e.g., arousal, initiation and termination of activity, sequencing, spatial operations, problem solving, generalization,

and concept formation) can be assessed through interview, observation of task performance, and other measures.[7] Some of the tests, such as psychometric and neuropsychological tests, have been "borrowed" from other disciplines. Many have been standardized and have normative data for older adults. Mental status measures, which really measure the cognitive portion of a much longer mental status assessment, include assessments such as the Mini-Mental State Exam (MMSE)[36] and the Short Portable Mental Status Questionnaire (SPMSQ).[73] These assessments are helpful as screening measures to quickly determine the possibility of dementia and possible deficits in cognitive components that can then be assessed in greater depth. These measures also serve to establish a baseline in cognitive function and can then be used grossly to measure change over time. Premorbid educational level is important; limited fluency with English can affect cutoff scores.

A measure that provides more in-depth **cognitive screening** without a large time expenditure is the COGNISTAT.[69] Unfortunately, assessing a cognitive component in isolation may not be useful in addressing concerns about impaired performance in functional activities.

PSYCHOSOCIAL SKILLS AND PSYCHOLOGICAL COMPONENTS. The OA's values, interests, and self-concept have been shaped by a lifetime of living and are certainly affected by all aspects (especially the temporal and environmental) of the performance context. Activities such as the life review process[17,18] or reminiscence may help the therapist learn about the individual's values, self-concept, and self-expressiveness. Depending on the affective nature of the information obtained, opportunities may be presented to assess coping skills, coping styles, and self-control. Eliciting stories about family, children, and friends provides information on the OA's perception of social relationships and interpersonal skills. Social and interpersonal aspects may also be observed in therapist-family interaction and in groups, by interviewing the family and care providers, and by watching task performance in a group, family, or one-to-one setting.

The language of Uniform Terminology[5] does not explicitly identify psychiatric symptoms and signs, the components of mental status that are important in detecting and monitoring mental disorders. The therapist must nonetheless be able to recognize disturbances in mood or affect (e.g., sad, anxious, irritable, or fatigued), suicidal or homicidal thoughts, disturbed thought content or processes, preoccupation, or substance use. These factors may significantly affect function and treatment compliance.

Questions about suicide must be asked directly; it is not possible to be indirect.[40] If the client is making veiled statements about ending his or her life, this cannot be ignored. The client must be asked, "Are you having thoughts of killing yourself?" Questions should be asked about frequency of the thoughts, intensity, specifics of a plan, access to means, and intention. The physician or a licensed mental health professional must then be contacted. A history of previous suicide attempts, family suicide, complaints of great pain, chronic illness, psychotic thoughts, and substance use are additional risk factors for suicide.

Determining Client's Prognosis (Potential)

The occupational therapist needs to estimate the client's likely potential to benefit from OT intervention; this is essential before setting realistic goals in collaboration with the client. The process of determining a client's potential is complex and requires consideration of many different factors. Some of these are the therapist's knowledge base and previous clinical experience, results of the OA's evaluation, and input from other health professionals treating the client. The occupational therapist compares the identified deficits with the client's past level of function, considering the client's level of motivation, social support, severity of deficits, history of recovery, emotional and psychological status, and the presence and degree of cognitive and perceptual deficits. If the potential cannot be determined immediately, the therapist provides a trial of therapy to see if the OA is able to make progress. The therapist is then better able to project what the client's status will be at the end of a given length of treatment and can justify ongoing treatment.

Determining potential is a complex process. The therapist must consider the OA's learning potential, determine the degree of motivation as affected by social and cultural context, and judge the severity of the physical deficits in relation to functional deficits. All these are considered within the larger context of age-related changes to be expected in the future.

Look again at the case of Mrs. Nelson (Boxes 51-3 and 51-4). The following questions may be considered in determining her potential for improvement:

- Will she be able to use the walker eventually without supervision?
- Will she learn to lock her wheelchair brakes consistently?
- To what extent can she improve her upper extremity strength?
- Can she improve on her limitations in upper and lower extremity range of motion sufficiently for independent dressing and bathing?
- Will she be able to learn how to cook from a wheelchair?
- Is she able to learn to use adaptive equipment?
- Are her depressive symptoms a chronic condition, and do they interfere (and to what extent) with optimal functional performance?

- Will she be able to continue to cope with future age- or disease-related physical and mental health changes?
- How does she imagine her life story changing as her abilities change and she grows older?
- Have she and her family looked at both the near and far future in terms of her functioning, care, and living situation with the family?

Mrs. Nelson is highly motivated. Her family has a desire to bring her home, and she is willing to modify her activities by doing meal preparation from a wheelchair. It is still not clear whether her memory problems are related to depression or to a cognitive deficit and whether she is able to compensate for the problems. This requires further evaluation and a trial of treatment to evaluate progress.

The occupational therapist may share evaluation results with other professionals to get a broader perspective. In Mrs. Nelson's case the occupational therapist may speak to the physical therapist regarding the client's potential to improve ambulation with the walker. The occupational therapist will discuss with the physical therapist the potential cognitive deficits that may affect safety and function.

Neuromusculoskeletal deficits should be approached cautiously because the joint limitations are of long standing. The hand deformities and duration of preexisting deficits suggest that OT treatment is unlikely to improve ROM; therefore compensatory strategies may be implemented. A gentle strengthening program may be appropriate if the client is motivated and not in an acute stage of inflammation and distress.

The complexity of such a case makes determination of potential cumbersome for the novice therapist, who may need to consider each goal carefully and review methodically whether the client has the potential to attain it. The novice may attempt to treat every problem even though improvement may not be possible. The expert clinician is more experienced in weighing multiple factors and has a "mental case file" against which this case may be compared. To the novice the expert may seem to work on an intuitive level, pulling together all of the factors that affect the client's rehabilitation potential. In fact, what looks like intuition is a series of clinical reasoning decisions based on evidence from evaluation and from previous cases and reports from the literature. Decisions are made as the evaluation is in progress.

Goal Setting

During evaluation the therapist identifies problems that have potential for improvement. Goal setting is always accomplished in collaboration with the OA and family or partner or with the care providers. Hoppes[44] indicates that collaborative goal setting may be the key to motivating a client. His survey found that clients will accomplish the goals set if they know specifically what those goals are. He also found that clients frequently feel they are not involved in choosing therapy goals, although the therapist has reported involving the client. The following are some suggestions to increase perceived control on the part of clients:

- Provide specific written goals.
- Design challenging goals.
- Make sure the client remembers the goals.

The therapist must also involve family members in goal setting, since the family members will be responsible for supervision and follow-through of the home program. Families may feel overwhelmed with this responsibility, but after providing some input into the treatment plan, they are frequently willing to develop the skills necessary to care for their family member. The novice clinician may *inform* the OA of the treatment goals, but the expert clinician will *collaborate* with OAs and their families in establishing goals. The expert clinician will be able to articulate the differences and the similarities between the client's and the therapist's goals and will negotiate agreement with the client. The novice clinician may have difficulty accepting a client's refusal to work on some treatment goals. The expert clinician accepts these differences in cultural and social values and focuses on the goals the client feels are pertinent.

Treatment

The treatment process involves teaching and learning. Adults have some specific learning needs. Integrating the learning needs of the adult into treatment will produce a more effective teaching session. Some of the assumptions in the following list are related to adult learning and are pertinent to OT treatment:

1. Adults need to understand the reasoning behind the learning.
2. The adult learner brings a breadth of experience and knowledge to learning situations.
3. Adults are willing and ready to learn those things that are necessary.
4. Adults are life centered with learning experiences and willing to learn those things that will help them with day-to-day experiences.
5. The greatest motivators are internal pressures.[51]

Knowles[51] also recommends an environment of mutual trust, respect, and acceptance of differences. The therapist must take the time during initial contacts with the OA to listen to and get to know the client.

By the time treatment begins, the occupational therapist will have an understanding of the client's learning style, deficits that may require specific types of teaching, and any cognitive or perceptual deficits that need to be considered. The pace and style of the treatment will be individualized to suit the client's learning needs.

Consider the case of Mrs. Nelson again. Her sensory deficits include mild vision impairment (correctable with glasses) and a mild hearing loss. Possible cognitive deficits involve an inability to concentrate and forgetfulness. To help Mrs. Nelson work with meal preparation from the wheelchair, the occupational therapist must make sure Mrs. Nelson is wearing her glasses. When speaking to Mrs. Nelson, the therapist should look at her to make sure she is hearing any instructions. So that Mrs. Nelson can better hear and concentrate, the meal preparation should occur in a quiet environment. To encourage generalization, the occupational therapist should match the environment to the home kitchen as much as possible. The therapist may review methods or techniques used from previous treatments at the beginning of each treatment session in order to create continuity and reinforce skills.

Involving the family is important because they will ultimately be responsible for following through with recommendations from the health care team. The health care team makes recommendations that frequently require planning by the family, such as modifying the bathroom, buying a shower seat, or hiring part-time help if the OA will need 24-hour supervision. If the family is not present during therapy sessions and visits the OA only at the end of the day when the OA is in bed, they may assume that the client is dependent in most activities. The OA may have a partner or spouse who is also older and has his or her own set of problems. The occupational therapist may indirectly evaluate the caregiver's ability to learn and to cope with new and complex situations; this helps determine to what degree the caregiver will be able to assist the client physically. During family training the occupational therapist will need to keep in mind the learning needs of the caregiver, who may need repetition and practice with new skills. If all the teaching is left until the day of discharge, the caregiver may become overwhelmed and retain little of what is taught.

Family training provides the opportunity for the occupational therapist to model for the family how to supervise and provide varying degrees of assistance. For example, with Mrs. Nelson the occupational therapist may ask the daughter to attend a session of bathing training. The occupational therapist may model how to assist the client minimally by making sure the items she needs (e.g., shampoo, long-handle sponge, shower hose, liquid soap with nylon scrubber, shower seat) are within reach. Mrs. Nelson will also be able to demonstrate the compensatory techniques she has learned to wash her hair, such as propping her elbows on her legs and bending her head forward. During the next treatment session the occupational therapist may step back and observe Mrs. Nelson's daughter providing minimal assistance with bathing. Transfer training, safety, and types of bathroom equipment needed at home may also be reviewed. The occupational therapist may ask the daughter and Mrs. Nelson how their home bathroom differs from the one at the skilled nursing facility and what needs to be done to ensure Mrs. Nelson can make the transition to the home setting with her newly learned skills. This approach takes into account the adult learning principles. The caregiver and client are able to provide input into their learning experience and make a plan of their own to use at home. The occupational therapist steps out of the role of authority and allows the caregiver and client to problem solve independently.

The occupational therapist may note problems with the caregiver's ability to cope and learn during family training sessions. This may cause concern for discharge plans and the client's safety. At that point the occupational therapist should be communicating with the social worker, discharge planner, and other team members to alert them to the potential problems.

Treatment requires ongoing reevaluation and modification of the original treatment plan. The expert clinician recognizes this and modifies the plan as needed. At some point in the treatment continuum the occupational therapist must determine if and how the OA will be able to problem solve in unique situations. It is important to see whether the client can function in a less predictable physical or social environment. The therapist may modify the physical or social environment to challenge the client and aid in the transfer of newly learned compensatory strategies and skills to a variety of settings.

Consider again the case of Mrs. Nelson. If the therapist continues to perform all treatment in the client's bedroom, where the bed setup is exactly the same, Mrs. Nelson may establish a routine within that environment in which she consistently locks the wheelchair brakes during transfers, when dressing in the wheelchair, and when getting on the toilet. This routine may transfer poorly to other settings. The expert clinician helps Mrs. Nelson begin to make the transition to other environments, such as using the bathroom in the activity room or in the therapy treatment room. The next step is to explore with Mrs. Nelson and her family how her bedroom at home is set up and how she will need to approach each activity in her home environment. Families and the OA client must learn to transfer skills to the home by modifying the environment or techniques learned and by establishing new routines.

Discharge Planning

Discharge planning requires a team effort, with some forethought given to the OA's and family members' needs. Discharge planning begins at the first meeting with the client. The occupational therapist has many opportunities to develop goals collaboratively with the OA and family and to discuss the frequency and duration of treatment and plans for discharge. Discharge planning may include recommending OT in the next setting. If an OA is leaving an acute care hospital and going to the skilled nursing facility, OT may be recommended with a justification of why the services are needed. The discharging occupational therapist makes sure that a discharge summary is sent to the next occupational therapist to identify what treatment has already been done and what progress has been made.

Discharge may be to the community. Community resources aid in the transition from one level of care to another and often provide the support families need to care for the OA at home. Typically, various members of the health care team recommend community resources based on the type of service each team member provides. The social worker or discharge planner may provide information about in-home meals and home health aide services. The physical therapist may refer the client to a community-based exercise class. The occupational therapist may encourage the client to attend the local senior center and may provide information on equipment loan closets. Often care providers are unaware of the many resources available. It is up to the health care team to provide OAs and their families with resource information and instruct them on how to obtain those services.

SUMMARY

The OA population continues to grow at a rapid pace. Many OAs will need rehabilitative services and the skills of occupational therapists. Gerontic OT, perhaps more than any other area of practice, demands a great deal from the therapist. Not only must the gerontic occupational therapist have the basic knowledge and skills to address occupation and performance, but he or she must have more advanced clinical reasoning skills to intervene with the complex, multidimensional issues that encompass occupational performance for the OA client. Collaborating with OA clients and their caregivers is essential in understanding the client's unique story of life and occupations. Defining problems, framing those problems, and determining what aspects of occupational performance to address depend on several key factors. These include the knowledge, experience, and attitudes of the therapist; the type of care setting and limitations imposed by the reimbursement source; and the particular life experiences, health status, illness experience, personal circumstances, and occupations of the client.

Procedural clinical reasoning (clinical reasoning that addresses primarily the client's pathological condition or addresses limited aspects of occupational performance) is not adequate to work effectively with the multidimensional problems of an OA adjusting to age-related changes and struggling with the onset of new disabilities. A more integrated approach to the evaluation and treatment of older adults has been presented here.

REVIEW QUESTIONS

1. What will be the demographic characteristics of a "typical" geriatric client seeking OT services in the year 2008?

2. Name seven age-related physical changes that a therapist would look for in a client who is 85 years of age, has had an inactive lifestyle, and has eaten a high-cholesterol diet.

3. A student comments that most persons 80 years of age and older are senile and immobile. Write what you would say in response. Include in your answer an understanding of the beliefs of the student, as well as the facts.

4. What behavioral indicators would suggest that a patient may be depressed and possibly suicidal? What actions should the therapist take?

5. Identify five aspects of performance components that you would immediately observe or screen for when meeting an OA client for the first time.

6. How might your initial evaluation and treatment plan be different if Mrs. Nelson were an African-American grandmother, with mild dementia, living in a single-family home, with a daughter who worked days and went to school at night, and grandchildren aged 7 and 8 years who came home after school?

7. Typically the client is evaluated and treated in a setting that will promote optimum performance. Why might the occupational therapist at times provide treatment of the client in circumstances that are slightly or considerably more challenging?

8. What other aspects of Mrs. Nelson's performance areas, components, or context might merit further consideration?

REFERENCES

1. Abrams R, Alexopoulis G, Young R: Geriatric depression and DSM-III-R personality disorder criteria, *J Am Geriatr Soc* 35(5):383-386, 1987.
2. Allen C: *Occupational therapy for psychiatric diseases: measurement and management of cognitive disabilities*, Boston, 1985, Little, Brown.
3. Allen C: *Allen Cognitive Level (ACL) test*, Rockville, Md, 1991, American Occupational Therapy Foundation.
4. American Association of Retired Persons: *A profile of older Americans 1999*, on-line at www.aoa dhhs.gov./aoa/stats/profile/, 1999, US Administration on Aging.
5. American Occupational Therapy Association: Uniform terminology for occupational therapy, *Am J Occup Ther* 48(11):1047-1054, 1994.
6. American Psychiatric Association: *Diagnostic and statistical manual of mental disorders*, ed 4, Washington, DC, 1994, American Psychiatric Association.
7. Asher I: *Occupational therapy assessment tools: an annotated index*, ed 2, Bethesda, Md, 1996, American Occupational Therapy Association.
8. Baum C: Activity profile. From *Handouts for managing cognitively impaired older adults*, California Occupational Therapy Association Conference, San Jose, Calif, 1994.
9. Beck AT, Ward CM, Mendelson M, et al: An inventory for measuring depression, *Arch Gen Psychiatry* 4:561-571, 1961.
10. Beech J, Harding L: *Assessment of the elderly*, Windsor, Ontario, 1990, NFER-NELSON.
11. Bennett J: Oral health maintenance. In Carnevali D, Patrick M, editors: *Nursing management*, San Mateo, Calif, 1979, Appleton & Lange.
12. Berkman C, Miller P: Falls interview schedule: comprehensive falls questionnaire for community-dwelling elders. In Miller P, editors: *Programs in occupational therapy*, New York, 1991, Columbia University.
13. Berlin E: *Guidelines for health practitioners* (DHHS Grant No. 5-UO1-PE-00053-04). Date Unknown, Stanford University Division of Family Medicine and the South Bay Area Health Education Center.
14. Blazer D, George L, Hughes D: The epidemiology of anxiety disorder. In Salzman C, Lebowitz BD, editors: *Anxiety and the elderly: treatment and research*, New York, 1991, Springer.
15. Brayne C, Gill C, Paykel E, et al: Cognitive decline in an elderly population: a two-wave study of change, *Psychol Med* 25(4):673-683, 1995.
16. Butin DN: *Psychosocial and psychological components*, ed 2, Bethesda, Md, 1996, American Occupational Therapy Association.
17. Butler R: The life review: an interpretation of reminiscence in the aged, *Psychiatry* 26:65-76, 1963.
18. Butler R, Lewis M: *Aging and mental health: positive psychosocial approaches*, ed 3, St Louis, 1982, Mosby.
19. Cantor M: Family and community: changing roles in an aging society, *Gerontologist* 31(3):337-339, 1991.
20. Clark F, Azen S, Zemke R, et al: Occupational therapy for independent living older adults, *JAMA* 278(16):1321-1326, 1997.
21. Clark F, Carlson M, Zemke R, et al: Life domains and adaptive strategy of a group of low-income, well older adults, *Am J Occup Ther* 50(2):106-107, 1996.
22. Cohen S, Edwards J: Personality characteristics as moderators of the relationship between stress and disorder. In Neufeld R, editor: *Advances in the investigation of psychological stress*, New York, 1989, Wiley.
23. Conwell Y: Suicide in elderly patients. In Schneider LS, Reynolds CF, Lebowitz BD, et al, editors: *Diagnosis and treatment of depression in late life*, Washington, DC, 1994, American Psychiatric Press.
24. Cook A: Prevention of falls in the elderly. In Pedretti LW, editor: *Role of occupational therapy with the elderly*, Bethesda, Md, 1996, American Occupational Therapy Association.
25. Costa P, McCrae R: Psychological stress and coping in old age. In Breznitz LGS, editor: *Handbook of stress: theoretical and clinical aspects*, New York, 1993, Free Press.
26. Craik F, Jennings J: Human memory. In Craik FC, Salthouse TA, editors: *The handbook of aging and cognition*, Hillsdale, NJ, 1992, Erlbaum.
27. Cristofala V: The destiny of cells: mechanisms and implications of senescence, *Gerontologist* 25:577-583, 1985.
28. Crook T, West R: Name recall performance across the adult life span, *Br J Psychol* 81(pt 3):335-349, 1990.
29. Deeg D, Kardaun J, Fozard J: Health, behavior and aging. In Birren JE, Schaie KW, editors: *Handbook of the psychology of aging*, San Diego, Calif, 1996, Academic Press.
30. Dittmann-Kohli F: The construction of meaning in old age: possibilities and constraints, *Aging and Society* 10:279-294, 1990.
31. Elias M, Elias J, Elias P: Biological and health influences on behavior. In Birren JE, Schaie KW, editors: *Handbook of the psychology of aging*, San Diego, 1990, Academic Press.
32. Elias M, Wolf P, D'Augustino R, et al: Untreated blood pressure is inversely related to cognitive functioning: the Framingham study, *Am J Epidemiol* 138(6):353-364, 1993.
33. Ewing J: Detecting alcoholism: the CAGE questionnaire, *JAMA* 252(14):1905-1907, 1984.
34. Ferrini AF, Ferrini RL: *Health in the later years*, ed 3, Boston, 2000, McGraw-Hill.
35. Fleming M: Procedural reasoning: addressing functional limitations. In Mattingly C, Fleming MH, editors: *Clinical reasoning: forms of inquiry in a therapeutic practice*, Philadelphia, 1994, FA Davis.

36. Folstein MF, Folstein MF, McHugh PR: Mini-Mental State: a practical method for grading the cognitive state of patients for the clinician, *J Psychiatr Res* 12(3):189-198, 1975.

37. Gallo J, Anthony J, Muthen B: Age differences in the symptoms of depression: a latent trait analysis, *J Gerontol* 49(6):P251-P264, 1994.

38. Gatz M, Kasl-Godley J, Karel M: Aging and mental disorders. In Birren JE, Schaie KW, editors: *Handbook of the psychology of aging,* San Diego, Calif, 1996, Academic Press.

39. Gatz M, Smyer M: The mental health system and older adults in the 1990s, *Am Psychol* 47(6):741-751, 1992.

40. Glogoski-Williams C: Recognition of depression in the older adult, *J Occup Ther Mental Health* (publication pending).

41. Hasher L, Zacks R: Working memory, comprehension and aging: a review and a new view. In Bower G, editor: *The psychology of learning and motivation: advances in research and theory,* San Diego, Calif, 1988, Academic Press.

42. Heidrich S, Ryff C: The role of social comparisons processes in the psychological adaptation of elderly adults, *J Gerontol* 48(3):P127-P136, 1993.

43. Himes C: Future caregivers projected family structures of older people, *J Gerontol* 47(1):S23-S26, 1992.

44. Hoppes S: Motivating clients through goal setting, *OT Practice,* June 1997, pp 22-27.

45. Johnson C: Personal meanings and long-term survivorship. In *Gerontological Society of America Meeting,* New Orleans, 1993, Gerontological Society.

46. Kausler D: *Experimental psychology, cognition and human aging,* ed 2, New York, 1990, Springer-Verlag.

47. Kausler D: *Experimental psychology, cognition and aging.* Summer institute at St Scholastica College, 1992, Sponsored by the National Science Foundation.

48. Kausler DH: *Learning and memory in normal aging,* San Diego, 1994, Academic Press.

49. Keller M, Leventhal E, Larson B: Aging: the lived experience, *Int J Aging Hum Dev* 29(1):67-82, 1989.

50. Kessler R, McGonagle K, Zhao S, et al: Life-time and 12-month prevalence of DSM-II-R psychiatric disorders in the United States: results from the national co-morbidity survey, *Arch Gen Psychiatry* 51(1):8-19, 1989.

51. Knowles M: *The adult learner: a neglected species,* Houston, 1984, Gulf Publishing.

52. Koening H, Blazer D: Mood disorders and suicide. In Birren JE, Sloane RB, Cohen GD, editors: *Handbook of mental health and aging,* San Diego, Calif, 1992, Academic Press.

53. Labouvie-Vief G, Hakim-Larson J, Hobart C: Age, ego level, and life span development of coping and defense processes, *Psychol Aging* 2(3):286-293, 1987.

54. Larson K: *Conceptual models of practice and frames of reference,* ed 2, Bethesda, Md, 1996, American Occupational Therapy Association.

55. Laver A: Module III—The occupational therapy assessment and evaluation of the older adult. In Pedretti LW, editor: *Role of occupational therapy and the elderly,* Bethesda, Md, 1996, American Occupational Therapy Association.

56. LeBarge E: A preliminary scale to measure degree of worry among mildly demented Alzheimer's disease patients, *Phys Occup Ther Geriatr* 11:43-57, 1993.

57. Lebowitz B, Pearson J, Schneider L: Diagnosis and treatment of depression in late life: consensus statement update, *JAMA* 278(14):1186-1190, 1997.

58. Leventhal H, Leventhal E, Schaeffer P: Vigilant coping and health behaviors. In Ory MG, Abeles RP, Lipman PD, editors: *Aging, health and behavior,* Newbury Park, Calif, 1992, Sage.

59. Levy L: *Adaptation and the aging adult,* ed 2, Bethesda, Md, 1992, American Occupational Therapy Association.

60. Levy L: *Mental disorders in aging adults,* ed 2, Bethesda, Md, 1996, American Occupational Therapy Association.

61. Levy L: *Health and impairment: the performance component,* Bethesda, Md, 1996, American Occupational Therapy Association.

62. Levy L: *Cognition and the aging adult,* ed 2, Bethesda, Md, 1996, American Occupational Therapy Association.

63. Levy L: Information processing and dementia. II. Cognitive disability in perspective, *OT Practice* December 4(10):CE-1-CE-8, 1999.

64. Lewis C: *Elder care in occupational therapy,* Thorofare, NJ, 1989, Slack.

65. Lindenberger U: Intellectual aging. In Steinberg RJ, editor: *Encyclopedia of intelligence,* New York, 1994, Macmillan.

66. Matsutsuyu J: Interest checklist, *Am J Occup Ther* 23(6):323-328, 1969.

67. Mattingly C: The narrative nature of clinical reasoning. In Mattingly C, Fleming MH, editors: *Clinical reasoning: forms of inquiry in a therapeutic practice,* Philadelphia, 1994, FA Davis.

68. Mossey J, Knott K, Craik R: The effects of persistent depressive symptoms on hip fracture recovery *J Gerontol* 45(5):M163-M168, 1990.

69. Northern California Neurobehavioral Group: *Cognistat,* Fairfax, Calif, 1995, The Group.

70. Orgel L: The maintenance of the accuracy of protein synthesis and its relevancy to aging, *Proc Natl Acad Sci USA* 49:517, 1963.

71. Orgel L: The maintenance of the accuracy of protein synthesis and its relevancy to aging, *Proc Natl Acad Sci* 67:1496, 1973.

72. Orr A: *Interest in aging and vision: a curriculum for university programs and in-service training,* New York, 1998, American Foundation for the Blind.

73. Pfeiffer E: SPMSQ: Short Portable Mental Status Questionnaire, *J Am Geriatr Soc* 23:433-441, 1975.

74. Reifler B: Depression: diagnosis and co-morbidity. In Schneider LS, Reynolds CF, Lebowitz BD, et al, editors: *Diagnosis and treatment of depression in late life,* Washington, DC, 1994, American Psychiatric Press.

75. Reifler B: Detection and treatment of mixed cognitive and affective symptoms in the elderly: is it dementia, depression or both? *Clin Geriatr* 6:17-33, 1998.

76. Rodin J, Langer E: Long-term effects of a control relevant intervention with the institutionalized aged, *J Pers Soc Psychol* 35(12):897-902, 1977.

77. Rogers J, Holm M: Occupational therapy diagnostic reasoning: a component of clinical reasoning, *Am J Occup Ther* 45(11):1045-1053, 1991.

78. Rott C, Thomae H: Coping in longitudinal perspective: findings from the Bonn Longitudinal Study on Aging, *J Cross-Cultural Gerontol* 6:23-40, 1991.

79. Rowe J, Kahn R: Human aging: usual and successful, *Science* 237(4811):143-149, 1987.

80. Rusting R: Why do we age? *Sci Am* 267(6):130-135, 138-141, 1987.

81. Ruth JE, Coleman P: Personality and aging: coping and management of the self in later life. In Birren JE, Schaie KW, editors: *Handbook of the psychology of aging,* San Diego, Calif, 1996, Academic Press.

82. Ryff C: In the eye of the beholder: views of psychological well-being among middle-aged and older adults, *Psychol Aging* 4(2):195-210, 1989.

83. Sadavcy J, Fogel F: Personality disorders in old age. In Birren JE, Sloane RB, Cohen GD, editors: *Handbook of mental health and aging,* San Diego, Calif, 1992, Academic Press.

84. Salthouse T, Babock R: Decomposing adult age differences in working memory, *Dev Psychol* 27:763-776, 1991.

85. Sands L, Merideth W: Intellectual functioning in late midlife, *J Gerontol Psychol Sci,* 47:81-84, 1992.

86. Schaie K, editor: *Intellectual development in adulthood,* San Diego, Calif, 1996, Academic Press.

87. Schell B: Clinical reasoning: the basis of practice. In Neistadt M, Crepeau E, editor: *Willard & Spackman's occupational therapy*, Philadelphia, 1998, Lippincott-Raven.

88. Schell B, Cervero R: Clinical reasoning in occupational therapy: an integrative review, *Am J Occup Ther* 47(7):605-610, 1993.

89. Seligman M: *Helplessness: on depression, development and death*, San Francisco, 1975, Freeman.

90. Siev E, Freishtat B, Zoltan B: *Perceptual and cognitive dysfunction in the adult stroke patient*, Thorofare, NJ, 1986, Slack.

91. Sinnott J: A model for solution of ill-structured problems: implications for everyday and abstract problem solving. In Sinnott JD, editor: *Everyday problem solving: theory and applications*, New York, 1989, Praeger.

92. Smith A, editor: *Memory*, San Diego, 1996, Academic Press.

93. Strehler B: A new age for aging, *Natural History* 2:8-85, 1973.

94. Sunderland T, Lawlor B, Martinez R, et al: Anxiety in the elderly: neurobiological and clinical interface. In Salzman C, Lebowitz BD, editors: *Anxiety and the elderly: treatment and research*, New York, 1991, Springer.

95. Thomae H: Emotion and personality. In Birren JE, Shane B, Cohen G, editors: *Handbook of mental health and aging*, San Diego, 1992, Academic Press.

96. Toglia J: A dynamic interactional approach to cognitive rehabilitation. In Katz N, editor: *Cognitive rehabilitation*, Boston, 1992, Andover Medical Publishers.

97. Toitman D, Katz N: Predictive validity of the Large Allen Cognitive Level tests using the Allen Diagnostic Module in an aged, non-disabled population, *Phys Occup Ther Geriatr* 14:43-53, 1996.

98. Trombly R: Anticipating the future: assessment of occupational function, *Am J Occup Ther* 47(3):253-257, 1994.

99. United States Bureau of the Census: Americans with disabilities: 1994-95, *Current Population Reports*, August 1997, P70-61.

100. United States Bureau of the Census: Household and family characteristics, *Current Population Reports*, March 1998, PPL-20-515.

101. United States Bureau of the Census: Population projections of the United States by age, sex, race and Hispanic origin: 1995-2050, *Current Population Reports*, 1998, P25-1130.

102. United States Bureau of the Census: Poverty in the United States: 1998, *Current Population Reports*, September 1999, P60-207.

103. Vaillant G: *Adaptation to life*, Boston, 1977, Little, Brown.

104. Walford R: The clinical promise of diet restriction, *Geriatrics* 45(4):81-83, 86-87, 1990.

105. Wallston K, Wallston B: Who is responsible for your health? In Sanders GS, Suls J, editors: *Social psychology of health and illness*, Hillsdale, NJ, 1982, Erlbaum.

106. Willis S: Everyday problem solving. In Birren JE, Schaie KW, editors: *Handbook of the psychology of aging*, San Diego, Calif, 1996, Academic Press.

107. Yeo G: The need for culturally competent models of long term care. In Stanford Geriatric Education Center: *AARP series on ethnicity and long term care*, 1997, Stanford Geriatric Education Center.

108. Yeo G, Hagan J, Levkoff S, et al: *Core curriculum in ethnogeriatrics* (Curriculum guide—Bureau of Health Professions Health Resources and Services Administration and U.S. Department of Health and Human Services Grant Report No. 97-0260), Stanford, Calif, 1999, Stanford Geriatric Education Center.

109. Yeo G, Hikoyeda N, Mcbride M, et al: *Cohort analysis as a tool in ethnogeriatrics: historical profiles of elders from eight ethnic populations in the United States*, ed 2, Stanford, Calif, 1998, Stanford Geriatric Education Center.

110. Yesavage JA, Brink TL, Rose TL, et al: Development and validation of a geriatric depression scale: a preliminary report, *J Psychiatr Res* 17(1):37-49, 1982-1983.

RECOMMENDED READING

Allen CK, Earhart CA, Blue T: *Occupational therapy treatment goals for the physically and cognitively disabled*, Rockville, Md, 1992, American Occupational Therapy Association.

Atchley R: A continuity theory of normal aging, *Gerontologist* 29(2):183-190, 1989.

Bachman D, Wolf P, Linn R: Incidence of dementia and probable Alzheimer's disease in a general population: the Framingham study, *Neurology* 43(3 pt 1):515-519, 1993.

Barrett J, Haley W, Harrell L, et al: Knowledge about Alzheimer's disease among primary care physicians, psychologists, nurses and social workers, *Alzheimer's Dis Assoc Disord* 11:99-106, 1997.

Berg S: Aging, behavior and cognitive decline. In Birren JE, Schaie KW, editors: *Handbook of the psychology of aging*, San Diego, Calif, 1996, Academic Press.

Chisolm D, Dolhi C, Schrieber J: Creating occupation-based opportunities in a medical model clinical practice setting, *OT Pract* January 2000, CE1-CE8.

Dey A: *Characteristics of elderly nursing home residents: data from the 1995 national nursing home survey*, Advance data from vital and health statistics, National Center for Health Statistics, 1997.

Ferrucci L, Guralnik S, Marchionni M, et al: Relationship between health status, fluid intelligence, and disability in a non-demented elderly population, *Aging* 5(6):435-443, 1993.

Fleming M: The therapist with three track mind, *Am J Occup Ther*, 45(11):1007-1014, 1991.

Hershey D, Walsh D, Read S, et al: The effects of expertise on financial problem solving, *Organizational Behavior and Human Decision Processes* 46:77-101, 1990.

Hinojosa J, Kramer P, editors: *Evaluation: obtaining and interpreting data*, Bethesda, Md, 1998, American Occupational Therapy Association.

Jorm A: *The epidemiology of Alzheimer's disease and related disorders*, London, 1990, Chapman & Hall.

Larson K, Stevens-Ratchford R, Pedretti L, et al, editors: *Role of occupational therapy with the elderly*, ed 2, Bethesda, Md, 1996, American Occupational Therapy Association.

McCann K: Home health rules published, *OT Week*, March 4: 8-10, 1999.

McCann K: The 2000 Medicare fee schedule, *OT Pract*, January 3: 8, 2000.

Neistadt M: Teaching clinical reasoning as a teaching frame, *Am J Occup Ther* 52(3):221-229, 1998.

Rosowsky E, Gurian B: Borderline personality disorder in late life, *Int Psychogeriatr* 3(1):39-52, 1991.

Salcido R, Moore R: Cost-effectiveness of subacute rehabilitation, *Rehabil Management*, August, September: 33-40, 1995.

Salthouse T: *Theoretical perspectives on cognitive aging*, Hillsdale, NJ, 1991, Erlbaum.

Salthouse T, Kausler D, Saults J: Age, self-assessed health status, and cognition, *J Gerontol B Psychol Sci Soc Sci* 45(4):P156-P160, 1990.

Stevens-Ratchford RG: *Occupational therapy services within the rehabilitation health care system*, ed 2, Bethesda, Md, 1996, American Occupational Therapy Association.

Strahan G: *An overview of nursing homes and their current residents: data from the 1995 national nursing home survey* (Pub. No. 280), 1997, National Center for Health Statistics.

United States Bureau of the Census: Marital status and living arrangements, *Current Population Reports*, March 1998, PPL-100.

HIV Infection and AIDS

LINDA GUTTERMAN

LEARNING OBJECTIVES

After studying this chapter the student or practitioner will be able to do the following:
1. Define HIV and AIDS.
2. Understand both the psychosocial issues and physical manifestations of AIDS.
3. Recognize the need to employ a wide range of treatment options, including pain and stress management.
4. Evaluate an individual with AIDS by addressing physical, psychosocial, and psychological concerns.
5. Develop an appropriate and relevant treatment plan for the individual with AIDS or HIV.

Worldwide, 33.4 million people are estimated to be living with the **human immunodeficiency virus** (HIV) and **acquired immune deficiency syndrome** (AIDS). Of these, over 27 million persons have no idea that they are infected. As of June 1998 the total number of AIDS cases reported in the United States was 665,357. Approximately 401,028 people have died of AIDS. Some 650,000 to 900,000 people in the United States are now living with HIV or AIDS. The number of new cases is rising among intravenous drug users and their sexual partners, racial and ethnic minority populations (especially women, who make up 20% of the AIDS population), and youth and children. Although the incidence of new infection had been falling among gay males, it has recently begun to rise; this group represented 60% of men diagnosed with AIDS in 1997.[2]

DEFINITION AND DIAGNOSIS OF HIV INFECTION AND AIDS

HIV infects white blood cells of the immune system. These white blood cells help to combat disease and are called CD4+ cells or T-helper cells. When HIV invades the T-helper cells, it eventually takes over and begins to reproduce more HIV. As the disease progresses, the immune system becomes compromised and the body is then susceptible to numerous infections, cancers, and other diseases and conditions. AIDS was first recognized in 1981. It is one aspect of a broad spectrum of disease related to HIV infection. The **Centers for Disease Control and Prevention** (CDC) determines what defines a case as HIV infection or AIDS. In 1993 the CDC updated its definition, which created two sets of three categories each. The first set relates to CD4+ cell count:
- Category 1: CD4+ cell counts of 500 or more cells per microliter of blood
- Category 2: counts from 200 to 499 CD4+ cells
- Category 3: counts below 200 CD4+ cells

The second set of categories relates to the expression of HIV from a clinical perspective:
- Category A: individuals who have been asymptomatic except for persistent, generalized lymphadenopathy seroconversion syndrome. This includes the initial acute onset of HIV exposure

- Category B: individuals who have never had an AIDS-defining illness but have had some symptoms of HIV infection such as candidiasis, fever, persistent diarrhea, oral hairy leukoplakia, herpes zoster, idiopathic thrombocytopenic purpura, peripheral neuropathy, cervical dysplasia, or pelvic inflammatory disease
- Category C: individuals who have or have had one or more of the AIDS-defining illnesses

An individual is determined to have HIV infection if one category from each set applies. For example, if an individual is designated C3, he or she has fewer than 200 CD4+ cells and has had at least one AIDS-defining illness. Categories 1 and 2 and A and B are considered HIV positive (a less grave condition), while categories 3 and C are defined as AIDS. These categories are used primarily to pinpoint where an individual is along the continuum of HIV infection.[9]

TRANSMISSION

The three primary routes of HIV infection are as follows:
1. Exposure to infected blood or blood products through a break in the skin or contact with a mucosal entry point
2. Intimate sexual contact with exchange or exposure to semen and vaginal secretions
3. Perinatal transmission from infected mother or exposure to breast milk

Groups at risk include men who have sex with men; men and women who have unsafe heterosexual contact; intravenous drug users; individuals with a hemophilia or coagulation disorder; individuals who have had blood transfusions or have received blood components or tissue; breastfeeding children; and health care workers exposed to blood or blood products.

RACE AND GENDER CONCERNS

In 1996 the following number (approximately) of people were newly diagnosed with AIDS:

African-American men	17,250
African-American women	6,750
Hispanic men	8,860
Hispanic women	2,210
White men	18,790
White women	2,390[3]

These statistics reveal a disproportionate impact of the epidemic on minority populations. Some of the issues that mostly affect women also apply to minority populations. For example, poor access to health care is a significant contributor to the overall mortality of women and minorities. Limited opportunity for education on prevention is a significant issue in certain communities, sometimes related to community values, fears and denial, and poverty. A closer look at the issue of women with AIDS suggests that although AIDS-related deaths per year in the general population have declined because of the new medication regimens and better medical management and prevention of opportunistic infections, the number of AIDS-related deaths among women has not decreased proportionally.[4]

Historically, women have had shorter survival times than men within the AIDS epidemic. This may reflect women's role of caring for others and not having enough support and time to care for themselves. Lower incomes of women and the lack of awareness by the medical profession of the unique needs of women also contribute. The AIDS epidemic came to the forefront in the 1980s; however, the CDC came to recognize symptoms and illnesses of AIDS specific to women only in 1993. Even when women are able to access adequate health care, the medication regimen may be prohibitive within a busy schedule that includes child care and caring for another family member with HIV infection while continuing to meet employment obligations and maintain health through multiple medical appointments. Women whose virus is detected early and who receive medical treatment survive as long as men with HIV infection; of course, this relates only to the use of medications as treatment for HIV infection.

From a sociopolitical standpoint, the history of the medical profession's approach to women's problems in general is revealing. Clinical trial studies have typically focused on men, although the results have been used for both men and women. Further explanations for the lag in care for women relative to men include attitudes of patients and providers, difficulties with adherence to medication regimens, a variety of adverse effects of medications, and imprecise dosage in relation to body mass.[4] Essentially, studies have shown that men and women do not always get the same kind of medical care, although they may at times have the same health issues. Additionally, the emotional response to learning of their HIV status has a role in delaying some women's attempts to receive medical treatment. Of course, women are not alone in having difficulty adjusting to learning they are HIV positive.

Permanency planning is the planning patients need to ensure care and education of their children in the event of the patients' disability or death. Although more men today are involved with their children than in the past, they are rarely the primary caretakers. Therefore the tremendous responsibility for permanency planning falls to the mother, further complicating the emotional aspect of being a woman with HIV infection. The ordeal of explaining their HIV status and the ramifications of that for their children is extremely painful for parents, yet necessary for the children's protection and future. Ideally the planning includes another family member who will parent the children after the mother's death or as she becomes too ill to fulfill parental responsibilities. Permanency planning may be addressed by a variety of health team members. Certainly, as someone with AIDS deteriorates, the occupational therapist can help the patient recognize that certain abilities are no longer present and that the help of others is needed to complete many daily life tasks for the family.

MEDICATION AND AIDS

In the last few years numerous medications have become available to address the AIDS virus. As the process of replication of the virus is studied, researchers continue to work with different points along the chain of replication at which pharmaceuticals may effectively interrupt the progression of the disease. Often patients are placed on two to five antiretroviral drugs at a time. This practice is called **highly active antiretroviral therapy** (HAART). Protease inhibitors are one class of such drugs and are perhaps best known to the public. Two others are nucleoside analogues and nonnucleoside analogues. Someone being treated with HAART is taking a combination of these medications. More recently, physicians and researchers have suggested that in addition to attempting to interfere with the replication process, treatment should address the rebuilding of the immune system—for example, by exploring the role of cytokines in the immunological response.[8] The discussion of medications becomes relevant to occupational therapists because of the range of side effects and their power to alter the **quality of life** for individuals with HIV and AIDS. In addition, some of the medications have complicated adherence regimens that can be significantly disruptive to daily life. Side effects may include diarrhea, muscle atrophy, rashes, pancreatitis, diabetes, peripheral neuropathy, nightmares, insomnia, lethargy, anxiety, nausea, an increase in liver enzymes, kidney stones (causing low back pain), and lipodystrophy syndrome (changes in body composition such as buffalo hump, truncal obesity, facial and peripheral fat atrophy, and breast enlargement in women). Lipodystrophy syndrome also includes insulin resistance, hyperglycemia, and hypertriglyceridemia. For some individuals with HIV and AIDS, lipodystrophy syndrome can add a cardiac precaution to treatment. Someone who has significant side effects that become too compromising may stop taking medications for a period of time. This is known as a "drug holiday."

ROLE OF THE OCCUPATIONAL THERAPIST

AIDS involves many diseases. Many opportunistic infections, cancers, conditions (e.g., developmental delay in children), and side effects of pharmaceuticals create tremendous havoc for the person living with AIDS. The range of psychiatric conditions, some of which may be preexisting and include substance use and chemical de-

pendency, further complicates the ability of individuals to engage adequately in their own health care.

Evaluation

Looking at the whole picture for any person living with AIDS, it is essential to evaluate the following:
1. *Physical ability*, including range of motion (ROM), strength, endurance, balance, coordination, sensation, functional ambulation, activities of daily living (ADL) (e.g., self-care and housekeeping), and **pain**
2. *Cognitive and behavioral status*
3. Presence and extent of *sleep disturbance*
4. Exploration of the individual's *ability to cope* and how the individual's lifestyle supports or does not support adequate coping and stress management
5. Place of *spirituality* in the individual's life
6. *Substance use history* and *addiction issues*
7. *Family role* or *responsibilities* and concerns of the individual in relation to family, such as childcare or caring for an adult with an illness
8. *Work history*
9. History of experience with "complementary" therapies and medicine and openness to incorporating these into a treatment program

An evaluation form similar to that in Fig. 52-1 may be used.

Impairment of functional abilities varies significantly with each individual, and the possible range of deficits is broad (see Case Study). Generally, HIV infection and AIDS may result in fatigue, muscle wasting and weakness, pain, sleep dysfunction, vision impairment, dementia or cognitive deficit, impaired mobility, and swallowing impairment. Some of these may be related to neurological sequelae. Further, most individuals have some degree of gastrointestinal complications from HIV infection and AIDS, which cause diarrhea and malabsorption and affect the freedom to leave the home. Many clients have spoken about the loss of bowel control in public that curtailed further venturing out of doors. All of these result in a loss of independence in ADL. Each of the preceding conditions can be attributed to different AIDS-related illnesses. For example, fatigue can be the result of anemia, which can also be caused by certain medications. Pain can be the result of the virus affecting the neurological or musculoskeletal system, or respiratory problems can cause musculoskeletal pain and tension. Sleep dysfunction can be caused by anxiety or depression or by certain medications.

The occupational therapist must not only consider the variety of conditions caused by impaired immune systems, but also respond to the range of medication side effects previously discussed. An occupational therapist treats what is, in effect, the individual's limit in function and facilitates the individual's maintenance of function. ADL training for the person with AIDS-related dementia

REHABILITATION AND HOLISTIC HEALTH SERVICE ASSESSMENT

Client name: _____ Date: _____

PHYSICAL STATUS

1. ( ) ROM-WNL   2. ( ) Strength-WNL   3. ( ) Coordination-WNL   4. ( ) Sensation-WNL
5. ( ) Balance-WNL   6. ( ) Endurance-WNL   7. ( ) Ambulation-WNL

Limitations/Impairments _____
_____
_____
_____
_____

( ) Cognition-WNL (R/L Discrimination, attention span, memory, judgement)

Impairments _____
_____
( ) Sleep-WNL _____
_____

( ) ADL Independent   ( ) IADL Independent
Assistance needed: _____
_____

Work history _____
_____
_____
_____

WELLNESS PROFILE on a scale of 1–10

1.   How well do you feel?

       _____
       1   10
       Don't feel well   Feel great

2.   How happy or sad are you?

       _____
       1   10
       Very sad   Very happy

3.   How much stress do you have?

       _____
       1   10
       No stress   Lots of stress

4.   What bothers you the most? _____
5.   What do you feel the best about? _____
6.   How do you handle the ups & downs of your life? _____
       _____

FIG. 52-1
Rehabilitation and holistic health service assessment. (Courtesy of Linda Gutterman, OTR.)

PAIN PROFILE (If indicated)
If you have pain on a scale from 1–10, how much pain do you have?

1	5	10
little pain	moderate pain	too much pain

Describe your pain and where it's located _____

COPING MECHANISMS

1.   Emotional support from friends, relatives, health professionals

_____

2.   Spiritual beliefs _____

3.   Self-medication (Drugs, ETOH) _____

4.   Meditation _____

5.   Participation in other meaningful activities _____

PREVIOUS TREATMENT (INCLUDE HX, FREQUENCY, DOSAGE WHERE INDICATED)

1. Acupuncture _____		6. Speech Therapy _____
2. Massage _____		7. Hypnosis/Meditation _____
3. Chiropractor _____		8. Herbal Intervention _____
4. Occupational Therapy _____		9. Other Pain/Stress Management _____
5. Physical Therapy _____		

REHABILITATION AND HOLISTIC HEALTH SERVICE

Problems/Issue/Needs Related to HIV/AIDS Illness Prioritized
by Clinician in Discussion With Client

_____

_____

_____

_____

_____

_____

_____

_____

Clinician Signature _____ Date _____

FIG. 52-1—cont'd
Rehabilitation and holistic health service assessment. (Courtesy of Linda Gutterman, OTR.)

may be no different from that for someone with dementia from Alzheimer's disease. However, with AIDS-related dementia the occupational therapist must consider whether the dementia is a sign of an opportunistic infection, such as toxoplasmosis, that is medically treatable, in which case the dementia may possibly resolve. Another consideration when determining the appropriateness of ADL training is the stage of the individual within the disease process. For example, at the end stage of disease, palliative care may be more appropriate, with ADL being the responsibility of a caretaker.

Psychological and Spiritual Aspects

Treating the whole individual requires that occupational therapists consider not only the physical components of disease, but also the psychiatric, psychosocial, and spiritual issues that may influence the expression of disease and the course of a disease process. Holistic medicine (such as traditional Chinese medicine, Ayurvedic medicine, or integrative medicine, as we sometimes refer to holistic medicine in the United States) views these aspects as interdependent. Physical pain is sometimes more effectively addressed when emotions are considered.

Stress in relation to HIV infection and AIDS is a major factor in quality-of-life issues. Negative stress and depletion of the immune system are known to be correlated.[1] The range of psychosocial issues extends beyond the obvious stresses of opportunistic infections and the knowledge of having a potentially life-threatening disease with a progressive and unpredictable course. A social **stigma**, in which a person with a disease is viewed as flawed or morally repulsive, may deter individuals from telling their families, friends, or employers that they are HIV positive or have AIDS. In addition, some may feel that they are bad and deserve AIDS or feel guilty over having infected others.[11] The initial diagnosis for some is terrifying; anxiety or anger may disrupt daily functioning, with ensuing loss of ability to fulfill occupational roles and expectations. For some, suicidal feelings will arise. As the disease progresses, changes in appearance can create issues in self-esteem and body image.[10] There may be discomfort or feelings of grief in needing assistance for self-care and housekeeping activities or needing someone else to bring the children to school. On the other hand, some individuals without social and financial supports have said that AIDS has not been the worst event in their lives and that it has afforded them housing and other benefits that have addressed previously unmet survival and social needs.[6] For others who have had adequate social and financial support and a comfortable standard of living, AIDS has caused more loss than gain. At times it has appeared that persons in the latter group have been less tolerant of the pain and the assault on self-image.

Some other psychosocial issues for the long-term survivor that cause major stress include the cumulative effect of the deaths of friends and family and wondering why "I have survived when all my friends have died," an inability to work consistently, permanency planning for the person's children, dealing with a chronic illness and compromising medications, coping with nonacceptance of the person's sexual preference, or fear of stigmatization by family or friends.

Four psychological states related to HIV infection and AIDS have been proposed.[5] An individual may experience any of these states at any time and fluctuate from one to another. First is the initial crisis state, when the HIV diagnosis is recent. Affective numbing, denial, and anxiety are characteristic. Second is the transitional state, occurring when the disease has been diagnosed for some time and the person is no longer paralyzed or in shock and begins to seek assistance. Feelings of anger, guilt, self-pity, and anxiety may arise, as well as (for some) suicidal ideation. Third is the acceptance state, occurring when the person has had a major clinical manifestation of the disease. In this state individuals may become more proactive about their health care, seeking changes in lifestyle, questioning medications and standard treatment, becoming more discerning about treatment, and using multiple providers. Fourth is the preparatory state, in which the person addresses fears of becoming dependent and dying and concern over legal issues. The person feels this is the end of life and may experience anxiety and control issues.

For individuals with substance abuse problems and preexisting psychiatric conditions, the psychosocial issues specific to HIV infection and AIDS further complicate the provision of health care. Common problems include denial, unsafe sexual practices, sharing needles, an inability to follow a medication regimen, an acute psychiatric disorder that precludes treatment for AIDS, and major drug use or relapse in which the individual stops all health care.

Occupational Therapy Goals

The goals of the occupational therapy (OT) program are to address such quality-of-life issues as pain and stress; to maintain strength, flexibility, mobility, and endurance; to maintain and increase independence in ADL; to improve lifestyle and coping mechanisms through counseling and education; to provide support and education to the family; and to facilitate the client's adjustment to diagnosis.

Treatment Methods

Pain and stress should be addressed immediately. The occupational therapist should be aware of any pain medications the person is taking and knowledgeable about the HIV medications that could also cause pain. The therapist should also know what stresses are current in the individual's life, since stress also plays a role in pain perception and tolerance.[7]

Occupational therapists can address pain or stress by using such methods as biofeedback or transcutaneous electrical stimulation, various bodywork modalities such as craniosacral balancing and myofascial release, therapeutic touch, massage and reflexology, proprioceptive neuromuscular facilitation, yoga, and t'ai chi. These methods should be used as part of any ROM programs and muscle strengthening and maintenance programs to meet goals of reduction in pain. Additionally, when appropriate for the individual it is important to include education in guided imagery and visualization, which gives the client the ability to self-treat as needed for pain and stress reduction. These techniques offer treatment on several levels simultaneously, which may enhance reduction of pain. Physical pain can be remediated for some when the emotional and spiritual components are acknowledged. Stress management and pain management may ameliorate issues of self-esteem and body image; as anxiety decreases, sleep disturbance may abate. Some modalities lend themselves well to group work, whereas others must be administered one on one. Although some of these modalities are not at present part of the core curriculum for OT students, they may contribute to the success of treatment. As part of treatment for pain and stress, occupational therapists can also offer time management intervention, development of skills to budget finances (often an area of stress), and energy-saving techniques (since reduced endurance and fatigue are extremely common among individuals with AIDS). As a result of decreased pain (and stress), mobility may improve, as well as energy and level of independence in ADL.

In AIDS, cognitive impairment most often manifests as memory loss, difficulty in attending, and poor judgment. In many cases these impairments can be attributed to the individual's feeling overwhelmed by his or her illness. When cognitive losses are attributed to actual changes in the brain and opportunistic infection (which may be treatable) has been ruled out, the occupational therapist should follow a protocol similar to that for other kinds of brain injury. In other words, the therapist would provide (1) training in compensatory techniques, (2) remediation as feasible, or (3) education of the individual and caregivers (e.g., family or home attendant) so as to facilitate the individual's functioning safely at home and in the community.

As health providers who deal with **mind, body, and spirit,** occupational therapists must become knowledgeable about health care options, including those outside traditional medicine. In the same way that we know when to refer an individual to the nurse, psychiatrist, or neurologist, therapists should also consider when to refer someone to the acupuncturist, chiropractor, massage therapist, herbalist, or other alternative source. More facilities are offering these services, and insurance companies are beginning to cover some of them (although this is not yet a widespread practice).

SUMMARY

HIV and AIDS is a complex disease with an uncertain course. Some long-term survivors may still use illegal drugs or alcohol. On the other extreme are individuals who work hard every day to survive, who watch their diet and their activities, and who meditate daily. An individual can experience severe and life-threatening opportunistic infection and 2 months later return to work. Parents can plan for the care of their children, expecting to soon be disabled or die, and then live for many years, leaving the plan dormant. Some individuals who have had AIDS since they were children are now entering college. Some in whom the disease is newly diagnosed believe that with all the new medications, such as protease inhibitors, the prognosis for HIV and AIDS is not as grave as it once was. AIDS continues to challenge all of us with constant change. Today's cutting-edge treatment may be replaced by new treatment protocols over the next few years. Occupational therapists should continue to study a broader range of modalities that will address the unique psychological and physical issues related to AIDS. With all the various therapies available, it is imperative that we continue to combine various approaches in order to afford the most compassionate and thorough treatment for our clients so that we may support their quality of life, resumption of roles, and creation of new roles.

CASE STUDY 52-1

CASE STUDY—MR. Z.

Mr. Z. is a 38-year-old Caucasian man who contracted HIV through homosexual sex. He received his diagnosis in 1987 through a routine health examination. He has a lover who lives in England with whom he has daily phone contact and whom he sees every other month. Mr. Z. lives in his own apartment in New York City. He spends considerable time and creative energy on his visual artwork, both painting and drawing. He has two siblings and remains close to his sister, who lives in a suburb outside of New York City. Both of his parents died from AIDS, his mother in 1991 and his father in 1985. His father was bisexual but lived in secrecy about this. Mr. Z. was sexually abused for a significant period of his childhood by both his father and his brother. His mother was physically abusive toward him. His father was physically abusive toward his mother. Mr. Z. has generalized anxiety disorder, depression, and mild histrionic and narcissistic traits, in addition to AIDS. At times he has been suicidal.

Over the past 2 years Mr. Z. has become weaker, has exhibited muscle atrophy in both hands and lower extremities, and has developed swallowing problems and slurred speech. The safety of his gait fluctuates because of his loss of strength. Ambulation is slowed and unsteady when he becomes fatigued. He has intermittent pain in the lower extremities, especially in his calves. The atrophy in his hands is more pronounced on the right side, where there is flattening of the thenar and hypothenar eminences. He has experienced some carpal tunnel pain in both wrists. Additionally, he shows muscle wasting on his face. A neurological examination has suggested the possibility that Mr. Z. also has amyotrophic lateral sclerosis; however, a definitive diagnosis has not been established.

Mr. Z. has had numerous medical appointments over the past 2 years. At times he has been unable to attend these on his own because of his extreme anxiety, and a staff member from his day treatment program has accompanied him to these appointments as an advocate. Before these physical issues, he was also beginning to deal with major psychological issues stemming from his childhood, which were and are compounding his anxiety response.

Occupational therapy (OT) was initiated to maintain strength, maintain independence in activities of daily living, monitor safety at home and in the community, provide stress and anxiety management and education, and provide emotional support and stability.

OT included an exercise program that Mr. Z. was able to perform both with the occupational therapist and on his own at home. He was given adapted equipment to enable him to continue writing, drawing, painting, and feeding himself. Clothing fastenings were adapted as needed. The occupational therapist went with Mr. Z. to a specialized shoe store to help select an appropriate shoe for his lower-extremity orthotics, so as to facilitate safe ambulation.

Mr. Z.'s bathroom was assessed for equipment, and he was provided with a nonskid material for the bottom of his bathtub and grab bars for the shower. Mr. Z. currently has a housekeeper who assists him with shopping, cleaning, and laundry. The occupational therapist and Mr. Z. have attended some medical appointments together. When Mr. Z. goes on his own, the occupational therapist works with him to develop a question list before the visit with his physician, so as to reduce anxiety and facilitate maintaining focus during the appointment. Further treatment by the therapist for anxiety and depression involved group ear acupuncture for relaxation, group training in visualization and guided imagery, the use of humor within supportive counseling, and referral by the occupational therapist to a massage therapist and chiropractor to further address pain issues.

Mr. Z. continues to deal with numerous losses in his life because of the degenerative nature of his disease. He continues to struggle to make sense of his childhood. OT has, in part, given him a greater sense of safety and independence and at times a sense of control, which has reduced his level of anxiety. He now has skills to help himself relax. He has a protocol in place that enables him to manage his medical appointments. He attends massage approximately one time each month and sees the chiropractor intermittently. He has been in psychotherapy for several years and continues to feel its benefits.

REVIEW QUESTIONS

1. What is the difference between HIV infection and AIDS?
2. What are the routes of transmission of HIV?
3. Name three significant side effects of HAART that affect quality-of-life issues.
4. Which groups of people represent the majority of those newly diagnosed, and why?
5. What role does psychiatric impairment play in complicating the success of treatment?
6. What are four goals of OT intervention?
7. Define permanency planning.
8. Name four disciplines to which the occupational therapist might refer someone for additional pain management.
9. List six areas the occupational therapist should evaluate.
10. List three individual treatments and three group treatments that could be used for someone with HIV infection or AIDS.

REFERENCES

1. Badgley L: *Healing AIDS naturally—natural therapies for the immune system*, Berkeley, Calif, 1986, Human Energy Press.
2. Centers for Disease Control and Prevention: *Basic Statistics*, December 1, 1998, www.cdc.gov.
3. Centers for Disease Control and Prevention: *Trends in the HIV: an AIDS epidemic*, 1998, www.cdc.gov.
4. Denenberg R: HIV infection in women: still untreated, still deadly, *Gay Men's Health Crisis Treatment Issues* 11(7-8), 1997.
5. Grimes R, Grimes D: Psychological states in HIV: disease and the nursing response, *J Assoc Nurses in AIDS Care* 6:25-32, 1995.
6. Gutterman L: A day treatment program for persons with AIDS, *Am J Occup Ther* 44(3):234-237, 1990.
7. Kabat-Zinn J: *Full catastrophe living: using the wisdom of your body and mind to face stress, pain, and illness*, New York, 1990, Dell Publishing.
8. Konlee M: The search for TH1, a consumer's guide to immune restoration, *Positive Health News*, West Allis, Wis, Report Number 18, Spring Issue, 1999.
9. McGovern T, Smith R: *Case definition of AIDS, encyclopedia of AIDS: a social, political, cultural and scientific record of the HIV epidemic*, Illinois, 1998, Fitzroy Dearborn Publishers.
10. Piemme J, Bolle J: Coping with grief in response to caring for persons with AIDS, *Am J Occup Ther* 44(3):266-269, 1990.
11. Williams J: Values and life goals: clinical intervention for people with AIDS. In Pizzi M, editor: *Productive living strategies for people with AIDS*, New York, 1990, Haworth Press.

APPENDIX

LORRAINE WILLIAMS PEDRETTI
MARY BETH EARLY

Included in this section are 12 case studies and a treatment plan form that may be reproduced for student use. These are provided as a resource for instructors and their students to use for classroom discussion or homework assignments.

Learning Objectives

1. To develop and practice clinical reasoning skills used in treatment planning
2. To analyze the effects of context on treatment planning
3. To increase skills in treatment planning

HOW TO USE THE APPENDIX

1. Select a case study.
2. Read the chapter on the patient's disability in Part 6, Treatment Applications.
3. Refer to chapters on occupational therapy process, treatment contexts, and evidence-based practice (Part 2). Refer to chapters on relevant assessments of occupational performance, performance areas (Part 3), and performance components (Part 4). Refer to chapters on relevant treatment interventions (Part 5).
4. Refer to the questions that guide clinical reasoning and the treatment planning guide in Chapter 6. For the case selected, write a client-centered, occupational performance-based treatment plan, that reflects a top-down approach to treatment. Use the treatment plan outline provided in this appendix. Reproduce as many copies of the outline as needed to complete your treatment plan.

CASE STUDIES

Case 1   Upper Extremity Amputation

Marilyn is a 29-year-old mother of two children, ages 3 and 6. She and her husband own a ranch and are responsible for the care of their animals and crops. Marilyn describes herself as having been independent in all aspects of daily life, including home management, childcare, ranch management, and leisure activities, before her accident. She suffered an extensive injury on the ranch in November while operating a post hole digger. The injury resulted in a traumatic below-elbow amputation of the dominant right arm. Two full-thickness skin grafts were performed during her 5-week hospitalization.

The following May Marilyn received a body-powered prosthesis. Comfortable socket fit was difficult to achieve, and she experienced numerous episodes of skin irritation that necessitated healing before resuming prosthesis usage. In November (one year postinjury) she was assessed by a different prosthetist, who prescribed and acquired approval for a myoelectric prosthesis with myoelectric hand and Greifer terminal devices (TDs). The prosthesis was fabricated and provided by the end of the month.

Marilyn perceives herself as an independent woman, confident, and very practical. She is interested in acquiring more proficiency in use of the new prosthesis to continue living the full life that she desires. Her interest is in fully resuming her ranch activities that include raking, operating a tractor, riding and training horses, and hauling heavy items. The majority of self-care, childcare, and home management tasks are presently performed to her satisfaction. She is referred to occupational therapy in January for prosthetic training.
Reference: Chapter 48
Case contributed by **Denise Keenan**

Case 2   Burn Injury

Bobby is a 3-year-old boy who sustained 50% TBSA full- and deep partial-thickness burns as a result of an explosion caused by an adult using gasoline to re-ignite a wood stove. The patient's anterior chest, face, neck, and circumferential upper extremities, including the hands, all required extensive grafting with donor sites from the patient's legs and back. Because of the depth of the dorsal hand burns, the patient developed finger web space tightness and Boutonnière contractures in all PIP joints. He also developed scar tightness in both axillae, elbows, anterior neck, face and oral commissures.

Bobby lives in a large family with limited resources, which makes it difficult to travel the long distance to visit the regional burn center. On initial interview, his mother reported behaviors that indicated possible preinjury developmental delays in motor planning and speech.

Bobby was referred to occupational therapy for treatment of deformities, reduction of scar tissue, pressure garments and splints as needed, maintenance of range of motion and strength in unaffected parts, psychosocial adjustment, activities of daily living, and developmental play activities.

Reference: Chapter 47
Case contributed by **Sandra Utley Reeves**

Case 3   Burn Injury

Erik is a 17-year-old boy who was burned in an auto accident. At the time of the accident he was a senior in high school, where his academic performance was above average. He plans to attend community college in the next academic year. He got along well with his peers and was liked by his teachers. He participated in intramural sports such as basketball and softball.

Erik lives with his mother, who is divorced from his father. His father was driving at the time of the accident and was injured but not burned. His mother holds her ex-husband responsible for Erik's plight and speaks of this to Erik.

Erik sustained superficial partial-thickness burns over the anterior surface of the left thigh and over the knee and deep partial-thickness burns to the dorsal surface of the left forearm and hand and left side of the face and neck. He will be treated with skin grafting to the face and neck and the dorsum of the hand. Erik was admitted to the burn unit of a city hospital. Occupational therapy has been called upon to treat him through all phases of rehabilitation.

Reference: Chapter 47

Case 4   Spinal Cord Injury

Jack is a 23-year-old man who suffered a spinal cord injury in an auto accident, resulting in C6 quadriplegia. He has complete trunk and lower extremity paralysis and partial paralysis of the arms. He was transferred from a hospital to a spinal cord injury center for active rehabilitation.

Before his injury, Jack was working as an assistant to an accountant. He had recently completed a college degree in accounting and was hoping to advance in this field. He is single and maintained a one-bedroom apartment independently. He drove a sports car and enjoyed dancing, playing baseball, movies, and theater. He has a steady girlfriend and supportive parents. He has been emotionally overwhelmed by this turn of events and still holds hope for a complete recovery in the near future.

Jack's injury is stabilized, and sitting tolerance is 4 hours a day. He has good shoulder function, good elbow flexion, and some wrist extension, but no hand function. Jack cannot grasp eating or writing utensils or manage the implements for oral hygiene (e.g., toothbrush, wash cloth, and shaver). He cannot hold a telephone or operate a typewriter, computer, or tape recorder. He is currently using a wheelchair owned by the treatment facility and needs to be evaluated for one that he will own permanently.

Jack was referred to occupational therapy for assessment of activities of daily living, mobility, vocational potential, and psychosocial adjustment.

Reference: Chapter 41

Case 5   Cerebrovascular Accident

Mrs. M. is a 68-year-old woman who had a right cerebrovascular accident affecting the middle cerebral artery (MCA), resulting in left hemiplegia, 2 weeks ago. She has been discharged home from the acute care facility and was referred to home care occupational therapy for evaluation and maximal functional restoration.

Mrs. M. is a garrulous woman who is cheerful and seems very determined to succeed. She has always worked hard in a rapid and perfectionistic manner. Before the stroke, she enjoyed housekeeping, cooking, baking, and cake decorating. She lives in a four-bedroom, two-story house with two single daughters and a sister, age 60. She was responsible for all of the housekeeping and cooking while the others worked outside of the home. Since the stroke, she has abdicated most of these responsibilities to her daughters and sister.

Mrs. M. ambulates slowly with the aid of a quad cane. She carries the left upper extremity (LUE) passively in a posture of shoulder adduction and internal rotation, elbow flexion, forearm pronation, and wrist and finger flexion. With great effort there is some voluntary synergistic movement (flexion) when she tries to reach her mouth. There is no voluntary spontaneous movement of the LUE. The patient can feed herself except for cutting meat, but she needs assistance with dressing because "I get the clothes all turned around when I try to dress." She requires assistance for bathing and has not yet attempted to transfer into the bathtub. She has not resumed any homemaking activities yet. Mrs. M. was referred to occupational therapy to increase independence in activities of daily living and mobility, assessment of home management skills, and psychosocial adjustment.

References: Chapter 37 and 51

Case 6   Alzheimer's Disease

Mr. L. is a 78-year-old man with Alzheimer's disease, in the middle stage. His wife is 70 and has realized the significant loss of function in her husband of 50 years. He cannot remember his friends' names or faces, and he cannot recall what he did or said a few minutes ago. His hygiene and grooming have become slovenly, and he requires considerable assistance with many self-care tasks to maintain his former standards of self-care. He can no longer walk about the neighborhood without becoming lost. He sometimes becomes very irritable and yells at his wife for what seems like a minor annoyance. Mr. L. is still ambulatory and has no significant motor impairment. There is an Alzheimer's day treatment program in the community, but his wife has been reluctant to allow his participation. She feels she should supervise him at all times.

Mr. L. was referred to occupational therapy for assessment of cognitive skills for function, activities of daily living, and assisting the caregiver to make adaptations in the home and in the daily schedule to allow her more time for herself.

References: Chapters 39 and 51
Case contributed by **Carolyn Glogoski**

Case 7   Multiple Sclerosis

Sally is a 25-year-old woman who works as a computer engineer. She is married and has a 2-year-old daughter, Carrie. Sally enjoys gardening, reading, swimming, and bicycling. She has not participated in these activities much since her daughter was born. Between work and home life she has little time for herself and participating in hobbies.

Sally recently had an episode at work of blurred vision, pain in her right eye, an overwhelming sense of fatigue, and loss of sensation in her right arm. She noted this problem while in the middle of presenting a report to her colleagues. She had difficulty focusing on her presentation notes and needed to sit to complete the presentation. She related her problems to her stress level from working many hours to complete this recent project, balancing her time with her daughter and family needs. She decided to take a couple of days off work to rest, and, if her symptoms didn't disappear, to call her doctor. Within a week Sally's symptoms were minimal, and she returned to work and did not call her doctor.

A couple of months later, Sally experienced the same symptoms, along with weakness in her legs. She felt unsteady when walking to her car, as she tried to balance her briefcase and laptop computer. When she picked her daughter up from day care, she was unable to carry her to the car. Sally was too fatigued to prepare dinner when she returned home. Sally's husband, Dirk, works fairly regular hours at a nearby automotive repair center and is home each evening by 5:30. Dirk usually unwinds after work by watching television. Although Sally typically prepares dinner, Dirk was willing to help out this night with the cooking.

The following day, Sally saw her primary physician, who referred her for a neurological consult. The neurologist informed Sally that there was a possibility that she had multiple sclerosis but advised her that the course of the disease varies between individuals.

Sally was quite depressed, because she has a 45-year-old cousin with multiple sclerosis who is unable to walk and needs attendant care. She talked to her husband about the probable diagnosis but insisted he not talk to his family or her family. She began to worry about work and whether she should tell her employer.

Sally's greatest concerns are how she will manage work or if she will need to quit, whether she and her husband can have a second child, and how she can take care of her daughter. Since her second exacerbation, she has been unable to keep up with her daughter when her daughter runs away from her, and she has been unable to carry her.

Sally lives in a two-story home with the main living area and a half bath on the bottom level. There are two steps to enter the home. The second floor contains the bedrooms and two bathrooms. The master bathroom has a shower stall and a sunken tub. Sally reports that she is able to manage the stairs with effort. There is a rail on one side of the indoor staircase. The steps to enter the house do not have any rails. The washer and dryer are located in the garage, which is detached from the house.

The neurologist recommended that Sally take a couple of weeks off for rest and referred her to physical therapy to evaluate the need for an assistive walking device and to occupational therapy for assessment of home management, instruction in energy conservation techniques, and facilitating psychosocial adjustment.

Reference: Chapter 39
Case contributed by **Diane Foti**

Case 8   Rheumatoid Arthritis

Rachel is a 21-year-old college junior with a recent diagnosis of rheumatoid arthritis. Symptoms have been appearing intermittently over the past year. Since Rachel participates in sports, symptoms were often dismissed as fatigue, sprains, or strains.

A recent episode involved the wrists, metacarpophalangeal joints, proximal interphalangeal joints, hips, and knees bilaterally with much pain and inflammation. This episode required a short hospitalization and resulted in slight losses of range of motion (ROM) and strength in the involved joints and associated muscle groups. Rachel has also experienced decreased physical endurance. There are no permanent deformities at this time, but vigilant care will be required to prevent potential deformity and contractures.

Rachel currently resides in a dormitory and shares a room. Meals are provided, but she is responsible for her own laundry, care of the room, and personal care, as well as school work. Rachel enjoys college life, including dating, volleyball, and studying business courses, her major. At the time of the hospitalization Rachel found that the pain and stiffness severely impaired her ability to write, ambulate, and lift and carry books. Participation in sports was impossible.

Since her release from the hospital, Rachel has returned to a limited schedule of classes and is living in the dorm again. Her roommate is helpful at times, but lives the "fast" life and is not patient with Rachel's slowness. Rachel is scheduled to graduate in a year and plans to apply for positions with financial investing firms. She plans to move into her own apartment upon graduation. Rachel is depressed and anxious over the pain, limited function, unpredictable disease process, and the future.

Rachel was referred as an outpatient to an occupational therapy clinic for training in joint protection and energy conservation suitable for the student role, increase or maintenance of ROM and strength, prevention of deformity, fabrication of splints and assistive devices as needed, vocational evaluation, and aid with adjustment to disability.

Reference: Chapter 43

Case 9   Hand Injury

Mr. G. is a 56-year-old man who has been an expert butcher all of his adult life. He is married and the father of three children. Two are married and out of the family home. The youngest is 17 years old and a senior in high school. Mrs. G. is alive and well and has been a homemaker and club woman all of her life. The family is stable and has been relatively happy and comfortable.

In a recent work-related accident, Mr. G. severed the flexor digitorum superficialis and flexor digitorum profundus tendons of the index and middle fingers and the flexor pollicis longus tendon of the thumb of the left hand with a butcher knife. The finger tendons were severed at the level of the proximal phalanx and the thumb tendon near its insertion just distal to the metacarpophalangeal joint. The tendons were sutured three weeks ago, and Mr. G. has been splinted since the surgery.

Mr. G. is very anxious about his future employment. He is receiving workman's compensation and disability insurance benefits at this time. He is in a state of denial and is shocked to disbelief that he could have had this self-inflicted accident after years as a skilled worker without a scratch. He is concerned that his vision, balance, and memory are failing.

The surgeon has given clearance for gentle motion to the fingers, within the limits of the treatment protocol for flexor

tendon injuries. The patient was referred to occupational therapy for remobilization of affected fingers; restoration of range of motion, strength, and hand function; assessment of cognitive functions; aid with adjustment to disability; and vocational assessment.
Reference: Chapter 44

Case 10   Guillain-Barré Syndrome

Lauren is a 28-year-old woman who is not married but does have a partner, with whom she lives and who is a strong support for her. She is employed as a clerk and editorial assistant at a local college. Her major life roles are those of being a worker, partner, friend, and confidant. Her leisure interests include writing, reading, dancing, video games, and board games.

A few weeks after receiving an influenza vaccine, Lauren began to experience the feeling that her hands and feet were falling asleep. Two days later she complained of progressive muscle weakness and was taken to the hospital by her partner. When she was admitted to the hospital, there was no movement in her lower extremities, and there was significant weakness in the upper extremities. A diagnosis of Guillain-Barré Syndrome secondary to influenza vaccine was made based on the symptoms and the increased protein in the cerebrospinal fluid. There was no apparent cranial nerve involvement or significant sensory loss at this time.

As a result of the dramatic onset of the disability and sudden total dependency, Lauren has begun to withdraw and is weeping frequently. She is fearful that she will not fully recover. Lauren was referred to occupational therapy (OT) during the acute phase of the disease. Initial contact was made at the bedside. She appeared alert and was articulate. She expressed a strong desire to "get back to normal." OT intervention is to continue through all phases of the recovery process, with the aims of training in energy conservation, training in activities of daily living, psychosocial support and aid with adjustment, vocational assessment, preventing contractures, maintaining range of motion, and increasing strength.
Reference: Chapter 42
Case contributed by **Regina M. Lehman**

Case 11   Hip Fracture

Mrs. Q. is an 80-year-old woman who fell in the shower and fractured her hip. She has had a total hip replacement. Before her fall, Mrs. Q. lived alone in a first-floor, one-bedroom apartment. She did her own cooking and cleaning. She enjoyed playing cards and socializing with friends one afternoon a week. She is a volunteer at the local library and helps arrange bake sales and book sales to benefit the library. She enjoyed tending house plants. She used to be an avid quilter, but recently her eyesight has been failing and she finds the fine stitching very difficult to do.

Mrs. Q. is not allowed to flex her hip more than 90° and has precautions to avoid hip adduction and external rotation for 6 to 12 weeks. She was referred to occupational therapy for learning hip precautions, increasing self-care independence, and home management assessment to determine the feasibility of living alone.
References: Chapter 45 and 51

Case 12   Low Back Injury with Nerve Root Involvement

Mr. S. is a 60-year-old man who had a low back injury 7 months ago that caused compression of the lumbosacral nerve roots. This resulted in bilateral lower extremity muscle weakness, more severe on the right side. There is partial weakness in hip flexors, abductors, adductors, and extensors; knee flexors and extensors; and ankle dorsiflexors. Generally, muscle grades in all affected groups are Fair+ (3+) on the right and good (4) on the left. Distal muscles are the weakest bilaterally. There has been slight improvement in strength since the initial injury and there is potential for further improvement.

Initially, Mr. S. ambulated with the aid of a walker and a short leg orthosis on the right leg. Muscle weakness resulted in poor balance and the patient was fearful of standing without support. Standing tolerance with support was 30 minutes.

The patient appears depressed. He is concerned about whether or not he should retire. He has worked as a fork lift operator in a box factory for many years and had very few leisure interests other than watching television and visiting his grandchildren. He is married and has two married children and three grandchildren who live nearby. His wife does all of the home management and is supportive of her husband. However, she sometime feels impatient with his depression and negative attitude and with caring for him and the home.

Mr. S. is independent in self-care, except for some difficulty in dressing the lower body (shoes, socks, and trousers), and with tub transfers.

Mr. S. was referred to occupational therapy as an outpatient for activities of daily living evaluation and training, vocational evaluation, exploration of leisure skills or other work substitutes, strengthening of leg musculature, improvement of standing balance and tolerance, functional ambulation, and aid with adjustment to disability.
References: Chapters 46 and 51

TREATMENT PLAN FORM

Case (number/name) _____

Patient's age _____ Diagnosis _____

Disability _____

OT treatment goals:

_____

_____

Treatment model(s)/treatment approach(s) (List which models or approaches to treatment you would use with this patient).

_____

_____

OT EVALUATION

(List assessments that could be used in each area)

Occupational performance

_____

_____

Performance areas

1. Activities of daily living _____

_____

2. Work and productive activities _____

_____

3. Play or leisure activities _____

_____

Performance contexts

1. Physical aspects_____

_____

2. Temporal aspects _____

_____

3. Sociocultural aspects _____

_____

Performance components

1. Sensorimotor _____

_____

2. Cognitive integration and cognitive _____

_____

3. Psychosocial skills and psychological _____

_____

Evaluation summary (On a separate page, write a summary based on the information in the case and the results of the assessments as you conceptualize them)

Problem list (List and number occupational performance problems.)

_____

_____

_____

Assets (List the intrinsic and extrinsic strengths in the circumstances.)

_____

_____

_____

Treatment plan
1. Problem (Identify the problem being addressed by name and number.)

_____

_____

_____

_____

2. Objective (Write a measurable objective for the problem.)

_____

_____

_____

_____

3. Methods (List and describe the intervention strategies you would use to address this problem.)

_____

_____

_____

_____

4. Grading (Describe how you would grade treatment as the patient improves or declines.)

_____

_____

_____

_____

Repeat 1 through 4 for as many problems as selected. This form may be reproduced for classroom/student use.

Index